Did you know that you can also...

Get access to www.identadrug.com

Get everything in this book, plus more - with powerful searches - updated daily

For details, see the last pages in this book or contact the publisher.

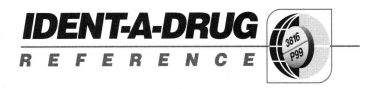

3120 W. March Lane
PO Box 8190
Stockton CA 95208
Tel: 209-472-2240
Fax: 209-472-2249
mail@identadrug.com
www.identadrug.com

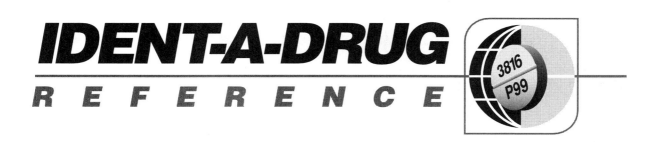

For Drug Tablet and Capsule Identification

Published by:

Therapeutic Research Center
3120 W. March Lane
PO Box 8190
Stockton, CA 95208

Tel: 209-472-2240
Fax: 209-472-2249
E-mail: mail@identadrug.com
www.identadrug.com

We wish to recognize some of the people who created this reference:

Timothy Swaim, Product Manager

Kay A. Shaver, Pharm.D.

Adam Marc Kaye, Pharm.D., FASCP

Stephen C. Burson, R.Ph.

Michelle Carlson, Project Manager

Jocosa Bottemiller

Therapeutic Research Center Faculty also publish:

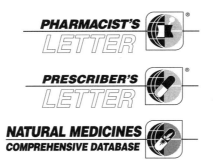

For information on obtaining additional copies of this issue
or to receive a subscription to the printed version of
Ident-A-Drug Reference, see the order form in the back of the book or contact:
Therapeutic Research Center, PO Box 8190, Stockton, CA 95208
TEL: 209-472-2240 • FAX: 209-472-2249 • E-MAIL: mail@identadrug.com
www.identadrug.com

Printed in the United States of America

ISBN # 0-9676136-5-5

Preface

Pharmaceutical tablets and capsules are imprinted with specific identification codes. This *Ident-A-Drug Reference* identifies drug products by the codes imprinted on them. Subscribers who receive each new issue of *Ident-A-Drug Reference* on a subscription basis will notice that this edition has many more products listed than previous issues. New products are coming out all the time. Often a seemingly identical product is marketed by different generic manufacturers, or different repackagers. In these instances the product often has a different identification code imprinted on it. All the various identification codes appear in this *Reference*.

This *Ident-A-Drug Reference* includes brand name products and generic products from the United States and Canada. It gives a description of each product's colors, shape, graphics, imprint code, etc. It shows the code that's imprinted on the front and the back of the tablet or capsule. The ingredients and strength of each ingredient are shown. *Ident-A-Drug Reference* also gives the national drug code (NDC #) as well as the drug class. If the drug is a narcotic or in one of the schedules determined by the Drug Enforcement Administration (DEA), the schedule is also shown.

This compilation of drug identification codes is the most comprehensive in existence. Our staff constantly adds data on newly introduced drugs, and new versions of older drugs. To see the very latest data, subscribe to **www.identadrug.com** which makes an excellent companion to this book. The website is updated all the time, and can be provided on a network for large organizations, and can be linked to consumer websites so that consumers can assure themselves of the medication they are taking or giving to a loved one.

There is a tremendous need for this *Reference*. The huge number of different generic and brand name drug products have different sizes, shapes, colors, and identification codes by each of the many pharmaceutical manufacturers. In addition, manufacturers often change the identification codes on their products. The need to identify medications is crucial...often with important legal or even life and death ramifications.

Pharmacists, physicians, and nurses frequently need to be able to identify tablets and capsules. Many times a patient will be admitted to a hospital, long-term care, or intermediate care facility and have some medication in their possession that needs to be identified.

Emergency medical personnel often have no medical information on a sick or injured person. Sometimes the only clue to the person's medical history is to identify the medication they carry.

Law enforcement officers find this *Reference* extremely useful.

Parents and school officials are also finding the need to identify various medications.

People often feel the need to check their own medications, or medications of loved ones.

This *Ident-A-Drug Reference* is a unique resource dedicated to promoting the health and well-being of people by helping make accurate identification of thousands of drug products. The publisher encourages any user of this *Reference* who is not a health professional to seek advice from an appropriate professional regarding drug or medical questions.

Jeff M. Jellin, Pharm.D.
Editor, *Pharmacist's Letter*
Editor, *Prescriber's Letter*
Editor, *Natural Medicines Comprehensive Database*

How to Use *IDENT-A-DRUG* *Reference*

Guidelines for Use:

To use the *Ident-A-Drug Reference*, start with the code that's imprinted on either side of the oral medication. Use the following rules:

- First look up the number or letter that is farthest to the left, then the number or letter next to it, etc.
- The entries are listed in typical dictionary or phonebook order. For example, 469 is followed by 47, is followed by 471, is followed by 4711, is followed by 48, etc.
- Letters follow numbers. For example, 469 would be followed by 46A. 999999 would be followed by A.
- Only letters and numerals are listed in the imprint column. When looking up a medication, ignore any spaces, dashes, slashes, periods, or other symbols. Logos are also not included in the imprint column. For example, if you're trying to find information on a tablet that's imprinted 345 33, look up 34533. For 0.5 look up 05. For 45/GG look up 45GG. For a Logo 25, look up 25. For imprints that do contain symbols other than numerals and letters, a more detailed description will be given in the Description column.
- Oral medications that have an imprint on the front and back are listed as two separate listings. In *Ident-A-Drug*, the symbol <> separates the code that is imprinted on the front of the tablet and the code that is imprinted on the back of the tablet. You should be able to find the medication by looking up either side and then verifying the alternate side's information.

Description of Columns:

Imprint: This column contains the numerical and alphabetical imprints on oral medications. Other symbols are omitted, i.e. dashes, periods, slashes, logos, etc. If a tablet has imprints on both sides, the information is listed separated by <>. Entries that include the front-back symbol (<>) are listed twice in the database; one listing for the imprint on the front and one listing for the imprint on the back.

Description: This column contains a physical description of the oral medication. The information occurs in the following order: Tab (for Tablet) or Cap (for Capsule), Color, Shape (if a tablet), and other information which may include scoring, embossing, debossing, etc. Clarification of the imprint information by including dashes, slashes, decimals, spaces, and logo information is also included in the description column.

Ingredient & Strength: This column contains a listing of the active ingredients and the amounts.

Brand (Or Equiv.) & Firm: This column lists the brand name of a product and the manufacturer in the following format: i.e. Zocor by Merck. For some generic drugs, the equivalent brand name is given in this column.

NDC#: The NDC number is given in the following format: 00000-0000. The third segment of the NDC code, the packaging information, is omitted because it is not necessary for the identification of an oral medication by imprint. Some older drugs or drugs no longer manufactured may not have an NDC# listed. Canadian drugs are indicated in this column. If Canadian drugs have an accompanying DIN#, it is included in this column.

Class; Schedule: This column contains the class of drug and the schedule assigned by the Drug Enforcement Agency (DEA) if the medication is a controlled substance. This schedule is shown in the following format: Schedule 2 is listed as C II, Schedule 3 as C III, and so forth. Canadian products do not contain a controlled substance rating, even if they are a controlled substance in the United States.

If you find a tablet or capsule that is not listed in *Ident-A-Drug Reference*, or if you find anything that you think should be changed, please alert the publisher. It's possible that a new drug has come on the market after this edition of the book. This information may be available on our website, **www.identadrug.com**, which is updated daily.

ID FRONT <> BACK	DESCRIPTION FRONT <> BACK	INGREDIENT & STRENGTH	BRAND (OR EQUIV.) & FIRM	NDC#	CLASS; SCH.
001 <> ETHEX	Cap, Red Print	Potassium Chloride 750 mg	Micro- K 10 by Ethex	58177-0001	Electrolytes
001 <> ETHEX	Cap	Potassium Chloride 750 mg	by Heartland	61392-0402	Electrolytes
0016 <> PAL	Cap, White Print	Acetaminophen 356.4 mg, Caffeine 30 mg, Dihydrocodeine Bitartrate 16 mg	Panlor DC by Pan Am	00525-0016	Analgesic; C III
0016 <> PAL	Cap	Acetaminophen 356.4 mg, Caffeine 30 mg, Dihydrocodeine Bitartrate 16 mg	by Mikart	46672-0267	Analgesic; C III
002 <> AMIDE	Tab, Orange, Pink & Purple, Pillow Shaped, Chewable	Ascorbic Acid 30 mg, Sodium Ascorbate 33 mg, Sodium Fluoride, Vitamin A Acetate, Vitamin D 400 Units	Tri Vitamin Fluoride by Schein	00364-0846	Vitamin
002 <> ETHEX	Cap, Orange & Purple	Disopyramide Phosphate	Norpace by Ethex	58177-0002	Antiarrhythmic
0025 <> PHARMICS	Tab, 00 over 25	Acetaminophen 500 mg, Hydrocodone Bitartrate 5 mg	by Quality Care	60346-0442	Analgesic; C III
003 <> 59743	Cap	Guaifenesin 300 mg, Pseudoephedrine HCl 60 mg	G Phed PD by Pharmafab	62542-0402	Cold Remedy
003 <> RPC25	Tab, RPC Above Score, 2.5 Below Score	Midodrine HCl 2.5 mg	Proamatine by Roberts	54092-0003	Antihypotension
003 <> RPC25	Tab, RPC Above Score, 2.5 Below Score	Midodrine HCl 2.5 mg	Proamatine by Nycomed	57585-0103	Antihypotension
0030 <> G	Tab, Off-White, Film Coated, 00 Over 30	Ranitidine HCl 168 mg	by Genpharm	55567-0030	Gastrointestinal
0031 <> G	Tab, Film Coated	Ranitidine HCl 336 mg	by Genpharm	55567-0031	Gastrointestinal
0034	Tab	Acetaminophen 300 mg, Codeine Phosphate 60 mg	by PDRX	55289-0916	Analgesic; C III
0034 <> G	Cap	Acyclovir 200 mg	by Genpharm	55567-0034	Antiviral
0037 <> G	Tab	Acyclovir 800 mg	by Genpharm	55567-0037	Antiviral
004 <> ETHEX	Cap, Lavender, Black Ink, Ex Release	Nitroglycerin 2.5 mg	Nitrobid by Ethex	58177-0004	Vasodilator
004 <> RPC5	Tab, RPC Above Score, 5 Below Score	Midodrine HCl 5 mg	Proamatine by Roberts	54092-0004	Antihypotension
004 <> RPC5	Tab, RPC Above Score, 5 Below Score	Midodrine HCl 5 mg	Proamatine by Nycomed	57585-0104	Antihypotension
0041 <> G	Cap	Nicardipine HCl 20 mg	by Genpharm	55567-0041	Antihypertensive
0042 <> G	Cap	Nicardipine HCl 30 mg	by Genpharm	55567-0042	Antihypertensive
005 <> ETHEX	Cap, Black Print	Nitroglycerin 6.5 mg	Nitrobid by Ethex	58177-0005	Vasodilator
0053	Tab, White, Round	Niacin 500 mg	Nicolar by H.L.Moore		Vitamin
0057	Cap, Maroon, Oval, Gelatin	Docusate Sodium 100 mg, Casanthranol 30 mg	Peri-Colace by UDL	51079-0039	Laxative
0057	Cap, Maroon, Oval, Gelatin	Docusate Sodium with Casanthranol 100 mg	Peri-Colace by Geneva	00781-2653	Laxative
0058 <> MAJOR	Cap	Chlorpheniramine Maleate 8 mg, Pseudoephedrine HCl 120 mg	Pseudo Chlor by Sovereign	58716-0014	Cold Remedy
005GEST <> 51479DURA	Cap, 005/Gest <> 51479/Dura	Guaifenesin 200 mg, Phenylephrine HCl 5 mg, Phenylpropanolamine HCl 45 mg	Dura Gest by Anabolic	00722-6060	Cold Remedy
005R	Tab, Coated	Acetaminophen 650 mg, Propoxyphene Napsylate 100 mg	by Med Pro	53978-5013	Analgesic; C IV
006 <> ETHEX	Cap, Black Print	Nitroglycerin 9 mg	Nitrobid by Ethex	58177-0006	Vasodilator
006 <> HOYT	Tab, Pink, Chewable	Sodium Fluoride 2.2 mg	Luride Cherry by Colgate Oral	00126-0006	Element
00631390	Tab, Peach, Round, 0063 / 1390	Hydralazine 25 mg, Hydrochlorothiazide 15 mg, Reserpine 0.1 mg	Ser-Ap-Es by Reid-Rowell		Antihypertensive
008 <> ACG	Tab, Light Pink, Round	Candesartan Cilexetil 8 mg	Atacand by Astra Merck	00186-0008	Antihypertensive
008 <> ACG	Tab	Candesartan Cilexetil 8 mg	by Astra AB	17228-0017	Antihypertensive
009 <> 51674	Cap, Green	Acetaminophen 325 mg, Butalbital 50 mg, Caffeine 40 mg	Anolor 300 by Blansett	51674-0009	Analgesic
009 <> DURA	Tab, Light Blue, 009 <> DU-RA	Guaifenesin 600 mg	Fenesin by Anabolic	00722-6139	Expectorant
01	Tab, White, Round, 0.1	Desmopressin Acetate 0.1 mg	DDAVP by Ferring	Canadian	Antidiuretic
01 <> BIOCRAFT	Cap, Buff & Carmel	Amoxicillin 250 mg	by Quality Care	60346-0655	Antibiotic
01 <> DAN5609	Tab, 0.1 <> Dan 5609	Clonidine HCl 0.1 mg	by Quality Care	60346-0786	Antihypertensive
01 <> DAN5609	Tab, 0.1 <> Dan 5609	Clonidine HCl 0.1 mg	by Danbury	00591-5609	Antihypertensive
010	Cap, Barr Logo	Tetracycline HCl 500 mg	by Apotheca	12634-0162	Antibiotic
010	Cap, Barr Logo	Tetracycline HCl 500 mg	by Major	00904-2407	Antibiotic
0100	Cap, Red	Amantadine HCl 100 mg	by Pharmascience	Canadian	Antiviral
0100	Tab, White	Flouride 3.75 mg, Calcium 145 mg	by Kremers Urban		Mineral
0100	Cap, Yellow	Vitamin A Palmitate 25,000 Units	by Richlyn		Vitamin
01001	Tab, Beige, Round	Pancreatin 425 mg	Pancreatin by Viobin Corporation		Gastrointestinal
0101	Cap, Yellow	Vitamin A Natural 25,000 Units	by Richlyn		Vitamin
0102	Cap, Red	Vitamin A Palmitate 50,000 Units	by Richlyn		Vitamin
0104	Cap, Yellow	Vitamin A Solubilized 25,000 Units	by Richlyn		Vitamin
0105	Tab, White, 0105/Mericon Logo	Flouride 3 mg, Calcium 250 mg	Monocal by Mericon		Mineral
0105	Cap, Red	Vitamin A Natural 50,000 Units	by Richlyn		Vitamin
0109	Cap, Yellow	Vitamin A Solubilized 50,000 Units	by Richlyn		Vitamin

ID FRONT <> BACK	DESCRIPTION FRONT <> BACK	INGREDIENT & STRENGTH	BRAND (OR EQUIV.) & FIRM	NDC#	CLASS; SCH.
011	Tab, Pink, Round, Schering Logo 011	Betamethasone 0.6 mg	Celestone by Schering	00085-0011	Steroid
011 <> 59743	Cap, White Print	Acetaminophen 500 mg, Hydrocodone Bitartrate 5 mg	Dolagesic by Alphagen	59743-0011	Analgesic; C III
0111	Tab, White, Round	Butalbital 50 mg, Acetaminophen 325 mg, Caffeine 40 mg	Fioricet by D.M. Graham		Analgesic
0115 <> 7001	Cap	Pancrelipase (Amylase,Lipase,Protease) 175.74 mg	Pancreatic Enzyme by Zenith Goldline	00182-1968	Gastrointestinal
0115 <> 7001	Cap	Pancrelipase (Amylase,Lipase,Protease) 175.74 mg	Protilase by Rugby	00536-4509	Gastrointestinal
01151110	Cap	Diphenhydramine HCl 25 mg	by Zenith Goldline	00182-0492	Antihistamine
01151111	Cap	Diphenhydramine HCl 50 mg	by Zenith Goldline	00182-0135	Antihistamine
01151142	Cap, Pink	Ephedrine Sulfate 0.75 gr	by Richlyn		Antiasthmatic
01151300	Cap, Yellow	Oxytetracycline 250 mg	Terramycin by Richlyn		Antibiotic
01151398	Cap, Orange & Yellow	Tetracycline 100 mg	Achromycin V by Richlyn		Antibiotic
01151400	Cap, Orange & Yellow, 0115/1400	Tetracycline HCl 250 mg	Achromycin V by Richlyn		Antibiotic
01151402	Cap, Black & Yellow, 0115/1402	Tetracycline HCl 500 mg	Achromycin V by Richlyn		Antibiotic
01151405	Cap, Black & Yellow, 0115/1405	Tetracycline HCl 250 mg	Achromycin V by Richlyn		Antibiotic
01152150	Tab, White, Round	Aminophylline 100 mg	Aminophyllin by Richlyn		Antiasthmatic
01152151	Tab, Beige, Round	Aminophylline 100 mg	Aminophyllin by Richlyn		Antiasthmatic
01152158	Tab, White, Round	Aminophylline 200 mg	Aminophyllin by Richlyn		Antiasthmatic
01152162	Tab, White, Round	Aminophylline 200 mg	Aminophyllin by Richlyn		Antiasthmatic
01152390	Tab, Maroon, Round	Sulfisoxazole 500 mg, Phenazopyridine HCl 50 mg	Azo-Gantrisin by Richlyn		Antibiotic; Urinary Analgesic
01152400	Tab, Green, Round	Phenobarbital 16.2 mg, Belladonna 10.8 mg	Bellophen by Richlyn		Gastrointestinal; C IV
01152758	Cap, Green & Yellow	Chlordiazepoxide HCl 5 mg	Librium by Richlyn		Antianxiety; C IV
01152760	Cap, Black & Green	Chlordiazepoxide HCl 10 mg	Librium by Richlyn		Antianxiety; C IV
01152762	Cap, Green & White	Chlordiazepoxide HCl 25 mg	Librium by Richlyn		Antianxiety; C IV
01152810	Tab, Yellow, Round	Chlorpheniramine Maleate 4 mg	Chlor-trimeton by Richlyn		Antihistamine
01152920	Tab, White, Round	Cortisone Acetate 25 mg	Cortone by Richlyn		Steroid
01153030	Tab, White, Round	Dehydrocholic Acid 250 mg	Decholin by Richlyn		Gastrointestinal
01153100	Tab, Blue, Pentagonal	Dexamethasone 0.75 mg	Decadron by Richlyn		Steroid
01153200	Cap, Blue	Decyclomine HCl 10 mg	Bentyl by Richlyn		Gastrointestinal
01153210	Cap, Blue & Clear	Decyclomine HCl 10 mg, Phenobarbital 15 mg	Bentyl with Pb by Richlyn		Gastrointestinal; C IV
01153220	Tab, Blue	Decyclomine HCl 20 mg	Bentyl by Richlyn		Gastrointestinal
01153225	Tab, White	Decyclomine HCl 20 mg, Phenobarbital 15 mg	Bentyl with Pb by Richlyn		Gastrointestinal; C IV
01153250	Tab, White, Round	Pepsin 250 mg, Pancreatin 300 mg, Dehydrocholic Acid 150 mg	Entozyme by Richlyn		Gastrointestinal
01153585	Tab, Yellow, Round	Folic Acid 1 mg	Folvite by Richlyn		Vitamin
01153660	Tab, Blue, Round	Hydralazine HCl 25 mg	Apresoline by Richlyn		Antihypertensive
01153662	Tab, Blue, Round	Hydralazine HCl 50 mg	Apresoline by Richlyn		Antihypertensive
01153670	Tab, Peach, Round	Hydrochlorothiazide 25 mg	Hydrodiuril by Richlyn		Diuretic
01153675	Tab, Peach, Round	Hydrochlorothiazide 50 mg	Hydrodiuril by Richlyn		Diuretic
01153677	Tab, Peach, Round	Hydrochlorothiazide 100 mg	Hydrodiuril by Richlyn		Diuretic
01153685	Tab, White, Round	Hydrocortisone 20 mg	Hydrocortone by Richlyn		Steroid
01153706	Tab, White, Round	Isoniazid 100 mg	by Richlyn		Antimycobacterial
01153888	Tab, White, Round	Meprobamate 200 mg	Equanil by Richlyn		Sedative/Hypnotic; C IV
01153890	Tab, White, Round	Meprobamate 400 mg	Equanil by Richlyn		Sedative/Hypnotic; C IV
01153900	Tab, White, Round	Methocarbamol 500 mg	Robaxin by Richlyn		Muscle Relaxant
01153902	Tab, White, Oblong	Methocarbamol 750 mg	Robaxin by Richlyn		Muscle Relaxant
01153975	Tab, Brown, Round	Methenamine Mandelate 250 mg	Mandelamine by Richlyn		Antibiotic; Urinary Tract
01153976	Tab, Brown, Oblong	Methenamine Mandelate 500 mg	Mandelamine by Richlyn		Antibiotic; Urinary Tract
01153977	Tab, Lavender, Oval	Methenamine Mandelate 1000 mg	Mandelamine by Richlyn		Antibiotic; Urinary Tract
01153982	Tab, Yellow, Oblong	Methyltestosterone SL 10 mg	Metandren by Richlyn		Hormone; C III
01153986	Tab, Yellow, Round	Methyltestosterone Oral 25 mg	Metandren by Richlyn		Hormone; C III
01154086	Tab, White, Round	Nicotinic Acid 500 mg	Niacin by Richlyn		Vitamin
01154214	Tab, Green, Round	Phenobarbital 15 mg	by Richlyn		Sedative/Hypnotic; C IV
01154214	Tab, White, Round	Phenobarbital 15 mg	by Richlyn		Sedative/Hypnotic; C IV

ID FRONT ⟷ BACK	DESCRIPTION FRONT ⟷ BACK	INGREDIENT & STRENGTH	BRAND (OR EQUIV.) & FIRM	NDC#	CLASS; SCH.
01154214	Tab, Pink, Round	Phenobarbital 15 mg	by Richlyn		Sedative/Hypnotic; C IV
01154233	Tab, Pink, Round	Phenobarbital 30 mg	by Richlyn		Sedative/Hypnotic; C IV
01154233	Tab, Green, Round	Phenobarbital 30 mg	by Richlyn		Sedative/Hypnotic; C IV
01154233	Tab, White, Round	Phenobarbital 30 mg	by Richlyn		Sedative/Hypnotic; C IV
01154252	Tab, White, Round	Piperazine Citrate 250 mg	by Richlyn		Antihistamine
01154280	Tab, Orange, Round	Prednisolone 5 mg	by Richlyn		Steroid
01154294	Tab, White, Round	Prednisone 5 mg	by Richlyn		Steroid
01154302	Tab, White, Oblong, 0115-4302	Colchicine 0.5 mg, Probenecid 500 mg	ColBenemid by Richlyn		Antigout
01154308	Tab, Peach, Round	Propantheline Bromide 15 mg	Probanthine by Richlyn		Gastrointestinal
01154322	Tab, White, Round	Propylthiouracil 50 mg	Propylthiouracil by Richlyn		Antithyroid
01154331	Tab, White, Round	Pseudoephedrine 60 mg, Triprolidine 2.5 mg	Actifed by Richlyn		Cold Remedy
01154332	Tab, White, Round	Pseudoephedrine HCl 60 mg	Sudafed by Richlyn		Decongestant
01154334	Tab, Dark Red, Round	Phenazopyridine HCl 100 mg	Pyridium by Richlyn		Urinary Analgesic
01154336	Tab, Dark Red, Round	Phenazopyridine HCl 200 mg	Pyridium by Richlyn		Urinary Analgesic
01154360	Tab, Yellow, Round	Pyrilamine Maleate 25 mg	by Richlyn		Antihistamine
01154380	Tab, White, Round	Quinidine Sulfate 200 mg	by Richlyn		Antiarrhythmic
01154400	Tab, Orange, Round	Rauwolfia Serpentina 50 mg	Raudixin by Richlyn		Antihypertensive
01154404	Tab, Orange, Round	Rauwolfia Serpentina 100 mg	Raudixin by Richlyn		Antihypertensive
01154423	Tab, White, Round, 0115-4423	Reserpine 0.25 mg	Serpasil by Qualitest		Antihypertensive
01154426	Tab, White, Round	Reserpine 0.1 mg	Serpasil by Richlyn		Antihypertensive
01154428	Tab, White, Round	Reserpine 0.25 mg	Serpasil by Richlyn		Antihypertensive
01154631	Tab, Pink, Round	Sodium Fluoride 2.2 mg	Luride by Richlyn		Element
01154652	Tab, White, Round	Hyoscyamine, Atropine, Scopolamine, Phenobarbital	Donnatal by Richlyn		Gastrointestinal; C IV
01154711	Tab, White, Round	Sulfadiazine 2.5 gr, Sulfamerazine 2.5 gr, Sulfamethazine 2.5 gr	Terfonyl by Richlyn		Antibiotic
01154714	Tab, White, Round	Sulfadiazine 500 mg	by Richlyn		Antibiotic
01154747	Tab, White, Round	Sulfisoxazole 500 mg	Gantrisin by Richlyn		Antibiotic
01154812	Tab, Beige, Round	Thyroglobulin 1 gr	Proloid by Richlyn		Thryoid
01154824	Tab, Beige, Round	Thyroid 1 gr	by Richlyn		Thyroid
01154825	Tab, Red, Round	Thyroid 1 gr	by Richlyn		Thyroid
01154826	Tab, Beige, Round	Thyroid 2 gr	by Richlyn		Thyroid
01154827	Tab, Red, Round	Thyroid 2 gr	by Richlyn		Thyroid
01154840	Tab, White, Round, 0115/4840	Triamcinolone 4 mg	Aristocort by Richlyn		Steroid
01154860	Tab, Light Blue, 0115/4860	Trichlormethiazide 4 mg	Aq 4B Aquazide by Jones	52604-9780	Diuretic
01154871	Tab, Blue, Round	Tripelennamine HCl 50 mg	PBZ by Richlyn		Antihistamine
01154895	Tab, Purple, Round	Benzoic A., Methenamine, Phenyl Sal., Atropine, Hyoscy	by Richlyn		Urinary Tract
01154900	Tab, Blue, Round	Benzoic A., Methen, Phenyl Sal., Atropine, Hyosc, M.Blu	Urised by Richlyn		Urinary Tract
01154902	Tab, Purple, Round	Benzoic A., Methen, Phenyl Sal., Atropine, Hyosc, M.Blu	Urised by Richlyn		Urinary Tract
01157003	Cap, Brown & Flesh	Amylase 33200 Units, Lipase 10000 Units, Protease 37500 Units	Lipram 10000 by Global	00115-7003	Gastrointestinal
01157017	Cap, Brown & Green	Minocycline HCl 50 mg	by Neuman Distr	64579-0305	Antibiotic
012	Tab, Green, Round	Chlorzoxazone 250 mg, Acetaminophen 300 mg	Parafon Forte by Amide		Muscle Relaxant
012 ⟷ ADAMS	Tab	Guaifenesin 600 mg	Humibid LA by Nat Pharmpak Serv	55154-5903	Expectorant
012 ⟷ MEDEVA	Tab, Light Green, Scored	Guaifenesin 600 mg	Humibid LA by Adams	53014-0012	Expectorant
012 ⟷ MEDEVA	Tab	Guaifenesin 600 mg	Humibid LA by Medeva	53014-0012	Expectorant
012 ⟷ MEDEVA	Tab	Guaifenesin 600 mg, Pseudoephedrine HCl 60 mg	Syn Rx by Adams	53014-0308	Cold Remedy
012 ⟷ PAR	Tab, Coated	Hydroxyzine HCl 10 mg	by Par	49884-0012	Antihistamine
0121	Tab, Ross Logo 0121	Prenatal, Folic Acid	Pramilet by Ross		Vitamin
0127 ⟷ LUNSCO	Tab, Film Coated	Acetaminophen 500 mg, Chlorpheniramine Maleate 8 mg, Phenylephrine HCl 40 mg	Protid by Lunsco	10892-0127	Cold Remedy
0127 ⟷ LUNSCO	Tab, Film Coated	Acetaminophen 500 mg, Chlorpheniramine Maleate 8 mg, Phenylephrine HCl 40 mg	by Mikart	46672-0161	Cold Remedy
013	Cap, Black & Clear	Niacin TD 125 mg	Nicobid by Time-Caps		Vitamin
013 ⟷ PAR	Tab, Coated	Hydroxyzine HCl 25 mg	by Par	49884-0013	Antihistamine
01312008	Tab, Peach, Oblong, 0131 20/08	Chlorpheniramine 2 mg, Pseudoephedrine 30 mg, Acetaminophen 325 mg	Codimal by Schwarz Pharma		Cold Remedy
01312008	Cap, Red & White, 0131 20/08	Pseudoephedrine 120 mg, Chlorpheniramine 8 mg	Codimal LA by Schwarz		Cold Remedy

ID FRONT <> BACK	DESCRIPTION FRONT <> BACK	INGREDIENT & STRENGTH	BRAND (OR EQUIV.) & FIRM	NDC#	CLASS; SCH.
014	Cap, Clear & Green	Niacin TD 250 mg	Nicobid by Time-Caps		Vitamin
014 <> AMIDE	Tab, Film Coated	Dexchlorpheniramine Maleate 4 mg	by Schein	00364-0585	Antihistamine
014 <> COP	Tab, Chewable	Sodium Fluoride 1.1 mg	Luride Half Strength by Colgate Oral	00126-0014	Element
014 <> PAR	Tab, Coated	Hydroxyzine HCl 50 mg	by Par	49884-0014	Antihistamine
014 <> THERRX	Tab, Yellow, Diamond Shaped, Film Coated	Ascorbic Acid 60 mg; Calcium Carbonate 200 mg; Iron 30 mg; Vitamin E 30 unt; Thiamine Mononitrate 3 mg; Riboflavin 3.4 mg; Niacinamide 20 mg; Pyridoxine HCl 50 mg; Folic Acid 1 mg; Magnesium Oxide 100 mg; Cyanocobalamin 12 mcg; Zinc Oxide 15 mg; Cupric Ox	Precare Conceive by Ther Rx	64011-0014	Vitamin
0140	Cap, Gelatin Coated, Graphic enclosed in an Inverted Triangle	Ergocalciferol 1.25 mg	Ergo D by Optimum	61298-0020	Vitamin
0140 <> P	Cap, Gelatin, P in a triangle	Ergocalciferol 1.25 mg	Vitamin D by Banner Pharmacaps	10888-0140	Vitamin
0147 <> CC	Cap, C-C is in a box	Phentermine HCl 30 mg	T Diet by Jones	52604-0010	Anorexiant; C IV
0149 0436 <> ENTEXLA	Tab	Guaifenesin 400 mg, Phenylpropanolamine HCl 75 mg	Entex LA by Leiner	59606-0641	Cold Remedy
01490008 <> MACRODANTIN50MG	Cap, 0149-0008 & Two Black Lines <> Macrodantin 50 mg	Nitrofurantoin 50 mg	Macrodantin by Thrift Drug	59198-0056	Antibiotic
01490008 <> MACRODANTIN50MG	Cap, 0149 over 0008 <> Macrodantin over 50 mg	Nitrofurantoin 50 mg	Macrodantin by Amerisource	62584-0008	Antibiotic
01490008 <> MACRODANTIN50MG	Cap, Yellow, Opaque, 0149-0008 <> 2 Black Lines & Macrodantin 50 mg	Nitrofurantoin 50 mg	Macrodantin by Quality Care	60346-0318	Antibiotic
01490009 <> MACRODANTIN100	Cap, 0149-0009 <> Macrodantin 100 mg, 3 Black Lines	Nitrofurantoin 100 mg	Macrodantin by Quality Care	60346-0651	Antibiotic
01490009 <> MACRODANTIN100	Cap	Nitrofurantoin 100 mg	Macrodantin by Pharmedix	53002-0273	Antibiotic
01490009 <> MACRODANTIN100	Cap, 3 Black Lines	Nitrofurantoin 100 mg	Macrodantin by Pharm Utilization	60491-0389	Antibiotic
01490009 <> MACRODANTIN100M	Cap, 0149 over 0009 & 3 Black Lines <> Macrodantin over 100 mg	Nitrofurantoin 100 mg	Macrodantin by Amerisource	62584-0009	Antibiotic
01490030	Cap, Orange & Tan, 0149/0300	Dantrolene Sodium 50 mg	by Procter & Gamble		Muscle Relaxant
01490033	Cap, Orange & Tan, 0149/0033	Dantrolene Sodium 100 mg	by Procter & Gamble		Muscle Relaxant
01490412 <> ENTEX	Cap	Guaifenesin 200 mg, Phenylephrine HCl 5 mg, Phenylpropanolamine HCl 45 mg	Entex by Amerisource	62584-0412	Cold Remedy
01490436 <> ENTEXLA	Tab	Guaifenesin 400 mg, Phenylpropanolamine HCl 75 mg	Entex LA by Amerisource	62584-0436	Cold Remedy
01490436 <> ENTEXLA	Tab	Guaifenesin 400 mg, Phenylpropanolamine HCl 75 mg	Entex LA by Quality Care	60346-0336	Cold Remedy
01490436 <> ENTEXLA	Tab	Guaifenesin 400 mg, Phenylpropanolamine HCl 75 mg	Entex LA by Caremark	00339-5128	Cold Remedy
01490436 <> ENTEXLA	Tab	Guaifenesin 400 mg, Phenylpropanolamine HCl 75 mg	Entex LA by Urgent Care Ctr	50716-0436	Cold Remedy
01490436 <> ENTEXLA	Tab	Guaifenesin 400 mg, Phenylpropanolamine HCl 75 mg	Entex LA by Nat Pharmpak Serv	55154-2303	Cold Remedy
014930 <> DANTRIUM25MG	Cap, Orange & Tan	Dantrolene Sodium 25 mg	Dantrium by Procter & Gamble	00149-0030	Muscle Relaxant
014931 <> DANTRIUM50MG	Cap, Orange & Tan	Dantrolene Sodium 50 mg	Dantrium by Procter & Gamble	00149-0031	Muscle Relaxant
015	Cap, Maroon & Pink	Niacin TD 400 mg	Nicobid by Time-Caps		Vitamin
015 <> AMIDE	Tab, Film Coated	Dexchlorpheniramine Maleate 6 mg	by Schein	00364-0586	Antihistamine
015 <> MEDEVA	Tab	Guaifenesin 400 mg, Pseudoephedrine HCl 120 mg	Deconsal LA by Medeva	53014-0015	Cold Remedy
015 <> MEDEVA	Tab	Guaifenesin 400 mg, Pseudoephedrine HCl 120 mg	Deconsal LA by Adams	53014-0015	Cold Remedy
015 <> PAR	Tab	Meclizine HCl 50 mg	by Par	49884-0015	Antiemetic
0150	Tab, Peach, Round, 0.150	Desogestrel 0.03 mg, Ethinyl Estradiol 0.15 mg	Ortho Cept by Ortho-McNeil	00062-1796	Oral Contraceptive
0158	Tab, Blue, Round, Scored, Duramed Logo-Diamond	Estradiol 1.5 mg	Gynodiol 1.5 mg by Heartland	61392-0042	Hormone
0158	Tab, Blue, Round, Scored	Gynodiol 1.5 mg	by Medicus	99207-0499	Hormone
016	Tab, Rugby Logo	Chlorpheniramine Maleate 4 mg	by Allscripts	54569-0243	Antihistamine
016 <> ACH	Tab, Light Pink, Round	Candesartan Cilexetil 16 mg	Atacand by Astra Merck	00186-0016	Antihypertensive
016 <> PAR	Tab	Chlorzoxazone 250 mg	by Par	49884-0016	Muscle Relaxant
017 <> MEDEVA	Tab	Guaifenesin 600 mg, Pseudoephedrine HCl 60 mg	Deconsal II by Adams	53014-0017	Cold Remedy
017 <> MEDEVA	Tab	Guaifenesin 600 mg, Pseudoephedrine HCl 60 mg	Deconsal II by Medeva	53014-0017	Cold Remedy

4

ID FRONT <> BACK	DESCRIPTION FRONT <> BACK	INGREDIENT & STRENGTH	BRAND (OR EQUIV.) & FIRM	NDC#	CLASS; SCH.
017 <> MEDEVA	Tab	Guaifenesin 600 mg, Pseudoephedrine HCl 60 mg	Syn Rx by Adams	53014-0308	Cold Remedy
018	Tab, Greek Letter Alpha	Guaifenesin 600 mg	by Pharmafab	62542-0700	Expectorant
018	Tab, Greek Letter Alpha	Guaifenesin 600 mg	Hip 600 by Sovereign	58716-0600	Expectorant
018 <> 0088	Tab, Peach, Oblong, Coated	Fexofenadine HCl 180 mg	Allegra by Aventis	00088-1109	Antihistamine
018 <> A	Cap	Chlordiazepoxide HCl 5 mg, Clidinium Bromide 2.5 mg	by Schein	00364-0559	Gastrointestinal; C IV
019 <> TCL	Cap	Papaverine HCl 150 mg	by UDL	51079-0010	Vasodilator
019 <> TCL	Cap, Black Print	Papaverine HCl 150 mg	Para Time by Time Caps	49483-0019	Vasodilator
019 <> THERRX	Tab, Blue, Oval, Film Coated	Calcium 200 mg, Folic Acid 1 mg, Vitamin B6 75 mg, Vitamin B12 12 mcg	by KV Pharmaceutical	64011-0019	Vitamin/Mineral
0198	Cap, Gray, Savage Logo 0198	Butalbital 50 mg, Acetaminophen 650 mg	Axocet by Savage	00281-0198	Analgesic
019TCL	Cap	Papaverine HCl 150 mg	by Schein	00364-0181	Vasodilator
01A	Cap, Ivory & Red	Dipyridamole 200 mg; Aspirin 25 mg	Aggrenox by Boehringer Ingelheim	12714-0125	Antiplatelet
01B	Tab, White, Round	Fenoterol 2.5 mg	by Boehringer Ingelheim	Canadian	Antiasthmatic
02	Tab, White, Round, 0.2	Desmopressin Acetate 0.2 mg	DDAVP by Ferring	Canadian	Antidiuretic
02 <> DAN5612	Tab, 0.2 <> Dan 5612	Clonidine HCl 0.2 mg	by Danbury	00591-5612	Antihypertensive
020	Cap, Pink & White, Advance Logo	Diphenhydramine HCl 25 mg	by Geneva	00781-2053	Antihistamine
020	Cap	Loperamide HCl 2 mg	by United Res	00677-1422	Antidiarrheal
020 <> WESTWARD	Tab	Aminophylline 100 mg	by Schein	00364-0004	Antiasthmatic
020N2	Cap	Loperamide HCl 2 mg	by Schein	00364-2481	Antidiarrheal
021	Tab	Thyroid 32.5 mg	by Time Caps	49483-0021	Thyroid
021MJ	Tab, 021/MJ	Estradiol 0.5 mg	by Caremark	00339-5464	Hormone
022 <> TCL	Tab	Thyroid 65 mg	by Time Caps	49483-0022	Thyroid
0221	Tab, Circa Logo	Glipizide 5 mg	by HL Moore	00839-7939	Antidiabetic
0221	Tab, Circa Logo	Glipizide 5 mg	by United Res	00677-1544	Antidiabetic
0221	Tab, Circa Logo	Glipizide 5 mg	by Circa	71114-0221	Antidiabetic
0222	Tab, Circa Logo	Glipizide 10 mg	by Circa	71114-0222	Antidiabetic
0222	Tab, Circa Logo	Glipizide 10 mg	by United Res	00677-1545	Antidiabetic
0222	Tab, Circa Logo	Glipizide 10 mg	by Schein	00364-2605	Antidiabetic
0222	Tab, Circa Logo	Glipizide 10 mg	by HL Moore	00839-7940	Antidiabetic
023	Tab, Purepac Logo	Aspirin 325 mg, Butalbital 50 mg, Caffeine 40 mg	by Quality Care	60346-0619	Analgesic; C III
023 <> R	Tab, White, Round	Aspirin 325 mg, Butalbital 50 mg, Caffeine 40 mg	by Purepac	00228-2023	Analgesic; C III
023 <> TLC	Tab	Thyroid 130 mg	by Time Caps	49483-0023	Thyroid
023R	Tab, 023/R	Aspirin 325 mg, Butalbital 50 mg, Caffeine 40 mg	by Allscripts	54569-0339	Analgesic; C III
024 <> ADAMS	Tab, 0/24 <> Adams	Atropine Sulfate 0.04 mg, Chlorpheniramine Maleate 8 mg, Hyoscyamine Sulfate 0.19 mg, Phenylephrine HCl 25 mg, Phenylpropanolamine HCl 50 mg, Scopolamine Hydrobromide 0.01 mg	Atrohist Plus by Drug Distr	52985-0227	Cold Remedy
024 <> ADAMS	Tab	Atropine Sulfate 0.04 mg, Chlorpheniramine Maleate 8 mg, Hyoscyamine Sulfate 0.19 mg, Phenylephrine HCl 25 mg, Phenylpropanolamine HCl 50 mg, Scopolamine Hydrobromide 0.01 mg	Atrohist Plus by Medeva	53014-0024	Cold Remedy
024 <> THX	Tab, Mottled Orange, Oval, Film Coated	Calcium 250 mg, Copper 2 mg, Folic Acid 1 mg, Iron 40 mg, Magnesium 50 mg, Vitamin B6 2 mg, Vitamin C 50 mg, Vitamin D3 6 mcg, Vitamin E 3.5 mg, Zinc 15 mg	by KV Pharmaceutical	64011-0024	Vitamin/Mineral
0245 <> ROCHE	Cap, Roche	Saquinavir Mesylate 200 mg	Invirase by Hoffmann La Roche	00004-0245	Antiviral
0245 <> ROCHE	Cap, Roche	Saquinavir Mesylate 200 mg	Invirase by Physicians Total Care	54868-3699	Antiviral
0245ROCHE	Cap, Green & Light Brown, 0245/Roche	Saquinavir 200 mg	by 3M Pharmaceuticals	Canadian	Antiviral
025	Cap	Amylase 20000 Units, Lipase 4000 Units, Protease 25000 Units	Pancreatic Enzyme by Zenith Goldline	00182-1554	Gastrointestinal
025 <> AP	Tab, White, Round	Estradiol 0.5 mg	by Apothecon	59772-0025	Hormone
025 <> ETHEX	Cap, Gelatin, White Print	Cyanocobalamin 25 mcg, Folic Acid 1 mg, Iron 150 mg	Fe Tinic 150 by KV	10609-1365	Vitamin
025 <> ETHEX	Cap, Gelatin, White Print	Cyanocobalamin 25 mcg, Folic Acid 1 mg, Iron 150 mg	Fe Tinic 150 by Ethex	58177-0025	Vitamin
025 <> N126	Tab, 0.25 <> N over 126	Alprazolam 0.25 mg	by Medirex	57480-0520	Antianxiety; C IV
025 <> N126	Tab, 0.25 <> N over 126	Alprazolam 0.25 mg	by PDRX	55289-0962	Antianxiety; C IV
025 <> N126	Tab, Coated, 0.25 <> N over 126	Alprazolam 0.25 mg	by Quality Care	60346-0876	Antianxiety; C IV
025 <> N126	Tab, White, Round, Scored, 0.25 <> N over 126	Alprazolam 0.25 mg	by Novopharm	55953-8131	Antianxiety; C IV

5

ID FRONT <> BACK	DESCRIPTION FRONT <> BACK	INGREDIENT & STRENGTH	BRAND (OR EQUIV.) & FIRM	NDC#	CLASS; SCH.
025 <> THERRX	Tab, Peach, Cap Shaped, Film Coated, Scored	Ascorbic Acid 50 mg; Calcium Carbonate 250 mg; Cyanocobalamin12 mcg; Cholecalciferol 6 mcg; Thiamine Mononitrate 3 mg; Riboflavin 3.4 mg; Niacinamide 20 mg; Pyridoxine HCl 20 mg; Folic Acid 1 mg; Magnesium Oxide 50 mg; Zinc Sulfate 15 mg; Cupric Sulfate 2	Precare Prenatal by Ther Rx	64011-0025	Vitamin
025 <> WESTWARD	Tab	Aminophylline 200 mg	by Schein	00364-0005	Antiasthmatic
0252240MG	Cap, Black Bands, RPR Logo over 240 mg	Diltiazem HCl 240 mg	Dilacor by RPR	00075-0252	Antihypertensive
0258	Cap, Maroon/Brown, Sav. Logo 0258	Vitamin, Iron	Chromagen FA by Savage	00281-0259	Vitamin
025ALG	Tab, Light Yellow, 0.25/AL/G	Alprazolam 0.25 mg	by Schein	00364-2582	Antianxiety; C IV
025AP	Tab	Estradiol 0.5 mg	by Bristol Myers	15548-0025	Hormone
026	Tab, Greek Letter Alpha	Hyoscyamine Sulfate 0.125 mg	by Pharmafab	62542-0350	Gastrointestinal
026 <> AP	Tab, Lavender, Round	Estradiol 1 mg	by Apothecon	59772-0026	Hormone
026 <> G	Cap	Piroxicam 10 mg	by Par	49884-0440	NSAID
026 <> G	Cap, Dark Green & Olive	Piroxicam 10 mg	by Genpharm	55567-0026	NSAID
026 <> R	Tab, White, Round, Scored	Phenobarbital 15 mg	by UDL	51079-0094	Sedative/Hypnotic; C IV
026 <> R	Tab, White, Round	Phenobarbital 15 mg	by Purepac	00228-2026	Sedative/Hypnotic; C IV
026 <> R	Tab	Phenobarbital 17.01 mg	by Vangard	00615-0420	Sedative/Hypnotic; C IV
0262	Cap, Brown, Sav. Logo 0262	Vitamin, Iron	Chromagen Forte by Savage	00281-0262	Vitamin
026AP	Tab	Estradiol 1 mg	by Bristol Myers	15548-0026	Hormone
026G	Cap, Powder Blue, 026/G	Piroxicam 10 mg	by Genpharm	Canadian	NSAID
026G	Cap, Black Print	Piroxicam 10 mg	by Quality Care	60346-0737	NSAID
027 <> 027	Tab, Purepac Logo	Alprazolam 0.25 mg	by Heartland	61392-0034	Antianxiety; C IV
027 <> AP	Tab, Turquoise, Round	Estradiol 2 mg	by Apothecon	59772-0027	Hormone
027 <> ETHEX	Cap, Maroon	Meperidine HCl 50 mg, Promethazine HCl 25 mg	Mepergan by Ethex	58177-0027	Analgesic; C II
027 <> ETHEX	Cap, White Print	Meperidine HCl 50 mg, Promethazine HCl 25 mg	by KV	10609-1398	Analgesic; C II
027 <> G	Cap	Piroxicam 20 mg	by Par	49884-0441	NSAID
027 <> G	Cap	Piroxicam 20 mg	by Genpharm	55567-0027	NSAID
027 <> R	Tab, White, Round, Scored	Alprazolam 0.25 mg	by Purepac	00228-2027	Antianxiety; C IV
027AP	Tab	Estradiol 2 mg	by Bristol Myers	15548-0027	Hormone
027G	Cap, Maroon, 027/G	Piroxicam 20 mg	by Genpharm	Canadian	NSAID
027G	Cap, Dark Green, Black Print	Piroxicam 20 mg	by Quality Care	60346-0676	NSAID
028 <> R	Tab, White, Round, Scored	Phenobarbital 30 mg		51079-0095	Sedative/Hypnotic; C IV
028 <> R	Tab, White, Round, Scored	Phenobarbital 30 mg	by Purepac	00228-2028	Sedative/Hypnotic; C IV
028 <> R	Tab	Phenobarbital 30 mg	by Vangard	00615-0421	Sedative/Hypnotic; C IV
029	Tab, Scored	Alprazolam 0.5 mg	by Heartland	61392-0035	Antianxiety; C IV
029 <> R	Tab, Peach, Round, Scored	Alprazolam 0.5 mg	by Purepac	00228-2029	Antianxiety; C IV
02C <> SEPTRADS	Tab	Sulfamethoxazole 800 mg, Trimethoprim 160 mg	Septra DS by Nat Pharmpak Serv	55154-0703	Antibiotic
03 <> DAN5613	Tab, 0.3 <> Dan 5613	Clonidine HCl 0.3 mg	by Danbury	00591-5613	Antihypertensive
03 <> DAN5613	Tab	Clonidine HCl 0.3 mg	by Allscripts	54569-2801	Antihypertensive
030 <> MEDEVA	Tab	Dextromethorphan Hydrobromide 30 mg, Guaifenesin 600 mg	Humibid DM by Medeva	53014-0030	Cold Remedy
030 <> MEDEVA	Tab, Dark Green	Dextromethorphan Hydrobromide 30 mg, Guaifenesin 600 mg	Humibid DM by Adams	53014-0030	Cold Remedy
0305 <> PAL	Cap, White	Dyphilline 200 mg, Guaifenesin 100 mg	Panfil G by Pan Am	00525-0305	Antiasthmatic
031 <> A	Tab, Chewable	Ascorbic Acid 34.5 mg, Cyanocobalamin 4.9 mcg, Folic Acid 0.35 mg, Niacinamide 14.16 mg, Pyridoxine HCl 1.1 mg, Riboflavin 1.2 mg, Sodium Ascorbate 32.2 mg, Sodium Fluoride 1.1 mg, Thiamine Mononitrate 1.15 mg, Vitamin A Acetate 5.5 mg, Vitamin D 0.194 mg, Vitamin E Acetate 15.75 mg	Poly Vitamins by Zenith Goldline	00182-1819	Vitamin
031 <> R	Tab, Blue, Round, Scored	Alprazolam 1 mg	by Purepac	00228-2031	Antianxiety; C IV
0310	Tab, Yellow, Oblong, Ascher logo 0310	Magnesium Salicylate 600 mg	Mobidin by B.F.Ascher		Analgesic
0310	Tab, White, Cap Shaped, Scored, Ascher Logo <> Ascher Logo	Magnesium Salicylate 600 mg	Mobidin by BFAscher	00225-0310	Analgesic
0311	Cap, White, Cap Shaped, Film Coated	Acetaminophen 500 mg	by UDL	51079-0396	Antipyretic
0319	Cap, Purple, Savage Logo 0319	Folic Acid 1 mg	Chromagen OB by Savage	00281-0319	Vitamin
032 <> ACL	Tab, Pink, Round	Candesartan Cilexetil 32 mg	Atacand by Astra Merck	00186-0032	Antihypertensive
032 <> ACL	Tab	Candesartan Cilexetil 32 mg	by Astra AB	17228-0032	Antihypertensive

ID FRONT <> BACK	DESCRIPTION FRONT <> BACK	INGREDIENT & STRENGTH	BRAND (OR EQUIV.) & FIRM	NDC#	CLASS; SCH.
032032 <> ENTEXPSE	Tab, Yellow, Scored, Film Coated	Guaifenesin 600 mg, Pseudoephedrine HCl 120 mg	Entex PSE by Dura	51479-0032	Cold Remedy
032032 <> ENTEXPSE	Tab, Film Coated, 032 over 032 <> Entex PSE	Guaifenesin 600 mg, Pseudoephedrine HCl 120 mg	Entex PSE by Welpharm	63375-6376	Cold Remedy
0321US	Tab, 0321/US	Magnesium Salicylate 600 mg, Phenyltoloxamine Citrate 25 mg	Magsal		Antiarthritic; C III
0321US	Tab, Green, Oval, 0321/US	Magnesium Salicylate 600 mg, Phenyltoloxamine Citrate 25 mg	Magsal by Nat Pharmpak Serv	55154-5238	Antiarthritic; C III
0321US	Tab, Green, Oblong, 0321/US	Magnesium Salicylate, Phenyltolaxamine	Magsal by US	52747-0321	Antiarthritic; C III
033 <> BARR	Cap, Black & Green	Chlordiazepoxide HCl 10 mg	Librium by UDL	51079-0375	Antianxiety; C IV
033 <> BARR	Cap, Barr Logo	Chlordiazepoxide HCl 10 mg	by Geneva	00781-2082	Antianxiety; C IV
033 <> BARR	Cap	Chlordiazepoxide HCl 10 mg	by Med Pro	53978-3175	Antianxiety; C IV
033033 <> ENTEXLA	Tab, Film Coated	Guaifenesin 400 mg, Phenylpropanolamine HCl 75 mg	Entex LA by Welpharm	63375-6377	Cold Remedy
033033 <> ENTEXLA	Tab, Orange, Scored	Guaifenesin 400 mg, Phenylpropanolamine HCl 75 mg	Entex LA by Dura	51479-0033	Cold Remedy
033033 <> ENTEXLA	Tab, Orange, Oblong, Scored, 033 033 <> Entex LA	Guaifenesin 400 mg, Phenylpropanolamine HCl 75 mg	Entex LA by Martec		Cold Remedy
033033ENTEXLA	Tab, Orange, 033 033/Entex LA	Guaifenesin 400 mg, Phenylpropanolamine HCl 75 mg	Entex LA by Dura		Cold Remedy
0331 <> MP	Tab, Red, Film Coated	Calcium Carbonate 312 mg, Cyanocobalamin 3 mcg, Ferric Polysaccharide Complex, Folic Acid 1 mg, Niacinamide 10 mg, Pyridoxine HCl 2 mg, Riboflavin 3 mg, Sodium Ascorbate, Thiamine Mononitrate 3 mg, Vitamin A 4000 Units, Vitamin D 400 Units	Nu Iron V	00131-2306	Vitamin/Mineral
0331 <> MP	Tab, Coated	Calcium Carbonate 312 mg, Cyanocobalamin 3 mcg, Ferric Polysaccharide Complex, Folic Acid 1 mg, Niacinamide 10 mg, Pyridoxine HCl 2 mg, Riboflavin 3 mg, Sodium Ascorbate, Thiamine Mononitrate 3 mg, Vitamin A 4000 Units, Vitamin D 400 Units	Nu Iron V by Merz	00259-0331	Vitamin/Mineral
034 <> PAR	Tab, Blue & White, Oval	Meclizine HCl 12.5 mg	Antivert by UDL	51079-0089	Antiemetic
034 <> PAR	Tab	Meclizine HCl 12.5 mg	by Schein	00364-0411	Antiemetic
034 <> PAR	Tab	Meclizine HCl 12.5 mg	by Vangard	00615-1553	Antiemetic
034 <> PAR	Tab, Blue & White	Meclizine HCl 12.5 mg	by Par	49884-0034	Antiemetic
03451032	Cap, Gray & Red	Propoxyphene 65 mg, Aspirin 389 mg, Caffeine 32.4 mg	Darvon Compound by Lemmon		Analgesic; C IV
035 <> PAR	Tab, Yellow & White, Football Shaped	Meclizine HCl 25 mg	Antivert by UDL	51079-0090	Antiemetic
035 <> PAR	Tab	Meclizine HCl 25 mg	by Schein	00364-0412	Antiemetic
035 <> PAR	Tab	Meclizine HCl 25 mg	by Par	49884-0035	Antiemetic
035 <> PAR	Tab	Meclizine HCl 25 mg	by Vangard	00615-1554	Antiemetic
036 <> TCL	Cap, Black Print	Chlorpheniramine Maleate 4 mg, Phenylephrine HCl 20 mg, Phenyltoloxamine Citrate 50 mg	Com Time by Time Caps	49483-0036	Cold Remedy; C III
0364 <> NIFEDIPINE10	Cap	Nifedipine 10 mg	by Nat Pharmpak Serv	55154-5206	Antihypertensive
0364 <> NIFEDIPINE10	Cap	Nifedipine 10 mg	by Amerisource	62584-0802	Antihypertensive
0364 <> NIFEDIPINE10	Cap	Nifedipine 10 mg	by Quality Care	60346-0803	Antihypertensive
0364 <> NIFEDIPINE20	Cap	Nifedipine 20 mg	by Schein	00364-2377	Antihypertersive
0364 <> NIFEDIPINE20	Cap, 0364 <> Nifedipine 20-0364	Nifedipine 20 mg	by Allscripts	54569-3122	Antihypertensive
0364 <> NIFEDIPINE20	Cap	Nifedipine 20 mg	by Amerisource	62584-0803	Antihypertensive
0364 <> VALPROIC250	Cap, Off-White	Valproic Acid 250 mg	by Schein	00364-0822	Anticonvulsant
037 <> ETHEX	Cap, Green, Opaque	Trimethobenzamide HCl 250 mg	Tigan by Ethex	58177-0037	Antiemetic
037 <> ETHEX	Cap	Trimethobenzamide HCl 250 mg	by KV	10609-1401	Antiemetic
0379 <> MR	Tab, Off-White, Film Coated	Guaifenesin 400 mg, Pseudoephedrine HCl 120 mg	Anatuss LA by Merz	00259-0379	Cold Remedy
038 <> TCL	Tab	Thyroid 195 mg	by Time Caps	49483-0038	Thyroid
039 <> TCL	Tab, Sugar Coated, White Print	Brompheniramine Maleate 12 mg, Phenylephrine HCl 15 mg, Phenylpropanolamine HCl 15 mg	Dime Time by Time Caps	49483-0039	Cold Remedy
03Z3636	Tab, White, Round, 0.3/Z 3636	Conjugated Estrogens 0.3 mg	Premarin by Zenith Goldline		Estrogen
04 <> WE	Cap	Brompheniramine Maleate 6 mg, Pseudoephedrine HCl 60 mg	Ultrabrom PD by Sovereign	58716-0026	Cold Remedy
0405 <> 0524	Tab	Allopurinol 100 mg	by Major	00904-2613	Antigout
041 <> TCL	Cap, Blue-Green, White Print	Chlorpheniramine Maleate 8 mg	by Time Caps	49483-0041	Antihistamine
0410 <> 0524	Tab	Allopurinol 300 mg	by Quality Care	60346-0638	Antigout
0410 <> 0524	Tab	Allopurinol 300 mg	by Major	00904-2614	Antigout
0410 <> 0524	Tab	Allopurinol 300 mg	by IDE Inter	00814-0511	Antigout
043 <> TCL	Cap, Blue-Green, Black Print	Chlorpheniramine Maleate 12 mg	by Time Caps	49483-0043	Antihistamine

ID FRONT <> BACK	DESCRIPTION FRONT <> BACK	INGREDIENT & STRENGTH	BRAND (OR EQUIV.) & FIRM	NDC#	CLASS; SCH.
0430 <> WALLACE	Tab, Yellow, Cap Shaped, Scored	Felbamate 400 mg	Felbatol by Wallace	00037-0430	Anticonvulsant
0431 <> WALLACE	Tab, Peach, Cap Shaped, Scored	Felbamate 600 mg	Felbatol by Wallace	00037-0431	Anticonvulsant
0431 <> WALLACE	Tab, Peach, Oblong, Scored	Felbamate 600 mg	Felbatol by Hoffmann La Roche	00004-6200	Anticonvulsant
044HD	Tab, White, Round	Meprobamate 400 mg	Neuramate by Halsey		Sedative/Hypnotic; C IV
0478 <> 5477	Tab	Atropine Sulfate 0.0194 mg, Hyoscyamine Sulfate 0.1037 mg, Phenobarbital 16.2 mg, Scopolamine Hydrobromide 0.0065 mg	Belladonna PB by Quality Care	60346-0042	Gastrointestinal; C IV
04785477	Tab, 0478-5477	Atropine Sulfate 0.0194 mg, Hyoscyamine Sulfate 0.1037 mg, Phenobarbital 16.2 mg, Scopolamine Hydrobromide 0.0065 mg	Rexatal by Shire Richwood	58521-0754	Gastrointestinal; C IV
04785477	Tab, 0478-5477	Atropine Sulfate 0.0194 mg, Hyoscyamine Sulfate 0.1037 mg, Phenobarbital 16.2 mg, Scopolamine Hydrobromide 0.0065 mg	Bellatal by Shire Richwood	58521-0162	Gastrointestinal; C IV
04785477	Tab, White, Round, Scored, 0478/5477	Phenobarbital 16.2 mg	by Physicians Total Care	54868-3720	Sedative/Hypnotic; C IV
048	Tab, Red, Cap Shaped, Film Coated	Calcium Pantothenate 10 mg, Cyanocobalamin 25 mcg, Ferrous Sulfate 525 mg, Folic Acid 800 mcg, Niacinamide 30 mg, Pyridoxine HCl 5 mg, Riboflavin 6 mg, Sodium Ascorbate 500 mg, Thiamine Mononitrate 6 mg	Multiret Folic 500 by Amide	52152-0048	Vitamin/Mineral
0497 <> 50MG	Cap	Minocycline HCl	Dynacin by Medicus	99207-0497	Antibiotic
049750MG <> MEDICIS	Cap	Minocycline HCl	Dynacin by Thrift Drug	59198-0276	Antibiotic
0497DYNACIN50MG	Cap	Minocycline HCl	Dynacin by Eckerd Drug	19458-0866	Antibiotic
0498100MG <> MEDICIS	Cap	Minocycline HCl	Dynacin by Medicis	99207-0498	Antibiotic
0498100MG <> MEDICIS	Cap	Minocycline HCl	Dynacin by Thrift Drug	59198-0277	Antibiotic
0498DYNACIN100M	Cap	Minocycline HCl	Dynacin by Eckerd Drug	19458-0867	Antibiotic
0498DYNACIN100M	Cap, Gray & White	Minocycline HCl 100 mg	Dynacin by Rx Pac	65084-0122	Antibiotic
0499 <> DYNACIN75MG	Cap, Gray, Opaque	Minocycline HCl 75 mg	Minocycline HCl by Neuman Distr	64579-0250	Antibiotic
0499DYNACIN	Cap, Gray	Minocycline HCl 75 mg	Dynacin by Thrift Services	59198-0330	Antibiotic
04A <> PURINETHOL	Tab	Mercaptopurine 50 mg	Purinethol by Catalytica	63552-0807	Antineoplastic
04A <> PURINETHOL	Tab	Mercaptopurine 50 mg	Purinethol by Glaxo	00173-0807	Antineoplastic
05 <> 180605240	Tab, 0.05 <> 1806.05-240	Lorazepam 0.5 mg	by Zenith Goldline	00182-1806	Sedative/Hypnotic; C IV
05 <> 240	Tab, Coated, 0.5 <> Royce Logo 240	Lorazepam 0.5 mg	by Quality Care	60346-0363	Sedative/Hypnotic; C IV
05 <> 240	Tab, 0.5 <> 240	Lorazepam 0.51 mg	by United Res	00677-1056	Sedative/Hypnotic; C IV
05 <> 240	Tab, 0.5/Royce Logo	Lorazepam 0.51 mg	by Qualitest	00603-4243	Sedative/Hypnotic; C IV
05 <> BIOCRAFT	Cap, Scarlet	Ampicillin Trihydrate	by Quality Care	60346-0082	Antibiotic
05 <> BIOCRAFT	Cap, Scarlet	Ampicillin Trihydrate	by Schein	00364-2001	Antibiotic
05 <> G	Tab, White, Oval, Scored, 0.5 <> G	Estradiol 0.51 mg	by Teva	00093-1057	Hormone
05 <> G	Tab, 0.5 <> G	Estradiol 0.51 mg	by AAI	27280-0004	Hormone
05 <> N127	Tab, 0.5 <> N over 127	Alprazolam 0.5 mg	by Medirex	57480-0521	Antianxiety; C IV
05 <> N127	Tab, 0.5 <> N over 127	Alprazolam 0.5 mg	by HL Moore	00839-7852	Antianxiety; C IV
05 <> N127	Tab, Orange, Round, Scored, 0.5 <> N over 127	Alprazolam 0.5 mg	by Novopharm	55953-8127	Antianxiety; C IV
05 <> NU	Tab, White, Round, 0.5 <> NU	Lorazepam 0.5 mg	by Nu-Pharm	Canadian DIN # 00865672	Sedative/Hypnotic
05 <> Z4232	Tab, Green, Round, Scored, 0.5 <> Z 4232	Bumetanide 0.5 mg	by Caraco	57664-0220	Diuretic
05 <> Z4232	Tab, 0.5 <> Z 4232	Bumetanide 0.5 mg	by Geneva	00781-1821	Diuretic
05 <> Z4232	Tab, Green, Round, 0.5 <> Z4232	Bumetanide 0.5 mg	Bumex by Zenith Goldline	00182-2615	Diuretic
05 <> Z4232	Tab, Scored, 0.5 <> Z over 4232	Bumetanide 0.5 mg	by HL Moore	00839-8011	Diuretic
05 <> Z4232	Tab, 0.5 <> Z 4232	Bumetanide 0.5 mg	by Major	00904-5102	Diuretic
051 <> R	Tab, White, Round, Scored	Diazepam 2 mg	by Purepac	00228-2051	Antianxiety; C IV
052	Tab, Purepac Logo 052	Diazepam 5 mg	by Quality Care	60346-0478	Antianxiety; C IV
052	Tab	Diazepam 5 mg	by Talbert Med	44514-0955	Antianxiety; C IV
052 <> R	Tab, Yellow, Round, Scored	Diazepam 5 mg	by Purepac	00228-2052	Antianxiety; C IV

ID FRONT <> BACK	DESCRIPTION FRONT <> BACK	INGREDIENT & STRENGTH	BRAND (OR EQUIV.) & FIRM	NDC#	CLASS; SCH.
052 <> R	Tab	Diazepam 5 mg	by Urgent Care Ctr	50716-0132	Antianxiety; C IV
0524 <> 0405	Tab	Allopurinol 100 mg	by Major	00904-2613	Antigout
0524 <> 0410	Tab	Allopurinol 300 mg	by Quality Care	60346-0638	Antigout
0524 <> 0410	Tab	Allopurinol 300 mg	by Major	00904-2614	Antigout
0524 <> 0410	Tab	Allopurinol 300 mg	by IDE Inter	00814-0511	Antigout
05240405	Tab	Allopurinol 100 mg	by Vangard	00615-1592	Antigout
05240405	Tab, 0524 over 0405	Allopurinol 100 mg	by Par	49884-0602	Antigout
05240405	Tab, Off-White, 0524 over 0405	Allopurinol 100 mg	by HJ Harkins Co	52959-0473	Antigout
05240405	Tab, White, Round, Scored, 0524 over 0405	Allopurinol 100 mg	by Apotheca	12634-0491	Antigout
05240405	Tab, 0524 over 0405	Allopurinol 100 mg	by BASF	10117-0602	Antigout
05240410	Tab, 0524 over 0410	Allopurinol 300 mg	by Par	49884-0603	Antigout
05240410	Tab, 0524 over 0410	Allopurinol 300 mg	by BASF	10117-0603	Antigout
0527 <> 1552	Cap	Aspirin 325 mg, Butalbital 50 mg, Caffeine 40 mg	by United Res	00677-1439	Analgesic; C III
05271152	Cap	Aspirin 325 mg, Butalbital 50 mg, Caffeine 40 mg	by Zenith Goldline	00182-0140	Analgesic; C III
05271552	Cap	Aspirin 325 mg, Butalbital 50 mg, Caffeine 40 mg	by Rugby	00536-3933	Analgesic; C III
05271552 <> LANNETT	Cap, Dark Green & Light Green, 0527/1552 <> Lannett	Aspirin 325 mg, Butalbital 50 mg, Caffeine 40 mg	by Novopharm	55953-0633	Analgesic; C III
05271552 <> LANNETT	Cap, 0527/1552 <> Lannett	Aspirin 325 mg, Butalbital 50 mg, Caffeine 40 mg	by Lannett	00527-1552	Analgesic; C III
053	Tab, Purepac Logo	Diazepam 10 mg	by United Res	00677-1050	Antianxiety; C IV
053 <> R	Tab, Blue, Round, Scored	Diazepam 10 mg	by Purepac	00228-2053	Antianxiety; C IV
05510123	Tab, 0551/0123	Dyphylline 200 mg, Guaifenesin 200 mg	Dyline GG by Seatrace	00551-0123	Antiasthmatic
058	Tab, Cream & Orange Specks, Round	Chewable Vitamin 1 mg, Fluoride 1 mg	PolyVi-Flor by Amide		Vitamin
059 <> BARR	Cap, Pink	Diphenhydramine HCl 50 mg	Benadryl by UDL	51079-0066	Antihistamine
05915238	Tab, White, Round	Meprobamate 400 mg	Miltown by Schein		Sedative/Hypnotic; C IV
05915239	Tab, White, Round	Meprobamate 200 mg	Miltown by Schein		Sedative/Hypnotic; C IV
05ALG	Tab, Dark Yellow, 0.5/AL/G	Alprazolam 0.5 mg	by Schein	00364-2583	Antianxiety; C IV
05MG <> F607	Cap, White, Red Band, 0.5 mg <> F 607	Tacrolimus 0.5 mg	Prograf by Fujisawa	00469-0607	Immunosuppressant
05MG <> F607	Cap, Yellow, Branded Red, 0.5 mg <> F607	Tacrolimus 0.5 mg	Prograf 0.5 mg by St. Marys Med	60760-0457	Immunosuppressant
06 <> 59	Tab, White, Oblong, Scored	Tramidol 50 mg	by Ultram		Analgesic
06 <> BIOCRAFT	Cap, Scarlet	Ampicillin Trihydrate	by Quality Care	60346-0593	Antibiotic
06 <> WE	Cap	Brompheniramine Maleate 12 mg, Pseudoephedrine HCl 120 mg	Ultrabrom by Sovereign	58716-0025	Cold Remedy
060 <> 59743	Cap, Clear & Green with White Beads	Brompheniramine Maleate 12 mg, Pseudoephedrine HCl 120 mg	by Quality Care	60346-0929	Cold Remedy
061 <> PAR	Tab, Film Coated	Fluphenazine HCl 1 mg	by Schein	00364-2265	Antipsychotic
061 <> PAR	Tab, Film Coated	Fluphenazine HCl 1 mg	by Qualitest	00603-3666	Antipsychotic
062 <> PAR	Tab, Coated	Fluphenazine HCl 2.5 mg	by Qualitest	00603-3667	Antipsychotic
062 <> PAR	Tab, Coated	Fluphenazine HCl 2.5 mg	by Schein	00364-2266	Antipsychotic
0625 <> PREMARIN	Tab, Coated, 0.625	Conjugated, Estrogens 0.625 mg	Premarin by Quality Care	60346-0599	Estrogen
0625 <> PREMARIN	Tab, Coated	Conjugated, Estrogens 0.625 mg	Premarin by Med Pro	53978-0189	Estrogen
0625Z2042	Tab, White, Round, 0.625 Z/2042	Conjugated, Estrogens 0.625 mg	Premarin by Zenith Goldline		Estrogen
063	Tab, White, Round, Scored, Purepac Logo	Lorazepam 2 mg	by Nat Pharmpak Serv	55154-0214	Sedative/Hypnotic; C IV
063 <> P	Tab, White, Round, Scored, Purepac Logo	Lorazepam 2 mg	by Nat Pharmpak Serv	55154-1050	Sedative/Hypnotic; C IV
063 <> P	Tab, Scored, 063 <> Purepac Logo	Lorazepam 2 mg	by Talbert Med	44514-0100	Sedative/Hypnotic; C IV
063 <> R	Tab, White, Round	Lorazepam 2 mg	by Purepac	00228-2063	Sedative/Hypnotic; C IV
063 <> R	Tab, White, Round	Lorazepam 2 mg	by Nat Pharmpak Serv	55154-0552	Sedative/Hypnotic; C IV
064 <> PAR	Tab, Film Coated	Fluphenazine HCl 10 mg	by Qualitest	00603-3669	Antipsychotic
064 <> PAR	Tab, Film Coated	Fluphenazine HCl 10 mg	by Schein	00364-2268	Antipsychotic
06554160	Cap	Lithium Carbonate 300 mg	by Major	00904-2912	Antipsychotic
0665 <> 4001	Tab	Medroxyprogesterone Acetate 10 mg	by Quality Care	60346-0571	Progestin
0665 <> 4001	Tab	Medroxyprogesterone Acetate 10 mg	by Int'l Lab	00665-4001	Progestin
0665 <> 4120	Cap, Black Print	Valproic Acid 250 mg	by Int'l Lab	00665-4120	Anticonvulsant
0665 <> 4160	Cap	Lithium Carbonate 300 mg	by Schein	00364-0855	Antipsychotic
0665 <> 4160	Cap, Red Print	Lithium Carbonate 300 mg	by Int'l Lab	00665-4160	Antipsychotic
0665 <> 4160	Cap	Lithium Carbonate 300 mg	by United Res	00677-1092	Antipsychotic

ID FRONT <> BACK	DESCRIPTION FRONT <> BACK	INGREDIENT & STRENGTH	BRAND (OR EQUIV.) & FIRM	NDC#	CLASS; SCH.
06654001	Tab	Medroxyprogesterone Acetate 10 mg	by Talbert Med	44514-0542	Progestin
06654120	Cap	Valproic Acid 250 mg	by Zenith Goldline	00182-1754	Anticonvulsant
06654120	Cap	Valproic Acid 250 mg	by Rugby	00536-4477	Anticonvulsant
06654120	Cap	Valproic Acid 250 mg	by Major	00904-2101	Anticonvulsant
06654120	Cap, Gelatin	Valproic Acid 250 mg	by United Res	00677-1079	Anticonvulsant
06654120	Cap, International Labs Logo	Valproic Acid 250 mg	by Geneva	00781-2203	Anticonvulsant
06654120	Cap	Valproic Acid 250 mg	by RP Scherer	11014-0790	Anticonvulsant
06654140	Cap, Green	Hydralazine HCl 25 mg, Hydrochlorothiazide 25 mg	Apresazide by Solvay		Antihypertensive
06654160	Cap	Lithium Carbonate 300 mg	Lithonate by Solvay	00032-7512	Antipsychotic
06654160	Cap	Lithium Carbonate 300 mg	by Zenith Goldline	00182-1781	Antipsychotic
06654160	Cap, White, 0665-4160	Lithium Carbonate 300 mg	by Mylan	00378-1242	Antipsychotic
06654160	Cap, 0665-4160 in Red Print	Lithium Carbonate 300 mg	by DRX	55045-2324	Antipsychotic
06654160	Cap, 0665 over 4160	Lithium Carbonate 300 mg	by Quality Care	60346-0799	Antipsychotic
06654160	Cap	Lithium Carbonate 300 mg	by Geneva	00781-2100	Antipsychotic
06654160	Cap, 0665-4160	Lithium Carbonate 300 mg	by Qualitest	00603-4220	Antipsychotic
06654160	Cap, Red Print	Lithium Carbonate 300 mg	by HL Moore	00839-7149	Antipsychotic
0698	Cap, Clear & Yellow, Gelatin, Oblong	Benzonatate 200 mg	Tessalonn Double Strength by Forest	00456-0698	Antitussive
07 <> SL	Tab, Sugar Coated, Black Print	Hydroxyzine HCl 10 mg	by Kaiser	00179-0294	Antihistamine
07 <> SL	Tab, White, Round, Sugar Coated	Hydroxyzine HCl 10 mg	Atarax by Sidmak	50111-0307	Antihistamine
07 <> SL	Tab, Sugar Coated	Hydroxyzine HCl 10 mg	by Qualitest	00603-3970	Antihistamine
07 <> SL	Tab, Sugar Coated	Hydroxyzine HCl 10 mg	by Talbert Med	44514-0418	Antihistamine
070	Tab, Coated	Ethinyl Estradiol 0.05 mg	by Amerisource	62584-0299	Oral Contraceptive
070	Tab, Pink, Round, Schering Logo 070	Ethinyl Estradiol 0.05 mg	Estinyl by Schering		Oral Contraceptive
070	Tab, RP Logo	Theophylline 300 mg	Quibron T Sr Accudose by Monarch	61570-0019	Antiasthmatic
073 <> RPC	Tab, Sugar Coated	Propantheline Bromide 7.5 mg	Pro Banthine by Roberts	54092-0073	Gastrointestinal
074 <> RPC	Tab, Sugar Coated	Propantheline Bromide 15 mg	Pro Banthine by Roberts	54092-0074	Gastrointestinal
0748 <> 0748	Tab, Blue, Scored	Estradiol 2.0 mg	Gynodiol by Heartland	61392-0081	Hormone
076	Tab, Green, Oval, Coated	Ascorbic Acid 500 mg, Calcium Pantothenate 18 mg, Cyanocobalamin 5 mcg, Folic Acid 0.5 mg, Niacinamide 100 mg, Pyridoxine HCl 4 mg, Riboflavin 15 mg, Thiamine Mononitrate 15 mg	Berocca by Amide	52152-0076	Vitamin
076 <> PAR	Tab, Film Coated	Fluphenazine HCl 5 mg	by Qualitest	00603-3668	Antipsychotic
076 <> PAR	Tab, Film Coated	Fluphenazine HCl 5 mg	by Schein	00364-2267	Antipsychotic
0765400 <> SCHEIN	Tab, Film Coated, 0765/400	Ibuprofen 400 mg	by Schein	00364-0765	NSAID
0766 <> SCHEIN600	Tab, Film Coated	Ibuprofen 600 mg	by Schein	00364-0766	NSAID
0768	Tab, Blue, Round, Scored	Estradiol 0.5 mg	Gynodiol by Heartland		Hormone
077	Tab, Yellow, Oval, Coated	Ascorbic Acid 500 mg, Biotin 0.15 mg, Chromic Nitrate 0.1 mg, Cupric Oxide, Cyanocobalamin 50 mcg, Ferrous Fumarate 27 mg, Folic Acid 0.8 mg, Magnesium Oxide 50 mg, Manganese Dioxide 5 mg, Niacin 100 mg, Pantothenic Acid 25 mg, Pyridoxine HCl 25 mg, Riboflavin 20 mg, Thiamine Mononitrate 20 mg, Vitamin A Acetate 5000 Units, Vitamin E Acetate 30 Units	Berocca Plus by Amide	52152-0077	Vitamin
077	Tab, Coated	Ascorbic Acid 500 mg, Biotin 0.15 mg, Chromic Nitrate 0.1 mg, Cupric Oxide, Cyanocobalamin 50 mcg, Ferrous Fumarate 27 mg, Folic Acid 0.8 mg, Magnesium Oxide 50 mg, Manganese Dioxide 5 mg, Niacin 100 mg, Pantothenic Acid 25 mg, Pyridoxine HCl 25 mg, Riboflavin 20 mg, Thiamine Mononitrate 20 mg, Vitamin A Acetate 5000 Units, Vitamin E Acetate 30 Units	Therapeutic Plus Vit by Rugby	00536-4746	Vitamin
077	Tab, Gray, Round, Sch. Logo 077	Perphenazine 16 mg	Trilafon by Schering		Antipsychotic
0770 <> S	Tab	Isosorbide Dinitrate 5 mg	Sorbitrate by Zeneca	00310-0770	Antianginal
0775 <> PAL	Tab, 07/75 <> Pal	Guaifenesin 600 mg, Pseudoephedrine HCl 90 mg	Panmist LA by Sovereign	58716-0658	Cold Remedy
0775 <> PAL	Tab, 07/75 <> Pal	Guaifenesin 600 mg, Pseudoephedrine HCl 90 mg	Panmist LA by Pan Am	00525-0775	Cold Remedy
0780 <> PAL	Tab, Green, Speckled	Chlorpheniramine Maleate 8 mg, Methscopolamine Nitrate 2.5 mg, Phenylpropanolamine HCl 75 mg	Pannaz by Pan Am	00525-0780	Cold Remedy

ID FRONT <> BACK	DESCRIPTION FRONT <> BACK	INGREDIENT & STRENGTH	BRAND (OR EQUIV.) & FIRM	NDC#	CLASS; SCH.
0780 <> PAL	Tab, White, Green Specks	Chlorpheniramine Maleate 8 mg, Methscopolamine Nitrate 2.5 mg, Phenylpropanolamine HCl 75 mg	Pannaz by Anabolic	00722-6337	Cold Remedy
079	Tab, White, Oblong	Aspirin SR 800 mg	Zorprin by Amide		Analgesic
07SL	Tab, White, Round, Film Coated	Hydroxyzine HCl 10 mg	by Mutual	53489-0126	Antihistamine
08 <> SL	Tab, Light Blue, Sugar Coated	Hydroxyzine HCl 25 mg	by Qualitest	00603-3971	Antihistamine
08 <> SL	Tab, White, Round, Sugar Coated	Hydroxyzine HCl 25 mg	Atarax by Sidmak	50111-0308	Antihistamine
08 <> SL	Tab, Sugar Coated, Black Print	Hydroxyzine HCl 25 mg	by Kaiser	00179-0295	Antihistamine
08 <> SL	Tab, Sugar Coated	Hydroxyzine HCl 25 mg	by Talbert Med	44514-0419	Antihistamine
080	Tab, Coated	Ascorbic Acid 500 mg, Calcium Pantothenate 18 mg, Cyanocobalamin 5 mcg, Folic Acid 0.5 mg, Niacinamide 100 mg, Pyridoxine HCl 4 mg, Riboflavin 15 mg, Thiamine Mononitrate 15 mg	Vitaplex by Amide	52152-0076	Vitamin
0822	Tab, Pink, Round	Sodium Fluoride Chewable 2.2 mg	Luride by Pharmafair		Element
08220405	Tab, White, Round, 0822/0405	Allopurinol 100 mg	Zyloprim by Boots		Antigout
08220410	Tab, Peach, Round, 0822/0410	Allopurinol 300 mg	Zyloprim by Boots		Antigout
08220430	Tab, White, Round, 0822/0430	Butalbital 50 mg, Aspirin 325 mg, Caffeine 40 mg	Fiorinal by Halsey		Analgesic
08220576	Tab, Pink, Round, 0822/0576	Meclizine HCl Chewable 25 mg	Bonine by Boots		Antiemetic
08220841	Tab, Pink, Round, 0822/0841	Sodium Fluoride Chewable 2.2 mg	Luride Lozi-tabs by Boots		Element
08221530	Tab, Pink, Round, 0822/1530	Levothyroxine Sodium. 300 mcg	Synthroid by Boots		Antithyroid
08221531	Tab, Green, Round, 0822/1531	Levothyroxine Sodium. 300 mcg	Synthroid by Boots		Antithyroid
08225	Tab, White, Round, 0822/5	Diphenoxylate 2.5 mg, Atropine 0.025 mg	Lomotil by Pharmafair		Antidiarrheal; C V
0832G536C	Cap, Yellow, 0832/G536C	Phentermine HCl 30 mg	by Forest Pharma	00456-0766	Anorexiant; C IV
0832G536C	Cap, Black, 0832/G536C	Phentermine HCl 30 mg	by Forest Pharma	00456-0606	Anorexiant; C IV
084 <> WC	Tab, White, Oval, Film Coated	Gemfibrozil 600 mg	by Allscripts	54569-3695	Antihyperlipidemic
084 <> WC	Tab, Elliptical, Film Coated	Gemfibrozil 600 mg	by Warner Chilcott	00047-0084	Antihyperlipidemic
084 <> WC	Tab, Film Coated, Blue Print	Gemfibrozil 600 mg	by Kaiser	00179-1171	Antihyperlipidemic
084WC	Tab, Film Coated	Gemfibrozil 600 mg	by Med Pro	53978-2033	Antihyperlipidemic
085 <> 085	Tab, Film Coated, Purepac Logo	Acetaminophen 650 mg, Propoxyphene Napsylate 100 mg	by Heartland	61392-0446	Analgesic; C IV
085 <> R	Tab, Pink, Cap Shaped, Film Coated	Acetaminophen 650 mg, Propoxyphene Napsylate 100 mg	by Purepac	00228-2085	Analgesic; C IV
0866	Cap, Red, Oblong, Gelatin	Docusate Calcium 240 mg	Surfak by UDL	51079-0071	Laxative
0866	Cap, Red, Oblong	Docusate Calcium 240 mg	Surfak by Scherer		Laxative
089 <> 93	Tab	Sulfamethoxazole 800 mg, Trimethoprim 160 mg	SMZ TMP DS by Quality Care	60346-0087	Antibiotic
0894	Tab, Light Brown, Scored	Hydrocodone Bitartrate 5 mg	by Rhone-Poulenc Rorer	Canadian	Analgesic; C III
0897	Cap, Orange, Oval, Gelatin	Docusate Sodium 100 mg	Colace by UDL	51079-0019	Laxative
0898	Cap, Orange, Oblong, Gelatin	Docusate Sodium 250 mg	Colace by UDL	51079-0048	Laxative
08980897	Cap, Red, 0898/0897	Docusate Na	by Scherer		Laxative
0920	Cap, Pink & Clear, Royce Logo	Isosorbide Dinitrate SR 40 mg	Dilatrate-SR by Eon		Antianginal
093 <> MIA	Tab	Chlorpheniramine Tannate 8 mg, Phenylephrine Tannate 25 mg, Pyrilamine Tannate 25 mg	Rhinatate by Major	00904-1669	Cold Remedy
093 <> MIA	Tab	Chlorpheniramine Tannate 8 mg, Phenylephrine Tannate 25 mg, Pyrilamine Tannate 25 mg	by Zenith Goldline	00182-1912	Cold Remedy
093 <> MIA	Tab	Chlorpheniramine Tannate 8 mg, Phenylephrine Tannate 25 mg, Pyrilamine Tannate 25 mg	Histatan by Zenith Goldline	00172-4376	Cold Remedy
095	Tab, Red, Oval, Schering Logo 095	Dexchlorpheniramine ER 4 mg	Polaramine by Schering		Antihistamine
0993	Cap, Orange	Acetaminophen 250 mg, Pseudoephedrine 30 mg, Guaifenesin 100 mg, DM 10 mg	by PFI		Cold Remedy
1	Tab, Orange, Oval	Dextrothyroxine Sodium 1 mg	Choloxin by Boots		Thyroid
1	Tab, Bright Pink, Round	Fluphenazine HCl 1 mg	Fluphenazine by Apotex	Canadian	Antipsychotic
1	Tab, White, Round	Nitro Tab 0.3 mg	by Novopharm	55953-0294	Vasodilator
1	Tab, White, Round	Nitro Tab 0.3 mg	by Novopharm	43806-0294	Vasodilator
1	Tab, White, Round	Nitroglycerin 0.3 mg (1/200 gr)	Nitrostat by Able Lab	53265-0249	Vasodilator
1	Tab	Nitroglycerin 1 mg	Sustachron ER Buccal by Forest	10418-0136	Vasodilator
1	Tab, White, Round	Nitroglycerin CR Buccal 1 mg	Nitrogard bussal by Forest		Vasodilator
1	Tab, Off-White, Round	Nitroglycerin 1 mg	by Forest Pharma	00456-0686	Vasodilator

ID FRONT <> BACK	DESCRIPTION FRONT <> BACK	INGREDIENT & STRENGTH	BRAND (OR EQUIV.) & FIRM	NDC#	CLASS; SCH.
1	Tab, Blue, Round	Trifluoperazine HCl 1 mg	Apo Trifluoperazine by Apotex	Canadian	Antipsychotic
1 <> 241	Tab, Royce Logo 241	Lorazepam 1 mg	by Quality Care	60346-0047	Sedative/Hypnotic; C IV
1 <> 241	Tab	Lorazepam 1 mg	by United Res	00677-1057	Sedative/Hypnotic; C IV
1 <> 241	Tab, 1/Royce Logo	Lorazepam 1 mg	by Qualitest	00603-4244	Sedative/Hypnotic; C IV
1 <> 5624DAN	Tab	Lorazepam 1 mg	by Quality Care	60346-0047	Sedative/Hypnotic; C IV
1 <> A	Tab, Light Yellow	Dextromethorphan Hydrobromide 30 mg, Guaifenesin 600 mg, Phenylephrine HCl 15 mg	Albatussin Sr by Anabolic	00722-6211	Cold Remedy
1 <> ETHEX	Cap, Clear, Gelatin	Potassium Chloride 750 mg	by Eckerd	19458-0877	Electrolytes
1 <> G	Tab, White, Hexagon, Scored	Estradiol 1 mg	by Teva	00093-1058	Hormone
1 <> G	Tab	Estradiol 1 mg	by AAI	27280-0005	Hormone
1 <> SEARLE	Tab	Mestranol 0.05 mg, Norethindrone 1 mg	Norinyl 1 50 21 Day by GD Searle	00025-0263	Oral Contraceptive
1 <> Z4233	Tab, Scored, 1 <> Z over 4233	Bumetanide 1 mg	by Nat Pharmpak Serv	55154-5819	Diuretic
1 <> Z4233	Tab, 1 <> Z over 4232	Bumetanide 1 mg	by Geneva	00781-1822	Diuretic
1 <> Z4233	Tab, 1 <> Z over 4233	Bumetanide 1 mg	by HL Moore	00839-8012	Diuretic
1 <> Z4233	Tab, Yellow, Round	Bumetanide 1 mg	Bumex by Zenith Goldline	00182-2616	Diuretic
1 <> Z4233	Tab, 1 <> Z over 4233	Bumetanide 1 mg	by Murfreesboro	51129-1337	Diuretic
1 <> Z4233	Tab, 1 <> Z over 4234	Bumetanide 1 mg	by Major	00904-5103	Diuretic
10	Tab, Blue, Round	Amitriptyline HCl 10 mg	Apo Amitriptyline by Apotex	Canadian	Antidepressant
10	Tab, Orange, Round	Bethanechol Chloride 10 mg	Duvoid by Roberts	Canadian	Urinary Tract
10	Tab, Red, Round, Scored	Chlorpheniramine Tannate 5 mg; Phenylephrine Tannate 10 mg; Carbetapentane Tannate 60 mg	Ricotuss by Rico Pharma	62453-0103	Cold Remedy
10	Tab, Red, Round, Scored	Chlorpheniramine Tannate 5 mg; Phenylephrine Tannate 10 mg; Carbetapentane Tannate 60 mg	Ricotuss by Pegasus Labs	55246-0055	Cold Remedy
10	Tab, Pale Yellow, Triangular	Clomipramine 10 mg	Apo Clomipramine by Apotex	Canadian	OCD
10	Tab, Blue, Round	Desipramine 10 mg	Desipramine by Apotex	Canadian	Antidepressant
10	Tab, Pink, Square	Famotidine 10 mg	Famotidine by Apotex	Canadian	Gastrointestinal
10	Tab, Light Brown, Round	Imipramine HCl 10 mg	Apo Imipramine by Apotex	Canadian	Antidepressant
10	Cap, Orange	Hydroxyzine HCl 10 mg	Apo Hydroxyzine by Apotex	Canadian	Antihistamine
10	Tab, Yellow, Oval, Dish Logo/10	Loratadine 10 mg	Claritin by Schering	Canadian	Antihistamine
10	Tab, Rose, Round	Nifedipine 10 mg	Adalat 10 by Bayer	Canadian	Antihypertensive
10	Tab, Gold, Round, Hourglass Logo <> 10	Prochlorperazine 10 mg	Compazine by Zenith Goldline	00172-3691	Antiemetic
10	Tab, Light Green, Round	Thioridazine HCl 10 mg	Apo Thioridazine by Apotex	Canadian	Antipsychotic
10	Tab, Blue, Round	Trifluoperazine HCl 10 mg	Apo Trifluoperazine by Apotex	Canadian	Antipsychotic
10	Tab	Yohimbine HCl 5.4 mg	by Jerome Stevens	50564-0509	Impotence Agent
10 <> 103	Tab, White, Oval, Scored	Torsemide 10 mg	Demadex by Natl Pharmpak	55154-0406	Diuretic
10 <> 103	Tab, White, Oval, 10 <> 103 Mannheim Boehringer Logo	Torsemide 10 mg	Demadex by Hoffmann La Roche	00004-0263	Diuretic
10 <> 255	Tab, Coated, 10/Royce Logo	Baclofen 10 mg	by Qualitest	00603-2408	Muscle Relaxant
10 <> 257	Tab, Coated, 10/Royce Logo <> 257	Cyclobenzaprine HCl 10 mg	by Qualitest	00603-3077	Muscle Relaxant
10 <> 335	Tab, Coated, 10/Royce Logo	Piroxicam 10 mg	by Qualitest	00603-5222	NSAID
10 <> 341	Tab, Coated, 10/Royce Logo	Pindolol 10 mg	by Qualitest	00603-5221	Antihypertensive
10 <> 4197	Tab, Salmon, Round	Enalapril Maleate 10 mg	Vasotec by Zenith Goldline	00172-4197	Antihypertensive
10 <> 832	Tab, Butterscotch Yellow, Sugar Coated	Chlorpromazine HCl 10 mg	by Schein	00364-0380	Antipsychotic
10 <> 832	Tab, Butterscotch Yellow, Sugar Coated	Chlorpromazine HCl 10 mg	by Qualitest	00603-2808	Antipsychotic
10 <> AD	Tab, Blue, Round, 1/0	Amphetamine Aspartate 2.5 mg, Amphetamine Sulfate 2.5 mg, Dextroamphetamine Saccharate 2.5 mg, Dextroamphetamine Sulfate 2.5 mg	Adderall by Shire Richwood	58521-0032	Stimulant; C II
10 <> AD	Tab	Amphetamine Aspartate 2.5 mg, Amphetamine Sulfate 2.5 mg, Dextroamphetamine Saccharate 2.5 mg, Dextroamphetamine Sulfate 2.5 mg	Adderall by Physicians Total Care	54868-3674	Stimulant; C II
10 <> AMIDE009	Tab, Amide 009	Isoxsuprine HCl 10 mg	by Qualitest	00603-4146	Vasodilator
10 <> ARICEPT	Tab, Yellow, Film Coated	Donepezil 10 mg	Arecept by Pfizer	Canadian DIN# 02232044	Antialzheimers
10 <> DAN5554	Tab	Propranolol HCl 10 mg	by Danbury	00591-5554	Antihypertensive

ID FRONT <> BACK	DESCRIPTION FRONT <> BACK	INGREDIENT & STRENGTH	BRAND (OR EQUIV.) & FIRM	NDC#	CLASS; SCH.
10 <> DAN5620	Tab, Light Blue	Diazepam 10 mg	by Quality Care	60346-0033	Antianxiety; C IV
10 <> DAN5620	Tab	Diazepam 10 mg	by St Marys Med	60760-0776	Antianxiety; C IV
10 <> DAN5620	Tab	Diazepam 10 mg	by Danbury	00591-5620	Antianxiety; C IV
10 <> DAN5643	Tab	Minoxidil 10 mg	by Danbury	00591-5643	Antihypertensive
10 <> DAN5730	Tab	Baclofen 10 mg	by Heartland	61392-0706	Muscle Relaxant
10 <> DAN5730	Tab, White, Round, Scored	Baclofen 10 mg	by Heartland Hlthcare	61392-0090	Muscle Relaxant
10 <> DAN5730	Tab	Baclofen 10 mg	by Amerisource	62584-0623	Muscle Relaxant
10 <> DAN5730	Tab	Baclofen 10 mg	by Danbury	00591-5730	Muscle Relaxant
10 <> DELTASONE	Tab	Prednisone 10 mg	Deltasone by Quality Care	60346-0721	Steriod
10 <> E	Tab, Red, Octagonal	Acetaminophen 400 mg, Hydrocodone Bitartrate 10 mg	Zydone by Allscripts	54569-4732	Analgesic; C III
10 <> E	Tab, Red, Octagonal	Acetaminophen 400 mg, Hydrocodone Bitartrate 10 mg	Zydone by Endo Labs	63481-0698	Analgesic; C III
10 <> E	Tab, Red, Octagonal	Acetaminophen 400 mg; Hydrocodone Bitartrate 10 mg	Zydone by West Pharm	52967-0275	Analgesic; C III
10 <> E246	Tab, Film Coated	Donepezil HCl 10 mg	Aricept by Eisai	62856-0246	Antialzheimers
10 <> E530	Tab, White, Round	Isoxsuprine HCl 10 mg	Vasodilan by Eon	00185-0530	Vasodilator
10 <> F	Tab, White	Medroxyprogesterone Acetate 10 mg	Proclim by Fournier Pharma	Canadian	Progestin
10 <> G1295	Tab, White, Round	Baclofen 10 mg	Lioresal by Zenith Goldline	00172-4096	Muscle Relaxant
10 <> GG455	Tab, Yellow, Round, Film Coated	Chlorpromazine HCl 10 mg	by Heartland Hlthcare	61392-0880	Antipsychotic
10 <> GG455	Tab, Butterscotch Yellow, Round, Film Coated	Chlorpromazine HCl 10 mg	Thorazine by Geneva	00781-1715	Antipsychotic
10 <> GG58	Tab, Lavender, Round, Film Coated	Trifluoperazine HCl 10mg	Stelazine by Geneva	00781-1036	Antipsychotic
10 <> INV276	Tab, Yellow, Round, Film Coated	Prochlorperazine Maleate 10 mg	by Invamed	52189-0276	Antiemetic
10 <> INV276	Tab, Yellow, Round, Film Coated	Prochlorperazine Maleate 10 mg	by Apotheca	12634-0676	Antiemetic
10 <> INV281	Tab, Purple, Round, Film Coated	Trifluoperazine HCl 10 mg	by Invamed	52189-0281	Antipsychotic
10 <> JANSSENP	Tab, 10 <> Janssen/P	Cisapride 10 mg	Propulsid by Janssen	50458-0430	Gastrointestinal
10 <> KU106	Tab, White	Isosorbide Mononitrate 10 mg	by Kremers Urban	62175-0106	Antianginal
10 <> KU106	Tab, White, Round, Scored	Isosorbide Mononitrate 10 mg	by Schwarz Pharma Mfg	00131-9106	Antianginal
10 <> LOTENSIN	Tab, Dark Yellow, Coated	Benazepril HCl 10 mg	Lotensin by PDRX	55289-0109	Antihypertensive
10 <> LOTENSIN	Tab, Dark Yellow, Coated	Benazepril HCl 10 mg	Lotensin by DRX	55045-2374	Antihypertensive
10 <> LOTENSIN	Tab, Coated	Benazepril HCl 10 mg	Lotensin by Quality Care	60346-0833	Antihypertensive
10 <> LOTENSIN	Tab, Coated	Benazepril HCl 10 mg	Lotensin by Amerisource	62584-0063	Antihypertensive
10 <> LOTENSIN	Tab, Dark Yellow, Coated	Benazepril HCl 10 mg	Lotensin by Pharm Utilization	60491-0383	Antihypertensive
10 <> LOTENSIN	Tab, Dark Yellow	Benazepril HCl 10 mg	Lotensin by Novartis	00083-0063	Antihypertensive
10 <> LOTENSIN	Tab, Coated	Benazepril HCl 10 mg	Lotensin by Allscripts	54569-3423	Antihypertensive
10 <> M	Tab, White, Round, Scored	Methylphenidate HCl 10 mg	Methylin by Neuman Distr	64579-0029	Stimulant; C II
10 <> M	Tab, White, Round, Scored	Methylphenidate HCl 10 mg	by Neuman Distr	64579-0022	Stimulant; C II
10 <> M	Tab, White, Round, Scored	Methylphenidate HCl 10 mg	Methylin ER by D M Graham	00756-0284	Stimulant; C II
10 <> M	Tab, White, Round, Scored	Methylphenidate HCl 10 mg	Methylin ER by Mallinckrodt Hobart	00406-1122	Stimulant; C II
10 <> M54	Tab, Orange, Round, Film Coated	Thioridazine HCl 10 mg	by Dixon Shane	17236-0318	Antipsychotic
10 <> M54	Tab, Orange, Round, Film Coated, 10 <> M over 54	Thioridazine HCl 10 mg	Mellaril by UDL	51079-0565	Antipsychotic
10 <> M54	Tab, Orange, Film Coated, 10 <> M over 54	Thioridazine HCl 10 mg	by Mylan	00378-0612	Antipsychotic
10 <> M54	Tab, Film Coated	Thioridazine HCl 10 mg	by Qualitest	00603-5992	Antipsychotic
10 <> M54	Tab, Coated	Thioridazine HCl 10 mg	by Vangard	00615-2504	Antipsychotic
10 <> MERIDIA	Cap, Blue & White	Sibutramine HCl 10 mg	Meridia by Knoll	00048-0610	Anorexiant; C IV
10 <> MERIDIA	Cap	Sibutramine HCl 10 mg	Meridia by Quality Care	62682-7049	Anorexiant; C IV
10 <> MERIDIA	Cap	Sibutramine HCl 10 mg	Meridia by DRX	55045-2555	Anorexiant; C IV
10 <> MERIDIA	Cap, -10-	Sibutramine HCl 10 mg	Meridia by BASF	10117-0610	Anorexiant; C IV
10 <> MERIDIA	Cap, Blue & White	Sibutramine HCl 10 mg	Meridia by Compumed	00403-5373	Anorexiant; C IV
10 <> MERIDIA	Cap, Blue & White	Sibutramine HCl 10 mg	Meridia by PDRX Pharms	55289-0375	Anorexiant; C IV
10 <> MERIDIA	Cap, Blue & White	Sibutramine HCl 10 mg	Meridia by Apotheca	12634-0534	Anorexiant; C IV
10 <> MJ543	Tab	Isoxsuprine HCl 10 mg	Vasodilan by Bristol Myers Squibb	00087-0543	Vasodilator
10 <> MYLAN182	Tab, Orange, Round, Scored, 10 <> Mylan over 182	Propranolol HCl 10 mg	Inderal by UDL	51079-0277	Antihypertensive
10 <> MYLAN182	Tab, Orange, 10 <> Mylan over 182	Propranolol HCl 10 mg	by Mylan	00378-0182	Antihypertensive
10 <> MYLAN182	Tab, 10 <> Mylan over 182	Propranolol HCl 10 mg	by Quality Care	60346-0570	Antihypertensive

13

ID FRONT <> BACK	DESCRIPTION FRONT <> BACK	INGREDIENT & STRENGTH	BRAND (OR EQUIV.) & FIRM	NDC#	CLASS; SCH.
10 <> N093	Tab	Pindolol 10 mg	by Med Pro	53978-2025	Antihypertensive
10 <> N131	Tab, Blue, Round, Scored, 1.0 <> N over 131	Alprazolam 1 mg	by Novopharm	55953-0131	Antianxiety; C IV
10 <> N131	Tab, 1.0 <> N over 131	Alprazolam 1 mg	by Medirex	57480-0522	Antianxiety; C IV
10 <> N171	Cap	Nifedipine 10 mg	by HL Moore	00839-7564	Antihypertensive
10 <> N171	Cap	Nifedipine 10 mg	by Warrick	59930-1618	Antihypertensive
10 <> N171	Cap, Brown, NovoPharm <> N over 171	Nifedipine 10 mg	by Novopharm	55953-0171	Antihypertensive
10 <> N171	Cap, Gelatin, 10 <> N over 171	Nifedipine 10 mg	by Quality Care	60346-0803	Antihypertensive
10 <> N525	Tab, White, Oval, Scored	Glipizide 10 mg	by Novopharm (CA)	43806-0525	Antidiabetic
10 <> N617	Cap	Piroxicam 10 mg	by Heartland	61392-0398	NSAID
10 <> N617	Cap	Piroxicam 10 mg	by HL Moore	00839-7773	NSAID
10 <> NU	Tab, Grayish-Pink, Round, Film Coated	Nifedipine 10 mg	by Nu Pharm	Canadian DIN# 02212102	Antihypertensive
10 <> OC	Tab, White, Round	Oxycodone HCl 10 mg	OxyContin by Purdue Frederick	Canadian	Analgesic; C II
10 <> OC	Tab, White, Round	Oxycodone HCl 10 mg	Oxycontin by PF Labs	48692-0670	Analgesic; C II
10 <> OC	Tab, White, Round	Oxycodone HCl 10 mg	Oxycontin by PF Labs	48692-0710	Analgesic; C II
10 <> OC	Tab, Film Coated	Oxycodone HCl 10 mg	Oxycontin by Physicians Total Care	54868-3813	Analgesic; C II
10 <> PAXIL	Tab, Film Coated	Paroxetine HCl	Paxil by SB	59742-3210	Antidepressant
10 <> PAXIL	Tab, Yellow, Oval	Paroxetine HCl 10 mg	Paxil by Phcy Care	65070-0144	Antidepressant
10 <> PAXIL	Tab, Yellow, Oval, Film Coated	Paroxetine HCl 10 mg	Paxil by SKB	00029-3210	Antidepressant
10 <> PD155	Tab, White, Elliptical, Film Coated	Atorvastatin 10 mg	Lipitor by Parke-Davis	Canadian DIN# 02230711	Antihyperlipidemic
10 <> PD155	Tab, Film Coated, PD155	Atorvastatin Calcium	Lipitor by Pharm Utilization	60491-0803	Antihyperlipidemic
10 <> PD155	Tab, White, Elliptical, Film Coated	Atorvastatin Calcium	Lipitor by Parke Davis	00071-0155	Antihyperlipidemic
10 <> PD155	Tab, Film Coated	Atorvastatin Calcium	Lipitor by Allscripts	54569-4466	Antihyperlipidemic
10 <> PD155	Tab, Film Coated	Atorvastatin Calcium	Lipitor by Goedecke	53869-0155	Antihyperlipidemic
10 <> PD530	Tab, Brown, Triangular, Coated	Quinapril HCl 10 mg	Accupril by Parke Davis	00071-0530	Antihypertensive
10 <> PD530	Tab, Coated	Quinapril HCl 10 mg	Accupril by Allscripts	54569-3984	Antihypertensive
10 <> PD530	Tab, Brown, Triangular, Film Coated, 10 <> PD/530	Quinapril 10 mg	Accupril by Park-Davis	Canadian DIN# 01947672	Antihypertensive
10 <> PD530	Tab, Brown, Triangle	Quinapril HCl 10 mg	Accupril by PDRX Pharms	55289-0553	Antihypertensive
10 <> PD530	Tab, Brown, Triangle	Quinapril HCl 10 mg	Accupril by Direct Dispensing	57866-4420	Antihypertensive
10 <> PERCOCET	Tab, Yellow, Oval	Acetaminophen 650 mg; Oxycodone HCl 10 mg	Percocet by Dupont Pharma	00056-0622	Analgesic; C II
10 <> PERCOCET	Tab, Yellow, Oval	Acetaminophen 650 mg; Oxycodone HCl 10 mg	Percocet by West Pharm	52967-0280	Analgesic; C II
10 <> PERCOCET	Tab, Yellow, Oval	Oxycodone HCl 10 mg, Acetaminophen 650 mg	Percocet by Endo	63481-0622	Analgesic; C II
10 <> PF	Tab, White, Round	Morphine Sulfate 10 mg	MS IR by Purdue Frederick	Canadian	Analgesic
10 <> SCHWARZ610	Tab, White, Scored	Isosorbide Mononitrate 10 mg	Monoket by Schwarz Pharma	00091-3610	Antianginal
10 <> SP2309	Tab, White, Cap Shaped, Film Coated, Scored	Ascorbic Acid, Calcium Carbonate, Cupric Oxide, Cyanocobalamin 12 mcg, Ergocalciferol, Ferric Polysaccharide Complex, Folic Acid 1 mg, Magnesium Oxide, Niacinamide 20 mg, Potassium Iodide, Pyridoxine HCl, Riboflavin 3.4 mg, Thiamine Mononitrate, Vitamin A Acetate, Vitamin E Acetate, Zinc Sulfate	Niferex PN Forte by Schwarz Pharma	00131-2309	Vitamin
10 <> U137	Tab, White, Round, Scored	Minoxidil 10 mg	by Pharmacia	Canadian DIN# 00514500	Antihypertensive
10 <> Z3691	Tab, Gold, Round	Prochlorperazine Mal 10 mg	Compazine by Zenith Goldline	00182-8211	Antiemetic
10 <> Z3927	Tab, Light Blue	Diazepam 10 mg	by Quality Care	60346-0033	Antianxiety; C IV
10 <> Z3927	Tab, Light Blue, Round	Diazepam 10 mg	Valium by Zenith Goldline	00172-3927	Antianxiety; C IV
10 <> Z4096	Tab, Z over 4096	Baclofen 10 mg	by Baker Cummins	63171-1295	Muscle Relaxant
10 <> Z4096	Tab, White, Round	Baclofen 10 mg	Lioresal by Zenith Goldline	00172-4096	Muscle Relaxant
10 <> Z4096	Tab, Z over 4096	Baclofen 10 mg	by Caremark	00339-5834	Muscle Relaxant

ID FRONT <> BACK	DESCRIPTION FRONT <> BACK	INGREDIENT & STRENGTH	BRAND (OR EQUIV.) & FIRM	NDC#	CLASS; SCH.
10 <> ZAROXOLYN	Tab	Metolazone 10 mg	Zaroxolyn by Medeva	53014-0835	Diuretic
10 <> ZYRTEC	Tab, White, Rectangular, Film Coated	Cetirizine HCl 10 mg	Zyrtec by Murfreesboro Ph	51129-1379	Antihistamine
100	Tab, White	Atenolol 100 mg	by Schein	Canadian	Antihypertensive
100	Tab, Peach, Round	Desipramine HCl 100 mg	Desioramine by Apotex	Canadian	Antidepressant
100	Tab, Yellow, Round	Ketoprofen 100 mg	Rhodis by Rhodiapharm	Canadian	NSAID
100	Tab, Yellow, Oblong	Levothyroxine Sodium 100 mcg	Levothroid by Murfreesboro	51129-1665	Antithyroid
100	Tab, Logo	Levothyroxine Sodium 100 mcg	by Nat Pharmpak Serv	55154-4007	Antithyroid
100	Tab	Levothyroxine Sodium 100 mcg	by Amerisource	62584-0014	Antithyroid
100	Tab, Blue, Oblong, Scored	Metoprolol Tartrate 100 mg	by Nu-Pharm	Canadian	Antihypertensive
100	Tab, Blue, Cap Shaped, Film Coated, Scored	Metoprolol Tartrate 100 mg	Metoprolol by Apotex	Canadian DIN# 00865613	Antihypertensive
100	Cap, ER, 100 Printed in Red Ink	Theophylline 100 mg	Slo Bid by Nat Pharmpak Serv	55154-4025	Antiasthmatic
100	Cap, White, Red Print	Theophylline 100 mg	Slo Bid by RPR	00801-0100	Antiasthmatic
100	Tab, Green, Round	Thioridazine HCl 100 mg	Apo Thioridazine by Apotex	Canadian	Antipsychotic
100	Tab, Pink, Round	Trimipramine 100 mg	Rhotrimine by Rhodiapharm	Canadian	Antidepressant
100 <> 105	Tab, Boehringer Mannheim Logo & 105	Torsemide 100 mg	Demadex by Hoffmann La Roche	00004-0265	Diuretic
100 <> 274INV	Tab, 274/INV	Captopril 100 mg	by Schein	00364-2631	Antihypertensive
100 <> 350	Tab, 100/Royce Logo <> 350	Captopril 100 mg	by Qualitest	00603-2558	Antihypertensive
100 <> 4360	Tab, Pale Yellow, Round, 100 <> Hourglass Logo 4360	Clozapine 100 mg	Clozaril by Zenith Goldline	00172-4360	Antipsychotic
100 <> 4364	Tab, Yellow, Round, 100 <> Hourglass Logo 4364	Labetalol HCl 100 mg	Normodyne & Trandate by Zenith Goldline	00172-4364	Antihypertensive
100 <> 734N	Tab, Film Coated, 734/N	Metoprolol Tartrate 100 mg	by Schein	00364-2561	Antihypertensive
100 <> 7767	Cap, White	Celecoxib 100 mg	Celebrex by Allscripts	54569-4671	NSAID
100 <> 7767	Cap, White w/ Blue Print	Celecoxib 100 mg	Celebrex by Pfizer	Canadian DIN# 02239941	NSAID
100 <> 832	Tab, Butterscotch Yellow, Sugar Coated	Chlorpromazine HCl 100 mg	by Schein	00364-0383	Antipsychotic
100 <> 832	Tab, Sugar Coated	Chlorpromazine HCl 100 mg	by United Res	00677-0456	Antipsychotic
100 <> 832	Tab, Butterscotch Yellow, Sugar Coated	Chlorpromazine HCl 100 mg	by Qualitest	00603-2811	Antipsychotic
100 <> ANZEMET	Tab, Film Coated	Dolasetron Mesylate Monohydrate 100 mg	Anzemet by Merrell	00068-1203	Antiemetic
100 <> BARR066	Tab, Debosse, Barr/066	Isoniazid 100 mg	Isoniazid by Rugby	00536-5901	Antimycobacterial
100 <> BARR066	Tab, Barr/066	Isoniazid 100 mg	Isoniazid by Barr	00555-0066	Antimycobacterial
100 <> BARR066	Tab	Isoniazid 100 mg	Isoniazid by Quality Care	60346-0203	Antimycobacterial
100 <> BARR066	Tab, Debossed	Isoniazid 100 mg	Isoniazid by Prepackage Spec	58864-0298	Antimycobacterial
100 <> BARR066	Tab, Barr/066	Isoniazid 100 mg	Isoniazid by Medirex	57480-0495	Antimycobacterial
100 <> BARR066	Tab, White, Round, Scored, 100 <> Barr Over 066	Isoniazid 100 mg	INH by UDL	51079-0082	Antimycobacterial
100 <> BARR324	Cap, 100 in Black Ink, Filled with Yellow Powder, Barr Over 324 in Black Ink	Hydroxyzine Pamoate	by Barr	00555-0324	Antihistamine
100 <> CIPRO	Tab, Film Coated	Ciprofloxacin HCl 116.4 mg	Ciprobay by Bayer	00026-8511	Antibiotic
100 <> CLOZARIL	Tab, Pale Yellow, Round, Scored	Clozapine 100 mg	Clozaril by Novartis	00078-0127	Antipsychotic
100 <> CLOZARIL	Tab	Clozapine 100 mg	Clozaril by Physicians Total Care	54868-3576	Antipsychotic
100 <> FL	Tab, Compressed, Logo FL	Levothyroxine Sodium 0.1 mg	by Kaiser	00179-0458	Antithyroid
100 <> FLINT	Tab	Levothyroxine Sodium 0.1 mg	Synthroid by Nat Pharmpak Serv	55154-0906	Antithyroid
100 <> FLINT	Tab	Levothyroxine Sodium 0.1 mg	Synthroid by Giant Food	11146-0305	Antithyroid
100 <> FLINT	Tab	Levothyroxine Sodium 0.1 mg	Synthroid by Rite Aid	11822-5193	Antithyroid
100 <> FLINT	Tab, 100 is Debossed Horizontally in Break of Vertical Score	Levothyroxine Sodium 0.1 mg	Synthroid by Allscripts	54569-0909	Antithyroid
100 <> FLINT	Tab, Yellow, Round, Scored	Levothyroxine Sodium 100 mcg	Synthroid by Knoll	00048-1070	Antithyroid
100 <> G	Tab	Atenolol 100 mg	by Par	49884-0457	Antihypertensive
100 <> GG34	Tab, Film Coated, GG 34	Thioridazine HCl 100 mg	by Heartland	61392-0144	Antipsychotic
100 <> GG34	Tab, Orange, Round, Film Coated	Thioridazine HCl 100 mg	Mellaril by Geneva	00781-1644	Antipsychotic
100 <> GG437	Tab, Coated	Chlorpromazine HCl 100 mg	by Haines	59564-0131	Antipsychotic

ID FRONT <> BACK	DESCRIPTION FRONT <> BACK	INGREDIENT & STRENGTH	BRAND (OR EQUIV.) & FIRM	NDC#	CLASS; SCH.
100 <> GG437	Tab, Butterscotch Yellow, Coated	Chlorpromazine HCl 100 mg	by Golden State	60429-0043	Antipsychotic
100 <> GG437	Tab, Butterscotch Yellow, Round, Film Coated	Chlorpromazine HCl 100 mg	Thorazine by Geneva	00781-1718	Antipsychotic
100 <> INV274	Tab, Scored	Captopril 100 mg	by Invamed	52189-0274	Antihypertensive
100 <> LAMICTAL	Tab, Peach, Hexagon, Scored	Lamotrigine 100 mg	Lamictal by Glaxo Wellcome	00173-0594	Anticonvulsant
100 <> M61	Tab, Orange, Round, Film Coated, 100 <> M over 61	Thioridazine HCl 100 mg	Mellaril by UDL	51079-0580	Antipsychotic
100 <> M61	Tab, Orange, Film Coated, M Over 61	Thioridazine HCl 100 mg	by Mylan	00378-0618	Antipsychotic
100 <> M61	Tab, Film Coated	Thioridazine HCl 100 mg	by Qualitest	00603-5995	Antipsychotic
100 <> M61	Tab, Orange, Round, Film Coated	Thioridazine HCl 100 mg	by Dixon Shane	17236-0305	Antipsychotic
100 <> M61	Tab, Film Coated	Thioridazine HCl 100 mg	by Vangard	00615-2508	Antipsychotic
100 <> MYLAN167	Tab, Beige, Film Coated, 100 <> Mylan over 167	Doxycycline Hyclate 100 mg	by Mylan	00378-0167	Antibiotic
100 <> MYLAN167	Tab, Beige, Round, Film Coated, 100<> Mylan over 167	Doxycycline Hyclate 100 mg	Vibra-Tabs by UDL	51079-0554	Antibiotic
100 <> MYLAN197	Tab, Green, Round, Scored, 100 <> Mylan over 197	Chlorpropamide 100 mg	Diabinese by UDL	51079-0202	Antidiabetic
100 <> MYLAN197	Tab, Green, Scored, 100 <> Mylan over 197	Chlorpropamide 100 mg	by Mylan	00378-0197	Antidiabetic
100 <> N135	Tab, Scored, 100 <> N over 135	Captopril 100 mg	by Medirex	57480-0841	Antihypertensive
100 <> N135	Tab, 100 <> N over 135	Captopril 100 mg	by Major	00904-5048	Antihypertensive
100 <> N135	Tab, White, Oval, 100 <> N over 135	Captopril 100 mg	by Novopharm	43806-0135	Antihypertensive
100 <> N401	Tab, 100 <> N over 401	Atenolol 100 mg	by Medirex	57480-0447	Antihypertensive
100 <> N401	Tab, 100 <> N over 401	Atenolol 100 mg	by Quality Care	60346-0914	Antihypertensive
100 <> N401	Tab, White, Round, 100 <> N over 401	Atenolol 100 mg	by Novopharm	55953-0401	Antihypertensive
100 <> N401	Tab, White, Round	Atenolol 100 mg	by Allscripts	54569-3654	Antihypertensive
100 <> N401	Tab, White, Round	Atenolol 100 mg	by Novopharm (US)	62528-0401	Antihypertensive
100 <> N577	Tab, Film Coated	Flurbiprofen 100 mg	by Warrick	59930-1772	NSAID
100 <> N577	Tab, Dark Blue, Round, Film Coated	Flurbiprofen 100 mg	by Allscripts	54569-3858	NSAID
100 <> N577	Tab, Coated	Flurbiprofen 100 mg	by Quality Care	60346-0968	NSAID
100 <> N577	Tab, Film Coated	Flurbiprofen 100 mg	by Qualitest	00603-3700	NSAID
100 <> N577	Tab, Film Coated	Flurbiprofen 100 mg	by HL Moore	00839-8004	NSAID
100 <> N734	Tab, Film Coated, N 734	Metoprolol Tartrate 100 mg	by Brightstone	62939-2221	Antihypertensive
100 <> N734	Tab, White, Cap-Shaped, Film Coated, Engraved	Metoprolol Tartrate 100 mg	by Novopharm	55953-0734	Antihypertensive
100 <> N734	Tab, Film Coated	Metoprolol Tartrate 100 mg	by Direct Dispensing	57866-6579	Antihypertensive
100 <> N734	Tab, Film Coated	Metoprolol Tartrate 100 mg	by Medirex	57480-0803	Antihypertensive
100 <> NU	Tab, White, Oval, Film Coated	Fluvoxamine Maleate 100 mg	by Nu Pharm	Canadian DIN# 02231193	OCD
100 <> SCHERING244	Tab, Brown, Round, Scored	Labetalol HCl 100 mg	Normodyne by Rightpak	65240-0705	Antihypertensive
100 <> TOPAMAX	Tab, Yellow, Coated	Topiramate 100 mg	Topamax by McNeil	00045-0641	Anticonvulsant
100 <> TOPAMAX	Tab, Coated	Topiramate 100 mg	Topamax by Ortho	00062-0641	Anticonvulsant
100 <> TOPAMAX	Tab, Coated	Topiramate 100 mg	Topamax by McNeil	52021-0641	Anticonvulsant
100 <> VIDEX	Tab, Mottled Off-White to Light Orange & Yellow, Orange Specks, Chewable	Didanosine 100 mg	Videx T by Bristol Myers Squibb	00087-6652	Antiviral
100 <> VOLTARENSR	Tab, Pink, Round, Film Coated	Diclofenac Sodium 100 mg	Voltaren SR by Novartis	Canadian DIN# 00590827	NSAID
100 <> VOLTARENXR	Tab, Pink, Round, Film Coated	Diclofenac Sodium 100 mg	Voltaren by HJ Harkins	52959-0472	NSAID
100 <> VOLTARENXR	Tab, 100 <> Voltaren-XR	Diclofenac Sodium 100 mg	Voltaren by Caremark	00339-6091	NSAID
100 <> VOLTARENXR	Tab, Light Pink, Round, Coated, 100 <> Voltaren-XR	Diclofenac Sodium 100 mg	Voltaren-XL by Novartis	00028-0205	NSAID
100 <> VOLTARENXR	Tab, 100 <> Voltaren-XR	Diclofenac Sodium 100 mg	Voltaren XR by Allscripts	54569-4513	NSAID
100 <> VOLTARENXR	Tab, Film Coated	Diclofenac Sodium 100 mg	Voltaren XR by Novartis	17088-0205	NSAID
100 <> WELLBUTRIN	Tab	Bupropion HCl 100 mg	Wellbutrin by Glaxo	00173-0178	Antidepressant
100 <> Z4362	Tab, Green, Oval	Flurbiprofen 100 mg	Ansaid by Zenith Goldline	00182-2621	NSAID
100 <> ZOLOFT	Tab, Yellow, Oblong	Sertraline HCl 100 mg	Zoloft by PDRX Pharms	55289-0550	Antidepressant
1000 <> BMS6071	Tab, White, Oval	Metformin HCl 1000 mg	Glucophage by Direct Dispensing	57866-9057	Antidiabetic
1000 <> BMS6071	Tab, White to Off-White, Oval, Scored, Film Coated	Metformin HCl 1000 mg	Glucophage by Bristol Myers Squibb	00087-6071	Antidiabetic

ID FRONT <> BACK	DESCRIPTION FRONT <> BACK	INGREDIENT & STRENGTH	BRAND (OR EQUIV.) & FIRM	NDC#	CLASS; SCH.
1000 <> BMS6071	Tab, White, Oval, Film Coated	Metformin HCl 1000 mg	Glucophage by Caremark	00339-6173	Antidiabetic
1000 <> KOS	Tab, Off-White, Cap Shaped, ER, Debossed	Niacin 1000 mg	Niaspan by KOS	60598-0003	Vitamin
1000 <> PROCANBID	Tab, Gray, Oval, Film Coated	Procainamide HCl 1000 mg	Procanbid by Monarch Pharms	61570-0071	Antiarrhythmic
1000 <> PROCANBID	Tab, Elliptical-Shaped, Film Coated	Procainamide HCl 1000 mg	Procanbid by Parke Davis	00071-0564	Antiarrhythmic
1001	Tab, White, Round	Aminophylline 100 mg	by Vortech		Antiasthmatic
10010 <> NU	Tab, Blue, Oval, Scored, 100 over 10 <> NU	Carbidopa 10 mg, Levodopa 100 mg	by Nu Pharm	Canadian DIN# 02182831	Antiparkinson
100100100 <> MJ796	Tab, Off-White, MJ 796	Trazodone HCl 300 mg	Desyrel by Bristol Myers Squibb	00087-0796	Antidepressant
100101 <> JACOBUS	Tab, 100/101 <> Jacobus	Dapsone 100 mg	by Jacobus	49938-0101	Antimycobacterial
100101 <> JACOBUS	Tab, Scored, 100 over 101 <> Jacobus	Dapsone 100 mg	by Physicians Total Care	54868-3801	Antimycobacterial
100105	Tab, White, Oval, 100/105	Torsemide 100 mg	Demadex by Boehringer Mannheim	Canadian	Diuretic
10010APO	Tab, Blue, Oval, 100 10/APO	Levodopa 100 mg, Carbidopa 10 mg	Levocarb by Apotex	Canadian	Antiparkinson
10010ENDO	Tab, Apple & Blue, Oval, 100/10/Endo	Levodopa 100 mg, Carbidopa 10 mg	by Altimed	Canadian	Antiparkinson
10025APO	Tab, Yellow, Oval, 100 25/APO	Levodopa 100 mg, Carbidopa 25 mg	Levocarb by Apotex	Canadian	Antiparkinson
10025ENDO	Tab, Yellow, Oval, 100/25/Endo	Levodopa 100 mg, Carbidopa 25 mg	by Altimed	Canadian	Antiparkinson
10025MG	Tab, White, Round, 100/25 mg	Atenolol 100 mg, Chlorthalidone 25 mg	Tenoretic by Zeneca	Canadian	Antihypertensive; Diuretic
100364 <> NIFEDIPINE	Cap, 10-0364	Nifedipine 10 mg	by Schein	00364-2376	Antihypertensive
10054862	Tab, White, 100/54/862	Morphine Sulfate 100 mg	Oramorph by Boehringer Ingelheim	Canadian	Analgesic
1008	Tab, Round	Dextroamphetamine Sulfate 5 mg	Oxydess by Vortech		Stimulant; C II
1009	Tab, Round	Digitoxin 0.2 mg	by Vortech		Cardiac Agent
100BARR066	Tab	Isoniazid 100 mg	Isoniazid by Zenith Goldline	00182-0559	Antimycobacterial
100CAPOTEN	Tab, White, Oval	Capoten 100 mg	Capoten by ER Squibb	00003-0485	Antihypertensive
100FLI	Tab, Yellow, Round, 100/FLI	Levothyroxine Sodium 100 mcg	Levothroid by Forest	00456-0323	Antithyroid
100LLA17	Tab, Blue, Heptagonal	Amoxapine 100 mg	Asendin by Lederle		Antidepressant
100LLT28	Tab, Orange, Round	Thioridazine HCl 100 mg	Mellaril by Lederle		Antipsychotic
100M	Tab	Levothyroxine Sodium 100 mcg	Levo T by MOVA	55370-0129	Antithyroid
100M10 <> MOVA	Tab, White, Cap Shaped	Captopril 100 mg	Capoten by MOVA	55370-0145	Antihypertensive
100MCG <> FLINT	Tab, Debossed	Levothyroxine Sodium 0.1 mg	Synthroid by Amerisource	62584-0070	Antithyroid
100MCG <> FLINT	Tab, Yellow, Round, Scored	Levothyroxine Sodium 0.1 mg	Synthroid by Wal Mart	49035-0194	Antithyroid
100MCG <> FLINT	Tab, Yellow, Round, Scored	Levothyroxine Sodium 0.1 mg	Synthroid by Rightpac	65240-0742	Antithyroid
100MG	Cap, White	Cyclosporine 100 mg	Gengraf by Abbott Labs	00074-6479	Immunosuppressant
100MG <> 2131	Cap, Pink & White	Nitrofurantoin 100 mg	by Direct Dispensing	57866-6590	Antibiotic
100MG <> ANSAID	Tab, Coated	Flurbiprofen 100 mg	Ansaid by Quality Care	60346-0099	NSAID
100MG <> BRISTOL3032	Cap, Moss Green	Lomustine 100 mg	Ceenu by Mead Johnson	00015-3032	Antineoplastic
100MG <> CLOZARIL	Tab, Pale Yellow, Round, Scored	Clozapine 100 mg	Clozaril by Novartis	Canadian DIN# 00894745	Antipsychotic
100MG <> KADIAN	Cap	Morphine Sulfate 100 mg	Kadian ER by Purepac	00228-2055	Analgesic; C II
100MG <> PF	Tab, Gray, Round	Morphine Sulfate 100 mg	MS Contin by Purdue Frederick	Canadian	Analgesic
100MG <> SCHWARZ4085	Cap, Amethyst & White, Opaque	Verapamil HCl 100 mg	Verelan PM by Schwarz Pharma	00091-4085	Antihypertensive
100MG <> T	Tab, Yellow, Round, Coated	Carbamazepine XR 100 mg	by Novartis	00083-0061	Anticonvulsant
100MG <> ZOLOFT	Tab, Yellow, Oblong, Film Coated, Scored	Sertraline HCl 100 mg	Zoloft by Natl Pharmpak	55154-2712	Antidepressant
100MG <> ZOLOFT	Tab, Film Coated, Engraved	Sertraline HCl 100 mg	Zoloft by Physicians Total Care	54868-2637	Antidepressent
100MG <> ZOLOFT	Tab, Film Coated	Sertraline HCl 100 mg	Zoloft by Allscripts	54569-3575	Antidepressent
100MG <> ZOLOFT	Tab, Film Coated	Sertraline HCl 100 mg	Zoloft by Amerisource	62584-0910	Antidepressent
100MG <> ZOLOFT	Tab, Film Coated	Sertraline HCl 100 mg	Zoloft by Direct Dispensing	57866-6305	Antidepressent

ID FRONT <> BACK	DESCRIPTION FRONT <> BACK	INGREDIENT & STRENGTH	BRAND (OR EQUIV.) & FIRM	NDC#	CLASS; SCH.
100MGFLUVOX	Tab, White, Oval, 100/mg/Fluvox	Fluvoxamine Maleate 100 mg	by AltiMed	Canadian DIN# 02218461	OCD
100MGLEDERLEM4	Orange & Purple	Minocycline HCl 100 mg	Minocin by Lederle		Antibiotic
100MGPI	Cap, Abbott Logo	Ritonavir 100 mg	Norvir by Abbott	00074-9492	Antiviral
100MGPI	Cap, Abbott Logo	Ritonavir 100 mg	Norvir by Physicians Total Care	54868-3782	Antiviral
100MGPI	Cap, Abbott Logo	Ritonavir 100 mg	Norvir by DRX	55045-2485	Antiviral
100MGSAMPLE <> MACRODANTIN	Cap, White w/ Yellow Powder, Opaque	Nitrofurantoin 100 mg	Macrodantin by Procter & Gamble	00149-0009	Antibiotic
100NORMODYNE <> SCHERING	Tab, Light Brown, Film Coated	Labetalol HCl 100 mg	Normodyne by Pharm Utilization	60491-0458	Antihypertensive
100NORMODYNE <> SCHERING244	Tab, Light Brown, Film Coated, 100 Normodyne <> Schering 244	Labetalol HCl 100 mg	Normodyne by Thrift Drug	59198-0080	Antihypertensive
100NORMODYNE <> SCHERING244	Tab, Film Coated	Labetalol HCl 100 mg	Normodyne by Nat Pharmpak Serv	55154-3511	Antihypertensive
100NORMODYNE <> SCHERING244	Tab, Film Coated	Labetalol HCl 100 mg	Normodyne by Amerisource	62584-0244	Antihypertensive
100NOVO	Tab, White, Round, 100/Novo	Acebutolol HCl 100 mg	by Novopharm	Canadian	Antihypertensive
100P <> DAN	Tab, White, Round, Scored	Phenobarbital 100 mg	by Schein	00364-0206	Sedative/Hypnotic; C IV
100TRPZSL44150	Tab, White, Trapezoidal, Scored, Compressed, SL 441 50/100 TRPZ	Trazodone HCl 150 mg	Desyrel by Geneva	00781-1826	Antidepressant
100WYETH	Tab, White, Round, 100/Wyeth	Acebutolol HCl 100 mg	by Wyeth-Ayerst	Canadian	Antihypertensive
101	Tab	Sulfasalazine 500 mg	Azulfidine by Amerisource	62584-0005	Gastrointestinal
101 <> GG	Tab, White, Compressed	Methocarbamol 750 mg	Robaxin by Geneva	00781-1750	Muscle Relaxant
101 <> KP	Tab, Gold, Compressed, KP Logo	Sulfasalazine 500 mg	Azulfidine by Thrift Drug	59198-0010	Gastrointestinal
101 <> KPH	Tab, Mustard	Sulfasalazine 500 mg	Azulfidine by Pharmacia & Upjohn	00013-0101	Gastrointestinal
101 <> KPH	Tab	Sulfasalazine 500 mg	Azulfidine by Pharmacia & Upjohn	59632-0101	Gastrointestinal
101 <> KPH	Tab, Orangish Yellow, Round, 101 <> KPh	Sulfasalazine 500 mg	by Pharmacia	Canadian DIN# 02064480	Gastrointestinal
101 <> KU	Tab, White, Scored	Hyoscyamine Sulfate 0.125 mg	by Schwarz Pharma Mfg	00131-9101	Gastrointestinal
101 <> KU	Tab, White	Hyoscyamine Sulfate 0.125 mg	by Kremers Urban	62175-0101	Gastrointestinal
101 <> MUTUAL	Cap	Indomethacin 25 mg	by Quality Care	60346-0684	NSAID
101 <> TENORMIN	Tab	Atenolol 100 mg	Tenormin by Pharm Utilization	60491-0629	Antihypertensive
101 <> TENORMIN	Tab, White, Round	Atenolol 100 mg	Tenormin by AstraZeneca	00310-0101	Antihypertensive
101010 <> 822	Tab, Pink, Trisected, MJ Logo	Buspirone HCl 30 mg	Buspar by Bristol Myers Squibb	00087-0824	Antianxiety
10103	Tab, White, Oval, 10/103	Torsemide 10 mg	Demadex by Boehringer Mannheim	Canadian	Diuretic
1011 <> STASON	Tab, 10/11	Captopril 12.5 mg	by Stason	60763-1011	Antihypertensive
1011 <> STASON	Tab, White, Diamond, 10/11 <> Stason	Captopril 12.5 mg	by Duramed	51285-0955	Antihypertensive
1012 <> STASON	Tab, Off-White, Diamond Shaped, Scored	Captopril 25 mg	by Stason Pharms	60763-1012	Antihypertensive
1013 <> STASON	Tab, White, Diamond Shaped, Scored	Captopril 50 mg	by Stason Pharms	60763-1013	Antihypertensive
101362	Cap, Yellow, 10-1362	Ephedrine 25 mg	by PDK Labs		Decongestant
1014 <> STASON	Tab, Oblong, Scored	Captopril 100 mg	by Stason Pharms	60763-1014	Antihypertensive
1014 <> STASON	Tab, White, Cap Shaped, 10/14 <> Stason	Captopril 100 mg	by Duramed	51285-0958	Antihypertensive
102 <> 5	Tab, Plus BM Logo	Torsemide 5 mg	Demadex by Boehringer Mannheim	12871-6477	Diuretic
102 <> KP	Tab, Gold, Elliptical-Shaped, Film Coated	Sulfasalazine 500 mg	Azulfidine EN by Thrift Drug	59198-0230	Gastrointestinal
102 <> KPH	Tab, Mustard, Film Coated	Sulfasalazine 500 mg	Azulfidine EN Tabs by Pharmacia & Upjohn	00013-0102	Gastrointestinal
102 <> KPH	Tab, Film Coated	Sulfasalazine 500 mg	Azulfidine EN Tabs by Pharmacia & Upjohn	59632-0102	Gastrointestinal

ID FRONT <> BACK	DESCRIPTION FRONT <> BACK	INGREDIENT & STRENGTH	BRAND (OR EQUIV.) & FIRM	NDC#	CLASS; SCH.
102 <> KPH	Tab, Orange, Elliptical, Enteric Coated, 102 <> KPh	Sulfasalazine 500 mg	by Pharmacia	Canadian DIN# 02064472	Gastrointestinal
102 <> KPH	Tab, Gold, Film Coated	Sulfasalazine 500 mg	Azulfidine EN Tabs by Wal Mart	49035-0167	Gastrointestinal
102 <> KPH	Tab, Yellow, Oval, Enteric Coated	Sulfasalazine 500 mg	Azulfidine by Natl Pharmpak	55154-2801	Gastrointestinal
102 <> KPH	Tab, Yellow	Sulfasalazine 500 mg	Azulfidine by Rx Pac	65084-0171	Gastrointestinal
102 <> KU	Tab, White, Round, Scored	Hyoscyamine Sulfate 0.125 mg	by Schwarz Pharma Mfg	00131-9102	Gastrointestinal
102 <> KU	Tab, White, Round, Scored, Sublingual	Hyoscyamine Sulfate 0.125 mg	by Kremers Urban	62175-0102	Gastrointestinal
1022 <> SOLVAY	Tab, Sugar Coated	Estrogens, Esterified 0.625 mg	by Apotheca	12634-0509	Hormone
1025	Tab, White, Oval, 102/5	Torsemide 5 mg	Demadex by Boehringer Mannheim	Canadian	Diuretic
10251025 <> VISKAZIDES	Tab, Peach, Round, Scored, 10/25 10/25 <> Viskazide S in a triangle	Hydrochlorothiazide 25 mg, Pindolol 10 mg	Viskazide by Sandoz	Canadian DIN# 00568627	Diuretic; Antihypertensive
103 <> 10	Tab, White, Oval, Scored	Torsemide 10 mg	Demadex by Natl Pharmpak	55154-0406	Diuretic
103 <> 10	Tab, White, Oval, 103 & Boehringer Logo <> 10	Torsemide 10 mg	Demadex by Hoffmann La Roche	00004-0263	Diuretic
103 <> PEC	Tab, Coated	Ascorbic Acid 120 mg, Calcium 250 mg, Cholecalciferol 400 Units, Copper 2 mg, Cyanocobalamin 12 mcg, Docusate Sodium 50 mg, Folic Acid 1 mg, Iodine 150 mcg, Iron 90 mg, Niacinamide 20 mg, Pyridoxine HCl 20 mg, Riboflavin 3.4 mg, Thiamine HCl 3 mg, Vitamin A 4000 Units, Vitamin E 30 Units, Zinc 25 mg	Maternity 90 Prenatal Vit & Min by Qualitest	00603-5355	Vitamin
1031	Tab	Carbetapentane Tannate 60 mg, Chlorpheniramine Tannate 5 mg, Ephedrine Tannate 10 mg, Phenylephrine Tannate 10 mg	Tri Tannate Plus by Rugby	00536-4394	Cold Remedy
1032	Tab, White, Round	Reserpine 0.25 mg	Serpasil by Vortech		Antihypertensive
1033	Tab, Round	Rauwolfia Serpentina 100 mg	Raudixin by Vortech		Antihypertensive
1039 <> NUMARK	Tab, Soluble	Chlorpheniramine Maleate 4 mg, Phenylephrine HCl 10 mg, Phenylpropanolamine HCl 50 mg, Pyrilamine Maleate 25 mg	Histalet Forte by Numark	55499-1039	Cold Remedy; C III
1039 <> NUMARK	Tab, Soluble, 10/39 <> Numark	Chlorpheniramine Maleate 4 mg, Phenylephrine HCl 10 mg, Phenylpropanolamine HCl 50 mg, Pyrilamine Maleate 25 mg	by Mikart	46672-0021	Cold Remedy; C III
104	Tab, Orange, Oval	Sulfasalazine 500 mg	by AltiMed	Canadian DIN# 00685925	Gastrointestinal
104	Tab, White, Oval, Scored, Boehringer Mannheim Logo	Torsemide 20 mg	Demadex by Teva	00480-0147	Diuretic
104 <> 20	Tab, Boehringer Mannheim Logo & 104	Torsemide 20 mg	Demadex by Hoffmann La Roche	00004-0264	Diuretic
104 <> 20	Tab, Boehringer Mannheim Logo and 104, Debossed	Torsemide 20 mg	Demadex by Caremark	00339-6012	Diuretic
104 <> 20	Tab, 104 and Boehringer Mannheim Logo	Torsemide 20 mg	Demadex by Nat Pharmpak Serv	55154-0405	Diuretic
104 <> PAR	Tab	Allopurinol 100 mg	by Quality Care	60346-0774	Antigout
1041 <> 93	Tab, Pink, Round, Film Coated	Diclofenac Sodium 100 mg	by Biovail	62660-0021	NSAID
1041 <> 93	Tab, Pink, Round	Diclofenac Sodium 100 mg	by Teva Pharms	00093-1041	NSAID
1043	Tab, Tan, Round	Thyroid 2 gr	by Vortech		Thyroid
1044	Tab, Tan, Round	Thyroid 1 gr	by Vortech		Thyroid
1045	Tab, Red, Round	Thyroid 1 gr	by Vortech		Thyroid
105 <> 100	Tab, Boehringer Mannheim Logo & 105	Torsemide 100 mg	Demadex by Hoffmann La Roche	00004-0265	Diuretic
105 <> BIOCRAFT	Tab	Sucralfate 1 gm	by Golden State	60429-0706	Gastrointestinal
105 <> BIOCRAFT	Tab	Sucralfate 1 gm	by Vangard	00615-4517	Gastrointestinal
105 <> BIOCRAFT	Tab, White, Oblong, Scored	Sucralfate 1 gm	by Allscripts	54569-4446	Gastrointestinal
105 <> CC	Tab, Blue, Cap-Shaped, Film Coated, Scored	Salsalate 750 mg	by Allscripts	54569-1712	NSAID
105 <> GG	Tab, White, Round, Scored	Haloperidol 0.5 mg	by Natl Pharmpak	55154-5412	Antipsychotic
105 <> GG	Tab	Haloperidol 0.5 mg	by PDRX	55289-0157	Antipsychotic
105 <> GG	Tab	Haloperidol 0.5 mg	by Med Pro	53978-3043	Antipsychotic
105 <> ICI	Tab, White, Round	Atenolol 50 mg	Tenormin by AstraZeneca	00310-0105	Antihypertensive
105 <> MUTUAL	Cap, Light Blue	Doxycycline Hyclate	by Quality Care	60346-0109	Antibiotic
105 <> TENORMIN	Tab, Scored	Atenolol 50 mg	Tenormin by Pharm Utilization	60491-0627	Antihypertensive
105 <> TENORMIN	Tab	Atenolol 50 mg	Tenormin by Wal Mart	49035-0166	Antihypertensive

ID FRONT <> BACK	DESCRIPTION FRONT <> BACK	INGREDIENT & STRENGTH	BRAND (OR EQUIV.) & FIRM	NDC#	CLASS; SCH.
105 <> TENORMIN	Tab, White, Round	Atenolol 50 mg	Tenormin by AstraZeneca	00310-0105	Antihypertensive
10501050 <> VISKAZIDES	Tab, Orange, Round, Scored, 10/50 10/50 <> Viskazide S in a triangle	Pindolol 10 mg, Hydrochlorothiazide 50 mg	Viskazide by Sandoz	Canadian DIN# 00568635	Antihypertensive
105105 <> BIOCRAFT	Tab, White, Oblong, Scored	Sucralfate 1 gm	by Murfreesboro Ph	51129-1266	Gastrointestinal
105105 <> BIOCRAFT	Tab, White, Oblong, Scored, 105/105 <> Biocraft	Sucralfate 1 gm	by Teva	00093-2210	Gastrointestinal
105105 <> BIOCRAFT	Tab, White, Oval Shaped, Scored, 105/105 <> Biocraft	Sucralfate 1 gm	Carafate by UDL	51079-0871	Gastrointestinal
105105 <> CARACO	Tab, Film Coated, 105/105 <> Caraco	Salsalate 750 mg	by Allscripts	54569-1712	NSAID
106 <> MUTUAL	Cap	Indomethacin 50 mg	by Quality Care	60346-0733	NSAID
107	Tab	Acetaminophen 500 mg, Chlorpheniramine Maleate 4 mg, Phenylpropanolamine 25 mg	Alumadrine by Fleming	00256-0107	Cold Remedy
107	Tab, Brown & Yellow, Round	Sulfasalazine 500 mg	Sulfasalazine by Kenral	Canadian	Gastrointestinal
107	Tab, Orange, Round	Sulfasalazine 500 mg	by AltiMed	Canadian DIN# 00685933	Gastrointestinal
107 <> A	Tab, Coated	Ascorbic Acid 120 mg, Calcium 200 mg, Copper 2 mg, Cyanocobalamin 12 mcg, Folic Acid 1 mg, Iron 65 mg, Niacinamide 20 mg, Pyridoxine HCl 10 mg, Riboflavin 3 mg, Thiamine Mononitrate 1.84 mg, Vitamin A 4000 Units, Vitamin D 400 Units, Vitamin E 22 mg, Zinc 25 mg	Prenatal Plus by Zenith Goldline	00182-4464	Vitamin
107 <> T	Tab, White, Round	Atenolol 25 mg	Tenormin by AstraZeneca	00310-0107	Antihypertensive
1077	Tab, Round	Chlorpheniramine Maleate 8 mg	Chlor-trimeton by Vortech		Antihistamine
1078	Tab, Round	Phenobarbital 15 mg, Belladonna 10 mg	Bellophen by Vortech		Gastrointestinal; C IV
1078212	Tab, White, Round, 10 78-212	Metaproterenol 10 mg	Metaprel by Sandoz		Antiasthmatic
1079	Tab, Round	Digitoxin 0.1 mg	by Vortech		Cardiac Agent
108 <> MIA	Tab	Acetaminophen 500 mg, Hydrocodone Bitartrate 5 mg	by Zenith Goldline	00172-5643	Analgesic; C III
108MIA	Tab, 108/MIA	Acetaminophen 500 mg, Hydrocodone Bitartrate 5 mg	by Schein	00364-0744	Analgesic; C III
109	Tab, Peach, Oblong, Star Logo 109	Ortho-Phosphate Formula 1 g	Uro-KP-Neutral by Star		Vitamin
109	Tab, Peach, Oblong	Ortho Phosphate 1g	URO-KP NEUT by Star Pharm		Vitamin
109 <> T	Tab	Carbamazepine 200 mg	by Baker Cummins	63171-1233	Anticonvulsant
1091 <> NUMARK	Tab	Hydrocodone Bitartrate 5 mg, Pseudoephedrine HCl 60 mg	P V Tussin by Numark	55499-1091	Analgesic; C III
1091 <> NUMARK	Tab, 10/91	Hydrocodone Bitartrate 5 mg, Pseudoephedrine HCl 60 mg	by Mikart	46672-0133	Analgesic; C III
1093	Tab, Red, Round	Thyroid 2 gr	by Vortech		Thyroid
1094	Tab, Round	Penicillin G 250,000 Units	Pentids by Vortech		Antibiotic
1098	Tab, Round	Prednisone 5 mg	by Vortech		Steroid
10ALG	Tab, 1.0/AL/G	Alprazolam 1 mg	by Schein	00364-2584	Antianxiety; C IV
10AMIDE009	Tab	Isoxsuprine HCl 10 mg	by Zenith Goldline	00182-1055	Vasodilator
10AMIDE009	Tab, White, Round, 10 and Amide 009	Isoxsuprine HCl 10 mg	Vasodilan by Amide	52152-0009	Vasodilator
10DAN5566	Tab, Yellowish Green, Triangular, 10/Dan 5566	Thioridazine HCl 10 mg	Mellaril by Danbury		Antipsychotic
10F	Tab, White, Round, 10/F	Tamoxifen Citrate 10 mg	Tamone by Pharmacia	Canadian	Antiestrogen
10LLC12	Tab, Yellow, Square	Leucovorin Calcium 10 mg	Leucovorin by Lederle		Antineoplastic
10M	Tab, White, 10/M	Benzoyl Peroxide 10 mg	Benoxyl by Stiefel	Canadian	Antiacne
10M	Tab, White, 10/M	Decyclomine 10 mg	by Hoechst Marion Roussel	Canadian	Gastrointestinal
10MG	Tab, Black Print	Glipizide 10 mg	Glucotrol XL by Direct Dispensing	57866-6303	Antidiabetic
10MG	Cap, Pamelor Logo <> Sandoz Logo 10 mg	Nortriptyline HCl 10 mg	Pamelor by Allscripts	54569-0225	Antidepressant
10MG	Cap, Blue	Pericyazine 10 mg	by Rhone-Poulenc Rorer	Canadian	Psychotropic Agent
10MG <> BRISTOL3030	Cap, Black Print, 10 mg <> Bristol Over 3030	Lomustine 10 mg	Ceenu by Mead Johnson	00015-3030	Antineoplastic
10MG <> BUSPAR	Tab, MJ Logo	Buspirone HCl 10 mg	by Med Pro	53978-3024	Antianxiety
10MG <> LOTENSIN	Tab, Dark Yellow	Benazepril HCl 10 mg	Lotensin by Southwood Pharms	58016-0420	Antihypertensive
10MG <> SONATA	Cap, Green	Zaleplon 10 mg	Sonata by Wyeth Pharms	52903-0926	Sedative/Hypnotic; C IV
10MG <> SONATA	Cap, Green & Opaque	Zaleplon 10 mg	Sonata by United Res	00677-1685	Sedative/Hypnotic; C IV
10MG <> SONATA	Cap, Green & Opaque	Zaleplon 10 mg	Sonata by United Res	00677-1689	Sedative/Hypnotic; C IV

ID FRONT <> BACK	DESCRIPTION FRONT <> BACK	INGREDIENT & STRENGTH	BRAND (OR EQUIV.) & FIRM	NDC#	CLASS; SCH.
10MG <> SONATA	Cap, Green	Zaleplon 10 mg	Sonata by Wyeth Labs	00008-0926	Sedative/Hypnotic; C IV
10MG <> WATSON370	Cap, White & Yellow	Loxapine Succinate 10 mg	by Dixon Shane	17236-0694	Antipsychotic
10MG <> WATSON370	Cap, White & Yellow, Opaque, 10 mg <> Watson over 370	Loxapine 10 mg	Loxitane by UDL	51079-0901	Antipsychotic
10MG <> WATSON370	Cap	Loxapine Succinate	by Watson	52544-0370	Antipsychotic
10MG <> WATSON370	Cap	Loxapine Succinate	by Zenith Goldline	00182-1306	Antipsychotic
10MG <> WATSON370	Cap	Loxapine Succinate	by Physicians Total Care	54868-2327	Antipsychotic
10MG <> WATSON370	Cap, 10 mg <> Watson Over 370	Loxapine Succinate	by UDL	51079-0678	Antipsychotic
10MG <> WATSON370	Cap	Loxapine Succinate	by Qualitest	00603-4269	Antipsychotic
10MG <> WATSON370	Cap	Loxapine Succinate	by Major	00904-2311	Antipsychotic
10MG <> WATSON370	Cap	Loxapine Succinate	by Geneva	00781-2711	Antipsychotic
10MG <> WATSON370	Cap	Loxapine Succinate	by HL Moore	00839-7496	Antipsychotic
10MG <> WATSON695	Cap	Doxepin HCl 11.25 mg	by Watson	52544-0695	Antidepressant
10MG <> WATSON712	Cap, Light Blue & White	Piroxicam 10 mg	by Allscripts	54569-3974	NSAID
10MG <> WATSON712	Cap, Filled with Off-White to Yellow Powder	Piroxicam 10 mg	by Watson	52544-0712	NSAID
10MG3344 <> 10MGSB	Cap, Ivory & Natural with White & Yellow Pellets	Prochlorperazine 10 mg	Compazine by Intl Processing	59885-3344	Antiemetic
10MG3513 <> 10MGSB	Cap, Brown & Clear	Dextroamphetamine Sulfate 10 mg	Dexedrine by DRX	55045-2616	Stimulant; C II
10MG3513 <> 10MGSB	Cap	Dextroamphetamine Sulfate 10 mg	Dexedrine by Physicians Total Care	54868-3811	Stimulant; C II
10MGLEDERLE12	Cap, Green & Yellow	Loxapine 10 mg	Loxitane by Lederle		Antipsychotic
10MGSB <> 10MG3344	Cap, Ivory & Natural with White & Yellow Pellets	Prochlorperazine 10 mg	Compazine by Intl Processing	59885-3344	Antiemetic
10MGSB <> 10MG3513	Cap	Dextroamphetamine Sulfate 10 mg	Dexedrine by Physicians Total Care	54868-3811	Stimulant; C II
10MGZAR	Tab, Yellow, Round, 10 mg/Zar	Metolazone 10 mg	Zaroxolyn by Medeva		Diuretic
10MJ <> BUSPAR	Tab, 10 over MJ <> Buspar	Buspirone HCl 10 mg	Buspar by Nat Pharmpak Serv	55154-2010	Antianxiety
10NOVO	Tab, Yellow, D-Shaped, 10/Novo	Cyclobenzaprine 10 mg	Novo Cycloprine by Novopharm	Canadian	Muscle Relaxant
10ROCHE <> VESANOID	Cap	Tretinoin 10 mg	Vesanoid by Hoffmann La Roche	00004-0250	Retinoid
10VVALIUM <> ROCHEVROCHE	Tab, 10 over V over Valium <> Roche V Roche	Diazepam 10 mg	Valium by Roche	00140-0006	Antianxiety; C IV
10XL	Tab, Pink, Oval	Oxybutynin Chloride 10 mg	Ditropan XL by Alza	17314-8501	Urinary
11	Tab, White, Round, Triangle Logo	Biperiden HCl 2 mg	Akineton by Knoll		Antiparkinson
11	Tab, Triangle Logo	Biperiden HCl 2 mg	Akineton by Physicians Total Care	54868-2432	Antiparkinson
11	Tab, White, Triangle Logo	Biperiden HCl 2 mg	Akineton by Knoll	Canadian	Antiparkinson
11 <> B	Tab, Light Green	Ethinyl Estradiol 0.03 mg, Ethinyl Estradiol 0.04 mg, Ethinyl Estradiol 0.03 mg, Levonorgestrel 0.05 mg, Levonorgestrel 0.125 mg, Levonorgestrel 0.075 mg	Tri-Levlen 28 by Berlex	50419-00111	Oral Contraceptive
11 <> B	Tab, Light Green, Film Coated	Ethinyl Estradiol 0.03 mg, Ethinyl Estradiol 0.04 mg, Ethinyl Estradiol 0.03 mg, Levonorgestrel 0.05 mg, Levonorgestrel 0.125 mg, Levonorgestrel 0.075 mg	Tri-Levlen 28 by Berlex	50419-0433	Oral Contraceptive
11 <> B	Tab, Light Green, Film Coated	Inert	Tri-Levlen 28 by Berlex	50419-0111	Placebo
11 <> DUPONT	Tab, Pale Yellow, Cap-Shaped, Coated	Naltrexone HCl 50 mg	Revia by Du Pont Pharma	00056-0011	Opiod Antagonist
11 <> P	Tab, Round, Dye Free, Chewable, 1.1 <> P	Sodium Fluoride 1.1 mg	Pharmaflur 1.1 by Pharmics	00813-0065	Element
11 <> SL	Tab, Sugar Coated	Dipyridamole 25 mg	by Sidmak	50111-0311	Antiplatelet
11 <> VP	Tab, White, Round	Ethambutol HCl 100 mg	by Versapharm	61748-0011	Antituberculosis
11 <> VP	Tab, White, Round, Film Coated	Ethambutol HCl 100 mg	by WestWard Pharm	00143-9100	Antituberculosis
110	Tab, Light Blue, Oblong	Butalbital 50 mg, Acetaminophen 650 mg	Cephadyn by Atley		Analgesic
110 <> AP	Tab, Light Blue, Cap Shaped, 110 <> A/P	Acetaminophen 650 mg, Butalbital 50 mg	Cephadyn by Atley	59702-0650	Analgesic
110 <> CSCOTT	Tab, Sugar Coated, C Scott	Thyroid 1 gr	by JMI Canton	00252-7007	Thyroid
110 <> MIA	Tab	Acetaminophen 325 mg, Butalbital 50 mg, Caffeine 40 mg	by Quality Care	60346-0703	Analgesic
1101 <> MYLAN	Cap	Prazosin HCl 1 mg	by Quality Care	60346-0572	Antihypertensive
1102 <> 60MG	Cap, Gelatin Coated	Fexofenadine HCl 60 mg	by Kaiser	62224-1114	Antihistamine
1102 <> 60MG	Cap, Pink & White	Fexofenadine HCl 60 mg	Allegra by DRX Pharm Consults	55045-2582	Antihistamine
1102 <> 60MG	Cap, Pink & White	Fexofenadine HCl 60 mg	Allegra by PDRX Pharms	55289-0456	Antihistamine
1102 <> 60MG	Cap, Gelatin Coated	Fexofenadine HCl 60 mg	Allegra by Kaiser	00179-1265	Antihistamine
1102 <> 60MG	Cap, Gelatin	Fexofenadine HCl 60 mg	Allegra by Hoechst Roussel	00088-1102	Antihistamine
1102 <> 60MG	Cap, Gelatin, Black Print	Fexofenadine HCl 60 mg	Allegra by Caremark	00339-6083	Antihistamine

ID FRONT <> BACK	DESCRIPTION FRONT <> BACK	INGREDIENT & STRENGTH	BRAND (OR EQUIV.) & FIRM	NDC#	CLASS; SCH.
1102 <> 60MG	Cap, Gelatin Coated	Fexofenadine HCl 60 mg	Allegra by Physicians Total Care	54868-3898	Antihistamine
110260MG <> 60MGALLEGRA	Cap, Gelatin Coated, Black Print	Fexofenadine HCl 60 mg	Allegra by Quality Care	62682-8004	Antihistamine
1105	Cap, Red, Oblong, Gelatin	Docusate Sodium 50 mg	Colace by UDL	51079-0521	Laxative
1105	Tab, Red, Oval	Docusate Sodium 50 mg	Colace by Scherer		Laxative
111 <> 93	Tab, White, Round, Film Coated	Cimetidine 200 mg	by Teva	00093-0111	Gastrointestinal
111 <> A	Tab, Brown, Oval, Film Coated, Scored	Methenamine Mandelate 500 mg	by Murfreesboro Ph	51129-1430	Antibiotic; Urinary Tract
111 <> COPLEY	Tab, Yellowish Tan, Coated	Ascorbic Acid 120 mg, Beta-Carotene 4.2 mg, Calcium Carbonate 490.76 mg, Cholecalciferol 0.49 mg, Cupric Oxide 2.5 mg, Cyanocobalamin 12 mcg, Ferrous Fumarate 197.75 mg, Folic Acid 1 mg, Niacinamide 21 mg, Pyridoxine HCl 10.5 mg, Riboflavin 3.15 mg, Thiamine Mononitrate 1.575 mg, Vitamin A Acetate 8.4 mg, Vitamin E Acetate 44 mg, Zinc Oxide 31.12 mg	Prenatal One Mg Plus Iron by Copley	38245-0111	Vitamin
111 <> PEC	Cap, Gray, Pink & White Beads	Chlorpheniramine Maleate 12 mg, Phenylpropanolamine HCl 75 mg	Ordrine by Mutual	53489-0302	Cold Remedy
111 <> SP	Tab, White, Round	Hyoscyamine Sulfate 0.125 mg	NuLev by Schwarz	00091-3111	Gastrointestinal
1114 <> BEACH	Tab, Film Coated	Methenamine Mandelate 500 mg, Sodium Phosphate, Monobasic, Monohydrate 500 mg	Uroqid Acid No 2 by Pharm Assoc	00121-0352	Antibiotic; Urinary Tract
1114 <> BEACH	Tab, Film Coated	Methenamine Mandelate 500 mg, Sodium Phosphate, Monobasic, Monohydrate 500 mg	Uroqid Acid No 2 by Beach	00486-1114	Antibiotic; Urinary Tract
1114 <> BEACH	Tab, Yellow, Oblong, Film Coated	Methenamine Mandelate 500 mg, Sodium Phosphate, Monobasic 500 mg	Uroqid by WestWard Pharm	00143-9023	Antibiotic; Urinary Tract
1115	Tab, Blue, Round, Savage Logo 1115	Dyphylline 200 mg	Dilor by Savage	00281-1115	Antiasthmatic
1116	Tab, White, Round, Savage Logo 1116	Dyphylline 400 mg	Dilor 400 by Savage	00281-1116	Antiasthmatic
1116	Tab, Large Triangle over Small Triangle 1116	Dyphylline 400 mg	Dilor-400 by Savage	00281-1116	Antiasthmatic
1118 <> 93	Tab, Light Blue	Etodolac 600 mg	by Teva Pharms	00093-1118	NSAID
112	Tab, Ex Release, 1 1/2	Nitroglycerin 1.5 mg	Sustachron ER Buccal by Forest	10418-0143	Vasodilator
112 <> 93	Tab, Film Coated	Cimetidine 300 mg	by Quality Care	60346-0944	Gastrointestinal
112 <> 93	Tab, Film Coated	Cimetidine 300 mg	by PDRX	55289-0799	Gastrointestinal
112 <> 93	Tab, White, Round, Film Coated	Cimetidine 300 mg	by Teva	00093-0112	Gastrointestinal
112 <> BIOCRAFT	Cap, Light Green	Cephradine Monohydrate 250 mg	by Quality Care	60346-0040	Antibiotic
112 <> FLINT	Tab	Levothyroxine Sodium 0.112 mg	Synthroid by Nat Pharmpak Serv	55154-0911	Antithyroid
112 <> FLINT	Tab, Rose, Round, Scored	Levothyroxine Sodium 112 mcg	Synthroid by Knoll	00048-1080	Antithyroid
1124	Tab, Pink, Round, Savage Logo 1124	Dyphylline 200 mg, Guaifenesin 200 mg	Dilor-G by Savage	00281-1124	Antiasthmatic
1125	Tab, Film Coated, Beach Logo	Potassium Phosphate (Monobasic 155 mg), Sodium Phosphate (Dibasic, Anhydrous 852 mg), Sodium Phosphate (Monobasic, Monohydrate 130 mg)	K Phos Neutral by Beach	00486-1125	Electrolytes
1125 <> BEACH	Tab, Film Coated	Potassium Phosphate (Monobasic 155 mg), Sodium Phosphate (Dibasic, Anhydrous 852 mg), Sodium Phosphate (Monobasic, Monohydrate 130 mg)	K Phos by Pharm Assoc	00121-0349	Electrolytes
1125 <> BEACH	Tab, Film Coated	Potassium Phosphate (Monobasic 155 mg), Sodium Phosphate (Dibasic, Anhydrous 852 mg), Sodium Phosphate (Monobasic, Monohydrate 130 mg)	K-Phos Neutral by Beach	00486-1125	Electrolytes
1127 <> BRL	Tab, Blue, Oblong, Scored	Sucralfate 1 gm	by Blue Ridge	59273-0001	Gastrointestinal
1127 <> BRL	Tab, Embossed	Sucralfate 1 gm	by Rugby	00536-1127	Gastrointestinal
1127 <> BRL	Tab	Sucralfate 1 gm	by Hoechst Roussel	00088-1127	Gastrointestinal
112FLI	Tab, Rose, Round, 112/FLI	Levothyroxine Sodium 112 mcg	by Forest	00456-0330	Antithyroid
112M	Tab	Levothyroxine Sodium 0.112 mg	Levo T by MOVA	55370-0161	Antithyroid
112M	Tab	Levothyroxine Sodium 0.112 mg	Euthyrox by Em Pharma	63254-0440	Antithyroid
112MCG	Tab	Levothyroxine Sodium 0.112 mg	Eltroxin by Glaxo	53873-0118	Antithyroid
112MCG	Tab, Rose	Levothyroxine Sodium 0.112 mg	Levoxyl by Physicians Total Care	54868-3849	Antithyroid
112MCG <> FLINT	Tab, Round, Scored	Levothyroxine Sodium 0.112 mg	Synthroid by Rightpac	65240-0743	Antithyroid
112MCG <> FLINT	Tab, Debossed	Levothyroxine Sodium 0.112 mg	Synthroid by Amerisource	62584-0080	Antithyroid
113 <> 93	Tab, Film Coated	Cimetidine 400 mg	by Quality Care	60346-0945	Gastrointestinal
113 <> 93	Tab, Film Coated	Cimetidine 400 mg	by Vangard	00615-3566	Gastrointestinal
113 <> BIOCRAFT	Cap, Light Green	Cephradine 500 mg	by Schein	00364-2142	Antibiotic
113 <> BIOCRAFT	Cap, Light Green	Cephradine Monohydrate 500 mg	by Quality Care	60346-0041	Antibiotic

ID FRONT <> BACK	DESCRIPTION FRONT <> BACK	INGREDIENT & STRENGTH	BRAND (OR EQUIV.) & FIRM	NDC#	CLASS; SCH.
113 <> COPLEY	Tab, Buff	Chlorpheniramine Tannate 8 mg, Phenylephrine Tannate 25 mg, Pyrilamine Tannate 25 mg	R-Tannate by Schein	00364-2196	Cold Remedy
1134 <> BEACH	Tab, Coated	Potassium Phosphate (Monobasic 305 mg), Sodium Phosphate (Monobasic 700 mg)	K Phos No 2 by Pharm Assoc	00121-0386	Electrolytes
1134 <> BEACH	Tab, White, Coated	Potassium Phosphate (Monobasic 305 mg), Sodium Phosphate (Monobasic 700 mg)	K-Phos No 2 by Beach	00486-1134	Electrolytes
1134 <> BEACH	Tab	Potassium Phosphate (Monobasic 500 mg)	K Phos Original by Pharm Assoc	00121-0382	Electrolytes
1134 <> BEACH	Tab, White, Oblong, Film Coated, Scored	Sodium Phosphate, Dibasic, Anhydrous 852 mg, Potassium Phosphate, Tribasic 155 mg; Sodium Phosphate, Monobasic, Monohydrate 130 mg	K Phos by WestWard Pharm	00143-9024	Electrolyte
1135 <> BEACH	Tab, White	Potassium Phosphate (Monobasic 155 mg), Sodium Phosphate (Monobasic 350 mg)	K Phos M F by Pharm Assoc	00486-1135	Electrolytes
1136 <> BEACH	Tab	Potassium Citrate Anhydrous 50 mg, Sodium Citrate, Anhydrous 950 mg	Citrolith by Beach	00486-1136	Electrolytes
1136 <> BEACH	Tab	Potassium Citrate Anhydrous 50 mg, Sodium Citrate, Anhydrous 950 mg	Citrolith by Pharm Assoc	00121-0374	Electrolytes
1136 <> BEACH	Tab, 11/36	Potassium Citrate Anhydrous 50 mg, Sodium Citrate, Anhydrous 950 mg	Citrolith by		Electrolytes
113GDC	Tab, White, Round	Calcium Carbonate 500 mg	Tums by Guardian		Vitamin/Mineral
114 <> COPLEY	Tab, Film Coated, Copley	Procainamide HCl 750 mg	by Murfreesboro	51129-1174	Antiarrhythmic
114 <> COPLEY	Tab, Film Coated	Procainamide HCl 750 mg	by Copley	38245-0114	Antiarrhythmic
114 <> COPLEY	Tab, Film Coated	Procainamide HCl 750 mg	by HL Moore	00839-7029	Antiarrhythmic
114 <> MP	Tab, White, Round, Coated, Scored	Trazodone HCl 100 mg	by Allscripts	54569-1999	Antidepressant
114 <> PAR	Tab, Coated, Debossed	Metronidazole 500 mg	by Quality Care	60346-0507	Antibiotic
115 <> MYLAN	Cap, Scarlet	Ampicillin Trihydrate	by Quality Care	60346-0082	Antibiotic
115 <> TENORETIC	Tab, White, Round	Atenolol 50 mg, Chlorthalidone 25 mg	Tenoretic 50 by AstraZeneca	00310-0115	Antihypertensive; Diuretic
115 <> TENORETIC	Tab	Atenolol 50 mg, Chlorthalidone 25 mg	Tenoretic 50 by Physicians Total Care	54868-0321	Antihypertensive; Diuretic
1155 <> MYLAN	Tab, White, Capsule Shaped, Film Coated	Propoxyphene Napsylate 100 mg, Acetaminophen 650 mg	Darvocet-N by UDL	51079-0934	Analgesic; C IV
1157018	Cap, Green & White	Minocycline HCl 100 mg	by Par Pharm	49884-0644	Antibiotic
1161	Tab	Furosemide 40 mg	by Med Pro	53978-5032	Diuretic
1166 <> COPLEY	Tab, Orange, Pink & Purple, Chewable	Ascorbic Acid 34.5 mg, Cyanocobalamin 4.9 mcg, Folic Acid 0.35 mg, Niacinamide 14.17 mg, Pyridoxine HCl 1.1 mg, Riboflavin 1.26 mg, Sodium Ascorbate 32.2 mg, Sodium Fluoride 2.21 mg, Thiamine Mononitrate 1.15 mg, Vitamin A Palmitate 5.5 mg, Vitamin D 0.194 mg, Vitamin E Acetate 15.75 mg	Polyvitamin by Schein	00364-1075	Vitamin
117	Cap, Green & Yellow	Vitamin B Complex, C	Allbee with C by Fresh		Vitamin
117 <> BIOCRAFT	Cap	Cephalexin Monohydrate	by Quality Care	60346-0055	Antibiotic
117 <> BVF	Tab, White, Oblong	Pentoxifylline 400 mg	by Vangard Labs	00615-4523	Anticoagulent
117 <> TENORETIC	Tab, White, Round	Atenolol 100 mg, Chlorthalidone 25 mg	Tenoretic 100 by AstraZeneca	00310-0117	Antihypertensive; Diuretic
1171 <> 75	Tab, Pink, Round	Clopidogrel Bisulfate 75 mg	Plavix by Natl Pharmpak	55154-2016	Antiplatelet
1177 <> 93	Tab, Off-White, Round	Neomycin Sulfate 500 mg	by UDL	51079-0015	Antibiotic
1177 <> 93	Tab, Off-White, Round	Neomycin Sulfate 500 mg	by Teva	00093-1177	Antibiotic
117COPLEY	Tab, Red, Oblong, 117/Copley	Procainamide HCl ER 1000 mg	PROCAN by Copley		Antiarrhythmic
118 <> 93	Tab, Blue, Oval	Etodolac 600 mg	by Teva Pharm	00480-1118	NSAID
1189500 <> G	Tab	Chlorzoxazone 500 mg	by Royce	51875-0239	Muscle Relaxant
119	Tab, Orange, Round, Schering Logo 119	Perphenazine 4 mg, Amitriptyline HCl 10 mg	Etrafon-A by Schering		Antipsychotic; Antidepressant
11DUPONT	Tab, Yellow, Oblong, 11/DuPont	Naltrexone HCl 50 mg	Revia by DuPont	Canadian	Opiod Antagonist
12	Cap	Oxacillin Sodium Monohydrate	by DRX	55045-2277	Antibiotic
12 <> 54169	Tab, 1 over 2 <> 54 169	Haloperidol 0.5 mg	by Murfreesboro	51129-1130	Antipsychotic
12 <> 54169	Tab, White, 1 over 2 <> 54/169	Haloperidol 0.5 mg	Haldol by Roxane	00054-8342	Antipsychotic
12 <> MEDEVA	Tab, Green, Oblong, Scored	Guaifenesin 600 mg	Humibid LA by Phy Total Care	54868-1777	Expectorant
12 <> MEDEVA	Tab, Green, Oblong, Scored	Guaifenesin 600 mg	Humabid LA by Adams Labs	63824-0012	Expectorant
12 <> MEDEVA	Tab, Green, Oblong, Scored	Guaifenesin 600 mg	Humibid LA by Compumed	00403-1009	Expectorant
12 <> MEDEVA	Tab, Green, Oblong, Scored	Guaifenesin 600 mg; Pseudoephedrine HCl 60 mg	Syn Rx by Adams Labs	63824-0308	Cold Remedy
12 <> MYKROX	Tab, 1/2	Metolazone 0.5 mg	Mykrox by Medeva	53014-0847	Diuretic

ID FRONT <> BACK	DESCRIPTION FRONT <> BACK	INGREDIENT & STRENGTH	BRAND (OR EQUIV.) & FIRM	NDC#	CLASS; SCH.
120	Tab, Ivory, Round, Hourglass Logo <> 120	Verapamil 120 mg	Calan SR / Isoptin Sr by Zenith Goldline	00172-4285	Antihypertensive
120	Tab, Ivory, Round, Film Coated	Verapamil HCl 120 mg	by Caremark	00339-5812	Antihypertensive
120 <> ANDRX687	Cap, White	Diltiazem HCl 120 mg	Cartia XT by Heartland Healthcare	61392-0957	Antihypertensive
120 <> IMDUR	Tab, White, Oval	Isosorbide Mononitrate 120 mg	Imdur by Schering	00085-1153	Antianginal
120 <> IMDUR	Tab	Isosorbide Mononitrate 120 mg	Imdur by Pharm Utilization	60491-0314	Antianginal
120 <> STARLIX	Tab, Yellow, Oval	Nateglinide 120 mg	Starlix by Novartis	00078-0352	Antidiabetic
120 <> W587	Tab, White, Oval, Scored	Isosorbide Mononitrate 120 mg	by Warrick Pharms	59930-1587	Antianginal
120 <> Z4238	Tab, White, Cap-Shaped	Nadolol 120 mg	Nadolol by Zenith Goldline	00172-4238	Antihypertensive
1202MJ <> M	Tab, 1202MG <> m	Fosinopril Sodium 40 mg	Monopril by Quality Care	62682-6027	Antihypertensive
1202MJ <> M	Tab	Fosinopril Sodium 40 mg	Monopril by Bristol Myers	15548-0202	Antihypertensive
1205 <> SOLVAY	Cap, Gelatin	Amylase 16600 Units, Lipase 5000 Units, Protease 18750 Units	Creon 5 by Solvay	00032-1205	Gastrointestinal
120MGBERLEX	Tab, White, Cap Shaped, Scored	Sotalol HCl 120 mg	Betapace by Berlex Labs	50419-0119	Antiarrhythmic
120MGBETAPACE	Tab, Light Blue, Cap Shaped, Scored	Sotalol HCl 120 mg	Betapace by Berlex	50419-0109	Antiarrhythmic
120WATSON662	Cap, Pink & White, 120/Watson/662	Diltiazem 120 mg	Dilacor XR by Watson		Antihypertensive
120Z4238	Tab, White, Cap-Shaped, 120/Z4238	Nadolol 120 mg	Corgard by Zenith Goldline	00172-4238	Antihypertensive
1210 <> SOLVAY	Cap	Amylase 33200 Units, Lipase 10000 Units, Protease 37500 Units	Creon 10 by Solvay	00032-1210	Gastrointestinal
1217L	Cab, Black	Separpanide 0.3 mg	by Smith Labs	23455-9311	Fibromyalgia
122	Cap, Green	Loperamide 2 mg	Imodium by OHM		Antidiarrheal
122 <> PEC	Cap, Orangish Clear & Orange, Opaque	Amylase 48,000 Units, Lipase 16,000 Units, Protease 48,000 Units	Pancrelipase 16,000 by Pecos	59879-0122	Gastrointestinal
122 <> PEC	Cap, Clear & Orange, Opaque	Amylase 48,000 Units, Lipase 16,000 Units, Protease 48,000 Units	Pancrelipase 16,000 by Lini	58215-0300	Gastrointestinal
122 <> PEC	Cap, Orangish Clear & Orange, Opaque	Amylase 48,000 Units, Lipase 16,000 Units, Protease 48,000 Units	Pancrelipase 16,000 by Mutual	53489-0247	Gastrointestinal
122 <> PEC	Cap, Clear & Orange, Opaque	Amylase 48,000 Units, Lipase 16,000 Units, Protease 48,000 Units	Pancrelipase 16,000 by United Res	00677-1543	Gastrointestinal
1220 <> SOLVAY	Cap	Amylase 66400 Units, Lipase 20000 Units, Protease 75000 Units	Creon 20 by Solvay	00032-1220	Gastrointestinal
1221 <> TCL	Cap	Nitroglycerin 2.5 mg	by Schein	00364-0174	Vasodilator
1221 <> TCL	Cap, Lavender, ER, Black Ink	Nitroglycerin 2.5 mg	Nitro Time by Time Caps	49483-0221	Vasodilator
12210	Cap, Yellow	D-Alpha Tocopheryl Acetate 100 Units	Epsilan-M by Adria		Vitamin
1222 <> TCL	Cap	Nitroglycerin 6.5 mg	by Schein	00364-0432	Vasodilator
1222 <> TCL	Cap, Black Print	Nitroglycerin 6.5 mg	Nitro Time by Time Caps	49483-0222	Vasodilator
1223 <> TCL	Cap	Nitroglycerin 9 mg	by Schein	00364-0664	Vasodilator
1223 <> TCL	Cap, Black Print	Nitroglycerin 9 mg	Nitro Time by Time Caps	49483-0223	Vasodilator
122GDC	Tab, Multi-Colored, Round, 122/GDC	Bismuth 262 mg	Pepto-Bismol by Guardian		Gastrointestinal
123 <> GG	Tab	Haloperidol 1 mg	by Golden State	60429-0087	Antipsychotic
123 <> GG	Tab, Yellow, Round, Scored	Haloperidol 1 mg	by Natl Pharmpak	55154-5413	Antipsychotic
123 <> GG	Tab	Haloperidol 1 mg	by Med Pro	53978-3004	Antipsychotic
1231 <> LAN	Tab	Primidone 250 mg	by Qualitest	00603-5370	Anticonvulsant
1237	Tab, Round	Pentaerythritol Tetranitrate 20 mg	Peritrate by Vortech		Antianginal
124 <> GG	Tab, Pink, Round, Scored	Haloperidol 2 mg	Haloperidol by Geneva	00781-1393	Antipsychotic
1242	Tab, Round	Prednisolone 5 mg	by Vortech		Steroid
125	Tab, Oval, Red, Enteric Coated	Divalproex Sodium 125 mg	by Nu Pharm	Canadian DIN# 02239517	Anticonvulsant
125	Tab, Purple, Round, Scored	Levothyroxine Sodium 125 mcg	by Murfreesboro	51129-1653	Antithyroid
125	Cap, White, Red Print	Theophylline 125 mg	Slo Bid by RPR	00801-1125	Antiasthmatic
125 <> 355	Tab, 12.5/Royce Logo <> 355	Captopril 12.5 mg	by Qualitest	00603-2555	Antihypertensive
125 <> AMOXIL	Tab, Chewable	Amoxicillin Trihydrate	by Quality Care	60346-0100	Antibiotic
125 <> CAPOTEN	Tab, Mottled White, Round, 12.5 <> Capoten	Captopril 12.5 mg	Capoten by ER Squibb	00003-0450	Antihypertensive
125 <> CAPOTEN	Tab, 12.5 <> Capoten	Captopril 12.5 mg	Capoten by Nat Pharmpak Serv	55154-3706	Antihypertensive
125 <> FAMVIR	Tab, Film Coated	Famciclovir 125 mg	Famvir by Apotheca	12634-0508	Antiviral
125 <> FAMVIR	Tab, Film Coated	Famciclovir 125 mg	Famvir by SKB	60351-4115	Antiviral
125 <> FAMVIR	Tab, White, Round, Film Coated	Famciclovir 125 mg	Famvir by Phy Total Care	54868-3882	Antiviral
125 <> FAMVIR	Tab, White, Film Coated	Famciclovir 125 mg	Famvir by SKB	00007-4115	Antiviral

ID FRONT <> BACK	DESCRIPTION FRONT <> BACK	INGREDIENT & STRENGTH	BRAND (OR EQUIV.) & FIRM	NDC#	CLASS; SCH.
125 <> FAMVIR	Tab, White, Round, Film Coated	Famciclovir 125 mg	Famvir by Novartis	00078-0366	Antiviral
125 <> FAMVIR	Tab, Film Coated	Famciclovir 125 mg	Famvir by Allscripts	54569-4533	Antiviral
125 <> FAMVIR	Tab, White, Round, Film Coated	Famciclovir 125 mg	by SmithKline SKB	Canadian DIN# 02229110	Antiviral
125 <> FL	Tab, Compressed, Logo	Levothyroxine Sodium 0.125 mg	by Kaiser	00179-1210	Antithyroid
125 <> FLINT	Tab	Levothyroxine Sodium 0.125 mg	Synthroid by Nat Pharmpak Serv	55154-0909	Antithyroid
125 <> FLINT	Tab	Levothyroxine Sodium 0.125 mg	Synthroid by Giant Food	11146-0303	Antithyroid
125 <> FLINT	Tab	Levothyroxine Sodium 0.125 mg	Synthroid by Rite Aid	11822-5285	Antithyroid
125 <> FLINT	Tab, Brown, Round, Scored	Levothyroxine Sodium 125 mcg	Synthroid by Knoll	00048-1130	Antithyroid
125 <> GRISPEG	Tab, Film Coated	Griseofulvin (Ultramicrosize) 125 mg	Gris Peg by Novartis	00043-0800	Antifungal
125 <> N	Cap, Pink	Amoxicillin Trihydrate 250 mg	by Southwood Pharms	58016-0103	Antibiotic
125 <> N132	Tab, White, Oval, Scored, 12.5 <> N over 132	Captopril 12.5 mg	by Novopharm	55953-0132	Antihypertensive
125 <> N132	Tab, Scored, 12.5 <> N over 132	Captopril 12.5 mg	by Medirex	57480-0838	Antihypertensive
125 <> N132	Tab, Scored, 12.5 <> N over 132	Captopril 12.5 mg	by Major	00904-5045	Antihypertensive
125 <> N132	Tab, White, Oval, Scored, 12.5 <> N over 132	Captopril 12.5 mg	by Novopharm	43806-0132	Antihypertensive
125 <> N342	Tab, White, Round, 1.25 <> N over 342	Glyburide 1.25 mg	by Novopharm	55953-0342	Antidiabetic
125 <> N342	Tab, 1.25 <> N 342	Glyburide 1.25 mg	by Warrick	59930-1592	Antidiabetic
125 <> N342	Tab, N/342	Glyburide 1.25 mg	by Brightstone	62939-3211	Antidiabetic
125 <> N342	Tab, 1.25 <> N over 342	Glyburide 1.25 mg	by Qualitest	00603-3762	Antidiabetic
125 <> N342	Tab, 1.25 <> N 342	Glyburide 1.25 mg	by HL Moore	00839-8039	Antidiabetic
125 <> N342	Tab, 1.25 <> N over 342	Glyburide 1.25 mg	by Zenith Goldline	00182-2645	Antidiabetic
125 <> N342	Tab, White, Round, 1.25 <> N/342	Glyburide 1.25 mg	by Novopharm	43806-0342	Antidiabetic
125 <> N342	Tab, 1.25 <> N 342	Glyburide 1.25 mg	by Major	00904-5075	Antidiabetic
125 <> N747	Tab, Pink, Round, 125 <> N over 747	Amoxicillin Trihydrate 125 mg	by Novopharm	43806-0747	Antibiotic
125 <> N747	Tab, Cherry & Rose, Chewable, 25 <> N over 747	Amoxicillin Trihydrate 155 mg	by Novopharm	55953-0747	Antibiotic
125 <> N747	Tab, Chew	Amoxicillin Trihydrate 155 mg	by Warrick	59930-1573	Antibiotic
125 <> N853	Tab, Light Yellow, Film Coated, 1.25	Indapamide 1.25 mg	by Novopharm	55953-0853	Diuretic
125 <> N853	Tab, Light Yellow, Film Coated, 1.25	Indapamide 1.25 mg	by Novopharm	43806-0853	Diuretic
125 <> NU	Tab, White, Cap Shaped, Scored, 12.5 <> NU	Captopril 12.5 mg	Nu Capto by Nu-Pharm	Canadian DIN# 01913824	Antihypertensive
125 <> Z4262	Tab, Orange, Round, 1.25 <> Z4262	Indapamide 1.25 mg	Lozol by Zenith Goldline	00182-8201	Diuretic
1253	Tab, Pink, Oblong	Hematinic Vitamin	Theragran by H.L.Moore		Vitamin
12530 <> WATSON	Tab, Pink, Round, 125/30 <> Watson	Ethinyl Estradiol 30 mcg; Levonorgestrel 0.25 mg	Trivora-28 by Watson	52544-0291	Oral Contraceptive
1259	Tab, Pink, Round, Scored	Estradiol 1 mg	Gynodiol by Heartland		Hormone
125CAPOTEN	Tab, 12.5 Capoten	Captopril 12.5 mg	by Med Pro	53978-0939	Antihypertensive
125DPI	Tab, 125/DPI	Estropipate 1.5 mg	by Schein	00364-2601	Hormone
125FLI	Tab, Purple, Round, 125/FLI Logo	Levothyroxine Sodium 125 mcg	by Forest	00456-0324	Antithyroid
125M	Tab	Levothyroxine Sodium 0.125 mg	Euthyrox by Em Pharma	63254-0441	Antithyroid
125M	Tab	Levothyroxine Sodium 0.125 mg	Levo T by MOVA	55370-0130	Antithyroid
125MCG <> FLINT	Tab, Brown, Round, Scored	Levothyroxine Sodium 0.125 mg	Synthroid by Rightpac	65240-0744	Antithyroid
125MCG <> FLINT	Tab, Debossed	Levothyroxine Sodium 0.125 mg	Synthroid by Amerisource	62584-0130	Antithyroid
125NAXEN	Tab, Green, Oval, 125/Naxen	Naproxen 125 mg	Navalbine by B.W. Inc	Canadian	NSAID
125Z2045	Tab, White, Round, 1.25 Z/2045	Conjugated Estrogens 1.25 mg	Premarin by Zenith		Estrogen
126	Tab, White, Round	Calcium Carbonate 500 mg	Tums by Guardian		Vitamin/Mineral
126	Tab, Blue, Alpha Sign	Hyoscyamine Sulfate 0.125 mg	HSS 0.125 O2 by Murfreesboro	51129-1506	Gastrointestinal
126 <> GG	Tab, Light Green, Round, Scored	Haloperidol 10 mg	Haloperidol by Geneva	00781-1397	Antipsychotic
126FLINT	Tab	Levothyroxine Sodium 0.125 mg	Synthroid by Med Pro	53978-1120	Antithyroid
127 <> R	Tab, Orange, Round	Clonidine HCl 0.1 mg	by Purepac	00228-2127	Antihypertensive
1276	Tab, Tan, Round	Thyroid 0.5 gr	by Vortech		Thyroid

ID FRONT <> BACK	DESCRIPTION FRONT <> BACK	INGREDIENT & STRENGTH	BRAND (OR EQUIV.) & FIRM	NDC#	CLASS; SCH.
127R	Tab	Clonidine HCl 0.1 mg	by Zenith Goldline	00182-1250	Antihypertensive
127R	Tab	Clonidine HCl 0.1 mg	by Med Pro	53978-0936	Antihypertensive
128	Tab, White, Ovoid, 128 <> Assyrian Lion	Pivampicillin 500 mg	Pondicillin by Leo	Canadian	Antibiotic
128 <> PEC	Tab, Film Coated	Ascorbic Acid 120 mg, Biotin 30 mcg, Calcium 200 mg, Chromium 25 mcg, Copper 2 mg, Cyanocobalamin 12 mcg, Folic Acid 1 mg, Iodine 150 mcg, Iron 27 mg, Magnesium 25 mg, Manganese 5 mg, Molybdenum 25 mcg, Niacinamide 20 mg, Pantothenic Acid 10 mg, Pyridoxine HCl 10 mg, Riboflavin 3.4 mg, Selenium 20 mcg, Thiamine HCl 3 mg, Vitamin A 5000 Units, Vitamin D 400 Units, Vitamin E 30 Units, Zinc 25 mg	Prenatal M New Form by Pecos	59879-0128	Vitamin
128R	Tab	Clonidine HCl 0.2 mg	by Zenith Goldline	00182-1251	Antihypertensive
129 <> MYLAN	Cap	Aspirin 389 mg, Caffeine 32.4 mg, Propoxyphene HCl 65 mg	by Qualitest	00603-5460	Analgesic; C IV
129R	Tab	Clonidine HCl 0.3 mg	by Zenith Goldline	00182-1252	Antihypertensive
12H <> DALLERGY	Tab, White, Cap Shaped, Scored	Chlorpheniramine Maleate 8 mg, Methscopolamine Nitrate 2.5 mg, Phenylephrine HCl 20 mg	Dallergy ER by Laser	00277-0180	Cold Remedy
13 <> GG220	Tab	Acetaminophen 300 mg, Codeine Phosphate 30 mg	by Med Pro	53978-2086	Analgesic; C III
13 <> KPI	Tab	Guaifenesin 600 mg	Monafed by Monarch	61570-0026	Expectorant
130	Tab, White	Methorixide 13 mg	by Chemaide	36678-5533	Analgesic
130 <> BL	Tab, White, Round, Scored	Albuterol 2 mg	by Teva	00093-2226	Antiasthmatic
130 <> BL	Tab	Albuterol Sulfate	by UDL	51079-0657	Antiasthmatic
130 <> EL	Tab	Hyoscyamine Sulfate 0.125 mg	by Anabolic	00722-6294	Gastrointestinal
130 <> MYLAN	Tab	Acetaminophen 650 mg, Propoxyphene HCl 65 mg	by Quality Care	60346-0909	Analgesic; C IV
130 <> MYLAN	Tab, Orange, Coated	Acetaminophen 650 mg, Propoxyphene HCl 65 mg	by Mylan	00378-0130	Analgesic; C IV
130 <> MYLAN	Tab	Acetaminophen 650 mg, Propoxyphene HCl 65 mg	by Qualitest	00603-5463	Analgesic; C IV
130 <> MYLAN	Tab, Orange, Cap Shaped, Film Coated	Acetaminophen 650 mg, Propoxyphene HCl 65 mg	Wygesic by UDL	51079-0741	Analgesic; C IV
130 <> ZESTRIL	Tab, Pink, Oblong	Lisinopril 5 mg	Zestril by Heartland Healthcare	61392-0929	Antihypertensive
130 <> ZESTRIL	Tab, Pink, Cap-Shaped, Biconvex	Lisinopril 5 mg	Zestril by Zeneca	00310-0130	Antihypertensive
130 <> ZESTRIL	Tab	Lisinopril 5 mg	Zestril by Caremark	00339-5618	Antihypertensive
130 <> ZESTRIL	Tab, Debossed	Lisinopril 5 mg	Lisinopril by Kaiser	00179-1168	Antihypertensive
130 <> ZESTRIL	Tab	Lisinopril 5 mg	Lisinopril by Med Pro	53978-3063	Antihypertensive
130 <> ZESTRIL	Tab	Lisinopril 5 mg	Zestril by Allscripts	54569-3771	Antihypertensive
130 <> ZESTRIL	Tab, Biconvex	Lisinopril 5 mg	Zestril by Pharm Utilization	60491-0711	Antihypertensive
130 <> ZESTRIL	Tab, 130 Bottom Half of Score	Lisinopril 5 mg	Lisinopril by Talbert Med	44514-0480	Antihypertensive
131 <> BL	Tab, White, Round, Scored	Albuterol 4 mg	by Teva	00093-2228	Antiasthmatic
131 <> BL	Tab	Albuterol Sulfate	by UDL	51079-0658	Antiasthmatic
131 <> ZESTRIL10	Tab, Pink, Round, Film Coated	Ketorolac Tromethamine 10 mg	by Compumed	00403-4136	NSAID
131 <> ZESTRIL10	Tab, Pink, Round	Lisinopril 10 mg	Zestril by Heartland Healthcare	61392-0930	Antihypertensive
131 <> ZESTRIL10	Tab, Pink, Round	Lisinopril 10 mg	Zestril by PDRX Pharms	55289-0509	Antihypertensive
131 <> ZESTRIL10	Tab, Zestril 10	Lisinopril 10 mg	Zestril by Murfreesboro	51129-1105	Antihypertensive
131 <> ZESTRIL10	Tab	Lisinopril 10 mg	Zestril by Caremark	00339-5638	Antihypertensive
131 <> ZESTRIL10	Tab, Debossed <> Zestril 10	Lisinopril 10 mg	Lisinopril by Kaiser	00179-1157	Antihypertensive
131 <> ZESTRIL10	Tab, Pink, Round, Biconvex	Lisinopril 10 mg	Zestril by Zeneca	00310-0131	Antihypertensive
131 <> ZESTRIL10	Tab, Zestril 10	Lisinopril 10 mg	Zestril by IPR	54921-0131	Antihypertensive
131 <> ZESTRIL10	Tab	Lisinopril 10 mg	Zestril by Med Pro	53978-1000	Antihypertensive
131 <> ZESTRIL10	Tab, Debossed	Lisinopril 10 mg	Zestril by Drug Distr	52985-0216	Antihypertensive
131 <> ZESTRIL10	Tab, Zestril 10	Lisinopril 10 mg	Zestril by Nat Pharmpak Serv	55154-6901	Antihypertensive
131 <> ZESTRIL10	Tab, Debossed	Lisinopril 10 mg	Zestril by DRX	55045-2389	Antihypertensive
131 <> ZESTRIL10	Tab, Debossed	Lisinopril 10 mg	Zestril by Repack Co of Amer	55306-0131	Antihypertensive
131 <> ZESTRIL10	Tab	Lisinopril 10 mg	Zestril by Quality Care	60346-0871	Antihypertensive
131 <> ZESTRIL10	Tab	Lisinopril 10 mg	Zestril by Eckerd Drug	19458-0835	Antihypertensive
131 <> ZESTRIL10MG	Tab, Pink, Round	Lisinopril 10 mg	Zestril by Promex Medcl	62301-0044	Antihypertensive

ID FRONT <> BACK	DESCRIPTION FRONT <> BACK	INGREDIENT & STRENGTH	BRAND (OR EQUIV.) & FIRM	NDC#	CLASS; SCH.
13105 <> SP2209	Tab, Blue, Film Coated, 131/05 <> SP 2209	Calcium Carbonate, Cyanocobalamin 3 mcg, Vitamin D 400 Units, Polysaccharide Iron Complex, Folic Acid 1 mg, Niacinamide 10 mg, Pyridoxine HCl 2 mg, Riboflavin 3 mg, Sodium Ascorbate 50, Thiamine Mononitrate 3 mg, Vitamin A 4000 Units, Zinc Sulfate Monohydrate	Niferex PN by Schwarz Pharma	00131-2209	Vitamin/Mineral
13120	Tab, Orange, Round	Aspirin 250 mg, Phenacetin 120 mg, Phenobarbital 15 mg	Axotal by Adria		Analgesic; C IV
132 <> M	Tab	Nadolol 80 mg	Nadolol by Qualitest	00603-4742	Antihypertensive
132 <> ZESTRIL20	Tab, Red, Round	Lisinopril 20 mg	Zestril by Heartland Healthcare	61392-0931	Antihypertensive
132 <> ZESTRIL20	Tab, Debossed, Zestril 20	Lisinopril 20 mg	Lisinopril by Kaiser	00179-1169	Antihypertensive
132 <> ZESTRIL20	Tab, Red, Round, Biconvex, Zestril 20	Lisinopril 20 mg	Zestril by Zeneca	00310-0132	Antihypertensive
132 <> ZESTRIL20	Tab	Lisinopril 20 mg	Zestril by Caremark	00339-5632	Antihypertensive
132 <> ZESTRIL20	Tab	Lisinopril 20 mg	Zestril by Med Pro	53978-1017	Antihypertensive
132 <> ZESTRIL20	Tab, Red-Pink, Zestril 20	Lisinopril 20 mg	Zestril by Murfreesboro	51129-1330	Antihypertensive
132 <> ZESTRIL20	Tab, Debossed	Lisinopril 20 mg	Zestril by Drug Distr	52985-0217	Antihypertensive
132 <> ZESTRIL20	Tab, Zestril 20	Lisinopril 20 mg	Zestril by Nat Pharmpak Serv	55154-6902	Antihypertensive
132 <> ZESTRIL20	Tab	Lisinopril 20 mg	Zestril by Repack Co of Amer	55306-0132	Antihypertensive
132 <> ZESTRIL20	Tab, Debossed	Lisinopril 20 mg	Zestril by PDRX	55289-0106	Antihypertensive
132 <> ZESTRIL20	Tab	Lisinopril 20 mg	Zestril by Quality Care	60346-0537	Antihypertensive
132 <> ZESTRIL20	Tab	Lisinopril 20 mg	Zestril by Eckerd Drug	19458-0830	Antihypertensive
132GG	Tab, White, Round, Scored, Film Coated, GG/132	Verapamil HCl 80 mg	Isoptin by Geneva	00781-1016	Antihypertensive
133	Tab, Tan, Round	Chlorpheniramine 2 mg, Phenylephrine 10 mg, Methscopolamine 1.25 mg	Extendryl Chews by Fleming		Cold Remedy
133 <> 133	Tab, Chewable	Chlorpheniramine Maleate 2 mg, Methscopolamine Nitrate 1.25 mg, Phenylephrine HCl 10 mg	Extendryl by Fleming	00256-0133	Cold Remedy
133 <> ASSYRIANLION	Tab, White, Circular	Bumetanide 1 mg	Burniex by Leo	Canadian	Diuretic
133 <> BL	Tab, Buff, Round, Scored	Metaproterenol Sulfate 20 mg	by Teva	00093-2232	Antiasthmatic
13308	Cap, Green, 13/308	Potassium Chloride 10 mEq	K-Lease by Adria		Electrolytes
1332	Tab, Round	Chlorpheniramine Maleate 4 mg	Chlor-trimeton by Vortech		Antihistamine
1332 <> MP53	Tab, Peach, Scored	Prednisone 20 mg	by Southwood Pharms	58016-0217	Steroid
1339	Tab, Round	Phenylprop 40 mg, Phenyleph 10 mg, Phentoloxamine 15 mg, Chlorpherirami 5 mg	Amaril by Vortech		Cold Remedy
134 <> E	Tab	Reserpine 0.25 mg	by Allscripts	54569-0597	Antihypertensive
134 <> GG	Tab, Coral, Round, Scored	Haloperidol 20 mg	Haloperidol by Geneva	00781-1398	Antipsychotic
134 <> ZESTRIL 40	Tab	Lisinopril 40 mg	Zestril by Caremark	00339-5636	Antihypertensive
134 <> ZESTRIL40	Tab, Yellow, Round	Lisinopril 40 mg	Zestril by Heartland Healthcare	61392-0932	Antihypertensive
134 <> ZESTRIL40	Tab	Lisinopril 40 mg	Lisinopril by Kaiser	00179-1203	Antihypertensive
134 <> ZESTRIL40	Tab	Lisinopril 40 mg	Zestril by Zeneca	00310-0134	Antihypertensive
134 <> ZESTRIL40	Tab, Debossed	Lisinopril 40 mg	Zestril by Quality Care	60346-0595	Antihypertensive
13411	Tab, Pink, Oblong	Magnesium Salicylate 650 mg	Magan by Adria		Analgesic
1342	Tab, Round	Penicillin G 400,000 Units	Pentids by Vortech		Antibiotic
135 <> ORTHO	Tab	Ethinyl Estradiol 0.035 mg, Norethindrone 1 mg	Ortho Novum 1 Plus 35 by Dept Health Central Pharm	53808-0031	Oral Contraceptive
135 <> ZESTRIL 212	Tab, 135 <> Zestril 2 1/2	Lisinopril 2.5 mg	Zestril by Zeneca	00310-0135	Antihypertensive
13511	Cap, Green, Oval	Docusate Sodium 100 mg	Modane Soft by Adria		Laxative
135COPLEY	Tab, White, Oval, 135/Copley	Doxylamine Succinate 25 mg	Unisom by Copley		Sleep Aid
136 <> BL	Tab, White, Oblong, Scored, 136 <> B/L	Cephalexin 250 mg	by Teva	00093-2238	Antibiotic
136 <> COPLEY	Tab	Metoprolol Tartrate 50 mg	by Copley	38245-0136	Antihypertensive
13685	Tab, White, Round, Hourglass Logo <> 1 3685	Doxazosin Mesylate 1 mg	Cardura by Zenith Goldline	00172-3685	Antihypertensive
136BL	Tab, Coated, 136/BL	Cephalexin Monohydrate	by Schein	00364-2292	Antibiotic
137	Tab, White, Round	Aspirin 325 mg	Aspirin by Granutec		Analgesic
137	Tab, White, 137 <> Assyrian Lion	Pivmecillinam HCl 200 mg	Selexid by Leo	Canadian	Antibiotic
137 <> BL	Tab, White, Oblong, Scored, 137 <> B/L	Cephalexin 500 mg	by Teva	00093-2240	Antibiotic
1375 <> DITROPAN	Tab, 13/75	Oxybutynin Chloride 5 mg	Ditropan by Hoechst Roussel	00088-1375	Urinary
1375 <> DITROPAN	Tab, 13/75	Oxybutynin Chloride 5 mg	Ditropan by Nat Pharmpak Serv	55154-2209	Urinary
137BL	Tab, Coated, 137/BL	Cephalexin Monohydrate	by Schein	00364-2293	Antibiotic

ID FRONT <> BACK	DESCRIPTION FRONT <> BACK	INGREDIENT & STRENGTH	BRAND (OR EQUIV.) & FIRM	NDC#	CLASS; SCH.
137FLI	Tab, Blue, Round, 137/FLI Logo	Levothyroxine Sodium 137 mcg	by Forest	00456-0331	Antithyroid
137MCG	Tab, Debossed	Levothyroxine Sodium 137 mcg	Eltroxin by Glaxo	53873-0119	Antithyroid
138 <> SQUIBB	Tab, White, Round, Scored	Sulfamethoxazole 400 mg, Trimethoprim 80 mg	by Mutual	53489-0145	Antibiotic
138 <> SQUIBB	Tab	Sulfamethoxazole 400 mg, Trimethoprim 80 mg	SMZ TMP 400/80 by Apothecon	59772-0139	Antibiotic
1381 <> DAYPRO	Tab, White, Cap-Shaped, Film Coated	Oxaprozin 600 mg	Daypro by GD Searle	00025-1381	NSAID
1381 <> DAYPRO	Tab, Film Coated, 13/81	Oxaprozin 600 mg	Daypro by GD Searle	00014-1381	NSAID
1381 <> DAYPRO	Tab, Film Coated	Oxaprozin 600 mg	Daypro by Caremark	00339-5881	NSAID
1381 <> DAYPRO	Tab, Film Coated	Oxaprozin 600 mg	Daypro by HJ Harkins Co	52959-0252	NSAID
1381 <> DAYPRO	Tab, Film Coated, 13/81	Oxaprozin 600 mg	Daypro by DRX	55045-2120	NSAID
1381 <> DAYPRO	Tab, Film Coated	Oxaprozin 600 mg	Daypro by Allscripts	54569-3702	NSAID
1381 <> DAYPRO	Tab, Film Coated	Oxaprozin 600 mg	Daypro by St Marys Med	60760-0381	NSAID
1381 <> DAYPRO	Tab, Film Coated, Debossed	Oxaprozin 600 mg	Daypro by Amerisource	62584-0381	NSAID
1381 <> DAYPRO	Tab, Film Coated	Oxaprozin 600 mg	Daypro by Prescription Dispensing	61807-0079	NSAID
1381 <> DAYPRO	Tab, Film Coated	Oxaprozin 600 mg	Daypro by Quality Care	60346-0722	NSAID
1381 <> DAYPRO	Cap, White, Scored, Film Coated	Oxaprozin 600 mg	by Pharmacia	Canadian DIN# 02027860	NSAID
1388	Tab, Blue, Round	Urinary Tract Combination	Uritabs by Vortech		Urinary Tract
1390	Tab, Round	Sodium Levothyroxine 0.2 mg	Synthroid by Vortech		Hormone
14	Tab, White, Round, Triangle Logo	Ephedrine 24 mg, Pb 24 mg, Theophylline 65 mg, Potassium Iodide 320 mg	Quadrinal by Knoll		Antiasthmatic; C IV
14 <> THERRX	Tab, Yellow, Diamond Shaped, Film Coated	Ascorbic Acid 60 mg; Calcium Carbonate 200 mg; Iron 30 mg; Vitamin E 30 Unt; Thiamine Mononitrate 3 mg; Riboflavin 3.4 mg; Niacinamide 20 mg; Pyridoxine HCl 50 mg; Folic Acid 1 mg; Magnesium Oxide 100 mg; Cyanocobalamin 12 mcg; Zinc Oxide 15 mg	Precare Conceive by KV Pharm	10609-1433	Vitamin
14 <> VP	Tab, White, Round, Film Coated	Ethambutol HCl 400 mg	by WestWard Pharm	00143-9101	Antituberculosis
140 <> BMP	Cap	Ampicillin Trihydrate	by Quality Care	60346-0082	Antibiotic
1400 <> 0115	Cap, Orange & Yellow	Tetracycline HCl 250 mg	by Global	00115-1400	Antibiotic
1402 <> 0115	Cap, Black & Yellow	Tetracycline HCl 500 mg	by Global	00115-1402	Antibiotic
14036	Tab, Hourglass Logo <> 1 4036	Estazolam 1 mg	Prosom by Zenith Goldline	00172-4036	Sedative/Hypnotic; C IV
141 <> ZESTORETIC	Tab, Debossed	Hydrochlorothiazide 12.5 mg, Lisinopril 10 mg	Zestoretic by IPR	54921-0141	Diuretic; Antihypertensive
141 <> ZESTORETIC	Tab, Peach, Round, Debossed	Hydrochlorothiazide 12.5 mg, Lisinopril 10 mg	Zestoretic by AstraZeneca	00310-0141	Diuretic; Antihypertensive
141 <> ZESTORETIC	Tab, Peach, Round, Convex	Lisinopril 10 mg, Hydrochlorothiazide 12.5 mg	Zestoretic by Mylan	00378-0378	Antihypertensive
142	Tab, White, Round	Acetaminophen 325 mg	Tylenol by Granutec		Antipyretic
142 <> ZESTORETIC	Tab, White, Round, Debossed	Hydrochlorothiazide 12.5 mg, Lisinopril 20 mg	Zestoretic 20 1 2.5 by AstraZeneca	00310-0142	Diuretic; Antihypertensive
142 <> ZESTORETIC	Tab, Debossed	Hydrochlorothiazide 12.5 mg, Lisinopril 20 mg	Zestoretic by IPR	54921-0142	Diuretic; Antihypertensive
1423 <> M	Tab, White, Round	Methylphenidate HCl 20 mg	Methylin ER by D M Graham	00756-0285	Stimulant; C II
1423 <> M	Tab, White, Round	Methylphenidate HCl 10 mg	by Mallinckrodt Hobart	00406-1423	Stimulant; C II
143	Tab	Carbenicillin Indanyl Sodium	Geocillin by Pharm Utilization	60491-0277	Antibiotic
143	Tab, Green, Orange, Pink or Yellow	Sodium Fluoride 2.21 mg	Luride T by Colgate Oral	00126-0143	Element
143 <> R	Tab, White, Round	Carbamazepine 200 mg	by Purepac	00228-2143	Anticonvulsant
143 <> R	Tab	Carbamazepine 200 mg	by Vangard	00615-3505	Anticonvulsant
1432 <> DANDAN5660	Tab, Yellow, Round, Scored, 14/32 <> Dan Dan 5660	Sulindac 200 mg	by St. Marys Med	60760-0330	NSAID
144 <> PD	Tab, White, D-Shaped	Ethinyl Estradiol 5 mcg, Norethindrone Acetate 1 mg	FemHRT by Pfizer	Canadian DIN# 02242531	Oral Contraceptive
145	Tab	Digoxin 0.125 mg	by Physicians Total Care	54868-2134	Cardiac Agent
145 <> ZESTORETIC	Tab, Peach, Round, Debossed	Hydrochlorothiazide 25 mg, Lisinopril 20 mg	Zestoretic 20 25 Mg by AstraZeneca	00310-0145	Diuretic; Antihypertensive

ID FRONT <> BACK	DESCRIPTION FRONT <> BACK	INGREDIENT & STRENGTH	BRAND (OR EQUIV.) & FIRM	NDC#	CLASS; SCH.
145 <> ZESTORETIC	Tab, Debossed	Hydrochlorothiazide 25 mg, Lisinopril 20 mg	Zestoretic by IPR	54921-0145	Diuretic; Antihypertensive
1451 <> M	Tab, White, Round	Methylphenidate HCl 20 mg	by Mallinckrodt Hobart	00406-1451	Stimulant; C II
1451 <> SEARLE	Tab	Misoprostol 100 mcg	Cytotec by GD Searle	00025-1451	Gastrointestinal
1451 <> SEARLE	Tab	Misoprostol 100 mcg	Cytotec by HJ Harkins Co	52959-0353	Gastrointestinal
1451 <> SEARLE	Tab	Misoprostol 200 mcg	Cytotec by GD Searle	00025-1461	Gastrointestinal
1451 <> SEARLE	Tab	Misoprostol 200 mcg	Cytotec by Nat Pharmpak Serv	55154-3613	Gastrointestinal
1458	Tab, Round	Allylbutylbarbituric Acid 50 mg, Aspirin 200 mg, Phenacetin 130 mg, Caffeine 40 mg	Marnal by Vortech		Analgesic
146 <> COPLEY	Tab, Off-White	Naproxen 250 mg	by Quality Care	60346-0816	NSAID
14611461	Tab, 1461 Debossed Above Line and Below Line	Misoprostol 200 mg	Cytotec by PDRX	55289-0698	Gastrointestinal
1463	Tab, Round	Conjugated Estrogens 0.625 mg	Premarin by Vortech		Estrogen
1468	Cap, Red	Ferrous Sulfate 325 mg	Feosol by Nutro Laboratories		Mineral
147 <> 93	Tab, Mottled Light Red	Naproxen 250 mg	by Brightstone	62939-8311	NSAID
147 <> 93	Tab, Mottled Light Red, Round	Naproxen 250 mg	by Allscripts	54569-3758	NSAID
147 <> 93	Tab, Mottled Light Red, Round	Naproxen 250 mg	by Teva	00093-0147	NSAID
147 <> 93	Tab	Naproxen 250 mg	by Quality Care	60346-0816	NSAID
147 <> 93	Tab	Naproxen 250 mg	by Heartland	61392-0289	NSAID
1472 <> SOLVAY	Tab, Coated	Ascorbic Acid 70 mg, Calcium 200 mg, Cyanocobalamin 2.2 mcg, Folic Acid 1 mg, Iodine 175 mcg, Iron 65 mg, Magnesium 100 mg, Niacin 17 mg, Pyridoxine HCl 2.2 mg, Riboflavin 1.6 mg, Thiamine Mononitrate 1.5 mg, Vitamin A 3000 Units, Vitamin D 400 Units, Vitamin E 10 Units, Zinc 15 mg	Zenate by Leiner	59606-0497	Vitamin
1472 <> SOLVAY	Tab, Coated	Ascorbic Acid 70 mg, Calcium 200 mg, Cyanocobalamin 2.2 mcg, Folic Acid 1 mg, Iodine 175 mcg, Iron 65 mg, Magnesium 100 mg, Niacin 17 mg, Pyridoxine HCl 2.2 mg, Riboflavin 1.6 mg, Thiamine Mononitrate 1.5 mg, Vitamin A 3000 Units, Vitamin D 400 Units, Vitamin E 10 Units, Zinc 15 mg	Zenate by Solvay	00032-1472	Vitamin
148	Tab, Red, Oval, Schering Logo 148	Dexchlorpheniramine ER 6 mg	Polaramine by Schering		Antihistamine
148 <> 93	Tab	Naproxen 375 mg	by Brightstone	62939-8321	NSAID
148 <> 93	Tab	Naproxen 375 mg	by Heartland	61392-0292	NSAID
148 <> 93	Tab	Naproxen 375 mg	by Quality Care	60346-0817	NSAID
148 <> 93	Tab, Mottled Peach, Oval	Naproxen 375 mg	by Teva	00093-0148	NSAID
1481	Tab, Peach, Oval	Prenatal Vitamins	Precare by Pecos Pharmaceuticals		Vitamin
149 <> 37	Tab, Light Red, Oblong, Mottled	Naproxen 500 mg	by Allscripts	54569-4255	NSAID
149 <> 93	Tab, Mottled Light Red, Oblong	Naproxen 500 mg	by Allscripts	54569-3760	NSAID
149 <> 93	Tab, Mottled Light Red, Oblong	Naproxen 500 mg	by Allscripts	54569-4255	NSAID
149 <> 93	Tab, Mottled Light Red, Oval	Naproxen 500 mg	by Teva	00093-0149	NSAID
149 <> 93	Tab	Naproxen 500 mg	by Heartland	61392-0295	NSAID
149 <> 93	Tab	Naproxen 500 mg	by Brightstone	62939-8331	NSAID
149 <> 93	Tab, Red, Oval	Naproxen 500 mg	by Vangard Labs	00615-3563	NSAID
149 <> BIOCRAFT	Cap	Clindamycin HCl	by Quality Care	60346-0018	Antibiotic
1490008 <> MACRODANTIN50MG	Cap, White & Yellow	Nitrofurantoin Macrocrystalline 50 mg	Macrodantin by Med-Pro	53978-3397	Antibiotic
1492	Tab, Peach, Round	Fosinopril Sodium 10 mg; Hydrochlorothiazide 12.5 mg	Monopril by Bristol Myers Squibb	00087-1492	Antihypertensive; Diuretic
1492	Tab, Peach, Round	Fosinopril Sodium 10 mg; Hydrochlorothiazide 12.5 mg	Monopril HCT by Bristol Myers Squibb	12698-1492	Antihypertensive; Diuretic
1493	Tab, Peach, Round, Scored	Fosinopril Sodium 20 mg; Hydrochlorothiazide 12.5 mg	Monopril by Bristol Myers Squibb	00087-1493	Antihypertensive; Diuretic
1493	Tab, Peach, Round, Scored	Fosinopril Sodium 20 mg; Hydrochlorothiazide 12.5 mg	Monopril HCT by Bristol Myers Squibb	12698-1493	Antihypertensive; Diuretic
15 <> 25	Tab, White, Round, 15 <> Hourglass Logo 25	Captopril 25 mg, Hydrochlorothiazide 15 mg	Capozide by Zenith Goldline	00172-2515	Antihypertensive; Diuretic

ID FRONT ⟷ BACK	DESCRIPTION FRONT ⟷ BACK	INGREDIENT & STRENGTH	BRAND (OR EQUIV.) & FIRM	NDC#	CLASS; SCH.
15 ⟷ 50	Tab, White, Oval, 15 ⟷ Hourglass Logo 50	Captopril 50 mg, Hydrochlorothiazide 15 mg	Capozide by Zenith Goldline	00172-5015	Antihypertensive; Diuretic
15 ⟷ 54782	Tab, White, Round, 15 ⟷ 54/782	Morphine Sulfate 15 mg	MS Contin by Roxane	00054-8790	Analgesic; C II
15 ⟷ 54782	Tab, White, Round, 54 Over 782	Morphine Sulfate 15 mg	MS Cortin by Roxane	00054-4790	Analgesic; C II
15 ⟷ 93	Tab, White, Oval	Nabumetone 500 mg	by Teva Pharm Inds	00480-1015	NSAID
15 ⟷ ACTOS	Tab, White, Round	Pioglitazone HCl 15 mg	Actos by Takeda Chem Inds	11532-0011	Antidiabetic
15 ⟷ BL	Tab, White, Round, Scored, 1 over 5 ⟷ BL	Penicillin V Potassium 250 mg	by Teva	00093-1171	Antibiotic
15 ⟷ BL	Tab, White, Round, Scored	Penicillin V Potassium 250 mg	Pen*Vee K by UDL	51079-0615	Antibiotic
15 ⟷ BL	Tab	Penicillin V Potassium	by Quality Care	60346-0414	Antibiotic
15 ⟷ BMS1964	Cap, Dark Red & Light Yellow, Black Print, 15 ⟷ BMS over 1964	Stavudine 15 mg	Zerit by Bristol Myers	00003-1964	Antiviral
15 ⟷ DORAL	Tab, Light Orange w/ White Speckles, Capsule-shaped, 15 ⟷ Doral	Quazepam 15 mg	Doral by Wallace	00037-9002	Sedative/Hypnotic; C IV
15 ⟷ DURA	Tab, White, Scored	Guaifenesin 600 mg; Pseudoephedrine HCl 120 mg	by DJ Pharma	64455-0015	Cold Remedy
15 ⟷ DURA	Tab, White, Oblong	Guaifenesin 600 mg; Pseudoephedrine HCl 120 mg	Guai Vent PSE by Anabolic Ca	00722-6310	Cold Remedy
15 ⟷ E652	Tab, Blue, Round	Morphine Sulfate 15 mg	by Endo Labs	60951-0652	Analgesic; C II
15 ⟷ E652	Tab, Blue, Round	Morphine Sulfate 15 mg	by Dupont Pharma	00056-0652	Analgesic; C II
15 ⟷ ETH	Tab, Partially Bisected	Morphine Sulfate 15 mg	by KV	10609-1405	Analgesic; C II
15 ⟷ ETHEX	Cap, Blue & Clear	Guaifenesin 300 mg; Pseudoephedrine HCl 60 mg	Pseudovent by Ethex	58177-0046	Cold Remedy
15 ⟷ ETHEX	Tab, Partially Bisected	Morphine Sulfate 15 mg	MSIR by Ethex	58177-0313	Analgesic; C II
15 ⟷ GG31	Tab, Orange, Round, Film Coated	Thioridazine HCl 15 mg	by Heartland Healthcare	61392-0464	Antipsychotic
15 ⟷ GG31	Tab, Film Coated, GG 31	Thioridazine HCl 15 mg	by Murfreesboro	51129-1110	Antipsychotic
15 ⟷ GG31	Tab, Orange, Round, Film Coated	Thioridazine HCl 15 mg	Mellaril by Geneva	00781-1614	Antipsychotic
15 ⟷ GG31	Tab, Film Coated, GG 31	Thioridazine HCl 15 mg	by Vangard	00615-2505	Antipsychotic
15 ⟷ MEDEVA	Tab, Blue, Scored	Guaifenesin 400 mg; Pseudoephedrine HCl 120 mg	Deconsal LA by Adams Labs	63824-0015	Cold Remedy
15 ⟷ MERIDIA	Cap, White & Yellow	Sibutramine HCl 15 mg	Meridia by PDRX Pharms	55289-0380	Anorexiant; C IV
15 ⟷ MERIDIA	Cap, White & Yellow	Sibutramine HCl 15 mg	Meridia by Apotheca	12634-0545	Anorexiant; C IV
15 ⟷ MERIDIA	Cap, Yellow & White	Sibutramine HCl 15 mg	Meridia by Knoll	00048-0615	Anorexiant; C IV
15 ⟷ MERIDIA	Cap	Sibutramine HCl 15 mg	Meridia by Quality Care	62682-7050	Anorexiant; C IV
15 ⟷ MERIDIA	Cap, -15-	Sibutramine HCl 15 mg	Meridia by BASF	10117-0615	Anorexiant; C IV
15 ⟷ MERIDIA	Cap, White & Yellow	Sibutramine HCl 15 mg	Meridia by Compumed	00403-5375	Anorexiant; C IV
15 ⟷ MSD	Tab, White, Round	Lisinopril 2.5 mg	by Allscripts	54569-4721	Antihypertensive
15 ⟷ N	Tab, White, Round	Codeine Phosphate 15 mg	by Altimed	Canadian DIN# 00779458	Analgesic
15 ⟷ WATSON365	Tab, Watson over 365	Clorazepate Dipotassium 15 mg	by Watson	52544-0365	Antianxiety; C IV
15 ⟷ WESTWARDFLURAZE	Cap	Flurazepam HCl 15 mg	by Quality Care	60346-0239	Hypnotic; C IV
150	Tab, Peach, Round, Schering Logo 150	Ethinyl Estradiol 0.5 mg	Estinyl by Schering		Oral Contraceptive
150	Tab, Symbol	Levothyroxine Sodium 150 mcg	by Nat Pharmpak Serv	55154-4008	Antithyroid
150	Tab	Levothyroxine Sodium 150 mcg	by Amerisource	62584-0015	Antithyroid
150	Tab, White, Round, Film Coated, Scored	Propafenone HCl 150 mg	Rythmol by Natl Pharmpak	55154-1608	Antiarrhythmic
150	Tab, Film Coated, 150 and Knoll Logo	Propafenone HCl 150 mg	Rythmol by Knoll	00044-5022	Antiarrhythmic
150	Tab, Film Coated, 150 and an Arched Triangle	Propafenone HCl 150 mg	Rythmol by Caremark	00339-6050	Antiarrhythmic
150	Tab, Film Coated, 150 and an Arched Triangle	Propafenone HCl 150 mg	Rythmol by Nat Pharmpak Serv	55154-1606	Antiarrhythmic
150	Tab, White, Round, Film, 150 and Knoll Logo	Propafenone HCl 150 mg	Rythmol by RX PAK	65084-0116	Antiarrhythmic
150 ⟷ COPLEY	Tab, Film Coated	Naproxen Sodium 550 mg	by Prescription Dispensing	61807-0021	NSAID
150 ⟷ COPLEY	Tab, White, Oblong	Naproxen 500 mg	by Southwood Pharms	58016-0289	NSAID
150 ⟷ COPLEY	Tab, Off-White	Naproxen 500 mg	by Quality Care	60346-0815	NSAID
150 ⟷ COPLEY	Tab, Off-White	Naproxen 500 mg	by Copley	38245-0150	NSAID
150 ⟷ COPLEY	Tab	Naproxen 500 mg	by Qualitest	00603-4732	NSAID
150 ⟷ FL	Tab, Compressed, Logo	Levothyroxine Sodium 150 mcg	by Kaiser	00179-0459	Antithyroid
150 ⟷ FLINT	Tab, Blue, Round, Scored	Levothyroxine Sodium 0.15 mg	Synthroid by Rx Pac	65084-0182	Antithyroid

ID FRONT <> BACK	DESCRIPTION FRONT <> BACK	INGREDIENT & STRENGTH	BRAND (OR EQUIV.) & FIRM	NDC#	CLASS; SCH.
150 <> FLINT	Tab	Levothyroxine Sodium 0.15 mg	Synthroid by Nat Pharmpak Serv	55154-0905	Antithyroid
150 <> FLINT	Tab	Levothyroxine Sodium 0.15 mg	Synthroid by Giant Food	11146-0304	Antithyroid
150 <> FLINT	Tab	Levothyroxine Sodium 0.15 mg	Synthroid by Rite Aid	11822-5210	Antithyroid
150 <> FLINT	Tab, Blue, Round, Scored	Levothyroxine Sodium 150 mcg	Synthroid by Knoll	00048-1090	Antithyroid
150 <> GXCJ7	Tab, Film Coated	Lamivudine 150 mg	Epivir by Glaxo	00173-0470	Antiviral
150 <> GXCJ7	Tab, Film Coated	Lamivudine 150 mg	Epivir by Allscripts	54569-4221	Antiviral
150 <> GXCJ7	Tab, White, Diamond, Film Coated	Lamivudine 150 mg	Epivir by Murfreesboro	51129-1619	Antiviral
150 <> GXCJ7	Tab, Film Coated	Lamivudine 150 mg	Epivir by Physicians Total Care	54868-3693	Antiviral
150 <> GXCJ7	Tab, Film Coated	Lamivudine 150 mg	Epivir by St Marys Med	60760-0470	Antiviral
150 <> GXCJ7	Tab, Film Coated	Lamivudine 150 mg	Epivir by Quality Care	62682-1016	Antiviral
150 <> GXCJ7	Tab, White, Diamond, Film Coated	Lamivudine 150 mg	Epivir by Compumed	00403-4977	Antiviral
150 <> N544	Tab, White, Round, Film Coated, 150 <> N over 544	Ranitidine HCl 150 mg	Zantac by UDL	51079-0879	Gastrointestinal
150 <> N544	Tab, White, Round, Film Coated	Ranitidine HCl	by Natl Pharmpak	55154-5581	Gastrointestinal
150 <> N544	Tab, Film Coated, N Over 544	Ranitidine HCl	by Allscripts	54569-4507	Gastrointestinal
150 <> N544	Tab, Film Coated, Novopharm Limited <> N Over 544	Ranitidine HCl	by Med Pro	53978-2075	Gastrointestinal
150 <> N544	Tab, White, Round, Film Coated, N Over 544	Ranitidine HCl	by Novopharm	55953-0544	Gastrointestinal
150 <> N544	Tab, White, Round, Film Coated, N Over 544	Ranitidine HCl	by Novopharm	43806-0544	Gastrointestinal
150 <> N544	Tab, White, Round, Film Coated	Ranitidine HCl 150 mg	by Murfreesboro Ph	51129-1197	Gastrointestinal
150 <> N544	Tab, White, Round	Ranitidine HCl 150 mg	by Phcy Care	65070-0053	Gastrointestinal
150 <> N739	Cap, Tan & Orange, Gelatin	Acetaminophen 400 mg, Hydrocodone Bitartrate 10 mg	by Allscripts	54569-4732	Analgesic; C III
150 <> N739	Cap, N Over 739	Mexiletine HCl 150 mg	by Physicians Total Care	54868-3776	Antiarrhythmic
150 <> N739	Cap	Mexiletine HCl 150 mg	by Brightstone	62939-2312	Antiarrhythmic
150 <> N739	Cap, 150 in Black Ink <> N Over 739 in Black Ink, Hard Gelatin Capsule with White Powder	Mexiletine HCl 150 mg	by Medirex	57480-0836	Antiarrhythmic
150 <> N739	Cap, Light Orange & Tan, in Black Ink, <> White Granular Powder	Mexiletine HCl 150 mg	by Novopharm	55953-0739	Antiarrhythmic
150 <> N739	Cap, Black Ink	Mexiletine HCl 150 mg	by Warrick	59930-1685	Antiarrhythmic
150 <> ORTHO	Tab	Ethinyl Estradiol 0.035 mg, Norgestimate 0.215 mg, Norgestimate 0.18 mg, Norgestimate 0.25 mg	Ortho Tri Cyclen 28 by Dept Health Central Pharm	53808-0043	Oral Contraceptive
150 <> ORTHO	Tab	Mestranol 0.05 mg, Norethindrone 1 mg	Ortho Novum 1 Plus 50 by Dept Health Central Pharm	53808-0030	Oral Contraceptive
150 <> PRIFTIN	Tab, Dark Pink	Rifapentine 150 mg	Priftin by Gruppo Lepetit	12522-8598	Antibiotic
150 <> PT	Cap	Chlorpheniramine Maleate 12 mg, Phenylpropanolamine HCl 75 mg	by Kaiser	00179-1136	Cold Remedy
150 <> PT	Cap, Clear, 150 <> P/T	Chlorpheniramine Maleate 12 mg, Phenylpropanolamine HCl 75 mg	Drize by Jones	52604-0405	Cold Remedy
150 <> VIDEX	Tab, Mottled Off-White to Light Orange & Yellow, Orange Specks, Chewable	Didanosine 150 mg	Videx T by Bristol Myers Squibb	00087-6653	Antiviral
150 <> WEFFEXORXR	Cap, Orange	Venlafaxine HCl 150 mg	Effexor XR by Wyeth Pharms	52903-0836	Antidepressant
150 <> WEFFEXORXR	Cap, Orange	Venlafaxine HCl 150 mg	Effexor XR by Murfreesboro Ph	51129-1677	Antidepressant
150 <> WEFFEXORXR	Cap, Orange	Venlafaxine HCl 150 mg	Effexor XR by Wyeth Labs	00008-0836	Antidepressant
150 <> XELODA	Tab, Film Coated	Capecitabine 150 mg	Xeloda by Hoffmann La Roche	00004-1100	Antineoplastic
150FLI	Tab, Light Blue, Round, 150/Flint Logo	Levothyroxine Sodium 150 mcg	by Forest	00456-0325	Antithyroid
150GXCJ7	Tab, White, Diamond, 150/GXCJ7	Lamivudine 150 mg	Epivir by Glaxo		Antiviral
150LLA18	Tab, Peach, Heptagonal	Amoxapine 150 mg	Asendin by Lederle		Antidepressant
150M	Tab	Levothyroxine Sodium 150 mcg	Euthyrox by Em Pharma	63254-0442	Antithyroid
150M	Tab	Levothyroxine Sodium 150 mcg	Levo T by MOVA	55370-0131	Antithyroid
150M	Tab	Levothyroxine Sodium 150 mcg	by Quality Care	60346-0801	Antithyroid
150MCG <> FLINT	Tab, Blue, Round, Scored	Levothyroxine Sodium 0.15 mg	Synthroid by Wal Mart	49035-0193	Antithyroid
150MCG <> FLINT	Tab, Debossed	Levothyroxine Sodium 0.15 mg	Synthroid by Amerisource	62584-0090	Antithyroid
150MG <> WATSON491	Cap, Light Brown, Ex Release	Mexiletine HCl 150 mg	by Watson	52544-0491	Antiarrhythmic
150WALLACE374001	Cap, Blue & White, 150 Wallace 37-4001	Methacycline HCl 150 mg	Rondomycin by Wallace		Analgesic
151 <> GXCJ7	Tab, White, Diamond, Film	Lamivudine 150 mg	Epivir by Murfreesboro	51129-1620	Antiviral

ID FRONT <> BACK	DESCRIPTION FRONT <> BACK	INGREDIENT & STRENGTH	BRAND (OR EQUIV.) & FIRM	NDC#	CLASS; SCH.
151 <> LUNSCO	Cap	Acetaminophen 300 mg, Phenyltoloxamine Citrate 20 mg, Salicylamide 200 mg	Anabar by Seatrace	00551-0151	Analgesic
151 <> LUNSCO	Cap	Acetaminophen 300 mg, Phenyltoloxamine Citrate 20 mg, Salicylamide 200 mg	Anabar by Lunsco	10892-0151	Analgesic
151 <> SEARLE	Tab, Placebo	Ethinyl Estradiol 35 mcg, Ethynodiol Diacetate 1 mg	Demulen 1/35-21 by Pharm Utilization	60491-0181	Oral Contraceptive
151 <> SEARLE	Tab, White, Round, 151 <> Searle Logo	Ethinyl Estradiol 35 mcg, Ethynodiol Diacetate 1 mg	Demulen 1/35-21 by GD Searle	00025-0181	Oral Contraceptive
151 <> SEARLE	Tab, White, Round, 151 <> Searle Logo	Ethinyl Estradiol 35 mcg, Ethynodiol Diacetate 1 mg	Demulen 1/35-28 by GD Searle	00025-0161	Oral Contraceptive
151 <> SEARLE	Tab	Ethinyl Estradiol 35 mcg, Ethynodiol Diacetate 1 mg	Demulen 1 35 28 by Nat Pharmpak Serv	55154-3612	Oral Contraceptive
151 <> SEARLE	Tab	Ethinyl Estradiol 35 mcg, Ethynodiol Diacetate 1 mg	Demulen by Physicians Total Care	54868-0404	Oral Contraceptive
151 <> SEARLE	Tab, White, Round	Ethinyl Estradiol 35 mcg; Ethynodiol Diacetate 1 mg	Demulen Compack by Rx Pac	65084-0219	Oral Contraceptive
152	Tab, Coated	Ascorbic Acid 500 mg, Biotin 0.15 mg, Chromic Nitrate 0.1 mg, Cupric Oxide, Cyanocobalamin 50 mcg, Ferrous Fumarate 27 mg, Folic Acid 0.8 mg, Magnesium Oxide 50 mg, Manganese Dioxide 5 mg, Niacin 100 mg, Pantothenic Acid 25 mg, Pyridoxine HCl 25 mg, Riboflavin 20 mg, Thiamine Mononitrate 20 mg, Vitamin A Acetate 5000 Units, Vitamin E Acetate 30 Units	B C w Folic Acid Plus by Geneva	00781-1102	Vitamin
152	Tab, Film Coated, White Print	Dexbrompheniramine Maleate 6 mg, Pseudoephedrine Sulfate 120 mg	by Sovereign	58716-0659	Cold Remedy
152 <> CARACO	Tab	Guaifenesin 600 mg	by Caraco	57664-0152	Expectorant
152 <> COPLEY	Tab, Film Coated	Ascorbic Acid 200 mg, Biotin 0.15 mg, Calcium Pantothenate 27.17 mg, Chromic Chloride 0.51 mg, Cupric Oxide 3.75 mg, Cyanocobalamin 50 mcg, Ferrous Fumarate 82.2 mg, Folic Acid 0.8 mg, Magnesium Oxide 82.89 mg, Manganese 50 mg, Manganese Sulfate 15.5 mg, Niacinamide Ascorbate 400 mg, Pyridoxine HCl 30.25 mg, Riboflavin 20 mg, Thiamine Mononitrate 20 mg, Vitamin A Acetate 10.75 mg, Vitamin E Acetate 30 mg, Zinc Oxide 27.99 mg	Berplex Plus by Schein	00364-0814	Vitamin
152 <> COPLEY	Tab, Golden Yellow, Film Coated	Ascorbic Acid 200 mg, Biotin 0.15 mg, Calcium Pantothenate 27.17 mg, Chromic Chloride 0.51 mg, Cupric Oxide 3.75 mg, Cyanocobalamin 50 mcg, Ferrous Fumarate 82.2 mg, Folic Acid 0.8 mg, Magnesium Oxide 82.89 mg, Manganese 50 mg, Manganese Sulfate 15.5 mg, Niacinamide Ascorbate 400 mg, Pyridoxine HCl 30.25 mg, Riboflavin 20 mg, Thiamine Mononitrate 20 mg, Vitamin A Acetate 10.75 mg, Vitamin E Acetate 30 mg, Zinc Oxide 27.99 mg	B Complex Vit Plus by Copley	38245-0152	Vitamin
152 <> GXCJ7	Tab, White, Diamond, Film Coated	Lamivudine 150 mg	Epivir by Murfreesboro	51129-1622	Antiviral
152 <> WPPH	Tab, Yellow, Round, Film Coated	Methyldopa 250 mg	by Endo	60951-0776	Antihypertensive
152 <> WPPH	Tab, Film Coated	Methyldopa 250 mg	by Quality Care	60346-0459	Antihypertensive
1520 <> WARRICK	Tab, White, Round, Scored	Albuterol Sulfate 2 mg	by Allscripts	54569-3409	Antiasthmatic
1520 <> WARRICK	Tab, White, Round, Scored	Albuterol Sulfate 2 mg	by Southwood Pharms	58016-0473	Antiasthmatic
153 <> WPPH	Tab, Film Coated	Hydrochlorothiazide 25 mg, Methyldopa 250 mg	by Merck	00006-0153	Diuretic; Antihypertensive
153 <> WPPH	Tab, Film Coated	Hydrochlorothiazide 25 mg, Methyldopa 250 mg	by West Point	59591-0153	Diuretic; Antihypertensive
153 <> WPPH	Tab, White, Round, Film Coated	Hydrochlorothiazide 25 mg, Methyldopa 250 mg	by Endo	60951-0779	Diuretic; Antihypertensive
1530 <> SCS	Tab	Ethinyl Estradiol 0.03 mg, Levonorgestrel 0.15 mg	Levora by Patheon	63285-0100	Oral Contraceptive
1530 <> WATSON	Tab, White, Round, 15/30 <> Watson	Levora 0,15 mg, 30 mcg	Nordette by Watson	52544-0279	Oral Contraceptive
1531	Tab, Round	Sulfisoxazole 500 mg	Gantrisin by Vortech		Antibiotic
1533	Tab, Round	Digoxin 0.25 mg	Lanoxin by Vortech		Cardiac Agent
154	Tab, Yellow, Scored	Sulindac 200 mg	by Kaiser Fdn	00179-1334	NSAID
154 <> 93	Tab, White, Oval, Film Coated	Ticlopidine HCl 250 mg	by UDL	51079-0920	Anticoagulant
154 <> CIBA	Cap, Caramel & Scarlet	Rifampin 300 mg	by Geneva	00781-2018	Antibiotic
154 <> WPPH	Tab, Bright Yellow, Hexagonal, Scored	Sulindac 200 mg	by Endo	60951-0781	NSAID
154 <> WPPH	Tab	Sulindac 200 mg	by Merck Sharp & Dohme	62904-0154	NSAID
154 <> WPPH	Tab	Sulindac 200 mg	by West Point	59591-0154	NSAID
154 <> WPPH	Tab	Sulindac 200 mg	by Quality Care	60346-0686	NSAID
155 <> ASSYRIANLION	Tab, White, Circular, Assyrian Lion Logo	Bumetanide 2 mg	Burinex by Leo	Canadian	Diuretic
155 <> MYLAN	Tab, Coated	Acetaminophen 650 mg, Propoxyphene Napsylate 100 mg	by Qualitest	00603-5466	Analgesic; C IV

ID FRONT <> BACK	DESCRIPTION FRONT <> BACK	INGREDIENT & STRENGTH	BRAND (OR EQUIV.) & FIRM	NDC#	CLASS; SCH.
155 <> MYLAN	Tab	Acetaminophen 650 mg, Propoxyphene Napsylate 100 mg	by Vangard	00615-0455	Analgesic; C IV
155 <> MYLAN	Tab, Pink, Coated	Acetaminophen 650 mg, Propoxyphene Napsylate 100 mg	by Mylan	00378-0155	Analgesic; C IV
155 <> MYLAN	Tab, Coated	Acetaminophen 650 mg, Propoxyphene Napsylate 100 mg	Propoxacet N by Quality Care	60346-0628	Analgesic; C IV
155 <> MYLAN	Tab, Coated	Acetaminophen 650 mg, Propoxyphene Napsylate 100 mg	by UDL	51079-0322	Analgesic; C IV
155 <> MYLAN	Tab, Coated	Acetaminophen 650 mg, Propoxyphene Napsylate 100 mg	by Allscripts	54569-0015	Analgesic; C IV
1552 <> 0527	Cap	Aspirin 325 mg, Butalbital 50 mg, Caffeine 40 mg	by United Res	00677-1439	Analgesic; C III
1554	Tab, Round	Dextroamphetamine Sulfate 10 mg	Oxydess II by Vortech		Stimulant; C II
156 <> A	Tab	Hyoscyamine Sulfate 0.375 mg	by Zenith Goldline	00182-2657	Gastrointestinal
156 <> WPPH	Tab, D Shaped, Film Coated	Cyclobenzaprine HCl 10 mg	by West Point	59591-0156	Muscle Relaxant
156 <> WPPH	Tab, Butterscotch Yellow, D-Shaped, Film Coated	Cyclobenzaprine HCl 10 mg	by Quality Care	60346-0581	Muscle Relaxant
156 <> WPPH	Tab, Yellow, D-Shaped, Film Coated	Cyclobenzaprine HCl 10 mg	by Endo	60951-0767	Muscle Relaxant
156 <> WPPH	Tab, D-Shaped, Film Coated	Cyclobenzaprine HCl 10 mg	by PDRX	55289-0567	Muscle Relaxant
156WPPH	Tab, Coated	Cyclobenzaprine HCl 10 mg	by Med Pro	53978-1035	Muscle Relaxant
157 <> CARACO	Tab	Guaifenesin 400 mg, Phenylpropanolamine HCl 75 mg	Miraphen LA by Caraco	57664-0157	Cold Remedy
157 <> WPPH	Cap	Indomethacin 75 mg	by Quality Care	60346-0687	NSAID
157 <> WPPH	Cap, Blue and White Beads	Indomethacin 75 mg	by West Point	59591-0157	NSAID
1571 <> 252	Tab	Phenobarbital 64.8 mg	by United Res	00677-0762	Sedative/Hypnotic; C IV
157WPPH	Cap	Indomethacin 75 mg	by Endo	60951-0774	NSAID
158 <> 879	Cap	Tetracycline HCl 250 mg	by Qualitest	00603-5919	Antibiotic
158 <> BARR	Cap, Green & Yellow	Chlordiazepoxide HCl 5 mg	Librium by UDL	51079-0374	Antianxiety; C IV
158 <> BARR	Cap, Qualitest Logo	Chlordiazepoxide HCl 5 mg	by Qualitest	00603-2666	Antianxiety; C IV
158 <> BARR	Cap, Barr Logo	Chlordiazepoxide HCl 5 mg	by Geneva	00781-2080	Antianxiety; C IV
158 <> BARR	Cap	Chlordiazepoxide HCl 5 mg	by Physicians Total Care	54868-2463	Antianxiety; C IV
158 <> COPLEY	Tab, Chewable	Ascorbic Acid 34.5 mg, Cyanocobalamin 4.9 mcg, Folic Acid 0.35 mg, Niacinamide 14.16 mg, Pyridoxine HCl 1.1 mg, Riboflavin 1.2 mg, Sodium Ascorbate 32.2 mg, Sodium Fluoride 1.1 mg, Thiamine Mononitrate 1.15 mg, Vitamin A Acetate 5.5 mg, Vitamin D 0.194 mg, Vitamin E Acetate 15.75 mg	Polyvitamin by Schein	00364-1157	Vitamin
158MJ <> M	Tab, Off-White to White	Fosinopril Sodium 10 mg	Monopril by Nat Pharmpak Serv	55154-2015	Antihypertensive
158MJ <> MONOPRIL10	Tab, Scored	Fosinopril Sodium 10 mg	Monopril by Bristol Myers Squibb	00087-0158	Antihypertensive
159 <> 879	Cap	Tetracycline HCl 500 mg	by Quality Care	60346-0435	Antibiotic
159 <> 879	Cap	Tetracycline HCl 500 mg	by Qualitest	00603-5920	Antibiotic
159 <> BARR	Cap, Green & White	Chlordiazepoxide HCl 25 mg	Libruim by UDL	51079-0141	Antianxiety; C IV
159 <> BARR	Cap, Green & White	Chlordiazepoxide HCl 25 mg	by PDRX	55289-0126	Antianxiety; C IV
159 <> COPLEY	Tab, Chewable	Cholecalciferol 0.194 mg, Cupric Oxide 1.25 mg, Cyanocobalamin 4.9 mcg, Ferrous Fumarate 36.5 mg, Folic Acid 0.35 mg, Niacinamide 14.17 mg, Pyridoxine HCl 1.1 mg, Riboflavin 1.26 mg, Sodium Ascorbate 32.2 mg, Sodium Fluoride 2.21 mg, Thiamine Mononitrate 1.15 mg, Vitamin A Acetate 5.5 mg, Vitamin E 15.75 mg, Zinc Oxide 12.5 mg	Polyvitamin by Schein	00364-0770	Vitamin
159 <> WPPH	Cap, Blue	Indomethacin 50 mg	by Southwood Pharms	58016-0236	NSAID
159 <> WPPH	Cap	Indomethacin 50 mg	by West Point	59591-0159	NSAID
159 WPPH	Cap	Indomethacin 50 mg	by Endo	60951-0773	NSAID
15ATASOL	Tab, Light Yellow, Round, 15/Atasol	Acetaminophen 325 mg, Codeine Phosphate 15 mg, Caffeine Citrate 30 mg	by Horner	Canadian	Analgesic
15BL	Tab	Penicillin V Potassium	by Med Pro	53978-5042	Antibiotic
15MG <> PF	Tab, Green, Round	Morphine Sulfate 15 mg	MS Contin by Purdue Frederick	Canadian	Analgesic
15MG3346 <> 15MGSB	Cap, White & Yellow Pellets	Prochlorperazine 15 mg	Compazine by Intl Processing	59885-3346	Antiemetic
15MG3346 <> 15MGSB	Cap, White & Yellow Pellets, 15 mg/3346 in White Print	Prochlorperazine Maleate 24.3 mg	Compazine by SKB	00007-3346	Antiemetic
15MG3514 <> 15MGSB	Cap, Brown & Natural	Dextroamphetamine Sulfate 15 mg	Dexedrine by Intl Processing	59885-3514	Stimulant; C II
15MGSB <> 15MG3346	Cap, White & Yellow Pellets	Prochlorperazine 15 mg	Compazine by Intl Processing	59885-3346	Antiemetic
15MGSB <> 15MG3346	Cap, White & Yellow Pellets, 15 mg/3346 in White Print	Prochlorperazine Maleate 24.3 mg	Compazine by SKB	00007-3346	Antiemetic
15MGSB <> 15MG3514	Cap, Brown & Natural	Dextroamphetamine Sulfate 15 mg	Dexedrine by Intl Processing	59885-3514	Stimulant; C II
15P <> DAN	Tab, White, Round, Scored	Phenobarbital 15 mg	by Schein	00364-2444	Sedative/Hypnotic; C IV

ID FRONT <> BACK	DESCRIPTION FRONT <> BACK	INGREDIENT & STRENGTH	BRAND (OR EQUIV.) & FIRM	NDC#	CLASS; SCH.
15SYCBMZ	Tab, White, Round, 1.5/Syc-BMZ	Bromazepam 1.5 mg	by Altimed	Canadian DIN# 02167808	Sedative
15XL	Tab, Gray, Oval	Oxybutynin Chloride 15 mg	Ditropan XL by Alza	17314-8502	Urinary
16	Tab, White, Round	Perphenazine 16 mg	Apo Perphenazine by Apotex	Canadian	Antipsychotic
16 <> ACH	Tab, White, Oval	Candesartan Cilexetil 16 mg	by Astra AB	17228-0016	Antihypertensive
16 <> BIOCRAFT	Tab, White, Oval	Penicillin V Potassium 250 mg	by Teva	00093-1172	Antibiotic
16 <> BIOCRAFT	Tab	Penicillin V Potassium	by Quality Care	60346-0414	Antibiotic
16 <> CIBA	Tab, White, Round, Film Coated	Methylphenidate HCl 20 mg	Ritalin by Novartis	Canadian DIN# 00632775	Stimulant
16 <> ETHEX	Cap, White	Guaifenesin 250 mg; Pseudoephedrine HCl 120 mg	Pseudovent by Ethex	58177-0045	Cold Remedy
160	Tab	Acetaminophen 160 mg	by Mead Johnson	Canadian DIN# 00876038	Antipyretic
160	Tab	Acetaminophen 160 mg	by Mead Johnson	Canadian DIN# 02231805	Antipyretic
160	Tab, Pink, Round, Schering Logo 160	Carisoprodol 350 mg	Rela by Schering		Muscle Relaxant
160	Tab, White, Round	Triprolidine HCl 2.5 mg, Pseudophedrine HCl 60 mg	Actifed by OHM		Cold Remedy
160 <> TY	Tab, Pink or Purple, Round, Scored, Chewable	Acetaminophen 160 mg	Jr. Streng Tylenol by McNeil	Canadian DIN# 02241361	Antipyretic
160 <> 59911	Cap, Blue & White	Propranolol HCl 160 mg	by ESI Lederle	59911-5479	Antihypertensive
160 <> TCMDM	Tab, Purple, Round, Scored, Chewable	Acetaminophen 160 mg, Chlorpheniramine Maleate 1 mg, Pseudoephedrine HCl 15 mg, Dextromethorphan Hydrobromide 7.5 mg	Junior Strength Tylenol Cold DM	Canadian DIN# 00890677	Cold Remedy
160 <> Z4239	Tab, White, Cap-Shaped	Nadolol 160 mg	Nadolol by Zenith Goldline	00172-4239	Antihypertensive
1605 <> W	Tab, Sugar-Coated	Perphenazine 8 mg	by Schein	00364-2625	Antipsychotic
160MGBERLEX	Tab, White, Cap Shaped, Scored	Sotalol HCl 160 mg	Betapace by Berlex Labs	50419-0116	Antiarrhythmic
160MGBETAPACE	Tab, Light Blue, Cap Shaped, Scored	Sotalol HCl 160 mg	Betapace by Berlex	50419-0106	Antiarrhythmic
160Z4239	Tab, White, Cap-Shaped, 160/Z4239	Nadolol 160 mg	Nadolol by Zenith Goldline	00172-4239	Antihypertensive
162	Tab, White & Yellow, Round	Aluminum 200 mg, Magnesium Hydroxide 200 mg	Maalox by Guardian		Gastrointestinal
162 <> ACS	Tab, Peach, Oval	Candesartan Cilexetil 16 mg; Hydrochlorothiazide 12.5 mg	Atacand HCT by Astra Zeneca	17228-0162	Antihypertensive; Diuretic
162 <> WPPH	Tab	Amiloride HCl 5 mg, Hydrochlorothiazide 50 mg	by West Point	59591-0162	Diuretic
162 <> WPPH	Tab, Peach, Diamond-Shaped, Scored	Amiloride HCl 5 mg, Hydrochlorothiazide 50 mg	by Endo	60951-0764	Diuretic
164PAR	Tab	Benztropine Mesylate 0.5 mg	by Schein	00364-0834	Antiparkinson
165 <> COPLEY	Tab, Film Coated	Ascorbic Acid 17.53 mg, Beta-Carotene 0.56 mg, Calcium Carbonate 249.41 mg, Calcium Pantothenate 4.18 mg, Cholecalciferol 0.25 mg, Cupric Oxide 2.02 mg, Ferrous Fumarate 82.15 mg, Magnesium Oxide 82.93 mg, Niacinamide Ascorbate 8.54 mg, Pyridoxine HCl 2.43 mg, Riboflavin 0.84 mg, Thiamine Mononitrate 1 mg, Vitamin A Acetate 2680 Units, Zinc Oxide 15.56 mg	Prenatal Rx by Copley	38245-0165	Vitamin
165PAR	Tab, 165/Par	Benztropine Mesylate 1 mg	by Schein	00364-0703	Antiparkinson
166	Tab, Brown, Oval	Methenamine Mandelate 500 mg	Mandelamine by PD		Antibiotic; Urinary Tract
166	Tab, Brown, Oblong	Methenamine Mandelate 0.5grams	Mandelamine by Warner Chilcott	00430-0166	Antibiotic; Urinary Tract
166	Tab	Metoprolol Tartrate 50 mg	by Caraco	57664-0166	Antihypertensive
166	Tab	Metoprolol Tartrate 100 mg	by Qualitest	00603-4628	Antihypertensive
166	Tab, White, Oblong, Convex, Scored	Metoprolol Tartrate 50 mg	by Neuman Distr	64579-0071	Antihypertensive
166PAR	Tab, 166/Par	Benztropine Mesylate 2 mg	by Schein	00364-0704	Antiparkinson
167	Tab, Purple, Oblong, Film Coated, Debossed	Methenamine Mandelate 1 gm	Mandelamine by Warner Chilcott	00430-0167	Antibiotic; Urinary Tract
167	Tab, White, Oblong, Convex, Scored	Metoprolol Tartrate 100 mg	by Neuman Distr	64579-0076	Antihypertensive

ID FRONT ⟷ BACK	DESCRIPTION FRONT ⟷ BACK	INGREDIENT & STRENGTH	BRAND (OR EQUIV.) & FIRM	NDC#	CLASS; SCH.
167	Tab	Metoprolol Tartrate 100 mg	by Caraco	57664-0167	Antihypertensive
168	Tab, Triangular	Nilutamide 50 mg	Nilandron by Hoechst Roussel	00088-1110	Antiandrogen
168	Tab, Triangular	Nilutamide 50 mg	Nilandron by Hoechst Roussel	12579-0808	Antiandrogen
17 ⟷ ADAMS	Tab	Guaifenesin 600 mg, Pseudoephedrine HCl 60 mg	Deconsal II by Nat Pharmpak Serv	55154-5901	Cold Remedy
17 ⟷ BL	Tab, White, Round, Scored	Penicillian-VK 500 mg	Pen*Vee K	51079-0616	Antibiotic
17 ⟷ BL	Tab	Penicillin V 500 mg	by Talbert Med	44514-0645	Antibiotic
17 ⟷ BL	Tab, Film Coated, 1/7 ⟷ BL	Penicillin V Potassium	by Quality Care	60346-0095	Antibiotic
17 ⟷ BL	Tab, White, Round, Scored, 1/7 ⟷ BL	Penicillin V Potassium 500 mg	by Teva	00093-1173	Antibiotic
17 ⟷ MEDEVA	Tab, Blue, Scored	Guaifenesin 600 mg; Pseudoephedrine HCl 60 mg	Deconsal LA by Adams Labs	63824-0017	Cold Remedy
17 ⟷ MEDEVA	Tab, Blue, Oblong, Scored	Guaifenesin 600 mg; Pseudoephedrine HCl 60 mg	Syn Rx by Adams Labs	63824-0308	Cold Remedy
170	Tab, Yellow	Sulindac 150 mg	by Kaiser Fdn	00179-1333	NSAID
170 ⟷ WPHH	Tab, Compressed	Sulindac 150 mg	by Merck Sharp & Dohme	62904-0170	NSAID
170 ⟷ WPPH	Tab	Sulindac 150 mg	by West Point	59591-0170	NSAID
170 ⟷ WPPH	Tab	Sulindac 150 mg	by Quality Care	60346-0044	NSAID
170 ⟷ WPPH	Tab, Bright Yellow, Round	Sulindac 150 mg	by Endo	60951-0780	NSAID
1705	Tab, White, Round	Diphenoxylate 2.5 mg, Atropine 0.025 mg	Lomotil by Vortech		Antidiarrheal; C V
171 ⟷ M	Tab	Nadolol 40 mg	Nadolol by Qualitest	00603-4741	Antihypertensive
171 ⟷ SQUIBB	Tab, White, Oval Shaped, Scored	Sulfamethoxazole 800 mg, Trimethoprim 160 mg	by Mutual	53489-0146	Antibiotic
171 ⟷ SQUIBB	Tab	Sulfamethoxazole 800 mg, Trimethoprim 160 mg	SMZ TMP 800/160 by Apothecon	59772-0174	Antibiotic
1712 ⟷ CARAFATE	Tab	Sucralfate 1 gm	Carafate by Heartland	61392-0606	Gastrointestinal
1712 ⟷ CARAFATE	Tab, Light Pink, 17 Over 12	Sucralfate 1 gm	Carafate by Quality Care	60346-0922	Gastrointestinal
1712 ⟷ CARAFATE	Tab	Sucralfate 1 gm	Carafate by Amerisource	62584-0712	Gastrointestinal
1712 ⟷ CARAFATE	Tab	Sucralfate 1 gm	Carafate by Giant Food	11146-0041	Gastrointestinal
1712 ⟷ CARAFATE	Tab	Sucralfate 1 gm	Carafate by Murfreesboro	51129-1166	Gastrointestinal
1712 ⟷ CARAFATE	Tab, Light Pink	Sucralfate 1 gm	Carafate by Hoechst Roussel	00088-1712	Gastrointestinal
1712 ⟷ CARAFATE	Tab, Light Pink	Sucralfate 1 gm	Carafate by HJ Harkins Co	52959-0052	Gastrointestinal
1712 ⟷ CARAFATE	Tab	Sucralfate 1 gm	Carafate by Allscripts	54569-0422	Gastrointestinal
1712 ⟷ CARAFATE	Tab	Sucralfate 1 gm	Carafate by Nat Pharmpak Serv	55154-2207	Gastrointestinal
1712 ⟷ CARAFATE	Tab	Sucralfate 1 gm	by Med Pro	53978-3070	Gastrointestinal
172 ⟷ GG	Tab, Yellow, Round, Scored, Compressed	Hydrochlorothiazide 50 mg, Triamterene 75 mg	Maxzide by Geneva	00781-1008	Diuretic
172 ⟷ WPPH	Cap	Indomethacin 25 mg	by West Point	59591-0172	NSAID
172 WPPH	Cap	Indomethacin 25 mg	by Endo	60951-0772	NSAID
173 ⟷ MSD	Tab, Green, Squared Cap Shape	Enalapril Maleate 5 mg, Hydrochlorothiazide 12.5 mg	Vaseretic 5 12.5 by Merck	00006-0173	Antihypertensive; Diuretic
1739	Tab, Round	Butabarbital Sodium 30 mg	Butisol by Vortech		Sedative; C III
174 ⟷ WPPH	Tab, Yellow, Round, Film Coated	Methyldopa 125 mg	by Endo	60951-0775	Antihypertensive
175	Cap, Red	Hexavitamin	by West-ward		Vitamin
175	Tab, Purple, Round, Scored	Levothyroxine Sodium 175 mcg	Synthroid by Murfreesboro	51129-1643	Antithyroid
175 ⟷ 175	Cap	Paromomycin Sulfate	by Caraco	57664-0175	Antibiotic
175 ⟷ FLINT	Tab, Lilac, Round, Scored	Levothyroxine Sodium 175 mcg	Synthroid by Knoll	00048-1100	Antithyroid
175 ⟷ FLINT	Tab, Purple, Round, Scored	Levothyroxine Sodium 175 mcg	Synthroid by Murfreesboro	51129-1652	Antithyroid
175 ⟷ NL	Tab, White, Oval	Guaifenesin 600 mg; Phenylpropanolamine HCl 37.5 mg	by Neil Labs	60242-0700	Cold Remedy
175M	Tab	Levothyroxine Sodium 175 mcg	Euthyrox by Em Pharma	63254-0443	Antithyroid
175M	Tab	Levothyroxine Sodium 175 mcg	Levo T by MOVA	55370-0162	Antithyroid
1757	Tab, Pink, Round	Phenobarbital 15 mg	by Vortech		Sedative/Hypnotic; C IV
1758	Tab, White, Round	Phenobarbital 15 mg	by Vortech		Sedative/Hypnotic; C IV
1759	Tab, Pink, Round	Phenobarbital 30 mg	by Vortech		Sedative/Hypnotic; C IV
175FLI	Tab, Turquoise, Round, 175/FLI Logo	Levothyroxine Sodium 175 mcg	by Forest	00456-0326	Antithyroid
175MCG	Tab, Debossed	Levothyroxine Sodium 175 mcg	Eltroxin by Glaxo	53873-0120	Antithyroid
175MCG ⟷ FLINT	Tab, Purple, Round, Scored	Levothyroxine Sodium 0.175 mg	Synthroid by Rightpac	65240-0758	Antithyroid
176 ⟷ WPPH	Tab, Film Coated	Methyldopa 500 mg	by Merck	00006-0176	Antihypertensive
176 ⟷ WPPH	Tab, Yellow, Round, Film Coated	Methyldopa 500 mg	by Endo	60951-0777	Antihypertensive

ID FRONT <> BACK	DESCRIPTION FRONT <> BACK	INGREDIENT & STRENGTH	BRAND (OR EQUIV.) & FIRM	NDC#	CLASS; SCH.
1761	Tab, White, Round	Phenobarbital 30 mg	by Vortech		Sedative/Hypnotic; C IV
1771 <> MARION	Tab, Coated	Diltiazem HCl 30 mg	Cardizem by Hoechst Roussel	00088-1771	Antihypertensive
1772	Tab, White, Round	Phenobarbital 16 mg	by Vortech		Sedative/Hypnotic; C IV
1772 <> MARION	Tab, Coated	Diltiazem HCl 60 mg	Cardizem by Drug Distr	52985-0191	Antihypertensive
1778	Tab, Round	Phenobarbital, Hyoscyamine, Atropine	Hypnaldyne by Vortech		Gastrointestinal; C IV
1779	Tab, Round	Colchicine 0.65 mg	Colsalide Improved by Vortech		Antigout
179 <> WPPH	Tab, Film Coated	Hydrochlorothiazide 15 mg, Methyldopa 250 mg	by Merck	00006-0179	Diuretic; Antihypertensive
179 <> WPPH	Tab, Salmon, Round, Film Coated	Hydrochlorothiazide 15 mg, Methyldopa 250 mg	by Endo	60951-0778	Diuretic; Antihypertensive
1796180MG	Cap, Blue & Light Blue	Diltiazem HCl CD 180 mg	Cardizem CD by Marion		Antihypertensive
1797240MG	Cap, Blue	Diltiazem HCl CD 240 mg	Cardizem CD by Marion		Antihypertensive
1798300MG	Cap, 1798/300 mg	Diltiazem HCl 300 mg	Cardizem CD by Murfreesboro	51129-9732	Antihypertensive
17BL	Tab, Film Coated	Penicillin V Potassium	by Med Pro	53978-5055	Antibiotic
18 <> BI	Tab, Sugar Coated	Dipyridamole 50 mg	Persantine by Nat Pharmpak Serv	55154-0402	Antiplatelet
18 <> BI	Tab, Reddish Orange, Sugar Coated	Dipyridamole 50 mg	Persantine-50 by Boehringer Ingelheim	00597-0018	Antiplatelet
18 <> BL	Tab, Off-White, Round	Neomycin Sulfate 500 mg	by Teva	00093-1177	Antibiotic
180 <> TIAZAC	Cap	Diltiazem HCl 180 mg	Tiazac by CVS	51316-0244	Antihypertensive
180010	Cap, Clear, 18-0010	Potassium Chloride CR 750 mg	K-Norm by Penwalt		Electrolytes
180605 <> G	Tab, 1806, 1806 0.5 <> G	Lorazepam 0.51 mg	by Royce	51875-0240	Sedative/Hypnotic; C IV
180605240 <> 005	Tab, 1806.05-240 <> 0.05	Lorazepam 0.5 mg	by Zenith Goldline	00182-1806	Sedative/Hypnotic; C IV
180605G	Tab	Lorazepam 1 mg	by Zenith Goldline	00182-1807	Sedative/Hypnotic; C IV
18071 <> G	Tab	Lorazepam 1 mg	by Royce	51875-0241	Sedative/Hypnotic; C IV
18082 <> G	Tab	Lorazepam 2 mg	by Royce	51875-0242	Sedative/Hypnotic; C IV
180MG <> ANDRX549	Cap, Gray & White	Diltiazem HCl 180 mg	by Kaiser Fdn	00179-1375	Antihypertensive
180MG <> ANDRX598	Cap, Yellow	Diltiazem HCl 180 mg	Cartia XT by Heartland Healthcare	61392-0958	Antihypertensive
180MG <> DILACORXR	Cap	Diltiazem HCl 180 mg	by Kaiser	62224-9339	Antihypertensive
180WATSON663	Cap, Pink & White, 180/Watson/663	Diltazem 180 mg	Dilacor XR by Watson		Antihypertensive
1812	Tab, Round	Benzthiazide 50 mg	Marazide by Vortech		Diuretic
183 <> R	Tab, Coated	Dipyridamole 50 mg	by Vangard	00615-1573	Antiplatelet
1840	Tab, Round	Nitrofurantoin 50 mg	Furatoin by Vortech		Antibiotic
184Q	Cap, Buff, 184/Q	Doxepin HCl 10 mg	Sinequan by Quantum		Antidepressant
185 <> BEECHAM	Tab	Penicillin V Potassium	by Quality Care	60346-0414	Antibiotic
185Q	Ivory & White, 185/Q	Doxepin HCl 25 mg	Sinequan by Quantum		Antidepressant
186 <> COP	Tab, Chewable	Fluoride Ion 0.25 mg, Sodium Fluoride 0.55 mg	Luride Vanilla by Colgate Oral	00126-0186	Mineral
186QPL	Cap, Ivory, 186/QPL	Doxepin HCl 50 mg	Sinequan by Quantum		Antidepressant
187 <> PAR	Tab, Film Coated	Hydrochlorothiazide 25 mg, Methyldopa 250 mg	by Par	49884-0187	Diuretic; Antihypertensive
1875 <> CC	Cap, 18.75 <> CC	Phentermine HCl 18.75 mg	by Quality Care	60346-0102	Anorexiant; C IV
1876	Tab, Round	Phentermine 8 mg	Phentrol by Vortech		Anorexiant; C IV
1879	Tab, Yellow, Round	Phendimetrazine 35 mg	Weightrol by Vortech		Anorexiant; C III
187Q	Cap, Green, 187/Q	Doxepin HCl 75 mg	Sinequan by Quantum		Antidepressant
188 <> COPLEY	Tab	Procainamide HCl 500 mg	by Zenith Goldline	00182-1708	Antiarrhythmic
188 <> COPLEY	Tab	Procainamide HCl 500 mg	by Copley	38245-0188	Antiarrhythmic
188 <> COPLEY	Cap	Procainamide HCl 500 mg	by Qualitest	00603-5411	Antiarrhythmic
188 <> COPLEY	Tab	Procainamide HCl 500 mg	by HL Moore	00839-7028	Antiarrhythmic
188 <> PAR	Tab, Coated	Hydrochlorothiazide 30 mg, Methyldopa 500 mg	by Par	49884-0188	Diuretic; Antihypertensive
1886	Tab, Round	Propantheline Bromide 15 mg	Probanthine by Vortech		Gastrointestinal
19 <> BI	Tab, Sugar Coated	Dipyridamole 75 mg	Persantine 75 by Boehringer Ingelheim	00597-0019	Antiplatelet

ID FRONT <> BACK	DESCRIPTION FRONT <> BACK	INGREDIENT & STRENGTH	BRAND (OR EQUIV.) & FIRM	NDC#	CLASS; SCH.
19 <> BL	Tab, Yellow, Round	Imipramine HCl 10 mg	by Teva	00093-2111	Antidepressant
19 <> THERRX	Tab, Blue, Oval	P 75 mg, Cyanocobalamin 12 mcg, Folic Acid 1 mg, Calcium 200 mg	Premesisrx by KV Pharm	10609-1444	Vitamin
190 <> GG	Tab, White, Round, Scored, Compressed	Methocarbamol 500 mg	Robaxin by Geneva	00781-1760	Muscle Relaxant
1908	Tab, White, Round	Orphenadrine Citrate 100 mg	Norflex by Vortech		Muscle Relaxant
191 <> GG	Tab, Blue, Round	Amoxapine 100 mg	Asendin by Geneva	00781-1846	Antidepressant
1915	Tab, Round	Hydrochlorothiazide 50 mg	Hydrodiuril by Vortech		Diuretic
1919PRINIVIL	Tab, White, Shield, 19/19 Prinivil	Lisonopril 5 mg	by MSD	Canadian	Antihypertensive
192 <> WPPH	Tab	Timolol Maleate 5 mg	by West Point	59591-0192	Antihypertensive
192 <> WPPH	Tab, Light Blue, Round	Timolol Maleate 5 mg	by Endo	60951-0782	Antihypertensive
1922	Tab, Round	Brompheniramine 12 mg, Phenyleph 15 mg, Phenylpropanolamine 15 mg	Normatane TD by Vortech		Cold Remedy
192Q	Cap, Green & White, 192-Q	Temazepam 15 mg	Restoril by Quantum		Sedative/Hypnotic; C IV
193 <> PAR	Cap	Flurazepam HCl 15 mg	by Qualitest	00603-3691	Hypnotic; C IV
1934	Cap, Red & Clear, Savage Logo 1934	Chlorpheniramine Maleate 8 mg, Pseudoephedrine HCl 120 mg	Brexin LA by Savage	00281-1934	Cold Remedy
193Q	Cap, White, 193-Q	Temazepam 30 mg	Restoril by Quantum		Sedative/Hypnotic; C IV
194 <> PAR	Cap	Flurazepam HCl 30 mg	by Qualitest	00603-3692	Hypnotic; C IV
194 <> WPPH	Tab	Timolol Maleate 10 mg	by West Point	59591-0194	Antihypertensive
194 <> WPPH	Tab, Light Blue, Round	Timolol Maleate 10 mg	by Endo	60951-0783	Antihypertensive
1945	Tab, Round	Trichlormethiazide 4 mg	Marazide II by Vortech		Diuretic
195 <> WPPH	Tab, Peach, Cap Shaped, Film Coated	Diflunisal 250 mg	by Endo	60951-0768	NSAID
196 <> WPPH	Tab, Film Coated	Diflunisal 500 mg	by Quality Care	60346-0053	NSAID
196 <> WPPH	Tab, Orange, Cap Shaped, Film Coated	Diflunisal 500 mg	by Endo	60951-0769	NSAID
196 <> WPPH	Tab, Orange, Oblong, Film Coated	Diflunisal 500 mg	by HJ Harkins	52959-0379	NSAID
197 <> COPLEY	Tab, Dark Red, Chewable	Ascorbic Acid 34.47 mg, Cholecalciferol 0.194 mg, Cupric Oxide 1.25 mg, Cyanocobalamin 4.9 mcg, Ferrous Fumarate 36.48 mg, Folic Acid 0.35 mg, Niacinamide 14.16 mg, Pyridoxine HCl 1.1 mg, Riboflavin 1.258 mg, Sodium Fluoride 1.1 mg, Thiamine Mononitrate 1.15 mg, Vitamin A Acetate 5.5 mg, Vitamin E Acetate 15.75 mg, Zinc Oxide 12.5 mg	Polyvitamin by Schein	00364-2506	Vitamin
1975	Tab, Round	Triprolidine HCl 2.5 mg, Pseudoephedrine 60 mg	Actifed by Vortech		Cold Remedy
1998	Tab, Oblong	Methocarbamol 750 mg	Robaxin by Vortech		Muscle Relaxant
19WYETH	Tab	Promethazine HCl 12.5 mg	Phenergan by Quality Care	60346-0712	Cold Remedy
1AHR <> TENEX	Tab, Pink, Diamond	Guanfacine HCl 1 mg	Tenex by Med Pro	53978-3364	Antihypertensive
1AHR <> TENEX	Tab, Pink, Diamond	Guanfacine HCl 1.0 mg	Tenex by Med Pro	53978-5027	Antihypertensive
1AHR <> TENEX	Tab	Guanfacine HCl 1.15 mg	Tenex by Leiner	59606-0748	Antihypertensive
1AHR <> TENEX	Tab	Guanfacine HCl 1.15 mg	Tenex by Amerisource	62584-0901	Antihypertensive
1AHR <> TENEX	Tab, Light Pink, #1 AHR <> Tenex	Guanfacine HCl 1.15 mg	Tenex by A H Robins	00031-8901	Antihypertensive
1AHRTENEX	Tab	Guanfacine HCl 1.15 mg	by Pharmedix	53002-1045	Antihypertensive
1D300	Cap	Chlorpheniramine Maleate 8 mg, Pseudoephedrine HCl 120 mg	De Congestine by Qualitest	00603-3143	Cold Remedy
1KLONOPIN <> ROCHE	Tab	Clonazepam 1 mg	by Allscripts	54569-2727	Anticonvulsant; C IV
1LLL11	Tab, Yellow, Round	Levothyroxine Sodium 0.1 mg	Synthroid by Lederle		Antithyroid
1MG <> 511	Tab, White, Pentagon	Lorazepam 1 mg	by Wyeth Pharms	52903-5812	Sedative/Hypnotic; C IV
1MG <> CARAFATE1712	Tab	Sucralfate 1 gm	Carafate by Med Pro	53978-0305	Gastrointestinal
1MG <> CARDURA	Tab, White, Oblong, 1/mg <> Cardura	Doxazosin Mesylate 1 mg	Cardura by Roerig	00049-2750	Antihypertensive
1MG <> ETH266	Tab, Light Purple, Oblong	Doxazosin Mesylate 1 mg	Cardura by Pfizer	58177-0266	Antihypertensive
1MG617	Cap, White, 1 mg/617	Anhydrous Tacrolimus 1 mg	Prograf by Fujisawa	Canadian	Immunosuppressant
1P96	Tab	Guaifenesin 400 mg, Phenylpropanolamine HCl 75 mg	by Major	00904-3264	Cold Remedy
1W	Tab, White, Round, 1/W	Lorazepam 1 mg	by Wyeth-Ayerst	Canadian	Sedative/Hypnotic
2	Tab, Yellow, Oval	Dextrothyroxine Sodium 2 mg	Choloxin by Boots		Thyroid
2	Tab, Yellow, Oblong	Doxazosin Mesylate 2 mg	Cardura by Roerig	00049-2760	Antihypertensive
2	Tab, Pink, Round	Fluphenazine HCl 2 mg	Fluphenazine by Apotex	Canadian	Antipsychotic
2	Tab, Yellow, Round	Methotrimeprazine Maleate 2 mg	Methoprazine by Apotex	Canadian	Antipsychotic
2	Tab, White, Round	Nitro Tab 0.4 mg	by Novopharm	55953-0295	Vasodilator
2	Tab, White, Round	Nitro Tab 0.4 mg	by Novopharm	43806-0295	Vasodilator

ID FRONT <> BACK	DESCRIPTION FRONT <> BACK	INGREDIENT & STRENGTH	BRAND (OR EQUIV.) & FIRM	NDC#	CLASS; SCH.
2	Tab, White, Round	Nitroglycerin 0.4 mg (1/150 gr)	Nitrostat by Able Lab	53265-0250	Vasodilator
2	Tab, Off-White, Round	Nitroglycerin 2 mg	Nitrogard 2 by Forest	00456-0687	Vasodilator
2	Tab	Nitroglycerin 2 mg	Sustachron ER Buccal by Forest	10418-0137	Vasodilator
2	Tab, White, Round	Perphenazine 2 mg	Apo Perphenazine by Apotex	Canadian	Antipsychotic
2	Tab, Gray, Round, Schering Logo/2	Perphenazine 2 mg	Trilafon by Schering	Canadian	Antipsychotic
2	Tab, Blue, Round	Trifluoperazine HCl 2 mg	Apo Trifluoperazine by Apotex	Canadian	Antipsychotic
2 <> 2063V	Tab	Acetaminophen 300 mg, Codeine Phosphate 15 mg	by PDRX	55289-0449	Analgesic; C III
2 <> 242	Tab, Royce Logo 242	Lorazepam 2 mg	by Quality Care	60346-0800	Sedative/Hypnotic; C IV
2 <> 242	Tab, 2/Royce Logo	Lorazepam 2 mg	by Qualitest	00603-4245	Sedative/Hypnotic; C IV
2 <> 256	Tab, White, Round	Betahistine HCl 8 mg	SERC by Solvay Pharma	Canadian DIN# 02240601	Antivertigo
2 <> 9350	Tab	Acetaminophen 300 mg, Codeine Phosphate 15 mg	by Quality Care	60346-0015	Analgesic; C III
2 <> 9350	Tab, White, Round, 2 <> 93 over 50	Acetaminophen 300 mg, Codeine Phosphate 15 mg	by Teva	00093-0050	Analgesic; C III
2 <> A	Tab, Blue, Round, Scored	Guaifenesin 1200 mg; Dextromethorphan Hydrobromide 60 mg	Aquatab DM by Adams Labs	63824-0002	Cold Remedy
2 <> CPI	Tab, CPI Logo	Phenobarbital 30 mg	by Century	00436-0870	Sedative/Hypnotic; C IV
2 <> CPI	Tab, CPI Logo	Phenobarbital 30 mg	by Century	00436-0129	Sedative/Hypnotic; C IV
2 <> CPI	Tab, CPI Logo	Phenobarbital 30 mg	by Century	00436-0869	Sedative/Hypnotic; C IV
2 <> DAN5621	Tab, White, Round, Scored	Diazepam 2 mg	by Vangard Labs	00615-1532	Antianxiety; C IV
2 <> DAN5621	Tab, 2 <> Dan over 5621	Diazepam 2 mg	by Quality Care	60346-0579	Antianxiety; C IV
2 <> DAN5621	Tab, White, Round, Scored	Diazepam 2 mg	by Murfreesboro Ph	51129-1302	Antianxiety; C IV
2 <> DAN5621	Tab	Diazepam 2 mg	by Danbury	00591-5621	Antianxiety; C IV
2 <> E	Tab, Blue, Round, Coated	Hydromorphone HCl 2 mg	Dilaudid by KV	10609-1366	Analgesic; C II
2 <> G	Tab, White, Round, Scored	Estradiol 2 mg	by Teva	00093-1059	Hormone
2 <> G	Tab	Estradiol 2 mg	by AAI	27280-0006	Hormone
2 <> GG53	Tab, Coated	Trifluoperazine HCl 2 mg	by Vangard	00615-3598	Antipsychotic
2 <> GG52	Tab, Lavender, Round, Film Coated	Trifluoperazine HCl 2 mg	Stelazine by Geneva	00781-1032	Antipsychotic
2 <> GG53	Tab, Coated	Trifluoperazine HCl 2 mg	by Med Pro	53978-2090	Antipsychotic
2 <> GG53	Tab, Lavender, Coated, Debossed	Trifluoperazine HCl 2 mg	by Golden State	60429-0192	Antipsychotic
2 <> GG53	Tab, Coated, Debossed	Trifluoperazine HCl 2 mg	by Heartland	61392-0822	Antipsychotic
2 <> INV279	Tab, Purple, Round, Film Coated	Trifluoperazine HCl 2 mg	by Invamed	52189-0279	Antipsychotic
2 <> M	Tab, White, Round	Hydromorphone HCl 2 mg	by Mallinckrodt Hobart	00406-3243	Analgesic; C II
2 <> MP111	Tab	Acetaminophen 300 mg, Codeine 15 mg	by United Res	00677-0611	Analgesic; C III
2 <> MP111	Tab	Acetaminophen 300 mg, Codeine Phosphate 15 mg	by Pharmedix	53002-0122	Analgesic; C III
2 <> MPIII	Tab	Acetaminophen 300 mg, Codeine Phosphate 15 mg	by Quality Care	60346-0015	Analgesic; C III
2 <> N	Cap	Loperamide HCl 2 mg	by Rugby	00536-3974	Antidiarrheal
2 <> N	Cap	Loperamide HCl 2 mg	by MOVA	55370-0169	Antidiarrheal
2 <> N	Cap, White	Loperamide HCl 2 mg	by Novopharm	55953-0020	Antidiarrheal
2 <> N	Cap	Loperamide HCl 2 mg	by HL Moore	00839-7623	Antidiarrheal
2 <> N020	Cap, N Over 020	Loperamide HCl 2 mg	by Martec	52555-0519	Antidiarrheal
2 <> N020	Cap, 2 <> N Over 020	Loperamide HCl 2 mg	by Allscripts	54569-3707	Antidiarrheal
2 <> N020	Cap, N Over 020	Loperamide HCl 2 mg	by Medirex	57480-0830	Antidiarrheal
2 <> N020	Cap, Opaque White	Loperamide HCl 2 mg	by Quality Care	60346-0046	Antidiarrheal
2 <> N020	Cap	Loperamide HCl 2 mg	by Heartland	61392-0336	Antidiarrheal
2 <> N020	Cap, N Over 020	Loperamide HCl 2 mg	by Amerisource	62584-0768	Antidiarrheal
2 <> N020	Cap, N Over 020	Loperamide HCl 2 mg	by Major	00904-7617	Antidiarrheal
2 <> N020	Cap	Loperamide HCl 2 mg	by DHHS Prog	11819-0036	Antidiarrheal
2 <> N125	Tab, White, 2 <> N over 125	Alprazolam 2 mg	by Novopharm	55953-8125	Antianxiety; C IV
2 <> N480	Tab	Albuterol Sulfate 2.4 mg	by Heartland	61392-0567	Antiasthmatic
2 <> N480	Tab, White, Round, 2 <> N over 480	Albuterol Sulfate 2.4 mg	by Novopharm	55953-0480	Antiasthmatic
2 <> U	Tab, White, Round	Pramipexole DiHCl 0.125 mg	Mirapex by Pharmacia & Upjohn	00009-0002	Antiparkinson
2 <> U	Tab	Pramipexole DiHCl 0.125 mg	Mirapex by Promex Med	62301-0026	Antiparkinson

ID FRONT <> BACK	DESCRIPTION FRONT <> BACK	INGREDIENT & STRENGTH	BRAND (OR EQUIV.) & FIRM	NDC#	CLASS; SCH.
2 <> XANAX	Tab, White, Oblong, Coated	Alprazolam 2 mg	Xanax by Pharmacia & Upjohn	00009-0094	Antianxiety; C IV
2 <> XANAX	Tab, White, Trisected	Alprazolam 2 mg	by Pharmacia	Canadian DIN# 00813958	Antianxiety
2 <> Z3925	Tab	Diazepam 2 mg	by Quality Care	60346-0579	Antianxiety; C IV
2 <> Z3925	Tab, 2 <> Z over 3925	Diazepam 2 mg	by Kaiser	00179-1085	Antianxiety; C IV
2 <> Z3925	Tab, White, Round	Diazepam 2 mg	Valium by Zenith Goldline	00172-3925	Antianxiety; C IV
2 <> Z4234	Tab, Peach, Round, Scored, 2 <> Z over 4234	Bumetanide 2 mg	by Caraco	57664-0222	Diuretic
2 <> Z4234	Tab, Peach, Round, Scored	Bumetanide 2 mg	by Murfreesboro Ph	51129-1383	Diuretic
2 <> Z4234	Tab, Scored	Bumetanide 2 mg	by Geneva	00781-1823	Diuretic
2 <> Z4234	Tab, Peach, Round	Bumetanide 2 mg	Bumex by Zenith Goldline	00182-2617	Diuretic
2 <> Z4234	Tab, Scored, 2 <> Z over 4234	Bumetanide 2 mg	by Major	00904-5104	Diuretic
20	Tab, Rose	Nifedipine 20 mg	Adalat 20 by Bayer	Canadian	Antihypertensive
20	Cap, Opaque & Pink	Omeprazole 20 mg	Losec by Astra	Canadian	Gastrointestinal
20	Tab, White, Oval, Scored	Torsemide 20 mg	Demadex by Compumed	00403-0715	Diuretic
20 <> 104	Tab, 104 and Boehringer Mannheim LOG	Torsemide 20 mg	Demadex by Hoffmann La Roche	00004-0264	Diuretic
20 <> 104	Tab, Debossed <> Boehringer Mannheim Logo and 104	Torsemide 20 mg	Demadex by Caremark	00339-6012	Diuretic
20 <> 104	Tab, 104 and Boehringer Mannheim LOG	Torsemide 20 mg	Demadex by Nat Pharmpak Serv	55154-0405	Diuretic
20 <> 256	Tab, 20/Royce Logo	Baclofen 20 mg	by Qualitest	00603-2409	Muscle Relaxant
20 <> 336	Cap, 20/Royce Logo	Piroxicam 20 mg	by Qualitest	00603-5223	NSAID
20 <> 336	Cap, Filled with Off-White to Light Yellow Powder <> Royce Logo and 336	Piroxicam 20 mg	by Quality Care	60346-0676	NSAID
20 <> 4198	Tab, Peach, Round	Enalapril Maleate 20 mg	Vasotec by Zenith Goldline	00172-4198	Antihypertensive
20 <> AD	Tab, Orange, Round	Amphetamine Aspartate 5 mg, Amphetamine Sulfate 5 mg, Dextroamphetamine Saccharate 5 mg, Dextroamphetamine Sulfate 5 mg	Adderall by Shire Richwood	58521-0033	Stimulant; C II
20 <> AMIDE010	Tab, Amide 010	Isoxsuprine HCl 20 mg	by Qualitest	00603-4147	Vasodilator
20 <> AO	Tab, Coated	Salsalate 750 mg	by Quality Care	60346-0034	NSAID
20 <> BL	Tab, Salmon, Round	Imipramine HCl 25 mg	by Teva	00093-2113	Antidepressant
20 <> BL	Tab, Salmon, Coated	Imipramine HCl 25 mg	by Schein	00364-0406	Antidepressant
20 <> BL	Tab, Salmon	Imipramine HCl 25 mg	by Allscripts	54569-0194	Antidepressant
20 <> BL	Tab, Salmon	Imipramine HCl 25 mg	by UDL	51079-0080	Antidepressant
20 <> BMS1965	Cap, Brown	Stavudine 20 mg	Zerit by Murfreesboro Ph	51129-1396	Antiviral
20 <> BMS1965	Cap, Light Brown, Black Print, 20 <> BMS over 1965	Stavudine 20 mg	Zerit by Bristol Myers	00003-1965	Antiviral
20 <> DAN5555	Tab, 20 <> Dan 5555	Propranolol HCl 20 mg	by Quality Care	60346-0598	Antihypertensive
20 <> DAN5555	Tab, Blue, Round, Scored	Propranolol HCl 20 mg	by Vangard Labs	00615-2562	Antihypertensive
20 <> DAN5555	Tab	Propranolol HCl 20 mg	by Danbury	00591-5555	Antihypertensive
20 <> DAN5731	Tab	Baclofen 20 mg	by Amerisource	62584-0624	Muscle Relaxant
20 <> DAN5731	Tab	Baclofen 20 mg	by Danbury	00591-5731	Muscle Relaxant
20 <> E531	Tab, White, Round	Isoxsuprine HCl 20 mg	Vasodilan by Eon	00185-0531	Vasodilator
20 <> EFF	Tab	Methazolamide 50 mg	by Mikart	46672-0109	Diuretic
20 <> G1296	Tab, White, Round, Film Coated	Baclofen 20 mg	Lioresal by Zenith Goldline	00172-4097	Muscle Relaxant
20 <> INV236	Tab, White, Round	Nadolol 20 mg	Corgard by Zenith Goldline	00182-2632	Antihypertensive
20 <> INV236	Tab	Nadolol 20 mg	Nadolol by Schein	00364-2652	Antihypertensive
20 <> INV236	Tab, Scored, 20 <> INV over 236	Nadolol 20 mg	Nadolol by Invamed	52189-0236	Antihypertensive
20 <> INV236	Tab, 20 <> INV/236	Nadolol 20 mg	Nadolol by Geneva	00781-1181	Antihypertensive
20 <> INV236	Tab	Nadolol 20 mg	Nadolol by HL Moore	00839-7869	Antihypertensive
20 <> INV236	Tab	Nadolol 20 mg	Nadolol by Major	00904-5069	Antihypertensive
20 <> KU107	Tab, White, Round, Scored	Isosorbide Mononitrate 20 mg	by Schwarz Pharma Mfg	00131-9107	Antianginal
20 <> KU107	Tab, 20 <> KU107	Isosorbide Mononitrate 20 mg	by Physicians Total Care	54868-3822	Antianginal
20 <> KU107	Tab, White	Isosorbide Mononitrate 20 mg	by Kremers Urban	62175-0107	Antianginal
20 <> LESCOL	Cap, Triangle Logo	Fluvastatin Sodium 20 mg	Lescol by Amerisource	62584-0176	Antihyperlipidemic
20 <> LESCOL	Cap, Brown & Light Brown, Triangle Logo 20 <> Lescol Logo	Fluvastatin Sodium 20 mg	Lescol by Novartis	00078-0176	Antihyperlipidemic

ID FRONT <> BACK	DESCRIPTION FRONT <> BACK	INGREDIENT & STRENGTH	BRAND (OR EQUIV.) & FIRM	NDC#	CLASS; SCH.
20 <> LESCOL	Cap, Sandoz Logo	Fluvastatin Sodium 20 mg	Lescol by Allscripts	54569-3821	Antihyperlipidemic
20 <> LOTENSIN	Tab, Coated	Benazepril HCl 20 mg	Lotensin by PDRX	55289-0086	Antihypertensive
20 <> LOTENSIN	Tab, Coated	Benazepril HCl 20 mg	Lotensin by Quality Care	60346-0892	Antihypertensive
20 <> LOTENSIN	Tab, Coated	Benazepril HCl 20 mg	Lotensin by Amerisource	62584-0079	Antihypertensive
20 <> LOTENSIN	Tab, Beige Pink	Benazepril HCl 20 mg	Lotensin by Novartis	00083-0079	Antihypertensive
20 <> LOTENSIN	Tab, Coated	Benazepril HCl 20 mg	Lotensin by Allscripts	54569-3359	Antihypertensive
20 <> M	Tab, White, Round, Scored, M inside square box	Methylphenidate HCl 20 mg	by Neuman Distr	64579-0023	Stimulant; C II
20 <> M	Tab, White, Round, Scored	Methylphenidate HCl 20 mg	Methylin ER by Mallinckrodt Hobart	00406-1124	Stimulant; C II
20 <> MC	Tab, M/C	Isoxsuprine HCl 20 mg	by Shire Richwood	58521-0576	Vasodilator
20 <> MJ544	Tab, 20 <> MJ544, Debossed	Isoxsuprine HCl 20 mg	Vasodilan by Bristol Myers Squibb	00087-0544	Vasodilator
20 <> MYLAN183	Tab, Blue, Round, Scored, 20 <> Mylan over 183	Propranolol HCl 20 mg	Inderal by UDL	51079-0278	Antihypertensive
20 <> MYLAN183	Tab, Blue, Mylan Over 183, Beveled Edge	Propranolol HCl 20 mg	by Mylan	00378-0183	Antihypertensive
20 <> N	Cap, Novopharm	Piroxicam 20 mg	by Prescription Dispensing	61807-0039	NSAID
20 <> N640	Cap, Dark Green	Piroxicam 20 mg	by Heartland	61392-0401	NSAID
20 <> N640	Cap	Piroxicam 20 mg	by HL Moore	00839-7774	NSAID
20 <> NU	Tab, Grayish-Pink, Round, Film Coated	Nifedipine 20 mg	by Nu Pharm	Canadian DIN# 02200937	Antihypertensive
20 <> OC	Tab, Pink, Round	Oxycodone HCl 20 mg	OxyContin by Purdue Frederick	Canadian	Analgesic; C II
20 <> OC	Tab, Pink, Round	Oxycodone HCl 20 mg	Oxycontin by PF Labs	48692-0711	Analgesic; C II
20 <> OC	Tab, Pink, Round	Oxycodone HCl 20 mg	Oxycontin by PF Labs	48692-0601	Analgesic; C II
20 <> OC	Tab, Film Coated	Oxycodone HCl 20 mg	Oxycontin by Physicians Total Care	54868-3814	Analgesic; C II
20 <> PAXIL	Tab, Film Coated	Paroxetine HCl	Paxil by Kaiser	00179-1182	Antidepressant
20 <> PAXIL	Tab, Film Coated	Paroxetine HCl	Paxil by Allscripts	54569-3810	Antidepressant
20 <> PAXIL	Tab, Film Coated	Paroxetine HCl	Paxil by Nat Pharmpak Serv	55154-4504	Antidepressant
20 <> PAXIL	Tab, Film Coated	Paroxetine HCl	Paxil by HJ Harkins Co	52959-0360	Antidepressant
20 <> PAXIL	Tab, Film Coated	Paroxetine HCl	Paxil by Amerisource	62584-0211	Antidepressant
20 <> PAXIL	Tab, Film Coated	Paroxetine HCl	Paxil by SB	59742-3211	Antidepressant
20 <> PAXIL	Tab, Film Coated	Paroxetine HCl	by Kaiser	62224-2340	Antidepressant
20 <> PAXIL	Tab, Pink, Oval, Film Coated	Paroxetine HCl 20 mg	Paxil by SKB	00029-3211	Antidepressant
20 <> PD156	Tab, White, Elliptical, Film Coated	Atorvastatin 20 mg	Lipitor by Parke-Davis	Canadian DIN# 02230713	Antihyperlipidemic
20 <> PD156	Tab, Film Coated	Atorvastatin Calcium	Lipitor by Pharm Utilization	60491-0804	Antihyperlipidemic
20 <> PD156	Tab, White, Elliptical, Film Coated	Atorvastatin Calcium	Lipitor by Parke Davis	00071-0156	Antihyperlipidemic
20 <> PD156	Tab, Film Coated	Atorvastatin Calcium	Lipitor by Allscripts	54569-4467	Antihyperlipidemic
20 <> PD156	Tab, Film Coated	Atorvastatin Calcium	Lipitor by Goedecke	53869-0156	Antihyperlipidemic
20 <> PD156	Tab, White	Atorvastatin Calcium 20 mg	Lipitor by Phy Total Care	54868-3946	Antihyperlipidemic
20 <> PD532	Tab, Brown, Round	Quinapril HCl 20 mg	Accupril by PDRX Pharms	55289-0554	Antihypertensive
20 <> PD532	Tab, Brown, Round, Coated	Quinapril HCl 20 mg	Accupril by Parke Davis	00071-0532	Antihypertensive
20 <> PD532	Tab, Coated	Quinapril HCl 20 mg	Accupril by Allscripts	54569-3985	Antihypertensive
20 <> PD532	Tab, Brown, Round, Film Coated, 20 <> PD/532	Quinapril 20 mg	Accupril by Park-Davis	Canadian DIN# 01947680	Antihypertensive
20 <> PF	Tab, White, Cap-Shaped	Morphine Sulfate 20 mg	MS IR by Purdue Frederick	Canadian	Analgesic
20 <> SCHWARZ620	Tab, White, Round, Scored	Isosorbide Mononitrate 20 mg	Monoket by Heartland Healthcare	61392-0630	Antianginal
20 <> SCHWARZ620	Tab, White, Round, Scored	Isosorbide Mononitrate 20 mg	Monoket by Schwarz Pharma Mfg	00131-3620	Antianginal
20 <> SCHWARZ620	Tab, White, Scored	Isosorbide Mononitrate 20 mg	Monoket by Schwarz Pharma	00091-3620	Antianginal
20 <> VISTA065	Tab, White, Round, Scored	Isoxsuprine HCl 20 mg	by Vista Pharms	61970-0066	Vasodilator
20 <> VISTA065	Tab, White, Round, Convex, Scored	Isoxsuprine HCl 20 mg	Tri Soxsuprine USP by Murfreesboro	51129-1587	Vasodilator
20 <> VISTA065	Tab, Coated, Embossed	Isoxsuprine HCl 20 mg	Tri Soxsuprine by Vista	61970-0065	Vasodilator
20 <> WATSON334	Tab, 2.0, <> Watson 334	Lorazepam 2 mg	by Quality Care	60346-0800	Sedative/Hypnotic; C IV

ID FRONT <> BACK	DESCRIPTION FRONT <> BACK	INGREDIENT & STRENGTH	BRAND (OR EQUIV.) & FIRM	NDC#	CLASS; SCH.
20 <> Z4097	Tab, Film Coated	Baclofen 20 mg	by Prescription Dispensing	61807-0131	Muscle Relaxant
20 <> Z4097	Tab, Film Coated, 20 <> Z Over 4097	Baclofen 20 mg	by Baker Cummins	63171-1296	Muscle Relaxant
20 <> Z4097	Tab, White, Round, Film Coated	Baclofen 20 mg	Lioresal by Zenith Goldline	00172-4097	Muscle Relaxant
20 <> Z4097	Tab, Film Coated, 20 <> Z over 4097	Baclofen 20 mg	by Med Pro	53978-3167	Muscle Relaxant
20 <> Z4097	Tab, Film Coated, 20 <> Z over 4097	Baclofen 20 mg	by UDL	51079-0669	Muscle Relaxant
200	Cap, White	Etodolac 200 mg	by ESI Lederle		NSAID
200	Tab, Yellow, Cap-Shaped	Ibuprofen 200 mg	Ibuprofen FC by Apotex	Canadian	NSAID
200	Tab, Pink, Round, Scored	Levothyroxine Sodium 200 mcg	by Murfreesboro	51129-1654	Antithyroid
200	Tab, Buff, Round, Savage Logo 200	Pancrelipase 400 mg, Lipase 400 mg, Protease NLT 400 mg, Amylase NLT 400 mg	Ilozyme by Savage	00281-2001	Gastrointestinal
200	Cap, White, Ex Release, Printed in Red	Theophylline 200 mg	Slo Bid by RPR	00801-0200	Antiasthmatic
200 <> 4266	Cap, Opaque	Acyclovir 200 mg	Zovirax by Zenith Goldline	00182-2666	Antiviral
200 <> 4266	Cap, White	Acyclovir 200 mg	Zovirax by Zenith Goldline	00172-4266	Antiviral
200 <> 4365	Tab, White, Round, 200 <> Hourglass Logo 4365	Labetalol HCl 200 mg	Normodyne & Trandate by Zenith Goldline	00172-4365	Antihypertensive
200 <> 599113606	Cap, White	Etodolac 200 mg	by Wyeth Pharms	52903-3606	NSAID
200 <> 599113606	Cap, White	Etodolac 200 mg	by Ayerst Lab (Div Wyeth)	00046-3606	NSAID
200 <> 7767	Cap, White	Celecoxib 200 mg	Celebrex by Pfizer	Canadian DIN# 02239942	NSAID
200 <> 7767	Cap, White	Celecoxib 200 mg	Celebrex by Phy Total Care	54868-4101	NSAID
200 <> 7767	Cap, White	Celecoxib 200 mg	Celebrax by Southwood Pharms	58016-0223	NSAID
200 <> 7767	Cap, White, Gold Print	Celecoxib 200 mg	Celeboxib by PP\rado	Canadian DIN# 02239941	NSAID
200 <> 832	Tab, Butterscotch Yellow, Sugar Coated	Chlorpromazine HCl 200 mg	by Schein	00364-0384	Antipsychotic
200 <> 832	Tab, Coated	Chlorpromazine HCl 200 mg	by United Res	00677-0787	Antipsychotic
200 <> 832	Tab, Butterscotch Yellow, Sugar Coated	Chlorpromazine HCl 200 mg	by Qualitest	00603-2812	Antipsychotic
200 <> A05	Cap, Blue	Acyclovir 200 mg	Zovirax by MOVA	55370-0557	Antiviral
200 <> A05	Cap, Black Print	Acyclovir 200 mg	by Martec	52555-0682	Antiviral
200 <> ALTI200	Tab, Pink, Round, Scored	Amiodarone HCl 200 mg	by Altimed	Canadian DIN# 02240071	Antiarrhythmic
200 <> C	Tab, Pink, Round	Amiodarone HCl 200 mg	Cordorone by Wyeth Pharms	52903-4188	Antiarrhythmic
200 <> DP	Tab	Levothyroxine Sodium 200 mcg	Levoxyl by Jones	52604-1112	Antithyroid
200 <> FL	Tab, Compressed, Logo FL	Levothyroxine Sodium 200 mcg	by Kaiser	00179-0460	Antithyroid
200 <> FLINT	Tab	Levothyroxine Sodium 0.2 mg	Synthroid by Giant Food	11146-0306	Antithyroid
200 <> FLINT	Tab, Pink, Round, Scored	Levothyroxine Sodium 0.2 mg	Synthroid by Rx Pac	65084-0160	Antithyroid
200 <> FLINT	Tab	Levothyroxine Sodium 0.2 mg	Synthroid by Wal Mart	49035-0172	Antithyroid
200 <> FLINT	Tab	Levothyroxine Sodium 0.2 mg	Synthroid by Nat Pharmpak Serv	55154-0907	Antithyroid
200 <> FLINT	Tab	Levothyroxine Sodium 0.2 mg	Synthroid by Rite Aid	11822-5194	Antithyroid
200 <> FLINT	Tab, Pink, Round, Scored	Levothyroxine Sodium 200 mcg	Synthroid by Knoll	00048-1140	Antithyroid
200 <> GG457	Tab, Yellow, Round, Film Coated	Chlorpomazine HCl 200 mg	by Murfreesboro Ph	51129-1370	Antipsychotic
200 <> GG457	Tab, Butterscotch Yellow, Film Coated	Chlorpromazine HCl 200 mg	by Physicians Total Care	54868-2465	Antipsychotic
200 <> GG457	Tab, Butterscotch Yellow, Round, Film Coated	Chlorpromazine HCl 200 mg	Thorazine by Geneva	00781-1719	Antipsychotic
200 <> N181	Tab, Green, Oval, Film Coated	Cimetidine 200 mg	by Novopharm	55953-0181	Gastrointestinal
200 <> N181	Tab, Coated	Cimetidine 200 mg	by Brightstone	62939-2111	Gastrointestinal
200 <> N181	Tab, Film Coated	Cimetidine 200 mg	by Darby Group	66467-3480	Gastrointestinal
200 <> N181	Tab, Coated	Cimetidine 200 mg	by United Res	00677-1527	Gastrointestinal
200 <> N214	Tab, Pink, Oval, Scored	Amiodarone HCl 200 mg	by Novopharm	55953-0214	Antiarrhythmic
200 <> N740	Cap, Light & Orange, Engraved in Black Ink <> White Granular Powder	Mexiletine HCl 200 mg	by Novopharm	55953-0740	Antiarrhythmic
200 <> N740	Cap	Mexiletine HCl 200 mg	by Brightstone	62939-2322	Antiarrhythmic

ID FRONT <> BACK	DESCRIPTION FRONT <> BACK	INGREDIENT & STRENGTH	BRAND (OR EQUIV.) & FIRM	NDC#	CLASS; SCH.
200 <> N740	Cap, Black Ink	Mexiletine HCl 200 mg	by Warrick	59930-1686	Antiarrhythmic
200 <> N740	Cap, N Over 740 in Black Ink Hard Gelatin with White Powder	Mexiletine HCl 200 mg	by Medirex	57480-0837	Antiarrhythmic
200 <> N940	Cap	Acyclovir 200 mg	by Warrick	59930-1538	Antiviral
200 <> N940	Cap, Blue, Gelatin	Acyclovir 200 mg	by Phy Total Care	54868-3996	Antiviral
200 <> N940	Cap, Blue, Gelatin	Acyclovir 200 mg	by Murfreesboro Ph	51129-1359	Antiviral
200 <> N940	Cap, Blue, Opaque, 200 <> N over 940	Acyclovir 200 mg	by UDL	51079-0876	Antiviral
200 <> N940	Cap	Acyclovir 200 mg	by Allscripts	54569-4482	Antiviral
200 <> N940	Cap	Acyclovir 200 mg	by Major	00904-5231	Antiviral
200 <> N940	Cap, Blue, 200 <> N Oover 940	Acyclovir 200 mg	by Novopharm	43806-0940	Antiviral
200 <> PD352	Tab, Yellow, Oval, Film Coated	Troglitazone 200 mg	Rezulin by Murfreesboro Ph	51129-1286	Antidiabetic
200 <> PD352	Tab, Yellow, Oval, Film Coated	Troglitazone 200 mg	Rezulin by Parke Davis	00071-0352	Antidiabetic
200 <> PF	Tab	Morphine Sulfate 200 mg	Ms Contin by Purdue Frederick	00034-0513	Analgesic; C II
200 <> SCHERING752	Tab, White, Round, Scored	Labetalol HCl 200 mg	Normodyne by Rightpak	65240-0706	Antihypertensive
200 <> SW	Tab	Tiludronate Disodium 240 mg	Skelid by Sanofi	00024-1800	Bisphosphonate
200 <> SW	Tab	Tiludronate Disodium 240 mg	Skelid by Sanofi Winthrop	53360-1800	Bisphosphonate
200 <> TOPAMAX	Tab, Coated	Topiramate 200 mg	Topamax by Ortho	00062-0642	Anticonvulsant
200 <> TOPAMAX	Tab, Salmon, Coated	Topiramate 200 mg	Topamax by McNeil	00045-0642	Anticonvulsant
200 <> TOPAMAX	Tab, Coated	Topiramate 200 mg	Topamax by McNeil	52021-0642	Anticonvulsant
200 <> WELLCOMEZOVIRAX	Cap	Acyclovir 200 mg	Zovirax by Catalytica	63552-0991	Antiviral
200 <> ZENITH4266	Cap, 200 <> Zenith Logo Zenith 4266	Acyclovir 200 mg	by Murfreesboro	51129-1252	Antiviral
200MG <> FLOXIN	Tab, Light Yellow, Film Coated, 200MG	Ofloxacin 200 mg	Floxin by Quality Care	60346-0647	Antibiotic
200NORMODYNE <> SCHERING 752	Tab, Film Coated	Labetalol HCl 200 mg	Normodyne by Schering	53922-0752	Antihypertensive
200ZPP	Cap, Clear & White	Phenylpropanolamine HCl 75 mg, Caramiphen Edisylate 40 mg	Tuss- by Pioneer		Cold Remedy
2002PP	Cap, Clear & White	Phenylpropanolamine 75 mg, Caraminephen Edisylate 40 mg	Tuss Ornade by Pioneer		Antitussive
200FLI	Tab, Pink, Round, 200/FLI Logo	Levothyroxine Sodium 200 mcg	by Forest	00456-0327	Antithyroid
200G60	Tab, White, Oval, 200/G 60	Cimetidine 200 mg	by Novopharm		Gastrointestinal
200M	Tab	Levothyroxine Sodium 200 mcg	Levo T by MOVA	55370-0132	Antithyroid
200MCG <> 283	Tab, Coated	Cerivastatin Sodium 0.2 mg	Baycol by Bayer	00026-2883	Antihyperlipidemic
200MCG <> FLINT	Tab, Debossed	Levothyroxine Sodium 0.2 mg	Synthroid by Amerisource	62584-0140	Antithyroid
200MG <> PF	Tab, Red, Cap-Shaped	Morphine Sulfate 200 mg	MS Contin by Purdue Frederick	Canadian	Analgesic
200MG <> SCHWARZ4086	Cap, Amethyst, Opaque	Verapamil HCl 200 mg	Verelan PM by Schwarz Pharma	00091-4086	Antihypertensive
200MG <> T	Tab, Pink, Round, Coated	Carbamazepine XR 200 mg	by Novartis	00083-0062	Anticonvulsant
200MG <> WATSON492	Cap	Mexiletine HCl 200 mg	by Watson	52544-0492	Antiarrhythmic
200MG <> ZENITH4171	Cap	Quinine Sulfate 200 mg	by Quality Care	60346-0808	Antimalarial
200MG4176	Cap, Light Gray, Gelatin, Red Print	Etodolac 200 mg	by Zenith Goldline	00172-4176	NSAID
200MG4176	Cap, Gelatin, Red Print, 2 Bands	Etodolac 200 mg	by Zenith Goldline	00182-2664	NSAID
200NOVO	Tab, White, Oval, 200/Novo	Acebutolol HCl 200 mg	by Novopharm	Canadian	Antihypertensive
200WYETH	Tab, White, Oval, 200/Wyeth	Acebutolol HCl 200 mg	by Wyeth-Ayerst	Canadian	Antihypertensive
201	Tab, Film Coated, Logo	Naproxen Sodium 412.5 mg	Naprelan by Elan	56125-0201	NSAID
201 <> U	Tab	Acetaminophen 650 mg, Hydrocodone Bitartrate 7.5 mg	Lorcet Plus by Amerisource	62584-0028	Analgesic; C III
201 <> U	Tab	Acetaminophen 650 mg, Hydrocodone Bitartrate 7.5 mg	Lorcet Plus by Med Pro	53978-2071	Analgesic; C III
201 <> U	Tab	Acetaminophen 650 mg, Hydrocodone Bitartrate 7.5 mg	by Mikart	46672-0025	Analgesic; C III
201 <> UU	Tab	Acetaminophen 650 mg, Hydrocodone Bitartrate 7.5 mg	Lorcet Plus by Quality Care	60346-0759	Analgesic; C III
201 <> UU	Tab, 201 <> U/U	Acetaminophen 650 mg, Hydrocodone Bitartrate 7.5 mg	Lorcet Plus by Nat Pharmpak Serv	55154-7302	Analgesic; C III
201 <> UU	Tab	Acetaminophen 650 mg, Hydrocodone Bitartrate 7.5 mg	Lorcet Plus by Murfreesboro	51129-0053	Analgesic; C III
201 <> UU	Tab, 201 <> U-U	Acetaminophen 650 mg, Hydrocodone Bitartrate 7.5 mg	Lorcet Plus by Allscripts	54569-0916	Analgesic; C III

ID FRONT <> BACK	DESCRIPTION FRONT <> BACK	INGREDIENT & STRENGTH	BRAND (OR EQUIV.) & FIRM	NDC#	CLASS; SCH.
201 <> UU	Tab, White, U/U	Acetaminophen 650 mg, Hydrocodone Bitartrate 7.5 mg	Lorcet Plus by UAD	00785-1122	Analgesic; C III
201 <>GG	Tab, White, Round, Scored	Furosemide 40 mg	Lasix by Geneva	00781-1966	Diuretic
2010 <> PENTASA250MG	Cap, Blue & Green, Pentagonal Starburst Logo and 2010 <> Pentsa 250 mg	Mesalamine 250 mg	Pentasa CR by Nat Pharmpak Serv	55154-5585	Gastrointestinal
2010	Cap, Blue & Green	Mesalamine 250 mg	Pentasa by Natl Pharmpak	55154-2216	Gastrointestinal
2011 <> G	Tab, White, Round	Orphenadrine Citrate 100 mg	by Global Pharms (Ca)	00115-2011	Muscle Relaxant
2013	Tab, Yellow, Round	Chlorpheniramine Maleate 4 mg	Chlor-Trimeton by Circa		Antihistamine
201NORMODYNE <> SCHERING752	Tab, Film Coated, 200 Normodyne <> Schering 752	Labetalol HCl 200 mg	Normodyne by Thrift Drug	59198-0081	Antihypertensive
201SEARLE	Tab, White to Off-White, Round, 201/Searle	Spironolactone 25 mg, Hydrochlorothiazide 25 mg	Aldactazide 25 by Searle	Canadian DIN# 00180408	Diuretic
202	Tab, Film Coated, Logo	Naproxen Sodium 550 mg	Naprelan by Elan	56125-0202	NSAID
2020	Tab, White with Specks, Oblong	Caffeine 175 mg	20-20 by B & M Labs		Stimulant
2020 <> MYLAN	Cap, Green	Piroxicam 20 mg	by Va Cmop	65243-0057	NSAID
2020 <> MYLAN	Cap	Piroxicam 20 mg	by Quality Care	60346-0676	NSAID
202NORMODYNE <> SCHERING752	Tab, Film Coated	Labetalol HCl 200 mg	Normodyne by Amerisource	62584-0752	Antihypertensive
2035	Cap	Chlordiazepoxide 10 mg	Librium by Vortech		Antianxiety; C IV
203A <> TEC	Tab, White to Off-White, Round, Scored	Doxazosin Mesylate 1 mg	by Altimed	Canadian DIN# 02243215	Antihypertensive
203A <> TEC	Tab, White to Off-White, Rectangular, Scored	Doxazosin Mesylate 2 mg	by Altimed	Canadian DIN# 02243216	Antihypertensive
203B	Tab, Green, Round	Amitriptyline HCl 25 mg	Elavil by Barr		Antidepressant
204 <> 400N	Tab, Light Green, Film Coated	Cimetidine 400 mg	by Quality Care	60346-0945	Gastrointestinal
204 <> 400N	Tab, Light Green, Coated, 400/N	Cimetidine 400 mg	by Schein	00364-2593	Gastrointestinal
204 <> M	Tab, White, Round	Diclofenac Sodium 50 mg	by Martec Pharms	65413-0001	NSAID
204 <> UAD	Tab	Guaifenesin 300 mg, Phenylephrine HCl 20 mg	by Mikart	46672-0145	Cold Remedy
205	Tab, Pink, Oval	Diphenhydramine 25 mg	Benadryl by Granutec		Antihistamine
205 <> INV	Tab, Film Coated	Hydrochlorothiazide 15 mg, Methyldopa 250 mg	by Qualitest	00603-4543	Diuretic; Antihypertensive
205 <> M	Tab, White, Round	Diclofenac Sodium 75 mg	by Martec Pharms	65413-0002	NSAID
205ETHEX	Tab	Guaifenesin 600 mg	by Quality Care	60346-0863	Expectorant
206 <> INV	Tab, Film Coated	Hydrochlorothiazide 25 mg, Methyldopa 250 mg	by Qualitest	00603-4544	Diuretic; Antihypertensive
2063V <> 2	Tab,	Acetaminophen 300 mg, Codeine Phosphate 15 mg	by PDRX	55289-0449	Analgesic; C III
2065V <> 4	Tab, 2065 over V <> 2	Acetaminophen 300 mg, Codeine Phosphate 60 mg	by Quality Care	60346-0632	Analgesic; C III
207	Tab, Scored	Nadolol 40 mg	Corgard by Rightpak	65240-0625	Antihypertensive
207	Tab, Scored	Nadolol 40 mg	Corgard by Novartis	17088-0003	Antihypertensive
207 <> TT	Tab	Guaifenesin 600 mg, Pseudoephedrine HCl 60 mg	by United Res	00677-1487	Cold Remedy
2078213	Tab, White, Round, 20 78-213	Metaproterenol 20 mg	Metaprel by Sandoz		Antiasthmatic
208 <> ETHEX	Tab, White, Oblong, Scored	Guaifenesin 600 mg; Pseudoephedrine HCl 120 mg	by Murfreesboro Ph	51129-1390	Cold Remedy
2083	Tab, Orange, Round, Scored	Hydrochlorothiazide 25 mg	by Va Cmop	65243-0039	Diuretic
2083	Tab, Orange, Round, Scored	Hydrochlorothiazide 25 mg	by Vangard Labs	00615-1561	Diuretic
2083	Tab, Orange, Round, Scored	Hydrochlorothiazide 25 mg	by Vangard Labs	00615-1561	Diuretic
2089	Tab, Orange, Round, Scored	Hydrochlorothiazide 50 mg	by Va Cmop	65243-0040	Diuretic
2095	Cap	Docusate Sodium 100 mg	Dio-Sul by Vortech		Laxative
209B	Tab, Pink, Round	Amitriptyline HCl 10 mg	Elavil by Barr		Antidepressant
20A	Tab, White, Round, 20A/Tower Symbol	Orciprenaline 20 mg	Alupent by Boehringer Ingelheim	Canadian	Antiasthmatic
20AMIDE010	Tab, White, Round, 20 and Amide 010	Isoxsuprine HCl 20 mg	Vasodilan by Amide	52152-0010	Vasodilator

ID FRONT <> BACK	DESCRIPTION FRONT <> BACK	INGREDIENT & STRENGTH	BRAND (OR EQUIV.) & FIRM	NDC#	CLASS; SCH.
20AMIDE10	Tab	Isoxsuprine HCl 20 mg	by Zenith Goldline	00182-1056	Vasodilator
20AO	Tab, Orange & Peach, Round, 20/AO	Dextroamphetamine Sacranate 5 mg	Adderall by Richwood		Stimulant; C II
20F	Tab, White, Round, 20/F	Tamoxifen Citrate 20 mg	Tamone by Pharmacia	Canadian	Antiestrogen
20LESCOL	Cap, Brown, 20/Lescol	Fluvastatin 20 mg	by Novartis	Canadian	Antihyperlipidemic
20M	Tab, White, 20/M	Benzoyl Peroxide 20 mg	Benoxyl by Stiefel	Canadian	Antiacne
20M	Tab, White, 20/M	Decyclomine 20 mg	by Hoechst Marion Roussel	Canadian	Gastrointestinal
20MG	Cap, Amethyst, Opaque, 2 Yellow Bands	Esomeprazole 20 mg	Nexium by AstraZeneca	00186-5020	Proton Pump Inhibitor
20MG	Cap, Amethyst, Opaque, 2 Yellow Bands	Esomeprazole 20 mg	Nexium by AstraZeneca	00186-5022	Proton Pump Inhibitor
20MG	Cap, Blue	Pericyazine 20 mg	by Rhone-Poulenc Rorer	Canadian	Psychotropic Agent
20MG <> FP	Tab, Pink, Oval, Film Coated, Scored	Citalopram Hydrobromide 20 mg	Celexa by Forest	00456-4020	Antidepressant
20MG <> KADIAN	Cap	Morphine Sulfate 20 mg	Kadian ER by Purepac	00228-2043	Analgesic; C II
20MG <> LILLY3220	Cap, Pink & Purple	Fluoxetine 20 mg	Sarafem by Lilly	00002-3220	Antidepressant
20MG <> PERIOSTAT	Cap, White, Opaque	Doxycycline Hyclate 20 mg	Periostat by H J Harkins Co	52959-0438	Antibiotic
20MG <> PERIOSTAT	Cap, White	Doxycycline Hyclate 20 mg	Periostat by H J Harkins Co	52959-0446	Antibiotic
20MG <> WATSON713	Cap, Filled with Off-White to Yellow Powder	Piroxicam 20 mg	by Watson	52544-0713	NSAID
20R <> RPR	Tab	Chlorthalidone 50 mg	Hygroton by RPR	00801-0020	Diuretic
20R <> RPR	Tab, 20 in raised H <> RPR Logo	Chlorthalidone 50 mg	Hygroton by RPR	00075-0020	Diuretic
20Z <> 4235	Tab, White Round	Nadolol 20 mg	Corgard by Zenith Goldline	00182-2632	Antihypertensive
20Z <> 4235	Tab, White, Round	Nadolol 20 mg	Corgard by Zenith Goldline	00172-4235	Antihypertensive
20Z4235	Tab, White, Round, 20Z/4235	Nadolol 20 mg	Corgard by Zenith Goldline	00172-4235	Antihypertensive
21	Cap, Advance Logo 21	Diphenhydramine HCl 50 mg	by Quality Care	60346-0045	Antihistamine
21	Cap, Pink, Red Band, Qualitest Logo	Diphenhydramine HCl 50 mg	by Allscripts	54569-0241	Antihistamine
21	Cap, Pink, Qualitest Logo	Diphenhydramine HCl 50 mg	by Allscripts	54569-0241	Antihistamine
21 <> 93	Cap, Pink & White	Diltiazem HCl 60 mg	by Allscripts	54569-3784	Antihypertensive
21 <> B	Tab, Light Orange	Ethinyl Estradiol 0.03 mg, Levonorgestrel 0.15 mg	Levlen 28 by Berlex	50419-0411	Oral Contraceptive
21 <> B	Tab, Light Orange	Ethinyl Estradiol 0.03 mg, Levonorgestrel 0.15 mg	Levlen 21 by Berlex	50419-0410	Oral Contraceptive
21 <> B	Tab, Light Orange	Ethinyl Estradiol 0.03 mg, Levonorgestrel 0.15 mg	Levlen 21 by Berlex	50419-0021	Oral Contraceptive
21 <> BL	Tab, Green, Round	Imipramine HCl 50 mg	by Teva	00093-2117	Antidepressant
21 <> BL	Tab	Imipramine HCl 50 mg	by UDL	51079-0081	Antidepressant
21 <> M	Tab, White, Round, Scored, M inside square	Methylphenidate HCl 20 mg	Methylin by Neuman Distr	64579-0034	Stimulant; C II
210	Tab, Yellow, Round, Schering Logo/2-10	Amitriptyline HCl 2 mg, Perphenazine 10 mg	Etrafon by Schering	Canadian	Antipsychotic
210	Tab, Yellow, Logo/2-10	Perphenazine 2 mg, Amitriptyline 10 mg	by Schering	Canadian	Antipsychotic; Antidepressant
210 <> 247	Tab, 2-10/Royce Logo <> 247	Amitriptyline HCl 25 mg, Perphenazine 2 mg	by Qualitest	00603-5115	Antipsychotic
210 <> ANTIVERT	Tab, Turquoise	Meclizine HCl 12.5 mg	Antivert by Roerig Pfizer	00662-2100	Antiemetic
2101V	Tab, Blue, Round, Film Coated	Amitriptyline HCl 10 mg	by Apothecon	59772-0386	Antidepressant
2101V	Tab, Blue, Round, Film Coated	Amitriptyline HCl 10 mg	Amitriptyline HCl by Astra Zeneca	00186-0452	Antidepressant
2101V	Tab, Blue, Round, Film Coated	Amitriptyline HCl 10 mg	by Vintage Pharms	00254-2101	Antidepressant
2102V	Tab, Pale Yellow, Coated	Amitriptyline 25 mg	Qualitest by Vintage Pharm		Antidepressant
2102V	Tab, Yellow, Round, Film Coated	Amitriptyline HCl 25 mg	by Apothecon	59772-0387	Antidepressant
2102V	Tab, Yellow, Round, Film Coated	Amitriptyline HCl 25 mg	Amitriptyline HCl by Astra Zeneca	00186-0707	Antidepressant
2102V	Tab, Yellow, Round, Film Coated	Amitriptyline HCl 25 mg	by Vintage Pharms	00254-2102	Antidepressant
2103V	Tab, Beige, Round, Film Coated	Amitriptyline HCl 50 mg	by Caremark	00339-6137	Antidepressant
21040	Tab, White, Round, 210/40	Furosemide 40 mg	Lasix by Martec		Diuretic
211	Tab, Coated	Amitriptyline HCl 12.5 mg, Chlordiazepoxide 5 mg	by Qualitest	00603-2690	Antianxiety; C IV
211 <> ANTIVERT	Tab, Layered	Meclizine HCl 25 mg	Antivert by Roerig Pfizer	00662-2110	Antiemetic
211 <> ANTIVERT	Tab, White & Yellow, Oval	Meclizine HCl 25 mg	Antivert by Rightpak	65240-0605	Antiemetic
211 <> INV	Cap	Amantadine HCl 100 mg	by Caremark	00339-5780	Antiviral
211 <> MYLAN	Tab, Green, Coated	Amitriptyline HCl 12.5 mg, Chlordiazepoxide 5 mg	by Mylan	00378-0211	Antianxiety; C IV
212	Tab, 2 1/2	Nitroglycerin 2.5 mg	Sustachron ER Buccal by Forest	10418-0138	Vasodilator
212	Tab, Blue, Round, Savage Logo 212	Potassium Chloride 600 mg	Kaon-CL 8 by Savage		Electrolytes
212 <> ZAROXOLYN	Tab, Pink, Round	Metolazone 2.5 mg	Zaroxolyn by Compumed	00403-1597	Diuretic

ID FRONT <> BACK	DESCRIPTION FRONT <> BACK	INGREDIENT & STRENGTH	BRAND (OR EQUIV.) & FIRM	NDC#	CLASS; SCH.
212 <> ZAROXOLYN	Tab, Debossed, 2 1/2 <> Zaroxolyn	Metolazone 2.5 mg	Zaroxolyn by Caremark	00339-5426	Diuretic
212 <> ZAROXOLYN	Tab, 2 1/2 <> Zaroxolyn	Metolazone 2.5 mg	Zaroxolyn by Nat Pharmpak Serv	55154-2504	Diuretic
212 <> ZAROXOLYN	Tab, Debossed, 2 1/2 <> Zaroxolyn	Metolazone 2.5 mg	Zaroxolyn by Medeva	53014-0975	Diuretic
212 <> ZAROXOLYN	Tab, Debossed, 2 1/2 <> Zaroxolyn	Metolazone 2.5 mg	Zaroxolyn by Amerisource	62584-0975	Diuretic
212 <> ZAROXOLYN	Tab, Debossed, 2 1/2 <> Zaroxolyn	Metolazone 2.5 mg	Zaroxolyn by Prestige Packaging	58056-0355	Diuretic
2120	Cap, White	Valproic Acid 250 mg	Depakene by Sidmak		Anticonvulsant
2120	Cap, White, Oblong, Gelatin	Valproic Acid 250 mg	Depakene by Sidmak	50111-0852	Anticonvulsant
2120V <> 3	Tab, White, Round, Scored	Aspirin 325 mg, Codeine Phosphate 30 mg	by Allscripts	54569-0300	Analgesic; C III
2120V <> 3	Tab, 2120/V <> 3	Aspirin 325 mg, Codeine Phosphate 30 mg	by Vintage	00254-2120	Analgesic; C III
2120V <> 3	Tab	Aspirin 325 mg, Codeine Phosphate 30 mg	by United Res	00677-0647	Analgesic; C III
2120V <> 3	Tab, 2120/V	Aspirin 325 mg, Codeine Phosphate 30 mg	by Qualitest	00603-2361	Analgesic; C III
2121V <> 4	Tab, 2121/V <> 4	Aspirin 325 mg, Codeine Phosphate 60 mg	by Vintage	00254-2121	Analgesic; C III
2121V <> 4	Tab, 2121/V	Aspirin 325 mg, Codeine Phosphate 60 mg	by Qualitest	00603-2362	Analgesic; C III
212COUMADIN <> DUPONT	Tab, Green, Round, Scored, 2 1/2 Coumadin <> Dupont	Warfarin Sodium 2.5 mg	Coumadin by Thrift Drug	59198-0349	Anticoagulant
213	Tab, White, Round	Acetaminophen 500 mg	Tylenol Ext. St. by Granutec		Antipyretic
213 <> 93	Cap	Tolmetin Sodium 492 mg	by Quality Care	60346-0615	NSAID
2130 <> 50MG	Cap, Opaque & Pink & White	Nitrofurantoin Macrocrystalline 50 mg	Nitrofurantoin by PDRX	55289-0055	Antibiotic
2130 <> ZENITH50MG	Cap, Zenith Logo	Nitrofurantoin 50 mg	by Caremark	00339-6037	Antibiotic
2130 <> ZENITH50MG	Cap	Nitrofurantoin 50 mg	by Allscripts	54569-0181	Antibiotic
2130 <> ZENITH50MG	Cap, Zenith Logo	Nitrofurantoin 50 mg	by Medirex	57480-0816	Antibiotic
2130 <> ZENITH50MG	Cap, 2130 with 2 lines <> Zenith 50 mg	Nitrofurantoin 50 mg	by Thrift Drug	59198-0242	Antibiotic
2130<> 50MG	Cap, Pink & White	Nitrofurantoin Macrocrystalline 50 mg	by Goldline Labs	00182-1944	Antibiotic
2130V	Tab, Light Brown, Round	Amitriptyline 50 mg	by Vintage		Antidepressant
2130ZENITH50MG	Cap, Pink & White, 2130/Zenith 50 mg	Nitrofurantoin 50 mg	by Par	49884-0724	Antibiotic
2130ZENITH50MG	Cap, Pink & White	Nitrofurantoin Macrocrystalline 50 mg	by Compumed	00403-1528	Antibiotic
2131 <> 100MG	Cap, Pink & White	Nitrofurantoin 100 mg	by Direct Dispensing	57866-6590	Antibiotic
2131 <> ZENITH100	Cap, ER	Nitrofurantoin 103 mg	by Prepackage Spec	58864-0371	Antibiotic
2131 <> ZENITH100MG	Cap, Zenith 100 mg	Nitrofurantoin 100 mg	by Quality Care	60346-0008	Antibiotic
2131 <> ZENITH100MG	Cap, 2131 with 3 lines <> Zenith 100 mg	Nitrofurantoin 100 mg	by Thrift Drug	59198-0243	Antibiotic
2131 <> ZENITH100MG	Cap, Zenith symbol	Nitrofurantoin 100 mg	by Medirex	57480-0817	Antibiotic
2131 <> ZENITH100MG	Cap, Logo and Zenith Over 100 mg	Nitrofurantoin 100 mg	Nitrofurant Macrcrys by HJ Harkins Co	52959-0405	Antibiotic
215Q	Cap, Ivory, 215/Q	Meclofenamate Sodium 50 mg	Meclomen by Quantum		NSAID
216 <> ETHEX	Tab, White, Oval, Coated	Ascorbic Acid 80 mg, Beta-Carotene 0.4 mg, Biotin 30 mcg, Calcium 200 mg, Copper 3 mg, Cyanocobalamin 2.5 mcg, Folic Acid 1 mg, Iron 60 mg, Magnesium 100 mg, Niacinamide 17 mg, Pantothenic Acid 7 mg, Pyridoxine HCl 4.86 mg, Riboflavin 1.6 mg, Thiamine 1.5 mg, Vitamin A 0.8 mg, Vitamin D 10 mcg, Vitamin E 10 mg, Zinc 25 mg	Prenatal Rx by Ethex	58177-0216	Vitamin
216Q	Cap, Yellow, 216/Q	Meclofenamate Sodium 100 mg	Meclomen by Quantum		NSAID
217	Tab, White	Aspirin 325 mg, Caffeine 30 mg	217 Tablets by Frosst	Canadian	Analgesic
217 <> ABANA	Cap, White & Green Beads <> with Logo	Phentermine HCl 37.5 mg	Obenix by Elge	58298-0952	Anorexiant; C IV
217 <> PAR	Cap, Buff	Doxepin HCl	by Qualitest	00603-3455	Antidepressant
217FORT	Tab, White	Aspirin 500 mg, Caffeine 30 mg	217 Strong Tablets by Frosst	Canadian	Analgesic
218 <> PAR	Cap	Doxepin HCl	by Qualitest	00603-3456	Antidepressant
218BARR	Tab, White, Round	Ergoloid Mesylates Sublingual 0.5 mg	Hydergine by Barr		Ergot
219	Tab, Yellow, Oblong, Scored, Film Coated	Choline Magnesium Trisalicylate 500 mg	by Compumed	00403-0544	NSAID
219 <> ARR	Tab, Coated	Erythromycin Stearate 500 mg	by Barr	00555-0219	Antibiotic
219 <> PAR	Cap	Doxepin HCl	by Qualitest	00603-3457	Antidepressant
21MG <> FP	Tab, Film Coated, F/P	Citalopram Hydrobromide 24.98 mg	Celexa by Forest	63711-0120	Antidepressent
22 <> 93	Cap	Diltiazem HCl 90 mg	by Allscripts	54569-3785	Antihypertensive
22 <> B	Tab, Round, Sugar Coated	Ethinyl Estradiol 0.02 mg, Levonorgestrel 0.1 mg	Levlite 28 by Berlex	50419-0408	Oral Contraceptive
22 <> B	Tab, Round, Sugar Coated	Ethinyl Estradiol 0.02 mg, Levonorgestrel 0.1 mg	Levlite 21 by Berlex	50419-0406	Oral Contraceptive

ID FRONT <> BACK	DESCRIPTION FRONT <> BACK	INGREDIENT & STRENGTH	BRAND (OR EQUIV.) & FIRM	NDC#	CLASS; SCH.
22 <> B	Tab, Sugar Coated	Ethinyl Estradiol 0.02 mg, Levonorgestrel 0.1 mg	Levlite by Schering	12866-1163	Oral Contraceptive
22 <> B	Tab, Pink, Round	Levonorgestrel 0.1 mg, Ethinyl Estradiol 0.02 mg	Levlite by Schering Productions	64259-1165	Oral Contraceptive
22 <> BL	Tab, Pink, Round, Coated	Amitriptyline HCl 10 mg	by Teva	00093-2120	Antidepressant
22 <> P	Tab, Round, Dye Free, Chewable, 2.2 <> P	Sodium Fluoride 2.21 mg	Pharmaflur by Pharmics	00813-0066	Element
220	Tab, Blue, Oblong, Scored, Film Coated	Choline Magnesium Trisalicylate 750 mg	by Compumed	00403-0561	NSAID
220 <> PAR	Cap, Green	Doxepin HCl	by Qualitest	00603-3458	Antidepressant
2200 <> MYLAN	Cap, Lavender, Opaque	Acyclovir 200 mg	by Allscripts	54569-4482	Antiviral
220MERICON	Cap, Pink, 220/Mericon	Zinc Sulfate 220 mg	ORAZINC by MERICON		Mineral Supplement
221	Tab, Pink, Oblong, Scored, Film Coated	Choline Magnesium Trisalicylate 1000 mg	by Compumed	00403-0694	NSAID
221 <> 3M	Tab, White, Round	Orphenadrine Citrate 100 mg	Norflex by Rx Pac	65084-0229	Muscle Relaxant
221 <> 3M	Tab, White, Round	Orphenadrine Citrate 100 mg	Norflex by HJ Harkins	52959-0178	Muscle Relaxant
221 <> 3M	Tab, White, Round	Orphenadrine Citrate 100 mg	Norflex by Rightpak	65240-0703	Muscle Relaxant
221 <> 3M	Tab, White, Round	Orphenadrine Citrate 100 mg	Norflex ER by 3M	00089-0221	Muscle Relaxant
221 <> 3M	Tab	Orphenadrine Citrate 100 mg	Norflex by Allscripts	54569-0839	Muscle Relaxant
221 <> 3M	Tab	Orphenadrine Citrate 100 mg	Norflex Sr by Nat Pharmpak Serv	55154-2907	Muscle Relaxant
221 <> 3M	Tab	Orphenadrine Citrate 100 mg	Norflex by PDRX	55289-0646	Muscle Relaxant
221 <> 3M	Tab	Orphenadrine Citrate 100 mg	Norflex by Quality Care	60346-0554	Muscle Relaxant
221 <> 3M	Tab	Orphenadrine Citrate 100 mg	Norflex by Amerisource	62584-0221	Muscle Relaxant
221 <> BL	Tab, White to Off-White, Oblong, Chewable	Amoxicillin 125 mg	by Teva	00093-2267	Antibiotic
221 <> BL	Tab, Chewable	Amoxicillin Trihydrate	by HL Moore	00839-7776	Antibiotic
221 <> P	Tab, Partially Bisected	Hydrochlorothiazide 25 mg	Hctz by Quality Care	60346-0184	Diuretic
221 <> R	Tab, Peach, Round, Scored	Hydrochlorothiazide 25 mg	by Purepac	00228-2221	Diuretic
22190	Tab, Coated, Debossed	Probenecid 500 mg	by PDRX	55289-0715	Antigout
221R	Tab, 221/R	Hydrochlorothiazide 25 mg	by Allscripts	54569-0547	Diuretic
222	Tab, White, Round, Scored	Acetaminophen 375 mg, Caffeine 30 mg, Cod. Phos 8 mg	222 by Johnson & Johnson	Canadian DIN# 00108162	Analgesic
222 <> BL	Tab, Chewable, 222 <> B/L	Amoxicillin Trihydrate	by St Marys Med	60760-0268	Antibiotic
222 <> BL	Tab, Chewable	Amoxicillin Trihydrate	by Quality Care	60346-0113	Antibiotic
222 <> BL	Tab, Chewable	Amoxicillin Trihydrate	by Casa De Amigos	62138-6005	Antibiotic
222 <> BL	Tab, Chewable, 222 <> B over L	Amoxicillin Trihydrate	by Allscripts	54569-3689	Antibiotic
222 <> BL	Tab, Chewable, 222 <> B/L	Amoxicillin Trihydrate	by DRX	55045-2004	Antibiotic
222 <> BL	Tab, White to Off-White, Oblong, Scored, Chewable, 222 <> B/L	Amoxicillin Trihydrate 250 mg	by Teva	00093-2268	Antibiotic
222 <> CARACO	Tab, Mottled Yellow, Round, Scored	Guaifenesin 600 mg, Phenylpropanolamine HCl 120 mg	Miraphen PSE by Med Pro	53978-3330	Cold Remedy
222 <> PAR	Cap	Doxepin HCl	by Schein	00364-2525	Antidepressant
222 <> PAR	Cap	Doxepin HCl	by Qualitest	00603-3460	Antidepressant
222 <> R	Tab, Peach, Round, Scored	Hydrochlorothiazide 50 mg	by Purepac	00228-2222	Diuretic
222BL	Tab, Chewable	Amoxicillin Trihydrate	by Pharmedix	53002-0207	Antibiotic
22425	Tab, White, Round, 224 / 2.5	Minoxidil 2.5 mg	Loniten by Royce		Antihypertensive
224ST2 <> 3850	Cap, Yellow	Ephedra, Colanut, White Willow Bark	by NVE Pharm		Supplement
225	Tab	Baclofen 10 mg	by Geneva	00781-1641	Muscle Relaxant
225	Cap, Maroon, Logo/225	Clindamycin HCl 150 mg	Dalacin C by Upjohn	Canadian	Antibiotic
225	Tab, White, Round, Film Coated, Scored	Propafenone HCl 225 mg	Rythmol by Murfreesboro Ph	51129-1362	Antiarrhythmic
225 <> COPLEY	Tab, Film Coated	Potassium Chloride 600 mg	by Schein	00364-0861	Electrolytes
225 <> ETHEX	Tab, Pink, Oval, Scored	Ascorbic Acid 120 mg, Calcium 200 mg, Copper 2 mg, Cyanocobalamin 12 mcg, Folic Acid 1 mg, Iron 27 mg, Niacinamide 20 mg, Pyridoxine HCl 10 mg, Riboflavin 3 mg, Thiamine HCl 1.84 mg, Vitamin A 4000 Units, Vitamin D 400 Units, Vitamin E 22 mg, Zinc 25 mg	Natalcare Plus by Ethex	58177-0225	Vitamin
225 <> ETHEX	Tab, Scored	Ascorbic Acid 120 mg, Calcium 200 mg, Copper 2 mg, Cyanocobalamin 12 mcg, Folic Acid 1 mg, Iron 27 mg, Niacinamide 20 mg, Pyridoxine HCl 10 mg, Riboflavin 3 mg, Thiamine HCl 1.84 mg, Vitamin A 4000 Units, Vitamin D 400 Units, Vitamin E 22 mg, Zinc 25 mg	Natalcare Plus by KV	10609-1382	Vitamin

ID FRONT <> BACK	DESCRIPTION FRONT <> BACK	INGREDIENT & STRENGTH	BRAND (OR EQUIV.) & FIRM	NDC#	CLASS; SCH.
225 <> GG	Tab, White, Round, Compressed	Promethazine HCl 25 mg	Phenergan by Geneva	00781-1830	Antiemetic; Antihistamine
225 <> PAR	Tab	Haloperidol 2 mg	by Zenith Goldline	00182-1264	Antipsychotic
22510	Tab, White, Round, 225 / 10	Minoxidil 10 mg	Loniten by Royce		Antihypertensive
225105	Tab, Coated, 225/105	Ascorbic Acid 100 mg, Cyanocobalamin 25 mcg, Ferrous Fumarate 600 mg	Tolfrinic by BFAscher	00225-0105	Vitamin
225245	Tab, 225/245 <> Ascher Logo	Hyoscyamine Sulfate 0.125 mg	Anaspaz by Sovereign	58716-0612	Gastrointestinal
225250	Tab, White, 225-250	Ethaverine HCl 100 mg	by B.F.Ascher		Vasodilator
225295	Tab, 225/295 <> Imprinted with the Ascher Logo	Hyoscyamine Sulfate 0.125 mg	Anaspaz by DRX	55045-2362	Gastrointestinal
225295	Tab, Pale Yellow, Round, Scored, 225/295 <> Ascher Logo	L-Hyoscyamine Sulfate 0.125 mg	Anaspaz by B F Ascher	00225-0295	Urinary Tract
225356	Tab, White, Round, Ascher logo 225/356	Magnesium Salicylate 325 mg, Phenyltoloxamine Citrate 30 mg	Mobigesic by B F Ascher		Analgesic
225356	Tab, White, Round, Scored, Ascher Logo <> 225/356	Magnesium Salicylate, Anhydrous, 325 mg, Phenyltoloxamine Citrate 30 mg	Mobigesic by B F Ascher	00225-0356	Analgesic
225405	Cap, 225/405	Chlorpheniramine Maleate 12 mg, Phenylpropranolamine 75 mg	by B.F.Ascher		Cold Remedy
225450	Tab, Scored, Ascher Logo	Acetaminophen 500 mg, Hydrocodone Bitartrate 5 mg	Hy Phen by		Analgesic; C III
225450	Tab, 225-450 <> 2 Ascher Logos	Acetaminophen 500 mg, Hydrocodone Bitartrate 5 mg	Hy-Phen by B F Ascher	00225-0450	Analgesic; C III
225470	Cap, Clear & White, 225/470	Phendimetrazine Tartrate 105 mg	by B.F.Ascher		Anorexiant; C III
225480	Cap, 225 over 480 <> Ascher Logo	Brompheniramine Maleate 12 mg, Pseudoephedrine HCl 120 mg	Allent by Pharmafab	62542-0154	Cold Remedy
225480	Cap, Ascher Logo 225-480	Brompheniramine Maleate 12 mg, Pseudoephedrine HCl 120 mg	Allent by BFAscher	00225-0480	Cold Remedy
225490	Cap, Gold & Tan, Oval, 225/490	Docusate Na 230 mg, Phenolphthalein 130 mg	Unilax by B.F.Ascher		Laxative
226	Tab, Orange, Round	Aspirin Enteric Coated 325 mg	Ecotrin by Granutec		Analgesic
226	Tab	Baclofen 20 mg	by Geneva	00781-1642	Muscle Relaxant
2263 <> 93	Tab, Off-White, Cap Shaped, Film Coated	Amoxicillin 500 mg	by Teva	55953-2263	Antibiotic
227	Tab, Invamed Logo	Metoclopramide 5 mg	by Med Pro	53978-2094	Gastrointestinal
227 <> GG	Tab, Green, Round, Scored, Compressed	Isosorbide Dinitrate 20 mg	Isordil by Geneva	00781-1695	Antianginal
227 <> WC	Tab, Light Buff, Round	Vitamin A 1000 Unt; Cholecalciferol 400 Unt; Vitamin E 11 Unt; Ascorbic Acid 120 mg; Folic Acid 1 mg; Thiamine Mononitrate 2 mg; Riboflavin 3 mg; Niacinamide 20 mg; Cyanocobalamin 12 mcg; Pyridoxine HCl 10 mg; Iron 29 mg	Natachew by Warner Chilcott W C	00430-0227	Vitamin
227 <> WC	Tab, Round	Vitamin A 1000 Unt, Cholecalciferol 400 Unt, Vitamin E 11 Unt, Ascorbic Acid 120 mg; Folic Acid 1 mg; Thiamine Mononitrate 2 mg; Riboflavin 3 mg; Niacinamide 20 mg; Cyanocobalamin 12 mcg, Pyridoxine HCl 10 mg, Iron 29 mg	Natachew by Amide Pharm	52152-0210	Vitamin
227 <> WYETH	Tab, Pink, Scored	Promethazine HCl 50 mg	Phenargan by Wyeth Pharms	52903-0227	Antiemetic; Antihistamine
227555	Tab, White, Oval	Ergoloid Mesylates Sublingual 1 mg	Hydergine by Barr		Ergot
228	Tab, Yellow, Round	Aspirin Enteric Coated 81 mg	Ecotrin by Granutec		Analgesic
228	Tab, White, Round, Schering Logo 228	Griseofulvin Ultramicrosize 125 mg	Fulvicin P/G by Schering		Antifungal
228QPL10	Tab, White, Round, 228/QPL/10	Minoxidil 10 mg	Loniten by Quantum		Antihypertensive
22905	Tab, White, Round, 229/0.5	Haloperidol 0.5 mg	Haldol by Royce		Antipsychotic
22R <> RPR	Tab, 22 in raised H <> RPR Logo	Chlorthalidone 25 mg	Hygroton by RPR	00075-0022	Diuretic
22R <> RPR	Tab	Chlorthalidone 25 mg	Hygroton by RPR	00801-0022	Diuretic
23 <> BL	Tab, Light Green, Round, Coated	Amitriptyline HCl 25 mg	by Teva	00093-2122	Antidepressant
230	Tab, Yellow, Round	Bisacodyl 5 mg	Dulcolax by BI		Gastrointestinal
230	Tab, Yellow, Round, Enteric, Sugar Coated	Bisacodyl DR 5mg	Dulcolax by UDL	51079-0907	Gastrointestinal
2301	Tab, Yellow, Round, 230/1	Haloperidol 1 mg	Haldol by Royce		Antipsychotic
231	Tab, Red, Round, Schering Logo 231	Dexbrompheniramine Maleate 6 mg, Pseudoephedrine Sulf 120 mg	Disophrol by Schering		Cold Remedy
231	Tab, White, Round, Savage Logo 231	Dexpanthenol 50 mg, Choline Bitartrate 25 mg	Ilopan-Choline by Savage	00281-2311	Paralyticlleus
231 <> M	Tab, Scored	Atenolol 50 mg	by Heartland	61392-0543	Antihypertensive
231 <> M	Tab	Atenolol 50 mg	by Quality Care	60346-0719	Antihypertensive
231 <> M	Tab, White, Scored	Atenolol 50 mg	by Mylan	00378-0231	Antihypertensive
231 <> M	Tab	Atenolol 50 mg	by Allscripts	54569-3432	Antihypertensive
231 <> M	Tab, White, Round, Scored	Atenolol 50 mg	Tenormin by UDL	51079-0684	Antihypertensive
2312	Tab, Purple, Round, 231/2	Haloperidol 2 mg	Haldol by Royce		Antipsychotic

ID FRONT <> BACK	DESCRIPTION FRONT <> BACK	INGREDIENT & STRENGTH	BRAND (OR EQUIV.) & FIRM	NDC#	CLASS; SCH.
232 <> ETHEX	Tab, Peach, Film Coated	Ascorbic Acid 50 mg, Calcium 250 mg, Copper 2 mg, Folic Acid 1 mg, Iron 40 mg, Magnesium 50 mg, Pyridoxine HCl 2 mg, Vitamin D 6 mcg, Vitamin E 3.5 mg, Zinc 15 mg	Natalcare by Ethex	58177-0232	Vitamin
232232	Tab, Chewable, Scored, 232 232 <> Clonmell Logo	Amoxicillin Trihydrate	by Clonmell	55190-0232	Antibiotic
232232	Tab, Pink, Oval, Chewable, 232 over 232 <> Mova Logo	Amoxicillin Trihydrate	Amoxil by MOVA	55370-0892	Antibiotic
232232	Tab, Oval, 232 over 232	Amoxicillin 250 mg	by Bayer	00280-0036	Antibiotic
2325	Tab, Green, Round, 232/5	Haloperidol 5 mg	Haldol by Royce		Antipsychotic
23280	Tab, White, Round, 232/80	Furosemide 80 mg	Lasix by Martec		Diuretic
23310	Tab, Bluish Green, Round, 233/10	Haloperidol 10 mg	Haldol by Royce		Antipsychotic
23420	Tab, Salmon, Round, 234/20	Haloperidol 20 mg	Haldol by Royce		Antipsychotic
235 <> 800N	Tab, Light Green, Coated, 800/N	Cimetidine 800 mg	by Schein	00364-2594	Gastrointestinal
23686	Tab, White, Round, Hourglass Logo <> 2 3686	Doxazosin Mesylate 2 mg	Cardura by Zenith Goldline	00172-3686	Antihypertensive
237 <> A	Tab, White to Off-White, Round	Diphenoxylate HCl 2.5 mg, Atropine Sulfate 0.025 mg	Lomotil by Able Lab	53265-0237	Antidiarrheal; C V
237 <> ETHEX	Tab, Orange, Oblong, Scored	Hyoscyamine Sulfate 0.375 mg	by Murfreesboro	51129-1500	Gastrointestinal
237 <> MYLAN	Tab, White, Film Coated	Etodolac 400 mg	by Mylan	00378-0237	NSAID
237 <> MYLAND	Tab, White, Oval, Film Coated	Etodolac 400 mg	by Allscripts	54569-4468	NSAID
2384	Cap	Hematinic Combination	Tri-Tinic by Vortech		Vitamin
239 <> SQUIBB	Cap	Cephalexin Monohydrate	by Quality Care	60346-0055	Antibiotic
239500	Tab, 239/500 <> Royce Logo	Chlorzoxazone 500 mg	by Quality Care	60346-0663	Muscle Relaxant
239500	Tab, Green, Oblong, Royce Logo 239 500	Chlorzoxazone 500 mg	Parafon DSC by Royce		Muscle relaxant
239500	Tab, Mortar and Pestle Logo	Chlorzoxazone 500 mg	by Royce	51875-0239	Muscle Relaxant
24 <> BL	Tab, Brown, Round, Coated	Amitriptyline HCl 50 mg	by Teva	00093-2124	Antidepressant
240 <> 05	Tab, Coated, Royce Logo 240 <> 0.5	Lorazepam 0.5 mg	by Quality Care	60346-0363	Sedative/Hypnotic; C IV
240 <> 05	Tab, 240 <> 0.5	Lorazepam 0.51 mg	by United Res	00677-1056	Sedative/Hypnotic; C IV
240 <> 05	Tab, 0.5/Royce Logo	Lorazepam 0.51 mg	by Qualitest	00603-4243	Sedative/Hypnotic; C IV
240 <> TIAZAC	Cap	Diltiazem HCl 240 mg	Tiazac by CVS	51316-0243	Antihypertensive
240 <> WPPH	Tab, White, Round, Scored	Chlorothiazide 250 mg	by Endo	60951-0765	Diuretic; Antihypertensive
240 <> WPPH	Tab, White, Scored	Chlorothiazide 250 mg	by Circa	71114-4207	Diuretic
240 <> WPPH	Tab	Chlorothiazide 250 mg	by Merck	00006-0240	Diuretic
24005	Tab, 240 0.5 <> Mortar and Pestle Logo	Lorazepam 0.51 mg	by Royce	51875-0240	Sedative/Hypnotic; C IV
24005	Tab, 240/0.5	Lorazepam 0.51 mg	by Talbert Med	44514-0098	Sedative/Hypnotic; C IV
24005	Tab, White, Round, Royce logo 240 / 0.5	Lorazepam 0.5 mg	Ativan by Royce		Sedative/Hypnotic; C IV
24005 <> WATSON	Tab, 240 Over 0.5, Beveled Edge	Lorazepam 0.51 mg	by Watson	52544-0240	Sedative/Hypnotic; C IV
24037	Tab, Salmon, Square, Hourglass Logo <> 2 4037	Estazolam 2 mg	Prosom by Zenith Goldline	00172-4037	Sedative/Hypnotic; C IV
2407Z <> 2407Z	Cap, in White Ink	Tetracycline HCl 500 mg	by Kaiser	00179-1021	Antibiotic
240MG <> ANDRX699	Cap, Brown & Orange	Diltiazem HCl 240 mg	Cartia XT by Heartland Healthcare	61392-0959	Antihypertensive
240MGBETAPACE	Tab, Light Blue, Cap Shaped, Scored	Sotalol HCl 240 mg	Betapace by Berlex	50419-0107	Antiarrhythmic
240WATSON664	Cap, Red & White, 240/Watson/664	Diltazem 240 mg	Dilacor XR by Watson		Antihypertensive
241	Tab	Nadolol 80 mg	Corgard by Leiner	59606-0626	Antihypertensive
241 <> 1	Tab, Royce Logo 241 <> 1	Lorazepam 1 mg	by Quality Care	60346-0047	Sedative/Hypnotic; C IV
241 <> 1	Tab	Lorazepam 1 mg	by United Res	00677-1057	Sedative/Hypnotic; C IV
241 <> 1	Tab, 1/Royce Logo	Lorazepam 1 mg	by Qualitest	00603-4244	Sedative/Hypnotic; C IV
241 <> WPPH	Tab	Hydrochlorothiazide 25 mg	by Merck	00006-0241	Diuretic
241 <> WPPH	Tab, Compressed	Hydrochlorothiazide 25 mg	by Endo	60951-0770	Diuretic
2410V	Tab, 2410 V	Carisoprodol 350 mg	by Qualitest	00603-2582	Muscle Relaxant
2410V	Tab	Carisoprodol 350 mg	by Vintage	00254-2410	Muscle Relaxant
2411	Tab, White, Round, Royce logo 241/1	Lorazepam 1 mg	Ativan by Royce		Sedative/Hypnotic; C IV
2411	Tab, 241 1 <> Mortar and Pestle Logo	Lorazepam 1 mg	by Royce	51875-0241	Sedative/Hypnotic; C IV
2411	Tab, 241 Over 1, Beveled Edge <> Royce Logo	Lorazepam 1 mg	by St Marys Med	60760-0241	Sedative/Hypnotic; C IV
2411	Tab, Scored	Lorazepam 1 mg	by Talbert Med	44514-0099	Sedative/Hypnotic; C IV
2411 <> WATSON	Tab, 241 Over 1, Beveled Edge	Lorazepam 1 mg	by Watson	52544-0241	Sedative/Hypnotic; C IV

ID FRONT <> BACK	DESCRIPTION FRONT <> BACK	INGREDIENT & STRENGTH	BRAND (OR EQUIV.) & FIRM	NDC#	CLASS; SCH.
2416 <> Z	Cap	Tetracycline HCl 250 mg	by Quality Care	60346-0609	Antibiotic
242 <> 2	Tab, Royce Logo 242 <> 2	Lorazepam 2 mg	by Quality Care	60346-0800	Sedative/Hypnotic; C IV
242 <> 2	Tab, 2/Royce Logo	Lorazepam 2 mg	by Qualitest	00603-4245	Sedative/Hypnotic; C IV
2422	Tab, White, Round, Flat, Scored, 242 and 2 <> Mortar and Pestle Logo	Lorazepam 2 mg	by Nat Pharmpak Serv	55154-0651	Sedative/Hypnotic; C IV
2422	Tab, White, Round, Scored	Lorazepam 2 mg	by Compumed	00403-0012	Sedative/Hypnotic; C IV
2422	Tab, White, Round, Royce logo 242/2	Lorazepam 2 mg	Ativan by Royce		Sedative/Hypnotic; C IV
2422	Tab, 242, 2 <> Mortar and Pestle Logo	Lorazepam 2 mg	by Royce	51875-0242	Sedative/Hypnotic; C IV
2422	Tab, 242 Over 2, Beveled Edge <> Royce Logo	Lorazepam 2 mg	by St Marys Med	60760-0242	Sedative/Hypnotic; C IV
2422 <> WATSON	Tab, 242 Over 2, Beveled Edge <> Beveled Edge	Lorazepam 2 mg	by Watson	52544-0242	Sedative/Hypnotic; C IV
2428	Cap	Phenytoin 100 mg	Di-Phen by Vortech		Anticonvulsant
243 <> WPPH	Tab	Hydrochlorothiazide 50 mg	by Merck	00006-0243	Diuretic
243 <> WPPH	Tab	Hydrochlorothiazide 50 mg	by Endo	60951-0771	Diuretic
243 <> WPPH	Tab	Hydrochlorothiazide 50 mg	Hctz by Quality Care	60346-0675	Diuretic
244 <> MYLAN	Tab, Blue, Oval, Film Coated	Verapamil HCl 120 mg	Isoptin SR by UDL	51079-0894	Antihypertensive
244 <> MYLAN	Tab, Film Coated	Verapamil HCl 120 mg	by Murfreesboro	51129-1298	Antihypertensive
244 <> MYLAN	Tab, Blue, Film Coated, Beveled Edge	Verapamil HCl 120 mg	by Mylan	00378-1120	Antihypertensive
244SEARLE	Tab, White to Off-White, Round, 244/Searle	Spironolactone 50 mg, Hydrochlorothiazide 50 mg	Aldactazide 50 by Searle	Canadian DIN# 00594377	Diuretic
245 <> MYLAN	Tab, Light Green	Bumetanide 0.5 mg	by Hoffmann La Roche	00004-0290	Diuretic
245 <> MYLAN	Tab, Light Green, Scored	Bumetanide 0.5 mg	by Mylan	00378-0245	Diuretic
245 <> WPPH	Tab, White, Round, Scored	Chlorothiazide 500 mg	by Endo	60951-0766	Diuretic
246 <> PAR	Tab, Lavender	Aspirin 325 mg, Carisoprodol 200 mg	by Schein	00364-2524	Analgesic; Muscle Relaxant
247 <> 210	Tab, 247 <> 2-10/Royce Logo	Amitriptyline HCl 25 mg, Perphenazine 2 mg	by Qualitest	00603-5115	Antipsychotic
2472	Cap	Diphenhydramine HCl 25 mg	Benadryl by Vortech		Antihistamine
247210	Tab, Coated	Amitriptyline HCl 10 mg, Perphenazine 2 mg	by Zenith Goldline	00182-1235	Antipsychotic
247210	Tab, Coated, 247 2-10 <> Mortar and Pestle Logo	Amitriptyline HCl 10 mg, Perphenazine 2 mg	by Royce	51875-0247	Antipsychotic
247210	Tab, Blue, Round, Royce logo 247/2-10	Perphenazine 2 mg, Amitriptyline 10 mg	Triavil by Royce		Antipsychotic; Antidepressant
2473	Cap	Diphenhydramine HCl 50 mg	Benadryl by Vortech		Antihistamine
248225	Tab	Amitriptyline HCl 25 mg, Perphenazine 2 mg	by Zenith Goldline	00182-1236	Antipsychotic
248225	Tab, 248 2-25, Mortar and Pestle Logo	Amitriptyline HCl 25 mg, Perphenazine 2 mg	by Royce	51875-0248	Antipsychotic
248225	Tab, Orange, Round, Royce logo 248/2-25	Perphenazine 2 mg, Amitriptyline 25 mg	Triavil by Royce		Antipsychotic; Antidepressant
249410	Tab	Amitriptyline HCl 10 mg, Perphenazine 4 mg	by Zenith Goldline	00182-1237	Antipsychotic
249410	Tab, Salmon, 249 4-10, Mortar and Pestle Logo	Amitriptyline HCl 10 mg, Perphenazine 4 mg	by Royce	51875-0249	Antipsychotic
249410	Tab, Salmon, Round, Royce logo 249/4-10	Perphenazine 4 mg, Amitriptyline 10 mg	Triavil by Royce		Antipsychotic; Antidepressant
25	Tab, Yellow, Round	Amitriptyline HCl 25 mg	Apo Amitriptyline by Apotex	Canadian	Antidepressant
25	Tab, White, Round	Bethanechol Chloride 25 mg	Duvoid by Roberts	Canadian	Urinary Tract
25	Tab, Pale Yellow, Round	Clomipramine 25 mg	Apo Clomipramine by Apotex	Canadian	OCD
25	Tab, Orangish Yellow, Round, Film Coated	Desipramine HCl 25 mg	Desipramine by Apotex	Canadian DIN# 02211947	Antidepressant
25	Tab, Yellow, Round, Coated	Diclofenac Sodium 25 mg	Apo Diclo by Apotex	Canadian DIN# 00886017	NSAID
25	Tab, Orange, Round	Dipyridamole 25 mg	Dipyridamole by Apotex	Canadian	Antiplatelet
25	Tab, Light Brown, Round	Imipramine 25 mg	Imipramine by Apotex	Canadian	Antidepressant

ID FRONT <> BACK	DESCRIPTION FRONT <> BACK	INGREDIENT & STRENGTH	BRAND (OR EQUIV.) & FIRM	NDC#	CLASS; SCH.
25	Tab, Blue, Round, Film Coated	Hydralazine HCl 25 mg	Hydralazine by Apotex	Canadian DIN# 02004828	Antihypertensive
25	Cap, Green	Hydroxyzine HCl 25 mg	Apo Hydroxyzine by Apotex	Canadian	Antihistamine
25	Tab, Pink, Round, Film Coated, 2.5	Indapamide 2.5 mg	Indapamide by Apotex	Canadian DIN# 02223597	Diuretic
25	Tab	Levothyroxine Sodium 0.025 mg	Synthroid by Nat Pharmpak Serv	55154-0910	Antithyroid
25	Cap, White	Pancreatic Enzyme 40 mg	Pancrease by Eurand		Gastrointestinal
25	Tab, Red, Round	Phenazopyridine HCl 100 mg	Pyridium by Breckenridge	51991-0520	Urinary Analgesic
25	Tab, White, Round	Terbutaline Sulfate 2.5 mg	Bricanyl by Astra	Canadian	Antiasthmatic
25	Tab, Brown, Round	Thioridazine HCl 25 mg	Apo Thioridazine by Apotex	Canadian	Antipsychotic
25	Tab, Pink, Round	Trimipramine Maleate 25 mg	Trimip by Apotex	Canadian	Antidepressant
25	Tab, Pink, Round, Film Coated	Trimipramine Maleate 25 mg	by Nu Pharm	Canadian DIN# 02020602	Antidepressant
25	Tab, Pink, Round	Trimipramine 25 mg	Rhotrimine by Rhodiapharm	Canadian	Antidepressant
25 <> 15	Tab, White, Round, Hourglass Logo 25 <> 15	Captopril 25 mg, Hydrochlorothiazide 15 mg	Capozide by Zenith Goldline	00172-2515	Antihypertensive; Diuretic
25 <> 25	Tab, Peach, Round, Hourglass Logo 25 <> 25	Captopril 25 mg, Hydrochlorothiazide 25 mg	Capozide by Zenith Goldline	00172-2525	Antihypertensive; Diuretic
25 <> 25	Tab, Peach, Round, 25 <> Hourglass Logo 25	Captopril 25 mg, Hydrochlorothiazide 25 mg	Capozide by Zenith Goldline	00172-2525	Antihypertensive; Diuretic
25 <> 310	Cap, Royce Logo	Doxepin HCl	by Quality Care	60346-0553	Antidepressant
25 <> 348	Tab, 25/Royce Logo <> 348	Captopril 25 mg	by Qualitest	00603-2556	Antihypertensive
25 <> 4195	Tab, Yellow, Round, 2.5 <> 4195	Enalapril Maleate 2.5 mg	Vasotec by Zenith Goldline	00172-4195	Antihypertensive
25 <> 4359	Tab, Pale Yellow, Round, 25 <> Hourglass Logo 4359	Clozapine 25 mg	Clozaril by Zenith Goldline	00172-4359	Antipsychotic
25 <> 50	Tab, Off-White, Oval, 25 <> Hourglass Logo 50	Captopril 50 mg, Hydrochlorothiazide 25 mg	Capozide by Zenith Goldline	00172-5025	Antihypertensive; Diuretic
25 <> 832	Tab, Butterscotch Yellow, Sugar Coated	Chlorpromazine HCl 25 mg	by Qualitest	00603-2809	Antipsychotic
25 <> BARR323	Cap, Barr Over 323 in Black Ink	Hydroxyzine Pamoate 42.61 mg	by Barr	00555-0323	Antihistamine
25 <> BARR323	Cap, in Black Ink <> Company Logo and 323 in Black Ink	Hydroxyzine Pamoate 42.61 mg	by Qualitest	00603-3994	Antihistamine
25 <> BL	Tab, Lavender, Round, Coated	Amitriptyline HCl 75 mg	by Teva	00093-2126	Antidepressant
25 <> CAPOTEN	Tab, Mottled	Captopril 25 mg	Capoten by ER Squibb	00003-0452	Antihypertensive
25 <> CAPOTEN	Tab	Captopril 25 mg	Capoten by Nat Pharmpak Serv	55154-3707	Antihypertensive
25 <> CLOZARIL	Tab, Yellow, Round, Scored	Clozapine 25 mg	Clozaril by Natl Pharmpak	55154-3412	Antipsychotic
25 <> CLOZARIL	Tab, Pale Yellow, Round, Scored	Clozapine 25 mg	Clozaril by Novartis	00078-0126	Antipsychotic
25 <> DAN5642	Tab, 2.5	Minoxidil 2.5 mg	by Danbury	00591-5642	Antihypertensive
25 <> DYNACIRC	Cap, 2.5 and Sandoz Logo	Isradipine 2.5 mg	Dynacirc by Caremark	00339-5719	Antihypertensive
25 <> F	Tab, Pink, 2.5 <> F	Medroxyprogesterone Aceate 2.5 mg	Proclim by Fournier Pharma	Canadian	Progestin
25 <> FLINT	Tab	Levothyroxine Sodium 0.025 mg	Synthroid by Rite Aid	11822-5287	Antithyroid
25 <> FLINT	Tab, Orange, Round, Scored	Levothyroxine Sodium 25 mcg	Synthroid by Knoll	00048-1020	Antithyroid
25 <> GG 476	Tab, Butterscotch, Coated, 25 <> GG 476	Chlorpromazine HCl 25 mg	by Heartland	61392-0040	Antipsychotic
25 <> GG 476	Tab, Butterscotch, Coated, 25 <> GG 476	Chlorpromazine HCl 25 mg	by Quality Care	62682-7045	Antipsychotic
25 <> GG32	Tab, Coated, 25 <> GG32	Thioridazine HCl 25 mg	by Heartland	61392-0463	Antipsychotic
25 <> GG32	Tab, Orange, Round, Film Coated	Thioridazine HCl 25 mg	Mellaril by Geneva	00781-1624	Antipsychotic
25 <> GG476	Tab, Butterscotch Yellow, Round, Film Coated	Chlorpromazine HCl 25 mg	Thorazine by Geneva	00781-1716	Antipsychotic
25 <> I	Tab, Coated	Sumatriptan Succinate 25 mg	Imitrex by Glaxo	00173-0460	Antimigraine
25 <> I	Tab, Coated	Sumatriptan Succinate 25 mg	Imitrex by Physicians Total Care	54868-3777	Antimigraine
25 <> INV272	Tab, INV over 272	Captopril 25 mg	by Schein	00364-2629	Antihypertensive
25 <> INV272	Tab, Quadrisected, 25 <> INV over 272	Captopril 25 mg	by Invamed	52189-0272	Antihypertensive
25 <> INV277	Tab, Yellow, Round, Film Coated	Prochlorperazine Maleate 25 mg	by Invamed	52189-0277	Antiemetic

ID FRONT <> BACK	DESCRIPTION FRONT <> BACK	INGREDIENT & STRENGTH	BRAND (OR EQUIV.) & FIRM	NDC#	CLASS; SCH.
25 <> LAMICTAL	Tab, White, Hexagon, Scored	Lamotrigine 25 mg	Lamictal by Glaxo Wellcome	00173-0594	Anticonvulsant
25 <> M58	Tab, Orange, Film Coated, M Over 58	Thioridazine HCl 25 mg	by Mylan	00378-0614	Antipsychotic
25 <> M58	Tab, Film Coated	Thioridazine HCl 25 mg	by Quality Care	60346-0839	Antipsychotic
25 <> M58	Tab, Orange, Round, Film Coated	Thioridazine HCl 25 mg	by Dixon Shane	17236-0301	Antipsychotic
25 <> M58	Tab, Coated	Thioridazine HCl 25 mg	by Vangard	00615-2506	Antipsychotic
25 <> M58	Tab, Orange, Round, Film Coated, 25 <> M over 58	Thioridazine HCl 25 mg	Mellaril by UDL	51079-0566	Antipsychotic
25 <> MJ504	Tab	Cyclophosphamide 25 mg	Cytoxan by Mead Johnson	00015-0504	Antineoplastic
25 <> MYLAN146	Tab, White, Mylan Above Score, 146 Below	Spironolactone 25 mg	by Mylan	00378-2146	Diuretic
25 <> MYLAN146	Tab	Spironolactone 25 mg	by Vangard	00615-1535	Diuretic
25 <> MYLAN146	Tab, White, Round, Scored, 25 <> Mylan over 146	Spironolactone 25 mg	Aldactone by UDL	51079-0103	Diuretic
25 <> MYLAN146	Tab, Mylan 146	Spironolactone 25 mg	by Heartland	61392-0083	Diuretic
25 <> MYLAN146	Tab	Spironolactone 25 mg	by Nat Pharmpak Serv	55154-5517	Diuretic
25 <> MYLAN146	Tab, Mylan 146	Spironolactone 25 mg	by Qualitest	00603-5766	Diuretic
25 <> N031	Cap, Bright Yellow & Deep Orange, 25 <> N over 031	Clomipramine HCl 25 mg	by Novopharm	55953-0031	OCD
25 <> N031	Cap, Bright Yellow & Deep Orange, 25 <> N over 031	Clomipramine HCl 25 mg	by Novopharm	43806-0031	OCD
25 <> N343	Tab, 2.5 <> N 343	Glyburide 2.5 mg	by Kaiser	62224-1331	Antidiabetic
25 <> N343	Tab, 2.5 <> N343	Glyburide 2.5 mg	by Warrick	59930-1622	Antidiabetic
25 <> N343	Tab, Peach, Round, 2.5 <> N over 343	Glyburide 2.5 mg	by Novopharm	55953-0343	Antidiabetic
25 <> N343	Tab, Scored, 2.5 <> N over 343	Glyburide 2.5 mg	by Medirex	57480-0408	Antidiabetic
25 <> N343	Tab, Peach, Round, Scored	Glyburide 2.5 mg	by Murfreesboro Ph	51129-1405	Antidiabetic
25 <> N343	Tab, 2.5 <> N Over 343	Glyburide 2.5 mg	by Quality Care	62682-5006	Antidiabetic
25 <> N343	Tab, Pale Peach, Round, Scored, 2.5 <> N 343	Glyburide 2.5 mg	by Allscripts	54569-3830	Antidiabetic
25 <> N343	Tab, Peach, Round	Glyburide 2.5 mg	by Heartland Healthcare	61392-0709	Antidiabetic
25 <> N343	Tab, 2.5 <> N/343	Glyburide 2.5 mg	by Brightstone	62939-3221	Antidiabetic
25 <> N343	Tab, 2.5 <> N over 343	Glyburide 2.5 mg	by Zenith Goldline	00182-2646	Antidiabetic
25 <> N343	Tab, 2.5 <> N 343	Glyburide 2.5 mg	by HL Moore	00839-8040	Antidiabetic
25 <> N343	Tab, Peach, Round, Scored, 2.5 <> N over 343	Glyburide 2.5 mg	Micronase by UDL	51079-0872	Antidiabetic
25 <> N343	Tab, Peach, Round, 2.5 <> N 343	Glyburide 2.5 mg	by Novopharm	43806-0343	Antidiabetic
25 <> N343	Tab, 2.5 <> N 343	Glyburide 2.5 mg	by Major	00904-5076	Antidiabetic
25 <> N420	Cap, Light Green	Indomethacin 25 mg	by Allscripts	54569-0277	NSAID
25 <> N420	Cap, Light Green	Indomethacin 25 mg	by Quality Care	60346-0684	NSAID
25 <> N420	Cap	Indomethacin 25 mg	by Apotheca	12634-0455	NSAID
25 <> N837	Tab, Film Coated, 2.5	Indapamide 2.5 mg	by Novopharm	55953-0837	Diuretic
25 <> N837	Tab, Film Coated, 2.5	Indapamide 2.5 mg	by Novopharm	43806-0837	Diuretic
25 <> NORVASC	Tab, White, Diamond Shaped, 2.5 <> Norvasc	Amlodipine Besylate	Norvasc by Pfizer	00069-1520	Antihypertensive
25 <> NORVASC	Tab, 2.5 <> Norvasc	Amlodipine Besylate	Norvasc by Murfreesboro	51129-1260	Antihypertensive
25 <> NORVASC	Tab, 2.5 <> Norvasc	Amlodipine Besylate	Norvasc by Physicians Total Care	54868-3853	Antihypertensive
25 <> NORVASC	Tab, 2.5 <> Norvasc	Amlodipine Besylate	Norvasc by DRX	55045-2377	Antihypertensive
25 <> PERCOCET	Tab, Pink, Oval	Acetaminophen 325 mg, Oxycodone HCl 2.5 mg	Percocet by Allscripts	54569-4695	Analgesic; C II
25 <> PERCOCET	Tab, White, Round, Scored	Clorazepate Dipotassium 15 mg	Percocet by Allscripts	54569-4586	Antianxiety; C IV
25 <> PERCOCET	Tab, Pink, Oval, Percocet <> 2.5	Oxycodone HCl 5 mg, Acetaminophen 325 mg	Percocet by West Pharm	52967-0278	Analgesic; C II
25 <> PERCOCET	Tab, Pink, Oval, 2.5 <> Percocet	Oxycodone HCl 2.5 mg, Acetaminophen 325 mg	Percocet by Endo	63481-0627	Analgesic; C II
25 <> PRECOSE	Tab	Acarbose 25 mg	Precose by Bayer	00026-2863	Antidiabetic
25 <> PREMARIN	Tab, Film Coated, 2.5	Estrogens, Conjugated 2.5 mg	Premarin by Quality Care	60346-0859	Hormone
25 <> PROVERA	Tab, 2.5 <> Upjohn	Medroxyprogesterone Acetate 2.5 mg	Provera by Quality Care	60346-0848	Progestin
25 <> SANDOZ	Tab, Red, Round, Sugar Coated	Mesoridazine Besylate 25 mg	Serentil by Novartis	Canadian DIN# 00027456	Antipsychotic
25 <> THERRX	Tab, Peach, Oblong, Film Coated, Scored	Ascorbic Acid 50 mg; Calcium Carbonate 250 mg; Cyanocobalamin 12 mcg; Cholecalciferol 6 mcg; Thiamine Mononitrate 3 mg; Riboflavin 3.4 mg; Niacinamide 20 mg; Pyridozine HCl 20 mg; Folic Acid 1 mg; Magnesium Oxide 50 mg; Zinc Sulfate 15 mg; Cupric sulfate	Precare Prenatal by KV Pharm	10609-1445	Vitamin

ID FRONT <> BACK	DESCRIPTION FRONT <> BACK	INGREDIENT & STRENGTH	BRAND (OR EQUIV.) & FIRM	NDC#	CLASS; SCH.
25 <> TOP	Tab, White, Coated	Topiramate 25 mg	Topamax by McNeil	00045-0639	Anticonvulsant
25 <> TOP	Tab, Coated	Topiramate 25 mg	Topamax by Ortho	00062-0639	Anticonvulsant
25 <> TOP	Tab, Coated	Topiramate 25 mg	Topamax by McNeil	52021-0639	Anticonvulsant
25 <> U121	Tab, White, Round, Scored, 2.5 <> U 121	Minoxidil 2.5 mg	by Pharmacia	Canadian DIN# 00514497	Antihypertensive
25 <> VIDEX	Tab, Mottled Off-White to Light Orange & Yellow, Orange Specks, Chewable	Didanosine 25 mg	Videx T by Bristol Myers Squibb	00087-6650	Antiviral
25 <> VOLTAREN	Tab, Yellow, Round, Enteric Coated	Diclofenac Sodium 25 mg	Voltaren by Novartis	Canadian DIN# 00514004	NSAID
25 <> ZAROXOLYN	Tab, Debossed, 2.5 <> Zaroxolyn	Metolazone 2.5 mg	Zaroxolyn by Drug Distr	52985-0218	Diuretic
250	Tab, Orange, Oval, Enteric Coated	Divalproex Sodium 250 mg	by Nu Pharm	Canadian DIN# 02239518	Anticonvulsant
250	Tab, Pink, Oblong	Niacin SR 250 mg	Slo Niacin by Upsher		Vitamin
250	Cap, Pink, Elongated	Polygel Controlled-Release Niacin 250 mg	Slo-Niacin by Upsher-Smith	00245-0062	Vitamin
250 <> 400	Tab, Red, Oblong	Amoxicillin 400 mg	Amoxil by Allscripts	54569-4791	Antibiotic
250 <> 7720	Tab, Film Coated	Cefprozil 250 mg	Cefzil by Bristol Myers Squibb	00087-7720	Antibiotic
250 <> ABANA	Cap	Guaifenesin 250 mg, Pseudoephedrine HCl 90 mg	Nasabid by Sovereign	58716-0005	Cold Remedy
250 <> AMOXIL	Tab, Chewable	Amoxicillin Trihydrate	by Quality Care	60346-0450	Antibiotic
250 <> AMOXIL	Tab, Chewable	Amoxicillin Trihydrate	by Allscripts	54569-0097	Antibiotic
250 <> AMOXILR	Cap, Navy Blue	Amoxicillin 250 mg	by Quality Care	60346-0655	Antibiotic
250 <> AMOXILR	Cap	Amoxicillin 250 mg	by Quality Care	60346-0655	Antibiotic
250 <> AMP	Cap, Light Blue & White	Ampicillin Trihydrate 250 mg	by Teva	00093-5145	Antibiotic
250 <> AP7491	Cap	Cefaclor Monohydrate	by Golden State	60429-0701	Antibiotic
250 <> AP7491	Cap	Cefaclor Monohydrate	by Apothecon	59772-7491	Antibiotic
250 <> CIPRO	Tab, Slightly Yellowish, Film Coated	Ciprofloxacin HCl	Cipro by HJ Harkins Co	52959-0171	Antibiotic
250 <> CIPRO	Tab, Yellow, Oblong	Ciprofloxacin HCl 250 mg	Cipro by Direct Dispensing	57866-6250	Antibiotic
250 <> CIPRO	Tab, Film Coated	Ciprofloxacin HCl 291.5 mg	Cipro by Amerisource	62584-0335	Antibiotic
250 <> CIPRO	Tab, Pale Yellow, Film Coated	Ciprofloxacin HCl 291.5 mg	Cipro by Quality Care	60346-0433	Antibiotic
250 <> CIPRO	Tab, Film Coated	Ciprofloxacin HCl 291.5 mg	Ciprobay by Bayer	00026-8512	Antibiotic
250 <> CIPRO	Tab, Film Coated	Ciprofloxacin HCl 291.5 mg	Cipro by Nat Pharmpak Serv	55154-4806	Antibiotic
250 <> CIPRO	Tab, Film Coated	Ciprofloxacin HCl 291.5 mg	Cipro by Apotheca	12634-0423	Antibiotic
250 <> FAMVIR	Tab, Film Coated	Famciclovir 250 mg	Famvir by SKB	60351-4116	Antiviral
250 <> FAMVIR	Tab, White, Round, Film Coated,	Famciclovir 250 mg	Famvir by SKB	00007-4116	Antiviral
250 <> FAMVIR	Tab, White, Round, Film Coated	Famciclovir 250 mg	Famvir by Novartis	00078-0367	Antiviral
250 <> FAMVIR	Tab, Film Coated	Famciclovir 250 mg	Famvir by Physicians Total Care	54868-3969	Antiviral
250 <> FAMVIR	Tab, White, Round, Film Coated	Famciclovir 250 mg	by SmithKline SKB	Canadian DIN# 02229129	Antiviral
250 <> GLAXO	Tab, White, Oblong	Cefuroxime Axetil 250 mg	Ceftin by Glaxo Wellcome	00173-7004	Antibiotic
250 <> GRISPEG	Tab, Film Coated, 250 <> Gris-Peg	Griseofulvin 250 mg	Gris Peg by Quality Care	60346-0953	Antifungal
250 <> GRISPEG	Tab, Film Coated, 250 <> Gris-Peg	Griseofulvin 250 mg	Gris Peg by Leiner	59606-0654	Antifungal
250 <> GRISPEG	Tab, Film Coated	Griseofulvin 250 mg	Gris Peg by Amerisource	62584-0773	Antifungal
250 <> GRISPEG	Tab, Film Coated	Griseofulvin 250 mg	Gris Peg by Novartis	00043-0801	Antifungal
250 <> GRISPEG	Tab, Film Coated	Griseofulvin 250 mg	Gris-Peg by Allergan	00023-0773	Antifungal
250 <> INV	Tab, White, Oblong, Film Coated	Hydroxychloroquine Sulfate 200 mg	by Murfreesboro Ph	51129-1426	Antimalarial
250 <> INV	Tab, White, Oblong, Film Coated	Hydroxychloroquine Sulfate 200 mg	by DRX Pharm Consults	55045-2766	Antimalarial
250 <> INV	Tab, Film Coated	Hydroxychloroquine Sulfate 200 mg	by Invamed	52189-0250	Antimalarial
250 <> LAMISIL	Tab, White To Off White, Round, Scored	Terbinafine HCl 250 mg	Lamisil by Novartis Pharms (CA)	61615-0100	Antifungal
250 <> LAMISIL	Tab, White to Yellow-Tinged White, Round	Terbinafine HCl 250 mg	Lamisil by Novartis	00078-0179	Antifungal

ID FRONT <> BACK	DESCRIPTION FRONT <> BACK	INGREDIENT & STRENGTH	BRAND (OR EQUIV.) & FIRM	NDC#	CLASS; SCH.
250 <> LAMISIL	Tab, Lamisil in Circular Form	Terbinafine HCl 250 mg	Lamisil by Novartis	17088-9586	Antifungal
250 <> LEVAQUIN	Tab, Pink, Square	Levofloxacin 250 mg	Levaquin by Allscripts	54569-4915	Antibiotic
250 <> LN72Y	Cap	Amoxicillin 250 mg	by Geneva	00781-2020	Antibiotic
250 <> MCNEIL1520	Tab, Terra Cotta Pink, Modified Rectangle, Film Coated	Levofloxacin 250 mg	Levaquin by Ortho	00062-1520	Antibiotic
250 <> MCNEIL1520	Tab, Coated	Levofloxacin 250 mg	Levaquin by McNeil	00045-1520	Antibiotic
250 <> MCNEIL1520	Tab, Film Coated	Levofloxacin 250 mg	Levaquin by Johnson & Johnson	59604-0520	Antibiotic
250 <> MYLAN106	Tab, Film Coated	Erythromycin Stearate	by Quality Care	60346-0580	Antibiotic
250 <> MYLAN106	Tab, Film Coated, 250 <> Mylan over 106	Erythromycin Stearate	by Diversified Hlthcare Serv	55887-0994	Antibiotic
250 <> MYLAN106	Tab, Film Coated, 250 <> Mylan over 106	Erythromycin Stearate	by Prescription Dispensing	61807-0013	Antibiotic
250 <> MYLAN106	Tab, Film Coated, 250 <> Mylan over 106	Erythromycin Stearate	by Mylan	00378-0106	Antibiotic
250 <> MYLAN210	Tab, Green, Scored, 250 <> Mylan over 210	Chlorpropamide 250 mg	by Mylan	00378-0210	Antidiabetic
250 <> MYLAN210	Tab	Chlorpropamide 250 mg	by Physicians Total Care	54868-0036	Antidiabetic
250 <> MYLAN210	Tab, Green, Round, Scored, 250 <> Mylan over 210	Chlorpropamide 250 mg	Diabinese by UDL	51079-0203	Antidiabetic
250 <> MYLAN217	Tab, White, Scored, 250 <> Mylan over 217	Tolazamide 250 mg	by Mylan	00378-0217	Antidiabetic
250 <> N084	Cap, N Over 084	Cephalexin Monohydrate	by St Marys Med	60760-0008	Antibiotic
250 <> N084	Cap, 250 <> N over 084	Cephalexin Monohydrate	by HJ Harkins Co	52959-0030	Antibiotic
250 <> N084	Cap, 250 <> N over 084	Cephalexin Monohydrate	by Apotheca	12634-0433	Antibiotic
250 <> N084	Cap, Gray & Swedish Orange, 250 <> N over 084	Cephalexin Monohydrate 541 mg	by Novopharm	43806-0114	Antibiotic
250 <> N084250	Cap, 250 <> N over 084	Cephalexin Monohydrate	by Prescription Dispensing	61807-0005	Antibiotic
250 <> N253	Cap, Light Orange & White	Cefaclor Monohydrate	by Novopharm	55953-0253	Antibiotic
250 <> N253	Cap, 250 <> N over 253	Cefaclor Monohydrate	by Qualitest	00603-2586	Antibiotic
250 <> N253	Cap	Cefaclor Monohydrate	by Rugby	00536-1365	Antibiotic
250 <> N253	Cap, 250 <> N over 253	Cefaclor Monohydrate	by HJ Harkins Co	52959-0367	Antibiotic
250 <> N253	Cap, Light Orange & White	Cefaclor Monohydrate	by Novopharm	43806-0253	Antibiotic
250 <> N253	Cap, 250 <> N over 253	Cefaclor Monohydrate	by Major	00904-5204	Antibiotic
250 <> N253	Cap, Bright Orange & White, Opaque, 250 <> N over 253	Cefaclor Monohydrate 250 mg	Ceclor by UDL	51079-0617	Antibiotic
250 <> N517	Tab, Light Yellow	Naproxen 250 mg	by Quality Care	60346-0816	NSAID
250 <> N517	Tab, Peach & Yellow, Oval, N Over 517	Naproxen 250 mg	by Novopharm	55953-0517	NSAID
250 <> N724	Cap, Buff & Caramel	Amoxicillin 250 mg	by Quality Care	60346-0655	Antibiotic
250 <> N724	Cap, 250 <> N over 724	Amoxicillin Trihydrate	by Qualitest	00603-2266	Antibiotic
250 <> N724	Cap, Buff & Caramel, 250 <> N over 724	Amoxicillin 250 mg	by Novopharm	43806-0724	Antibiotic
250 <> N724	Cap, 250 <> N over 724	Amoxicillin 250 mg	by Apotheca	12634-0185	Antibiotic
250 <> N741	Cap, Dark Green & Light Orange, Engraved in Black Ink <> White Granular Powder	Mexiletine HCl 250 mg	by Novopharm	55953-0741	Antiarrhythmic
250 <> N741	Cap, Black Ink	Mexiletine HCl 250 mg	by Warrick	59930-1687	Antiarrhythmic
250 <> N741	Cap	Mexiletine HCl 250 mg	by Brightstone	62939-2332	Antiarrhythmic
250 <> N751	Tab, Pink, Rond, Scored, 250 <> N over 751	Amoxicillin Trihydrate 250 mg	by Novopharm	43806-0751	Antibiotic
250 <> N751	Tab, Cherry & Rose, Chewable, 250 <> N over 751	Amoxicillin Trihydrate 310 mg	by Novopharm	55953-0751	Antibiotic
250 <> N751	Tab, Chewable, N/751	Amoxicillin Trihydrate 310 mg	by Warrick	59930-1611	Antibiotic
250 <> NAPROSYN	Tab	Naproxen 250 mg	Naprosyn by HJ Harkins Co	52959-0110	NSAID
250 <> NORTRIPTYLINE10	Cap, Green & White	Nortriptyline HCl 10 mg	by HJ Harkins	52959-0358	Antidepressant
250 <> SYCTCP	Tab, White, Oval, Film Coated, 250 <> Syc-TCP	Ticlopidine HCl 250 mg	by Altimed	Canadian DIN# 02194422	Anticoagulant
250 <> TICLID	Tab, Film Coated, Printed in Blue	Ticlopidine HCl 250 mg	Ticlid by Wal Mart	49035-0165	Anticoagulant
250 <> TICLID	Tab, Film Coated, Printed in Blue	Ticlopidine HCl 250 mg	by Med Pro	53978-3027	Anticoagulant
250 <> TICLID	Tab, Film Coated, Printed in Blue	Ticlopidine HCl 250 mg	Ticlid by Physicians Total Care	54868-3783	Anticoagulant
250 <> TICLID	Tab, Film Coated, Printed in Blue	Ticlopidine HCl 250 mg	Ticlid by Quality Care	60346-0702	Anticoagulant
250 <> TICLID	Tab, Film Coated, Printed in Blue	Ticlopidine HCl 250 mg	Ticlid by Hoffmann La Roche	00004-0018	Anticoagulant
250 <> TICLID	Tab, Film Coated, Printed in Blue	Ticlopidine HCl 250 mg	Ticlid by Syntex	18393-0431	Anticoagulant
250 <> UCB	Tab, Blue, Oblong, Scored, Film Coated	Levetiracetam 250 mg	Keppra by UCB Pharma	50474-0591	Anticonvulsant

ID FRONT <> BACK	DESCRIPTION FRONT <> BACK	INGREDIENT & STRENGTH	BRAND (OR EQUIV.) & FIRM	NDC#	CLASS; SCH.
2500V	Cap	Chlorpheniramine Maleate 8.8 mg	by Vintage	00254-2500	Antihistamine
250125 <> AUGMENTIN	Tab, White, Oval	Amoxicillin Trihydrate 500 mg; Clavulanate Potassium 125 mg	Augmentin by Southwood Pharms	58016-0107	Antibiotic
250125 <> AUGMENTIN	Tab, Film Coated	Amoxicillin Trihydrate, Clavulanate Potassium	Augmentin by Casa De Amigos	62138-6075	Antibiotic
250125 <> AUGMENTIN	Tab, Film Coated	Amoxicillin Trihydrate, Clavulanate Potassium	Augmentin by Pharmedix	53002-0250	Antibiotic
2501V	Cap	Chlorpheniramine Maleate 12 mg	by Vintage	00254-2501	Antihistamine
25025 <> NU	Tab, Blue, Oval, Scored, 250 over 50 <> NU	Carbidopa 25 mg, Levodopa 250 mg	by Nu Pharm	Canadian DIN# 02182831	Antiparkinson
25025APO	Tab, Blue, Oval, 250/25/APO	Levodopa 250 mg, Carbidopa 25 mg	Levocarb by Apotex	Canadian	Antiparkinson
25025ENDO	Tab, Apple & Blue, Oval, 250/25/Endo	Endo Levodopa 250 mg, Carbidopa 25 mg	by Altimed	Canadian	Antiparkinson
250425	Tab	Amitriptyline HCl 25 mg, Perphenazine 4 mg	by Zenith Goldline	00182-1238	Antipsychotic
250425	Tab, 250 4-25 <> Mortar and Pestle Logo	Amitriptyline HCl 25 mg, Perphenazine 4 mg	by Royce	51875-0250	Antipsychotic
250425	Tab, Yellow, Round, Royce logo 250/4-25	Perphenazine 4 mg, Amitriptyline 25 mg	Triavil by Royce		Antipsychotic; Antidepressant
250BRISTOL7375	Cap, Blue & Purple, 250/Bristol 7375	Cephalexin 250 mg	Keflex by BMS		Antibiotic
250CP	Cap, Branded Nortriptyline	Nortriptyline 10 mg	by HL Moore	00839-7798	Antidepressant
250GLAXO	Tab, White, Oblong, 250/Glaxo	Cefuroxime Axetil 250 mg	by Glaxo	Canadian	Antibiotic
250M25 <> MOVA	Tab	Naproxen 250 mg	by Caremark	00339-5870	NSAID
250M25 <> MOVA	Tab	Naproxen 250 mg	by Martec	52555-0712	NSAID
250M25 <> MOVA	Tab, Rose, Round	Naproxen 250 mg	Naprosyn by MOVA	55370-0139	NSAID
250MG <> 7375BRISTOL	Cap, Printed in White Ink	Cephalexin Monohydrate 250 mg	by Golden State	60429-0036	Antibiotic
250MG <> ATRAL	Cap	Tetracycline HCl 250 mg	by Quality Care	60346-0609	Antibiotic
250MG <> AUGMENTIN	Tab, Film Coated	Amoxicillin Trihydrate, Clavulanate Potassium	Augmentin by Quality Care	60346-0074	Antibiotic
250MG <> EMYCIN	Tab, 250 mg <> E-Mycin	Erythromycin 250 mg	by Quality Care	60346-0630	Antibiotic
250MG <> VIRACEPT	Tab, Light Blue	Nelfinavir Mesylate	Viracept by MOVA	55370-0560	Antiviral
250MG <> VIRACEPT	Tab	Nelfinavir Mesylate	Viracept by Physicians Total Care	54868-3947	Antiviral
250MG <> VIRACEPT	Tab, Blue, Oblong	Nelfinavir Mesylate 250 mg	Viracept by Allscripts	54569-4543	Antiviral
250MG <> VIRACEPT	Tab	Nelfinavir Mesylate 292.25 mg	Viracept by Circa	71114-4206	Antiviral
250MG <> VIRACEPT	Tab	Nelfinavir Mesylate 292.25 mg	Viracept by Patheon	63285-0010	Antiviral
250MG <> VIRACEPT	Tab, Light Blue	Nelfinavir Mesylate 292.25 mg	Viracept by Agouron	63010-0010	Antiviral
250MG <> WATSON493	Cap	Mexiletine HCl 250 mg	by Watson	52544-0493	Antiarrhythmic
250MG <> Z4760CEFACLOR	Cap, 250 mg <> Zenith Logo 4760 Cefaclor	Cefaclor Monohydrate 250 mg	by Allscripts	54569-3901	Antibiotic
250MLA05	Cap, Blue & White, 250ML-A05	Cefaclor 250 mg	Ceclor by MOVA	55370-0894	Antibiotic
250MLA07	Cap, Green & White, 250ML-A07	Cephalexin 250 mg	Keflex by MOVA	55370-0900	Antibiotic
250MYLAN106	Tab, Film Coated	Erythromycin Stearate	by Med Pro	53978-5029	Antibiotic
250NAXEN	Tab, Yellow, Oval, 250/Naxen	Naproxen 250 mg	Navalbine by B.W. Inc	Canadian	NSAID
251	Tab, Orange, Round, Schering Logo 251	Halazepam 20 mg	Paxipam by Schering		Antianxiety; C IV
251	Tab, Red, Round	Pseudoephedrine HCl 30 mg	Sudafed by Granutec		Decongestant
251 <> NORTRIPTYLINE25	Cap, Green & White	Nortriptyline HCl 25 mg	by HJ Harkins	52959-0359	Antidepressant
25102 <> JACOBUS	Tab, 25/102 <> Jacobus	Dapsone 25 mg	by Jacobus	49938-0102	Antimycobacterial
25102 <> JACOBUS	Tab, 25 over 102 <> Jacobus	Dapsone 25 mg	by PDRX	55289-0188	Antimycobacterial
251CP	Cap, Branded Nortriptyline 25MG	Nortriptyline HCl 25 mg	by HL Moore	00839-7799	Antidepressant
251CP <> NORTRIPTYLINE25	Cap, Imprinted in Black Ink <> Imprinted in White Ink	Nortriptyline HCl 25 mg	by Prescription Dispensing	61807-0142	Antidepressant
252	Tab, Film Coated, Barr Logo	Dipyridamole 25 mg	by Kaiser	00179-1153	Antiplatelet
252 <> 1571	Tab	Phenobarbital 64.8 mg	by United Res	00677-0762	Sedative/Hypnotic; C IV
252 <> B	Tab, Film Coated, Barr Logo	Dipyridamole 25 mg	by Quality Care	60346-0789	Antiplatelet
252 <> B	Tab, Film Coated	Dipyridamole 25 mg	by Heartland	61392-0549	Antiplatelet

ID FRONT <> BACK	DESCRIPTION FRONT <> BACK	INGREDIENT & STRENGTH	BRAND (OR EQUIV.) & FIRM	NDC#	CLASS; SCH.
252 <> B	Tab, Film Coated, Barr Logo	Dipyridamole 25 mg	by Geneva	00781-1890	Antiplatelet
252 <> B	Tab, Film Coated, Schein Logo	Dipyridamole 25 mg	by Schein	00364-2491	Antiplatelet
252 <> B	Tab, Film Coated, Barr Logo	Dipyridamole 25 mg	by Barr	00555-0252	Antiplatelet
252 <> B	Tab, White, Round, Film Coated	Dipyridamole 25 mg	Persantine by UDL	51079-0068	Antiplatelet
252 <> INV	Tab, Film Coated	Cyclobenzaprine HCl 10 mg	by Physicians Total Care	54868-1110	Muscle Relaxant
2520220	Tab, Natural, Round, 252/0220	Thyroid 130 mg	by Jones		Thyroid
2520400	Tab	Phenobarbital 16.2 mg	by United Res	00677-0236	Sedative/Hypnotic; C IV
2520400	Tab, 252/0400	Phenobarbital 16.2 mg	by JMI Canton	00252-6712	Sedative/Hypnotic; C IV
2520400	Tab, 252/0400, Compressed	Phenobarbital 16.2 mg	by Kaiser	00179-0602	Sedative/Hypnotic; C IV
2520400	Tab, 252/0400	Phenobarbital 16.2 mg	by Jones	52604-6712	Sedative/Hypnotic; C IV
2520400	Tab, 252/0400	Phenobarbital 16.2 mg	by HL Moore	00839-1478	Sedative/Hypnotic; C IV
2520401	Tab, 252/0401	Phenobarbital 30 mg	by Rugby	00536-4224	Sedative/Hypnotic; C IV
2520401	Tab, 252/0401, Compressed Powder	Phenobarbital 30 mg	by Kaiser	00179-0601	Sedative/Hypnotic; C IV
2520401	Tab	Phenobarbital 30 mg	by Zenith Goldline	00182-0292	Sedative/Hypnotic; C IV
2520401	Tab, 252/0401	Phenobarbital 30 mg	by JMI Canton	00252-6722	Sedative/Hypnotic; C IV
2520401	Tab, 252/0401	Phenobarbital 30 mg	by Jones	52604-6722	Sedative/Hypnotic; C IV
2520401	Tab, White, Round, Scored, Debossed 252 0401	Phenobarbital 30 mg	by Physicians Total Care	54868-3903	Sedative/Hypnotic; C IV
2520401	Tab, 252/0401	Phenobarbital 30 mg	by HL Moore	00839-1484	Sedative/Hypnotic; C IV
2520494	Tab, Natural, Round, 252/0494	Thyroid 32 mg	by Jones		Thyroid
2520495	Tab, Natural, Round, 252/0495	Thyroid 65 mg	by Jones		Thyroid
2521571	Tab, 252/1571, Compressed	Phenobarbital 64.8 mg	by Kaiser	00179-1019	Sedative/Hypnotic; C IV
2521571	Tab	Phenobarbital 64.8 mg	by Zenith Goldline	00182-0590	Sedative/Hypnotic; C IV
2521571	Tab, 252/1571	Phenobarbital 64.8 mg	by JMI Canton	00252-6731	Sedative/Hypnotic; C IV
2521571	Tab, 252/0401	Phenobarbital 64.8 mg	by Jones	52604-6731	Sedative/Hypnotic; C IV
2521571	Tab, 252/1571	Phenobarbital 64.8 mg	by HL Moore	00839-6257	Sedative/Hypnotic; C IV
252252 <> PROVENTIL2	Tab, Off-White, Round, 252 over 252 <> Proventil 2	Albuterol Sulfate 2.41 mg	Proventil by Schering	00085-0252	Antiasthmatic
2523089	Tab	Phenobarbital 30 mg	by United Res	00677-0237	Sedative/Hypnotic; C IV
2523089	Tab, 252/3089	Phenobarbital 97.2 mg	by JMI Canton	00252-6740	Sedative/Hypnotic; C IV
2523089	Tab, 252/3089	Phenobarbital 97.2 mg	by Jones	52604-6740	Sedative/Hypnotic; C IV
2523089	Tab	Phenobarbital 97.2 mg	by United Res	00677-0238	Sedative/Hypnotic; C IV
25237	Tab, Chew, 252/37	Sodium Fluoride 2.2 mg	by JMI Canton	00252-7928	Element
25237	Tab, Chew, 252-37	Sodium Fluoride 2.2 mg	by Quality Care	60346-0263	Element
25237	Tab	Sodium Fluoride 2.2 mg	by United Res	00677-0132	Element
252389	Tab, White, Round, 252-389	Phenobarbital 100 mg	by Bowman		Sedative/Hypnotic; C IV
2525	Cap	Butalbital 50 mg, Aspirin 200 mg, Phenacetin 130 mg, Caffeine 40 mg	Marnal by Vortech		Analgesic; C III
2525	Tab, Ivory, Round, 25/25	Hydrochlorothiazide 25 mg, Spironolactone 25 mg	Novo Spirozine by Novopharm	Canadian	Diuretic; Antihypertensive
25255050 <> MP168	Tab, 25 in 2 quadrants and 50 in 2 quadrants	Trazodone HCl 150 mg	by Rugby	00536-4691	Antidepressant
25255050 <> MP168	Tab, White, Round, Scored, 25 in the Two top quadrants, 50 in the Two bottom quadrants <> MP 168	Trazodone HCl 150 mg	by Teva	00480-0319	Antidepressant
25255050 <> MP168	Tab, 25 25 / 50 50	Trazodone HCl 150 mg	by Allscripts	54569-3732	Antidepressant
253 <> MIA	Cap, White Print	Acetaminophen 325 mg, Dichloralantipyrine 100 mg, Isomeptene Mucate (2:1) 65 mg	Midrin by Carnrick	00086-0120	Analgesic
253 <> MIA	Cap, White Print	Acetaminophen 325 mg, Dichloralantipyrine 100 mg, Isometheptene Mucate (1:1) 65 mg	Migratine by Major	00904-7622	Analgesic
254	Tab, White, Round	Triprolidine HCl 2.5 mg, Pseudoephedrine 60 mg	Actifed by Granutec		Cold Remedy
255	Tab, Yellow, Round	Chlorpheniramine 4 mg	Chlor-Trimeton by Granutec		Antihistamine
255 <> 10	Tab, 10/Royce Logo	Baclofen 10 mg	by Qualitest	00603-2408	Muscle Relaxant
2550	Tab, Peach, Round, 25/50	Triamterene 25 mg, Hydrochlorothiazide 50 mg	Novo Triamzide by Novopharm	Canadian	Diuretic
25510	Tab, White, Oval, Royce Logo 255/10	Baclofen 10 mg	Lioresal by Royce		Muscle Relaxant
25510	Tab, 255 10 <> Mortar and Pestle Logo	Baclofen 10 mg	by Royce	51875-0255	Muscle Relaxant

ID FRONT <> BACK	DESCRIPTION FRONT <> BACK	INGREDIENT & STRENGTH	BRAND (OR EQUIV.) & FIRM	NDC#	CLASS; SCH.
256 <> 2	Tab, White, Round	Betahistine HCl 8 mg	SERC by Solvay Pharma	Canadian DIN# 02240601	Antivertigo
256 <> 20	Tab, 20/Royce Logo	Baclofen 20 mg	by Qualitest	00603-2409	Muscle Relaxant
256 <> S	Tab, White to Off-White, Round	Betahistine Dihydrochloride 8 mg	by Solvay	Canadian DIN# 02240601	Antivertigo
25620	Tab, White, Round, Royce Logo 256/20	Baclofen 20 mg	Lioresal by Royce		Muscle Relaxant
25620	Tab, 256 20 <> Mortar and Pestle Logo	Baclofen 20 mg	by Royce	51875-0256	Muscle Relaxant
25650 <> WATSON	Tab, Light Aqua, Cap-Shaped, 25/650 <> Watson	Pentazocine 25 mg, Acetaminohen 650 mg	Talacen by Watson	52544-0396	Analgesic; C IV
257 <> 10	Tab, Coated, 257 <> 10/Royce Logo	Cyclobenzaprine HCl 10 mg	by Qualitest	00603-3077	Muscle Relaxant
25710	Tab, Coated, 257 over 10 <> Mortar and Pestle Logo	Cyclobenzaprine HCl 10 mg	by Royce	51875-0257	Muscle Relaxant
25710	Tab, Dark Yellow, Film Coated, 257/10 <> Royce Logo	Cyclobenzaprine HCl 10 mg	by Quality Care	60346-0581	Muscle Relaxant
258	Tab, Blue, Round	Diphenhydramine 25 mg	by Granutec		Antihistamine
258	Tab, Blue, Round, Sch. Logo 258	Pseudoephedrine Sulfate 120 mg	Afrinol by Schering		Decongestant
259 <> BARR	Tab, Coated	Erythromycin Ethylsuccinate	by Barr	00555-0259	Antibiotic
259 <> GG	Tab, Pink, Round, Scored, Compressed	Isosorbide Dinitrate 5 mg	Isordil by Geneva	00781-1635	Antianginal
259 <> INV	Tab	Atenolol 25 mg	by Apothecon	62269-0259	Antihypertensive
259 <> INV	Tab	Atenolol 25 mg	by Invamed	52189-0259	Antihypertensive
25DAN5542	Tab, Beige, Triangular, 25/Dan 5542	Thioridazine HCl 25 mg	Mellaril by Danbury		Antipsychotic
25FLI	Tab, Orange, Round, 25/FLI Logo	Levothyroxine Sodium 25 mcg	by Forest	00456-0320	Antithyroid
25FLINT	Tab	Levothyroxine Sodium 0.025 mg	Synthroid by Med Pro	53978-1221	Antithyroid
25LLA13	Tab, White, Heptagonal	Amoxapine 25 mg	Asendin by Lederle		Antidepressant
25M	Tab, Mova	Levothyroxine Sodium 25 mcg	Euthyrox by Em Pharma	63254-0435	Antithyroid
25M	Tab	Levothyroxine Sodium 25 mcg	Levo T by MOVA	55370-0125	Antithyroid
25MCG	Tab	Levothyroxine Sodium 25 mcg	Eltroxin by Glaxo	53873-0104	Antithyroid
25MCG <> FLINT	Tab, Orange, Round, Scored	Levothyroxine Sodium 0.025 mg	Synthroid by Rightpac	65240-0739	Antithyroid
25MCG <> FLINT	Tab, Debossed	Levothyroxine Sodium 0.025 mg	Synthroid by Amerisource	62584-0020	Antithyroid
25MG	Cap, White	Cyclosporine 25 mg	Gengraf by Abbott Labs	00074-6463	Immunosuppressant
25MG <> CLOZARIL	Tab, Pale Yellow, Round, Scored	Clozapine 25 mg	Clozaril by Novartis	Canadian DIN# 00894737	Antipsychotic
25MG <> NEORAL	Cap	Cyclosporine 25 mg	Sandimmun Neoral B63 by RP Scherer	11014-1197	Immunosuppressant
25MG <> WATSON371	Cap, Green & White	Loxapine Succinate 25 mg	by Dixon Shane	17236-0695	Antipsychotic
25MG <> WATSON371	Cap, Green & White, Opaque, 25 mg <> Watson over 371	Loxapine 25 mg	Loxitane by UDL	51079-0902	Antipsychotic
25MG <> WATSON371	Cap	Loxapine Succinate	by Physicians Total Care	54868-2478	Antipsychotic
25MG <> WATSON371	Cap, 25mg <> Watson Over 371	Loxapine Succinate	by UDL	51079-0679	Antipsychotic
25MG <> WATSON371	Cap	Loxapine Succinate	by Geneva	00781-2712	Antipsychotic
25MG <> WATSON371	Cap	Loxapine Succinate	by HL Moore	00839-7497	Antipsychotic
25MG <> WATSON371	Cap	Loxapine Succinate	by Major	00904-2312	Antipsychotic
25MG <> WATSON371	Cap	Loxapine Succinate	by United Res	00677-1320	Antipsychotic
25MG <> WATSON594	Cap	Clomipramine HCl 25 mg	by Watson	52544-0594	OCD
25MG <> WATSON696	Cap	Doxepin HCl 28.35 mg	by Watson	52544-0696	Antidepressant
25MG <> WATSON696	Cap	Doxepin HCl 28.35 mg	by Martec	52555-0295	Antidepressant
25MG <> ZOLOFT	Tab, Light Green, Cap-Shaped, Film Coated	Sertraline HCl	Zoloft by Roerig	00049-4960	Antidepressant
25MG <> ZOLOFT	Tab, Light Green, Film Coated	Sertraline HCl	Zoloft by Murfreesboro	51129-1333	Antidepressant
25MG <> ZOLOFT	Tab, Film Coated	Sertraline HCl	Zoloft by Allscripts	54569-4529	Antidepressant
25MG <> ZOLOFT	Tab, Light Green, Oblong, Scored	Sertraline HCl 25 mg	Zoloft by Phcy Care	65070-0210	Antidepressant
25MG <> ZOLOFT	Tab, Light Green, Oblong, Scored	Sertraline HCl 25 mg	Zoloft by Direct Dispensing	57866-1057	Antidepressant
25MGLEDERLEL3	Cap, Green	Loxapine 25 mg	Loxitane by Lederle		Antipsychotic
25MGSAMPLE <> MACRODANTIN	Cap, White w/ Yellow Powder, Opaque	Nitrofurantoin 25 mg	Macrodantin by Procter & Gamble	00149-0007	Antibiotic

ID FRONT <> BACK	DESCRIPTION FRONT <> BACK	INGREDIENT & STRENGTH	BRAND (OR EQUIV.) & FIRM	NDC#	CLASS; SCH.
25NOVO	Tab, Beige, Round, 25/Novo	Clomipramine HCl 25 mg	Novo Clopamine by Novopharm	Canadian	OCD
25W <> 701	Tab	Venlafaxine HCl	Effexor by Quality Care	62682-7029	Antidepressant
25Z2160	Tab, White, Round, 2.5 Z/2160	Conjugated Estrogens 2.5 mg	Premarin by Zenith		Estrogen
26 <> BL	Tab, Orange, Round, Coated, Scored	Amitriptyline HCl 100 mg	by Teva	00093-2128	Antidepressant
26 <> GG	Tab, White, Round, Scored, Compressed	Isosorbide Dinitrate 10 mg	Isordil by Geneva	00781-1556	Antianginal
260 <> DBETHEX	Tab, Coated, Scored	Ascorbic Acid 100 mg, Biotin 30 mcg, Calcium Carbonate, Precipitated 250 mg, Chromic Chloride 25 mcg, Cupric Oxide 2 mg, Cyanocobalamin 12 mcg, Ferrous Fumarate 60 mg, Folic Acid 1 mg, Magnesium Oxide 25 mg, Manganese Sulfate 5 mg, Niacinamide 20 mg, Pantothenic Acid 10 mg, Potassium Iodide 150 mcg, Pyridoxine HCl 10 mg, Riboflavin 3.4 mg, Sodium Molybdate 25 mcg, Thiamine HCl 3 mg, Vitamin A 5000 Units, Vitamin D 400 Units, Vitamin E 30 Units, Zinc Oxide 25 mg	Prenatal Mtr by KV	10609-1351	Vitamin
260 <> WESTWARD	Tab, White, Round	Isoniazid 100 mg	by Allscripts	54569-2942	Antimycobacterial
260 <> WESTWARD	Tab, White, Round	Isoniazid 100 mg	Isoniazid by West Ward	00143-1260	Antimycobacterial
260 <> WESTWARD	Tab	Isoniazid 100 mg	Isoniazid by Versapharm	61748-0016	Antimycobacterial
260 <> WESTWARD	Tab	Isoniazid 100 mg	Isoniazid by Amerisource	62584-0759	Antimycobacterial
260R <> 384	Tab, White, Round	Quinine Sulfate 260 mg	Quinamm by Zenith Goldline	00172-3001	Antimalarial
260R <> 384	Tab, White, Round	Quinine Sulfate 260 mg	Quinamm by Zenith Goldline	00182-8615	Antimalarial
261 <> INV	Tab, White, Round	Methazolamide 25 mg	by Invamed	52189-0261	Diuretic
261 <> INV	Tab, White, Round	Methazolamide 25 mg	by Apothecon	62269-0261	Diuretic
261 <> WESTWARD	Tab	Isoniazid 300 mg	Isoniazid by Versapharm	61748-0013	Antimycobacterial
2614SCHEIN <> CEFACLOR250MG	Cap, Purple	Cefaclor 250 mg	by Schein	00364-2614	Antibiotic
2615SCHEIN <> CEFACLOR500MG	Cap, Purple & Yellow	Cefaclor 500 mg	by Schein	00364-2615	Antibiotic
262	Tab, White, Round	Dimenhydrinate 50 mg	Dramamine by Granutec		Antiemetic
262 <> BARR	Tab, Coated, Debossed	Thioridazine HCl 50 mg	by Barr	00555-0262	Antipsychotic
263 <> BARR	Tab, Coated, Debossed	Thioridazine HCl 100 mg	by Barr	00555-0263	Antipsychotic
265 <> PAR	Tab, Coated	Amitriptyline HCl 14.145 mg, Chlordiazepoxide 5 mg	by Par	49884-0265	Antianxiety; C IV
266 <> CP	Tab, Coated, Imprinted in Black Ink	Thioridazine HCl 25 mg	by Heartland	61392-0463	Antipsychotic
266 <> MRK	Tab, Pale Pink, Cap-Shaped	Rizatriptan Benzoate 7.265 mg	Maxalt by Merck	00006-0266	Antimigraine
266 <> MRK	Tab	Rizatriptan Benzoate 7.265 mg	by Merck Sharp & Dohme	60312-0266	Antimigraine
266 <> PAR	Tab, Coated	Amitriptyline HCl 25 mg, Chlordiazepoxide 10 mg	by Par	49884-0266	Antianxiety; C IV
269	Tab, UDL Logo	Metoclopramide HCl 10 mg	by UDL	51079-0283	Gastrointestinal
269 <> R	Tab, White, Round, Scored	Metoclopramide HCl 10 mg	Reglan by UDL	51079-0283	Gastrointestinal
269 <> R	Tab, White, Round, Scored	Metoclopramide HCl 10 mg	by Purepac	00228-2269	Gastrointestinal
2690V	Tab, 2960 over V	Diethylpropion HCl 75 mg	by Quality Care	60346-0689	Antianorexiant; C IV
2690V	Tab	Diethylpropion HCl 75 mg	Durad by Macnary	55982-0008	Antianorexiant; C IV
2690V	Tab, White, Oval	Diethylpropion HCl 75 mg	by PDRX Pharms	55289-0368	Antianorexiant; C IV
2690V	Tab	Diethylpropion HCl 75 mg	by 3M	00089-0212	Antianorexiant; C IV
2690V	Tab	Diethylpropion HCl 75 mg	by United Res	00677-0436	Antianorexiant; C IV
2690V	Tab	Diethylpropion HCl 75 mg	by Qualitest	00603-3290	Antianorexiant; C IV
2690V	Tab	Diethylpropion HCl 75 mg	by Allscripts	54569-0396	Antianorexiant; C IV
27 <> 27TEGRETOL	Tab	Carbamazepine 200 mg	by Allscripts	54569-0163	Anticonvulsant
27 <> R	Tab, Orange, Round	Propranolol HCl 10 mg	by Purepac	00228-2327	Antihypertensive
270 <> CP	Tab, Coated	Thioridazine HCl 200 mg	by Creighton Prod	50752-0270	Antipsychotic
271 <> INV	Tab, Scored	Captopril 12.5 mg	by Schein	00364-2628	Antihypertensive
271 <> INV	Tab, Scored	Captopril 12.5 mg	by Invamed	52189-0271	Antihypertensive
2715	Cap	Nitrogylcerine SA 6.5 mg	Nitrobid by Vortech		Antianginal
2718	Cap	Nitrogylcerine SA 2.5 mg	Nitrobid by Vortech		Antianginal
272 <> DMSP	Tab	Carbidopa 25 mg, Levodopa 100 mg	by Murfreesboro	51129-1127	Antiparkinson

ID FRONT <> BACK	DESCRIPTION FRONT <> BACK	INGREDIENT & STRENGTH	BRAND (OR EQUIV.) & FIRM	NDC#	CLASS; SCH.
272 <> TEMAZEPAM15MG	Cap, 272 and Creighton's Logo <> Imprint in Red Ink	Temazepam 15 mg	Tem by Kaiser	00179-1106	Sedative/Hypnotic; C IV
2727 <> TEGRETOL	Tab, Pink, Cap Shaped, Scored, 27/27 <> Tegretol	Carbamazepine 200 mg	Tegretol by Novartis	00083-0027	Anticonvulsant
2727 <> TEGRETOL	Tab	Carbamazepine 200 mg	by Quality Care	60346-0777	Anticonvulsant
2727 <> TEGRETOL	Tab	Carbamazepine 200 mg	by Nat Pharmpak Serv	55154-1012	Anticonvulsant
272CP <> TEMAZEPAM15MG	Cap	Temazepam 15 mg	Tem by Creighton Prod	50752-0272	Sedative/Hypnotic; C IV
272CP <> TEMAZEPAM15MG	Cap, Body, CP <> Cap, Temazepam 15 mg is printed around the Cap in Red Ink	Temazepam 15 mg	Tem by Quality Care	60346-0668	Sedative/Hypnotic; C IV
2732 <> V	Cap	Chlordiazepoxide HCl 5 mg, Clidinium Bromide 2.5 mg	by Quality Care	60346-0780	Gastrointestinal; C IV
2732V	Cap	Chlordiazepoxide HCl 5 mg, Clidinium Bromide 2.5 mg	by Vintage	00254-2732	Gastrointestinal; C IV
273CP <> TEMAZEPAM30MG	Cap	Temazepam 30 mg	Tem by Creighton Prod	50752-0273	Sedative/Hypnotic; C IV
273CP <> TEMAZEPAM30MG	Cap, Around the Capsule in Red Ink, Body <> Around the Capsule in Red Ink	Temazepam 30 mg	Tem by Quality Care	60346-0005	Sedative/Hypnotic; C IV
273INV <> 50	Tab, 273/INV	Captopril 50 mg	by Schein	00364-2630	Antihypertensive
274 <> ETH	Tab, Coated	Hyoscyamine Sulfate 0.125 mg	by KV	10609-1352	Gastrointestinal
274 <> ETH	Tab, White, Ovaloid, Coated, Debossed, Partially Bisected	Hyoscyamine Sulfate 0.125 mg	Levsin by Ethex	58177-0274	Gastrointestinal
274 <> GG	Tab, White, Round, Scored, Compressed	Isoxsuprine HCl 10 mg	Vasodilan by Geneva	00781-1840	Vasodilator
274 <> ROCHE	Tab, Light Blue, Oval, Film Coated	Naproxen Sodium 275 mg	Anaprox by Allscripts	54569-0264	NSAID
274 <> ROCHE	Tab, Light Blue, Film Coated	Naproxen Sodium 275 mg	Anaprox by Syntex	18393-0274	NSAID
274 <> SYNTEX	Tab, Film Coated	Naproxen Sodium 275 mg	Anaprox by Allscripts	54569-0264	NSAID
274 <> SYNTEX	Tab, Light Blue, Film Coated	Naproxen Sodium 275 mg	Anaprox by Quality Care	60346-0727	NSAID
274INV <> 100	Tab, 274/INV	Captopril 100 mg	by Schein	00364-2631	Antihypertensive
275 <> CP	Tab, Creighton Logo	Acetaminophen 325 mg, Butalbital 50 mg, Caffeine 40 mg	by Quality Care	60346-0703	Analgesic
275 <> CP	Tab	Acetaminophen 325 mg, Butalbital 50 mg, Caffeine 40 mg	Fiorpap by Creighton Prod	50752-0275	Analgesic
275 <> ETHEX	Tab, White, Film Coated	Ascorbic Acid 70 mg, Calcium 200 mg, Cyanocobalamin 2.2 mcg, Folic Acid 1 mg, Iodine 175 mcg, Iron 65 mg, Magnesium 100 mg, Niacin 17 mg, Pyridoxine HCl 2.2 mg, Riboflavin 1.6 mg, Thiamine HCl 1.5 mg, Vitamin A 3000 Units, Vitamin D 400 Units, Vitamin E 10 Units, Zinc 15 mg	Prenatal Z by Ethex	58177-0275	Vitamin
275 <> ETHEX	Tab, Film Coated	Ascorbic Acid 70 mg, Calcium 200 mg, Cyanocobalamin 2.2 mcg, Folic Acid 1 mg, Iodine 175 mcg, Iron 65 mg, Magnesium 100 mg, Niacin 17 mg, Pyridoxine HCl 2.2 mg, Riboflavin 1.6 mg, Thiamine HCl 1.5 mg, Vitamin A 3000 Units, Vitamin D 400 Units, Vitamin E 10 Units, Zinc 15 mg	Prenatal Z by KV	10609-1360	Vitamin
275 <> N531	Tab, White, Round, Coated, N Over 531	Naproxen Sodium 275 mg	by Novopharm	55953-0531	NSAID
275 <> N531	Tab, Film Coated	Naproxen Sodium 275 mg	by HL Moore	00839-7889	NSAID
275 <> N531	Tab, Film Coated	Naproxen Sodium 275 mg	by Major	00904-5040	NSAID
2768	Cap	Tetracycline HCl 250 mg	Nor-Tet by Vortech		Antibiotic
277	Tab, Coated	Amitriptyline HCl 25 mg, Chlordiazepoxide 10 mg	by Qualitest	00603-2691	Antianxiety; C IV
277 <> MYLAN	Tab, White, Coated	Amitriptyline HCl 25 mg, Chlordiazepoxide 10 mg	by Mylan	00378-0277	Antianxiety; C IV
2771	Tab, White, Oval	Irbesartan 75 mg	Avapro by Sanofi	Canadian	Antihypertensive
2771	Tab, Debossed with a Heart Shape	Irbesartan 75 mg	Avapro by Bristol Myers Squibb	00087-2771	Antihypertensive
2772	Tab, White, Oval	Irbesartan 150 mg	Avapro by Sanofi	Canadian	Antihypertensive
2772	Tab, Debossed with a Heart Shape	Irbesartan 150 mg	Avapro by Bristol Myers Squibb	00087-2772	Antihypertensive
2772	Tab, White, Oval	Irbesartan 150 mg	Avapro by Murfreesboro	51129-1557	Antihypertensive
2772	Tab, Heart Shape	Irbesartan 150 mg	Avapro by Murfreesboro	51129-1339	Antihypertensive
2773	Tab, White, Oval	Irbesartan 300 mg	Avapro by Sanofi	Canadian	Antihypertensive
2773	Tab, Debossd with a Heart Shape	Irbesartan 300 mg	Avapro by Bristol Myers Squibb	00087-2773	Antihypertensive
2773	Tab, White, Oval	Irbesartan 300 mg	Avapro by Murfreesboro	51129-1558	Antihypertensive
2775	Tab, Peach, Oval, Convex, Heart Debossed	Hydrochlorothiazide 12.5 mg, Irbestartan 150 mg	Avalide by Murfreesboro	51129-1320	Diuretic
278 <> BRISTOL	Cap, Salmon	Amoxicillin 250 mg	by Quality Care	60346-0655	Antibiotic
278 <> INV	Tab, Purple, Round, Film Coated	Trifluoperazine HCl 1 mg	by Apothecon	62269-0278	Antipsychotic

ID FRONT <> BACK	DESCRIPTION FRONT <> BACK	INGREDIENT & STRENGTH	BRAND (OR EQUIV.) & FIRM	NDC#	CLASS; SCH.
278 <> INV	Tab, Purple, Round, Film Coated	Trifluoperazine HCl 1 mg	by Invamed	52189-0278	Antipsychotic
2790 <> 0115	Tab, White, Round	Chloroquine Phosphate 250 mg	by Global	00115-2790	Antimalarial
27TEGRETAL27	Tab	Carbamazepine 200 mg	by Med Pro	53978-1070	Anticonvulsant
27TEGRETOL <> 27	Tab	Carbamazepine 200 mg	by Allscripts	54569-0163	Anticonvulsant
28 <> B	Tab, Pink	Inert	Levlen 28 by Berlex	50419-0028	Placebo
28 <> M	Tab	Nadolol 20 mg	Nadolol by Qualitest	00603-4740	Antihypertensive
281	Tab, White, Oblong	Acetaminophen 500 mg	Tylenol Ext. St. by Granutec		Antipyretic
2813	Tab, Pink & White, Scored, Logo	Aspirin 325 mg, Methocarbamol 400 mg	by Allscripts	54569-2893	Analgesic; Muscle Relaxant
282	Tab, White, Round, Schering Logo 282	Azatadine Maleate 1 mg	Optimine by Schering	00085-0282	Antihistamine
282MEP	Tab, White	Acetaminophen 350 mg, Caffeine 30 mg, Codeine Phosphate 15 mg	by Frosst	Canadian	Analgesic
283	Tab, Bluish White, Round	Nadolol 40 mg, Bendroflumethiazide 5 mg	Corzide by Apothecon		Antihypertensive
283	Tab, Bluish White, Roumd	Nadolol 40 mg, Bendroflumethiazide 5 mg	Corzide by Apothecon		Antihypertensive
283 <> 200MCG	Tab, Coated	Cerivastatin Sodium 0.2 mg	Baycol by Bayer	00026-2883	Antihyperlipidemic
2832 <> THEO24100MGUCB	Cap, Clear & Orangish Yellow, Theo-24 100 mg ucb <> 2832	Theophylline Anhydrous ER 100 mg	Theo-24 by UCB Pharma	50474-0100	Antiasthmatic
283200MCG	Tab, Light Yellow-Brown, Round, 283/200 mcg	Cerivastatin 0.2 mg	Baycol by Bayer	Canadian	Antihyperlipidemic
284	Tab, Bluish White, Round	Nadolol 80 mg, Bendroflumethiazide 5 mg	Corzide by Apothecon		Antihypertensive
284	Tab, Bluish White, Round	Nadolol 80 mg, Bendroflumethiazide 5 mg	Corzide by Apothecon		Antihypertensive
284 <> 300MCG	Tab, Coated	Cerivastatin Sodium 0.3 mg	Baycol by Bayer	00026-2884	Antihyperlipidemic
284 <> GG	Tab, White, Round, Scored, Compressed	Isoxsuprine HCl 20 mg	Vasodilan by Geneva	00781-1842	Vasodilator
2842 <> THEO24200MG	Cap, Orange & Red, Ex Release	Theophylline Anhydrous 200 mg	Theo 24 ER by DRX	55045-2354	Antiasthmatic
2842 <> THEO24200MGUCB	Cap, Clear & Orangish Red, Theo-24 200 mg ucb <> 2842	Theophylline Anhydrous ER 300 mg	Theo-24 by UCB Pharma	50474-0200	Antiasthmatic
284300MCG	Tab, Yellow-Brown, Round, 284/300 mcg	Cerivastatin 0.3 mg	Baycol by Bayer	Canadian	Antihyperlipidemic
285	Tab, Film Coated	Dipyridamole 50 mg	by Baker Cummins	63171-1569	Antiplatelet
285	Tab, Film Coated, Barr Logo	Dipyridamole 50 mg	by Kaiser	00179-1057	Antiplatelet
285 <> 400MCG	Tab, Yellow, Round	Cerivastatin Sodium 0.4 mg	Baycol by Carlsbad	61442-0112	Antihyperlipidemic
285 <> 400MCG	Tab, Brown, Round	Cerivastatin Sodium 0.4 mg	Baycol by Carlsbad	61442-0113	Antihyperlipidemic
285 <> 400MCG	Tab, Yellow	Cerivastatin Sodium 0.4 mg	Baycol by Catalytica	63552-0031	Antihyperlipidemic
285 <> B	Tab, Film Coated	Dipyridamole 50 mg	by Heartland	61392-0552	Antiplatelet
285 <> B	Tab, Film Coated	Dipyridamole 50 mg	by Amerisource	62584-0370	Antiplatelet
285 <> B	Tab, Film Coated	Dipyridamole 50 mg	by Barr	00555-0285	Antiplatelet
285 <> B	Tab, Film Coated, Barr Logo	Dipyridamole 50 mg	by Geneva	00781-1678	Antiplatelet
285 <> B	Tab, White, Round, Film Coated	Dipyridamole 50 mg	Persantine by UDL	51079-0069	Antiplatelet
285 <> B	Tab, Film Coated	Dipyridamole 50 mg	by Allscripts	54569-0468	Antiplatelet
285 <> BARR	Tab, White, Round, Film Coated	Dipyridamole 50 mg	by Allscripts	54569-0468	Antiplatelet
2852 <> THEO24300MGUCB	Cap, Clear & Red, Theo-24 300 mg ucb <> 2852	Theophylline Anyhdrous ER 300 mg	Thea-24 by UCB Pharma	50474-0300	Antiasthmatic
286	Tab, Film Coated, Barr Logo	Dipyridamole 75 mg	by Kaiser	00179-1162	Antiplatelet
286 <> 800MCG	Tab, Brown	Cerivastatin Sodium 0.8 mg	Baycol by Bayer	00026-2886	Antihyperlipidemic
286 <> BARR	Tab, Film Coated	Dipyridamole 75 mg	by Heartland	61392-0142	Antiplatelet
286 <> BARR	Tab, Film Coated	Dipyridamole 75 mg	by Heartland	61392-0553	Antiplatelet
286 <> BARR	Tab, Film Coated	Dipyridamole 75 mg	by Nat Pharmpak Serv	55154-5817	Antiplatelet
286 <> BARR	Tab, Film Coated	Dipyridamole 75 mg	by Quality Care	60346-0790	Antiplatelet
286 <> BARR	Tab, White, Round, Film Coated	Dipyridamole 75 mg	by Natl Pharmpak	55154-9304	Antiplatelet
286 <> BARR	Tab, Film Coated	Dipyridamole 75 mg	by Zenith Goldline	00182-1570	Antiplatelet
286 <> BARR	Tab, Film Coated	Dipyridamole 75 mg	by Schein	00364-2493	Antiplatelet
286 <> BARR	Tab, Sugar Coated	Dipyridamole 75 mg	by Qualitest	00603-3385	Antiplatelet
286 <> BARR	Tab, Film Coated	Dipyridamole 75 mg	by Barr	00555-0286	Antiplatelet
286 <> BARR	Tab, Film Coated	Dipyridamole 75 mg	by Geneva	00781-1478	Antiplatelet

ID FRONT <> BACK	DESCRIPTION FRONT <> BACK	INGREDIENT & STRENGTH	BRAND (OR EQUIV.) & FIRM	NDC#	CLASS; SCH.
286 <> BARR	Tab, White, Round, Film Coated	Dipyridamole 75 mg	Persantine by UDL	51079-0070	Antiplatelet
286 <> BARR	Tab, Film Coated	Dipyridamole 75 mg	by Allscripts	54569-0470	Antiplatelet
286 <> BARR	Tab, Film Coated	Dipyridamole 75 mg	by Major	00904-1088	Antiplatelet
2867	Cap	Tetracycline HCl 500 mg	Nor-Tet by Vortech		Antibiotic
2869	Cap	Propoxyphene HCl 65 mg	Margesic by Vortech		Analgesic; C IV
287	Tab, Pink, Round	Acetaminophen 325 mg, Pseudoephedrine HCl 30 mg	Sinutab by Granutec		Cold Remedy
287	Tab, Yellow, Round, Schering Logo 287	Perphenazine 2 mg, Amitriptyline HCl 10 mg	Etrafon by Schering		Antipsychotic; Antidepressant
2874	Cap	Decyclomine HCl 10 mg	Bentyl by Vortech		Gastrointestinal
289 <> PAR	Tab	Megestrol Acetate 20 mg	by Schein	00364-2235	Progestin
29	Tab, Purepac Logo 29	Propranolol HCl 20 mg	by Quality Care	60346-0598	Antihypertensive
29 <> B	Tab, Round, Sugar Coated	Ethinyl Estradiol 0.02 mg, Levonorgestrel 0.1 mg	Levlite 28 by Berlex	50419-0408	Oral Contraceptive
290 <> PAR	Tab	Megestrol Acetate 40 mg	by Schein	00364-2234	Progestin
2902 <> THEO24400MGUCB	Cap, Clear & Pink, Theo-24 400 mg ucb <> 2902	Theophylline Anhydrous ER 400 mg	Theo 24 by UCB	50474-0400	Antiasthmatic
2908	Tab, White, Oval	Furosemide 20 mg	by Kaiser Fdn	00179-1373	Diuretic
2908 <> Z	Tab	Furosemide 20 mg	by Quality Care	60346-0761	Diuretic
2909	Cap, Green & White	Hydroxyzine Pamoate 50 Mg	by Vangard Labs	00615-0332	Antihistamine
2909	Cap, Green & White	Hydroxyzine Pamoate 50 mg	Hydroxyzine Pamoate by Murfreesboro	51129-1485	Antihistamine
2909 <> Z	Cap	Hydroxyzine Pamoate	by Schein	00364-0484	Antihistamine
291291 <> S	Tab, White, Round, Scored, Film Coated	Fluvoxamine Maleate 50 mg	Luvox by Solvay Pharma	Canadian DIN# 01919342	OCD
291BARR	Tab, Off-White, Round	Metronidazole 250 mg	Flagyl by Barr		Antibiotic
292 <> 93	Tab	Carbidopa 10 mg, Levodopa 100 mg	by Baker Cummins	63171-1948	Antiparkinson
292 <> ETHEX	Tab, Beige, Oval, Film Coated	Ascorbic Acid 120 mg, Calcium 200 mg, Cholecalciferol 400 Units, Copper 2 mg, Cyanocobalamin 12 mcg, Docusate Sodium 50 mg, Folic Acid 1 mg, Iodine 150 mcg, Iron 90 mg, Niacinamide 20 mg, Pyridoxine HCl 20 mg, Riboflavin 3.4 mg, Thiamine HCl 3 mg, Vitamin A 2700 Units, Vitamin E 30 Units, Zinc 25 mg	Ultra Natalcare by Ethex	58177-0292	Vitamin
292 <> ETHEX	Tab, Film Coated, Scored	Ascorbic Acid 120 mg, Calcium 200 mg, Cholecalciferol 400 Units, Copper 2 mg, Cyanocobalamin 12 mcg, Docusate Sodium 50 mg, Folic Acid 1 mg, Iodine 150 mcg, Iron 90 mg, Niacinamide 20 mg, Pyridoxine HCl 20 mg, Riboflavin 3.4 mg, Thiamine HCl 3 mg, Vitamin A 2700 Units, Vitamin E 30 Units, Zinc 25 mg	Ultra Natalcare by KV	10609-1358	Vitamin
292BARR	Tab, Off-White, Oblong	Metronidazole 500 mg	Flagyl by Barr		Antibiotic
293	Cap, Duramed Logo 293	Guaifenesin 200 mg, Phenylephrine HCl 5 mg, Phenylpropanolamine HCl 45 mg	Enomine by Quality Care	60346-0725	Cold Remedy
293 <> 93	Tab	Carbidopa 25 mg, Levodopa 100 mg	by Vangard	00615-3561	Antiparkinson
29350	Tab, 2/93/50	Acetaminophen 300 mg, Codeine Phosphate 15 mg	by Allscripts	54569-0311	Analgesic; C III
294	Tab, Red, Round	Pseudoephedrine 30 mg	Pseudoval Plus by Granutec		Decongestant
295DP	Tab, Duramed Logo	Guaifenesin 400 mg, Phenylpropanolamine HCl 75 mg	by Schein	00364-2138	Cold Remedy
2975	Cap	Propoxyphene HCl 65 mg, Aspirin 227 mg, Phenacetin 162 mg, Caffeine 32 mg	Margesic Comp. 65 by Vortech		Analgesic; C IV
298	Tab, Coated	Ethinyl Estradiol 0.02 mg	by Amerisource	62584-0298	Hormone
298	Tab, Beige, Round, Schering Logo 298	Ethinyl Estradiol 0.02 mg	Estinyl by Schering		Hormone
298 <> ETHEX	Tab, Blue, Coated	Hydromorphone HCl 2 mg	Dilaudid by Ethex	58177-0298	Analgesic; C II
2985	Cap, Blue	Doxycycline Hyclate 100 mg	by H J Harkins Co	52959-0463	Antibiotic
2985 <> Z	Cap, Light Blue	Doxycycline Hyclate	by Quality Care	60346-0109	Antibiotic
298B	Tab, Orange, Round	Hydroxyzine HCl 25 mg	Atarax by Barr		Antihistamine
298ER	Tab, Beige, Oblong	Ethinyl Estradiol 0.02 mg	Estinyl by Heartland	61392-0799	Hormone
299BARR	Tab, Orange, Round	Hydroxyzine HCl 50 mg	Atarax by Barr		Antihistamine
2AHRTENEX	Tab	Guanfacine HCl 2.3 mg	by Pharmedix	53002-1052	Antihypertensive
2AMPM <> VERSACAP	Cap, 2-AM over PM <> Versacap	Guaifenesin 300 mg, Pseudoephedrine HCl 60 mg	Versacaps by Pharmafab	62542-0403	Cold Remedy
2ATIVAN	Tab, White, Ovoid, 2/Ativan	Lorazepam 2 mg	by Wyeth-Ayerst	Canadian	Sedative/Hypnotic

ID FRONT <> BACK	DESCRIPTION FRONT <> BACK	INGREDIENT & STRENGTH	BRAND (OR EQUIV.) & FIRM	NDC#	CLASS; SCH.
2C	Tab, Pink, Oval	Clonidine 0.1 mg, Chlorthalidone 15 mg	Combipres by Boehringer Ingelheim	Canadian	Antihypertensive; Diuretic
2LLL12	Tab, Pink, Round	Levothyroxine Sodium 0.2 mg	Synthroid by Lederle		Antithyroid
2MG <> 511	Tab, White, Pentagon	Lorazepam 2 mg	by Wyeth Pharms	52903-5813	Sedative/Hypnotic; C IV
2MG <> ETH267	Tab, Yellow, Oblong	Doxazosin Mesylate 2 mg	Cardura by Pfizer	58177-0267	Antihypertensive
2NS	Tab, Purple, Oblong	Divalproex Sodium 500 mg	Depakote by Heartland Healthcare	61392-0610	Anticonvulsant
2RORER142	Tab, White, Round	Aspirin 325 mg, Codeine Phosphate 15 mg, Maalox 150 mg	Ascriptin Codeine #2 by Rorer		Analgesic; C III
2VVALIUM <> ROCHEVROCHE	Tab, 2 over V Logo Valium <> Roche V Roche	Diazepam 2 mg	Valium by Roche	00140-0004	Antianxiety; C IV
2W	Tab, Blue, Round, 2/W	Lorazepam 2 mg	by Wyeth-Ayerst	Canadian	Sedative/Hypnotic
2XANAX	Tab, White, 2/Xanax	Alprazolam 2 mg	by Pharmacia	Canadian	Antianxiety
3	Tab, White, Round	Nitro Tab 0.5 mg	by Novopharm	55953-0296	Vasodilator
3	Tab, White, Round	Nitro Tab 0.5 mg	by Novopharm	43806-0296	Vasodilator
3	Tab, White, Round	Nitroglycerin 0.6 mg (1/100 gr)	Nitrostat by Able Lab	53265-0250	Vasodilator
3	Tab, Off-White, Round	Nitroglycerin 3 mg	Nitrogard Buccal 3 by Forest	00456-0683	Vasodilator
3	Tab	Nitroglycerin 3 mg	Sustachron ER Buccal by Forest	10418-0139	Vasodilator
3 <> 2120V	Tab, White, Round, Scored	Aspirin 325 mg, Codeine Phosphate 30 mg	by Allscripts	54569-0300	Analgesic; C III
3 <> 2120V	Tab	Aspirin 325 mg, Codeine Phosphate 30 mg	by United Res	00677-0647	Analgesic; C III
3 <> 2120V	Tab, 3 <> 2120/V	Aspirin 325 mg, Codeine Phosphate 30 mg	by Vintage	00254-2120	Analgesic; C III
3 <> 2120V	Tab, 2120/V	Aspirin 325 mg, Codeine Phosphate 30 mg	by Qualitest	00603-2361	Analgesic; C III
3 <> 3984	Tab	Aspirin 325 mg, Codeine Phosphate 30 mg	by DRX	55045-2307	Analgesic; C III
3 <> 93150	Tab, 3 <> 93 over 150	Acetaminophen 300 mg, Codeine Phosphate 30 mg	by Nat Pharmpak Serv	55154-5548	Analgesic; C III
3 <> 93150	Tab, 93 Over 150	Acetaminophen 300 mg, Codeine Phosphate 30 mg	by Quality Care	60346-0059	Analgesic; C III
3 <> 93150	Tab, White, Round, 3 <> 93 over 150	Acetaminophen 300 mg, Codeine Phosphate 30 mg	by UDL	51079-0161	Analgesic; C III
3 <> 93150	Tab, 93-150	Acetaminophen 300 mg, Codeine Phosphate 30 mg	by Murfreesboro	51129-0089	Analgesic; C III
3 <> 93150	Tab, White, Round, 3 <> 93 over 150	Acetaminophen 300 mg, Codeine Phosphate 30 mg	by Teva	00093-0150	Analgesic; C III
3 <> 93150	Tab	Acetaminophen 300 mg, Codeine Phosphate 30 mg	by Urgent Care Ctr	50716-0465	Analgesic; C III
3 <> 93150	Tab	Acetaminophen 300 mg, Codeine Phosphate 30 mg	by Pharmedix	53002-0101	Analgesic; C III
3 <> A	Tab, Pink, Round, Film Coated, Scored	Guaifenesin 1200 mg; Phenylpropanolamine HCl 75 mg	Aquatab D by Adams Labs	63824-0003	Cold Remedy
3 <> A	Tab, Film Coated	Indapamide 2.5 mg	by Arcola	00070-3000	Diuretic
3 <> A	Tab, White, Octagon-Shaped, Film Coated	Indapamide 2.5 mg	Indapamide by RPR	00801-3000	Diuretic
3 <> BARR198	Tab, 3 <> Barr/198	Acetaminophen 300 mg, Codeine Phosphate 30 mg	by Barr	00555-0198	Analgesic; C III
3 <> BARR198	Tab	Acetaminophen 300 mg, Codeine Phosphate 30 mg	by Pharmedix	53002-0101	Analgesic; C III
3 <> BIOCRAFT	Tab	Sulfamethoxazole 800 mg, Trimethoprim 160 mg	by Zenith Goldline	00182-8844	Antibiotic
3 <> BIOCRAFT	Tab	Sulfamethoxazole 800 mg, Trimethoprim 160 mg	by Nat Pharmpak Serv	55154-5805	Antibiotic
3 <> BIOCRAFT3	Tab	Sulfamethoxazole 800 mg, Trimethoprim 160 mg	by Allscripts	54569-0075	Antibiotic
3 <> DPI	Tab	Acetaminophen 300 mg, Codeine Phosphate 30 mg	by Quality Care	60346-0059	Analgesic; C III
3 <> ETH	Tab, White, Rectangle	Nitroglycerin 0.3 mg	Nitroquick by PDRX	55289-0308	Vasodilator
3 <> ETH	Tab, White, Ovaloid	Nitroglycerin 0.3 mg	Nitroquick by Ethex	58177-0323	Vasodilator
3 <> GG 220	Tab	Acetaminophen 300 mg, Codeine Phosphate 30 mg	by Golden State	60429-0500	Analgesic; C III
3 <> GG220	Tab	Acetaminophen 300 mg, Codeine Phosphate 30 mg	by Quality Care	60346-0059	Analgesic; C III
3 <> LOGO001	Tab, Logo 001	Acetaminophen 300 mg, Codeine Phosphate 30 mg	by Quality Care	60346-0059	Analgesic; C III
3 <> MP122	Tab	Acetaminophen 300 mg, Codeine 30 mg	by United Res	00677-0612	Analgesic; C III
3 <> MP122	Tab, 3 <> MP over 122	Acetaminophen 300 mg, Codeine Phosphate 30 mg	by Quality Care	60346-0059	Analgesic; C III
3 <> P001	Tab, Purepac Logo	Acetaminophen 300 mg, Codeine Phosphate 30 mg	by Talbert Med	44514-0223	Analgesic; C III
3 <> R001	Tab	Acetaminophen 300 mg, Codeine Phosphate 30 mg	by Vangard	00615-0430	Analgesic; C III
3 <> R001	Tab	Acetaminophen 300 mg, Codeine Phosphate 30 mg	by Purepac	00228-2001	Analgesic; C III
3 <> R001	Tab, Purepac Logo	Acetaminophen 300 mg, Codeine Phosphate 30 mg	by Pharmedix	53002-0101	Analgesic; C III
3 <> R20	Tab, White, Round	Acetaminophen 300 mg, Codeine Phosphate 30 mg	by Purepac	00228-3020	Analgesic; C III
3 <> Z3984	Tab	Aspirin 325 mg, Codeine Phosphate 30 mg	by Quality Care	60346-0560	Analgesic; C III
3 <> Z3984	Tab	Aspirin 325 mg, Codeine Phosphate 30 mg	by Allscripts	54569-0300	Analgesic; C III
3 <> Z3984	Tab	Aspirin 325 mg, Codeine Phosphate 30 mg	by Pharmedix	53002-0109	Analgesic; C III

ID FRONT <> BACK	DESCRIPTION FRONT <> BACK	INGREDIENT & STRENGTH	BRAND (OR EQUIV.) & FIRM	NDC#	CLASS; SCH.
30 <> ACTOS	Tab, White, Round	Pioglitazone HCl 30 mg	Actos by Takeda Chem Inds	11532-0012	Antidiabetic
30 <> ADALACCC	Tab, Pink, Round	Nifedipine 30 mg	Adalat CC by DRX Pharm Consults	55045-2788	Antihypertensive
30 <> ADALATCC	Tab, Pink, Round	Nifedipine 30 mg	Adalat CC by Va Cmop	65243-0053	Antihypertensive
30 <> ADALATCC	Tab, Pink, Round	Nifedipine 30 mg	Adalat CC by Southwood Pharms	58016-0120	Antihypertensive
30 <> ADALATCC	Tab, Film Coated	Nifedipine 30 mg	Adalat CC by Bayer	00026-8841	Antihypertensive
30 <> ADALATCC	Tab, Film Coated	Nifedipine 30 mg	Adalat CC by Amerisource	62584-0841	Antihypertensive
30 <> ADALATCC	Tab, Pink, Round, Film Coated	Nifedipine 30 mg	Adalat CC by Compumed	00403-4957	Antihypertensive
30 <> ADALATCC	Tab, Pink, Round, Film Coated	Nifedipine 30 mg	Adalat CC by Eckerd	19458-0878	Antihypertensive
30 <> ADALATCC	Tab, Film Coated	Nifedipine 30 mg	by Talbert Med	44514-0701	Antihypertensive
30 <> ADALATCC	Tab, Film Coated	Nifedipine 30 mg	Adalat CC by Nat Pharmpak Serv	55154-4805	Antihypertensive
30 <> ADALATCC	Tab, Pink, Round, Film Coated	Nifedipine 30 mg	Adalat CC by Par	49884-0621	Antihypertensive
30 <> ADALATCC	Tab, Film Coated	Nifedipine 30 mg	Adalat CC by Wal Mart	49035-0154	Antihypertensive
30 <> ADALATCC	Tab, Film Coated	Nifedipine 30 mg	Adalat CC by Allscripts	54569-3891	Antihypertensive
30 <> ADALATCC	Tab, Film Coated	Nifedipine 30 mg	by Med Pro	53978-3033	Antihypertensive
30 <> ADALATCC	Tab, Film Coated	Nifedipine 30 mg	Adalat CC by Smiths Food & Drug	58341-0058	Antihypertensive
30 <> ADALATCC	Tab, Film Coated	Nifedipine 30 mg	Adalat CC by Quality Care	62682-6020	Antihypertensive
30 <> ADAMS	Tab	Dextromethorphan Hydrobromide 30 mg, Guaifenesin 600 mg	Humibid DM by Nat Pharmpak Serv	55154-5902	Cold Remedy
30 <> BLANSETT	Cap, Red Print	Guaifenesin 250 mg, Pseudoephedrine HCl 120 mg	Nalex by Sovereign	58716-0010	Cold Remedy
30 <> BMS1966	Cap, Dark Orange & Light Orange, Black Print, 30 <> BMS over 1966	Stavudine 30 mg	Zerit by Bristol Myers	00003-1966	Antiviral
30 <> E653	Tab, Green, Round	Morphine Sulfate 30 mg	by Dupont Pharma	00056-0653	Analgesic; C II
30 <> E653	Tab, Green, Round	Morphine Sulfate 30 mg	by Endo Labs	60951-0653	Analgesic; C II
30 <> ETHEX	Tab, White, Scored	Morphine Sulfate 30 mg	MSIR by Ethex	58177-0314	Analgesic; C II
30 <> ETHEX	Tab, Scored	Morphine Sulfate 30 mg	by KV	10609-1406	Analgesic; C II
30 <> G	Tab, White, Round, Film Coated	Ranitidine HCl 150 mg	by Mylan Pharms	00378-3252	Gastrointestinal
30 <> IMDUR	Tab, Rose	Isosorbide Mononitrate 30 mg	Imdur ER by Schering	00085-3306	Antianginal
30 <> MEDEVA	Tab, Green, Oblong, Scored	Guaifenesin 600 mg; Dextromethorphan Hydrobromide 30 mg	Humibid DM by Adams Labs	63824-0030	Cold Remedy
30 <> PAXIL	Tab, Coated	Paroxetine HCl	Paxil by Physicians Total Care	54868-3526	Antidepressant
30 <> PAXIL	Tab, Coated	Paroxetine HCl	Paxil by SB	59742-3212	Antidepressant
30 <> PAXIL	Tab, Blue, Oval, Coated	Paroxetine HCl 30 mg	Paxil by SKB	00029-3212	Antidepressant
30 <> PF	Tab, White, Cap-Shaped	Morphine Sulfate 30 mg	MS IR by Purdue Frederick	Canadian	Analgesic
30 <> PROCARDIAXL	Tab, Pink, Round, Procardia XL	Nifedipine 30 mg	Procardia XL by Pfizer	00069-2650	Antihypertensive
30 <> PROCARDIAXL	Tab, Procardia XL	Nifedipine 30 mg	Procardia XL by Amerisource	62584-0650	Antihypertensive
30 <> PROCARDIAXL	Tab, Procardia XL	Nifedipine 30 mg	Procardia XL by Nat Pharmpak Serv	55154-2706	Antihypertensive
30 <> PROCARDIAXL30	Tab	Nifedipine 30 mg	by Med Pro	53978-1107	Antihypertensive
30 <> WESTWARD	Cap	Flurazepam HCl 30 mg	by Quality Care	60346-0762	Hypnotic; C IV
300	Tab, Red, Round	Ferrous Sulfate 300 mg	Ferrous by Apotex	Canadian	Mineral
300	Cap, White	Etodolac 300 mg	by ESI Lederle		NSAID
300	Tab, Peach, Round, Logo/300	Penicillan V Potassium 300 mg	by Nadeau	Canadian	Antibiotic
300	Tab, White, Round, Scored, Film, Arched Triangle	Propafenone HCl 300 mg	Rythmol by Ranbaxy	63304-0691	Antiarrhythmic
300	Tab, White, Oblong	Theophylline 300 mg	Theo SR by Rhone-Poulenc Rorer	Canadian	Antiasthmatic
300	Cap, White, ER, Printed in Red	Theophylline 300 mg	Slo Bid by RPR	00801-0300	Antiasthmatic
300 <> 4364	Tab, Green, Round, 300 <> Hourglass Logo 4364	Labetalol HCl 300 mg	Normodyne & Trandate by Zenith Goldline	00172-4366	Antihypertensive
300 <> 599223607	Cap, White	Etodolac 300 mg	by Wyeth Pharms	52903-3607	NSAID
300 <> BARR071	Tab, Debossed <> Barr/071 Debossed	Isoniazid 300 mg	Isoniazid by Rugby	00536-3941	Antimycobacterial
300 <> BARR071	Tab, Debossed, 300 <> Barr/071	Isoniazid 300 mg	Isoniazid by Schein	00364-0151	Antimycobacterial
300 <> BARR071	Tab, Barr/071	Isoniazid 300 mg	Isoniazid by Barr	00555-0071	Antimycobacterial
300 <> BARR071	Tab	Isoniazid 300 mg	Isoniazid by Quality Care	60346-0483	Antimycobacterial
300 <> BARR071	Tab, White, Round, Scored, 300 <> Barr Over 071	Isoniazid 300 mg	INH by UDL	51079-0083	Antimycobacterial
300 <> FLINT	Tab, Debossed	Levothyroxine Sodium 0.3 mg	Synthroid by CVS	51316-0246	Antithyroid

ID FRONT <> BACK	DESCRIPTION FRONT <> BACK	INGREDIENT & STRENGTH	BRAND (OR EQUIV.) & FIRM	NDC#	CLASS; SCH.
300 <> FLINT	Tab, Debossed, Score is Vertical with 300 running horizontal through break in Score <> Debossed	Levothyroxine Sodium 0.3 mg	Synthroid by Thrift Drug	59198-0298	Antithyroid
300 <> FLINT	Tab, Debossed	Levothyroxine Sodium 0.3 mg	Synthroid by Amerisource	62584-0170	Antithyroid
300 <> FLINT	Tab, Green, Round, Scored	Levothyroxine Sodium 300 mcg	Synthroid by Knoll	00048-1170	Antithyroid
300 <> GXCW3	Tab, Film Coated	Zidovudine 300 mg	Retrovir by Catalytica	63552-0501	Antiviral
300 <> GXCW3	Tab, Film Coated	Zidovudine 300 mg	Retrovir by Glaxo	00173-0501	Antiviral
300 <> GXCW3	Tab, Film Coated	Zidovudine 300 mg	Retrovir by DRX	55045-2488	Antiviral
300 <> ID	Cap	Chlorpheniramine Maleate 8 mg, Pseudoephedrine HCl 120 mg	Deconomed Sr by Sovereign	58716-0044	Cold Remedy
300 <> N192	Tab, Light Green, Film Coated	Cimetidine 300 mg	by Quality Care	60346-0944	Gastrointestinal
300 <> N192	Tab, Film Coated	Cimetidine 300 mg	by Medirex	57480-0813	Gastrointestinal
300 <> N192	Tab, Film Coated	Cimetidine 300 mg	by Warrick	59930-1801	Gastrointestinal
300 <> N192	Tab, Dark Green, Oval, Film Coated	Cimetidine 300 mg	by Novopharm	55953-0192	Gastrointestinal
300 <> N192	Tab, Coated, N/192	Cimetidine 300 mg	by Brightstone	62939-2121	Gastrointestinal
300 <> N192	Tab, Coated	Cimetidine 300 mg	by United Res	00677-1528	Gastrointestinal
300 <> N192	Tab, Green, Oval, Film Coated	Cimetidine 300 mg	by Nat Pharmpak Serv	55154-9303	Gastrointestinal
300 <> N192	Tab, Film Coated	Cimetidine 300 mg	by DRX	55045-2272	Gastrointestinal
300 <> N192	Tab, Green, Oval, Film Coated	Cimetidine 300 mg	by Dixon Shane	17236-0171	Gastrointestinal
300 <> N547	Tab, Film Coated, N Over 547	Ranitidine HCl 336 mg	by UDL	51079-0880	Gastrointestinal
300 <> N547	Tab, Film Coated, N Over 547	Ranitidine HCl 336 mg	by Allscripts	54569-4508	Gastrointestinal
300 <> N547	Tab, White, Cap-Shaped, Film Coated, N Over 547	Ranitidine HCl 336 mg	by Novopharm	55953-0547	Gastrointestinal
300 <> N547	Tab, White, Cap-Shaped, Film Coated	Ranitidine HCl 336 mg	by Novopharm	43806-0547	Gastrointestinal
300 <> PD357	Tab, White, Oval, Film Coated	Troglitazone 300 mg	Rezulin by Murfreesboro Ph	51129-1423	Antidiabetic
300 <> PD357	Tab, White, Oval, Film Coated, Debossed	Troglitazone 300 mg	Rezulin by Parke Davis	00071-0357	Antidiabetic
300 <> SCHERING438	Tab, Blue, Round	Labetalol HCl 300 mg	Normdyne by Rightpak	65240-0670	Antihypertensive
300 <> TAGAMETSB	Tab, Film Coated	Cimetidine 300 mg	Tagamet by HJ Harkins Co	52959-0270	Gastrointestinal
300 <> TIAZAC	Cap, Purple & White	Diltiazem HCl 300 mg	Tiazac by Rx Pac	65084-0134	Antihypertensive
300 <> WATSON	Tab, White, Round	Furosemide 20 mg	by Allscripts	54569-0572	Diuretic
3000	Tab, White, Round	Quinidine Gluconate 324 mg	Quinaglute by Roxane		Antiarrhythmic
3000 <> MYLAN	Cap, Coral	Meclofenamate Sodium	by Quality Care	60346-0350	NSAID
3001	Tab, White, Round	Quinine Sulfate 260 mg	Quinamm by Zenith Goldline	00172-3001	Antimalarial
300490MG <> LILLY	Cap, Clear & Green, Opaque	Fluoxetine 90 mg	Prozac by Lilly	00002-3004	Antidepressant
3007 <> Z	Tab, Coated	Metronidazole 500 mg	by Quality Care	60346-0507	Antibiotic
300BARR	Tab, Orange, Round	Hydroxyzine HCl 100 mg	Atarax by Barr		Antihistamine
300FLI	Tab, Lime Green, Round, 300/FLI Logo	Levothyroxine Sodium 300 mcg	by Forest	00456-0328	Antithyroid
300M	Tab	Levothyroxine Sodium 300 mcg	Euthyrox by Em Pharma	63254-0445	Antithyroid
300M	Tab	Levothyroxine Sodium 300 mcg	Levo T by MOVA	55370-0134	Antithyroid
300M30 <> MOVA	Tab, White, Round, Film Coated, 300/M30 <> Mova	Cimetidine 300 mg	by Compumed	00403-1340	Gastrointestinal
300M30 <> MOVA	Tab, White, Round	Cimetidine 300 mg	Tagamet by MOVA	55370-0135	Gastrointestinal
300MCG <> 284	Tab, Coated	Cerivastatin Sodium 0.3 mg	Baycol by Bayer	00026-2884	Antihyperlipidemic
300MG <> FLOXIN	Tab, Film Coated	Ofloxacin 300 mg	Ofloxacin by Med Pro	53978-3018	Antibiotic
300MG <> FLOXIN	Tab, Coated	Ofloxacin 300 mg	Floxin by Quality Care	60346-0716	Antibiotic
300MG <> SCHWARZ4087	Cap, Amethyst & Lavender, Opaque	Verapamil HCl 300 mg	Verelan PM by Schwarz Pharma	00091-4087	Antihypertensive
300MG4177	Cap, Gelatin, Red Print	Etodolac 300 mg	by Zenith Goldline	00172-4177	NSAID
300MG4177	Cap, Gelatin, Red Print, 2 Bands	Etodolac 300 mg	by Zenith Goldline	00182-2665	NSAID
300NORMODYNE <> SCHERING438	Tab, Coated, 300 Normodyne <> Schering 438	Labetalol HCl 300 mg	Normodyne by Thrift Drug	59198-0082	Antihypertensive
300SB <> TAGAMET	Tab, Light Green, Film Coated	Cimetidine 300 mg	Tagamet by Quality Care	60346-0001	Gastrointestinal
300SKF <> TAGAMET	Tab, Film Coated	Cimetidine 300 mg	by Pharmedix	53002-0328	Gastrointestinal
300WALLACE374101	Cap, Blue & White, 300 Wallace 37-4101	Methacycline HCl 300 mg	Rondomycin by Wallace		Analgesic
301 <> DP	Tab, Duramed Logo	Methylprednisolone 4 mg	by Quality Care	60346-0608	Steroid
301 <> ETHEX	Tab, White, Round, Film Coated	Ketorolac Tromethamine 10 mg	by Murfreesboro Ph	51129-1437	NSAID

ID FRONT <> BACK	DESCRIPTION FRONT <> BACK	INGREDIENT & STRENGTH	BRAND (OR EQUIV.) & FIRM	NDC#	CLASS; SCH.
301 <> ETHEX	Tab, Film Coated, Red Ink	Ketorolac Tromethamine 10 mg	by Allscripts	54569-4494	NSAID
301 <> ETHEX	Tab, White, Film Coated, in Red Ink	Ketorolac Tromethamine 10 mg	Toradol by Ethex	58177-0301	NSAID
301 <> ETHEX	Tab, White, Round, Film Coated	Ketorolac Tromethamine 10 mg	by Compumed	00403-4136	NSAID
301 <> ETHEX	Tab, Film Coated, Red Print	Ketorolac Tromethamine 10 mg	by Syntex	18393-0301	NSAID
301 <> HOPE	Tab	Scopolamine Hydrobromide 0.4 mg	Scopace by Hope	60267-0301	Antiemetic
301 <> HOPE	Tab	Scopolamine Hydrobromide 0.4 mg	by Anabolic	00722-6383	Antiemetic
301 <> ID	Cap	Brompheniramine Maleate 12 mg, Pseudoephedrine HCl 120 mg	Iofed by Sovereign	58716-0045	Cold Remedy
301 <> ID	Cap	Brompheniramine Maleate 12 mg, Pseudoephedrine HCl 120 mg	Iofed by Physicians Total Care	54868-3989	Cold Remedy
301 <> RS	Tab, White, Round	Diphenoxylate HCl 2.5 mg; Atropine Sulfate 0.025 mg	by Corepharma	64720-0301	Antidiarrheal; C V
301 <> RS	Tab, White, Round	Diphenoxylate HCl 2.5 mg; Atropine Sulfate 0.025 mg	by R & S Pharma	65162-0301	Antidiarrheal; C V
301 <> WATSON	Tab, White, Round	Furosemide 40 mg	by Allscripts	54569-0574	Diuretic
30102	Cap, Orange & White, 3 Mericon Logo/0102	Flouride 3.74 mg, Calcium 145 mg	FLORICAL by MERICON		Mineral
301B	Tab, Yellow, Round	Hydroxyzine HCl 10 mg	Atarax by Barr		Antihistamine
302 <> BARR50	Cap, Yellow Powder <> Barr/50 Over 302 Black Ink	Hydroxyzine Pamoate 85.22 mg	by Barr	00555-0302	Antihistamine
302 <> BARR50	Cap, in Black Ink	Hydroxyzine Pamoate 85.22 mg	by Qualitest	00603-3995	Antihistamine
302 <> ETHEX	Tab	Naproxen 375 mg	by Syntex	18393-0257	NSAID
302 <> ETHEX	Tab	Naproxen 375 mg	by Allscripts	54569-4523	NSAID
302 <> ID	Cap	Brompheniramine Maleate 6 mg, Pseudoephedrine HCl 60 mg	Iofed PD by Sovereign	58716-0046	Cold Remedy
303 <> ETHEX	Tab	Naproxen 500 mg	by Allscripts	54569-4520	NSAID
303 <> ETHEX	Tab	Naproxen 500 mg	by PDRX	55289-0307	NSAID
303 <> ETHEX	Tab	Naproxen 500 mg	by Syntex	18393-0258	NSAID
3030	Tab, Blue, Oblong, 30/30	Caffeine 200 mg	by B & M Labs		Stimulant
3030 <> IMDUR	Tab, Rose	Isosorbide Mononitrate 30 mg	Imdur by Caremark	00339-6002	Antianginal
3030 <> IMDUR	Tab	Isosorbide Mononitrate 30 mg	Imdur by Astra AB	17228-3306	Antianginal
303303 <> GILGIL	Tab, White, Oval	Guaifenesin 600 mg; Dextromethorphan Hydrobromide 30 mg; Phenylephrine HCl 20 mg	Giltuss by Gil Pharm	58552-0303	Cold Remedy
303303 <> GILGIL	Tab, White, Oval, Scored	Guaifenesin 600 mg; Dextromethorphan Hydrobromide 30 mg; Phenylephrine HCl 20 mg	Giltuss by Sovereign Pharms	58716-0646	Cold Remedy
303325	Cap, White, Royce logo 303/325	Quinine Sulfate 324 mg	by Royce		Antimalarial
303325	Cap, White, Royce logo 303/325	Quinine Sulfate 324 mg	by Royce		Antimalarial
305 <> PFIZER	Cap	Azithromycin Dihydrate	Zithromax by Quality Care	60346-0670	Antibiotic
305 <> TRIADUAD	Cap, White, 305 <> Triad/UAD	Acetaminophen 325 mg, Butalbital 50 mg, Caffeine 40 mg	Triad by UAD	00785-2305	Analgesic
3054090	Tab, White, 30/54/090	Morphine Sulfate 30 mg	Oramorph SR by Boehringer Ingelheim	Canadian	Analgesic
306 <> PFIZER	Tab, Red, Film Coated	Azithromycin Dihydrate	Zithromax by Pfizer	00069-3060	Antibiotic
306 <> PFIZER	Tab, Film Coated	Azithromycin Dihydrate	Zithromax by Allscripts	54569-4522	Antibiotic
306 <> PFIZER	Tab, Pink, Cap Shaped, Film Coated, Scored	Azithromycin Dihydrate 250 mg	Zithromax by Pfizer	Canadian DIN# 02212021	Antibiotic
306 <> PFIZER	Tab, Red, Oblong	Azithromycin Dihydrate 250 mg	ZPAK by Phy Total Care	54868-4183	Antibiotic
3061	Cap	Cefaclor Anhydrous 250 mg	Ceclor by Lilly	00110-3061	Antibiotic
3062	Cap	Cefaclor Monohydrate 500 mg	Ceclor by Lilly	00110-3062	Antibiotic
308 <> 93	Tab	Clemastine Fumarate 2.68 mg	by HJ Harkins Co	52959-0501	Antihistamine
308 <> ETHEX	Tab, White, Film Coated, Scored	Guaifenesin 1200 mg	Guaifenex G by Ethex	58177-0308	Expectorant
308 <> ETHEX	Tab, Film Coated, Scored	Guaifenesin 1200 mg	Guaifenex G by KV	10609-1397	Expectorant
308 <> ETHEX	Tab, White, Oblong, Scored, Film Coated	Guaifenex 1200 mg	by Med Pro	53978-3362	Expectorant
308 <> ID	Cap	Trimethobenzamide HCl 250 mg	by Sovereign	58716-0055	Antiemetic
308 <> PFIZER	Tab, White, Cap Shaped, Film Coated	Azithromycin Dihydrate 600 mg	Zithromax by Pfizer	Canadian DIN# 02231143	Antibiotic

ID FRONT <> BACK	DESCRIPTION FRONT <> BACK	INGREDIENT & STRENGTH	BRAND (OR EQUIV.) & FIRM	NDC#	CLASS; SCH.
308US	Tab, Film Coated	Calcium Pantothenate 10 mg, Copper Sulfate, Cu-64, Cyanocobalamin 15 mcg, Ferrous Fumarate 324 mg, Folic Acid 1 mg, Magnesium Sulfate, Manganese Sulfate, Niacinamide 30 mg, Pyridoxine HCl 5 mg, Riboflavin 6 mg, Sodium Ascorbate 200 mg, Thiamine Mononitrate 10 mg, Zinc Sulfate	Hemocyte Plus by U.S. Pharmaceuticala Corp.	52747-0308	Vitamin/Mineral
308US	Tab, Film Coated	Calcium Pantothenate 10 mg, Copper Sulfate, Cu-64, Cyanocobalamin 15 mcg, Ferrous Fumarate 324 mg, Folic Acid 1 mg, Magnesium Sulfate, Manganese Sulfate, Niacinamide 30 mg, Pyridoxine HCl 5 mg, Riboflavin 6 mg, Sodium Ascorbate 200 mg, Thiamine Mononitrate 10 mg, Zinc Sulfate	Hemocyte Plus by Opti Med	63369-0308	Vitamin/Mineral
309 <> MEDEVA	Tab	Dextromethorphan Hydrobromide 30 mg, Guaifenesin 600 mg, Pseudoephedrine HCl 60 mg	Syn Rx DM by Medeva	53014-0311	Cold Remedy
309 <> MEDEVA	Tab	Dextromethorphan Hydrobromide 30 mg, Guaifenesin 600 mg, Pseudoephedrine HCl 60 mg	Syn Rx DM by Adams	53014-0311	Cold Remedy
309 <> MEDEVA	Tab, Yellow, Oblong, Scored	Guaifenesin 600 mg; Pseudoephedrine HCl 60 mg; Dextromethorphan Hydrobromide 30 mg	Syn Rx by Adams Labs	63824-0311	Cold Remedy
309 <> SL	Tab, White, Round, Sugar Coated	Hydroxyzine HCl 50 mg	by Allscripts	54569-0409	Antihistamine
309 <> SL	Tab, White, Round, Sugar Coated	Hydroxyzine HCl 50 mg	Atarax by Sidmak	50111-0309	Antihistamine
309 <> SL	Tab, White, Round	Hydroxyzine HCl 50 mg	by Murfreesboro	51129-1477	Antihistamine
309 <> SL	Tab, Sugar Coated	Hydroxyzine HCl 50 mg	by Qualitest	00603-3972	Antihistamine
30910	Cap, Scarlet, 309 10 <> Mortar and Pestle Logo	Doxepin HCl	by Royce	51875-0309	Antidepressant
30910	Cap, Pink & Scarlet, Royce Logo 309/10	Doxepin HCl 10 mg	Sinequan by Royce		Antidepressant
30ATASOL	Tab, Green, Round, 30/Atasol	Acetaminophen 325 mg, Codeine Phosphate 30 mg, Caffeine Citrate 30 mg	by Horner	Canadian	Analgesic
30MG <> PF	Tab, Violet, Round	Morphine Sulfate 30 mg	MS Contin by Purdue Frederick	Canadian	Analgesic
30MG <> RSN	Tab, White, Oval, Film Coated	Risedronate Sodium 30 mg	Actonel by Procter & Gamble	Canadian DIN# 02239146	Bisphosphonate
30MG <> RSN	Tab, Yellow, Oval, Film Coated	Risedronate Sodium 30 mg	Actonel by Procter & Gamble	00149-0470	Bisphosphonate
30P <> DAN	Tab, White, Round, Scored	Phenobarbital 30 mg	by Schein	00364-0203	Sedative/Hypnotic; C IV
31 <> BMS100	Tab	Nefazodone HCl 100 mg	Serzone by Kaiser	00179-1241	Antidepressant
31 <> BMS50	Tab	Nefazodone HCl 50 mg	Serzone by Murfreesboro	51129-1106	Antidepressant
31 <> G	Tab, White, Oblong, Film Coated	Ranitidine HCl 300 mg	by Mylan Pharms	00378-3254	Gastrointestinal
310	Tab	Hematinic	Trihemic 600 by Marlop		Vitamin
310	Tab, Yellow, Oblong, Ascher logo 310	Magnesium Salicylate 600 mg	Mobidin by B.F.Ascher		Analgesic
310 <> 25	Cap, Royce Logo 310	Doxepin HCl	by Quality Care	60346-0553	Antidepressant
310 <> MEDEVA	Tab	Dextromethorphan Hydrobromide 30 mg, Guaifenesin 600 mg, Pseudoephedrine HCl 60 mg	Syn Rx DM by Medeva	53014-0311	Cold Remedy
310 <> MEDEVA	Tab	Dextromethorphan Hydrobromide 30 mg, Guaifenesin 600 mg, Pseudoephedrine HCl 60 mg	Syn Rx DM by Adams	53014-0311	Cold Remedy
310 <> MEDEVZ	Tab, Blue, Oblong, Scored	Guaifenesin 600 mg; Pseudoephedrine HCl 60 mg; Dextromethorphan Hydrobromide 30 mg	Syn Rx by Adams Labs	63824-0311	Cold Remedy
3100	Cap, Yellow	Phentermine 30 mg	Phentrol #4 by Vortech		Anorexiant; C IV
3101	Cap, Blue & White, Pulvule	Nabilone 1 mg	by Lilly	Canadian	Antiemetic
3101 <> BRL30	Tab, Blue, Round, Scored	Diltiazem HCl 30 mg	by Blue Ridge	59273-0002	Antihypertensive
3102 <> BRL60	Tab, White, Round, Scored	Diltiazem HCl 60 mg	by Blue Ridge	59273-0003	Antihypertensive
31025	Cap, Mortar and Pestle Logo	Doxepin HCl	by Royce	51875-0310	Antidepressant
31025	Cap, Blue & Pink, Royce Logo 310/25	Doxepin HCl 25 mg	Sinequan by Royce		Antidepressant
3103 <> BRL90	Tab, Blue, Oblong, Scored	Diltiazem HCl 90 mg	by Blue Ridge	59273-0004	Antihypertensive
3104 <> BRL120	Tab, White, Oblong, Scored	Diltiazem HCl 120 mg	by Blue Ridge	59273-0005	Antihypertensive
3104PROZAC10	Cap, Green, 3104/Prozac 10	Fluoxetine HCl 10 mg	Prozac by Lilly		Antidepressant
3105	Cap, Off-White, Gelatin Coated	Fluoxetine 20 mg	Prozac by Nat Pharmpak Serv	55154-0802	Antidepressant
3105PROZAC20	Cap, Green & Yellow, 3105/Prozac 20	Fluoxetine HCl 20 mg	Prozac by Lilly		Antidepressant
3109 <> RUGBY	Tab	Clomiphene Citrate 50 mg	by Rugby	00536-3109	Infertility
311	Tab, Brown	Hematinic	Pronemia by Marlop		Vitamin

ID FRONT <> BACK	DESCRIPTION FRONT <> BACK	INGREDIENT & STRENGTH	BRAND (OR EQUIV.) & FIRM	NDC#	CLASS; SCH.
311	Tab, White, Round, Sch. Logo 311	Methyltestosterone 10 mg	Oreton by Schering		Hormone; C III
311 <> 50	Cap, Flesh, Royce Logo 311	Doxepin HCl	by Quality Care	60346-0269	Antidepressant
311 <> ID	Cap	Chlorpheniramine Maleate 8 mg	by Sovereign	58716-0051	Antihistamine
311 <> WATSON	Tab	Furosemide 20 mg	by Golden State	60429-0078	Diuretic
311 <> WATSON	Tab	Furosemide 20 mg	Delone by Macnary	55982-0010	Diuretic
311 <> WATSON	Tab	Furosemide 20 mg	by Watson	52544-0311	Diuretic
311 <> WATSON	Tab	Furosemide 20 mg	by DRX	55045-1553	Diuretic
311 <> WATSON	Tab	Furosemide 20 mg	by Major	00904-1580	Diuretic
3111DARVONCOMP65	Cap, Gray & Red, 3111/Darvon Comp 65	Propoxyphene HCl 65 mg, Aspirin 389 mg, Caffeine 324 mg	Darvon by Lilly		Analgesic; C IV
3113	Cap, Gray & White	Codeine Phosphate 30 mg, Aspirin 380 mg, Caffeine 30 mg	A.S.A. by Lilly		Analgesic; C III
3115	Cap, Black	Phentermine 30 mg	Phentrol #5 by Vortech		Anorexiant; C IV
31150	Cap, Flesh, Mortar and Pestle Logo	Doxepin HCl	by Royce	51875-0311	Antidepressant
31150	Cap, Flesh & Pink, Royce Logo 311/50	Doxepin HCl 50 mg	Sinequan by Royce		Antidepressant
312	Tab	Therapeutic Multivitamin	Berocca by Marlop		Vitamin
312 <> ID	Cap	Chlorpheniramine Maleate 12 mg	by Sovereign	58716-0049	Antihistamine
312 <> SL	Tab, Sugar Coated	Dipyridamole 50 mg	by Sidmak	50111-0312	Antiplatelet
3123 <> 93	Cap, Light Green & Green, Oval	Dicloxacillin Sodium 250 mg	by Allscripts	54569-0384	Antibiotic
3125 <> 93	Cap, Green	Dicloxacillin Sodium 500 mg	by Allscripts	54569-1889	Antibiotic
3125 <> VANCOCINHCL125M	Cap	Vancomycin HCl	by Eli Lilly	00002-3125	Antibiotic
3126 <> VANCOCINHCL250M	Cap	Vancomycin HCl	by Eli Lilly	00002-3126	Antibiotic
313	Tab, Gray, Round, Schering Logo 313	Perphenazine 8 mg	Trilafon by Schering		Antipsychotic
313	Tab	Therapeutic Multivitamin, Minerals	Berocca Plus by Marlop		Vitamin
313 <> SL	Tab, Sugar Coated	Dipyridamole 75 mg	by Sidmak	50111-0313	Antiplatelet
3131	Tab, White, Round, Savage Logo 3131	Potassium Chloride 750 mg	Kaon-CL 10 by Savage	00281-3131	Electrolytes
3131	Tab, Film Coated	Potassium Chloride 750 mg	Kaon CL by Savage	00281-3131	Electrolytes
313313 <> S	Tab, White, Oval, Scored, Film Coated	Fluvoxamine Maleate 100 mg	Luvox by Solvay Pharma	Canadian DIN# 01919369	OCD
314 <> 93	Tab, White, Round, Film Coated	Ketorolac Tromethamine 10 mg	by Teva	00093-0314	NSAID
314 <> 93	Tab, White, Round, Film-Coated	Ketorolac Tromethamine 10 mg	By Allscripts	54569-4494	NSAID
314 <> 93	Tab, White, Round	Ketorolac Tromethamine 10 mg	by Southwood Pharms	58016-0247	NSAID
3142 <> WESTWARD	Cap	Doxycycline Hyclate	by Quality Care	60346-0109	Antibiotic
3144	Cap, Yellow, Pulvule	Nizatidine 150 mg	by Lilly	Canadian	Gastrointestinal
3144 <> AXID150MG	Cap, Symbol/3144 <> Axid 150 mg	Nizatidine 150 mg	Axid by Nat Pharmpak Serv	55154-1803	Gastrointestinal
3145	Cap, Brown & Yellow, Pulvule	Nizatidine 300 mg	by Lilly	Canadian	Gastrointestinal
315	Cap, Red	Hematinic	Pronemia by Marlop		Vitamin
315 <> ETH	Tab, Orange & Rust, Partially Bisected, Beveled Edge	Oxycodone HCl 5 mg	Roxicodone by Ethex	58177-0315	Analgesic; C II
315 <> ETH	Tab, Partially Bisected, Beveled Edge	Oxycodone HCl 5 mg	by KV	10609-1419	Analgesic; C II
315 <> UCB	Cap, Black & Orange	Niacinamide 25 mg, Vitamin A 8000 unt, Magnesium Sulfate 70 mg, Zinc Sulfate 80 mg; Ascorbic Acid 150 mg; Vitamin E 50 unt; Thiamine Mononitrate 10 mg; Calcium Pantothenate 10 mg; Riboflavin 5 mg; Manganese Chloride 4 mg, Pyridoxine HCl 2 mg, Folic Acid	Vicon Forte by Rx Pac	65084-0211	Vitamin
316	Tab, Red, Oval, Schering Logo 316	Fluphenazine HCl 10 mg	Permitil by Schering	00085-0316	Antipsychotic
316 <> ETHEX	Tab, Tan, Oval, Film Coated, Scored	Ascorbic Acid 120 mg, Biotin 30 mcg, Calcium 200 mg, Chromium 25 mcg, Copper 2 mg, Cyanocobalamin 12 mcg, Folic Acid 1 mg, Iodine 150 mcg, Iron 27 mg, Magnesium 25 mg, Manganese 5 mg, Molybdenum 25 mcg, Niacinamide 20 mg, Pantothenic Acid 10 mg, Pyridoxine HCl 10 mg, Riboflavin 3.4 mg, Selenium 20 mcg, Thiamine HCl 3 mg, Vitamin A 5000 Units, Vitamin D 400 Units, Vitamin E 30 mg, Zinc 25 mg	Prenatal Mtr by Ethex	58177-0316	Vitamin

ID FRONT <> BACK	DESCRIPTION FRONT <> BACK	INGREDIENT & STRENGTH	BRAND (OR EQUIV.) & FIRM	NDC#	CLASS; SCH.
316 <> ETHEX	Tab, Film Coated, Scored	Ascorbic Acid 120 mg, Biotin 30 mcg, Calcium 200 mg, Chromium 25 mcg, Copper 2 mg, Cyanocobalamin 12 mcg, Folic Acid 1 mg, Iodine 150 mcg, Iron 27 mg, Magnesium 25 mg, Manganese 5 mg, Molybdenum 25 mcg, Niacinamide 20 mg, Pantothenic Acid 10 mg, Pyridoxine HCl 10 mg, Riboflavin 3.4 mg, Selenium 20 mcg, Thiamine HCl 3 mg, Vitamin A 5000 Units, Vitamin D 400 Units, Vitamin E 30 mg, Zinc 25 mg	Prenatal Mtr by KV	10609-1412	Vitamin
316 <> UCB	Cap	Ascorbic Acid 150 mg, Calcium Pantothenate 10 mg, Cyanocobalamin 10 mcg, Folic Acid 1 mg, Magnesium Sulfate 70 mg, Manganese Chloride 4 mg, Niacinamide 25 mg, Pyridoxine HCl 2 mg, Riboflavin 5 mg, Thiamine Mononitrate 10 mg, Vitamin A 8000 Units, Vitamin E 50 Units, Zinc Sulfate 80 mg	Vicon Forte by Eckerd Drug	19458-0847	Vitamin
317 <> M	Tab, Film Coated	Cimetidine 300 mg	by Quality Care	60346-0944	Gastrointestinal
317 <> M	Tab, Film Coated	Cimetidine 300 mg	by Nat Pharmpak Serv	55154-5560	Gastrointestinal
317 <> M	Tab, Green, Film Coated	Cimetidine 300 mg	by Mylan	00378-0317	Gastrointestinal
317 <> M	Tab, Green, Pentagonal, Film Coated	Cimetidine 300 mg	Tagamet by UDL	51079-0807	Gastrointestinal
317 <> M	Tab, Pentagonal, Film Coated	Cimetidine 300 mg	by HJ Harkins Co	52959-0345	Gastrointestinal
317 <> M	Tab, Film Coated	Cimetidine 300 mg	by Murfreesboro	51129-1181	Gastrointestinal
3170LORABID200MG	Cap, Blue & Gray, 3170/Lorabid 200 mg	Loracarbef 200 mg	Lorabid by Lilly		Antibiotic
3171	Cap	Loracarbef 400 mg	Lorabid by Lilly	00110-3171	Antibiotic
3171	Cap, Coated	Loracarbef 400 mg	Lorabid by DRX	55045-2259	Antibiotic
3171LORABID400MG	Cap, Blue & Pink, 3171/Lorabid 400 mg	Loracarbef 400 mg	Lorabid by Lilly		Antibiotic
317B	Tab, White, Oblong	Propoxyphene Napsylate 50 mg, Acetaminophen 325 mg	Darvocet-N by Barr		Analgesic; C IV
3186 <> V	Tab, Coated	Codeine Phosphate 10 mg, Guaifenesin 300 mg	by Vintage	00254-3186	Analgesic; C III
3186 <> V	Tab, Red, Oblong	Guaifenesin 300 mg; Codeine Phosphate 10 mg	by Qualitest Pharms	00603-3781	Analgesic; C III
3189V	Tab, Film Coated, V-Scored	Guaifenesin 600 mg, Pseudoephedrine HCl 120 mg	by Vintage	00254-3189	Cold Remedy
318BARR	Tab, White, Oblong	Propoxyphene Napsylate 100 mg, Acetaminophen 650 mg	Darvocet-N by Barr		Analgesic; C IV
318BARR	Tab, Orange, Oblong	Propoxyphene Napsylate 100 mg, Acetaminophen 650 mg	Darvocet-N by Barr		Analgesic; C IV
32 <> BL	Tab	Sulfamethoxazole 400 mg, Trimethoprim 80 mg	SMX TMP SS by PDRX	55289-0457	Antibiotic
32 <> BMS100	Tab, White	Nefazodone HCl 100 mg	Serzone by Bristol Myers Squibb	00087-0032	Antidepressant
32 <> BMS100	Tab	Nefazodone HCl 100 mg	Serzone by Quality Care	60346-0172	Antidepressant
32 <> BMS100	Tab	Nefazodone HCl 100 mg	Serzone by Bristol Myers	15548-0032	Antidepressant
32 <> PAL	Tab, Purple, Oval, Scored	Acetaminophen 712.8 mg; Caffeine 60 mg; Dihydrocodeine Bitartrate 32 mg	by Mikart	46672-0141	Analgesic; C III
32 <> PAL	Tab, Purple, Oval, Scored	Acetaminophen 712.8 mg; Caffeine 60 mg; Dihydrocodeine Bitartrate 32 mg	Panlor SS by Pan Am Labs	00525-0032	Analgesic; C III
321 <> M	Tab, Beveled Edge	Lorazepam 0.5 mg	by Mylan	00378-0321	Sedative/Hypnotic; C IV
321 <> M	Tab	Lorazepam 0.5 mg	by Murfreesboro	51129-1344	Sedative/Hypnotic; C IV
321 <> M	Tab	Lorazepam 0.5 mg	by Vangard	00615-0450	Sedative/Hypnotic; C IV
321 <> M	Tab, White, Round	Lorazepam, C-IV .50 mg	Ativan by UDL	51079-0417	Sedative/Hypnotic; C IV
321 <> R	Tab, Pink, Round	Propranolol HCl 60 mg	by Purepac	00228-2321	Antihypertensive
322 <> ACJ	Tab, Yellow, Oval	Candesartan Cilexetil 32 mg; Hydrochlorothiazide 12.5 mg	Atacand HCT by Astra Zeneca	17228-0322	Antihypertensive; Diuretic
323	Cap, Maroon	Piroxicam 20 mg	Feldene by Rx Pac	65084-0156	NSAID
323	Cap, Maroon	Piroxicam 20 mg	Feldene by Rightpak	65240-0648	NSAID
325	Tab, White, Round	Acetaminophen 325 mg	Apo Asa by Apotex	Canadian	Antipyretic
325 <> R303	Cap, Clear	Quinine Sulfate 325 mg	Quinine Sulfate by Zenith Goldline	00172-4172	Antimalarial
325 <> RSTSM	Cap, Green, Film Coated	Acetaminophen 325 mg, Pseudoephedrine HCl 30 mg	Regular Tylenol Sinus	Canadian DIN# 00778400	Cold Remedy
325 <> TCM	Cap, Yellow, Film Coated	Acetaminophen 325 mg, Chlorpheniramine Maleate 2mg, Pseudoephedrine HCl 30 mg, Dextromethorphan Hydrobromide 15 mg	Regular Tylenol Cold Nighttime	Canadian DIN# 00574007	Cold Remedy
325 <> TCMND	Cap, Yellow, Film Coated	Acetaminophen 325 mg, Pseudoephedrine HCl 30 mg, Dextromethorphan Hydrobromide 15 mg	Regular Tylenol Daytime	Canadian DIN# 00743283	Cold Remedy

ID FRONT ⟷ BACK	DESCRIPTION FRONT ⟷ BACK	INGREDIENT & STRENGTH	BRAND (OR EQUIV.) & FIRM	NDC#	CLASS; SCH.
325 ⟷ TYLENOL	Tab, White, Round, Scored	Acetaminophen 325 mg	Tylenol by McNeil	Canadian DIN# 00559393	Antipyretic
325 ⟷ TYLENOL	Cap, White, Film Coated, Scored	Acetaminophen 325 mg	Tylenol by McNeil	Canadian DIN# 00723894	Antipyretic
325MG ⟷ WATSON716	Cap, Filled with White Powder	Quinine Sulfate 325 mg	by Watson	52544-0716	Antimalarial
325MG ⟷ WATSON716	Cap	Quinine Sulfate 325 mg	by Golden State	60429-0242	Antimalarial
32BL	Tab	Sulfamethoxazole 400 mg, Trimethoprim 80 mg	SMZ TMP by Quality Care	60346-0559	Antibiotic
33	Tab, Purepac Logo	Clonazepam 0.5 mg	by Med Pro	53978-3300	Anticonvulsant; C IV
33 ⟷ BIOCRAFT	Tab	Sulfamethoxazole 800 mg, Trimethoprim 160 mg	SMZ TMP DS by Quality Care	60346-0087	Antibiotic
33 ⟷ BIOCRAFT	Tab	Sulfamethoxazole 800 mg, Trimethoprim 160 mg	SMX TMP by Vangard	00615-0170	Antibiotic
33 ⟷ BMS200	Tab, Light Yellow	Nefazodone HCl 200 mg	Serzone by Bristol Myers Squibb	00087-0033	Antidepressant
33 ⟷ BMS200	Tab	Nefazodone HCl 200 mg	Serzone by Kaiser	00179-1243	Antidepressant
33 ⟷ BMS200	Tab, Light Yellow	Nefazodone HCl 200 mg	Serzone by Quality Care	60346-0175	Antidepressant
33 ⟷ BMS200	Tab	Nefazodone HCl 200 mg	Serzone by Bristol Myers	15548-0033	Antidepressant
33 BIOCRAFT	Tab	Sulfamethoxazole 800 mg, Trimethoprim 160 mg	SMZ TMP DS by Diversified Hlthcare Serv	55887-0983	Antibiotic
33 BIOCRAFT	Tab	Sulfamethoxazole 800 mg, Trimethoprim 160 mg	SMX TMP DS by Prepackage Spec	58864-0478	Antibiotic
330 ⟷ GRISACTIN	Tab	Griseofulvin, Ultramicrosize 330 mg	Grisactin Ultra by Pharm Utilization	60491-0290	Antifungal
330 ⟷ MYLAN	Tab, White, Coated	Amitriptyline HCl 10 mg, Perphenazine 2 mg	by Mylan	00378-0330	Antipsychotic
33110	Tab	Lorazepam 1 mg	by Zenith Goldline	00182-1807	Sedative/Hypnotic; C IV
33205 ⟷ WATSON	Tab, 332 Over 0.5	Lorazepam 0.5 mg	by UDL	51079-0417	Sedative/Hypnotic; C IV
33205 ⟷ WATSON	Tab, White, Round, Scored	Lorazepam 0.5 mg	by Murfreesboro Ph	51129-1410	Sedative/Hypnotic; C IV
3328 ⟷ G150MG	Cap	Clindamycin HCl	by Quality Care	60346-0018	Antibiotic
333 ⟷ R	Tab, Yellow, Round	Propranolol HCl 80 mg	by Purepac	00228-2333	Antihypertensive
333 ⟷ SL	Tab, Film Coated	Metronidazole 250 mg	by Diversified Hlthcare Serv	55887-0978	Antibiotic
33310 ⟷ WATSON	Tab, 333 1.0	Lorazepam 1 mg	by Quality Care	60346-0047	Sedative/Hypnotic; C IV
33310 ⟷ WATSON	Tab, 333 Over 1.0	Lorazepam 1 mg	by UDL	51079-0386	Sedative/Hypnotic; C IV
33420	Tab	Lorazepam 2 mg	by Zenith Goldline	00182-1808	Sedative/Hypnotic; C IV
33420 ⟷ WATSON	Tab, 334 Over 2.0	Lorazepam 2 mg	by UDL	51079-0387	Sedative/Hypnotic; C IV
334410MG ⟷ SB10MG	Cap, Ivory & Natural, White & Yellow Pellets	Prochlorperazine Maleate 16.2 mg	Compazine by SKB	00007-3344	Antiemetic
335 ⟷ 10	Cap, 10/Royce Logo	Piroxicam 10 mg	by Qualitest	00603-5222	NSAID
33510	Cap, Blue & White, Royce logo 335/10	Piroxicam 10 mg	Feldene by Royce		NSAID
33510	Cap, 335/10	Piroxicam 10 mg	by Mutual	53489-0441	NSAID
3358 ⟷ M	Tab, White, Round	Orphenadrine Citrate 100 mg	by Phy Total Care	54868-4102	Muscle Relaxant
336 ⟷ 20	Cap, 20/Royce Logo	Piroxicam 20 mg	by Qualitest	00603-5223	NSAID
336 ⟷ 20	Cap, Royce Logo, Capsules Filled with Off-White to Light Yellow Powder	Piroxicam 20 mg	by Quality Care	60346-0676	NSAID
33620	Cap, Blue, Royce logo 336/20	Piroxicam 20 mg	Feldene by Royce		NSAID
33620	Cap, 335/20	Piroxicam 20 mg	by Mutual	53489-0442	NSAID
33620	Cap	Piroxicam 20 mg	by Med Pro	53978-1255	NSAID
3367 ⟷ RUGBY	Cap	Decyclomine HCl 10 mg	by Chelsea	46193-0105	Gastrointestinal
3367RUGBY	Cap, Clear & Dark Blue	Decyclomine HCl 10 mg	by Quality Care	60346-0911	Gastrointestinal
3367RUGBY	Cap, Clear & Dark Blue	Decyclomine HCl 10 mg	by Caremark	00339-6054	Gastrointestinal
337 ⟷ R	Tab, Peach, Round	Prednisone 20 mg	by Purepac	00228-2337	Steroid
3377 ⟷ RUGBY	Tab	Decyclomine HCl 20 mg	by Heartland	61392-0041	Gastrointestinal
3377 ⟷ RUGBY	Tab	Decyclomine HCl 20 mg	by Quality Care	60346-0912	Gastrointestinal
3377 ⟷ RUGBY	Tab	Decyclomine HCl 20 mg	by DRX	55045-1467	Gastrointestinal
3377 ⟷ RUGBY	Tab	Dicyclomine HCl 20 mg	by Allscripts	54569-0419	Gastrointestinal

ID FRONT <> BACK	DESCRIPTION FRONT <> BACK	INGREDIENT & STRENGTH	BRAND (OR EQUIV.) & FIRM	NDC#	CLASS; SCH.
3377RUGBY	Tab	Decyclomine HCl 20 mg	by Kaiser	62224-9222	Gastrointestinal
338	Tab, Purepac Logo	Prednisone 10 mg	by Quality Care	60346-0058	Steroid
338 <> R	Tab, White, Round	Prednisone 10 mg	by Purepac	00228-2338	Steroid
3399	Cap	Chlorpheniramine 12 mg, Phenylpropanolamine HCl 75 mg	Oraminic Spancap by Vortech		Cold Remedy
34	Tab, White, Round, Scored, Purepac Logo 34	Clonazepam 1 mg	by DHHS Prog	11819-0028	Anticonvulsant; C IV
34	Tab, Med Pro Logo	Clonazepam 1 mg	by Med Pro	53978-3185	Anticonvulsant; C IV
34 <> BIOCRAFT	Tab, White, Round, Scored, 3 over 4 <> Biocraft	Trimethoprim 100 mg	by Teva	00093-2158	Antibiotic
34 <> BIOCRAFT	Tab, 3 4 <> Debossed	Trimethoprim 100 mg	by Murfreesboro	51129-1204	Antibiotic
340 <> 5	Tab, 5/Royce Logo	Pindolol 5 mg	by Qualitest	00603-5220	Antihypertensive
3405	Tab, 340 Above Bisect, 5 Below <> Mortar and Pestle Logo	Pindolol 5 mg	by Royce	51875-0340	Antihypertensive
3405	Tab, White, Round, 340/5 Royce logo	Pindolol 5 mg	Visken by Royce		Antihypertensive
341 <> 10	Tab, 10/Royce Logo	Pindolol 10 mg	by Qualitest	00603-5221	Antihypertensive
34110	Tab, White, Round, 341/10 Royce logo	Pindolol 10 mg	Visken by Royce		Antihypertensive
342 <> 3M	Tab, White, Round, Scored	Theophylline 125 mg	Theolair by 3M	00089-0342	Antiasthmatic
342 <> SL	Tab	Sulfamethoxazole 800 mg, Trimethoprim 160 mg	SMZ TMP DS by Quality Care	60346-0087	Antibiotic
3438 <> A	Tab, Coated, Apotex Logo	Selegiline HCl 5 mg	by Caraco	57664-0172	Antiparkinson
3438 <> A	Tab, White, Round, Coated, Apotex Logo	Selegiline HCl 5 mg	by Apotex	60505-3438	Antiparkinson
344	Tab, Coated, Debossed Watson 344	Verapamil HCl 80 mg	by Watson	52544-0344	Antihypertensive
344	Tab, Coated, Debossed Watson 344	Verapamil HCl 80 mg	by HL Moore	00839-7267	Antihypertensive
344	Tab, Coated, Debossed Watson 344	Verapamil HCl 80 mg	by IDE Inter	00814-8280	Antihypertensive
34510	Tab, Orange, Round, Royce logo 345/10	Hydroxyzine HCl 10 mg	Atarax by Royce		Antihistamine
34510	Tab, Film Coated, Mortar and Pestle Logo	Hydroxyzine HCl 10 mg	by Royce	51875-0345	Antihistamine
34510	Tab, Film Coated, Debossed <> Royce Logo	Hydroxyzine HCl 10 mg	by Quality Care	60346-0795	Antihistamine
346	Tab, Coated, Debossed Watson 346	Verapamil HCl 120 mg	by Watson	52544-0346	Antihypertensive
346	Tab, Coated, Debossed Watson 346	Verapamil HCl 120 mg	by IDE Inter	00814-8281	Antihypertensive
346	Tab, Coated, Debossed Watson 346	Verapamil HCl 120 mg	by HL Moore	00839-7268	Antihypertensive
34625	Tab, Film Coated, Mortar and Pestle Logo	Hydroxyzine HCl 25 mg	by Royce	51875-0346	Antihistamine
34625	Tab, Green, Round, Royce logo 346/25	Hydroxyzine HCl 25 mg	Atarax by Royce		Antihistamine
34625	Tab, Film Coated, Royce	Hydroxyzine HCl 25 mg	by Prescription Dispensing	61807-0032	Antihistamine
34625 <> R	Tab, Film Coated, 346 25 <> Royce Logo	Hydroxyzine HCl 25 mg	by Quality Care	60346-0086	Antihistamine
34750	Tab, Yellow, Round, Royce logo 347/50	Hydroxyzine HCl 50 mg	Atarax by Royce		Antihistamine
34750	Tab, Film Coated, Mortar and Pestle Logo	Hydroxyzine HCl 50 mg	by Royce	51875-0347	Antihistamine
347BARR	Tab, White, Round	Chlorpropamide 100 mg	Diabinese by Barr		Antidiabetic
348 <> 25	Tab, 348 <> 25/Royce Logo	Captopril 25 mg	by Qualitest	00603-2556	Antihypertensive
348 <> R	Tab, White, Round, Scored	Propylthiouracil 50 mg	by Purepac	00228-2348	Antithyroid
34825	Tab, White, Round, Royce Logo 348/25	Captopril 25 mg	Capoten by Royce		Antihypertensive
34825	Tab	Captopril 25 mg	by Zenith Goldline	00182-2623	Antihypertensive
34825	Tab, 348 25 <> Mortar and Pestle Logo	Captopril 25 mg	by Royce	51875-0348	Antihypertensive
349 <> 50	Tab, 349 <> 50/Royce Logo	Captopril 50 mg	by Qualitest	00603-2557	Antihypertensive
34950	Tab	Captopril 50 mg	by Zenith Goldline	00182-2624	Antihypertensive
34950	Tab, White, Oval, Royce Logo 349/50	Captopril 50 mg	Capoten by Royce		Antihypertensive
349WATSON	Tab, White, Cap Shaped	Acetaminophen 500 mg, Hydrocodone Bitartrate 5 mg	by Quality Care	60346-0442	Analgesic; C III
35	Tab, White, Round, Scored, Purepac Logo 35	Clonazepam 2 mg	by DHHS Prog	11819-0052	Anticonvulsant; C IV
35 <> BL	Tab, White, Round, Scored	Trimethoprim 200 mg	by Teva	00093-2159	Antibiotic
35 <> ORTHO	Tab	Ethinyl Estradiol 0.035 mg, Norethindrone 0.5 mg, Norethindrone 1 mg, Norethindrone 0.75 mg	Ortho Novum 777 by Dept Health Central Pharm	53808-0032	Oral Contraceptive
35 <> ORTHO	Tab	Norethindrone 0.35 mg	Micronor 28 by Dept Health Central Pharm	53808-0029	Oral Contraceptive
35 <> X	Tab, White, Round	Phendimetrazine Tartrate 35 mg	by Allscripts	54569-2668	Anorexiant; C III
350 <> 100	Tab, 350 <> 100/Royce Logo	Captopril 100 mg	by Qualitest	00603-2558	Antihypertensive
350100	Tab, White, Oval, Royce Logo 350/100	Captopril 100 mg	Capoten by Royce		Antihypertensive
350100	Tab	Captopril 100 mg	by Zenith Goldline	00182-2625	Antihypertensive

ID FRONT <> BACK	DESCRIPTION FRONT <> BACK	INGREDIENT & STRENGTH	BRAND (OR EQUIV.) & FIRM	NDC#	CLASS; SCH.
351	Tab, RPR Logo Over 351	Theophylline 100 mg	Slo Phyllin by Novartis	00067-0351	Antiasthmatic
351	Tab, RPR Logo Over 351	Theophylline 100 mg	Slo Phyllin by RPR	00075-0351	Antiasthmatic
351 <> ETHEX	Tab, White, Round	Vitamin A 1000 unt, Cholecalciferol 400 unt, Vitamin E 11 unt, Ascorbic Acid 120 mg; Folic Acid 1 mg; Thiamine Mononitrate 2 mg; Riboflavin 3 mg; Niacinamide 20 mg; Pyridoxine HCl 10 mg; Cyanocobalamin 12 mcg, Iron 29 mg	Nutrinate Chewable with Iron by KV Pharm	10609-1459	Vitamin
351 <> ETHEX	Tab, White, Round	Vitamin A 1000 unt, Cholecalciferol 400 unt, Vitamin E 11 unt, Ascorbic Acid 120 mg; Folic Acid 1 mg; Thiamine Mononitrate 2 mg; Riboflavin 3 mg; Niacinamide 20 mg; Pyridoxine HCl 10 mg; Cyanocobalamin 12 mcg, Iron 29 mg	Nutrinate Chewable with Iron by Ethex	58177-0351	Vitamin
351 <> RPR	Tab, White, Round	Theophylline 100 mg	Slo-Phyllin by RPR	00801-0351	Bronchodilator
351310MG <> SB10MG	Cap, Ivory & Natural, 3513/10 mg	Dextroamphetamine Sulfate 10 mg	Dexedrine by SKB	00007-3513	Stimulant; C II
352	Tab, RPR Logo Over 352	Theophylline 200 mg	Slo Phyllin by Novartis	00067-0352	Antiasthmatic
352	Tab, RPR Logo Over 352	Theophylline 200 mg	Slo Phyllin by RPR	00075-0352	Antiasthmatic
352 <> FULVICINPG	Tab, Off-White, Fulvicin P/G	Griseofulvin, Ultramicrocrystalline 330 mg	Fulvicin P G 330 by Pharm Utilization	60491-0275	Antifungal
352 <> RPR	Tab, White, Round	Theophylline 200 mg	Slo-Phyllin by RPR	00801-0352	Bronchodilator
3535 <> GEIGY	Tab	Hydrochlorothiazide 25 mg, Metoprolol Tartrate 50 mg	Lopressor HCT by Novartis	00028-0035	Diuretic; Antihypertensive
3549IL	Tab, Ex Release, 3459 IL	Isosorbide Dinitrate 40 mg	by Schein	00364-0401	Antianginal
3549IL	Tab, Diamond Shape, ER, 3549 IL	Isosorbide Dinitrate 40 mg	by Murfreesboro	51129-1329	Antianginal
355 <> 125	Tab, 355 <> 12.5/Royce Logo	Captopril 12.5 mg	by Qualitest	00603-2555	Antihypertensive
355 <> C	Tab, Green, Oblong	Guaifenesin 600 mg; Dextromethorphan Hydrobromide 30 mg	by Caraco Pharm	57664-0355	Cold Remedy
355 <> FOREST	Cap, Blue & Pink	Racemethionine 200 mg	Pedameth by Forest	00456-0355	Urinary
355125	Tab, White, Oblong, Royce Logo 355/12.5	Captopril 12.5 mg	Capoten by Royce		Antihypertensive
355125	Tab	Captopril 12.5 mg	by Zenith Goldline	00182-2622	Antihypertensive
357 <> MYLAN	Tab, Lavender, Film Coated	Pentoxifylline 400 mg	by Mylan	00378-0357	Anticoagulent
357 <> MYLAN	Tab, Lavender, Capsule Shaped, Film Coated	Pentoxifylline 400 mg	Trental by UDL	51079-0889	Anticoagulent
357HRMAGNUM	Cap, Pink & White, 357 HR/Magnum	Caffeine 200 mg	357 Magnum by BDI		Stimulant
357MAGNUM	Tab, Pink, Bullet Shaped	Caffeine 200 mg	by B & M Labs		Stimulant
358 <> 550	Tab	Amiloride HCl 5 mg, Hydrochlorothiazide 50 mg	by United Res	00677-1223	Diuretic
3581 <> IL	Tab, ER	Theophylline 300 mg	by Schein	00364-0660	Antiasthmatic
3583 <> IL	Tab, ER	Theophylline 200 mg	by Schein	00364-0681	Antiasthmatic
3584 IL	Tab, ER, 3584 IL	Theophylline 100 mg	by Schein	00364-0680	Antiasthmatic
358550	Tab, Peach, Round, Royce Logo 358 5-50	Amiloride HCl 5 mg, Hydrochlorothiazide 50 mg	Moduretic 5/50 by Royce		Diuretic
358550	Tab, 358 5-50 <> Mortar and Pestle Logo	Amiloride HCl 5 mg, Hydrochlorothiazide 50 mg	by Royce	51875-0358	Diuretic
358R	Tab, 358/R	Hydrochlorothiazide 25 mg, Propranolol HCl 40 mg	by Schein	00364-0838	Diuretic; Antihypertensive
3591V	Tab, 35/91 V	Acetaminophen 555 mg, Hydrocodone Bitartrate 2.5 mg	by Qualitest	00603-3880	Analgesic; C III
3591V	Tab, White, Red Specks, 35/91 V	Acetaminophen 555 mg, Hydrocodone Bitartrate 2.5 mg	by Vintage	00254-3591	Analgesic; C III
3592 <> V	Tab, 35/92	Acetaminophen 500 mg, Hydrocodone Bitartrate 5 mg	by Kaiser	00179-1026	Analgesic; C III
3592 <> V	Tab, 35 92	Acetaminophen 500 mg, Hydrocodone Bitartrate 5 mg	by Quality Care	60346-0442	Analgesic; C III
3592 <> V	Tab, White, Oblong, Scored	Hydrocodone Bitartrate 5 mg, Acetaminophen 500 mg	by Vangard Labs	00615-0400	Analgesic; C III
3592V	Tab	Acetaminophen 500 mg, Hydrocodone Bitartrate 5 mg	by Pharmedix	53002-0119	Analgesic; C III
3594V	Tab, 35/94 V	Acetaminophen 500 mg, Hydrocodone Bitartrate 7.5 mg	by St Marys Med	60760-0594	Analgesic; C III
3594V	Tab, White with Green Specks, 35/94 V	Acetaminophen 500 mg, Hydrocodone Bitartrate 7.5 mg	by Quality Care	60346-0012	Analgesic; C III
3594V	Tab, White, Green Specks, 35/94 V	Acetaminophen 500 mg, Hydrocodone Bitartrate 7.5 mg	by Vintage	00254-3594	Analgesic; C III
3594V	Tab, White, Green Specks, 35/94 V	Acetaminophen 500 mg, Hydrocodone Bitartrate 7.5 mg	by Murfreesboro	51129-1381	Analgesic; C III
3595V	Tab, White, Oblong	Hydrocodone Bitartrate 7.5 mg, Acetaminophen 650 mg	by ESI Lederle		Analgesic; C III
3596V	Tab, 35/96V	Acetaminophen 750 mg, Hydrocodone Bitartrate 7.5 mg	by Vintage	00254-3596	Analgesic; C III
3596V	Tab, White, Oblong, Scored, 35/96 V	Acetaminophen 750 mg, Hydrocodone Bitartrate 7.5 mg	Hydrocodone APAP by American Pharm	58605-0521	Analgesic; C III
3597V	Tab, 35/97 V	Acetaminophen 650 mg, Hydrocodone Bitartrate 10 mg	by Vintage	00254-3597	Analgesic; C III
3597V	Tab, Light Blue, 35/97 V	Acetaminophen 650 mg, Hydrocodone Bitartrate 10 mg	by Qualitest	00603-3885	Analgesic; C III
3597V	Tab, 35/97 V	Acetaminophen 650 mg, Hydrocodone Bitartrate 10 mg	by Martec	52555-0672	Analgesic; C III
36 <> SL	Tab, Light Yellow, Sugar Coated	Desipramine HCl 25 mg	by Schein	00364-2209	Antidepressant

ID FRONT <> BACK	DESCRIPTION FRONT <> BACK	INGREDIENT & STRENGTH	BRAND (OR EQUIV.) & FIRM	NDC#	CLASS; SCH.
36 <> SL	Tab, Light Yellow, Round, Sugar Coated	Desipramine HCl 25 mg	Norpramin by Sidmak	50111-0436	Antidepressant
3601V	Tab, Yellow, Oblong	Acetaminophen 325 mg, Hydrocodone Bitartrate 10 mg	by Vintage		Analgesic; C III
3607 <> IL	Cap, Lavender, ER	Indomethacin 75 mg	by Schein	00364-2211	NSAID
3607 <> IL	Cap, Clear & Lavender, ER	Indomethacin 75 mg	by Quality Care	60346-0687	NSAID
3607 <> IL	Cap, Lavender, ER	Indomethacin 75 mg	by Qualitest	00603-4070	NSAID
3608 <> 59911	Tab, White, Oval	Etodolac 400 mg	by ESI Lederle	59911-3608	NSAID
3608 <> 59911	Tab, White, Oval, Film Coated	Etodolac 400 mg	by Wyeth Pharms	52903-3608	NSAID
3609 <> IL	Cap, ER	Propranolol HCl 60 mg	by Qualitest	00603-5497	Antihypertensive
361 <> M	Tab, Blue, Oblong, Scored	Hydrocodone Bitartrate 10 mg, Acetaminophen 650 mg	by Southwood Pharms	58016-0232	Analgesic; C III
3610	Cap, Opaque Blue & Clear, ER, with Off-White Beads	Propranolol HCl 80 mg	by United Res	00677-1364	Antihypertensive
3610 <> IL	Cap, ER	Propranolol HCl 80 mg	by Qualitest	00603-5498	Antihypertensive
3611	Cap, ER	Propranolol HCl 120 mg	by United Res	00677-1365	Antihypertensive
3611 <> IL	Cap, ER	Propranolol HCl 120 mg	by Qualitest	00603-5499	Antihypertensive
3611V	Tab, Bisected V	Hydromorphone HCl 2 mg	by Vintage	00254-3611	Analgesic; C II
3612V	Tab, Bisected V	Hydromorphone HCl 4 mg	by Vintage	00254-3612	Analgesic; C II
3613 <> IL	Tab, Peach, Round, Scored	Isosorbide Dinitrate 40 mg	by Allscripts	54569-0454	Antianginal
36154	Tab, White, Round, 361/5.4 Royce logo	Yohimbine HCl 5.4 mg	Yocon by Royce		Impotence Agent
36154	Tab, 361, 5.4 <> Mortar and Pestle Logo	Yohimbine HCl 5.4 mg	by Royce	51875-0361	Impotence Agent
3626 <> Z	Cap	Doxycycline Hyclate	by Quality Care	60346-0449	Antibiotic
363025	Tab, White, Oval, Royce Logo 363/0.25	Alprazolam 0.25 mg	Xanax by Royce		Antianxiety; C IV
364 <> DPI	Cap, Scarlet, Black Print	Acetaminophen 325 mg, Dichloralantipyrine 100 mg, Isometheptene Mucate (1:1) 65 mg	Duradrin by Kaiser	00179-1222	Cold Remedy
364 <> DPI	Cap, Scarlet, DPI or DP	Acetaminophen 325 mg, Dichloralantipyrine 100 mg, Isometheptene Mucate (1:1) 65 mg	Midchlor by Schein	00364-2342	Cold Remedy
3640061	Cap, Clear & Light Green	Chloral Hydrate 500 mg	by RP Scherer	11014-0913	Sedative/Hypnotic; C IV
36405	Tab, Peach, Oval, Royce Logo, 364/0.5	Alprazolam 0.5 mg	Xanax by Royce		Antianxiety; C IV
3642	Cap	Papaverine HCl 150 mg	Pavabid by Vortech		Vasodilator
364364 <> GLYBUR	Tab, 364 364	Glyburide 5 mg	by Quality Care	60346-0938	Antidiabetic
364364 <> GLYBUR	Tab	Glyburide 5 mg	by PDRX	55289-0892	Antidiabetic
364364 <> GLYBUR	Tab, Blue, Oblong, Scored	Glyburide 5 mg	by Blue Ridge	59273-0015	Antidiabetic
364364 <> GLYBUR	Tab	Glyburide 5 mg	by Merrell	00068-3202	Antidiabetic
364364 <> GLYBUR	Tab	Glyburide 5 mg	by Allscripts	54569-3831	Antidiabetic
364364 <> GLYBUR	Tab	Glyburide 5 mg	by Copley	38245-0364	Antidiabetic
364COPLEY	Tab, Blue, Oblong, 364/Copley	Glyburide 5.0 mg	DIABETA by Copley		Antidiabetic
3651	Tab, Blue, Oval, Scored, 365 over 1 <> Royce Logo	Alprazolam 1 mg	by Apotheca	12634-0522	Antianxiety; C IV
3651	Tab, Blue, Oval, Royce Logo 365/1	Alprazolam 1 mg	Xanax by Royce		Antianxiety; C IV
367 <> C	Tab, Red, Oblong, Film Coated	Guaifenesin 300 mg, Codeine Phosphate 10 mg	by Martec	52555-0160	Analgesic; C III
3678	Cap, Clear Yellow	Benzonatate 200 mg	by Inwood	00258-3678	Antitussive
3678	Cap	Phentermine 30 mg	Phentrol #6 by Vortech		Anorexiant; C IV
368 <> SL	Tab, Brown, Round, Film Coated	Amitriptyline HCl 50 mg	Elavil by Sidmak	50111-0368	Antidepressant
3685 <> 0115	Tab, White, Oval	Hydrocortisone 20 mg	by Global	00115-3685	Steroid
369 <> 54	Cap, Green	Loperamide HCl 2 mg	Imodium A-D by Roxane	00054-8537	Antidiarrheal
369 <> 54	Cap	Loperamide HCl 2 mg	by Nat Pharmpak Serv	55154-4912	Antidiarrheal
36SL	Tab, Sugar Coated	Desipramine HCl 25 mg	by Med Pro	53978-2076	Antidepressant
37 <> 149	Tab, Light Red, Oblong, Mottled	Naproxen 500 mg	by Allscripts	54569-4255	NSAID
370 <> MYLAN	Tab, Yellow, Round	Bumetanide 1 mg	by UDL	51079-0892	Diuretic
370 <> MYLAN	Tab, Yellow, Scored	Bumetanide 1 mg	by Mylan	00378-0370	Diuretic
37046 <> BUTIBEL	Tab, Red, Round, 37 over 046 <> Butibel	Belladonna Extract 15 mg, Butabarbital Sodium 15 mg	Butibel by Wallace	00037-0046	Gastrointestinal; C IV
370B	Tab, White, Round	Lorazepam 0.5 mg	Ativan by Barr		Sedative/Hypnotic; C IV
371001 <> WALLACE	Tab, White, Round, Scored, 37-1001 <> Wallace	Meprobamate 400 mg	Miltown by Wallace	00037-1001	Sedative/Hypnotic; C IV
371101 <> WALLACE	Tab, White, Round, Sugar Coated, 37-1101 <> Wallace	Meprobamate 200 mg	Miltown by Wallace	00037-1101	Sedative/Hypnotic; C IV

ID FRONT <> BACK	DESCRIPTION FRONT <> BACK	INGREDIENT & STRENGTH	BRAND (OR EQUIV.) & FIRM	NDC#	CLASS; SCH.
37112 <> BUTISOLSODIUM	Tab, Lavender, Scored, 37 over 112 <> Butisol Sodium	Butabarbital Sodium 15 mg	Butisol Sodium by Wallace	00037-0112	Sedative; C III
37113 <> BUTISOLSODIUM	Tab, Green, Scored, 37 over 113 <> Butisol Sodium	Butabarbital Sodium 30 mg	Butisol Sodium by Wallace	00037-0113	Sedative; C III
37114 <> BUTISOLSODIUM	Tab, Orange, Scored, 37 over 114 <> Butisol Sodium	Butabarbital Sodium 50 mg	Butisol Sodium by Wallace	00037-0114	Sedative; C III
371B	Tab, White, Round	Lorazepam 1 mg	Ativan by Barr		Sedative/Hypnotic; C IV
372 <> M	Tab, Film Coated	Cimetidine 400 mg	by Quality Care	60346-0945	Gastrointestinal
372 <> M	Tab, Film Coated, Scored	Cimetidine 400 mg	by Nat Pharmpak Serv	55154-5555	Gastrointestinal
372 <> M	Tab, Green, Pentagonal, Coated, Scored	Cimetidine 400 mg	by Allscripts	54569-3838	Gastrointestinal
372 <> M	Tab, Green, Film Coated, Scored	Cimetidine 400 mg	by Mylan	00378-0372	Gastrointestinal
372 <> M	Tab, Pentagonal, Film Coated, Scored	Cimetidine 400 mg	by HJ Harkins Co	52959-0375	Gastrointestinal
372 <> M	Tab, Green, Pentagonal, Film Coated	Cimetidine 400 mg	Tagamet by UDL	51079-0808	Gastrointestinal
372 <> M	Tab, Film Coated, Scored	Cimetidine 400 mg	by Murfreesboro	51129-1179	Gastrointestinal
3725 <> MYLAN	Tab, 37 to Left, 25 to Right of Score, Beveled Edge	Hydrochlorothiazide 25 mg, Triamterene 37.5 mg	Maxzide 25 by Mylan	00378-3725	Diuretic
372BARR	Tab, White, Round	Lorazepam 2 mg	Ativan by Barr		Sedative/Hypnotic; C IV
373 <> M	Tab, Film Coated	Hydroxychloroquine 155 mg	by Mylan	00378-0373	Antimalarial
3737	Tab, White, Oblong, 37/37	Dyphylline 400 mg	Lufyllin by Lemmon		Antiasthmatic
3737 <> UU	Tab, White, Round, 37 Twice <> U Twice	Pramipexole DiHCl 1.5 mg	Mirapex by Pharmacia & Upjohn	00009-0037	Antiparkinson
373BARR	Tab, Yellow, Round	Oxazepam 15 mg	Serax by Barr		Sedative/Hypnotic; C IV
373WATSON	Tab, Film Coated, Watson 373	Maprotiline HCl 25 mg	by Watson	52544-0373	Antidepressant
373WATSON	Tab, Film Coated, Watson 373	Maprotiline HCl 25 mg	by Medirex	57480-0493	Antidepressant
373WATSON	Tab, Film Coated, Watson 373	Maprotiline HCl 25 mg	by Geneva	00781-1631	Antidepressant
373WATSON	Tab, Film Coated, Watson 373	Maprotiline HCl 25 mg	by Zenith Goldline	00182-1882	Antidepressant
374401	Tab, White, Ellipsoid, 37/4401	Penicillamine 250 mg	by Horner	Canadian	Chelating Agent
374401 <> WALLACE	Tab, White, Oval, Scored, 37 Over 4401 <> Wallace	Penicillamine 250 mg	Depen Titratable by Wallace	00037-4401	Chelating Agent
375 <> ECNAPROSYN	Tab, DR	Naproxen 375 mg	Naprosyn by Syntex	18393-0255	NSAID
375 <> ECNAPROSYN	Tab, DR, EC Naprosyn	Naproxen 375 mg	EC Naprosyn by Allscripts	54569-3981	NSAID
375 <> ECNAPROSYN	Tab, DR, EC Naprosyn	Naproxen 375 mg	E C Naprosyn by PDRX	55289-0267	NSAID
375 <> ECNAPROSYN	Tab, DR	Naproxen 375 mg	EC Naprosyn by DRX	55045-2425	NSAID
375 <> FLAGYL	Cap	Metronidazole 375 mg	Flagyl by GD Searle	00025-1942	Antibiotic
375 <> FLAGYL	Cap, Light Green	Metronidazole 375 mg	Flagyl by Physicians Total Care	54868-3786	Antibiotic
375 <> N518	Tab, Pink, Oval, N Over 518	Naproxen 375 mg	by Novopharm	55953-0518	NSAID
375 <> N518	Tab, N Over 518	Naproxen 375 mg	by Medirex	57480-0834	NSAID
375 <> NAPROSYN	Tab	Naproxen 375 mg	Naprosyn by Nat Pharmpak Serv	55154-3803	NSAID
375 <> NAPROSYN	Tab	Naproxen 375 mg	Naprosyn by Amerisource	62584-0273	NSAID
375 <> NAPROSYN	Tab	Naproxen 375 mg	Naprosyn by Quality Care	60346-0636	NSAID
375 <> NAPROSYN	Tab, Debossed	Naproxen 375 mg	Naprosyn by Syntex	18393-0273	NSAID
375 <> NAPROSYN	Tab, Peach, Oblong	Naproxen 375 mg	Naprosyn by Rightpak	65240-0700	NSAID
375 <> NAPROSYN	Tab	Naproxen 375 mg	Naprosyn by Allscripts	54569-0293	NSAID
375 <> NAPROSYN	Tab	Naproxen 375 mg	Naprosyn by HJ Harkins Co	52959-0192	NSAID
375 <> NAPROSYN	Tab, Debossed	Naproxen 375 mg	Naprosyn by Thrift Drug	59198-0238	NSAID
375 <> NAPROXEN	Tab	Naproxen 375 mg	by Quality Care	60346-0817	NSAID
375 <> SIDMAK	Tab	Nystatin 100000 Units	by Qualitest	00603-4831	Antifungal
375 <> SIDMAK	Tab, Off-White, Oval	Nystatin Vaginal 100000 Units	Mycostatin by Sidmak	50111-0375	Antifungal
375 <> WATSON363	Tab, 3.75 <> Watson 363	Clorazepate Dipotassium 3.75 mg	by Quality Care	60346-0409	Antianxiety; C IV
375 <> WEEFEXORXR	Cap, Gray & Peach	Venlafaxine HCl 37.5 mg	Effexor XR by Wyeth Pharms	52903-0837	Antidepressant
375 <> WEEFEXORXR	Cap, Gray & Peach	Venlafaxine HCl 37.5 mg	Effexor XR y Murfreesboro Ph	51129-1678	Antidepressant
375 <> WEEFEXORXR	Cap, Gray & Peach	Venlafaxine HCl 37.5 mg	Effexor XR by Wyeth Labs	00008-0837	Antidepressant
375M37 <> MOVA	Tab, 375 M37	Naproxen 375 mg	by Caremark	00339-5872	NSAID
375M37 <> MOVA	Tab, White, Cap Shaped	Naproxen 375 mg	Naprosyn by MOVA	55370-0140	NSAID
375M37 <> MOVA	Tab, 375 M37 <> Mova	Naproxen 375 mg	by Martec	52555-0713	NSAID

ID FRONT <> BACK	DESCRIPTION FRONT <> BACK	INGREDIENT & STRENGTH	BRAND (OR EQUIV.) & FIRM	NDC#	CLASS; SCH.
375NAXEN	Tab, Peach, Oblong, 375/Naxen	Naproxen 375 mg	Navalbine by B.W. Inc	Canadian	NSAID
375W <> 781	Tab, Shield-Shaped	Venlafaxine HCl	Effexor by Allscripts	54569-4131	Antidepressant
375W <> 781	Tab, Shield-Shaped	Venlafaxine HCl	Effexor by Caremark	00339-6035	Antidepressant
376	Tab, White, Round	Genaced	Excedrin by Granutec		Antibiotic
3762	Cap	Diphenhydramine HCl 50 mg	by Quality Care	60346-0045	Antihistamine
377 <> MYLAN	Tab, White	Naproxen 250 mg	by Mylan	00378-0377	NSAID
377 <> MYLAN	Tab	Naproxen 250 mg	by Kaiser	00179-1186	NSAID
377 <> MYLAN	Tab, White, Round	Naproxen 250 mg	Naprosyn by UDL	51079-0793	NSAID
377 <> MYLAN	Tab	Naproxen 250 mg	by HJ Harkins Co	52959-0190	NSAID
377 <> MYLAN	Tab	Naproxen 250 mg	by Allscripts	54569-3758	NSAID
377 <> MYLAN	Tab	Naproxen 250 mg	by Quality Care	60346-0816	NSAID
377 <> MYLAN	Tab, White, Round	Naproxen 250 mg	by Dixon Shane	17236-0076	NSAID
3770008	Tab, White, Round, 377-0008	Aminophylline 100 mg	by Vale		Antiasthmatic
3770106	Tab, Yellow, Round, 377-0106	Chlorpheniramine 1 mg, Pyrilamine 12.5 mg, Phenylephrine 5 mg	Duphrene by Vale		Cold Remedy
3770109	Tab, Yellow, Round, 377-0109	Ephedrine 16.2 mg, Sodium Phenobarbital 24.3 mg	by Vale		Antiasthmatic; C IV
3770125	Tab, White, Round, 377-0125	Guaifenesin 100 mg	Glycotuss by Vale		Expectorant
3770167	Tab, White, Round, 377-0167	Pyrilamine Maleate 25 mg	Nisaval by Vale		Antihistamine
3770187	Tab, Pink, Round, 377-0187	Phenobarbital 15 mg	by Vale		Sedative/Hypnotic; C IV
3770188	Tab, White, Round, 377-0188	Phenobarbital 15 mg	by Vale		Sedative/Hypnotic; C IV
3770189	Tab, Green, Round, 377-0189	Phenobarbital 15 mg	by Vale		Sedative/Hypnotic; C IV
3770192	Tab, White, Round, 377-0192	Phenobarbital 30 mg	by Vale		Sedative/Hypnotic; C IV
3770193	Tab, Pink, Round, 377-0193	Phenobarbital 30 mg	by Vale		Sedative/Hypnotic; C IV
3770196	Tab, White, Round, 377-0196	Phenobarbital 90 mg	by Vale		Sedative/Hypnotic; C IV
3770214	Tab, Red, Round, 377-0214	Rauwolfia Serpentina 50 mg	Raudixin by Vale		Antihypertensive
3770215	Tab, Pink, Round, 377-0215	Rauwolfia Serpentina 100 mg	Raudixin by Vale		Antihypertensive
3770216	Tab, Green & White Mottled, Round, 377-0216	Phenylephrine 5 mg, Chlorpheniramine 2 mg, Salicylamide 250 mg, Acetaminophen 150 mg	Rhinogesic by Vale		Cold Remedy
3770217	Tab, Green & White Mottled, Round, 377-0217	Phenylephrine 2 mg, Chlorpheniramine 1 mg, Salicylamide 90 mg, Acetaminophen 60 mg	Rhinogesic JR by Vale		Cold Remedy
3770232	Tab, Pink, Round, 377-0232	Sodium Butabarbital 15 mg	Butisol by Vale		Sedative/Hypnotic; C III
3770233	Tab, Green, Round, 377-0233	Sodium Butabarbital 30 mg	Butisol by Vale		Sedative/Hypnotic; C III
3770238	Tab, Pink, Round, 377-0238	Sodium Salicylate 324 mg	by Vale		Analgesic
3770240	Tab, Red, Round, 377-0240	Sodium Salicylate 324 mg	by Vale		Analgesic
3770242	Tab, Purple, Round, 377-0242	Sodium Salicylate 324 mg	by Vale		Analgesic
3770272	Tab, Tan, Round, 377-0272	Thyroid 30 mg	by Vale		Thyroid
3770277	Tab, Pink, Round, 377-0277	Sulfadiazine 167 mg, Sulfamerazine 167 mg, Sulfamethazine 167 mg	Triple Sulfoid by Vale		Antibiotic
3770290	Tab, Orange, Round, 377-0290	Diphenhydramine HCl 50 mg	Valdrene by Vale		Antihistamine
3770311	Tab, Green & White, Round, 377-0311	Phenyleph 5, Chlorphenir 2, Salicylamide 250, Acetaminophen 150, Guaifen 100	Rhinogesic GG by Vale		Cold Remedy
3770332	Tab, Tan, Round, 377-0332	Pepsin 259 mg, Pancreatin 32 mg, Diastase 2 mg	Pepsin & Pancreatin by Vale		Gastrointestinal
3770349	Tab, Yellow, Round, 377-0349	Magnesium Trisilicate 500 mg	Trioval by Vale		Antiarthritic
3770351	Tab, Yellow, Round, 377-0351	Phendimetrazine Tartrate 35 mg	Obeval by Vale		Anorexiant; C III
3770358	Tab, Green, Round, 377-0358	Pseudoephedrine 60 mg	Sudafed by Vale		Decongestant
3770359	Tab, Mottled White, Round, 377-0359	Guaifenesin 100 mg, Pseudoephedrine HCl 30 mg	Glycofed by Vale		Cold Remedy
3770365	Tab, Green, Round, 377-0365	Phenobarbital, Hyoscyamine, Scopolamine, Atropine	Barbeloid by Vale		Gastrointestinal; C IV
3770396	Tab, Green, Round, 377-0396	Thyroid 65 mg	by Vale		Thyroid
3770498	Tab, Yellow, Round, 377-0498	Phenobarbital, Hyoscyamine, Scopolamine, Atropine	Barbeloid by Vale		Gastrointestinal; C IV
3770630	Tab, Blue & White, Round, 377-0630	Dover's Pwd 24 mg, Aspirin 324 mg, Caffeine 32 mg	Dovacet by Vale		Analgesic
3770636	Tab, Red, Round, 377-0636	Dover's Pwd 15 mg, Aspirin 162 mg, Caffeine 8.1 mg	Acedoval by Vale		Analgesic
3770642	Tab, Yellow, Round, 377-0642	Phenobarbital, Hyoscyamine, Scopolamine, Camphor, Valerian, Passif	Nevrotose #3 by Vale		Gastrointestinal; C IV
3770650	Tab, Blue, Round, 377-0650	Barbital, Hyoscyamine, Scopolamine, Passiflora, Valeri	Barbatose #2 by Vale		Gastrointestinal
377200	Tab, White, Oval. Royce Logo 377/200	Hydroxychloroquine Sulfate 200 mg	Plaquenil by Royce		Antimalarial
377200	Tab, Coated, 377/200 <> Royce Logo	Hydroxychloroquine Sulfate 200 mg	by Schein	00364-2627	Antimalarial

ID FRONT <> BACK	DESCRIPTION FRONT <> BACK	INGREDIENT & STRENGTH	BRAND (OR EQUIV.) & FIRM	NDC#	CLASS; SCH.
377200	Tab, White, Oval, Scored, 377,200 Royce Logo	Hydroxychloroquine Sulfate 200 mg	Plaquenil Sulfate by Martec	52555-0642	Antimalarial
377200	Tab, Coated, Partial Score <> Royce Logo	Hydroxychloroquine Sulfate 200 mg	by Royce	51875-0377	Antimalarial
377200	Tab, Coated, 377 200 <> Royce Logo	Hydroxychloroquine Sulfate 201 mg	by Major	00904-5107	Antimalarial
377200	Tab, Coated, Partial Score <> Royce Logo	Hydroxychloroquine Sulfate 201 mg	by Qualitest	00603-3944	Antimalarial
377200 <> ROYCE	Tab, Coated, 377, 200, and A Partial Score <> Royce Logo	Hydroxychloroquine Sulfate 200 mg	by Zenith Goldline	00182-2609	Antimalarial
3774280	Tab, Orange, Round, 377-4280	Prednisolone 5 mg	by Vale		Steroid
3774294	Tab, White, Round, 377-4294	Prednisone 5 mg	by Vale		Steroid
378 <> PFIZER	Tab, Blue, Round	Trovafloxacin 100 mg	Trovan by Pfizer	Canadian DIN# 02239191	Antibiotic
378 <> PFIZER	Tab, Blue, Round, DR	Trovafloxacin Mesylate	Trovan by Roerig	00049-3780	Antibiotic
379	Tab	Amoxapine 25 mg	by Watson	52544-0379	Antidepressant
379 <> PFIZER	Tab, Blue, Oval	Trovafloxacin 200 mg	Trovan by Pfizer	Canadian DIN# 02239192	Antibiotic
379 <> PFIZER	Tab, Blue, DR, Modified IV	Trovafloxacin Mesylate	Trovan by Roerig	00049-3790	Antibiotic
3796	Cap	Dextroamphetamine Sulfate 15 mg	Spancap #1 by Vortech		Stimulant; C II
37WALLACE <> SOMA	Tab	Carisoprodol 350 mg	Soma by Nat Pharmpak Serv	55154-4102	Muscle Relaxant
37WALLACE2001	Tab, White, Round, 37-Wallace 2001	Carisoprodol 350 mg	Soma by Horner	Canadian	Muscle Relaxant
37WALLACE2001 <> SOMA	Tab, White, Round	Carisoprodol 350 mg	Soma by Rightpac	65240-0738	Muscle Relaxant
37WALLACE2001 <> SOMA	Tab, White, Round	Carisoprodol 350 mg	Soma by Thrift Services	59198-0361	Muscle Relaxant
37WALLACE2001 <> SOMA	Tab, White, Round, 37-Wallace 2001 <> Soma	Carisoprodol 350 mg	Soma by Wallace	00037-2001	Muscle Relaxant
37WALLACE2001 <> SOMA	Tab, White, Round, 37-Wallace 2001 <> Soma	Carisoprodol 350 mg	Soma by Caremark	00339-6145	Muscle Relaxant
37WALLACE4312	Tab, Rose, Round, 37 over Wallace over 4312	Guaifenesin 200 mg	Organidin NR by Wallace	00037-4312	Expectorant
38 <> 832	Tab	Oxybutynin Chloride 5 mg	by Rosemont	00832-0038	Urinary
38 <> 832	Tab, White, Round, Scored, 3/8 <> 832	Oxybutynin Chloride 5 mg	Ditropan by UDL	51079-0628	Urinary
38 <> 832	Tab, White, Round, Scored	Oxybutynin Chloride 5 mg	by Dixon Shane	17236-0850	Urinary
38 <> G	Cap, Gray	Etodolac 200 mg	by Genpharm	55567-0038	NSAID
38 <> GG	Tab, Lavender, Film Coated	Hydroxyzine HCl 25 mg	by Quality Care	60346-0086	Antihistamine
381	Tab	Amoxapine 100 mg	by Watson	52544-0381	Antidepressant
381 <> ORGANON	Cap	Amylase 30000 Units, Lipase 8000 Units, Protease 30000 Units	Cotazym by Physicians Total Care	54868-3793	Gastrointestinal
381381 <> COPLEY	Tab, Green, Hexagon, Scored	Glyburide 1.5 mg	by Blue Ridge	59273-0016	Antidiabetic
381381 <> COPLEY	Tab, Green, Hexagon, Scored	Glyburide 3 mg	by Blue Ridge	59273-0017	Antidiabetic
381381 <> COPLEY	Tab	Glyburide 3 mg	Micronized by DRX	55045-2267	Antidiabetic
381381 <> COPLEY	Tab, Light Green, Rounded Hexagon	Glyburide 3 mg	Micronized by Copley	38245-0381	Antidiabetic
381B	Tab, 381 Over b	Meperidine HCl 50 mg	by Barr	00555-0381	Analgesic; C II
382	Tab	Amoxapine 150 mg	by Watson	52544-0382	Antidepressant
382 <> BARR	Tab, Debossed	Meperidine HCl 100 mg	by Barr	00555-0382	Analgesic; C II
384 <> 260R	Tab, White, Round	Quinine Sulfate 260 mg	Quinamm by Zenith Goldline	00172-3001	Antimalarial
384 <> 260R	Tab, White, Round	Quinine Sulfate 260 mg	Quinamm by Zenith Goldline	00182-8615	Antimalarial
3840 <> RUGBY	Tab	Furosemide 20 mg	by Rugby	00536-3840	Diuretic
3841 <> RUGBY	Tab	Furosemide 40 mg	by Rugby	00536-3841	Diuretic
384260	Tab, White, Round, 384/260 Royce logo	Quinine Sulfate 260 mg	Quinamm by Royce		Antimalarial
384260	Tab, 384, 260 <> Mortar and Pestle Logo	Quinine Sulfate 260 mg	by Royce	51875-0384	Antimalarial
384260R	Tab, White, Round	Quinine Sulfate 260 mg	Quinamm by Zenith Goldline	00182-1213	Antimalarial
386	Cap, Maroon	Phenylpropanolamine HCl 75 mg, Brompheniramine Sulfate 12 mg	Dimetapp Gelcaps by Granutec		Cold Remedy
38625500	Tab, Scored, 386 Left of Score, 2.5 over 500 Right of Score <> Royce Logo	Acetaminophen 500 mg, Hydrocodone Bitartrate 2.5 mg	by Royce	51875-0386	Analgesic; C III

ID FRONT <> BACK	DESCRIPTION FRONT <> BACK	INGREDIENT & STRENGTH	BRAND (OR EQUIV.) & FIRM	NDC#	CLASS; SCH.
38625500	Tab, White, Oblong, Royce Logo 386 2.5/500	Hydrocodone Bitartrate 2.5 mg, Acetaminophen 500 mg	Lortab by Royce		Analgesic; C III
387 <> GLAXO	Tab, Film Coated	Cefuroxime Axetil	Ceftin by Amerisource	62584-0325	Antibiotic
387 <> GLAXO	Tab, Film Coated	Cefuroxime Axetil	Ceftin by Glaxo	00173-0387	Antibiotic
387 <> GLAXO	Tab, Film Coated	Cefuroxime Axetil	Ceftin by Glaxo	51952-1347	Antibiotic
387 <> GLAXO	Tab, Film Coated	Cefuroxime Axetil	Ceftin by Nat Pharmpak Serv	55154-1109	Antibiotic
387 <> GLAXO	Tab, Light Blue, Film Coated	Cefuroxime Axetil	by Med Pro	53978-2088	Antibiotic
387 <> GLAXO	Tab, Light Blue, Film Coated	Cefuroxime Axetil 250 mg	Ceftin by Quality Care	60346-0369	Antibiotic
387 <> GLAXO	Tab, Blue, Oblong	Cefuroxime Axetil 250 mg	Ceftin by Allscripts	54569-1792	Antibiotic
387 <> GLAXO	Tab, Film Coated	Cefuroxime Axetil 250 mg	Ceftin by Glaxo	51947-8121	Antibiotic
387 <> SL	Tab, Film Coated, Debossed	Ibuprofen 400 mg	by Sidmak	50111-0387	NSAID
387 <> WATSON	Tab	Acetaminophen 750.6 mg, Hydrocodone Bitartrate 7.5 mg	by Quality Care	60346-0106	Analgesic; C III
3875500	Tab, Scored, 387 Left of the Score, 5 over 500 Right of the Score <> Royce Logo	Acetaminophen 500 mg, Hydrocodone Bitartrate 5 mg	by Royce	51875-0387	Analgesic; C III
3875500	Tab, White, Oblong, Royce Logo 387 5/500	Hydrocodone Bitartrate 5 mg, Acetaminophen 500 mg	Lortab by Royce		Analgesic; C III
3875500	Tab, 387 5 over 500	Acetaminophen 500 mg, Hydrocodone Bitartrate 5 mg	by Quality Care	60346-0442	Analgesic; C III
388 <> SL	Tab, Film Coated	Ibuprofen 600 mg	by Sidmak	50111-0388	NSAID
38832	Tab, White, Round, Scored, 38/832	Oxybutynin Chloride 5 mg	Ditropan by Martec	52555-0685	Urinary
38875500	Tab, Scored, 388 Left of Score, 7.5 over 500 Right of Score <> Royce Logo	Acetaminophen 500 mg, Hydrocodone Bitartrate 7.5 mg	by Zenith Goldline	00182-0691	Analgesic; C III
38875500	Tab, Scored, 388 Left of Score, 7.5 over 500 Right of Score <> Royce Logo	Acetaminophen 500 mg, Hydrocodone Bitartrate 7.5 mg	by Royce	51875-0388	Analgesic; C III
38875500	Tab, Scored, 388 Left of Score, 7.5 over 500 Right of Score <> Royce Logo	Acetaminophen 500 mg, Hydrocodone Bitartrate 7.5 mg	by Martec	52555-0652	Analgesic; C III
38875500	Tab, White, Oblong, Royce Logo 388 7.5/500	Hydrocodone Bitartrate 7.5 mg, Acetaminophen 500 mg	Lortab by Royce		Analgesic; C III
38975650	Tab, Scored, 389 Right of Score, 7.5 over 650 Left of the Score <> Royce Logo	Acetaminophen 650 mg, Hydrocodone Bitartrate 7.5 mg	by Zenith Goldline	00182-0692	Analgesic; C III
38975650	Tab, Scored, 389 Left of Score, 7.5 over 650 Right of Score <> Royce Logo	Acetaminophen 650 mg, Hydrocodone Bitartrate 7.5 mg	by Qualitest	00603-3884	Analgesic; C III
38975650	Tab, Scored, 389 Left of Score & 7.5 over 650 Right of Score <> Royce Logo	Acetaminophen 650 mg, Hydrocodone Bitartrate 7.5 mg	by Royce	51875-0389	Analgesic; C III
38975650	Tab, Scored, 389 Left of Score, 7.5 over 650 Right of Score <> Royce Logo	Acetaminophen 650 mg, Hydrocodone Bitartrate 7.5 mg	by Martec	52555-0653	Analgesic; C III
38975650	Tab, White, Oblong, Royce Logo 389 7.5/650	Hydrocodone Bitartrate 7.5 mg, Acetaminophen 650 mg	Lorcet Plus by Royce		Analgesic; C III
39	Tab, White	Naltrexone HCl 50 mg	by Drugabuse	65694-0100	Opiod Antagonist
39 <> BMS150	Tab, Peach	Nefazodone HCl 150 mg	Serzone by Bristol Myers Squibb	00087-0039	Antidepressant
39 <> BMS150	Tab	Nefazodone HCl 150 mg	Serzone by Kaiser	00179-1242	Antidepressant
39 <> BMS150	Tab	Nefazodone HCl 150 mg	Serzone by Allscripts	54569-4127	Antidepressant
39 <> BMS150	Tab	Nefazodone HCl 150 mg	Serzone by Bristol Myers	15548-0039	Antidepressant
39 <> G	Cap, Gray	Etodolac 300 mg	by Genpharm	55567-0039	NSAID
39 <> SB	Tab, Film Coated	Carvedilol 3.125 mg	Coreg by Murfreesboro	51129-1126	Antihypertensive
390 <> WYETH	Tab	Penicillin V Potassium	Pen Vee K by Casa De Amigos	62138-0390	Antibiotic
3900 <> P	Cap, Gelatin	Guaifenesin 90 mg, Theophylline 150 mg	Bronchial by Banner Pharmacaps	10888-3900	Antiasthmatic
39010650	Tab, Scored, 390 Left of Score, 10 over 650 Right of Score <> Royce Logo	Acetaminophen 650 mg, Hydrocodone Bitartrate 10 mg	by Zenith Goldline	00182-0034	Analgesic; C III
39010650	Tab, Scored, 390 Left of Score, 10 over 650 Right of Score <> Royce Logo	Acetaminophen 650 mg, Hydrocodone Bitartrate 10 mg	by Royce	51875-0390	Analgesic; C III
39010650	Tab, Scored, 390 Left of Score, 10 over 650 Right of Score <> Royce Logo	Acetaminophen 650 mg, Hydrocodone Bitartrate 10 mg	Hycomed by Med Tek	52349-0202	Analgesic; C III
39010650	Tab, White, Oblong, Royce Logo 390 10/650	Hydrocodone Bitartrate 10 mg, Acetaminophen 650 mg	Lortab by Royce		Analgesic; C III
3911V	Tab, Peach, Round	Levothyroxine Sodium 25 mcg	by Direct Dispensing	57866-5503	Antithyroid
3911V	Tab, Bisected V	Levothyroxine Sodium 25 mcg	by Vintage	00254-3911	Antithyroid
3911V	Tab, Peach, Round, Scored	Levothyroxine Sodium 25 mcg	by United Res	00677-1648	Antithyroid

ID FRONT <> BACK	DESCRIPTION FRONT <> BACK	INGREDIENT & STRENGTH	BRAND (OR EQUIV.) & FIRM	NDC#	CLASS; SCH.
3912V	Tab, Bisected V	Levothyroxine Sodium 50 mcg	by Vintage	00254-3912	Antithyroid
3912V	Tab, White, Round, Scored	Levothyroxine Sodium 50 mcg	by United Res	00677-1649	Antithyroid
3913	Tab, Purple, Round, Scored	Levothyroxine Sodium 75 mcg	by Direct Dispensing	57866-5505	Antithyroid
3913 <> V	Tab, Bluish Purple, Round, Scored	Levothyroxine Sodium 0.075 mg	by Allscripts	54569-4157	Antithyroid
3913V	Tab, Bisected V	Levothyroxine Sodium 75 mcg	by Vintage	00254-3913	Antithyroid
3913V	Tab, Purple, Round, Scored	Levothyroxine Sodium 75 mcg	by United Res	00677-1650	Antithyroid
3914 <> RUGBY	Tab	Acetaminophen 500 mg, Hydrocodone Bitartrate 7.5 mg	by Rugby	00536-5507	Analgesic; C III
3914V	Tab, Bisected V	Levothyroxine Sodium 100 mcg	by Vintage	00254-3914	Antithyroid
3914V	Tab, Yellow, Round, Scored, 3914/V	Levothyroxine Sodium 100 mcg	by Murfreesboro	51129-1649	Antithyroid
3914V	Tab, 3914/V	Levothyroxine Sodium 100 mcg	by Heartland	61392-0201	Antithyroid
3914V	Tab, Yellow, Oval	Levothyroxine Sodium 25 mcg	by Direct Dispensing	57866-3953	Antithyroid
3915V	Tab, 3915/V <> Coded	Levothyroxine Sodium 150 mcg	by PDRX	55289-0084	Antithyroid
3915V	Tab, 3915 V	Levothyroxine Sodium 150 mcg	by Quality Care	60346-0801	Antithyroid
3916	Tab, Bisected V	Levothyroxine Sodium 200 mcg	by Vintage	00254-3916	Antithyroid
3916V	Tab, Pink, Round	Levothyroxine Sodium 200 mcg	by Direct Dispensing	57866-4381	Antithyroid
39175750	Tab, Scored, 391 Left of Score, 7.5 over 750 Right of Score <> Royce Logo	Acetaminophen 750 mg, Hydrocodone Bitartrate 7.5 mg	by Zenith Goldline	00182-0681	Analgesic; C III
39175750	Tab, Scored, 391 Left of Score 7.5 over 750 Right of Score <> Royce Logo	Acetaminophen 750.6 mg, Hydrocodone Bitartrate 7.5 mg	by Royce	51875-0391	Analgesic; C III
39175750	Tab, White, Oblong, Royce Logo 391 7.5/750	Hydrocodone Bitartrate 7.5 mg, Acetaminophen 750 mg	Vicodin ES by Royce		Analgesic; C III
3917V	Tab, Green, Round, Scored	Levothyroxine Sodium 300 mcg	by Direct Dispensing	57866-3958	Antithyroid
3917V	Tab, Bisected V	Levothyroxine Sodium 300 mcg	by Vintage	00254-3917	Antithyroid
3917V	Tab, Green, Round, Scored	Levothyroxine Sodium 300 mcg	by United Res	00677-0769	Antithyroid
3918 <> RUGBY	Tab, 39/18	Hyoscyamine Sulfate 0.125 mg	by Anabolic	00722-6286	Gastrointestinal
3919V	Tab, 3919/V	Levothyroxine Sodium 0.125 mg	by Vintage	00254-3919	Antithyroid
3919V	Tab, Brown, Round	Levothyroxine Sodium 0.125 mg	by United Res	00677-1637	Antithyroid
3920 <> RUGBY	Tab	Atropine Sulfate 0.0194 mg, Hyoscyamine Sulfate 0.1037 mg, Phenobarbital 16.2 mg, Scopolamine Hydrobromide 0.0065 mg	Belladonna PB by Quality Care	60346-0042	Gastrointestinal; C IV
3922 <> RUGBY	Tab	Hydrochlorothiazide 25 mg	by Heartland	61392-0011	Diuretic
3925	Cap, Blue & Clear	Phentermine 30 mg	Phentrol #2 by Vortech		Anorexiant; C IV
3938	Cap, Blue & Pink	Phentermine 15 mg	Phentrol #3 by Vortech		Anorexiant; C IV
394	Tab, Scored	Chlorpropamide 250 mg	Diabinese by Rightpak	65240-0634	Antidiabetic
394	Tab, Peach, Round, Sch. Logo 394	Reserpine 0.1 mg, Trichlormethiazide 4 mg	Naquival by Schering		Antihypertensive
394 <> GLAXO	Tab, Film Coated	Cefuroxime Axetil	Ceftin by Glaxo	00173-0394	Antibiotic
394 <> GLAXO	Tab, Film Coated	Cefuroxime Axetil	Ceftin by Nat Pharmpak Serv	55154-1111	Antibiotic
39465650	Tab, 394 65 over 650 <> Royce Logo	Acetaminophen 650.7 mg, Propoxyphene HCl 65 mg	by Royce	51875-0394	Analgesic; C IV
39465650	Tab, Orange, Oblong, 394 65/650 Royce logo	Propoxyphene HCl 65 mg, Acetaminophen 650 mg	Wygesic by Royce		Analgesic; C IV
395 <> GLAXO	Tab, Film Coated	Cefuroxime Axetil	Ceftin by Glaxo	00173-0395	Antibiotic
3955005	Tab, Green, Oblong, 395/50/0.5 Royce logo	Pentazocine HCl 50 mg, Naloxone HCl 0.5 mg	Talwin by Royce		Analgesic; C IV
3955005 <> WATSON	Tab, Green, Oblong, Scored	Pentazocine HCl 50 mg, Naloxone HCl 0.5 mg	by Watson Labs	52544-0395	Analgesic; C IV
3966	Tab, White, Round, Hourglass over 3966	Atropine Sulfate 0.025 mg, Diphenoxylate HCl 2.5 mg	Lomotil by Zenith Goldline	00406-0463	Antidiarrheal; C V
3966	Tab, White, Round, Hourglass Logo 3966	Diphenoxylate HCl 2.5 mg, Atropine Sulfate 0.025 mg	Lomotil by Zenith Goldline	00172-3966	Antidiarrheal; C V
3984 <> 0115	Tab, White, Round	Methyltestosterone 10 mg	Methitest by Global	00115-7037	Hormone; C III
3984 <> 0115	Tab, White, Round	Methyltestosterone 10 mg	Methitest by Global	00115-3984	Hormone; C III
3984 <> 3	Tab	Aspirin 325 mg, Codeine Phosphate 30 mg	by DRX	55045-2307	Analgesic; C III
3985 <> 4	Tab	Aspirin 325 mg, Codeine Phosphate 60 mg	by DRX	55045-2355	Analgesic; C III
3986 <> 0115	Tab, Yellow, Round	Methyltestosterone 25 mg	by Global	00115-3986	Hormone; C III
399	Tab, Yellow, Round	Caffeine 200 mg	Vivarin by Granutec		Stimulant
39SB	Tab, Film Coated	Carvedilol 3.125 mg	Coreg by SB	59742-4139	Antihypertensive
39SB	Tab, White, Oval, 39/SB	Carvedilol 3.125 mg	by SmithKline SKB	Canadian	Antihypertensive
39SB	Tab, White, Oval, Film Coated	Carvedilol 3.125 mg	Famvir by SKB	00007-4139	Antihypertensive
3LLL13	Tab, Green, Round	Levothyroxine Sodium 0.3 mg	Synthroid by Lederle		Antithyroid

ID FRONT <> BACK	DESCRIPTION FRONT <> BACK	INGREDIENT & STRENGTH	BRAND (OR EQUIV.) & FIRM	NDC#	CLASS; SCH.
3M <> 221	Tab, White, Round	Orphenadrine Citrate 100 mg	Norflex by HJ Harkins	52959-0178	Muscle Relaxant
3M <> 221	Tab, White, Round	Orphenadrine Citrate 100 mg	Norflex by Rx Pac	65084-0229	Muscle Relaxant
3M <> 221	Tab, White, Round	Orphenadrine Citrate 100 mg	Norflex by Rightpak	65240-0703	Muscle Relaxant
3M <> 221	Tab, White, Round	Orphenadrine Citrate 100 mg	by Perrigo	00113-0381	Muscle Relaxant
3M <> 221	Tab, White, Round	Orphenadrine Citrate 100 mg	Norflex ER by 3M	00089-0221	Muscle Relaxant
3M <> 221	Tab, ER	Orphenadrine Citrate 100 mg	Norflex Sr by Nat Pharmpak Serv	55154-2907	Muscle Relaxant
3M <> 221	Tab, ER	Orphenadrine Citrate 100 mg	Norflex by Allscripts	54569-0839	Muscle Relaxant
3M <> 221	Tab, ER	Orphenadrine Citrate 100 mg	Norflex by PDRX	55289-0646	Muscle Relaxant
3M <> 221	Tab, ER	Orphenadrine Citrate 100 mg	Norflex by Amerisource	62584-0221	Muscle Relaxant
3M <> 221	Tab, ER	Orphenadrine Citrate 100 mg	Norflex by Quality Care	60346-0554	Muscle Relaxant
3M <> 342	Tab, White, Round, Scored	Theophylline 125 mg	Theolair by 3M	00089-0342	Antiasthmatic
3M <> ALUCAP	Cap, Green & Red, 3M <> Alu-Cap	Aluminum Hydroxide 400 mg	Alu-Cap by 3M	00089-0105	Gastrointestinal
3M <> DISALCID	Tab, Aqua, Round, Bisected, Film Coated	Salsalate 500 mg	Disalcid by 3M	00089-0149	NSAID
3M <> DISALCID	Cap, Aqua & White	Salsalate 500 mg	Disalcid by 3M	00089-0148	NSAID
3M <> DISALCID750	Tab, Blue, Oblong, Film Coated, Bisected	Salsalate 750 mg	Disalcid by Rx Pac	65084-0212	NSAID
3M <> DISALCID750	Tab, Aqua, Cap-Shaped, Bisected, Film Coated, Disalcid 750	Salsalate 750 mg	Disalcid by 3M	00089-0151	NSAID
3M <> DISALCID750	Tab, Disalcid 750, Film Coated	Salsalate 750 mg	Disalcid by Nat Pharmpak Serv	55154-2902	NSAID
3M <> DISALCID750	Tab, Disalcid 750, Film Coated	Salsalate 750 mg	Disalcid by Thrift Drug	59198-0121	NSAID
3M <> DISALCID750	Tab, Film Coated	Salsalate 750 mg	Disalcid by Leiner	59606-0635	NSAID
3M <> DISALCID750	Tab, Film Coated, Embossed	Salsalate 750 mg	Disalcid by Amerisource	62584-0151	NSAID
3M <> NORGESIC	Tab, White & Yellow, Round	Aspirin 385 mg, Caffeine 30 mg, Orphenadrine Citrate 25 mg	Norgesic by 3M	00089-0231	Analgesic; Muscle Relaxant
3M <> NORGESIC	Tab	Aspirin 770 mg, Caffeine 60 mg, Orphenadrine Citrate 50 mg	Norgesic Forte by Nat Pharmpak Serv	55154-2905	Analgesic
3M <> NORGESICFORTE	Tab, Green & White & Yellow, 3M <> Norgesic over Forte	Aspirin 770 mg, Caffeine 60 mg, Orphenadrine Citrate 50 mg	Norgesic Forte by Quality Care	60346-0185	Analgesic
3M <> NORGESICFORTE	Tab, Light Green, 3M <> Norgesic over Forte	Aspirin 770 mg, Caffeine 60 mg, Orphenadrine Citrate 50 mg	Norgesic Forte by Amerisource	62584-0233	Analgesic
3M <> NORGESICFORTE	Tab, Green & White, Cap Shaped, Scored	Aspirin 770 mg, Caffeine 60 mg, Orphenadrine Citrate 50 mg	Norgesic Forte by 3M	00089-0233	Analgesic
3M <> NORGESICFORTE	Tab, Green & White	Aspirin 770 mg, Caffeine 60 mg, Orphenadrine Citrate 50 mg	Norgesic Forte by Nat Pharmpak Serv	55154-2905	Analgesic
3M <> NORGESICFORTE	Tab, Light Green, White & Yellow	Aspirin 770 mg, Caffeine 60 mg, Orphenadrine Citrate 50 mg	Norgesic Forte by CVS	51316-0050	Analgesic
3M <> NORGESICFORTE	Tab, Yellow,	Aspirin 770 mg, Caffeine 60 mg, Orphenadrine Citrate 50 mg	Norgesic Forte by Allscripts	54569-0840	Analgesic
3M <> NORGESICFORTE	Tab, Light Green & White & Yellow, Layered: 3 Layers	Aspirin 770 mg, Caffeine 60 mg, Orphenadrine Citrate 50 mg	Norgesic Forte by Thrift Drug	59198-0158	Analgesic
3M <> NORGESICFORTE	Tab	Aspirin 770 mg, Caffeine 60 mg, Orphenadrine Citrate 50 mg	Norgesic Forte by CVS Revco	00894-6767	Analgesic
3M <> NORGESICFORTE	Tab, White & Yellow, Oblong	Orphenadrine Citrate 50 mg, Aspirin 770 mg, Caffeine 60 mg	by 3M Pharma	Canadian	Muscle Relaxant
3M <> NORGESICFORTE	Tab, White & Yellow, Oblong	Orphenadrine Citrate 50 mg; Caffeine 60 mg; Aspirin 770 mg	Norgesic Forte by Med-Pro	53978-3384	Muscle Relaxant
3M <> SR200	Tab, ER	Theophylline 200 mg	by Urgent Care Ctr	50716-0505	Antiasthmatic
3M <> SR200	Tab, White, Round, Scored	Theophylline 200 mg	Theolair SR by 3M	00089-0341	Antiasthmatic
3M <> SR250	Tab, White, Round, Scored	Theophylline 250 mg	Theolair SR by 3M	00089-0345	Antiasthmatic
3M <> SR300	Tab, White, Oval, Scored	Theophylline 300 mg	Theolair SR by 3M	00089-0343	Antiasthmatic
3M <> SR500	Tab, White, Cap Shaped, Scored	Theophylline 500 mg	Theolair SR by 3M	00089-0347	Antiasthmatic
3M <> THEOLAIR250	Tab, White, Cap-Shaped, Scored	Theophylline 250 mg	Theolair by 3M	00089-0344	Antiasthmatic
3M <> TR100	Tab, White, Round, Scored	Flecainide 100 mg	Tambocor by 3M	00089-0307	Antiarrhythmic
3M <> TR150	Tab, White, Oval, Scored	Flecainide 150 mg	Tambocor by 3M	00089-0314	Antiarrhythmic
3M <> TR150	Tab, White, Round, Scored	Flecainide Acetate 150 mg	Tambocor by Integrity	64731-0945	Antiarrhythmic

ID FRONT ⬦ BACK	DESCRIPTION FRONT ⬦ BACK	INGREDIENT & STRENGTH	BRAND (OR EQUIV.) & FIRM	NDC#	CLASS; SCH.
3M ⬦ TR50	Tab, White, Round	Flecainide 50 mg	Tambocor by 3M	00089-0305	Antiarrhythmic
3M ⬦ TR50	Tab, White, Round	Flecainide Acetate 50 mg	Tambocor by Murfreesboro Ph	51129-1378	Antiarrhythmic
3M ⬦ UREX	Tab, White, Cap-Shaped, Scored	Methenamine Hippurate 1 g	Urex by 3M	00089-0371	Antibiotic; Urinary Tract
3M107	Tab, Green, Oblong, 3M/107	Aluminum Hydroxide 600 mg	Alu-Tab by 3M		Gastrointestinal
3M161	Tab, Green, Round, 3M/161	Orphenadrine HCl 50 mg	by 3M Pharmaceuticals	Canadian	Muscle Relaxant
3M221	Tab, White, 3M/221	Orphenadrine Citrate 100 mg	by 3M Pharmaceuticals	Canadian	Muscle Relaxant
3M342	Tab, White, Round	Theophylline 125 mg	Theolair by 3M		Antiasthmatic
3M342	Tab, White, Round, 3M/342	Theophylline Anhydrous 125 mg	by Theolair	Canadian	Antiasthmatic
3MDISALCID	Tab, Aqua, Round, 3M/Disalcid	Salsalate 500 mg	by 3M Pharmaceuticals	Canadian	NSAID
3MDISALCID750	Tab, Aqua, Oblong, 3M/Disalcid 750	Salsalate 750 mg	by 3M Pharmaceuticals	Canadian	NSAID
3MSR250	Tab, White, Round, 3M/SR 250	Theophylline SR 250 mg	Theolair-SR by 3M		Antiasthmatic
3MSR250	Tab, White, Round, 3M/SR-250	Theophylline Anhydrous 250 mg	by 3M Pharmaceuticals	Canadian	Antiasthmatic
3MSR300	Tab, White, Oval, 3M/SR 300	Theophylline SR 300 mg	Theolair-SR by 3M		Antiasthmatic
3MSR300	Tab, White, Oval, 3M/SR-300	Theophylline Anhydrous 300 mg	by 3M Pharmaceuticals	Canadian	Antiasthmatic
3MSR500	Tab, White, Oblong, 3M/SR 500	Theophylline SR 500 mg	Theolair-SR by 3M		Antiasthmatic
3MSR500	Tab, White, Oblong, 3M/SR-500	Theophylline Anhydrous 500 mg	by 3M Pharmaceuticals	Canadian	Antiasthmatic
3MTR100	Tab, White, Round, 3M/TR 100	Flecainide Acetate 100 mg	Tambocor by 3M Pharmaceuticals	Canadian	Antiarrhythmic
3MTR100	Tab, White, Round	Flecainide Acetate 100 mg	Tambocor by 3M		Antiarrhythmic
3MTR150	Tab, White, Oval, 3M/TR150	Flecainide Acetate 150 mg	Tambocor by 3M		Antiarrhythmic
3MTR50	Tab, White, Round, 3M/TR 50	Flecainide Acetate 50 mg	Tambocor by 3M Pharmaceuticals	Canadian	Antiarrhythmic
3MTR50	Tab, White, Round, 3M/TR50	Flecainide Acetate 50 mg	Tambocor by 3M		Antiarrhythmic
3P1153	Tab, Purple, Round	Levothyroxine Sodium 0.175 mg	Synthroid by Wal Mart	49035-0191	Antithyroid
3PT ⬦ GLYNASE	Tab, Coated	Glyburide 3 mg	Glynase Prestab by Nat Pharmpak Serv	55154-3909	Antidiabetic
3RORER143	Tab, White, Round	Aspirin 325 mg, Codeine Phosphate 30 mg, Maalox 150 mg	Ascriptin Codeine #3 by Rorer		Analgesic; C III
3SYCBMZ	Tab, Pink, Cylindrical, 3/Syc-BMZ	Bromazepam 3 mg	by Altimed	Canadian DIN# 02167816	Sedative
4	Tab, White, Oval	Dextrothyroxine Sodium 4 mg	Choloxin by Boots		Thyroid
4	Tab, Film Coated	Ibuprofen 400 mg	by Quality Care	60346-0430	NSAID
4	Tab, White, Round, Film Coated	Ibuprofen 400 mg	by Goldline Labs	00182-1809	NSAID
4	Tab, White, Round	Ibuprofen 400 mg	Motrin by Norton		NSAID
4	Tab, White, Round	Ibuprofen 400 mg	Ibuprofen by Murfreesboro	51129-1522	NSAID
4	Tab, White, Round	Perphenazine 4 mg	Apo Perphenazine by Apotex	Canadian	Antipsychotic
4	Tab, Gray, Round, Schering Logo/4	Perphenazine 4 mg	Trilafon by Schering	Canadian	Antipsychotic
4 ⬦ 2065V	Tab, 2065 over V	Acetaminophen 300 mg, Codeine Phosphate 60 mg	by Quality Care	60346-0632	Analgesic; C III
4 ⬦ 2121V	Tab, 4 ⬦ 2121/V	Aspirin 325 mg, Codeine Phosphate 60 mg	by Vintage	00254-2121	Analgesic; C III
4 ⬦ 2121V	Tab, 2121/V	Aspirin 325 mg, Codeine Phosphate 60 mg	by Qualitest	00603-2362	Analgesic; C III
4 ⬦ 3985	Tab	Aspirin 325 mg, Codeine Phosphate 60 mg	by DRX	55045-2355	Analgesic; C III
4 ⬦ 93350	Tab, 93 350	Acetaminophen 300 mg, Codeine Phosphate 60 mg	by Quality Care	60346-0632	Analgesic; C III
4 ⬦ 93350	Tab, White, Round, 4 ⬦ 93 over 350	Acetaminophen 300 mg, Codeine Phosphate 60 mg	by Teva	00093-0350	Analgesic; C III
4 ⬦ 93350	Tab, White, Round, 4 ⬦ 93 over 350	Acetaminophen 300 mg, Codeine Phosphate 60 mg	by UDL	51079-0106	Analgesic; C III
4 ⬦ 93350	Tab	Acetaminophen 300 mg, Codeine Phosphate 60 mg	by Murfreesboro	51129-6662	Analgesic; C III
4 ⬦ 93350	Tab, White, Round	Acetaminophen 300 mg; Codeine Phosphate 60 mg	by Southwood Pharms	58016-0272	Analgesic; C III
4 ⬦ A	Tab, Yellow, Round, Scored	Guaifenesin 1200 mg; Phenylpropanolamine HCl 75 mg; Dextromethorphan Hydrobromide 60 mg	Aquatab D by Adams Labs	63824-0004	Cold Remedy
4 ⬦ BARR229	Tab	Acetaminophen 300 mg, Codeine Phosphate 60 mg	by Pharmedix	53002-0103	Analgesic; C III
4 ⬦ COPLEY717	Tab	Guanabenz Acetate 5.14 mg	by Copley	38245-0717	Antihypertensive
4 ⬦ CPI	Tab, CPI Logo	Phenobarbital 16.2 mg	by Century	00436-0867	Sedative/Hypnotic; C IV
4 ⬦ CPI	Tab, CPI Logo	Phenobarbital 16.2 mg	by Century	00436-0866	Sedative/Hypnotic; C IV
4 ⬦ DPI	Tab	Acetaminophen 300 mg, Codeine Phosphate 60 mg	by Quality Care	60346-0632	Analgesic; C III
4 ⬦ E	Tab, Tan, Coated	Hydromorphone HCl 4 mg	Dilaudid by Ethex	58177-0299	Analgesic; C II
4 ⬦ E	Tab, Coated	Hydromorphone HCl 4 mg	by KV	10609-1367	Analgesic; C II

ID FRONT <> BACK	DESCRIPTION FRONT <> BACK	INGREDIENT & STRENGTH	BRAND (OR EQUIV.) & FIRM	NDC#	CLASS; SCH.
4 <> ETH	Tab, White, Rectangle	Nitroglycerin 0.4 mg	Nitroquick by PDRX	55289-0309	Vasodilator
4 <> ETH	Tab, White, Ovaloid	Nitroglycerin 0.4 mg	Nitroquick by Ethex	58177-0324	Vasodilator
4 <> G3327	Tab, White, Oval, Scored	Methylprednisolone 4 mg	by Pharmacia & Upjohn	00009-3327	Steroid
4 <> GG	Tab	Atropine Sulfate 0.025 mg, Diphenoxylate HCl 2.5 mg	Lonox by Quality Care	60346-0437	Antidiarrheal; C V
4 <> GLAXO	Tab, White, Oval, Film Coated	Ondansetron HCl	Zofran by Glaxo Wellcome	00173-0446	Antiemetic
4 <> M	Tab, White, Triangular, Film Coated	Fluphenazine HCl 1 mg	Prolixin by UDL	51079-0485	Antipsychotic
4 <> M	Tab, White, Coated	Fluphenazine HCl 1 mg	by Mylan	00378-6004	Antipsychotic
4 <> M	Tab, White, Round	Hydromorphone HCl 4 mg	by Mallinckrodt Hobart	00406-3244	Analgesic; C II
4 <> MP127	Tab	Acetaminophen 300 mg, Codeine 60 mg	by United Res	00677-0632	Analgesic; C III
4 <> N499	Tab, White, Round, Scored	Albuterol 4 mg	by Allscripts	54569-2874	Antiasthmatic
4 <> N499	Tab, White, Round, 4 <> N over 499	Albuterol Sulfate 4.8 mg	by Novopharm	55953-0499	Antiasthmatic
4 <> N499	Tab	Albuterol Sulfate 4.8 mg	by Medirex	57480-0423	Antiasthmatic
4 <> N499	Tab, Coated, 4 <> N 499	Albuterol Sulfate 4.8 mg	by Quality Care	60346-0285	Antiasthmatic
4 <> N499	Tab	Albuterol Sulfate 4.8 mg	by Heartland	61392-0570	Antiasthmatic
4 <> N499	Tab, 4 <> N over 499	Albuterol Sulfate 4.8 mg	by DRX	55045-2283	Antiasthmatic
4 <> PROVENTIL	Tab, Film Coated	Albuterol 4 mg	Proventil by Nat Pharmpak Serv	55154-3507	Antiasthmatic
4 <> R003	Tab	Acetaminophen 300 mg, Codeine Phosphate 60 mg	by Purepac	00228-2003	Analgesic; C III
4 <> R21	Tab, White, Round	Acetaminophen 300 mg, Codeine Phosphate 60 mg	by Purepac	00228-3021	Analgesic; C III
4 <> RPC5	Tab, Orange, Round, Scored	Midodrine HCl 5 mg	Proamatine by Murfreesboro Ph	51129-1433	Antihypotension
4 <> SAMPLE	Tab, Film Coated	Ondansetron HCl	Zofran by Glaxo Wellcome	00173-0446	Antiemetic
4 <> VOLMAX	Tab, Blue, Hexagonal	Albuterol Sulfate 4 mg	Volmax by Med-Pro	53978-2026	Antiasthmatic
4 <> VOLMAX	Tab, Dark Blue Print	Albuterol Sulfate 4.8 mg	Volmax by Muro	00451-0398	Antiasthmatic
4 <> VOLMAX	Tab, Dark Blue Print	Albuterol Sulfate 4.8 mg	Volmax by CVS	51316-0240	Antiasthmatic
4 <> VOLMAX	Tab	Albuterol Sulfate 4.8 mg	Volmax by Wal Mart	49035-0159	Antiasthmatic
4 <> VOLMAX	Tab, Dark Blue Print	Albuterol Sulfate 4.8 mg	Volmax by Nat Pharmpak Serv	55154-4304	Antiasthmatic
4 <> VOLMAX	Tab, Dark Blue Print	Albuterol Sulfate 4.8 mg	Volmax by Eckerd Drug	19458-0848	Antiasthmatic
4 <> Z36684	Tab, Film Coated, Zenith Logo Over 3668 Over 4	Perphenazine 4 mg	by Quality Care	60346-0835	Antipsychotic
4 <> ZOFRAN	Tab, White, Oval, Film Coated	Ondansetron HCl	Zofran by Glaxo Wellcome	00173-0446	Antiemetic
40	Tab, Blue, Round, 40(triangle)	Verapamil HCl 40 mg	Isoptin by Knoll		Antihypertensive
40	Tab, Film Coated, Surrounded by the Knoll Triangle	Verapamil HCl 40 mg	by Med Pro	53978-3076	Antihypertensive
40 <> BMS1967	Cap, Dark Orange, Black Print, 40 <> BMS over 1967	Stavudine 40 mg	Zerit by Bristol Myers	00003-1967	Antiviral
40 <> BMS1967	Cap, Orange	Stavudine 40 mg	Zerit by Squibb Mfg	12783-0967	Antiviral
40 <> CALAN	Tab, Pink, Round, Coated	Verapamil HCl 40 mg	Calan by GD Searle	00025-1771	Antihypertensive
40 <> DAN5556	Tab	Propranolol HCl 40 mg	by Danbury	00591-5556	Antihypertensive
40 <> DAN5556	Tab, Green, Round, Scored	Propranolol HCl 40 mg	by Vangard Labs	00615-2563	Antihypertensive
40 <> ELAVIL	Tab, Blue, Round, Film Coated	Amitriptyline HCl 10 mg	Elavil by HJ Harkins	52959-0396	Antidepressant
40 <> ELAVIL	Tab, Coated	Amitriptyline HCl 10 mg	Elavil by Zeneca	00310-0040	Antidepressant
40 <> G	Tab, Orange, Oval, Film Coated	Etodolac 400 mg	by Genpharm	55567-0040	NSAID
40 <> INV237	Tab, White, Round	Nadolol 40 mg	Corgard by Zenith Goldline	00182-2633	Antihypertensive
40 <> INV237	Tab	Nadolol 40 mg	Nadolol by Schein	00364-2653	Antihypertensive
40 <> INV237	Tab, Scored, 40 <> INV over 237	Nadolol 40 mg	Nadolol by Invamed	52189-0237	Antihypertensive
40 <> INV237	Tab	Nadolol 40 mg	Nadolol by Major	00904-5070	Antihypertensive
40 <> INV237	Tab	Nadolol 40 mg	Nadolol by HL Moore	00839-7870	Antihypertensive
40 <> INV237	Tab	Nadolol 40 mg	Nadolol by Geneva	00781-1182	Antihypertensive
40 <> LESCOL	Cap, Brown & Gold, Triangle Logo 40 <> Lescol Logo	Fluvastatin Sodium 40 mg	Lescol by Novartis	00078-0234	Antihyperlipidemic
40 <> LOTENSIN	Tab, Red, Round	Benazepril HCl 40 mg	Lotensin by Phy Total Care	54868-2352	Antihypertensive
40 <> LOTENSIN	Tab, Dark Rose	Benazepril HCl 40 mg	Lotensin by Novartis	00083-0094	Antihypertensive
40 <> MEGACE	Tab, Light Blue, Flat-faced and Beveled-Edged	Megestrol Acetate 40 mg	Megace by Mead Johnson	00015-0596	Progestin
40 <> MYLAN 216	Tab	Furosemide 40 mg	by Kaiser	62224-1222	Diuretic
40 <> MYLAN184	Tab, Green, Mylan Over 184, Beveled Edge	Propranolol HCl 40 mg	by Mylan	00378-0184	Antihypertensive
40 <> MYLAN184	Tab, Green, Round, Scored, Mylan over 184 <> 40	Propranolol HCl 40 mg	Inderal by UDL	51079-0279	Antihypertensive
40 <> MYLAN216	Tab	Furosemide 40 mg	by Allscripts	54569-0574	Diuretic

ID FRONT <> BACK	DESCRIPTION FRONT <> BACK	INGREDIENT & STRENGTH	BRAND (OR EQUIV.) & FIRM	NDC#	CLASS; SCH.
40 <> MYLAN216	Tab	Furosemide 40 mg	by Quality Care	60346-0487	Diuretic
40 <> MYLAN216	Tab, White, Round, Scored	Furosemide 40 mg	by Murfreesboro Ph	51129-1389	Diuretic
40 <> MYLAN216	Tab, White, Scored, 40 <> Mylan over 216	Furosemide 40 mg	by Mylan	00378-0216	Diuretic
40 <> MYLAN216	Tab, White, Round, Scored, 40 <> Mylan over 216	Furosemide 40 mg	Laxis by UDL	51079-0073	Diuretic
40 <> OC	Tab, Yellow, Round	Oxycodone HCl 40 mg	OxyContin by Purdue Frederick	Canadian	Analgesic; C II
40 <> OC	Tab, Yellow, Round	Oxycodone HCl 40 mg	Oxycontin by PF Labs	48692-0712	Analgesic; C II
40 <> OC	Tab, Yellow, Round	Oxycodone HCl 40 mg	Oxycontin by PF Labs	48692-0672	Analgesic; C II
40 <> OC	Tab, Film Coated	Oxycodone HCl 40 mg	Oxycontin by Physicians Total Care	54868-3815	Analgesic; C II
40 <> PAXIL	Tab, Film Coated	Paroxetine HCl	Paxil by SB	59742-3213	Antidepressant
40 <> PAXIL	Tab, Green, Oval, Film Coated	Paroxetine HCl 40 mg	Paxil by SKB	00029-3213	Antidepressant
40 <> PD157	Tab, White, Elliptical, Film Coated	Atorvastatin 40 mg	Lipitor by Parke-Davis	Canadian DIN# 02230714	Antihyperlipidemic
40 <> PD157	Tab, White, Elliptical, Film Coated	Atorvastatin Calcium	Lipitor by Parke Davis	00071-0157	Antihyperlipidemic
40 <> PD157	Tab, Film Coated	Atorvastatin Calcium	Lipitor by Goedecke	53869-0157	Antihyperlipidemic
40 <> PD157	Tab, White, Oval, Film Coated	Atorvastatin Calcium 40 mg	Lipitor by Murfreesboro Ph	51129-1424	Antihyperlipidemic
40 <> PD157	Tab, White	Atorvastatin Calcium 40 mg	Lipitor by Phy Total Care	54868-4229	Antihyperlipidemic
40 <> PD535	Tab, Brown	Quinapril HCl 40 mg	Accupril by PDRX Pharms	55289-0555	Antihypertensive
40 <> PD535	Tab, Brown, Elliptical-Shaped, Coated	Quinapril HCl 40 mg	Accupril by Parke Davis	00071-0535	Antihypertensive
40 <> PD535	Tab, Brown, Elliptical, Film Coated, 40 <> PD/535	Quinapril 40 mg	Accupril by Park-Davis	Canadian DIN# 01947699	Antihypertensive
400	Tab, Geneva Logo	Caffeine 100 mg, Ergotamine Tartrate 1 mg	Ercaf by Quality Care	60346-0958	Analgesic
400	Tab, Upjohn Logo and 400, Film Coated	Ibuprofen 400 mg	by Quality Care	60346-0430	NSAID
400 <> 250	Tab, Red, Oblong	Amoxicillin 400 mg	Amoxil by Allscripts	54569-4791	Antibiotic
400 <> 4175	Tab	Etodolac 400 mg	by Qualitest	00603-3570	NSAID
400 <> 4175	Tab, White, Oblong, Film	Etodolac 400 mg	by Heartland	61392-0917	NSAID
400 <> 4175	Tab, White, Round, Film Coated	Etodolac 400 mg	Lodine by Zenith Goldline	00172-4175	NSAID
400 <> 4267	Tab, White, Round	Acyclovir 400 mg	Zovirax by Zenith Goldline	00172-4267	Antiviral
400 <> 4267	Tab, White, Round	Acyclovir 400 mg	Zovirax by Zenith Goldline	00182-8200	Antiviral
400 <> A02	Tab, White, Oval	Acyclovir 400 mg	Zovirax by MOVA	55370-0555	Antiviral
400 <> A02	Tab	Acyclovir 400 mg	by Martec	52555-0683	Antiviral
400 <> A04	Tab, White, Elliptical	Etodolac 400 mg	Lodine by MOVA	55370-0552	NSAID
400 <> FLOXIN	Tab, Pale Gold, Film Coated	Ofloxacin 400 mg	Floxin by Quality Care	60346-0400	Antibiotic
400 <> IBU	Tab, Film Coated	Ibuprofen 400 mg	by Quality Care	60346-0430	NSAID
400 <> IP131	Tab, Film Coated, IP 131	Ibuprofen 400 mg	by Quality Care	60346-0430	NSAID
400 <> IP131	Tab, White, Round, Film Coated	Ibuprofen 400 mg	by Goldline Labs	00182-1809	NSAID
400 <> IP131	Tab, Coated	Ibuprofen 400 mg	by Golden State	60429-0092	NSAID
400 <> IP131	Tab, Coated	Ibuprofen 400 mg	by Prescription Dispensing	61807-0027	NSAID
400 <> IP138	Tab, White, Round	Ibuprofen 400 mg	by Breckenridge	51991-0720	NSAID
400 <> MEDEVA	Cap	Chlorpheniramine Maleate 4 mg, Pseudoephedrine HCl 60 mg	Atrohist Ped by Medeva	53014-0400	Cold Remedy
400 <> MEDEVA	Cap	Chlorpheniramine Maleate 4 mg, Pseudoephedrine HCl 60 mg	Atrohist Ped by Adams	53014-0400	Cold Remedy
400 <> MEDEVA	Cap, White & Yellow	Pseudoephedrine HCl 60 mg, Chlorpheniramine Maleate 4 mg	Atrohist by Adams Labs	63824-0400	Cold Remedy
400 <> N204	Tab, Film Coated, Scored	Cimetidine 400 mg	by Medirex	57480-0814	Gastrointestinal
400 <> N204	Tab, Film Coated, N Vertical Bisect 204	Cimetidine 400 mg	by Warrick	59930-1802	Gastrointestinal
400 <> N204	Tab, Green, Oval, Film Coated, Scored	Cimetidine 400 mg	by Novopharm	55953-0204	Gastrointestinal
400 <> N204	Tab, Film Coated, Scored	Cimetidine 400 mg	by Prescription Dispensing	61807-0066	Gastrointestinal
400 <> N204	Tab, Coated, N/204	Cimetidine 400 mg	by Brightstone	62939-2131	Gastrointestinal
400 <> N204	Tab, Coated	Cimetidine 400 mg	by United Res	00677-1529	Gastrointestinal
400 <> N815	Cap, Red	Tolmetin Sodium 400 mg	by Allscripts	54569-3730	NSAID
400 <> N815	Cap, N Over 815 <> 400	Tolmetin Sodium 492 mg	by Quality Care	60346-0615	NSAID
400 <> N815	Cap, Red, N Over 815	Tolmetin Sodium 492 mg	by Novopharm	43806-0815	NSAID

ID FRONT <> BACK	DESCRIPTION FRONT <> BACK	INGREDIENT & STRENGTH	BRAND (OR EQUIV.) & FIRM	NDC#	CLASS; SCH.
400 <> N815	Cap, N Over 815	Tolmetin Sodium 492 mg	by United Res	00677-1424	NSAID
400 <> N943	Tab	Acyclovir 400 mg	by Warrick	59930-1576	Antiviral
400 <> N943	Tab, Deep Blue, Cap Shaped, 400 <> N over 943	Acyclovir 400 mg	by Novopharm	55953-0943	Antiviral
400 <> N943	Tab, Blue, Oblong	Acyclovir 400 mg	by Allscripts	54569-4765	Antiviral
400 <> N943	Tab, Blue, Cap Shaped, 400 <> N over 943	Acyclovir 400 mg	by UDL	51079-0877	Antiviral
400 <> N943	Tab	Acyclovir 400 mg	by Major	00904-5232	Antiviral
400 <> N943	Tab, Deep Blue, Cap Shaped, 400 <> N over 943	Acyclovir 400 mg	by Novopharm	43806-0943	Antiviral
400 <> NU	Tab, Pink, Cap Shaped	Pentoxifylline 400 mg	by Nu Pharm	Canadian DIN# 02230401	Anticoagulent
400 <> PAR162	Tab, Film Coated	Ibuprofen 400 mg	by PDRX	55289-0590	NSAID
400 <> PAR162	Tab, White, Round, Film Coated, 400 <> Par over 162	Ibuprofen 400 mg	Rufen/Motrin by UDL	51079-0281	NSAID
400 <> PAR162	Tab, Film Coated	Ibuprofen 400 mg	by Zenith Goldline	00172-4018	NSAID
400 <> PAR162	Tab, Film Coated, Par Over 162	Ibuprofen 400 mg	by Par	49884-0162	NSAID
400 <> PAR162	Tab, Film Coated, Debossed	Ibuprofen 400 mg	by Amerisource	62584-0746	NSAID
400 <> PAR162	Tab, Film Coated	Ibuprofen 400 mg	by Quality Care	60346-0430	NSAID
400 <> PAR162	Tab, Coated	Ibuprofen 400 mg	by Prescription Dispensing	61807-0027	NSAID
400 <> PAR162	Tab, White, Round, Film Coated	Ibuprofen 400 mg	by Goldline Labs	00182-1809	NSAID
400 <> PD353	Tab, Tan, Oval, Coated	Troglitazone 400 mg	Rezulin by Parke Davis	00071-0353	Antidiabetic
400 <> TOLMETIN	Cap	Tolmetin Sodium 492 mg	by Quality Care	60346-0615	NSAID
400000LLP17	Tab, White, Round, 400/000 LL P17	Penicillin G Potassium 400,000 Units	Pentids by Lederle		Antibiotic
4001 <> 0665	Tab	Medroxyprogesterone Acetate 10 mg	by Int'l Lab	00665-4001	Progestin
4001 <> 0665	Tab	Medroxyprogesterone Acetate 10 mg	by Quality Care	60346-0571	Progestin
4001 <> 6666	Tab	Medroxyprogesterone Acetate 10 mg	by Apotheca	12634-0108	Progestin
4005R	Tab, 4005 and R Printed in A Diamond Shape	Meprobamate 200 mg	by Rugby	00536-4005	Sedative/Hypnotic; C IV
4005R	Tab, 4005 and R Printed in A Diamond Shape	Meprobamate 200 mg	by Chelsea	46193-0902	Sedative/Hypnotic; C IV
4006R	Tab, 4006 and R Printed in A Diamond Shape	Meprobamate 400 mg	by Rugby	00536-4006	Sedative/Hypnotic; C IV
4006R	Tab, 4006 and R Printed in A Diamond Shape	Meprobamate 400 mg	by Chelsea	46193-0901	Sedative/Hypnotic; C IV
400G	Tab	Ibuprofen 400 mg	by Allscripts	54569-3820	NSAID
400M40 <> MOVA	Tab, White, Oblong, Film Coated, 400/M40 <> Mova	Cimetidine 400 mg	by Compumed		Gastrointestinal
400M40 <> MOVA	Tab, Coated, 400/M40 <> Mova	Cimetidine 400 mg	by Rosemont	00832-0103	Gastrointestinal
400M40 <> MOVA	Tab, White, Round, Film Coated, Scored, 400 over M40 <> Mova	Cimetidine 400 mg	by Compumed	00403-1067	Gastrointestinal
400M40 <> MOVA	Tab, White, Cap Shaped, Scored	Cimetidine 400 mg	Tagamet by MOVA	55370-0136	Gastrointestinal
400MG <> MOTRIN	Tab, Coated	Ibuprofen 400 mg	Motrin by Allscripts	54569-0284	NSAID
400MG <> T	Tab, Film Coated	Carbamazepine 400 mg	by Physicians Total Care	54868-3862	Anticonvulsant
400MG <> T	Tab, Brown, Round, Coated	Carbamazepine XR 400 mg	by Novartis	00083-0060	Anticonvulsant
400MONITAN	Tab, White, Oblong, 400/Monitan	Acebutolol HCl 400 mg	by Wyeth-Ayerst	Canadian	Antihypertensive
400N <> 204	Tab, Light Green, Film Coated	Cimetidine 400 mg	by Quality Care	60346-0945	Gastrointestinal
400N <> 204	Tab, Light Green, Coated, 400/N	Cimetidine 400 mg	by Schein	00364-2593	Gastrointestinal
400NOVO	Tab, White, Oval, 400/Novo	Acebutolol HCl 400 mg	by Novopharm	Canadian	Antihypertensive
400SB <> TAGAMET	Tab, Light Green, Film Coated	Cimetidine 400 mg	Tagamet by Quality Care	60346-0706	Gastrointestinal
401 <> MYLAN	Tab, Coated, Beveled Edge	Ibuprofen 400 mg	by Mylan	00378-0401	NSAID
4010 <> MYLAN	Cap, Peach	Temazepam 15 mg	by Natl Pharmpak	55154-5591	Sedative/Hypnotic; C IV
4012 <> RUGBY	Tab, Film Coated	Etodolac 400 mg	by Rugby	00536-4012	NSAID
4012 <> RUGBY	Tab, Film Coated	Etodolac 400 mg	by Chelsea	46193-0584	NSAID
402	Cap, Green & Yellow, Schering Logo 402	Theophylline LA 125 mg	Theovent by Schering		Antiasthmatic
402 <> MEDEVA	Cap, Clear & Green	Guaifenesin 300 mg	Humibid by Adams Labs	63824-0402	Expectorant
402 <> MEDEVA	Cap	Guaifenesin 300 mg	Humibid Ped by Medeva	53014-0402	Expectorant
402 <> MEDEVA	Cap	Guaifenesin 300 mg	Humibid Ped by Adams	53014-0402	Expectorant
402 <> P&G	Tab, P & G	Etidronate Disodium 200 mg	Didronel by Pharm Utilization	60491-0801	Calcium Metabolism
402 <> PANDG	Tab	Etidronate Disodium 200 mg	Didronel by DRX	55045-2326	Calcium Metabolism

ID FRONT <> BACK	DESCRIPTION FRONT <> BACK	INGREDIENT & STRENGTH	BRAND (OR EQUIV.) & FIRM	NDC#	CLASS; SCH.
402 <> PG	Tab, White, Rectangular	Etidronate Disodium 200 mg	Didronel by Procter & Gamble	Canadian DIN# 01997629	Calcium Metabolism
402 <> PG	Tab, White, Pillow shaped, 402 <> P & G	Etidronate Disodium 200 mg	Didronel by Procter & Gamble	00149-0405	Calcium Metabolism
402400	Tab, Yellow, Oblong, Royce Logo 402/400	Etodolac 400 mg	Lodine by Royce		NSAID
4025 <> RUGBY	Tab	Methyclothiazide 5 mg	by Chelsea	46193-0525	Diuretic
4029	Green, Oblong	Indomethacin 25 mg	by Kaiser Fdn	00179-1059	NSAID
4029 <> Z	Cap	Indomethacin 25 mg	by Quality Care	60346-0684	NSAID
403	Tab, Red, Round	Pseudoephedrine 30 mg	Sudafed by OHM		Decongestant
4030	Green, Oblong	Indomethacin 50 mg	by Kaiser Fdn	00179-1060	NSAID
4030 <> Z	Cap	Indomethacin 50 mg	by Quality Care	60346-0733	NSAID
4040 <> LESCOL	Cap, Brown & Gold, Logo 40 Logo 40 <> Lescol	Acetaminophen 500 mg, Hydrocodone Bitartrate 7.5 mg	by Allscripts	54569-4761	Analgesic; C III
4058 <> 500MG	Cap, Clear & White	Cefadroxil 500 mg	by Caremark	00339-6155	Antibiotic
4058 <> 500MG	Cap	Cefadroxil Hemihydrate	by Quality Care	60346-0022	Antibiotic
4058 <> 500MG	Cap, White to Yellowish Powder	Cefadroxil Hemihydrate	by HJ Harkins Co	52959-0428	Antibiotic
4058 <> Z500MG	Cap	Cefadroxil Hemihydrate	by Pharmedix	53002-0229	Antibiotic
4058500MG	Cap	Cefadroxil Hemihydrate	by CVS Revco	00894-5133	Antibiotic
405HD	Tab, Pink, Round	Amitriptyline HCl 10 mg	Elavil by Halsey		Antidepressant
406	Cap	Indomethacin 50 mg	by United Res	00677-0873	NSAID
406 <> NE	Tab	Etidronate Disodium 400 mg	Didronel by Pharm Utilization	60491-0802	Calcium Metabolism
406 <> NE	Tab, White, Cap Shaped, Scored	Etidronate Disodium 400 mg	Didronel by Procter & Gamble	00149-0406	Calcium Metabolism
406 <> SL	Cap	Indomethacin 25 mg	by Quality Care	60346-0684	NSAID
4067	Tab, White, Round	Codeine Phosphate 30 mg, Aspirin 380 mg, Caffeine 30 mg	A.S.A. by Lilly		Analgesic; C III
4068	Cap, Zenith Logo	Prazosin HCl	by Quality Care	60346-0805	Antihypertensive
406HD	Tab, Green, Round	Amitriptyline HCl 25 mg	Elavil by Halsey		Antidepressant
4073 <> Z	Cap, Gray & Red	Cephalexin Monohydrate 250 mg	by Zenith Goldline	00172-4073	Antibiotic
4074 <> Z	Cap, Logo	Cephalexin Monohydrate	by Quality Care	60346-0055	Antibiotic
4074 <> Z	Cap, Red	Cephalexin Monohydrate 500 mg	by Zenith Goldline	00172-4074	Antibiotic
407HD	Tab, Brown, Round	Amitriptyline HCl 50 mg	Elavil by Halsey		Antidepressant
408HD	Tab, Purple, Round	Amitriptyline HCl 75 mg	Elavil by Halsey		Antidepressant
409HD	Tab, Orange, Round	Amitriptyline HCl 100 mg	Elavil by Halsey		Antidepressant
40LESCOL	Cap, Brown & Gold, 40/Lescol	Fluvastatin 40 mg	by Novartis	Canadian	Antihyperlipidemic
40MG	Cap, Amethyst, Opaque with 3 Yellow Radial Bars	Esomeprazole 40 mg	Nexium by AstraZeneca	00186-5042	Proton Pump Inhibitor
40MG	Cap, Amethyst, Opaque with 3 Yellow Radial Bars	Esomeprazole 40 mg	Nexium by AstraZeneca	00186-5040	Proton Pump Inhibitor
40MG <> BRISTOL3031	Cap, Moss Green, 40 mg <> Bristol Over 3031	Lomustine 40 mg	Ceenu by Mead Johnson	00015-3031	Antineoplastic
40MG <> FP	Tab, White, Oval, Film Coated, Scored	Citalopram Hydrobromide 40 mg	Celexa by Forest	00456-4040	Antidepressant
40MG <> FP	Tab, Film Coated, F/P	Citalopram Hydrobromide 49.96 mg	Celexa by Forest	63711-0140	Antidepressant
40Z <> 4236	Tab, White, Round	Nadolol 40 mg	Corgard by Zenith Goldline	00172-4236	Antihypertensive
40Z4236	Tab, White, Round, 40Z/4236	Nadolol 40 mg	Corgard by Zenith Goldline	00172-4236	Antihypertensive
41 <> BMS250	Tab, White	Nefazodone HCl 250 mg	Serzone by Bristol Myers Squibb	00087-0041	Antidepressant
41 <> BMS250	Tab	Nefazodone HCl 250 mg	Serzone by Kaiser	00179-1244	Antidepressant
41 <> BMS250	Tab	Nefazodone HCl 250 mg	Serzone by Bristol Myers	15548-0041	Antidepressant
41 <> ELAVIL	Tab, Beige, Round, Film	Amitriptyline 50 mg	Elavil by Apothecon	59772-0364	Antidepressant
41 <> ELAVIL	Tab, Film Coated	Amitriptyline HCl 50 mg	Elavil by Zeneca	00310-0041	Antidepressant
4107 <> Z	Tab	Naproxen 250 mg	by Quality Care	60346-0816	NSAID
411 <> COPLEY	Tab, Shallow Concave	Methazolamide 25 mg	by Copley	38245-0411	Diuretic
411 <> PFIZER	Tab	Glipizide 5 mg	Glucotrol by Allscripts	54569-0206	Antidiabetic
411 <> USE	Tab, Scored, 411 <> US Over E	Nitroglycerin 2.6 mg	Nitrong by RPR	00075-0221	Vasodilator
4115 <> LILLY	Tab, White, Round	Olanzapine 5 mg	Zyprexa by Lilly Del Caribe	00110-4115	Antipsychotic
4115 <> LILLY	Tab, White, Round	Olanzapine 5 mg	Zyprexa by PDRX	55289-0462	Antipsychotic
4115LILLY	Tab, White, Round, Film Coated	Olanzapine 5 mg	Zyprexa by Heartland Healthcare	61392-0858	Antipsychotic
412	Tab, Pink, Oblong, Savage Logo 412	Magnesium Salicylate 545 mg	Magan by Adria		Analgesic

ID FRONT <> BACK	DESCRIPTION FRONT <> BACK	INGREDIENT & STRENGTH	BRAND (OR EQUIV.) & FIRM	NDC#	CLASS; SCH.
412 <> PFIZER	Tab	Glipizide 5 mg	Glucotrol by Med Pro	53978-0226	Antidiabetic
412 <> USE	Tab, Scored, 412 <> US Over E	Nitroglycerin 6.5 mg	Nitrong by RPR	00075-0274	Vasodilator
4120 <> 0665	Cap, ER, in Black Ink	Valproic Acid 250 mg	by Int'l Lab	00665-4120	Anticonvulsant
4125 <> WYETH	Tab, Light Green, Ex Release	Isosorbide Dinitrate 40 mg	Isordil by Wyeth Labs	00008-4125	Antianginal
4131	Tab, Ivory, Rectangular, 4131/Logo	Pergolide Mesylate 0.05 mg	Permax by Draxis Health	Canadian	Antiparkinson
4133	Tab, Green, Rectangular, 4133/Logo	Pergolide Mesylate 0.25 mg	Permax by Draxis Health	Canadian	Antiparkinson
4135	Tab, Pink, Rectangular, 4135/Logo	Pergolide Mesylate 1 mg	Permax by Draxis Health	Canadian	Antiparkinson
4135	Tab, Pink, Rectangle, Draxis Logo	Pergolide Mesylate 1 mg	Permax by Draxis	Canadian	Antiparkinson
4140 <> V	Tab, Double Layered	Meclizine HCl 12.5 mg	by Qualitest	00603-4319	Antiemetic
4140SB	Tab, Film Coated	Carvedilol 6.25 mg	Coreg by SB	59742-4140	Antihypertensive
4140SB	Tab, White, Oval, 4140/SB	Carvedilol 6.25 mg	by SmithKline SKB	Canadian	Antihypertensive
4140SB	Tab, White, Film Coated	Carvedilol 6.25 mg	Coreg by SKB	00007-4140	Antihypertensive
4141SB	Tab, Film Coated	Carvedilol 12.5 mg	Coreg by SB	59742-4141	Antihypertensive
4141SB	Tab, White, Oval, 4141/SB	Carvedilol 12.5 mg	by SmithKline SKB	Canadian	Antihypertensive
4141SB	Tab, Film Coated	Carvedilol 12.5 mg	Coreg by SKB	00007-4141	Antihypertensive
4142SB	Tab, Film Coated	Carvedilol 25 mg	Coreg by SB	59742-4142	Antihypertensive
4142SB	Tab, White, Oval, 4142/SB	Carvedilol 25 mg	by SmithKline SKB	Canadian	Antihypertensive
4142SB	Tab, Film Coated	Carvedilol 25 mg	Coreg by SKB	00007-4142	Antihypertensive
4160 <> 0665	Cap	Lithium Carbonate 300 mg	by Schein	00364-0855	Antipsychotic
4160 <> 0665	Cap	Lithium Carbonate 300 mg	by United Res	00677-1092	Antipsychotic
4160 <> 0665	Cap, in Red Ink	Lithium Carbonate 300 mg	by Int'l Lab	00665-4160	Antipsychotic
417 <> COPLEY	Tab, Light Blue	Metoprolol Tartrate 100 mg	by Copley	38245-0417	Antihypertensive
417 <> MYLAN	Tab, Peach, Scored	Bumetanide 2 mg	by Mylan	00378-0417	Diuretic
4172	Cap, Natural Clear	Quinine Sulfate 325 mg	by Zenith Goldline	00172-4172	Antimalarial
4174 <> 500	Tab, White, Cap Shaped	Etodolac 500 mg	Lodine by Zenith Goldline	00172-4174	NSAID
4175 <> 400	Tab	Etodolac 400 mg	by Qualitest	00603-3570	NSAID
4175 <> 400	Tab, White, Round, Film Coated	Etodolac 400 mg	Lodine by Zenith Goldline	00172-4175	NSAID
418 <> WATSON	Tab, Film Coated	Cyclobenzaprine HCl 10 mg	by Watson	52544-0418	Muscle Relaxant
418 <> WATSON	Tab, Film Coated	Cyclobenzaprine HCl 10 mg	by Major	00904-7809	Muscle Relaxant
418 <> WATSON	Tab, Film Coated	Cyclobenzaprine HCl 10 mg	by DHHS Prog	11819-0069	Muscle Relaxant
418 <> WATSON	Tab, Film Coated	Cyclobenzaprine HCl 10 mg	by Prepackage Spec	58864-0128	Muscle Relaxant
418 <> WATSON	Tab, Film Coated	Cyclobenzaprine HCl 10 mg	by Quality Care	60346-0581	Muscle Relaxant
418 <> WATSON	Tab, White, Round	Cyclobenzaprine HCl 10 mg	by Apotheca	12634-0528	Muscle Relaxant
4191 <> WYETH	Cap	Aspirin 356.4 mg, Caffeine 30 mg, Dihydrocodeine Bitartrate 16 mg	Synalgos DC by Quality Care	60346-0303	Analgesic; C III
4191 <> WYETH	Cap	Aspirin 356.4 mg, Caffeine 30 mg, Dihydrocodeine Bitartrate 16 mg	Synalgos DC by Wyeth Labs	00008-4191	Analgesic; C III
4194 <> 500	Tab, Blue, Oblong	Cefaclor 500 mg	by Ceclor	00172-4194	Antibiotic
4195 <> 25	Tab, Yellow, Round, 4195 <> 2.5	Enalapril Maleate 2.5 mg	Vasotec by Zenith Goldline	00172-4195	Antihypertensive
4196 <> 5	Tab, White, Round	Enalapril Maleate 5 mg	Vasotec by Zenith Goldline	00172-4196	Antihypertensive
4197 <> 10	Tab, Salmon, Round	Enalapril Maleate 10 mg	Vasotec by Zenith Goldline	00172-4197	Antihypertensive
4198 <> 20	Tab, Peach, Round	Enalapril Maleate 20 mg	Vasotec by Zenith Goldline	00172-4198	Antihypertensive
42 <> ELAVIL	Tab, Film Coated	Amitriptyline HCl 75 mg	Elavil by Zeneca	00310-0042	Antidepressant
42 <> GG	Tab	Imipramine HCl 50 mg	by Allscripts	54569-0196	Antidepressant
42 <> GG	Tab, Coated, Debossed	Imipramine HCl 50 mg	by Golden State	60429-0097	Antidepressant
4216V <> 4	Tab, White, Oval	Methylprednisolone 4 mg	by Vintage		Steroid
420	Tab, White, Round	Ibuprofen 200 mg	Advil by OHM		NSAID
420	Tab, White, Round, Sugar-Coated, 420 Circled	Ibuprofen 200 mg	Motrin IB/Advil by UDL	51079-0731	NSAID
420BARR	Tab, White, Oval	Ibuprofen 600 mg	Motrin by Barr		NSAID
421 <> MYLAN	Tab, Beige, Capsule-Shaped, Film-Coated	Methyldopa 500 mg	Aldomet by UDL	51079-0201	Antihypertensive
421 <> MYLAN	Tab, Beige, Coated, Beveled Edge	Methyldopa 500 mg	by Mylan	00378-0421	Antihypertensive
4220	Tab	Cefaclor 375 mg	Ceclor CD by Lilly	00110-4220	Antibiotic
4220	Tab	Cefaclor 375 mg	Ceclor CD by Dura	51479-0036	Antibiotic
4221	Tab	Cefaclor 500 mg	Ceclor CD by Lilly	00110-4221	Antibiotic

ID FRONT <> BACK	DESCRIPTION FRONT <> BACK	INGREDIENT & STRENGTH	BRAND (OR EQUIV.) & FIRM	NDC#	CLASS; SCH.
4221	Tab	Cefaclor 500 mg	Ceclor CD by Dura	51479-0035	Antibiotic
4226 <> Z	Tab	Guanabenz Acetate 4 mg	by Zenith Goldline	00172-4226	Antihypertensive
4227 <> Z	Tab	Guanabenz Acetate 8 mg	by Zenith Goldline	00172-4227	Antihypertensive
423205 <> Z	Tab, Green, Round, 4232 0.5 <> Z	Bumetanide 0.5 mg	Bumex by Zenith Goldline	00172-4232	Diuretic
42331 <> Z	Tab, Yellow, Round, 4233 1 <> Z	Bumetanide 1 mg	Bumex by Zenith Goldline	00172-4233	Diuretic
42342 <> Z	Tab, Peach, Round, 4234 2 <> Z	Bumetanide 2 mg	Bumex by Zenith Goldline	00172-4234	Diuretic
4235 <> 20Z	Tab	Nadolol 20 mg	Nadolol by Zenith Goldline	00182-2632	Antihypertensive
4235 <> 20Z	Tab, White, Round	Nadolol 20 mg	Corgard by Zenith Goldline	00172-4235	Antihypertensive
4236 <> 40Z	Tab, White, Round	Nadolol 40 mg	Corgard by Zenith Goldline	00172-4236	Antihypertensive
4237 <> 80Z	Tab	Nadolol 80 mg	Nadolol by Zenith Goldline	00182-2634	Antihypertensive
4237 <> 80Z	Tab, White, Round	Nadolol 80 mg	Corgard by Zenith Goldline	00172-4237	Antihypertensive
425 <> WATSON	Cap	Aspirin 325 mg, Butalbital 50 mg, Caffeine 40 mg, Codeine Phosphate 30 mg	by Watson	52544-0425	Analgesic; C III
425 <> WATSON	Cap	Aspirin 325 mg, Butalbital 50 mg, Caffeine 40 mg, Codeine Phosphate 30 mg	by Rugby	00536-5754	Analgesic; C III
425 <> WATSON	Cap	Aspirin 325 mg, Butalbital 50 mg, Caffeine 40 mg, Codeine Phosphate 30 mg	by HL Moore	00839-6689	Analgesic; C III
425 <> WATSON	Cap	Aspirin 325 mg, Butalbital 50 mg, Caffeine 40 mg, Codeine Phosphate 30 mg	by Major	00904-5140	Analgesic; C III
425 <> WATSON	Cap, Blue & Yellow	Butalbital 50 mg; Aspirin 325 mg; Caffeine 40 mg; Codeine Phosphate 30 mg	by Phy Total Care	54868-1037	Analgesic; C III
425 <> WATSON425	Cap	Aspirin 325 mg, Butalbital 50 mg, Caffeine 40 mg, Codeine Phosphate 30 mg	by Zenith Goldline	00182-0036	Analgesic; C III
4259 <> Z	Tab, Coated	Indapamide 2.5 mg	Lozol by Zenith Goldline	00172-4259	Diuretic
4259 <> Z	Tab, Coated, Debossed	Indapamide 2.5 mg	by Physicians Total Care	54868-3106	Diuretic
4259 <> Z	Tab, Coated, Debossed	Indapamide 2.5 mg	by Major	00904-5074	Diuretic
4259 <> Z	Tab, Coated	Indapamide 2.5 mg	by Qualitest	00603-4061	Diuretic
4259 <> Z	Tab, Coated, Debossed	Indapamide 2.5 mg	by Geneva	00781-1051	Diuretic
4259 <> Z	Tab, Coated, Debossed	Indapamide 2.5 mg	by Qualitest	00603-4161	Diuretic
42616	Tab, White, Round	Aspirin 325 mg	by Pennex Laboratories		Analgesic
42616	Tab, White, Round	Aspirin 325 mg	by Pennex Laboratories		Analgesic
4266 <> 200	Cap, Opaque	Acyclovir 200 mg	Zovirax by Zenith Goldline	00182-2666	Antiviral
4266 <> 200	Cap, White	Acyclovir 200 mg	Zovirax by Zenith Goldline	00172-4266	Antiviral
4267 <> 400	Tab, White, Round, Flat Beveled	Acyclovir 400 mg	by Amerisource	62584-0606	Antiviral
4267 <> 400	Tab, White, Round	Acyclovir 400 mg	Zovirax by Zenith Goldline	00172-4267	Antiviral
4267 <> 400	Tab, White, Round	Acyclovir 400 mg	Zovirax by Zenith Goldline	00182-8200	Antiviral
4268 <> 800	Tab, White, Oval	Acyclovir 800 mg	Zovirax by Zenith Goldline	00172-4268	Antiviral
4268 <> 800	Tab, White, Oval	Acyclovir 800 mg	Zovirax by Zenith Goldline	00182-2667	Antiviral
427 <> MYLAN	Tab, Yellowish Orange	Sulindac 150 mg	by Mylan	00378-0427	NSAID
427 <> MYLAN	Tab, Yellow-Orange, Round	Sulindac 150 mg	Clinoril by UDL	51079-0666	NSAID
427 <> MYLAN	Tab	Sulindac 150 mg	by Quality Care	60346-0044	NSAID
427 <> ZANTAC150	Tab, Efferv	Ranitidine HCl 168 mg	Zantac Efferdose by Glaxo	00173-0427	Gastrointestinal
427 <> ZANTAC150	Tab, Efferv	Ranitidine HCl 168 mg	Zantac Efferdose by Glaxo	60937-0427	Gastrointestinal
4270V	Cap	Acetaminophen 325 mg, Dichloralantipyrine 100 mg, Isometheptene Mucate 65 mg	Migquin by Vintage	00254-4270	Cold Remedy
427COPLEY	Tab, Pink, Round, 427/Copley	Diclofenac Sodium 75 mg	Voltaren by Copley		NSAID
4285	Cap, Dark Red, Opaque, Gelatin, Scherer Logo 4285	Ascorbic Acid 250 mg, Cyanocobalamin 10 mcg, Ferrous Fumarate 200 mg, Stomach Extract 100 mg	Chromagen by RP Scherer	11014-0222	Vitamin
4285	Cap, Maroon, Savage Logo 4285	Vitamin, Iron	Chromagen by Savage	00281-4285	Vitamin
4288 <> ZG20MG	Cap, White, Opaque	Nicardipine HCl 20 mg	Cardene by Zenith Goldline	00172-4288	Antihypertensive
4289 <> ZG30MG	Cap, Light Blue, Opaque	Nicardipine HCl 30 mg	Cardene by Zenith Goldline	00172-4289	Antihypertensive
429	Tab, Pink, Round, Convex, Scored	Fludrocortisone Acetate 0.1 mg	Florinef Acetate USP by Integrity	64731-0947	Steroid
429 <> GG	Tab, Green, Cap Shaped, Film Coated	Cimetidine 400 mg	Tagamet by Geneva	00781-1449	Gastrointestinal
43 <> ELAVIL	Tab, Film Coated	Amitriptyline HCl 100 mg	Elavil by Zeneca	00310-0043	Antidepressant
43 <> ELAVIL	Tab, Film Coated	Amitriptyline HCl 100 mg	Elavil by Merck	00006-0435	Antidepressant
430 <> GG	Tab, Green, Cap Shaped	Cimetidine 800 mg	Tagamet by Geneva	00781-1444	Gastrointestinal
4306 <> 0115	Tab	Promethazine HCl 25 mg	by Global	00115-4306	Antiemetic; Antihistamine
431	Tab, Film Coated, Schering Trademark and 431	Albuterol 4 mg	Proventil by Thrift Drug	59198-0318	Antiasthmatic

ID FRONT <> BACK	DESCRIPTION FRONT <> BACK	INGREDIENT & STRENGTH	BRAND (OR EQUIV.) & FIRM	NDC#	CLASS; SCH.
431	Tab, Film Coated, Branded in Red with Schering TM	Albuterol 4 mg	Proventil by Leiner	59606-0771	Antiasthmatic
431	Tab, Film Coated	Albuterol 4 mg	by Med Pro	53978-0820	Antiasthmatic
431	Tab, Film Coated, Schering Logo/431	Albuterol 4 mg	Proventil by Allscripts	54569-0387	Antiasthmatic
431	Tab, Film Coated	Albuterol 4 mg	Proventil by Pharmedix	53002-1036	Antiasthmatic
431	Tab, Schering Logo in Red Print	Albuterol Sulfate 4.8 mg	Proventil by Quality Care	60346-0665	Antiasthmatic
431COPLEY	Tab, Pink, Round, 431/Copley	Diclofenac Sodium 25 mg	Voltaren by Copley		NSAID
4324RUGBY	Tab	Prednisone 5 mg	by Pharmedix	53002-0352	Steriod
4328 <> RUGBY	Tab, White, Scored	Prednisone 50 mg	by Allscripts	54569-0333	Steriod
433 <> M	Tab, Peach, Round, Film Coated	Bupropion 75 mg	Wellbutrin by UDL	51079-0943	Antidepressant
433433 <> GLYBUR	Tab	Glyburide 2.5 mg	by Coventry	61372-0577	Antidiabetic
433433 <> GLYBUR	Tab, Pink, Oblong, Scored	Glyburide 2.5 mg	by Blue Ridge	59273-0014	Antidiabetic
433433 <> GLYBUR	Tab	Glyburide 2.5 mg	by Merrell	00068-3201	Antidiabetic
433433 <> GLYBUR	Tab	Glyburide 2.5 mg	by Allscripts	54569-3830	Antidiabetic
433433 <> GLYBUR	Tab	Glyburide 2.5 mg	by Copley	38245-0433	Antidiabetic
433433 <> GLYBUR	Tab, Pink, Oblong, Scored	Glyburide 5 mg	by Blue Ridge	59273-0015	Antidiabetic
433COPLEY	Tab, Pink, Oblong, 433/Copley	Glyburide 2.5 mg	Diabeta by Copley		Antidiabetic
435 <> M	Tab, Light Blue, Round, Film Coated	Bupropion 100 mg	Wellbutrin by UDL	51079-0944	Antidepressant
4354	Tab, White, Round, Scored	Isoniazid 100 mg	by Southwood Pharms	58016-0912	Antimycobacterial
4359 <> 25	Tab, Pale Yellow, Round, Hourglass Logo 4359 <> 25	Clozapine 25 mg	Clozaril by Zenith Goldline	00172-4359	Antipsychotic
4359 <> 25	Tab	Clozapine 25 mg	by Dixon	17236-0357	Antipsychotic
4360 <> 100	Tab, Pale Yellow, Round, Hourglass Logo 4360 <> 100	Clozapine 100 mg	by Zenith Goldline	00172-4360	Antipsychotic
4360 <> 100	Tab, Yellow, Round, Scored, 2 Triangles	Clozapine 100 mg	by Dixon	17236-0356	Antipsychotic
4364 <> 100	Tab, Yellow, Round, Hourglass Logo 4364 <> 100	Labetalol HCl 100 mg	Normodyne & Trandate by Zenith Goldline	00172-4364	Antihypertensive
4364 <> 300	Tab, Green, Round, Hourglass Logo 4364 <> 300	Labetalol HCl 300 mg	Normodyne & Trandate by Zenith Goldline	00172-4366	Antihypertensive
4365 <> 200	Tab, White, Round, Hourglass Logo 4365 <> 200	Labetalol HCl 200 mg	Normodyne & Trandate by Zenith Goldline	00172-4365	Antihypertensive
43687	Tab, Orange, Round, Hourglass Logo <> 4 3687	Doxazosin Mesylate 4 mg	Cardura by Zenith Goldline	00172-3687	Antihypertensive
437 <> SL	Tab, Light Green, Sugar Coated	Desipramine HCl 50 mg	by Schein	00364-2210	Antidepressant
437 <> SL	Tab, Light Green, Round, Sugar Coated	Desipramine HCl 50 mg	Norpramin by Sidmak	50111-0437	Antidepressant
43797007	Tab, Green, Hexagonal, 43797-007	Hyoscyamine Sulfate 0.125 mg	Gastrosed by Hauck		Gastrointestinal
438 <> GG	Tab, White, Round, Scored, Compressed	Pindolol 5 mg	Visken by Geneva	00781-1168	Antihypertensive
438 <> SL	Tab, Light Orange, Sugar Coated	Desipramine HCl 75 mg	by Schein	00364-2243	Antidepressant
438 <> SL	Tab, Light Orange, Round, Sugar Coated	Desipramine HCl 75 mg	Norpramin by Sidmak	50111-0438	Antidepressant
4382 <> R	Cap, R in A Diamond	Propoxyphene HCl 65 mg	by Teva	00093-0741	Analgesic; C IV
439	Tab, Film Coated, Purepac Logo and 439	Trazodone HCl 50 mg	by Nat Pharmpak Serv	55154-1910	Antidepressant
439 <> GG	Tab, White, Round, Scored, Compressed	Pindolol 10 mg	Visken by Geneva	00781-1169	Antihypertensive
439 <> R	Tab	Trazodone HCl 50 mg	by UDL	51079-0427	Antidepressant
439 <> R	Tab, White, Round, Film Coated	Trazodone HCl 50 mg	by Purepac	00228-2439	Antidepressant
439 <> R	Tab, Coated	Trazodone HCl 50 mg	by Vangard	00615-2578	Antidepressant
439R	Tab, Film Coated	Trazodone HCl 50 mg	by Med Pro	53978-0495	Antidepressant
44 <> UU	Tab, White, Oval	Pramipexole DiHCl 0.25 mg	Mirapex by Pharmacia & Upjohn	00009-0004	Antiparkinson
441 <> R	Tab, White, Round, Film Coated	Trazodone HCl 100 mg	by Purepac	00228-2441	Antidepressant
441 <> R	Tab	Trazodone HCl 100 mg	by UDL	51079-0428	Antidepressant
441 <> R	Tab, Coated	Trazodone HCl 100 mg	by Vangard	00615-2579	Antidepressant
44104	Tab, White, Round	Acetaminophen 325 mg	Tylenol by LNK		Antipyretic
44107	Cap, 44-107	Diphenhydramine HCl 25 mg	by Heartland	61392-0220	Antihistamine
44107 <> 44107	Cap, White, with Red Bands, 44-107, <> 44-107	Diphenhydramine HCl 25 mg	by Quality Care	60346-0589	Antihistamine
44107 <> 44107	Cap, White, with Red Bands, 44-107, <> 44-107	Diphenhydramine HCl 25 mg	by Quality Care	60346-0589	Antihistamine
44111	Tab, White, Round	Pseudoephedrine 60 mg	Pseudoval Plus by LNK		Decongestant
44111	Tab, White, Round	Pseudoephedrine 60 mg	Pseudoval Plus by LNK		Decongestant

ID FRONT <> BACK	DESCRIPTION FRONT <> BACK	INGREDIENT & STRENGTH	BRAND (OR EQUIV.) & FIRM	NDC#	CLASS; SCH.
44148	Tab, White, Round, 44/148	Acetaminophen 500 mg	by LNK		Analgesic
4415 <> LILLY4415	Tab, Blue, Oval, Lilly Over 4415	Olanzapine 15 mg	Zyprexa by PDRX	55289-0458	Antipsychotic
44156	Tab, Orange, Round	Acetaminophen 325 mg, Phenyltoloxamine Citrate 30 mg	Percogesic by LNK		Analgesic
44157 <> ASPIRIN	Tab, White, Round, Film Coated, 44 over 157 <> Aspirin	Aspirin 325 mg	Aspirin by UDL	51079-0005	Analgesic
44159	Tab, White, Round	Acetaminophen 250 mg, Aspirin 250 mg, Caffeine 65 mg	by LNK		Analgesic
44160	Tab, White, Round	Aspirin, Magnesium, Alum. Hydroxide	Ascriptin by LNK		Analgesic
44163	Tab, White & Yellow, Round	Decongestant Combination	Dristan by LNK		Cold Remedy
44165	Tab, White, Oblong	Aspirin, Antacid	Ascriptin AD by LNK		Analgesic
44165	Tab, White, Round	Aspirin, Magnesium, Aluminum Hydroxide	Ascriptin AD by LNK		Analgesic
44175	Cap, White	Acetaminophen 500 mg	by LNK		Antipyretic
44183	Tab, White, Round	Aspirin Buffered 325 mg	Bufferin by LNK		Analgesic
44184	Cap, Red & White	Acetaminophen 500 mg	Tylenol by LNK		Antipyretic
44184	Tab, Pink, Round	Acetaminophen 80 mg	Tylenol Chewable by LNK		Antipyretic
44189	Tab, Blue, Round	Diphenhydramine 25 mg	Sominex by LNK		Antihistamine
44191	Tab, Pink, Oval, Film Coated	Diphenhydramine HCL 25 mg	Benadryl by UDL	51079-0862	Antihistamine
44191	Tab, Pink, Oblong	Diphenhydramine 25 mg	Benadryl by LNK		Antihistamine
44194	Tab, Yellow, Round	Chlorpheniramine Maleate 4 mg	Chlor-trimeton by LNK		Antihistamine
44194	Tab, Yellow, Round, Scored, 44/194	Chlorpheniramine Maleate 4 mg	by Circa	71114-4208	Antihistamine
44194	Tab, Yellow, Round, Scored	Chlorpheniramine Maleate 4 mg	by Allscripts	54569-0243	Antihistamine
44194	Tab, Yellow, Round, Scored, 44 over 194	Chlorpheniramine Maleate 4 mg	Chlor-Trimeton by UDL	51079-0163	Antihistamine
44197	Tab, Blue, Round	Brompheniramine 12 mg, Phenylephrine 15 mg, Phenylpropanolamine 15 mg	Dimetapp by LNK		Cold Remedy
44198	Tab, White, Round	Dimenhydrinate 50 mg	Dramamine by LNK		Antiemetic
442	Tab, Orange, Oval, Schering Logo 442	Fluphenazine HCl 2.5 mg	Permitil by Schering	00085-0442	Antipsychotic
442	Tab, Pink, Round, Savage Logo 442	Phenolphthalein 65 mg, Docusate Sodium 100 mg	Modane Plus by Adria		Gastrointestinal
442	Tab, Pink, Round	Phenolphthalein 65 mg, Docusate Sodium 100 mg	by Perrigo	00113-0442	Gastrointestinal
442 <> MYLAN	Tab, Purple, Coated	Amitriptyline HCl 25 mg, Perphenazine 2 mg	by Mylan	00378-0442	Antipsychotic
44201	Tab, White, Round	Aluminum 200 mg, Magnesium Hydroxide 200 mg	Maalox by LNK		Gastrointestinal
44218	Tab, Orange, Round, White Specks	Aspirin 81 mg	by LNK		Analgesic
44222	Tab, White, Round	Aspirin 81 mg	by LNK		Analgesic
44225	Tab, Yellow, Round	Aspirin 81 mg	Bayer by LNK		Analgesic
44236	Cap, White, Oblong	Aspirin 500 mg	by Rite-Aid		Analgesic
44243	Tab, Red, Round	Aspirin Enteric Coated 500 mg	Ecotrin Max-Strength by LNK		Analgesic
44255	Tab, Yellow, Round, 44/255	Enteric Coated Aspirin 81 mg	Aspirin Enteric by LNK		Analgesic
44290 <> 44290	Cap, 44-290 <> 44-290	Diphenhydramine HCl 50 mg	by Quality Care	60346-0045	Antihistamine
44290 <> 44290	Cap, 44-290 <> 44-290	Diphenhydramine HCl 50 mg	by Quality Care	60346-0045	Antihistamine
443 <> COPLEY	Tab, Off-White	Naproxen 375 mg	by Quality Care	60346-0817	NSAID
443 <> COPLEY	Tab, Off-White	Naproxen 375 mg	by Copley	38245-0443	NSAID
443 <> COPLEY	Tab	Naproxen 375 mg	by Qualitest	00603-4731	NSAID
443 <> COPLEY	Tab, White, Oblong	Naproxen 375 mg	by Southwood Pharms	58016-0267	NSAID
4432 <> RUGBY	Tab	Quinidine Sulfate 200 mg	by Quality Care	60346-0627	Antiarrhythmic
4441W	Cap, Yellow	Temilian 10 mg	by LentLife	73245-5679	Cold Remedy
445 <> GG	Tab, Yellow, Round, Scored	Enalapril 2.5 mg	Vasotec by Geneva	00781-1229	Antihypertensive
4455RUGBY	Tab, Tan, Round, 4455/Rugby	Ranitidine 150 mg	by Rugby		Gastrointestinal
446	Tab	Polythiazide 2 mg, Reserpine 0.25 mg	Renese R by Pfizer	00069-4460	Duiretic; Antihypertensive
446 <> BARR	Tab	Tamoxifen Citrate 10 mg	by Zeneca	00310-0446	Antiestrogen
446 <> BARR	Tab	Tamoxifen Citrate 10 mg	by Haines	59564-0144	Antiestrogen
44MAG	Cap, Red	Caffeine 200 mg	44 Magnum by BDI		Stimulant
45 <> ACTOS	Tab, White, Round	Pioglitazone HCl 45 mg	Actos by Takeda Chem Inds	11532-0013	Antidiabetic
45 <> ELAVIL	Tab, Yellow, Round, Film	Amitriptyline 25 mg	Elavil by Apothecon	59772-0369	Antidepressant
45 <> ELAVIL	Tab, Yellow, Round, Film Coated	Amitriptyline HCl 25 mg	by Allscripts	54569-0174	Antidepressant
45 <> ELAVIL	Tab, Yellow, Round	Amitriptyline HCl 25 mg	Elavil by Rightpak	65240-0637	Antidepressant

ID FRONT <> BACK	DESCRIPTION FRONT <> BACK	INGREDIENT & STRENGTH	BRAND (OR EQUIV.) & FIRM	NDC#	CLASS; SCH.
45 <> ELAVIL	Tab, Film Coated	Amitriptyline HCl 25 mg	Elavil by Zeneca	00310-0045	Antidepressant
45 <> ELAVIL	Tab, Yellow, Round, Film	Amitriptyline HCl 25 mg	Elavil by Astra Zeneca	00186-0709	Antidepressant
45 <> ELAVIL	Tab, Film Coated	Amitriptyline HCl 25 mg	Elavil by Physicians Total Care	54868-0409	Antidepressant
450	Cap, Brown & Light Green	Hypericum perforatum 450 mg	Alterra by Upsher-Smith	00245-0450	Gastrointestinal
450 <> MD	Tab	Diethylpropion HCl 75 mg	by Jones	52604-9160	Antianorexiant; C IV
450 <> PLENDIL	Tab, Green, Round, Film	Felodipine 2.5 mg	Plendil by Horizon	59630-0170	Antihypertensive
450 <> PLENDIL	Tab, Sugar Coated	Felodipine 2.5 mg	Plendil by Merck	00006-0450	Antihypertensive
450 <> PLENDIL	Tab, Green, Round	Felodipine 2.5 mg	Plendil ER by Hoffmann La Roche	00004-6310	Antihypertensive
450 <> PLENDIL	Tab, Sage Green, Round	Felodipine 2.5 mg	Plendil by AstraZeneca	00186-0450	Antihypertensive
450 <> PLENDIL	Tab, Sugar Coated	Felodipine 2.5 mg	Plendil by Murfreesboro	51129-1248	Antihypertensive
450MD	Tab, White, Oval	Diethylpropion HCl SA 75 mg	Tenuate Dosepan by MD		Antianorexiant; C IV
451 <> MYLAN	Tab	Naproxen 500 mg	by Kaiser	00179-1188	NSAID
451 <> MYLAN	Tab	Naproxen 500 mg	by Murfreesboro	51129-1314	NSAID
451 <> MYLAN	Tab	Naproxen 500 mg	by Allscripts	54569-3760	NSAID
451 <> MYLAN	Tab, White, Capsule-Shaped	Naproxen 500 mg	Naprosyn by UDL	51079-0795	NSAID
451 <> MYLAN	Tab	Naproxen 500 mg	by Allscripts	54569-4255	NSAID
451 <> MYLAN	Tab, White	Naproxen 500 mg	by Mylan	00378-0451	NSAID
451 <> MYLAN	Tab	Naproxen 500 mg	by St Marys Med	60760-0451	NSAID
451 <> MYLAN	Tab	Naproxen 500 mg	by Kaiser	62224-2119	NSAID
451 <> MYLAN	Tab	Naproxen 500 mg	by Quality Care	60346-0815	NSAID
451 <> MYLAN	Tab, White, Oblong	Naproxen 500 mg	by Dixon Shane	17236-0078	NSAID
451 <> MYLAN	Tab	Naproxen 500 mg	by Talbert Med	44514-0651	NSAID
451 <> PLENDIL	Tab, Red-Brown, Ex Release	Felodipine 5 mg	Plendil by Promex Med	62301-0029	Antihypertensive
451 <> PLENDIL	Tab, Red, Round	Felodipine 5 mg	by Va Cmop	65243-0028	Antihypertensive
451 <> PLENDIL	Tab, Red, Round	Felodipine 5 mg	Plendil ER by Hoffmann La Roche	00004-6416	Antihypertensive
451 <> PLENDIL	Tab, Red, Round	Felodipine 5 mg	Plendil ER by Hoffmann La Roche	00004-6311	Antihypertensive
451 <> PLENDIL	Tab, Light Reddish Brown, Round	Felodipine 5 mg	Plendil by AstraZeneca	00186-0451	Antihypertensive
451 <> SL	Tab, Film Coated, Debossed	Ibuprofen 800 mg	by Sidmak	50111-0451	NSAID
4519	Tab, Pink, Ross logo 4519	Multivitamin Chewable	Vi-Daylin by Ross		Vitamin
452 <> PLENDIL	Tab, Red, Round	Felodipine 10 mg	Plendil ER by Hoffmann La Roche	00004-6415	Antihypertensive
452 <> PLENDIL	Tab, Reddish Brown, Round	Felodipine 10 mg	Plendil by AstraZeneca	00186-0452	Antihypertensive
452 <> PLENDIL	Tab	Felodipine 10 mg	Plendil by Allscripts	54569-3719	Antihypertensive
452 <> PLENDIL	Tab	Felodipine 10 mg	Plendil ER by Physicians Total Care	54868-2168	Antihypertensive
4520	Tab, Orange, Ross logo 4520	Multivitamin, Iron Chewable	Vi-Daylin by Ross		Vitamin
454 <> M	Tab, Round	Pindolol 5 mg	by Merckle	58107-0004	Antihypertensive
45435	Cap, Green, Oval, 45-435	Chloral Hydrate 500 mg	Noctec by Chase		Sedative/Hypnotic; C IV
455	Cap, One-Piece Gelatin Capsule	Ipodate Sodium 500 mg	Oragrafin Sodium by Bracco	00270-0455	Diagnostic
455 <> M	Tab, Round	Pindolol 10 mg	by Merckle	58107-0005	Antihypertensive
4556	Tab, Yellow, Round	Phenylpropanolamine 50 mg, Pheniramine 25 mg, Pyrilamine 25 mg	by Eon		Cold Remedy
457 <> MYLAN	Tab	Lorazepam 1 mg	by Vangard	00615-0451	Sedative/Hypnotic; C IV
458 <> CLARITIN10	Tab, White, Round	Loratadine 10 mg	Claritin by Neuman Distbtrs	64579-0251	Antihistamine
458 <> CLARITIN10	Tab, White, Round	Loratadine 10 mg	Claritin by Natl Pharmpak	55154-3513	Antihistamine
458 <> CLARITIN10	Tab, White	Loratadine 10 mg	Claritin by Patient 1st	57575-0100	Antihistamine
458 <> CLARITIN10	Tab, White, Oblong	Loratadine 10 mg	Claritin by Southwood Pharms	58016-0560	Antihistamine
458 <> CLARITIN10	Tab	Loratadine 10 mg	Claritin DR by Schering	00085-0458	Antihistamine
458 <> CLARITIN10	Tab, Off-White, ER, <> Claritin 10	Loratadine 10 mg	Claritin by Urgent Care Ctr	50716-0267	Antihistamine
458 <> CLARITIN10	Tab, DR	Loratadine 10 mg	Claritin by HJ Harkins Co	52959-0452	Antihistamine
458 <> CLARITIN10	Tab, DR	Loratadine 10 mg	Claritin by Allscripts	54569-3738	Antihistamine
458 <> CLARITIN10	Tab, ER, Claritin 10	Loratadine 10 mg	Claritin by Direct Dispensing	57866-3500	Antihistamine
458 <> CLARITIN10	Tab, ER	Loratadine 10 mg	Claritin by Amerisource	62584-0458	Antihistamine
458 <> CLARITIN10	Tab, ER, Claritin Over 10	Loratadine 10 mg	Claritin by Quality Care	60346-0941	Antihistamine
458 <> CLARITIN10	Tab, White, Round	Loratadine 10 mg	Claritin by Compumed	00403-4369	Antihistamine

ID FRONT <> BACK	DESCRIPTION FRONT <> BACK	INGREDIENT & STRENGTH	BRAND (OR EQUIV.) & FIRM	NDC#	CLASS; SCH.
458B	Tab, White, Oblong	Amitriptyline HCl 150 mg	Elavil by Barr		Antidepressant
4600	Cap, Yellow, Gelatin	Benzonatate 100 mg	Tessalon Perles by Sidmak	50111-0851	Antitussive
4600 <> P	Cap, Gelatin, P in a triangle	Benzonatate 100 mg	by Banner Pharmacaps	10888-4600	Antitussive
4617 <> RUGBY	Tab, Partial Score	Sulfasalazine 500 mg	by Murfreesboro	51129-1338	Gastrointestinal
463 <> 54	Cap	Lithium Carbonate 300 mg	by Roxane	00054-8527	Antipsychotic
467 <> PAR	Tab, Film Coated	Ibuprofen 400 mg	by Quality Care	60346-0430	NSAID
467 <> SL	Tab	Propranolol HCl 10 mg	by Zenith Goldline	00182-1812	Antihypertensive
467HD	Tab, White, Round	Dipyridamole 75 mg	Persantine by Halsey		Antiplatelet
468 <> MJ	Tab, Chewable	Ascorbic Acid 60 mg, Cholecalciferol 400, Cyanocobalamin 4.5 mcg, Folic Acid 0.3 mg, Niacin 13.5 mg, Niacinamide, Pyridoxine HCl, Riboflavin Phosphate Sodium, Sodium Fluoride, Thiamine Mononitrate, Vitamin A Acetate, Vitamin E 15 Units	Poly Vi Flor by Bristol Myers Squibb	00087-0468	Vitamin
468 <> PAR	Tab, Elongated Shape, Film Coated	Ibuprofen 600 mg	by Quality Care	60346-0556	NSAID
468 <> SL	Tab	Propranolol HCl 20 mg	by Zenith Goldline	00182-1813	Antihypertensive
469 <> PAR	Tab, Film Coated	Ibuprofen 400 mg	by Quality Care	60346-0030	NSAID
469 <> SL	Tab	Propranolol HCl 40 mg	by Zenith Goldline	00182-1814	Antihypertensive
47 <> A	Cap, Green & Yellow	Phendimetrazine Tartrate 105 mg	Bontril SR by Amarin Pharms	65234-0047	Anorexiant; C III
47 <> ELAVIL	Tab, Film Coated	Amitriptyline HCl 150 mg	Elavil by Zeneca	00310-0047	Antidepressant
47 <> GG	Tab, Film Coated	Imipramine HCl 25 mg	by Direct Dispensing	57866-3930	Antidepressant
47 <> GG	Tab, Film Coated, Debossed	Imipramine HCl 25 mg	by Golden State	60429-0096	Antidepressant
470BARR	Tab, Pink, Oblong, 470/Barr	Propoxyphene Napsylate 100 mg, Acetaminophen 650 mg	Darvocet-N by Barr		Analgesic; C IV
471 <> SL	Tab	Propranolol HCl 80 mg	by Zenith Goldline	00182-1815	Antihypertensive
4719RUGBY	Tab	Triazolam 0.25 mg	by Chelsea	46193-0978	Sedative/Hypnotic; C IV
473 <> PAR	Tab, Green & White, Oblong, Scored	Orphenadrine Citrate 50 mg; Aspirin 770 mg; Caffeine 60 mg	Orphengesic Forte by Par Pharm	49884-0473	Muscle Relaxant
473 <> R	Tab, White, Round, Bisected, Film Coated	Verapamil HCl 80 mg	by Purepac	00228-2473	Antihypertensive
473 <> WESTWARD	Tab	Prednisone 10 mg	by Quality Care	60346-0058	Steroid
474 <> MJ	Tab, Orange, Pink & Purple, Pillow Shaped, Chewable	Ascorbic Acid 60 mg, Cyanocobalamin 4.5 mcg, Fluoride Ion 1 mg, Folic Acid 0.3 mg, Niacin 13.5 mg, Pyridoxine HCl 1.05 mg, Riboflavin 1.2 mg, Thiamine 1.05 mg, Vitamin A 2500 Units, Vitamin D 400 Units, Vitamin E 15 Units	Poly Vi Flo by Bristol Myers Squibb	00087-0474	Vitamin
474COPLEY	Tab, Pink, Round, 474/Copley	Diclofenac Sodium 50 mg	Voltaren by Copley		NSAID
475	Tab, Imprint Begins West-Ward	Prednisone 5 mg	Sterapred by Merz	00259-0390	Steroid
475	Tab, Film Coated, Purepac Logo Precedes 475	Verapamil HCl 120 mg	by Quality Care	60346-0296	Antihypertensive
475	Tab, Purepac Logo, Film Coated	Verapamil HCl 120 mg	by PDRX	55289-0481	Antihypertensive
475 <> R	Tab, White, Round, Bisected, Film Coated	Verapamil HCl 120 mg	by Purepac	00228-2475	Antihypertensive
476 <> MJ	Tab, Pillow-Shaped, Chewable	Ascorbic Acid 60 mg, Copper 1 mg, Cyanocobalamin 4.5 mcg, Fluoride Ion 1 mg, Folic Acid 0.3 mg, Iron 12 mg, Niacin 13.5 mg, Pyridoxine HCl 1.05 mg, Riboflavin 1.2 mg, Thiamine 1.05 mg, Vitamin A 2500 Units, Vitamin D 400 Units, Vitamin E 15 Units, Zinc 10 mg	Poly Vi Flor Iron by Bristol Myers Squibb	00087-0476	Vitamin
4761CEFACLOR <> 500MG	Cap, Zenith Logo	Cefaclor Monohydrate 500 mg	by DRX	55045-2337	Antibiotic
477 <> MJ	Tab, Orange, Pink & Purple, Pillow Shaped, Chewable	Ascorbic Acid 60 mg, Cholecalciferol 400 Units, Sodium Fluoride, Vitamin A Acetate 2500 Units	Tri Vi Flor by Bristol Myers Squibb	00087-0477	Vitamin
477477 <> GLYBUR	Tab	Glyburide 1.25 mg	by Coventry	61372-0576	Antidiabetic
477477 <> GLYBUR	Tab, White, Oblong, Scored	Glyburide 1.25 mg	by Blue Ridge	59273-0013	Antidiabetic
477477 <> GLYBUR	Tab, 477/477 <> Glybur	Glyburide 1.25 mg	by Merrell	00068-3200	Antidiabetic
477477 <> GLYBUR	Tab, 477/477 <> Glybur	Glyburide 1.25 mg	by Copley	38245-0477	Antidiabetic
477477 <> GLYBUR	Tab, White, Oblong, Scored	Glyburide 5 mg	by Blue Ridge	59273-0015	Antidiabetic
477COPLEY	Tab, White, Oblong, 477/Copley	Glyburide 1.25 mg	Diabeta by Copley		Antidiabetic
479HD	Tab, White, Round	Dipyridamole 50 mg	Persantine by Halsey		Antiplatelet
48	Tab, Fushchia, Film Coated	Calcium Pantothenate 10 mg, Cyanocobalamin 25 mcg, Ferrous Sulfate 525 mg, Folic Acid 800 mcg, Niacinamide 30 mg, Pyridoxine HCl 5 mg, Riboflavin 6 mg, Sodium Ascorbate 500 mg, Thiamine Mononitrate 6 mg	Generet 500 Folic Acid by Zenith Goldline	00182-4333	Vitamin/Mineral
480 <> P	Tab, Film Coated, Purepac Symbol	Tolmetin Sodium 735 mg	by Physicians Total Care	54868-2421	NSAID

ID FRONT <> BACK	DESCRIPTION FRONT <> BACK	INGREDIENT & STRENGTH	BRAND (OR EQUIV.) & FIRM	NDC#	CLASS; SCH.
480 <> R	Tab, White, Oval, Film Coated	Tolmetin Sodium 600 mg	by Purepac	00228-2480	NSAID
4804	Cap, Blue & White	Oxazepam 10 mg	by PF	48692-0094	Sedative/Hypnotic; C IV
4804	Cap, Blue & White	Oxazepam 10 mg	by PF	48692-0030	Sedative/Hypnotic; C IV
4805 <> 4805	Tab, Clear, Oval, Logo	Oxazepam 15 mg	by PF	48692-0106	Sedative/Hypnotic; C IV
481BARR	Tab, Aqua, Round	Haloperidol 10 mg	Haldol by Barr		Antipsychotic
482 <> GG	Tab, White, Round, Scored	Enalapril 5 mg	Vasotec by Geneva	00781-1231	Antihypertensive
482 <> MJ	Tab, Pillow-Shaped, Chewable	Ascorbic Acid 60 mg, Copper 1 mg, Cyanocobalamin 4.5 mcg, Fluoride Ion 0.5 mg, Folic Acid 0.3 mg, Iron 12 mg, Niacin 13.5 mg, Pyridoxine HCl 1.05 mg, Riboflavin 1.2 mg, Thiamine 1.05 mg, Vitamin A 2500 Units, Vitamin D 400 Units, Vitamin E 15 Units, Zinc 10 mg	Poly Vi Flor Iron by Bristol Myers Squibb	00087-0482	Vitamin
482BARR	Tab, Salmon, Round	Haloperidol 20 mg	Haldol by Barr		Antipsychotic
4832V	Cap, 4832/V	Acetaminophen 500 mg, Oxycodone HCl 5 mg	by Vintage	00254-4832	Analgesic; C II
4832V	Cap, 4832/V	Acetaminophen 500 mg, Oxycodone HCl 5 mg	by Qualitest	00603-4997	Analgesic; C II
4839V	Tab	Acetaminophen 325 mg, Oxycodone HCl 5 mg	by Zenith Goldline	00182-1465	Analgesic; C II
4839V	Tab	Acetaminophen 325 mg, Oxycodone HCl 5 mg	by Qualitest	00603-4998	Analgesic; C II
4839V	Tab, 4839 V	Acetaminophen 325 mg, Oxycodone HCl 5 mg	by Vintage	00254-4839	Analgesic; C II
484 <> B	Tab, White, Round, 484 <> B	Leucovorin Calcium	Wellcovoring by UDL	51079-0581	Antineoplastic
484 <> B	Tab	Leucovorin Calcium	by Barr	00555-0484	Antineoplastic
484 <> B	Tab, Debossed Company Logo	Leucovorin Calcium	by Rugby	00536-4148	Antineoplastic
484 <> B	Tab, Company Logo Debossed	Leucovorin Calcium	by Supergen	62701-0900	Antineoplastic
484 <> B	Tab, 484 <> b	Leucovorin Calcium	by Major	00904-2315	Antineoplastic
484 <> B	Tab, Debossed	Leucovorin Calcium	by Qualitest	00603-4183	Antineoplastic
4840 <> RUGBY	Tab, Film Coated	Cyclobenzaprine HCl 10 mg	by Quality Care	60346-0581	Muscle Relaxant
4841	Tab, White, Round	Neomycin Sulfate 500 mg	Neomycin by Eon		Antibiotic
4843 <> RUGBY	Tab	Naproxen 375 mg	by Quality Care	60346-0817	NSAID
485 <> B	Tab, Pale Green, Round, 485 <> B	Leucovorin Calcium	Wellcovoring by UDL	51079-0582	Antineoplastic
485 <> B	Tab, Debossed <> in Lower Case Letter	Leucovorin Calcium	by Barr	00555-0485	Antineoplastic
485 <> B	Tab, Company Logo Debossed	Leucovorin Calcium	by Supergen	62701-0901	Antineoplastic
485 <> B	Tab, Debossed	Leucovorin Calcium	by Qualitest	00603-4184	Antineoplastic
4853V	Tab, 4853 and V Separated by Horizontal Line	Oxybutynin Chloride 5 mg	by Vintage	00254-4835	Urinary
4853V	Tab, 4853 and V Separated by Horizontal Line	Oxybutynin Chloride 5 mg	by Qualitest	00603-4975	Urinary
487 <> MJ	Tab, Orange, Pink & Purple, Chewable	Cyanocobalamin 4.5 mcg, Folic Acid 0.3 mg, Niacinamide, Pyridoxine HCl 1.05 mg, Riboflavin 1.2 mg, Sodium Ascorbate, Sodium Fluoride, Thiamine Mononitrate, Vitamin A Acetate, Vitamin D 400 Units, Vitamin E Acetate	Poly Vi Flo by Bristol Myers Squibb	00087-0487	Vitamin
488 <> MJ	Tab, Chewable	Cupric Oxide, Cyanocobalamin 4.5 mcg, Ferrous Fumarate, Folic Acid 0.3 mg, Niacinamide, Pyridoxine HCl 1.05 mg, Riboflavin 1.2 mg, Sodium Ascorbate, Sodium Fluoride, Thiamine Mononitrate, Vitamin A Acetate, Vitamin D 400 Units, Vitamin E Acetate, Zinc Oxide	Poly Vi Flor Iron by Bristol Myers Squibb	00087-0488	Vitamin
4890 <> SB	Tab, White, Pentagon, Film	Ropinirole HCl 0.25 mg	Requip by RX PAK	65084-0202	Antiparkinson
4892 <> SB	Tab, Green, Pentagon, Film	Ropinirole HCl 1 mg	Requip by RX PAK	65084-0203	Antiparkinson
49 <> BIOCRAFT	Tab, Film Coated	Penicillin V Potassium	by Quality Care	60346-0095	Antibiotic
49 <> BIOCRAFT	Tab, White, Oval, Scored, 4/9 <> Biocraft	Penicillin V Potassium 500 mg	by Teva	00093-1174	Antibiotic
490 <> 93	Tab, Coated	Acetaminophen 650 mg, Propoxyphene Napsylate 100 mg	Propoxy N APAP by Quality Care	60346-0610	Analgesic; C IV
494HD	Tab, White, Round	Dipyridamole 25 mg	Persantine by Halsey		Antiplatelet
496 <> SCHERING	Tab, White, Mortar and Pestle to Right of Schering	Griseofulvin, Microsize 500 mg	Fulvicin-U/F by Schering	00085-0496	Antifungal
497	Cap, Yellow	Nifedipine 10 mg	Procardia by Novopharm		Antihypertensive
497 <> DYNACIN50MG	Cap, White	Minocycline HCl 50 mg	Dynacin by Natl Pharmpak	55154-9102	Antibiotic
4971V	Tab, Maroon, Round	Phenazopyridine HCl 100 mg	by Direct Dispensing	57866-4388	Urinary Analgesic
4971V	Tab, Coated, Embossed	Phenazopyridine HCl 100 mg	by Kaiser	00179-0542	Urinary Analgesic
4971V	Tab, Maroon, Round, Scored	Phenazopyridine HCl 100 mg	by Pharmafab	62542-0917	Urinary Analgesic
4971V	Tab, Maroon, Round	Phenazopyridine HCl 200 mg	by Direct Dispensing	57866-4392	Urinary Analgesic
4972 <> V	Tab, Maroon, Round, Scored	Phenazopyridine HCl 200 mg	by Physicians Total Care	54868-0879	Urinary Analgesic

ID FRONT <> BACK	DESCRIPTION FRONT <> BACK	INGREDIENT & STRENGTH	BRAND (OR EQUIV.) & FIRM	NDC#	CLASS; SCH.
4972V	Tab, Burgundy, Sugar Coated	Phenazopyridine HCl 200 mg	by Kaiser	00179-0545	Urinary Analgesic
498 <> DYNACIN	Cap, Gray & White	Minocycline HCl 100 mg	Dynacin by Natl Pharmpak	55154-9101	Antibiotic
498 <> DYNACIN100MG	Cap, Gray & White	Minocycline HCl 100 mg	Dynacin by WalMart	49035-0186	Antibiotic
4980	Tab, Pink, Cap-Shaped, Hourglass Logo 4980	Propoxy NAPS 100 mg, Acetaminophen 650 mg	Darvocet-N-100 by Zenith Goldline	00172-4980	Analgesic; C IV
499	Tab, Peach, Round, Sch. Logo 499	Methyltestosterone 25 mg	Oreton by Schering		Hormone; C III
499 <> DYNACIN75MG	Cap, Gray	Minocycline HCl 75 mg	Dynacin by Rx Pac	65084-0236	Antibiotic
499 <> DYNACIN75MG	Cap, Gray	Minocycline HCl 75 mg	Dynacin by Eckerd	19458-0914	Antibiotic
4G87C879	Tab	Aspirin 325 mg, Codeine Phosphate 60 mg	by United Res	00677-0676	Analgesic; C III
4LLA39	Tab, White, Round	Acetaminophen 300 mg, Codeine 60 mg	Tylenol #4 by Lederle		Analgesic; C III
4MG <> CARDURA	Tab	Doxazosin Mesylate 4 mg	Cardura by Nat Pharmpak Serv	55154-3216	Antihypertensive
4MG <> CARDURA	Tab, Orange, Oblong, 4/mg <> Cardura	Doxazosin Mesylate 4 mg	Cardura by Roerig	00049-2770	Antihypertensive
4MG <> ETH268	Tab, Pink, Oblong, Scored	Doxazosin Mesylate 4 mg	Cardura by Pfizer	58177-0268	Antihypertensive
5	Tab, Yellow, Round	Bisacodyl 5 mg	Bisacodyl by Apotex	Canadian	Gastrointestinal
5	Tab, White, Round	Fluphenazine HCl 5 mg	Fluphenazine by Apotex	Canadian	Antipsychotic
5	Tab, White, Oblong, 5/Logo	Glyburide 5 mg	Albert Glyburide by Albert Pharma	Canadian DIN# 01900935	Antidiabetic
5	Tab, White, Oblong, 5 Albert Logo	Glyburide 5 mg	by Altimed	Canadian	Antidiabetic
5	Tab, Pink, Round	Isosorbide Dinitrate 5 mg	Apo Isdn by Apotex	Canadian	Antianginal
5	Tab, Pink, Round	Lisinopril 5 mg	Zestril by Zeneca	Canadian	Antihypertensive
5	Tab, Yellow, Round	Methotrimeprazine Maleate 5 mg	Methoprazine by Apotex	Canadian	Antipsychotic
5	Cap, Mustard	Nifedipine 5 mg	Apo Nifed by Apotex	Canadian	Antihypertensive
5	Tab, ER	Nitroglycerin 5 mg	Sustachron ER Buccal by Forest	10418-0140	Vasodilator
5	Tab, Gold, Round, Hourglass Logo <> 5	Prochlorperazine 5 mg	Compazine by Zenith Goldline	00172-3690	Antiemetic
5	Tab, White, Round	Terbutaline Sulfate 5 mg	Bricanyl by Astra	Canadian	Antiasthmatic
5	Tab, Blue, Round	Trifluoperazine HCl 5 mg	Apo Trifluoperazine by Apotex	Canadian	Antipsychotic
5	Tab	Warfarin Sodium 5 mg	Coumadin by Pharmedix	53002-1048	Anticoagulant
5 <> 102	Tab, BM Logo	Torsemide 5 mg	Demadex by Boehringer Mannheim	12871-6477	Diuretic
5 <> 340	Tab, 5/Royce Logo	Pindolol 5 mg	by Qualitest	00603-5220	Antihypertensive
5 <> 4196	Tab, White, Round	Enalapril Maleate 5 mg	Vasotec by Zenith Goldline	00172-4196	Antihypertensive
5 <> 511	Tab, White, Pentagon	Lorazepam 0.5 mg	by Wyeth Pharms	52903-5811	Sedative/Hypnotic; C IV
5 <> A660	Tab, A Over 660	Selegiline HCl 5 mg	Atapryl by Athena	59075-0660	Antiparkinson
5 <> AD	Tab, Blue, Round	Amphetamine Aspartate 1.25 mg, Amphetamine Sulfate 1.25 mg, Dextroamphetamine Saccharate 1.25 mg, Dextroamphetamine Sulfate 1.25 mg	Adderall by Shire Richwood	58521-0031	Stimulant; C II
5 <> ARICEPT	Tab, White, Film Coated	Donepezil 5 mg	Arecept by Pfizer	Canadian DIN# 02232043	Antialzheimers
5 <> DAN5619	Tab, 5 <> Dan over 5619	Diazepam 5 mg	by Quality Care	60346-0478	Antianxiety; C IV
5 <> DAN5619	Tab	Diazepam 5 mg	by St Marys Med	60760-0775	Antianxiety; C IV
5 <> DAN5619	Tab	Diazepam 5 mg	by Danbury	00591-5619	Antianxiety; C IV
5 <> DAN5619	Tab, Yellow, Round, Scored	Diazepam 5 mg	by Vangard Labs	00615-1533	Antianxiety; C IV
5 <> E	Tab, Yellow, Octagonal	Acetaminophen 400 mg; Hydrocodone Bitartrate 5 mg	Zydone by West Pharm	52967-0273	Analgesic; C III
5 <> E	Tab, Yellow, Octagonal	Acetaminophen 500 mg, Hydrocodone Bitartrate 5 mg	Zydone by Endo Labs	63481-0668	Analgesic; C III
5 <> E	Tab	Lisinopril 2.5 mg	Prinivil by Allscripts	54569-4721	Antihypertensive
5 <> E245	Tab, Film Coated	Donepezil HCl 5 mg	Aricept by Eisai	62856-0245	Antialzheimers
5 <> EPI132	Tab, EPI Over 132	Oxycodone HCl 5 mg	Percolone by Du Pont Pharma	00056-0132	Analgesic; C II
5 <> EPI132	Tab, White, Round, Scored, 5 <> EPI Over 132	Oxycodone HCl 5 mg	Percolone by Endo	63481-0132	Analgesic; C II
5 <> F	Tab, Blue	Medroxyprogesterone Acetate 5 mg	Proclim by Fournier Pharma	Canadian	Progestin
5 <> GG55	Tab, Coated, Debossed	Trifluoperazine HCl 5 mg	by Med Pro	53978-2089	Antipsychotic
5 <> GG55	Tab, Lavender, Coated, Debossed	Trifluoperazine HCl 5 mg	by Golden State	60429-0193	Antipsychotic
5 <> GG55	Tab, Coated, GG 55	Trifluoperazine HCl 5 mg	by Quality Care	62682-7031	Antipsychotic

ID FRONT <> BACK	DESCRIPTION FRONT <> BACK	INGREDIENT & STRENGTH	BRAND (OR EQUIV.) & FIRM	NDC#	CLASS; SCH.
5 <> GG55	Tab, Lavender,Round, Film Coated	Trifluoperazine HCl 5 mg	Stelazine by Geneva	00781-1034	Antipsychotic
5 <> INV275	Tab, Yellow, Round, Film Coated	Prochlorperazine Maleate 5 mg	by Invamed	52189-0275	Antiemetic
5 <> INV275	Tab, Yellow, Round, Film Coated	Prochlorperazine Maleate 5 mg	by Murfreesboro Ph	51129-1427	Antiemetic
5 <> INV280	Tab, Purple, Round, Film Coated	Trifluoperazine HCl 5 mg	by Invamed	52189-0280	Antipsychotic
5 <> INV280	Tab, Purple, Round, Film Coated	Trifluoperazine HCl 5 mg	by Apothecon	62269-0280	Antipsychotic
5 <> LOTENSIN	Tab, Light Yellow	Benazepril HCl 5 mg	Lotensin by Novartis	00083-0059	Antihypertensive
5 <> M	Tab, White, Round, M Inside Square Company Logo	Methylphenidate HCl 5 mg	by Neuman Distr	64579-0021	Stimulant; C II
5 <> M	Tab, White, Round, M Inside the Box	Methylphenidate HCl 5 mg	Methylin by Neuman Distr	64579-0024	Stimulant; C II
5 <> M	Tab, White, Round	Methylphenidate HCl 5 mg	Ritalin by Mallinckrodt Hobart	00406-1121	Stimulant; C II
5 <> MERIDIA	Cap, Blue & Yellow	Sibutramine HCl 5 mg	Meridia by Knoll	00048-0605	Anorexiant; C IV
5 <> MERIDIA	Cap	Sibutramine HCl 5 mg	Meridia by Quality Care	62682-7048	Anorexiant; C IV
5 <> MERIDIA	Cap, Blue & Yellow	Sibutramine HCl 5 mg	Meridia by Compumed	00403-5371	Anorexiant; C IV
5 <> MERIDIA	Cap, -5-	Sibutramine HCl 5 mg	Meridia by BASF	10117-0605	Anorexiant; C IV
5 <> MERIDIA	Cap, Blue & Yellow	Sibutramine HCl 5 mg	Meridia by PDRX Pharms	55289-0377	Anorexiant; C IV
5 <> MJ822	Tab, White, Rectangular, Scored	Buspirone HCl 15 mg	Buspar by Murfreesboro Ph	51129-1375	Antianxiety
5 <> MOXY	Tab, White, Round, Scored, M-Oxy	Oxycodone HCl 5 mg	M-OXY by Pharmacia & Upjohn	00009-5014	Analgesic; C II
5 <> MOXY	Tab, White, Round, Scored, M-Oxy <> 5	Oxycodone HCl 5 mg	Roxicodone/Percolone by Mallinckrodt Hobart	00406-0552	Analgesic; C II
5 <> N179	Tab, N Over 179	Selegiline HCl 5 mg	by Warrick	59930-1537	Antiparkinson
5 <> N179	Tab, White, Round, Beveled Edged, <> N Over 179	Selegiline HCl 5 mg	by Novopharm	55953-0179	Antiparkinson
5 <> N179	Tab	Selegiline HCl 5 mg	by Major	00904-5206	Antiparkinson
5 <> N179	Tab, White, Round, Beveled Edged, <> N Over 179	Selegiline HCl 5 mg	by Novopharm	43806-0179	Antiparkinson
5 <> N344	Tab	Glyburide 5 mg	by Talbert Med	44514-0385	Antidiabetic
5 <> N344	Tab, Light Green, Round, Scored	Glyburide 5 mg	by Novopharm	43806-0344	Antidiabetic
5 <> N344	Tab, Light Green, Round, Scored, 5 <> N over 344	Glyburide 5.1 mg	by Novopharm	55953-0344	Antidiabetic
5 <> N344	Tab, Light Green, Round, Scored, 5 <> N over 344	Glyburide 5.1 mg	by Novopharm	62528-0344	Antidiabetic
5 <> N344	Tab, Scored, 5 <> N over 344	Glyburide 5 mg	by Medirex	57480-0409	Antidiabetic
5 <> N344	Tab, Scored, 5 <> N over 344	Glyburide 5 mg	by PDRX	55289-0892	Antidiabetic
5 <> N344	Tab	Glyburide 5 mg	by Warrick	59930-1639	Antidiabetic
5 <> N344	Tab, N/344	Glyburide 5 mg	by Brightstone	62939-3231	Antidiabetic
5 <> N344	Tab, Green, Round, Scored	Glyburide 5 mg	by Murfreesboro Ph	51129-1288	Antidiabetic
5 <> N344	Tab, Light Green, Round, Scored	Glyburide 5 mg	by Allscripts	54569-3831	Antidiabetic
5 <> N344	Tab, N/344	Glyburide 5 mg	by Kaiser	00179-1205	Antidiabetic
5 <> N344	Tab	Glyburide 5 mg	by HL Moore	00839-8041	Antidiabetic
5 <> N344	Tab	Glyburide 5 mg	by Qualitest	00603-3764	Antidiabetic
5 <> N344	Tab, 5 <> N over 344	Glyburide 5 mg	by Zenith Goldline	00182-2647	Antidiabetic
5 <> N344	Tab, Light Green, Round, Scored, 5 <> N over 344	Glyburide 5 mg	Micronase by UDL	51079-0873	Antidiabetic
5 <> N344	Tab	Glyburide 5 mg	by Major	00904-5077	Antidiabetic
5 <> N524	Tab, White, Oval, Scored	Glipizide 5 mg	by Novopharm (CA)	43806-0524	Antidiabetic
5 <> NORVASAC	Tab	Amlodipine Besylate	Norvasc by Nat Pharmpak Serv	55154-2708	Antihypertensive
5 <> PD527	Tab, Brown	Quinapril HCl 5 mg	Accupril by PDRX Pharms	55289-0552	Antihypertensive
5 <> PD527	Tab, Brown, Elliptical-Shaped, Coated	Quinapril HCl 5 mg	Accupril by Parke Davis	00071-0527	Antihypertensive
5 <> PD527	Tab, Coated	Quinapril HCl 5 mg	Accupril by Pharm Utilization	60491-0001	Antihypertensive
5 <> PD527	Tab, Brown, Elliptical, Scored, Film Coated, 5 <> PD/527	Quinapril 5 mg	Accupril by Pfizer	Canadian DIN# 01947664	Antihypertensive
5 <> PF	Tab, White, Round	Morphine Sulfate 5 mg	MS IR by Purdue Frederick	Canadian	Analgesic
5 <> PROVERA	Tab	Medroxyprogesterone Acetate 5 mg	Provera by Quality Care	60346-0603	Progestin
5 <> S	Tab, White, Shield-Shaped	Selegiline HCl 5 mg	Eldepryl by Watson	52544-0136	Antiparkinson
5 <> SAL	Tab, White, Round, Film Coated	Pilocarpine HCl 5 mg	by Pharmacia	Canadian DIN# 02216345	Cholinergic Agonist

ID FRONT <> BACK	DESCRIPTION FRONT <> BACK	INGREDIENT & STRENGTH	BRAND (OR EQUIV.) & FIRM	NDC#	CLASS; SCH.
5 <> Z3690	Tab, Gold, Round	Prochlorperazine Mal 5 mg	Compazine by Zenith Goldline	00182-8210	Antiemetic
5 <> Z3926	Tab	Diazepam 5 mg	by Quality Care	60346-0478	Antianxiety; C IV
5 <> Z3926	Tab, Yellow, Round	Diazepam 5 mg	Valium by Zenith Goldline	00172-3926	Antianxiety; C IV
5 <> Z3926	Tab	Diazepam 5 mg	by Qualitest	00603-3217	Antianxiety; C IV
5 <> Z3926	Tab	Diazepam 5 mg	by Pharmedix	53002-0334	Antianxiety; C IV
5 <> Z4232	Tab, Green, Round, Scored	Bumetanide 0.5 mg	by Vangard Labs	00615-4541	Diuretic
5 <> ZAROXOLYN	Tab	Metolazone 5 mg	Zaroxolyn by Nat Pharmpak Serv	55154-2505	Diuretic
5 <> ZAROXOLYN	Tab	Metolazone 5 mg	Zaroxolyn by Medeva	53014-0850	Diuretic
5 <> ZAROXOLYN	Tab, Debossed	Metolazone 5 mg	Zaroxolyn by Amerisource	62584-0850	Diuretic
5 <> ZAROXOLYN	Tab	Metolazone 5 mg	Zaroxolyn by Prestige Packaging	58056-0356	Diuretic
5 <> ZAROXOLYN	Tab	Metolazone 5 mg	Zaroxolyn by Quality Care	62682-6023	Diuretic
5 <> ZAROXOLYN	Tab, Blue, Round	Metolazone 5 mg	by Compumed	00403-1603	Diuretic
5 <> ZAROXOLYN	Tab, Blue, Round, Scored	Metolazone 5 mg	Zaroxolyn by Caremark	00339-5428	Diuretic
5 <> ZYRTEC	Tab, White, Rectangular, Film Coated	Cetirizine HCl 5 mg	Zyrtec by Murfreesboro Ph	51129-1192	Antihistamine
5C33	Tab, Yellow, Round	Leucovorin Calcium 5 mg	Leucovorin by Lederle		Antineoplastic
5MG	Tab, White, Circular, Scored	Bumetanide 5 mg	Burinex by Leo	Canadian	Diuretic
50	Tab, Brown, Round	Amitriptyline HCl 50 mg	Apo Amitriptyline by Apotex	Canadian	Antidepressant
50	Tab, Tab, Round	Bethanechol Chloride 50 mg	Duvoid by Roberts	Canadian	Urinary Tract
50	Tab, White, Biconvex	Atenolol 50 mg	by Schein	Canadian	Antihypertensive
50	Tab, Green, Round, Film Coated	Desipramine HCl 50 mg	Desipramine by Apotex	Canadian DIN# 02211955	Antidepressant
50	Tab, Light Brown, Round, Coated	Diclofenac Sodium 50 mg	Apo Diclo by Apotex	Canadian DIN# 00886025	NSAID
50	Tab, Light Brown, Round	Imipramine 50 mg	Apo Imipramine by Apotex	Canadian	Antidepressant
50	Cap, Red	Hydroxyzine HCl 50 mg	Apo Hydroxyzine by Apotex	Canadian	Antihistamine
50	Tab, Pink, Round, Film Coated	Hydralazine HCl 50 mg	Apo Hydralazine by Apotex	Canadian DIN# 02004836	Antihypertensive
50	Tab, Yellow, Round	Ketoprofen 50 mg	by Nu-Pharm	Canadian	NSAID
50	Tab, Yellow, Round	Ketoprofen 50 mg	Rhodis by Rhodiapharm	Canadian	NSAID
50	Tab, Yellow, Round	Ketoprofen 50 mg	Keto-E by Apotex	Canadian	NSAID
50	Tab, Yellow, Round	Ketoprofen 50 mg	Apo Keto E by Apotex	Canadian	NSAID
50	Tab	Levothyroxine Sodium 0.05 mg	Synthroid by Nat Pharmpak Serv	55154-0903	Antithyroid
50	Tab, White, Oval	Levothyroxine Sodium 0.05 mg	Levoxyl by Murfreesboro	51129-1657	Antithyroid
50	Tab, White	Levothyroxine Sodium 50 mcg	by Direct Dispensing	57866-5400	Antithyroid
50	Tab, Symbol	Levothyroxine Sodium 50 mcg	by Nat Pharmpak Serv	55154-4006	Antithyroid
50	Tab	Levothyroxine Sodium 50 mcg	by Quality Care	60346-0979	Antithyroid
50	Tab	Levothyroxine Sodium 50 mcg	by Amerisource	62584-0013	Antithyroid
50	Tab, Pink, Cap Shaped, Film Coated, Scored	Metoprolol Tartrate 50 mg	Metoprolol by Apotex	Canadian DIN# 00865605	Antihypertensive
50	Tab, Pink, Oblong	Metoprolol Tartrate 50 mg	by Nu-Pharm	Canadian	Antihypertensive
50	Tab, White, Round	Thioridazine HCl 50 mg	Apo Thioridazine by Apotex	Canadian	Antipsychotic
50	Cap, White, ER, Printed in Red	Theophylline 50 mg	Slo Bid by RPR	00801-0057	Antiasthmatic
50	Tab, Pink, Round, Film Coated	Trimipramine Maleate 50 mg	by Nu Pharm	Canadian DIN# 02020599	Antidepressant
50	Tab, Pink, Round	Trimipramine 50 mg	Rhotrimine by Rhodiapharm	Canadian	Antidepressant
50 <> 15	Tab, White, Oval, Hourglass Logo 50 <> 15	Captopril 50 mg, Hydrochlorothiazide 15 mg	Capozide by Zenith Goldline	00172-5015	Antihypertensive; Diuretic

ID FRONT <> BACK	DESCRIPTION FRONT <> BACK	INGREDIENT & STRENGTH	BRAND (OR EQUIV.) & FIRM	NDC#	CLASS; SCH.
50 <> 25	Tab, Off-White, Oval, Hourglass Logo 50 <> 25	Captopril 50 mg, Hydrochlorothiazide 25 mg	Capozide by Zenith Goldline	00172-5025	Antihypertensive; Diuretic
50 <> 273INV	Tab, 273/INV	Captopril 50 mg	by Schein	00364-2630	Antihypertensive
50 <> 311	Cap, Flesh, <> Royce Logo 311	Doxepin HCl	by Quality Care	60346-0269	Antidepressant
50 <> 349	Tab, 50/Royce Logo <> 349	Captopril 50 mg	by Qualitest	00603-2557	Antihypertensive
50 <> 727N	Tab, 727/N	Metoprolol Tartrate 50 mg	by Schein	00364-2560	Antihypertensive
50 <> 832	Tab, Butterscotch Yellow, Sugar Coated	Chlorpromazine HCl 50 mg	by Qualitest	00603-2810	Antipsychotic
50 <> 832	Tab, Sugar Coated	Chlorpromazine HCl 50 mg	by Schein	00364-0382	Antipsychotic
50 <> 832	Tab, Sugar Coated	Chlorpromazine HCl 50 mg	by United Res	00677-0455	Antipsychotic
50 <> CAPOTEN	Tab	Captopril 50 mg	Capoten by Nat Pharmpak Serv	55154-3708	Antihypertensive
50 <> CAPOTEN	Tab, Mottled Oval	Captopril 50 mg	Capoten by ER Squibb	00003-0482	Antihypertensive
50 <> CATAFLAM	Tab, Coated	Diclofenac Potassium 50 mg	Cataflam by PDRX	55289-0818	NSAID
50 <> CATAFLAM	Tab, Coated	Diclofenac Potassium 50 mg	Cataflam by Quality Care	60346-0975	NSAID
50 <> CATAFLAM	Tab, Coated	Diclofenac Potassium 50 mg	Cataflam by Direct Dispensing	57866-1182	NSAID
50 <> CATAFLAM	Tab, Brown, Round	Diclofenac Potassium 50 mg	Cataflam by HJ Harkins	52959-0344	NSAID
50 <> CATAFLAM	Tab, Light Brown, Round	Diclofenac Potassium 50 mg	Cataflam by Novartis	00028-0151	NSAID
50 <> CATAFLAM	Tab, Coated	Diclofenac Potassium 50 mg	Cataflam by Allscripts	54569-3823	NSAID
50 <> CATAFLAM	Tab, Coated	Diclofenac Potassium 50 mg	Cataflam by DRX	55045-2225	NSAID
50 <> CATAFLAM	Tab, Coated	Diclofenac Potassium 50 mg	Cataflam by Novartis	17088-0151	NSAID
50 <> FL	Tab, Compressed, <> Logo FL	Levothyroxine Sodium 50 mcg	by Kaiser	00179-0457	Antithyroid
50 <> FLINT	Tab	Levothyroxine Sodium 0.05 mg	Synthroid by Physicians Total Care	54868-1011	Antithyroid
50 <> FLINT	Tab	Levothyroxine Sodium 0.05 mg	Synthroid by Knoll BV	55445-0104	Antithyroid
50 <> FLINT	Tab	Levothyroxine Sodium 0.05 mg	Synthroid by Giant Food	11146-0301	Antithyroid
50 <> FLINT	Tab, White, Round, Scored	Levothyroxine Sodium 50 mcg	Synthroid by Knoll	00048-1040	Antithyroid
50 <> G	Tab	Atenolol 50 mg	by Par	49884-0456	Antihypertensive
50 <> GG33	Tab, Film Coated, Debossed <> GG 33	Thioridazine HCl 50 mg	by Heartland	61392-0819	Antipsychotic
50 <> GG33	Tab, Orange, Round, Film Coated	Thioridazine HCl 50 mg	Mellaril by Geneva	00781-1634	Antipsychotic
50 <> GG407	Tab, Butterscotch Yellow, Round, Film Coated	Chlorpromazine HCl 50 mg	Thorazine by Geneva	00781-1717	Antipsychotic
50 <> GG407	Tab, Butterscotch, Film Coated, Debossed	Chlorpromazine HCl 50 mg	by Golden State	60429-0042	Antipsychotic
50 <> GG407	Tab, Yellow, Round, Film Coated	Chlorpromazine HCl 50 mg	by Murfreesboro Ph	51129-1361	Antipsychotic
50 <> GG407	Tab, Yellow, Round, Film Coated	Chlorpromazine HCl 50 mg	by Haines Pharms	59564-0130	Antipsychotic
50 <> IMITREX	Tab, Coated	Sumatriptan Succinate 50 mg	Imitrex by Physicians Total Care	54868-3852	Antimigraine
50 <> IMITREX	Tab, Coated	Sumatriptan Succinate 50 mg	Imitrex by Pharm Utilization	60491-0318	Antimigraine
50 <> IMITREX	Tab, Coated	Sumatriptan Succinate 50 mg	Imitrex by Glaxo	00173-0459	Antimigraine
50 <> IMURAN	Tab, Off-White to Yellow, Shape is Overlapping Circle	Azathioprine 50 mg	Imuran by Catalytica	63552-0597	Immunosuppressant
50 <> INV273	Tab, Scored	Captopril 50 mg	by Invamed	52189-0273	Antihypertensive
50 <> M59	Tab, Orange, Film Coated, M Over 59	Thioridazine HCl 50 mg	by Mylan	00378-0616	Antipsychotic
50 <> M59	Tab, Orange, Round, Film Coated, 50 <> M over 59	Thioridazine HCl 50 mg	Mellaril by UDL	51079-0567	Antipsychotic
50 <> M59	Tab, Film Coated, M Over 59	Thioridazine HCl 50 mg	by Quality Care	60346-0840	Antipsychotic
50 <> M59	Tab, Orange, Round, Film Coated	Thioridazine HCl 50 mg	by Dixon Shane	17236-0302	Antipsychotic
50 <> M59	Tab, Film Coated	Thioridazine HCl 50 mg	by Qualitest	00603-5994	Antipsychotic
50 <> M59	Tab, Film Coated	Thioridazine HCl 50 mg	by Vangard	00615-2507	Antipsychotic
50 <> MJ503	Tab	Cyclophosphamide 50 mg	Cytoxan by Mead Johnson	00015-0503	Antineoplastic
50 <> N032	Cap, Bright Yellow & Turquoise, 50 <> N over 032	Clomipramine HCl 50 mg	by Novopharm	55953-0032	OCD
50 <> N032	Cap, Bright Yellow & Turquoise, 50 <> N over 032	Clomipramine HCl 50 mg	by Novopharm	43806-0032	OCD
50 <> N039	Tab, White, Round, 50 <> N over 039	Atenolol 50 mg	by Novopharm	55953-0039	Antihypertensive
50 <> N039	Tab, 50 <> N over 039	Atenolol 50 mg	by Medirex	57480-0446	Antihypertensive
50 <> N039	Tab, 50 <> N over 039	Atenolol 50 mg	by Quality Care	60346-0719	Antihypertensive
50 <> N039	Tab, White, Round, Scored	Atenolol 50 mg	by Novopharm (US)	62528-0039	Antihypertensive
50 <> N039	Tab, 50 <> N over 039	Atenolol 50 mg	by DRX	55045-1860	Antihypertensive
50 <> N039	Tab, 50 <> N over 039	Atenolol 50 mg	by Apotheca	12634-0436	Antihypertensive
50 <> N134	Tab, Scored, 50 <> N over 134	Captopril 50 mg	by HL Moore	00839-7996	Antihypertensive

93

ID FRONT <> BACK	DESCRIPTION FRONT <> BACK	INGREDIENT & STRENGTH	BRAND (OR EQUIV.) & FIRM	NDC#	CLASS; SCH.
50 <> N134	Tab, 50 <> N over 134	Captopril 50 mg	by Major	00904-5047	Antihypertensive
50 <> N134	Tab, White, Oval, 50 <> N over 134	Captopril 50 mg	by Novopharm	43806-0134	Antihypertensive
50 <> N134	Tab, Scored, 50 <> N over 134	Captopril 50 mg	by Medirex	57480-0840	Antihypertensive
50 <> N134	Tab, White, Oval, 50 <> N over 134	Captopril 50 mg	by Novopharm	55953-0134	Antihypertensive
50 <> N439	Cap, Green	Indomethacin 50 mg	by Allscripts	54569-0275	NSAID
50 <> N573	Tab, Film Coated	Flurbiprofen 50 mg	by Warrick	59930-1771	NSAID
50 <> N573	Tab, Film Coated	Flurbiprofen 50 mg	by HL Moore	00839-8003	NSAID
50 <> N727	Tab, White, Oblong, Scored	Metoprolol Tartrate 50 mg	by Va Cmop	65243-0048	Antihypertensive
50 <> N727	Tab, White, Cap-Shaped, Film Coated	Metoprolol Tartrate 50 mg	by Novopharm	55953-0727	Antihypertensive
50 <> N727	Tab, Film Coated, N 727	Metoprolol Tartrate 50 mg	by Brightstone	62939-2211	Antihypertensive
50 <> N727	Tab, Film Coated	Metoprolol Tartrate 50 mg	by Medirex	57480-0802	Antihypertensive
50 <> N727	Tab, Film Coated, Engraved N 727	Metoprolol Tartrate 50 mg	by Major	00904-7946	Antihypertensive
50 <> N735	Tab, Dark Orange, Round, Film Coated	Diclofenac Sodium 50 mg	by Allscripts	54569-4165	NSAID
50 <> NU	Tab, White, Round, Film Coated	Fluvoxamine Maleate 50 mg	by Nu Pharm	Canadian DIN# 02231192	OCD
50 <> PRECOSE	Tab, Whitish Yellow	Acarbose 50 mg	Precose by Physicians Total Care	54868-3823	Antidiabetic
50 <> ROBERTS103	Tab	Bethanechol Chloride 50 mg	Duvoid by Pharm Utilization	60491-0221	Urinary Tract
50 <> S	Tab, Orange, Round, Film Coated, 50 <> S over Triangle	Pinaverium Bromide 50 mg	Dicetel by Solvay Pharma	Canadian DIN# 01950592	Gastrointestinal
50 <> UAD63	Tab, Light Blue, UAD/63	Acetaminophen 650 mg, Hydrocodone Bitartrate 10 mg	Lorcet by UAD	00785-6350	Analgesic; C III
50 <> VIDEX	Tab, Mottled Off-White to Light Orange & Yellow, Orange Specks, Round, Chewable	Didanosine 50 mg	Videx T by Bristol Myers Squibb	00087-6651	Antiviral
50 <> VOLTAREN	Tab, Light Brown, Round, Enteric Coated	Diclofenac Sodium 50 mg	Voltaren by Novartis	Canadian DIN# 00514012	NSAID
50 <> WATSON372	Cap	Loxapine Succinate	by Major	00904-2313	Antipsychotic
50LLT27	Tab, Orange, Round	Thioridazine HCl 50 mg	Mellaril by Lederle		Antipsychotic
500	Tab, Oval, Pink, Enteric Coated	Divalproex Sodium 500 mg	by Nu Pharm	Canadian DIN# 02239519	Anticonvulsant
500	Tab, Coated	Metformin HCl 500 mg	Glucophage by Lipha	64130-1010	Antidiabetic
500	Cap, Gray & Green	Metronidazole 500 mg	Flagyl by Rhone-Poulenc Rorer	Canadian	Antibiotic
500	Cap, Pink, Elongated	Polygel Controlled-Release Niacin 500 mg	Slo-Niacin by Upsher-Smith	00245-0063	Vitamin
500 <> 4174	Tab, White, Cap Shaped	Etodolac 500 mg	Lodine by Zenith Goldline	00172-4174	NSAID
500 <> 4194	Tab, Blue, Oblong	Cefaclor 500 mg	by Ceclor	00172-4194	Antibiotic
500 <> 7721	Tab, Film Coated	Cefprozil 500 mg	Cefzil by Bristol Myers Squibb	00087-7721	Antibiotic
500 <> AMP	Cap, Light Blue & White	Ampicillin Trihydrate 500 mg	by Teva	00093-5146	Antibiotic
500 <> AP7494	Cap	Cefaclor Monohydrate	by Golden State	60429-0702	Antibiotic
500 <> AP7494	Cap	Cefaclor Monohydrate	by Apothecon	59772-7494	Antibiotic
500 <> BMS6060	Tab, White to Off-White, Round, Film Coated	Metformin HCl 500 mg	Glucophage by Bristol Myers Squibb	00087-6060	Antidiabetic
500 <> BMS6060	Tab, Film Coated, 500 across the face <> BMS 6060 around the Periphery of the Tab	Metformin HCl 500 mg	Glucophage by PDRX	55289-0211	Antidiabetic
500 <> BMS6060	Tab, Around the Periphery of the Tab Coated	Metformin HCl 500 mg	Glucophage by Heartland	61392-0717	Antidiabetic
500 <> CIPRO	Tab, Film Coated	Ciprofloxacin HCl	Cipro by HJ Harkins Co	52959-0037	Antibiotic
500 <> CIPRO	Tab, Yellow, Oblong, Film Coated	Ciprofloxacin HCl 500 mg	Cipro by Allscripts	54569-4820	Antibiotic
500 <> CIPRO	Tab, Film Coated	Ciprofloxacin HCl 583 mg	Cipro by Amerisource	62584-0336	Antibiotic
500 <> CIPRO	Tab, Pale Yellow, Film Coated	Ciprofloxacin HCl 583 mg	Cipro by Quality Care	60346-0031	Antibiotic
500 <> CIPRO	Tab, Film Coated	Ciprofloxacin HCl 583 mg	Cipro by Prescription Dispensing	61807-0035	Antibiotic
500 <> CIPRO	Tab, Film Coated	Ciprofloxacin HCl 583 mg	Ciprobay by Bayer	00026-8513	Antibiotic
500 <> CIPRO	Tab, Slightly Yellowish, Film Coated	Ciprofloxacin HCl 583 mg	by Med Pro	53978-3075	Antibiotic

ID FRONT <> BACK	DESCRIPTION FRONT <> BACK	INGREDIENT & STRENGTH	BRAND (OR EQUIV.) & FIRM	NDC#	CLASS; SCH.
500 <> CIPRO	Tab, Coated	Ciprofloxacin HCl 583 mg	Cipro by Physicians Total Care	54868-0939	Antibiotic
500 <> CIPRO	Tab, Film Coated	Ciprofloxacin HCl 583 mg	Cipro by Nat Pharmpak Serv	55154-4801	Antibiotic
500 <> CIPRO	Tab, Coated	Ciprofloxacin HCl 583 mg	Cipro by HJ Harkins Co	52959-0036	Antibiotic
500 <> CIPRO	Tab, Film Coated	Ciprofloxacin HCl 583 mg	Cipro by PDRX	55289-0371	Antibiotic
500 <> ECNAPROSYN	Tab, DR, EC Naprosyn	Naproxen 500 mg	EC Naprosyn by Allscripts	54569-3982	NSAID
500 <> ECNAPROSYN	Tab, DR, EC Naprosyn	Naproxen 500 mg	Naprosyn EC by HJ Harkins Co	52959-0456	NSAID
500 <> ECNAPROSYN	Tab, DR	Naproxen 500 mg	EC Naprosyn by DRX	55045-2441	NSAID
500 <> ECNAPROSYN	Tab, DR, EC Naprosyn	Naproxen 500 mg	EC Naprosyn by Quality Care	60346-0334	NSAID
500 <> ECNAPROSYN	Tab, White, Oblong	Naproxen 500 mg	Naprosyn EC by Compumed	00403-0717	NSAID
500 <> ECNAPROSYN	Tab, DR	Naproxen 500 mg	Naprosyn by Syntex	18393-0256	NSAID
500 <> ESTAC	Cap, Blue, Film Coated	Acetaminophen	Extra Strength Tylenol Aches & Strains by McNeil	Canadian DIN# 02155214	Antipyretic
500 <> FAMVIR	Tab, Film Coated	Famciclovir 500 mg	Famvir by SKB	60351-4117	Antiviral
500 <> FAMVIR	Tab, White, Round, Film Coated	Famciclovir 500 mg	Famvir by SKB	00007-4117	Antiviral
500 <> FAMVIR	Tab, White, Round, Film Coated	Famciclovir 500 mg	Famvir by Novartis	00078-0368	Antiviral
500 <> FAMVIR	Tab, Film Coated	Famciclovir 500 mg	Famvir by Allscripts	54569-4534	Antiviral
500 <> FAMVIR	Tab, White, Oval, Film Coated	Famciclovir 500 mg	by SmithKline SKB	Canadian DIN# 02177102	Antiviral
500 <> FLAGYL	Tab, Film Coated	Metronidazole 500 mg	Flagyl by GD Searle	00025-1821	Antibiotic
500 <> FLAGYL	Tab, Film Coated, Debossed	Metronidazole 500 mg	Flagyl by Thrift Drug	59198-0030	Antibiotic
500 <> GL	Tab, Coated	Metformin HCl 500 mg	Glucophage by Allscripts	54569-4202	Antidiabetic
500 <> GLAXO	Tab, White, Oblong	Cefuroxime Axetil 500 mg	Ceftin by Glaxo Wellcome	00173-7005	Antibiotic
500 <> KEFTAB	Tab, Dark-Green, Elliptical, Coated	Cephalexin HCl	Keftab by Quality Care	60346-0650	Antibiotic
500 <> KOS	Tab, White, Oblong	Niacin 500 mg	Niaspan by DRX Pharm Consults	55045-2767	Vitamin
500 <> KOS	Tab, Off-White, Cap-Shaped, Debossed, ER	Niacin 500 mg	Niaspan by KOS	60598-0001	Vitamin
500 <> LEVAQUIN	Tab, Peach, Rectangle	Levofloxacin 500 mg	Levaquin by Phy Total Care	54868-3923	Antibiotic
500 <> MCNEIL1525	Tab, Film Coated	Levofloxacin 500 mg	Levaquin by McNeil	00045-1525	Antibiotic
500 <> MCNEIL1525	Tab, Peach, Modified Rectangle, Film Coated	Levofloxacin 500 mg	Levaquin by Ortho	00062-1525	Antibiotic
500 <> MCNEIL1525	Tab, Film Coated	Levofloxacin 500 mg	Levaquin by Allscripts	54569-4489	Antibiotic
500 <> MCNEIL1525	Tab, Film Coated	Levofloxacin 500 mg	Levaquin by Johnson & Johnson	59604-0525	Antibiotic
500 <> MPC	Tab	Acetohydroxamic Acid 250 mg	Lithostat by Mission	00178-0500	Analgesic
500 <> MSTSM	Cap, Green, Film Coated	Acetaminophen 500 mg, Pseudoephedrine HCl 30 mg	Extra Strength Tylenol Sinus	Canadian DIN# 00663980	Cold Remedy
500 <> MYLAN156	Tab, Yellow, Film Coated	Probenecid 500 mg	by Mylan	00378-0156	Antigout
500 <> MYLAN107	Tab, Coated	Erythromycin Stearate	by PDRX	55289-0705	Antibiotic
500 <> MYLAN107	Tab, Coated	Erythromycin Stearate	by Quality Care	60346-0645	Antibiotic
500 <> MYLAN107	Tab, Film Coated, 500 <> Mylan over 107	Erythromycin Stearate	by St Marys Med	60760-0107	Antibiotic
500 <> MYLAN107	Tab, Film Coated, 500 <> Mylan over 107	Erythromycin Stearate	by Prescription Dispensing	61807-0015	Antibiotic
500 <> MYLAN107	Tab, Coated	Erythromycin Stearate	by Direct Dispensing	57866-0265	Antibiotic
500 <> MYLAN107	Tab, Film Coated, 500 <> Mylan over 107	Erythromycin Stearate	by Mylan	00378-0107	Antibiotic
500 <> MYLAN107	Tab, Film Coated	Erythromycin Stearate	by Med Pro	53978-0026	Antibiotic
500 <> MYLAN107	Tab, Film Coated, Mylan over 107	Erythromycin Stearate	by DRX	55045-1113	Antibiotic
500 <> MYLAN156	Tab, Film Coated	Probenecid 500 mg	by Med Pro	53978-0014	Antigout
500 <> MYLAN156	Tab, Film Coated, Mylan 156	Probenecid 500 mg	by Quality Care	60346-0768	Antigout
500 <> N	Cap, Brown	Amoxicillin 500 mg	by Natl Pharmpak	55154-1750	Antibiotic
500 <> N	Cap	Cephalexin Monohydrate 541 mg	by Prescription Dispensing	61807-0006	Antibiotic
500 <> N114	Cap	Cephalexin Monohydrate	by Quality Care	60346-0055	Antibiotic
500 <> N114	Cap, 500 <> N over 114	Cephalexin Monohydrate	by Apotheca	12634-0434	Antibiotic
500 <> N114	Cap, Swedish Orange, 500 <> N over 114	Cephalexin Monohydrate 541 mg	by Novopharm	55953-0114	Antibiotic

ID FRONT <> BACK	DESCRIPTION FRONT <> BACK	INGREDIENT & STRENGTH	BRAND (OR EQUIV.) & FIRM	NDC#	CLASS; SCH.
500 <> N114	Cap, 500 <> N over 114	Cephalexin Monohydrate 541 mg	by HJ Harkins Co	52959-0031	Antibiotic
500 <> N251	Cap	Cefaclor Monohydrate	by Warrick	59930-1536	Antibiotic
500 <> N251	Cap	Cefaclor Monohydrate	by Rugby	00536-1375	Antibiotic
500 <> N251	Cap, 500 <> N over 251	Cefaclor Monohydrate	by Qualitest	00603-2587	Antibiotic
500 <> N251	Cap, Gray & Light Orange, 500 <> N over 251	Cefaclor Monohydrate	by Novopharm	43806-0251	Antibiotic
500 <> N251	Cap, 500 <> N over 251	Cefaclor Monohydrate	by Major	00904-5205	Antibiotic
500 <> N251	Cap, Bright Orange & Gray, Opaque, 500 <> N over 251	Cefaclor Monohydrate 500 mg	Ceclor by UDL	51079-0618	Antibiotic
500 <> N520	Tab, N Over 520	Naproxen 500 mg	by Medirex	57480-0835	NSAID
500 <> N520	Tab, Peach & Yellow, Oval, N Over 520	Naproxen 500 mg	by Novopharm	55953-0520	NSAID
500 <> N520	Tab, Light Yellow, N Over 520	Naproxen 500 mg	by Quality Care	60346-0815	NSAID
500 <> N716	Cap, Buff, Opaque, 500 <> N over 716	Amoxicillin 500 mg	by Novopharm	43806-0716	Antibiotic
500 <> N716	Cap	Amoxicillin Trihydrate	by Qualitest	00603-2267	Antibiotic
500 <> N716	Cap, 500 <> N over 716	Amoxicillin 500 mg	by St Marys Med	60760-0716	Antibiotic
500 <> N716	Cap, Buff & Opaque	Amoxicillin 500 mg	by Quality Care	60346-0634	Antibiotic
500 <> N716	Cap	Amoxicillin 500 mg	by Casa De Amigos	62138-0601	Antibiotic
500 <> NAPROSYN	Tab	Naproxen 500 mg	Naprosyn by HJ Harkins Co	52959-0111	NSAID
500 <> NAPROSYN	Tab, Yellow, Round, Scored	Naproxen 500 mg	by HJ Harkins	52959-0516	NSAID
500 <> NAPROSYN	Tab, Yellow, Oblong	Naproxen 500 mg	Naprosyn by Rightpak	65240-0701	NSAID
500 <> NAPROSYN	Tab	Naproxen 500 mg	Naprosyn by Allscripts	54569-0294	NSAID
500 <> NAPROSYN	Tab, Debossed	Naproxen 500 mg	Naprosyn by Thrift Drug	59198-0239	NSAID
500 <> NAPROSYN	Tab	Naproxen 500 mg	Naprosyn by Nat Pharmpak Serv	55154-3804	NSAID
500 <> NAPROSYN	Tab	Naproxen 500 mg	Naprosyn by Quality Care	60346-0637	NSAID
500 <> NAPROSYN	Tab, Bone	Naproxen 500 mg	Naprosyn by Syntex	18393-0277	NSAID
500 <> P	Cap, Purepac Logo	Prazosin HCl 1 mg	by Quality Care	60346-0572	Antihypertensive
500 <> PROCANBID	Tab, Elliptical Shaped, Film Coated	Procainamide HCl 500 mg	Procanbid by Parke Davis	00071-0562	Antiarrhythmic
500 <> RELAFEN	Tab, Film Coated	Nabumetone 500 mg	Relafen by Amerisource	62584-0851	NSAID
500 <> RELAFEN	Tab, Oval, Film Coated	Nabumetone 500 mg	Relafen by SKB	00029-4851	NSAID
500 <> RELAFEN	Tab, Film Coated	Nabumetone 500 mg	Relafen by HJ Harkins Co	52959-0227	NSAID
500 <> RELAFEN	Tab, Film Coated	Nabumetone 500 mg	Relafen by Nat Pharmpak Serv	55154-4505	NSAID
500 <> RELAFEN	Tab, Film Coated	Nabumetone 500 mg	Relafen by Quality Care	60346-0316	NSAID
500 <> RELAFEN	Tab, Oval, Film Coated	Nabumetone 500 mg	Relafen by SB	59742-4851	NSAID
500 <> TAS	Cap, Yellow, Film Coated	Acetaminophen 500 mg, Chlorpheniramine Maleate 2mg, Pseudoephedrine HCl 30 mg	Extra Strength Tylenol Allergy Sinus by McNeil	Canadian DIN# 01933728	Cold Remedy
500 <> TCM	Cap, Yellow, Film Coated	Acetaminophen 500 mg, Chlorpheniramine Maleate 2mg, Pseudoephedrine HCl 30 mg, Dextromethorphan Hydrobromide 15 mg	Extra Strength Tylenol Cold Nighttime	Canadian DIN# 00743275	Cold Remedy
500 <> TCMND	Cap, Yellow, Film Coated	Acetaminophen 500 mg, Pseudoephedrine HCl 30 mg, Dextromethorphan Hydrobromide 15 mg	Extra Strength Tylenol Cold Daytime by McNeil	Canadian DIN# 00743267	Cold Remedy
500 <> TYCOF	Cap, Red, Film Coated	Acetaminophen 500 mg, Dextromethorphan Hydrobromide	Extra Strength Tylenol Cough	Canadian DIN# 02017377	Cold Remedy
500 <> TYLENOL	Cap, White, Film Coated	Acetaminophen 500 mg	ES Tylenol by McNeil	Canadian DIN# 00723908	Antipyretic
500 <> TYLENOL	Tab, White, Round	Acetaminophen 500 mg	ES Tylenol by McNeil	Canadian DIN# 00559407	Antipyretic
500 <> UCB	Tab	Aspirin 500 mg, Hydrocodone Bitartrate 5 mg	Lortab ASA by UCB	50474-0500	Analgesic; C III
500 <> UCB	Tab, Yellow, Oblong, Scored, Film Coated	Levetiracetam 500 mg	Keppra by UCB Pharma	50474-0592	Anticonvulsant
500 <> XELODA	Tab, Film Coated	Capecitabine 500 mg	Xeloda by Hoffmann La Roche	00004-1101	Antineoplastic

ID FRONT <> BACK	DESCRIPTION FRONT <> BACK	INGREDIENT & STRENGTH	BRAND (OR EQUIV.) & FIRM	NDC#	CLASS; SCH.
500 <> ZENITH4058	Cap	Cefadroxil Monohydrate	by Prescription Dispensing	61807-0123	Antibiotic
500 <>TYME	Cap, Peach, Film Coated	Acetaminophen 500 mg, Pamabrom 25 mg, Pyrilamine Maleate15 mg	Extra Strength Tylenol Menstrual	Canadian DIN# 02231239	Cold Remedy
5000	Cap, 5000 Proceeded By Eon Logo <> Blue & White Pellets	Phentermine HCl 30 mg	by Quality Care	62682-7025	Anorexiant; C IV
500125	Tab, White, Oval, Film Coated	Amoxicillin Trihydrate 500 mg; Clavulanate Potassium 125 mg	Augmentin by Allscripts	54569-1959	Antibiotic
500125 <> AUGMENTIN	Tab, White, Oval, Film Coated	Amoxicillin Trihydrate 500 mg; Clavulanate Potassium 125 mg	Augmentin by PDRX Pharms	55289-0296	Antibiotic
500125 <> AUGMENTIN	Tab, Film Coated	Amoxicillin Trihydrate, Clavulanate Potassium	Augmentin by Casa De Amigos	62138-6080	Antibiotic
500125 <> AUGMENTIN	Tab, Film Coated, 500/125	Amoxicillin Trihydrate, Clavulanate Potassium	Augmentin by Amerisource	62584-0312	Antibiotic
500125 <> AUGMENTIN	Tab, Yellow, Round, Film Coated, 500/125 <> Augmentin	Amoxicillin Trihydrate, Clavulanate Potassium	Augmentin by SKB	00029-6080	Antibiotic
500125 <> AUGMENTIN	Tab, Film Coated	Amoxicillin Trihydrate, Clavulanate Potassium	Augmentin by Pharmedix	53002-0239	Antibiotic
500125 <> AUGMENTIN	Tab, Film Coated, 500/125	Amoxicillin Trihydrate, Clavulanate Potassium	Augmentin by HJ Harkins Co	52959-0021	Antibiotic
500222AF	Cap, White, 500/222 AF	Acetaminophen 500 mg	by Johnson & Johnson	Canadian	Antipyretic
5002DAN	Cap, Clear & Pink	Diphenhydramine HCl 25 mg	by Schein	00364-0116	Antihistamine
5003DAN	Cap, Pink	Diphenhydramine HCl 50 mg	by Schein	00364-0117	Antihistamine
5005 <> SP2104	Tab, White, Scored	Acetaminophen 500 mg, Hydrocodone Bitartrate 5 mg	Co Gesic by	00131-2104	Analgesic; C III
500A	Tab, Film Coated, 500/A	Salsalate 500 mg	by Schein	00364-0832	NSAID
500BRISTOL7376	Cap, Blue, 500 Bristol 7376	Cephalexin 500 mg	Keflex by BMS		Antibiotic
500CIPRO	Tab, Film Coated	Ciprofloxacin HCl 583 mg	Cipro by Pharmedix	53002-0264	Antibiotic
500GLAXO	Tab, White, Oblong, 500/Glaxo	Cefuroxime Axetil 500 mg	by Glaxo	Canadian	Antibiotic
500M50 <> MOVA	Tab, Rose, Cap Shaped	Naproxen 500 mg	Naprosyn by Mova	55370-0141	NSAID
500M50 <> MOVA	Tab	Naproxen 500 mg	by Martec	52555-0714	NSAID
500M50 <> MOVA	Tab, Pink, Oblong	Naproxen 500 mg	by Opti Med	63369-0560	NSAID
500M50 <> MOVA	Tab, 500 M50	Naproxen 500 mg	by Caremark	00339-5874	NSAID
500M50 <> MOVA	Tab, Rose	Naproxen 500 mg	by Quality Care	60346-0815	NSAID
500M50 <> MOVA	Tab, Pink, Oblong	Naproxen 500 mg	by Compumed	00403-1442	NSAID
500MG	Tab, Green	Cephalexin 500 mg	Keftabs by HJ Harkins	52959-0086	Antibiotic
500MG <> 4058	Cap	Cefadroxil Hemihydrate	by Quality Care	60346-0022	Antibiotic
500MG <> 4058	Cap, White to Yellowish Powder	Cefadroxil Hemihydrate	by HJ Harkins Co	52959-0428	Antibiotic
500MG <> 4761CEFACLOR	Cap, Zenith Logo	Cefaclor Monohydrate 500 mg	by DRX	55045-2337	Antibiotic
500MG <> 7376BRISTOL	Cap, Blue, White Print	Cephalexin Monohydrate	by Golden State	60429-0037	Antibiotic
500 MG	Cap	Tetracycline HCl 500 mg	by Quality Care	60346-0435	Antibiotic
500MG <> AUGMENTIN	Tab, Film Coated	Amoxicillin Trihydrate, Clavulanate Potassium	Augmentin by Quality Care	60346-0364	Antibiotic
500MG <> BRISTOL7376	Cap, 500 mg <> Bristol over 7376	Cephalexin Monohydrate	by Quality Care	60346-0055	Antibiotic
500MG <> TRYPTAN	Tab, White, Oval, Film Coated	L-Tryptophan 500 mg	by Altimed	Canadian DIN# 02240333	Supplement
500MG <> Z4761CEFACLOR	Cap	Cefaclor Monohydrate 500 mg	by Zenith Goldline	00172-4761	Antibiotic
500MG <> Z4761CEFACLOR	Cap, 500 mg <> Zenith Logo 4761 Cefaclor	Cefaclor Monohydrate 500 mg	by Allscripts	54569-3902	Antibiotic
500MG <> ZENITH	Cap, Yellowish White Powder	Cefadroxil Hemihydrate	by Physicians Total Care	54868-3742	Antibiotic
500MGCALSAN	Cap, White, 500 mg/Calsan	Calcium Carbonate 500 mg	by Novartis	Canadian DIN# 02232482	Vitamin/Mineral
500MLA06	Cap, Blue & Gray, 500ML-A06	Cefaclor 500 mg	Ceclor by Mova	55370-0895	Antibiotic
500MLA08	Cap, Light Green & Dark Green, 500ML-A08	Cephalexin 500 mg	Keflex by Mova	55370-0901	Antibiotic
500POLY	Cap, Blue Print	Acetaminophen 500 mg, Hydrocodone Bitartrate 5 mg	Polygesic by Poly	50991-0005	Analgesic; C III

ID FRONT <> BACK	DESCRIPTION FRONT <> BACK	INGREDIENT & STRENGTH	BRAND (OR EQUIV.) & FIRM	NDC#	CLASS; SCH.
501	Tab, Round, Lavender, Scored, Martec Logo 501	Estradiol 0.5 mg	Estrace by Martec	52555-0716	Hormone
501 <> DP	Tab, Lavender, Round, Duramed Logo	Estradiol 0.5 mg	by Duramed	51285-0501	Hormone
501 <> M	Tab, Orange, Round, Film Coated	Bisoprolol Fumarate 2.5 mg, Hydrochlorothiazide 6.25 mg	Ziac by UDL	51079-0954	Antihypertensive; Diuretic
50100 <> SL441	Tab	Trazodone HCl 150 mg	by Physicians Total Care	54868-1959	Antidepressant
50100 <> SL441	Tab, 50/100 <> SL/441	Trazodone HCl 150 mg	by Heartland	61392-0179	Antidepressant
50100 <> SL441	Tab, White, Trapezoid, Scored	Trazodone HCl 150 mg	Desyrel by Sidmak	50111-0441	Antidepressant
5012 <> V	Tab, White, Round	Phenobarbital 30 mg	by Vangard Labs	00615-0463	Sedative/Hypnotic; C IV
5012 <> V	Tab, White, Round, Convex	Phenobarbital 30 mg	by Physicians Total Care	54868-3866	Sedative/Hypnotic; C IV
5012V	Tab, White, Round	Phenobarbital 30 mg	by PDRX Pharms	55289-0535	Sedative/Hypnotic; C IV
5013 <> V	Tab, White, Round, Convex	Phenobarbital 64.8 mg	by Physicians Total Care	54868-3933	Sedative/Hypnotic; C IV
5013V	Tab, 5013/V	Phenobarbital 64.8 mg	by Heartland	61392-0392	Sedative/Hypnotic; C IV
5013VV	Tab	Phenobarbital 64.8 mg	by DRX	55045-2387	Sedative/Hypnotic; C IV
5014 <> V	Tab, White, Round, Convex	Phenobarbital 97.2 mg	by Physicians Total Care	54868-3958	Sedative/Hypnotic; C IV
502	Tab, Pink, Round	Estrace 1 mg	Estrace by Duramed		Hormone
502	Tab, Round, Rose, Scored, Martec Logo 502	Estradiol 1 mg	Estrace by Martec	52555-0717	Hormone
502 <> 502	Cap, Purepac Logo	Prazosin HCl	by Heartland	61392-0112	Antihypertensive
502 <> DP	Tab, Pink, Round, Scored, 502 <> D over P	Estradiol 1 mg	by Heartland	61392-0178	Hormone
502 <> DP	Tab, Rose, Round, Duramed Logo	Estradiol 1 mg	by Duramed	51285-0502	Hormone
502 <> MD	Tab, Dark Green	Dextromethorphan Hydrobromide 30 mg, Guaifenesin 600 mg	Humigen DM by MD	43567-0502	Cold Remedy
5025	Tab, White, Round, 50/25	Atenolol 50 mg, Chlorthalidone 25 mg	Tenoretic by Zeneca	Canadian	Antihypertensive; Diuretic
50252550 <> NU150	Tab, Pale Orange, Rectangular, Scored, 50 over 25 over 25 over 50 <> NU-150	Trazodone HCl 150 mg	by Nu Pharm	Canadian DIN# 02165406	Antidepressant
5026DAN	Cap, Yellow	Procainamide HCl 250 mg	by Schein	00364-0219	Antiarrhythmic
5028DAN	Cap, Clear	Quinine Sulfate 5 gr	by Schein	00364-0230	Antimalarial
503 <> M	Tab, Blue, Round, Film Coated	Bisoprolol Fumarate 5 mg; Hydrochlorothiazide 6.25 mg	Ziac by UDL	51079-0955	Antihypertensive; Diuretic
5030 <> WATSON	Tab, Blue, Round, 50/30 <> Watson	Ethinyl Estradiol 30 mcg; Levonorgestrel 0.05 mg	Trivora-28 by Watson	52544-0291	Oral Contraceptive
503HD	Tab, Blue, Round	Chlorpropamide 250 mg	Diabinese by Halsey		Antidiabetic
504	Tab, Round, Blue, Scored, Martec Logo 504	Estradiol 2 mg	Estrace by Martec	52555-0718	Hormone
504 <> DP	Tab, Blue, Round, Duramed Logo	Estradiol 2 mg	by Duramed	51285-0504	Hormone
5040 <> BMS	Tab	Atenolol 50 mg	by Quality Care	60346-0719	Antihypertensive
5044 <> 5044	Tab, Pink, Oval, Scored	Eprosartan Mesylate 400 mg	Teveten by SKB Pharms (UK)	60351-5044	Antihypertensive
5044 <> 5044	Tab, Pink, Oval, Scored	Eprosartan Mesylate 400 mg	Teveten by Halsey Drug	00904-5342	Antihypertensive
505 <> M	Tab, White, Round, Film Coated	Bisoprolol Fumarate 10 mg; Hydrochlorothiazide 6.25 mg	Ziac by UDL	51079-0956	Antihypertensive; Diuretic
505 <> PEC	Cap	Amylase 33200 Units, Lipase 10000 Units, Protease 37500 Units	Pancrelipase 10000 by Mutual	53489-0246	Gastrointestinal
505 <> PEC	Cap	Amylase 33200 Units, Lipase 10000 Units, Protease 37500 Units	Pancreatin 10 by HL Moore	00839-8016	Gastrointestinal
5050	Tab, White, Cap Shaped, Scored	Ephedrine HCL 25 mg, Guaifenesin 400 mg	Ephedrine Formula 400 by D & E Pharma		Cold Remedy
5050	Tab, White, Round, 50/50	Hydrochlorothiazide 50 mg, Spironolactone 50 mg	Novo Spirozine by Novopharm	Canadian	Diuretic; Antihypertensive
5050 <> DAN	Tab, Orange, Round, Film Coated	Hydralazine HCl 25 mg	by Schein	00364-0144	Antihypertensive
505050 <> MJ778	Tab, Orange, Scored	Trazodone HCl 150 mg	Desyrel by Rx Pac	65084-0221	Antidepressant
505050 <> MJ778	Tab	Trazodone HCl 150 mg	Desyrel Dividose by Bristol Myers Squibb	00087-0778	Antidepressant
505050 <> MJ778	Tab, 50 50 50 <> MJ 778	Trazodone HCl 150 mg	Desyrel by Nat Pharmpak Serv	55154-2011	Antidepressant
505050 <> MJ778	Tab	Trazodone HCl 150 mg	Desyrel by Physicians Total Care	54868-2549	Antidepressant
505050 <> MJ778	Tab	Trazodone HCl 150 mg	Desyrel Dividose by Amerisource	62584-0778	Antidepressant
505050 <> MJ778	Tab, Dividose	Trazodone HCl 150 mg	Desyrel by Pharm Utilization	60491-0912	Antidepressant

ID FRONT <> BACK	DESCRIPTION FRONT <> BACK	INGREDIENT & STRENGTH	BRAND (OR EQUIV.) & FIRM	NDC#	CLASS; SCH.
505050 <> MJ778	Tab	Trazodone HCl 150 mg	Desyrel by Leiner	59606-0631	Antidepressant
505050 <> SL441	Tab, 50/50/50	Trazodone HCl 100 mg	by Major	00904-3991	Antidepressant
505050 <> SL441	Tab, 50/50/50	Trazodone HCl 100 mg	by Qualitest	00603-6145	Antidepressant
505050 <> SL441	Tab, 50/50/50	Trazodone HCl 150 mg	by Warner Chilcott	00047-0716	Antidepressant
505050 <> SL441	Tab, 50/50/50	Trazodone HCl 150 mg	by Schein	00364-2300	Antidepressant
505050 <> SL441	Tab, 50/50/50	Trazodone HCl 150 mg	by Parmed	00349-8824	Antidepressant
505050 <> SL441	Tab, 50/50/50	Trazodone HCl 150 mg	by Zenith Goldline	00182-1298	Antidepressant
505050 <> SL441	Tab, 50/50/50	Trazodone HCl 150 mg	by Martec	52555-0132	Antidepressant
505050 <> SL441	Tab, 50/50/50	Trazodone HCl 150 mg	by Geneva	00781-1826	Antidepressant
505050 <> SL441	Tab, 50/50/50	Trazodone HCl 150 mg	by Major	00904-3992	Antidepressant
505050 <> SL441	Tab, 50/50/50	Trazodone HCl 150 mg	by Qualitest	00603-6146	Antidepressant
505050 <> SL441	Tab, 50/50/50	Trazodone HCl 150 mg	by United Res	00677-1302	Antidepressant
505050 <> SL441	Tab, White, Trapezoid, Scored, 50 50 50 <> Debossed	Trazodone HCl 150 mg	Desyrel by Sidmak	50111-0441	Antidepressant
505050 <> SL441	Tab, 50/50/50	Trazodone HCl 150 mg	by HL Moore	00839-7507	Antidepressant
505050 <> SL443	Tab, 50/50/50	Trazodone HCl 100 mg	by Rugby	00536-4688	Antidepressant
5052 <> DAN	Tab	Prednisone 5 mg	by Nat Pharmpak Serv	55154-5208	Steroid
5052 <> DANDAN	Tab	Prednisone 5 mg	by Vangard	00615-0536	Steroid
5052 <> DANDAN	Tab, White, Round, Scored	Prednisone 10 mg	by Southwood Pharms	58016-0216	Steroid
5052 <> DANDAN	Tab	Prednisone 10 mg	by Vangard	00615-3593	Steroid
5052 <> DANDAN	Tab	Prednisone 5 mg	by Danbury	00591-5052	Steroid
5052 <> DANDAN	Tab, White, Round, Scored	Prednisone 5 mg	by Schein	00364-0218	Steroid
5052 <> DANDAN	Tab	Prednisone 5 mg	by Vedco	50989-0601	Steroid
5052 <> DANDAN	Tab	Prednisone 5 mg	by Danbury	61955-0218	Steroid
5052 <> DANDAN	Tab	Prednisone 5 mg	by Heartland	61392-0408	Steroid
5052 <> DANDAN	Tab	Prednisone 5 mg	by Quality Care	60346-0515	Steroid
5052 <> DANDAN	Tab	Prednisone 5 mg	by WA Butler	11695-1801	Steroid
5052JMI	Tab, Yellow, Round	Chlorpheniramine 4 mg	by JMI Canton		Antihistamine
5052V	Tab, 5052/V	Guaifenesin 400 mg, Phenylpropanolamine HCl 75 mg	Enomine LA by Quality Care	60346-0339	Cold Remedy
5052V	Tab, Film Coated, 5052/V	Guaifenesin 400 mg, Phenylpropanolamine HCl 75 mg	Guaitex LA by Vintage	00254-5052	Cold Remedy
5053 <> V	Tab	Guaifenesin 600 mg, Phenylpropanolamine HCl 75 mg	Guaivent by Qualitest	00603-3778	Cold Remedy
5053 <> V	Tab, 50/53 <> V	Guaifenesin 600 mg, Phenylpropanolamine HCl 75 mg	Guaivent by Vintage	00254-5053	Cold Remedy
5055 <> DAN	Tab, Orange, Round, Film Coated	Hydralazine HCl 50 mg	by Schein	00364-0145	Antihypertensive
5058 <> DANDAN	Tab, Blue-Green, Round, Scored	Tripelennamine HCl 50 mg	by Schein	00364-0281	Antihistamine
5059 <> DANDAN	Tab, Dan Dan	Prednisolone 5 mg	by Darby Group	66467-4346	Steroid
5059 <> DANDAN	Tab, Peach, Round, Scored	Prednisolone 5 mg	by Schein	00364-0217	Steroid
506HD	Tab, White, Round	Metronidazole 250 mg	Flagyl by Halsey		Antibiotic
507	Tab, Goldline Labs Logo	Folic Acid 1 mg	by Zenith Goldline	00182-0507	Vitamin
507	Tab, White, Round, Schering Logo 507	Griseofulvin Ultramicrosize 250 mg	Fulvicin P/G by Schering		Antifungal
507 <> MYLAN	Tab, Green, Coated, Beveled Edge	Hydrochlorothiazide 15 mg, Methyldopa 250 mg	by Mylan	00378-0507	Diuretic; Antihypertensive
507 <> WATSON	Tab	Ethinyl Estradiol 0.035 mg, Norethindrone 0.5 mg	Necon 0.5 35 21 by Watson	52544-0507	Oral Contraceptive
507 <> WATSON	Tab	Ethinyl Estradiol 0.035 mg, Norethindrone 0.5 mg	Necon 0.5 35 28 by Watson	52544-0550	Oral Contraceptive
507 <> WATSON	Tab	Ethinyl Estradiol 0.035 mg, Norethindrone 0.5 mg, Norethindrone 1 mg	Necon 10 11 21 by Watson	52544-0553	Oral Contraceptive
507 <> WATSON	Tab	Ethinyl Estradiol 0.035 mg, Norethindrone 0.5 mg, Norethindrone 1 mg	Necon 10 11 28 by Watson	52544-0554	Oral Contraceptive
507HD	Cap, Green	Indomethacin 25 mg	Indocin by Halsey		NSAID
508	Cap, Off-White & Red	Acetaminophen 325 mg, Dichloralphenazone 100 mg, Isometheptane Mucate 65 mg	by Jerome Stevens Pharm		Analgesic
508 <> WATSON	Tab	Ethinyl Estradiol 0.035 mg, Norethindrone 0.5 mg, Norethindrone 1 mg	Necon 10 11 21 by Watson	52544-0553	Oral Contraceptive
508 <> WATSON	Tab	Ethinyl Estradiol 0.035 mg, Norethindrone 0.5 mg, Norethindrone 1 mg	Necon 10 11 28 by Watson	52544-0554	Oral Contraceptive
508 <> WATSON	Tab	Ethinyl Estradiol 0.035 mg, Norethindrone 1 mg	Necon 1 35 21 by Watson	52544-0508	Oral Contraceptive
508 <> WATSON	Tab	Ethinyl Estradiol 0.035 mg, Norethindrone 1 mg	Necon 1 35 28 by Watson	52544-0552	Oral Contraceptive
508HD	Cap, Green	Indomethacin 50 mg	Indocin by Halsey		NSAID
50902 <> B	Tab, 50/902 <> Barr Logo	Naltrexone HCl 50 mg	Naltrexone Hydrochloride by Barr	00555-0902	Opiod Antagonist

ID FRONT <> BACK	DESCRIPTION FRONT <> BACK	INGREDIENT & STRENGTH	BRAND (OR EQUIV.) & FIRM	NDC#	CLASS; SCH.
5097V	Tab, Coated, Scored	Ascorbic Acid 80 mg, Beta-Carotene, Biotin 0.03 mg, Calcium Carbonate, Cholecalciferol 400 Units, Cupric Oxide, Cyanocobalamin 2.5 mcg, Ferrous Fumarate, Folic Acid 1 mg, Magnesium Oxide, Niacinamide 17 mg, Pantothenic Acid 7 mg, Pyridoxine HCl 4 mg, Riboflavin 1.6 mg, Thiamine Mononitrate 1.5 mg, Vitamin A Acetate, Vitamin E Acetate 15 mg, Zinc Oxide	Prenatal Rx by Vintage	00254-5097	Vitamin
5097V	Tab, Coated, Scored	Ascorbic Acid 80 mg, Beta-Carotene, Biotin 0.03 mg, Calcium Carbonate, Cholecalciferol 400 Units, Cupric Oxide, Cyanocobalamin 2.5 mcg, Ferrous Fumarate, Folic Acid 1 mg, Magnesium Oxide, Niacinamide 17 mg, Pantothenic Acid 7 mg, Pyridoxine HCl 4 mg, Riboflavin 1.6 mg, Thiamine Mononitrate 1.5 mg, Vitamin A Acetate, Vitamin E Acetate 15 mg, Zinc Oxide	Prenatal Rx by Physicians Total Care	54868-3828	Vitamin
50DAN5568	Tab, White, Triangular, 50/Dan 5568	Thioridazine HCl 50 mg	Mellaril by Danbury		Antipsychotic
50FLI	Tab, White, Round, 50/FLI Logo	Levothyroxine Sodium 50 mcg	by Forest	00456-0321	Antithyroid
50LLA15	Tab, Orange, Heptagonal	Amoxapine 50 mg	Asendin by Lederle		Antidepressant
50M	Tab, Mova Logo	Levothyroxine Sodium 50 mcg	Euthyrox by Em Pharma	63254-0436	Antithyroid
50M	Tab	Levothyroxine Sodium 50 mcg	Levo T by MOVA	55370-0126	Antithyroid
50MCG	Tab, Color Coded	Levothyroxine Sodium 50 mcg	by Med Pro	53978-3022	Antithyroid
50MCG <> FLINT	Tab, Debossed	Levothyroxine Sodium 0.05 mg	Synthroid by Amerisource	62584-0040	Antithyroid
50MCG <> FLINT	Tab, White, Round, Scored	Levothyroxine Sodium 0.05 mg	Synthroid by Rightpac	65240-0740	Antithyroid
50MG <> 0497	Cap	Minocycline HCl	Dynacin by Medicis	99207-0497	Antibiotic
50MG <> 2130	Cap, Pink & White	Nitrofurantoin Macrocrystalline 50 mg	by Goldline Labs	00182-1944	Antibiotic
50MG <> KADIAN	Cap	Morphine Sulfate 50 mg	Kadian ER by Purepac	00228-2045	Analgesic; C II
50MG <> SANDOZ	Cap	Cyclosporine 50 mg	Sandimmun Neoral B17 by RP Scherer	11014-1196	Immunosuppressant
50MG <> WATSON372	Cap, Blue & White	Loxapine Succinate 50 mg	by Murfreesboro Ph	51129-1351	Antipsychotic
50MG <> WATSON372	Cap, Blue & White	Loxapine Succinate 50 mg	by Dixon Shane	17236-0696	Antipsychotic
50mg <> WATSON372	Cap, Blue & White, Opaque, 50 mg <> Watson over 372	Loxapine 50 mg	Loxitane by UDL	51079-0903	Antipsychotic
50MG <> WATSON372	Cap	Loxapine Succinate	by Watson	52544-0372	Antipsychotic
50MG <> WATSON372	Cap	Loxapine Succinate	by Zenith Goldline	00182-1308	Antipsychotic
50MG <> WATSON372	Cap, 50 mg <> Watson Over 372	Loxapine Succinate	by UDL	51079-0680	Antipsychotic
50MG <> WATSON372	Cap	Loxapine Succinate	by Physicians Total Care	54868-2479	Antipsychotic
50MG <> WATSON372	Cap	Loxapine Succinate	by Geneva	00781-2713	Antipsychotic
50MG <> WATSON372	Cap	Loxapine Succinate	by HL Moore	00839-7498	Antipsychotic
50MG <> WATSON595	Cap, Gelatin	Clomipramine HCl 50 mg	by Watson	52544-0595	OCD
50MG <> WATSON697	Cap, Flesh	Doxepin HCl 56.7 mg	by Watson	52544-0697	Antidepressant
50MG <> WATSON697	Cap	Doxepin HCl 56.7 mg	by Martec	52555-0296	Antidepressant
50MG <> ZOLOFT	Tab, Light Blue, Cap-Shaped, Film Coated, 50MG	Sertraline HCl	Zoloft by Roerig	00049-4900	Antidepressant
50MG <> ZOLOFT	Tab, Film Coated	Sertraline HCl	Zoloft by Nat Pharmpak Serv	55154-2709	Antidepressant
50MG <> ZOLOFT	Tab, Film Coated	Sertraline HCl	by Med Pro	53978-3019	Antidepressant
50MG <> ZOLOFT	Tab, Film Coated	Sertraline HCl	Zoloft by Allscripts	54569-3724	Antidepressant
50MG <> ZOLOFT	Tab, Film Coated	Sertraline HCl	Zoloft by Direct Dispensing	57866-6304	Antidepressant
50MG <> ZOLOFT	Tab, Light Blue, Film Coated	Sertraline HCl	Zoloft by Amerisource	62584-0900	Antidepressant
50MG <> ZOLOFT	Tab, Blue, Oblong, Film Coated, Scored	Sertraline HCl 50 mg	Zoloft by Heartland Healthcare	61392-0629	Antidepressant
50MG <> ZOLOFT	Tab, Blue, Oblong, Film Coated, Scored	Sertraline HCl 50 mg	Zoloft by Compumed	00403-4721	Antidepressant
50MG <> ZOLOFT	Tab, Blue, Oblong, Scored	Sertraline HCl 50 mg	Zoloft by Phcy Care	65070-0035	Antidepressant
50MG <> ZOLOFT	Tab, Blue, Scored	Sertraline HCl 50 mg	Zoloft by Southwood Pharms	58016-0366	Antidepressant
50MGFLUVOX	Tab, White, Round, 50/mg/Fluvox	Fluvoxamine 50 mg	by Altimed	Canadian	OCD
50MGFLUVOX	Tab, White, Round, 50/mg/Fluvox	Fluvoxamine Maleate 50 mg	by AltiMed	Canadian DIN# 02218453	OCD
50MGLEDERLEL4	Cap, Blue & Green	Loxapine 50 mg	Loxitane by Lederle		Antipsychotic
50MGLEDERLEM2	Cap, Orange	Minocycline HCl 50 mg	Minocin by Lederle		Antibiotic
50MGSAMPLE <> MACRODANTIN	Cap, White w/ Yellow Powder, Opaque	Nitrofurantoin 50 mg	Macrodantin by Procter & Gamble	00149-0008	Antibiotic

ID FRONT <> BACK	DESCRIPTION FRONT <> BACK	INGREDIENT & STRENGTH	BRAND (OR EQUIV.) & FIRM	NDC#	CLASS; SCH.
50MO <> MOVA	Tab, Debossed	Captopril 50 mg	by Quality Care	60346-0868	Antihypertensive
50MO5 <> MOVA	Tab, White, Cap Shaped	Captopril 50 mg	Capoten by Mova	55370-0144	Antihypertensive
50N <> 727	Tab, Film Coated	Metoprolol Tartrate 50 mg	by Zenith Goldline	00182-1987	Antihypertensive
50NOVO	Tab, White, Round, 50/Novo	Clomipramine HCl 50 mg	Novo Clopamine by Novopharm	Canadian	OCD
51 <> C	Tab	Atenolol 50 mg, Chlorthalidone 25 mg	by IPR	54921-0115	Antihypertensive; Diuretic
51 <> RP	Tab, Yellow, Round	Dextroamphetamine Sulfate 5 mg	Dextrostat by Shire Richwood	58521-0451	Stimulant; C II
510 <> WATSON	Tab	Mestranol 0.05 mg, Norethindrone 1 mg	Necon 1 50 21 by Watson	52544-0510	Oral Contraceptive
510 <> WATSON	Tab	Mestranol 0.05 mg, Norethindrone 1 mg	Necon 1 50 28 by Watson	52544-0556	Oral Contraceptive
510 <> WATSON	Tab, Blue, Round	Norethindrone 1 mg, Mestranol 0.05 mg	Necon by DRX Pharm Consults	55045-2722	Oral Contraceptive
510 <> WATSON	Tab, Blue, Round	Norethidrone 1 mg, Mestranol 50 mcg	Necon by PDRX	55289-0379	Oral Contraceptive
5100 <> RPR	Tab, Film Coated, 5100 <> RPR Logo	Enoxacin Sesquihydrate	Penetrex by RPR	00075-5100	Antibiotic
5100 <> RPR	Tab, Light Blue, Oblong	Enoxacin Sesquihydrate	Penetrex by RPR	00801-5100	Antibiotic
511 <> 05	Tab, White, Pentagon, 511 <> 0.5	Lorazepam 0.5 mg	by Mylan	55160-0129	Sedative/Hypnotic; C IV
511 <> 1MG	Tab, White, Pentagon	Lorazepam 1 mg	Ativan by Nat Pharmpak Serv	55154-1914	Sedative/Hypnotic; C IV
511 <> 1MG	Tab, White, Pentagon	Lorazepam 1 mg	by ESI Lederle	59911-5812	Sedative/Hypnotic; C IV
511 <> 1MG	Tab, White, Pentagon	Lorazepam 1 mg	by Wyeth Pharms	52903-5812	Sedative/Hypnotic; C IV
511 <> 2MG	Tab, White, Pentagon	Lorazepam 2 mg	by Wyeth Pharms	52903-5813	Sedative/Hypnotic; C IV
511 <> 2MG	Tab, White, Pentagon	Lorazepam 2 mg	Ativan by Nat Pharmpak Serv	55154-2002	Sedative/Hypnotic; C IV
511 <> 2MG	Tab, White, 5 Sided	Lorazepam 2 mg	by ESI Lederle	59911-5813	Sedative/Hypnotic; C IV
511 <> 5	Tab, White, Pentagon	Lorazepam 0.5 mg	by Wyeth Pharms	52903-5811	Sedative/Hypnotic; C IV
511 <> A75	Tab, White, Round	Acyclovir 400 mg	by ESI Lederle	59911-3163	Antiviral
511 <> A77	Tab, White, Oval	Acyclovir 800 mg	by ESI Lederle	59911-3164	Antiviral
511 <> E1	Tab, White, Round	Estradiol 0.5 mg	by ESI Lederle	59911-5879	Hormone
511 <> E1	Tab, White, Round, Scored	Estradiol 0.5 mg	by Ayerst Lab (Div Wyeth)	00046-5879	Hormone
511 <> E7	Tab, White, Round	Estradiol 1 mg	by ESI Lederle	59911-5880	Hormone
511 <> E77	Tab, White, Round	Estradiol 2 mg	by ESI Lederle	59911-5882	Hormone
511 <> E77	Tab, White, Round, 511 <> E over 77	Estradiol 2 mg	by Ayerst		Hormone
511 <> E77	Tab, White, Round, Scored	Estradiol 2 mg	by Ayerst Lab (Div Wyeth)	00046-5882	Hormone
511 <> LODOSYN	Tab, Orange, Round, Scored	Carbidopa 25 mg	Lodosyn by Dupont Pharma	00056-0511	Antiparkinson
511 <> MX	Tab, Yellow, Round, Scored	Methotrexate Sodium 2.5 mg	by Lederle Pharm	00005-5874	Antineoplastic
511 <> MX	Tab, Yellow, Round, Scored	Methotrexate Sodium 2.5 mg	by ESI Lederle	59911-5874	Antineoplastic
511 <> P77	Tab, White, Oblong	Pentoxifylline 400 mg	by ESI Lederle	59911-3290	Anticoagulent
511 <> SELEGILINEHCL5MG	Cap, White	Selegiline HCl 5 mg	Selegiline HCl by Sanofi	00024-2775	Antiparkinson
511 <> SELEGILINEHCL5MG	Cap, White	Selegiline HCl 5 mg	Selegiline HCl by SB	59742-3158	Antiparkinson
51105	Tab, White, 5 Sided, 511/0.5	Lorazepam 0.5 mg	by ESI Lederle		Sedative/Hypnotic; C IV
5112 <> V	Tab, Coated	Acetaminophen 650 mg, Propoxyphene Napsylate 100 mg	by Vintage	00254-5112	Analgesic; C IV
5112 <> V	Tab, Coated	Acetaminophen 650 mg, Propoxyphene Napsylate 100 mg	by Qualitest	00603-5466	Analgesic; C IV
5112V	Tab, Orange, Oblong, Film Coated	Acetaminophen 650 mg, Propoxyphene Napsylate 100 mg	by 3M	00089-1231	Analgesic; C IV
5112V	Tab, Orange, Oblong	Propoxyphene Napsylate 100 mg, Acetaminophen 650 mg	by Direct Dispensing	57866-4361	Analgesic; C IV
5113 <> V	Tab, Coated	Acetaminophen 650 mg, Propoxyphene Napsylate 100 mg	by Vintage	00254-5113	Analgesic; C IV
5113V	Tab, White, Oblong, Film Coated	Acetaminophen 650 mg, Propoxyphene Napsylate 100 mg	by 3M	00089-1233	Analgesic; C IV
5113V	Tab, Coated	Acetaminophen 650 mg, Propoxyphene Napsylate 100 mg	by Qualitest	00603-5467	Analgesic; C IV
5113V	Tab, Coated	Acetaminophen 650 mg, Propoxyphene Napsylate 100 mg	by Rugby	00536-4361	Analgesic; C IV
5113V	Tab, White, Oblong	Propoxyphene Napsylate 100 mg, Acetaminophen 650 mg	by Direct Dispensing	57866-4361	Analgesic; C IV
5114 <> V	Tab, Coated	Acetaminophen 650 mg, Propoxyphene Napsylate 100 mg	by Vintage	00254-5114	Analgesic; C IV
5114 <> V	Tab, Coated	Acetaminophen 650 mg, Propoxyphene Napsylate 100 mg	by Qualitest	00603-5468	Analgesic; C IV
5114V	Tab, Pink, Oblong, Film Coated	Acetaminophen 650 mg, Propoxyphene Napsylate 100 mg	by AAI	27280-0007	Analgesic; C IV
5114V	Tab, Pink, Cap Shaped, Coated	Acetaminophen 650 mg, Propoxyphene Napsylate 100 mg	Famvir by Allscripts	54569-0015	Analgesic; C IV
5114V	Tab, Film Coated	Acetaminophen 650 mg, Propoxyphene Napsylate 100 mg	by Amerisource	62584-0840	Analgesic; C IV

ID FRONT <> BACK	DESCRIPTION FRONT <> BACK	INGREDIENT & STRENGTH	BRAND (OR EQUIV.) & FIRM	NDC#	CLASS; SCH.
5114V	Tab, Pink, Oblong	Propoxyphene Napsylate 100 mg, Acetaminophen 650 mg	by Direct Dispensing	57866-4361	Analgesic; C IV
511MX	Tab, Yellow, Round, 511/MX	Methotrexate 2.5 mg	by ESI Lederle		Antineoplastic
511P77	Tab, White, Oval, 511/P77	Pentoxifylline 400 mg	by ESI Lederle		Anticoagulent
512	Tab, White, Round, Scored	Acetaminophen 325 mg, Oxycodone HCl 5 mg	Tylox by Mallinckrodt Hobart	00406-0512	Analgesic; C II
512 <> HD	Tab	Acetaminophen 325 mg, Oxycodone HCl 5 mg	by Schein	00364-0605	Analgesic; C II
512 <> MILES	Tab, Film Coated	Ciprofloxacin HCl 291.5 mg	Cipro by Quality Care	60346-0433	Antibiotic
5123	Tab, White, Round, Scored	Captopril 50 mg	Captopril USP by Caremark	00339-6116	Antihypertensive
513	Tab, Red, Round, Sav. Logo 513	Phenolphthalein 130 mg	Modane by Savage	00281-0298	Gastrointestinal
513 <> JSP	Tab, Peach, Round, Scored	Levothyroxine Sodium 25 mg	Unithroid by Watson	52544-0902	Antithyroid
513 <> MILES	Tab, Pale Yellow, Film Coated	Ciprofloxacin HCl 583 mg	Cipro by Quality Care	60346-0031	Antibiotic
513 <> MILES	Tab, Film Coated	Ciprofloxacin HCl 583 mg	Ciprobay by Bayer	00026-8513	Antibiotic
513 <> MILES	Tab, Film Coated	Ciprofloxacin HCl 583 mg	Cipro by Nat Pharmpak Serv	55154-4801	Antibiotic
514 <> JSP	Tab, White, Round, Scored	Levothyroxine Sodium 50 mg	Unithroid by Watson	52544-0903	Antithyroid
5140 <> RPR	Tab, Film Coated, 5140 <> RPR Logo	Enoxacin Sesquihydrate	Penetrex by RPR	00075-5140	Antibiotic
5140 <> RPR	Tab, Dark Blue, Oblong	Enoxacin Sesquihydrate	Penetrex by RPR	00801-5140	Antibiotic
51479005 <> DURAGEST	Cap, 51479005 <> Dura-Gest	Guaifenesin 200 mg, Phenylephrine HCl 5 mg, Phenylpropanolamine HCl 45 mg	Enomine by Quality Care	60346-0725	Cold Remedy
51479019	Cap, Gray & Red	Cycloserine 250 mg	Seromycin by Lilly		Antibiotic
51479019	Cap, Gray & Red	Cycloserine 250 mg	Seromycin by Dura	51479-0019	Antibiotic
51479030 <> ENTEX	Cap	Guaifenesin 200 mg, Phenylephrine HCl 5 mg, Phenylpropanolamine HCl 45 mg	Entex by Welpharm	63375-6378	Cold Remedy
51479DURA <> 005GEST	Cap, 51479/Dura <> 005/Gest	Guaifenesin 200 mg, Phenylephrine HCl 5 mg, Phenylpropanolamine HCl 45 mg	Dura Gest by Anabolic	00722-6060	Cold Remedy
515	Cap, Green, Oval, Savage Logo 515	Docusate Sodium 100 mg	Modane Soft by Savage	00281-5111	Laxative
515 <> JSP	Tab, Purple, Round, Scored	Levothyroxine Sodium 75 mg	Unithroid by Watson	52544-0904	Antithyroid
5151 <> GEIGY	Tab, Coated	Metoprolol Tartrate 50 mg	Lopressor by Novartis	00028-0051	Antihypertensive
5151 <> GEIGY	Tab, Coated	Metoprolol Tartrate 50 mg	Lopressor by Caremark	00339-5213	Antihypertensive
5151 <> GEIGY	Tab, Coated	Metoprolol Tartrate 50 mg	Lopressor by Nat Pharmpak Serv	55154-1009	Antihypertensive
5151 <> GEIGY	Tab, Light Red, Cap Shaped, Film Coated, Scored	Metoprolol Tartrate 50 mg	Lopresor by Novartis	Canadian DIN# 00397423	Antihypertensive
5151 <> GEIGY	Tab, Coated, 51/51	Metoprolol Tartrate 50 mg	Lopressor by Wal Mart	49035-0179	Antihypertensive
5156	Cap, ER, Logo 5156	Papaverine HCl 150 mg	by DRX	55045-1629	Vasodilator
516 <> JSP	Tab	Levothyroxine Sodium 0.1 mg	by Jones	52604-7701	Antithyroid
516 <> JSP	Tab, Yellow, Round, Scored	Levothyroxine Sodium 100 mg	Unithroid by Watson	52544-0906	Antithyroid
5162DAN	Cap, Orange & Yellow	Tetracycline HCl 250 mg	by Schein	00364-2026	Antibiotic
51674 <> 009	Cap, Green	Acetaminophen 325 mg, Butalbital 50 mg, Caffeine 40 mg	Anolor 300 by Blansett	51674-0009	Analgesic
517 <> GG	Cap, Light Green	Indomethacin 25 mg	by Quality Care	60346-0684	NSAID
517 <> MYLAN	Tab, White, Film Coated, Scored	Gemfibrozil 600 mg	by Mylan	00378-0517	Antihyperlipidemic
518MD	Tab, Blue, Round	Diethylpropion HCl 25 mg	Tenuate by MD		Antianorexiant; C IV
519 <> JSP	Tab, Tan, Round, Scored	Levothyroxine Sodium 125 mg	Unithroid by Watson	52544-0908	Antithyroid
5196DAN	Cap, Brown & Clear	Papaverine HCl 150 mg	by Schein	00364-0181	Vasodilator
51H	Tab, White, Oblong, Scored	Telmisartan 40 mg	Micardis by Boehringer Ingelheim	12714-0109	Antihypertensive
51H	Tab, White, Oblong, Scored	Telmisartan 40 mg	Micardis by Boehringer Pharms	00597-0040	Antihypertensive
52 <> MP	Tab, White, Round, Scored	Prednisone 10 mg	by Allscripts	54569-0331	Steroid
52 <> MP	Tab, White, Round, Scored	Prednisone 10 mg	by Allscripts	54569-3302	Steroid
52 <> RP	Tab, Yellow, Round	Dextroamphetamine Sulfate 10 mg	Dextrostat by Shire Richwood	58521-0452	Stimulant; C II
52 <> TEGRETOL	Tab, Chew	Carbamazepine 100 mg	by Basel	58887-0052	Anticonvulsant
52 <> TEGRETOL	Tab, Pink, Round, Scored	Carbamazepine 100 mg	Tegretol Chewable by Allscripts	54569-0165	Anticonvulsant
520 <> JSP	Tab	Levothyroxine Sodium 0.15 mg	by JMI Canton	00252-7700	Antithyroid
520 <> JSP	Tab, Debossed	Levothyroxine Sodium 0.15 mg	Estre by Macnary	55982-0015	Antithyroid
520 <> JSP	Tab, Blue, Round, Scored	Levothyroxine Sodium 150 mg	Unithroid by Watson	52544-0909	Antithyroid
520 <> N517	Tab, Film Coated	Naproxen Sodium 550 mg	by United Res	00677-1514	NSAID

ID FRONT <> BACK	DESCRIPTION FRONT <> BACK	INGREDIENT & STRENGTH	BRAND (OR EQUIV.) & FIRM	NDC#	CLASS; SCH.
521	Tab, Peach, Oval, Scored	Carbidopa 50 mg, Levodopa 200 mg	Sinemet CR by DuPont Pharma	00056-0521	Antiparkinson
521 <> DP	Tab, Orange, Round	Prochlorperazine 5 mg	by Duramed Pharms	51285-0521	Antiemetic
521 <> MYLAN	Tab, Coated	Acetaminophen 650 mg, Propoxyphene Napsylate 100 mg	by Mylan	00378-0521	Analgesic; C IV
521 <> SINEMENTCR	Tab, Peach, Oval, Scored	Carbidopa 50 mg, Levodopa 200 mg	Sinemet CR by Caremark	00339-6141	Antiparkinson
521 <> SINEMENTCR	Tab, Peach, Oval, Scored	Carbidopa 50 mg, Levodopa 200 mg	Sinemet CR by Caremark	00339-6142	Antiparkinson
521 <> SINEMETCR	Tab, Ex Release, 521 <> Sinemet over CR	Carbidopa 50 mg, Levodopa 200 mg	Sinemet CR by Nat Pharmpak Serv	55154-7705	Antiparkinson
521 <> SINEMETCR	Tab, Peach, Oval, Score	Carbidopa 50 mg, Levodopa 200 mg	Sinemet CR by Dupont Pharma	00056-0521	Antiparkinson
521 <> SINEMETCR	Tab, Peach, Oval, Scored	Carbidopa 50 mg; Levodopa 200 mg	Sinemet by WalMart	49035-0189	Antiparkinson
5216 <> DANDAN	Tab	Folic Acid 1 mg	by Quality Care	60346-0697	Vitamin
5216 <> DANDAN	Tab	Folic Acid 1 mg	by Vangard	00615-0664	Vitamin
5216 <> DANDAN	Tab	Folic Acid 1 mg	by Danbury	00591-5216	Vitamin
5216 <> DANDAN	Tab, Yellow, Round, Scored	Folic Acid 1 mg	by Schein	00364-0137	Vitamin
522 <> DP	Tab, Yellow, Round, Debossed <> Logo	Prochlorperazine 10 mg	by Duramed	51285-0522	Antiemetic
522 <> JSP	Tab, Pink, Round, Scored	Levothyroxine Sodium 200 mg	Unithroid by Watson	52544-0911	Antithyroid
52273111Q	Tab, Yellow, Diamond, 52273-111/Q	Nystatin Vaginal 100,000 Units	Mycostatin by Quantum		Antifungal
522HD	Tab, Blue, Round	Chlorpropamide 100 mg	Diabinese by Halsey		Antidiabetic
523 <> 54	Cap	Mexiletine HCl 150 mg	by Roxane	00054-2616	Antiarrhythmic
523 <> 54	Cap	Mexiletine HCl 150 mg	by Roxane	00054-8616	Antiarrhythmic
523 <> JSP	Tab, Green, Round, Scored	Levothyroxine Sodium 300 mg	Unithroid by Watson	52544-0912	Antithyroid
524HD	Tab, White, Round	Cyproheptadine HCl 4 mg	Periactin by Halsey		Antihistamine
525 <> 879	Cap	Doxycycline Hyclate	by United Res	00677-0598	Antibiotic
525 <> SCHWARZ	Cap, White	Pancrelipase (Amylase 30000 unt, Lipase 8000 unt, Protease 8000 unt)	Kuzyme HP by Schwarz Pharma Mfg	00131-3525	Gastrointestinal
5250 <> BMS	Tab, Coated	Diltiazem HCl 30 mg	by Quality Care	60346-0960	Antihypertensive
5250 <> BMS	Tab, Coated, Mottled	Diltiazem HCl 30 mg	by ER Squibb	00003-5250	Antihypertensive
5252 <> TEGRETOL	Tab, Red Specks, Scored, Chewable	Carbamazepine 100 mg	by Nat Pharmpak Serv	55154-1011	Anticonvulsant
5252 <> TEGRETOL	Tab, Pink, Round, Scored	Carbamazepine 100 mg	Tegretol by Neuman Distbtrs	64579-0325	Anticonvulsant
5252 <> TEGRETOL	Tab, Pink with Red Specks, Round, Scored	Carbamazepine 100 mg	by Novartis	00083-0052	Anticonvulsant
526 <> 879	Cap, Light Blue	Doxycycline Hyclate	by Quality Care	60346-0109	Antibiotic
526 <> 879	Cap, Opaque Blue	Doxycycline Hyclate	by Quality Care	60346-0109	Antibiotic
526 <> 879	Cap, Blue	Doxycycline Hyclate 100 mg	by Dixon Shane	17236-0527	Antibiotic
526 <> DANDAN	Tab, White, Round, Scored	Isoniazid 300 mg	by Schein	00364-0151	Antimycobacterial
5271043	Tab, Round, 527/1043	Isobutylallylbarbituric Acid 50 mg, Caff. 40 mg, Aspirin 200 mg, Phenacetin 130 mg	Lanorinal by Lannett		Analgesic
5271053	Tab, White, Round, 527/1053	Phenobarbital 0.25 g	Phenobarbital by Lannett		Sedative/Hypnotic; C IV
5271053	Tab, Pink, Round, 527/1053	Phenobarbital 0.25 g	Phenobarbital by Lannett		Sedative/Hypnotic; C IV
5271053	Tab, Green, Round, 527/1053	Phenobarbital 0.25 g	Phenobarbital by Lannett		Sedative/Hypnotic; C IV
5271054	Tab, White, Round, 527/1054	Phenobarbital 0.5 g	Phenobarbital by Lannett		Sedative/Hypnotic; C IV
5271054	Tab, Green, Round, 527/1054	Phenobarbital 0.5 g	Phenobarbital by Lannett		Sedative/Hypnotic; C IV
5271054	Tab, Pink, Round, 527/1054	Phenobarbital 0.5 g	Phenobarbital by Lannett		Sedative/Hypnotic; C IV
5271055	Tab, Pink, Round, 527/1055	Phenobarbital 1.5 g	Phenobarbital by Lannett		Sedative/Hypnotic; C IV
5271055	Tab, White, Round, 527/1055	Phenobarbital 1.5 g	Phenobarbital by Lannett		Sedative/Hypnotic; C IV
5271057	Tab, White, Round, 527/1057	Phenobarbital 1 g	Phenobarbital by Lannett		Sedative/Hypnotic; C IV
5271060	Tab, White, Round, 527/1060	Glutethimide 500 mg	Doriden by Lannett		Hypnotic
5271088	Tab, White, Round, 527/1088	Glutethimide 250 mg	Doriden by Lannett		Hypnotic
5271123	Tab, Green, Round, 527/1123	Dextroamphetamine Sulfate 15 mg	by Lannett		Stimulant; C II
5271138	Tab, Round, 527/1138	Amphetamine Sulfate 5 mg	by Lannett		Stimulant; C II
5271139	Tab, Round, 527/1139	Amphetamine Sulfate 10 mg	by Lannett		Stimulant; C II
5271143	Tab, Yellow, Round, 527/1143	Dextroamphetamine Sulfate 5 mg	by Lannett		Stimulant; C II
5271151	Tab, White, Round, 527/1151	Acetaminophen 325 mg, Phenobarbital 16 mg	by Lannett		Analgesic; C IV
5271170	Tab, White, Round, 527/1170	Diphenoxylate HCl 2.5 mg, Atropine Sulfate 0.025 mg	Lofene by Lannett		Antidiarrheal; C V
5271179	Tab, Lavender, Round, 527/1179	Butabarbital Sodium 0.25 gr	Butisol by Lannett		Sedative; C III
5271180	Tab, Green, Round, 527/1180	Butabarbital Sodium 0.5 gr	Butisol by Lannett		Sedative; C III
5271184	Tab, Pink, Round, 527/1184	Butabarbital Sodium 1.5 gr	Butisol by Lannett		Sedative; C III

ID FRONT <> BACK	DESCRIPTION FRONT <> BACK	INGREDIENT & STRENGTH	BRAND (OR EQUIV.) & FIRM	NDC#	CLASS; SCH.
5271219	Tab, Orange, Round, 527/1219	Dextroamphetamine Sulfate 10 mg	by Lannett		Stimulant; C II
5271224	Tab, White, Round, 527/1224	Meprobamate 400 mg	Equanil by Lannett		Sedative/Hypnotic; C IV
5271250	Tab, White, Round, 527/1250	Meprobamate 200 mg	Equanil by Lannett		Sedative/Hypnotic; C IV
5271252	Tab, Green, Round, 527/1252	Phendimetrazine Tartrate 35 mg	Obalan by Lannett		Anorexiant; C III
5271269	Tab, Oval, Speckled, 527/1269	Phendimetrazine Tartrate 35 mg	P-D-M Ovals by Lannett		Anorexiant; C III
5271270	Tab, Pink, Round, 527/1270	Phendimetrazine Tartrate 35 mg	P-D-M by Lannett		Anorexiant; C III
5271271	Tab, Yellow, Round, 527/1271	Phendimetrazine Tartrate 35 mg	P-D-M by Lannett		Anorexiant; C III
5271272	Tab, Gray, Round, 527/1272	Phendimetrazine Tartrate 35 mg	P-D-M by Lannett		Anorexiant; C III
5271273	Tab, White, Round, 527/1273	Phendimetrazine Tartrate 35 mg	P-D-M by Lannett		Anorexiant; C III
5271274	Tab, Speckled Green & White, Round, 527/1274	Phendimetrazine Tartrate 35 mg	P-D-M by Lannett		Anorexiant; C III
527155 <> LANNETT	Cap, Dark Green & Light Green	Aspirin 325 mg, Butalbital 50 mg, Caffeine 40 mg	by Duramed	51285-0908	Analgesic; C III
527508	Cap, Yellow, 527/508	Pentobarbital Sodium 1.5 gr	by Lannett		Sedative/Hypnotic; C II
527510	Cap, Black, 527/510	Phendimetrazine Tartrate 35 mg	P-D-M by Lannett		Anorexiant; C III
527511	Cap, Clear & Yellow, 527/511	Pentobarbital Sodium 0.75 gr	by Lannett		Sedative/Hypnotic; C II
527515	Cap, Blue, 527/515	Amobarbital Sodium 3 gr	Amytal by Lannett		Sedative/Hypnotic; C II
527535	Cap, 527/535	Secobarbital Sodium 0.5 g, Butalbital Sodium 0.5 g, Pb 0.5 g	Tribarb by Lannett		Sedative/Hypnotic; C IV
527544	Cap, Reddish-Orange, 527/544	Secobarbital Sodium 1.5 gr	Seconal by Lannett		Sedative/Hypnotic; C II
527546	Cap, Reddish-Orange, 527/546	Secobarbital Sodium 0.75 gr	Seconal by Lannett		Sedative/Hypnotic; C II
527549	Cap, Brown & Clear, 527/549	Phentermine HCl 30 mg	by Lannett		Anorexiant; C IV
527549	Cap, Blue & Clear, 527/549	Phentermine HCl 30 mg	by Lannett		Anorexiant; C IV
527549	Cap, Red & Yellow, 527/549	Phentermine HCl 30 mg	by Lannett		Anorexiant; C IV
527549	Cap, Clear & Green, 527/549	Phentermine HCl 30 mg	by Lannett		Anorexiant; C IV
527549	Cap, Yellow, 527/549	Phentermine HCl 30 mg	by Lannett		Anorexiant; C IV
527549	Cap, Black, 527/549	Phentermine HCl 30 mg	by Lannett		Anorexiant; C IV
527557	Cap, Green, 527/557	Chloral Hydrate 500 mg	Noctec by Lannett		Sedative/Hypnotic; C IV
527558	Cap, Blue & White, 527/558	Glutethimide 500 mg	by Lannett		Hypnotic
527561	Cap, Pink & White, 527/561	Dover's Pwd., Phenacetin, Aspirin, Camphor, Caff., Atropine	Doverin by Lannett		Analgesic
527566	Cap, Blue & Orange, 527/566	Amobarbital Sodium 0.75 gr, Secobarbital Sodium 0.75 gr	Lanabarb No.1 by Lannett		Sedative/Hypnotic; C II
527567	Cap, Blue & Orange, 527/567	Amobarbital Sodium 1.5 gr, Secobarbital Sodium 1.5 gr	Lanabarb No.2 by Lannett		Sedative/Hypnotic; C II
527568	Cap, Blue & Gold, 527/568	Dover's Pwd., Phenacetin, Aspirin, Camphor, Caff., Atropine	Doverin by Lannett		Analgesic
527584	Cap, Gray & Red, 527/584	Propoxyphene Compound 65	Darvon Compound 65 by Lannett		Analgesic; C IV
527591	Cap, Green & Yellow, 527/591	Chlordiazepoxide HCl 5 mg	Librium by Lannett		Antianxiety; C IV
527592	Cap, Black & Green, 527/592	Chlordiazepoxide HCl 10 mg	Librium by Lannett		Antianxiety; C IV
527593	Cap, Green & White, 527/593	Chlordiazepoxide HCl 25 mg	Librium by Lannett		Antianxiety; C IV
527595	Cap, Pink, 527/595	Propoxyphene HCl 65 mg	Darvon by Lannett		Analgesic; C IV
527625	Cap, Yellow, 527/625	Phendimetrazine Tartrate 35 mg	P-D-M by Lannett		Anorexiant; C III
527626	Cap, Blue & Clear, 527/626	Phendimetrazine Tartrate 35 mg	P-D-M by Lannett		Anorexiant; C III
527627	Cap, Brown & Clear, 527/627	Phendimetrazine Tartrate 35 mg	P-D-M by Lannett		Anorexiant; C III
527628	Cap, Clear & Green, 527/628	Phendimetrazine Tartrate 35 mg	P-D-M by Lannett		Anorexiant; C III
527637	Cap, Brown & Clear, 527/637	Phendimetrazine Tartrate 35 mg	Obalan by Lannett		Anorexiant; C III
527638	Cap, Red & Yellow, 527/638	Phendimetrazine Tartrate 35 mg	Obalan by Lannett		Anorexiant; C III
527639	Cap, Clear & Green, 527/639	Phendimetrazine Tartrate 35 mg	Obalan by Lannett		Anorexiant; C III
527900	Tab, White, Round, 527/900	Acetaminophen 300 mg, Codeine 30 mg	Tylenol #3 by Lannett		Analgesic; C III
527903	Tab, Orange, Round, 527/903	Codeine 8 mg, Salicylamide 230 mg, Acetaminophen 150 mg, Caffeine 30 mg	Codalan No.1 by Lannett		Analgesic; C III
527904	Tab, White, Round, 527/904	Codeine 15 mg, Salicylamide 230 mg, Acetaminophen 150 mg, Caffeine 30 mg	Codalan No.2 by Lannett		Analgesic; C III
527905	Tab, Green, Round, 527/905	Codeine 30 mg, Salicylamide 230 mg, Acetaminophen 150 mg, Caffeine 30 mg	Codalan No.3 by Lannett		Analgesic; C III
529MD	Tab, White, Round	Glutethimide 500 mg	Doriden by MD		Hypnotic
52H	Tab, White, Oblong, Scored	Telmisartan 80 mg	Micardis by Boehringer Ingelheim	12714-0110	Antihypertensive
52H	Tab, White, Oblong, Scored	Telmisartan 80 mg	Micardis by Boehringer Pharms	00597-0041	Antihypertensive
53 <> M	Tab, House-Shaped, Film Coated	Cimetidine 200 mg	by Heartland	61392-0194	Gastrointestinal
53 <> M	Tab, Film Coated	Cimetidine 200 mg	by Murfreesboro	51129-1177	Gastrointestinal
53 <> M	Tab, Green, Film Coated	Cimetidine 200 mg	by Mylan	00378-0053	Gastrointestinal

ID FRONT <> BACK	DESCRIPTION FRONT <> BACK	INGREDIENT & STRENGTH	BRAND (OR EQUIV.) & FIRM	NDC#	CLASS; SCH.
53 <> M	Tab, Pentagonal, Film Coated	Cimetidine 200 mg	by HJ Harkins Co	52959-0374	Gastrointestinal
53 <> MP	Tab, Peach, Round, Scored	Prednisone 20 mg	by Allscripts	54569-0332	Steriod
530	Cap, Reddish Brown, Purepac Logo 530	Nifedipine 20 mg	by HJ Harkins Co	52959-0488	Antihypertensive
530 <> MD	Tab, Light Blue, Round, Scored	Hethylphenidate HCl 10 mg	by Altimed	Canadian DIN# 02230321	CNS Stimulant
530 <> MD	Tab, Blue, Round, Scored	Methylphenidate HCl 10 mg	by Apothecon	59772-8841	Stimulant; C II
530 <> MD	Tab	Methylphenidate HCl 10 mg	by Qualitest	00603-4570	Stimulant; C II
5307 <> DANDAN	Tab, White, Round, Scored	Promethazine HCl 25 mg	by Schein	00364-0222	Antiemetic; Antihistamine
5307 <> DANDAN	Tab	Promethazine HCl 25 mg	by Danbury	00591-5307	Antiemetic; Antihistamine
5307 <> DANDAN	Tab	Promethazine HCl 25 mg	by Allscripts	54569-1754	Antiemetic; Antihistamine
5307 <> DANDAN	Tab	Promethazine HCl 25 mg	by Quality Care	60346-0085	Antiemetic; Antihistamine
5307DAN	Tab	Promethazine HCl 25 mg	by Pharmedix	53002-0402	Antiemetic; Antihistamine
530MD	Tab, Blue-Green	Methylphenidate HCl 10 mg	by Caremark	00339-4096	Stimulant; C II
530MD	Tab, Pale Blue/Green	Methylphenidate HCl 10 mg	by Int'l Med Systems	00548-7010	Stimulant; C II
530MD	Tab	Methylphenidate HCl 10 mg	by Zenith Goldline	00182-1066	Stimulant; C II
530MD	Tab, Pale Blue	Methylphenidate HCl 10 mg	by Schein	00364-0479	Stimulant; C II
530MD	Tab, Pale Blue/Green	Methylphenidate HCl 10 mg	by Caremark	00339-4093	Stimulant; C II
530MD	Tab, Pale Blue/Green	Methylphenidate HCl 10 mg	by Medeva	53014-0530	Stimulant; C II
530MD	Tab, Pale Blue/Green	Methylphenidate HCl 10 mg	by MD	43567-0530	Stimulant; C II
531 <> MD	Tab	Methylphenidate HCl 5 mg	by Qualitest	00603-4569	Stimulant; C II
531 <> SCHWARZ	Tab, White, Scored	Hyoscyamine Sulfate 0.125 mg	Levsin by Schwarz Pharma	00091-3531	Gastrointestinal
531 <> SCHWARZ	Tab	Hyoscyamine Sulfate 0.125 mg	Levsin by Prestige Packaging	58056-0351	Gastrointestinal
531 <> SCHWARZ	Tab	Hyoscyamine Sulfate 0.125 mg	Levsin by Thrift Drug	59198-0287	Gastrointestinal
5311 <> V	Tab, Green, Oblong, Scored	Dextromethorphan Hydrobromide 30 mg, Guaifenesin 600 mg	Q Bid DM by DRX	55045-2623	Cold Remedy
5311V	Tab, Film Coated, 5311/V	Dextromethorphan Hydrobromide 30 mg, Guaifenesin 600 mg	by Quality Care	60346-0182	Cold Remedy
5311V	Tab, Film Coated	Dextromethorphan Hydrobromide 30 mg, Guaifenesin 600 mg	by PDRX	55289-0625	Cold Remedy
5311V	Tab, Film Coated, V-Scored	Dextromethorphan Hydrobromide 30 mg, Guaifenesin 600 mg	Guaibid DM by Vintage	00254-5311	Cold Remedy
5311V	Tab, Green, Oblong, Scored, Film	Guaifenesin 600 mg, Dextromethorphan Hydrobromide 30 mg	Q Bid DM SR by Med Pro	53978-3312	Cold Remedy
5312	Tab, Light Green, Delayed Release, 5312	Guaifenesin 600 mg	by Quality Care	60346-0863	Expectorant
5312 <> V	Tab, Green, Oblong, Scored, Debossed 5312 <> Debossed V	Guaifenesin 600 mg	Q Bid LA by Lederle	59911-5897	Expectorant
5312V	Tab, V-Scored	Guaifenesin 600 mg	Guaibid LA by Vintage	00254-5312	Expectorant
5312V	Tab, Green, Oblong, Scored	Guaifenesin 600 mg	by Vangard Labs	00615-4524	Expectorant
5319 <> DAN	Tab	Promethazine HCl 50 mg	by Danbury	00591-5319	Antiemetic; Antihistamine
5319 <> DAN	Tab, White, Round	Promethazine HCl 50 mg	by Schein	00364-0345	Antiemetic; Antihistamine
531MD	Tab	Methylphenidate HCl 5 mg	by MD	43567-0531	Stimulant; C II
531MD	Tab, Yellow, Round, Scored	Methylphenidate HCl 5 mg	by Apothecon	59772-8840	Stimulant; C II
531MD	Tab	Methylphenidate HCl 5 mg	by Schein	00364-0561	Stimulant; C II
531MD	Tab, Debossed	Methylphenidate HCl 5 mg	by Int'l Med Systems	00548-7005	Stimulant; C II
531MD	Tab	Methylphenidate HCl 5 mg	by Zenith Goldline	00182-1173	Stimulant; C II
531MD	Tab	Methylphenidate HCl 5 mg	by Caremark	00339-4097	Stimulant; C II
531MD	Tab	Methylphenidate HCl 5 mg	by Medeva	53014-0531	Stimulant; C II
532 <> MD	Tab, Orange, Round, Scored	Methylphenidate HCl 20 mg	by Apothecon	59772-8842	Stimulant; C II
532 <> MD	Tab, Orange, Round, Scored	Methylphenidate HCl 20 mg	by Altimed	Canadian DIN# 02230322	Stimulant

ID FRONT <> BACK	DESCRIPTION FRONT <> BACK	INGREDIENT & STRENGTH	BRAND (OR EQUIV.) & FIRM	NDC#	CLASS; SCH.
532 <> SCHWARZ	Tab, Pale Blue-Green	Hyoscyamine Sulfate 0.125 mg	Levsin Sl by Quality Care	60346-0998	Gastrointestinal
532 <> SCHWARZ	Tab, Blue-Green, Embossed	Hyoscyamine Sulfate 0.125 mg	Levsin Sl by Prestige Packaging	58056-0352	Gastrointestinal
532 <> SCHWARZ	Tab, Green, Octagon, Scored	Hyoscyamine Sulfate 0.125 mg	Levsin SL by Natl Pharmpak	55154-0952	Gastrointestinal
532 <> SCHWARZ	Tab, Blue, Octagon, Scored	Hyoscyamine Sulfate 0.125 mg	Levsin SL by Med-Pro	53978-3372	Gastrointestinal
532 <> SCHWARZ	Tab, White, Octagonal, Scored	Hyoscyamine Sulfate 0.125 mg	Levsin SL by Schwarz Pharma	00091-3532	Gastrointestinal
532 <> SCHWARZ	Tab, Pale Blue-Green	Hyoscyamine Sulfate 0.125 mg	Levsin Sl by Physicians Total Care	54868-1767	Gastrointestinal
532 <> SCHWARZ	Tab, Pale Blue-Green	Hyoscyamine Sulfate 0.125 mg	Levsin Sl by Thrift Drug	59198-0173	Gastrointestinal
532 <> SCHWARZ	Tab	Hyoscyamine Sulfate 0.125 mg	Levsin Sl by Amerisource	62584-0007	Gastrointestinal
5321 <> DANDAN	Tab, White, Round, Scored	Primidone 250 mg	by Schein	00364-0366	Anticonvulsant
5321 <> DANDAN	Tab	Primidone 250 mg	by Danbury	00591-5321	Anticonvulsant
5321 <> DANDAN	Tab	Primidone 250 mg	by Vangard	00615-2521	Anticonvulsant
5325 <> DANDAN	Tab, White, Cap Shaped, Scored	Colchicine 0.5 mg, Probenecid 500 mg	by Schein	00364-0315	Antigout
5325 <> DANDAN	Tab	Colchicine 0.5 mg, Probenecid 500 mg	Col Probenecid by Danbury	00591-5325	Antigout
5325V	Tab, Ex Release, Debossed, Appears As 53/25V	Atropine Sulfate 0.04 mg, Chlorpheniramine Maleate 8 mg, Hyoscyamine Sulfate 0.19 mg, Phenylephrine HCl 25 mg, Phenylpropanolamine HCl 50 mg, Scopolamine Hydrobromide 0.01 mg	Pro Tuss by Quality Care	60346-0287	Cold Remedy
5325V	Tab, 53/25V	Atropine Sulfate 0.04 mg, Chlorpheniramine Maleate 8 mg, Hyoscyamine Sulfate 0.19 mg, Phenylephrine HCl 25 mg, Phenylpropanolamine HCl 50 mg, Scopolamine Hydrobromide 0.01 mg	Deconhist LA by Zenith Goldline	00172-4375	Cold Remedy
5325V	Tab	Atropine Sulfate 0.04 mg, Chlorpheniramine Maleate 8 mg, Hyoscyamine Sulfate 0.19 mg, Phenylephrine HCl 25 mg, Phenylpropanolamine HCl 50 mg, Scopolamine Hydrobromide 0.01 mg	Q Tuss by Qualitest	00603-5549	Cold Remedy
532HD	Tab, Red & White	Oxycodone 5 mg, Acetaminophen 500 mg	Tylox by Halsey		Analgesic; C II
532MD	Tab, Orange, Round, 532/MD	Methylphenidate HCl 20 mg	by Pharmascience	Canadian	Stimulant
532MD	Tab	Methylphenidate HCl 20 mg	by Caremark	00339-4098	Stimulant; C II
532MD	Tab	Methylphenidate HCl 20 mg	by Schein	00364-0562	Stimulant; C II
532MD	Tab	Methylphenidate HCl 20 mg	by Caremark	00339-4094	Stimulant; C II
532MD	Tab	Methylphenidate HCl 20 mg	by Int'l Med Systems	00548-7020	Stimulant; C II
532MD	Tab	Methylphenidate HCl 20 mg	by Medeva	53014-0532	Stimulant; C II
532MD	Tab	Methylphenidate HCl 20 mg	by MD	43567-0532	Stimulant; C II
5333DAN	Cap, Orange & Yellow	Procainamide HCl 500 mg	by Schein	00364-0344	Antiarrhythmic
5335 <> DANDAN	Tab, White, Round, Scored	Trihexyphenidyl HCl 2 mg	by Heartland Healthcare	61392-0634	Antiparkinson
5335 <> DANDAN	Tab, White, Round, Scored	Trihexyphenidyl HCl 2 mg	by Schein	00364-0408	Antiparkinson
5335 <> DANDAN	Tab	Trihexyphenidyl HCl 2 mg	by Vangard	00615-0675	Antiparkinson
5335 <> DANDAN	Tab	Trihexyphenidyl HCl 2 mg	by Danbury	00591-5335	Antiparkinson
5335 <> DANDAN	Tab	Trihexyphenidyl HCl 2 mg	by Amerisource	62584-0886	Antiparkinson
5335 <> DANDAN	Tab	Trihexyphenidyl HCl 2 mg	by Quality Care	60346-0844	Antiparkinson
5335 <> DANDAN	Tab	Trihexyphenidyl HCl 2 mg	by Octofoil	63467-0301	Antiparkinson
5335 <> DANDAN	Tab	Trihexyphenidyl HCl 2 mg	by Danbury	61955-0408	Antiparkinson
5337 <> DANDAN	Tab, White, Round, Scored	Trihexyphenidyl HCl 5 mg	by Schein	00364-0409	Antiparkinson
5337 <> DANDAN	Tab	Trihexyphenidyl HCl 5 mg	by Danbury	00591-5337	Antiparkinson
5337 <> DANDAN	Tab	Trihexyphenidyl HCl 5 mg	by Amerisource	62584-0887	Antiparkinson
5337 <> DANDAN	Tab	Trihexyphenidyl HCl 5 mg	by Danbury	61955-0409	Antiparkinson
533HD	Cap, Blue	Flurazepam HCl 30 mg	Dalmane by Halsey		Hypnotic; C IV
534 <> SCHWARZ	Tab, Pink	Hyoscyamine Sulfate 0.125 mg, Phenobarbital 15 mg	Levsin Phenobarb by Schwarz Pharma	00091-3534	Gastrointestinal; C IV
5342 <> DANDAN	Tab, White, Round, Scored	Nylidrin 6 mg	by Schein	00364-0391	Vasodilator
5345 <> DANDAN	Tab	Hydrochlorothiazide 50 mg	by Talbert Med	44514-0411	Diuretic
5345 <> DANDAN	Tab, Peach, Round, Scored	Hydrochlorothiazide 50 mg	by Schein	00364-0328	Diuretic
5347 <> DANDAN	Tab, Yellow, Cap-Shaped, Film Coated, Scored	Probenecid 500 mg	by Schein	00364-0314	Antigout
5347 <> DANDAN	Tab	Probenecid 500 mg	by Danbury	00591-5347	Antigout
534HD	Cap, Blue & White	Flurazepam HCl 15 mg	Dalmane by Halsey		Hypnotic; C IV
535 <> GG	Cap	Nitrofurantoin 50 mg	by Quality Care	60346-0616	Antibiotic

ID FRONT <> BACK	DESCRIPTION FRONT <> BACK	INGREDIENT & STRENGTH	BRAND (OR EQUIV.) & FIRM	NDC#	CLASS; SCH.
535 <> MD	Tab	Atropine Sulfate 0.025 mg, Diphenoxylate HCl 2.5 mg	Lonox by Quality Care	60346-0437	Antidiarrheal; C V
5350DAN	Cap, Orange & White	Procainamide HCl 375 mg	by Schein	00364-0343	Antiarrhythmic
53511	Tab, White, Oblong, Scored, Accucaps Logo 535/11	Acetaminophen 325 mg, Butalbital 50 mg, Caffeine 40 mg	Esgic by Accucaps	61474-4073	Analgesic
53511	Tab, Debossed 535-11 <> Gilbert Logo	Acetaminophen 325 mg, Butalbital 50 mg, Caffeine 40 mg	Esgic by Amerisource	62584-0630	Analgesic
53511	Tab, White, Oblong, Scored, Logo	Butalbital 50 mg; Acetaminophen 325 mg; Caffeine 40 mg	Esgic by Thrift Services	59198-0331	Analgesic
53511 <> G	Tab, Gilbert Logo	Acetaminophen 325 mg, Butalbital 50 mg, Caffeine 40 mg	Esgic by Nat Pharmpak Serv	55154-4601	Analgesic
53511 <> GL	Tab, 535-11 <> Gilbert Logo G with Overlayed L	Acetaminophen 325 mg, Butalbital 50 mg, Caffeine 40 mg	Esgic by Prestige Packaging	58056-0354	Analgesic
53511 <> GL	Tab, White, Oblong, Scored	Butalbital 50 mg; Acetaminophen 325 mg; Caffeine 40 mg	Esgic by Rx Pac	65084-0126	Analgesic
53512	Cap, Opaque & White, Logo and 535-12 in Kelly Green	Acetaminophen 325 mg, Caffeine 40 mg, Butalbital 50 mg	Esgic by Accucaps	61474-4074	Analgesic
5353 <> GEIGY	Tab	Hydrochlorothiazide 25 mg, Metoprolol Tartrate 100 mg	Lopressor HCT by Novartis	00028-0053	Diuretic; Antihypertensive
5353 <> GEIGY	Tab, Pink & White	Hydrochlorothiazide 25 mg, Metoprolol Tartrate 100 mg	Lopressor HCT by Pharm Utilization	60491-0371	Diuretic; Antihypertensive
535HD	Tab, Pink, Round	Hydralazine HCl 10 mg	Apresoline by Halsey		Antihypertensive
535II	Tab, Gilbert Logo	Acetaminophen 325 mg, Butalbital 50 mg, Caffeine 40 mg	Esgic by Leiner	59606-0643	Analgesic
536 <> 93	Tab, White to Off-White, Oval, Film Coated	Naproxen Sodium 275 mg	by Allscripts	54569-3761	NSAID
536 <> 93	Tab, Film Coated	Naproxen Sodium 275 mg	by Kaiser	00179-1206	NSAID
536 <> 93	Tab, White to Off-White, Oval, Film Coated	Naproxen Sodium 275 mg	by Teva	00093-0536	NSAID
536 <> 93	Tab, Off-White, Oval, Film Coated	Naproxen Sodium 275 mg	by Brightstone	62939-8431	NSAID
536 <> GG	Cap	Nitrofurantoin 100 mg	by Quality Care	60346-0008	Antibiotic
5361 <> DAN075	Tab, Light Blue, Both Sides <> Dan 0.75	Dexamethasone 0.75 mg	by Quality Care	60346-0550	Steroid
5361 <> DAN075	Tab, Light Blue, Round, Scored, 5361 <> Dan 0.75	Dexamethasone 0.75 mg	by Schein	00364-0098	Steroid
5363 <> ANEXSIA	Tab	Acetaminophen 660 mg, Hydrocodone Bitartrate 10 mg	Anexsia by Mallinckrodt Hobart	00406-5363	Analgesic; C III
5368 <> DANDAN	Tab, Off-White, Round, Scored	Disulfiram 500 mg	by Schein	00364-0337	Antialcoholism
5369 <> DANDAN	Tab, White, Round, Scored	Bethanechol Chloride 10 mg	by Schein	00364-0349	Urinary Tract
5369 <> DANDAN	Tab	Bethanechol Chloride 10 mg	by Danbury	00591-5369	Urinary Tract
536HD	Tab, Peach, Round	Hydralazine HCl 25 mg	Apresoline by Halsey		Antihypertensive
537 <> 93	Tab, Off-White, Oval, Film Coated	Naproxen Sodium 550 mg	by Brightstone	62939-8441	NSAID
537 <> 93	Tab, Film Coated	Naproxen Sodium 550 mg	by Quality Care	60346-0826	NSAID
537 <> 93	Tab, Film Coated	Naproxen Sodium 550 mg	by Kaiser	00179-1223	NSAID
537 <> 93	Tab, White to Off-White, Oval	Naproxen Sodium 550 mg	by Teva	00093-0537	NSAID
537 <> KREMERSURBANE	Cap	Hyoscyamine Sulfate 0.375 mg	Levsinex by Drug Distr	52985-0228	Gastrointestinal
537 <> M	Tab, Light Blue, Film Coated, Beveled Edge	Naproxen Sodium 275 mg	by Mylan	00378-0537	NSAID
537 <> M	Tab, Film Coated	Naproxen Sodium 275 mg	by Allscripts	54569-3761	NSAID
537 <> M	Tab, Light Blue, Film Coated	Naproxen Sodium 275 mg	by HJ Harkins Co	52959-0357	NSAID
537 <> SCHWARZ	Cap, Brown & Clear	Hyoscyamine Sulfate 0.375 mg	Levsinex by Thrift Drug	59198-0288	Gastrointestinal
5373 <> DAN	Tab	Isosorbide Dinitrate 10 mg	by Danbury	00591-5373	Antianginal
5373 <> DANDAN	Tab, White, Round, Scored	Isosorbide Dinitrate 10 mg	by Schein	00364-0341	Antianginal
5373 <> DANDAN	Tab	Isosorbide Dinitrate 10 mg	by Quality Care	60346-0577	Antianginal
5374 <> DANDAN	Tab	Isosorbide Dinitrate 5 mg	by Danbury	00591-5374	Antianginal
5374 <> DANDAN	Tab, White, Round, Scored	Isosorbide Dinitrate 5 mg	by Schein	00364-0340	Antianginal
5375 <> MYLAN	Cap	Doxepin HCl	by PDRX	55289-0258	Antidepressant
537HD	Tab, Orange, Round	Hydralazine HCl 50 mg	Apresoline by Halsey		Antihypertensive
538	Tab, White, Round, Schering Logo 538	Halazepam 40 mg	Paxipam by Schering		Antianxiety; C IV
538 <> R	Tab, Mottled Dark Blue, Round, Scored	Carbidopa 10 mg, Levodopa 100 mg	by Purepac	00228-2538	Antiparkinson
538 <> R	Tab	Carbidopa 10 mg, Levodopa 100 mg	by Murfreesboro	51129-1301	Antiparkinson
5381 <> DANDAN	Tab, White, Round, Scored	Methocarbamol 500 mg	by Schein	00364-0346	Muscle Relaxant
5381 <> DANDAN	Tab	Methocarbamol 500 mg	by Danbury	00591-5381	Muscle Relaxant
5381 <> DANDAN	Tab	Methocarbamol 500 mg	by Kaiser	00179-0446	Muscle Relaxant
5381 <> DANDAN	Tab	Methocarbamol 500 mg	by Quality Care	60346-0080	Muscle Relaxant
5381 <> DANDAN	Tab	Methocarbamol 500 mg	by Talbert Med	44514-0557	Muscle Relaxant

ID FRONT <> BACK	DESCRIPTION FRONT <> BACK	INGREDIENT & STRENGTH	BRAND (OR EQUIV.) & FIRM	NDC#	CLASS; SCH.
5382 <> DANDAN	Tab	Methocarbamol 750 mg	by Danbury	00591-5382	Muscle Relaxant
5382 <> DANDAN	Tab	Methocarbamol 750 mg	by Kaiser	00179-0447	Muscle Relaxant
5382 <> DANDAN	Tab, White, Cap-Shaped, Scored	Methocarbamol 750 mg	by Schein	00364-0347	Muscle Relaxant
5382 <> DANDAN	Tab	Methocarbamol 750 mg	by Allscripts	54569-0843	Muscle Relaxant
5382 <> DANDAN	Tab	Methocarbamol 750 mg	by Talbert Med	44514-0558	Muscle Relaxant
5385 <> DAN	Tab	Isosorbide Dinitrate 5 mg	by Danbury	00591-5385	Antianginal
5385 <> DAN	Tab, White, Round	Isosorbide Dinitrate 5 mg	by Schein	00364-0368	Antianginal
5387 <> DAN	Tab	Isosorbide Dinitrate 2.5 mg	by Danbury	00591-5387	Antianginal
5387 <> DAN	Tab, Yellow, Round	Isosorbide Dinitrate 2.5 mg	by Schein	00364-0367	Antianginal
5388 <> DANDAN	Tab, White, Cap Shaped, Scored	Triamcinolone 4 mg	by Schein	00364-0352	Steroid
538HD	Tab, Orange, Round	Hydralazine HCl 100 mg	Apresoline by Halsey		Antihypertensive
539 <> R	Tab, Mottled Yellow, Round, Scored	Carbidopa 25 mg, Levodopa 100 mg	by Purepac	00228-2539	Antiparkinson
5390 <> DANDAN	Tab, White, Round, Scored	Nylidrin 12 mg	by Schein	00364-0392	Vasodilator
54 <> 369	Cap	Loperamide HCl 2 mg	by Roxane	00054-8537	Antidiarrheal
54 <> 369	Cap	Loperamide HCl 2 mg	by Nat Pharmpak Serv	55154-4912	Antidiarrheal
54 <> 463	Cap, Flesh	Lithium Carbonate 300 mg	Eskalith Lithonate by Roxane	00054-8527	Antipsychotic
54 <> 523	Cap, Carmel & Red	Mexiletine HCl 150 mg	Mexitil by Roxane	00054-2616	Antiarrhythmic
54 <> 523	Cap, Carmel & Red	Mexiletine HCl 150 mg	Mexitil by Roxane	00054-8616	Antiarrhythmic
54 <> 643	Tab, Beige, Round	Naproxen 250 mg	Naprosyn by Roxane	00054-8641	NSAID
54 <> 899	Tab	Prednisone 10 mg	by Med Pro	53978-3037	Steroid
54 <> PAR	Tab, Yellow, Triangular, Sugar Coated	Imipramine 10 mg	by Allscripts	54569-2726	Antidepressant
54 <> PAR	Tab, Sugar Coated	Imipramine HCl 10 mg	by Par	49884-0054	Antidepressant
54 <> PAR	Tab, Sugar Coated	Imipramine HCl 10 mg	by Quality Care	60346-0718	Antidepressant
54839	Tab, Delayed Release, 54 839	Diclofenac Sodium 75 mg	by Quality Care	60346-0463	NSAID
540 <> R	Tab, Mottled Light Blue, Round, Scored	Carbidopa 25 mg, Levodopa 250 mg	by Purepac	00228-2540	Antiparkinson
540 <> R	Tab	Carbidopa 25 mg, Levodopa 250 mg	by Murfreesboro	51129-1292	Antiparkinson
54009	Tab, White, Round, 54-009	Propranolol HCl 20 mg	Inderal by Roxane		Antihypertensive
5401 <> AMB5	Tab, Pink, Cap-Shaped, Film Coated	Zolpidem Tartrate 5 mg	Ambien by GD Searle	00025-5401	Sedative/Hypnotic; C IV
5401 <> AMB5	Tab, Film Coated	Zolpidem Tartrate 5 mg	Ambien by Caremark	00339-4064	Sedative/Hypnotic; C IV
5401 <> AMB5	Tab, Film Coated	Zolpidem Tartrate 5 mg	Ambien by Nat Pharmpak Serv	55154-3617	Sedative/Hypnotic; C IV
5401 <> AMB5	Tab, Film Coated	Zolpidem Tartrate 5 mg	Ambien by Allscripts	54569-3827	Sedative/Hypnotic; C IV
5401 <> AMB5	Tab, Film Coated	Zolpidem Tartrate 5 mg	Ambien by HJ Harkins Co	52959-0362	Sedative/Hypnotic; C IV
5401 <> AMB5	Tab, Film Coated	Zolpidem Tartrate 5 mg	Ambien by Quality Care	60346-0867	Sedative/Hypnotic; C IV
54010	Tab, Orange, Oblong	Diflunisal 250 mg	Dolobid by Roxane	00054-8210	NSAID
54012	Tab, White, Round, 54-012	Amitriptyline 25 mg	Elavil by Roxane		Antidepressant
54013	Tab, Yellow, Round, 54-013	Leucovorin Calcium 25 mg	Wellcovorin by Roxane	00054-8499	Antineoplastic
54019	Tab, Yellow, Round, 54-019	Chlorpheniramine Maleate 4 mg	Chlor-trimeton by Roxane		Antihistamine
5402 <> DANDAN	Tab, Yellow, Round, Scored	Bethanechol Chloride 25 mg	by Schein	00364-0410	Urinary Tract
5402 <> DANDAN	Tab	Bethanechol Chloride 25 mg	by Danbury	00591-5402	Urinary Tract
54039	Tab, Beige, Oblong, 54-039	Naproxen 500 mg	Naproxyn by Roxane	00054-8643	NSAID
54043	Tab, 54/043	Azathioprine 50 mg	by Roxane	00054-8084	Immunosuppressant
54043	Tab, Yellow, Round, 54/043	Azathioprine 50 mg	Imuran by Roxane	00054-4084	Immunosuppressant
54050	White, Hexagon, Scored, 54 050	Haloperidol 1 mg	by Merck & Sharp & Dohme	60312-0072	Antipsychotic
54050	Tab, 54 050	Haloperidol 1 mg	by Amerisource	62584-0725	Antipsychotic
54050	Tab	Haloperidol 1 mg	by Roxane	00054-8343	Antipsychotic
54050	Tab	Haloperidol 1 mg	by Nat Pharmpak Serv	55154-4924	Antipsychotic
540501	Tab, White, Hexagonal, 54-050 1	Haloperidol 1 mg	Haldol by Roxane	00054-8343	Antipsychotic
54053300	Tab, White, Round, 54-053 300	Quinidine Sulfate 300 mg	Lin-Qin, Quinova by Roxane	00054-8735	Antiarrhythmic
5406 <> DANDAN	Tab, Green, Round, Scored	Reserpine 0.125 mg, Hydrochlorothiazide 25 mg	by Schein	00364-0354	Antihypertensive
54062	Tab, Round, 54-062	Propranolol HCl 60 mg	Inderal by Roxane		Antihypertensive
54063	Tab, White, Round, 54-063	Acetaminophen 325 mg	Tylenol by Roxane	00054-8014	Antipyretic
5407 <> DANDAN	Tab, Green, Round, Scored	Reserpine 0.125 mg, Hydrochlorothiazide 50 mg	by Schein	00364-0355	Antihypertensive

ID FRONT <> BACK	DESCRIPTION FRONT <> BACK	INGREDIENT & STRENGTH	BRAND (OR EQUIV.) & FIRM	NDC#	CLASS; SCH.
54072	Cap, Green, Scored	Hydroxyurea 500 mg	by Natl Pharmpak	55154-4930	Antineoplastic
54072	Cap, Flesh & Green, 54-072	Hydroxyurea 500 mg	Hydrea by Roxane	00054-8247	Antineoplastic
54072 <> 54072	Cap, Green & Opaque & Tan	Hydroxyurea 500 mg	by Murfreesboro	51129-1470	Antineoplastic
54080	Tab, White, Round	Prednisone 25 mg	Prednisone by Roxane		Steroid
5409030	Tab, White, Round	Morphine Sulfate SR 30 mg	MS Contin by Roxane	00054-8805	Analgesic; C II
54092	Tab, White, Scored	Prednisone 1 mg	by Allscripts	54569-1469	Steroid
54092	Tab, White, Round, 54/092	Prednisone 1 mg	Deltasone by Roxane	00054-8739	Steroid
54092	Tab	Prednisone 1 mg	by Pharmedix	53002-0483	Steroid
54092	Tab	Prednisone 1 mg	by Nat Pharmpak Serv	55154-4926	Steroid
54093	Tab, Orange, Oblong	Diflunisal 500 mg	Dolobid by Roxane	00054-8220	NSAID
54099	Tab, White, Round, 54-099	Amitriptyline 50 mg	Elavil by Roxane		Antidepressant
540HD	Tab, White, Round	Metronidazole 500 mg	Flagyl by Halsey		Antibiotic
54103	Tab, Round, 54-103	Bisacodyl 5 mg	Dulcolax by Roxane		Gastrointestinal
54140	Tab, White, Round, 54-140	Diclofenac Sodium DR 25 mg	Voltaren by Roxane	00054-8223	NSAID
54142	Tab, White, Round, 54/142	Methadone HCl 10 mg	Methadone by Roxane	00054-8554	Analgesic; C II
54143	Tab, White, Round, 54-143	Amitriptyline 100 mg	Elavil by Roxane		Antidepressant
54162	Tab, White, Round	Methadone HCl 5 mg	by Roxane	00054-4216	Analgesic; C II
54163	Tab, White, Round	Meperidine HCl 100 mg	Demerol by Roxane	00054-8596	Analgesic; C II
54169	Tab	Haloperidol 0.5 mg	by Nat Pharmpak Serv	55154-4923	Antipsychotic
54169 <> 12	Tab, 54 169 <> 1 over 2	Haloperidol 0.5 mg	by Murfreesboro	51129-1130	Antipsychotic
54169 <> 12	Tab, White, Hexagonal, 54/169 <> 1 over 2	Haloperidol 0.5 mg	Haldol by Roxane	00054-8342	Antipsychotic
54179	Cap, Reddish Orange, 54-179	Chloral Hydrate 500 mg	Noctec by Roxane	00054-8140	Sedative/Hypnotic; C IV
54180	Tab, Blue, Oval, 54-180	Naproxen Sodium 275 mg	Anaprox by Roxane	00054-8638	NSAID
54183	Tab, White, Round, 54-183	Prednisolone 5 mg	by Roxane		Steroid
54193	Tab, Embossed 54 193 with a Single Bisect	Nevirapine 200 mg	by Roxane	00054-8647	Antiviral
54193	Tab, Scored	Nevirapine 200 mg	Viramune by Roxane	00054-4647	Antiviral
54193	Tab, Scored	Nevirapine 200 mg	Viramune by Boehringer Ingelheim	00597-0045	Antiviral
54193	Tab, 54/193	Nevirapine 200 mg	Viramune by Physicians Total Care	54868-3844	Antiviral
54199	Tab, Light Blue, Round, 54/199	Oxycodone HCl 30 mg	by Roxane		Analgesic; C II
5421 <> AMB10	Tab, Film Coated	Zolpidem Tartrate 10 mg	Ambien by Allscripts	54569-3828	Sedative/Hypnotic; C IV
5421 <> AMB10	Tab, Film Coated	Zolpidem Tartrate 10 mg	Ambien by HJ Harkins Co	52959-0363	Sedative/Hypnotic; C IV
5421 <> AMB10	Tab, Film Coated	Zolpidem Tartrate 10 mg	Ambien by PDRX	55289-0792	Sedative/Hypnotic; C IV
5421 <> AMB10	Tab, Film Coated	Zolpidem Tartrate 10 mg	Ambien by Quality Care	60346-0949	Sedative/Hypnotic; C IV
5421 <> AMB10	Tab, White, Cap-Shaped, Film Coated	Zolpidem Tartrate 10 mg	Ambien by GD Searle	00025-5421	Sedative/Hypnotic; C IV
5421 <> AMB10	Tab, Film Coated, Searle	Zolpidem Tartrate 10 mg	Ambien by Caremark	00339-4065	Sedative/Hypnotic; C IV
54210	Tab, White, Round, 54-210	Methadone HCl 5 mg	Methadone by Roxane	00054-8553	Analgesic; C II
54212	Tab, White, Round, 54-212	Neomycin Sulfate 500 mg	by Roxane	00054-8600	Antibiotic
54213	Cap, Opaque	Lithium Carbonate 150 mg	Eskalith Lithonate by Roxane	00054-8526	Antipsychotic
54213	Cap	Lithium Carbonate 150 mg	by Quality Care	62682-7030	Antipsychotic
54223	Cap, Pink, 54-223	Diphenhydramine HCl 50 mg	Benadryl by Roxane		Antihistamine
54249	Tab, White, Round, 54-249	Propranolol HCl 80 mg	Inderal by Roxane		Antihypertensive
54252	Tab, White, Round, 54-252	Acetaminophen 500 mg	Tylenol by Roxane	00054-8016	Antipyretic
54253	Tab, White, Oblong	Sulfamethoxazole 400 mg, Trimethoprim 80 mg	Septra by Roxane		Antibiotic
54259	Tab, Red, Round, 54/259	Ferrous Sulfate 300 mg	by Roxane	00054-8284	Mineral
54262	Tab, White, Round, 54/262	Morphine Sulfate 30 mg	Morphine Sulfate by Roxane	00054-8583	Analgesic; C II
54263	Tab, White, Round, 54-263	Phenobarbital 100 mg	by Roxane	00054-8707	Sedative/Hypnotic; C IV
5428 <> DAN	Tab, Light Yellow, Round	Reserpine 0.1 mg, Hydralazine HCl 25 mg, Hydrochlorothiazide 15 mg	by Schein	00364-0361	Antihypertensive
54280	Tab, White, Round, 54-280	Dihydrotachysterol 0.125 mg	DHT by Roxane	00054-8172	Vitamin
54293	Tab, White, Round, 54-293	Leucovorin Calcium 5 mg	Wellcovorin by Roxane	00054-8496	Antineoplastic
54299	Tab, Yellow, Round, Scored	Dexamethasone 0.5 mg	by Roxane	00054-4179	Steroid
54299	Tab, Yellow, Round, 54-299	Dexamethasone 0.5 mg	Decadron by Roxane	00054-8179	Steroid
5430 <> DANDAN	Tab	Acetazolamide 250 mg	by Quality Care	60346-0734	Diuretic

ID FRONT <> BACK	DESCRIPTION FRONT <> BACK	INGREDIENT & STRENGTH	BRAND (OR EQUIV.) & FIRM	NDC#	CLASS; SCH.
5430 <> DANDAN	Tab, White, Round, Scored	Acetazolamide 250 mg	by Schein	00364-0400	Diuretic
5430 <> DANDAN	Tab	Acetazolamide 250 mg	by Danbury	00591-5430	Diuretic
54302	Tab, White, Oblong, 54-302	Calcium Carbonate 1250 mg	Caltrate by Roxane	00054-8120	Vitamin/Mineral
54303	Tab, White, 54/303	Propantheline Bromide 15 mg	Pro-Banthine by Roxane	00054-8737	Gastrointestinal
54303	Tab, Coated, in Black Ink 54/303	Propantheline Bromide 15 mg	by Kaiser	00179-0627	Gastrointestinal
5432	Tab, Blue, Round	Amphetamine, Dextroamphetamine Combination	Obetrol-10 by Richwood		Stimulant; C II
54323	Tab, Yellow, Round, 54-323	Methotrexate 2.5 mg	Rheumatrex by Roxane	00054-8550	Antineoplastic
54329	Cap, Green, 54-329	Indomethacin 50 mg	Indocin by Roxane		NSAID
54333	Tab, White, Round, 54-333	Propranolol HCl 40 mg	Inderal by Roxane		Antihypertensive
54339	Tab, White, Round, 54/339	Prednisone 2.5 mg	Deltasone by Roxane	00054-8740	Steroid
54339	Tab	Prednisone 2.5 mg	by Nat Pharmpak Serv	55154-4918	Steroid
54343	Tab, White, Round, 54/343	Prednisone 50 mg	Deltasone by Roxane	00054-8729	Steroid
54343	Tab, Identified 54 343	Prednisone 50 mg	by DRX	55045-1928	Steroid
54343	Tab	Prednisone 50 mg	by Qualitest	00603-5022	Steroid
54343	Tab, White, Scored	Prednisone 50 mg	by Allscripts	54569-0333	Steriod
54352	Tab, White, Round, 54-352	Megesterol Acetate 40 mg	Megace by Roxane	00054-8604	Progestin
54360	Tab, White, Round, 54-360	Amitriptyline 75 mg	Elavil by Roxane		Antidepressant
54372	Tab, White, Oblong, 54-372	Calcium Gluconate 500 mg	Caltrate by Roxane	00054-8121	Vitamin/Mineral
5438 <> DANDAN	Tab	Quinidine Sulfate 200 mg	by Danbury	00591-5438	Antiarrhythmic
5438 <> DANDAN	Tab, White, Round, Scored	Quinidine Sulfate 200 mg	by Schein	00364-0229	Antiarrhythmic
5438210	Tab, White, Hexagonal, 54-382 10	Haloperidol 10 mg	Haldol by Roxane	00054-8343	Antipsychotic
54383	Tab, Beige, Round, 54-383	Methyldopa 500 mg	Aldomet by Roxane		Antihypertensive
54392	Cap, Red & White	Oxycodone 5 mg, Acetaminophen 500 mg	Tylox by Roxane	00054-2795	Analgesic; C II
543HD	Tab, White, Round	Butalbital 50 mg, Acetaminophen 325 mg	Fioricet by Halsey		Analgesic
54403	Tab, Off-White, Round	Hydromorphone HCl 8 mg	Dilaudid by Roxane	00054-4370	Analgesic; C II
54409	Tab, White, Round	Morphine Sulfate SR 30 mg	Oramorph SR by Roxane		Analgesic; C II
5440DAN	Cap, Blue	Doxycycline Hyclate 100 mg	by Schein	00364-2033	Antibiotic
54410	Tab, White, Round, 54-410	Levorphanol 2 mg	Levo-Dromoran by Roxane	00054-8494	Analgesic; C II
54412	Tab, White, Round, 54-412	Codeine Sulfate 60 mg	by Roxane	00054-8157	Analgesic;C II
54413	Tab, White, Oblong, 54-413	Aluminum Hydroxide 500 mg	by Roxane		Gastrointestinal
5442 <> DANDAN	Tab	Prednisone 10 mg	by Danbury	00591-5442	Steroid
5442 <> DANDAN	Tab, White, Round, Scored	Prednisone 10 mg	by Schein	00364-0461	Steroid
5442 <> DANDAN	Tab	Prednisone 10 mg	by Allscripts	54569-0331	Steroid
5442 <> DANDAN	Tab	Prednisone 10 mg	by Med Pro	53978-3037	Steroid
5442 <> DANDAN	Tab	Prednisone 10 mg	by Nat Pharmpak Serv	55154-5215	Steroid
5442 <> DANDAN	Tab	Prednisone 10 mg	by Allscripts	54569-3302	Steroid
5442 <> DANDAN	Tab	Prednisone 10 mg	by Danbury	61955-0461	Steroid
5442 <> DANDAN	Tab, 5442 <> Dan/Dan	Prednisone 10 mg	by Quality Care	60346-0058	Steroid
5442 <> DANDAN	Tab	Prednisone 10 mg	by Heartland	61392-0417	Steroid
54422	Cap, 54-422	Indomethacin 25 mg	Indocin by Roxane		NSAID
5443	Tab	Prednisone 20 mg	by Nat Pharmpak Serv	55154-5209	Steroid
5443 <> DANDAN	Tab	Prednisone 20 mg	by Danbury	61955-0442	Steroid
5443 <> DANDAN	Tab, 5443 <> Dan/Dan	Prednisone 20 mg	by Quality Care	60346-0094	Steroid
5443 <> DANDAN	Tab	Prednisone 20 mg	by WA Butler	11695-1802	Steroid
5443 <> DANDAN	Tab	Prednisone 20 mg	by Danbury	00591-5443	Steroid
5443 <> DANDAN	Tab, Peach, Round, Scored	Prednisone 20 mg	by Schein	00364-0442	Steroid
5443 <> DANDAN	Tab	Prednisone 20 mg	by Vangard	00615-1542	Steroid
5443 <> DANDAN	Tab	Prednisone 20 mg	by Allscripts	54569-0332	Steroid
5443 <> DANDAN	Tab	Prednisone 20 mg	by HJ Harkins Co	52959-0127	Steroid
5443 <> DANDAN	Tab	Prednisone 20 mg	by Vedco	50989-0602	Steroid
5443 <> DANDAN	Tab, Peach, Round, Scored	Prednisone 20 mg	by Allscripts	54569-3043	Steroid
5444 <> DAN	Tab, White, Round, Scored	Chlorothiazide 250 mg	by Schein	00364-0389	Diuretic

ID FRONT <> BACK	DESCRIPTION FRONT <> BACK	INGREDIENT & STRENGTH	BRAND (OR EQUIV.) & FIRM	NDC#	CLASS; SCH.
54452	Tab, White, Round	Lithium Carbonate 300 mg	Eskalith Lithane by Roxane	00054-8531	Antipsychotic
54452	Tab, White, Round, Scored	Lithium Carbonate 300 mg	by Mylan	00378-1914	Antipsychotic
54452	Tab, White, Scored	Lithium Carbonate 300 mg	by Roxane	00054-8528	Antipsychotic
54452 <> 54452	Cap, Tan, Scored	Lithium Carbonate 300 mg	by Mylan	00378-1910	Antipsychotic
54460	Tab, Green, Oval	Cimetidine 800 mg	Tagamet by Roxane	00054-8226	Gastrointestinal
54463	Cap, Flesh	Lithium Carbonate 300 mg	by Direct Dispensing	57866-6523	Antipsychotic
54463	Cap, Pink	Lithium Carbonate 300 mg	by Mylan	00378-1912	Antipsychotic
54463	Cap	Lithium Carbonate 300 mg	by Med Pro	53978-0523	Antipsychotic
54463	Cap	Lithium Carbonate 300 mg	by Nat Pharmpak Serv	55154-4920	Antipsychotic
54463	Cap, Flesh	Lithium Carbonate 300 mg	by Heartland	61392-0131	Antipsychotic
54472	Cap, Blue, 54-472	Piroxicam 10 mg	Feldene by Roxane	00054-8660	NSAID
54479	Cap, Blue, 54-479	Piroxicam 20 mg	Feldene by Roxane	00054-8661	NSAID
54489	Tab, Yellow, Round, 54-489	Dexamethasone 1 mg	Decadron by Roxane	00054-8174	Steroid
5449 <> DAN025	Tab, Orange, Pentagonal, Scored, 5449 <> Dan 0.25	Dexamethasone 0.25 mg	by Schein	00364-0397	Steroid
54492	Tab, White, Round, 54-492	Amitriptyline 150 mg	Elavil by Roxane		Antidepressant
54499	Tab, Peach, Round, 54-499	Hydrochlorothiazide 50 mg	Hydrodiuril by Roxane		Diuretic
544HD5	Tab, Yellow, Round	Diazepam 5 mg	Valium by Halsey		Antianxiety; C IV
545 <> BARR	Cap	Cephalexin Monohydrate	by Warner Chilcott	00047-0938	Antibiotic
545 <> R	Tab, Purepac Logo 545 <> R	Diflunisal 250 mg	by Purepac	00228-2545	NSAID
5450 <> DAN050	Tab, Yellow, Pentagonal, Scored, 5450 <> Dan 0.50	Dexamethasone 0.5 mg	by Schein	00364-0398	Steroid
54503	Tab, White, Round, 54-503	Phenobarbital 15 mg	by Roxane	00054-8703	Sedative/Hypnotic; C IV
5451	Tab, Yellow, Round	Dextroamphetamine Sulfate 10 mg	Dexedrine by Richwood		Stimulant; C II
5451 <> DAN15	Tab, White, Pentagonal, Scored, 5451 <> Dan 1.5	Dexamethasone 1.5 mg	by Schein	00364-0399	Steroid
54512	Tab, White, Oval, 54/512	Alprazolam 1 mg	Xanax by Roxane	00054-8104	Antianxiety; C IV
54519	Tab, White, 54-519	Triazolam 0.125 mg	Halcion by Roxane	00054-8748	Sedative/Hypnotic; C IV
5452	Tab, Yellow, Round	Dextroamphetamine Sulfate 5 mg	Dexedrine by Richwood		Stimulant; C II
54523	Cap	Mexiletine HCl 150 mg	by Ridgebury	60921-0066	Antiarrhythmic
54529	Tab, Yellow, Round	Thiethylperazine Maleate 10 mg	by Roxane	00054-8748	Antiemetic
54532	Tab, White, Round, 54-532	Pseudoephedrine 60 mg	Sudafed by Roxane	00054-8744	Decongestant
54533	Tab, White, Round, 54/583	Furosemide 80 mg	Lasix by Roxane	00054-8301	Diuretic
54533	Tab	Furosemide 80 mg	by Med Pro	53978-0927	Diuretic
54533	Tab, 54/533	Furosemide 80 mg	by Nat Pharmpak Serv	55154-4909	Diuretic
5454 <> DANDAN	Tab	Quinidine Sulfate 300 mg	by Danbury	00591-5454	Antiarrhythmic
5454 <> DANDAN	Tab, White, Round, Scored	Quinidine Sulfate 300 mg	by Schein	00364-0582	Antiarrhythmic
54543	Tab, White, Round, Scored	Oxycodone HCl 5 mg, Acetaminophen 325 mg	Roxicet by Boehringer Ingelheim	Canadian	Analgesic; C II
54543	Tab, White, Round	Oxycodone HCl 5 mg, Acetaminophen 325 mg	Percocet by Roxane	00054-8650	Analgesic; C II
54549	Tab, White, Round	Methadone HCl 10 mg	by Roxane	00054-4217	Analgesic; C II
5455	Tab, Pink, Round	Methamphetamine HCl 5 mg	by Richwood		Stimulant; C II
5455 <> DANDAN	Tab, Blue, Tab, Blue, Round, Scored	Chlorpropamide 250 mg	by Schein	00364-0510	Antidiabetic
5456	Tab, Pink, Round	Methamphetamine HCl 10 mg	by Richwood		Stimulant; C II
5457	Tab, Blue, Round	Phendimetrazine Tartrate 35 mg	X-Trozine by Richwood		Anorexiant; C III
5457	Tab, Yellow, Round	Phendimetrazine Tartrate 35 mg	X-Trozine by Richwood		Anorexiant; C III
5457	Tab, Pink, Round	Phendimetrazine Tartrate 35 mg	X-Trozine by Richwood		Anorexiant; C III
5457	Tab, Green, Round	Phendimetrazine Tartrate 35 mg	X-Trozine by Richwood		Anorexiant; C III
545702	Tab, White, Hexagonal, 54-570 2	Haloperidol 2 mg	Haldol by Roxane	00054-8344	Antipsychotic
54572	Tab, White, Round, 54-572	Phenobarbital 30 mg	by Roxane	00054-8705	Sedative/Hypnotic; C IV
54582	Tab, White, Round, 54/582	Oxycodone HCl 5 mg	by Roxane	00054-8657	Analgesic; C II
54583	Tab, White, Scored	Furosemide 40 mg	by JB	51111-0481	Diuretic
54583	Tab, 54/583	Furosemide 40 mg	Lasix by Roxane	00054-4299	Diuretic
54583	Tab, 54/583	Furosemide 40 mg	by Nat Pharmpak Serv	55154-4908	Diuretic
54583	Tab, White, Round	Furosemide 40 mg	by Med Pro	53978-5032	Diuretic
54592	Tab	Diclofenac Sodium 50 mg	by Quality Care	60346-0238	NSAID

ID FRONT <> BACK	DESCRIPTION FRONT <> BACK	INGREDIENT & STRENGTH	BRAND (OR EQUIV.) & FIRM	NDC#	CLASS; SCH.
54592	Tab, White, Round, 54/592	Diclofenac Sodium 50 mg	Voltaren by Roxane	00054-8221	NSAID
54599	Tab, White, Oval, 54-599	Alprazolam 0.5 mg	Xanax by Roxane	00054-8105	Antianxiety; C IV
546 <> SL	Tab, Peach, Round, Film Coated	Diclofenac Sodium 50 mg	Voltaren by Sidmak Labs	50111-0546	NSAID
5460	Tab, Yellow, Round	Phendimetrazine Tartrate 35 mg	Plegine by Richwood		Anorexiant; C III
54603	Tab, Blue, Oblong, 54-603	Naproxen Sodium 550 mg	Anaprox by Roxane	00054-8639	NSAID
54609	Tab	Hydromorphone HCl 4 mg	by Roxane	00054-8394	Analgesic; C II
546094	Tab, White, Round, 54 609/4	Hydromorphone 4 mg	Hydromorphone by MSD	Canadian	Analgesic
546094	Tab, White, Round, 54-609 4	Hydromorphone HCl 4 mg	Dilaudid by Roxane	00054-8394	Analgesic; C II
54612	Tab, White, Round, 54/612	Prednisone 5 mg	Deltasone by Roxane	00054-8724	Steroid
54612	Tab, Flat-face, Beveled with 54/612	Prednisone 5 mg	by Kaiser	00179-0610	Steriod
54612	Tab	Prednisone 5 mg	by Caremark	00339-5292	Steriod
54612	Tab	Prednisone 5 mg	by Murfreesboro	51129-1307	Steroid
54612	Tab	Prednisone 5 mg	by Med Pro	53978-0060	Steroid
54612 <> 54612	Tab, White, Round, Scored	Prednisone 5 mg	by Southwood Pharms	58016-0218	Steroid
54613	Tab, White, Round, 54-613	Codeine Sulfate 15 mg	by Roxane	00054-8155	Analgesic; C III
5462	Cap, Brown & Clear	Phendimetrazine Tartrate 105 mg	X-Trozine LA-105 by Richwood		Anorexiant; C III
54620	Tab, Blue, Oval, 54-620	Triazolam 0.25 mg	Halcion by Roxane	00054-4859	Sedative/Hypnotic; C IV
54622	Tab, Beige, Round	Methyldopa 250 mg	Aldomet by Roxane		Antihypertensive
546233	Tab, White, Round, 54-623 3	Acetaminophen 300 mg, Codeine 30 mg	Tylenol #3 by Roxane	00054-8022	Analgesic; C III
5463	Cap, Red & White	Phendimetrazine Tartrate 35 mg	X-Trozine by Richwood		Anorexiant; C III
5463	Cap, Blue	Phendimetrazine Tartrate 35 mg	X-Trozine by Richwood		Anorexiant; C III
54632	Cap, Red, 54/632	Mexiletine HCl 200 mg	Mexitil by Roxane	00054-2617	Antiarrhythmic
54632	Cap, Red, 54/632	Mexiletine HCl 200 mg	Mexitil by Roxane	00054-8617	Antiarrhythmic
54632	Cap	Mexiletine HCl 200 mg	by Ridgebury	60921-0067	Antiarrhythmic
54639	Tab, Light Blue, Round, 54/639	Cyclophosphamide 25 mg	Cytoxan, Neosar by Roxane	00054-8089	Antineoplastic
54639	Tab, Blue, Round	Cyclophosphamide 25 mg	by Roxane	00054-4129	Antineoplastic
54643	Tab	Naproxen 250 mg	by Nat Pharmpak Serv	55154-5907	NSAID
54650	Tab, Yellow, Round, 54-650	Leucovorin Calcium 15 mg	Wellcovorin by Roxane	00054-8498	Antineoplastic
54662	Tab, White, Scored	Dexamethasone 2 mg	by DRX	55045-2605	Steroid
54662	Tab	Dexamethasone 2 mg	by Quality Care	62682-5000	Steroid
54662	Tab, White, Round, 54/662	Dexamethasone 2 mg	by Roxane	00054-8176	Steroid
54662	Tab	Dexamethasone 2 mg	by Nat Pharmpak Serv	55154-4914	Steroid
54662	Tab	Dexamethasone 2 mg	by Allscripts	54569-0336	Steroid
5468	Cap, Yellow	Phentermine HCl 30 mg	Oby-Trim 30 by Richwood		Anorexiant; C IV
5468	Cap, Black	Phentermine HCl 30 mg	Oby-Trim 30 by Richwood		Anorexiant; C IV
54680	Tab, White, Round	Vitamin C 500 mg	by Roxane		Vitamin
5469020	Tab, White, Hexagonal, 54-690 20	Haloperidol 20 mg	Haldol by Roxane	00054-8347	Antipsychotic
546HD2	Tab, White, Round	Diazepam 2 mg	Valium by Halsey		Antianxiety; C IV
547 <> SL	Tab, Beige, Round, Film Coated	Diclofenac Sodium 75 mg	Voltaren by Sidmak Labs	50111-0547	NSAID
54702	Cap, Flesh & White	Lithium Carbonate 600 mg	Eskalith Lithonate by Roxane	00054-8531	Antipsychotic
54703	Tab, Coral, Round, 54-703	Imipramine HCl 50 mg	Tofranil by Roxane		Antidepressant
54710	Tab, Green, Round, 54/710	Oxycodone HCl 15 mg	by Roxane		Analgesic; C II
54730	Tab, White, Oblong, 54-730	Oxycodone 5 mg, Acetaminophen 500 mg	by Roxane	00054-8784	Analgesic; C II
54732	Tab, White, Round, 54-732	Diphenoxylate 2.5 mg, Atropine 0.025 mg	Lomotil by Roxane		Antidiarrheal; C V
54733	Tab, White, Round, 54/733	Morphine Sulfate 15 mg	MSIR by Roxane	00054-8582	Analgesic; C II
54733	Tab	Morphine Sulfate 15 mg	by Physicians Total Care	54868-3191	Analgesic; C II
547432	Tab, White, Round, 54 743/2	Hydromorphone 2 mg	Hydromorphone by MSD	Canadian	Analgesic
547432	Tab, White, Round	Hydromorphone HCl 2 mg	Dilaudid by Roxane	00054-8392	Analgesic; C II
54760	Tab, White, Round, 54/670	Prednisone 20 mg	Deltasone by Roxane	00054-8726	Steroid
54760	Tab	Prednisone 20 mg	by Med Pro	53978-0084	Steroid
54760	Tab, Roxane	Prednisone 20 mg	by PDRX	55289-0352	Steroid
54760	Tab, 54/760	Prednisone 20 mg	by Nat Pharmpak Serv	55154-4905	Steroid

ID FRONT <> BACK	DESCRIPTION FRONT <> BACK	INGREDIENT & STRENGTH	BRAND (OR EQUIV.) & FIRM	NDC#	CLASS; SCH.
54763	Tab, White, Round, 54-763	Megesterol Acetate 20 mg	Megace by Roxane	00054-8603	Progestin
54769	Tab, Aqua, Round, 54-769	Dexamethasone 6 mg	Decadron by Roxane	00054-8183	Steroid
5477 <> 0478	Tab	Atropine Sulfate 0.0194 mg, Hyoscyamine Sulfate 0.1037 mg, Phenobarbital 16.2 mg, Scopolamine Hydrobromide 0.0065 mg	Belladonna PB by Quality Care	60346-0042	Gastrointestinal; C IV
54772	Tab, White, Round, 54-772	Dihydrotachysterol 0.4 mg	Hytakerol by Roxane	00054-4191	Vitamin
547735	Tab, White, Hexagonal, 54-773 5	Haloperidol 5 mg	Haldol by Roxane	00054-8345	Antipsychotic
54779	Tab, White, Round, 54-779	Phenobarbital 60 mg	by Roxane	00054-8708	Sedative/Hypnotic; C IV
54782 <> 15	Tab, ER, 54/782 <> 15	Morphine Sulfate 15 mg	Oramorph SR by Roxane	00054-8790	Analgesic; C II
54782 <> 15	Tab, ER, 54 Over 782	Morphine Sulfate 15 mg	Oramorph by Roxane	00054-4790	Analgesic; C II
54783	Tab, White, Round, 54-783	Codeine Sulfate 30 mg	by Roxane	00054-8156	Analgesic; C III
54799	Tab	Cimetidine 400 mg	Tagamet by Roxane	00054-8225	Gastrointestinal
5479DAN	Cap, Red & Ivory	Erythromycin Estolate 250 mg	by Schein	00364-0530	Antibiotic
548	Cap, Green & Tan	Hydroxyurea 500 mg	by Murfreesboro	51129-1469	Antineoplastic
548	Cap, Green & Tan	Hydroxyurea 500 mg	by United Res	00677-1680	Antineoplastic
548	Cap, Green & Tan	Hydroxyurea 500 mg	by Qualitest Pharms	00603-3946	Antineoplastic
54810	Tab, White, Round, 54-810	Propranolol HCl 90 mg	Inderal by Roxane		Antihypertensive
54819	Tab, White, Oblong, 54-819	Acetaminophen 650 mg	Tylenol by Roxane	00054-8015	Antipyretic
54820	Tab, 54 over 820	Ranitidine HCl 300 mg	by Eon	00185-0136	Gastrointestinal
54820	Tab, 54 Over 820	Ranitidine HCl 336 mg	Zantac by Roxane	00054-4854	Gastrointestinal
54820	Tab, 54 over 820	Ranitidine HCl 336 mg	by Ridgebury	60921-0098	Gastrointestinal
54822	Tab, White, Oblong	Sulfamethoxazole 800 mg, Trimethoprim 160 mg	Septra DS by Roxane		Antibiotic
54823	Tab, White, Round, 54-823	Pseudoephedrine 30 mg	Sudafed by Roxane		Decongestant
54823	Tab, White, Round	Pseudoephedrine 30 mg	Sudafed by Roxane	00054-8743	Decongestant
54839	Tab, White, Round, 54/839	Diclofenac Sodium 75 mg	Voltaren by Roxane	00054-8222	NSAID
54839	Tab, White, Round, Enteric Coated	Diclofenac Sodium 75 mg	by Murfreesboro Ph	51129-1348	NSAID
54840	Tab	Furosemide 20 mg	by PDRX	55289-0593	Diuretic
54840	Tab, 54/840	Furosemide 20 mg	Lasix by Roxane	00054-8297	Diuretic
54840	Tab	Furosemide 20 mg	by Murfreesboro	51129-1275	Diuretic
54840	Tab, 54/840	Furosemide 20 mg	by Nat Pharmpak Serv	55154-4906	Diuretic
54840	Tab	Furosemide 20 mg	by Med Pro	53978-5031	Diuretic
54840	Tab, White	Furosemide 20 mg	by JB	51111-0484	Diuretic
54843	Tab, Square, 54-843	Methadone HCl 40 mg	Methadone by Roxane	00054-4547	Analgesic; C II
54853	Tab, Beige, Round, 54-853	Methyldopa 125 mg	Aldomet by Roxane		Antihypertensive
54859	Tab, White, Round, 54-859	Aminophylline 100 mg	Aminophyllin by Roxane	00054-8025	Antiasthmatic
54860	Tab, White, Oval, 54-860	Alprazolam 1 mg	Xanax by Roxane	00054-8107	Antianxiety; C IV
5486210	Tab, White, Round	Morphine Sulfate SR 100 mg	MS Contin by Roxane	00054-8793	Analgesic; C II
54879	Tab, White, Round	Meperidine HCl 50 mg	Demerol by Roxane	00054-8595	Analgesic; C II
54880	Tab, Coral, Round, 54-880	Imipramine HCl 25 mg	Tofranil by Roxane		Antidepressant
54883	Tab, Debossed	Methadone HCl 40 mg	by Eli Lilly	00002-2153	Analgesic; C II
54883	Tab, Light Pinkish-Orange, Pillow-Shaped, 54-883	Methadone HCl 40 mg	by Roxane	00054-4538	Analgesic; C II
54892	Tab, Green, Round, 54/892	Dexamethasone 4 mg	by Roxane	00054-8175	Steroid
54892	Tab, 54/892	Dexamethasone 4 mg	by Med Pro	53978-2057	Steroid
54892	Tab	Dexamethasone 4 mg	by Allscripts	54569-0324	Steroid
54892	Tab, 54 over 892	Dexamethasone 4 mg	by Nat Pharmpak Serv	55154-4901	Steroid
54899	Tab, White, Round, 54/889	Prednisone 10 mg	Deltasone by Roxane	00054-8725	Steriod
54899	Tab, Flat-faced, Beveled Edge, Compressed, 54/899	Prednisone 10 mg	by Kaiser	00179-1154	Steriod
54899	Tab	Prednisone 10 mg	by Nat Pharmpak Serv	55154-4919	Steriod
54902	Tab, White, Round, 54-902	Oxycodone HCl 4.5 mg, Oxycodone Terephthalate 0.38 mg, Aspirin 325 mg	Percodan by Roxane	00054-8653	Analgesic; C II
54903	Tab, Pink, Round, 54-903	Dihydrotachysterol 0.2 mg	DHT by Roxane	00054-8182	Vitamin
54912	Tab, Light Green, Round	Cimetidine 300 mg	Tagamet by Roxane	00054-8224	Gastrointestinal
54919	Tab, Orange, Round, 54 Over 919	Ranitidine HCl 168 mg	Zantac by Roxane	00054-4853	Gastrointestinal
54919	Tab, 54 Over 919	Ranitidine HCl 168 mg	by Ridgebury	60921-0097	Gastrointestinal

ID FRONT <> BACK	DESCRIPTION FRONT <> BACK	INGREDIENT & STRENGTH	BRAND (OR EQUIV.) & FIRM	NDC#	CLASS; SCH.
54923	Cap, Blue, 54/923	Acyclovir 200 mg	Zovirax by Roxane	00054-2080	Antiviral
54923	Cap, Blue, 54/923	Acyclovir 200 mg	Zovirax by Roxane	00054-8080	Antiviral
54930	Tab, White, Round, 54-930	Aminophylline 200 mg	Aminophyllin by Roxane	00054-8026	Antiasthmatic
54932	Tab, White, Round, 54-932	Acetaminophen 300 mg, Codeine 60 mg	Tylenol #4 by Roxane		Analgesic; C III
54933	Tab, White, Round	Morphine Sulfate SR 60 mg	MS Contin by Roxane	00054-8792	Analgesic; C II
54939	Tab, Coral, Round, 54-939	Imipramine HCl 10 mg	Tofranil by Roxane		Antidepressant
54942	Tab, White, Round, 54-942	Leucovorin Calcium 10 mg	Wellcovorin by Roxane	00054-8497	Antineoplastic
54943	Tab, Pink, Round, Scored	Dexamethasone 1.5 mg	by DRX	55045-2591	Steroid
54943	Tab, Pink, Round, 54-943	Dexamethasone 1.5 mg	Decadron by Roxane	00054-8181	Steroid
54949	Tab, 54 Over 949	Ranitidine HCl 150 mg	by Eon	00185-0135	Gastrointestinal
54959	Cap, Aqua & Green & Red, 54/959	Mexiletine HCl 250 mg	Mexitil by Roxane	00054-2618	Antiarrhythmic
54959	Cap, Aqua & Green & Red, 54/959	Mexiletine HCl 250 mg	Mexitil by Roxane	00054-8618	Antiarrhythmic
54959	Cap	Mexiletine HCl 250 mg	by Ridgebury	60921-0068	Antiarrhythmic
5496 <> DANDAN	Tab, Buff, Round, Scored	Spironolactone 25 mg, Hydrochlorothiazide 25 mg	by Schein	00364-0513	Diuretic
54960	Tab, Pale Blue, Round, 54/960	Dexamethasone 0.75 mg	Decadron by Roxane	00054-8180	Steroid
54960	Tab, 54/960	Dexamethasone 0.75 mg	by Allscripts	54569-0322	Steroid
54969	Tab, Round, 54-969	Diazepam 2 mg	Valium by Roxane		Antianxiety; C IV
54970	Tab, White, Round, 54-970	Propranolol HCl 10 mg	Inderal by Roxane		Antihypertensive
54972	Cap, Pink, 54-972	Propoxyphene HCl 65 mg	Darvon by Roxane		Analgesic; C IV
549735	Tab, Peach, Round, 54-973 5	Diazepam 5 mg	Valium by Roxane		Antianxiety; C IV
54979	Tab	Quinidine Sulfate 200 mg	by PDRX	55289-0222	Antiarrhythmic
54979200	Tab, White, Round, 54-979 200	Quinidine Sulfate 200 mg	Lin-Qin, Quinova by Roxane	00054-8733	Antiarrhythmic
54980	Tab, Light Blue, Round, 54/980	Cyclophosphamide 50 mg	Cytoxan, Neosar by Roxane	00054-8130	Antineoplastic
54980	Tab, Blue, Round	Cyclophosphamide, Anhydrous 50 mg	by Roxane	00054-4130	Antineoplastic
5498210	Tab, Peach, Round	Diazepam 10 mg	Valium by Roxane		Antianxiety; C IV
54983	Tab, White, Round, 54-983	Amitriptyline 10 mg	Elavil by Roxane		Antidepressant
54989	Cap, Green	Phendimetrazine Tartrate 105 mg	by Allscripts	54569-0395	Anorexiant; C III
54989	Cap, Celery & Green	Phendimetrazine Tartrate 105 mg	by Roxane	00054-2719	Anorexiant; C III
54992	Tab, Pink, Oblong, 54-992	Naproxen 375 mg	Naproxyn by Roxane	00054-8642	NSAID
549HD10	Tab, Blue, Round	Diazepam 10 mg	Valium by Halsey		Antianxiety; C IV
55 <> PAR	Tab, Sugar Coated	Imipramine HCl 25 mg	by Par	49884-0055	Antidepressant
55 50 <> BMS	Tab, Coated, Slightly Mottled	Diltiazem HCl 30 mg	by Golden State	60429-0061	Antihypertensive
550	Tab, Pinkish Purple, Oval, Schering Logo 550	Fluphenazine HCl 5 mg	Permitil by Schering	00085-0550	Antipsychotic
550 <> 358	Tab	Amiloride HCl 5 mg, Hydrochlorothiazide 50 mg	by United Res	00677-1223	Diuretic
550 <> N533	Tab, Light Blue, Coated	Naproxen Sodium 550 mg	by HL Moore	00839-7890	NSAID
550 <> N533	Tab, Film Coated	Naproxen Sodium 550 mg	by Major	00904-5041	NSAID
550 <> N533	Tab, Film Coated, N Over 533	Naproxen Sodium 550 mg	by Quality Care	60346-0826	NSAID
550 <> N533	Tab, White, Oval, Film Coated, N Over 533	Naproxen Sodium 550 mg	by Novopharm	55953-0533	NSAID
550 <> PFIZER	Tab, White, Rectangular	Cetirizine HCl 5 mg	Zyrtec by Pfizer	00069-5500	Antihistamine
550 <> R	Tab, White, Round, Enteric Coated	Diclofenac Sodium 50 mg	DR by Purepac	00228-2550	NSAID
550 <> SCS	Tab, White, Round, 5/50 <> SCS	Ogestral (Norgestrel 0.5 mg Ethinyl Estradiol .05 mg)	Ovral by Watson	52544-0848	Hormone
5500MG <> WATSON737	Cap, 5-500 mg <> Watson over 737	Acetaminophen 500 mg, Oxycodone HCl 5 mg	by Watson	52544-0737	Analgesic; C II
5501 <> DAN	Tab, White, Oval, Sublingual	Ergoloid Mesylates 1 mg	by Schein	00364-0446	Ergot
5502 <> DAN	Tab, White, Round, Sublingual	Ergoloid Mesylates 0.5 mg	by Schein	00364-0415	Ergot
5503 <> DAN	Tab, Amber-Yellow, Round	Sulfasalazine 500 mg	by Schein	00364-0444	Gastrointestinal
5504 <> DAN	Tab, White, Round	Ergoloid Mesylates 1 mg	by Schein	00364-0622	Ergot
5507 <> DAN	Tab, Yellow, Round	Chlorthalidone 25 mg	by Schein	00364-0564	Diuretic
5507 <> DAN	Tab, Orange, Round	Chlorthalidone 25 mg	by Schein	00364-0592	Diuretic
5508 <> DANDAN	Tab, White, Round, Scored	Tolbutamide 500 mg	by Schein	00364-0477	Antidiabetic
550HD	Tab, White, Round	Glutethimide 500 mg	Doriden by Halsey		Hypnotic
551 <> PFIZER	Tab, Rectangle Shape with Rounded Edges, Film Coated	Cetirizine HCl 10 mg	Zyrtec by Quality Care	60346-0036	Antihistamine

ID FRONT <> BACK	DESCRIPTION FRONT <> BACK	INGREDIENT & STRENGTH	BRAND (OR EQUIV.) & FIRM	NDC#	CLASS; SCH.
551 <> PFIZER	Tab, Rounded Rectangle, Film Coated	Cetirizine HCl 10 mg	Zyrtec by PDRX	55289-0108	Antihistamine
551 <> PFIZER	Tab, White, Rectangular, Film Coated	Cetirizine HCl 10 mg	Zyrtec by Pfizer	00069-5510	Antihistamine
551 <> PFIZER	Tab, Rectangular, Film Coated	Cetirizine HCl 10 mg	Zyrtec by Caremark	00339-6097	Antihistamine
551 <> PFIZER	Tab, Film Coated	Cetirizine HCl 10 mg	Zyrtec by Allscripts	54569-4290	Antihistamine
551 <> PFIZER	Tab, Rounded Rectangular,Film Coated	Cetirizine HCl 10 mg	Zyrtec by Physicians Total Care	54868-3876	Antihistamine
551 <> R	Tab, White, Round, Enteric Coated	Diclofenac Sodium 75 mg	DR by Purepac	00228-2551	NSAID
5513 <> DAN	Tab, White, Round	Carisoprodol 350 mg	by Kaiser Fdn	00179-1349	Muscle Relaxant
5513 <> DAN	Tab, White, Round	Carisoprodol 350 mg	by Schein	00364-0475	Muscle Relaxant
5513 <> DAN	Tab	Carisoprodol 350 mg	by Danbury	00591-5513	Muscle Relaxant
5513 <> DAN	Tab	Carisoprodol 350 mg	by Urgent Care Ctr	50716-0202	Muscle Relaxant
5513 <> DAN	Tab	Carisoprodol 350 mg	by Allscripts	54569-3403	Muscle Relaxant
5513 <> DAN	Tab	Carisoprodol 350 mg	by Allscripts	54569-1709	Muscle Relaxant
5513 <> DAN	Tab	Carisoprodol 350 mg	by Quality Care	60346-0635	Muscle Relaxant
5515 <> DANDAN	Tab	Bethanechol Chloride 50 mg	by Danbury	00591-5515	Urinary Tract
5515 <> DANDAN	Tab, Yellow, Round, Scored	Bethanechol Chloride 50 mg	by Schein	00364-0590	Urinary Tract
5516 <> DAN	Tab, White, Round	Quinine Sulfate 260 mg	by Schein	00364-0560	Antimalarial
5518 <> DAN	Tab, Light Blue, Round	Chlorthalidone 50 mg	by Schein	00364-0593	Diuretic
5518 <> DAN	Tab, Light Green, Round	Chlorthalidone 50 mg	by Schein	00364-0528	Diuretic
5520DAN	Cap, Black & Yellow	Tetracycline HCl 500 mg	by Schein	00364-2029	Antibiotic
5522 <> DAN	Tab, Coated	Hydroxyzine HCl 10 mg	by Danbury	00591-5522	Antihistamine
5522 <> DAN	Tab, Orange, Round, Film Coated	Hydroxyzine HCl 10 mg	by Schein	00364-0494	Antihistamine
5522 <> DAN	Tab, Coated	Hydroxyzine HCl 10 mg	by Heartland	61392-0012	Antihistamine
5523 <> DAN	Tab, Green, Round, Film Coated	Hydroxyzine HCl 25 mg	by Schein	00364-0495	Antihistamine
5523 <> DAN	Tab, Film Coated	Hydroxyzine HCl 25 mg	by Quality Care	60346-0086	Antihistamine
5523 <> DAN	Tab, Film Coated	Hydroxyzine HCl 25 mg	by Heartland	61392-0013	Antihistamine
5523 <> DAN	Tab, Film Coated	Hydroxyzine HCl 25 mg	by Vangard	00615-1526	Antihistamine
5523 <> DAN	Tab, Film Coated	Hydroxyzine HCl 25 mg	by Danbury	00591-5523	Antihistamine
5535DAN	Cap, Blue & White	Doxycycline Hyclate 50 mg	by Schein	00364-2032	Antibiotic
5538 <> DAN	Tab	Quinidine Gluconate 324 mg	by Danbury	00591-5538	Antiarrhythmic
5538 <> DAN	Tab, Off-White, Round	Quinidine Gluconate 324 mg	by Schein	00364-0604	Antiarrhythmic
554 <> R	Tab, Film Coated	Metoprolol Tartrate 50 mg	by Vangard	00615-3552	Antihypertensive
5540 <> DAN	Tab	Metronidazole 250 mg	by Danbury	00591-5540	Antibiotic
5540 <> DAN	Tab, Off-White to White, Round	Metronidazole 250 mg	by Schein	00364-0595	Antibiotic
5540 <> DAN	Tab	Metronidazole 250 mg	by Nat Pharmpak Serv	55154-5212	Antibiotic
5540 <> DAN	Tab	Metronidazole 250 mg	by Allscripts	54569-0965	Antibiotic
5542 <> DAN25	Tab, Beige, Triangular, Film Coated	Thioridazine HCl 25 mg	by Schein	00364-0662	Antipsychotic
5543 <> DANDAN	Tab	Allopurinol 100 mg	by Quality Care	60346-0774	Antigout
5543 <> DANDAN	Tab	Allopurinol 100 mg	by Danbury	61955-0632	Antigout
5543 <> DANDAN	Tab, White, Round, Scored	Allopurinol 100 mg	by Natl Pharmpak	55154-5239	Antigout
5543 <> DANDAN	Tab	Allopurinol 100 mg	by Danbury	00591-5543	Antigout
5543 <> DANDAN	Tab, White, Round, Scored	Allopurinol 100 mg	by Schein	00364-0632	Antigout
5544	Tab	Allopurinol 300 mg	by Nat Pharmpak Serv	55154-5216	Antigout
5544 <> DANDAN	Tab	Allopurinol 300 mg	by Danbury	61955-0633	Antigout
5544 <> DANDAN	Tab, Orange, Round, Scored	Allopurinol 300 mg	by Schein	00364-0633	Antigout
5544 <> DANDAN	Tab	Allopurinol 300 mg	by Danbury	00591-5544	Antigout
5544DAN	Tab	Allopurinol 300 mg	by Med Pro	53978-5001	Antigout
5546 <> DANDAN	Tab, White, Round, Scored	Sulfamethoxazole 400 mg, Trimethoprim 80 mg	by Schein	00364-2068	Antibiotic
5546 <> DANDAN	Tab	Sulfamethoxazole 400 mg, Trimethoprim 80 mg	by Danbury	00591-5546	Antibiotic
5546 <> DANDAN	Tab	Sulfamethoxazole 400 mg, Trimethoprim 80 mg	by Allscripts	54569-0269	Antibiotic
5547 <> DAN	Tab, White, Oval, Scored	Sulfamethoxazole 800 mg, Trimethoprim 160 mg	by Va Cmop	65243-0067	Antibiotic
5547 <> DANDAN	Tab	Sulfamethoxazole 800 mg, Trimethoprim 160 mg	by Danbury	00591-5547	Antibiotic
5547 <> DANDAN	Tab, White, Oval, Scored	Sulfamethoxazole 800 mg, Trimethoprim 160 mg	by Schein	00364-2069	Antibiotic

ID FRONT ◇ BACK	DESCRIPTION FRONT ◇ BACK	INGREDIENT & STRENGTH	BRAND (OR EQUIV.) & FIRM	NDC#	CLASS; SCH.
5547 ◇ DANDAN	Tab	Sulfamethoxazole 800 mg, Trimethoprim 160 mg	Trimeth Sulfa DS by Pharmedix	53002-0210	Antibiotic
5548 ◇ DANDAN	Tab, White, Round, Scored	Chloroquine Phosphate 250 mg	by Schein	00364-0470	Antimalarial
5549 ◇ DAN	Tab, White, Round, Film Coated	Chloroquine Phosphate 500 mg	by Schein	00364-2431	Antimalarial
555 ◇ 822	Tab, White, Trisected, MJ Logo	Buspirone HCl 15 mg	Buspar by Bristol Myers Squibb	00087-0822	Antianxiety
555 ◇ MJ822	Tab, White, Rectangle, Scored	Buspirone HCl 15 mg	Buspar by WalMart	49035-0188	Antianxiety
555 ◇ MYLAN	Tab	Naproxen 375 mg	by Kaiser	62224-4552	NSAID
555 ◇ MYLAN	Tab, Mylan	Naproxen 375 mg	by Quality Care	60346-0817	NSAID
555 ◇ MYLAN	Tab, White, Oblong	Naproxen 375 mg	by Dixon Shane	17236-0077	NSAID
555 ◇ MYLAN	Tab, White	Naproxen 375 mg	by Mylan	00378-0555	NSAID
555 ◇ MYLAN	Tab	Naproxen 375 mg	by Kaiser	00179-1187	NSAID
555 ◇ MYLAN	Tab	Naproxen 375 mg	by Allscripts	54569-3759	NSAID
555 ◇ MYLAN	Tab, White, Capsule-Shaped	Naproxen 375 mg	Naprosyn by UDL	51079-0794	NSAID
555 ◇ MYLAN	Tab	Naproxen 375 mg	by HJ Harkins Co	52959-0191	NSAID
5550 ◇ BMS	Tab, Coated, Mottled	Diltiazem HCl 60 mg	by ER Squibb	00003-5550	Antihypertensive
5550 ◇ BMS	Tab, Coated, Bisect Bar	Diltiazem HCl 60 mg	by Golden State	60429-0062	Antihypertensive
5550 ◇ BMS	Tab, Mottled Clear, Film Coated, Scored	Diltiazem HCl 60 mg	by Med Pro	53978-1235	Antihypertensive
555013 ◇ BARR	Tab, Coated	Erythromycin Stearate 250 mg	by Barr	00555-0013	Antibiotic
555013BARR	Tab, Red, Round, 555/013 Barr	Erythromycin Stearate 250 mg	Erythrocin by Barr		Antibiotic
555064	Tab, Orange, Round, 555/064	Hydralazine HCl 25 mg	Apresoline by Barr		Antihypertensive
555065	Tab, Orange, Round, 555/065	Hydralazine HCl 50 mg	Apresoline by Barr		Antihypertensive
555089	Tab, White, Round, 555/089	Propylthiouracil 50 mg	by Barr		Antithyroid
555126	Tab, Blue, Round, 555/126	Decyclomine HCl 20 mg	Bentyl by Barr		Gastrointestinal
555153LLP21	Tab, White, Round, 555/153 LL P21	Phenobarbital 30 mg	by Lederle		Sedative/Hypnotic; C IV
555157BARR	Tab, Peach, Round, 555/157 Barr	Prednisone 20 mg	Deltasone by Barr		Steroid
555163 ◇ BARR	Tab, White, Round, Scored	Diazepam 2 mg	by Southwood Pharms	58016-0274	Antianxiety; C IV
555163 ◇ BARR	Tab, 555/163 ◇ Barr	Diazepam 2 mg	by Barr	00555-0163	Antianxiety; C IV
555164 ◇ BARR	Tab, 555/164	Diazepam 10 mg	by Quality Care	60346-0033	Antianxiety; C IV
555164 ◇ BARR	Tab, Blue, Round, Scored	Diazepam 10 mg	by Southwood Pharms	58016-0273	Antianxiety; C IV
555164 ◇ BARR	Tab, 555/164 ◇ Barr	Diazepam 10 mg	by Barr	00555-0164	Antianxiety; C IV
555169BARR	Tab, White, Round, 555/169 Barr	Furosemide 40 mg	Lasix by Barr		Diuretic
555174	Tab, Pink, Round, 555/174	Isosorbide Dinitrate 5 mg	Isordil by Barr		Antianginal
555175	Tab, White, Round, 555/175	Isosorbide Dinitrate 10 mg	Isordil by Barr		Antianginal
555186	Tab, Green, Round, 555/186	Isosorbide Dinitrate 20 mg	Isordil by Barr		Antianginal
555188BARR	Tab, White, Round, 555/188 Barr	Quinidine Sulfate 200 mg	by Barr		Antiarrhythmic
55519	Tab, Flat-faced, Bevel-edged, 555/19	Hydrochlorothiazide 25 mg	by Barr	00555-0019	Diuretic
555192BARR	Tab, Peach, Round, 555/192 Barr	Hydrochlorothiazide HCl 100 mg	Hydrodiuril by Barr		Diuretic
5552 ◇ DAN	Tab	Metronidazole 500 mg	by Nat Pharmpak Serv	55154-5234	Antibiotic
5552 ◇ DANDAN	Tab, Off-White to White, Round	Metronidazole 500 mg	by Schein	00364-0687	Antibiotic
5552 ◇ DANDAN	Tab	Metronidazole 500 mg	by Danbury	00591-5552	Antibiotic
55520	Tab, 555/20	Hydrochlorothiazide 50 mg	by Barr	00555-0020	Diuretic
555200	Tab, White, Round, 555/200	Diphenoxylate HCl 2.5 mg, Atropine Sulfate 0.025 mg	Lomotil by Barr		Antidiarrheal; C V
555210	Tab, Brown, Round, 555/210	Amitriptyline HCl 50 mg	Elavil by Barr		Antidepressant
555211	Tab, Purple, Round, 555/211	Amitriptyline HCl 75 mg	Elavil by Barr		Antidepressant
555212	Tab, Orange & Red, Round	Amitriptyline HCl 100 mg	Elavil by Barr		Antidepressant
555233	Tab, 555/233	Prednisone 10 mg	by Barr	00555-0233	Steroid
555241BARR	Tab, White, Round, 555/241 Barr	Allopurinol 100 mg	Zyloprim by Barr		Antigout
555242	Tab, Peach, Round, 555/242	Allopurinol 300 mg	Zyloprim by Barr		Antigout
555251	Tab, White, Round, 555/251	Tolbutamide 500 mg	Orinase by Barr		Antidiabetic
555255	Tab, Green, Round, 555/255	Chlorzoxazone 250 mg, Acetaminophen 300 mg	Parafon Forte by Barr		Muscle Relaxant
55526	Tab, White, Round, 555/26	Prednisone 5 mg	Deltasone by Barr		Steroid
555265	Tab, 555/265 Debossed	Hydrochlorothiazide 25 mg, Spironolactone 25 mg	by Barr	00555-0265	Diuretic; Antihypertensive

ID FRONT <> BACK	DESCRIPTION FRONT <> BACK	INGREDIENT & STRENGTH	BRAND (OR EQUIV.) & FIRM	NDC#	CLASS; SCH.
555266	Tab, 555/266 Debossed	Spironolactone 25 mg	by Barr	00555-0266	Diuretic
555271 <> BARR	Tab, 555/271 Debossed	Sulfinpyrazone 100 mg	by Barr	00555-0271	Uricosuric
555278	Tab, 555/278	Acetaminophen 325 mg, Oxycodone HCl 5 mg	by Barr	00555-0278	Analgesic; C II
555279	Tab, Blue, Round, 555/279	Isosorbide Dinitrate 30 mg	Isordil by Barr		Antianginal
555288	Tab, Green, Round, 555/288	Isosorbide Dinitrate Oral 40 mg	Isordil by Barr		Antianginal
555293BARR	Tab, Yellow, Round, 555/293 Barr	Oxycodone HCl 4.5 mg, Oxycodone Terephthalate 0.38 mg, Aspirin 325	Percodan by Barr		Analgesic; C II
5553 <> DAN	Tab, Light Orange, Round, Film Coated	Doxycycline Hyclate 100 mg	by Schein	00364-2063	Antibiotic
5553 <> DAN	Tab, Orange, Round, Film Coated	Doxycycline Hyclate	by Murfreesboro Ph	51129-1357	Antibiotic
5553 <> DAN	Tab, Film Coated	Doxycycline Hyclate	by Danbury	00591-5553	Antibiotic
55535	Tab, White, Round, 555/35	Meprobamate 200 mg	Miltown by Barr		Sedative/Hypnotic; C IV
55536	Tab, 555/36 Debossed	Meprobamate 400 mg	by Barr	00555-0036	Sedative/Hypnotic; C IV
555363 <> BARR	Tab, 555/363	Diazepam 5 mg	by Quality Care	60346-0478	Antianxiety; C IV
555363 <> BARR	Tab, Yellow, Round, Scored	Diazepam 5 mg	by Southwood Pharms	58016-0275	Antianxiety; C IV
555363 <> BARR	Tab, 555/363	Diazepam 5 mg	by Barr	00555-0363	Antianxiety; C IV
555365	Tab, Peach, Round, 555/365	Propranolol 10 mg	Inderal by Barr		Antihypertensive
555366	Tab, Blue, Round, 555/366	Propranolol 20 mg	Inderal by Barr		Antihypertensive
555367	Tab, Green, Round, 555/367	Propranolol 40 mg	Inderal by Barr		Antihypertensive
555368	Tab, Pink, Round, 555/368	Propranolol 60 mg	Inderal by Barr		Antihypertensive
555369	Tab, Yellow, Round, 555/369	Propranolol 80 mg	Inderal by Barr		Antihypertensive
5553DAN	Tab, Film Coated	Doxycycline Hyclate	by Allscripts	54569-0118	Antibiotic
5554 <> DAN10	Tab, Orange, Round, Scored	Propranolol HCl 10 mg	by Schein	00364-0756	Antihypertensive
555424B	Tab, White, Round, 555/424 B	Metoclopramide 10 mg	Reglan by Barr		Gastrointestinal
555427 <> BARR	Tab, 555/427 Debossed	Hydrochlorothiazide 25 mg, Propranolol HCl 40 mg	by Barr	00555-0427	Diuretic; Antihypertensive
555428 <> BARR	Tab, 555/428 Debossed	Hydrochlorothiazide 25 mg, Propranolol HCl 80 mg	by Barr	00555-0428	Diuretic; Antihypertensive
555429	Tab, White, Round, 555/429	Trimethoprim 100 mg	Trimpex by Barr		Antibiotic
555430	Tab, White, Round, 555/430	Trimethoprim 200 mg	Trimpex by Barr		Antibiotic
555444 <> BARR	Tab, 555/444 <> Debossed	Hydrochlorothiazide 50 mg, Triamterene 75 mg	by Rugby	00536-4927	Diuretic
555444 <> BARR	Tab, 555/444 Debossed	Hydrochlorothiazide 50 mg, Triamterene 75 mg	by Barr	00555-0444	Diuretic
555444 <> BARR	Tab	Hydrochlorothiazide 50 mg, Triamterene 75 mg	by PDRX	55289-0488	Diuretic
555444 <> BARR	Tab, 555/444	Hydrochlorothiazide 50 mg, Triamterene 75 mg	by Quality Care	60346-0704	Diuretic
555444 <> BARR	Tab, 555/444 Debossed <> Company Logo Debossed	Hydrochlorothiazide 50 mg, Triamterene 75 mg	by Major	00904-1965	Diuretic
555483 <> BARR	Tab, Light Yellow, 555/483 <> Barr	Amiloride HCl 5 mg, Hydrochlorothiazide 50 mg	by Barr	00555-0483	Diuretic
555489 <> BARR	Tab, White, Round, Scored, 555 over 489 <> Barr	Trazodone HCl 50 mg	Desyrel by UDL	51079-0427	Antidepressant
555489 <> BARR	Tab, 555/489 Debossed	Trazodone HCl 50 mg	by Barr	00555-0489	Antidepressant
555489 <> BARR	Tab, Debossed 555/489	Trazodone HCl 50 mg	by Rugby	00536-4715	Antidepressant
555489 <> BARR	Tab, Film Coated, 555/489	Trazodone HCl 50 mg	by Nat Pharmpak Serv	55154-1406	Antidepressant
555490 <> BARR	Tab, Debossed 555/490	Trazodone HCl 100 mg	by Rugby	00536-4688	Antidepressant
555490 <> BARR	Tab, 555/490 Debossed	Trazodone HCl 100 mg	by Barr	00555-0490	Antidepressant
555490 <> BARR	Tab, White, Round, Scored, 555 over 490 <> Barr	Trazodone HCl 100 mg	Desyrel by UDL	51079-0428	Antidepressant
555490 <> BARR	Tab, 555 Over 490 <> B Printed as Small B with 6-Sided Ring Instead of Circle	Trazodone HCl 100 mg	by Murfreesboro	51129-1131	Antidepressant
555490 <> BARR	Tab, Film Coated, 555/490	Trazodone HCl 100 mg	by Quality Care	60346-0014	Antidepressant
5555 <> DAN20	Tab, Blue, Round, Scored	Propranolol HCl 20 mg	by Schein	00364-0757	Antihypertensive
555585 <> BARR	Tab, Light Green, 555/585	Chlorzoxazone 500 mg	by Quality Care	60346-0663	Muscle Relaxant
555585 <> BARR	Tab, Stylized Barr	Chlorzoxazone 500 mg	by PDRX	55289-0633	Muscle Relaxant
555585 <> BARR	Tab, Green, Round, Scored	Chlorzoxazone 500 mg	by Direct Dispensing	57866-3444	Muscle Relaxant
555585 <> BARR	Tab, Light Green, Round, Scored, 555 over 585 <> Barr	Chlorzoxazone 500 mg	Parafon Forte by UDL	51079-0476	Muscle Relaxant
555585 <> BARR	Tab, 555/585	Chlorzoxazone 500 mg	by Barr	00555-0585	Muscle Relaxant
5556 <> DAN40	Tab, Green, Round, Scored	Propranolol HCl 40 mg	by Schein	00364-0758	Antihypertensive
555606 <> B	Tab, White, Round, Scored, 555 Over 606 <> B	Megestrol Acetate 20 mg	Megace by UDL	51079-0434	Progestin

ID FRONT <> BACK	DESCRIPTION FRONT <> BACK	INGREDIENT & STRENGTH	BRAND (OR EQUIV.) & FIRM	NDC#	CLASS; SCH.
555606 <> B	Tab, 555/606 <> Barr Logo	Megestrol Acetate 20 mg	by Barr	00555-0606	Progestin
555606 <> B	Tab, Debossed, 555/606 <> Barr Logo	Megestrol Acetate 20 mg	by Major	00904-3570	Progestin
555607	Tab, Debossed, Barr Logo	Megestrol Acetate 40 mg	by United Res	00677-1206	Progestin
555607 <> B	Tab, Debossed as 555/607	Megestrol Acetate 20 mg	by Supergen	62701-0920	Progestin
555607 <> B	Tab, White, Round, Scored, 555 Over 607 <> B	Megestrol Acetate 40 mg	Megace by UDL	51079-0435	Progestin
555607 <> BARR	Tab, Debossed, 555/607 <> Barr	Megestrol Acetate 40 mg	by Warner Chilcott	00047-0108	Progestin
555607 <> BARR	Tab, 555/607 Debossed	Megestrol Acetate 40 mg	by Rugby	00536-4822	Progestin
555607 <> BARR	Tab, 555/607 Debossed	Megestrol Acetate 40 mg	by Barr	00555-0607	Progestin
555607 <> BARR	Tab, Debossed	Megestrol Acetate 40 mg	by CVS	51316-0239	Progestin
555607 <> BARR	Tab, 555 Over 607 <> Barr	Megestrol Acetate 40 mg	by CVS Revco	00894-6651	Progestin
555607 <> BARR	Tab, 555/607	Megestrol Acetate 40 mg	by Qualitest	00603-4392	Progestin
555607 <> BARR	Tab, 555/607 Beveled	Megestrol Acetate 40 mg	by Major	00904-3571	Progestin
555643 <> BARR	Tab, 555/643 Debossed <> Barr Logo	Hydrochlorothiazide 25 mg, Triamterene 37.5 mg	by Barr	00555-0643	Diuretic
5557 <> DAN80	Tab, Yellow, Round, Scored	Propranolol HCl 80 mg	by Schein	00364-0760	Antihypertensive
555779 <> B	Tab, White, Round, Convex, Scored, 555/779 <> Barr Logo	Medroxyprogesterone Acetate 10 mg	by Nat Pharmpak Serv	55154-5575	Progestin
555779 <> B	Tab, Coated, 555/779 <> b with Carbon Ring	Medroxyprogesterone Acetate 10 mg	by Barr	00555-0779	Progestin
555779 <> B	Tab, Coated, 555/779 Debossed <> Barr Logo	Medroxyprogesterone Acetate 10 mg	by Qualitest	00603-4367	Progestin
555779 <> B	Tab, Coated, Debossed, 555/779	Medroxyprogesterone Acetate 10 mg	by United Res	00677-1619	Progestin
555779 <> B	Tab, Coated, Debossed <> Barr Logo	Medroxyprogesterone Acetate 10 mg	by Major	00904-2690	Progestin
555831 <> BARR	Tab, 555/831, Beveled Edge <> in Lower Case	Warfarin Sodium 1 mg	by Barr	00555-0831	Anticoagulant
555832 <> BARR	Tab, 555/832, Beveled Edge <> in Lower Case	Warfarin Sodium 2.5 mg	by Barr	00555-0832	Anticoagulant
555833 <> BARR	Tab, 555/833	Warfarin Sodium 5 mg	by Barr	00555-0833	Anticoagulant
555834 <> BARR	Tab, 555/834	Warfarin Sodium 7.5 mg	by Barr	00555-0834	Anticoagulant
555835 <> BARR	Tab, 555/835	Warfarin Sodium 10 mg	by Barr	00555-0835	Anticoagulant
555869 <> BARR	Tab, Lavender, Beveled Edge, 555/869, <> in Lower Case	Warfarin Sodium 2 mg	by Barr	00555-0869	Anticoagulant
555872	Tab, Coated, 555/872 <> Barr Logo	Medroxyprogesterone Acetate 2.5 mg	by Barr	00555-0872	Progestin
555872	Tab, White, Round, Convex, Scored, 555/872 <> Barr Logo	MedroxyproGesterone Acetate 2.5 mg	by Nat Pharmpak Serv	55154-5569	Hormone
555872 <> 6	Tab, White, Round, Scored	Medroxyprogesterone Acetate 2.5 mg	by Southwood Pharms	58016-0374	Progestin
555872 <> B	Tab, White, Round, Scored	Medroxyprogesterone Acetate 2.5 mg	by Murfreesboro Ph	51129-1373	Progestin
555872 <> B	Tab, Coated, Debossed 555/872 <> Company Logo	Medroxyprogesterone Acetate 2.5 mg	by United Res	00677-1617	Progestin
555872 <> B	Tab, Coated, Debossed, 555/872	Medroxyprogesterone Acetate 2.5 mg	by Qualitest	00603-4365	Progestin
555873	Tab, White, Round, Convex, Scored, 555/873 <> Barr Logo	MedroxyproGesterone Acetate 5 mg	by Nat Pharmpak Serv	55154-5571	Progestin
555873	Tab, Coated, Debossed <> Barr Logo	Medroxyprogesterone Acetate 5 mg	by Major	00904-5228	Progestin
555873 <> B	Tab, Coated, 555/873 <> b with Carbon Ring as Circle	Medroxyprogesterone Acetate 5 mg	by Barr	00555-0873	Progestin
555873 <> B	Tab, Coated, 555/873 <> b with Carbon Ring as Circle	Medroxyprogesterone Acetate 5 mg	by Qualitest	00603-4366	Progestin
555873 <> B	Tab, Coated, Debossed <> Company Logo	Medroxyprogesterone Acetate 5 mg	by United Res	00677-1618	Progestin
555874 <> BARR	Tab, 555/874	Warfarin Sodium 4 mg	by Barr	00555-0874	Anticoagulant
5560DAN	Cap, Orange, Opaque	Disopyramide Phosphate 100 mg	by Schein	00364-0739	Antiarrhythmic
5561DAN	Cap, Brown, Opaque	Disopyramide Phosphate 150 mg	by Schein	00364-0740	Antiarrhythmic
5562 <> DAN	Tab, White, Oval, Film Coated, Ex Release	Procainamide HCl 250 mg	by Schein	00364-0715	Antiarrhythmic
5562 <> DAN	Tab, Film Coated	Procainamide HCl 250 mg	by Danbury	00591-5562	Antiarrhythmic
5563 <> DANDAN	Tab, White, Oval, Film Coated, Scored, Ex Release	Procainamide HCl 500 mg	by Schein	00364-0716	Antiarrhythmic
5564 <> DANDAN	Tab, White, Oval, Film Coated, Scored, Ex Release	Procainamide HCl 750 mg	by Schein	00364-0717	Antiarrhythmic
5565 <> DAN	Tab, Yellow, Round, Film Coated	Hydroxyzine HCl 50 mg	by Schein	00364-0496	Antihistamine
5565 <> DAN	Tab, Sugar Coated	Hydroxyzine HCl 50 mg	by Allscripts	54569-0409	Antihistamine
5565 <> DAN	Tab, Coated	Hydroxyzine HCl 50 mg	by Med Pro	53978-3186	Antihistamine
5565 <> DAN	Tab, Coated	Hydroxyzine HCl 50 mg	by Quality Care	60346-0796	Antihistamine
5565 <> DAN	Tab, Coated	Hydroxyzine HCl 50 mg	by Danbury	00591-5565	Antihistamine
5566 <> DAN10	Tab, Yellow-Green, Triangular	Thioridazine HCl 10 mg	by Schein	00364-2317	Antipsychotic
5568 <> DAN50	Tab, White, Triangular, Film Coated	Thioridazine HCl 50 mg	by Schein	00364-2318	Antipsychotic
5569 <> DAN	Tab, Orange, Round, Film Coated	Thioridazine HCl 100 mg	by Schein	00364-0670	Antipsychotic
557 <> SL	Tab, Debossed	Naproxen 500 mg	by Sidmak	50111-0557	NSAID

ID FRONT <> BACK	DESCRIPTION FRONT <> BACK	INGREDIENT & STRENGTH	BRAND (OR EQUIV.) & FIRM	NDC#	CLASS; SCH.
557HD	Tab, White, Round	Ibuprofen 200 mg	Advil by Halsey		NSAID
5571 <> DANDAN	Tab, White, Oval, Scored	Trimethoprim 100 mg	by Schein	00364-0649	Antibiotic
5571 <> DANDAN	Tab	Trimethoprim 100 mg	by Danbury	00591-5571	Antibiotic
5572 <> DAN	Tab, White, Round, Film Coated	Thioridazine HCl 15 mg	by Schein	00364-0669	Antipsychotic
5574 <> RUGBY	Cap	Nicardipine HCl 30 mg	by Chelsea	46193-0560	Antihypertensive
5575 <> DANDAN	Tab, White, Round, Scored	Furosemide 40 mg	by Schein	00364-0514	Diuretic
5576 <> DAN	Tab, White, Round	Furosemide 20 mg	by Schein	00364-0568	Diuretic
55779 <> B	Tab, White, Round, Convex, Scored	MedroxyproGesterone Acetate 10 mg	by Nat Pharmpak Serv	55154-5579	Progestin
5579 <> DANDAN	Tab, Blue, Round, Scored	Chlorpropamide 100 mg	by Schein	00364-0699	Antidiabetic
5580 <> DAN	Tab, Orange, Round, Film Coated	Thioridazine HCl 150 mg	by Schein	00364-0723	Antipsychotic
5581 <> DAN	Tab, Orange, Round, Film Coated	Thioridazine HCl 200 mg	by Schein	00364-0724	Antipsychotic
5582 <> DANDAN	Tab, White, Round, Scored	Tolazamide 250 mg	by Schein	00364-0720	Antidiabetic
5584 <> DAN	Tab, White, Round, Film Coated	Ibuprofen 400 mg	by Schein	00364-0765	NSAID
5585 <> DAN	Tab, White, Round, Film Coated	Ibuprofen 200 mg	by Schein	00364-2145	NSAID
5586 <> DAN	Tab, White, Oval, Film Coated	Ibuprofen 600 mg	by Schein	00364-0766	NSAID
5587 <> DAN	Tab, White, Round, Film Coated	Methyldopa 500 mg	by Schein	00364-0708	Antihypertensive
5588 <> DAN	Tab, White, Round, Film Coated	Methyldopa 250 mg	by Schein	00364-0707	Antihypertensive
5589 <> DANDAN	Tab	Metoclopramide HCl	by Quality Care	60346-0802	Gastrointestinal
5589 <> DANDAN	Tab	Metoclopramide HCl	by Danbury	00591-5589	Gastrointestinal
5589 <> DANDAN	Tab, White, Round, Scored	Metoclopramide HCl 10 mg	by Schein	00364-0769	Gastrointestinal
559HD	Tab, White, Round	Ibuprofen 400 mg	Motrin by Halsey		NSAID
5590 <> DANDAN	Tab, White, Round, Scored	Tolazamide 500 mg	by Schein	00364-0722	Antidiabetic
5591 <> DANDAN	Tab, White, Round, Scored	Tolazamide 100 mg	by Schein	00364-0721	Antidiabetic
5592DAN	Cap, Light Green, Opaque	Thiothixene 2 mg	by Schein	00364-2167	Antipsychotic
5593DAN	Cap, Yellow, Opaque	Thiothixene 1 mg	by Schein	00364-2166	Antipsychotic
5594DAN	Cap, White, Opaque	Thiothixene 10 mg	by Schein	00364-2169	Antipsychotic
5595DAN	Tab, Orange, Opaque	Thiothixene 5 mg	by Schein	00364-2168	Antipsychotic
5597 <> DANDAN	Tab, White, Cap Shaped, Scored	Acetohexamide 500 mg	by Schein	00364-2233	Antidiabetic
5597 <> DANDAN	Tab	Acetohexamide 500 mg	by Danbury	00591-5597	Antidiabetic
5598 <> DANDAN	Tab, White, Cap Shaped, Scored	Acetohexamide 250 mg	by Schein	00364-2232	Antidiabetic
5598 <> DANDAN	Tab	Acetohexamide 250 mg	by Danbury	00591-5598	Antidiabetic
5599 <> DANDAN	Tab, White, Round, Film Coated, Scored	Trazodone HCl 100 mg	by Schein	00364-2110	Antidepressant
5599 <> DANDAN	Tab, Coated	Trazodone HCl 100 mg	by Danbury	00591-5599	Antidepressant
56 <> PAR	Tab, Sugar Coated	Imipramine HCl 50 mg	by Par	49884-0056	Antidepressant
56 <> PAR	Tab, Sugar Coated, Printed in Black	Imipramine HCl 50 mg	by Amerisource	62584-0751	Antidepressant
56 <> PAR	Tab, Sugar Coated	Imipramine HCl 50 mg	by Quality Care	60346-0709	Antidepressant
56 <> WYETH	Tab	Ethinyl Estradiol 0.05 mg, Norgestrel 0.5 mg	Ovral by Quality Care	60346-0715	Oral Contraceptive
56 <> WYETH	Tab	Ethinyl Estradiol 0.05 mg, Norgestrel 0.5 mg	Ovral by PDRX	55289-0245	Oral Contraceptive
56 <> WYETH	Tab	Ethinyl Estradiol 0.05 mg, Norgestrel 0.5 mg	Ovral by MS Dept Hlth	50596-0026	Oral Contraceptive
560	Tab, White, Cap Shaped, Ascher Logo <> 560	Acetaminophen 500 mg, Melatonin 1.5 mg	Melagesic by B F Ascher	00225-0560	Analgesic, Supplement
560 <> WYETH	Cap	Amoxicillin Trihydrate	Wymox by Allscripts	54569-1509	Antibiotic
560 HD	Tab, White, Oval	Ibuprofen 600 mg	Motrin by Halsey		NSAID
5600 <> DAN	Tab, Film Coated	Trazodone HCl 50 mg	by Allscripts	54569-1470	Antidepressant
5600 <> DANDAN	Tab, Coated	Trazodone HCl 50 mg	by Danbury	00591-5600	Antidepressant
5600 <> DANDAN	Tab, White, Round, Film Coated, Scored	Trazodone HCl 50 mg	by Schein	00364-2109	Antidepressant
5600 <> DANDAN	Tab, Coated	Trazodone HCl 50 mg	by Quality Care	60346-0620	Antidepressant
5601 <> DAN	Tab, Film Coated	Verapamil HCl 80 mg	by Nat Pharmpak Serv	55154-5227	Antihypertensive
5601 <> DANDAN	Tab, White, Round, Film Coated, Scored	Verapamil HCl 80 mg	by Schein	00364-2111	Antihypertensive
5601 <> DANDAN	Tab, Film Coated	Verapamil HCl 80 mg	by Amerisource	62584-0888	Antihypertensive
5601 <> DANDAN	Tab, Film Coated	Verapamil HCl 80 mg	by Danbury	00591-5601	Antihypertensive
5602 <> DANDAN	Tab, 5602 <> Dan/Dan	Clonidine HCl 0.2 mg	by Nat Pharmpak Serv	55154-5229	Antihypertensive
5602 <> DANDAN	Tab, White, Round, Coated, Scored	Verapamil HCl 120 mg	by Schein	00364-2112	Antihypertensive

ID FRONT <> BACK	DESCRIPTION FRONT <> BACK	INGREDIENT & STRENGTH	BRAND (OR EQUIV.) & FIRM	NDC#	CLASS; SCH.
5602 <> DANDAN	Tab, Coated	Verapamil HCl 120 mg	by Amerisource	62584-0889	Antihypertensive
5602 <> DANDAN	Tab, Coated	Verapamil HCl 120 mg	by Danbury	00591-5602	Antihypertensive
5603 <> DAN2	Tab, Yellow, Round, Scored	Haloperidol 2 mg	by Schein	00364-2206	Antipsychotic
5604 <> DAN1	Tab, Peach, Round, Scored	Haloperidol 1 mg	by Schein	00364-2205	Antipsychotic
5605 <> DAN05	Tab, White, Round, Scored, 5605 <> Dan 0.5	Haloperidol 0.5 mg	by Schein	00364-2204	Antipsychotic
5606 <> DAN5	Tab, Blue, Round, Scored	Haloperidol 5 mg	by Schein	00364-2207	Antipsychotic
5607 <> DAN15	Tab, White, Round, Film Coated	Methyldopa 250 mg, Hydrochlorothiazide 15 mg	by Schein	00364-0827	Antihypertensive
5608 <> DAN25	Tab, White, Round, Film Coated	Methyldopa 250 mg, Hydrochlorothiazide 25 mg	by Schein	00364-0828	Antihypertensive
5609 <> DAN01	Tab, White, Pentagonal, Scored, 5609 <> Dan 0.1	Clonidine HCl 0.1 mg	by Schein	00364-0820	Antihypertensive
561 <> JSP	Tab, Olive, Round, Scored	Levothyroxine Sodium 88 mg	Unithroid by Watson	52544-0905	Antithyroid
561HD	Tab, White, Oblong	Metoclopramide HCl 10 mg	Reglan by Halsey		Gastrointestinal
5610 <> DAN50	Tab, White, Round, Film Coated, Scored	Methyldopa 500 mg, Hydrochlorothiazide 50 mg	by Schein	00364-2401	Antihypertensive
5611 <> DAN30	Tab, White, Round, Film Coated	Methyldopa 500 mg, Hydrochlorothiazide 30 mg	by Schein	00364-2400	Antihypertensive
5612 <> DAN02	Tab, Light Yellow, Pentagonal, Scored, 5612 <> Dan 0.2	Clonidine HCl 0.2 mg	by Schein	00364-0821	Antihypertensive
5613 <> DAN03	Tab, Light Blue, Pentagonal, Scored, 5613 <> Dan 0.3	Clonidine HCl 0.3 mg	by Schein	00364-0824	Antihypertensive
5614DAN	Cap, Blue & White	Flurazepam HCl 15 mg	by Schein	00364-0801	Hypnotic; C IV
5615DAN	Cap, Blue	Flurazepam HCl 30 mg	by Schein	00364-0802	Hypnotic; C IV
5616DAN	Cap, Red	Oxazepam 15 mg	by Schein	00364-2152	Sedative/Hypnotic; C IV
5617DAN	Cap, White	Oxazepam 10 mg	by Schein	00364-2154	Sedative/Hypnotic; C IV
5618DAN	Cap, Maroon	Oxazepam 30 mg	by Schein	00364-2153	Sedative/Hypnotic; C IV
5619 <> DAN5	Tab, Yellow, Round, Scored	Diazepam 5 mg	by Schein	00364-0775	Antianxiety; C IV
561MD	Tab, White, Oval	Methylphenidate HCl 10 mg	Metadate by Medeva Pharms	53014-0593	Stimulant; C II
561MD	Tab, White, Oval	Methylphenidate HCl 10 mg	Metadate ER by Medeva Pharms Ca	43567-0561	Stimulant; C II
562 <> JSP	Tab, Rose, Round, Scored	Levothyroxine Sodium 112 mg	Unithroid by Watson	52544-0907	Antithyroid
5620 <> DAN10	Tab, Light Blue, Round, Scored	Diazepam 10 mg	by Schein	00364-0776	Antianxiety; C IV
5621 <> DAN2	Tab, White, Round, Scored	Diazepam 2 mg	by Schein	00364-0774	Antianxiety; C IV
5622 <> DAN2	Tab, White, Round, Scored	Lorazepam 2 mg	by Schein	00364-0795	Sedative/Hypnotic; C IV
5624 <> DAN1	Tab, White, Round, Scored	Lorazepam 1 mg	by Schein	00364-0794	Sedative/Hypnotic; C IV
5624DAN <> 1	Tab	Lorazepam 1 mg	by Quality Care	60346-0047	Sedative/Hypnotic; C IV
5625 <> DAN05	Tab, White, Round, Scored, 5625 <> Dan 0.5	Lorazepam 0.5 mg	by Schein	00364-0793	Sedative/Hypnotic; C IV
5629DAN	Cap, Buff	Doxepin HCl 10 mg	by Schein	00364-2113	Antidepressant
562HD	Tab, Peach, Round	Brompheniramine Maleate 4 mg	Dimetane by Halsey		Antihistamine
562MD	Tab, White, Round	Methylphenidate HCl 20 mg	Metadate by Medeva Pharms	53014-0594	Stimulant; C II
562MD	Tab	Methylphenidate HCl 20 mg	by Caremark	00339-4099	Stimulant; C II
562MD	Tab	Methylphenidate HCl 20 mg	by Int'l Med Systems	00548-7029	Stimulant; C II
562MD	Tab	Methylphenidate HCl 20 mg	by MD	43567-0562	Stimulant; C II
563 <> JSP	Tab, Lilac, Round, Scored	Levothyroxine Sodium 175 mg	Unithroid by Watson	52544-0910	Antithyroid
563 <> SL	Tab, Yellow, Round, Film Coated	Cyclobenzaprine HCl 10 mg	Flexeril by Sidmak	50111-0563	Muscle Relaxant
5630DAN	Cap, Ivory, Opaque	Doxepin HCl 25 mg	by Schein	00364-2114	Antidepressant
5631DAN	Cap, Ivory, Opaque	Doxepin HCl 50 mg	by Schein	00364-2115	Antidepressant
5632DAN	Cap, Green, Opaque	Doxepin HCl 75 mg	by Schein	00364-2116	Antidepressant
5633DAN	Cap, Green, Opaque	Doxepin HCl 100 mg	by Schein	00364-2117	Antidepressant
5636DAN	Cap, Coral	Meclofenamate Sodium 50 mg	by Schein	00364-2155	NSAID
5637 <> DAN	Cap, Coraled	Meclofenamate Sodium	by Quality Care	60346-0350	NSAID
5637DAN	Cap, Coral & White	Meclofenamate Sodium 100 mg	by Schein	00364-2156	NSAID
5642 <> DAN25	Tab, White, Round, Scored, 5642 <> Dan 2.5	Minoxidil 2.5 mg	by Schein	00364-2172	Antihypertensive
5643 <> DAN10	Tab, White, Round, Scored	Minoxidil 10 mg	by Schein	00364-2173	Antihypertensive
5644 <> DAN	Tab, White, Oval, Film Coated	Ibuprofen 800 mg	by Schein	00364-2137	NSAID
5658 <> DAN	Tab, White, Round, Film Coated	Cyclobenzaprine HCl 10 mg	by Schein	00364-2348	Muscle Relaxant
5658 <> DAN	Tab, Film Coated	Cyclobenzaprine HCl 10 mg	by Danbury	00591-5658	Muscle Relaxant
5658 <> DAN	Tab, Film Coated	Cyclobenzaprine HCl 10 mg	by Vangard	00615-3520	Muscle Relaxant
5658 <> DAN	Tab, Film Coated	Cyclobenzaprine HCl 10 mg	by Nat Pharmpak Serv	55154-5217	Muscle Relaxant

ID FRONT <> BACK	DESCRIPTION FRONT <> BACK	INGREDIENT & STRENGTH	BRAND (OR EQUIV.) & FIRM	NDC#	CLASS; SCH.
5658 <> DAN	Tab, Film Coated	Cyclobenzaprine HCl 10 mg	by Heartland	61392-0830	Muscle Relaxant
5658 <> DAN	Tab, Film Coated	Cyclobenzaprine HCl 10 mg	by Amerisource	62584-0354	Muscle Relaxant
5658 <> DAN	Tab, Film Coated	Cyclobenzaprine HCl 10 mg	by Heartland	61392-0098	Muscle Relaxant
5658 <> DAN	Tab, Film Coated	Cyclobenzaprine HCl 10 mg	by PDRX	55289-0567	Muscle Relaxant
5658 <> DAN	Tab, Film Coated	Cyclobenzaprine HCl 10 mg	by Quality Care	60346-0581	Muscle Relaxant
5658 <> DAN	Tab, White, Round	Cyclobenzaprine HCl 10 mg	by Southwood Pharms	58016-0234	Muscle Relaxant
5659 <> DANDAN	Tab, White, Round, Scored	Furosemide 80 mg	by Schein	00364-0700	Diuretic
565HD05	Tab, White, Round, 565 HD 0.5	Lorazepam 0.5 mg	Ativan by Halsey		Sedative/Hypnotic; C IV
5660 <> 60	Tab, Yellow, Round, Scored	Isosorbide Mononitrate 60 mg	by Zenith Goldline	00172-5660	Antianginal
5660 <> DANDAN	Tab	Sulindac 200 mg	by Danbury	00591-5660	NSAID
5660 <> DANDAN	Tab, Yellow, Round, Scored	Sulindac 200 mg	by Schein	00364-2442	NSAID
5660 <> DANDAN	Tab	Sulindac 200 mg	by Allscripts	54569-4032	NSAID
5660 <> DANDAN	Tab	Sulindac 200 mg	by HJ Harkins Co	52959-0195	NSAID
5660 <> DANDAN	Tab	Sulindac 200 mg	by St Marys Med	60760-0424	NSAID
5660 <> DANDAN	Tab	Sulindac 200 mg	by PDRX	55289-0930	NSAID
5660 <> DANDAN	Tab, 56/60 <> Dan/Dan	Sulindac 200 mg	by Quality Care	60346-0686	NSAID
5661 <> DAN	Tab	Sulindac 150 mg	by Danbury	00591-5661	NSAID
5661 <> DAN	Tab, Yellow, Round	Sulindac 150 mg	by Schein	00364-2441	NSAID
5661 <> DAN	Tab	Sulindac 150 mg	by Quality Care	60346-0044	NSAID
5661 <> DAN	Tab	Sulindac 150 mg	by Direct Dispensing	57866-4621	NSAID
5662 <> DAN	Tab, Off-White, Oval, Scored	Nalidixic Acid 1 gm	by Schein	00364-2325	Antibiotic
5663 <> RUGBY	Tab, Film Coated	Cimetidine 400 mg	by Quality Care	60346-0945	Gastrointestinal
566HD	Tab, White, Round	Butalbital 50 mg, Aspirin 325 mg, Caffeine 40 mg	Fiorinal by Halsey		Analgesic
567 <> HD	Tab	Acetaminophen 325 mg, Butalbital 50 mg, Caffeine 40 mg	by Schein	00364-2297	Analgesic
5677 <> DANDAN	Tab, Off-White, Round, Scored	Nalidixic Acid 500 mg	by Schein	00364-2324	Antibiotic
5678 <> DAN	Tab, White, Round, Film Coated	Chlordiazepoxide 10 mg, Amitriptyline 25 mg	by Schein	00364-2158	Antianxiety; C IV
5679 <> DAN	Tab, Light Green, Round, Film Coated	Chlordiazepoxide 5 mg, Amitriptyline 12.5 mg	by Schein	00364-2157	Antianxiety; C IV
5682 <> DAN	Tab, Yellow, Round, Scored	Triamterene 75 mg, Hydrochlorothiazide 50 mg	by Schein	00364-2242	Diuretic
5693DANPRAZOSIN	Cap, Orange, Opaque	Prazosin 5 mg	by Schein	00364-2391	Antihypertensive
5694DANMINOCYCL	Cap, Yellow, Opaque	Minocycline HCl 50 mg	by Schein	00364-2497	Antibiotic
5695DANMINO CYCLINE100	Cap, Gray & Yellow, Opaque	Minocycline HCl 100 mg	by Schein	00364-2498	Antibiotic
5696DANPRAZOSIN	Cap, Dark Gray, Opaque	Prazosin 2 mg	by Schein	00364-2390	Antihypertensive
5697DANPRAZOSIN	Cap, Yellow, Opaque	Prazosin 1 mg	by Schein	00364-2389	Antihypertensive
57	Tab	Aspirin 800 mg	Zorprin by BASF	10117-0057	Analgesic
57	Tab, White, Round, Scored, Purepac Logo 57	Lorazepam 0.5 mg	by Mylan	55160-0130	Sedative/Hypnotic; C IV
57 <> LOTENSINHCT	Tab, White, Oblong, Scored	Benazepril HCl 5 mg, Hydrochlorothiazide 6.25 mg	Lotensin HCT by Novartis	00083-0057	Antihypertensive; Diuretic
57 <> M	Tab, White, Oblong, Scored	Sucralfate 1000 mg	by Warrick Pharms	59930-1532	Gastrointestinal
57 <> M	Tab, Round	Sucralfate 1000 mg	by Merckle	58107-0001	Gastrointestinal
57 <> P	Tab, White, Round, Scored, Purepac Logo	Lorazepam 0.5 mg	by Nat Pharmpak Serv	55154-1116	Sedative/Hypnotic; C IV
57 <> P	Tab, Coated, Purepac Logo	Lorazepam 0.5 mg	by Quality Care	60346-0363	Sedative/Hypnotic; C IV
57 <> R	Tab, Coated, Engraved	Lorazepam 0.5 mg	by Kaiser	00179-1174	Sedative/Hypnotic; C IV
57 <> R	Tab, White, Round, Coated	Lorazepam 0.5 mg	by Purepac	00228-2057	Sedative/Hypnotic; C IV
570 <> DP	Tab, White, Round	Desogestrel 0.15 mg; Ethinyl Estradiol 0.03 mg	Apri by Allscripts	54569-4878	Oral Contraceptive
5704 <> DANDAN	Tab, White, Cap Shaped, Film Coated, Scored	Fenoprofen Calcium 600 mg	by Schein	00364-2316	NSAID
5706 <> DAN500	Tab, Light Green, Round, Scored	Chlorzoxazone 500 mg	by Schein	00364-2255	Muscle Relaxant
5708DAN	Cap, Gray & Pink, Opaque	Clindamycin HCl 150 mg	by Schein	00364-2337	Antibiotic
571	Tab, White, Round, Film Coated	Indapamide 2.5 mg	by Caremark	00339-6183	Diuretic
571 <> R	Tab, White, Round, Coated	Indapamide 2.5 mg	by Purepac	00228-2571	Diuretic
5710 <> DAN2	Tab, White, Round, Scored	Albuterol 2 mg	by Schein	00364-2438	Antiasthmatic
5711 <> DAN4	Tab, White, Round, Scored	Albuterol 4 mg	by Schein	00364-2439	Antiasthmatic

ID FRONT <> BACK	DESCRIPTION FRONT <> BACK	INGREDIENT & STRENGTH	BRAND (OR EQUIV.) & FIRM	NDC#	CLASS; SCH.
5713 <> DAN25	Tab	Amoxapine 25 mg	by Danbury	00591-5713	Antidepressant
5713 <> DAN25	Tab, White, Round, Scored	Amoxapine 25 mg	by Schein	00364-2432	Antidepressant
5714 <> DAN50	Tab	Amoxapine 50 mg	by Danbury	00591-5714	Antidepressant
5714 <> DAN50	Tab, Orange, Round, Scored	Amoxapine 50 mg	by Schein	00364-2433	Antidepressant
5715 <> DAN100	Tab	Amoxapine 100 mg	by Danbury	00591-5715	Antidepressant
5715 <> DAN100	Tab, Blue, Round, Scored	Amoxapine 100 mg	by Schein	00364-2434	Antidepressant
5716 <> DAN150	Tab, Orange, Round, Scored	Amoxapine 150 mg	by Schein	00364-2435	Antidepressant
5716 <> DAN150	Tab	Amoxapine 150 mg	by Danbury	00591-5716	Antidepressant
572	Tab, Coated, Debossed, Barr Logo	Methotrexate 2.5 mg	by Rugby	00536-3998	Antineoplastic
572	Tab, Coated, Debossed, Barr Logo	Methotrexate 2.5 mg	by United Res	00677-1610	Antineoplastic
572 <> B	Tab, Coated	Methotrexate 2.5 mg	by Qualitest	00603-4499	Antineoplastic
5721 <> RUGBY	Tab, Film Coated	Ketorolac Tromethamine 10 mg	by Rugby	00536-5721	NSAID
5721 <> RUGBY	Tab, Film Coated	Ketorolac Tromethamine 10 mg	by Chelsea	46193-0564	NSAID
5721DAN	Cap, Flesh & Pink	Fenoprofen Calcium 300 mg	by Schein	00364-2315	NSAID
5724 <> DAN10	Tab, White, Round, Scored	Metaproterenol Sulfate 10 mg	by Schein	00364-2283	Antiasthmatic
5725 <> DAN20	Tab, White, Round, Scored	Metaproterenol Sulfate 20 mg	by Schein	00364-2284	Antiasthmatic
5725 <> RUGBY	Cap	Acyclovir 200 mg	by Rugby	00536-5725	Antiviral
5725 <> RUGBY	Cap	Acyclovir 200 mg	by Chelsea	46193-0569	Antiviral
5726 <> DAN	Cap, Dark Green & Light Green	Hydroxyzine Pamoate 25 mg	by Schein	00364-0483	Antihistamine
5726 <> DAN	Cap, Light Green & Dark Green	Hydroxyzine Pamoate 43 mg	by Quality Care	60346-0208	Antihistamine
572HD1	Tab, White, Round	Lorazepam 1 mg	Ativan by Halsey		Sedative/Hypnotic; C IV
573 <> PROVENTIL4	Tab, Film Coated	Albuterol 4 mg	Proventil by PDRX	55289-0634	Antiasthmatic
573 <> PROVENTIL4	Tab, Film Coated	Albuterol 4 mg	Proventil by Amerisource	62584-0463	Antiasthmatic
573HD2	Tab, White, Round	Lorazepam 2 mg	Ativan by Halsey		Sedative/Hypnotic; C IV
5730 <> DAN10	Tab, White, Round, Scored	Baclofen 10 mg	by Schein	00364-2312	Muscle Relaxant
5731 <> DAN20	Tab, White, Round, Scored	Baclofen 20 mg	by Schein	00364-2313	Muscle Relaxant
57344 <> 033	Tab, White, Oblong	Diphenhydramine 50 mg	by AAN Pharm.		Antihistamine
573573 <> PROVENTIL4	Tab, Off-White, Round, 573/573 <> Proventil 4	Albuterol Sulfate 4.8 mg	Proventil by Schering	00085-0573	Antiasthmatic
5736 <> DAN5	Tab, White, Round	Timolol Maleate 5 mg	by Schein	00364-2357	Antihypertensive
5737 <> DAN10	Tab, White, Round, Scored	Timolol Maleate 10 mg	by Schein	00364-2358	Antihypertensive
5738 <> DAN20	Tab, White, Cap Shaped, Scored	Timolol Maleate 20 mg	by Schein	00364-2359	Antihypertensive
574 <> MYLAN	Tab, Orange, Film Coated	Amitriptyline HCl 25 mg, Perphenazine 4 mg	by Mylan	00378-0574	Antipsychotic
574HD	Tab, White, Oblong	Hydrocodone Bitartrate 5 mg, Acetaminophen 500 mg	Vicodin by Halsey		Analgesic; C III
575 <> DP	Tab, Pink, Round	Desogestrel 0.15 mg; Ethinyl Estradiol 0.03 mg	Apri by Allscripts	54569-4878	Oral Contraceptive
5751V	Tab, Tan, Oval	Chlorpheniramine Tannate 8 mg, Phenylephrine Tannate 25 mg, Pyrilamine Tannate 25 mg	by Vintage Pharms		Cold Remedy
5752 <> SCS	Cap, Orange	Piroxicam 10 mg	by Quality Care	60346-0737	NSAID
5752 <> SCS	Cap	Piroxicam 10 mg	by SCS	00905-5752	NSAID
5762 <> SCS	Cap	Piroxicam 20 mg	by SCS	00905-5762	NSAID
5770 <> BMS	Tab, Coated, Mottled	Diltiazem HCl 90 mg	by ER Squibb	00003-5770	Antihypertensive
5777	Tab	Atenolol 50 mg	by Nat Pharmpak Serv	55154-5211	Antihypertensive
5777 <> DAN50	Tab	Atenolol 50 mg	by Danbury	61955-2513	Antihypertensive
5777 <> DAN50	Tab, White, Round, Scored	Atenolol 50 mg	by Schein	00364-2513	Antihypertensive
5777 <> DAN50	Tab	Atenolol 50 mg	by Danbury	00591-5777	Antihypertensive
5778 <> DAN100	Tab, White, Round	Atenolol 100 mg	by Schein	00364-2514	Antihypertensive
5778DAN100	Tab	Atenolol 100 mg	by Danbury	61955-2514	Antihypertensive
5782 <> DAN	Tab, White, Round, Scored	Atenolol 50 mg, Chlorthalidone 25 mg	by Schein	00364-2527	Antihypertensive; Diuretic
5783 <> DAN	Tab, White, Round	Atenolol 100 mg, Chlorthalidone 25 mg	by Schein	00364-2528	Antihypertensive; Diuretic

ID FRONT <> BACK	DESCRIPTION FRONT <> BACK	INGREDIENT & STRENGTH	BRAND (OR EQUIV.) & FIRM	NDC#	CLASS; SCH.
58	Tab, Green, Elongated, Boots Logo 58	Phenyleph 25 mg, Phenylpro 50 mg, Chlorphen 8 mg, Hyosc 0.19 mg, Atro 0.04 mg, Scop 0.01 mg	Ru- by Eon		Cold Remedy
5811V	Tab, Film Coated, 5811/V	Salsalate 500 mg	by Vintage	00254-5811	NSAID
5812 <> V	Tab, Turquoise, Coated, 58 to Left 12 to Right	Salsalate 750 mg	by Quality Care	60346-0034	NSAID
5812V	Tab, Film Coated, 5812/V	Salsalate 750 mg	by Vintage	00254-5812	NSAID
5815 <> 59911	Tab, White, Oblong, Scored	Metoclopramide 10 mg	by A H Robins Co	00031-5815	Gastrointestinal
5816 <> DAN250	Cap, Light Green, Round	Naproxen 250 mg	by Schein	00364-2562	NSAID
5816 <> DAN250	Tab, Green, Round	Naproxen 250 mg	by Danbury Pharma	00591-5816	NSAID
5817 <> DAN375	Tab, Purple, Oblong	Naproxen 375 mg	by Danbury Pharma	00591-5817	NSAID
5817 <> DAN375	Tab, Lavender, Cap Shaped	Naproxen 375 mg	by Schein	00364-2563	NSAID
5818 <> DAN500	Tab, Light Green, Cap Shaped	Naproxen 500 mg	by Schein	00364-2564	NSAID
5818 <> DAN500	Tab, Green, Oblong	Naproxen 500 mg	by Danbury Pharma	00591-5818	NSAID
581HD	Tab, White, Round	Acetaminophen 500 mg	Tylenol by Halsey		Antipyretic
582HD	Tab, White, Round	Quinidine Gluconate 324 mg	Quinaglute by Halsey		Antiarrhythmic
583 <> MJ	Tab, MJ Logo	Ethinyl Estradiol 0.035 mg, Norethindrone 0.4 mg	Ovcon 35 28 by Bristol Myers Squibb	00087-0578	Oral Contraceptive
583 <> MJ	Tab	Ethinyl Estradiol 0.035 mg, Norethindrone 0.4 mg	Ovcon 35 21 by Bristol Myers Squibb	00087-0583	Oral Contraceptive
583 <> MJ	Tab	Ethinyl Estradiol 0.035 mg, Norethindrone 0.4 mg	Ovcon 35 by Physicians Total Care	54868-0509	Oral Contraceptive
584 <> BARR	Cap, Clear & Green	Erythromycin 250 mg	by Murfreesboro Ph	51129-1392	Antibiotic
584 <> MJ	Tab, MJ Logo	Ethinyl Estradiol 0.05 mg, Norethindrone 1 mg	Ovcon 50 28 by Bristol Myers Squibb	00087-0579	Oral Contraceptive
584 <> MJ	Tab	Ethinyl Estradiol 0.05 mg, Norethindrone 1 mg	Ovcon 50 by Physicians Total Care	54868-3772	Oral Contraceptive
584 <> MJ	Tab	Ethinyl Estradiol 0.05 mg, Norethindrone 1 mg	Ovcon 50 28 by Bristol Myers	15548-0579	Oral Contraceptive
5840 <> 59911	Tab, Coated	Guanfacine HCl 1.15 mg	by ESI Lederle	59911-5840	Antihypertensive
5840 <> 59911	Tab, Coated	Guanfacine HCl 1.15 mg	by A H Robins	00031-5840	Antihypertensive
5841 <> 59911	Tab, Coated	Guanfacine HCl 2.3 mg	by ESI Lederle	59911-5841	Antihypertensive
5841 <> 59911	Tab, Light Yellow, Coated	Guanfacine HCl 2.3 mg	by A H Robins	00031-5841	Antihypertensive
5850 <> BMS	Tab, Coated, Mottled	Diltiazem HCl 120 mg	by ER Squibb	00003-5850	Antihypertensive
5858 <> DAN50	Tab, White, Round, Scored	Captopril 50 mg	by Schein	00364-2630	Antihypertensive
5859 <> DAN100	Tab, White, Round, Quadrisected	Captopril 100 mg	by Schein	00364-2631	Antihypertensive
5870 <> 59911	Cap, Transparent	Minocycline HCl	by Quality Care	60346-0831	Antibiotic
5871 <> 59911	Tab, White, Scored	Promethazine HCl 12.5 mg	by Wyeth Pharms	52903-5871	Antiemetic; Antihistamine
5871 <> 59911	Tab, White, Scored	Promethazine HCl 12.5 mg	by ESI Lederle	59911-5871	Antiemetic; Antihistamine
5872 <> 59911	Tab, White, Scored	Promethazine HCl 25 mg	by Wyeth Pharms	52903-5872	Antiemetic; Antihistamine
5873 <> 59911	Tab, White, Scored	Promethazine HCl 50 mg	by Wyeth Pharms	52903-5873	Antiemetic; Antihistamine
5873 <> 59911	Tab, White	Promethazine HCl 50 mg	by ESI Lederle	59911-5873	Antiemetic; Antihistamine
5876 <> 59911	Cap, Pink & White	Oxazepam 10 mg	by Wyeth Pharms	52903-5876	Sedative/Hypnotic; C IV
5876 <> 59911	Cap, Pink & White	Oxazepam 10 mg	by ESI Lederle	59911-5876	Sedative/Hypnotic; C IV
5877 <> 59911	Cap, Orange & White	Oxazepam 15 mg	by Wyeth Pharms	52903-5877	Sedative/Hypnotic; C IV
5877 <> 59911	Cap, Orange & White	Oxazepam 15 mg	by ESI Lederle	59911-5877	Sedative/Hypnotic; C IV
5878 <> 59911	Cap, Blue & White	Oxazepam 30 mg	by Wyeth Pharms	52903-5878	Sedative/Hypnotic; C IV
5878 <> 59911	Cap, Blue & White	Oxazepam 30 mg	by ESI Lederle	59911-5878	Sedative/Hypnotic; C IV
5882 <> DAN5	Tab, Purple, Round	Methylphenidate HCl 5 mg	by Danbury	00591-5882	Stimulant; C II
5882 <> DAN5	Tab, Purple, Round	Methylphenidate HCl 5 mg	by Schein	00364-0561	Stimulant; C II
5883 <> DAN10	Tab, Green, Round, Scored	Methylphenidate HCl 10 mg	by Schein	00364-0479	Stimulant; C II
5883 <> DAN10	Tab, Green, Round, Scored	Methylphenidate HCl 10 mg	by Danbury	00591-5883	Stimulant; C II
5884 <> DAN20	Tab, Peach, Round, Scored	Methylphenidate HCl 20 mg	by Danbury	00591-5884	Stimulant; C II
5884 <> DAN20	Tab, Peach, Round, Scored	Methylphenidate HCl 20 mg	by Schein	00364-0562	Stimulant; C II
5887 <> 59911	Cap, Blue & Green	Ketoprofen 100 mg	by Wyeth Pharms	52903-5887	NSAID

ID FRONT <> BACK	DESCRIPTION FRONT <> BACK	INGREDIENT & STRENGTH	BRAND (OR EQUIV.) & FIRM	NDC#	CLASS; SCH.
5888 <> 59911	Cap, Blue & Yellow	Ketoprofen 150 mg	by Wyeth Pharms	52903-5888	NSAID
5889 <> 59911	Cap, Blue & White	Ketoprofen 200 mg	by Wyeth Pharms	52903-5889	NSAID
5899 <> 59911	Cap	Potassium Chloride 750 mg	by Quality Care	60346-0112	Electrolytes
59	Tab, White, Round, Scored, Purepac Logo 59	Lorazepam 1 mg	by Mylan	55160-0131	Sedative/Hypnotic; C IV
59 <> 06	Tab, White, Oblong, Scored	Tramidol 50 mg	by Ultram		Analgesic
59 <> 59	Tab, Wyeth	Penicillin V Potassium	Pen Vee K by Casa De Amigos	62138-0059	Antibiotic
59 <> P	Tab, White, Round, Scored, Purepac Logo	Lorazepam 1 mg	by Nat Pharmpak Serv	55154-1115	Sedative/Hypnotic; C IV
59 <> R	Tab, White, Round, Scored	Lorazepam 0.5 mg	by Allscripts	54569-2687	Sedative/Hypnotic; C IV
59 <> R	Tab, White, Round	Lorazepam 1 mg	by Purepac	00228-2059	Sedative/Hypnotic; C IV
59 <> WYETH	Tab, Flat-faced, Beveled Edges	Penicillin V Potassium	by Kaiser	00179-0081	Antibiotic
59010240	Tab, Light Blue, Cap Shaped, Scored	Acetaminophen 650 mg, Butalbital 50 mg	Bupap by ECR	00095-0240	Analgesic
59010240	Tab, 59010/240	Acetaminophen 650 mg, Butalbital 50 mg	by Mikart	46672-0098	Analgesic
5912 <> DAN	Tab, Blue, Oval, Scored	Captopril 50 mg, Hydrochlorothiazide 25 mg	by Schein	00364-2640	Antihypertensive; Diuretic
591A	Tab, White, Round, Scored, 591-A	Meprobamate 400 mg	by Schein	00364-0161	Sedative/Hypnotic; C IV
591A	Tab, 591-A	Meprobamate 400 mg	by Danbury	00591-5238	Sedative/Hypnotic; C IV
591A	Tab	Meprobamate 400 mg	by Quality Care	62682-7032	Sedative/Hypnotic; C IV
591B	Tab, White, Round, Scored, 591-B	Meprobamate 200 mg	by Schein	00364-0160	Sedative/Hypnotic; C IV
591B	Tab	Meprobamate 200 mg	by Danbury	00591-5239	Sedative/Hypnotic; C IV
591B	Tab, 591-B	Meprobamate 200 mg	by Quality Care	60346-0119	Sedative/Hypnotic; C IV
591C	Tab, White, Round, 591 - C	Phenobarbital 15 mg	by Danbury		Sedative/Hypnotic; C IV
591D	Tab, White, Round, 591 - D	Phenobarbital 30 mg	by Danbury		Sedative/Hypnotic; C IV
591F	Tab, White, Round, 591-F	Butalbital 50 mg, Acetaminophen 325 mg	Fioricet by Danbury		Analgesic
591O	Tab, White, Round, 591 - O	Phenobarbital 100 mg	by Danbury		Sedative/Hypnotic; C IV
591V	Tab, White, Round, 591 - V	Phenobarbital 60 mg	by Danbury		Sedative/Hypnotic; C IV
5925 <> RUGBY	Tab, White, Round	Diethylpropion HCl 25 mg	by Blue Ridge	59273-0007	Antianorexiant; C IV
594	Tab, White, Round, Scored, with an A shaped logo above the 594	Tizanidine 4 mg	Zanaflex by Athena		Muscle Relaxant
597	Tab, Orange, Round, Film Coated	Indapamide 1.25 mg	by Caremark	00339-6182	Diuretic
597 <> R	Tab, Orange, Round, Coated	Indapamide 1.25 mg	by Purepac	00228-2597	Diuretic
59743 <> 003	Cap, Ex Release	Guaifenesin 300 mg, Pseudoephedrine HCl 60 mg	G Phed PD by Pharmafab	62542-0402	Cold Remedy
59743 <> 011	Cap, in White Ink	Acetaminophen 500 mg, Hydrocodone Bitartrate 5 mg	Dolagesic by Alphagen	59743-0011	Analgesic; C III
59743 <> 060	Cap, Clear & Green, Ex Release, with White Beads, 597 43	Brompheniramine Maleate 12 mg, Pseudoephedrine HCl 120 mg	Nasal Decongestant TR by Quality Care	60346-0929	Cold Remedy
59743002	Cap	Guaifenesin 250 mg, Pseudoephedrine HCl 120 mg	G Phed by Pharmafab	62542-0451	Cold Remedy
59743050	Tab, 59743 over 050	Guaifenesin 600 mg, Pseudoephedrine HCl 60 mg	Desal II by Pharmafab	62542-0740	Cold Remedy
59743053	Cap	Chlorpheniramine Maleate 8 mg, Pseudoephedrine HCl 120 mg	D Amine Sr by Pharmafab	62542-0251	Cold Remedy
59743054	Tab, 59743/054	Dextromethorphan Hydrobromide 30 mg, Guaifenesin 600 mg	Aquabid DM by Pharmafab	62542-0720	Cold Remedy
59743060	Cap	Brompheniramine Maleate 12 mg, Pseudoephedrine HCl 120 mg	Pseubrom by Alphagen	59743-0060	Cold Remedy
59743060	Cap, Off-White to White Beads	Brompheniramine Maleate 12 mg, Pseudoephedrine HCl 120 mg	Pseubrom by Pharmafab	62542-0153	Cold Remedy
59743060	Cap	Brompheniramine Maleate 12 mg, Pseudoephedrine HCl 120 mg	by Zenith Goldline	00182-1053	Cold Remedy
59743060 <> CLEAR	Cap	Brompheniramine Maleate 12 mg, Pseudoephedrine HCl 120 mg	by Qualitest	00603-2505	Cold Remedy
59743061	Cap	Brompheniramine Maleate 6 mg, Pseudoephedrine HCl 60 mg	Pseubrom PD by DRX	55045-2297	Cold Remedy
59743061	Cap, Blue-Green, White Beads	Brompheniramine Maleate 6 mg, Pseudoephedrine HCl 60 mg	Pseubrom PD by Pharmafab	62542-0103	Cold Remedy
59743061	Cap	Brompheniramine Maleate 6 mg, Pseudoephedrine HCl 60 mg	by Zenith Goldline	00182-1054	Cold Remedy
598	Tab, Pink, Round, Schering Logo 598	Perphenazine 2 mg, Amitriptyline HCl 25 mg	Etrafon by Schering		Antipsychotic; Antidepressant
599	Tab, Film Coated, Logo 599	Etodolac 400 mg	by Caremark	00339-5986	NSAID
59911 <> 160	Cap, Blue & White	Propranolol HCl 160 mg	by ESI Lederle	59911-5479	Antihypertensive
59911 <> 3608	Tab, White, Oval	Etodolac 400 mg	by ESI Lederle	59911-3608	NSAID
59911 <> 3608	Tab, White, Oval, Film Coated	Etodolac 400 mg	by Wyeth Pharms	52903-3608	NSAID
59911 <> 3608	Tab, White, Oval, Film Coated	Etodolac 400 mg	Lodine by Hoffmann La Roche	00004-0292	NSAID
59911 <> 3608	Tab, White, Oval, Film	Etodolac 400 mg	by Hoffmann La Roche	00004-0256	NSAID
59911 <> 5815	Tab, White, Oblong, Scored	Metoclopramide 10 mg	by A H Robins Co	00031-5815	Gastrointestinal

ID FRONT <> BACK	DESCRIPTION FRONT <> BACK	INGREDIENT & STRENGTH	BRAND (OR EQUIV.) & FIRM	NDC#	CLASS; SCH.
59911 <> 5840	Tab, Coated	Guanfacine HCl 1.15 mg	by ESI Lederle	59911-5840	Antihypertensive
59911 <> 5840	Tab, Coated	Guanfacine HCl 1.15 mg	by A H Robins	00031-5840	Antihypertensive
59911 <> 5841	Tab, Coated	Guanfacine HCl 2.3 mg	by ESI Lederle	59911-5841	Antihypertensive
59911 <> 5841	Tab, Light Yellow, Coated	Guanfacine HCl 2.3 mg	by A H Robins	00031-5841	Antihypertensive
59911 <> 5870	Cap, Clear	Minocycline HCl	by Quality Care	60346-0831	Antibiotic
59911 <> 5871	Tab, White, Scored	Promethazine HCl 12.5 mg	by ESI Lederle	59911-5871	Antiemetic; Antihistamine
59911 <> 5871	Tab, White, Scored	Promethazine HCl 12.5 mg	by Wyeth Pharms	52903-5871	Antiemetic; Antihistamine
59911 <> 5872	Tab, White, Scored	Promethazine HCl 25 mg	by Wyeth Pharms	52903-5872	Antiemetic; Antihistamine
59911 <> 5873	Tab, White, Scored	Promethazine HCl 50 mg	by Wyeth Pharms	52903-5873	Antiemetic; Antihistamine
59911 <> 5873	Tab, White	Promethazine HCl 50 mg	by ESI Lederle	59911-5873	Antiemetic; Antihistamine
59911 <> 5876	Cap, Pink & White	Oxazepam 10 mg	by Wyeth Pharms	52903-5876	Sedative/Hypnotic; C IV
59911 <> 5876	Cap, Pink & White	Oxazepam 10 mg	by ESI Lederle	59911-5876	Sedative/Hypnotic; C IV
59911 <> 5877	Cap, Orange & White	Oxazepam 15 mg	by Wyeth Pharms	52903-5877	Sedative/Hypnotic; C IV
59911 <> 5877	Cap, Orange & White	Oxazepam 15 mg	by ESI Lederle	59911-5877	Sedative/Hypnotic; C IV
59911 <> 5878	Cap, Blue & White	Oxazepam 30 mg	by Wyeth Pharms	52903-5878	Sedative/Hypnotic; C IV
59911 <> 5878	Cap, Blue & White	Oxazepam 30 mg	by ESI Lederle	59911-5878	Sedative/Hypnotic; C IV
59911 <> 5887	Cap, Blue & Green	Ketoprofen 100 mg	by Wyeth Pharms	52903-5887	NSAID
59911 <> 5887	Cap, Blue & Green & Opaque	Ketoprofen 100 mg	Ketoprofen by Murfreesboro	51129-1598	NSAID
59911 <> 5887	Cap, Blue & Green & Opaque	Ketoprofen ER 100 mg	Oruvail by Murfreesboro	51129-1601	NSAID
59911 <> 5888	Cap, Blue & Yellow	Ketoprofen 150 mg	by Wyeth Pharms	52903-5888	NSAID
59911 <> 5888	Cap, Blue & Opaque & Yellow	Ketoprofen 150 mg	Ketoprofen by Murfreesboro	51129-1599	NSAID
59911 <> 5888	Cap, Blue & Opaque & Yellow	Ketoprofen ER 150.0 mg	Oruvail by Murfreesboro	51129-1602	NSAID
59911 <> 5889	Cap, Blue & White	Ketoprofen 200 mg	by Wyeth Pharms	52903-5889	NSAID
59911 <> 5889	Cap, Blue & Opaque & White	Ketoprofen 200 mg	Ketoprofen by Murfreesboro	51129-1600	NSAID
59911 <> 5889	Cap, Blue & Opaque & White	Ketoprofen ER 200 mg	Oruvail by Murfreesboro	51129-1603	NSAID
59911 <> 5895	Tab, White	Quinidine Sulfate 300 mg	by ESI Lederle	59911-5895	Antiarrhythmic
59911 <> 5899	Cap	Potassium Chloride 750 mg	by Quality Care	60346-0112	Electrolytes
59911 <> 60	Cap, White	Propranolol HCl 60 mg	by RPR	00801-1101	Antihypertensive
59911 <> 60	Cap, White	Propranolol HCl 60 mg	by Vangard Labs	00615-1331	Antihypertensive
59911 <> 80	Cap, Blue & White	Propranolol HCl 80 mg	by ESI Lederle	59911-5471	Antihypertensive
59911 <> 80	Cap, Blue & White	Propranolol HCl 80 mg	by RX PAK	65084-0100	Antihypertensive
599113607 <> 300	Cap, Cream, Oblong	Etodollac 300 mg	by Lederle	59911-3607	NSAID
59911120	Cap, Dark Blue	Propranolol HCl 120 mg	by Caremark	00339-5756	Antihypertensive
59911120	Cap	Propranolol HCl 120 mg	by ESI Lederle	59911-5473	Antihypertensive
59911120 <> 59911120	Cap, White	Propranolol HCl 120 mg	by Ayerst Lab (Div Wyeth)	00046-5473	Antihypertensive
59911120 <> 59911120	Cap, White	Propranolol HCl 120 mg	by Wyeth Pharms	52903-5473	Antihypertensive
59911160	Cap, Blue & White	Propranolol HCl LA 160 mg	Inderal LA by ESI Lederle		Antihypertensive
59911160 <> 59911160	Cap, White	Propranolol HCl 160 mg	by Wyeth Pharms	52903-5479	Antihypertensive
59911160 <> 59911160	Cap, White	Propranolol HCl 160 mg	by Ayerst Lab (Div Wyeth)	00046-5479	Antihypertensive
599113606 <> 200	Cap, White, 59911/3606 <> 200 and One Red Band	Etodolac 200 mg	Lodine by Heartland	61392-0906	NSAID
599113606 <> 200	Cap, White	Etodolac 200 mg	Etodolac by Heartland	61392-0862	NSAID
599113606 <> 200	Cap, White	Etodolac 200 mg	by Wyeth Pharms	52903-3606	NSAID
599113606 <> 200	Cap, White	Etodolac 200 mg	by Ayerst Lab (Div Wyeth)	00046-3606	NSAID
599113607 <> 300	Cap, White, 59911/3607 <> 300	Etodolac 300 mg	Lodine by Heartland	61392-0907	NSAID
599113607 <> 300	Cap, White	Etodolac 300 mg	by Wyeth Pharms	52903-3607	NSAID
599113608	Tab, White, Oval	Etodolac 400 mg	by ESI Lederle		NSAID
599113767	Tab, White, Oval	Etodolac 500 mg	by ESI Lederle		NSAID

ID FRONT <> BACK	DESCRIPTION FRONT <> BACK	INGREDIENT & STRENGTH	BRAND (OR EQUIV.) & FIRM	NDC#	CLASS; SCH.
599113787	Tab, White	Etodolac 500 mg	Etodolac by Heartland	61392-0872	NSAID
599113787	Tab, White, Oval, Film Coated	Etodolac 500 mg	by Wyeth Pharms	52903-3787	NSAID
599113787	Tab, White	Etodolac 500 mg	Lodine by Hoffmann La Roche	00004-0800	NSAID
599115805	Tab, White, Square	Griseofulvin Ultramicrosize 250 mg	Grisactin Ultra by ESI Lederle		Antifungal
599115806	Tab, White, Oval	Griseofulvin Ultramicrosize 330 mg	Grisactin Ultra by ESI Lederle		Antifungal
599115807	Cap, Opaque & White	Griseofulvin 250 mg	by ESI Lederle		Antifungal
599115808	Tab, White, Round	Griseofulvin 500 mg	by ESI Lederle		Antifungal
599115814	Tab, White, Elliptical	Metoclopramide 5 mg	Reglan by ESI Lederle		Gastrointestinal
599115814	Tab, A White, Oval, Scored	Metoclopramide 5 mg	by A H Robins Co	00031-5814	Gastrointestinal
599115814	Tab, White, Oval	Metoclopramide 5 mg	by ESI Lederle	59911-5814	Gastrointestinal
599115815	Tab, White, Oblong	Metoclopramide 10 mg	Reglan by ESI Lederle		Gastrointestinal
599115815	Tab, White, Oblong, Scored	Metoclopramide 10 mg	by ESI Lederle	59911-5815	Gastrointestinal
599115842	Cap, Blue & Pink	Acebutolol HCl 200 mg	Sectral by ESI Lederle		Antihypertensive
599115842	Cap, Blue & Pink	Acebutolol HCl 200 mg	by ESI Lederle	59911-5842	Antihypertensive
599115842	Cap, Blue & Pink	Acebutolol HCl 200 mg	by Wyeth Pharms	52903-5842	Antihypertensive
599115844	Cap, Pink & Red	Acebutolol HCl 400 mg	by ESI Lederle	59911-5844	Antihypertensive
599115844	Cap, Pink & Rose	Acebutolol HCl 400 mg	Sectral by ESI Lederle		Antihypertensive
599115844	Cap, Pink & Red	Acebutolol HCl 400 mg	by Wyeth Pharms	52903-5844	Antihypertensive
599115869	Cap, Yellow	Minocycline 50 mg	Minocin by ESI Lederle		Antibiotic
599115869	Cap, Yellow	Minocycline HCl 50 mg	by ESI Lederle	59911-5869	Antibiotic
599115870	Cap, Green & Yellow	Minocycline 100 mg	Minocin by ESI Lederle		Antibiotic
599115870	Cap, Green & Yellow	Minocycline HCl 100 mg	by Murfreesboro Ph	51129-1414	Antibiotic
599115870	Cap, Green & Yellow	Minocycline HCl 100 mg	by ESI Lederle	59911-5870	Antibiotic
599115871	Tab, White, Round	Promethazine 12.5 mg	Phenergan by ESI Lederle		Antiemetic; Antihistamine
599115872	Tab, White, Round	Promethazine 25 mg	Phenergan by ESI Lederle		Antiemetic; Antihistamine
599115872	Tab, White, Scored	Promethazine HCl 25 mg	by ESI Lederle	59911-5872	Antiemetic; Antihistamine
599115873	Tab, White, Round	Promethazine 50 mg	Phenergan by ESI Lederle		Antiemetic; Antihistamine
599115876	Cap, Pink & White	Oxazepam 10 mg	by ESI Lederle		Sedative/Hypnotic; C IV
599115877	Cap, Orange & White	Oxazepam 15 mg	by Murfreesboro Ph	51129-1676	Sedative/Hypnotic; C IV
599115877	Cap, Orange & White	Oxazepam 15 mg	by ESI Lederle		Sedative/Hypnotic; C IV
599115878	Cap, Blue & White	Oxazepam 30 mg	by ESI Lederle		Sedative/Hypnotic; C IV
599115895	Tab, White, Scored	Quinidine Sulfate 300 mg	by A H Robins Co	00031-5895	Antiarrhythmic
599115895	Tab, White, Round	Quinidine Sulfate ER 300 mg	Quinidex by ESI Lederle		Antiarrhythmic
599115899	Cap, White	Potassium Chloride 750 mg	by A H Robins Co	00031-5899	Electrolytes
599115899	Cap	Potassium Chloride 750 mg	by Caremark	00339-6119	Electrolytes
5991160	Cap	Propranolol HCl 60 mg	by Caremark	00339-5752	Antihypertensive
5991160	Cap	Propranolol HCl 60 mg	by ESI Lederle	59911-5470	Antihypertensive
5991160 <> 5991160	Cap, White	Propranolol HCl 60 mg	by Wyeth Pharms	52903-5470	Antihypertensive
5991160 <> 5991160	Cap, White	Propranolol HCl 60 mg	by Ayerst Lab (Div Wyeth)	00046-5470	Antihypertensive
5991180	Cap, Light Blue	Propranolol HCl 80 mg	by Caremark	00339-5754	Antihypertensive
5991180 <> 5991180	Cap, White	Propranolol HCl 80 mg	by Wyeth Pharms	52903-5471	Antihypertensive
5991180 <> 5991180	Cap, White	Propranolol HCl 80 mg	by Ayerst Lab (Div Wyeth)	00046-5471	Antihypertensive
59911PLUS	Tab, Yellow, Oval, 59911/Plus	Prenatal	by ESI Lederle		Vitamin
5AYGESTIN	Tab, White, Oval, 5 over Aygestin	Aygestin 5 mg	by ESI Lederle	59911-5849	Hormone
5DAN5606	Tab	Haloperidol 5 mg	by Allscripts	54569-2883	Antipsychotic
5MG	Cap, Blue	Pericyazine 5 mg	by Rhone-Poulenc Rorer	Canadian	Psychotropic Agent
5MG <> LOTENSIN	Tab, Yellow	Benazepril HCl 5 mg	Lotensin by Southwood Pharms	58016-0264	Antihypertensive

ID FRONT <> BACK	DESCRIPTION FRONT <> BACK	INGREDIENT & STRENGTH	BRAND (OR EQUIV.) & FIRM	NDC#	CLASS; SCH.
5MG <> RSN	Tab, Yellow, Oval, Film Coated	Risedronate Sodium 5 mg	Actonel by Procter & Gamble	Canadian DIN# 02242518	Bisphosphonate
5MG <> RSN	Tab, Yellow, Oval, Film Coated	Risedronate Sodium 5 mg	Actonel by Procter Gamble Pharm	00149-0471	Bisphosphonate
5MG <> SONATA	Cap, Green	Zaleplon 5 mg	Sonata by Wyeth Pharms	52903-0925	Sedative/Hypnotic; C IV
5MG <> SONATA	Cap, Green	Zaleplon 5 mg	Sonata by Wyeth Labs	00008-0925	Sedative/Hypnotic; C IV
5MG <> SONATA	Cap, Green & Opaque	Zaleplon 5 mg	Sonata by United Res	00677-1684	Sedative/Hypnotic; C IV
5MG <> WATSON369	Cap, White	Losapine Succinate 5 mg	by Dixon Shane	17236-0698	Antipsychotic/Antimanic
5MG <> WATSON369	Cap, White, Opaque, 5 mg <> Watson over 369	Loxapine Succinate	Loxitane by UDL	51079-0900	Antipsychotic
5MG <> WATSON369	Cap	Loxapine Succinate	by Watson	52544-0369	Antipsychotic
5MG <> WATSON369	Cap	Loxapine Succinate	by Zenith Goldline	00182-1305	Antipsychotic
5MG <> WATSON369	Cap, 5 mg <> Watson Over 369	Loxapine Succinate	by UDL	51079-0677	Antipsychotic
5MG <> WATSON369	Cap	Loxapine Succinate	by HL Moore	00839-7495	Antipsychotic
5MG <> WATSON369	Cap	Loxapine Succinate	by Major	00904-2310	Antipsychotic
5MG3512 <> 5MGSB	Cap, Brown & Clear	Dextroamphetamine Sulfate 5 mg	Dexedrine by Intl Processing	59885-3512	Stimulant; C II
5MG657	Cap, Gray & Red, 5 mg/657	Anhydrous Tacrolimus 5 mg	Prograf by Fujisawa	Canadian	Immunosuppressant
5MGLEDERLEL1	Cap, Green	Loxapine 5 mg	Loxitane by Lederle		Antipsychotic
5MGSB <> 5MG3512	Cap, Brown & Clear	Dextroamphetamine Sulfate 5 mg	Dexedrine by Intl Processing	59885-3512	Stimulant; C II
5MGSB <> 5MG3512	Cap, Brown & Natural	Dextroamphetamine Sulfate 5 mg	Dexedrine Spansule by SKB	00007-3512	Stimulant; C II
5MGZAR	Tab, Blue, Round, 5 mg/Zar	Metolazone 5 mg	Zaroxolyn by Medeva		Diuretic
5MMDC	Tab, White, Square, 5/MMDC	Metoclopramide 5 mg	by Hoechst Marion Roussel	Canadian	Gastrointestinal
5VALIUM <> ROCHE	Tab, V Design	Diazepam 5 mg	Valium by PDRX	55289-0117	Antianxiety; C IV
5VALIUM <> ROCHEROCHE	Tab, Round with Cut Out V Design	Diazepam 5 mg	Valium by Quality Care	60346-0439	Antianxiety; C IV
5VALIUM <> ROCHEROCHE	Tab, V Design	Diazepam 5 mg	Valium by Caremark	00339-4073	Antianxiety; C IV
5VALIUM <> ROCHEROCHE	Tab, Scored, V over Valium <> Roche over Roche	Diazepam 5 mg	Valium by Allscripts	54569-0948	Antianxiety; C IV
5VVALIUM <> ROCHEVROCHE	Tab, 5 over V Logo Valium <> Roche V Roche	Diazepam 5 mg	Valium by Roche	00140-0005	Antianxiety; C IV
5XL	Tab, Yellow, Oval	Oxybutynin Chloride 5 mg	Ditropan XL by Alza	17314-8500	Urinary
5Z2941	Tab, Light Lavender, Sugar-Coated, 5/Z2941	Trifluoperazine HCl	by Physicians Total Care	54868-1352	Antipsychotic
6	Tab, Green, Oval	Dextrothyroxine Sodium 6 mg	Choloxin by Boots		Thyroid
6	Tab, White, Oval	Ibuprofen 600 mg	Motrin by Norton		NSAID
6	Tab, Film Coated, Norton	Ibuprofen 600 mg	by Med Pro	53978-5006	NSAID
6	Tab, Film Coated	Ibuprofen 600 mg	by Quality Care	60346-0556	NSAID
6 <> 555872	Tab, White, Round, Scored	Medroxyprogesterone Acetate 2.5 mg	by Southwood Pharms	58016-0374	Progestin
6 <> ADAMS	Tab, Yellow, Oblong, Scored	Pseudoephedrine HCl 120 mg; Methscopolamine Nitrate 2.5 mg; Chlorpheniramine Maleate 8 mg; Methscopolamine Nitrate 2.5 mg	Allerx by Adams Labs	63824-0067	Cold Remedy
6 <> ETH	Tab, White, Rectangle	Nitroglycerin 0.6 mg	Nitroquick by PDRX	55289-0302	Vasodilator
6 <> ETH	Tab, White, Ovaloid	Nitroglycerin 0.6 mg	Nitroquick by Ethex	58177-0325	Vasodilator
6 <> SEARLE	Tab, Underlined 6 <> Searle	Ethinyl Estradiol 0.035 mg, Norethindrone 0.5 mg	Brevicon 21 Day by GD Searle	00025-0252	Oral Contraceptive
6 <> SEARLE	Tab	Ethinyl Estradiol 0.035 mg, Norethindrone 0.5 mg, Norethindrone 1 mg	Tri Norinyl 21 Day by GD Searle	00025-0272	Oral Contraceptive
60	Tab, Peach, Round	Fexofenadine HCl 60 mg	by Hoechst Marion Roussel	Canadian	Antihistamine
60	Cap, Gray, Oval	Terazosin HCl 1 mg	by Teva Pharms	00093-0760	Antihypertensive
60	Cap, Gray	Terazosin HCl 1 mg	by Scherer Rp North	11014-1218	Antihypertensive
60 <> 5660	Tab, Yellow, Round, Scored	Isosorbide Mononitrate 60 mg	by Zenith Goldline	00172-5660	Antianginal
60 <> 59911	Cap, White	Propranolol HCl 60 mg	by Vangard Labs	00615-1331	Antihypertensive
60 <> ADALATCC	Tab, Pink, Round	Nifedipine 60 mg	Adalat CC by Va Cmop	65243-0054	Antihypertensive
60 <> ADALATCC	Tab, Film Coated	Nifedipine 60 mg	Adalat CC by Bayer	00026-8851	Antihypertensive
60 <> ADALATCC	Tab, Pink, Round, Film Coated	Nifedipine 60 mg	Adalat CC by Par	49884-0622	Antihypertensive
60 <> ADALATCC	Tab, Pink, Round, Film Coated	Nifedipine 60 mg	by Par	49884-0631	Antihypertensive

ID FRONT <> BACK	DESCRIPTION FRONT <> BACK	INGREDIENT & STRENGTH	BRAND (OR EQUIV.) & FIRM	NDC#	CLASS; SCH.
60 <> ADALATCC	Tab, Film Coated	Nifedipine 60 mg	Adalat CC by Nat Pharmpak Serv	55154-4809	Antihypertensive
60 <> ADALATCC	Tab, Film Coated	Nifedipine 60 mg	Adalat CC by Wal Mart	49035-0155	Antihypertensive
60 <> ADALATCC	Tab, Film Coated	Nifedipine 60 mg	by Med Pro	53978-3034	Antihypertensive
60 <> ADALATCC	Tab, Yellowish Pink, Film Coated	Nifedipine 60 mg	Adalat CC by Quality Care	62682-6021	Antihypertensive
60 <> ADALATCC	Tab, Film Coated	Nifedipine 60 mg	Adalat CC by Amerisource	62584-0006	Antihypertensive
60 <> ADALATCC	Tab, Film Coated	Nifedipine 60 mg	Adalat CC by Smiths Food & Drug	58341-0059	Antihypertensive
60 <> ADALATCC	Tab, Film Coated	Nifedipine 60 mg	by Talbert Med	44514-0761	Antihypertensive
60 <> E655	Tab, Orange, Round	Morphine Sulfate 60 mg	by Endo Pharms	60951-0655	Analgesic; C II
60 <> E655	Tab, Orange, Oblong	Morphine Sulfate 60 mg	by Dupont Pharma	00056-0655	Analgesic; C II
60 <> IMDUR	Tab	Isosorbide Mononitrate 60 mg	Imdur by Caremark	00339-6003	Antianginal
60 <> IMDUR	Tab	Isosorbide Mononitrate 60 mg	Imdur by Caremark	00339-6004	Antianginal
60 <> IMDUR	Tab	Isosorbide Mononitrate 60 mg	Imdur by Nat Pharmpak Serv	55154-3512	Antianginal
60 <> IMDUR	Tab, Yellow	Isosorbide Mononitrate 60 mg	Imdur ER by Schering	00085-4110	Antianginal
60 <> M	Tab, White, Coated, Beveled Edge, 6 on Left, 0 on Right of Score	Maprotiline HCl 25 mg	by Mylan	00378-0060	Antidepressant
60 <> PROCARDIAXL	Tab, Pink, Round, ER, Procardia XL	Nifedipine 60 mg	Procardia XL by Pfizer	00069-2660	Antihypertensive
60 <> PROCARDIAXL	Tab, ER, Procardia XL	Nifedipine 60 mg	Procardia XL by Nat Pharmpak Serv	55154-2707	Antihypertensive
60 <> PROCARDIAXL	Tab, ER, Procardia XL	Nifedipine 60 mg	Procardia XL by Amerisource	62584-0660	Antihypertensive
60 <> STARLIX	Tab, Pink, Round	Nateglinide 60 mg	Starlix by Novartis	00078-0351	Antidiabetic
600	Tab, Film Coated, Upjohn Logo and 600	Ibuprofen 600 mg	by Quality Care	60346-0556	NSAID
600 <> AP0034	Tab, White, Oval, Film Coated	Gemfibrozil 600 mg	by Major Pharms	00904-5379	Antihyperlipidemic
600 <> APO034	Tab, White, Oval, Coated	Gemfibrozil 600 mg	by Apotex	60505-0034	Antihyperlipidemic
600 <> APO034	Tab, Coated	Gemfibrozil 600 mg	by Torpharm	62318-0034	Antihyperlipidemic
600 <> G	Tab, Film Coated	Ibuprofen 600 mg	by Quality Care	60346-0556	NSAID
600 <> IP132	Tab, Film Coated	Ibuprofen 600 mg	by Urgent Care Ctr	50716-0743	NSAID
600 <> IP132	Tab, Film Coated, IP 132	Ibuprofen 600 mg	by Quality Care	60346-0556	NSAID
600 <> IP132	Tab, Coated	Ibuprofen 600 mg	by Golden State	60429-0093	NSAID
600 <> IP132	Tab, Coated, Interpharm	Ibuprofen 600 mg	by Prescription Dispensing	61807-0011	NSAID
600 <> IP132	Tab, White, Oval, Film Coated	Ibuprofen 600 mg	by Major Pharms	00904-5186	NSAID
600 <> MPC	Tab, ER	Potassium Citrate 540 mg	Urocit K by Mission	00178-0600	Electrolytes
600 <> PAR163	Tab, White, Oval, Film Coated, 600 <> Par over 163	Ibuprofen 600 mg	Rufen/Motrin by UDL	51079-0282	NSAID
600 <> PAR163	Tab, Film Coated	Ibuprofen 600 mg	by Zenith Goldline	00172-3646	NSAID
600 <> PAR163	Tab, Film Coated	Ibuprofen 600 mg	by Par	49884-0163	NSAID
600 <> PAR163	Tab, Film Coated	Ibuprofen 600 mg	by Pharmedix	53002-0301	NSAID
600 <> PAR163	Tab, Film Coated	Ibuprofen 600 mg	by Quality Care	60346-0556	NSAID
600 <> SCHEIN0766	Tab, Film Coated	Ibuprofen 600 mg	by Quality Care	60346-0556	NSAID
600 <> WALLACE371601	Tab, Wallace Over 37-1601	Meprobamate 600 mg	Miltown by Wallace	00037-1601	Sedative/Hypnotic; C IV
600 <> Z4141	Tab, Film Coated, 600 and Zenith Logo	Fenoprofen Calcium 691.8 mg	by Quality Care	60346-0233	NSAID
600 <> ZL	Tab, White, Oval, Film Coated, Scored	Zileuton 600 mg	Zyflo by Murfreesboro Ph	51129-1380	Antiasthmatic
600 <> ZL	Tab, White, Ovaloid, Scored, 600 <> ZL over Abbott Logo	Zileuton 600 mg	Zyflo by Abbott	00074-8036	Antiasthmatic
60030 <> TRINITY	Tab, Film Coated, Scored	Dextromethorphan Hydrobromide 30 mg, Guaifenesin 600 mg	by United Res	00677-1486	Cold Remedy
600MG	Tab, Yellow, Round	Potassium Chloride 600 mg	Klor Con by Phcy Care	65070-0067	Electrolytes
600ZL	Tab, Film Coated, Abbott Logo and ZL	Zileuton 600 mg	Zyflo by Abbott	00074-8036	Antiasthmatic
601 <> MYLAN	Tab, Beveled Edge, Coated	Ibuprofen 600 mg	by Mylan	00378-0601	NSAID
601 <> SINEMETCR	Tab, Pink, Oval	Carbidopa 25 mg, Levodopa 100 mg	Sinemet CR by DuPont Pharma	00056-0601	Antiparkinson
602	Tab, Endo	Acetaminophen 325 mg, Oxycodone HCl 5 mg	by Rugby	00536-5670	Analgesic; C II
60274120MG	Cap, Yellow, Hard Gel, 60274 Above 120 mg in Black Ink	Verapamil HCl 120 mg	Verelan Sustained Release by Teva	00480-0948	Antihypertensive
60274180MG	Cap, Gray & Yellow, Hard Gel, 60274 Above 180 mg in Black Ink	Verapamil HCl 180 mg	Verelan Sustained Release by Teva	00480-0956	Antihypertensive
60274240MG	Cap, Blue & Yellow, Hard Gel, 60274 Above 240 mg in Black Ink	Verapamil HCl 240 mg	Verelan Sustained Release by Teva	00480-0958	Antihypertensive
60274360MG	Cap, Purple & Yellow, Hard Gel, 60274 Above 360 mg in Black Ink	Verapamil HCl 360 mg	Verelan Sustained Release by Teva	00480-0960	Antihypertensive
604 <> SL	Tab, Green, Oval, Film Coated, Scored	Guaifenesin 600 mg, Pseudoephedrine HCl 120 mg	Entex PSE by Sidmak	50111-0604	Cold Remedy
6054933	Tab, White, 60/54/933	Morphine Sulfate 60 mg	Oramorph SR by Boehringer Ingelheim	Canadian	Analgesic

ID FRONT <> BACK	DESCRIPTION FRONT <> BACK	INGREDIENT & STRENGTH	BRAND (OR EQUIV.) & FIRM	NDC#	CLASS; SCH.
606 <> P	Tab, Purepac Symbol	Acyclovir 400 mg	by Golden State	60429-0712	Antiviral
606 <> PRILOSEC10	Cap	Omeprazole 10 mg	Prilosec by Merck	00006-0606	Gastrointestinal
606 <> PRILOSEC10	Cap	Omeprazole 10 mg	Prilosec by Astra Merck	00186-0606	Gastrointestinal
606 <> PRILOSEC10	Cap	Omeprazole 10 mg	Omeprazole by Kaiser	62224-2226	Gastrointestinal
606 <> PRILOSEC10	Cap, Opaque & Peach & Purple	Omeprazole 10 mg	Prilosec by PDRX	55289-0475	Gastrointestinal
606 <> R	Tab, White, Round, Purepac Logo, Scrolled P with Arm Extension	Acyclovir 400 mg	by Purepac	00228-2606	Antiviral
606PRILOSEC 10	Cap, Amethysed & Apricot	Omeprazole 10 mg	Prilosec by AstraZeneca	00186-0606	Gastrointestinal
6060500 <> BMS	Tab, White, Round, Film Coated	Metformin HCl 500 mg	by Allscripts	54569-4202	Antidiabetic
606HD	Tab, White, Round	Methyldopa 125 mg	Aldomet by Halsey		Antihypertensive
6072 <> BMS	Tab, Pale Yellow, Cap Shaped, Film Coated	Glyburide 1.25mg, Metformin 250 mg	Glucovance by Bristol-Myers	00087-6072	Antidiabetic
6073 <> BMS	Tab, Pale Orange, Cap Shaped, Film Coated	Glyburide 2.50mg, Metformin HCl 500 mg	Glucovance by Bristol-Myers	00087-6073	Antidiabetic
6074 <> BMS	Tab. Yellow, Cap Shaped	Glyburide 5 mg, Metformin HCl 500 mg	Gluconance by Bisto-Myers	00088-6074	Antidiabetic
6074 <> BMS	Tab, Yellow	Glyburide 5 mg; Metformin HCl 500 mg	Glucovance by Bristol Myers Squibb	12783-0074	Antidiabetic
607HD	Tab, White, Round	Methyldopa 250 mg	Aldomet by Halsey		Antihypertensive
607OR	Tab, Light Pink, Round, OR <> 607	Ranitidine HCl 75 mg	by Schein	00364-none	Gastrointestinal
608 <> SL	Tab, White, Round, Film Coated	Ketorolac Tromethamine 10 mg	Toradol by Sidmak Labs	50111-0608	NSAID
608HD	Tab, White, Round	Methyldopa 500 mg	Aldomet by Halsey		Antihypertensive
609MJ <> M	Tab, Lower Case M	Fosinopril Sodium 20 mg	Monopril by Quality Care	62682-6026	Antihypertensive
60ADALATCC <> 885MILES60	Tab, Salmon, Film Coated, 885/Miles 60	Nifedipine 60 mg	Adalat CC by Allscripts	54569-3892	Antihypertensive
60MG <> 1102	Cap, Gelatin Coated, 60 MG	Fexofenadine HCl 60 mg	by Kaiser	62224-1114	Antihistamine
60MG <> 1102	Cap, Opaque & Pink & White	Fexofenadine HCl 60 mg	Allegra by Integrity	64731-0532	Antihistamine
60MG <> 1102	Cap, Opaque & Pink & White	Fexofenadine HCl 60 mg	Allegra by Integrity	64731-0300	Antihistamine
60MG <> 1102	Cap, Opaque & Pink & White	Fexofenadine HCl 60 mg	by Integrity	64731-0275	Antihistamine
60MG <> 1102	Cap, Opaque & Pink & White	Fexofenadine HCl 60 mg	Allegra by Integrity	64731-0575	Antihistamine
60MG <> 1102	Cap, Pink & White	Fexofenadine HCl 60 mg	Allegra by DRX Pharm Consults	55045-2582	Antihistamine
60MG <> 1102	Cap, Pink & White	Fexofenadine HCl 60 mg	Allegra by PDRX Pharms	55289-0456	Antihistamine
60MG <> 1102	Cap, Gelatin Coated	Fexofenadine HCl 60 mg	Allegra by Kaiser	00179-1265	Antihistamine
60MG <> 1102	Cap, Gelatin, Black Print	Fexofenadine HCl 60 mg	Allegra by Caremark	00339-6083	Antihistamine
60MG <> 1102	Cap, Gelatin Coated	Fexofenadine HCl 60 mg	Allegra by Physicians Total Care	54868-3898	Antihistamine
60MG <> ALLEGRA	Cap, Pink & White	Fexofenadine HCl 60 mg	Allegra by DRX Pharm Consults	55045-2582	Antihistamine
60MG <> ALLEGRA	Cap, Pink & White	Fexofenadine HCl 60 mg	Allegra by PDRX Pharms	55289-0456	Antihistamine
60MG <> ALLEGRA	Cap, Pink & White	Fexofenadine HCl 60 mg	Allegra by Va Cmop	65243-0029	Antihistamine
60MG <> PF	Tab, Orange, Round	Morphine Sulfate 60 mg	MS Contin by Purdue Frederick	Canadian	Analgesic
60MGALLEGRA <> 110260MG	Cap, Gelatin Coated, Black Print	Fexofenadine HCl 60 mg	Allegra by Quality Care	62682-8004	Antihistamine
60P <> DAN	Tab, White, Round, Scored	Phenobarbital 60 mg	by Schein	00364-0697	Sedative/Hypnotic; C IV
61	Cap, Yellow	Terazosin HCl 2 mg	by Scherer Rp North	11014-1212	Antihypertensive
61	Cap, Yellow, Oval	Terazosin HCl 2 mg	by Teva Pharms	00093-0761	Antihypertensive
61 <> SEARLE	Tab	Atropine Sulfate 0.025 mg, Diphenoxylate HCl 2.5 mg	Lomotil by Amerisource	62584-0027	Antidiarrheal; C V
61 <> SEARLE	Tab	Atropine Sulfate 0.025 mg, Diphenoxylate HCl 2.5 mg	Lomotil by St Marys Med	60760-0061	Antidiarrheal; C V
61 <> SEARLE	Tab	Atropine Sulfate 0.025 mg, Diphenoxylate HCl 2.5 mg	Lomotil by GD Searle	00014-0061	Antidiarrheal; C V
61 <> SEARLE	Tab	Atropine Sulfate 0.025 mg, Diphenoxylate HCl 2.5 mg	Lomotil by GD Searle	00025-0061	Antidiarrheal; C V
61 <> SEARLE	Tab	Atropine Sulfate 0.025 mg, Diphenoxylate HCl 2.5 mg	Lomotil by Med Pro	53978-3088	Antidiarrheal; C V
61 <> SEARLE	Tab	Atropine Sulfate 0.025 mg, Diphenoxylate HCl 2.5 mg	Lomotil by Nat Pharmpak Serv	55154-3614	Antidiarrheal; C V
61 <> SEARLE	Tab, White, Round	Diphenoxylate HCl 2.5 mg	Lomotil by Searle	Canadian DIN# 00036323	Antidiarrheal
610	Tab, Endo Logo	Aspirin 325 mg, Oxycodone HCl 4.5 mg, Oxycodone Terephthalate 0.38 mg	by Rugby	00536-5671	Analgesic; C II
610 <> MISSION	Tab	Potassium Citrate 1080 mg	Urocit K by Mission	00178-0610	Electrolytes
610HD	Tab, White, Oblong	Propoxyphene Napsylate 50 mg, Acetaminophen 325 mg	Darvocet N by Halsey		Analgesic; C IV
611	Tab, Film Coated, Logo 611	Pentoxifylline 400 mg	by Caremark	00339-5278	Anticoagulent

ID FRONT <> BACK	DESCRIPTION FRONT <> BACK	INGREDIENT & STRENGTH	BRAND (OR EQUIV.) & FIRM	NDC#	CLASS; SCH.
611 <> MYLAN	Tab, Beige, Round, Film Coated	Methyldopa 250 mg	by Allscripts	54569-0508	Antihypertensive
611 <> MYLAN	Tab, Beige, Round, Film Coated	Methyldopa 250 mg	Aldomet by UDL	51079-0200	Antihypertensive
611 <> MYLAN	Tab, Beige, Film Coated, Beveled Edge	Methyldopa 250 mg	by Mylan	00378-0611	Antihypertensive
611 <> MYLAN	Tab, Film Coated	Methyldopa 250 mg	by Murfreesboro	51129-1293	Antihypertensive
611 <> R	Tab, Film Coated, Purepac Logo	Pentoxifylline 400 mg	by Murfreesboro	51129-1121	Anticoagulent
611 <> R	Tab, Yellow, Oblong, Film Coated	Pentoxifylline 400 mg	ER by Purepac	00228-2611	Anticoagulent
612 <> UCB	Tab, Film Coated	Guaifenesin 600 mg, Pseudoephedrine HCl 120 mg	by Mikart	46672-0126	Cold Remedy
612 <> UCB	Tab, Film Coated	Guaifenesin 600 mg, Pseudoephedrine HCl 120 mg	Duratuss by Nat Pharmpak Serv	55154-7203	Cold Remedy
612 <> UCB	Tab, White, Oval, Film Coated, Scored	Guaifenesin 600 mg, Pseudoephedrine HCl 120 mg	Duratuss by UCB Pharma	50474-0612	Cold Remedy
612 <> UCB	Tab, Film Coated	Guaifenesin 600 mg, Pseudoephedrine HCl 120 mg	Duratuss by Paco	53668-0237	Cold Remedy
612 <> UCB	Tab, White, Oval, Scored	Pseudoephedrine HCl 120 mg; Guaifenesin 600 mg	Duratuss by Phy Total Care	54868-3943	Cold Remedy
612 <> WHITBY	Tab, Film Coated	Guaifenesin 600 mg, Pseudoephedrine HCl 120 mg	Duratuss by UCB	50474-0612	Cold Remedy
612 <> WHITBY	Tab, Film Coated	Guaifenesin 600 mg, Pseudoephedrine HCl 120 mg	Duratuss by CVS	51316-0238	Cold Remedy
6121 <> PAL	Tab, White, Oblong, Scored	Carbinoxamine Maleate 8 mg; Pseudoephedrine HCl 90 mg	Palgic D by Pan Am Labs	00525-6121	Cold Remedy
613	Cap, Dark Green & Light Green, Eon Logo 613	Hydroxyzine Pamoate 43 mg	by Quality Care	60346-0208	Antihistamine
613 <> R	Tab, White, Oval, Film Coated	Ticlopidine HCl 250 mg	by Purepac	00228-2613	Anticoagulant
617 <> R	Tab, Yellow, Cap Shaped, Black Print	Naproxen 375 mg	DR by Purepac	00228-2617	NSAID
618 <> R	Tab, Yellow, Cap Shaped, Black Print	Naproxen 500 mg	DR by Purepac	00228-2618	NSAID
6180100	Tab, White, Round, 6180/100	Labetalol HCl 100 mg	by Bristol-Myers		Antihypertensive
6181200	Tab, White, Round, 6181/200	Labetalol HCl 200 mg	by Bristol-Myers		Antihypertensive
6182300	Tab, White, Round, 6182/300	Labetalol HCl 300 mg	by Bristol-Myers		Antihypertensive
61SEARLE	Tab	Atropine Sulfate 0.025 mg, Diphenoxylate HCl 2.5 mg	Lomotil by Allscripts	54569-0221	Antidiarrheal; C V
62	Cap, Red	Terazosin HCl 5 mg	by Scherer Rp North	11014-1213	Antihypertensive
62	Cap, Red, Oval	Terazosin HCl 5 mg	by Teva Pharms	00093-0762	Antihypertensive
62 <> RPC	Cap	Phendimetrazine Tartrate 105 mg	X Trozine LA by Shire Richwood	58521-0105	Anorexiant; C III
620	Tab, Blue, Round, Scored, Logo and 620	Isosorbide Mononitrate 20 mg	by Murfreesboro	51129-1577	Antianginal
6211V	Tab	Guaifenesin 600 mg, Pseudoephedrine HCl 120 mg	Enomine PSE by Quality Care	60346-0933	Cold Remedy
622HD	Tab, White, Oblong	Ibuprofen 800 mg	Motrin by Halsey		NSAID
625	Cap, Yellow	Docusate Potassium 100 mg, Casanthranol 30 mg	Dialose Plus by OHM		Laxative
625DPI	Tab, Light Orange, 625/DPI	Estropipate 0.75 mg	by Schein	00364-2600	Hormone
63	Cap, Blue, Oval	Terazosin HCl 10 mg	by Teva Pharms	00093-0763	Antihypertensive
63	Cap, Blue	Terazosin HCl 10 mg	by Scherer Rp North	11014-1219	Antihypertensive
63 <> R	Tab, White, Round, Scored	Lorazepam 2 mg	by Compumed	00403-0012	Sedative/Hypnotic; C IV
630 <> SJ	Cap, Blue Print, 630 <> S-J	Acetaminophen 500 mg, Hydrocodone Bitartrate 5 mg	Ugesic by Stewart Jackson	45985-0630	Analgesic; C III
630HD	Tab, Pink, Oblong	Propoxyphene Napsylate 100 mg, Acetaminophen 650 mg	Wygesic by Halsey		Analgesic; C IV
631	Tab, Blue, Round, Scored, Logo 631	Isosorbide Mononitrate 10 mg	by Murfreesboro	51129-1576	Antianginal
631 <> ENDO	Tab, Film Coated	Cimetidine 300 mg	by Quality Care	60346-0944	Gastrointestinal
631PAR	Tab, White, Oval	Penicillin V Potassium 250 mg	by Pharmafab	62542-0710	Antibiotic
632HD	Cap, Flesh & Lavender	Fenoprofen Calcium 200 mg	Nalfon by Halsey		NSAID
632PAR	Tab, White, Oval	Penicillin V Potassium 500 mg	by Pharmafab	62542-0723	Antibiotic
6330 <> VAD	Tab, Blue, Oblong, Scored	Acetaminophen 650 mg; Hydrocodone Bitartrate 10 mg	Lorcet by HJ Harkins	52959-0403	Analgesic; C III
633HD	Cap, Flesh & Orange	Fenoprofen Calcium 300 mg	Nalfon by Halsey		NSAID
634HD	Tab, Peach, Oblong	Fenoprofen Calcium 600 mg	Nalfon by Halsey		NSAID
635	Tab, White, Ellipsoid	Chlorambucil 2 mg	Leukeran by B.W. Inc	Canadian	Antineoplastic
635	Tab, Sugar Coated	Chlorambucil 2 mg	Leukeran by Catalytica	63552-0635	Antineoplastic
635	Tab, Sugar Coated, Black Print	Chlorambucil 2 mg	Leukeran by Glaxo	00173-0635	Antineoplastic
6350 <> UAD	Tab	Acetaminophen 650 mg, Hydrocodone Bitartrate 10 mg	Lorcet by Nat Pharmpak Serv	55154-7301	Analgesic; C III
6350 <> UAD	Tab	Acetaminophen 650 mg, Hydrocodone Bitartrate 10 mg	Lorcet by Quality Care	60346-0955	Analgesic; C III
6350 <> UAD	Tab	Acetaminophen 650 mg, Hydrocodone Bitartrate 10 mg	Lorcet by Amerisource	62584-0021	Analgesic; C III
6350 <> UAD	Tab	Acetaminophen 650 mg, Hydrocodone Bitartrate 10 mg	Lorcet 10-650 by DRX	55045-2122	Analgesic; C III
6350 <> UAD	Tab	Acetaminophen 650 mg, Hydrocodone Bitartrate 10 mg	Lorcet 10-650 by Allscripts	54569-3782	Analgesic; C III
6350 <> UAD	Tab	Acetaminophen 650 mg, Hydrocodone Bitartrate 10 mg	Lorcet by Med Pro	53978-2068	Analgesic; C III

ID FRONT <> BACK	DESCRIPTION FRONT <> BACK	INGREDIENT & STRENGTH	BRAND (OR EQUIV.) & FIRM	NDC#	CLASS; SCH.
6350 <> UAD	Tab	Acetaminophen 650 mg, Hydrocodone Bitartrate 10 mg	by Mikart	46672-0103	Analgesic; C III
6350 <> UAD	Tab, Blue, Oblong, Scored	Hydrocodone Bitartrate 10 mg, Acetaminophen 650 mg	by Southwood Pharms	58016-0232	Analgesic; C III
6377V	Tab, 6377/V	Yohimbine HCl 5.4 mg	by Zenith Goldline	00172-4368	Impotence Agent
638 <> 93	Tab	Trazodone HCl 100 mg	by Allscripts	54569-1999	Antidepressant
639500 <> WATSON	Tab	Chlorzoxazone 500 mg	by Martec	52555-0263	Muscle Relaxant
64 <> BI	Cap, Celery	Phendimetrazine Tartrate 105 mg	Prelu 2 by Quality Care	60346-0621	Anorexiant; C III
640	Cap, Eon Logo 640	Phentermine HCl 30 mg	by Quality Care	62682-7025	Anorexiant; C IV
643 <> 250	Tab	Naproxen 250 mg	by Roxane	00054-8641	NSAID
643 <> COPLEY	Tab, Film Coated, Debossed	Prochlorperazine 5 mg	by Qualitest	00603-5418	Antiemetic
643 <> COPLEY	Tab, Film Coated, Debossed	Prochlorperazine Maleate	by UDL	51079-0541	Antiemetic
643 <> COPLEY	Tab, Film Coated	Prochlorperazine Maleate 8.26 mg	by HJ Harkins Co	52959-0511	Antiemetic
643 <> COPLEY	Tab, Film Coated	Prochlorperazine Maleate 8.26 mg	by Quality Care	62682-7046	Antiemetic
643 <> COPLEY	Tab, Film Coated	Prochlorperazine Maleate 8.26 mg	by Copley	38245-0643	Antiemetic
644 <> DPI	Cap	Acetaminophen 500 mg, Oxycodone HCl 5 mg	by Schein	00364-2395	Analgesic; C II
647	Cap, Eon Logo 647	Phentermine HCl 30 mg	by Quality Care	62682-7025	Anorexiant; C IV
647 <> SINEMET	Tab, Dark Dapple Blue, Oval	Carbidopa 10 mg, Levodopa 100 mg	Sinemet by Dupont Pharma	00056-0647	Antiparkinson
647HD	Cap, Blue & White	Codeine 30 mg, Butalbital 50 mg, Caffeine 40 mg, Aspirin 325 mg	Fiorinal #3 by Halsey		Analgesic; C III
648HD	Cap, Gray & White	Codeine 15 mg, Butalbital 50 mg, Caffeine 40 mg, Aspirin 325 mg	Fiorinal #2 by Halsey		Analgesic; C III
650 <> ICN	Cap, Gelatin Coated	Methoxsalen 10 mg	Oxsoralen Ultra by RP Scherer	11014-1123	Dermatologic
650 <> ICN	Cap	Methoxsalen 10 mg	Oxsoralen Ultra by Banner Pharmacaps	10888-4554	Dermatologic
650 <> R	Tab, Yellow, Cap Shaped, Film Coated	Bisoprolol Fumarate 2.5 mg, Hydrochlorothiazide 6.25 mg	by Purepac	00228-2650	Antihypertensive; Diuretic
650 <> SINEMET	Tab, Yellow, Oval	Carbidopa 25 mg, Levodopa 100 mg	Sinemet by Dupont Pharma	00056-0650	Antiparkinson
651 <> R	Tab, Pink, Cap Shaped, Film Coated	Bisoprolol Fumarate 5 mg, Hydrochlorothiazide 6.25 mg	by Purepac	00228-2651	Antihypertensive; Diuretic
652 <> COPLEY	Tab, Debossed	Prochlorperazine 10 mg	by Qualitest	00603-5419	Antiemetic
652 <> COPLEY	Tab, Film Coated, Debossed	Prochlorperazine Maleate	by UDL	51079-0542	Antiemetic
652 <> COPLEY	Tab, Yellow, Round, Film Coated	Prochlorperazine Maleate 10 mg	by Phy Total Care	54868-1082	Antiemetic
652 <> COPLEY	Tab, Film Coated	Prochlorperazine Maleate 16.53 mg	by HJ Harkins Co	52959-0476	Antiemetic
652 <> COPLEY	Tab, Film Coated	Prochlorperazine Maleate 16.53 mg	by Copley	38245-0652	Antiemetic
652 <> R	Tab, White, Cap Shaped, Film Coated	Bisoprolol Fumarate 10 mg, Hydrochlorothiazide 6.25 mg	by Purepac	00228-2652	Antihypertensive; Diuretic
654 <> SINEMET	Tab, Light Dapple Blue, Oval	Carbidopa 25 mg, Levodopa 250 mg	Sinemet by Dupont Pharma	00056-0654	Antiparkinson
655 <> SQUIBB	Cap	Tetracycline HCl	by Prepackage Spec	58864-0493	Antibiotic
655 <> SQUIBB	Cap	Tetracycline HCl 250 mg	by Quality Care	60346-0609	Antibiotic
656HD	Cap, Green	Chlordiazepoxide HCl 5 mg, Clidinium Bromide 2.5 mg	Librax by Halsey		Gastrointestinal; C IV
659 <> MCNEIL	Tab, Film Coated	Tramadol HCl 50 mg	Ultram by Ortho	00062-0659	Analgesic
659 <> MCNEIL	Tab, Film Coated	Tramadol HCl 50 mg	Ultram by Caremark	00339-6099	Analgesic
659 <> MCNEIL	Tab, Film Coated	Tramadol HCl 50 mg	Ultram by DRX	55045-2219	Analgesic
659 <> MCNEIL	Tab, Film Coated	Tramadol HCl 50 mg	Ultram by McNeil	52021-0659	Analgesic
659 <> MCNEIL	Tab, Film Coated	Tramadol HCl 50 mg	Ultram by Allscripts	54569-4089	Analgesic
659 <> MCNEIL	Tab, Film Coated	Tramadol HCl 50 mg	Ultram by HJ Harkins Co	52959-0414	Analgesic
659 <> MCNEIL	Tab, Film Coated	Tramadol HCl 50 mg	Ultram by Prescription Dispensing	61807-0128	Analgesic
659 <> MCNEIL	Tab, Film Coated	Tramadol HCl 50 mg	Ultram by Heartland	61392-0625	Analgesic
659 <> MCNEIL	Tab, Film Coated	Tramadol HCl 50 mg	Ultram by PDRX	55289-0650	Analgesic
659 <> MCNEIL	Tab, Film Coated	Tramadol HCl 50 mg	Ultram by Northeast	58163-0659	Analgesic
659 <> MCNEIL	Tab, Film Coated	Trazodone HCl 50 mg	by Nat Pharmpak Serv	55154-1910	Antidepressant
65B	Cap, White, Opaque, Gelatin w/ Dark Blue Print, Organon Logo 65B	Amylase 30,000 USP, Bile Salts 65 mg, Cellulase 2 mg, Lipase 8,000 USP, Proteasse 30,000 USP	Cotazym ECS 65B by Organon	Canadian DIN# 00456233	Gastrointestinal
66 <> MP	Tab, Off-White, ER	Quinidine Gluconate 324 mg	by Quality Care	60346-0555	Antiarrhythmic
66 <> SL	Tab, Film Coated	Amitriptyline HCl 10 mg	by Vangard	00615-0828	Antidepressant

ID FRONT <> BACK	DESCRIPTION FRONT <> BACK	INGREDIENT & STRENGTH	BRAND (OR EQUIV.) & FIRM	NDC#	CLASS; SCH.
66 <> SL	Tab, Pink, Round, Film Coated	Amitriptyline HCl 10 mg	Elavil by Sidmak	50111-0366	Antidepressant
66 <> UU	Tab, White, Round	Pramipexole DiHCl 1 mg	Mirapex by Pharmacia & Upjohn	00009-0006	Antiparkinson
663 <> 93	Tab, White, Oval, Film Coated	Indapamide 1.25 mg	by Teva	00093-0663	Diuretic
6666 <> 4001	Tab	Medroxyprogesterone Acetate 10 mg	by Apotheca	12634-0108	Progestin
667400 <> WATSON	Tab, 667 over 400 <> Watson	Etodolac 400 mg	by Rugby	00536-3623	NSAID
667400 <> WATSON	Tab, 667 over 400 <> Watson	Etodolac 400 mg	by Qualitest	00603-3570	NSAID
667400 <> WATSON	Tab, 667 over 400 <> Watson	Etodolac 400 mg	by Watson	52544-0667	NSAID
667400 <> WATSON	Tab, 667 over 400 <> Watson	Etodolac 400 mg	by Major	00904-5246	NSAID
67 <> SL	Tab, Film Coated	Amitriptyline HCl 25 mg	by Nat Pharmpak Serv	55154-5814	Antidepressant
67 <> SL	Tab, Film Coated	Amitriptyline HCl 25 mg	by Kaiser	00179-1275	Antidepressant
67 <> SL	Tab, Film Coated	Amitriptyline HCl 25 mg	by Zenith Goldline	00182-1019	Antidepressant
67 <> SL	Tab, Film Coated	Amitriptyline HCl 25 mg	by Vangard	00615-0829	Antidepressant
67 <> SL	Tab, Green, Round, Film Coated	Amitriptyline HCl 25 mg	Elavil by Sidmak	50111-0367	Antidepressant
670 <> 93	Tab, Film Coated	Gemfibrozil 600 mg	by Med Pro	53978-2033	Antihyperlipidemic
67093	Tab, White, Oval, 670/93	Gemfibrozil 500 mg	by Genpharm	Canadian	Antihyperlipidemic
670L	Tab	Quinine Sulfate 260 mg	Quinamm by Zenith Goldline	00182-8615	Antimalarial
672 <> PENTOX	Tab, White, Oblong, Film Coated	Pentoxifylline 400 mg	by Blue Ridge	59273-0018	Anticoagulent
672 <> PENTOX	Tab, Film Coated	Pentoxifylline 400 mg	by Merrell	00068-0672	Anticoagulent
672 <> PENTOX	Tab, Film Coated	Pentoxifylline 400 mg	by Copley	38245-0672	Anticoagulent
672COPLEY	Tab, White, Oval, 672/Copley	Pentoxifylline 400 mg	TRENTAL by Copley		Anticoagulent
673WC	Tab	Penicillin V Potassium	by Pharmedix	53002-0202	Antibiotic
675 <> POLYVENT	Tab, 6 over 75 <> Poly-vent	Guaifenesin 600 mg, Phenylpropanolamine HCl 75 mg	Poly Vent by Pharmafab	62542-0780	Cold Remedy
675 <> POLYVENT	Tab, 6 over 75 <> Poly-Vent	Guaifenesin 600 mg, Phenylpropanolamine HCl 75 mg	Poly Vent by Poly	50991-0408	Cold Remedy
678 <> FOREST	Tab	Acetaminophen 500 mg, Butalbital 50 mg, Caffeine 40 mg	Esgic-Plus by Quality Care	60346-0957	Analgesic
678 <> FOREST	Tab	Acetaminophen 500 mg, Butalbital 50 mg, Caffeine 40 mg	Esgic Plus by Nat Pharmpak Serv	55154-4602	Analgesic
678 <> FOREST	Tab	Acetaminophen 500 mg, Butalbital 50 mg, Caffeine 40 mg	Esgic Plus by PDRX	55289-0264	Analgesic
678 <> FOREST	Tab, White, Oblong, Scored	Acetaminophen 500 mg; Butalbital 50 mg; Caffeine 40 mg	Esgic Plus by Rx Pac	65084-0195	Analgesic
678 <> FOREST	Tab, White, Oblong, Scored	Acetaminophen 500 mg; Butalbital 50 mg; Caffeine 40 mg	Esgic Plus by Rightpak	65240-0644	Analgesic
6792 <> JMI	Tab	Atropine Sulfate 0.0194 mg, Hyoscyamine Sulfate 0.1037 mg, Phenobarbital 16.2 mg, Scopolamine Hydrobromide 0.0065 mg	Belladonna PB by Quality Care	60346-0042	Gastrointestinal; C IV
682025 <> WATSON	Tab, White, Oval, Scored, 682 0.25 <> Watson	Alprazolam 0.25 mg	by Allscripts	54569-3755	Antianxiety; C IV
682025 <> WATSON	Tab, 682 over 0.25 <> Watson	Alprazolam 0.25 mg	by Watson	52544-0682	Antianxiety; C IV
68305 <> WATSON	Tab, Peach, Oval, Scored	Alprazolam 0.5 mg	by Allscripts	54569-3756	Antianxiety; C IV
68305 <> WATSON	Tab, Scored, 683 over 0.5 <> Watson	Alprazolam 0.5 mg	by Watson	52544-0683	Antianxiety; C IV
6841 <> WATSON	Tab, Blue, Oval, Scored, 684 over 1 <> Watson	Alprazolam 1 mg	by Apotheca	12634-0523	Antianxiety; C IV
68410 <> WATSON	Tab, Scored, 684 over 1.0 <> Watson	Alprazolam 1 mg	by Watson	52544-0684	Antianxiety; C IV
68410 <> WATSON	Tab, Blue, Oval, Scored, 684 1.0 <> Watson	Alprazolam 1 mg	by Allscripts	54569-4619	Antianxiety; C IV
685550 <> WATSON	Tab	Amiloride HCl 5 mg, Hydrochlorothiazide 50 mg	by Qualitest	00603-2188	Diuretic
685550 <> WATSON	Tab, Scored, 685 over 5-50 <> Watson	Amiloride HCl 5 mg, Hydrochlorothiazide 50 mg	by Watson	52544-0685	Diuretic
685550 <> WATSON	Tab, 685 over 5-50 <> Watson	Amiloride HCl 5 mg, Hydrochlorothiazide 50 mg	by Martec	52555-0338	Diuretic
685550 <> WATSON	Tab	Amiloride HCl 5 mg, Hydrochlorothiazide 50 mg	by Major	00904-2114	Diuretic
686 <> 93	Cap	Aspirin 389 mg, Caffeine 32.4 mg, Propoxyphene HCl 65 mg	Propoxyphene Compd 65 by Quality Care	60346-0682	Analgesic; C IV
68610 <> WATSON	Tab, 686 Over 10	Baclofen 10 mg	by Supremus Med	62114-0120	Muscle Relaxant
68610 <> WATSON	Tab, White, Oval, Scored	Baclofen 10 mg	by Murfreesboro Ph	51129-1409	Muscle Relaxant
68610 <> WATSON	Tab, White, Oval, Scored	Baclofen 10 mg	by DRX Pharm Consults	55045-2724	Muscle Relaxant
68610 <> WATSON	Tab, 686/10 <> Watson	Baclofen 10 mg	by Watson	52544-0686	Muscle Relaxant
68610 <> WATSON	Tab, 686/10 <> Watson	Baclofen 10 mg	by Major	00904-5216	Muscle Relaxant
68610 <> WATSON	Tab, 686/10 <> Watson	Baclofen 10 mg	by HL Moore	00839-7472	Muscle Relaxant
687	Tab, Blue, Round, 68-7	Desipramine HCl 10 mg	Norpramin by Marion Merrell Dow	Canadian	Antidepressant
687	Tab, Blue, Round, 68-7	Desipramine HCl 10 mg	Norpramin by Hoechst Marion Roussel	00068-0007	Antidepressant
68720 <> WATSON	Tab, 687/20	Baclofen 20 mg	by Supremus Med	62114-0122	Muscle Relaxant

ID FRONT <> BACK	DESCRIPTION FRONT <> BACK	INGREDIENT & STRENGTH	BRAND (OR EQUIV.) & FIRM	NDC#	CLASS; SCH.
68720 <> WATSON	Tab, 687/20 <> Watson	Baclofen 20 mg	by Watson	52544-0687	Muscle Relaxant
68720 <> WATSON	Tab, 687/20 <> Watson	Baclofen 20 mg	by Major	00904-5222	Muscle Relaxant
688125 <> WATSON	Tab, White, Oblong, Scored	Captopril 12.5 mg	by Allscripts	54569-4593	Antihypertensive
688125 <> WATSON	Tab, 688 12.5 <> Watson	Captopril 12.5 mg	by Qualitest	00603-2555	Antihypertensive
688125 <> WATSON	Tab, 688 12.5 <> Watson	Captopril 12.5 mg	by Watson	52544-0688	Antihypertensive
688125 <> WATSON	Tab, 688 12.5 <> Watson	Captopril 12.5 mg	by Major	00904-5045	Antihypertensive
68925	Tab, White, Round, Scored	Captopril 25 mg	by Southwood Pharms	58016-0166	Antihypertensive
68925 <> WATSON	Tab	Captopril 25 mg	by Qualitest	00603-2556	Antihypertensive
68925 <> WATSON	Tab	Captopril 25 mg	by Watson	52544-0689	Antihypertensive
68925 <> WATSON	Tab	Captopril 25 mg	by Major	00904-5046	Antihypertensive
69 <> M	Tab, Pink, Film Coated	Indapamide 1.25 mg	by Mylan	00378-0069	Diuretic
690	Tab, White, Round	Testolactone 50 mg	Teslac by Bristol Myers	64747-0690	Hormone
69050 <> WATSON	Tab	Captopril 50 mg	by Qualitest	00603-2557	Antihypertensive
69050 <> WATSON	Tab, Football Shaped	Captopril 50 mg	by Watson	52544-0690	Antihypertensive
69050 <> WATSON	Tab	Captopril 50 mg	by Major	00904-5047	Antihypertensive
691 <> WATSON	Tab	Captopril 100 mg	by Major	00904-5048	Antihypertensive
6910AP10MEQ	Tab, Light Orange, Round	Potassium Chloride	Klotrix by Apothecon	59772-6910	Electrolytes
6910AP10MEQ	Tab, Film Coated	Potassium Chloride 750 mg	by Mead Johnson	00015-6910	Electrolytes
6910AP10MEQ	Tab, Film Coated	Potassium Chloride 750 mg	by Caremark	00339-6120	Electrolytes
691100 <> WATSON	Tab	Captopril 100 mg	by Watson	52544-0691	Antihypertensive
693500 <> WATSON	Tab, Green, Cap Shaped, Scored, 693,500 <> Watson	Chlorzoxazone 500 mg	by Allscripts	54569-1970	Muscle Relaxant
693500 <> WATSON	Tab, Scored	Chlorzoxazone 500 mg	by Watson	52544-0693	Muscle Relaxant
693500 <> WATSON	Tab	Chlorzoxazone 500 mg	by Major	00904-0302	Muscle Relaxant
698200 <> WATSON	Tab, White, Oval, Scored	Hydroxychloroquine Sulfate 201 mg	by Allscripts	54569-4981	Antimalarial
698200 <> WATSON	Tab, Coated	Hydroxychloroquine Sulfate 201 mg	by Martec	52555-0642	Antimalarial
698200 <> WATSON	Tab, Coated	Hydroxychloroquine Sulfate 201 mg	by Watson	52544-0698	Antimalarial
698200 <> WATSON	Tab, Coated	Hydroxychloroquine Sulfate 201 mg	by Major	00904-5107	Antimalarial
698200 <> WATSON	Tab, Coated	Hydroxychloroquine Sulfate 201 mg	by Qualitest	00603-3944	Antimalarial
698200 <> WATSON	Tab, Coated	Hydroxychloroquine Sulfate 201 mg	by HL Moore	00839-7963	Antimalarial
69910 <> WATSON	Tab	Hydroxyzine HCl 10 mg	by Watson	52544-0699	Antihistamine
69910 <> WATSON	Tab	Hydroxyzine HCl 10 mg	Rezine by Martec	52555-0557	Antihistamine
6SYCBMZ	Tab, Green, Cylindrical, 6/Syc-BMZ	Bromazepam 6 mg	by Altimed	Canadian DIN# 02167824	Sedative
7 <> A	Tab, Orange, Octagon-Shaped, Film Coated	Indapamide 1.25 mg	Indapamide by RPR	00801-0777	Diuretic
7 <> A	Tab, Film Coated	Indapamide 1.25 mg	by Arcola	00070-0777	Diuretic
7 <> A	Tab, Film Coated	Indapamide 1.25 mg	by Caremark	00339-6084	Diuretic
7 <> ADAMS	Tab, Blue, Oblong, Scored	Pseudoephedrine HCl 120 mg; Methscopolamine Nitrate 2.5 mg; Chlorpheniramine Maleate 8 mg; Methscopolamine Nitrate 2.5 mg	Allerx by Adams Labs	63824-0067	Cold Remedy
7 <> LLM	Tab, White, Round, Scored, Film Coated	Ethambutol HCl 400 mg	Myambutol by Dura	51479-0047	Antituberculosis
7 <> R	Tab, Film Coated	Indapamide 1.25 mg	Lozol by Amerisource	62584-0700	Diuretic
7 <> R	Tab, Film Coated	Indapamide 1.25 mg	Lozol by Thrift Drug	59198-0263	Diuretic
7 <> R	Tab, Orange, Octagon-Shaped, Film Coated	Indapamide 1.25 mg	Lozol by RPR	00801-0700	Diuretic
7 <> R	Tab, Film Coated	Indapamide 1.25 mg	Lozol by RPR	00075-0700	Diuretic
7 <> SEARLE	Tab, Yellowish Green	Ethinyl Estradiol 0.035 mg, Norethindrone 0.5 mg, Norethindrone 1 mg	Tri Norinyl 21 Day by GD Searle	00025-0272	Oral Contraceptive
7 <> SEARLE	Tab, Yellowish Green	Ethinyl Estradiol 0.035 mg, Norethindrone 1 mg	Norinyl 1 35 21 Day by GD Searle	00025-0257	Oral Contraceptive
700 <> PU	Tab	Cabergoline 0.5 mg	Dostinex by Pharmacia & Upjohn	00013-7001	Antiparkinson
700 <> PU	Tab	Cabergoline 0.5 mg	Dostinex by Pharmacia & Upjohn	10829-7001	Antiparkinson
700 <> PU	Tab, White, Cap Shaped, Scored	Cabergoline 0.5 mg	by Pharmacia	Canadian DIN# 02242471	Antiparkinson
7001 <> 0115	Cap, White	Lipram 4500 units	by Global	00115-7001	Gastrointestinal

ID FRONT <> BACK	DESCRIPTION FRONT <> BACK	INGREDIENT & STRENGTH	BRAND (OR EQUIV.) & FIRM	NDC#	CLASS; SCH.
7001 <> 0115	Cap	Pancrelipase (Amylase,Lipase,Protease) 175.74 mg	Pancreatic Enzyme by Zenith Goldline	00182-1968	Gastrointestinal
7001 <> 0115	Cap	Pancrelipase (Amylase,Lipase,Protease) 175.74 mg	Protilase by Rugby	00536-4509	Gastrointestinal
70025 <> WATSON	Tab	Hydroxyzine HCl 25 mg	by Martec	52555-0558	Antihistamine
70025 <> WATSON	Tab	Hydroxyzine HCl 25 mg	by Watson	52544-0700	Antihistamine
7004 <> 0115	Cap, White	Lipram 4500 units	by Global	00115-7004	Gastrointestinal
7005 <> 0115	Tab, White, Round	Mephobarbital 32 mg	by Global	00115-7005	Sedative/Hypnotic; C IV
7006 <> 0115	Tab, White, Round	Mephobarbital 50 mg	by Global	00115-7006	Sedative/Hypnotic; C IV
7007 <> 0115	Tab, White, Round	Mephobarbital 100 mg	by Global	00115-7007	Sedative/Hypnotic; C IV
7008 <> 0115	Tab, Pale Blue-Green, Compressed	Hyoscyamine 0.125 mg	by Global	00115-7008	Gastrointestinal
7009 <> 0115	Tab, White, Compressed	Hyoscyamine 0.125 mg	by Global	00115-7009	Gastrointestinal
701 <> 25W	Tab	Venlafaxine HCl	Effexor by Quality Care	62682-7029	Antidepressant
7011 <> 0115	Tab, White, Round	Aminobenzoate Potassium 0.5 mg	by Global	00115-7011	Antifibrotic
7012 <> 0115	Cap, Light Gray	Aminobenzoate Potassium 0.5 mg	by Global	00115-7012	Antifibrotic
7013 <> 0115	Tab, Orange, Oblong	Guaifenesin 600 mg, Pseudoephedrine 120 mg	by Global	00115-7013	Cold Remedy
7017 <> 0115	Cap, Brown & Olive	Minocycline HCl 50 mg	by Global	00115-7017	Antibiotic
7018 <> 0115	Cap, Olive & White	Minocycline HCl 100 mg	by Global	00115-7018	Antibiotic
701W25	Tab, Peach, Pentagonal, 701/W25	Venlafaxine HCl 25 mg	Effexor by Wyeth		Antidepressant
702 <> MJ	Tab, White, Coated, Speckled	Ascorbic Acid 80 mg, Biotin 0.03 mg, Calcium 200 mg, Copper 3 mg, Cyanocobalamin 2.5 mcg, Folic Acid 1 mg, Iron 54 mg, Magnesium 100 mg, Niacin 17 mg, Pantothenic Acid 7 mg, Pyridoxine HCl 4 mg, Riboflavin 1.6 mg, Thiamine 1.5 mg, Vitamin A 4000 Units, Vitamin D 400 Units, Vitamin E 15 Units, Zinc 25 mg	Natalins Tablets Rx by Bristol Myers Squibb	00087-0702	Vitamin
7023 <> 0115	Cap, Fleshed	Lipram-PN16 16,000 units	by Global	00115-7023	Gastrointestinal
7024 <> 0115	Cap, Brown & White	Lipram-CR20 20,000 units	by Global	00115-7024	Gastrointestinal
7025 <> 0115	Tab, Light Orange, Compressed	Hyoscyamine 0.375 mg	by Global	00115-7025	Gastrointestinal
7026 <> 0115	Tab, White, Round	Oxycodone HCl 5 mg	by Global	00115-7026	Analgesic; C II
7029 <> 0115	Tab, Tan, Round	Pancrelipase 8000 units	by Global	00115-7029	Gastrointestinal
7038 <> 0115	Tab, Yellow, Round	Methyltestosterone 25 mg	by Global	00115-7038	Hormone; C III
703W50	Tab, Peach, Pentagonal, 703/W50	Venlafaxine HCl 50 mg	Effexor by Wyeth		Antidepressant
704 <> 75W	Tab	Venlafaxine HCl	Effexor by Quality Care	60346-0807	Antidepressant
704 <> 75W	Tab, Shield-Shaped	Venlafaxine HCl	Effexor by Caremark	00339-6034	Antidepressant
704 <> R	Tab, Green, Cap Shaped, Film Coated	Fluvoxamine Maleate 25 mg	by Purepac	00228-2704	OCD
704 <> W75	Tab, Shield-Shaped	Venlafaxine HCl	Effexor by Allscripts	54569-4132	Antidepressant
7040 <> 0115	Cap, Brown & Clear	Lipram-PN10 10,000 units	by Global	00115-7040	Gastrointestinal
7041 <> 0115	Cap, Fleshed & White	Lipram-PN18 18,000 units	by Global	00115-7041	Gastrointestinal
7042 <> 0115	Cap, Clear & White	Lipram-PN12 12,000 units	by Global	00115-7042	Gastrointestinal
7043 <> 0115	Cap, Browned	Lipram-PN20 20,000 units	by Global	00115-7043	Gastrointestinal
7045 <> AP	Tab, Scored	Captopril 12.5 mg	by Nat Pharmpak Serv	55154-7601	Antihypertensive
7045 <> AP	Tab, Slightly Mottled	Captopril 12.5 mg	by Apothecon	59772-7045	Antihypertensive
7045 <> AP	Tab, White, Round, Scored	Captopril 12.5 mg	by Caremark	00339-5860	Antihypertensive
7045 <> AP	Tab	Captopril 12.5 mg	by Bristol Myers	15548-0045	Antihypertensive
70450 <> WATSON	Tab	Hydroxyzine HCl 50 mg	by Watson	52544-0704	Antihistamine
70450 <> WATSON	Tab	Hydroxyzine HCl 50 mg	by Martec	52555-0559	Antihistamine
705	Tab, Gray, Round, Schering Logo 705	Perphenazine 2 mg	Trilafon by Schering		Antipsychotic
705 <> MGI	Tab, Film Coated	Pilocarpine HCl 5 mg	Salagen by MGI	58063-0705	Cholinergic Agonist
705W100	Tab, Peach, Pentagonal, 705/W100	Venlafaxine HCl 100 mg	Effexor by Wyeth		Antidepressant
707 <> SP75	Tab, Pink, Film Coated, Scored, 707 <> SP 7.5	Moexipril HCl 7.5 mg	Univasc by Schwarz Pharma	00091-3707	Antihypertensive
707 <> TONOCARD	Tab, Yellow, Oval, Score, Film	Tocainide HCl 400 mg	Tonocard by Teva	00480-0089	Antiarrhythmic
707225 <> WATSON	Tab, Light Orange, 707 2-25 <> Watson	Amitriptyline HCl 25 mg, Perphenazine 2 mg	by Watson	52544-0707	Antipsychotic
707225 <> WATSON	Tab	Amitriptyline HCl 25 mg, Perphenazine 2 mg	by Major	00904-1825	Antipsychotic
709 <> TONOCARD	Tab, Yellow, Oblong, Scored, Film	Tocainide HCl 600 mg	Tonocard by Teva	00480-0090	Antiarrhythmic
71 <> C	Tab	Atenolol 100 mg, Chlorthalidone 25 mg	by IPR	54921-0117	Antihypertensive; Diuretic

ID FRONT <> BACK	DESCRIPTION FRONT <> BACK	INGREDIENT & STRENGTH	BRAND (OR EQUIV.) & FIRM	NDC#	CLASS; SCH.
71 <> SEARLE	Tab	Ethinyl Estradiol 50 mcg, Ethynodiol Diacetate 1 mg	Demulen 1 50 28 by Pharm Utilization	60491-0183	Oral Contraceptive
71 <> SEARLE	Tab, White, Round	Ethinyl Estradiol 50 mcg, Ethynodiol Diacetate 1 mg	Demulen 1/50-21 by GD Searle	00025-0071	Oral Contraceptive
71 <> SEARLE	Tab	Ethinyl Estradiol 50 mcg, Ethynodiol Diacetate 1 mg	Demulen by Physicians Total Care	54868-3790	Oral Contraceptive
7105 <> WATSON	Tab, 710 over 5	Pindolol 5 mg	by Watson	52544-0710	Antihypertensive
7105 <> WATSON	Tab, 710 Over 5	Pindolol 5 mg	by Qualitest	00603-5220	Antihypertensive
7105 <> WATSON	Tab, 710 Over 5	Pindolol 5 mg	by Major	00904-7893	Antihypertensive
7105 <> WATSON	Tab, 710 Over 5	Pindolol 5 mg	by HL Moore	00839-7761	Antihypertensive
711	Tab, Beige, Oval, Scored	Isosorbide Mononitrate 60 mg	by Vangard Labs	00615-4544	Antianginal
711	Tab, Beige, Oval, Scored, Film, Logo and 711	Isosorbide Mononitrate 60 mg	by Murfreesboro	51129-1572	Antianginal
711 <> 93	Tab, Coated	Flurbiprofen 100 mg	by Quality Care	60346-0968	NSAID
711 <> MYLAN	Tab, Green, Coated, Beveled Edge	Hydrochlorothiazide 25 mg, Methyldopa 250 mg	by Mylan	00378-0711	Diuretic; Antihypertensive
711 <> MYLAN	Tab, Coated	Hydrochlorothiazide 25 mg, Methyldopa 250 mg	by Allscripts	54569-0513	Diuretic; Antihypertensive
7111 <> Z200	Tab, Coated	Cimetidine 200 mg	by Zenith Goldline	00172-7111	Gastrointestinal
71110 <> WATSON	Tab, 711 Over 10	Pindolol 10 mg	by Watson	52544-0711	Antihypertensive
7113 <> M	Tab, White, Round, Scored	Meperidine HCl 50 mg	by D M Graham	00756-0286	Analgesic; C II
7113 <> M	Tab, Yellow, Cap Shaped, Scored	Meperidine HCl 50 mg	Demerol by Mallinckrodt Hobart	00406-7113	Analgesic; C II
7115 <> M	Tab, Yellow, Cap Shaped, Scored	Meperidine HCl 100 mg	Demerol by Mallinckrodt Hobart	00406-7115	Analgesic; C II
7117 <> Z300	Tab, Film Coated	Cimetidine 300 mg	by Quality Care	60346-0944	Gastrointestinal
7117 <> Z300	Tab, White, Round, Coated	Cimetidine 300 mg	Tagamet by Zenith Goldline	00172-7117	Gastrointestinal
711ENDO	Tab	Glipizide 5 mg	by Dupont Pharma	00056-0711	Antidiabetic
712 <> COPLEY	Tab	Atenolol 50 mg	by Copley	38245-0712	Antihypertensive
712 <> SP	Tab, Yellow, Film Coated, Scored	Hydrochlorothiazide 12.5 mg, Moexipril HCl 7.5 mg	Uniretic by Schwarz Pharma	00091-3712	Diuretic; Antihypertensive
712 <> SP	Tab, Yellow, Film Coated	Hydrochlorothiazide 12.5 mg, Moexipril HCl 7.5 mg	Uniretic by Schwarz	51217-3712	Diuretic; Antihypertensive
712 <> VASOTEC	Tab	Enalapril Maleate 5 mg	by Med Pro	53978-0176	Antihypertensive
7122212	Tab, Brown, Round, 7122 212	Senna Concentrate 8.6 mg	by Scherer	11014-1214	Gastrointestinal
713	Tab, White, Oval, Scored, Film, Logo 713	Isosorbide Mononitrate 30 mg	by Murfreesboro	51129-1571	Antianginal
713 <> COPLEY	Tab	Atenolol 100 mg	by Copley	38245-0713	Antihypertensive
71465650 <> WATSON	Tab, Orange, Cap Shaped, Film Coated	Acetaminophen 650 mg, Propoxyphene HCl 6.5 mg	by Allscripts	54569-2588	Analgesic; C IV
71465650 <> WATSON	Tab, 714/65 650	Acetaminophen 650 mg, Propoxyphene HCl 65 mg	by Qualitest	00603-5463	Analgesic; C IV
71465650 <> WATSON	Tab, 714 65 over 650 <> Watson	Acetaminophen 650 mg, Propoxyphene HCl 65 mg	by Watson	52544-0714	Analgesic; C IV
715 <> SP15	Tab, Salmon, Film Coated, Scored	Moexipril HCl 15 mg	Univasc by Schwarz Pharma	00091-3715	Antihypertensive
715 <> SP15	Tab, Salmon, Film Coated	Moexipril HCl 15 mg	Univasc by Allscripts	54569-4276	Antihypertensive
715250 <> WATSON	Tab	Quinine Sulfate 260 mg	by Watson	52544-0715	Antimalarial
715260 <> WATSON	Tab, White, Round	Quinine Sulfate 260 mg	by Rx Pak	65084-0143	Antimalarial
7171 <> GEIGY	Tab, Film Coated	Metoprolol Tartrate 100 mg	Lopressor by Novartis	00028-0071	Antihypertensive
7171 <> GEIGY	Tab, Light Blue, Cap Shaped, Film Coated, Scored	Metoprolol Tartrate 100 mg	Lopresor by Novartis	Canadian DIN# 00397431	Antihypertensive
7171 <> Z400	Tab, Film Coated	Cimetidine 400 mg	by Golden State	60429-0047	Gastrointestinal
7171 <> Z400	Tab, Film Coated, Zenith	Cimetidine 400 mg	by Quality Care	60346-0945	Gastrointestinal
7171 <> Z400	Tab, White, Cap Shaped, Film Coated	Cimetidine 400 mg	Tagamet by Zenith Goldline	00172-7171	Gastrointestinal
7171 <> Z400	Tab, Film Coated	Cimetidine 400 mg	by Med Pro	53978-2009	Gastrointestinal
7171 <> Z400	Tab, Film Coated, Scored	Cimetidine 400 mg	by Murfreesboro	51129-1336	Gastrointestinal
7172 <> 93	Tab, Gray	Etodolac 500 mg	by Teva Pharm	00480-7172	NSAID
7172 <> 93	Tab, Gray, Oval, Film Coated	Etodolac 500 mg	by Teva Pharms	00093-7172	NSAID
71754 <> WATSON	Tab, White, Round, Scored	Yohimbine HCl 5.4 mg	by Southwood Pharms	58016-0890	Impotence Agent
71754 <> WATSON	Tab, 717 Over 5.4	Yohimbine HCl 5.4 mg	by Watson	52544-0717	Impotence Agent
71754 <> WATSON	Tab, 717 5.4 <> Watson	Yohimbine HCl 5.4 mg	by Martec	52555-0538	Impotence Agent

ID FRONT <> BACK	DESCRIPTION FRONT <> BACK	INGREDIENT & STRENGTH	BRAND (OR EQUIV.) & FIRM	NDC#	CLASS; SCH.
72 <> LOTENSINHCT	Tab, Light Pink, Oblong, Scored	Benazepril HCl 10 mg, Hydrochlorothiazide 12.5 mg	Lotensin HCT by Novartis	00083-0072	Antihypertensive; Diuretic
720	Tab, Red, Round, Schering Logo 720	Perphenazine 4 mg, Amitriptyline HCl 25 mg	Etrafon-Forte by Schering		Antipsychotic; Antidepressant
720VASERETIC	Tab, Red, Squared-Oblong, 720/Vaseretic	Enalapril Maleate 10 mg	by Frosst	Canadian	Antihypertensive
721 <> ENDO	Tab, Coated	Captopril 12.5 mg	by Dupont Pharma	00056-0721	Antihypertensive
724 <> GG	Tab	Naproxen 250 mg	by Quality Care	60346-0816	NSAID
724 <> PAR	Cap, Green & Opaque & Pink	Hydroxyurea 500 mg	Hydroxyurea by Murfreesboro	51129-1472	Antineoplastic
725 <> HD	Cap	Doxycycline Hyclate	by Quality Care	60346-0449	Antibiotic
725 <> SP	Tab, Yellow, Film Coated, Scored	Hydrochlorothiazide 25 mg, Moexipril HCl 15 mg	Uniretic by Schwarz Pharma	00091-3725	Diuretic; Antihypertensive
725 <> SP	Tab, Yellow, Film Coated	Hydrochlorothiazide 25 mg, Moexipril HCl 15 mg	Uniretic by Schwarz	51217-3725	Diuretic; Antihypertensive
725725 <> COPLEY	Tab, Pink, Hexagon, Scored	Glyburide 1.5 mg	by Blue Ridge	59273-0016	Antidiabetic
725725 <> COPLEY	Tab, Rounded Hexagon	Glyburide 1.5 mg	Micronized by Merrell	00068-3203	Antidiabetic
725725 <> COPLEY	Tab, Rounded Hexagon	Glyburide 1.5 mg	Micronized by Copley	38245-0725	Antidiabetic
72650 <> WATSON	Tab, 726 Over 50	Meperidine HCl 50 mg	by Watson	52544-0726	Analgesic; C II
726Z	Tab, Buff, Shield, 726/Z	Simvastatin 5 mg	by Frosst	Canadian	Antihyperlipidemic
727 <> 50N	Tab, Film Coated	Metoprolol Tartrate 50 mg	by Zenith Goldline	00182-1987	Antihypertensive
727 <> MYLAN	Tab, Blue, Film Coated	Amitriptyline HCl 10 mg, Perphenazine 4 mg	by Mylan	00378-0042	Antipsychotic
727100 <> WATSON	Tab, 727 Over 100	Meperidine HCl 100 mg	by Watson	52544-0727	Analgesic; C II
7279 <> BRISTOL	Cap, Burgundy & Salmon	Amoxicillin 500 mg	by Quality Care	60346-0634	Antibiotic
727N <> 50	Tab, Film Coated, 727/N	Metoprolol Tartrate 50 mg	by Schein	00364-2560	Antihypertensive
728500 <> WATSON	Tab, Blue, Oblong, Film Coated	Etodolac 500 mg	by Watson Labs	52544-0728	NSAID
73 <> MYLAN	Tab, Purple, Coated	Amitriptyline HCl 50 mg, Perphenazine 4 mg	by Mylan	00378-0073	Antipsychotic
73 <> RPC	Tab, White, Round	Propantheline Bromide 7.5 mg	Pro Banthine by Compumed	00403-5167	Gastrointestinal
7300	Tab, Film Coated, Baker Norton	Verapamil HCl 240 mg	by Rugby	00536-4823	Antihypertensive
7300	Tab, Film Coated, 7300 & 2 Triangle, 1 Inverted on Other	Verapamil HCl 240 mg	by Schein	00364-2567	Antihypertensive
7300	Tab, Film Coated	Verapamil HCl 240 mg	by Zenith Goldline	00182-1970	Antihypertensive
7300	Tab, Film Coated, Hourglass Logo	Verapamil HCl 240 mg	by Kaiser	00179-1161	Antihypertensive
7300	Tab, Ivory, Film Coated, Baker Norton Logo	Verapamil HCl 240 mg	by Allscripts	54569-3691	Antihypertensive
7300	Tab, Film Coated, Hourglass Shaped Logo	Verapamil HCl 240 mg	by Golden State	60429-0198	Antihypertensive
7300	Tab, Film Coated, Hourglass Shaped Logo	Verapamil HCl 240 mg	by Kaiser	62224-8551	Antihypertensive
7300	Tab, Film Coated	Verapamil HCl 240 mg	by Talbert Med	44514-0905	Antihypertensive
7300	Tab, Ivory, Oblong, Film Coated, Scored	Verapamil HCl 240 mg	by Caremark	00339-5808	Antihypertensive
7300	Tab, Ivory, Oblong, Hourglass Logo <> 7300	Verapamil 240 mg	Calan SR / Isoptin Sr by Zenith Goldline	00172-4280	Antihypertensive
7300	Tab, Film Coated, Baker Norton Logo	Verapamil 240 mg	by Quality Care	60346-0959	Antihypertensive
7301	Tab, Orange, Oblong	Verapamil 180 mg	Calan SR/ Isoptin St by Zenith Goldline	00172-4286	Antihypertensive
7301	Tab, Light Orange, Film Coated, 7301 & 2 Triangles, 1 Inverted on Other <>	Verapamil HCl 180 mg	by Schein	00364-2590	Antihypertensive
7301	Tab, Film Coated, Hourglass Logo	Verapamil HCl 180 mg	by Kaiser	00179-1196	Antihypertensive
7301	Tab, Film Coated, Baker Norton	Verapamil HCl 180 mg	by Rugby	00536-5630	Antihypertensive
7301	Tab, Film Coated, Debossed <> Hourglass Shape	Verapamil HCl 180 mg	by Golden State	60429-0237	Antihypertensive
7301	Tab, Film Coated, Baker Norton's Logo on the Other Side	Verapamil HCl 180 mg	by Quality Care	60346-0781	Antihypertensive
7301	Tab, Light Orange, Film Coated, <> Baker Norton's Logo	Verapamil HCl 180 mg	by United Res	00677-1518	Antihypertensive
7301	Tab, Orange, Oblong, Film Coated, Scored	Verapamil HCl 180 mg	by Caremark	00339-5810	Antihypertensive
7301 <> X	Tab, Film Coated, Hourglass Shape	Verapamil HCl 180 mg	by Heartland	61392-0345	Antihypertensive
731731MEVACOR	Tab, Light Blue, Octagon, 731/731/Mevacor	Lovastatin 20 mg	Mevacor by MSD	Canadian	Antihyperlipidemic
732MEVACOR	Tab, Green, Octagon, 732/Mevacor	Lovastatin 40 mg	Mevacor by MSD	Canadian	Antihyperlipidemic
733 <> MYLAN	Tab, Film Coated	Naproxen Sodium 550 mg	by Quality Care	60346-0826	NSAID
733 <> MYLAN	Tab, Light Blue, Film Coated, Beveled Edge	Naproxen Sodium 550 mg	by Mylan	00378-0733	NSAID
733 <> MYLAN	Tab, Film Coated	Naproxen Sodium 550 mg	by Allscripts	54569-3762	NSAID

ID FRONT <> BACK	DESCRIPTION FRONT <> BACK	INGREDIENT & STRENGTH	BRAND (OR EQUIV.) & FIRM	NDC#	CLASS; SCH.
734N <> 100	Tab, Film Coated, 734/N	Metoprolol Tartrate 100 mg	by Schein	00364-2561	Antihypertensive
735Z	Tab, Peach, Shield, 735/Z	Simvastatin 10 mg	by Frosst	Canadian	Antihyperlipidemic
737	Cap	Ascorbic Acid 150 mg, Calcium Pantothenate 10 mg, Cyanocobalamin 10 mcg, Folic Acid 1 mg, Magnesium Sulfate 70 mg, Manganese Chloride 4 mg, Niacinamide 25 mg, Pyridoxine HCl 2 mg, Riboflavin 5 mg, Thiamine Mononitrate 10 mg, Vitamin A 8000 Units, Vitamin E 50 Units, Zinc Sulfate 80 mg	Therapeutic Vit & Min by Contract	10267-0737	Vitamin
737	Cap, Black & Orange	Vitamin A 8000 IU, Vitamin E 50 IU, Ascorbic Acid 150 mg, Zinc Sulfate 80 mg, Magnesium Sulfate 70 mg	Vitacon Forte by Breckenridge	51991-0645	Vitamin
7373 <> GEIGY	Tab	Hydrochlorothiazide 50 mg, Metoprolol Tartrate 100 mg	Lopressor HCT by Novartis	00028-0073	Diuretic; Antihypertensive
7375BRISTOL	Cap, Blue & Purple, 7375 over Bristol	Cephalexin 250 mg	by Apothecon	00087-7375	Antibiotic
7375BRISTOL <> 250MG	Cap, Printed in White Ink	Cephalexin Monohydrate 250 mg	by Golden State	60429-0036	Antibiotic
7376BRISTOL	Cap, Blue, 7376 over Bristol	Cephalexin 500 mg	by Apothecon	00087-7376	Antibiotic
7376BRISTOL <> 500MG	Cap, Blue, Blue Body Printed in White Ink <> Blue Cap Written in White Ink	Cephalexin Monohydrate	by Golden State	60429-0037	Antibiotic
739 <> GG	Tab, Delayed Release	Diclofenac Sodium 75 mg	by Quality Care	60346-0463	NSAID
74 <> LOTENSINHCT	Tab, Grayish Violet, Oblong, Scored	Benazepril HCl 20 mg, Hydrochlorothiazide 12.5 mg	Lotensin HCT by Novartis	00083-0074	Antihypertensive; Diuretic
74 <> M	Tab, Green, Triangular, Film Coated	Fluphenazine HCl 5 mg	Prolixin by UDL	51079-0487	Antipsychotic
74 <> M	Tab, Light Green, Coated	Fluphenazine HCl 5 mg	by Mylan	00378-6074	Antipsychotic
74 <> ZA	Tab, White	Terazosin 1 mg	by Altimed	Canadian DIN# 02218941	Antihypertensive
74 <> ZB	Tab, Orange	Terazosin 2 mg	by Altimed	Canadian DIN# 02218968	Antihypertensive
74 <> ZC	Tab, Tan	Terazosin 5 mg	by Altimed	Canadian DIN# 02218976	Antihypertensive
74 <> ZD	Tab, Blue	Terazosin 10 mg	by Altimed	Canadian DIN# 02218984	Antihypertensive
74 <> ZE	Tab, Film Coated	Erythromycin 500 mg	by Quality Care	60346-0646	Antibiotic
740 <> EL	Cap, Ex Release	Chlorpheniramine Maleate 8 mg, Pseudoephedrine HCl 120 mg	Colfed A by Pharmafab	62542-0253	Cold Remedy
740 <> EL	Cap	Chlorpheniramine Maleate 8 mg, Pseudoephedrine HCl 120 mg	N D Clear by Seatrace	00551-0147	Cold Remedy
740Z	Tab, Tan, Shield, 740/Z	Simvastatin 20 mg	by Frosst	Canadian	Antihyperlipidemic
741 <> COPLEY	Tab, Light Blue, Film Coated	Naproxen Sodium 275 mg	by Copley	38245-0741	NSAID
741LUCHEM	Tab, Blue & White Specks, Oblong, 7/41 LuChem	Phenylpropanolamine HCl 75 mg, Guaifenesin LA 400 mg	Banex LA by LuChem		Cold Remedy
742 <> HOPE	Tab	Atropine Sulfate 0.4 mg	by Anabolic	00722-6685	Gastrointestinal
742 <> PRILOSEC20	Cap, DR	Omeprazole 20 mg	Prilosec by Allscripts	54569-3267	Gastrointestinal
742 <> PRILOSEC20	Cap, DR	Omeprazole 20 mg	Omeprazole by Med Pro	53978-1129	Gastrointestinal
742 <> PRILOSEC20	Cap, Purple	Omeprazole 20 mg	Prilosec by Amerisource Hlth	62584-0451	Gastrointestinal
742 <> PRILOSEC20	Cap, Purple	Omeprazole 20 mg	Prilosec by Southwood Pharms	58016-0327	Gastrointestinal
742 <> PRILOSEC20	Cap, DR	Omeprazole 20 mg	Omeprazole by Kaiser	00179-1245	Gastrointestinal
742 <> PRILOSEC20	Cap, DR	Omeprazole 20 mg	Prilosec by Caremark	00339-5695	Gastrointestinal
742 <> PRILOSEC20	Cap, Purple	Omeprazole 20 mg	Prilosec by PDRX	55289-0477	Gastrointestinal
742 <> PRILOSEC20	Cap, DR	Omeprazole 20 mg	Prilosec by Quality Care	62682-4001	Gastrointestinal
742 <> PRILOSEC20	Cap, DR	Omeprazole 20 mg	Prilosec by Kaiser	62224-8111	Gastrointestinal
742PRILOSEC20	Cap, Amethyst	Omeprazole 20 mg	Prilosec by AstraZeneca	00186-0742	Gastrointestinal
743 <> PRILOSEC40	Cap	Omeprazole 40 mg	Prilosec by Merck	00006-0743	Gastrointestinal
743 <> PRILOSEC40	Cap	Omeprazole 40 mg	Prilosec by Astra Merck	00186-0743	Gastrointestinal

ID FRONT <> BACK	DESCRIPTION FRONT <> BACK	INGREDIENT & STRENGTH	BRAND (OR EQUIV.) & FIRM	NDC#	CLASS; SCH.
743 <> PRILOSEC40	Tab, Opaque & Purple, Oval	Omeprazole 40 mg	Prilosec by PDRX	55289-0476	Gastrointestinal
743 PRILOSEC 40	Cap, Apricot & Amethyst	Omeprazole 40 mg	Prilosec by AstraZeneca	00186-0743	Gastrointestinal
744 <> COPLEY	Tab, Film Coated, Debossed	Naproxen Sodium 550 mg	by St Marys Med	60760-0744	NSAID
744 <> COPLEY	Tab, Film Coated	Naproxen Sodium 550 mg	by Copley	38245-0744	NSAID
7441 <> WATSON	Tab, White, Diamond Shaped, Scored, 744/1 <> Watson	Estazolam 1 mg	Prosom by Watson	52544-0744	Sedative/Hypnotic; C IV
7452 <> WATSON	Tab, Pink, Diamond Shaped, Scored, 745/2 <> Watson	Estazolam 2 mg	Prosom by Watson	52544-0745	Sedative/Hypnotic; C IV
749Z	Tab, Red, Shield, 749/Z	Simvastatin 40 mg	by Frosst	Canadian	Antihyperlipidemic
74XX	Tab, Film Coated	Potassium Chloride 750 mg	by Kaiser	00179-1235	Electrolytes
74XX	Tab, Film Coated	Potassium Chloride 750 mg	by Abbott	60692-7763	Electrolytes
74ZA	Tab, White, Round, 74/ZA	Terazosin 1 mg	by Altimed	Canadian	Antihypertensive
74ZB	Tab, Orange, Round, 74/ZB	Terazosin 2 mg	by Altimed	Canadian	Antihypertensive
74ZC	Tab, Tan, Round, 74/ZC	Terazosin 5 mg	by Altimed	Canadian	Antihypertensive
74ZD	Tab, Blue, Round, 74/ZD	Terazosin 10 mg	by Altimed	Canadian	Antihypertensive
74ZE	Tab, Mottled Pink, Oval	Erythromycin Ethylsuccinate 400 mg	by Abbott	00074-2589	Antibiotic
74ZZ	Tab, Brown, Oval, Abbott Logo	Potassium Chloride ER 600 mg	by Abbott		Electrolytes
75	Tab, Orange, Round	Amitriptyline HCl 75 mg	Apo Amitriptyline by Apotex	Canadian	Antidepressant
75	Tab, Film Coated	Clopidogrel Bisulfate 97.875 mg	Plavix by Bristol Myers Squibb	63653-1171	Antiplatelet
75	Tab, Film Coated	Clopidogrel Bisulfate 97.875 mg	by Sanofi Winthrop	53360-1171	Antiplatelet
75	Tab, Orange, Round	Desipramine 75 mg	Desipramine by Apotex	Canadian	Antidepressant
75	Gray	Levothyroxine Sodium 75 mcg	Levothroid by Murfreesboro	51129-1644	Antithyroid
75	Tab, Pink, Shield-Shaped	Ranitidine HCl 75 mg	Ranitidine by Apotex	Canadian	Gastrointestinal
75	Cap, White, Ex Release, Printed in Red	Theophylline 75 mg	Slo Bid by RPR	00801-1075	Antiasthmatic
75 <> 1171	Tab, Pink, Round	Clopidogrel Bisulfate 75 mg	Plavix by Natl Pharmpak	55154-2016	Antiplatelet
75 <> 1171	Tab, Pink, Round, Film Coated	Clopidogrel bisulfate 75 mg	Plavix by BMS	63653-1171	Antiplatelet
75 <> DORAL	Tab, Light Orange w/ White Specks, Cap Shaped, 7.5 <> Doral	Quazepam 7.5 mg	Doral by Wallace	00037-9000	Sedative/Hypnotic; C IV
75 <> DORAL	Tab, Slightly White Specks: Impressed with 7.5	Quazepam 7.5 mg	Doral by Quality Care	60346-0865	Sedative/Hypnotic; C IV
75 <> E	Tab, White, 7.5 <> E	Acyclovir 800 mg	Zydone by Allscripts	54569-4724	Antiviral
75 <> E	Tab, Blue, Octagonal, 7.5 <> E	Acetaminophen 400 mg, Hydrocodone Bitartrate 7.5 mg	Zydone by Endo Labs	63481-0669	Analgesic; C III
75 <> E	Tab, Blue, Octagonal, 7.5 <> E	Acetaminophen 400 mg; Hydrocodone Bitartrate 7.5 mg	Zydone by West Pharm	52967-0274	Analgesic; C III
75 <> FLINT	Tab	Levothyroxine Sodium 0.075 mg	Synthroid by Nat Pharmpak Serv	55154-0904	Antithyroid
75 <> FLINT	Tab	Levothyroxine Sodium 0.075 mg	Synthroid by Rite Aid	11822-5286	Antithyroid
75 <> FLINT	Tab	Levothyroxine Sodium 0.075 mg	Synthroid by Giant Food	11146-0302	Antithyroid
75 <> FLINT	Tab, Violet, Round, Scored	Levothyroxine Sodium 75 mcg	Synthroid by Knoll	00048-1050	Antithyroid
75 <> LOTENSINHCT	Tab, Red, Oblong, Scored	Benazepril HCl 20 mg, Hydrochlorothiazide 25 mg	Lotensin HCT by Novartis	00083-0075	Antihypertensive; Diuretic
75 <> N033	Cap, Bright Yellow, 75 <> N over 033	Clomipramine HCl 75 mg	by Novopharm	55953-0033	OCD
75 <> N033	Cap, Bright Yellow, 75 <> N over 033	Clomipramine HCl 75 mg	by Novopharm	43806-0033	OCD
75 <> N737	Tab, 75 <> N over 737	Diclofenac Sodium 75 mg	by DRX	55045-2247	NSAID
75 <> N737	Tab, 75 <> N over 737	Diclofenac Sodium 75 mg	by HJ Harkins Co	52959-0423	NSAID
75 <> N737	Tab, White, Round	Diclofenac Sodium 75 mg	by Novopharm	43806-0737	NSAID
75 <> N737	Tab, 75 <> N over 737	Diclofenac Sodium 75 mg	by Warrick	59930-1642	NSAID
75 <> N737	Tab, Delayed Release	Diclofenac Sodium 75 mg	by Prescription Dispensing	61807-0088	NSAID
75 <> N737	Tab, White, Round, Film Coated	Diclofenac Sodium 75 mg	by Allscripts	54569-4166	NSAID
75 <> PERCOCET	Tab, Peach, Cap Shaped, 7.5 <> Percocet	Oxycodone HCl 7.5 mg, Acetaminophen 500 mg	Percocet by Endo	63481-0621	Analgesic; C II
75 <> PERCOCET	Tab, Peach, Oblong	Oxycodone HCl 7.5 mg, Acetaminophen 500 mg	Percocet by West Pharm	52967-0279	Analgesic; C II
75 <> WEFFEXORXR	Cap, Peach	Venlafaxine HCl 75 mg	Effexor XR by Wyeth Pharms	52903-0833	Antidepressant
75 <> WEFFEXORXR	Cap, Peach	Venlafaxine HCl 75 mg	Effexor XR by Wyeth Labs	00008-0833	Antidepressant
75 <> WELLBUTRIN	Tab	Bupropion HCl 75 mg	Wellbutrin by Catalytica	63552-0177	Antidepressant
75 <> WELLBUTRIN	Tab	Bupropion HCl 75 mg	Wellbutrin by Glaxo	00173-0177	Antidepressant
750	Cap, Pink, Elongated	Polygel Controlled-Release Niacin 750 mg	Slo-Niacin by Upsher-Smith	00245-0064	Vitamin
750 <> A	Tab, Coated	Salsalate 750 mg	by Quality Care	60346-0034	NSAID
750 <> CIPRO	Tab, Film Coated	Ciprofloxacin HCl	Cipro by Nat Pharmpak Serv	55154-4807	Antibiotic

ID FRONT <> BACK	DESCRIPTION FRONT <> BACK	INGREDIENT & STRENGTH	BRAND (OR EQUIV.) & FIRM	NDC#	CLASS; SCH.
750 <> CIPRO	Tab, Film Coated	Ciprofloxacin HCl 874.5 mg	Ciprobay by Bayer	00026-8514	Antibiotic
750 <> CIPRO	Tab, Film Coated	Ciprofloxacin HCl 874.5 mg	Cipro by Physicians Total Care	54868-1184	Antibiotic
750 <> KOS	Tab, Off-White, Cap-Shaped	Niacin 750 mg	Niaspan by KOS	60598-0002	Vitamin
750 <> RELAFEN	Tab, Beige, Oval, Film Coated	Nabumetone 750 mg	Relafen by SKB	00029-4852	NSAID
750 <> RELAFEN	Tab, Film Coated	Nabumetone 750 mg	Relafen by HJ Harkins Co	52959-0373	NSAID
750 <> RELAFEN	Tab, Film Coated	Nabumetone 750 mg	Relafen by Quality Care	60346-0925	NSAID
750 <> RELAFEN	Tab, Film Coated	Nabumetone 750 mg	Relafen by SB	59742-4852	NSAID
750 <> RELAFEN	Tab, Film Coated	Nabumetone 750 mg	Relafen by DRX	55045-2440	NSAID
750 <> UCB	Tab, Orange, Oblong, Scored, Film Coated	Levetiracetam 750 mg	Keppra by UCB Pharma	50474-0593	Anticonvulsant
750A	Tab, Film Coated, 750/A	Salsalate 750 mg	by Schein	00364-0833	NSAID
750MG <> SP2164	Tab, Pink, Scored	Salsalate 750 mg	Mono-Gesic by Schwarz Pharma	00131-2164	NSAID
751 <> M	Tab, Film Coated	Cyclobenzaprine HCl 10 mg	by Kaiser	00179-1140	Muscle Relaxant
751 <> M	Tab, Butterscotch Yellow, Film Coated	Cyclobenzaprine HCl 10 mg	by Mylan	00378-0751	Muscle Relaxant
751 <> M	Tab, Film Coated	Cyclobenzaprine HCl 10 mg	by Allscripts	54569-3193	Muscle Relaxant
751 <> M	Tab, Film Coated	Cyclobenzaprine HCl 10 mg	by Physicians Total Care	54868-1110	Muscle Relaxant
751 <> M	Tab, Film Coated	Cyclobenzaprine HCl 10 mg	by Allscripts	54569-2573	Muscle Relaxant
751 <> M	Tab, Butterscotch Yellow, Round, Film Coated	Cyclobenzaprine HCl 10 mg	Flexeril by UDL	51079-0644	Muscle Relaxant
751 <> M	Tab, Film Coated	Cyclobenzaprine HCl 10 mg	by Kaiser	62224-7559	Muscle Relaxant
751 <> M	Tab, Butterscotch Yellow, Film Coated	Cyclobenzaprine HCl 10 mg	by Quality Care	60346-0581	Muscle Relaxant
751 <> M	Tab, Film Coated	Cyclobenzaprine HCl 10 mg	by PDRX	55289-0567	Muscle Relaxant
751 <> M	Tab, Yellow, Round	Cyclobenzaprine HCl 10 mg	by Va Cmop	65243-0022	Muscle Relaxant
7522	Tab, 752 and 2	Hydromorphone HCl 2 mg	by Dupont Pharma	00056-0752	Analgesic; C II
7522	Tab, White, Round 752 2	Hydromorphone HCl 2 mg	by Endo	60951-0752	Analgesic; C II
753	Cap, Green & Clear, Schering Logo 753	Theophylline LA 250 mg	Theovent by Schering		Antiasthmatic
7540 <> WATSON	Tab, White, Round, 75/40 <> Watson	Ethinyl Estradiol 40 mcg; Levonorgestrel 0.075 mg	Trivora-28 by Watson	52544-0291	Oral Contraceptive
75493	Tab, Blue, Oblong, Film Coated, 754/93	Diflunisal 250 mg	by Teva	00093-0754	NSAID
755 <> 93	Tab, Film Coated	Diflunisal 500 mg	by Quality Care	60346-0053	NSAID
755 <> 93	Tab, Film Coated	Diflunisal 500 mg	by Schein	00364-2537	NSAID
755 <> MJ	Tab	Estradiol 1 mg	by Quality Care	60346-0375	Hormone
75593	Tab, Film Coated	Diflunisal 500 mg	by Medirex	57480-0479	NSAID
75593	Tab, Film Coated	Diflunisal 500 mg	by PDRX	55289-0460	NSAID
75593	Tab, Blue, Oblong, Film Coated	Diflunisal 500 mg	by Murfreesboro Ph	51129-1684	NSAID
75593	Tab, Blue, Oblong, Film Coated, 755/93	Diflunisal 500 mg	by Teva	00093-0755	NSAID
75593	Tab, Film Coated	Diflunisal 500 mg	by Zenith Goldline	00182-1954	NSAID
75593	Tab, Film Coated	Diflunisal 500 mg	by Pharmedix	53002-0303	NSAID
75593	Tab, Film Coated, 755/93	Diflunisal 500 mg	by UDL	51079-0754	NSAID
75593	Tab, Film Coated	Diflunisal 500 mg	by Allscripts	54569-3658	NSAID
75593	Tab, Blue, Oblong, Film Coated	Diflunisal 500 mg	Diflunisal by Duramed	51285-0684	NSAID
755MJ	Tab, 755 MJ <> Bristol	Estradiol 1 mg	by Kaiser	62224-0330	Hormone
755MJ	Tab, Purple, Round	Estradiol 1 mg	Estrace by Rx Pac	65084-0181	Hormone
755MJ	Tab	Estradiol 1 mg	by Amerisource	62584-0755	Hormone
755MJ	Tab	Estradiol 1 mg	by CVS	51316-0229	Hormone
756 <> 93	Cap, Olive	Piroxicam 10 mg	by Quality Care	60346-0737	NSAID
756 <> MJ	Tab, Blue, Round, Scored	Estradiol 2 mg	Estrace by Rx Pac	65084-0187	Hormone
756MJ	Tab, Turquoise Blue, 756 MJ <>	Estradiol 2 mg	by Quality Care	60346-0029	Hormone
756MJ	Tab, Tuquoise, 756 MJ <>	Estradiol 2 mg	by Kaiser	62224-0333	Hormone
756MJ	Tab,	Estradiol 2 mg	by Physicians Total Care	54868-0495	Hormone
756PPP <> 756PPP	Cap	Procainamide HCl 375 mg	Pronestyl by ER Squibb	00003-0756	Antiarrhythmic
757 <> M	Tab	Atenolol 100 mg	by Quality Care	60346-0914	Antihypertensive
757 <> M	Tab	Atenolol 100 mg	by Diversified Hlthcare Serv	55887-0998	Antihypertensive
757 <> M	Tab, White	Atenolol 100 mg	by Mylan	00378-0757	Antihypertensive
757 <> M	Tab, White, Round	Atenolol 100 mg	Tenormin by UDL	51079-0685	Antihypertensive

ID FRONT <> BACK	DESCRIPTION FRONT <> BACK	INGREDIENT & STRENGTH	BRAND (OR EQUIV.) & FIRM	NDC#	CLASS; SCH.
757 <> M	Tab	Atenolol 100 mg	by Allscripts	54569-3654	Antihypertensive
7574	Tab	Hydromorphone HCl 4 mg	by Dupont Pharma	00056-0757	Analgesic; C II
7574	Tab, Light Yellow, Round	Hydromorphone HCl 4 mg	by Endo	60951-0757	Analgesic; C II
7575 <> DURA	Tab, 7.5/7.5 <> Dura	Guaifenesin 600 mg, Phenylpropanolamine HCl 75 mg	Dura Vent by Anabolic	00722-6051	Cold Remedy
7575 <> DURA	Tab, 7.5/7.5 <> Dura	Guaifenesin 600 mg, Phenylpropanolamine HCl 75 mg	by DHHS Prog	11819-0049	Cold Remedy
7575 <> DURA	Tab, White, Oblong, Scored, 7.5/7.5 <> Dura	Guaifenesin 600 mg, Phenylpropanolamine HCl 75 mg	Dura Vent by Med Pro	53978-3337	Cold Remedy
7575 <> DURA	Tab, 7.5/7.5 <> Dura	Guaifenesin 600 mg, Phenylpropanolamine HCl 75 mg	Dura Vent by CVS	51316-0242	Cold Remedy
7575 <> DURA	Tab, White, Scored, 7.5/7.5 <> Dura	Phenylpropanolamine HCl 75 mg, Guaifenesin 600 mg	DuraVent by Prepackage Spec	58864-0100	Cold Remedy
7575DURA	Tab, White, Oval, 7.5/7.5 Dura	Phenylpropanolamine 75 mg, Guaifenesin 600 mg	Dura-Vent by Dura		Cold Remedy
757PPP <> 757PPP	Cap, in Black Ink	Procainamide HCl 500 mg	Pronestyl by ER Squibb	00003-0757	Antiarrhythmic
758 <> 758	Cap, Yellow	Procainamide HCl 250 mg	Pronestyl by Quality Care	60346-0907	Antiarrhythmic
758PPP <> 758PPP	Cap	Procainamide HCl 250 mg	Pronestyl by ER Squibb	00003-0758	Antiarrhythmic
75A <> SEARLE1421	Tab, White to Off-White, Round, A around the circumference, 75 in the middle <> Searle over 1421	Diclofenac Sodiummisoprostol 75 mg	by Pharmacia	Canadian DIN# 02229837	NSAID
75FLI	Tab, Gray, Round, 75/FLI Logo	Levothyroxine Sodium 75 mcg	by Forest	00456-0322	
75FLINT	Tab	Levothyroxine Sodium 0.075 mg	Synthroid by Med Pro	53978-2034	Antithyroid
75M	Tab	Levothyroxine Sodium 75 mcg	Euthyrox by Em Pharma	63254-0437	Antithyroid
75M	Tab	Levothyroxine Sodium 75 mcg	Levo T by Mova	55370-0127	Antithyroid
75M	Tab	Levothyroxine Sodium 75 mcg	by Allscripts	54569-4157	Antithyroid
75MCG <> FLINT	Tab, Debossed	Levothyroxine Sodium 0.075 mg	Synthroid by Amerisource	62584-0050	Antithyroid
75MG <> WATSON596	Cap, Gelatin	Clomipramine HCl 75 mg	by Watson	52544-0596	OCD
75W <> 704	Tab	Venlafaxine HCl	Effexor by Quality Care	60346-0807	Antidepressant
75W <> 704	Tab, Shield-Shaped	Venlafaxine HCl	Effexor by Caremark	00339-6034	Antidepressant
76 <> GG	Tab, Coated	Flurbiprofen 100 mg	by Quality Care	60346-0968	NSAID
760 <> WATSON	Tab, Beige, Round	Ranitidine 150 mg	Zantac By Watson	52544-0760	Gastrointestinal
761 <> WATSON	Tab, Beige, Cap-Shaped	Ranitidine 300 mg	Zantac By Watson	52544-0761	Gastrointestinal
762 <> PAL	Tab, White, Oblong	Pseudoephedrine HCl 45 mg, Guaifenesin 600 mg	Panmist Jr by Sovereign Pharms	58716-0680	Cold Remedy
762 <> PAL	Tab, White, Oblong	Pseudoephedrine HCl 45 mg, Guaifenesin 600 mg	Panmist JR by Pan Am Labs	00525-0762	Cold Remedy
7663	Tab, Light Gray to Off-White, Round	Exemestane 25 mg	by Pharmacia	Canadian DIN# 02242705	Aromatase Inhibitor
7663	Tab, White, Round	Exemestane 25 mg	Aromasin by Pharmacia Upjohn (IT)	10829-7663	Aromatase Inhibitor
7663	Tab, White, Round	Exemestane 25 mg	Aromasin by Pharmacia & Upjohn	00009-7663	Aromatase Inhibitor
769PPP	Tab, Green, Round	Rauwolfia Serpentina 50 mg, Bendroflumethiazide 4 mg	Rauzide by BMS		Antihypertensive
77	Tab, Coated	Ascorbic Acid 500 mg, Biotin 0.15 mg, Chromic Nitrate 0.1 mg, Cupric Oxide, Cyanocobalamin 50 mcg, Ferrous Fumarate 27 mg, Folic Acid 0.8 mg, Magnesium Oxide 50 mg, Manganese Dioxide 5 mg, Niacin 100 mg, Pantothenic Acid 25 mg, Pyridoxine HCl 25 mg, Riboflavin 20 mg, Thiamine Mononitrate 20 mg, Vitamin A Acetate 5000 Units, Vitamin E Acetate 30 Units	Therobec Plus by Qualitest	00603-5970	Vitamin
770	Cap, White	Acetaminophen 500 mg	by ABG	60999-0902	Antipyretic
770	Tab, White, Oblong	Acetaminophen 500 mg	Tylenol by JB Labs		Antipyretic
771 <> WWW	Tab, White, Round	Isosorbide Dinitrate 10 mg	Isordil by West Ward	00143-1771	Antianginal
7711 <> 800	Tab, White, Oval, Scored	Cimetidine 800 mg	by Direct Dispensing	57866-6753	Gastrointestinal
7711 <> SR180	Tab, Film Coated	Verapamil 180 mg	by Qualitest	00603-6359	Antihypertensive
7711 <> SR180	Tab, Off-White, Film Coated	Verapamil HCl 180 mg	by Quality Care	60346-0781	Antihypertensive
7711 <> Z800	Tab, Coated	Cimetidine 800 mg	by Golden State	60429-0048	Gastrointestinal
7711 <> Z800	Tab, White, Oval, Coated	Cimetidine 800 mg	Tagamet by Zenith Goldline	00172-7711	Gastrointestinal
7711875 <> WATSON	Tab, White, Round, Scored, 771 over 18.75 <> Watson	Pemoline 18.75 mg	by Watson	52544-0771	Stimulant; C IV
772 <> WWW	Tab, Green, Round	Isosorbide Dinitrate 20 mg	Isordil by West Ward	00143-1772	Antianginal
7720 <> 250	Tab, Light Orange, Film Coated	Cefprozil 250 mg	Cefzil by BMS	00087-7720	Antibiotic
7720 BMS250	Tab, Orange	Cefprozil 250 mg	Cefzil by BMS	00087-7720	Antibiotic

ID FRONT <> BACK	DESCRIPTION FRONT <> BACK	INGREDIENT & STRENGTH	BRAND (OR EQUIV.) & FIRM	NDC#	CLASS; SCH.
7720BMS250	Cap, Light Orange, 7720/BMS 250	Anhydrous Cefprozil 250 mg	by Bristol-Myers	Canadian	Antibiotic
7721 <> 500	Tab, White, Film Coated	Cefprozil 500 mg	Cefzil by Bristol Myers Squibb	00087-7721	Antibiotic
7721 BMS500	Tab, White, Oblong	Cefprozil 500 mg	Cefzil by BMS	00087-7721	Antibiotic
7721BMS250	Cap, White, 7721/BMS 250	Anhydrous Cefprozil 500 mg	by Bristol-Myers	Canadian	Antibiotic
7722 <> SR240	Tab, Off-White, Film Coated	Verapamil HCl 240 mg	by DRX	55045-2321	Antihypertensive
7722 <> SR240	Tab, Film Coated	Verapamil HCl 240 mg	by Qualitest	00603-6360	Antihypertensive
7722 <> SR240	Tab, Film Coated	Verapamil HCl 240 mg	by United Res	00677-1453	Antihypertensive
7722 <> SR240	Tab, Off-White, Film Coated	Verapamil 240 mg	by Quality Care	60346-0959	Antihypertensive
772375 <> WATSON	Tab, Peach, Round, Scored, 772 over 37.5 <> Watson	Pemoline 37.5 mg	by Watson	52544-0772	Stimulant; C IV
772WESTWARD	Tab	Isosorbide Dinitrate 20 mg	by Schein	00364-0509	Antianginal
773	Tab, White, Round	Hyoscyamine Sulfate 0.125 mg	Levsin by Marlop		Gastrointestinal
773 <> S	Tab	Isosorbide Dinitrate 30 mg	Sorbitrate by Zeneca	00310-0773	Antianginal
7731875 <> WATSON	Tab, Yellow, Round, Scored, 773 over 18.75 <> Watson	Pemoline 75 mg	by Watson	52544-0773	Stimulant; C IV
774 <> S	Tab, Light Blue	Isosorbide Dinitrate 40 mg	Sorbitrate by Zeneca	00310-0774	Antianginal
774 <> WATSON	Tab, White, Round, Scored	Oxycodone HCl 5 mg	Percolone by Watson	52544-0774	Analgesic; C II
7747BRL	Tab, Blue, 77/47/BRL	Oxybutynin Chloride 5 mg	by Parke-Davis	Canadian DIN# 02220067	Urinary
775 <> DESYRELMJ	Tab, Film Coated	Trazodone HCl 50 mg	Desyrel by Quality Care	60346-0504	Antidepressant
7767 <> 100	Cap, White	Celecoxib 100 mg	Celebrex by Allscripts	54569-4671	NSAID
7767 <> 100	Cap, White, Blue Print	Celecoxib 100 mg	Celebrex by Pfizer	Canadian DIN# 02239941	NSAID
7767 <> 100	Cap, White	Celecoxib 100 mg	Celebrex by Caremark	00339-6160	NSAID
7767 <> 100	Cap, White, 2 Blue Bands	Celecoxib 100 mg	Celebrex by Caremark	00339-6158	NSAID
7767 <> 100	Cap, White	Celecoxib 100 mg	Celebrex by Caremark	00339-6165	NSAID
7767 <> 100	Cap, White	Celecoxib 100 mg	Celebrex by Caremark	00339-6163	NSAID
7767 <> 200	Cap, White	Celecoxib 200 mg	Celebrex by Pfizer	Canadian DIN# 02239942	NSAID
7767 <> 200	Cap, White	Celecoxib 200 mg	Celebrax by Southwood Pharms	58016-0223	NSAID
7767 <> 200	Cap, White	Celecoxib 200 mg	Celebrex by Phy Total Care	54868-4101	NSAID
7767 <> 200	Cap, White, Gold Print	Celecoxib 200 mg	Celecoxib by Pfizer	Canadian DIN# 02239941	NSAID
7767 <> 200	Cap, White	Celecoxib 200 mg	Celebrex by Caremark	00339-6159	NSAID
7767 <> 200	Cap, White	Celecoxib 200 mg	Celebrex by Caremark	00339-6162	NSAID
7767 <> 200	Cap, White	Celecoxib 200 mg	Celebrex by Caremark	00339-6164	NSAID
7767 <> 200	Cap, White	Celecoxib 200 mg	Celebrex by Caremark	00339-6161	NSAID
7767100	Cap, White	Celecoxib 100 mg	Celebrex by GD Searle	00025-1520	NSAID
7767100	Cap, White w/ Blue Print, 7767 100	Celecoxib 100 mg	by Pharmacia	Canadian DIN# 02239941	NSAID
7767200	Cap, White	Celecoxib 200 mg	Celebrex by GD Searle	00025-1525	NSAID
7767200	Cap, White, w/ Gold Markings	Celecoxib 200 mg	Celebrex by Lederle	Canadian DIN# 02239942	NSAID
777 <> MYLAN	Tab	Lorazepam 2 mg	by Vangard	00615-0452	Sedative/Hypnotic; C IV
778 <> 9393	Tab, Pink with Red Specks, Round, Scored, Chewable, 778 <> 93 over 93	Carbamazepine 100 mg	by Teva	00093-0778	Anticonvulsant
778 <> 9393	Tab, Pink, with Red Specks, Round, Scored, 778 <> 93 over 93	Carbamazepine 100 mg, Chewable	Tegretol by UDL	51079-0870	Anticonvulsant

ID FRONT <> BACK	DESCRIPTION FRONT <> BACK	INGREDIENT & STRENGTH	BRAND (OR EQUIV.) & FIRM	NDC#	CLASS; SCH.
78 <> WYETH	Tab	Ethinyl Estradiol 0.03 mg, Norgestrel 0.3 mg	Lo Ovral 28 by Dept Health Central Pharm	53808-0028	Oral Contraceptive
78 <> WYETH	Tab	Ethinyl Estradiol 0.03 mg, Norgestrel 0.3 mg	Lo Ovral by PDRX	55289-0246	Oral Contraceptive
780 <> GG	Tab, White, Round, Film Coated	Methylphenidate HCl 20 mg	by Caremark	00339-4103	Stimulant; C II
780 <> PAL	Tab, Green, Oblong, Scored	Methscopolamine Nitrate 2.5 mg; Chlorpheniramne Maleate 8 mg; Phenylpropanolamine HCl 75 mg	Pannaz by Murfreesboro Ph	51129-1429	Cold Remedy
780 <> S	Tab	Isosorbide Dinitrate 10 mg	Sorbitrate by Zeneca	00310-0780	Antianginal
781 <> 375W	Tab, Shield-Shaped	Venlafaxine HCl	Effexor by Caremark	00339-6035	Antidepressant
781 <> 375W	Tab, Shield-Shaped, 37.5 W	Venlafaxine HCl	Effexor by Allscripts	54569-4131	Antidepressant
781W375	Tab, Peach, Pentagonal, 781/W37.5	Venlafaxine HCl 37.5 mg	Effexor by Wyeth		Antidepressant
782 <> S	Tab, Light Green, Coated, 78-2 <> S in Triangle	Thioridazine HCl 10 mg	Mellaril by Novartis	00078-0002	Antipsychotic
78240	Cap, 78/240 <> MMD Logo	Cyclosporine 25 mg	Sandimmune by Nat Pharmpak Serv	55154-3415	Immunosuppressant
78240	Cap, Pink, Gelatin, 78/240	Cyclosporine 25 mg	Sandimmune by Novartis	00078-0240	Immunosuppressant
78241	Cap, Dusty Rose, Gelatin, 78/241	Cyclosporine 100 mg	Sandimmune by Novartis	00078-0241	Immunosuppressant
78242	Cap, Yellow, Gelatin, 78/242	Cyclosporine 50 mg	Sandimmune by Novartis	00078-0242	Immunosuppressant
7827	Tab, Green, Orange & White, Round, 78-27	Bellafoline 0.25 mg, Phenobarbital 50 mg	Belladenal-S by Sandoz		Gastrointestinal; C IV
7828	Tab, White, Round, 78-28	Bellafoline 0.25 mg, Phenobarbital 50 mg	Belladenal by Sandoz		Gastrointestinal; C IV
783 <> GG	Tab, Yellow, Round	Methylphenidate HCl 5 mg	by Caremark	00339-4100	Stimulant; C II
783 <> WATSON	Tab, White, Round	Diethylpropion HCl 25 mg	by Blue Ridge	59273-0007	Antianorexiant; C IV
7831	Tab, Green, Orange & Yellow, Round, 78-31	Bellafoline 0.2 mg, Phenobarbital 40 mg, Ergotamine Tartrate 0.6 mg	Bellergal-S by Sandoz		Gastrointestinal; C IV
7840 <> AHR2	Tab, White, Round, Scored	Glycopyrrolate 2 mg	Robinul Forte by Lederle	59911-3787	Gastrointestinal
785	Tab	Ursodiol 250 mg	Urso by Schwarz Pharma		Gastrointestinal
785	Tab, Film Coated	Ursodiol 250 mg	Urso by Schering	00982-0785	Gastrointestinal
785 <> WATSON	Cap, Green & Yellow	Chlordiazepoxide HCl 5 mg	by Blue Ridge	59273-0045	Antianxiety; C IV
785 <> WESTWARD	Tab, West-Ward	Aspirin 325 mg, Butalbital 50 mg, Caffeine 40 mg	by Quality Care	60346-0619	Analgesic; C III
785 <> WESTWARD	Tab	Aspirin 325 mg, Butalbital 50 mg, Caffeine 40 mg	by Schein	00364-0677	Analgesic; C III
7854 <> SANDOZ	Tab, Purple, Round, 78-54	Methylergonovine Maleate 0.2 mg	Methergine by Neuman Distr	64579-0020	Ergot
7854 <> SANDOZ	Tab, Purple, Round	Methylergonovine Maleate 0.2 mg	Methergine by Novartis Pharms (Ca)	61615-0107	Ergot
7854 <> SANDOZ	Tab, Orchid, Coated, 78-54 in Black Ink	Methylergonovine Maleate 0.2 mg	Methergine by Kaiser	00179-0432	Ergot
7854 <> SANDOZ	Tab, Coated	Methylergonovine Maleate 0.2 mg	Methergine by Allscripts	54569-3920	Ergot
7854 <> SANDOZ	Tab, Coated	Methylergonovine Maleate 0.2 mg	Methergine by Allscripts	54569-0973	Ergot
7854 <> SANDOZ	Tab, Coated, 78-54	Methylergonovine Maleate 0.2 mg	Methergine by Quality Care	60346-0028	Ergot
7854 <> SANDOZ	Tab, Coated	Methylergonovine Maleate 0.2 mg	Methergine by PDRX	55289-0708	Ergot
7858 <> SANDOZ	Tab, 78-58 <> Sandoz	Methysergide Maleate 2 mg	Sansert by Novartis	00078-0058	Antimigraine
7866 <> SANDOZ	Tab, White, Round, Scored	Mazindol 2 mg	Sanorex by Nat Pharmpak Serv	55154-5545	Anorexiant
7871 <> SANOREX	Tab, White, Eliptical, 78-71 <> Sanorex	Mazindol 1 mg	by Allscripts	54569-4517	Anorexiant
788 <> 93	Tab	Selegiline HCl 5 mg	by Murfreesboro	51129-1111	Antiparkinson
788 <> 93	Tab, White to Off-White, Round	Selegiline HCl 5 mg	by Teva	00093-0788	Antiparkinson
788 <> 93	Tab, Flat	Selegiline HCl 5 mg	by Vangard	00615-4516	Antiparkinson
788 <> 93	Tab, Debossed, Beveled	Selegiline HCl 5 mg	by Teva	17372-0788	Antiparkinson
789 <> GG	Tab, Green, Round, Scored	Methylphenidate HCl 10 mg	by Caremark	00339-4101	Stimulant; C II
789 <> RESPA	Cap	Brompheniramine Maleate 6 mg, Pseudoephedrine HCl 60 mg	Respahist by Pharmafab	62542-0102	Cold Remedy
79	Tab, Coated	Ascorbic Acid 500 mg, Calcium Pantothenate 18 mg, Cyanocobalamin 5 mcg, Folic Acid 0.5 mg, Niacinamide 100 mg, Pyridoxine HCl 4 mg, Riboflavin 15 mg, Thiamine Mononitrate 15 mg	Therobec by Qualitest	00603-5969	Vitamin
793 <> WATSON	Tab, White	Naproxen Sodium 550 mg	by Blue Ridge	59273-0041	NSAID
79410 <> WATSON	Cap, Dark Blue	Dicyclomine HCl 10 mg	Bentyl by Watson	52544-0794	Gastrointestinal
795	Tab, Pink, Round	Anisindione 50 mg	Miradon by Schering	00085-0795	Anticoagulant
79520 <> WATSON	Tab, Blue, Round	Dicyclomine HCl 20 mg	Bentyl by Watson	52544-0795	Gastrointestinal
7992	Cap	Ampicillin Trihydrate	by Apotheca	12634-0417	Antibiotic
7992 <> BRISTOL	Cap	Ampicillin Trihydrate	by Quality Care	60346-0082	Antibiotic
7993 <> BRISTOL	Cap	Ampicillin Trihydrate	by Quality Care	60346-0593	Antibiotic

ID FRONT <> BACK	DESCRIPTION FRONT <> BACK	INGREDIENT & STRENGTH	BRAND (OR EQUIV.) & FIRM	NDC#	CLASS; SCH.
79B <> TEC	Tab, Beige, D-Shaped, Film Coated, Scored	Famotidine 20 mg	by Altimed	Canadian DIN# 02242327	Gastrointestinal
79B <> TEC	Tab, Brown, D-Shaped, Film Coated, Scored	Famotidine 40 mg	by Altimed	Canadian DIN# 02242328	Gastrointestinal
8	Tab, Green, Oblong	Doxazosin Mesylate 8 mg	Cardura by Roerig	00049-2780	Antihypertensive
8	Tab, Coated	Ibuprofen 800 mg	by Zenith Goldline	00182-1297	NSAID
8	Tab, Embossed, Double Knoll Triangle	Hydromorphone HCl 8 mg	Dilaudid by Knoll	00044-1028	Analgesic; C II
8	Tab, Film Coated	Ibuprofen 400 mg	by Quality Care	60346-0030	NSAID
8	Tab, White, Oval	Ibuprofen 800 mg	Mortin by Norton		NSAID
8	Tab, White, Round	Perphenazine 8 mg	Apo Perphenazine by Apotex	Canadian	Antipsychotic
8 <> 93	Tab, White, Round, Film Coated	Indapamide 2.5 mg	by Teva	00093-0008	Diuretic
8 <> COPLEY711	Tab	Guanabenz Acetate 10.28 mg	by Copley	38245-0711	Antihypertensive
8 <> GLAXO	Tab, Yellow, Oval	Ondansetron HCl 8 mg	Zofran by Glaxo Wellcome	00173-0447	Antiemetic
8 <> R	Tab, Film Coated	Indapamide 2.5 mg	Lozol by RPR	00075-0082	Diuretic
8 <> R	Tab, Film Coated	Indapamide 2.5 mg	Lozol by Drug Distr	52985-0062	Diuretic
8 <> R	Tab, Film Coated	Indapamide 2.5 mg	Lozol by Nat Pharmpak Serv	55154-4011	Diuretic
8 <> R	Tab, Film Coated	Indapamide 2.5 mg	Lozol by Allscripts	54569-0579	Diuretic
8 <> R	Tab, Film Coated	Indapamide 2.5 mg	Lozol by Thrift Drug	59198-0174	Diuretic
8 <> R	Tab, Film Coated	Indapamide 2.5 mg	Lozol by Pharm Utilization	60491-0382	Diuretic
8 <> R	Tab, White, Octagon-Shaped, Film Coated	Indapamide 2.5 mg	Lozol by RPR	00801-0082	Diuretic
8 <> SAMPLE	Tab	Ondansetron HCl 8 mg	Zofran by Glaxo Wellcome	00173-0447	Antiemetic
8 <> USL	Tab, Dark Blue, Film Coated	Potassium Chloride 600 mg	by Quality Care	60346-0453	Electrolytes
8 <> VOLMAX	Tab, White, Hexagon	Albuterol Sulfate 8 mg	Volmax by Thrift Services	59198-0355	Antiasthmatic
8 <> VOLMAX	Tab	Albuterol Sulfate 9.6 mg	Volmax by Muro	00451-0399	Antiasthmatic
8 <> VOLMAX	Tab, Dark Blue Print	Albuterol Sulfate 9.6 mg	Volmax by Eckerd Drug	19458-0849	Antiasthmatic
8 <> Z36698	Tab, Sugar Coated, Zenith Logo Over 3669 Over 8	Perphenazine 8 mg	by Quality Care	60346-0990	Antipsychotic
8 <> ZOFRAN	Tab, Yellow, Oval	Ondansetron HCl 8 mg	Zofran by Glaxo Wellcome	00173-0447	Antiemetic
80	Tab, Blue	Acetaminophen 80 mg	by Bayer	Canadian	Antipyretic
80	Tab	Acetaminophen 80 mg	by Mead Johnson	Canadian DIN# 00884561	Antipyretic
80 <> 59911	Cap, Blue & White	Propranolol HCl 80 mg	by ESI Lederle	59911-5471	Antihypertensive
80 <> CALAN	Tab, Film Coated	Verapamil HCl 80 mg	Calan by Nat Pharmpak Serv	55154-3603	Antihypertensive
80 <> CALAN	Tab, Peach, Oval, Film Coated	Verapamil HCl 80 mg	Calan by GD Searle	00025-1851	Antihypertensive
80 <> CALAN	Tab, Film Coated	Verapamil HCl 80 mg	Calan by Amerisource	62584-0852	Antihypertensive
80 <> CALAN	Tab, Film Coated, Debossed	Verapamil HCl 80 mg	Calan by Thrift Drug	59198-0015	Antihypertensive
80 <> DAN5557	Tab	Propranolol HCl 80 mg	by Danbury	00591-5557	Antihypertensive
80 <> INV238	Tab	Nadolol 80 mg	Nadolol by Schein	00364-2654	Antihypertensive
80 <> INV238	Tab	Nadolol 80 mg	Nadolol by Zenith Goldline	00182-2634	Antihypertensive
80 <> INV238	Tab	Nadolol 80 mg	Nadolol by Invamed	52189-0238	Antihypertensive
80 <> INV238	Tab	Nadolol 80 mg	Nadolol by Geneva	00781-1183	Antihypertensive
80 <> INV238	Tab	Nadolol 80 mg	Nadolol by Major	00904-5071	Antihypertensive
80 <> INV238	Tab	Nadolol 80 mg	Nadolol by HL Moore	00839-7871	Antihypertensive
80 <> LESCOLXL	Tab, Yellow, Round, Film Coated	Fluvastatin Sodium 80 mg	Lescol XL by Novartis	00078-0354	Antihyperlipidemic
80 <> M	Tab, White, Coated, Bevel-edged	Indapamide 2.5 mg	by Mylan	00378-0080	Diuretic
80 <> M	Tab, White, Round, Film-Coated, 80 <> M	Indapamide 2.5 mg	Lozol by UDL	51079-0868	Diuretic
80 <> M	Tab, Coated	Indapamide 2.5 mg	by DRX	55045-2385	Diuretic
80 <> MSD543	Tab, Brick Red, Cap-Shaped, Film Coated	Simvastatin 80 mg	Zocor by Merck	00006-0543	Antihyperlipidemic
80 <> MSD543	Tab, Film Coated	Simvastatin 80 mg	Simvastatin by Merck Sharp and Dohme	60312-0543	Antihyperlipidemic
80 <> MYLAN185	Tab, Yellow, Round, Scored, 80 <> Mylan over 185	Propranolol HCl 80 mg	Inderal by UDL	51079-0280	Antihypertensive

ID FRONT <> BACK	DESCRIPTION FRONT <> BACK	INGREDIENT & STRENGTH	BRAND (OR EQUIV.) & FIRM	NDC#	CLASS; SCH.
80 <> MYLAN185	Tab, Yellow, Beveled Edge, Mylan Over 185	Propranolol HCl 80 mg	by Mylan	00378-0185	Antihypertensive
80 <> MYLAN232	Tab, White, Round, Scored, 80 <> Mylan over 232	Furosemide 80 mg	Lasix by UDL	51079-0527	Diuretic
80 <> MYLAN232	Tab, White, 80 <> Mylan over 232	Furosemide 80 mg	by Mylan	00378-0232	Diuretic
80 <> OC	Tab, Green, Round	Oxycodone HCl 80 mg	Oxycontin by Phy Total Care	54868-3986	Analgesic; C II
80 <> OC	Tab	Oxycodone HCl 80 mg	Oxycontin by PF	48692-0005	Analgesic; C II
80 <> OC	Tab	Oxycodone HCl 80 mg	Oxycontin by Purdue Pharma	59011-0107	Analgesic; C II
80 <> TYLENOL	Tab, Pink or Purple, Round, Scored, Chewable	Acetaminophen	Children's Tylenol Chewable by McNeil	Canadian DIN# 02229539	Antipyretic
80 <> TYLENOLCOLD	Tab, Pink or Orange, Round, Scored, Chewable	Acetaminophen 80 mg, Chlorpheniramine Maleate 0.5 mg, Pseudoephedrine HCl 7.5 mg	Children's Tylenol by McNeil	Canadian DIN# 00743224	Cold Remedy
80 <> TYLENOLCOLDDM	Tab, Pink or Purple, Round, Chewable	Acetaminophen 80 mg, Chlorpheniramine Maleate 0.5 mg, Pseudoephedrine HCl 7.5 mg, Dextrometh 3.75 mg	Children's Tylenol by McNeil	Canadian DIN# 00870455	Cold Remedy
800	Tab, Film Coated	Ibuprofen 400 mg	by Quality Care	60346-0030	NSAID
800 <> 4268	Tab, White, Oval	Acyclovir 800 mg	Zovirax by Zenith Goldline	00172-4268	Antiviral
800 <> 4268	Tab, White, Oval	Acyclovir 800 mg	Zovirax by Zenith Goldline	00182-2667	Antiviral
800 <> 7711	Tab, White, Oval, Scored	Cimetidine 800 mg	by Direct Dispensing	57866-6753	Gastrointestinal
800 <> A03	Tab	Acyclovir 800 mg	by Martec	52555-0684	Antiviral
800 <> A03	Tab, White, Oval	Acyclovir 800 mg	Zovirax by Mova	55370-0556	Antiviral
800 <> G	Tab, Film Coated	Ibuprofen 400 mg	by Quality Care	60346-0030	NSAID
800 <> IP137	Tab, Film Coated	Ibuprofen 800 mg	by Urgent Care Ctr	50716-0726	NSAID
800 <> IP137	Tab, Coated	Ibuprofen 800 mg	by Golden State	60429-0094	NSAID
800 <> IP137	Tab, Coated	Ibuprofen 800 mg	by Prescription Dispensing	61807-0012	NSAID
800 <> IP137	Tab, White, Film Coated	Ibuprofen 800 mg	by Major Pharms	00904-5187	NSAID
800 <> IP137	Tab, Film Coated	Ibuprofen 400 mg	by Quality Care	60346-0030	NSAID
800 <> MP99	Tab, Film Coated	Ibuprofen 800 mg	by United Res	00677-1119	NSAID
800 <> N235	Tab, Film Coated, Scored	Cimetidine 800 mg	by Warrick	59930-1803	Gastrointestinal
800 <> N235	Tab, Coated, N/235	Cimetidine 800 mg	by Brightstone	62939-2141	Gastrointestinal
800 <> N235	Tab, Coated	Cimetidine 800 mg	by United Res	00677-1530	Gastrointestinal
800 <> N947	Tab, White, Cap Shaped	Acyclovir 800 mg	by Allscripts	54569-4724	Antiviral
800 <> N947	Tab, Off-White to White, Cap Shaped, 800 <> N over 947	Acyclovir 800 mg	by UDL	51079-0878	Antiviral
800 <> N947	Tab, White, Cap Shaped, 800 <> N over 947	Acyclovir 800 mg	by Novopharm	43806-0947	Antiviral
800 <> N947	Tab, White to Off-White, Cap Shaped	Acyclovir 800 mg	by Novopharm	55953-0947	Antiviral
800 <> N947	Tab	Acyclovir 800 mg	by Warrick	59930-1584	Antiviral
800 <> PAR216	Tab, Film Coated	Ibuprofen 800 mg	by Zenith Goldline	00172-3648	NSAID
800 <> PAR216	Tab, Coated, Debossed, Par Over 216	Ibuprofen 800 mg	by Zenith Goldline	00182-1297	NSAID
800 <> PAR216	Tab, Film Coated, Par Over 216	Ibuprofen 800 mg	by PDRX	55289-0140	NSAID
800 <> PAR216	Tab, Coated	Ibuprofen 800 mg	by Par	49884-0216	NSAID
800 <> PAR216	Tab, Coated, Par Over 216	Ibuprofen 800 mg	by Nat Pharmpak Serv	55154-5565	NSAID
800 <> PAR216	Tab, White, Capsule Shaped, Film-Coated, 800 <> Par Over 216	Ibuprofen 800 mg	Rufen/Motrin by UDL	51079-0596	NSAID
800 <> PAR216	Tab, Film Coated	Ibuprofen 400 mg	by Quality Care	60346-0030	NSAID
800 <> PAR216	Tab, Coated, Par Over 216	Ibuprofen 800 mg	by Baker Cummins	63171-1297	NSAID
800 <> SCHEIN2137	Tab, Film Coated	Ibuprofen 400 mg	by Quality Care	60346-0030	NSAID
800 <> ZOVIRAX	Tab, Light Blue	Acyclovir 800 mg	Zovirax by Quality Care	60346-0735	Antiviral
800M80 <> MOVA	Tab, White, Cap Shaped, Scored	Cimetidine 800 mg	Tagamet by Mova	55370-0137	Gastrointestinal
800M8C <> MOVA	Tab, White, Oblong, Film Coated, 800/M8C <> Mova	Cimetidine 800 mg	by Compumed		Gastrointestinal
800MCG <> 286	Tab, Brown	Cerivastatin Sodium 0.8 mg	Baycol by Bayer	00026-2886	Antihyperlipidemic
800MG	Tab	Ibuprofen 800 mg	Motrin by Rite Aid	11822-5213	NSAID
800MG <> MOTRIN	Tab, Apricot, Coated	Ibuprofen 800 mg	Motrin by Quality Care	60346-0855	NSAID
800N <> 235	Tab, Light Green, Coated, 800/N	Cimetidine 800 mg	by Schein	00364-2594	Gastrointestinal

ID FRONT <> BACK	DESCRIPTION FRONT <> BACK	INGREDIENT & STRENGTH	BRAND (OR EQUIV.) & FIRM	NDC#	CLASS; SCH.
801 <> MYLAN	Tab, Coated, Beveled Edge	Ibuprofen 800 mg	by Mylan	00378-0801	NSAID
801 <> WATSON	Cap, Green & White	Hydroxyzine Pamoate 50 mg	by Blue Ridge	59273-0044	Antihistamine
801 <> WATSON	Tab, Green & Opaque & White	Hydroxyzine Pamoate 50 mg	by Murfreesboro	51129-1486	Antihistamine
80MG <> BETAPACE	Tab, Light Blue	Sotalol HCl 80 mg	by Caremark	00339-6051	Antiarrhythmic
80MG <> BETAPACE	Tab, Light Blue	Sotalol HCl 80 mg	by Nat Pharmpak Serv	55154-0305	Antiarrhythmic
80MGBERLEX	Tab, White, Cap Shaped, Scored	Sotalol HCl 80 mg	Betapace by Berlex Labs	50419-0115	Antiarrhythmic
80MGBETAPACE	Tab, Light Blue, Cap Shaped, Scored	Sotalol HCl 80 mg	Betapace by Berlex	50419-0105	Antiarrhythmic
80Z <> 4237	Tab, White, Round	Nadolol 80 mg	Corgard by Zenith Goldline	00172-4237	Antihypertensive
80Z <> 4237	Tab	Nadolol 80 mg	Nadolol by Zenith Goldline	00182-2634	Antihypertensive
80Z4237	Tab, White, Round, 80Z/4237	Nadolol 80 mg	Nadolol by Zenith Goldline	00172-4237	Antihypertensive
810 <> S	Tab, Chew	Isosorbide Dinitrate 5 mg	Sorbitrate by Zeneca	00310-0810	Antianginal
812	Cap, Blue & White	Butalbital 50 mg, Acetaminophen 325 mg, Caffeine 40 mg	Fiogesic by Marlop		Analgesic
814	Tab	Ibuprofen 400 mg	Motrin by Marlop		NSAID
815	Tab, Chew	Isosorbide Dinitrate 10 mg	Sorbitrate by Pharmedix	53002-1061	Antianginal
815 <> S	Tab, Chew	Isosorbide Dinitrate 10 mg	Sorbitrate by Zeneca	00310-0815	Antianginal
82	Tab, White, Round	Indapamide 2.5 mg	Lozol by RPR		Diuretic
820	Tab, Red, Oval, 820 <> Schering Logo	Dexchlorpheniramine 2 mg	Polaramine by Schering	00085-0820	Antihistamine
820 <> S	Tab	Isosorbide Dinitrate 20 mg	Sorbitrate by Zeneca	00310-0820	Antianginal
820 <> S	Tab	Isosorbide Dinitrate 20 mg	Sorbitrate by Nat Pharmpak Serv	55154-4402	Antianginal
822 <> 101010	Tab, Pink, Trisected, MJ Logo	Buspirone HCl 30 mg	Buspar by Bristol Myers Squibb	00087-0824	Antianxiety
822 <> 555	Tab, White, Trisected, MJ Logo	Buspirone HCl 15 mg	Buspar by Bristol Myers Squibb	00087-0822	Antianxiety
822 <> MJ	Tab, White, Scored	Buspirone HCl 15 mg	Buspar by Direct Dispensing	57866-0904	Antianxiety
830	Cap	Hydroxyurea 500 mg	Hydrea by Bristol Myers Squibb	17101-0830	Antineoplastic
8311 <> BARR	Tab, Pink, Oval, Scored	Warfarin Sodium 1 mg	by UDL	51079-0908	Anticoagulant
8311 <> BARR	Tab, Pink, Oval, Flat, Scored, 831/1 <> Barr	Warfarin Sodium 1 mg	by UCB		Anticoagulant
831BM05	Tab	Benztropine Mesylate 0.5 mg	by Rosemont	00832-1080	Antiparkinson
832 <> 10	Tab, Butterscotch Yellow, Sugar Coated	Chlorpromazine HCl 10 mg	by Schein	00364-0380	Antipsychotic
832 <> 10	Tab, Butterscotch Yellow, Sugar Coated	Chlorpromazine HCl 10 mg	by Qualitest	00603-2808	Antipsychotic
832 <> 100	Tab, Butterscotch Yellow, Sugar Coated	Chlorpromazine HCl 100 mg	by Schein	00364-0383	Antipsychotic
832 <> 100	Tab, Butterscotch Yellow, Sugar Coated	Chlorpromazine HCl 100 mg	by Qualitest	00603-2811	Antipsychotic
832 <> 100	Tab, Sugar Coated	Chlorpromazine HCl 100 mg	by United Res	00677-0456	Antipsychotic
832 <> 200	Tab, Butterscotch Yellow, Sugar Coated	Chlorpromazine HCl 200 mg	by Schein	00364-0384	Antipsychotic
832 <> 200	Tab, Coated	Chlorpromazine HCl 200 mg	by United Res	00677-0787	Antipsychotic
832 <> 200	Tab, Butterscotch Yellow, Sugar Coated	Chlorpromazine HCl 200 mg	by Qualitest	00603-2812	Antipsychotic
832 <> 25	Tab, Butterscotch Yellow, Sugar Coated	Chlorpromazine HCl 25 mg	by Qualitest	00603-2809	Antipsychotic
832 <> 38	Tab, White, Round, Scored, 832 <> 3/8	Oxybutynin Chloride 5 mg	Ditropan by UDL	51079-0628	Urinary
832 <> 38	Tab	Oxybutynin Chloride 5 mg	by Rosemont	00832-0038	Urinary
832 <> 38	Tab, White, Round, Scored	Oxybutynin Chloride 5 mg	by Dixon Shane	17236-0850	Urinary
832 <> 50	Tab, Sugar Coated	Chlorpromazine HCl 50 mg	by Schein	00364-0382	Antipsychotic
832 <> 50	Tab, Sugar Coated	Chlorpromazine HCl 50 mg	by United Res	00677-0455	Antipsychotic
832 <> 50	Tab, Butterscotch Yellow, Sugar Coated	Chlorpromazine HCl 50 mg	by Qualitest	00603-2810	Antipsychotic
832 <> G359	Tab	Fluoxymesterone 10 mg	by Qualitest	00603-3645	Steroid; C III
832 <> G463	Tab	Medroxyprogesterone Acetate 10 mg	by Quality Care	60346-0571	Progestin
832 <> G463	Tab	Medroxyprogesterone Acetate 10 mg	by Qualitest	00603-4368	Progestin
8320420	Tab, Green, Round, 832-0420	Hydroflumethiazide 50 mg, Reserpine 0.125 mg	Salutensin by Rosemont		Diuretic; Antihypertensive
83205	Tab, Pink, Round, 832/05	Oxybutynin Chloride 5 mg	Ditropan by Rosemont		Urinary
83210	Tab, Butterscotch Yellow, Round, Sugar Coated, 832 over 10	Chlorpromazine HCl 10 mg	Thorazine by UDL	51079-0518	Antipsychotic
83210	Tab, Yellow, Sugar Coated	Chlorpromazine HCl 10 mg	by Rosemont	00832-0300	Antipsychotic
83210	Cap, 832 Over 10	Chlordiazepoxide HCl 10 mg	by Quality Care	60346-0052	Antianxiety; C IV
832100	Tab, Butterscotch Yellow, Round, Sugar Coated, 832 over 100	Chlorpromazine HCl 100 mg	Thorazine by UDL	51079-0516	Antipsychotic
832100	Tab, Butterscotch Yellow, Sugar Coated	Chlorpromazine HCl 100 mg	by Zenith Goldline	00182-0476	Antipsychotic

ID FRONT <> BACK	DESCRIPTION FRONT <> BACK	INGREDIENT & STRENGTH	BRAND (OR EQUIV.) & FIRM	NDC#	CLASS; SCH.
832100	Tab, Sugar Coated, 832 over 100	Chlorpromazine HCl 100 mg	by Rosemont	00832-0303	Antipsychotic
83210C	Tab, Blue, Round, 832/10C	Diazepam 10 mg	Valium by Rosemont		Antianxiety; C IV
8322	Tab, Lavender, Round, 832/2	Warfarin Sodium 2 mg	Coumadin by Rosemont		Anticoagulant
832200	Tab, Butterscotch Yellow, Round, Sugar Coated, 832 over 200	Chlorpromazine HCl 200 mg	Thorazine by UDL	51079-0517	Antipsychotic
832200	Tab, Butterscotch Yellow, Sugar Coated	Chlorpromazine HCl 200 mg	by Zenith Goldline	00182-0477	Antipsychotic
832200	Tab, Sugar Coated, 832 over 200	Chlorpromazine HCl 200 mg	by Rosemont	00832-0304	Antipsychotic
832212 <> BARR	Tab, Green, Oval, Flat, Scored, 832/2/1/2 <> Barr	Warfarin Sodium 2.5 mg	by UCB		Anticoagulant
83225	Cap, 832 over 25	Chlordiazepoxide HCl 25 mg	by Qualitest	00603-2668	Antianxiety; C IV
83225	Tab, Butterscotch Yellow, Round, Sugar Coated, 832 over 25	Chlorpromazine HCl 25 mg	Thorazine by UDL	51079-0519	Antipsychotic
83225	Tab, Butterscotch Yellow, Sugar Coated	Chlorpromazine HCl 25 mg	by Zenith Goldline	00182-0474	Antipsychotic
83225	Tab, Sugar Coated	Chlorpromazine HCl 25 mg	by Rosemont	00832-0301	Antipsychotic
83225	Cap, 832 over 25	Chlordiazepoxide HCl 25 mg	by Quality Care	60346-0260	Antianxiety; C IV
83225	Tab, Orange, Round, 832/2.5	Warfarin Sodium 2.5 mg	Coumadin by Rosemont		Anticoagulant
8322C	Tab, White, Round, 832/2C	Diazepam 2 mg	Valium by Rosemont		Antianxiety; C IV
8322L	Tab, White, Round, Coated	Cimetidine 200 mg	by Rosemont	00832-0101	Gastrointestinal
8322L	Tab, Coated	Cimetidine 200 mg	by Lek	48866-0101	Gastrointestinal
8322L	Tab, Coated	Cimetidine 200 mg	by Martec	52555-0708	Gastrointestinal
83238	Tab, Debossed	Oxybutynin Chloride 5 mg	by Major	00904-5223	Urinary
8323L	Tab, Coated	Cimetidine 300 mg	by Lek	48866-0102	Gastrointestinal
8323L	Tab, Coated	Cimetidine 300 mg	by Martec	52555-0709	Gastrointestinal
8323L	Tab, White, Round, Coated	Cimetidine 300 mg	Tagamet by Rosemont	00832-0102	Gastrointestinal
8325	Cap, Green & Yellow, 832/5	Chlordiazepoxide HCl 5 mg	Librium by Rosemont		Antianxiety; C IV
8325	Tab, Pink, Round, 832/5	Warfarin Sodium 5 mg	Coumadin by Rosemont		Anticoagulant
83250	Tab, Sugar Coated, 832 50	Chlorpromazine HCl 50 mg	by Quality Care	62682-7027	Antipsychotic
83250	Tab, Butterscotch Yellow, Round, Sugar Coated, 832 over 50	Chlorpromazine HCl 50 mg	Thorazine by UDL	51079-0130	Antipsychotic
83250	Tab, Butterscotch Yellow, Sugar Coated	Chlorpromazine HCl 50 mg	by Zenith Goldline	00182-0475	Antipsychotic
83250	Tab, Sugar Coated	Chlorpromazine HCl 50 mg	by Rosemont	00832-0302	Antipsychotic
8325C	Tab, Yellow, Round, 832/5C	Diazepam 5 mg	Valium by Rosemont		Antianxiety; C IV
8326113	Tab, White, Round, 832/6113	Carbamazepine 200 mg	Tegretol by Rosemont		Anticonvulsant
8328375C	Tab, Yellow, Round, 832/8375C	Phentermine HCl 37.5 mg	Adipex P by Rosemont		Anorexiant; C IV
83286	Tab	Fluoxymesterone 10 mg	by United Res	00677-0934	Steroid; C III
8328L	Tab, White	Cimetidine 800 mg	Tagamet by Rosemont		Gastrointestinal
8328L	Tab, Coated	Cimetidine 800 mg	by Lek	48866-0104	Gastrointestinal
8328L	Tab, Coated, 832 8L	Cimetidine 800 mg	by Schein	00364-2594	Gastrointestinal
8328L	Tab, Coated, 832/8L	Cimetidine 800 mg	by Rosemont	00832-0104	Gastrointestinal
8328L	Tab	Cimetidine 800 mg	by United Res	00677-1530	Gastrointestinal
8328L	Tab, Coated	Cimetidine 800 mg	by Martec	52555-0711	Gastrointestinal
8328L	Tab, Coated	Cimetidine 800 mg	by Apotheca	12634-0497	Gastrointestinal
8328L	Tab, White, Oval, Scored	Cimetidine 800 mg	by Dixon Shane	17236-0172	Gastrointestinal
832A5	Tab	Amiloride HCl 5 mg	Midamor by Rosemont		Diuretic
832BAC10	Tab, 832/BAC10	Baclofen 10 mg	by Qualitest	00603-2408	Muscle Relaxant
832BAC10	Tab	Baclofen 10 mg	by Rosemont	00832-1024	Muscle Relaxant
832BAC10	Tab, 832/BAC10	Baclofen 10 mg	by United Res	00677-1259	Muscle Relaxant
832BC20	Tab, White, Round, Scored, 832 BC20	Baclofen 20 mg	by Boca Pharmacal	64376-0501	Muscle Relaxant
832BC20	Tab, 832/BC20	Baclofen 20 mg	by United Res	00677-1260	Muscle Relaxant
832BC20	Tab	Baclofen 20 mg	by Rosemont	00832-1025	Muscle Relaxant
832BC20	Tab, 832/BC20	Baclofen 20 mg	by Qualitest	00603-2409	Muscle Relaxant
832BM05	Tab, White, Round, Scored, 832 over BM05	Benztropine Mesylate 0.5 mg	Cogentin by UDL	51079-0220	Antiparkinson
832BM05	Tab, White, Round, Scored, 832 over BM05	Benztropine Mesylate 0.5 mg	Cogentin by Martec	52555-0676	Antiparkinson
832BM1	Tab, White, Oval, Scored 832/BM1	Benztropine Mesylate 1 mg	Cogentin by UDL	51079-0221	Antiparkinson
832BM1	Tab, White, Round	Benztropine Mesylate 1 mg	Cogentin by Rosemont	00832-1081	Antiparkinson
832BM1	Tab, White, Oval, Scored, 832 over BM1	Benztropine Mesylate 1 mg	Cogentin by Martec	52555-0677	Antiparkinson

ID FRONT ‹› BACK	DESCRIPTION FRONT ‹› BACK	INGREDIENT & STRENGTH	BRAND (OR EQUIV.) & FIRM	NDC#	CLASS; SCH.
832BM1	Tab, White, Oval, Scored	Benztropine Mesylate 1 mg	by Dixon Shane	17236-0847	Antiparkinson
832BM2	Tab	Benztropine Mesylate 2 mg	by Quality Care	60346-0699	Antiparkinson
832BM2	Tab, White, Round, Scored, 832 BM2	Benztropine Mesylate 2 mg	by Bryant	63629-0351	Antiparkinson
832BM2	Tab, White, Round, Scored, 832 over BM2	Benztropine Mesylate 2 mg	Cogentin by UDL	51079-0222	Antiparkinson
832BM2	Tab, White, Round	Benztropine Mesylate 2 mg	Cogentin by Rosemont	00832-1082	Antiparkinson
832BM2	Tab, White, Round, Scored, 832 over BM2	Benztropine Mesylate 2 mg	Cogentin by Martec	52555-0678	Antiparkinson
832BM2	Tab, White, Scored	Benztropine Mesylate 2 mg	by Dixon Shane	17236-0848	Antiparkinson
832C5C	Cap, Blue & Green, 832/C5C	Chlordiazepoxide HCl 5 mg, Clidinium Bromide 2.5 mg	Librax by Rosemont		Gastrointestinal; C IV
832D25	Tab, White, Round, 832/D25	Dipyridamole 25 mg	Persantine by Rosemont		Antiplatelet
832D50	Tab, White, Round, 832/D50	Dipyridamole 50 mg	Persantine by Rosemont		Antiplatelet
832D75	Tab, White, Round, 832/D75	Dipyridamole 75 mg	Persantine by Rosemont		Antiplatelet
832FC500	Tab, Peach, Oblong, 832/FC500	Fenoprofen Calcium 600 mg	Nalfon by Rosemont		NSAID
832G133	Tab, White, Round, 832/G133	Carbamazepine 200 mg	Tegretol by Rosemont		Anticonvulsant
832G197	Tab, Blue, Round	Chlopropamide 250 mg	Diabinese by Rosemont		Antidiabetic
832G198	Tab, Blue, Round, 832/G198	Chlorpropamide 100 mg	Diabinese by Rosemont		Antidiabetic
832G203	Tab, Orange, Round, 832/G203	Chlorthalidone 25 mg	Hygroton by Rosemont		Diuretic
832G204	Tab, Blue, Round, 832/G204	Chlorthalidone 50 mg	Hygroton by Rosemont		Diuretic
832G220C	Cap, White, 832/G220C	Clorazepate Dipotassium 30.75 mg	Tranxene by Rosemont		Antianxiety; C IV
832G221C	Cap, White, 832/G221C	Clorazepate Dipotassium 7.5 mg	Tranxene by Rosemont		Antianxiety; C IV
832G222C	Cap, White, 832/G222C	Clorazepate Dipotassium 15 mg	Tranxene by Rosemont		Antianxiety; C IV
832G254	Tab, Lavender, Round, 832/G254	Desipramine HCl 25 mg	Norpramin by Rosemont		Antidepressant
832G255	Tab, Blue, Round, 832/G255	Desipramine HCl 50 mg	Norpramin by Rosemont		Antidepressant
832G256	Tab, White, Round, 832/G256	Desipramine HCl 75 mg	Norpramin by Rosemont		Antidepressant
832G257	Tab, Butterscotch Yellow, Round, 832/G257	Desipramine HCl 100 mg	Norpramin by Rosemont		Antidepressant
832G31	Tab, White, Oblong, 832/G31	Acetohexamide 250 mg	Dymelor by Rosemont		Antidiabetic
832G32	Tab, White, Oblong, 832/G32	Acetohexamide 500 mg	Dymelor by Rosemont		Antidiabetic
832G359	Tab, 832/G359 Rosemont	Fluoxymesterone 10 mg	by Rugby	00536-3826	Steroid; C III
832G366C	Cap, Blue & White, 832/G366C	Flurazepam HCl 15 mg	Dalmane by Rosemont		Hypnotic; C IV
832G367C	Cap, Blue, 832/G367C	Flurazepam HCl 30 mg	Dalmane by Rosemont		Hypnotic; C IV
832G368	Tab	Folic Acid 1 mg	Folic Acid by Rosemont		Vitamin
832G420	Tab, Green, Round, 832/G420	Hydroflumethiazide 50 mg, Reserpine 0.125 mg	Serpasil by Rosemont		Diuretic; Antihypertensive
832G423	Tab, Purple, Round, 832/G423	Hydroxyzine HCl 10 mg	Atarax by Rosemont		Antihistamine
832G424	Tab, Purple, Round, 832/G424	Hydroxyzine HCl 25 mg	Atarax by Rosemont		Antihistamine
832G425	Tab, Lavender, Round, 832/G425	Hydroxyzine HCl 50 mg	Atarax by Rosemont		Antihistamine
832G463	Tab, White, Round, 832 over G463	Medroxyprogesterone Acetate 10 mg	Provera by Martec	52555-0463	Progestin
832G463	Tab, Coated, 832/G463	Medroxyprogesterone Acetate 10 mg	by Major	00904-2690	Progestin
832G463	Tab, 832/G463	Medroxyprogesterone Acetate 10 mg	by United Res	00677-0803	Progestin
832G506	Tab, Brown, Round, 832/G506	Nystatin 500,000 Units	Mycostatin by Rosemont		Antifungal
832G528C	Tab, Green, Round, 832/G528C	Phendimetrazine HCl 35 mg	Melfiat by Rosemont		Anorexiant; C III
832G528C	Tab, Orange, Round, 832/G528C	Phendimetrazine HCl 35 mg	Melfiat by Rosemont		Anorexiant; C III
832G528C	Tab, Yellow, Round, 832/G528C	Phendimetrazine HCl 35 mg	Melfiat by Rosemont		Anorexiant; C III
832G531C	Tab, White, Round, 832 / G531C	Phenobarbital 15 mg	Phenobarbital by Rosemont		Sedative/Hypnotic; C IV
832G532C	Tab, White, Round, 832 / G532C	Phenobarbital 30 mg	Phenobarbital by Rosemont		Sedative/Hypnotic; C IV
832G533C	Tab, White, Round, 832/G533C	Phenobarbital 60 mg	by Rosemont		Sedative/Hypnotic; C IV
832G536C	Cap, Blue & Clear, 832/G536C	Phentermine HCl 30 mg	Fastin by Rosemont		Anorexiant; C IV
832G536C	Cap, Black, 832/G536C	Phentermine HCl 30 mg	Fastin by Forest		Anorexiant; C IV
832G536C	Cap, Yellow, 832/G536C	Phentermine HCl 30 mg	Ionamin by Forest		Anorexiant; C IV
832G55C	Tab, White, Round, 832/G55C	Chlordiazepoxide 5 mg, Amitriptyline 12.5 mg	Limbitrol by Rosemont		Antianxiety; C IV
832G56C	Tab, Green, Round, 832/G56C	Chlordiazepoxide 10 mg, Amitriptyline 25 mg	Limbitrol by Rosemont		Antianxiety; C IV
832G602	Tab, White, Oblong, 832/G602	Sulfamethoxazole 400 mg, Trimethoprim 80 mg	Bactrim by Rosemont		Antibiotic
832G603	Tab, White, Oblong, 832/G603	Sulfamethoxazole 800 mg, Trimethoprim 160 mg	Bactrim by Rosemont		Antibiotic

ID FRONT <> BACK	DESCRIPTION FRONT <> BACK	INGREDIENT & STRENGTH	BRAND (OR EQUIV.) & FIRM	NDC#	CLASS; SCH.
832G613	Tab, Tan, Round, 832/G613	Thyroid 30 mg	Thyroid by Rosemont		Thyroid
832G614	Tab, Tan, Round, 832/G614	Thyroid 60 mg	Thyroid by Rosemont		Thyroid
832G615	Tab, Tan, Round, 832/G615	Thyroid 120 mg	Thyroid by Rosemont		Thyroid
832G616	Tab, Tan, Round, 832/G616	Thyroid 180 mg	Thyroid by Rosemont		Thyroid
832G618	Tab, White, Round, 832/G618	Tolazamide 100 mg	Tolinase by Rosemont		Antidiabetic
832G621	Tab, White, Round, 832/G621	Tolazamide 500 mg	Tolinase by Rosemont		Antidiabetic
832G622	Tab, White, Round, 832/G622	Tolazamide 250 mg	Tolinase by Rosemont		Antidiabetic
832GC100	Tab, White, Round, 832/GC100	Chlorthalidone 100 mg	Hygroton by Rosemont		Diuretic
832L01	Tab, Yellow, Round	Levothyroxine Sodium 0.1 mg	Synthroid by Rosemont		Antithyroid
832L02	Tab, White, Round	Levothyroxine Sodium 0.2 mg	Synthroid by Rosemont		Antithyroid
832L03	Tab, Green, Round	Levothyroxine Sodium 0.3 mg	Synthroid by Rosemont		Antithyroid
832L15	Tab, Blue, Round	Levothyroxine Sodium 0.15 mg	Synthroid by Rosemont		Antithyroid
832L300	Cap, White, 832/L-300	Lithium Carbonate 300 mg	Lithane by Rosemont		Antipsychotic
832LR1C	Tab, White, Round, 832/LR1C	Lorazepam 1 mg	Ativan by Rosemont		Sedative/Hypnotic; C IV
832LR2C	Tab, White, Round, 832/LR2C	Lorazepam 2 mg	Ativan by Rosemont		Sedative/Hypnotic; C IV
832M400	Tab, Yellow, Round, 832/M400	Tridihexethyl Chloride 25 mg, Meprobamate 400 mg	Pathibamate by Rosemont		Antispasmodic
832M5	Tab, Orange, Round	Methyclothiazide 5 mg	Enduron by Rosemont		Diuretic
832M510	Tab, White, Round, 832/M 510	Metoproterenol 10 mg	Alupent by Rosemont		Antiasthmatic
832M520	Tab, White, Round, 832/M 520	Metoproterenol 20 mg	Alupent by Rosemont		Antiasthmatic
832MC100	Cap, Maroon & White, 832/MC100	Meclofenamate Sodium 100 mg	Meclomen by Rosemont		NSAID
832MC50	Cap, Maroon & Pink, 832/MC50	Meclofenamate Sodium 50 mg	Meclomen by Rosemont		NSAID
832MS	Tab, Rosemont	Methyclothiazide 5 mg	by Pharmedix	53002-1044	Diuretic
832MS10	Tab, White, Round, 832/MS10	Metaproterenol Sulfate 10 mg	Alupent by Rosemont		Antiasthmatic
832MS20	Tab, White, Round, 832/MS20	Metaproterenol Sulfate 20 mg	Alupent by Rosemont		Antiasthmatic
832P10C	Cap, Green & White, 832/P10C	Prazepam 10 mg	Centrax by Rosemont		Sedative/Hypnotic; C IV
832P19C	Tab, White, Oblong, 832/P19C	Hydrocodone Bitartrate 5 mg, Acetaminophen 500 mg	Vicodin by Rosemont		Analgesic; C III
832P375C	Tab, Yellow, Round, 832/P37.5C	Phentermine HCl 37.5 mg	by Rosemont		Anorexiant; C IV
832P375C	Tab, Blue & White, Round, 832/P37.5C	Phentermine HCl 37.5 mg	Adipex P by Rosemont		Anorexiant; C IV
832P5C	Cap, Green & White, 832/P5C	Prazepam 5 mg	Centrax by Rosemont		Sedative/Hypnotic; C IV
832PPPC	Tab, White, Round, with Red Mottles, 832/PPPC	Phenylprop. 40 mg, Phenyleph. 10 mg, Phenyltolox. 15 mg, Chlorphenir. 5 mg	Nalspan SR by Rosemont		Cold Remedy
832PPPC	Tab, White, Round, 832/PPPC	Phenylprop. 40 mg, Phenyleph. 10 mg, Phenyltolox. 15 mg, Chlorphenir. 5 mg	Naldecon by Rosemont		Cold Remedy
832S500	Tab, Blue, Round	Salsalate 500 mg	Disalcid by Rosemont		NSAID
832S500	Tab, Yellow, Round	Salsalate 500 mg	Disalcid by Rosemont		NSAID
832S750	Tab, Blue, Oblong	Salsalate 750 mg	Disalcid by Rosemont		NSAID
832S750	Tab, Yellow, Oblong	Salsalate 750 mg	Disalcid by Rosemont		NSAID
832T10	Tab, Green, Round, 832/T10	Timolol Maleate 10 mg	Blocadren by Rosemont		Antihypertensive
832T20	Tab, Green, Round, 832/T20	Timolol Maleate 20 mg	Blocadren by Rosemont		Antihypertensive
832T5	Tab, Green, Round, 832/T5	Timolol Maleate 5 mg	Blocadren by Rosemont		Antihypertensive
832TEM15	Cap, Green & White, 832/Tem15	Temazepam 15 mg	Restoril by Rosemont		Sedative/Hypnotic; C IV
832TEM30	Cap, White, 832/Tem30	Temazepam 30 mg	Restoril by Rosemont		Sedative/Hypnotic; C IV
832TM100	Cap, Brown & Green, 832/TM100	Trimipramine Maleate 100 mg	Surmontil by Rosemont		Antidepressant
832TM25	Cap, Orange & Purple, 832/TM25	Trimipramine Maleate 25 mg	Surmontil by Rosemont		Antidepressant
832TM50	Cap, Pink & White, 832/TM50	Trimipramine Maleate 50 mg	Surmontil by Rosemont		Antidepressant
832X25	Tab, White, Round, 832/X25	Minoxidil 2.5 mg	Loniten by Rosemont		Antihypertensive
833	Tab, White, Oblong, Film Coated, Compumed Logo 833	Choline Magnesium Trisalicylate 750 mg	by Compumed	00403-0694	NSAID
8335 <> BARR	Tab, Peach, Oval, Scored	Warfarin Sodium 5 mg	by UDL	51079-0913	Anticoagulant
8335 <> BARR	Tab, Peach, Oval, Scored	Warfarin Sodium 5 mg	by Allscripts	54569-4934	Anticoagulant
8335 <> BARR	Tab, Peach, Oval, Flat, Scored, 833/5 <> Barr	Warfarin Sodium 5 mg	by UCB	50474-0935	Anticoagulant
834712 <> BARR	Tab, Yellow, Oval, Scored	Warfarin Sodium 7.5 mg	by UDL	51079-0915	Anticoagulant
834712 <> BARR	Tab, Yellow, Oval, Flat, Scored, Debossed with 834/71/2	Warfarin Sodium 7.5 mg	by UDL	51079-0891	Anticoagulant
83510 <> BARR	Tab, White, Oval, Scored	Warfarin Sodium 10 mg	by UDL	51079-0916	Anticoagulant
83510 <> BARR	Tab, White, Oval, Flat, Scored, Debossed with 835/10	Warfarin Sodium 10 mg	by UDL	51079-0893	Anticoagulant

ID FRONT <> BACK	DESCRIPTION FRONT <> BACK	INGREDIENT & STRENGTH	BRAND (OR EQUIV.) & FIRM	NDC#	CLASS; SCH.
835375 <> WATSON	Tab, Blue, Triangular, Scored	Clorazepate Dipotassium 3.75 mg	by Watson Labs	52544-0835	Antianxiety; C IV
836750 <> WATSON	Tab, Peach, Triangular, Scored	Clorazepate Dipotassium 7.5 mg	by Watson Labs	52544-0836	Antianxiety; C IV
83688	Tab, Green, Round, Hourglass Logo <> 8 3688	Doxazosin Mesylate 8 mg	Cardura by Zenith Goldline	00172-3688	Antihypertensive
83715 <> WATSON	Tab, Purple, Triangular, Scored	Clorazepate Dipotassium 15 mg	by Watson Labs	52544-0837	Antianxiety; C IV
843	Tab, White, Round, Sch. Logo 843	Prednisone 1 mg	Meticorten by Schering		Steroid
85 <> WYETH	Tab, Coated	Acetaminophen 650 mg, Propoxyphene HCl 65 mg	Wygesic by Wyeth Labs	00008-0085	Analgesic; C IV
850 <> BMS6070	Tab, White, Round, Film Coated	Metformin HCl 850 mg	Glucophage by Squibb Mfg	12783-0070	Antidiabetic
850 <> BMS6070	Tab, White, Round	Metformin HCl 850 mg	Glucophage by Kaiser Fdn	00179-1378	Antidiabetic
850 <> BMS6070	Tab, White, Round	Metformin HCl 850 mg	Glucophage by Direct Dispensing	57866-9058	Antidiabetic
850 <> BMS6070	Tab, White to Off-White, Round, Film Coated	Metformin HCl 850 mg	Glucophage by Bristol Myers Squibb	00087-6070	Antidiabetic
850 <> BMS6070	Tab, Film Coated, Debossed Across the Face <> Debossed Around Periphery	Metformin HCl 850 mg	Glucophage by Caremark	00339-6085	Antidiabetic
850 <> MJ	Tab, MJ Logo	Ethinyl Estradiol 0.035 mg, Norethindrone 0.4 mg	Ovcon 35 28 by Bristol Myers Squibb	00087-0578	Oral Contraceptive
850 <> MJ	Tab	Ethinyl Estradiol 0.035 mg, Norethindrone 0.4 mg	Ovcon 35 by Physicians Total Care	54868-0509	Oral Contraceptive
850 <> MJ	Tab	Ethinyl Estradiol 0.05 mg, Norethindrone 1 mg	Ovcon 50 28 by Bristol Myers Squibb	00087-0579	Oral Contraceptive
850 <> MJ	Tab	Ethinyl Estradiol 0.05 mg, Norethindrone 1 mg	Ovcon 50 by Physicians Total Care	54868-3772	Oral Contraceptive
850 <> MJ	Tab	Inert	Ovcon 50 28 by Bristol Myers	15548-0579	Placebo
850 <> NU	Tab, White, Cap Shaped	Meftormin HCl 850 mg	by Nu Pharm	Canadian DIN# 02229517	Antidiabetic
851 <> 93	Tab, White, Round	Metronidazole 250 mg	by MS State Health	50596-0027	Antibiotic
851 <> 93	Tab, White, Round	Metronidazole 250 mg	by Teva	00093-0851	Antibiotic
851 <> 93	Tab, White, Round	Metronidazole 250 mg	Flagyl by UDL	51079-0122	Antibiotic
851 <> 93	Tab	Metronidazole 250 mg	by Golden State	60429-0128	Antibiotic
851 <> 93	Tab	Metronidazole 250 mg	by Nat Pharmpak Serv	55154-5509	Antibiotic
851 <> 93	Tab	Metronidazole 250 mg	by Quality Care	60346-0592	Antibiotic
85193	Tab, Lemmon	Metronidazole 250 mg	by Pharmedix	53002-0221	Antibiotic
852 <> 9393	Tab, White, Oblong, Scored, 852 <> 93/93	Metronidazole 500 mg	Flagyl by UDL	51079-0126	Antibiotic
852 <> 9393	Tab, White, Oblong, Scored	Metronidazole 500 mg	Metronidazole by Family Hlth Phcy	65149-0126	Antibiotic
852 <> 9393	Tab, White, Oblong, Scored, 852 <> 93-93	Metronidazole 500 mg	by Allscripts	54569-0967	Antibiotic
852 <> 9393	Tab, White, Oblong, Scored	Metronidazole 500 mg	by Natl Pharmpak	55154-5566	Antibiotic
852 <> 9393	Tab, Debossed	Metronidazole 500 mg	by Prepackage Spec	58864-0355	Antibiotic
852 <> 9393	Tab, Coated, Debossed	Metronidazole 500 mg	by Quality Care	60346-0507	Antibiotic
852 <> 9393	Tab, 93-93	Metronidazole 500 mg	by Golden State	60429-0129	Antibiotic
852<> 9393	Tab, White, Oblong, Scored, 852 <> 93/93	Metronidazole 500 mg	by Teva	00093-0852	Antibiotic
853 <> S	Tab	Isosorbide Dinitrate 2.5 mg	Sorbitrate by Zeneca	00310-0853	Antianginal
85WMH	Tab, Red, Round, 85-WMH	Dexbrompheniramine Maleate 6 mg, Pseudoephedrine Sulf 120 mg	Disophrol by Schering		Cold Remedy
860 <> EL	Cap	Guaifenesin 250 mg, Pseudoephedrine HCl 120 mg	Guaibid D by Econolab	55053-0860	Cold Remedy
860 <> EL	Cap	Guaifenesin 250 mg, Pseudoephedrine HCl 120 mg	by United Res	00677-1503	Cold Remedy
8631	Tab, White, Round	Theophylline Anhydrous 100 mg	Theo-X by Carnrick		Antiasthmatic
8632	Tab, White, Oval	Theophylline Anhydrous 200 mg	Theo-X by Carnrick		Antiasthmatic
8633	Tab, White, Oblong	Theophylline Anhydrous 300 mg	Theo-X by Carnrick		Antiasthmatic
8633UNIMED	Tab, White	Oxymetholone 50 mg	Anadrol 50 by Unimed	00051-8633	Steroid
8633UNIMED	Tab	Oxymetholone 50 mg	Anadrol 50 by Oread	63015-0007	Steroid
863PPP	Tab, White, Round	Fluphenazine HCl 1 mg	Prolixin by BMS		Antipsychotic
8648 <> C	Tab, Layered	Phendimetrazine Tartrate 35 mg	Bontril PDM by Carnrick	00086-0048	Anorexiant; C III
864PPP	Tab, Blue, Round	Fluphenazine HCl 2.5 mg	Prolixin by BMS		Antipsychotic
8650 <> C	Tab, Pale Violet	Acetaminophen 325 mg, Butalbital 50 mg	Phrenilin by Quality Care	60346-0915	Analgesic
8650 <> C	Tab	Acetaminophen 325 mg, Butalbital 50 mg	Phrenilin by Carnrick	00086-0050	Analgesic
8650 <> C	Tab, Purple, Oblong, Scored	Acetaminophen 325 mg; Butalbital 50 mg	Phrenilin by Thrift Services	59198-0364	Analgesic
8651	Tab, White, Oval	Phenylpropanolamine 25 mg	Propagest by Carnrick		Decongestant; Appetite Suppressant

ID FRONT <> BACK	DESCRIPTION FRONT <> BACK	INGREDIENT & STRENGTH	BRAND (OR EQUIV.) & FIRM	NDC#	CLASS; SCH.
8656 <> C	Cap	Acetaminophen 650 mg, Butalbital 50 mg	Phrenilin Forte by Carnrick	00086-0056	Analgesic
8656 <> C	Cap, Purple	Butalbital 50 mg; Acetaminophen 650 mg	Phrenilin Forte by Thrift Services	59198-0365	Analgesic
8657 <> C	Cap	Acetaminophen 500 mg, Hydrocodone Bitartrate 5 mg	Hydrocet by Carnrick	00086-0057	Analgesic; C III
866	Tab, White with Blue, Round, Schering Logo 866	Dexbrompheniramine Maleate 2 mg, Pseudoephedrine Sulf 60 mg	Disophrol by Schering		Cold Remedy
866	Cap, Red	Docusate Calcium 240 mg	Surfak by Scherer		Laxative
866	Tab, White, Round	Phenolphthalein 65 mg, Docusate Sodium 100 mg	by Perrigo		Gastrointestinal
8662 <> C	Tab, Pink, Oblong, Scored	Metaxalone 400 mg	Skelaxin by Thrift Services	59198-0367	Muscle Relaxant
8662 <> C	Tab, Pink, Scored	Metaxalone 400 mg	Skelaxin by HJ Harkins	52959-0410	Muscle Relaxant
8662 <> C	Tab, Pink, Oblong, Scored	Metaxalone 400 mg	Skelaxin by Rx Pac	65084-0167	Muscle Relaxant
8662 <> C	Tab, Lavender, 86 Over 62 <> C with Dot on Top Tip	Metaxalone 400 mg	Skelaxin by Carnrick	00086-0062	Muscle Relaxant
8662 <> C	Tab	Metaxalone 400 mg	Skelaxin by Drug Distr	52985-0226	Muscle Relaxant
8662 <> C	Tab, Pale Rose	Metaxalone 400 mg	Skelaxin by Allscripts	54569-0855	Muscle Relaxant
8662 <> C	Tab	Metaxalone 400 mg	Skelaxin by CVS	51316-0231	Muscle Relaxant
8662 <> C	Tab, Red, Round, Scored	Metaxalone 400 mg	Skelaxin by Nat Pharmpak Serv	55154-5588	Muscle Relaxant
8662 <> C	Tab, Pale Rose	Metaxalone 400 mg	Skelaxin by Amerisource	62584-0033	Muscle Relaxant
8662 <> C	Tab	Metaxalone 400 mg	Skelaxin by Direct Dispensing	57866-4637	Muscle Relaxant
8662 <> C	Tab, Pale Rose	Metaxalone 400 mg	Skelaxin by Quality Care	60346-0057	Muscle Relaxant
8662 <> C	Tab, Pink, Scored	Metaxalone 400 mg	Skelaxin by Nat Pharmpak Serv	55154-5590	Muscle Relaxant
8673 <> C	Tab, White with Blue Specks	Guaifenesin 400 mg, Phenylpropanolamine HCl 75 mg	Exgest LA by Carnrick	00086-0063	Cold Remedy
8673 <> C	Tab, White, Oval, Scored	Phenylpropanolamine HCl 75 mg, Guaifenesin 400 mg	Exgest by Eckerd	19458-0832	Cold Remedy
8674 <> C	Tab	Atropine 0.025 mg, Difenoxin HCl 1 mg	Motofen by Physicians Total Care	54868-3510	Antidiarrheal; C IV
8674 <> C	Tab, White, Pentagonal, Scored	Difenoxin HCl 1 mg; Atropine Sulfate 0.025 mg	Motofen by DRX Pharm Consults	55045-2771	Antidiarrheal; C IV
8674 <> C	Tab, White, Scored	Difenoxin HCl 1 mg; Atropine Sulfate 0.025 mg	Motofen by West Ward Pharm	00143-9031	Antidiarrheal; C IV
8692 <> BARR	Tab, Purple, Oval, Scored	Warfarin Sodium 2 mg	by UDL	51079-0909	Anticoagulant
8692 <> BARR	Tab, Purple, Oval, Flat, Scored, Debossed with 869/2 <> Barr	Warfarin Sodium 2 mg	by UCB		Anticoagulant
87 <> M	Tab, Blue, Round, Film Coated, Scored	Maprotiline HCl 50 mg	by Murfreesboro Ph	51129-1679	Antidepressant
87 <> M	Tab, Blue, Coated, Beveled Edge	Maprotiline HCl 50 mg	by Mylan	00378-0087	Antidepressant
870 <> EL	Cap, Ex Release, White Beads	Guaifenesin 300 mg, Pseudoephedrine HCl 60 mg	Guaibid D Ped by Pharmafab	62542-0401	Cold Remedy
872	Cap	Nifedipine 10 mg	by Geneva	00781-2504	Antihypertensive
872 <> CARACO	Cap, RP Scherer Logo 872	Nifedipine 10 mg	by Quality Care	60346-0803	Antihypertensive
8733UNIMED	Tab, White, Round, 87 33/Unimed	Oxymetuclor 50 mg	Anadrol by Unimed		Steroid
8744 <> BARR	Tab, Blue, Oval, Scored	Warfarin Sodium 4 mg	by UDL	51079-0912	Anticoagulant
8744 <> BARR	Tab, Blue, Oval, Flat, Scored, 874/4 <> Barr	Warfarin Sodium 4 mg	by UCB		Anticoagulant
877PPP	Tab, Green, Round	Fluphenazine HCl 5 mg	Prolixin by BMS		Antipsychotic
879	Tab	Acetaminophen 300 mg, Codeine Phosphate 60 mg	by Pharmedix	53002-0103	Analgesic; C III
879	Tab, White, Round	Codeine Sulfate 30 mg	by Halsey		Analgesic; C III
879 <> 158	Cap	Tetracycline HCl 250 mg	by Qualitest	00603-5919	Antibiotic
879 <> 159	Cap	Tetracycline HCl 500 mg	by Quality Care	60346-0435	Antibiotic
879 <> 159	Cap	Tetracycline HCl 500 mg	by Qualitest	00603-5920	Antibiotic
879 <> 525	Cap, Halsey Drug	Doxycycline Hyclate	by United Res	00677-0598	Antibiotic
879 <> 526	Cap, Light Blue	Doxycycline Hyclate	by Quality Care	60346-0109	Antibiotic
879 <> 526	Cap, Blue	Doxycycline Hyclate 100 mg	by Dixon Shane	17236-0527	Antibiotic
8790155	Cap, Pink	Propoxyphene HCl 65 mg	Prophene-65 by Halsey		Analgesic; C IV
8790158	Cap	Tetracycline HCl 250 mg	by Halsey Drug	00879-0158	Antibiotic
8790158	Cap	Tetracycline HCl 250 mg	by HL Moore	00839-1656	Antibiotic
879027	Cap, Yellow	Pentobarbital Sodium 100 mg	Nembutal by Halsey		Sedative/Hypnotic; C II
8790364	Cap	Chlordiazepoxide HCl 5 mg	by Zenith Goldline	00182-0977	Antianxiety; C IV
8790365	Cap	Chlordiazepoxide HCl 10 mg	by Zenith Goldline	00182-0978	Antianxiety; C IV
8790365	Cap	Chlordiazepoxide HCl 10 mg	by Pharmedix	53002-0450	Antianxiety; C IV
8790365 <> 8790365	Cap, 879/0365 <> 879/0365	Chlordiazepoxide HCl 10 mg	by Kaiser	00179-0134	Antianxiety; C IV
8790366	Cap, Green & White	Chlordiazepoxide 25 mg	Librium by Halsey		Antianxiety; C IV
879129	Tab, White, Round	Prednisone 5 mg	Cortan by Halsey		Steroid

ID FRONT <> BACK	DESCRIPTION FRONT <> BACK	INGREDIENT & STRENGTH	BRAND (OR EQUIV.) & FIRM	NDC#	CLASS; SCH.
879130	Tab, White, Round	Propylthiouracil 50 mg	by Halsey		Antithyroid
879159	Cap	Tetracycline HCl 500 mg	by Halsey Drug	00879-0159	Antibiotic
879159	Cap	Tetracycline HCl 500 mg	by HL Moore	00839-5075	Antibiotic
879317	Tab, Yellow, Round	Dextroamphetamine Sulfate 10 mg	by Halsey		Stimulant; C II
879341	Tab	Isoniazid 300 mg	Isoniazid by Quality Care	60346-0483	Antimycobacterial
879341	Tab	Isoniazid 300 mg	Isoniazid by Halsey Drug	00879-0341	Antimycobacterial
879358	Tab, White, Round	Quinidine Sulfate 200 mg	by Halsey		Antiarrhythmic
879360	Tab, White, Round	Triprolidine HCl 2.5 mg, Pseudoephedrine HCl 60 mg	Triposed by Halsey		Cold Remedy
879364	Cap, Green & Yellow	Chlordiazepoxide 5 mg	Librium by Halsey		Antianxiety; C IV
879365	Cap, Black & Green	Chlordiazepoxide 10 mg	Librium by Halsey		Antianxiety; C IV
879366	Cap, Green & White	Chlordiazepoxide 25 mg	Librium by Halsey		Antianxiety; C IV
879452	Cap, Red & White	Acetaminophen 500 mg	Tylenol by Halsey		Antipyretic
879453	Tab, White	Acetaminophen 500 mg	Tylenol by Halsey		Antipyretic
879501	Cap, White	Chlordiazepoxide HCl 5 mg, Clidinium Bromide 2.5 mg	Clinoxide by Halsey		Gastrointestinal; C IV
879525 <> AP0837	Cap	Doxycycline Hyclate	by Rachelle	00196-0552	Antibiotic
879526	Cap, 879/526	Doxycycline Hyclate	by Halsey Drug	00879-0526	Antibiotic
879526	Cap, 879/526	Doxycycline Hyclate	by Apotheca	12634-0169	Antibiotic
879526	Cap, 879/526	Doxycycline Hyclate 100 mg	by Prepackage Spec	58864-0190	Antibiotic
879526 <> 879526	Cap	Doxycycline Hyclate	by Urgent Care Ctr	50716-0522	Antibiotic
879G10C2	Tab, White, Round	Acetaminophen 300 mg, Codeine Phosphate 15 mg	Tylenol #2 by Halsey		Analgesic; C III
879G11C3	Tab, White, Round	Acetaminophen 300 mg, Codeine Phosphate 30 mg	Tylenol #3 by Halsey		Analgesic; C III
879G122C	Tab, Green, Round	Butabarbital Sodium 30 mg	Sarisol #2 by Halsey		Sedative; C III
879G12C4	Tab, White, Round	Acetaminophen 300 mg, Codeine Phosphate 60 mg	Tylenol #4 by Halsey		Analgesic; C III
879G180	Tab, Green, Round	Chlorpheniramine Maleate 4 mg	Chlor-trimeton by Halsey		Antihistamine
879G20C	Tab	Acetaminophen 325 mg, Oxycodone HCl 5 mg	by Zenith Goldline	00182-1465	Analgesic; C II
879G302	Cap, Clear & Pink	Diphenhydramine HCl 25 mg	Benadryl by Halsey		Antihistamine
879G303	Cap, Pink	Diphenhydramine HCl 50 mg	Benadryl by Halsey		Antihistamine
879G368	Tab, Yellow, Round	Folic Acid 1 mg	Folvite by Halsey		Vitamin
879G406	Tab, Peach, Round	Hydrochlorothiazide 25 mg	Hydro-D by Halsey		Diuretic
879G407	Tab, Peach, Round	Hydrochlorothiazide 50 mg	Hydro-D by Halsey		Diuretic
879G41	Tab, White, Round	Aminophylline 100 mg	Aminophyllin by Halsey		Antiasthmatic
879G468C	Tab, White, Round	Meperidine HCl 50 mg	Pethadol by Halsey		Analgesic; C II
879G469C	Tab, White, Round	Meperidine HCl 100 mg	Pethadol by Halsey		Analgesic; C II
879G471C	Tab, White, Round, 879 /G471C	Meprobamate 400 mg	Miltown by Halsey		Sedative/Hypnotic; C IV
879G545	Tab, Orange, Round	Prednisolone 5 mg	Cortalone by Halsey		Steroid
879G549	Tab, Peach, Round	Prednisone 20 mg	Cortan by Halsey		Steroid
879G587	Tab, Red, Round	Rauwolfia Serpentina 100 mg	Raudixin by Halsey		Antihypertensive
879G594C	Cap, Reddish-Orange	Secobarbital Sodium 100 mg	Seconal by Halsey		Sedative/Hypnotic; C II
879G650C	Tab, Yellow, Round	Oxycodone HCl 4.5 mg, Oxycodone Terephthalate 0.38 mg, Aspirin 325 mg	Percodan by Halsey		Analgesic; C II
879G85C2	Tab, White, Round	Aspirin 325 mg, Codeine Phosphate 15 mg	Empirin #2 by Halsey		Analgesic; C III
879G86C3	Tab, White, Round	Aspirin 325 mg, Codeine Phosphate 30 mg	Empirin #3 by Halsey		Analgesic; C III
879G87C4	Tab, White, Round	Aspirin 325 mg, Codeine Phosphate 60 mg	Empirin #4 by Halsey		Analgesic; C III
879G88C	Tab, White, Round	Diphenoxylate HCl 2.5 mg, Atropine Sulfate 0.025 mg	Lomotil by Halsey		Antidiarrheal; C V
879G90C	Tab, White, Round	Phenobarbital, Belladonna Alkaloids	Susano by Halsey		Gastrointestinal; C IV
88	Tab, Green, Round, Scored	Levothyroxine Sodium 0.088 mg	Synthroid by Murfreesboro	51129-1642	Antithyroid
88 <> FLINT	Tab, Green, Round, Scored	Levothyroxine Sodium 0.088 mg	Synthroid by Phy Total Care	54868-2705	Antithyroid
88 <> FLINT	Tab, Olive, Round, Scored	Levothyroxine Sodium 88 mcg	Synthroid by Knoll	00048-1060	Antithyroid
88 <> FLINT	Tab, Green, Round, Scored	Levothyroxine Sodium 88 mcg	Synthroid by Murfreesboro	51129-1650	Antithyroid
88 <> UU	Tab, White, Oval	Pramipexole DiHCl 0.5 mg	Mirapex by Pharmacia & Upjohn	00009-0008	Antiparkinson
8818 <> AP	Tab	Buspirone HCl 5 mg	by Apothecon	59772-8818	Antianxiety
8819 <> AP	Tab	Buspirone HCl 10 mg	by Apothecon	59772-8819	Antianxiety
884 <> MILES30	Tab, Pink	Nifedipine 30 mg	Adalat CC by Direct Dispensing	57866-6719	Antihypertensive

ID FRONT <> BACK	DESCRIPTION FRONT <> BACK	INGREDIENT & STRENGTH	BRAND (OR EQUIV.) & FIRM	NDC#	CLASS; SCH.
884 <> MILES30	Tab, Film Coated	Nifedipine 30 mg	Adalat CC by Caremark	00339-5976	Antihypertensive
885 <> MILES60	Tab, Film Coated	Nifedipine 60 mg	Adalat CC by Pharm Utilization	60491-0010	Antihypertensive
885MILES60 <> 60ADALATCC	Tab, Salmon, Film Coated	Nifedipine 60 mg	Adalat CC by Allscripts	54569-3892	Antihypertensive
8861 <> B	Tab, Purple, Oval, Scored	Estradiol 1 mg	by DRX Pharm Consults	55045-2739	Hormone
8861 <> B	Tab, Purple, Oval, Scored, 886/1 <> B	Estradiol 1 mg	Estradiol USP by Halsey Drug	00904-5442	Hormone
8872 <> B	Tab, Green, Oval, Scored, 887/2 <> B	Estradiol 2 mg	Estradiol USP by Halsey Drug	00904-7738	Hormone
889	Cap, Red & Yellow	Phentermine HCl 30 mg	Fastin by Marlop		Anorexiant; C IV
88FLI	Tab, Mint Green, Round, 88/FLI Logo	Levothyroxine Sodium 88 mcg	by Forest	00456-0329	Antithyroid
88M	Tab	Levothyroxine Sodium 88 mcg	Euthyrox by Em Pharma	63254-0438	Antithyroid
88M	Tab	Levothyroxine Sodium 88 mcg	Levo T by MOVA	55370-0160	Antithyroid
88MCG	Tab, Olive, Oval	Levothyroxine Sodium 88 mcg	Levoxyl by Phy Total Care	54868-4177	Antithyroid
88MCG	Tab	Levothyroxine Sodium 88 mcg	Eltroxin by Glaxo	53873-0117	Antithyroid
88MCG <> FLINT	Tab, Olive, Round, Scored	Levothyroxine Sodium 0.088 mg	Synthroid by Rightpac	65240-0757	Antithyroid
89 <> TARO	Tab, Blue, Oval, Film Coated	Etodolac 500 mg	by Taro Pharm (IS)	52549-4036	NSAID
89 <> TARO	Tab, Blue, Oval, Film Coated	Etodolac 500 mg	by Taro Pharms US	51672-4036	NSAID
890	Cap, Black	Phendimetrazine Tartrate 105 mg	Prelu-2 by Marlop		Anorexiant; C III
890 <> 93	Tab, Film Coated	Acetaminophen 650 mg, Propoxyphene Napsylate 100 mg	by Heartland	61392-0446	Analgesic; C IV
890 <> 93	Tab, Coated	Acetaminophen 650 mg, Propoxyphene Napsylate 100 mg	Propoxacet N by Quality Care	60346-0628	Analgesic; C IV
890 <> 93	Tab, Pink, Oblong, Film Coated	Acetaminophen 650 mg, Propoxyphene Napsylate 100 mg	by Teva	00093-0890	Analgesic; C IV
891 <> G	Tab	Levonorgestrel 0.25 mg, Ethinyl Estradiol 0.05 mg	Preven Emergency Contraceptive by Gynetics	63955-0020	Oral Contraceptive
891 <> G	Tab	Levonorgestrel 0.25 mg, Ethinyl Estradiol 0.05 mg	by Barr	00555-0891	Oral Contraceptive
891 <> ZENECA10	Tab, Oyster, Round	Nisoldipine 10 mg	Sular by AstraZeneca	00310-0891	Antihypertensive
891 <> ZENECA10	Tab	Nisoldipine 10 mg	Sular by Bayer AG	12527-0891	Antihypertensive
892 <> 93	Tab, Film Coated	Etodolac 400 mg	by Teva	17372-0892	NSAID
892 <> 93	Tab, Pink, Oblong, Film Coated	Etodolac 400 mg	by Teva	00093-0892	NSAID
892 <> ZENECA20	Tab, Yellow Cream, Round	Nisoldipine 20 mg	Sular by AstraZeneca	00310-0892	Antihypertensive
892 <> ZENECA20	Tab	Nisoldipine 20 mg	Sular E R by Murfreesboro	51129-1278	Antihypertensive
892 <> ZENECA20	Tab	Nisoldipine 20 mg	Sular by Bayer AG	12527-0892	Antihypertensive
893 <> ZENECA30	Tab, Mustard, Round	Nisoldipine 30 mg	Sular by AstraZeneca	00310-0893	Antihypertensive
893 <> ZENECA30	Tab	Nisoldipine 30 mg	Sular Er by Murfreesboro	51129-1334	Antihypertensive
893 <> ZENECA30	Tab	Nisoldipine 30 mg	Sular by Bayer AG	12527-0893	Antihypertensive
894 <> ZENECA40	Tab, Burnt Orange, Round	Nisoldipine 40 mg	Sular by AstraZeneca	00310-0894	Antihypertensive
894 <> ZENECA40	Tab, Orange, Round, Film	Nisoldipine 40 mg	Sular by Par	49884-0657	Antihypertensive
894 <> ZENECA40	Tab	Nisoldipine 40 mg	Sular by Bayer AG	12527-0894	Antihypertensive
899 <> 54	Tab	Prednisone 10 mg	by Med Pro	53978-3037	Steroid
89912 <> B	Tab, White, Oval, Flat, Scored, 899 over 1/2 <> B	Estradiol 0.5 mg	Estradiol USP by Hawthorn	63717-0301	Hormone
8A	Tab, White, Triangular, Bisected, 8a Knoll Double Triangle	Hydromorphone HCl 8 mg	Dilaudid by Knoll	00044-1028	Analgesic; C II
8ATASOL	Tab, Light Peach, Round, 8/Atasol	Acetaminophen 325 mg, Codeine Phosphate 8 mg, Caffeine Citrate 30 mg	by Horner	Canadian	Analgesic
8GLAXO	8/Glaxo	Ondansetron 8 mg	by Glaxo	Canadian	Antiemetic
8MG <> ETH269	Tab, Blue, Oblong	Doxazosin Mesylate 8 mg	Cardura by Pfizer	58177-0269	Antihypertensive
8R	Tab, Film Coated, 8 Over R	Indapamide 2.5 mg	Lozol by Quality Care	60346-0946	Diuretic
9 <> M	Tab, Yellow, Triangular, Film Coated	Fluphenazine HCl 2.5 mg	Prolixin by UDL	51079-0486	Antipsychotic
9 <> M	Tab, Yellow	Fluphenazine HCl 2.5 mg	by Mylan	00378-6009	Antipsychotic
90	Tab, Blue, Elongated, Triangle Logo	Guaifenesin 600 mg, Pseudoephedrine HCl 120 mg	Ru-Tuss DE by Knoll		Cold Remedy
90 <> ADALATCC	Tab, Film Coated	Nifedipine 90 mg	Adalat CC by Bayer	00026-8861	Antihypertensive
90 <> ADALATCC	Tab, Film Coated	Nifedipine 90 mg	by Med Pro	53978-3044	Antihypertensive
901 <> UCB	Tab, White, Oblong, Scored	Hydrocodone Bitartrate 2.5 mg, Acetaminophen 500 mg	Lortab by Murfreesboro Ph	51129-1399	Analgesic; C III
901 <> W	Tab, Film Coated	Naproxen Sodium 412.5 mg	Naprelan 375 by Wyeth Labs	00008-0901	NSAID
901 <> W	Tab, Film Coated	Naproxen Sodium 412.5 mg	Naprelan by Physicians Total Care	54868-3974	NSAID
901 <> W	Tab, Film Coated	Naproxen Sodium 412.5 mg	Naprelan by Quality Care	62682-2000	NSAID

ID FRONT <> BACK	DESCRIPTION FRONT <> BACK	INGREDIENT & STRENGTH	BRAND (OR EQUIV.) & FIRM	NDC#	CLASS; SCH.
902 <> UCB	Tab, White, Blue Specks, Cap Shaped, Scored	Acetaminophen 500 mg, Hydrocodone Bitartrate 5 mg	Lortab 5/500 by UCB	50474-0902	Analgesic; C III
902 <> UCB	Tab, White, Blue Specks, Oblong, Scored	Acetaminophen 500 mg, Hydrocodone Bitartrate 5 mg	by Allscripts	54569-0956	Analgesic; C III
902 <> W	Tab, Film Coated	Naproxen Sodium 550 mg	Naprelan by Physicians Total Care	54868-3973	NSAID
902 <> W	Tab, Film Coated	Naproxen Sodium 550 mg	Naprelan by Quality Care	62682-2001	NSAID
902 <> W	Tab, White, Oblong	Naproxen Sodium 550 mg	Naprelan by PDRX Pharms	55289-0304	NSAID
902 <> W	Tab, Film Coated	Naproxen Sodium 550 mg	Naprelan by Wyeth Labs	00008-0902	NSAID
902 <> W	Tab, Film Coated	Naproxen Sodium 550 mg	Naprelan 500 by Caremark	00339-6102	NSAID
902 <> WHITBY	Tab, White, Blue Specks	Acetaminophen 500 mg, Hydrocodone Bitartrate 5 mg	Lortab 5/500 by UCB	50474-0902	Analgesic; C III
903 <> UCB	Tab, White, Green Specks, Cap Shaped, Scored	Acetaminophen 500 mg, Hydrocodone Bitartrate 7.5 mg	by Allscripts	54569-0957	Analgesic; C III
903 <> UCB	Tab, White, Green Specks, Cap Shaped, Scored	Acetaminophen 500 mg, Hydrocodone Bitartrate 7.5 mg	Lortab 7.5 500 by UCB	50474-0907	Analgesic; C III
903 <> WHITBY	Tab, White, Oblong, Green Specks	Acetaminophen 500 mg, Hydrocodone Bitartrate 7.5 mg	Lortab by Allscripts	54569-4761	Analgesic; C III
904 <> BARR	Tab, Debossed	Tamoxifen Citrate 20 mg	by Zeneca	00310-0904	Antiestrogen
904 <> BARR	Tab	Tamoxifen Citrate 20 mg	by Barr	00555-0904	Antiestrogen
907	Tab, Green, Round, Duramed Logo	Belladonna Alkaloids 0.2 mg, Ergotamine Tartrate 0.6 mg, Phenobarbital 40 mg	Duragal S by Duramed	51285-0907	Gastrointestinal; C IV
91 <> GG	Tab, White, Round	Lorazepam 0.5 mg	by Heartland Healthcare	61392-0455	Sedative/Hypnotic; C IV
91 <> GG	Tab, White, Round	Lorazepam 0.5 mg	by Allscripts	54569-2687	Sedative/Hypnotic; C IV
910 <> STSS	Tab, White, Round, ST/SS	Sulfamethoxazole 400 mg, Trimethoprim 80 mg	by Teva	00093-0088	Antibiotic
910 <> UCB	Tab, Pink, Cap Shaped, Scored	Acetaminophen 500 mg, Hydrocodone Bitartrate 10 mg	Lortab 10/500 by UCB	50474-0910	Analgesic; C III
9111 <> VIOKASE	Tab	Amylase 30000 Units, Lipase 8000 Units, Protease 30000 Units	Viokase by Paddock	00574-9111	Gastrointestinal
9111 <> VIOKASE	Tab	Amylase 30000 Units, Lipase 8000 Units, Protease 30000 Units	Viokase by Eckerd Drug	19458-0871	Gastrointestinal
913 <> WATSON	Tab, White, Orange Specks, Cap Shaped, Scored	Acetaminophen 325 mg, Hydrocodone Bitartrate 5 mg	Norco 5/325 by Watson	52544-0913	Analgesic; C III
92 <> BL	Tab, White, Round	Metoclopramide HCl 5 mg	by Murfreesboro Ph	51129-1683	Gastrointestinal
92 <> BL	Tab, White, Round, Scored	Metoclopramide HCl 5 mg	by Teva	00093-2204	Gastrointestinal
92 <> BL	Tab, White, Round	Metoclopramide HCl 5 mg	Reglan by UDL	51079-0629	Gastrointestinal
92 <> BL	Tab, Debossed	Metoclopramide HCl	by Rugby	00536-4038	Gastrointestinal
92 <> GG	Tab, White, Round, Scored	Lorazepam 1 mg	by Allscripts	54569-1585	Sedative/Hypnotic; C IV
92 <> M	Tab, White, Coated, Beveled Edge	Maprotiline HCl 75 mg	by Mylan	00378-0092	Antidepressant
9200	Tab, White, Round	Glipizide 10 mg	Glucotrol by Zenith Goldline	00172-3650	Antidiabetic
9200	Tab, White, Round	Glipizide 10 mg	Glucotrol by Zenith Goldline	00182-1995	Antidiabetic
9200 <> DITROPAN	Tab, Blue, 92-00 <> Ditropan	Oxybutynin Chloride 5 mg	Ditropan by Alza	17314-9200	Urinary
9201	Tab, White, Round	Glipizide 5 mg	Glucotrol by Zenith Goldline	00172-3649	Antidiabetic
9201	Tab, White, Round	Glipizide 5 mg	Glucotrol by Zenith Goldline	00182-1994	Antidiabetic
9253 <> BARR	Tab, Tan, Oval, Scored	Warfarin Sodium 3 mg	by UDL	51079-0911	Anticoagulant
9253 <> BARR	Tab, Tan, Oval, Flat, Scored	Warfarin Sodium 3 mg	Warfarin Sodium by Truett	11312-0128	Anticoagulant
9253 <> BARR	Tab, Tan, Oval, Flat, Scored, Debossed with 925/3	Warfarin Sodium 3 mg	by UDL	51079-0899	Anticoagulant
9266 <> BARR	Tab, Green, Oval, Flat, Scored, Debossed with 926/6	Warfarin Sodium 6 mg	by UDL	51079-0898	Anticoagulant
9266 <> BARR	Tab, Blue, Oval, Flat, Scored	Warfarin Sodium 6 mg	Warfarin Sodium by UCB	50474-0612	Anticoagulant
93 <> 089	Tab	Sulfamethoxazole 800 mg, Trimethoprim 160 mg	SMZ TMP DS by Quality Care	60346-0087	Antibiotic
93 <> 1041	Tab, Pink, Round, Film Coated	Diclofenac Sodium 100 mg	by Biovail	62660-0021	NSAID
93 <> 1041	Tab, Pink, Round	Diclofenac Sodium 100 mg	by Teva Pharms	00093-1041	NSAID
93 <> 111	Tab, White, Round, Film Coated	Cimetidine 200 mg	by Teva	00093-0111	Gastrointestinal
93 <> 1118	Tab, Light Blue	Etodolac 600 mg	by Teva Pharms	00093-1118	NSAID
93 <> 112	Tab, Film Coated	Cimetidine 300 mg	by Quality Care	60346-0944	Gastrointestinal
93 <> 112	Tab, Film Coated	Cimetidine 300 mg	by PDRX	55289-0799	Gastrointestinal
93 <> 112	Tab, White, Round, Film Coated	Cimetidine 300 mg	by Teva	00093-0112	Gastrointestinal
93 <> 113	Tab, Film Coated	Cimetidine 400 mg	by Quality Care	60346-0945	Gastrointestinal
93 <> 113	Tab, Film Coated	Cimetidine 400 mg	by Vangard	00615-3566	Gastrointestinal
93 <> 1177	Tab, Off-White, Round	Neomycin Sulfate 500 mg	by UDL	51079-0015	Antibiotic
93 <> 1177	Tab, Off-White, Round	Neomycin Sulfate 500 mg	by Teva	00093-1177	Antibiotic
93 <> 129	Tab, White, Oval	Estazolam 1 mg	by Halsey Drug	00904-5438	Sedative/Hypnotic; C IV
93 <> 147	Tab, Mottled Light Red	Naproxen 250 mg	by Brightstone	62939-8311	NSAID
93 <> 147	Tab, Mottled Light Red, Round	Naproxen 250 mg	by Allscripts	54569-3758	NSAID

ID FRONT <> BACK	DESCRIPTION FRONT <> BACK	INGREDIENT & STRENGTH	BRAND (OR EQUIV.) & FIRM	NDC#	CLASS; SCH.
93 <> 147	Tab, Mottled Light Red, Round	Naproxen 250 mg	by Teva	00093-0147	NSAID
93 <> 147	Tab	Naproxen 250 mg	by Quality Care	60346-0816	NSAID
93 <> 147	Tab	Naproxen 250 mg	by Heartland	61392-0289	NSAID
93 <> 148	Tab	Naproxen 375 mg	by Heartland	61392-0292	NSAID
93 <> 148	Tab	Naproxen 375 mg	by Quality Care	60346-0817	NSAID
93 <> 148	Tab	Naproxen 375 mg	by Brightstone	62939-8321	NSAID
93 <> 148	Tab, Mottled Peach, Oval	Naproxen 375 mg	by Teva	00093-0148	NSAID
93 <> 148	Tab, Mottled Peach, Oval	Naproxen 375 mg	Naproxen by Otsuka	46602-0004	NSAID
93 <> 149	Tab, Mottled Light Red, Oval	Naproxen 500 mg	by Teva	00093-0149	NSAID
93 <> 149	Tab, Mottled Light Red, Oblong	Naproxen 500 mg	by Allscripts	54569-3760	NSAID
93 <> 149	Tab, Mottled Light Red, Oblong	Naproxen 500 mg	by Allscripts	54569-4255	NSAID
93 <> 149	Tab	Naproxen 500 mg	by Brightstone	62939-8331	NSAID
93 <> 149	Tab	Naproxen 500 mg	by Heartland	61392-0295	NSAID
93 <> 149	Tab, Mottled Red, Oval	Naproxen 500 mg	by Novopharm	55953-0399	NSAID
93 <> 149	Tab, Red, Oval	Naproxen 500 mg	by Vangard Labs	00615-3563	NSAID
93 <> 149	Tab, Mottled Red, Oval	Naproxen 500 mg	Naproxen by Par	49884-0458	NSAID
93 <> 15	Tab, White, Oval	Nabumetone 500 mg	by Teva Pharms	00093-1015	NSAID
93 <> 154	Tab, White, Oval, Film Coated	Ticlopidine HCl 250 mg	by UDL	51079-0920	Anticoagulant
93 <> 154	Tab, White, Oval, Film	Ticlopidine HCl 250 mg	Ticlopidine HCl by Teva	00093-5145	Anticoagulant
93 <> 21	Cap, Pink & White	Diltiazem HCl 60 mg	by Allscripts	54569-3784	Antihypertensive
93 <> 213	Cap	Tolmetin Sodium 492 mg	by Quality Care	60346-0615	NSAID
93 <> 22	Cap	Diltiazem HCl 90 mg	by Allscripts	54569-3785	Antihypertensive
93 <> 2263	Tab, Off-White, Cap Shaped, Film Coated	Amoxicillin 500 mg	by Teva	55953-2263	Antibiotic
93 <> 292	Tab	Carbidopa 10 mg, Levodopa 100 mg	by Baker Cummins	63171-1948	Antiparkinson
93 <> 293	Tab	Carbidopa 25 mg, Levodopa 100 mg	by Vangard	00615-3561	Antiparkinson
93 <> 308	Tab	Clemastine Fumarate 2.68 mg	by HJ Harkins Co	52959-0501	Antihistamine
93 <> 3123	Cap, Light Green & Green, Oval	Dicloxacillin Sodium 250 mg	by Allscripts	54569-0384	Antibiotic
93 <> 3125	Cap, Green	Dicloxacillin Sodium 500 mg	by Allscripts	54569-1889	Antibiotic
93 <> 314	Tab, White, Round, Film	Ketorolac Tromethamine 10 mg	by Murfreesboro	51129-1604	NSAID
93 <> 314	Tab, White, Round, Film-Coated	Ketorolac Tromethamine 10 mg	By Allscripts	54569-4494	NSAID
93 <> 314	Tab, White, Round	Ketorolac Tromethamine 10 mg	by Southwood Pharms	58016-0247	NSAID
93 <> 314	Tab, White, Round, Film Coated	Ketorolac Tromethamine 10 mg	by Teva	00093-0314	NSAID
93 <> 3145	Cap, Gray & Orange	Cephalexin 250 mg	by Caremark	00339-6166	Antibiotic
93 <> 490	Tab, Coated	Acetaminophen 650 mg, Propoxyphene Napsylate 100 mg	Propoxy N APAP by Quality Care	60346-0610	Analgesic; C IV
93 <> 536	Tab, White to Off-White, Oval, Film Coated	Naproxen Sodium 275 mg	by Allscripts	54569-3761	NSAID
93 <> 536	Tab, Film Coated	Naproxen Sodium 275 mg	by Kaiser	00179-1206	NSAID
93 <> 536	Tab, White to Off-White, Oval, Film Coated	Naproxen Sodium 275 mg	by Teva	00093-0536	NSAID
93 <> 536	Tab, Off-White, Film Coated	Naproxen Sodium 275 mg	by Brightstone	62939-8431	NSAID
93 <> 537	Tab, Off-White, Film Coated	Naproxen Sodium 550 mg	by Brightstone	62939-8441	NSAID
93 <> 537	Tab, Off-White, Film Coated	Naproxen Sodium 550 mg	by Quality Care	60346-0826	NSAID
93 <> 537	Tab, Film Coated	Naproxen Sodium 550 mg	by Kaiser	00179-1223	NSAID
93 <> 537	Tab, White to Off-White, Oval	Naproxen Sodium 550 mg	by Teva	00093-0537	NSAID
93 <> 638	Tab	Trazodone HCl 100 mg	by Allscripts	54569-1999	Antidepressant
93 <> 663	Tab, White, Oval, Film Coated	Indapamide 1.25 mg	by Teva	00093-0663	Diuretic
93 <> 670	Tab, Film Coated	Gemfibrozil 600 mg	by Med Pro	53978-2033	Antihyperlipidemic
93 <> 686	Cap	Aspirin 389 mg, Caffeine 32.4 mg, Propoxyphene HCl 65 mg	Propoxyphene Compd 65 by Quality Care	60346-0682	Analgesic; C IV
93 <> 711	Tab, Coated	Flurbiprofen 100 mg	by Quality Care	60346-0968	NSAID
93 <> 7172	Tab, Gray, Oval, Film Coated	Etodolac 500 mg	by Teva Pharms	00093-7172	NSAID
93 <> 755	Tab, Film Coated	Diflunisal 500 mg	by Quality Care	60346-0053	NSAID
93 <> 755	Tab, Film Coated	Diflunisal 500 mg	by Schein	00364-2537	NSAID
93 <> 756	Cap, Olive	Piroxicam 10 mg	by Quality Care	60346-0737	NSAID

ID FRONT <> BACK	DESCRIPTION FRONT <> BACK	INGREDIENT & STRENGTH	BRAND (OR EQUIV.) & FIRM	NDC#	CLASS; SCH.
93 <> 788	Tab	Selegiline HCl 5 mg	by Murfreesboro	51129-1111	Antiparkinson
93 <> 788	Tab, White to Off-White, Round	Selegiline HCl 5 mg	by Teva	00093-0788	Antiparkinson
93 <> 788	Tab, Flat	Selegiline HCl 5 mg	by Vangard	00615-4516	Antiparkinson
93 <> 788	Tab, Beveled, Debossed	Selegiline HCl 5 mg	by Teva	17372-0788	Antiparkinson
93 <> 788	Tab, White, Round, Beveled	Selegiline HCl 5 mg	Selegiline HCl by Schein	00364-2830	Antiparkinson
93 <> 8	Tab, White, Round, Film Coated	Indapamide 2.5 mg	by Teva	00093-0008	Diuretic
93 <> 833	Tab, Mottled Green, Round, Scored	Clonazepam 1 mg	by DHHS Prog	11819-0044	Anticonvulsant; C IV
93 <> 834	Tab, White, Round, Scored	Clonazepam 2 mg	by DHHS Prog	11819-0068	Anticonvulsant; C IV
93 <> 851	Tab, White, Round	Metronidazole 250 mg	by MS State Health	50596-0027	Antibiotic
93 <> 851	Tab, White, Round	Metronidazole 250 mg	by Teva	00093-0851	Antibiotic
93 <> 851	Tab White, Round	Metronidazole 250 mg	Flagyl by UDL	51079-0122	Antibiotic
93 <> 851	Tab	Metronidazole 250 mg	by Golden State	60429-0128	Antibiotic
93 <> 851	Tab	Metronidazole 250 mg	by Nat Pharmpak Serv	55154-5509	Antibiotic
93 <> 851	Tab	Metronidazole 250 mg	by Quality Care	60346-0592	Antibiotic
93 <> 890	Tab, Pink, Oblong, Film Coated	Acetaminophen 650 mg, Propoxyphene Napsylate 100 mg	by Teva	00093-0890	Analgesic; C IV
93 <> 890	Tab, Film Coated	Acetaminophen 650 mg, Propoxyphene Napsylate 100 mg	by Heartland	61392-0446	Analgesic; C IV
93 <> 890	Tab, Coated	Acetaminophen 650 mg, Propoxyphene Napsylate 100 mg	Propoxacet N by Quality Care	60346-0628	Analgesic; C IV
93 <> 890	Tab, Pink, Oblong, Film Coated	Propoxyphene Napsylate 100 mg, Acetaminophen 650 mg	by Ranbaxy	63304-0714	Analgesic; C IV
93 <> 892	Tab, Pink, Oblong, Film Coated	Etodolac 400 mg	by TEVA	00480-0892	NSAID
93 <> 892	Tab, Film Coated	Etodolac 400 mg	by Teva	17372-0892	NSAID
93 <> 892	Tab, Pink, Oblong, Film Coated	Etodolac 400 mg	by Heartland	61392-0911	NSAID
93 <> 892	Tab, Pink, Oblong, Film Coated	Etodolac 400 mg	by Teva	00093-0892	NSAID
93 <> 93778	Tab, Chewable, 93 <> 93/778	Carbamazepine 100 mg	by Major	00904-3854	Anticonvulsant
93 <> 983	Tab, Film Coated	Nystatin 500,000 Units	by Schein	00364-2051	Antifungal
93 <> 983	Tab, Brown, Round, Film Coated	Nystatin 500,000 Units	by Teva	00093-0983	Antifungal
93 <> 983	Tab, Film Coated	Nystatin 500,000 Units	by Quality Care	60346-0652	Antifungal
93 <> BL	Tab, White, Round, Scored	Metoclopramide HCl 10 mg	by Neuman Distr	64579-0049	Gastrointestinal
93 <> BL	Tab, White, Round, Scored	Metoclopramide HCl 10 mg	by Teva	00093-2203	Gastrointestinal
93 <> M	Tab, Coated	Flurbiprofen 100 mg	by Quality Care	60346-0968	NSAID
93019	Cap, Blue & White	Phentermine HCl 37.5 mg	Adipex-P by Lemmon		Anorexiant; C IV
93037	Tab, White, Round, 93/037	Clemastine 1.34 mg	Tavist-1 by Lemmon		Antihistamine
93044	Cap, Dark Blue, 93 over 044	Acyclovir 200 mg	by Teva	00093-0044	Antiviral
93064	Cap, Orange & Yellow, 93-064	Tetracycline HCl 250 mg	Achromycin V by Lemmon		Antibiotic
93088	Tab, White, Round, Scored	Sulfamethoxazole 400 mg , Trimethoprim 80 mg	Cotrim by Sovereign	58716-0676	Antibiotic
93088	Tab, White, Round, Scored	Sulfamethoxazole 400 mg, Trimethoprim 80 mg	by St. Marys Med	60760-0046	Antibiotic
93088	Tab, White, Round, Scored	Sulfamethoxazole 400mg, Trimethoprim 80 mg	by Allscripts	54569-0269	Antibiotic
93088	Tab, White, Round, Scored, 93 over 088	Sulfamethoxazole 80 mg, Trimethoprim 400 mg	by Teva	00093-0088	Antibiotic
93089	Tab	Sulfamethoxazole 800 mg, Trimethoprim 160 mg	by Murfreesboro	51129-1335	Antibiotic
93089	Tab, White, Oblong, Scored, 93 over 089	Sulfamethoxazole 160 mg, Trimethoprim 800 mg	by Teva	00093-0089	Antibiotic
93089	Tab, White, Oblong, Scored, 93/089	Sulfamethoxazole 160 mg, Trimethoprim 80 mg	by Teva	17372-0089	Antibiotic
93089	Tab, Oblong, Scored	Sulfamethoxazole 800 mg, Trimethoprim 160 mg	Cotrim DS by St. Marys Med	60760-0135	Antibiotic
93089	Tab	Sulfamethoxazole 800 mg, Trimethoprim 160 mg	by Golden State	60429-0170	Antibiotic
93089	Tab, White, Oblong, Scored	Sulfamethoxazole 800 mg, Trimethoprim 160 mg	by St. Marys Med	60760-0079	Antibiotic
93089	Tab, White, Oval, Scored	Sulfamethoxazole 800 mg, Trimethoprim 160 mg	by Allscripts	54569-0075	Antibiotic
93089	Tab, White, Oblong, Scored	Sulfamethoxazole 800 mg, Trimethoprim 160 mg	by Hj Harkins	52959-0144	Antibiotic
93089	Tab, White, Oblong, Scored	Sulfamethoxazole 800 mg, Trimethoprim 160 mg	by Heartland Healthcare	61392-0947	Antibiotic
93090	Tab, White, Round, 93-090	Carbamazepine 200 mg	Epitol by Lemmon		Anticonvulsant
931	Tab, Yellow, D-Shaped	Cyclobenzaprine 10 mg	Flexeril by Frosst	Canadian	Muscle Relaxant
9310	Tab, Blue, Round	Chlorpropamide 100 mg	Diabinese by Lemmon		Antidiabetic
93100	Tab, Pink, Round, Concave, Scored, Film	Labetalol HCl 100 mg	Labetalol HCl by Murfreesboro	51129-1612	Antihypertensive
93100	Tab, Light Pink, Round, Film Coated, Scored, 93 over 100	Labetolol HCl 100 mg	by Teva	00093-0100	Antihypertensive
93102	Tab, White, Round, Concave, Scored, Film	Labetalol HCl 200 mg	Labetalol HCl by Murfreesboro	51129-1613	Antihypertensive

ID FRONT <> BACK	DESCRIPTION FRONT <> BACK	INGREDIENT & STRENGTH	BRAND (OR EQUIV.) & FIRM	NDC#	CLASS; SCH.
93102	Tab, Off-White, Round, Film Coated, Scored, 93 over 102	Labetolol HCl 200 mg	by Teva	00093-0102	Antihypertensive
93106	Tab, Purple, Round, Concave, Film	Labetalol HCl 300 mg	Labetalol HCl by Murfreesboro	51129-1614	Antihypertensive
93106	Tab, Light Purple, Round, Film Coated, 93 over 106	Labetolol HCl 300 mg	by Teva	00093-0106	Antihypertensive
931060	Tab, Light Blue, Oval, Scored, 93/1060	Sotalol HCl 120 mg	by Teva Pharms	00093-1060	Antiarrhythmic
931060	Tab, Blue, Oval, Scored	Sotalol HCl 120 mg	by Teva Pharm Inds	00480-1060	Antiarrhythmic
93109	Tab	Carbamazepine 200 mg	by Teva	17372-0109	Anticonvulsant
93113	Tab, White, Oblong, Film Coated, Scored, 93/113	Cimetidine 400 mg	by Teva	00093-0113	Gastrointestinal
93122	Tab, White, Oblong, Film Coated, Scored, 93/122	Cimetidine 800 mg	by Teva	00093-0122	Gastrointestinal
93123	Tab, White, Round, 93 12/3	Aspirin 325 mg, Codeine 30 mg	Empirin #3 by Lemmon		Analgesic; C III
93129	Tab, White, Oval, Scored, 93/129	Estazolam 1 mg	by Teva	00093-0129	Sedative/Hypnotic; C IV
93130	Tab, Coral, Oval, Scored, 93/130	Estazolam 2 mg	by Teva	00093-0130	Sedative/Hypnotic; C IV
93132	Tab, Caramel & White	Acetaminophen 300 mg, Codeine 15 mg	Tylenol #2 by Lemmon		Analgesic; C III
93134	Tab, White, Round, 93 13/4	Aspirin 325 mg, Codeine 60 mg	Empirin #4 by Lemmon		Analgesic; C III
93138	Cap, Clear & Pink	Diphenhydramine HCl 25 mg	Benadryl by Lemmon		Antihistamine
93139	Cap, Pink	Diphenhydramine HCl 50 mg	Benadryl by Lemmon		Antihistamine
93143	Tab, Lavender, Round, 93-143	Warfarin Sodium 2 mg	Sofarin by Lemmon		Anticoagulant
93144	Tab, Orange, Round, 93-144	Warfarin Sodium 2.5 mg	Sofarin by Lemmon		Anticoagulant
93145	Tab, Pink, Round, 93-145	Warfarin Sodium 5 mg	Sofarin by Lemmon		Anticoagulant
93147	Tab	Naproxen 250 mg	by Zenith Goldline	00182-1971	NSAID
93147	Tab, Mottled Red, Round	Naproxen 250 mg	by Novopharm	62528-0734	NSAID
93147	Tab, Red, Round, Convex	Naproxen 250 mg	Naproxen by Otsuka	46602-0002	NSAID
93148	Tab	Naproxen 375 mg	by Zenith Goldline	00182-1972	NSAID
93149	Tab	Naproxen 500 mg	by Zenith Goldline	00182-1973	NSAID
93149	Tab, Light Red, 93 149 <>	Naproxen 500 mg	by St Marys Med	60760-0149	NSAID
93149	Tab, Light Red, 93 149 <>	Naproxen 500 mg	by Quality Care	60346-0815	NSAID
93150 <> 3	Tab, White, Round, 93 over 150 <> 3	Acetaminophen 300 mg, Codeine 30 mg	Acetaminophen W COD by ABG	60999-0903	Analgesic; C III
93150 <> 3	Tab, White, Round, 93 over 150 <> 3	Acetaminophen 300 mg, Codeine Phosphate 30 gm	by Teva	00093-0150	Analgesic; C III
93150 <> 3	Tab, 93 over 150 <> 3	Acetaminophen 300 mg, Codeine Phosphate 30 mg	by Nat Pharmpak Serv	55154-5548	Analgesic; C III
93150 <> 3	Tab, 93 Over 150	Acetaminophen 300 mg, Codeine Phosphate 30 mg	by Quality Care	60346-0059	Analgesic; C III
93150 <> 3	Tab, White, Round, 93 over 150 <> 3	Acetaminophen 300 mg, Codeine Phosphate 30 mg	by UDL	51079-0161	Analgesic; C III
93150 <> 3	Tab, 93-150	Acetaminophen 300 mg, Codeine Phosphate 30 mg	by Murfreesboro	51129-0089	Analgesic; C III
93150 <> 3	Tab	Acetaminophen 300 mg, Codeine Phosphate 30 mg	by Pharmedix	53002-0101	Analgesic; C III
93150 <> 3	Tab	Acetaminophen 300 mg, Codeine Phosphate 30 mg	by Urgent Care Ctr	50716-0465	Analgesic; C III
931503	Tab	Acetaminophen 300 mg, Codeine 30 mg	by Major	00904-0175	Analgesic; C III
931503	Tab, White, Round, 93-150 3	Acetaminophen 300 mg, Codeine Phosphate 30 mg	by Allscripts	54569-0025	Analgesic; C III
931504	Tab, White, Round, 93-350 4	Acetaminophen 300 mg, Codeine Phosphate 60 mg	by Allscripts	54569-0302	Analgesic; C III
93152	Cap, Coral & Scarlet	Acetaminophen 300 mg, Codeine 30 mg	Phenaphen #3 by Lemmon		Analgesic; C III
93157	Tab, White, Round	Diethylpropion HCl 25 mg	Tenuate by Lemmon		Antianorexiant; C IV
93172	Cap, Brown & Gray	Acetaminophen 300 mg, Codeine 60 mg	Tylenol #4 by Lemmon		Analgesic; C III
93176	Tab, White, Round, Scored, 93 over 176	Captopril 25 mg, Hydrochlorothiazide 15 mg	by Teva	00093-0176	Antihypertensive; Diuretic
93177	Tab, Tan, Round, Scored, 93 over 177	Captopril 25 mg, Hydrochlorothiazide 25 mg	by Teva	00093-0177	Antihypertensive; Diuretic
93181	Tab, White, Oval, Scored, 93/181	Captopril 50 mg, Hydrochlorothiazide 15 mg	by Teva	00093-0181	Antihypertensive; Diuretic
93182	Tab, Tan, Oval, Scored, 93/182	Captopril 50 mg, Hydrochlorothiazide 25 mg	by Teva	00093-0182	Antihypertensive; Diuretic
93188	Tab, White, Round	Sulfamethoxazole 400 mg, Trimethoprim 80 mg	Cotrim by Lemmon		Antibiotic
93189	Tab, White, Oval	Sulfamethoxazole 800 mg, Trimethoprim 160 mg	Cotrim DS by Lemmon		Antibiotic
932	Tab	Atenolol 50 mg	by Heartland	61392-0543	Antihypertensive
93208	Cap, Orange, Opaque, 93 over 208	Zinc Acetate 50 mg	Galzin by Teva	00093-0208	Mineral Supplement
93208	Cap, Orange, Opaque, 93-208	Zinc Acetate 50 mg	Galzin by Gate	57844-0208	Mineral Supplement

ID FRONT <> BACK	DESCRIPTION FRONT <> BACK	INGREDIENT & STRENGTH	BRAND (OR EQUIV.) & FIRM	NDC#	CLASS; SCH.
9321	Cap, Pink & White, 93 over 21	Diltiazem HCl 60 mg	by Teva	00093-0021	Antihypertensive
9321 <> 9321	Cap, Ex Release, 93-21	Diltiazem HCl 60 mg	by Quality Care	62682-6034	Antihypertensive
9321 <> 9321	Cap, Pink & White	Diltiazem HCl 60 mg	by Eisai	11071-0812	Antihypertensive
93213 <> 93213	Cap, 93 Over 213	Tolmetin Sodium 492 mg	by Teva	00093-0213	NSAID
93214	Tab, Coated	Tolmetin Sodium 735 mg	by Teva	00093-0214	NSAID
93214	Tab, Coated	Tolmetin Sodium 735 mg	by Teva	17372-0214	NSAID
93215	Cap, Aqua Blue, Opaque, 93 over 215	Zinc Acetate 25 mg	Galzin by Teva	00093-0215	Mineral Supplement
93215	Cap, Aqua Blue, 93-215	Zinc Acetate 25 mg	Galzin by Gate	57844-0215	Mineral Supplement
93218	Tab, White, Round	Phenobarbital 30 mg	by Lemmon		Sedative/Hypnotic; C IV
9322	Cap, Pink & Yellow, 93 over 22	Diltiazem HCl 90 mg	by Teva	00093-0022	Antihypertensive
9322 <> 9322	Cap, Ex Release, 93-22	Diltiazem HCl 90 mg	by Quality Care	62682-6035	Antihypertensive
932264	Tab, Off-White, Cap Shaped, Film Coated, Scored	Amoxicillin875 mg	by Teva	55953-2264	Antibiotic
9323	Cap, Orange & Pink	Diltiazem HCl ER 120 mg	Cardizem by Lemmon		Antihypertensive
9323	Cap, Orange & Pink, 93 over 23	Diltiazem HCl 120 mg	by Teva	00093-0023	Antihypertensive
93241	Tab, White, Round	Phenobarbital 15 mg	by Lemmon		Sedative/Hypnotic; C IV
9326	Tab, Yellow, Oval, Scored, 93/26	Enalapril Maleate 2.5 mg	by Teva Pharms	00093-0026	Antihypertensive
9327	Tab, White, Oval, Scored, 93/27	Enalapril Maleate 5 mg	by Teva Pharms	00093-0027	Antihypertensive
9328	Tab, Pink, Oval, 93 over 28	Enalapril Maleate 10 mg	by Teva Pharms	00093-0028	Antihypertensive
93280 <> 93280	Tab, Yellow, Round, Film Coated	Bupropion HCl 75 mg	Bupropion HCl by Caremark	00339-4056	Antidepressant
93290	Tab, Pink, Round, Film Coated	Bupropion HCl 100 mg	Bupropion HCl by Caremark	00339-4104	Antidepressant
93292	Tab, Mottled Blue, Round, Scored, 93 over 292	Carbidopa 10 mg, Levodopa 100 mg	by Teva	00093-0292	Antiparkinson
93292	Tab	Carbidopa 10 mg, Levodopa 100 mg	by Zenith Goldline	00182-1948	Antiparkinson
93292	Tab, Mottled Blue	Carbidopa 10 mg, Levodopa 100 mg	by Med Pro	53978-3059	Antiparkinson
93292	Tab, Mottled Blue, Round, Scored, 93 over 292	Carbidopa 10 mg, Levodopa 100 mg	Sinemet by UDL	51079-0755	Antiparkinson
93292	Tab	Carbidopa 10 mg, Levodopa 100 mg	by Teva	17372-0292	Antiparkinson
93292	Tab, Mottled Blue, Round, Scored, 93-292	Carbidopa 10 mg, Levodopa 100 mg	Carbidopa , Levodopa by Caremark	00339-6135	Antiparkinson
93292	Tab	Carbidopa 10 mg, Levodopa 100 mg	by Medirex	57480-0807	Antiparkinson
93292	Tab	Carbidopa 10 mg, Levodopa 100 mg	by Amerisource	62584-0641	Antiparkinson
93293	Tab, 93/293	Carbidopa 25 mg, Levodopa 100 mg	by Nat Pharmpak Serv	55154-5816	Antiparkinson
93293	Tab	Carbidopa 25 mg, Levodopa 100 mg	by Medirex	57480-0808	Antiparkinson
93293	Tab, 93 293	Carbidopa 25 mg, Levodopa 100 mg	by Amerisource	62584-0642	Antiparkinson
93293	Tab, Mottled Yellow, Round, Scored, 93 over 293	Carbidopa 25 mg, Levodopa 100 mg	by Teva	00093-0293	Antiparkinson
93293	Tab, 93/293	Carbidopa 25 mg, Levodopa 100 mg	by Zenith Goldline	00182-1949	Antiparkinson
93293	Tab, 93/293	Carbidopa 25 mg, Levodopa 100 mg	by Caremark	00339-6028	Antiparkinson
93293	Tab, Mottled Yellow, Round, Scored, 93 over 293	Carbidopa 25 mg, Levodopa 100 mg	Sinemet by UDL	51079-0756	Antiparkinson
93293	Tab	Carbidopa 25 mg, Levodopa 100 mg	by Teva	17372-0293	Antiparkinson
93293	Tab, Mottled Yellow, Round, Scored, 93 293	Carbidopa 25 mg, Levodopa 100 mg	Carbidopa, Levodopa by Caremark	00339-6136	Antiparkinson
93294	Tab, Mottled Blue	Carbidopa 25 mg, Levodopa 250 mg	by Nat Pharmpak Serv	55154-5536	Antiparkinson
93294	Tab	Carbidopa 25 mg, Levodopa 250 mg	by Medirex	57480-0476	Antiparkinson
93294	Tab, 93-294	Carbidopa 25 mg, Levodopa 250 mg	by Amerisource	62584-0643	Antiparkinson
93294	Tab	Carbidopa 25 mg, Levodopa 250 mg	by Zenith Goldline	00182-1950	Antiparkinson
93294	Tab, Mottled Blue, Round, Scored, 93 over 294	Carbidopa 25 mg, Levodopa 250 mg	by Teva	00093-0294	Antiparkinson
93294	Tab	Carbidopa 25 mg, Levodopa 250 mg	by Vangard	00615-4504	Antiparkinson
93294	Tab, Mottled Blue, Round, Scored, 93 over 294	Carbidopa 25 mg, Levodopa 250 mg	Sinemet by UDL	51079-0783	Antiparkinson
93294	Tab	Carbidopa 25 mg, Levodopa 250 mg	by Teva	17372-0294	Antiparkinson
93294	Tab, Mottled Blue, Round, Scored	Carbidopa 25 mg, Levodopa 250 mg	by Caremark	00339-6138	Antiparkinson
93307	Tab, 93/307	Clemastine Fumarate 1.34 mg	by Teva	00093-0307	Antihistamine
93308	Tab, 93 over 308	Clemastine Fumarate 2.68 mg	by Northeast	58163-0072	Antihistamine
93308	Tab, White, Round, Scored, 93 over 308	Clemastine Fumarate 2.68 mg	by Teva	00093-0308	Antihistamine
93308	Tab	Clemastine Fumarate 2.68 mg	by Zenith Goldline	00182-1936	Antihistamine
933107	Cap, Buff & Caramel, 93-3107	Amoxicillin 250 mg	Amoxil/Polymox by UDL	51079-0600	Antibiotic
933107	Cap, Buff & Caramel, 93 over 3107	Amoxicillin Trihydrate 250 mg	by Teva	00093-3107	Antibiotic

ID FRONT <> BACK	DESCRIPTION FRONT <> BACK	INGREDIENT & STRENGTH	BRAND (OR EQUIV.) & FIRM	NDC#	CLASS; SCH.
933107	Cap, Buff & Caramel	Amoxicillin 250 mg	by Teva	17372-0613	Antibiotic
933109	Cap, Buff, 93 over 3109	Amoxicillin Trihydrate 500 mg	by Teva	00093-3109	Antibiotic
933109	Cap, Teva	Amoxicillin 500 mg	by Quality Care	60346-0634	Antibiotic
933109	Cap, Buff, 93-3109	Amoxicillin 500 mg	Amoxil/Polymox by UDL	51079-0601	Antibiotic
93311	Cap	Loperamide 2 mg	by Zenith Goldline	00182-1505	Antidiarrheal
93311	Cap, Light Brown & Dark Brown	Loperamide HCl 2 mg	by Allscripts	54569-3707	Antidiarrheal
93311	Cap, Dark Brown & Light Brown, Opaque, 93 over 311	Loperamide HCl 2 mg	by Teva	00093-0311	Antidiarrheal
93311	Cap, Dark Brown & Brown, Opaque, 93-311	Loperamide HCl 2 mg	by Quality Care	60346-0046	Antidiarrheal
933111	Cap, 93-3111	Ampicillin Trihydrate	by HL Moore	00839-5087	Antibiotic
933111	Cap, Gray & Scarlet, 93 over 3111	Ampicillin Trihydrate 250 mg	by Teva	00093-3111	Antibiotic
933111 <> 933111	Cap, 93-3111	Ampicillin Trihydrate	by UDL	51079-0602	Antibiotic
933113	Cap, Gray & Scarlet, 93 over 3113	Ampicillin Trihydrate 500 mg	by Teva	00093-3113	Antibiotic
933115	Cap, Blue, Opaque, 93 over 3115	Oxacillin Sodium Monohydrate 250 mg	by Teva	00093-3115	Antibiotic
933117	Cap, Blue, Opaque, 93 over 3117	Oxacillin Sodium Monohydrate 500 mg	by Teva	00093-3117	Antibiotic
933119	Cap, Green & Red	Cloxacillin Sodium Monohydrate 250 mg	by HJ Harkins	52959-0468	Antibiotic
933119	Cap, Dark Green & Scarlet, 93 over 3119	Cloxacillin Sodium Monohydrate 250 mg	by Teva	00093-3119	Antibiotic
933121	Cap, Dark Green & Scarlet, 93 over 3121	Cloxacillin Sodium 500 mg	by Teva	00093-3121	Antibiotic
933123	Cap, Light Green, 93 over 3123	Dicloxacillin Sodium 250 mg	by Teva	00093-3123	Antibiotic
933123 <> 933123	Cap, Light Green, 93-3123 <> 93-3123	Dicloxacillin Sodium	by UDL	51079-0610	Antibiotic
933123 <> 933123	Cap, Green, 93 over 3123 <> 93 over 3123	Dicloxacillin Sodium 250 mg	by DRX		Antibiotic
933125	Cap, Light Green, 93 over 3125	Dicloxacillin Sodium 500 mg	by Teva	00093-3125	Antibiotic
933125 <> 933125	Cap, Light Green, 93-3125 <> 93-3125	Dicloxacillin Sodium 500 mg	by UDL	51079-0611	Antibiotic
933127	Cap, Blue & Scarlet, 93 over 3127	Disopyramide Phosphate 100 mg	by Teva	00093-3127	Antiarrhythmic
933129	Cap, Buff & Scarlet, 93 over 3129	Disopyramide Phosphate 150 mg	by Teva	00093-3129	Antiarrhythmic
933145	Cap, Gray & Orange, 93-3145	Cephalexin 250 mg	Keflex by UDL	51079-0604	Antibiotic
933145	Cap, Gray & Orange, 93 over 3145	Cephalexin 250 mg	by Teva	00093-3145	Antibiotic
933147	Cap, Orange, 93 over 3147	Cephalexin 500 mg	by Teva	00093-3147	Antibiotic
933147	Cap, Orange, 93-3147	Cephalexin Monohydrate 500 mg	Keflex by UDL	51079-0605	Antibiotic
933153	Cap, Light Green & Pink, 93 over 3153	Cephradine 250 mg	by Teva	00093-3153	Antibiotic
933153 <> 933153	Cap, Light Green, 93-3153 <> 93-3153	Cephradine 250 mg	by UDL	51079-0606	Antibiotic
933155	Cap, Light Green, Opaque, 93 over 3155	Cephradine 500 mg	by Teva	00093-3155	Antibiotic
933155	Cap, 93-3155	Cephradine 500 mg	by HJ Harkins Co	52959-0032	Antibiotic
933155 <> 933155	Cap, 93-3155	Cephradine 500 mg	by UDL	51079-0607	Antibiotic
933165	Cap, Pink, 93 over 3165	Minocycline HCl 50 mg	by Teva	00093-3165	Antibiotic
933167	Cap, Maroon & Pink, 93 over 3167	Minocycline HCl 100 mg	by Teva	00093-3167	Antibiotic
933169	Cap, Red, 93-3169	Clindamycin HCl 75 mg	by Teva	00093-3169	Antibiotic
933171	Cap, Blue & Red, 93-3171	Clindamycin HCl 150 mg	by Teva	00093-3171	Antibiotic
93318	Tab, Light Orange, Round	Diltiazem HCl 30 mg	Cardizem by Lemmon		Antihypertensive
93318	Tab, Light Orange, Round, Film Coated, 93 over 318	Diltiazem HCl 30 mg	by Teva	00093-0318	Antihypertensive
93318	Tab, Orange, Round, Film Coated	Diltiazem HCl 30 mg	Diltiazem HCl by Fielding	00421-0768	Antihypertensive
93319	Tab, Orange, Round	Diltiazem HCl 60 mg	Cardizem by Lemmon		Antihypertensive
93319	Tab, Orange, Round, Film Coated, Scored, 93 over 319	Diltiazem HCl 60 mg	by Teva	00093-0319	Antihypertensive
93319	Tab, Orange, Round, Scored, Film Coated	Diltiazem HCl 60 mg	Diltiazem HCl by Fielding	00421-1259	Antihypertensive
933193	Cap, Blue & Light Blue, 93 over 3193	Ketoprofen 50 mg	by Teva	00093-3193	NSAID
933195	Cap, Blue & White, 93 over 3195	Ketoprofen 75 mg	by Teva	00093-3195	NSAID
933195 <> 933195	Cap, Blue & White	Ketoprofen 75 mg	by Southwood Pharms	58016-0380	NSAID
93320	Tab, Orange, Oblong, Scored, Film, 93/320	Diltiazem HCl 90 mg	Diltiazem HCl by Fournier Pharma	63924-0002	Antihypertensive
93320	Tab, Light Orange	Diltiazem HCl 90 mg	Cardizem by Lemmon		Antihypertensive
93320	Tab, Light Orange, Oblong, Film Coated, Scored, 93/320	Diltiazem HCl 90 mg	by Teva	00093-0320	Antihypertensive
93321	Tab, Orange, Oblong, Scored, Film, Debossed	Diltiazem HCl 120 mg	Diltiazem HCl by Fournier Pharma	63924-0003	Antihypertensive
93321	Tab, Orange, Oblong	Diltiazem HCl 120 mg	Cardizem by Lemmon		Antihypertensive
93321	Tab, Orange, Oblong, Film Coated, Scored, 93/321	Diltiazem HCl 120 mg	by Teva	00093-0321	Antihypertensive

ID FRONT <> BACK	DESCRIPTION FRONT <> BACK	INGREDIENT & STRENGTH	BRAND (OR EQUIV.) & FIRM	NDC#	CLASS; SCH.
93325	Tab, Lavender, Round, 93-325	Desipramine HCl 25 mg	Norpramin by Lemmon		Antidepressant
93326	Tab, Blue, Round, 93-326	Desipramine HCl 50 mg	Norpramin by Lemmon		Antidepressant
93327	Tab, White, Round, 93-327	Desipramine HCl 75 mg	Norpramin by Lemmon		Antidepressant
93328	Tab, Butterscotch Yellow, Round, 93-328	Desipramine HCl 100 mg	Norpramin by Lemmon		Antidepressant
93350 <> 4	Tab, 93 350	Acetaminophen 300 mg, Codeine Phosphate 60 mg	by Quality Care	60346-0632	Analgesic; C III
93350 <> 4	Tab, White, Round, 93 over 350 <> 4	Acetaminophen 300 mg, Codeine Phosphate 60 mg	by Teva	00093-0350	Analgesic; C III
93350 <> 4	Tab, White, Round, 93 over 350 <> 4	Acetaminophen 300 mg, Codeine Phosphate 60 mg	by UDL	51079-0106	Analgesic; C III
93350 <> 4	Tab	Acetaminophen 300 mg, Codeine Phosphate 60 mg	by Murfreesboro	51129-6662	Analgesic; C III
93350 <> 4	Tab, White, Round	Acetaminophen 300 mg; Codeine Phosphate 60 mg	by Southwood Pharms	58016-0272	Analgesic; C III
933504	Tab, 93-350 4	Acetaminophen 300 mg, Codeine Phosphate 60 mg	by St Marys Med	60760-0350	Analgesic; C III
933504	Tab	Acetaminophen 300 mg, Codeine Phosphate 60 mg	by Geneva	00781-1654	Analgesic; C III
933DP	Tab, White, Oblong, Scored	Hyoscyamine Sulfate 0.375 mg	by Sovereign Pharms	58716-0668	Gastrointestinal
9341	Tab, White, Round, Scored, 93 over 41	Clomiphene Citrate 50 mg	by Teva	00093-0041	Infertility
93431	Tab, Blue, Round	Chlorthalidone 50 mg	Hygroton by Lemmon		Diuretic
93433	Tab, White, Round	Chlorthalidone 100 mg	Hygroton by Lemmon		Diuretic
93484	Tab, Orange, Round	Doxycycline Hyclate 100 mg	Vibra-Tab by Lemmon		Antibiotic
93486	Tab, White, Round	Ibuprofen 200 mg	Nuprin by Lemmon		NSAID
93490	Tab, White, Oblong, Film Coated, 93-490	Acetaminophen 650 mg, Propoxyphene Napsylate 100 mg	by Teva	00093-0490	Analgesic; C IV
93490	Tab, White, Oblong, Film, 93-490	Propoxyphene Napsylate 100 mg, Acetaminophen 650 mg	APAP by Reese	10956-0745	Analgesic; C IV
93490	Tab, White, Oblong, Film Coated	Propoxyphene Napsylate 100 mg	by HJ Harkins	52959-0335	Analgesic; C IV
93491	Tab, White, Round, 93-491	Ibuprofen 400 mg	Motrin by Lemmon		NSAID
93492	Tab, White, Oval, 93-492	Ibuprofen 600 mg	Motrin by Lemmon		NSAID
93498	Tab, White, Oblong, 93-498	Ibuprofen 800 mg	Motrin by Lemmon		NSAID
935	Tab, White to Off-White w/ Blue Ink Enteric Imprint, 93-5	Naproxen DR 375 mg	by Teva	00093-1005	NSAID
935	Tab, White, Oblong	Naproxen DR 375 mg	Naproxen by Par	49884-0490	NSAID
9350 <> 2	Tab, 93 50	Acetaminophen 300 mg, Codeine Phosphate 15 mg	by Quality Care	60346-0015	Analgesic; C III
9350 <> 2	Tab, White, Round, 93 over 50 <> 2	Acetaminophen 300 mg, Codeine Phosphate 15 mg	by Teva	00093-0050	Analgesic; C III
93525	Tab, Pink, Round	Amitriptyline HCl 10 mg	Elavil by Lemmon		Antidepressant
93527	Tab, Green, Round	Amitriptyline HCl 25 mg	Elavil by Lemmon		Antidepressant
93529	Tab, Brown, Round	Amitriptyline HCl 50 mg	Elavil by Lemmon		Antidepressant
93531	Tab, Purple, Round	Amitriptyline HCl 75 mg	Elavil by Lemmon		Antidepressant
93533	Tab, Orange, Round	Amitriptyline HCl 100 mg	Elavil by Lemmon		Antidepressant
93535	Tab, Peach, Round	Amitriptyline HCl 150 mg	Elavil by Lemmon		Antidepressant
93536	Tab, Coated	Naproxen Sodium 275 mg	by Zenith Goldline	00182-1974	NSAID
93536	Tab, Film Coated	Naproxen Sodium 550 mg	by Zenith Goldline	00182-1975	NSAID
93536	Tab, White, Oval, Film, 93 536	Naproxen Sodium 275 mg	Naproxen Sodium by Par	49884-0549	NSAID
93537	Tab, Film Coated, 93 537	Naproxen Sodium 550 mg	by HJ Harkins Co	52959-0271	NSAID
93537	Tab, White, Oval, Scored	Naproxen Sodium 550 mg	by Direct Dispensing	57866-6613	NSAID
93537	Tab, White, Oval, Film, 93 537	Naproxen Sodium 550 mg	Naproxen Sodium by Par	49884-0550	NSAID
93541	Cap, Dark Orange & Gray, 93 Over 541	Cephalexin Monohydrate 250 mg	by Teva	00093-0541	Antibiotic
93542	Tab, 93 Over 542	Chlorzoxazone 500 mg	by Quality Care	60346-0663	Muscle Relaxant
93542	Tab, White, Oblong, Scored, 93/542	Chlorzoxazone 500 mg	by Teva	00093-0542	Muscle Relaxant
93542	Tab, 93/542	Chlorzoxazone 500 mg	by Allscripts	54569-1970	Muscle Relaxant
93543	Cap, Orange, 93 Over 543	Cephalexin Monohydrate 500 mg	by Teva	00093-0543	Antibiotic
93545	Tab, Green, Round	Chlorzoxazone 250 mg, Acetaminophen 300 mg	Parafon Forte by Lemmon		Muscle Relaxant
93548	Cap, Yellow, 93-548	Amantadine HCl 100 mg	Symmetrel by Lemmon		Antiviral
93585	Cap, Green	Indomethacin 25 mg	Indocin by Lemmon		NSAID
93587	Cap, Green	Indomethacin 50 mg	Indocin by Lemmon		NSAID
93590	Tab, White	Propoxyphene Napsylate 100 mg, Acetaminophen 650 mg	Propacet 100 by Lemmon		Analgesic; C IV
936	Tab, White to Off-White w/ Blue Ink Enteric Imprint, 93-6	Naproxen DR 500 mg	by Teva	00093-1006	NSAID
936	Tab, White, Oblong, 93-6	Naproxen DR 500 mg	Naproxen by Par	49884-0495	NSAID
9361	Tab, Light Blue, Oval, Scored, 93/61	Sotalol HCl 80 mg	by Teva Pharms	00093-1061	Antiarrhythmic

159

ID FRONT <> BACK	DESCRIPTION FRONT <> BACK	INGREDIENT & STRENGTH	BRAND (OR EQUIV.) & FIRM	NDC#	CLASS; SCH.
9361	Tab, Blue, Oval, Scored	Sotalol HCl 80 mg	by Teva Pharm Inds	00480-1061	Antiarrhythmic
93613	Cap, Caramel & Ivory, 93-613	Amoxicillin 250 mg	Amoxil by Lemmon		Antibiotic
93615	Cap, Ivory, 93-615	Amoxicillin 500 mg	Amoxil by Lemmon		Antibiotic
93617	Cap, White	Chlordiazepoxide HCl 5 mg, Clidinium Bromide 2.5 mg	Librax by Lemmon		Gastrointestinal; C IV
9362	Tab, Light Blue, Oval, Scored, 93/62	Sotalol HCl 160 mg	by Teva Pharms	00093-1062	Antiarrhythmic
9362	Tab, Blue, Oval, Scored	Sotalol HCl 60 mg	by Teva Pharm Inds	00480-1062	Antiarrhythmic
93620	Tab, Blue, Round	Propranolol 20 mg	Inderal by Lemmon		Antihypertensive
93628	Cap, Clear & Lavender, 93-628	Indomethacin ER 75 mg	Indocin SR by Lemmon		NSAID
9363	Tab, Light Blue, Oval, Scored, 93/63	Sotalol HCl 240 mg	by Teva Pharms	00093-1063	Antiarrhythmic
9363	Tab, Blue, Oval, Scored	Sotalol HCl 240 mg	by Teva Pharm Inds	00480-1063	Antiarrhythmic
93637	Tab, White, Round, Scored, Film, 93 637	Trazodone HCl 50 mg	Trazodone HCl by Teva	00480-0320	Antidepressant
93637	Tab, White, Round, Film Coated, Scored, 93 over 637	Trazodone HCl 50 mg	by Teva	00093-0637	Antidepressant
93637	Tab, Coated, 93 637	Trazodone HCl 50 mg	by Quality Care	60346-0620	Antidepressant
93638	Tab, White, Round, Scored, Film	Trazodone HCl 100 mg	Trazodone HCl by Teva	00480-0321	Antidepressant
93638	Tab, White, Round, Film Coated, Scored, 93 over 638	Trazodone HCl 100 mg	by Teva	00093-0638	Antidepressant
93638	Tab, Film Coated, 93 Over 638	Trazodone HCl 100 mg	by Quality Care	60346-0014	Antidepressant
93640	Tab, Green, Round	Propranolol 40 mg	Inderal by Lemmon		Antihypertensive
93653	Cap, Blue, 93-653	Doxycycline Hyclate 100 mg	Vibramycin by Lemmon		Antibiotic
93665	Tab, White, Round, Scored, 93 over 665	Albuterol 2 mg	by Teva	00093-0665	Antiasthmatic
93666	Tab, White, Round, Scored, 93 over 666	Albuterol 4 mg	by Teva	00093-0666	Antiasthmatic
93670	Tab, Off-White to White, Film Coated, 93 670	Gemfibrozil 600 mg	by Heartland	61392-0093	Antihyperlipidemic
93670	Tab, Film Coated	Gemfibrozil 600 mg	by Medirex	57480-0809	Antihyperlipidemic
93670	Tab, White, Oval, Scored	Gemfibrozil 600 mg	by Va Cmop	65243-0035	Antihyperlipidemic
93670	Tab, Film Coated, 93 Over 670	Gemfibrozil 600 mg	by Baker Cummins	63171-1956	Antihyperlipidemic
93670	Tab, Film Coated	Gemfibrozil 600 mg	by Zenith Goldline	00182-1956	Antihyperlipidemic
93670	Tab, White, Oval, Scored, Film Coated, 93-670	Gemfibrozil 600 mg	by Kaiser	00179-1293	Antihyperlipidemic
93670	Tab, White to Off-White, Oval, Film Coated, Scored, 93/670	Gemfibrozil 600 mg	by Teva	00093-0670	Antihyperlipidemic
93670	Tab, Film Coated	Gemfibrozil 600 mg	by Nat Pharmpak Serv	55154-5231	Antihyperlipidemic
93670	Tab, Film Coated	Gemfibrozil 600 mg	by Allscripts	54569-3695	Antihyperlipidemic
93670	Tab, Off-White to White, Oval, Film Coated, Scored, 93/670	Gemfibrozil 600 mg	Lopid by UDL	51079-0787	Antihyperlipidemic
93670	Tab, White, Oval, Scored, Film Coated, 93 670	Gemfibrozil 600 mg	Gemfibrozil by Kaiser	00179-1294	Antihyperlipidemic
93686	Cap	Aspirin 389 mg, Caffeine 32.4 mg, Propoxyphene HCl 65 mg	Propoxyphene Compound 65 by Pharmedix	53002-0535	Analgesic; C IV
93686	Cap, Grey & Red, 93/686	Aspirin 389 mg, Caffeine 32.4 mg, Propoxyphene HCl 65 mg	by Allscripts	54569-0301	Analgesic; C IV
93686	Cap	Aspirin 389 mg, Caffeine 32.4 mg, Propoxyphene HCl 65 mg	Propoxyphene Compound 65 by Zenith Goldline	00182-1673	Analgesic; C IV
93686	Cap, Gray & Red, 93 over 686	Aspirin 389 mg, Caffeine 32.4 mg, Propoxyphene HCl 65 mg	Propoxyphene Compound 65 by Teva	00093-0686	Analgesic; C IV
93691	Cap, Brown & Clear, 93-691	Propranolol HCl ER 60 mg	Inderal LA by Lemmon		Antihypertensive
93692	Cap, Blue & Clear, 93-692	Propranolol HCl ER 80 mg	Inderal LA by Lemmon		Antihypertensive
93693	Cap, Blue & Clear, 93-693	Propranolol HCl ER 120 mg	Inderal LA by Lemmon		Antihypertensive
93694	Cap, Blue & Clear, 93-694	Propranolol HCl ER 160 mg	Inderal LA by Lemmon		Antihypertensive
93695	Tab, Coated, Debossed, Appears as 93-695	Trazodone HCl 150 mg	by Teva	00093-0695	Antidepressant
93695	Tab, White, Round	Trazodone HCl 150 mg	by Teva Pharm Inds	00480-0695	Antidepressant
93695	Cap, Coated, Debossed, Appears as 93-695	Trazodone HCl 150 mg	by Teva	17372-0695	Antidepressant
937	Tab, Blue, Round	Chlorpropamide 250 mg	Diabinese by Lemmon		Antidiabetic
93711	Tab, Blue, Round, Film Coated	Flurbiprofen 100 mg	by HJ Harkins	52959-0346	NSAID
93711	Tab, Blue, Round, Film Coated, 93 Over 711	Flurbiprofen 100 mg	by Teva	00093-0711	NSAID
93711	Tab, Blue, Round, Film Coated, 93 over 711	Flurbiprofen 100 mg	by Invamed	52189-0394	NSAID
93711	Tab, Blue, Round, Film Coated	Flurbiprofen 100 mg	by Major Pharms	00904-5019	NSAID
93727	Cap, Brown & Clear	Papaverine HCl 150 mg	Pavabid by Lemmon		Vasodilator
93728	Tab, Yellow, Round	Sulindac 150 mg	Clinoril by Lemmon		NSAID
93729	Tab, Yellow, Round	Sulindac 200 mg	Clinoril by Lemmon		NSAID

ID FRONT <> BACK	DESCRIPTION FRONT <> BACK	INGREDIENT & STRENGTH	BRAND (OR EQUIV.) & FIRM	NDC#	CLASS; SCH.
93733	Tab, Pink, Round, Convex, Scored, Film, 93 734	Metoprolol Tartrate	by Neuman Distr	64579-0096	Antihypertensive
93733	Tab, Pink, Round, Film Coated, Scored, 93 over 733	Metoprolol Tartrate 50 mg	by Teva	00093-0733	Antihypertensive
93733	Tab, Film Coated, 93 733	Metoprolol Tartrate 50 mg	by Quality Care	60346-0523	Antihypertensive
93734	Tab, Blue, Round, Convex, Scored, Film, 93 734	Metoprolol Tartrate 100 mg	by Neuman Distr	64579-0099	Antihypertensive
93734	Tab, Blue, Round, Scored	Metoprolol Tartrate 100 mg	by Caremark	00339-6191	Antihypertensive
93734	Tab, Mottled Blue, Round, Film Coated, Scored, 93 over 734	Metoprolol Tartrate 100 mg	by Teva	00093-0734	Antihypertensive
93741	Cap, 93/741, Lemmon	Propoxyphene HCl 65 mg	by Rugby	00536-4382	Analgesic; C IV
93741	Cap, Pink, Opaque, 93 over 741	Propoxyphene HCl 65 mg	by Teva	00093-0741	Analgesic; C IV
93741	Cap	Propoxyphene HCl 65 mg	by Pharmedix	53002-0574	Analgesic; C IV
93741	Cap, 93 731	Propoxyphene HCl 65 mg	by Allscripts	54569-0223	Analgesic; C IV
93741	Cap, 93 and 741	Propoxyphene HCl 65 mg	by Med Pro	53978-0531	Analgesic; C IV
93741	Cap, Coated, 93-741	Propoxyphene HCl 65 mg	by Quality Care	60346-0693	Analgesic; C IV
93741 <> 93741	Cap, 93/741 in Black Ink	Propoxyphene HCl 65 mg	by Kaiser	00179-0679	Analgesic; C IV
93742	Cap, Blue & White	Doxycycline Hyclate 50 mg	Vibramycin by Lemmon		Antibiotic
93743	Cap, Blue	Doxycycline Hyclate 100 mg	Vibramycin by Lemmon		Antibiotic
93752	Tab, 93 Above and 752 Below the Score	Atenolol 50 mg	by Quality Care	60346-0719	Antihypertensive
93752	Tab, White, Round, Scored, 93 over 752	Atenolol 50 mg	by Teva	00093-0752	Antihypertensive
93752	Tab	Atenolol 50 mg	by Med Pro	53978-1199	Antihypertensive
93752	Tab	Atenolol 50 mg	by Teva	17372-0752	Antihypertensive
93753	Tab, 93 753	Atenolol 100 mg	by Quality Care	60346-0914	Antihypertensive
93753	Tab, White, Round, 93 over 753	Atenolol 100 mg	by Teva	00093-0753	Antihypertensive
93753	Tab	Atenolol 100 mg	by Teva	17372-0753	Antihypertensive
93754	Cap, Blue & Lavender	Diflunisal 250 mg	Dolobid by Lemmon		NSAID
93755	Tab, Film Coated, 93/755 Teva	Diflunisal 500 mg	by Rugby	00536-5563	NSAID
93756	Cap	Piroxicam 10 mg	Feldene by Zenith Goldline	00182-1933	NSAID
93756	Cap, Dark Green & Olive, 93 over 756	Piroxicam 10 mg	by Teva	00093-0756	NSAID
93756 <> 93756	Cap, Green, 93 756	Piroxicam 10 mg	by Promeco SA	64674-0011	NSAID
93757	Cap, Dark Green, 93 Over 757	Piroxicam 20 mg	by Teva	00093-0757	NSAID
93757	Cap, 93-757	Piroxicam 20 mg	Feldene by Zenith Goldline	00182-1934	NSAID
93757	Cap, Dark Green	Piroxicam 20 mg	by Quality Care	60346-0676	NSAID
93757	Cap	Piroxicam 20 mg	by Major	00904-5063	NSAID
93757 <> 93757	Cap, Green, 93 757	Piroxicam 20 mg	by Promeco SA	64674-0017	NSAID
93758EPITOL	Tab, Pink, Round, Red Speckles, 93-758 Epitol	Carbamazepine Chewable 100 mg	Epitol by Lemmon		Anticonvulsant
9376	Tab, Yellow, Round, Film Coated, Scored, 93 over 76	Isosorbide Mononitrate 20 mg	by Teva	00093-0076	Antianginal
9376	Tab, Yellow, Round, Convex, Scored, Film	Isosorbide Mononitrate 20 mg	by Murfreesboro	51129-1578	Antianginal
93777	Tab, Peach, Round	Hydrochlorothiazide 25 mg	Hydrodiuril by Lemmon		Diuretic
93778 <> 93	Tab, Pink, Round, Scored, Red Specks, 93 over 778	Carbamazepine Chewable 100 mg	Epitol by Caremark	00339-6134	Anticonvulsant
93778 <> 93	Tab, Chewable, 93/778 <> 93	Carbamazepine 100 mg	by Major	00904-3854	Anticonvulsant
93779	Tab, Peach, Round	Hydrochlorothiazide 50 mg	Hydrodiuril by Lemmon		Diuretic
93783	Cap, Pink	Propoxyphene 65 mg	Darvon by Lemmon		Analgesic; C IV
93789	Tab, Gray, Round, 93-789	Perphenazine 2 mg	Trilafon by Lemmon		Antipsychotic
93790	Tab, Gray, Round, 93-790	Perphenazine 4 mg	Trilafon by Lemmon		Antipsychotic
93791	Tab, Gray, Round, 93-791	Perphenazine 8 mg	Trilafon by Lemmon		Antipsychotic
93792	Tab, Gray, Round, 93-792	Perphenazine 16 mg	Trilafon by Lemmon		Antipsychotic
93793	Cap, Aqua Blue & White, Gelatin Coated, Opaque, 93 over 793	Nicardipine HCl 20 mg	by Teva	00093-0793	Antihypertensive
93794	Cap, Light Blue & White, Gelatin Coated, Opaque, 93 over 794	Nicardipine HCl 30 mg	by Teva	00093-0794	Antihypertensive
93798	Cap, Green, 93-798	Indomethacin 25 mg	Indocin by Lemmon		NSAID
93799	Cap, Green, 93-799	Indomethacin 50 mg	Indocin by Lemmon		NSAID
938	Tab, White, Round	Indapamide 2.5 mg	Lozol by Lemmon		Diuretic
93802	Cap, Clear & Green	Phenobarbital, Hyoscyamine, Atropine, Scopolamine	Donnatal by Lemmon		Gastrointestinal; C IV
93804	Cap, Black & Scarlet	Phentermine HCl 30 mg	by Lemmon		Anorexiant; C IV
93810	Cap, Orange & White, 93 over 810	Nortriptyline HCl 10 mg	by Teva	00093-0810	Antidepressant

ID FRONT <> BACK	DESCRIPTION FRONT <> BACK	INGREDIENT & STRENGTH	BRAND (OR EQUIV.) & FIRM	NDC#	CLASS; SCH.
93810	Cap	Nortriptyline HCl 10 mg	by Zenith Goldline	00182-1190	Antidepressant
93810 <> 93810	Cap	Nortriptyline HCl 10 mg	by Allscripts	54569-4146	Antidepressant
93810 <> 93810	Cap, 93-810 <> 93-810	Nortriptyline HCl 10 mg	by Major	00904-7939	Antidepressant
93811	Cap, Orange & White, 93 over 811	Nortriptyline HCl 25 mg	by Teva	00093-0811	Antidepressant
93811	Cap	Nortriptyline HCl 25 mg	by Zenith Goldline	00182-1191	Antidepressant
93811	Cap	Nortriptyline HCl 25 mg	by Major	00904-7940	Antidepressant
93811 <> 93811	Cap, 93-811	Nortriptyline HCl 25 mg	by PDRX	55289-0099	Antidepressant
93811 <> 93811	Cap, Orange & White	Nortriptyline HCl 25 mg	by Quality Care	60346-0757	Antidepressant
93812	Cap, White, 93 over 812	Nortriptyline HCl 50 mg	by Teva	00093-0812	Antidepressant
93812	Cap	Nortriptyline HCl 50 mg	by Zenith Goldline	00182-1192	Antidepressant
93812	Cap	Nortriptyline HCl 50 mg	by Major	00904-7941	Antidepressant
93812 <> 93812	Cap, White	Nortriptyline HCl 50 mg	by HJ Harkins	52959-0519	Antidepressant
93813	Cap, Orange, 93 over 813	Nortriptyline HCl 75 mg	by Teva	00093-0813	Antidepressant
93813	Cap	Nortriptyline HCl 75 mg	by Zenith Goldline	00182-1193	Antidepressant
93813	Cap	Nortriptyline HCl 75 mg	by Major	00904-7942	Antidepressant
93816	Tab, White, Round	Belladonna Alkaloids, Phenobarbital	by Lemmon		Gastrointestinal; C IV
93821	Tab, White, Round	Reserpine 0.25 mg	by Lemmon		Antihypertensive
93824	Tab, White, Round	Pseudoephedrine HCl 60 mg	Sudafed by Lemmon		Decongestant
93827	Tab, White, Round	Reserpine 0.1 mg	by Lemmon		Antihypertensive
93828	Tab, Blue, Round	Urinary Antiseptic Comb.	Urinary Antiseptic 3 by Lemmon		Urinary Tract
93832	Tab, Coated, 93-832, Debossed	Clonazepam 0.5 mg	by Heartland	61392-0825	Anticonvulsant; C IV
93832	Tab, Yellow, Round, Scored, 93 over 832	Clonazepam 0.5 mg	by Teva	00093-0832	Anticonvulsant; C IV
93832	Tab, Coated	Clonazepam 0.5 mg	by Vangard	00615-0456	Anticonvulsant; C IV
93832	Tab, Coated, 93-832	Clonazepam 0.5 mg	by Caremark	00339-4091	Anticonvulsant; C IV
93832	Tab, Coated	Clonazepam 0.5 mg	by Physicians Total Care	54868-3854	Anticonvulsant; C IV
93832	Tab, Yellow, Round, Scored, 93 832	Clonazepam 0.5 mg	Clonazepam by DHHS Prog	11819-0096	Anticonvulsant; C IV
93833	Tab, Green, Round, Scored, 93-833	Clonazepam 1 mg	by Apotheca	12634-0677	Anticonvulsant; C IV
93833	Tab, Mottled Green, Round, Coated, Scored, 93 over 833	Clonazepam 1 mg	by Teva	00093-0833	Anticonvulsant; C IV
93833	Tab, Coated	Clonazepam 1 mg	by Vangard	00615-0457	Anticonvulsant; C IV
93833	Tab, Coated, 93-833	Clonazepam 1 mg	by Caremark	00339-4000	Anticonvulsant; C IV
93833	Tab, Mottled Green, Coated	Clonazepam 1 mg	by Physicians Total Care	54868-3855	Anticonvulsant; C IV
93833	Tab, Coated	Clonazepam 1 mg	by Teva	17372-0833	Anticonvulsant; C IV
93833	Tab, Green, Round, Scored, 93-833	Clonazepam 1 mg	by DHHS Prog	11819-0090	Anticonvulsant; C IV
93833	Tab, Mottled Green, Round, Scored	Clonazepam 1 mg	Clonazepam by DHHS Prog	11819-0098	Anticonvulsant; C IV
93834	Tab, Coated	Clonazepam 0.5 mg	by Teva	17372-0832	Anticonvulsant; C IV
93834	Tab, White to Off-White, Round, Scored, 93 over 834	Clonazepam 2 mg	by Teva	00093-0834	Anticonvulsant; C IV
93834	Tab, White, Round, Scored	Clonazepam 2 mg	by D M Graham	00756-0265	Anticonvulsant; C IV
93834	Tab, Coated	Clonazepam 2 mg	by Physicians Total Care	54868-3861	Anticonvulsant; C IV
93834	Tab, Coated, 93-834	Clonazepam 2 mg	by Teva	17372-0834	Anticonvulsant; C IV
93834	Tab, White, Round, Scored	Clonazepam 2 mg	Clonazepam by DHHS Prog	11819-0099	Anticonvulsant; C IV
93835	Tab, Purple, Round	Urinary Antiseptic Comb. (Veterinary)	Urinary Antiseptic by Lemmon		Veterinary
93841	Cap, Blue	Decyclomine HCl 10 mg	Bentyl by Lemmon		Gastrointestinal
93845	Tab, Purple, Round	Urinary Antiseptic Combination	Urinary Antiseptic 2 by Lemmon		Urinary Tract
93848	Tab, White, Round	Triprolidine HCl 2.5 mg, Pseudoephedrine HCl 60 mg	Actifed by Lemmon		Cold Remedy
93851	Tab, White, Round	Metronidazole 250 mg	by Allscripts	54569-0965	Antibiotic
93851 <> 93851	Tab, White, Round, Convex	Metronidazole 250 mg	by Neuman Distr	64579-0181	Antibiotic
93852	Tab, White, Oblong, 93-852	Metronidazole 500 mg	Flagyl by Lemmon		Antibiotic
93860	Cap, Yellow	Phentermine HCl 30 mg	by Lemmon		Anorexiant; C IV
93872	Tab, Purple, Round	Butabarbital Sodium 15 mg	Butisol by Lemmon		Sedative; C III
93873	Tab, Green, Round	Butabarbital Sodium 30 mg	Butisol by Lemmon		Sedative; C III
93888	Cap, Black	Phentermine HCl 30 mg	by Lemmon		Anorexiant; C IV
93890	Tab, Film Coated, Teva Logo	Acetaminophen 650 mg, Propoxyphene Napsylate 100 mg	by PDRX		Analgesic; C IV

ID FRONT <> BACK	DESCRIPTION FRONT <> BACK	INGREDIENT & STRENGTH	BRAND (OR EQUIV.) & FIRM	NDC#	CLASS; SCH.
93890	Tab, Film Coated	Acetaminophen 650 mg, Propoxyphene Napsylate 100 mg	by Zenith Goldline	00182-0317	Analgesic; C IV
93890	Tab, Pink, Oblong, Film Coated	Propoxyphene Napsylate 100 mg	by HJ Harkins	52959-0335	Analgesic; C IV
93891	Tab, Blue, Round	Decyclomine HCl 20 mg	Bentyl by Lemmon		Gastrointestinal
9390	Tab	Carbamazepine 200 mg	Epitol by Teva	17372-0090	Anticonvulsant
93900	Tab, White, Round, Scored, 93 over 900	Ketoconazole 200 mg	by Teva	00093-0900	Antianginal
9391	Tab, White, Oval, Scored, 93/91	Captopril 12.5 mg	by Teva	00093-0091	Antihypertensive
9391110	Tab, White, Round, 93 911/10	Isoxsuprine HCl 10 mg	Vasodilan by Lemmon		Vasodilator
9391320	Tab, White, Round, 93 913/20	Isoxsuprine HCl 20 mg	Vasodilan by Lemmon		Vasodilator
9392	Tab, White, Round, Scored, 93 over 92	Captopril 25 mg	by Teva	00093-0092	Antihypertensive
9393 <> 778	Tab, Pink with Red Specks, Round, Scored, Chewable, 93 over 93 <> 778	Carbamazepine 100 mg	by Teva	00093-0778	Anticonvulsant
9393 <> 778	Tab, Pink, with Red Specks, Round, Scored, 93 over 93 <> 778	Carbamazepine 100 mg, Chewable	Tegretol by UDL	51079-0870	Anticonvulsant
9393 <> 852	Tab, White, Oblong, Scored	Metronidazole 500 mg	Metronidazole by Family Hlth Phcy	65149-0126	Antibiotic
9393 <> 852	Tab, White, Oblong, Scored, 93/93 <> 852	Metronidazole 500 mg	Flagyl by UDL	51079-0126	Antibiotic
9393 <> 852	Tab, White, Oblong, Scored	Metronidazole 500 mg	by Natl Pharmpak	55154-5566	Antibiotic
9393 <> 852	Tab, White, Oblong, Scored, 93-93 <> 852	Metronidazole 500 mg	by Allscripts	54569-0967	Antibiotic
9393 <> 852	Tab, White, Oblong, Scored, 93 93	Metronidazole 500 mg	Metronidazole by Neuman Distr	64579-0103	Antibiotic
9393 <> 852	Tab, White, Oblong, Scored, 93/93 <> 852	Metronidazole 500 mg	by Teva	00093-0852	Antibiotic
9393 <> 852	Tab, White, Oblong, Scored, 93 93	Metronidazole 500 mg	by Neuman Distr	64579-0169	Antibiotic
9393 <> 852	Tab, Coated, Debossed	Metronidazole 500 mg	by Quality Care	60346-0507	Antibiotic
9393 <> 852	Tab, Debossed	Metronidazole 500 mg	by Prepackage Spec	58864-0355	Antibiotic
9393 <> 852	Tab, 93-93	Metronidazole 500 mg	by Golden State	60429-0129	Antibiotic
9393 <> COTRIM	Tab, 93 on Left, 93 on Right	Sulfamethoxazole 400 mg, Trimethoprim 80 mg	SMZ TMP by Quality Care	60346-0559	Antibiotic
9393 <> COTRIM	Tab, White, Round, Scored, 93 over 93 <> Cotrim	Sulfamethoxazole 400 mg, Trimethorprim 80 mg	Cotrim by Teva	00093-0188	Antibiotic
9393 <> COTRIMDS	Tab, 93 on Left, 93 on Right <> Cotrim DS	Sulfamethoxazole 800 mg, Trimethoprim 160 mg	SMZ TMP DS by Quality Care	60346-0087	Antibiotic
9393 <> COTRIMDS	Tab, White, Oblong, Scored, 93/93 <> Cotrim DS	Sulfamethoxazole 800 mg, Trimethorprim 160 mg	Cotrim DS by Teva	00093-0189	Antibiotic
9393 <> EPITOL	Tab, White, Round, Scored, 93 over 93 <> Epitol	Carbamazepine 200 mg	Epitol by Teva	00093-0090	Anticonvulsant
9393778	Tab, Pink, Chew, with Red Specks, 93.93/778	Carbamazepine 100 mg	by Heartland	61392-0029	Anticonvulsant
9393778	Tab, Chew, with Red Specks, 93 93/778 <>	Carbamazepine 100 mg	by Quality Care	62682-7026	Anticonvulsant
9393778	Tab, Red Specks, Chewable	Carbamazepine 100 mg	by Zenith Goldline	00182-1331	Anticonvulsant
9393778	Tab, Chewable, 93-93/778	Carbamazepine 100 mg	by Vangard	00615-4515	Anticonvulsant
9393852	Tab, White, Oblong, Scored, 93 93	Metronidazole 500 mg	by Neuman Distr	64579-0107	Antibiotic
9393852	Tab, Lemmon	Metronidazole 500 mg	by Pharmedix	53002-0247	Antibiotic
93943	Tab, Yellow, Diamond, 93-943	Nystatin Vaginal 100,000 Units	Mycostatin by Lemmon		Antifungal
93948	Tab, Orange, Round, Film Coated	Diclofenac Potassium 50 mg	Diclofenac Potassium by DRX	55045-2680	NSAID
93948	Tab, Orange, Round	Diclofenac Potassium 50 mg	by Allscripts	54569-4770	NSAID
93948	Tab, Orange, Round, Film Coated, 93 over 948	Diclofenac Potassium 50 mg	by Teva	00093-0948	NSAID
93948	Tab, Film Coated	Diclofenac Potassium 50 mg	by Teva	17372-0948	NSAID
93956	Cap, Medium Orange & White, 93 over 956	Clomipramine HCl 25 mg	by Teva	00093-0956	OCD
93956	Cap	Clomipramine HCl 25 mg	by Teva	17372-0956	OCD
93956 <> 93956	Cap, Orange & White	Clomipramine HCl 25 mg	Clomipramine HCl by D M Graham	00756-0215	OCD
93957	Cap, Green & Yellow	Chlordiazepoxide HCl 5 mg	Librium by Lemmon		Antianxiety; C IV
93958	Cap, Light Blue & White, 93 over 958	Clomipramine HCl 50 mg	by Teva	00093-0958	OCD
93958 <> 93958	Cap, White	Clomipramine HCl 50 mg	Clomipramine HCl by D M Graham	00756-0263	OCD
93958 <> 93958	Cap, Light Blue	Clomipramine HCl 50 mg	by Teva	17372-0958	OCD
93959	Cap, Black & Green	Chlordiazepoxide HCl 10 mg	Librium by Lemmon		Antianxiety; C IV
93960	Cap, Carmel & White, 93 over 960	Clomipramine HCl 75 mg	by Teva	00093-0960	OCD
93960	Cap, Brown & White	Clomipramine HCl 75 mg	Clomipramine HCl by D M Graham	00756-0264	OCD
93960 <> 93960	Cap	Clomipramine HCl 75 mg	by Teva	17372-0960	OCD
93961	Cap, Green & White	Chlordiazepoxide HCl 25 mg	Librium by Lemmon		Antianxiety; C IV
9397	Tab, White, Round, Scored, 93 Over 97	Captopril 50 mg	by Teva	00093-0097	Antihypertensive
9398	Tab, White, Round	Captopril 100 mg	Capoten by Lemmon		Antihypertensive

ID FRONT <> BACK	DESCRIPTION FRONT <> BACK	INGREDIENT & STRENGTH	BRAND (OR EQUIV.) & FIRM	NDC#	CLASS; SCH.
9398	Tab, White, Round, Scored, 93 over 98	Captopril 100 mg	by Teva	00093-0098	Antihypertensive
93983	Tab, Brown, Film Coated, 93-983	Nystatin 500,000 units	by Allscripts	54569-0270	Antifungal
93COTRIM	Tab, White, Round	Sulfamethoxazole 400 mg, Trimethoprim 80 mg	Cotrim by Lemmon		Antibiotic
93COTRIMDS	Tab, White, Round	Sulfamethoxazole 800 mg, Trimethoprim 160 mg	Cotrim DS by Lemmon		Antibiotic
93DOXY	Tab, Film Coated	Doxycycline Hyclate	by Teva	00093-0750	Antibiotic
93EPITOL	Tab, White, Round	Carbamazepine 200 mg	Epitol by Lemmon		Anticonvulsant
94 <> MYLAN	Tab, Purple, Oval, Scored, 9/4 <> Mylan	Carbidopa 50 mg; Levodopa 200 mg, ER	by UDL	51079-0923	Antiparkinson
940	Tab, Gray, Round, Sch. Logo 940	Perphenazine 4 mg	Trilafon by Schering		Antipsychotic
941	Tab, Yellow, Hexagonal	Sulindac 150 mg	by Frosst	Canadian	NSAID
942	Tab, Yellow, Hexagonal	Sulindac 200 mg	by Frosst	Canadian	NSAID
944 <> DAN	Tab	Colchicine 0.6 mg	by Heartland	61392-0174	Antigout
944 <> DAN	Tab	Colchicine 0.6 mg	by Danbury	00591-0944	Antigout
944 <> DAN	Tab, White, Round	Colchicine 0.6 mg	by Schein	00364-0074	Antigout
944 <> DAN	Tab	Colchicine 0.6 mg	by Allscripts	54569-0236	Antigout
948	Tab, White, Mortar and Pestle to Right of Schering Logo 948	Griseofulvin, Microsize 250 mg	Fulvicin UF by Schering	00085-0948	Antifungal
95 <> B	Tab, Brown, Film Coated	Ethinyl Estradiol 0.03 mg, Ethinyl Estradiol 0 mg, Levonorgestrel 0.125 mg, Levonorgestrel 0.050 mg	Tri-Levlen 28 by Berlex	50419-0195	Oral Contraceptive
95 <> B	Tab	Ethinyl Estradiol 0.03 mg, Ethinyl Estradiol 0.04 mg, Ethinyl Estradiol 0.03 mg, Levonorgestrel 0.05 mg, Levonorgestrel 0.125 mg, Levonorgestrel 0.075 mg	Tri Levlen 28 by Nat Pharmpak Serv	55154-0304	Oral Contraceptive
95 <> B	Tab, Brown	Ethinyl Estradiol 0.03 mg, Ethinyl Estradiol 0.04 mg, Ethinyl Estradiol 0.03 mg, Levonorgestrel 0.05 mg, Levonorgestrel 0.125 mg, Levonorgestrel 0.075 mg	Tri Levlen 28 by Pharm Utilization	60491-0653	Oral Contraceptive
95 <> B	Tab, Brown, Film Coated	Ethinyl Estradiol 0.03 mg, Ethinyl Estradiol 0.04 mg, Ethinyl Estradiol 0.03 mg, Levonorgestrel 0.05 mg, Levonorgestrel 0.125 mg, rel 0.050 mg	Tri Levlen 21 by Berlex	50419-0195	Oral Contraceptive
951 <> MRK	Tab, Light Green, Tear Drop Shaped, Film Coated	Losartan Potassium 25 mg	Cozaar by Merck	00006-0951	Antihypertensive
951 <> MRK	Tab, Light Green, Tear Drop Shaped, Film Coated	Losartan Potassium 25 mg	Cozaar by Nat Pharmpak Serv	55154-5009	Antihypertensive
951MRK	Tab, Light Green, Tear Drop Shaped, Film Coated, 951/MRK	Losartan Potassium 25 mg	by MSD	Canadian	Antihypertensive
952 <> MRK	Tab, Light Green, Tear Drop Shaped, Film Coated	Losartan Potassium 50 mg	Cozaar by Merck	00006-0952	Antihypertensive
9531	Tab, White, Round	Methenamine 300 mg, Sodium Biphosphate 500 mg	Uro-Phosphate by Poythress		Antibiotic; Urinary Tract
9532	Tab, White, Round	Potassium Iodide 195 mg, Aminophylline 130 mg	Mudrane-2 by Poythress		Antiasthmatic
9533	Tab, Green, Round	Aminophylline 130 mg, Guaifenesin 100 mg	Mudrane GG-2 by Poythress		Antiasthmatic
9540	Tab, Yellow, Round	Atropine Sulfate 0.195 mg, Phenobarbital 16 mg	Anthrocol by Poythress		Gastrointestinal; C IV
9550	Tab, Yellow, Round	Potassium Iodide 195 mg, Aminophylline 130 mg, Phenobarbital 8 mg, Ephedrine 16 mg	Mudrane by Poythress		Antiasthmatic; C IV
9551	Tab, Mottled Yellow, Round	Aminophylline 130 mg, Ephedrine 16 mg, Pb 8 mg, Guaifenesin 100 mg	Mudrane GG by Poythress		Antiasthmatic; C IV
956PPP	Tab, Pink, Round	Fluphenazine HCl 10 mg	Prolixin by BMS		Antipsychotic
96 <> B	Tab, Off-White	Ethinyl Estradiol 0.03 mg, Ethinyl Estradiol 0.04 mg, Ethinyl Estradiol 0.03 mg, Levonorgestrel 0.05 mg, Levonorgestrel 0.125 mg, Levonorgestrel 0.075 mg	Tri Levlen 28 by Pharm Utilization	60491-0653	Oral Contraceptive
96 <> B	Tab, Off-White to White, Film Coated	Ethinyl Estradiol 0.04 mg, Ethinyl Estradiol 0.04 mg, Ethinyl Estradiol 0.03 mg, Levonorgestrel 0.05 mg, Levonorgestrel 0.125 mg, Levonorgestrel 0.075 mg	Tri Levlen 21 by Berlex	50419-0196	Oral Contraceptive
96 <> B	Tab, Off-White to White, Film Coated	Ethinyl Estradiol 0.04 mg, Ethinyl Estradiol 0.04 mg, Ethinyl Estradiol 0.03 mg, Levonorgestrel 0.05 mg, Levonorgestrel 0.125 mg, Levonorgestrel 0.075 mg	Tri-Levlen 28 by Berlex	50419-0196	Oral Contraceptive
968	Tab, Salmon, Round, Schering Logo 968	Acetophenazine Maleate 20 mg	Tindal by Schering		Antipsychotic
97 <> B	Tab, Light Yellow	Ethinyl Estradiol 0.03 mg, Ethinyl Estradiol 0.04 mg, Ethinyl Estradiol 0.03 mg, Levonorgestrel 0.05 mg, Levonorgestrel 0.125 mg, Levonorgestrel 0.075 mg	Tri Levlen 28 by Pharm Utilization	60491-0653	Oral Contraceptive
97 <> B	Tab, Light Yellow, Film Coated	Ethinyl Estradiol 0.03 mg, Ethinyl Estradiol 0.04 mg, Ethinyl Estradiol 0.03 mg, Levonorgestrel 0.05 mg, Levonorgestrel 0.125 mg, Levonorgestrel 0.125 mg	Tri Levlen 21 by Berlex	50419-0197	Oral Contraceptive
97 <> B	Tab, Light Yellow, Film Coated	Ethinyl Estradiol 0.03 mg, Ethinyl Estradiol 0.04 mg, Ethinyl Estradiol 0.03 mg, Levonorgestrel 0.05 mg, Levonorgestrel 0.125 mg, Levonorgestrel 0.125 mg	Tri-Levlen 28 by Berlex	50419-0197	Oral Contraceptive
97 <> M	Tab, Orange, Triangular, Film Coated	Fluphenazine HCl 10 mg	Prolixin by UDL	51079-0488	Antipsychotic
97 <> M	Tab, Orange, Coated	Fluphenazine HCl 10 mg	by Mylan	00378-6097	Antipsychotic
970	Tab, Duramed Logo over 970	Digoxin 0.125 mg	by Murfreesboro	51129-1102	Cardiac Agent

ID FRONT <> BACK	DESCRIPTION FRONT <> BACK	INGREDIENT & STRENGTH	BRAND (OR EQUIV.) & FIRM	NDC#	CLASS; SCH.
970	Tab, Duramed Logo on Top of 970	Digoxin 0.125 mg	by Murfreesboro	51129-1113	Cardiac Agent
970	Tab, Lavender, Oval, Sch. Logo 970	Methyltestosterone Buccal 10 mg	Oreton Buccal by Schering		Hormone; C III
970 <> M	Tab, White, Round	Acetaminophen 325 mg; Caffeine 40 mg; Butalbital 50 mg	by Mallinckrodt Hobart	00406-0970	Analgesic
971	Tab, Logo 971	Digoxin 0.25 mg	by Quality Care	60346-0607	Cardiac Agent
983 <> 93	Tab, Brown, Round, Film Coated	Nystatin 500,000 Units	by Teva	00093-0983	Antifungal
983 <> 93	Tab, Film Coated	Nystatin 500000 Units	by Schein	00364-2051	Antifungal
983 <> 93	Tab, Film Coated	Nystatin 500000 Units	by Quality Care	60346-0652	Antifungal
99 <> ADIPEXP	Tab, Blue & White, Oblong, Scored, 9/9 <> Adipex-P	Phentermine HCl 37.5 mg	Adipex P by Teva	00093-0009	Anorexiant; C IV
99 <> LEMMON	Tab, Blue & White, Oblong, Scored, 9/9 <> Lemmon	Phentermine HCl 37.5 mg	Adipex P by Teva	00093-0009	Anorexiant; C IV
99 <> LEMMON	Tab, Mottled Blue & White	Phentermine HCl 37.5 mg	Adipex P by Allscripts	54569-1718	Anorexiant; C IV
99 <> LEMMON	Tab, Mottled Blue & White	Phentermine HCl 37.5 mg	Adipex P by Gate	57844-0009	Anorexiant; C IV
A	Tab, Orange, Round, Schering Logo/A	Amitriptyline HCl 4 mg, Perphenazine 10 mg	Etrafon by Bayer	Canadian	Antipsychotic
A	Tab, White, Scored	Disulfiram 500 mg	by Wyeth-Ayerst	Canadian	Antialcoholism
A	Tab, White, Round	Disulfuram 250 mg	Antabuse by Wyeth-Ayerst	Canadian	Antialcoholism
A	Tab, White, Round	Nylidrin 12 mg	by Rhone-Poulenc Rorer	Canadian	Vasodilator
A	Tab, White, Round	Nylidrin 6 mg	by Rhone-Poulenc Rorer	Canadian	Vasodilator
A	Tab, Deep Maroon, Round, Film Coated	Phenazopyridine HCl 95 mg	Pyridium by Able Lab	53265-0095	Urinary Analgesic
A	Tab, Orange, Logo/A	Perphenazine 4 mg, Amitriptyline 10 mg	by Schering	Canadian	Antipsychotic; Antidepressant
A	Tab, Yellow, Round	Phenylpropanolamine HCl 25 mg, Brompheniramine Sulfate 4 mg	Porcupine by PFI		Cold Remedy
A	Tab, Peach, Round, Uncoated	Phenylpropanolamine HCl 75 mg	Acutrim 12 TR by Physicians Total Care	54868-4099	Decongestant; Appetite Suppressant
A	Tab, Pink, Round	Trimipramine Maleate 12.5 mg	Trimip by Apotex	Canadian	Antidepressant
A <> 003	Tab, Pink, Round	Phenylpropanolamine HCl 75 mg, Guaifenesin 1200 mg	Aquatab D by Prepackage Spec	58864-0074	Cold Remedy
A <> 004	Tab, Yellow, Round, Scored	Phenylpropanolamine HCl 75 mg, Dextromethorphan Hydrobromide 60 mg, Guaifenesin 1200 mg	Aquatab C by Prepackage Spec	58864-0033	Cold Remedy
A <> 018	Cap	Chlordiazepoxide HCl 5 mg, Clidinium Bromide 2.5 mg	by Schein	00364-0559	Gastrointestinal; C IV
A <> 031	Tab, Chewable	Ascorbic Acid 34.5 mg, Cyanocobalamin 4.9 mcg, Folic Acid 0.35 mg, Niacinamide 14.16 mg, Pyridoxine HCl 1.1 mg, Riboflavin 1.2 mg, Sodium Ascorbate 32.2 mg, Sodium Fluoride 1.1 mg, Thiamine Mononitrate 1.15 mg, Vitamin A Acetate 5.5 mg, Vitamin D 0.194 mg, Vitamin E Acetate 15.75 mg	Poly Vitamins by Zenith Goldline	00182-1819	Vitamin
A <> 1	Tab, Light Yellow	Dextromethorphan Hydrobromide 30 mg, Guaifenesin 600 mg, Phenylephrine HCl 15 mg	Albatussin Sr by Anabolic	00722-6211	Cold Remedy
A <> 107	Tab, Coated	Ascorbic Acid 120 mg, Calcium 200 mg, Copper 2 mg, Cyanocobalamin 12 mcg, Folic Acid 1 mg, Iron 65 mg, Niacinamide 20 mg, Pyridoxine HCl 10 mg, Riboflavin 3 mg, Thiamine Mononitrate 1.84 mg, Vitamin A 4000 Units, Vitamin D 400 Units, Vitamin E 22 mg, Zinc 25 mg	Prenatal Plus by Zenith Goldline	00182-4464	Vitamin
A <> 111	Tab, Brown, Oval, Film Coated, Scored	Methenamine Mandelate 500 mg	by Murfreesboro Ph	51129-1430	Antibiotic; Urinary Tract
A <> 156	Tab, ER	Hyoscyamine Sulfate 0.375 mg	by Zenith Goldline	00182-2657	Gastrointestinal
A <> 2	Tab, Blue, Round, Scored	Guaifenesin 1200 mg; Dextromethorphan Hydrobromide 60 mg	Aquatab DM by Adams Labs	63824-0002	Cold Remedy
A <> 237	Tab, White to Off-White, Round	Diphenoxylate HCl 2.5 mg, Atropine Sulfate 0.025 mg	Lomotil by Able Lab	53265-0237	Antidiarrheal; C V
A <> 3	Tab, Pink, Round, Film Coated, Scored	Guaifenesin 1200 mg; Phenylpropanolamine HCl 75 mg	Aquatab D by Adams Labs	63824-0003	Cold Remedy
A <> 3	Tab, Film Coated	Indapamide 2.5 mg	by Arcola	00070-3000	Diuretic
A <> 3	Tab, White, Octagon Shaped, Film Coated	Indapamide 2.5 mg	Indapamide by RPR	00801-3000	Diuretic
A <> 3438	Tab, White, Round, Coated, Apotex Logo	Selegiline HCl 5 mg	by Apotex	60505-3438	Antiparkinson
A <> 3438	Tab, Coated, Apotex Logo	Selegiline HCl 5 mg	by Caraco	57664-0172	Antiparkinson
A <> 4	Tab, Yellow, Round, Scored	Guaifenesin 1200 mg; Phenylpropanolamine HCl 75 mg; Dextromethorphan Hydrobromide 60 mg	Aquatab D by Adams Labs	63824-0004	Cold Remedy
A <> 47	Cap, Green & Yellow	Phendimetrazine Tartrate 105 mg	Bontril SR by Amarin Pharms	65234-0047	Anorexiant; C III
A <> 7	Tab, Orange, Octagon Shaped, Film Coated	Indapamide 1.25 mg	Indapamide by RPR	00801-0777	Diuretic
A <> 7	Tab, Film Coated	Indapamide 1.25 mg	by Arcola	00070-0777	Diuretic
A <> 7	Tab, Film Coated	Indapamide 1.25 mg	by Caremark	00339-6084	Diuretic

ID FRONT <> BACK	DESCRIPTION FRONT <> BACK	INGREDIENT & STRENGTH	BRAND (OR EQUIV.) & FIRM	NDC#	CLASS; SCH.
A <> 750	Tab, Coated	Salsalate 750 mg	by Quality Care	60346-0034	NSAID
A <> ADX1	Tab, Film Coated, A Arrow Logo <> ADX 1	Anastrozole 1 mg	Arimidex by Murfreesboro	51129-1122	Antineoplastic
A <> ADX1	Tab, White, Film Coated, Arrow Logo	Anastrozole 1 mg	Arimidex by AstraZeneca	00310-0201	Antineoplastic
A <> AR	Cap, White, Abbott Logo	Fenofibrate 134 mg	Tricor by ICN	00187-4052	Antihyperlipidemic
A <> CIBA	Tab, White, Round, Film Coated, Scored	Oxprenolol HCl 40 mg	Trasicor by Novartis	Canadian DIN# 00402575	Antihypertensive
A <> EB	Tab, Film Coated, Abbott Logo	Erythromycin Stearate	by Apotheca	12634-0163	Antibiotic
A <> EK	Tab, Delayed Release, Abbott Symbol	Erythromycin 500 mg	PCE by Quality Care	60346-0445	Antibiotic
A <> KL	Tab, Yellow, Oval, Film Coated	Clarithromycin 500 mg	Biaxin by Promex Medcl	62301-0037	Antibiotic
A <> KTAB	Tab, K-Tab, Film Coated	Potassium Chloride 750 mg	K Tab by Abbott	00074-7804	Electrolytes
A <> PCE	Tab, Pink Specks, Abbott Logo	Erythromycin 333 mg	PCE by Pharmedix	53002-0253	Antibiotic
A <> SEARLE1411	Tab, White to Off-White, Round, A around the circumference <> Searle over 1411	Diclofenac Sodiummisoprostol 50 mg	by Pharmacia	Canadian DIN# 01917056	NSAID
A <> TD	Tab, Tan, Round, A over Mortar and Pestle Logo <> TD	Dessicated Thyroid 30 mg	Armour Thyroid USP by DRX	55045-1325	Thyroid
A <> TD	Tab	Levothyroxine 19 mcg, Liothyronine 4.5 mcg	Armour Thyroid by Amerisource	62584-0457	Antithyroid
A <> TF	Tab, Tan, Round, Convex, Mortar and Pestle Logo	Levothyroxine 76 mcg, Liothyronine 18 mcg	Armour Thyroid USP by Murfreesboro	51129-1638	Antithyroid
A <> TF	Tab	Levothyroxine 76 mcg, Liothyronine 18 mcg	Armour Thyroid by Amerisource	62584-0461	Antithyroid
A <> US	Tab, White, Round	Amiodarone HCl 200 mg	by Heartland Hlthcare	61392-0935	Antiarrhythmic
A <> US200	Tab, White, Round	Amiodarone 200 mg	Cordarone by Geneva	00781-1203	Antiarrhythmic
A <> US200	Tab, White, Round, Scored	Amiodarone HCl 200 mg	by Upsher Smith	00245-1480	Antiarrhythmic
A <> WYETH64	Tab, Raised A <> Wyeth 64	Lorazepam 1 mg	Ativan by Physicians Total Care	54868-1339	Sedative/Hypnotic; C IV
A <> WYETH64	Tab, Raised A <> Wyeth 64	Lorazepam 1 mg	Ativan by Med Pro	53978-3086	Sedative/Hypnotic; C IV
A <> WYETH64	Tab, White, Scored	Lorazepam 1 mg	Ativan by Natl Pharmapk	55154-4204	Sedative/Hypnotic; C IV
A <> WYETH64	Tab, Raised A <> Wyeth 64	Lorazepam 1 mg	Ativan by Wyeth Labs	00008-0064	Sedative/Hypnotic; C IV
A <> WYETH65	Tab, Raised A <> Wyeth 65	Lorazepam 2 mg	Ativan by Wyeth Labs	00008-0065	Sedative/Hypnotic; C IV
A <> WYETH81	Tab, Raised A <> Wyeth 81	Lorazepam 0.5 mg	Ativan by Wyeth Labs	00008-0081	Sedative/Hypnotic; C IV
A <> WYETH81	Tab, Raised A	Lorazepam 0.5 mg	Ativan by Med Pro	53978-3085	Sedative/Hypnotic; C IV
A002	Tab, Orange, Pink & Purple, Chewable	Ascorbic Acid 30 mg, Sodium Ascorbate 33 mg, Sodium Fluoride, Vitamin A Acetate, Vitamin D 400 Units	Tri Vita B by Amide	52152-0002	Vitamin
A002	Tab, Chewable	Ascorbic Acid 30 mg, Sodium Ascorbate 33 mg, Sodium Fluoride, Vitamin A Acetate, Vitamin D 400 Units	Tri-Vit/Fl Chew by Qualitest	00603-6300	Vitamin
A003	Tab, Brown, Round, Scored	Phenazopyridine HCl 100 mg	by Murfreesboro Ph	51129-1431	Urinary Analgesic
A003	Tab, Sugar Coated	Phenazopyridine HCl 100 mg	by Zenith Goldline	00182-0138	Urinary Analgesic
A003	Tab, Maroon, Round	Phenazopyridine HCl 100 mg	by Physicians Total Care	54868-0138	Urinary Analgesic
A003	Tab, Maroon, Round, Sugar Coated	Phenazopyridine HCl 100 mg	Pyridium by Amide	52152-0003	Urinary Analgesic
A003	Tab, Maroon, Round, Sugar Coated	Phenazopyridine HCl 100 mg	Pyridium by Geneva	00781-1510	Urinary Analgesic
A004	Tab, Sugar Coated	Phenazopyridine HCl 200 mg	by Zenith Goldline	00182-0904	Urinary Analgesic
A004	Tab, Maroon, Round, Sugar Coated	Phenazopyridine HCl 200 mg	Pyridium by Amide	52152-0004	Urinary Analgesic
A004	Tab, Sugar Coated	Phenazopyridine HCl 200 mg	by Apotheca	12634-0189	Urinary Analgesic
A004	Tab, Maroon, Round, Sugar Coated	Phenazopyridine HCl 200 mg	Pyridium by Geneva	00781-1512	Urinary Analgesic
A018	Cap, A-Levonorgest A-018	Chlordiazepoxide HCl 5 mg, Clidinium Bromide 2.5 mg	by Quality Care	60346-0780	Gastrointestinal; C IV
A018	Cap	Chlordiazepoxide HCl 5 mg, Clidinium Bromide 2.5 mg	by Zenith Goldline	00182-1856	Gastrointestinal; C IV
A018	Cap	Chlordiazepoxide HCl 5 mg, Clidinium Bromide 2.5 mg	by United Res	00677-1247	Gastrointestinal; C IV
A018	Cap, Green, A-018	Chlordiazepoxide HCl 5 mg, Clidinium Bromide 2.5 mg	Librax by Amide	52152-0018	Gastrointestinal; C IV
A019	Pink, Scored, Alpha 019	Guaifenesin 200 mg	GFN 200 00 by Lee	23558-5401	Expectorant
A019	Tab, Yellow, Round, Film Coated	Salsalate 500 mg	Disalcid by Martec	52555-0629	NSAID
A019	Tab, Blue or Yellow, Round, Coated	Salsalate 500 mg	Amigesic by Amide	52152-0019	NSAID
A02 <> 400	Tab, White, Oval	Acyclovir 400 mg	by Amerisource	62584-0817	Antiviral
A02 <> 400	Tab, White, Oval	Acyclovir 400 mg	Zovirax by Mova	55370-0555	Antiviral
A02 <> 400	Tab	Acyclovir 400 mg	by Martec	52555-0683	Antiviral

ID FRONT <> BACK	DESCRIPTION FRONT <> BACK	INGREDIENT & STRENGTH	BRAND (OR EQUIV.) & FIRM	NDC#	CLASS; SCH.
A020	Tab, Yellow, Oblong	Salsalate 750 mg	Disalcid by Martec	52555-0630	NSAID
A020	Tab, Blue or Yellow, Round	Salsalate 750 mg	Amigesic by Amide	52152-0020	NSAID
A025	Cap, White	Pancrelipase EC	Pancrease by Amide		Gastrointestinal
A027	Tab, White, Round	Calcium Carbonate 420 mg	Titralac by Amide		Vitamin/Mineral
A028	Tab, Oblong, Scored, Alpha Sign Over 028	Guaifenesin 1200 mg	by Lederle	59911-5886	Expectorant
A028	Tab, White, Oblong, Scored, Alpha Sign over 028	Guaifenesin 1200 mg	GFN 1200 05 by Eli Lilly	00002-3056	Expectorant
A03 <> 800	Tab	Acyclovir 800 mg	by Martec	52555-0684	Antiviral
A03 <> 800	Tab, White, Oval	Acyclovir 800 mg	Zovirax by Mova	55370-0556	Antiviral
A031	Tab, Chewable	Ascorbic Acid 60 mg, Cyanocobalamin 4.5 mcg, Fluoride Ion 0.5 mg, Folic Acid 0.3 mg, Niacin 13.5 mg, Pyridoxine HCl 1.05 mg, Riboflavin 1.2 mg, Thiamine Mononitrate 1.05 mg, Vitamin A 2500 Units, Vitamin D 400 Units, Vitamin E 15 Units	Multi-Vit-Fluoride by Qualitest	00603-4711	Vitamin
A031	Tab, Chewable	Ascorbic Acid 60 mg, Cyanocobalamin 4.5 mcg, Fluoride Ion 0.5 mg, Folic Acid 0.3 mg, Niacin 13.5 mg, Pyridoxine HCl 1.05 mg, Riboflavin 1.2 mg, Thiamine Mononitrate 1.05 mg, Vitamin A 2500 Units, Vitamin D 400 Units, Vitamin E 15 Units	Multi Vita Bets by Amide	52152-0031	Vitamin
A031	Tab, Chewable	Ascorbic Acid 60 mg, Cyanocobalamin 4.5 mcg, Fluoride Ion 0.5 mg, Folic Acid 0.3 mg, Niacin 13.5 mg, Pyridoxine HCl 1.05 mg, Riboflavin 1.2 mg, Thiamine Mononitrate 1.05 mg, Vitamin A 2500 Units, Vitamin D 400 Units, Vitamin E 15 Units	Multivite W Fl by Major	00904-5274	Vitamin
A031	Tab, Multicolor, Square	Multivitamin, Fluoride Chewable	Poly-Vi-Flor by Amide	52152-0031	Vitamin
A037	Tab, Pink, Rectangular	Chewable Vitamins, Fluoride, Iron	Poly-Vi-Flor with Fe by Amide		Vitamin
A038	Tab, Chewable	Ascorbic Acid 60 mg, Cupric Oxide 1 mg, Cyanocobalamin 4.5 mcg, Ferrous Fumarate 12 mg, Folic Acid 0.3 mg, Niacin 13.5 mg, Pyridoxine HCl 1.05 mg, Riboflavin 1.2 mg, Sodium Fluoride 1 mg, Thiamine Mononitrate 1.05 mg, Vitamin A Acetate 2500 Units, Vitamin D 400 Units, Vitamin E Acetate 15 Units, Zinc Oxide 10 mg	Multi Vita Bets by Amide	52152-0038	Vitamin
A039 <> AMIDE039	Cap, Red & White, A-039 <> Amide 039	Sodium Fluoride 2.2 mg	Amidrine by Allscripts	54569-2871	Element
A04 <> 400	Tab, White, Elliptical	Etodolac 400 mg	Lodine by Mova	55370-0552	NSAID
A04 <> 400	Tab, White, Oblong	Etodolac 400 mg	by Hoechst Marion Roussel	64734-0003	NSAID
A040	Tab, White, Round	Dimenhydrinate 50 mg	Dramamine by Amide		Antiemetic
A041	Cap, Red & White	Oxycodone 5 mg, Acetaminophen 500 mg	Tylox by Amide	52152-0041	Analgesic; C II
A048	Tab, Film Coated	Calcium Pantothenate 10 mg, Cyanocobalamin 25 mcg, Ferrous Sulfate 525 mg, Folic Acid 800 mcg, Niacinamide 30 mg, Pyridoxine HCl 5 mg, Riboflavin 6 mg, Sodium Ascorbate 500 mg, Thiamine Mononitrate 6 mg	Multi Ferrous Folic 500 by United Res	00677-0990	Vitamin/Mineral
A05	Tab, Red, Round	Potassium Chloride 300 mg	by Lilly		Electrolytes
A05 <> 200	Cap, Black Print	Acyclovir 200 mg	by Martec	52555-0682	Antiviral
A05 <> 200	Cap, Blue	Acyclovir 200 mg	Zovirax by Mova	55370-0557	Antiviral
A056	Tab, Yellow, Round, Scored	Chlorpheniramine Maleate 4 mg	Chlortrimenton by Geneva	00781-1148	Antihistamine
A056	Tab, Yellow, Round, Scored, Coated	Chlorpheniramine Maleate 4 mg	Chlortrimeton by Geneva		Antihistamine
A056	Tab, Yellow, Round	Chlorpheniramine Maleate 4 mg	Chlor-trimeton by Amide		Antihistamine
A057	Tab, Orange, Cap-Shaped	Vitamins & Minerals	Prenatal Care by Amide	52152-0057	Vitamin
A058	Tab, Blue, Cap Shaped	Guaifenesin 400 mg, Phenylpropanolamine HCl 75 mg	Amitex LA by Amide	52152-0058	Cold Remedy
A059	Cap	Guaifenesin 200 mg, Phenylephrine HCl 5 mg, Phenylpropanolamine HCl 45 mg	Quintex by Qualitest	00603-5665	Cold Remedy
A059	Cap, Orange & White, A-059	Guaifenesin 200 mg, Phenylephrine HCl 5 mg, Phenylpropanolamine HCl 45 mg	Ami Tex by Amide	52152-0059	Cold Remedy
A059	Cap	Guaifenesin 200 mg, Phenylephrine HCl 5 mg, Phenylpropanolamine HCl 45 mg	Guiatex by Rugby	00536-4459	Cold Remedy
A059	Cap, Orange	Phenylephrine HCl 5 mg, Phenylpropanolamine HCl 45 mg, Guasifenesin 200 mg	Quintex by Physicians Total Care	54868-4098	Cold Remedy
A059 <> A059	Cap	Guaifenesin 200 mg, Phenylephrine HCl 5 mg, Phenylpropanolamine HCl 45 mg	Enomine by Quality Care	60346-0725	Cold Remedy
A06	Tab, Red, Round	Potassium Iodide 300 mg	by Lilly		Antithyroid
A060	Cap, Pink & White, A-060	Ursodiol 300 mg	by Amide Pharm	52152-0060	Gastrointestinal
A060	Cap, Pink & White	Ursodiol 300 mg	by Qualitest Pharms	00603-6320	Gastrointestinal
A07	Tab, White, Round	Ketoconazole 200 mg	Nizoral by Mova	55370-0558	Antifungal
A071	Tab, White, Oblong	Prenatal Vitamin	Zenate by Amide		Vitamin
A07PB	Tab, White, Oblong, A07/pB	Hydrocodone Bitartrate 5 mg, Acetaminophen 500 mg	Vicodin by Martec		Analgesic; C III
A089	Cap, Red & Yellow	Docusate Sodium 250 mg	Colace by Amide		Laxative

ID FRONT <> BACK	DESCRIPTION FRONT <> BACK	INGREDIENT & STRENGTH	BRAND (OR EQUIV.) & FIRM	NDC#	CLASS; SCH.
A1	Tab, Coated	Ascorbic Acid 120 mg, Calcium 250 mg, Cholecalciferol 400 Units, Copper 2 mg, Cyanocobalamin 12 mcg, Docusate Sodium 50 mg, Folic Acid 1 mg, Iodine 150 mcg, Iron 90 mg, Niacinamide 20 mg, Pyridoxine HCl 20 mg, Riboflavin 3.4 mg, Thiamine HCl 3 mg, Vitamin A 4000 Units, Vitamin E 30 Units, Zinc 25 mg	Maternity 90 Prenatal Vit & Min by Qualitest	00603-5355	Vitamin
A1	Tab, Coated	Ascorbic Acid 120 mg, Calcium 250 mg, Cholecalciferol 400 Units, Copper 2 mg, Cyanocobalamin 12 mcg, Docusate Sodium 50 mg, Folic Acid 1 mg, Iodine 150 mcg, Iron 90 mg, Niacinamide 20 mg, Pyridoxine HCl 20 mg, Riboflavin 3.4 mg, Thiamine HCl 3 mg, Vitamin A 4000 Units, Vitamin E 30 Units, Zinc 25 mg	Prenatal Fe 90 by HL Moore	00839-8093	Vitamin
A1	Tab	Guanfacine HCl	by Qualitest	00603-3774	Antihypertensive
A1	Tab, White, Round	Guanfacine HCl	Tenex by Amide	52152-0118	Antihypertensive
A1	Tab	Guanfacine HCl	by Warner Chilcott	00047-0312	Antihypertensive
A1 <> F	Tab	Triamcinolone 1 mg	Aristocort by Fujisawa	00469-5121	Steroid
A10	Tab, Grayish Pink, Round	Nifedipine 10 mg	Adalat PA by Miles		Antihypertensive
A10 <> LL	Tab, White, Round, A/10 <> LL	Aminocaproic Acid 500 mg	Amicar by Immunex	58406-0612	Hemostatic
A100	Cap, Red	Amantadine HCl 100 mg	Gen Amantadine by Genpharm	Canadian	Antiviral
A100 <> G	Tab, A over 100 <> G	Atenolol 100 mg	by Amerisource	62584-0621	Antihypertensive
A105	Tab, Yellow, Cap-Shaped	Naltrexone HCl 50 mg	Revia by Amide	52152-0105	Opiod Antagonist
A105	Tab, Yellow, Cap Shaped, Film Coated, Scored	Naltrexone HCl 50 mg	Revia by Amide	00406-1170	Opiod Antagonist
A106	Tab, Green, Scored	Guaifenesin 600 mg	by Lederle	59911-5889	Expectorant
A106	Tab	Guaifenesin 600 mg	by Zenith Goldline	00182-1188	Expectorant
A106	Tab, Green, Cap Shaped	Guaifenesin 600 mg	Humibid LA by Amide	52152-0106	Expectorant
A11	Tab, Pink, Oval, Scored, A/11	Isosorbide Mononitrate ER 30 mg	by Murfreesboro	51129-1579	Antianginal
A11	Tab, Red, Oval, Scored	Isosorbide Mononitrate 30 mg	by Warrick Pharms	59930-1502	Antianginal
A11	Tab, Red, Oval, Scored	Isosorbide Mononitrate 30 mg	by Murfreesboro	51129-1567	Antianginal
A111	Tab, Film Coated	Methenamine Mandelate 500 mg	Mandelamine by Warner Chilcott	00430-0166	Antibiotic; Urinary Tract
A111	Tab, Brown, Oval, Film Coated	Methenamine Mandelate 500 mg	Mandelamine by Amide	52152-0111	Antibiotic; Urinary Tract
A112	Tab, Purple, Oval	Methenamine Mandelate 1000 mg	Mandelamine by Amide		Antibiotic; Urinary Tract
A115	Tab, Quadrisected	Belladonna Alkaloids 0.2 mg, Ergotamine Tartrate 0.6 mg, Phenobarbital 40 mg	Bellamine S by DRX	55045-2417	Gastrointestinal; C IV
A115	Tab, Green, Quadrisected, Scored	Belladonna Alkaloids 0.2 mg, Ergotamine Tartrate 0.6 mg, Phenobarbital 40 mg	Bellargal-S by Geneva	00781-1701	Gastrointestinal; C IV
A115	Tab, Quadrisected	Belladonna Alkaloids 0.2 mg, Ergotamine Tartrate 0.6 mg, Phenobarbital 40 mg	Bellaspas by Qualitest	00603-2424	Gastrointestinal; C IV
A115	Tab, Green, Round	Belladonna Alkaloids 0.2 mg, Ergotamine Tartrate 0.6 mg, Phenobarbital 40 mg	Bellamine S by Amide	52152-0115	Gastrointestinal; C IV
A117	Tab, Green, Round, Scored	Phenobarbital 40 mg, Ergotamine Tartrate 0.6 mg, Belladonna Alkaloids 0.2 mg	Bellamine S by Murfreesboro Ph	51129-1374	Antimigraie; C IV
A121	Tab, Pink, Round	Meclizine HCl 25 mg	Bonine by Amide	52152-0117	Antiemetic
A122	Tab, White, Round	Phenylpropanolamine HCl 25 mg	by Amide		Decongestant; Appetite Suppressant
A124	Tab, Yellow, Round	Phenylpropanolamine HCl 50 mg	by Amide		Decongestant; Appetite Suppressant
A127	Tab, Light Peach, Chew	Sodium Fluoride	by Amide	52152-0124	Element
A127	Tab	Sodium Fluoride 1.1 mg	by Rugby	00536-4548	Element
A127	Tab	Sodium Fluoride 1.1 mg	by Qualitest	00603-3622	Element
A128	Tab, Purple, Round	Sodium Fluoride 1.1 mg	Luride by Amide	52152-0127	Element
A128	Tab, Multi-Colored, Round, Chewable	Sodium Fluoride 2.2 mg	by Allscripts	54569-2871	Element
A128	Tab, Chew	Sodium Fluoride 2.2 mg	by Qualitest	00603-3623	Element
A13	Tab, Round, Chew, Assorteds	Sodium Fluoride 2.2 mg	Luride by Amide	52152-0128	Element
A136	Tab, Coated, Abbott Logo	Erythromycin Stearate	by Apotheca	12634-0170	Antibiotic
A136	Tab, Red & White, Round	Carisoprodol 350 mg	Soma by Amide	52152-0136	Muscle Relaxant
A137	Tab, White, Round	Carisoprodol 350 mg	by Southwood Pharms	58016-0261	Muscle Relaxant
A138	Tab, Red & White, Round	Carisoprodol 200 mg, Aspirin 325 mg	Soma by Amide	52152-0137	Muscle Relaxant
A139	Tab, White & Yellow, Round	Carisoprodol 200 mg, Aspirin 325 mg, Codeine Phosphate 16 mg	Soma Compound w/ Codeine by Amide	52152-0138	Analgesic; C III
A139	Tab	Dextromethorphan Hydrobromide 30 mg, Guaifenesin 600 mg	Guiadrine DM by HL Moore	00839-7897	Cold Remedy
A139	Tab, Green, Cap Shaped	Dextromethorphan Hydrobromide 30 mg, Guaifenesin 600 mg	Amibid DM by Amide	52152-0139	Cold Remedy
	Tab, Green, Oblong	Guaifenesin 600 mg, Dextromethorphan Hydrobromide 30 mg	Guaifenesin DM by Med Pro	53978-3092	Cold Remedy

ID FRONT <> BACK	DESCRIPTION FRONT <> BACK	INGREDIENT & STRENGTH	BRAND (OR EQUIV.) & FIRM	NDC#	CLASS; SCH.
A14	Tab, Red, Round	Thyroid 30 mg	by Lilly		Thyroid
A143	Tab	Hyoscyamine Sulfate 0.125 mg	by Qualitest	00603-4003	Gastrointestinal
A143	Tab, White, Round	Hyoscyamine Sulfate 0.125 mg	Levsin by Amide	52152-0143	Gastrointestinal
A145	Tab	Digoxin 0.125 mg	by Kaiser	00179-1251	Cardiac Agent
A145	Tab	Digoxin 0.125 mg	by Rugby	00536-5708	Cardiac Agent
A145	Tab	Digoxin 0.125 mg	by Qualitest	00603-3314	Cardiac Agent
A145	Tab, Yellow, Round	Digoxin 0.125 mg	Lanoxin by Amide	52152-0145	Cardiac Agent
A145	Tab, Yellow, Round, Scored	Digoxin 0.125 mg	by Compumed	00403-1194	Cardiac Agent
A146	Tab	Digoxin 0.25 mg	by PDRX	55289-0626	Cardiac Agent
A146	Tab	Digoxin 0.25 mg	by Kaiser	00179-1254	Cardiac Agent
A146	Tab	Digoxin 0.25 mg	by Rugby	00536-5709	Cardiac Agent
A146	Tab	Digoxin 0.25 mg	by Qualitest	00603-3313	Cardiac Agent
A146	Tab, White, Round	Digoxin 0.25 mg	Lanoxin by Amide	52152-0146	Cardiac Agent
A146	Tab, White, Scored	Digoxin 0.25 mg	by Compumed	00403-1196	Cardiac Agent
A147	Tab	Digoxin 0.5 mg	by Amide	52152-0147	Cardiac Agent
A15	Tab, Red, Round	Thyroid 60 mg	by Lilly		Thyroid
A15 <> LL50	Tab	Amoxapine 50 mg	Asendin by Lederle	00005-5390	Antidepressant
A155	Tab	Hyoscyamine Sulfate 0.125 mg	by United Res	00677-1536	Gastrointestinal
A155	Tab, Blue, Round	Hyoscyamine Sulfate 0.125 mg	by Murfreesboro	51129-1495	Gastrointestinal
A155	Tab, Blue, Round	Hyoscyamine Sulfate 0.125 mg	Levbid by Amide	52152-0155	Gastrointestinal
A156	Tab, Orange, Oblong, Scored	Hyoscyamine Sulfate 0.375 mg	by Murfreesboro	51129-1496	Gastrointestinal
A156	Tab, Orange, Oblong	Hyoscyamine Sulfate 0.375 mg	by United Res	00677-1717	Gastrointestinal
A156	Tab	Hyoscyamine Sulfate 0.375 mg	by Qualitest	00603-4005	Gastrointestinal
A156	Tab, Orange, Oblong	Hyoscyamine Sulfate 0.375 mg	by Amide Pharm	52152-0156	Gastrointestinal
A157	Tab, White, Round	Meperidine HCl 100 mg	Demerol by Amide	52152-0157	Analgesic; C II
A158	Tab, White, Round	Meperidine HCl 50 mg	Demerol by Amide	52152-0158	Analgesic; C II
A159	Tab, White, with Blue Specks	Phentermine HCl 37.5 mg	by Superior	00144-0740	Anorexiant; C IV
A159	Tab, White, Oval, with Blue Specks	Phentermine HCl 37.5 mg	Adipex by Amide	52152-0159	Anorexiant; C IV
A159	Tab, White w/ Blue Specks, Oval, Scored	Phentermine 37.5 mg	by Allscripts	54569-3203	Anorexiant; C IV
A159	Tab, White, with Blue Specks	Phentermine HCl 37.5 mg	by Qualitest	00603-5191	Anorexiant; C IV
A159	Tab, White, with Blue Specks	Phentermine HCl 37.5 mg	by United Res	00677-0829	Anorexiant; C IV
A160 <> A160	Cap, Yellow	Phentermine HCl 30 mg	Fastin by Amide	52152-0160	Anorexiant; C IV
A161	Tab, Peach, Round, Scored	Pemoline 37.5 mg	by Amide Pharm	52152-0161	Stimulant; C IV
A161	Tab, Peach, Round, Scored	Pemoline 37.5 mg	Cytert by Amide	00406-1558	Stimulant; C IV
A162	Tab, Peach, Round, Scored	Pemoline 75 mg	by Amide Pharm	52152-0162	Stimulant; C IV
A162	Tab, Peach, Round, Scored	Pemoline 75 mg	Cytert by Amide	00406-1552	Stimulant; C IV
A163	Tab	Hyoscyamine Sulfate 0.375 mg	by Zenith Goldline	00182-1993	Gastrointestinal
A163	Cap, Clear, ER	Hyoscyamine Sulfate 0.375 mg	Levsinex by Amide	52152-0163	Gastrointestinal
A163	Cap, Clear	Hyoscyamine Sulfate 0.375 mg	by United Res	00677-1718	Gastrointestinal
A166	Cap	Trimethobenzamide HCl 250 mg	by Rugby	00536-4727	Antiemetic
A166	Cap	Trimethobenzamide HCl 250 mg	by Zenith Goldline	00182-1396	Antiemetic
A166	Cap, Aqua Blue & Light Blue	Trimethobenzamide HCl 250 mg	Tigan by Amide	52152-0166	Antiemetic
A166	Cap	Trimethobenzamide HCl 250 mg	by Major	00904-3291	Antiemetic
A166 <> A166	Cap, Aqua & Blue	Trimethobenzamide HCl 250 mg	by HJ Harkins	52959-0479	Antiemetic
A167 <> A167	Cap, Opaque Blue & Opaque White	Phentermine 37.5 mg	by Physicians Total Care	54868-4064	Anorexiant; C IV
A167 <> A167	Cap, Blue & White	Phentermine HCl 37.5 mg	Adipex P by Amide	52152-0167	Anorexiant; C IV
A168	Tab, White, Oblong	Prenatal Vitamin, Iron	Prenate 90 by Amide		Vitamin
A16A16 <> ALTIMED	Tab, White, Round, Scored, A16 over A16 <> Altimed	Clobazam 10 mg	by Altimed	Canadian DIN# 02238797	Anticonvulsant

ID FRONT <> BACK	DESCRIPTION FRONT <> BACK	INGREDIENT & STRENGTH	BRAND (OR EQUIV.) & FIRM	NDC#	CLASS; SCH.
A171	Tab, White, Oval, Coated	Ascorbic Acid 80 mg, Biotin 0.03 mg, Calcium 200 mg, Copper 3 mg, Cyanocobalamin 2.5 mcg, Folic Acid 1 mg, Iron 54 mg, Magnesium 100 mg, Niacin 17 mg, Pantothenic Acid 7 mg, Pyridoxine HCl 4 mg, Riboflavin 1.6 mg, Thiamine 1.5 mg, Vitamin A 4000 Units, Vitamin D 400 Units, Vitamin E 15 Units, Zinc 25 mg	Prenatal Rx by Amide	52152-0171	Vitamin
A172	Tab, Red, Cap Shaped, Coated	Codeine Phosphate 10 mg, Guaifenesin 300 mg	Brontex by Amide	52152-0172	Cold Remedy; C III
A177	Tab, White, Cap Shaped, Film Coated	Ascorbic Acid 70 mg, Calcium 200 mg, Cyanocobalamin 2.2 mcg, Folic Acid 1 mg, Iodine 175 mcg, Iron 65 mg, Magnesium 100 mg, Niacin 17 mg, Pyridoxine HCl 2.2 mg, Riboflavin 1.6 mg, Thiamine HCl 1.5 mg, Vitamin A 3000 Units, Vitamin D 400 Units, Vitamin E 10 Units, Zinc 15 mg	New Adv Form Prenatal Z by Amide	52152-0177	Vitamin
A178	Tab, Yellow, Oval, Coated	Ascorbic Acid 120 mg, Calcium 200 mg, Copper 2 mg, Cyanocobalamin 12 mcg, Folic Acid 1 mg, Iron 27 mg, Niacinamide 20 mg, Pyridoxine HCl 10 mg, Riboflavin 3 mg, Thiamine HCl 1.84 mg, Vitamin A 4000 Units, Vitamin D 400 Units, Vitamin E 22 mg, Zinc 25 mg	Prenatal Plus w 27 Mg Iron by Amide	52152-0178	Vitamin
A179	Tab, White, Round	Betaxolol HCl 10 mg	Kerlone by Amide	52152-0179	Antihypertensive
A180	Tab, White, Round	Betaxolol HCl 20 mg	Kerlone by Amide	52152-0180	Antihypertensive
A186	Tab, Peach, Square, Scored, Chewable	Pemoline 37.5 mg	Cytert by Amide	00406-8854	Stimulant; C IV
A19	Tab, Red, Round	Diethylstilbestrol 0.1 mg	by Lilly		Hormone
A197	Tab, White, Round, Scored	Pemoline 18.75 mg	by Amide Pharm	52152-0197	Stimulant; C IV
A197	Tab, White, Round, Scored	Pemoline 18.75 mg	Cytert by Amide	00406-1552	Stimulant; C IV
A19LL	Tab, White, Round, A/19-LL	Acetaminophen 500 mg	Tylenol by Lederle		Antipyretic
A2	Tab, Off-White, A/2	Chlorpheniramine Maleate 8 mg, Methscopolamine Nitrate 2.5 mg, Phenylephrine HCl 20 mg	Phenacon TR by Anabolic	00722-6227	Cold Remedy
A2	Tab	Guanfacine HCl	by Qualitest	00603-3775	Antihypertensive
A2	Tab, Yellow, Round	Guanfacine HCl	Tenex by Amide	52152-0119	Antihypertensive
A2	Tab	Guanfacine HCl	by Warner Chilcott	00047-0313	Antihypertensive
A2 <> M	Tab, White, Round	Atenolol 25 mg	Tenormin by UDL	51079-0759	Antihypertensive
A200	Cap, White	Ibuprofen 200 mg	Actiprofen by Bayer	Canadian	NSAID
A200	Tab, White, Oblong	Ibuprofen 200 mg	Actiprofen by Sanofi		NSAID
A20A20	Tab, White, Round, A20/A20	Orciprenaline Sulfate 20 mg	Alupent by BI		Antiasthmatic
A21LL	Tab, White, Round, A/21-LL	Acetaminophen 325 mg	Tylenol by Lederle		Antipyretic
A22	Tab, Red, Round	Diethylstilbestrol 1 mg	by Lilly		Hormone
A22 <> DAN	Tab, Yellow, Round, Film Coated	Ranitidine HCl 150 mg	by Schein	00364-2633	Gastrointestinal
A22DAN	Tab, Yellow, Round	Ranitidine 150 mg	by Dandury Pharmacal		Gastrointestinal
A22LL	Tab, White, Oblong, A22-LL	Acetaminophen 500 mg	Tylenol by Lederle		Antipyretic
A23 <> DAN	Tab, Yellow, Cap-Shaped, Film Coated	Ranitidine HCl 300 mg	by Schein	00364-2634	Gastrointestinal
A23DAN	Tab, Yellow, Oblong	Ranitidine 300 mg	by Danbury Pharmacal		Gastrointestinal
A252	Tab, White, Round, A/252	Dipyridamole 25 mg	Persantine by Schein		Antiplatelet
A285	Tab, White, Round	Dipyridamole 50 mg	Persantine by Schein		Antiplatelet
A2909	Cap	Hydroxyzine Pamoate 85 mg	by Geneva	00781-2254	Antihistamine
A2A <> ALKERAN	Tab	Melphalan 2 mg	Alkeran by Glaxo	00173-0045	Antineoplastic
A2C	Cap	Digoxin 0.05 mg	Lanoxicaps by Catalytica	63552-0270	Cardiac Agent
A2C	Cap	Digoxin 0.05 mg	Lanoxicaps by Murfreesboro	51129-1112	Cardiac Agent
A2C	Cap, Red	Digoxin 0.05 mg	Lanoxicaps by Glaxo	00173-0270	Cardiac Agent
A2C <> A2C	Cap, Clear & Dark Red	Digoxin 0.05 mg	Lanoxicaps by RP Scherer	11014-0747	Cardiac Agent
A2L	Tab, Pink, A2/L	Triamcinolone 2 mg	Aristocort by Stiefel	Canadian	Steroid
A3	Tab, White, Round	Indapamide 2.5 mg	Lozol by Arcola Labs		Diuretic
A3	Tab, White, Round, Film	Indapamide 2.5 mg	by Murfreesboro	51129-1537	Diuretic
A31	Tab, Red, Round	Potassium Chloride 1000 mg	by Lilly		Electrolytes
A33	Tab, Red, Round	Diethylstilbestrol 5 mg	by Lilly		Hormone
A33	Tab, White, Circular, A/33	Metoprolol Tartrate 50 mg	by Astra	Canadian	Antihypertensive
A3A <> DARAPRIM	Tab	Pyrimethamine 25 mg	Daraprim by Catalytica	63552-0201	Antiprotozoal

ID FRONT <> BACK	DESCRIPTION FRONT <> BACK	INGREDIENT & STRENGTH	BRAND (OR EQUIV.) & FIRM	NDC#	CLASS; SCH.
A3A <> DARAPRIM	Tab	Pyrimethamine 25 mg	Daraprim by Glaxo	00173-0201	Antiprotozoal
A4 <> F	Tab	Triamcinolone 4 mg	Aristocort by Lederle	00005-4419	Steroid
A4 <> F	Tab	Triamcinolone 4 mg	Aristocort by Fujisawa	00469-5124	Steroid
A415	Tab, White, Oval	Ergoloid Mesylates 1 mg	by B.F.Ascher		Ergot
A49 <> LL	Tab	Atenolol 50 mg	by Kaiser	62224-7224	Antihypertensive
A49 <> LL	Tab, A/49 <> Lederle Logo	Atenolol 50 mg	by Quality Care	60346-0719	Antihypertensive
A49 <> LL	Tab	Atenolol 50 mg	by Baker Cummins	63171-1004	Antihypertensive
A49 <> LL	Tab, Kaiser Logo	Atenolol 50 mg	by Kaiser	00179-1165	Antihypertensive
A49 <> LL	Tab	Atenolol 50 mg	by Vangard	00615-3532	Antihypertensive
A49 <> LL	Tab	Atenolol 50 mg	by UDL	51079-0684	Antihypertensive
A4L	Tab, White, A4/L	Triamcinolone 4 mg	Aristocort by Stiefel	Canadian	Steroid
A5	Tab, White, Round	Oxycodone HCl 5 mg	Roxicodone by Amide	52152-0165	Analgesic; C II
A50 <> G	Tab, A 50	Atenolol 50 mg	by Quality Care	60346-0719	Antihypertensive
A50 <> G	Tab, A Over 50	Atenolol 50 mg	by Amerisource	62584-0620	Antihypertensive
A500	Tab, Film Coated, A/500	Salsalate 500 mg	by Superior	00144-1305	NSAID
A500	Tab, Film Coated	Salsalate 500 mg	by Rugby	00536-4522	NSAID
A500	Tab, Light Turquoise, Cap Shaped, Film Coated, Scored	Salsalate 500 mg	by Able	53265-0132	NSAID
A500	Tab, Film Coated	Salsalate 500 mg	by Able	53265-0187	NSAID
A51 <> LL	Tab	Alprazolam 0.25 mg	by Nat Pharmpak Serv	55154-5553	Antianxiety; C IV
A51 <> LL	Tab, Coated, A 51 <> Lederle Logo	Alprazolam 0.25 mg	by Quality Care	60346-0876	Antianxiety; C IV
A51 <> LL	Tab	Alprazolam 0.25 mg	by Vangard	00615-0426	Antianxiety; C IV
A51 <> LL	Tab, A/51	Alprazolam 0.25 mg	by UDL	51079-0788	Antianxiety; C IV
A512	Tab, Pink, Round	Phenolphthalein 60 mg	Modane Mild by Adria		Gastrointestinal
A513	Tab, Red, Round	Phenolphthalein 130 mg	Modane by Adria		Gastrointestinal
A515	Tab, Orange, Round	Phenolphthalein 65 mg, Docusate Sodium 100 mg	Modane Plus by Adria		Gastrointestinal
A52 <> LL	Tab	Alprazolam 0.5 mg	by Vangard	00615-0401	Antianxiety; C IV
A52 <> LL	Tab	Alprazolam 0.5 mg	by Caremark	00339-4057	Antianxiety; C IV
A52 <> LL	Tab, A/52	Alprazolam 0.5 mg	by UDL	51079-0789	Antianxiety; C IV
A53 <> LL	Tab, A/53	Alprazolam 1 mg	by UDL	51079-0790	Antianxiety; C IV
A53 <> LL	Tab	Alprazolam 1 mg	by Caremark	00339-4054	Antianxiety; C IV
A554	Tab, White, Round, Scored, A over 554	Carbamazepine 200 mg	by Teva	00093-0109	Anticonvulsant
A554 <> A554	Tab	Carbamazepine 200 mg	Atretol by Athena	59075-0554	Anticonvulsant
A585	Tab, Mottled Yellow, Round	Carbidopa 25 mg, Levodopa 100 mg	Sinemet by Lemmon		Antiparkinson
A58525100MG <> A58525100MG	Tab	Carbidopa 25 mg, Levodopa 100 mg	Atamet by Athena	59075-0585	Antiparkinson
A587	Tab, Mottled Blue, Round	Carbidopa 25 mg, Levodopa 250 mg	Sinemet by Lemmon		Antiparkinson
A58725250MG <> A58725250MG	Tab	Carbidopa 25 mg, Levodopa 250 mg	Atamet by Athena	59075-0587	Antiparkinson
A59025MG <> A59025MG	Tab, A590 2.5 mg	Bromocriptine Mesylate	by Athena	59075-0590	Antiparkinson
A615	Tab, Ivory, Round, Scored	Pergolide 0.05 mg	Permax by Lilly	00002-0615	Antiparkinson
A615	Tab, Ivory, Rectangular	Pergolide Mesylate 0.05 mg	Permax by Lilly		Antiparkinson
A615	Tab	Pergolide Mesylate 0.05 mg	Permax by Athena	59075-0615	Antiparkinson
A625	Tab, Green, Round	Pergolide 0.25 mg	Permax by Lilly	00002-0625	Antiparkinson
A625	Tab, Green, Rectangular	Pergolide Mesylate 0.25 mg	Permax by Lilly		Antiparkinson
A625	Tab	Pergolide Mesylate 0.25 mg	Permax by Athena	59075-0625	Antiparkinson
A625 <> UC5337	Tab, Green, Round, Scored	Pergolide Mesylate 0.25 mg	Epermax by Phcy Care	65070-0513	Antiparkinson
A630	Tab, Pink, Round	Pergolide 1 mg	Permax by Lilly	00002-0630	Antiparkinson
A630	Tab	Pergolide Mesylate 1 mg	Permax by Pharm Utilization	60491-0508	Antiparkinson
A630	Tab	Pergolide Mesylate 1 mg	Permax by Athena	59075-0630	Antiparkinson
A660 <> 5	Tab, A Over 660	Selegiline HCl 5 mg	Atapryl by Athena	59075-0660	Antiparkinson
A7	Tab, Orange, Octagon, Film	Indapamide 1.25 mg	by Murfreesboro	51129-1536	Diuretic

ID FRONT <> BACK	DESCRIPTION FRONT <> BACK	INGREDIENT & STRENGTH	BRAND (OR EQUIV.) & FIRM	NDC#	CLASS; SCH.
A7	Tab, Orange, Octagonal	Indapamide 1.25 mg	Lozol by Arcola Labs		Diuretic
A7 <> DAN25	Tab, White, Round, Scored	Captopril 25 mg	by Schein	00364-2629	Antihypertensive
A7 <> LL	Tab	Atenolol 25 mg	by Nat Pharmpak Serv	55154-5511	Antihypertensive
A7 <> LL	Tab	Atenolol 25 mg	by Med Pro	53978-3055	Antihypertensive
A71 <> LL	Tab, Lederle Logo	Atenolol 100 mg	by Quality Care	60346-0914	Antihypertensive
A71 <> LL	Tab	Atenolol 100 mg	by Kaiser	62224-7331	Antihypertensive
A71 <> LL	Tab, Kaiser Logo	Atenolol 100 mg	by Kaiser	00179-1166	Antihypertensive
A71 <> LL	Tab, A over 71 <> LL	Atenolol 100 mg	by UDL	51079-0685	Antihypertensive
A75	Tab, White, Round	Oxycodone 5 mg, Acetaminophen 325 mg	Percocet by Amide	52152-0075	Analgesic; C II
A75 <> 511	Tab, White, Round	Acyclovir 400 mg	by ESI Lederle	59911-3163	Antiviral
A75 <> 511	Tab, White, Round	Acyclovir 400 mg	by ESI Lederle		Antiviral
A750	Tab, Film Coated, A Over 750	Salsalate 750 mg	by Superior	00144-1307	NSAID
A750	Tab, Film Coated	Salsalate 750 mg	by Able	53265-0188	NSAID
A750	Tab, Light Turquoise, Round, Film Coated, Scored	Salsalate 750 mg	by Able	53265-0133	NSAID
A77	Tab, White, Oval	Acyclovir 800 mg	by ESI Lederle		Antiviral
A77 <> 511	Tab, White, Oval	Acyclovir 800 mg	by ESI Lederle	59911-3164	Antiviral
A77 <> W	Tab, Film Coated, Black Print	Chloroquine Phosphate 500 mg	Aralen Phosphate by Sanofi	00024-0084	Antimalarial
A77 <> W	Tab, Film Coated, Black Print	Chloroquine Phosphate 500 mg	Aralen Phosphate by Bayer	00280-0084	Antimalarial
A77 <> W	Tab, Film Coated	Chloroquine Phosphate 500 mg	Aralen by Allscripts	54569-3777	Antimalarial
A7DAN25	Tab, White, Round, Scored	Captopril 25 mg	Captopril USP by Caremark	00339-5791	Antihypertensive
A7LL	Tab	Atenolol 25 mg	by Zenith Goldline	00182-1001	Antihypertensive
A9L	Cap, Blue	Trihexyphenidyl HCl 5 mg	Artane Sequels by Lederle		Antiparkinson
AA	Tab, White, Oblong	Aspirin SR 800 mg	Zorprin by Able Labs		Analgesic
AA	Tab, Peach, Round, Abbott Logo	Chlorthalidone 25 mg	Hygroton by Abbott		Diuretic
AA	Tab, White, Oval, A/A	Phenylpropanolamine 50 mg, Pyrilamine 25 mg, Chlorphen 4 mg, Phenylep 10 mg	Vanex Forte by Abana		Cold Remedy
AA <> 150	Tab, Pink, Oblong, A/A <> 150	Choline Magnesium Trisalicylate 500 mg	Trilisate by Schein	00364-3150	NSAID
AA <> 151	Tab, White, Oblong, A/A <> 151	Choline Magnesium Trisalicylate 750 mg	Trilisate by Schein	00364-3151	NSAID
AA <> 152	Tab, Red, Oblong, A/A <> 152	Choline Magnesium Trisalicylate 1000 mg	Trilisate by Schein	00364-3152	NSAID
AAA	Cap, Clear & Dark Red	Vitamin A 18.334 mg	Vitamin A by RP Scherer	11014-1085	Vitamin
AAAA50 <> SEARLE1411	Tab, White, Round, A's around 50 <> Searle 1411	Diclofenac Sodium 50 mg, Misoprostol 200 mcg	Arthrotec by DRX	55045-2700	NSAID
AAAA50 <> SEARLE1411	Tab, Round, Searle 1411 <> A's around 50	Diclofenac Sodium 50 mg, Misoprostol 200 mcg	Arthrotec 50 by DRX	55045-2706	NSAID
AAAA50 <> SEARLE1411	Tab, Film Coated, A's around 50 <> Searle 1411	Diclofenac Sodium 50 mg, Misoprostol 200 mcg	Arthrotec 50 by GD Searle	00014-1411	NSAID
AAAA50 <> SEARLE1411	Tab, Off-White, Round, Film Coated, A's around 50 <> Searle 1411	Diclofenac Sodium 50 mg, Misoprostol 200 mcg	Arthrotec 50 by GD Searle	00025-1411	NSAID
AAAA50 <> SEARLE1411	Tab, Film Coated, A's around 50 <> Searle 1411	Diclofenac Sodium 50 mg, Misoprostol 200 mcg	Arthrotec 50 by Searle	51227-6169	NSAID
AAAA75 <> SEARLE1421	Tab, Off-White, Round, Film Coated, A's around 75 <> Searle 1421	Diclofenac Sodium 75 mg, Misoprostol 200 mcg	Arthrotec 75 by GD Searle	00025-1421	NSAID
AAAA75 <> SEARLE1421	Tab, Film Coated, A's around 75 <> Searle 1421	Diclofenac Sodium 75 mg, Misoprostol 200 mcg	Arthrotec 75 by GD Searle	00014-1421	NSAID
AAAA75 <> SEARLE1421	Tab, White, Round, Convex, Film, A's Encircling 75 <> Searle 1421	Diclofenac Sodium 75 mg, Misoprostol 200 mcg	Arthrotec 75 by DRX		NSAID
AAAA75 <> SEARLE1421	Tab, Film Coated, A's around 75 <> Searle 1421	Diclofenac Sodium 75 mg, Misoprostol 200 mcg	Arthrotec 75 by Searle	51227-6179	NSAID
AAB	Cap, Clear & Dark Red	Vitamin A 36.7 mg	Vitamin A by RP Scherer	11014-1084	Vitamin
AARP263	Tab, White, Round	Magnesium Hydroxide 311 mg	by PFI		Mineral
AARP556	Tab, Green, Oval	Magnesium Salicylate 325 mg	by PFI		Analgesic
AARP562	Tab, White, Round	Ibuprofen 200 mg	Advil by Danbury		NSAID
AARP173	Tab, Beige, Round	Ferrous Sulfate 325 mg	Feosol by AARP		Mineral

ID FRONT <> BACK	DESCRIPTION FRONT <> BACK	INGREDIENT & STRENGTH	BRAND (OR EQUIV.) & FIRM	NDC#	CLASS; SCH.
AARP174	Tab, White, Oblong	Ascorbic Acid 1000 mg	Formla 174 by AARP Pharmacy		Vitamin
AARP201	Tab, White, Round	Aluminum 200 mg, Magnesium Hydroxides 200 mg	by PFI		Gastrointestinal
AARP242	Tab, White, Round	Calcium Carbonate 420 mg	by PFI		Vitamin/Mineral
AARP247	Tab, Off-White, Round	Aluminum 80 mg, Magnesium Hydroxides 80 mg, Sodium Bicarbonate 200 mg	by PFI		Gastrointestinal
AARP400	Tab, Beige, Round	Docusate Sodium 100 mg, Phenophthalein 65 mg	Correctol by PFI		Laxative
AARP428	Tab, White & Yellow, Round	Acetaminophen 325 mg, Phenylephrine 5 mg, Chlorpheniramine 2 mg	by PFI		Cold Remedy
AARP5625	Tab, White	Ibuprofen 200 mg	Advil by Danbury		NSAID
AARP685	Cap, White	Acetaminophen 650 mg	Tylenol by AARP		Antipyretic
AB	Tab, Lavender, Round, Abbott Logo	Chlorthalidone 50 mg	Hygroton by Abbott		Diuretic
AB	Tab, White, Round, Film Coated, Scored	Metoprolol Succinate 25 mg	Toprol-XL by AstraZeneca	00186-1088	Antihypertensive
AB <> CIBA	Tab, Pale Blue, Round, Scored	Methylphenidate HCl 10 mg	Ritalin by Novartis	Canadian DIN# 00005606	Stimulant
ABANA <> 217	Cap, White, with Green Beads	Phentermine HCl 37.5 mg	Obenix by Elge	58298-0952	Anorexiant; C IV
ABANA <> 250	Cap, Ex Release	Guaifenesin 250 mg, Pseudoephedrine HCl 90 mg	Nasabid by Sovereign	58716-0005	Cold Remedy
ABANA217	Cap, Clear & Green	Phentermine HCl 37.5 mg	Obenix by Abana		Anorexiant; C IV
ABB	Tab, White, Round, A/BB	Metoprolol Tartrate 50 mg	Betaloc by Astra	Canadian	Antihypertensive
ABB	Tab, White, Circular, A/BB	Metoprolol Tartrate 50 mg	by Pharmascience	Canadian	Antihypertensive
ABBOTTLOGO	Cap, Dark Red, Round, Abbott Logo	Ethchlorvynol 200 mg	Placidyl by Abbott	00074-6661	Hypnotic; C IV
ABCD <> AMIDE001	Tab, Chewable	Ascorbic Acid 60 mg, Cyanocobalamin 4.5 mcg, Folic Acid 0.3 mg, Niacinamide, Pyridoxine HCl 1.05 mg, Riboflavin 1.2 mg, Sodium Fluoride, Thiamine Mononitrate, Vitamin A Acetate, Vitamin D 400 Units, Vitamin E Acetate	Multi-Vit/Fl Chew by Qualitest	00603-4712	Vitamin
ABCD <> AMIDE001	Tab, Orange, Pink & Purple, Round, Chewable	Ascorbic Acid 60 mg, Cyanocobalamin 4.5 mcg, Folic Acid 0.3 mg, Niacinamide, Pyridoxine HCl 1.05 mg, Riboflavin 1.2 mg, Sodium Fluoride, Thiamine Mononitrate, Vitamin A Acetate, Vitamin D 400 Units, Vitamin E Acetate	Multi Vita Bets by Amide	52152-0001	Vitamin
ABCD <> AMIDE001	Tab, Chewable	Ascorbic Acid 60 mg, Cyanocobalamin 4.5 mcg, Folic Acid 0.3 mg, Niacinamide, Pyridoxine HCl 1.05 mg, Riboflavin 1.2 mg, Sodium Fluoride, Thiamine Mononitrate, Vitamin A Acetate, Vitamin D 400 Units, Vitamin E Acetate	Multivite W Fl by Major	00904-5275	Vitamin
ABCIBA	Tab, Blue, Round, AB/Ciba	Methylphenidate HCl 10 mg	Ritalin by Ciba	Canadian	Stimulant; C II
ABG <> 100	Tab, Gray, Round, Convex	Morphine Sulfate 100 mg	by Novartis	00043-0143	Analgesic; C II
ABG <> 15	Tab, Blue, Round, Convex, Film	Morphine Sulfate 15 mg	by Neuman Distr	64579-0349	Analgesic; C II
ABG <> 200	Tab, Green, Oblong, Convex, Film Coated	Morphine Sulfate 200 mg	by Novartis	00043-0148	Analgesic; C II
ABG <> 30	Tab, Purple, Round, Convex, Film Coated	Morphine Sulfate 30 mg	by Neuman Distr	64579-0350	Analgesic; C II
ABG <> 60	Tab, Orange, Round, Convex, Film Coated	Morphine Sulfate 60 mg	by Neuman Distr	64579-0358	Analgesic; C II
AC10	Tab, Film Coated, AC/10	Salicylate 1000 mg	by Rugby	00536-3470	NSAID
AC150GLAXO	Tab, Coated	Ranitidine HCl 150 mg	by Med Pro	53978-0101	Gastrointestinal
AC200 <> G	Cap, Orange & Purple	Acebutolol HCl 200 mg	by Alphapharm	57315-0025	Antihypertensive
AC200 <> G	Cap, Orange & Purple	Acebutolol HCl 200 mg	by Par Pharm	49884-0587	Antihypertensive
AC200 <> G	Cap, Orange & Purple	Acebutolol HCl 200 mg	by Genpharm	55567-0089	Antihypertensive
AC400 <> G	Cap, Orange & Purple	Acebutolol HCl 400 mg	by Alphapharm	57315-0026	Antihypertensive
AC400 <> G	Cap, Orange & Purple	Acebutolol HCl 400 mg	by Genpharm	55567-0090	Antihypertensive
AC400 <> G	Cap, Orange & Purple	Acebutolol HCl 400 mg	by Par Pharm	49884-0588	Antihypertensive
AC50	Tab, White, Oblong	Choline Magnesium Trisalicylate 500 mg	Trilisate by Able Labs		NSAID
AC50	Tab, Yellow, Oblong	Choline Magnesium Trisalicylate 500 mg	Trilisate by Able Labs		NSAID
AC58	Tab	Guaifenesin 400 mg, Phenylpropanolamine HCl 75 mg	by Pharmedix	53002-0323	Cold Remedy
AC75	Tab, Blue, Oblong	Choline Magnesium Trisalicylate 750 mg	Trilisate by Able Labs		NSAID
AC75	Tab, White, Oblong	Choline Magnesium Trisalicylate 750 mg	Trilisate by Able Labs		NSAID
ACCOLATE20 <> ZENECA	Tab, White, Round, Film Coated	Zafirlukast 20 mg	Accolate by AstraZeneca	00310-0402	Antiasthmatic
ACCOLATE20 <> ZENECA	Tab, Film Coated	Zafirlukast 20 mg	Accolate by IPR	54921-0402	Antiasthmatic
ACCUTANE10ROCHE	Cap, Accutane Over 10 Roche	Isotretinoin 10 mg	Accutane by Hoffmann La Roche	00004-0155	Dermatologic

ID FRONT <> BACK	DESCRIPTION FRONT <> BACK	INGREDIENT & STRENGTH	BRAND (OR EQUIV.) & FIRM	NDC#	CLASS; SCH.
ACCUTANE20ROCHE	Cap, Accutane Over 20 Roche	Isotretinoin 20 mg	Accutane by Hoffmann La Roche	00004-0169	Dermatologic
ACCUTANE40ROCHE	Cap, Accutane Over 40 Roche	Isotretinoin 40 mg	Accutane by Hoffmann La Roche	00004-0156	Dermatologic
ACEON2 <> SLVSLV	Tab, White, Oblong, Scored	Perindopril Erbumine 2 mg	Aceon by Pharmafab	62542-0783	Antihypertensive
ACEON2 <> SLVSLV	Tab, White, Oblong, Scored	Perindopril Erbumine 2 mg	Aceon by Pharmafab	62542-0782	Antihypertensive
ACEON4 <> SLV	Tab, Pink, Oblong	Perindopril Erbumine 4 mg	Aceon by Solvay Pharms	00032-1102	Antihypertensive
ACEON4 <> SLVSLV	Tab, Pink, Oblong, Scored	Perindopril Erbumine 4 mg	Aceon by Rhone Poulenc (PR)	00801-1102	Antihypertensive
ACEON8 <> SLV	Tab, Orange, Oblong, Scored	Perindopril Erbumine 8 mg	Aceon by Rhone Poulenc (PR)	00801-1103	Antihypertensive
ACET2	Tab, White, Round, Acet-2	Acetaminophen 300 mg, Codeine Phosphate 15 mg, Caffeine 15 mg	Acet-2 by Pharmascience	Canadian	Analgesic
ACET3	Tab, White, Round, Acet-3	Acetaminophen 300 mg, Codeine Phosphate 30 mg, Caffeine 15 mg	Acet-3 by Pharmascience	Canadian	Analgesic
ACET30CODEINE	Tab, Salmon, Round, Acet-30 Codeine	Acetaminophen 300 mg, Codeine Phosphate 30 mg	Acet Codeine 30 by Pharmascience	Canadian	Analgesic
ACET60CODEINE	Tab, White, Round, Acet-60 Codeine	Acetaminophen 300 mg, Codeine Phosphate 60 mg	Acet Codeine 60 by Pharmascience	Canadian	Analgesic
ACF <> 004	Tab, Off-White to White, Round	Candesartan Cilexetil 4 mg	Atacand" by AstraZeneca	00186-0004	Antihypertensive
ACG <> 008	Tab, Light Pink, Round	Candesartan Cilexetil 8 mg	Atacand" by AstraZeneca	00186-0008	Antihypertensive
ACG <> 008	Tab, Light Pink, Round	Candesartan Cilexetil 8 mg	Atacand by Astra Merck	00186-0008	Antihypertensive
ACG <> 008	Tab	Candesartan Cilexetil 8 mg	by Astra AB	17228-0017	Antihypertensive
ACG <> 016	Tab, Pink, Round	Candesartan Cilexetil 16 mg	Atacand" by AstraZeneca	00186-0016	Antihypertensive
ACG <> 032	Tab, Round	Candesartan Cilexetil 32 mg	Atacand" by AstraZeneca	00186-0032	Antihypertensive
ACH <> 016	Tab, Light Pink, Round	Candesartan Cilexetil 16 mg	Atacand by Astra Merck	00186-0016	Antihypertensive
ACH <> 16	Tab	Candesartan Cilexetil 16 mg	by Astra AB	17228-0016	Antihypertensive
ACJ <> 322	Tab, Yellow, Oval	Candesartan Cilexetil 32 mg; Hydrochlorothiazide 12.5 mg	Atacand HCT by Astra Zeneca	17228-0322	Antihypertensive; Diuretic
ACL <> 032	Tab, Pink, Round	Candesartan Cilexetil 32 mg	Atacand by Astra Merck	00186-0032	Antihypertensive
ACL <> 032	Tab	Candesartan Cilexetil 32 mg	by Astra AB	17228-0032	Antihypertensive
ACS <> 162	Tab, Peach, Oval	Candesartan Cilexetil 16 mg; Hydrochlorothiazide 12.5 mg	Atacand HCT by Astra Zeneca	17228-0162	Antihypertensive; Diuretic
ACTIFEDA2F	Tab, White	Triprolidine HCl 2.5 mg, Pseudoephedrine 60 mg, Dextromethorphan 30 mg	Actifed DM by Warner Wellcome	Canadian	Cold Remedy
ACTIFEDM2A	Tab	Triprolidine HCl 2.5 mg, Pseudoephedrene HCl 60 mg	Actifed by Warner Wellcome	Canadian	Cold Remedy
ACTIGALL300MG	Cap	Ursodiol 300 mg	Actigall by Summit	57267-0153	Gastrointestinal
ACTOS <> 15	Tab, White, Round, Convex	Pioglitazone HCl 15 mg	Actos by Prestige	58056-0337	Antidiabetic
ACTOS <> 15	Tab, White, Round	Pioglitazone HCl 15 mg	Actos by Takeda Chem Inds	11532-0011	Antidiabetic
ACTOS <> 30	Tab, White, Round, Flat, Scored	Pioglitazone HCl 30 mg	Actos by Prestige	58056-0338	Antidiabetic
ACTOS <> 30	Tab, White, Round	Pioglitazone HCl 30 mg	Actos by Takeda Chem Inds	11532-0012	Antidiabetic
ACTOS <> 45	Tab, White, Round, Flat	Pioglitazone HCl 45 mg	Actos by Prestige	58056-0339	Antidiabetic
ACTOS <> 45	Tab, White, Round	Pioglitazone HCl 45 mg	Actos by Takeda Chem Inds	11532-0013	Antidiabetic
ACV200	Tab, Pink, Round, ACV/200	Acyclovir 200 mg	by Avirax	Canadian DIN# 02078635	Antiviral
ACV400	Tab, Pink, Round, ACV/400	Acyclovir 400 mg	by Avirax	Canadian DIN# 02078635	Antiviral
ACV800	Tab, Blue, Oval, ACV/800	Acyclovir 800 mg	by Avirax	Canadian DIN# 02078651	Antiviral
ACY200	Cap	Acyclovir 200 mg	by Lek	48866-1220	Antiviral
ACY200	Cap	Acyclovir 200 mg	by Schein	00364-2692	Antiviral
ACY200	Cap	Acyclovir 200 mg	by Par	49884-0460	Antiviral
ACY200	Cap, White	Acyclovir 200 mg	by Compumed	00403-2360	Antiviral
ACY200 <> ACY200	Cap, Opaque & White	Acyclovir 200 mg	by Amerisource	62584-0369	Antiviral
ACY200 <> ACY200	Cap, White	Acyclovir 200 mg	by HJ Harkins	52959-0517	Antiviral
ACY200 <> ACY200	Cap	Acyclovir 200 mg	by Apotheca	12634-0506	Antiviral
ACY400	Tab, White, Oval	Acyclovir 400 mg	by Amerisource	62584-0371	Antiviral
ACY400	Tab, White, Oval	Acyclovir 400 mg	by Amerisource	62584-0795	Antiviral

ID FRONT <> BACK	DESCRIPTION FRONT <> BACK	INGREDIENT & STRENGTH	BRAND (OR EQUIV.) & FIRM	NDC#	CLASS; SCH.
ACY400	Tab, White, Oval	Acyclovir 400 mg	by Amerisource	62584-0663	Antiviral
ACY400	Tab, Off-White	Acyclovir 400 mg	by Quality Care	62682-1020	Antiviral
ACY400	Tab	Acyclovir 400 mg	by Lek	48866-1140	Antiviral
ACY400	Tab	Acyclovir 400 mg	by Schein	00364-2689	Antiviral
ACY400	Tab	Acyclovir 400 mg	by Par	49884-0487	Antiviral
ACY800	Tab, Bar Shaped	Acyclovir 800 mg	by Lek	48866-1180	Antiviral
ACY800	Tab	Acyclovir 800 mg	by Mylan	00378-1468	Antiviral
ACY800	Tab	Acyclovir 800 mg	by Schein	00364-2690	Antiviral
ACY800	Tab	Acyclovir 800 mg	by Par	49884-0474	Antiviral
ACY800	Tab, White, Rectangle	Acyclovir 800 mg	by Amerisource	62584-0674	Antiviral
ACYCLOVIR200 <> STASON	Cap, Opaque & Blue	Acyclovir 200 mg	Acyclovir by Amerisource	62584-0784	Antiviral
ACYCLOVIR200 <> COPLEY299	Cap	Acyclovir 200 mg	by Copley	38245-0299	Antiviral
AD	Tab, White, Round, Abbott Logo	Ethotoin 250 mg	Pegaby Abbott		Anticonvulsant
AD <> 10	Tab, Blue, Round	Amphetamine Aspartate 2.5 mg, Amphetamine Sulfate 2.5 mg, Dextroamphetamine Saccharate 2.5 mg, Dextroamphetamine Sulfate 2.5 mg	Adderall by Shire Richwood	58521-0032	Stimulant; C II
AD <> 10	Tab	Amphetamine Aspartate 2.5 mg, Amphetamine Sulfate 2.5 mg, Dextroamphetamine Saccharate 2.5 mg, Dextroamphetamine Sulfate 2.5 mg	Adderall by Physicians Total Care	54868-3674	Stimulant; C II
AD <> 10	Tab, Blue, Round, Scored	Dextroamphetamine Sacranate 10 mg	Adderall by DRX	55045-2607	Stimulant; C II
AD <> 20	Tab, Orange, Round	Amphetamine Aspartate 5 mg, Amphetamine Sulfate 5 mg, Dextroamphetamine Saccharate 5 mg, Dextroamphetamine Sulfate 5 mg	Adderall by Shire Richwood	58521-0033	Stimulant; C II
AD <> 20	Tab, Orange, Round, Scored	Dextroamphetamine Sacranate 20 mg	Adderall by DRX	55045-2608	Stimulant; C II
AD <> 30	Tab, Orange, Round	Dextroamphetamine Saccharate 7.5 mg, Amphetamine Aspartate 7.5 mg, Dextroamphetamine Sulfate 7.5 mg, Amphetamine Sulfate 7.5 mg	Adderall by Shire Richwood	58521-0034	Stimulant; C II
AD <> 5	Tab, Blue, Round	Amphetamine Aspartate 1.25 mg, Amphetamine Sulfate 1.25 mg, Dextroamphetamine Saccharate 1.25 mg, Dextroamphetamine Sulfate 1.25 mg	Adderall by Shire Richwood	58521-0031	Stimulant; C II
AD <> 5	Tab, Blue, Round, Scored	Dextroamphetamine Sacranate 5 mg	Adderall by DRX	55045-2606	Stimulant; C II
ADALACCC <> 30	Tab, Pink, Round	Nifedipine 30 mg	Adalat CC by DRX Pharm Consults	55045-2788	Antihypertensive
ADALAT	Cap, Brown & Yellow, Adalat/Bayer Cross	Nifedipine 10 mg	Adalat by Bayer	Canadian	Antihypertensive
ADALAT <> MILES811	Cap	Nifedipine 10 mg	Adalat by Bayer	00026-8811	Antihypertensive
ADALAT <> MILES811	Cap	Nifedipine 10 mg	Adalat by Nat Pharmpak Serv	55154-4803	Antihypertensive
ADALAT <> MILES821	Cap	Nifedipine 20 mg	by Med Pro	53978-2050	Antihypertensive
ADALAT20	Tab, Dusty Rose, Round	Nifedipine 20 mg	Adalat XL by Bayer	Canadian	Antihypertensive
ADALAT30	Tab, Rose	Nifedipine 30 mg	Adalat XL by Bayer	Canadian	Antihypertensive
ADALAT5	Cap, Brown & Yellow, Adalat 5/Bayer Cross	Nifedipine 5 mg	Adalat by Bayer	Canadian	Antihypertensive
ADALAT60	Tab, Dusty Rose, Round	Nifedipine 60 mg	Adalat XL by Bayer	Canadian	Antihypertensive
ADALAT10	Cap, Adalat/10	Nifedipine 10 mg	Adalat by RP Scherer	11014-0802	Antihypertensive
ADALAT20	Cap, Pale Orange & Rust Brown, Adalat/20	Nifedipine 20 mg	Adalat by RP Scherer	11014-0894	Antihypertensive
ADALAT811	Cap	Nifedipine 10 mg	by Med Pro	53978-2048	Antihypertensive
ADALATCC <> 30	Tab, Pink, Round	Nifedipine 30 mg	Adalat CC by Southwood Pharms	58016-0120	Antihypertensive
ADALATCC <> 30	Tab, Pink, Round	Nifedipine 30 mg	Adalat CC by Va Cmop	65243-0053	Antihypertensive
ADALATCC <> 30	Tab, Film Coated	Nifedipine 30 mg	Adalat CC by Bayer	00026-8841	Antihypertensive
ADALATCC <> 30	Tab, Film Coated	Nifedipine 30 mg	Adalat CC by Smiths Food & Drug	58341-0058	Antihypertensive
ADALATCC <> 30	Tab, Film Coated	Nifedipine 30 mg	by Talbert Med	44514-0701	Antihypertensive
ADALATCC <> 30	Tab, Pink, Round, Film Coated	Nifedipine 30 mg	Adalat CC by Compumed	00403-4957	Antihypertensive
ADALATCC <> 30	Tab, Pink, Round, Film Coated	Nifedipine 30 mg	Adalat CC by Eckerd	19458-0878	Antihypertensive
ADALATCC <> 30	Tab, Film Coated	Nifedipine 30 mg	Adalat CC by Wal Mart	49035-0154	Antihypertensive
ADALATCC <> 30	Tab, Film Coated	Nifedipine 30 mg	Adalat CC by Allscripts	54569-3891	Antihypertensive
ADALATCC <> 30	Tab, Film Coated	Nifedipine 30 mg	by Med Pro	53978-3033	Antihypertensive
ADALATCC <> 30	Tab, Film Coated	Nifedipine 30 mg	Adalat CC by Nat Pharmpak Serv	55154-4805	Antihypertensive
ADALATCC <> 30	Tab, Film Coated	Nifedipine 30 mg	Adalat CC by Amerisource	62584-0841	Antihypertensive

ID FRONT <> BACK	DESCRIPTION FRONT <> BACK	INGREDIENT & STRENGTH	BRAND (OR EQUIV.) & FIRM	NDC#	CLASS; SCH.
ADALATCC <> 30	Tab, Film Coated	Nifedipine 30 mg	Adalat CC by Quality Care	62682-6020	Antihypertensive
ADALATCC <> 60	Tab, Pink, Round	Nifedipine 60 mg	Adalat CC by Va Cmop	65243-0054	Antihypertensive
ADALATCC <> 60	Tab, Film Coated	Nifedipine 60 mg	Adalat CC by Bayer	00026-8851	Antihypertensive
ADALATCC <> 60	Tab, Film Coated	Nifedipine 60 mg	Adalat CC by Wal Mart	49035-0155	Antihypertensive
ADALATCC <> 60	Tab, Film Coated	Nifedipine 60 mg	Adalat CC by Nat Pharmpak Serv	55154-4809	Antihypertensive
ADALATCC <> 60	Tab, Film Coated	Nifedipine 60 mg	by Med Pro	53978-3034	Antihypertensive
ADALATCC <> 60	Tab, Film Coated	Nifedipine 60 mg	Adalat CC by Amerisource	62584-0006	Antihypertensive
ADALATCC <> 60	Tab, Yellowish Pink, Film Coated	Nifedipine 60 mg	Adalat CC by Quality Care	62682-6021	Antihypertensive
ADALATCC <> 60	Tab, Film Coated	Nifedipine 60 mg	Adalat CC by Smiths Food & Drug	58341-0059	Antihypertensive
ADALATCC <> 60	Tab, Film Coated	Nifedipine 60 mg	by Talbert Med	44514-0761	Antihypertensive
ADALATCC <> 90	Tab, Film Coated	Nifedipine 90 mg	Adalat CC by Bayer	00026-8861	Antihypertensive
ADALATCC <> 90	Tab, Film Coated	Nifedipine 90 mg	by Med Pro	53978-3044	Antihypertensive
ADAMS <> 012	Tab	Guaifenesin 600 mg	Humibid LA by Nat Pharmpak Serv	55154-5903	Expectorant
ADAMS <> 024	Tab	Atropine Sulfate 0.04 mg, Chlorpheniramine Maleate 8 mg, Hyoscyamine Sulfate 0.19 mg, Phenylephrine HCl 25 mg, Phenylpropanolamine HCl 50 mg, Scopolamine Hydrobromide 0.01 mg	Atrohist Plus by Medeva	53014-0024	Cold Remedy
ADAMS <> 024	Tab, Adams <> 0/24	Atropine Sulfate 0.04 mg, Chlorpheniramine Maleate 8 mg, Hyoscyamine Sulfate 0.19 mg, Phenylephrine HCl 25 mg, Phenylpropanolamine HCl 50 mg, Scopolamine Hydrobromide 0.01 mg	Atrohist Plus by Drug Distr	52985-0227	Cold Remedy
ADAMS <> 17	Tab	Guaifenesin 600 mg, Pseudoephedrine HCl 60 mg	Deconsal II by Nat Pharmpak Serv	55154-5901	Cold Remedy
ADAMS <> 30	Tab	Dextromethorphan Hydrobromide 30 mg, Guaifenesin 600 mg	Humibid DM by Nat Pharmpak Serv	55154-5902	Cold Remedy
ADAMS <> 6	Tab, Yellow, Oblong, Scored	Pseudoephedrine HCl 120 mg; Methscopolamine Nitrate 2.5 mg; Chlorpheniramine Maleate 8 mg; Methscopolamine Nitrate 2.5 mg	Allerx by Adams Labs	63824-0067	Cold Remedy
ADAMS <> 7	Tab, Blue, Oblong, Scored	Pseudoephedrine HCl 120 mg; Methscopolamine Nitrate 2.5 mg; Chlorpheniramine Maleate 8 mg; Methscopolamine Nitrate 2.5 mg	Allerx by Adams Labs	63824-0067	Cold Remedy
ADAMS012	Tab, Adams/012	Guaifenesin 600 mg	Humibid LA by Amerisource	62584-0012	Expectorant
ADAMS015	Tab, Blue, Oblong	Guaifenesin 400 mg, Pseudoephedrine 120 mg	Deconsal LA by Adams		Cold Remedy
ADAMS017	Tab, Dark Blue	Guaifenesin 600 mg, Pseudoephedrine HCl 60 mg	Deconsal II by Quality Care	60346-0937	Cold Remedy
ADAMS018	Cap, Clear & Green	Guaifenesin 300 mg	Humibid Sprinkle by Adams		Expectorant
ADAMS019	Cap, Blue & Clear	Phenylephrine 10 mg, Guaifenesin 300 mg	Deconsal Sprinkle by Adams		Cold Remedy
ADAMS022	Cap, Clear & Yellow	Brompheniramine 2 mg, Phenyltoloxamine 25 mg, Phenylephrine 10 mg	Atrohist Sprinkle by Adams		Cold Remedy
ADAMS024	Tab, Adams/024	Atropine Sulfate 0.04 mg, Chlorpheniramine Maleate 8 mg, Hyoscyamine Sulfate 0.19 mg, Phenylephrine HCl 25 mg, Phenylpropanolamine HCl 50 mg, Scopolamine Hydrobromide 0.01 mg	Atrohist Plus by Vintage	00254-2162	Cold Remedy
ADAMS024	Tab	Atropine Sulfate 0.04 mg, Chlorpheniramine Maleate 8 mg, Hyoscyamine Sulfate 0.19 mg, Phenylephrine HCl 25 mg, Phenylpropanolamine HCl 50 mg, Scopolamine Hydrobromide 0.01 mg	Atrohist Plus by Eckerd Drug	19458-0839	Cold Remedy
ADAMS030	Tab, Adams/030	Dextromethorphan Hydrobromide 30 mg, Guaifenesin 600 mg	Humibid DM by Amerisource	62584-0030	Cold Remedy
ADAMS030	Tab	Dextromethorphan Hydrobromide 30 mg, Guaifenesin 600 mg	Humibid DM by Drug Distr	52985-0206	Cold Remedy
ADAMS034	Cap, Clear & Green	Guaifenesin 300 mg, Dextromethorphan Hydrobromide 15 mg	Humibid DM Sprinkle by Adams		Cold Remedy
ADAMS309	Tab, Oblong	Guaifenesin 600 mg, Pseudoephedrine 30 mg	Syn-RX DM by Adams		Cold Remedy
ADAMS310	Tab, Oblong	Guaifenesin 600 mg, Pseudoephedrine 60 mg	Syn-RX DM by Adams		Cold Remedy
ADEFLORM <> KENWOOD	Tab	Ascorbic Acid 100 mg, Calcium 250 mg, Calcium Pantothenate 10 mg, Cyanocobalamin 2 mcg, Fluorides 1 mg, Iron 30 mg, Niacinamide 20 mg, Pyridoxine HCl 10 mg, Riboflavin 2.5 mg, Thiamine Mononitrate 1.5 mg, Vitamin A 6000 Units, Vitamin D 400 Units	Adeflor M by Kenwood	00482-0115	Vitamin
ADH	Tab, Gray, Round, Schering Logo ADH	Perphenazine 2 mg	Trilafon by Schering		Antipsychotic
ADIPEXP <> 99	Tab, Blue & White, Oblong, Scored, Adipex-P <> 9/9	Phentermine HCl 37.5 mg	Adipex P by Teva	00093-0009	Anorexiant; C IV
ADIPEXP375	Cap, Bright Blue & White with 2 Dark Blue Stripes, Opaque, Adipex-P over 37.5	Phentermine HCl 37.5 mg	Adipex P by Teva	00093-0019	Anorexiant; C IV
ADIPEXP375	Cap, Blue & White, Adipex-P 37.5	Phentermine HCl 37.5 mg	Adipex P by Gate	57844-0019	Anorexiant; C IV
ADIPEXP99	Tab, Blue & White, Oblong, Scored, Adipex-P 9 9	Phentermine HCl 37.5 mg	by Allscripts	54569-1718	Anorexiant; C IV

ID FRONT <> BACK	DESCRIPTION FRONT <> BACK	INGREDIENT & STRENGTH	BRAND (OR EQUIV.) & FIRM	NDC#	CLASS; SCH.
ADIPEXP99	Cap, Blue & White, Scored, Adipex-P 99	Phentermine HCl 37.5 mg	Adipex P by Gate	57844-0009	Anorexiant; C IV
ADJ	Tab, Gray, Round, Schering Logo ADJ	Perphenazine 8 mg	Trilafon by Schering		Antipsychotic
ADK	Tab, Gray, Round, Schering Logo ADK	Perphenazine 4 mg	Trilafon by Schering		Antipsychotic
ADM	Tab, Gray, Round, Schering Logo ADM	Perphenazine 16 mg	Trilafon by Schering		Antipsychotic
ADRIA130	Tab, White, Oblong, Adria/130	Butalbital 50 mg, Aspirin 650 mg	Axotal by Adria		Analgesic
ADRIA200	Tab, Beige, Round, Adria/200	Pancrelipase, Lipase, Protease NLT, Amylase NLT	Ilozyme by Adria		Gastrointestinal
ADRIA217	Tab, Red, Round	Phenolphthalein 130 mg	Evac-Q-Tab by Adria		Gastrointestinal
ADRIA230	Tab, Yellow, Octagonal, Adria/230	Metoclopramide 10 mg	Octamide by Adria		Gastrointestinal
ADRIA231	Tab, White, Round, Adria/231	Dexpanthenol 50 mg, Choline Bitartrate 25 mg	Ilopan-Choline by Adria		Antiflatulent
ADRIA304	Tab, Green, Oblong, Adria/304	Potassium Chloride 10 mEq	Kaon Cl-10 by Adria		Electrolytes
ADRIA307	Tab, Yellow, Round, Adria/307	Potassium Chloride 6.7 mEq	Kaon-Cl by Adria		Electrolytes
ADRIA312	Tab, Purple, Round, Adria/312	Potassium Gluconate 5 mEq	Kaon by Adria		Electrolytes
ADRIA412	Tab, Pink, Oblong, Adria/412	Magnesium Salicylate 545 mg	Magan by Adria		Analgesic
ADRIA420	Tab, Yellow, Oblong, Adria/420	Magnesium Lactate 7 mEq	Mag-Tab by Adria		Mineral
ADRIA648	Tab, Peach, Oval	Cyclothiazide 2 mg	Fluidil by Adria		Diuretic
ADS100	Cap, White	Ritonavir 100 mg	Norvir by Scherer Rp North	11014-1233	Antiviral
ADVIL	Tab, Brown, Round	Ibuprofen 200 mg	Advil by Whitehall-Robbins		NSAID
ADVIL	Cap, Light Brown	Ibuprofen 200 mg	Advil by Whitehall-Robbins		NSAID
ADVILCOLDSINUS	Cap, Butterscotch, Oval, Advil Cold & Sinus	Ibuprofen 200 mg, Pseudoephedrine 30 mg	Advil by Whitehall-Robbins		Cold Remedy
ADX1 <> A	Tab, Film Coated, ADX 1 <> A Arrow Logo	Anastrozole 1 mg	Arimidex by Murfreesboro	51129-1122	Antineoplastic
ADX1 <> A	Tab, White, Film Coated, Arrow Logo	Anastrozole 1 mg	Arimidex by AstraZeneca	00310-0201	Antineoplastic
ADX1A	Tab, White, Biconvex, ADX 1/A	Anastrazole 1 mg	by Zeneca	Canadian	Antineoplastic
AE	Tab, White, Round, Abbott Logo	Ethotoin 500 mg	Pegaby Abbott		Anticonvulsant
AEB	Tab, Coated, Abbott Logo	Erythromycin 250 mg	by Apotheca	12634-0425	Antibiotic
AEC	Tab, Abbott Logo	Erythromycin 250 mg	by Dept Health Central Pharm	53808-0015	Antibiotic
AEE	Tab, Coated, A-EE	Erythromycin Ethylsuccinate	EES Filmtabs by Allscripts	54569-0127	Antibiotic
AEH	Tab, Abbott Logo	Erythromycin 333 mg	Ery Tab by Apotheca	12634-0407	Antibiotic
AF	Tab, White, Round	Colchicine 0.6 mg	by Abbott	00074-3781	Antigout
AF	Tab, Yellow, Round, AF over Abbott Logo	Colchicine 0.6 mg	by Abbott	00074-3781	Antigout
AF1	Tab, White & Yellow, Round, AF-1	Phenylephrine 5 mg, Chlorpheniramine 2 mg, Acetaminophen 325 mg	by Perrigo	00113-0414	Cold Remedy
AF2	Tab, Round	Sodium Fluoride 2.2 mg	Luride by Able Labs		Element
AFA	Tab, White	Acetaminophen 325 mg	A.F. Anacin by Whitehall-Robbins	Canadian	Antipyretic
AFA500	Tab, White, AFA/500	Acetaminophen 500 mg	A.F. Anacin ES by Whitehall-Robbins	Canadian	Antipyretic
AFE	Tab, Brown & Red, Circular, A/FE	Felodipine 10 mg	Plendil by Astra	Canadian	Antihypertensive
AFE10	Tab, Brown & Red, Round	Felodipine 10 mg	Plendil by Astra	Canadian	Antihypertensive
AFL25	Tab, Yellow, Circular, A/FL/2.5	Felodipine 2.5 mg	Plendil by Astra	Canadian	Antihypertensive
AFL25	Tab, Yellow, Round, A FL 2.5	Felodipine 2.5 mg	Plendil by Astra	Canadian	Antihypertensive
AFM	Tab, Pink, Circular, A/FM	Felodipine 5 mg	Plendil by Astra	Canadian	Antihypertensive
AFM5	Tab, Pink, Round	Felodipine 5 mg	Plendil by Astra	Canadian	Antihypertensive
AGA	Tab, Red, Oval, Schering Logo AGA	Dexchlorpheniramine ER 4 mg	Polaramine by Schering		Antihistamine
AGB	Tab, Red, Oval, Schering Logo AGB	Dexchlorpheniramine ER 6 mg	Polaramine by Schering		Antihistamine
AGT	Tab, Red, Oval, Schering Logo AGT	Dexchlorpheniramine 2 mg	Polaramine by Schering		Antihistamine
AH	Tab, Rose, Round, Abbott Logo	Hydrochlorothiazide 25 mg, Deserpidine 0.125 mg	Oreticyl by Abbott		Diuretic; Antihypertensive
AH <> TOURO	Cap, Ex Release, A & H	Brompheniramine Maleate 6 mg, Pseudoephedrine HCl 60 mg	Touro A & H by Sovereign	58716-0030	Cold Remedy
AH1K	Tab, Pink, Round, AH/1K	Salbutamol Sulfate 2 mg	Ventolin by Glaxo	Canadian	Antiasthmatic
AH2K	Tab, Pink, Round, AH/2K	Salbutamol Sulfate 4 mg	Ventolin by Glaxo	Canadian	Antiasthmatic
AHK	Cap, Abbott Logo and HK	Terazosin HCl 5 mg	Hytrin by Nat Pharmpak Serv	55154-0116	Antihypertensive
AHR	Cap, Black & Yellow	Acetaminophen 325 mg, Phenobarbital 16.2 mg, Codeine Phosphate 16.2 mg	Phenaphen by Wyeth-Ayerst	Canadian	Analgesic
AHR	Tab, Pink, Round, Schering Logo AHR	Carisoprodol 350 mg	Rela by Schering		Muscle Relaxant
AHR	Cap, Yellow	Attapulgite 300 mg, Pectin 71.4 mg, Opium 12 mg	Donnagel PG by Wyeth-Ayerst	Canadian	Antidiarrheal
AHR	Tab, Green, Round, Scored	Brom Mal 4 mg, Phen Hydr 5 mg, Phenpro Hydr 5 mg, Dextro Hybrom 15 mg	Dimetapp by Whitehall-Robbins		Cold Remedy

ID FRONT <> BACK	DESCRIPTION FRONT <> BACK	INGREDIENT & STRENGTH	BRAND (OR EQUIV.) & FIRM	NDC#	CLASS; SCH.
AHR	Tab, Peach	Brompheniramine Maleate 4 mg	Dimetane by Whitehall-Robbins	Canadian	Antihistamine
AHR	Tab	Glycopyrrolate 1 mg	by Pharm Packaging Ctr	54383-0081	Gastrointestinal
AHR	Tab, Blue, Round, Scored	Phen Hydro 5 mg, Phenpro Hydro 5 mg, Acetaminophen 325 mg	Dimetapp by Whitehall-Robbins		Cold Remedy
AHR	Tab, White	Pseudoephedrine HCl 60 mg	Robidrine by Whitehall-Robbins	Canadian	Decongestant
AHR	Tab, White, Round, Bisect	Pseudoephedrine HCl 60 mg	Robidrine by Whitehall-Robbins		Decongestant
AHR <> DONNATAL	Tab, Film Coated	Atropine Sulfate 0.0582 mg, Hyoscyamine Sulfate 0.3111 mg, Phenobarbital 48.6 mg, Scopolamine Hydrobromide 0.0195 mg	Antispasmotic by Pharmedix	53002-0449	Gastrointestinal; C IV
AHR <> DONNATALEXTENTAB	Tab, Pale Green, Film Coated	Atropine Sulfate 0.0582 mg, Hyoscyamine Sulfate 0.3111 mg, Phenobarbital 48.6 mg, Scopolamine Hydrobromide 0.0195 mg	Donnatal by Thrift Drug	59198-0233	Gastrointestinal; C IV
AHR <> ROBAXIN750	Tab, Film Coated, Robaxin 750	Methocarbamol 750 mg	Robaxin by A H Robins	00031-7449	Muscle Relaxant
AHR <> ROBAXIN750	Tab, Film Coated, Robaxin-750	Methocarbamol 750 mg	Robaxin by Thrift Drug	59198-0182	Muscle Relaxant
AHR <> ROBAXIN750	Tab, Film Coated, Robaxin Over 750	Methocarbamol 750 mg	Robaxin by Amerisource	62584-0450	Muscle Relaxant
AHR <> ROBAXIN750	Tab, Film Coated	Methocarbamol 750 mg	Robaxin 750 by Leiner	59606-0730	Muscle Relaxant
AHR <> TENEX	Tab, Pink, Diamond	Guanfacine HCl 1.15 mg	Tenex by Rightpac	65240-0748	Antihypertensive
AHR 2290	Tab, Purple	Brompheniramine Maleate 1 mg, Phenylpropanolamine 6.25 mg	by Whitehall-Robbins	Canadian	Cold Remedy
AHR0677	Tab, Orange, Elliptical	B Complex, Ascorbic Acid, Vitamin E	Allbee C-800 by Robins		Vitamin
AHR0678	Tab, Red, Elliptical	B Complex, Ascorbic Acid, Vitamin E, Iron	Allbee C-800 Plus FE by Robins		Vitamin
AHR1 <> TENEX	Tab	Guanfacine HCl 1.15 mg	Tenex by Nat Pharmpak Serv	55154-3008	Antihypertensive
AHR10 <> REGLAN	Tab	Metoclopramide HCl 10 mg	Reglan by A H Robins	00031-6701	Gastrointestinal
AHR10 <> REGLAN	Tab	Metoclopramide HCl 10 mg	Reglan by Wal Mart	49035-0157	Gastrointestinal
AHR10 <> REGLAN	Tab	Metoclopramide HCl 10 mg	Reglan by Thrift Drug	59198-0099	Gastrointestinal
AHR10 <> REGLAN	Tab	Metoclopramide HCl 10 mg	Reglan by Nat Pharmpak Serv	55154-3004	Gastrointestinal
AHR1007141	Tab, White, Round, AHR/100 7141	Amoxicillin Veterinary Tablets 100 mg	by Biocraft		Antibiotic
AHR1535	Tab, Yellow, Round	Calcium Polycarbophil 500 mg	Mitrolan by A.H.Robins		Vitamin/Mineral
AHR1843	Tab, Round	Brompheniramine Maleate 12 mg	Dimetane by A.H.Robins		Antihistamine
AHR1857	Tab, Round	Brompheniramine Maleate 4 mg	Dimetane by A.H.Robins		Antihistamine
AHR1868	Tab, Round	Brompheniramine Maleate 8 mg	Dimetane by A.H.Robins		Antihistamine
AHR2007151	Tab, White, Round, AHR/200 7151	Amoxicillin Veterinary Tablets 200 mg	by Biocraft		Antibiotic
AHR2255I	Tab, Purple & Red, Oval	Brom Maleat 4 mg, Phenylpropanolamine HCl 25 mg	Dimetapp by Whitehall-Robbins		Cold Remedy
AHR2279	Tab, Orange & Red, Oval	Brom Mal 4 mg, Phenylpro HCl 25 mg, Dextro HBr 20 mg	Dimetapp by Whitehall-Robbins		Cold Remedy
AHR27840	Tab, Pink, Round, AHR 2/7840	Glycopyrrolate 2 mg	Robinul Forte by A.H.Robins		Gastrointestinal
AHR4007171	Tab, White, Round, AHR/400 7171	Amoxicillin Veterinary Tablets 400 mg	by Biocraft		Antibiotic
AHR4207	Cap, Green & White	Phenobarbital, Hyoscyamine, Atropine, Scopolamine	Donnatal by A.H.Robins		Gastrointestinal; C IV
AHR4649	Tab, Green, Round	Combination Enzyme, Antispasmodic	Donnazyme by A.H.Robins		Digestant
AHR5 <> MICROK10	Cap	Potassium Chloride 750 mg	by Med Pro	53978-5044	Electrolytes
AHR5049	Tab, White, Round	Pancreatin 300 mg, Pepsin 250 mg, Bile Salts 150 mg	Entozyme by A.H.Robins		Gastrointestinal
AHR507131	Tab, White, Round, AHR/50 7131	Amoxicillin Veterinary Tablets 50 mg	by Biocraft		Antibiotic
AHR5449	Tab, Yellow, Round	Benzthiazide 50 mg	Exna by A.H.Robins		Diuretic
AHR5720 <> MICROK	Cap	Potassium Chloride 600 mg	Micro K by A H Robins	00031-5720	Electrolytes
AHR5720 <> MICROK	Cap, AHR 5720 <> Micro-K	Potassium Chloride 600 mg	by Med Pro	53978-0155	Electrolytes
AHR5720 <> MICROK	Cap	Potassium Chloride 600 mg	Micro K by Thrift Drug	59198-0310	Electrolytes
AHR5720 <> MICROK	Cap, AHR/5720 <> Micro-K	Potassium Chloride 600 mg	Micro K by Nat Pharmpak Serv	55154-3010	Electrolytes
AHR5730 <> MICROK	Cap, AHR/5730 <> Micro-K	Potassium Chloride 750 mg	Micro K 10 by Allscripts	54569-0660	Electrolytes
AHR5730 <> MICROK	Cap	Potassium Chloride 600 mg	Micro K by Leiner	59606-0691	Electrolytes
AHR5730 <> MICROK10	Cap, ER	Potassium Chloride 750 mg	Micro K 10 by A H Robins	00031-5730	Electrolytes
AHR5730 <> MICROK10	Cap, ER, AHR/5730, Micro-K 10	Potassium Chloride 750 mg	Micro K 10 by Wal Mart	49035-0153	Electrolytes
AHR5730 <> MICROK10	Cap, ER	Potassium Chloride 750 mg	Micro K by Nat Pharmpak Serv	55154-3012	Electrolytes
AHR5730 <> MICROK10	Cap, ER	Potassium Chloride 750 mg	Micro K by PDRX	55289-0899	Electrolytes

ID FRONT <> BACK	DESCRIPTION FRONT <> BACK	INGREDIENT & STRENGTH	BRAND (OR EQUIV.) & FIRM	NDC#	CLASS; SCH.
AHR5730 <> MICROK10	Cap, ER, AHR/5730 <> Micro-K 10	Potassium Chloride 750 mg	Micro K 10 by Leiner	59606-0772	Electrolytes
AHR5730 <> MICROK10	Cap, ER	Potassium Chloride 750 mg	Micro K 10 by Amerisource	62584-0730	Electrolytes
AHR5730 <> MICROK10	Cap, ER	Potassium Chloride 750 mg	Micro K 10 by Thrift Drug	59198-0229	Electrolytes
AHR5816	Tab, Yellow, Round	Sodium Salicylate 300 mg, Sodium Aminobenzoate 300 mg	Pabalate by A.H.Robins		Analgesic
AHR5883	Tab, Rose, Round	Potassium Salicylate 300 mg, Potassium Aminobenzoate 300 mg	Pabalate SF by A.H.Robins		Dermatological
AHR6242	Cap, Black & Yellow	Acetaminophen 325 mg, Codeine 15 mg	Phenaphen #2 by A.H.Robins		Analgesic; C III
AHR6251	Tab, White, Oblong	Acetaminophen 650 mg, Codeine 30 mg	Phenaphen 650 c Cod. by A.H.Robins		Analgesic; C III
AHR6257	Cap	Acetaminophen 325 mg, Codeine Phosphate 30 mg	Phenaphen Codeine No 3 by Allscripts	54569-1775	Analgesic; C III
AHR6257 <> AHR6257	Cap	Acetaminophen 325 mg, Codeine Phosphate 30 mg	Phenaphen Codeine No 3 by A H Robins	00031-6257	Analgesic; C III
AHR6274	Cap, Green & White	Acetaminophen 325 mg, Codeine 60 mg	Phenaphen #4 by A.H.Robins		Analgesic; C III
AHR6447	Tab, Orange, Round	Fenfluramine HCl 20 mg	Pondimin by A.H.Robins		Anorexiant; C IV
AHR7824	Tab, Pink, Round	Glycopyrrolate 1 mg	Robinul by A.H.Robins		Gastrointestinal
AHR8600	Cap, Red, Oval, AHR-8600	Guaifenesin 200 mg, Dextromethorp HBr 10 mg, Pseudophedrine HBr 30 mg	Robitussin by Whitehall-Robbins		Cold Remedy
AHR8602	Cap, Amber, Oval, AHR-8602	Guaifenesin 100 mg, Dextromethorp HBr 10 mg, Pseudo HCl 30 mg, Acetam 250 mg	Robitussin by Whitehall-Robbins		Cold Remedy
AHRDONNATAL	Tab, Light Green, Film Coated	Atropine Sulfate 0.0582 mg, Hyoscyamine Sulfate 0.3111 mg, Phenobarbital 48.6 mg, Scopolamine Hydrobromide 0.0195 mg	Donnatal by A H Robins	00031-4235	Gastrointestinal; C IV
AHRDONNATAL EXTENTABS	Tab, Pale Green, Film Coated, AHR over Donnatal Extentabs	Atropine Sulfate 0.0582 mg, Hyoscyamine Sulfate 0.3111 mg, Phenobarbital 48.6 mg, Scopolamine Hydrobromide 0.0195 mg	Donnatal by Quality Care	60346-0857	Gastrointestinal; C IV
AHRROBICAP8417	Cap	Tetracycline 250 mg	Robitet 250mg by A.H.Robins		Antibiotic
AHRROBICAP8427	Cap	Tetracycline 500 mg	Robitet 500mg by A.H.Robins		Antibiotic
AHT	Tab, Peach, Round, Schering Logo AHT	Reserpine 0.1 mg, Trichlormethiazide 4 mg	Naquival by Schering		Antihypertensive
AHY	Cap, Abbott Symbol and Abbott Code HY	Terazosin HCl 2 mg	Hytrin by PDRX	55289-0042	Antihypertensive
AI	Tab, Rose, Round, Abbott Logo	Hydrochlorothiazide 50 mg, Deserpidine 0.125 mg	Oreticyl by Abbott		Diuretic; Antihypertensive
AID	Tab, Yellow, Oval, Scored	Isosorbide Mononitrate ER 60 mg	by Murfreesboro	51129-1580	Antianginal
AID	Tab, Yellow, Oval, A/ID	Isosorbide-5-Mononitrate 60 mg	Imdur by Astra	Canadian	Antianginal
AID	Tab, Yellow, Oval, Scored	Isosorbide Mononitrate 60 mg	by Warrick Pharms	59930-1549	Antianginal
AID	Tab, Yellow, Oval, Scored	Isosorbide Mononitrate 60 mg	by Murfreesboro	51129-1568	Antianginal
AJ	Tab, Red, Oval, Film Coated	Ferrous Sulfate 525 mg, Folic Acid 80 mg, Vitamin C 500 mg	Fero-Folic 500 by Abbott	00074-7079	Mineral
AK	Tab, Red, Oval, Film Coated, AK over Abbott Logo	Ferrous Sulfate, Vitamin C, B-Complex, Folic Acid	Iberet-Folic 500 by Abbott	00074-7125	Mineral
AK	Tab, Red, Oblong, Film Coated	Sodium Ascorbate; Pyridoxine HCl 5 mg; Riboflavin 6 mg; Thiamine Mononitrate 6 mg; Cyanocobalamin 25 mcg; Niacinamide 30 mg; Ferrous Sulfate 525 mg; Folic Acid 800 mcg; Calcium Pantothenate 10 mg	Iberet Folic by Abbott Health	60692-7125	Vitamin
AKT	Tab, Film Coated, Abbott Logo Plus KT	Clarithromycin 250 mg	Biaxin by Quality Care	60346-0195	Antibiotic
AL	Tab, Blue, Round, Scored	Clorazepate Dipotassium 3.75 mg	by Novopharm	55953-0981	Antianxiety; C IV
AL	Tab	Clorazepate Dipotassium 3.75 mg	by Quality Care	60346-0409	Antianxiety; C IV
AL	Tab, Mottled Blue, Round, Scored	Clorazepate Dipotassium 3.75 mg	Tranxene by Able Lab	53265-0048	Antianxiety; C IV
AL	Tab	Clorazepate Dipotassium 3.75 mg	by Geneva	00781-1865	Antianxiety; C IV
AL	Tab, Scored	Clorazepate Dipotassium 3.75 mg	Clorazepate Dipotassium by DHHS Prog	11819-0143	Antianxiety; C IV
AL	Tab, Blue, Round	Clorazepate Dipotassium 3.75 mg	by Novopharm	43806-0981	Antianxiety; C IV
AL <> G2	Tab, White, Oblong, Scored	Alprazolam 2 mg	by Par Pharm	49884-0400	Antianxiety; C IV
AL <> G2	Tab, White, Oblong, /A/L <> /G/2/	Alprazolam 2 mg	Alprazolam by Apotheca	12634-0524	Antianxiety; C IV
AL025 <> G	Tab, Light Yellow, Coated, AL/0.25	Alprazolam 0.25 mg	by Quality Care	60346-0876	Antianxiety; C IV
AL025 <> G	Tab	Alprazolam 0.25 mg	by Par	49884-0448	Antianxiety; C IV
AL025G	Tab, White, Oval, AL/0.25/G	Alprazolam 0.25 mg	Gen Alprazolam by Genpharm	Canadian	Antianxiety
AL025MGG	Tab, Yellow, Oval, AL/0.25 mg G	Alprazolam 0.25 mg	Xanax by Par		Antianxiety; C IV

ID FRONT <> BACK	DESCRIPTION FRONT <> BACK	INGREDIENT & STRENGTH	BRAND (OR EQUIV.) & FIRM	NDC#	CLASS; SCH.
AL025MGG	Tab, AL/0.25MGG	Alprazolam 0.25 mg	by Qualitest	00603-2346	Antianxiety; C IV
AL05 <> G	Tab	Alprazolam 0.5 mg	by Par	49884-0449	Antianxiety; C IV
AL05G	Tab, Orange, Oval, AL/0.5/G	Alprazolam 0.5 mg	Gen Alprazolam by Genpharm	Canadian	Antianxiety
AL05MGG	Tab, Yellow, Oval, AL/0.5 mg G	Alprazolam 0.5 mg	Xanax by Par		Antianxiety; C IV
AL05MGG	Tab, AL/0.5MGG	Alprazolam 0.5 mg	by Qualitest	00603-2347	Antianxiety; C IV
AL10 <> G	Tab	Alprazolam 1 mg	by Par	49884-0450	Antianxiety; C IV
AL10 <> G	Tab, AL 1.0 <> G	Alprazolam 1 mg	by Alphapharm	57315-0008	Antianxiety; C IV
AL10 <> G	Tab, AL 1.0 <> G	Alprazolam 1 mg	by Direct Dispensing	57866-4636	Antianxiety; C IV
AL10MGG	Tab, White, Oval, AL/1.0 mg G	Alprazolam 1 mg	Xanax by Par		Antianxiety; C IV
AL10MGG	Tab, AL/1.0MGG	Alprazolam 1 mg	by Qualitest	00603-2348	Antianxiety; C IV
ALBERT <> GLYGLY	Tab, White, Round, Scored, Albert Logo <> Gly over Gly	Glyburide 2.5 mg	by Altimed	Canadian DIN# 01900927	Antidiabetic
ALDACTAZIDE25 <> SEARE1011	Tab, Tan, Round	Spironolactone 25 mg; Hydrochlorothiazide 25 mg	Aldactazide by Med-Pro	53978-3382	Diuretic
ALDACTAZIDE25 <> SEARLE1011	Tab, Tan, Round, Film Coated, Aldactazide 25 <> Searle 1011	Hydrochlorothiazide 25 mg, Spironolactone 25 mg	Aldactazide by GD Searle	00025-1011	Diuretic; Antihypertensive
ALDACTAZIDE25 <> SEARLE1011	Tab, Film Coated, Aldactazide 25 <> Searle 1011	Hydrochlorothiazide 25 mg, Spironolactone 25 mg	Aldactazide by Nat Pharmpak Serv	55154-3601	Diuretic; Antihypertensive
ALDACTAZIDE25 <> SEARLE1011	Tab, Film Coated, Debossed, Aldactazide 25 <> Searle 1011	Hydrochlorothiazide 25 mg, Spironolactone 25 mg	Aldactazide by Thrift Drug	59198-0170	Diuretic; Antihypertensive
ALDACTAZIDE25 <> SEARLE1011	Tab, Film Coated	Hydrochlorothiazide 25 mg, Spironolactone 25 mg	Aldactazide by Amerisource	62584-0011	Diuretic; Antihypertensive
ALDACTAZIDE50 <> SEARLE1021	Tab, Tan, Oblong, Film Coated, Aldactazide 50 <> Searle 1021	Hydrochlorothiazide 50 mg, Spironolactone 50 mg	Aldactazide by GD Searle	00025-1021	Diuretic; Antihypertensive
ALDACTAZIDE50 <> SEARLE1021	Tab, Tan, Oblong, Scored	Spironolactone 25 mg; Hydrochlorothiazide 25 mg	Aldactazide by Rightpak	65240-0600	Diuretic
ALDACTONE <> SEARLE	Tab, Film Coated	Spironolactone 25 mg	Aldactone by Nat Pharmpak Serv	55154-3602	Diuretic
ALDACTONE100 <> SEARLE1031	Tab, Peach, Round, Coated, Aldactone 100 <> Searle 1031	Spironolactone 100 mg	Aldactone by GD Searle	00025-1031	Diuretic
ALDACTONE25 <> SEARLE1001	Tab, Yellow, Round, Film Coated	Spironolactone 25 mg	Aldactone by Rx Pac	65084-0106	Diuretic
ALDACTONE25 <> SEARLE1001	Tab, Yellow, Round	Spironolactone 25 mg	Aldactone by Rightpak	65240-0601	Diuretic
ALDACTONE25 <> SEARLE1001	Tab, Light Yellow, Round, Film Coated, Aldacton 25 <> Searle 1001	Spironolactone 25 mg	Aldactone by GD Searle	00025-1001	Diuretic
ALDACTONE25 <> SEARLE1001	Tab, Light Yellow, Film Coated	Spironolactone 25 mg	Aldactone by Caremark	00339-5531	Diuretic
ALDACTONE25 <> SEARLE1001	Tab, Film Coated, Debossed	Spironolactone 25 mg	Aldactone by Thrift Drug	59198-0001	Diuretic
ALDACTONE25 <> SEARLE1001	Tab, Film Coated, Debossed	Spironolactone 25 mg	Aldactone by Amerisource	62584-0001	Diuretic
ALDACTONE25 <> SEARLE1001	Tab, Yellow, Round, Film Coated	Spironolactone 25 mg	Aldactone by DRX Pharm Consults	55045-2716	Diuretic
ALDACTONE50 <> SEARLE1041	Tab, Light Orange, Oval, Coated, Aldactone 50 <> Searle 1041	Spironolactone 50 mg	Aldactone by GD Searle	00025-1041	Diuretic
ALDOMET <> MSD401	Tab, Yellow, Round, Film Coated	Methyldopa 250 mg	Aldomet by Merck	00006-0401	Antihypertensive
ALDOMET <> MSD516	Tab, Yellow, Round, Film Coated	Methyldopa 500 mg	Aldomet by Merck	00006-0516	Antihypertensive
ALDOMETMSD135	Tab, Yellow, Biconvex, Aldomet/MSD 135	Methyldopa 125 mg	Aldomet by MSD	Canadian	Antihypertensive
ALDORIL <> MSD423	Tab, Salmon, Round, Film Coated	Hydrochlorothiazide 15 mg, Methyldopa 250 mg	Aldoril 15 by Merck	00006-0423	Diuretic; Antihypertensive

ID FRONT <> BACK	DESCRIPTION FRONT <> BACK	INGREDIENT & STRENGTH	BRAND (OR EQUIV.) & FIRM	NDC#	CLASS; SCH.
ALKERAN <> A2A	Tab	Melphalan 2 mg	Alkeran by Glaxo	00173-0045	Antineoplastic
ALKERANA2A	Tab, White, Alkeran/A2A	Melphalan 2 mg	by Glaxo	Canadian	Antineoplastic
ALKERANA2A	Tab	Melphalan 2 mg	Alkeran by Catalytica	63552-0045	Antineoplastic
ALLEGRA <> 60MG	Cap, Opaque Pink & White	Fexofenadine HCl 60 mg	Allegra by Integrity	64731-0576	Antihistamine
ALLEGRA <> 60MG	Cap, Opaque Pink & White	Fexofenadine HCl 60 mg	Allegra by Integrity	64731-0305	Antihistamine
ALLEGRA <> 60MG	Cap, Pink & White	Fexofenadine HCl 60 mg	Allegra by DRX Pharm Consults	55045-2582	Antihistamine
ALLEGRA <> 60MG	Cap, Pink & White	Fexofenadine HCl 60 mg	Allegra by PDRX Pharms	55289-0456	Antihistamine
ALLEGRA <> 60MG	Cap, Pink & White	Fexofenadine HCl 60 mg	Allegra by Va Cmop	65243-0029	Antihistamine
ALLEGRAD	Tan & White, Film, Allegra-D	Fexofenadine HCl 60 mg, Pseudoephedrine HCl 120 mg	Allegra D ER by Integrity	64731-0295	Antihistamine
ALLEGRAD	Tab, Film Coated, Allegra-D	Fexofenadine HCl 60 mg, Pseudoephedrine HCl 120 mg	Allegra D by Hoechst Roussel	00088-1090	Antihistamine
ALLERGY <> TOURO	Cap, Ex Release	Brompheniramine Maleate 5.75 mg, Pseudoephedrine HCl 60 mg	Touro Allergy by Pharmafab	62542-0106	Cold Remedy
ALLERGY <> TOURO	Cap, Ex Release	Brompheniramine Maleate 5.75 mg, Pseudoephedrine HCl 60 mg	Touro Allergy by Dartmouth	58869-0401	Cold Remedy
ALLFEN <> MCR513	Tab, White, Oblong	Guaifenesin 1000 mg	Allfen by AM Pharms	58605-0513	Expectorant
ALLFEN <> MCR513	Tab, White, Oblong, Scored	Guaifenesin 1000 mg	by Pfab	62542-0907	Expectorant
ALOR5 <> AP	Tab, Scored	Aspirin 500 mg, Hydrocodone Bitartrate 5 mg	Alor 5 500 by Atley	59702-0550	Analgesic; C III
ALRA <> K10	Tab, Film Coated, Debossed, Alra <> K+10	Potassium Chloride 750 mg	by PDRX	55289-0359	Electrolytes
ALRA <> K10	Tab, Film Coated, Alra <> K+10	Potassium Chloride 750 mg	K Plus 10 by Quality Care	62682-6025	Electrolytes
ALRA <> K10	Tab, Film Coated, K+10	Potassium Chloride 750 mg	by Golden State	60429-0215	Electrolytes
ALRA <> K8	Tab, Film Coated, K+8	Potassium Chloride 600 mg	by Golden State	60429-0158	Electrolytes
ALRA 215	Tab, Orange, Round	Ibuprofen 200 mg	Advil by Alra		NSAID
ALRAGN	Tab, Green, Round	Clorazepate Dipotassium 15 mg	Tranxene by Alra		Antianxiety; C IV
ALRAGT	Tab, Yellow, Round	Clorazepate Dipotassium 7.5 mg	Tranxene by Alra		Antianxiety; C IV
ALRAGX	Tab, Gray, Round	Clorazepate Dipotassium 30.75 mg	Tranxene by Alra		Antianxiety; C IV
ALRAIF400	Tab, Orange, Round	Ibuprofen 400 mg	Motrin by Alra		NSAID
ALRAIF600	Tab, Orange, Oval	Ibuprofen 600 mg	Motrin by Alra		NSAID
ALRAIF800	Tab, Light Peach, Oval	Ibuprofen 800 mg	Motrin by Alra		NSAID
ALTACE10	Cap, Blue & White, Altace/10	Ramipril 10 mg	Altace by Hoechst-Roussel	Canadian	Antihypertensive
ALTACE10MG <> HOECHST	Cap, Blue, Hard Gel	Ramipril 10 mg	Altace by Monarch Pharms	61570-0120	Antihypertensive
ALTACE10MG <> HOECHST	Cap, Blue, Gelatin Coated	Ramipril 10 mg	Altace by Hoechst Roussel	00039-0106	Antihypertensive
ALTACE10MG <> HOECHST	Cap, Gelatin Coated, Altace 10 mg	Ramipril 10 mg	Altace by Hoechst Roussel	00088-0106	Antihypertensive
ALTACE10MG <> HOECHST	Cap, ER, Altace Over 10 mg	Ramipril 10 mg	Altace by Caremark	00339-6047	Antihypertensive
ALTACE10MG <> HOECHST	Cap, ER	Ramipril 10 mg	Altace by Physicians Total Care	54868-3846	Antihypertensive
ALTACE10MG <> MP	Cap, Blue	Ramipril 10 mg	Altace by Natl Pharmpak	55154-1211	Antihypertensive
ALTACE125	Cap, White & Yellow, Altace/1.25	Ramipril 1.25 mg	Altace by Hoechst-Roussel	Canadian	Antihypertensive
ALTACE125HOECHST	Cap, Yellow, Altace 1.25/Hoechst	Ramipril 1.25 mg	Altace by Hoechst Roussel	00039-0103	Antihypertensive
ALTACE125MG <> HOECHST	Cap, Yellow, Altace1.25 mg <> Hoechst, Hard Gel	Ramipril 1.25 mg	Altace by Monarch Pharms	61570-0110	Antihypertensive
ALTACE125MG <> HOECHST	Cap, Gelatin Coated, Altack 1.25 mg	Ramipril 1.25 mg	Altace by Hoechst Roussel	00088-0103	Antihypertensive
ALTACE25	Cap, Orange & White, Altace/2.5	Ramipril 2.5 mg	Altace by Hoechst-Roussel	Canadian	Antihypertensive
ALTACE25MG <> HOECHST	Cap, Orange	Ramipril 2.5 mg	Altace by Rx Pac	65084-0234	Antihypertensive
ALTACE25MG <> HOECHST	Cap, Orange, Gelatin Coated, Altace 2.5 mg <> Hoechst	Ramipril 2.5 mg	Altace by Hoechst Roussel	00039-0104	Antihypertensive
ALTACE25MG <> HOECHST	Cap, Gelatin Coated, Altace 2.5 mg	Ramipril 2.5 mg	Altace by Hoechst Roussel	00088-0104	Antihypertensive

ID FRONT <> BACK	DESCRIPTION FRONT <> BACK	INGREDIENT & STRENGTH	BRAND (OR EQUIV.) & FIRM	NDC#	CLASS; SCH.
ALTACE25MG <> HOECHST	Cap, ER, Altace 2.5 mg	Ramipril 2.5 mg	Altace by Allscripts	54569-3713	Antihypertensive
ALTACE5	Cap, Red & White, Altace/5	Ramipril 5 mg	Altace by Hoechst-Roussel	Canadian	Antihypertensive
ALTACE5HOECHST	Cap, Red, Altace 5/Hoechst	Ramipril 5 mg	Altace by Hoechst Roussel	00039-0105	Antihypertensive
ALTACE5HOECHST	Cap, Red, Altace 5/Hoechst	Ramipril 5 mg	Altace by Monarch	61570-0112	Antihypertensive
ALTACE5MG <> HOECHST	Cap, Red	Ramipril 5 mg	Altace by Rx Pac	65084-0235	Antihypertensive
ALTACE5MG <> HOECHST	Cap, Gelatin Coated	Ramipril 5 mg	Altace by Hoechst Roussel	00039-0105	Antihypertensive
ALTACE5MG <> HOECHST	Cap, Gelatin Coated	Ramipril 5 mg	Altace by Hoechst Roussel	00088-0105	Antihypertensive
ALTACE5MG <> HOECHST	Cap	Ramipril 5 mg	Altace by Allscripts	54569-3714	Antihypertensive
ALTACE5MG <> HOECHST	Cap, ER	Ramipril 5 mg	Altace by Quality Care	60346-0618	Antihypertensive
ALTACE5MG <> MP	Cap, Red, Gelatin	Ramipril 5 mg	by Allscripts	54569-3714	Antihypertensive
ALTI200	Tab, Blue, Round	Acyclovir 200 mg	by Altimed	Canadian DIN# 02229707	Antiviral
ALTI200 <> 200	Tab, Pink, Round, Scored	Amiodarone HCl 200 mg	by Altimed	Canadian DIN# 02240071	Antiarrhythmic
ALTI400	Tab, Blue, Round	Acyclovir 400 mg	by Altimed	Canadian DIN# 02229708	Antiviral
ALTI50	Tab, Off-White & Yellow, Circle	Azathioprine 50 mg	by Altimed	Canadian DIN# 02236799	Immunosuppressant
ALTI800	Tab, Blue, Oval	Acyclovir 800 mg	by Altimed	Canadian DIN# 02229709	Antiviral
ALTIDILT120MG	Cap, Light Turquoise, Alti-Dilt 120 mg	Diltiazem 120 mg	by AltiMed	Canadian	Antihypertensive
ALTIDILT180MG	Cap, Light Turquoise, Alti-Dilt 180 mg	Diltiazem 180 mg	by AltiMed	Canadian	Antihypertensive
ALTIDILT240MG	Cap, Light Blue, Alti-Dilt 240 mg	Diltiazem 240 mg	by AltiMed	Canadian	Antihypertensive
ALTIDILT300MG	Cap, Light Blue & Light Gray, Alti-Dilt 300 mg	Diltiazem 300 mg	by AltiMed	Canadian	Antihypertensive
ALTIDILTCD120MG	Cap, Light Turquoise, Alti-Dilt CD 120 mg	Diltiazem CD 120 mg	by Altimed	Canadian DIN# 02229781	Antihypertensive
ALTIDILTCD180MG	Cap, Light Blue, Alti-Dilt CD 180 mg	Diltiazem CD 180 mg	by Altimed	Canadian DIN# 02229782	Antihypertensive
ALTIDILTCD240MG	Cap, Light Blue, Alti-Dilt CD 240 mg	Diltiazem CD 240 mg	by Altimed	Canadian DIN# 02229783	Antihypertensive
ALTIDILTCD300MG	Cap, Light Blue & Light Gray, Alti-Dilt CD 300 mg	Diltiazem CD 300 mg	by Altimed	Canadian DIN# 02229784	Antihypertensive
ALTIMED <> A16A16	Tab, White, Round, Scored, A16 over A16 <> Altimed	Clobazam 10 mg	by Altimed	Canadian DIN# 02238797	Anticonvulsant

ID FRONT <> BACK	DESCRIPTION FRONT <> BACK	INGREDIENT & STRENGTH	BRAND (OR EQUIV.) & FIRM	NDC#	CLASS; SCH.
ALTIMEDM2MIN50MG	Cap, Orange w/ Yellow Powder, AltiMed M2 Min 50 mg	Minocycline HCl 50 mg	by Altimed	Canadian DIN# 01914138	Antibiotic
ALTIMEDM4MIN100MG	Cap, Orange & Purple, Altimed/M4/Min 100 mg	Minocycline 100 mg	by Altimed	Canadian DIN# 01914146	Antibiotic
ALTIMEDPC150	Cap, Lavender & Maroon, Gelatin Altimed, PC 150	Clindamycin HCl 150 mg	by Altimed	Canadian DIN# 02130033	Antibiotic
ALTIMEDPC300	Cap, Light Blue, Gelatin, Altimed, PC 300	Clindamycin HCl 300 mg	by Altimed	Canadian DIN# 02192659	Antibiotic
ALTIPENTOX	Tab, Pink, Oblong, Alti/Pentox	Pentoxyfylline 400 mg	by Altimed	Canadian DIN# 01968432	Anticoagulent
ALTITRYP1GM	Tab, White, Oval, Alti-Tryp/1gm	Tryptophan 1g	by Altimed	Canadian DIN# 02237250	Herbal; Neutraceutical
ALTO 401	Cap, Blue & Pink	Zinc Sulfate 220 mg	by Alto	00731-0401	Mineral Supplement
ALUCAP <> 3M	Cap, Green & Red, Alu-Cap <> 3M	Aluminum Hydroxide 400 mg	Alu-Cap by 3M	00089-0105	Gastrointestinal
ALUCAPRIKER	Cap, Green & Red, Alu-Cap/Riker	Aluminum Hydroxide 400 mg	Alu-Cap by 3M		Gastrointestinal
ALZA10	Tab, Pink, Oval	Oxybutynin Chloride 10 mg	Ditropan XL by Alza	17314-8501	Urinary
ALZA15	Tab, Gray, Oval	Oxybutynin Chloride 15 mg	Ditropan XL by Alza	17314-8502	Urinary
ALZA18	Tab, Yellow	Methylphenidate HCl 18 mg	Concerta by Alza	17314-5850	Stimulant; C II
ALZA36	Tab, White	Methylphenidate HCl 36 mg	Concerta by Alza	17314-5851	Stimulant; C II
ALZA5	Tab, Yellow, Oval	Oxybutynin Chloride 5 mg	Ditropan XL by Alza	17314-8500	Urinary
ALZA54	Tab, Brownish-Red	Methylphenidate HCl 54 mg	Concerta by Alza	17314-5852	Stimulant; CII
AM	Tab, Peach, Round, Scored	Clorazepate Dipotassium 7.5 mg	by Novopharm	55953-0982	Antianxiety; C IV
AM	Tab, Mottled Peach, Round, Scored	Clorazepate Dipotassium 7.5 mg	Tranxene by Able Lab	53265-0049	Antianxiety; C IV
AM	Tab	Clorazepate Dipotassium 7.5 mg	by Geneva	00781-1866	Antianxiety; C IV
AM	Tab, Peach, Scored	Clorazepate Dipotassium 7.5 mg	Clorazepate Dipotassium by DHHS Prog	11819-0145	Antianxiety; C IV
AM	Tab, Peach, Round	Clorazepate Dipotassium 7.5 mg	by Novopharm	43806-0982	Antianxiety; C IV
AM	Cap, White, Abbott Logo	Trimethadione 300 mg	Tridione by Abbott		Anticonvulsant
AM1	Tab, Purple, Oval, Film Coated	Methenamine Mandelate 1 GM	by Nat Pharmpak Serv	55154-9305	Antibiotic; Urinary Tract
AM1	Tab, Purple, Oval, Film Coated	Methenamine Mandelate 1 gm	Mandelamine by Amide	52152-0112	Antibiotic; Urinary Tract
AM102004	Tab, Sugar Coated	Phenazopyridine HCl 200 mg	by Pharmedix	53002-0315	Urinary Analgesic
AM200 <> G	Tab, White, Round, Scored	Amiodarone HCl 200 mg	Amiodarone HCl by Apotheca	12634-0553	Antiarrhythmic
AM200 <> G	Tab, White, Round, Scored	Amiodarone HCl 200 mg	Amiodarone HCl by Apotheca	12634-0551	Antiarrhythmic
AM200 <> G	Tab, White, Round, Scored	Amiodarone HCl 200 mg	by Apotheca	12634-0555	Antiarrhythmic
AMARYL	Tab, Pink, Oblong, Scored, Hoechst Logo AMA RYL <> Hoechst Logo	Glimepiride 1 mg	Amaryl by Hoechst Roussel	00039-0221	Antidiabetic
AMARYL	Tab, Scored, AMA RYL <> Hoechst Logo Hoechst Logo	Glimepiride 1 mg	Amaryl by Murfreesboro	51129-1366	Antidiabetic
AMARYL	Tab, Pink, Oblong, Scored	Glimepiride 1 mg	Amaryl by Aventis Pharms	00088-0221	Antidiabetic
AMARYL	Tab, Green, Oblong, Scored, Hoechst Logo AMA RYL <> Hoechst Logo	Glimepiride 2 mg	Amaryl by Hoechst Roussel	00039-0222	Antidiabetic
AMARYL	Tab, Green, Oblong, Scored	Glimepiride 2 mg	Amaryl by Aventis Pharms	00088-0222	Antidiabetic
AMARYL	Tab, AMA RYL <> A Arrow Logo	Glimepiride 4 mg	Amaryl by Murfreesboro	51129-1114	Antidiabetic
AMARYL	Tab, Blue, Oblong, Hoechst Logo AMA RYL <> Hoechst Logo	Glimepiride 4 mg	Amaryl by Hoechst Roussel	00039-0223	Antidiabetic
AMARYL	Tab, AMA/RYL <> Hoechst Logo/Hoechst Logo	Glimepiride 4 mg	Amaryl by Caremark	00339-6113	Antidiabetic
AMARYL	Tab, Blue, Oblong, Scored	Glimepiride 4 mg	Amaryl by Aventis Pharms	00088-0223	Antidiabetic
AMB10 <> 5421	Tab, Film Coated	Zolpidem Tartrate 10 mg	Ambien by HJ Harkins Co	52959-0363	Sedative/Hypnotic; C IV

ID FRONT <> BACK	DESCRIPTION FRONT <> BACK	INGREDIENT & STRENGTH	BRAND (OR EQUIV.) & FIRM	NDC#	CLASS; SCH.
AMB10 <> 5421	Tab, Film Coated	Zolpidem Tartrate 10 mg	Ambien by Allscripts	54569-3828	Sedative/Hypnotic; C IV
AMB10 <> 5421	Tab, Film Coated	Zolpidem Tartrate 10 mg	Ambien by PDRX	55289-0792	Sedative/Hypnotic; C IV
AMB10 <> 5421	Tab, Film Coated	Zolpidem Tartrate 10 mg	Ambien by Quality Care	60346-0949	Sedative/Hypnotic; C IV
AMB10 <> 5421	Tab, White, Oblong, Film	Zolpidem Tartrate 10 mg	Ambien by United Res	00677-1707	Sedative/Hypnotic; C IV
AMB10 <> 5421	Tab, White, Cap-Shaped, Film Coated	Zolpidem Tartrate 10 mg	Ambien by GD Searle	00025-5421	Sedative/Hypnotic; C IV
AMB10 <> 5421	Tab, Film Coated, Searle Logo	Zolpidem Tartrate 10 mg	Ambien by Caremark	00339-4065	Sedative/Hypnotic; C IV
AMB5 <> 5401	Tab, Pink, Cap-Shaped, Film Coated	Zolpidem Tartrate 5 mg	Ambien by GD Searle	00025-5401	Sedative/Hypnotic; C IV
AMB5 <> 5401	Tab, Film Coated	Zolpidem Tartrate 5 mg	Ambien by Caremark	00339-4064	Sedative/Hypnotic; C IV
AMB5 <> 5401	Tab, Film Coated	Zolpidem Tartrate 5 mg	Ambien by Nat Pharmpak Serv	55154-3617	Sedative/Hypnotic; C IV
AMB5 <> 5401	Tab, Film Coated	Zolpidem Tartrate 5 mg	Ambien by Allscripts	54569-3827	Sedative/Hypnotic; C IV
AMB5 <> 5401	Tab, Film Coated	Zolpidem Tartrate 5 mg	Ambien by HJ Harkins Co	52959-0362	Sedative/Hypnotic; C IV
AMB5 <> 5401	Tab, Film Coated	Zolpidem Tartrate 5 mg	Ambien by Quality Care	60346-0867	Sedative/Hypnotic; C IV
AMD	Tab, White, Oval, A/MD	Metoprolol Tartrate 200 mg	Betaloc by Astra	Canadian	Antihypertensive
AME	Tab, Sugar Coated	Hyoscyamine Sulfate 0.12 mg, Methenamine 81.6 mg, Methylene Blue 10.8 mg, Phenyl Salicylate 36.2 mg, Sodium Phosphate, Monobasic 40.8 mg	Disurex DS by Advanced Med	55495-0100	Gastrointestinal
AME	Tab, White, Round, A/ME	Metoprolol Tartrate 100 mg	Betaloc by Astra	Canadian	Antihypertensive
AMEN	Tab, Layered	Medroxyprogesterone Acetate 10 mg	Amen by Carnrick	00086-0049	Progestin
AMEN <> C	Tab	Medroxyprogesterone Acetate 10 mg	Amen by Eckerd Drug	19458-0831	Progestin
AMIDE <> 002	Tab, Orange, Pink & Purple, Pillow Shaped, Chewable	Ascorbic Acid 30 mg, Sodium Ascorbate 33 mg, Sodium Fluoride, Vitamin A Acetate, Vitamin D 400 Units	Tri Vitamin Fluoride by Schein	00364-0846	Vitamin
AMIDE <> 014	Tab, Film Coated	Dexchlorpheniramine Maleate 4 mg	by Schein	00364-0585	Antihistamine
AMIDE <> 015	Tab, Film Coated	Dexchlorpheniramine Maleate 6 mg	by Schein	00364-0586	Antihistamine
AMIDE 014	Tab, Yellow, Oval, Film Coated	Dexchlorpheniramine Maleate 4 mg	Polaramine by Amide	52152-0014	Antihistamine
AMIDE001	Tab, Orange & Pink & Purple, Round	Multivitamin, Fluoride 1 mg	Poly-Vi-Flor by Amide		Vitamin
AMIDE001 <> ABCD	Tab, Chewable	Ascorbic Acid 60 mg, Cyanocobalamin 4.5 mcg, Folic Acid 0.3 mg, Niacinamide, Pyridoxine HCl 1.05 mg, Riboflavin 1.2 mg, Sodium Fluoride, Thiamine Mononitrate, Vitamin A Acetate, Vitamin D 400 Units, Vitamin E Acetate	Multi-Vit/Fl Chew by Qualitest	00603-4712	Vitamin
AMIDE001 <> ABCD	Tab, Orange, Pink & Purple, Round, Chewable	Ascorbic Acid 60 mg, Cyanocobalamin 4.5 mcg, Folic Acid 0.3 mg, Niacinamide, Pyridoxine HCl 1.05 mg, Riboflavin 1.2 mg, Sodium Fluoride, Thiamine Mononitrate, Vitamin A Acetate, Vitamin D 400 Units, Vitamin E Acetate	Multi Vita Bets by Amide	52152-0001	Vitamin
AMIDE001 <> ABCD	Tab, Chewable	Ascorbic Acid 60 mg, Cyanocobalamin 4.5 mcg, Folic Acid 0.3 mg, Niacinamide, Pyridoxine HCl 1.05 mg, Riboflavin 1.2 mg, Sodium Fluoride, Thiamine Mononitrate, Vitamin A Acetate, Vitamin D 400 Units, Vitamin E Acetate	Multivite W Fl by Major	00904-5275	Vitamin
AMIDE003	Tab, Sugar Coated	Phenazopyridine HCl 100 mg	by Pharmedix	53002-0463	Urinary Analgesic
AMIDE003	Tab, Sugar Coated	Phenazopyridine HCl 100 mg	by United Res	00677-0575	Urinary Analgesic
AMIDE004	Tab, Sugar Coated	Phenazopyridine HCl 200 mg	by Allscripts	54569-0197	Urinary Analgesic
AMIDE004	Tab, Sugar Coated	Phenazopyridine HCl 200 mg	by United Res	00677-0804	Urinary Analgesic
AMIDE0046	Tab, Buff	Chlorpheniramine Tannate 8 mg, Phenylephrine Tannate 25 mg, Pyrilamine Tannate 25 mg	Tri Tannate by Amide	52152-0046	Cold Remedy
AMIDE009 <> 10	Tab	Isoxsuprine HCl 10 mg	by Qualitest	00603-4146	Vasodilator
AMIDE010 <> 20	Tab	Isoxsuprine HCl 20 mg	by Qualitest	00603-4147	Vasodilator
AMIDE013	Tab, White, Round	Ephedrine 25 mg, Theophylline 130 mg, Hydroxyzine HCl 10 mg	Marax by Amide		Antiasthmatic
AMIDE013	Tab	Ephedrine Sulfate 25 mg, Hydroxyzine HCl 10 mg, Theophylline 130 mg	by Zenith Goldline	00182-1344	Antiasthmatic
AMIDE013	Tab	Ephedrine Sulfate 25 mg, Hydroxyzine HCl 10 mg, Theophylline 130 mg	Hydrophed by Rugby	00536-3906	Antiasthmatic
AMIDE013	Tab	Ephedrine Sulfate 25 mg, Hydroxyzine HCl 10 mg, Theophylline 130 mg	Hydroxy Compound by Qualitest	00603-3948	Antiasthmatic
AMIDE013	Tab	Ephedrine Sulfate 25 mg, Hydroxyzine HCl 10 mg, Theophylline 130 mg	Ami Rax by Amide	52152-0013	Antiasthmatic
AMIDE014	Tab, Film Coated	Dexchlorpheniramine Maleate 4 mg	by Zenith Goldline	00182-1014	Antihistamine
AMIDE014	Tab, Film Coated	Dexchlorpheniramine Maleate 4 mg	by Rugby	00536-3578	Antihistamine
AMIDE014	Tab, Film Coated	Dexchlorpheniramine Maleate 4 mg	by Qualitest	00603-3198	Antihistamine
AMIDE015	Tab, Film Coated	Dexchlorpheniramine Maleate 6 mg	by Zenith Goldline	00182-1015	Antihistamine
AMIDE015	Tab, Film Coated	Dexchlorpheniramine Maleate 6 mg	by Qualitest	00603-3199	Antihistamine
AMIDE015	Tab, Film Coated	Dexchlorpheniramine Maleate 6 mg	by Rugby	00536-3590	Antihistamine

ID FRONT <> BACK	DESCRIPTION FRONT <> BACK	INGREDIENT & STRENGTH	BRAND (OR EQUIV.) & FIRM	NDC#	CLASS; SCH.
AMIDE015	Tab, White, Oval, Film Coated	Dexchlorpheniramine Maleate 6 mg	Polaramine by Amide	52152-0015	Antihistamine
AMIDE019	Tab, Yellow, Round, Film Coated	Salsalate 500 mg	Disalcid by Geneva	00781-1108	NSAID
AMIDE020	Tab, Yellow, Cap-Shaped, Scored, Film Coated	Salsalate 750 mg	Disalcid by Geneva	00781-1109	NSAID
AMIDE022	Tab, Yellow, Oval	Prenatal Vitamins, Beta-Carotene	Stuartnatal by Amide		Vitamin
AMIDE024	Tab	Guaifenesin 300 mg, Phenylephrine HCl 20 mg	Quindal by Qualitest	00603-5571	Cold Remedy
AMIDE024	Tab, White, Cap Shaped	Guaifenesin 300 mg, Phenylephrine HCl 20 mg	Amidal by Amide	52152-0024	Cold Remedy
AMIDE025	Tab, Green, Cap Shaped	Chlorzoxazone 500 mg	Parafon Forte by Amide	52152-0025	Muscle Relaxant
AMIDE026	Tab, Orange & Pink & Purple, Round	Multivitamin, Fluoride DF 1 mg	Poly-Vi-Flor by Amide		Vitamin
AMIDE032	Tab, White, Round	Yohimbine HCl 5.4 mg	Yocon by Amide	52152-0032	Impotence Agent
AMIDE032	Tab	Yohimbine HCl 5.4 mg	by Amide	52152-0032	Impotence Agent
AMIDE035	Tab, White, Round	Theophylline 130 mg, Ephedrine HCl 24 mg, Phenobarbital 8 mg	Tedral by Amide		Antiasthmatic
AMIDE039	Cap	Acetaminophen 325 mg, Dichloralantipyrine 100 mg, Isometheptene Mucate 65 mg	Migquin by Qualitest	00603-4664	Cold Remedy
AMIDE039	Cap, Maroon or Red & White	Acetaminophen 325 mg, Dichloralantipyrine 100 mg, Isometheptene Mucate 65 mg	Midrin by Amide	52152-0039	Cold Remedy
AMIDE039 <> A039	Cap, Red & White, Amide 039 <> A-039	Sodium Fluoride 2.2 mg	Amidrine by Allscripts	54569-2871	Element
AMIDE043	Tab, Coated	Ascorbic Acid 120 mg, Calcium 200 mg, Copper 2 mg, Cyanocobalamin 12 mcg, Folic Acid 1 mg, Iron 65 mg, Niacinamide 20 mg, Pyridoxine HCl 10 mg, Riboflavin 3 mg, Thiamine Mononitrate 1.5 mg, Vitamin A Acetate 4000 Units, Vitamin E Acetate 11 Units, Zinc 25 mg	Prenatal 1 Plus 1 by Zenith Goldline	00182-4457	Vitamin
AMIDE043	Tab, Yellow, Oval	Vitamin, Minerals	Stuartnatal 1+1 by Amide		Vitamin
AMIDE045	Tab, Coated	Ascorbic Acid 80 mg, Beta-Carotene, Biotin 0.03 mg, Calcium Carbonate, Calcium Pantothenate, Cupric Oxide, Cyanocobalamin 2.5 mcg, Ergocalciferol, Ferrous Fumarate, Folic Acid 1 mg, Magnesium Hydroxide, Niacinamide, Pyridoxine HCl 4 mg, Riboflavin 1.6 mg, Thiamine Mononitrate 1.5 mg, Vitamin A Acetate, Vitamin E Acetate, Zinc Oxide	Prenatal Rx by Zenith Goldline	00182-4456	Vitamin
AMIDE046	Tab, Tan, Oblong, Scored	Chlorpheniramine Tannate 8 mg, Phenylephrine Tannate 25 mg, Pyrilamine Tannate 25 mg	Tri Tannate by Compumed		Cold Remedy
AMIDE046	Tab, Buff, Oblong	Phenylephrine 25 mg, Chlorpheniramine 8 mg, Pyrilamine 25 mg	Rynatan by Amide		Cold Remedy
AMIDE053	Tab	Chlorzoxazone 250 mg	by Zenith Goldline	00182-1780	Muscle Relaxant
AMIDE053	Tab, Peach, Round	Chlorzoxazone 250 mg	Para-Flex by Amide	52152-0053	Muscle Relaxant
AMIDE074	Tab, Pink, Round	Phenindamine 24 mg, Chlorpheniramine 4 mg, Phenylpropanolamine 50 mg	Nolamine by Amide		Cold Remedy
AMIDE076	Tab, Coated	Ascorbic Acid 500 mg, Calcium Pantothenate 18 mg, Cyanocobalamin 5 mcg, Folic Acid 0.5 mg, Niacinamide 100 mg, Pyridoxine HCl 4 mg, Riboflavin 15 mg, Thiamine Mononitrate 15 mg	B Plex by Zenith Goldline	00182-4062	Vitamin
AMIDE077	Tab, Coated	Ascorbic Acid 500 mg, Biotin 0.15 mg, Chromic Nitrate 0.1 mg, Cupric Oxide, Cyanocobalamin 50 mcg, Ferrous Fumarate 27 mg, Folic Acid 0.8 mg, Magnesium Oxide 50 mg, Manganese Dioxide 5 mg, Niacin 100 mg, Pantothenic Acid 25 mg, Pyridoxine HCl 25 mg, Riboflavin 20 mg, Thiamine Mononitrate 20 mg, Vitamin A Acetate 5000 Units, Vitamin E Acetate 30 Units	B Plex Plus by Zenith Goldline	00182-4064	Vitamin
AMIDE077	Tab, Mustard, Oval, Film Coated	Ascorbic Acid 500 mg, Biotin 0.15 mg, Chromic Nitrate 0.1 mg, Cupric Oxide, Cyanocobalamin 50 mcg, Ferrous Fumarate 27 mg, Folic Acid 0.8 mg, Magnesium Oxide 50 mg, Manganese Dioxide 5 mg, Niacin 100 mg, Pantothenic Acid 25 mg, Pyridoxine HCl 25 mg, Riboflavin 20 mg, Thiamine Mononitrate 20 mg, Vitamin A Acetate 5000 Units, Vitamin E Acetate 30 Units	Berroca Plus by Geneva	00781-1102	Vitamin
AMIDE078	Cap	Ascorbic Acid 150 mg, Calcium Pantothenate 10 mg, Cyanocobalamin 10 mcg, Folic Acid 1 mg, Magnesium Sulfate 70 mg, Manganese Chloride 4 mg, Niacinamide 25 mg, Pyridoxine HCl 2 mg, Riboflavin 5 mg, Thiamine Mononitrate 10 mg, Vitamin A 8000 Units, Vitamin E 50 Units, Zinc Sulfate 80 mg	Vica-Forte by Qualitest	00603-6381	Vitamin
AMIDE078	Cap, Black & Orange	Ascorbic Acid 150 mg, Calcium Pantothenate 10 mg, Cyanocobalamin 10 mcg, Folic Acid 1 mg, Magnesium Sulfate 70 mg, Manganese Chloride 4 mg, Niacinamide 25 mg, Pyridoxine HCl 2 mg, Riboflavin 5 mg, Thiamine Mononitrate 10 mg, Vitamin A 8000 Units, Vitamin E 50 Units, Zinc Sulfate 80 mg	Vicon Forte by Amide	52152-0078	Vitamin
AMIDE082	Cap, Blue	Cyclandelate 200 mg	Cyclospasmol by Amide		Vasodilator

ID FRONT <> BACK	DESCRIPTION FRONT <> BACK	INGREDIENT & STRENGTH	BRAND (OR EQUIV.) & FIRM	NDC#	CLASS; SCH.
AMIDE083	Cap, Blue & Red	Cyclandelate 400 mg	Cyclospasmol by Amide		Vasodilator
AMIDE084	Tab, Film Coated	Salicylate 500 mg	Choline Magnesium Trisalicylate by Zenith Goldline	00182-1899	NSAID
AMIDE084	Tab, Peach, Cap-Shaped, Film Coated	Salicylate 500 mg	Choline Magnesium Trisalicylate by Amide	52152-0084	NSAID
AMIDE085	Tab, Film Coated	Salicylate 750 mg	Choline Magnesium Trisalicylate by Zenith Goldline	00182-1895	NSAID
AMIDE085	Tab, White, Cap-Shaped, Film Coated	Salicylate 750 mg	Choline Magnesium Trisalicylate by Amide	52152-0085	NSAID
AMO	Tab, Film Coated, A Over MO	Metoprolol Succinate 47.5 mg	Toprol XL by Physicians Total Care	54868-3587	Antihypertensive
AMO	Tab, Film Coated, A Over MO	Metoprolol Succinate 47.5 mg	Toprol XL by Astra AB	17228-0109	Antihypertensive
AMO	Tab, White, Round, Convex, Scored, Film, A Over MO	Metoprolol Succinate 50 mg	Toprol XL by Neuman Distr	64579-0058	Antihypertensive
AMO	Tab, White, Round, Film Coated	Metoprolol Succinate 50 mg	Toprol XL by Astra	00186-1090	Antihypertensive
AMOX500	Cap, Yellow	Amoxicillin 500 mg	by Mova Pharms	55370-0920	Antibiotic
AMOX500 <> BC	Cap	Amoxicillin 500 mg, Amoxicillin Trihydrate 574 mg	by Biochemie	43858-0355	Antibiotic
AMOXIL <> 125	Tab, Pink, Oval	Amoxicillin 125 mg	Amoxil Chewable by Barr	00555-0727	Antibiotic
AMOXIL <> 125	Tab, Chew	Amoxicillin Trihydrate	by Quality Care	60346-0100	Antibiotic
AMOXIL <> 250	Tab, Chew	Amoxicillin Trihydrate	by Quality Care	60346-0450	Antibiotic
AMOXIL <> 250	Tab, Chewable	Amoxicillin Trihydrate	by Allscripts	54569-0097	Antibiotic
AMOXIL <> 250	Tab, Pink, Oval	Amoxicillin Trihydrate 250 mg	Amoxil Chewable by Bayer	00280-1060	Antibiotic
AMOXIL125	Tab, Pink, Oval	Amoxicillin 125 mg	Amoxil by SKB	00029-6004	Antibiotic
AMOXIL125	Tab, Chewable	Amoxicillin Trihydrate	by Pharmedix	53002-0283	Antibiotic
AMOXIL125	Tab, Rose, Oval, Amoxil/125	Amoxicillin Trihydrate 250 mg	Amoxil by Wyeth-Ayerst	Canadian	Antibiotic
AMOXIL200	Tab, Pale Pink, Round	Amoxicillin 200 mg	Amoxil by SKB	00029-6044	Antibiotic
AMOXIL250	Tab, Pink, Oval	Amoxicillin 250 mg	Amoxil by SKB	00029-6005	Antibiotic
AMOXIL250	Cap, Royal Blue	Amoxicillin 250 mg	Amoxil by SKB	00029-6006	Antibiotic
AMOXIL250	Tab, Rose, Oval, Amoxil/250	Amoxicillin Trihydrate 250 mg	by Wyeth-Ayerst	Canadian	Antibiotic
AMOXIL250	Cap	Amoxicillin Trihydrate	by Urgent Care Ctr	50716-0606	Antibiotic
AMOXIL400	Tab, Pale Pink, Round	Amoxicillin 400 mg	Amoxil by SKB	00029-6045	Antibiotic
AMOXIL500	Cap, Royal Blue	Amoxicillin 500 mg	Amoxil by SKB	00029-6007	Antibiotic
AMOXIL500	Tab, Pink, Cap Shaped, Amoxil over 500	Amoxicillin 500 mg	Amoxil by SKB	00029-6046	Antibiotic
AMOXIL875	Tab, Pink, Cap Shaped, Amoxil over 875	Amoxicillin 875 mg	Amoxil by SKB	00029-6047	Antibiotic
AMOXIL875	Tab, Coated, Amoxil over 875	Amoxicillin 875 mg	by SKB	00029-6047	Antibiotic
AMOXILR <> 250	Cap, Navy Blue, Amoxil <>	Amoxicillin 250 mg	by Quality Care	60346-0655	Antibiotic
AMP <> 250	Cap, Light Blue & White	Ampicillin Trihydrate 250 mg	by Teva	00093-5145	Antibiotic
AMP <> 500	Cap, Light Blue & White	Ampicillin Trihydrate 500 mg	by Teva	00093-5146	Antibiotic
AMP250	Cap, Blue & Gray	Ampicillin Trihydrate 250 mg	by Par Pharm	49884-0627	Antibiotic
AMP250	Cap, Opaque Blue & White	Ampicillin 250 mg	Ampicillin Trihyd by Bertek	62794-0027	Antibiotic
AMP250	Cap, Light Blue & White	Ampicillin 250 mg	by Allscripts	54569-1719	Antibiotic
AMP500	Cap, Blue & White	Ampicillin Trihydrate 500 mg	by Par Pharm	49884-0628	Antibiotic
AMP500	Cap, Light Blue & White, Opaque	Ampicillin 500 mg	by Allscripts	54569-2411	Antibiotic
AMP500	Cap, Opaque Blue & White	Ampicillin 500 mg	Ampicillin Trihyd by Bertek	62794-0072	Antibiotic
AMPHOJEL	Tab, White	Aluminum Hydroxide 600 mg	Amphojel by Axcan Pharma	Canadian	Gastrointestinal
AMPHOJEL PLUS	Tab, White	Aluminum Hydroxide 300 mg, Magnesium Carbonate 300 mg	Amphojel Plus by Axcan Pharma	Canadian	Gastrointestinal
AMPI250 <> BC	Cap	Ampicillin Trihydrate 288.7 mg	by Biochemie	43858-0282	Antibiotic
AMPI500 <> BC	Cap	Ampicillin Trihydrate	by Biochemie	43858-0285	Antibiotic
AMPM	Tab, AM over PM	Guaifenesin 500 mg, Pseudoephedrine HCl 120 mg	V Dec M by Pharmafab	62542-0901	Cold Remedy
AMPM	Tab, AM over PM	Guaifenesin 500 mg, Pseudoephedrine HCl 120 mg	V Dec M by Seatrace	00551-0170	Cold Remedy
AMS	Tab, White, Round, Film Coated	Metoprolol Succinate 100 mg	Toprol-XL by AstraZeneca	00186-1092	Antihypertensive
AMS	Tab, Film Coated, A Over MS	Metoprolol Succinate 95 mg	Toprol XL by Astra AB	17228-0110	Antihypertensive
AMX250	Cap, Orange & Peach	Amoxicillin 250 mg	by Barr	00555-0732	Antibiotic
AMX250	Cap, Yellow, Hard Shell	Amoxicillin 250 mg	Amoxil by Geneva	00781-2020	Antibiotic

ID FRONT <> BACK	DESCRIPTION FRONT <> BACK	INGREDIENT & STRENGTH	BRAND (OR EQUIV.) & FIRM	NDC#	CLASS; SCH.
AMX500	Cap, Yellow, Hard Shell	Amoxicillin 500 mg	Amoxil by Geneva	00781-2613	Antibiotic
AMX500	Cap, Orange & White	Amoxicillin 500 mg	by Barr	00555-0733	Antibiotic
AMY	Tab, Film Coated, A Over MY	Metoprolol Succinate 190 mg	Toprol XL by Caremark	00339-5782	Antihypertensive
AMY	Tab, Film Coated, A Over MY	Metoprolol Succinate 190 mg	Toprol XL by Astra	59252-0111	Antihypertensive
AMY	Tab, Film Coated, A Over MY	Metoprolol Succinate 190 mg	Toprol XL by Astra AB	17228-0111	Antihypertensive
AMY	Tab, White, Round, Film Coated	Metoprolol Succinate 200 mg	Toprol-XL by AstraZeneca	00186-1094	Antihypertensive
AN	Tab, White, Round, Scored	Clorazepate Dipotassium 15 mg	by Novopharm	55953-0983	Antianxiety; C IV
AN	Tab	Clorazepate Dipotassium 15 mg	by Quality Care	60346-0549	Antianxiety; C IV
AN	Tab, White, Round, Scored	Clorazepate Dipotassium 15 mg	Tranxene by Able Lab	53265-0050	Antianxiety; C IV
AN	Tab	Clorazepate Dipotassium 15 mg	by Geneva	00781-1867	Antianxiety; C IV
AN	Tab, White, Scored	Clorazepate Dipotassium 15 mg	Clorazepate Dipotassium by DHHS Prog	11819-0149	Antianxiety; C IV
AN	Tab, White, Round	Clorazepate Dipotassium 15 mg	by Novopharm	43806-0983	Antianxiety; C IV
AN	Tab, White, Round, Abbott Logo	Dicumarol 25 mg	by Abbott	00074-3794	Anticoagulant
AN25	Tab, White, Round, AN over 25 <> Abbott Logo	Dicumarol 25 mg	by Abbott	00074-3794	Anticoagulant
ANA	Tab, Yellow, Round, Schering Logo ANA	Perphenazine 2 mg, Amitriptyline HCl 10 mg	Etrafon by Schering		Antipsychotic; Antidepressant
ANACIN	Tab, White	Aspirin 325 mg, Caffeine 32 mg	by Whitehall-Robins	Canadian	Analgesic
ANACIN	Cap, White	Aspirin 325 mg, Caffeine 32 mg	by Whitehall-Robins	Canadian	Analgesic
ANACIN500	Tab, White	Aspirin 500 mg, Caffeine 32 mg	Anacin by Whitehall-Robbins	Canadian	Analgesic
ANACIN500	Cap, White	Aspirin 500 mg, Caffeine 32 mg	Anacin by Whitehall-Robbins	Canadian	Analgesic
ANAFRANIL50MG	Cap	Clomipramine HCl 50 mg	Anafranil by Pharm Utilization	60491-0035	OCD
ANAMINE1234	Cap, Black Print	Chlorpheniramine Maleate 8 mg, Pseudoephedrine HCl 120 mg	Anamine TD by Merz	00259-1234	Cold Remedy
ANANDRON100	Tab, White, Biconvex, Anandron/100	Nilutamide 100 mg	Anandron by Hoechst-Roussel	Canadian	Antiandrogen
ANANDRON50	Tab, White, Biconvex, Anandron/50	Nilutamide 50 mg	Anandron by Hoechst-Roussel	Canadian	Antiandrogen
ANAPROX <> ROCHE	Tab, Film Coated	Naproxen Sodium 275 mg	Anaprox by HJ Harkins Co	52959-0015	NSAID
ANAPROXDS	Tab, Film Coated	Naproxen Sodium 550 mg	Anaprox DS by Amerisource	62584-0276	NSAID
ANAPROXDS <> ROCHE	Tab, Dark Blue, Film Coated	Naproxen Sodium 550 mg	Anaprox DS by HJ Harkins Co	52959-0016	NSAID
ANAPROXDS <> ROCHE	Tab, Dark Blue, Film Coated	Naproxen Sodium 550 mg	Anaprox DS by Syntex	18393-0276	NSAID
ANAPROXDS <> ROCHE	Tab, Dark Blue, Film Coated, Debossed	Naproxen Sodium 550 mg	Anaprox DS by Thrift Drug	59198-0244	NSAID
ANAPROXDS <> ROCHE	Tab, Film Coated	Naproxen Sodium 550 mg	Anaprox DS by Quality Care	60346-0035	NSAID
ANAPROXDS <> ROCHE	Tab, Film Coated	Naproxen Sodium 550 mg	Anaprox DS by Nat Pharmpak Serv	55154-3805	NSAID
ANAPROXDS <> ROCHE	Tab, Blue, Oblong	Naproxen Sodium 550 mg	Anaprox DS by Rightpak	65240-0603	NSAID
ANAPROXDS <> ROCHE	Tab, Blue, Oblong	Naproxen Sodium 550 mg	Anaprox DS by Med-Pro	53978-3369	NSAID
ANAPROXDS <> ROCHE	Tab, Film Coated	Naproxen Sodium 550 mg	Anaprox DS by Allscripts	54569-1763	NSAID
ANAPROXDS <> SYNTEX	Tab, Film Coated	Naproxen Sodium 550 mg	Anaprox DS by Quality Care	60346-0035	NSAID
ANB	Tab, Orange, Round, Schering Logo ANB	Perphenazine 4 mg, Amitriptyline HCl 10 mg	Etrafon-A by Schering		Antipsychotic; Antidepressant
ANC	Tab, Pink, Round, Schering Logo ANC	Perphenazine 2 mg, Amitriptyline HCl 25 mg	Etrafon by Schering		Antipsychotic; Antidepressant
ANDRX510 <> 100MG	Cap, White, Opaque	Ketoprofen ER 100 mg	Ketoprofen by Andrx	62037-0510	NSAID
ANDRX515 <> 150MG	Cap, Light Turquoise & White, Opaque	Ketoprofen ER 150 mg	Ketoprofen by Andrx	62037-0515	NSAID
ANDRX520 <> 200MG	Cap, Light Turquoise	Ketoprofen ER 200 mg	Ketoprofen by Andrx	62037-0520	NSAID

ID FRONT <> BACK	DESCRIPTION FRONT <> BACK	INGREDIENT & STRENGTH	BRAND (OR EQUIV.) & FIRM	NDC#	CLASS; SCH.
ANDRX548	Cap, White	Diltiazem HCl 120 mg	Diltia XT by Andrx	62037-0548	Antihypertensive
ANDRX548 <> 120MG	Cap, White	Diltiazem HCl 120 mg	Diltia XT by F Hoffmann La Roche	12783-0060	Antihypertensive
ANDRX549	Cap, Gray & White	Diltiazem HCl 180 mg	Diltia XT by Andrx	62037-0549	Antihypertensive
ANDRX549 <> 180MG	Cap, Gray & White	Diltiazem HCl 180 mg	Diltia XT by F Hoffmann La Roche	12806-0800	Antihypertensive
ANDRX549 <> 180MG	Cap, Gray & White	Diltiazem HCl 180 mg	by Kaiser Fdn	00179-1375	Antihypertensive
ANDRX550	Cap, Gray	Diltiazem HCl 240 mg	Diltia XT by Andrx	62037-0550	Antihypertensive
ANDRX550 <> 240MG	Cap, Gray	Diltiazem HCl 240 mg	Diltia XT by Faulding	50564-0507	Antihypertensive
ANDRX597	Cap, Orange & White	Diltiazem ER HCl 120 mg	Cartia XT by Andrx	62037-0597	Antihypertensive
ANDRX598	Cap, Orange & Yellow	Diltiazem ER HCl 180 mg	Cartia XT by Andrx	62037-0598	Antihypertensive
ANDRX598 <> 180MG	Cap, Yellow	Diltiazem HCl 180 mg	Cartia XT by Heartland Healthcare	61392-0958	Antihypertensive
ANDRX599	Cap, Brown & Orange	Diltiazem ER HCl 240 mg	Cartia XT by Andrx	62037-0599	Antihypertensive
ANDRX600	Cap, Orange	Diltiazem ER HCl 300 mg	Cartia XT by Andrx	62037-0600	Antihypertensive
ANDRX687 <> 120	Cap, White	Diltiazem HCl 120 mg	Cartia XT by Heartland Healthcare	61392-0957	Antihypertensive
ANDRX699 <> 240MG	Cap, Brown	Diltiazem HCl 240 mg	Cartia XT by Heartland Healthcare	61392-0959	Antihypertensive
ANE	Tab, Yellow, Oblong	Niacin 500 mg	Nicolar by RPR		Vitamin
ANE	Tab, Red, Round, Schering Logo ANE	Perphenazine 4 mg, Amitriptyline HCl 25 mg	Etrafon-Forte by Schering		Antipsychotic; Antidepressant
ANEXSIA <> 5363	Tab	Acetaminophen 660 mg, Hydrocodone Bitartrate 10 mg	Anexsia by Mallinckrodt Hobart	00406-5363	Analgesic; C III
ANEXSIA <> MPC188	Tab	Acetaminophen 650 mg, Hydrocodone Bitartrate 7.5 mg	Anexsia by Nat Pharmpak Serv	55154-7101	Analgesic; C III
ANEXSIA <> MPC188	Tab	Acetaminophen 650 mg, Hydrocodone Bitartrate 7.5 mg	Anexsia by King	60793-0843	Analgesic; C III
ANEXSIA <> MPC188	Tab	Acetaminophen 650 mg, Hydrocodone Bitartrate 7.5 mg	Anexsia by Mallinckrodt Hobart	00406-5362	Analgesic; C III
ANEXSIA <> MPC188	Tab	Acetaminophen 650 mg, Hydrocodone Bitartrate 7.5 mg	Anexsia by Med Pro	53978-3309	Analgesic; C III
ANEXSIA <> MPC207	Tab	Acetaminophen 500 mg, Hydrocodone Bitartrate 5 mg	Anexsia 5/500 by King	60793-0842	Analgesic; C III
ANEXSIA <> MPC207	Tab	Acetaminophen 500 mg, Hydrocodone Bitartrate 5 mg	Anexsia by Mallinckrodt Hobart	00406-5361	Analgesic; C III
ANK	Tab, Pink, Round, Schering Logo ANK	Anisindione 50 mg	Miradon by Schering	00085-0795	Anticoagulant
ANR	Tab, Peach, Oval	Divalproex Sodium 250 mg	Depakote by Allscripts	54569-0261	Anticonvulsant
ANSAID	Tab, Blue, Elliptical, Film Coated, Ansaid Logo	Flurbiprofen 100 mg	by Pharmacia	Canadian DIN# 00600792	NSAID
ANSAID	Tab, White, Elliptical, Film Coated, Ansaid Logo	Flurbiprofen 50 mg	by Pharmacia	Canadian DIN# 00647942	NSAID
ANSAID <> 100MG	Tab, Coated, 100 mg	Flurbiprofen 100 mg	Ansaid by Quality Care	60346-0099	NSAID
ANSAID100MG	Tab, Coated	Flurbiprofen 100 mg	Ansaid by Amerisource	62584-0305	NSAID
ANSAID100MG	Tab, Blue, Oval	Flurbiprofen 100 mg	Ansaid by Med-Pro	53978-3379	NSAID
ANSAID100MG	Tab, Coated	Flurbiprofen 100 mg	Ansaid by Leiner	59606-0604	NSAID
ANSAID100MG	Tab, Coated	Flurbiprofen 100 mg	Ansaid by Pharmacia & Upjohn	00009-0305	NSAID
ANSAID100MG	Tab, Light Blue, Coated	Flurbiprofen 100 mg	Ansaid by Thrift Drug	59198-0125	NSAID
ANSAID100MG	Tab, Coated	Flurbiprofen 100 mg	Ansaid by Allscripts	54569-2413	NSAID
ANSAID100MG <> ANSAID100MG	Tab, Blue, Oval, Film Coated	Flurbiprofen 100 mg	Ansaid by Invamed	52189-0393	NSAID
ANTIVERT <> 210	Tab, Turquoise	Meclizine HCl 12.5 mg	Antivert by Roerig Pfizer	00662-2100	Antiemetic
ANTIVERT <> 211	Tab, White & Yellow, Oval	Meclizine HCl 25 mg	Antivert by Rightpak	65240-0605	Antiemetic
ANTIVERT <> 211	Tab, Layered	Meclizine HCl 25 mg	Antivert by Roerig Pfizer	00662-2110	Antiemetic
ANTIVERT210	Tab, Blue, Oval	Meclizine HCl 12.5 mg	Antivert by Rightpak	65240-0659	Antiemetic
ANZEMET <> 100	Tab, Pink, Oval, Film Coated	Dolasetron Mesylate Monohydrate 100 mg	Anzemet by Hoechst Roussel	00088-1203	Antiemetic
ANZEMET100	Tab, Pink, Oval, Anzemet/100	Dolasetron Mesylate Monohydrate 100 mg	Anzemet by Hoechst Marion Roussel	Canadian	Antiemetic
ANZEMET50	Tab, Light Pink, Round, Anzemet/50	Dolasetron Mesylate Monohydrate 50 mg	Anzemet by Hoechst Marion Roussel	Canadian	Antiemetic
ANZEMET50	Tab, Light Pink, Round, Film Coated	Dolasetron Mesylate Monohydrate 50 mg	Anzemet by Hoechst Roussel	00088-1202	Antiemetic
ANZEMET50	Tab, Film Coated	Dolasetron Mesylate Monohydrate 50 mg	Anzemet by Merrell	00068-1202	Antiemetic
AO	Tab, Pink, Round, Abbott Logo	Dicumarol 50 mg	by Abbott		Anticoagulant
AO <> 20	Tab, Coated	Salsalate 750 mg	by Quality Care	60346-0034	NSAID

ID FRONT <> BACK	DESCRIPTION FRONT <> BACK	INGREDIENT & STRENGTH	BRAND (OR EQUIV.) & FIRM	NDC#	CLASS; SCH.
AO58	Tab, Ex Release, AO Over 58	Guaifenesin 400 mg, Phenylpropanolamine HCl 75 mg	Enomine LA by Quality Care	60346-0339	Cold Remedy
AP <> 110	Tab, Light Blue, Cap Shaped, A/P Debossed	Acetaminophen 650 mg, Butalbital 50 mg	Cephadyn by Atley	59702-0650	Analgesic
AP <> 7045	Tab, Slightly Mottled	Captopril 12.5 mg	by Apothecon	59772-7045	Antihypertensive
AP <> 7045	Tab, Scored	Captopril 12.5 mg	by Nat Pharmpak Serv	55154-7601	Antihypertensive
AP <> 7045	Tab	Captopril 12.5 mg	by Bristol Myers	15548-0045	Antihypertensive
AP <> 8818	Tab	Buspirone HCl 5 mg	by Apothecon	59772-8818	Antianxiety
AP <> 8819	Tab	Buspirone HCl 10 mg	by Apothecon	59772-8819	Antianxiety
AP <> ALOR5	Tab, A Bisect P	Aspirin 500 mg, Hydrocodone Bitartrate 5 mg	Alor 5 500 by Atley	59702-0550	Analgesic; C III
AP <> SUDAL60	Tab, White, Cap Shaped, Ex Release	Guaifenesin 500 mg, Pseudoephedrine HCl 60 mg	Sudal by Atley	59702-0060	Cold Remedy
AP <> SUDAL60	Tab, A over P <> Sudal 60	Guaifenesin 500 mg, Pseudoephedrine HCl 60 mg	Sudal by Anabolic	00722-6395	Cold Remedy
AP <> SUDAL60	Tab, White, Oblong, Scored, A over P <> Sudal 60	Guaifenesin 500 mg, Pseudoephedrine HCl 60 mg	GFN 500 PSEH 60 by Martec		Cold Remedy
AP <> SUDALDM	Tab, White, Oblong, Scored, A over P <> Sudal DM	Guaifenesin 500 mg, Dextromethorphan Hydriodide 30 mg	GFN 500 DTMH 30 by Martec		Cold Remedy
AP025	Tab, White, Round	Estradiol 0.5 mg	Estrace by BMS		Hormone
AP026	Tab, Lavender, Round	Estradiol 1 mg	Estrace by BMS		Hormone
AP027	Tab, Turquoise, Round	Estradiol 2 mg	Estrace by BMS		Hormone
AP0812	Tab, Light Orange, Round, Film Coated	Doxycycline Hyclate 100 mg	by Mutual	53489-0120	Antibiotic
AP0812	Tab, Film Coated	Doxycycline Hyclate	by Apothecon	59772-0803	Antibiotic
AP0812	Tab, Film Coated	Doxycycline Hyclate	by ER Squibb	00003-0812	Antibiotic
AP0814	Cap, Light Blue,Opaque	Doxycycline Hyclate 100 mg	by Mutual	53489-0119	Antibiotic
AP0814	Cap	Doxycycline Hyclate	by Apothecon	59772-0940	Antibiotic
AP0814 <> AP0814	Cap	Doxycycline Hyclate	by ER Squibb	00003-0814	Antibiotic
AP0837	Cap, Blue & White	Doxycycline Hyclate 50 mg	by ER Squibb	00003-8708	Antibiotic
AP0837	Cap, Light Blue & White, Opaque	Doxycycline Hyclate 50 mg	by Mutual	53489-0118	Antibiotic
AP0837	Cap	Doxycycline Hyclate	by Apothecon	59772-0808	Antibiotic
AP0837 <> 879525	Cap	Doxycycline Hyclate	by Rachelle	00196-0552	Antibiotic
AP1	Tab, Sugar Coated	Phenazopyridine HCl 100 mg	by Superior	00144-1105	Urinary Analgesic
AP1	Tab, Sugar Coated	Phenazopyridine HCl 100 mg	by Schein	00364-0286	Urinary Analgesic
AP1	Tab, Maroon, Round, Sugar Coated	Phenazopyridine HCl 100 mg	Pyridium by Able	53265-0196	Urinary Analgesic
AP1	Tab, Sugar Coated	Phenazopyridine HCl 100 mg	by Alphagen	59743-0013	Urinary Analgesic
AP2	Tab, Deep Maroon, Round, Coated	Phenazopyridine 200 mg	by Allscripts	54569-0797	Urinary Analgesic
AP2	Tab, Deep Maroon, Round, Film Coated	Phenazopyridine HCl 200 mg	by Allscripts	54569-0197	Urinary Analgesic
AP2	Tab, Sugar Coated	Phenazopyridine HCl 200 mg	by Schein	00364-0321	Urinary Analgesic
AP2	Tab, Sugar Coated	Phenazopyridine HCl 200 mg	by Superior	00144-1210	Urinary Analgesic
AP2	Tab, Maroon, Round, Sugar Coated	Phenazopyridine HCl 200 mg	Pyridium by Able	53265-0197	Urinary Analgesic
AP2	Tab, Sugar Coated	Phenazopyridine HCl 200 mg	by Alphagen	59743-0014	Urinary Analgesic
AP2461	Tab	Nadolol 20 mg	Nadolol by Apothecon	59772-2461	Antihypertensive
AP2462	Tab, AP Over 2462	Nadolol 40 mg	Nadolol by Mead Johnson	00015-2462	Antihypertensive
AP2462	Tab	Nadolol 40 mg	Nadolol by Apothecon	59772-2462	Antihypertensive
AP2463	Tab	Nadolol 80 mg	Nadolol by Apothecon	59772-2463	Antihypertensive
AP2464	Tab	Nadolol 120 mg	Nadolol by Apothecon	59772-2464	Antihypertensive
AP2465	Tab	Nadolol 160 mg	Nadolol by Apothecon	59772-2465	Antihypertensive
AP2472	Tab, White, Round	Nadolol 40 mg, Bendroflumethiazide 5 mg	Corzide by Apothecon		Antihypertensive
AP2472	Tab, White, Round	Nadolol 40 mg, Bendroflumethiazide 5 mg	by Apothecon	59772-2472	Antihypertensive
AP2473	Tab, White, Round	Nadolol 80 mg, Bendroflumethiazide 5 mg	Corzide by Apothecon		Antihypertensive
AP2473	Tab, White, Round	Nadolol 80 mg, Bendroflumethiazide 5 mg	by Apothecon	59772-2473	Antihypertensive
AP3171505050	Tab, White, Rectangular, AP 3171 50-50-50	Trazodone HCl 150 mg	Desyrel by BMS		Antidepressant
AP35	Cap, Red & Yellow	Docusate Sodium 240 mg	by Advance		Laxative
AP35	Cap, Red & Yellow	Docusate Sodium 250 mg	Modane Soft		Laxative
AP4165	Tab, White, Round	Acyclovir 400 mg	Zovirax by BMS		Antiviral
AP4166	Tab, White, Oblong	Acyclovir 800 mg	Zovirax by BMS		Antiviral
AP4168	Cap, Blue & White	Acyclovir 200 mg	Zovirax by BMS		Antiviral

ID FRONT <> BACK	DESCRIPTION FRONT <> BACK	INGREDIENT & STRENGTH	BRAND (OR EQUIV.) & FIRM	NDC#	CLASS; SCH.
AP5160	Tab, Mottled Orange & White, Square	Captopril 25 mg, Hydrochlorothiazide 15 mg	Capozide by ER Squibb	00003-0338	Antihypertensive; Diuretic
AP5161	Tab, Peach, Square	Captopril 25 mg, Hydrochlorothiazide 25 mg	Capozide by ER Squibb	00003-0349	Antihypertensive; Diuretic
AP5162	Tab, Mottled Orange & White, Square	Captopril 50 mg, Hydrochlorothiazide 15 mg	Capozide by ER Squibb	00003-0384	Antihypertensive; Diuretic
AP5163	Tab, Peach, Square	Captopril 50 mg, Hydrochlorothiazide 25 mg	Capozide by ER Squibb	00003-0390	Antihypertensive; Diuretic
AP6910	Tab, Orange, Round	Potassium Chloride 10 mEq	K-Tab by BMS		Electrolytes
AP7045	Tab	Captopril 12.5 mg	by Med Pro	53978-0939	Antihypertensive
AP7046	Tab	Captopril 25 mg	by Nat Pharmpak Serv	55154-7602	Antihypertensive
AP7046	Tab, Slightly Mottled	Captopril 25 mg	by Apothecon	59772-7046	Antihypertensive
AP7046	Tab, White, Round, Scored	Captopril 25 mg	by Southwood Pharms	58016-0166	Antihypertensive
AP7046	Tab, White, Round, Scored	Captopril 25 mg	by Caremark	00339-5877	Antihypertensive
AP7046	Tab	Captopril 25 mg	by Allscripts	54569-4246	Antihypertensive
AP7046	Tab	Captopril 25 mg	by Med Pro	53978-0236	Antihypertensive
AP7046	Tab	Captopril 25 mg	by Bristol Myers	15548-0046	Antihypertensive
AP7047	Tab	Captopril 50 mg	by Murfreesboro	51129-1309	Antihypertensive
AP7047	Tab	Captopril 50 mg	by Bristol Myers	15548-0047	Antihypertensive
AP7047	Tab, Slightly Mottled	Captopril 50 mg	by Apothecon	59772-7047	Antihypertensive
AP7047	Tab, White, Round, Scored	Captopril 50 mg	by Southwood Pharms	58016-0165	Antihypertensive
AP7048	Tab, Slightly Mottled	Captopril 100 mg	by Apothecon	59772-7048	Antihypertensive
AP7048	Tab	Captopril 100 mg	by Bristol Myers	15548-0048	Antihypertensive
AP7491 <> 250	Cap	Cefaclor Monohydrate	by Apothecon	59772-7491	Antibiotic
AP7491 <> 250	Cap	Cefaclor Monohydrate	by Golden State	60429-0701	Antibiotic
AP7491250MG	Cap, Blue & White, AP 7491/250 mg	Cefaclor 250 mg	Ceclor by Apothecon		Antibiotic
AP7494 <> 500	Cap	Cefaclor Monohydrate	by Apothecon	59772-7494	Antibiotic
AP7494 <> 500	Cap	Cefaclor Monohydrate	by Golden State	60429-0702	Antibiotic
AP7494500MG	Cap, Blue & Gray, AP 7494/500 mg	Cefaclor 500 mg	Ceclor by Apothecon		Antibiotic
AP778	Tab, Orange, Rectangular	Trazodone HCl 150 mg	Dividose by Apothecon	59772-3171	Antidepressant
AP812	Tab, Beige, Round	Doxycycline Hyclate 100 mg	Vibramycin by BMS		Antibiotic
AP8819	Tab, White, Round	Buspirone HCl 10 mg	by Bristol-Myers		Antianxiety
AP908	Tab, White, Round	Selegiline 5 mg	Eldepryl by BMS		Antiparkinson
APCE	Tab, Pink Speckled, Abbott Logo	Erythromycin 333 mg	PCE by Quality Care	60346-0163	Antibiotic
APHRODYNE	Tab, Blue, Cap-Shaped	Yohimbine HCl 5.4 mg	Aphrodyne by Star	00076-0401	Impotence Agent
APISBULL <> NOVO288	Tab, White, Round, Film Coated	Estradiol 1 mg; Norethindrone Acetate 0.5 mg	Activella by Novo Nordisk	00420-5174	Hormone
APISBULL <> NOVO288	Tab, White, Round, Film Coated	Estradiol 1 mg; Norethindrone Acetate 0.5 mg	Activella by Pharmacia & Upjohn	00009-5174	Hormone
APO018	Tab, Green, Round	Cimetidine 200 mg	by Apotex	60505-0018	Gastrointestinal
APO019	Tab, Green, Round	Cimetidine 300 mg	by Apotex	60505-0019	Gastrointestinal
APO020	Tab, Green, Oval	Cimetidine 400 mg	by Apotex	60505-0020	Gastrointestinal
APO021	Tab, Green, Oval	Cimetidine 800 mg	by Apotex	60505-0021	Gastrointestinal
APO10	Cap, Black & Green	Chlordiazepoxide 10 mg	Chlordiazepoxide by Apotex	Canadian	Antianxiety
APO10	Cap, Gray & Green	Fluoxetine 10 mg	Fluoxetine by Apotex	Canadian	Antidepressant
APO100	Cap, Pale Blue	Doxycycline Hyclate 100 mg	Apo Doxy by Apotex	Canadian	Antibiotic
APO100	Cap, White	Fenofibrate 100 mg	Fenofibrate by Apotex	Canadian	Antihyperlipidemic
APO	Tab, Pink, Trapezoid	Fluconazole 100 mg	Fluconazole by Apotex	Canadian	Antifungal
APO100	Tab, White, Oval	Fluvoxamine Maleate 100 mg	Fluvoxamine by Apotex	Canadian	OCD
APO10MG	Tab, White, Ovoid, Scored	Cetirizine 10 mg	Cetirizine by Apotex	Canadian	Antihistamine
APO120	Cap, Light Turquoise	Diltiazem HCl 120 mg	Diltiaz CD by Apotex	Canadian	Antihypertensive
APO15	Cap, Ivory & Orange	Flurazepam HCl 15 mg	Apo Flurazepam by Apotex	Canadian	Hypnotic

ID FRONT <> BACK	DESCRIPTION FRONT <> BACK	INGREDIENT & STRENGTH	BRAND (OR EQUIV.) & FIRM	NDC#	CLASS; SCH.
APO 20	Cap, Green & Ivory	Fluoxetine 20 mg	Fluoxetine by Apotex	Canadian	Antidepressant
APO200	Tab, Blue, Round	Acyclovir 200 mg	Acyclovir by Apotex	Canadian	Antiviral
APO200	Cap, Dark Gray & Light Gray	Etodolac 200 mg	Etodolac by Apotex	Canadian	NSAID
APO240	Cap, Light Blue	Diltiazem HCl 240 mg	Diltiaz CD by Apotex	Canadian	Antihypertensive
APO25	Cap, Green & White	Chlordiazepoxide 25 mg	Chlordiazepoxide by Apotex	Canadian	Antianxiety
APO25	Cap, Blue & Pink	Doxepin HCl 25 mg	Apo Doxepin by Apotex	Canadian	Antidepressant
APO250	Cap, Purple & White	Cefaclor 250 mg	Cefaclor by Apotex	Canadian	Antibiotic
APO250	Cap, Black & Red	Ampicillin Trihydrate	Ampi by Apotex	Canadian	Antibiotic
APO250	Tab, White, Oval	Chlorpropamide 250 mg	Apo Chlorpropam by Apotex	Canadian	Antidiabetic
APO250	Cap, Clear & Orange	Erythromycin 250 mg	Apo Erythro E-C by Apotex	Canadian	Antibiotic
APO30	Cap, Ivory & Red	Flurazepam HCl 30 mg	Apo Flurazepam by Apotex	Canadian	Hypnotic
APO300	Cap, Light Gray	Etodolac 300 mg	Etodolac by Apotex	Canadian	NSAID
APO325	Tab, White, Round	Acetaminophen 325 mg	Acetaminophen by Apotex	Canadian	Antipyretic
APO333	Cap, Clear & Yellow	Erythromycin 333 mg	Erythro E-C by Apotex	Canadian	Antibiotic
APO333	Cap, Clear & Yellow	Erythromycin 333 mg	by Parke-Davis	Canadian	Antibiotic
APO40	Tab, Light Brown, D-Shaped	Famotidine 40 mg	Famotidine by Apotex	Canadian	Gastrointestinal
APO400	Tab, Pink, Round	Acyclovir 400 mg	Acyclovir by Apotex	Canadian	Antiviral
APO5	Cap, Caramel & White	Bromocriptine 5 mg	Bromocriptine by Apotex	Canadian	Antiparkinson
APO5	Cap, Green & Yellow	Chlordiazepoxide 5 mg	Chlordiazepoxide by Apotex	Canadian	Antianxiety
APO50	Tab, Pink, Trapezoid	Fluconazole 50 mg	Fluconazole by Apotex	Canadian	Antifungal
APO50	Tab, White, Round	Fluvoxamine Maleate 50 mg	Fluvoxamine by Apotex	Canadian	OCD
APO500	Cap, Black & Red	Ampicillin Trihydrate 500 mg	Ampli by Apotex	Canadian	Antibiotic
APO500	Cap, Gray & Purple	Cefaclor 500 mg	Cefaclor by Apotex	Canadian	Antibiotic
APO60	Cap, Chocolate Brown & Ivory	Diltiazem HCl 60 mg	Diltiaz SR by Apotex	Canadian	Antihypertensive
APO75	Tab, Pink, Triangular	Diclofenac Sodium 75 mg	Diclo SR by Apotex	Canadian	NSAID
APO800	Tab, Blue, Oval	Acyclovir 800 mg	Acyclovir by Apotex	Canadian	Antiviral
APO01	Tab, White, Round, APO/0.1	Clonidine HCl 0.1 mg	Apo Clonidine by Apotex	Canadian	Antihypertensive
APO016 <> APO016	Cap, Brown & White, Ex Release	Diltiazem HCl 240 mg	by Apotex	60505-0016	Antihypertensive
APO016 <> APO016	Cap, Ex Release	Diltiazem HCl 240 mg	by Torpharm	62318-0016	Antihypertensive
APO018	Tab, Green, Round, Film Coated, APO over 018	Cimetidine 200 mg	Cimetidine USP by Compumed	00403-1209	Gastrointestinal
APO019	Tab, Green, Round, Film Coated, APO over 019	Cimetidine 300 mg	Cimetidine USP by Compumed	00403-1312	Gastrointestinal
APO02	Tab, White, Round, APO/0.2	Clonidine HCl 0.2 mg	Apo Clonidine by Apotex	Canadian	Antihypertensive
APO020	Tab, Green, Oval, Film Coated	Cimetidine 400 mg	Cimetidine USP by Compumed	00403-1334	Gastrointestinal
APO021	Tab, Green, Oval, Film Coated	Cimetidine 800 mg	Cimetidine USP by Compumed	00403-1335	Gastrointestinal
APO025	Tab, White, Round, Film Coated	Ranitidine HCl 150 mg	by Apothecon	59772-6511	Gastrointestinal
APO025	Tab, Film Coated	Ranitidine HCl 150 mg	by Golden State	60429-0704	Gastrointestinal
APO025	Tab, Off-White to White, Film Coated	Ranitidine HCl 150 mg	by Torpharm	62318-0025	Gastrointestinal
APO025	Tab, White, Round, Film Coated	Ranitidine HCl 150 mg	by Zenith Goldline	00172-4357	Gastrointestinal
APO025	Tab, White, Round, Film Coated	Ranitidine HCl 150 mg	by Major Pharms	00904-5261	Gastrointestinal
APO025	Tab, Off-White, Round, Film Coated	Ranitidine HCl 150 mg	by Apotex	60505-0025	Gastrointestinal
APO025	Tab, Powder Blue, Oval, APO/0.25	Triazolam 0.25 mg	Apo Triazo by Apotex	Canadian	Sedative/Hypnotic
APO027	Tab, White, Oval, Convex, Film Coated	Ticlopidine HCl 250 mg	Ticlopidine HCl by Teva	00093-5146	Anticoagulant
APO027	Tab, White, Oval	Ticlopidine HCl 250 mg	by Apotex	60505-0027	Anticoagulant
APO033	Tab, White, Oval, Convex, Film Coated	Pentoxifylline 400 mg	Pentoxifylline ER by Pharmafab	62542-0744	Anticoagulent
APO033	Tab, White, Oval, Extended Release	Pentoxifylline 400 mg	by Apotex	60505-0033	Anticoagulent
APO034 <> 600	Tab, White, Oval, Coated	Gemfibrozil 600 mg	by Apotex	60505-0034	Antihyperlipidemic
APO034 <> 600	Tab, Coated	Gemfibrozil 600 mg	by Torpharm	62318-0034	Antihyperlipidemic
APO034 <> 600	Tab, White, Oval, Film Coated	Gemfibrozil 600 mg	by Major Pharms	00904-5379	Antihyperlipidemic
APO05	Tab, Peach, Oval, APO/0.5	Alprazolam 0.5 mg	Apo Alpraz by Apotex	Canadian	Antianxiety
APO05	Tab, White, Round, APO/0.5	Haloperidol 0.5 mg	Apo Haloperidol by Apotex	Canadian	Antipsychotic
APO05	Tab, White, Round, APO/0.5	Lorazepam 0.5 mg	Apo by Apotex	Canadian	Sedative/Hypnotic; C IV
APO055	Cap, Opaque Blue & White	Selegiline HCl 5 mg	Selegiline HCl by SB	59742-3159	Antiparkinson

ID FRONT <> BACK	DESCRIPTION FRONT <> BACK	INGREDIENT & STRENGTH	BRAND (OR EQUIV.) & FIRM	NDC#	CLASS; SCH.
APO055	Cap, Aqua Blue & White	Selegiline HCl 5 mg	by Apotex	60505-0055	Antiparkinson
APO1	Tab, Yellow, Round, APO/1	Haloperidol 1 mg	Apo Haloperidol by Apotex	Canadian	Antipsychotic
APO1	Cap, White	Lorazepam 1 mg	Apo by Apotex	Canadian	Sedative/Hypnotic
APO1	Tab, White, Round, APO/1	Prednisone 1 mg	by AltiMed	Canadian	Steroid
APO1	Tab, White, Round, APO/1	Prednisone 1 mg	Apo Prednisone by Apotex	Canadian	Steroid
APO10	Tab, Yellow, D-Shaped, APO/10	Cyclobenzaprine 10 mg	Cyclobenzaprine by Apotex	Canadian	Muscle Relaxant
APO10	Tab, Blue, Round, APO/10	Diazepam 10 mg	Apo Diazepam by Apotex	Canadian	Antianxiety
APO10	Tab, Blue, Round	Diazepam 10 mg	Valium by Apotex		Antianxiety; C IV
APO10	Tab, White, Round	Domperidone 10 mg	Domperidone by Apotex	Canadian	Gastrointestinal
APO10	Cap, Pink & Scarlet	Doxepin HCl 10 mg	Apo Doxepin by Apotex	Canadian	Antidepressant
APO10	Tab, Pale Yellow, Round, APO/10	Guanethidine Monosulfate 10 mg	Apo Guanethidine by Apotex	Canadian	Antihypertensive
APO10	Tab, Light Green, Round, APO/10	Haloperidol 10 mg	Apo Haloperidol by Apotex	Canadian	Antipsychotic
APO10	Tab, White, Round, APO/10	Isosorbide Dinitrate 10 mg	Apo Isdn by Apotex	Canadian	Antianginal
APO10	Tab, White, Round	Ketorolac 10 mg	Ketorolac by Apotex	Canadian	NSAID
APO10	Tab, Grayish Pink, Round	Nifedipine 10 mg	Nifed PA by Apotex	Canadian	Antihypertensive
APO10	Cap, Mustard	Nifedipine 10 mg	Apo Nifed by Apotex	Canadian	Antihypertensive
APO10	Cap, White & Yellow	Nortriptyline HCl 10 mg	Nortriptyline by Apotex	Canadian	Antidepressant
APO10	Tab, Yellow, Round, APO/10	Oxazepam 10 mg	Apo Oxazepam by Apotex	Canadian	Sedative/Hypnotic; C IV
APO10	Cap, Blue & Maroon	Piroxicam 10 mg	Apo Piroxicam by Apotex	Canadian	NSAID
APO10	Tab, Orange, Round, APO/10	Propranolol HCl 10 mg	Apo Propranolol by Apotex	Canadian	Antihypertensive
APO100	Tab, White, Round, APO/100	Acebutolol HCl 100 mg	Apo Acebutolol by Apotex	Canadian	Antihypertensive
APO100	Tab, White, Biconvex, APO/200	Allopurinol 100 mg	Apo Allopurinol by Apotex	Canadian	Antigout
APO100	Tab, White, Oval, APO/100	Captopril 100 mg	Apo Capto by Apotex	Canadian	Antihypertensive
APO100	Tab, White, Round, APO/100	Chlorpropamide 100 mg	Apo Chlorpropam by Apotex	Canadian	Antidiabetic
APO100	Tab, White, Round, APO/100	Chlorthalidone 100 mg	Apo Chlorthalidone by Apotex	Canadian	Diuretic
APO100	Tab, White, Round, APO/100	Diclofenac Sodium 100 mg	Apo Diclo SR by Apotex	Canadian	NSAID
APO100	Cap, Blue & Flesh	Doxepin HCl 100 mg	Apo Doxepin by Apotex	Canadian	Antidepressant
APO100	Tab, Blue, Oval, APO-100	Flurbiprofen 100 mg	Apo Flurbiprofen by Apotex	Canadian	NSAID
APO100	Tab, Pink, Round, APO/100	Hydrochlorothiazide 100 mg	Apo Hydro by Apotex	Canadian	Diuretic
APO100	Tab, Yellow, Round, APO/100	Ketoprofen 100 mg	Apo Keto-E by Apotex	Canadian	NSAID
APO100	Cap, Orange & Purple	Minocycline HCl 100 mg	Apo Minocycline by Apotex	Canadian	Antibiotic
APO100	Tab, Orange, Oval	Moclobemide 100 mg	Moclobemide by Apotex	Canadian	Antidepressant
APO100	Tab, Pink, Round, APO/100	Oxtriphylline 100 mg	Apo Oxtriphylline by Apotex	Canadian	Antiasthmatic
APO100	Tab, White, Round, APO/100	Sulfinpyrazone 100 mg	Apo Sulfinpyrazone by Apotex	Canadian	Uricosuric
APO100	Tab, White, Round, APO/100	Theophylline 100 mg	Apo Theo LA by Apotex	Canadian	Antiasthmatic
APO100	Tab, Pink, Round, APO/100	Trimipramine 100 mg	Trimip by Apotex	Canadian	Antidepressant
APO100	Cap, Opaque & White	Zidovudine 100 mg	Apo Zidovudine by Apotex	Canadian	Antiviral
APO120	Cap, Carmel & Chocolate Brown	Diltiazem HCl 120 mg	Diltiaz SR by Apotex	Canadian	Antihypertensive
APO120	Tab, Rose, Round, APO/120	Propranolol HCl 120 mg	Apo Propanolol by Apotex	Canadian	Antihypertensive
APO120	Tab, White, Oblong, APO/120	Terfenadine 120 mg	Apo Terfenadine by Apotex	Canadian	Antihistamine
APO125	Tab, White, Oblong, APO/12.5	Captopril 12.5 mg	Capto by Apotex	Canadian	Antihypertensive
APO125	Tab, Yellow, Round, APO/125	Methyldopa 125 mg	Apo Methyldopa by Apotex	Canadian	Antihypertensive
APO125	Tab, Light Green, Oval	Naproxen 125 mg	Apo Naproxen by Apotex	Canadian	NSAID
APO125	Tab, White, Round, APO/125	Primidone 125 mg	Apo Primidone by Apotex	Canadian	Anticonvulsant
APO125	Tab, Violet, Oval, APO/.125	Triazolam 0.125 mg	Apo Triazo by Apotex	Canadian	Sedative/Hypnotic
APO15	Cap, Gray & Gray	Clorazepate Dipotassium 15 mg	Apo Clorazepate by Apotex	Canadian	Antianxiety
APO15	Tab, Pink, Round, APO/15	Methyldopa, Hydrochlorothiazide 15 mg	Apo Methazide by Apotex	Canadian	Antihypertensive
APO15	Tab, Orange & Yellow, Round, APO/15	Oxazepam 15 mg	Apo Oxazepam by Apotex	Canadian	Sedative/Hypnotic; C IV
APO15	Cap, Flesh & Maroon	Temazepam 15 mg	Temazepam by Apotex	Canadian	Sedative/Hypnotic
APO150	Cap, Pink	Doxepin HCl 150 mg	Apo Doxepin by Apotex	Canadian	Antidepressant
APO150	Tab, Pale Yellow, Oval	Moclobemide 150 mg	Moclobemide by Apotex	Canadian	Antidepressant
APO150	Cap, Dark Yellow & Pale Yellow	Nizatidine 150 mg	Nizatidine by Apotex	Canadian	Gastrointestinal

ID FRONT <> BACK	DESCRIPTION FRONT <> BACK	INGREDIENT & STRENGTH	BRAND (OR EQUIV.) & FIRM	NDC#	CLASS; SCH.
APO150	Tab, White, Round, APO/150	Ranitidine HCl 150 mg	Apo Ranitidine by Apotex	Canadian	Gastrointestinal
APO150	Tab, Yellow, Hexagonal, APO/150	Sulindac 150 mg	Apo Sulin by Apotex	Canadian	NSAID
APO15050252550	Tab, Pale Orange, Rectangular, APO-150 50 25 25 50	Trazodone HCl 150 mg	Trazodone by Apotex	Canadian	Antidepressant
APO160	Cap, Blue	Nadolol 160 mg	Apo Nadol by Apotex	Canadian	Antihypertensive
APO160	Tab, White, Oval	Megestrol Acetate 160 mg	Megestrol by Apotex	Canadian	Progestin
APO160	Tab, Blue, Oblong, APO-160	Sotalol HCl 160 mg	Sotalol by Apotex	Canadian	Antiarrhythmic
APO180	Cap, Light Blue & Light Turquoise	Diltiazem HCl 180 mg	Diltiaz CD by Apotex	Canadian	Antihypertensive
APO1g	Tab, White, Oblong, APO-1 g	Sucralfate 1g	Apo Sucralfate by Apotex	Canadian	Gastrointestinal
APO2	Tab, White, Round, APO/2	Benztropine Mesylate 2 mg	Apo Benztropine by Apotex	Canadian	Antiparkinson
APO2	Tab, White, Round, APO/2	Diazepam 2 mg	Apo Diazepam by Apotex	Canadian	Antianxiety
APO2	Tab, Pink, Round, APO/2	Haloperidol 2 mg	Apo Haloperidol by Apotex	Canadian	Antipsychotic
APO2	Tab, White, Oval	Lorazepam 2 mg	Apo by Apotex	Canadian	Sedative/Hypnotic
APO2	Cap, Light Green	Loperamide HCl 2 mg	Loperamide by Apotex	Canadian	Antidiarrheal
APO2	Tab, Light Purple, Round, APO/2	Salbutamol Sulfate 2 mg	Salvent by Apotex	Canadian	Antiasthmatic
APO20	Tab, Beige, D-Shaped, APO/20	Famotidine 20 mg	Apo Famotidine by Apotex	Canadian	Gastrointestinal
APO20	Tab, White, Round, APO/20	Furosemide 20 mg	Apo Furosemide by Apotex	Canadian	Diuretic
APO20	Tab, Grayish Pink, Round	Nifedipine 20 mg	Nifed PA by Apotex	Canadian	Antihypertensive
APO20	Cap, Maroon	Piroxicam 20 mg	Apo Piroxicam by Apotex	Canadian	NSAID
APO20	Tab, Blue, Hexagonal, APO/20	Propranolol HCl 20 mg	Apo Propanolol by Apotex	Canadian	Antihypertensive
APO20	Tab, Yellow, Oval, APO/20	Tenoxicam 20 mg	Tenoxicam by Apotex	Canadian	NSAID
APO20	Tab, Blue, Round, APO/20	Trifluoperazine HCl 20 mg	Apo Trifluoperaz by Apotex	Canadian	Antipsychotic
APO200	Tab, White, Oval, APO/200	Acebutolol 200 mg	Apo Acebutolol by Apotex	Canadian	Antihypertensive
APO200	Tab, Peach, Round, APO/200	Allopurinol 200 mg	Apo Allopurinol by Apotex	Canadian	Antigout
APO200	Tab, White, Round, APO/200	Carbamazepine 200 mg	Apo Carbamazepine by Apotex	Canadian	Anticonvulsant
APO200	Tab, Pale Green, Round, APO/200	Cimetidine 200 mg	Apo Cimetidine by Apotex	Canadian	Gastrointestinal
APO200	Tab, Yellow, Round, APO/200	Ibuprofen 200 mg	Apo Ibuprofen by Apotex	Canadian	NSAID
APO200	Tab, Slightly Gray, Round, APO-200	Ketoconazole 200 mg	Ketoconazole by Apotex	Canadian	Antifungal
APO200	Tab, White, Round	Ketoprofen 200 mg	Keto-SR by Apotex	Canadian	NSAID
APO200	Tab, Light Yellow, Oval	Ofloxacin 200 mg	Oflox by Apotex	Canadian	Antibiotic
APO200	Tab, Yellow, Round, APO/200	Oxtriphylline 200 mg	Apo Oxtriphylline by Apotex	Canadian	Antiasthmatic
APO200	Tab, White, Round, APO/200	Quinidine Sulfate 200 mg	Apo Quinidine by Apotex	Canadian	Antiarrhythmic
APO200	Tab, White, Round, APO/200	Sulfinpyrazone 200 mg	Apo Sulfinpyrazone by Apotex	Canadian	Uricosuric
APO200	Tab, Yellow, Hexagonal, APO/200	Sulindac 200 mg	Apo Sulindac by Apotex	Canadian	NSAID
APO200	Tab, White, Oval	Theophylline 200 mg	Apo Theo LA by Apotex	Canadian	Antiasthmatic
APO200	Tab, White, Round, APO/200	Tiaprofenic Acid 200 mg	Apo Tiaprofenic by Apotex	Canadian	NSAID
APO25	Tab, White, Oval, APO/.25	Alprazolam 0.25 mg	Apo Alpraz by Apotex	Canadian	Antianxiety
APO25	Tab, White, Oval, APO/2.5	Bromocriptine 2.5 mg	Apo Bromocriptine by Apotex	Canadian	Antiparkinson
APO25	Tab, White, Square, APO/25	Captopril 25 mg	Apo Capto by Apotex	Canadian	Antihypertensive
APO25	Tab, Yellow, Round, APO/2.5	Enalapril Maleate 2.5 mg	Apo Enalapril by Apotex	Canadian	Antihypertensive
APO25	Tab, White, Round, APO/2.5	Glyburide 2.5 mg	Apo Glyburide by Apotex	Canadian	Antidiabetic
APO25	Tab, Pale Pink, Round, APO/25	Hydrochlorothiazide 25 mg	Apo Hydro by Apotex	Canadian	Diuretic
APO25	Cap, Blue	Indomethacin 25 mg	Apo Indomethacin by Apotex	Canadian	NSAID
APO25	Tab, White, Round, APO/25	Methyldopa, Hydrochlorothiazide 25 mg	Apo Methazide by Apotex	Canadian	Antihypertensive
APO25	Tab, Yellow, Round	Methotrimeprazine Maleate 25 mg	Methoprazine by Apotex	Canadian	Antipsychotic
APO25	Cap, Yellow & White	Nortriptyline HCl 25 mg	Nortriptyline by Apotex	Canadian	Antidepressant
APO250	Tab, White, Round, APO/250	Acetazolamide 250 mg	Apo Acetazolamid by Apotex	Canadian	Diuretic
APO250	Cap, Gold & Scarlet, APO/250	Amoxicillin Trihydrate 250 mg	Apo Amoxi by Apotex	Canadian	Antibiotic
APO250	Tab, Orange, Oblong, APO-250	Cephalexin 250 mg	Apo Cephalex by Apotex	Canadian	Antibiotic
APO250	Cap, Black & Orange	Cloxacillin Sodium 250 mg	Apo Cloxi by Apotex	Canadian	Antibiotic
APO250	Tab, Pink, Oval, APO-250	Erythromycin 250 mg	Apo Erythro Base by Apotex	Canadian	Antibiotic
APO250	Tab, Pink, Round, APO/250	Erythromycin Stearate 250 mg	Apo Erythro-S by Apotex	Canadian	Antibiotic
APO250	Tab, White, Round, APO/250	Metronidazole 250 mg	Apo Metronidazole by Apotex	Canadian	Antibiotic

ID FRONT <> BACK	DESCRIPTION FRONT <> BACK	INGREDIENT & STRENGTH	BRAND (OR EQUIV.) & FIRM	NDC#	CLASS; SCH.
APO250	Cap, Blue & Yellow	Mefenamic Acid 250 mg	Mefenamic by Apotex	Canadian	NSAID
APO250	Tab, Yellow, Round, APO/250	Methyldopa 250 mg	Apo Methyldopa by Apotex	Canadian	Antihypertensive
APO250	Tab, Yellow, Oval, APO-250	Naproxen 250 mg	Apo Naproxen by Apotex	Canadian	NSAID
APO250	Tab, White, Round, APO/250	Primidone 250 mg	Apo Primidone by Apotex	Canadian	Anticonvulsant
APO250	Cap, Yellow	Procainamide HCl 250 mg	Apo Procainamide by Apotex	Canadian	Antiarrhythmic
APO250	Cap, Orange & Yellow	Tetracycline HCl 250 mg	Apo Tetra by Apotex	Canadian	Antibiotic
APO250	Tab, White, Oval	Ticlopidine HCl 250 mg	Ticlopidine by Apotex	Canadian	Anticoagulant
APO250	Cap, Orange, Gel, Colorless Liquid-Filled	Valproic Acid 250 mg	Valproic Acid by Apotex	Canadian	Anticonvulsant
APO26	Tab, White, Oblong, Film Coated	Ranitidine HCl 300 mg	by Apothecon	59772-6512	Gastrointestinal
APO26	Tab, Off-White, Cap-Shaped, Film Coated	Ranitidine HCl 300 mg	by Apotex	60505-0026	Gastrointestinal
APO26	Tab, Off-White to White, Film Coated	Ranitidine HCl 300 mg	by Torpharm	62318-0026	Gastrointestinal
APO26	Tab, White, Oblong, Film Coated	Ranitidine HCl 300 mg	by Zenith Goldline	00172-4358	Gastrointestinal
APO26	Tab, White, Oblong, Film Coated	Ranitidine HCl 300 mg	by Major Pharms	00904-5262	Gastrointestinal
APO275	Tab, Blue, Oval, APO-275	Naproxen Sodium 275 mg	Napro-Na by Apotex	Canadian	NSAID
APO30	Tab, White, Round, APO/30	Oxazepam 30 mg	Apo Oxazepam by Apotex	Canadian	Sedative/Hypnotic; C IV
APO30	Cap, Blue & Maroon	Temazepam 30 mg	Temazepam by Apotex	Canadian	Sedative/Hypnotic
APO300	Tab, Orange, Round, APO/300	Allopurinol 300 mg	Apo Allopurinol by Apotex	Canadian	Antigout
APO300	Tab, Pale Green, Round, APO/300	Cimetidine 300 mg	Apo Cimetidine by Apotex	Canadian	Gastrointestinal
APO300	Cap, Light Blue & Light Gray	Diltiazem HCl 300 mg	Diltiaz CD by Apotex	Canadian	Antihypertensive
APO300	Tab, Pale Green, Round, APO/300	Ferrous Gluconate 300 mg	Apo Ferrous Gluco by Apotex	Canadian	Mineral
APO300	Cap, Maroon & White	Gemfibrozil 300 mg	Apo Gemfibrozil by Apotex	Canadian	Antihyperlipidemic
APO300	Tab, White, Round, APO/300	Ibuprofen 300 mg	Apo Ibuprofen by Apotex	Canadian	NSAID
APO300	Tab, White, Oval	Ofloxacin 300 mg	Oflox by Apotex	Canadian	Antibiotic
APO300	Cap, Reddish Brown & Pale Yellow	Nizatidine 300 mg	Nizatidine by Apotex	Canadian	Gastrointestinal
APO300	Tab, White, Round, APO/300	Oxtriphylline 300 mg	Apo Oxtriphylline by Apotex	Canadian	Antiasthmatic
APO300	Tab, Orange, Round, APO/300	Penicillan V Potassium 300 mg	Apo Pen VK by Apotex	Canadian	Antibiotic
APO300	Tab, White, Oblong, APO-300	Ranitidine HCl 300 mg	Apo Ranitidine by Apotex	Canadian	Gastrointestinal
APO300	Tab, White, Oblong	Theophylline 300 mg	Apo Theo LA by Apotex	Canadian	Antiasthmatic
APO300	Tab, White, Round, APO/300	Tiaprofenic Acid 300 mg	Apo Tiaprofenic by Apotex	Canadian	NSAID
APO325	Tab, White, Round, APO/325	Acetaminophen 325 mg	Apo Acetaminoph by Apotex	Canadian	Antipyretic
APO375	Cap, Gray & White, APO/3.75	Clorazepate Dipotassium 3.75 mg	Apo Clorazepate by Apotex	Canadian	Antianxiety
APO375	Tab, Peach, Oblong	Naproxen 375 mg	Apo Naproxen by Apotex	Canadian	NSAID
APO375	Cap, Orange & White	Procainamide HCl 375 mg	Apo Procainamide by Apotex	Canadian	Antiarrhythmic
APO4	Tab, Light Purple, Round, APO/4	Salbutamol Sulfate 4 mg	Salvent by Apotex	Canadian	Antiasthmatic
APO40	Tab, Yellow, Round, APO/40	Furosemide 40 mg	Apo Furosemide by Apotex	Canadian	Diuretic
APO40	Tab, Light Blue, Round, APO/40	Megestrol Acetate 40 mg	Megestrol by Apotex	Canadian	Progestin
APO40	Tab, Green, Round, APO/40	Propranolol HCl 40 mg	Apo Propanolol by Apotex	Canadian	Antihypertensive
APO400	Tab, White, Oblong, APO/400	Acebutolol 400 mg	Apo Acebutolol by Apotex	Canadian	Antihypertensive
APO400	Tab, Pale Green, Oblong, APO-400	Cimetidine 400 mg	Apo Cimetidine by Apotex	Canadian	Gastrointestinal
APO400	Tab, Orange, Round, APO/400	Ibuprofen 400 mg	Apo Ibuprofen by Apotex	Canadian	NSAID
APO400	Tab, Pink, Oblong, APO/400	Pentoxifylline 400 mg	Pentoxifylline SR by Apotex	Canadian	Anticoagulent
APO400	Tab, Yellow, Oval	Ofloxacin 400 mg	Oflox by Apotex	Canadian	Antibiotic
APO400	Tab, White, Oval	Norfloxacin 400 mg	Norflox by Apotex	Canadian	Antibiotic
APO40080	Tab, White, Round, APO/400-80	Sulfamethoxazole 400 mg, Trimethoprim 80 mg	Apo Sulfatrim by Apotex	Canadian	Antibiotic
APO5	Tab, Yellow, Round, APO/5	Diazepam 5 mg	Apo Diazepam by Apotex	Canadian	Antianxiety
APO5	Tab, Yellow, Round, APO/5	Folic Acid 5 mg	Apo Folic by Apotex	Canadian	Vitamin
APO5	Cap, White	Glyburide 5 mg	Apo Glyburide by Apotex	Canadian	Antidiabetic
APO5	Tab, Green, Round, APO/5	Haloperidol 5 mg	Apo Haloperidol by Apotex	Canadian	Antipsychotic
APO5	Tab, Blue	Oxybutynin Chloride 5 mg	Oxybutynin by Apotex	Canadian	Urinary
APO5	Tab, White, Round, APO/5	Prednisone 5 mg	Apo Prednisone by Apotex	Canadian	Steroid
APO5	Tab, White, Round, APO/5	Trihexyphenidyl HCl 5 mg	Apo Trihex by Apotex	Canadian	Antiparkinson
APO50	Tab, White, Oval, APO/50	Captopril 50 mg	Apo Capto by Apotex	Canadian	Antihypertensive

ID FRONT ⟷ BACK	DESCRIPTION FRONT ⟷ BACK	INGREDIENT & STRENGTH	BRAND (OR EQUIV.) & FIRM	NDC#	CLASS; SCH.
APO50	Tab, Yellow, Round, APO/50	Chlorthalidone 50 mg	Apo Chlorthalidone by Apotex	Canadian	Diuretic
APO50	Tab, White, Round, APO/50	Clomipramine 50 mg	Apo Clomipramine by Apotex	Canadian	OCD
APO50	Tab, Orange, Round, APO/50	Dimenhydrinate 50 mg	Apo Dimenhydrin by Apotex	Canadian	Antiemetic
APO50	Cap, Flesh & Pink	Doxepin HCl 50 mg	Apo Doxepin by Apotex	Canadian	Antidepressant
APO50	Tab, White, Oval, APO-50	Flurbiprofen 50 mg	Apo Flurbiprofen by Apotex	Canadian	NSAID
APO50	Tab, Pink, Round, APO/50	Hydrochlorothiazide 50 mg	Apo Hydro by Apotex	Canadian	Diuretic
APO50	Cap, Blue & White	Indomethacin 50 mg	Indomethacin by Apotex	Canadian	NSAID
APO50	Cap, Green & Ivory	Ketoprofen 50 mg	Apo Keto by Apotex	Canadian	NSAID
APO50	Tab, Yellow, Round	Methotrimeprazine Maleate 50 mg	Methoprazine by Apotex	Canadian	Antipsychotic
APO50	Cap, Orange, APO/50	Minocycline HCl 50 mg	Apo Minocycline by Apotex	Canadian	Antibiotic
APO50	Tab, White, Round, APO/50	Prednisone 50 mg	Apo Prednisone by Apotex	Canadian	Steroid
APO50	Tab, Rose, Round	Trimipramine Maleate 50 mg	Trimip by Apotex	Canadian	Antidepressant
APO500	Tab, White, Round	Acetaminophen 500 mg	Acetaminophen by Apotex	Canadian	Antipyretic
APO500	Tab, White, Round, APO/500	Acetaminophen 500 mg	Apo Acetaminophen by Apotex	Canadian	Antipyretic
APO500	Cap, Gold & Scarlet, APO/500	Amoxicillin Trihydrate 500 mg	Apo Amoxi by Apotex	Canadian	Antibiotic
APO500	Cap, Orange	Cephalexin 250 mg	Cephalex by Apotex	Canadian	Antibiotic
APO500	Cap, Black & Orange	Cloxacillin 500 mg	Cloxi by Apotex	Canadian	Antibiotic
APO500	Tab, White, Oval, APO-500	Erythromycin 500 mg	Erythro S by Apotex	Canadian	Antibiotic
APO500	Tab, White, Modified Oval	Nabumetone 500 mg	Nabumetone by Apotex	Canadian	NSAID
APO500	Tab, Yellow, Round, APO/500	Methyldopa 500 mg	Apo Methyldopa by Apotex	Canadian	Antihypertensive
APO500	Tab, Yellow, Oblong	Naproxen 500 mg	Apo Naproxen by Apotex	Canadian	NSAID
APO500	Cap, Orange & Yellow	Procainamide HCl 500 mg	Apo Procainamide by Apotex	Canadian	Antiarrhythmic
APO5025	Tab, Yellow, Round, APO-50-25	Triamterene 50 mg, Hydrochlorothiazide 25 mg	Apo Triazide by Apotex	Canadian	Diuretic
APO550	Tab, Peach, Diamond, APO/5/50	Hydrochlorothiazide 50 mg, Amiloride 5 mg	Apo Amilzide by Apotex	Canadian	Diuretic; Antihypertensive
APO550	Tab, Blue, Oval, APO-550	Naproxen Sodium 550 mg	Napro-Na by Apotex	Canadian	NSAID
APO60	Tab, White, Round, APO/60	Terfenadine 60 mg	Apo Terfenadine by Apotex	Canadian	Antihistamine
APO600	Tab, Pale Green, Oblong, APO-600	Cimetidine 600 mg	Apo Cimetidine by Apotex	Canadian	Gastrointestinal
APO600	Tab, Yellow, Oval, APO-600	Erythromycin 600 mg	Apo Erythro-ES by Apotex	Canadian	Antibiotic
APO600	Tab, White, Oval, APO-600	Gemfibrozil 600 mg	Apo Gemfibrozil by Apotex	Canadian	Antihyperlipidemic
APO600	Tab, Light Orange, Oval, APO-600	Ibuprofen 600 mg	Apo Ibuprofen FC by Apotex	Canadian	NSAID
APO75	Cap, Gray & Maroon, APO 7.5	Clorazepate Dipotassium 7.5 mg	Apo Clorazepate by Apotex	Canadian	Antianxiety
APO75	Cap, Flesh & Flesh	Doxepin HCl 75 mg	Apo Doxepin by Apotex	Canadian	Antidepressant
APO75	Tab, Light Brown, Round, APO/75	Imipramine 75 mg	Imipramine by Apotex	Canadian	Antidepressant
APO75	Cap, Pink	Trimipramine Maleate 75 mg	Apo Trimip by Apotex	Canadian	Antidepressant
APO75	Tab, Blue, Oval, APO 7.5	Zopiclone 7.5 mg	Zopiclone by Apotex	Canadian	Hypnotic
APO750	Tab, Peach, Cap-Shaped	Naproxen 750 mg	Naproxen SR by Apotex	Canadian	NSAID
APO80	Cap, Yellow, APO/80	Furosemide 80 mg	Apo Furosemide by Apotex	Canadian	Diuretic
APO80	Tab, Yellow, Round, APO/80	Propranolol HCl 80 mg	Apo Propanolol by Apotex	Canadian	Antihypertensive
APO80	Tab, Blue, Oblong, APO-80	Sotalol HCl 80 mg	Satalol by Apotex	Canadian	Antiarrhythmic
APO800	Tab, Pale Green, Oblong, APO-800	Cimetidine 800 mg	Apo Cimetidine by Apotex	Canadian	Gastrointestinal
APO850	Tab, White, Oblong, APO/850	Metformin 850 mg	Metformin by Apotex	Canadian	Antidiabetic
APO90	Cap, Chocolate Brown & Gold	Diltiazem HCl 90 mg	Diltiaz SR by Apotex	Canadian	Antihypertensive
APOA100	Tab, White, Round, APO/A100	Atenolol 100 mg	Apo Atenol by Apotex	Canadian	Antihypertensive
APOA50	Tab, White, Round, APO/A50	Atenolol 50 mg	Apo Atenol by Apotex	Canadian	Antihypertensive
APOB10	Tab, White, Oval, APO/B10	Baclofen 10 mg	Apo Baclofen by Apotex	Canadian	Muscle Relaxant
APOB15	Tab, White, Round, APO/B-1.5	Bromazepam 1.5 mg	Bromazepam by Apotex	Canadian	Sedative
APOB20	Tab, White, Oblong, APO/B20	Baclofen 20 mg	Apo Baclofen by Apotex	Canadian	Muscle Relaxant
APOB3	Tab, Pink, Round, APO/B-3	Bromazepam 3 mg	Bromazepam by Apotex	Canadian	Sedative
APOB6	Tab, Green, Round, APO/B-6	Bromazepam 6 mg	Bromazepam by Apotex	Canadian	Sedative
APOC05	Tab, Orange, Round, APO/C-0.5	Clonazepam 0.5 mg	Clonazepam by Apotex	Canadian	Anticonvulsant
APOC2	Tab, White, Round, APO/C-2	Clonazepam 2 mg	Clonazepam by Apotex	Canadian	Anticonvulsant

ID FRONT <> BACK	DESCRIPTION FRONT <> BACK	INGREDIENT & STRENGTH	BRAND (OR EQUIV.) & FIRM	NDC#	CLASS; SCH.
APOCAL	Tab, Light Green, Biconvex, APO/CAL	Calcium 250 mg	Apo Cal by Apotex	Canadian	Vitamin/Mineral
APOCAL	Tab, Light Green, Oblong, APO/CAL	Calcium 500 mg	Apo Cal by Apotex	Canadian	Vitamin/Mineral
APOD250	Cap, Light Orange, APO/D250	Diflunisal 250 mg	Apo Diflunisal by Apotex	Canadian	NSAID
APOD30	Tab, Light Green, Round, APO/D30	Diltiazem HCl 30 mg	Apo Diltiaz by Apotex	Canadian	Antihypertensive
APOD500	Cap, Orange, APO/D500	Diflunisal 500 mg	Apo Diflunisal by Apotex	Canadian	NSAID
APOD60	Tab, Yellow, Round, APO/D60	Diltiazem HCl 60 mg	Apo Diltiaz by Apotex	Canadian	Antihypertensive
APODOXY100	Tab, Orange, Round, APO-Doxy 100	Doxycycline Hyclate 100 mg	Apo Doxy Tabs by Apotex	Canadian	Antibiotic
APODS	Tab, White, Oblong	Sulfamethoxazole 800 mg, Trimethoprim 160 mg	Sulfatrim by Apotex	Canadian	Antibiotic
APOE10	Tab, Pink & Red, Barrel, APO/E10	Enalapril Maleate 10 mg	Apo Enalapril by Apotex	Canadian	Antihypertensive
APOE20	Tab, Peach, Barrel, APO/E20	Enalapril Maleate 20 mg	Apo Enalapril by Apotex	Canadian	Antihypertensive
APOE5	Tab, White, Barrel, APO/E5	Enalapril Maleate 5 mg	Apo Enalapril by Apotex	Canadian	Antihypertensive
APOH10	Tab, Yellow, Round, APO/H10	Hydralazine HCl 10 mg	Apo Hydralazine by Apotex	Canadian	Antihypertensive
APOI30	Tab, White, Round, APO/I30	Isosorbide Dinitrate 30 mg	Apo Isdn by Apotex	Canadian	Antianginal
APOK600	Tab, Orange, Round, APO/K600	Potassium Chloride 600 mg	Apo K by Apotex	Canadian	Electrolytes
APOL5	Tab, Pink, Oval, APO/L5	Lisonopril 5 mg	Lisinopril by Apotex	Canadian	Antihypertensive
APOLOVA20	Tab, Light Blue, Octagonal, APO/Lova 20	Lovastatin 20 mg	Lovastatin by Apotex	Canadian	Antihyperlipidemic
APOLOVA40	Tab, Light Green, Octagonal, APO/Lova 40	Lovastatin 40 mg	Lovastatin by Apotex	Canadian	Antihyperlipidemic
APOLOX10	Tab, Green, Round	Loxapine 10 mg	Loxapine by Apotex	Canadian	Antipsychotic
APOLOX25	Tab, Pink, Round	Loxapine 25 mg	Loxapine by Apotex	Canadian	Antipsychotic
APOLOX5	Tab, Yellow, Round	Loxapine 5 mg	Loxapine by Apotex	Canadian	Antipsychotic
APOLOX50	Tab, White, Round	Loxapine 50 mg	Loxapine by Apotex	Canadian	Antipsychotic
APOM10	Tab, White, Round, APO/M10	Metoclopramide HCl 10 mg	Apo Metoclop by Apotex	Canadian	Gastrointestinal
APOM100	Tab, White, Round, APO/M100	Metoprolol Tartrate 100 mg	Apo Metoprolol by Apotex	Canadian	Antihypertensive
APOM5	Tab, White, Square, APO/M5	Metoclopramide HCl 5 mg	Apo Metoclop by Apotex	Canadian	Gastrointestinal
APOM50	Tab, White, Round, APO/M50	Metoprolol Tartrate 50 mg	Apo Metoprolol by Apotex	Canadian	Antihypertensive
APOM500	Tab, White, Round, APO/M500	Metformin HCl 500 mg	Metformin by Apotex	Canadian	Antidiabetic
APON40	Tab, White, Round, APO/N40	Nadolol 40 mg	Apo Nadol by Apotex	Canadian	Antihypertensive
APON80	Tab, White, Round, APO/N80	Nadolol 80 mg	Apo Nadol by Apotex	Canadian	Antihypertensive
APOP1	Tab, Peach, Oblong	Prazosin HCl 1 mg	Apo Prazo by Apotex	Canadian	Antihypertensive
APOP10	Tab, White, Round, APO/P10	Pindolol 10 mg	Apo Pindol by Apotex	Canadian	Antihypertensive
APOP15	Tab, White, Round, APO/P15	Pindolol 15 mg	Apo Pindol by Apotex	Canadian	Antihypertensive
APOP2	Tab, White, Round, APO/P2	Prazosin HCl 2 mg	Apo Prazo by Apotex	Canadian	Antihypertensive
APOP5	Tab, White, Round, APO/P5	Pindolol 5 mg	Apo Pindol by Apotex	Canadian	Antihypertensive
APOP5	Tab, White, Diamond, APO/P5	Prazosin HCl 5 mg	Apo Prazo by Apotex	Canadian	Antihypertensive
APOPED	Tab, White, Round, APO/PED	Sulfamethoxazole 100 mg, Trimethoprim 20 mg	Sulfatrim by Apotex	Canadian	Antibiotic
APOT1	Tab, White, Round	Terazosin HCl 1 mg	Terazosin by Apotex	Canadian	Antihypertensive
APOT10	Tab, White, Round, APO/T10	Tamoxifen Citrate 10 mg	Apo Tamox by Apotex	Canadian	Antiestrogen
APOT10	Tab, Blue, Round	Terazosin HCl 10 mg	Terazosin by Apotex	Canadian	Antihypertensive
APOT10	Tab, Light Blue, Round, APO/T10	Timolol Maleate 10 mg	Apo Timol by Apotex	Canadian	Antihypertensive
APOT100	Tab, White, APO/T100	Trazodone HCl 100 mg	Trazodone by Apotex	Canadian	Antidepressant
APOT2	Tab, Orange, Round	Terazosin HCl 2 mg	Terazosin by Apotex	Canadian	Antihypertensive
APOT20	Tab, White, Octagonal, APO/T20	Tamoxifen Citrate 20 mg	Apo Tamox by Apotex	Canadian	Antiestrogen
APOT20	Tab, Light Blue, Oblong, APO/T20	Timolol Maleate 20 mg	Apo Timol by Apotex	Canadian	Antihypertensive
APOT5	Tab, Tab, Round	Terazosin HCl 5 mg	Terazosin by Apotex	Canadian	Antihypertensive
APOT5	Tab, White, Round, APO/T5	Timolol Maleate 5 mg	Apo Timol by Apotex	Canadian	Antihypertensive
APOT50	Tab, Round, APO/T50	Trazodone HCl 50 mg	Trazodone by Apotex	Canadian	Antidepressant
APOTOL	Tab, White, Round, APO/TOL	Tolbutamide 500 mg	Apo Tolbutamide by Apotex	Canadian	Antidiabetic
APOTRM	Tab, White, Round, APO/TRM	Trihexyphenidyl HCl 2 mg	Apo Trihex by Apotex	Canadian	Antiparkinson
APOV120	Tab, White, Round, APO/V120	Verapamil HCl 120 mg	Apo Verap by Apotex	Canadian	Antihypertensive
APOV80	Tab, Yellow, Round, APO/V80	Verapamil HCl 80 mg	Apo Verap by Apotex	Canadian	Antihypertensive
APP784 <> DURICEF500	Cap	Cefadroxil 500 mg	Duricef by Pharmedix	53002-0284	Antibiotic

ID FRONT <> BACK	DESCRIPTION FRONT <> BACK	INGREDIENT & STRENGTH	BRAND (OR EQUIV.) & FIRM	NDC#	CLASS; SCH.
APSE	Tab	Guaifenesin 600 mg, Pseudoephedrine HCl 120 mg	Enomine PSE by Quality Care	60346-0933	Cold Remedy
APSE	Tab, Yellow, Cap Shaped	Guaifenesin 600 mg, Pseudoephedrine HCl 120 mg	Amitex PSE by Amide	52152-0130	Cold Remedy
APSE	Tab, Yellow, Round, Scored	Pseudoephedrine HCl 120 mg; Guaifenesin 600 mg	by HJ Harkins	52959-0397	Cold Remedy
APT <> JMI	Tab, Sugar Coated	Thyroid 3 gr	Westhroid Apt 2 by JMI Canton	00252-7505	Thyroid
APT <> JMI	Tab, Sugar Coated	Thyroid 3 gr	Westhroid Apt 2 by Jones	52604-7505	Thyroid
AR	Cap, White, AR over Abbott Logo	Fenofibrate Micronized 134 mg	TriCor by Abbott	00074-6447	Antihyperlipidemic
ARACEPT10	Tab, Yellow, Aracept/10	Donepezil HCl 10 mg	by Pfizer	Canadian	Antialzheimers
ARACEPT5	Tab, White, Aracept/5	Donepezil HCl 5 mg	by Pfizer	Canadian	Antialzheimers
ARCOLA <> THEOPHYLLINEXR	Cap, Arcola <>Theophylline-XR 100	Theophylline Anhydrous 100 mg	by Arcola	00070-2340	Antiasthmatic
ARCOLA <> THEOPHYLLINEXR	Cap, Arcola <>Theophylline-XR 125	Theophylline Anhydrous 125 mg	by Arcola	00070-2341	Antiasthmatic
ARCOLA <> THEOPHYLLINEXR	Cap, ER, ALSO 200	Theophylline Anhydrous 200 mg	by DRX	55045-2279	Antiasthmatic
ARCOLA <> THEOPHYLLINEXR1	Cap, White	Theophylline Anhydrous 100 mg	Theophylline by RPR	00801-2340	Antiasthmatic
ARCOLA <> THEOPHYLLINEXR1	Cap, White	Theophylline Anhydrous 125 mg	by Murfreesboro Ph	51129-1670	Antiasthmatic
ARCOLA <> THEOPHYLLINEXR1	Cap, White	Theophylline Anhydrous 125 mg	Theophylline by RPR	00801-2341	Antiasthmatic
ARCOLA <> THEOPHYLLINEXR2	Cap, Arcola <>Theophylline-XR 200	Theophylline Anhydrous 200 mg	by Arcola	00070-2342	Antiasthmatic
ARCOLA <> THEOPHYLLINEXR2	Cap, White, ER	Theophylline Anhydrous 200 mg	Theophylline by RPR	00801-2342	Antiasthmatic
ARCOLA <> THEOPHYLLINEXR3	Cap, White	Theophylline Anhydrous 300 mg	Theophylline by RPR	00801-2343	Antiasthmatic
ARCOLA <> THEOPHYLLINEXR3	Cap, Arcola <>Theophylline-XR 300	Theophylline Anhydrous 300 mg	by Arcola	00070-2343	Antiasthmatic
ARICEPT <> 10	Tab, Yellow, Film Coated	Donepezil 10 mg	Arecept by Pfizer	Canadian DIN# 02232044	Antialzheimers
ARICEPT <> 5	Tab, White, Film Coated	Donepezil 5 mg	Arecept by Pfizer	Canadian DIN# 02232043	Antialzheimers
ARM	Tab, Yellow, Oblong, Caplet	Pseudoephedrine HCl 60 mg, Chlorpheniramine Maleate 4 mg	ARM by B F Ascher	00225-0575	Cold Remedy
ARMOURATO	Tab, Tan, Round, Armour A/ TO	Thyroid 30 mg	Thyrar by RPR		Thyroid
ARMOURATP	Tab, Tan, Round, Armour A/ TP	Thyroid 60 mg	Thyrar by RPR		Thyroid
ARR <> 219	Tab, Coated	Erythromycin Stearate 500 mg	by Barr	00555-0219	Antibiotic
ARTANE2 <> LLA11	Tab, Artane 2 <> LL A 11	Trihexyphenidyl HCl 2 mg	Artane by Lederle	00005-4434	Antiparkinson
ARTANE2 <> LLA11	Tab, Artane Over 2 <> LL Over A11	Trihexyphenidyl HCl 2 mg	by UDL	51079-0115	Antiparkinson
ARTANE2 <> LLA11	Tab, Artane Above 2 <> LL Above A11	Trihexyphenidyl HCl 2 mg	Artane by Amerisource	62584-0434	Antiparkinson
ARTANE2 <> LLALL	Tab, Artane 2 <> LL ALL	Trihexyphenidyl HCl 2 mg	Artane by Thrift Drug	59198-0006	Antiparkinson
ARTANE5 <> LLA12	Tab, Artane Over 5 <> LL Over A12	Trihexyphenidyl HCl 5 mg	by UDL	51079-0124	Antiparkinson
ARTANE5 <> LLA12	Tab, Artane Over 5 <> LL Over A12	Trihexyphenidyl HCl 5 mg	Artane by Lederle	00005-4436	Antiparkinson
ASACOLNE	Tab, Red-Brown, Cap Shaped	Mesalamine 400 mg	Asacol DR by Procter & Gamble	00149-0752	Gastrointestinal
ASACOLNE	Tab	Mesalamine 400 mg	Asacol by Caremark	00339-6026	Gastrointestinal
ASCOLD	Tab, Blue, Oblong, AS + Cold	Acetaminophen 325 mg, Chlorpheniramine Maleate 2 mg, Pseudoeniramine 30 mg	Alka Seltzer Plus Liquid Gels Cold Medicine	53014-0004	Cold Remedy
ASF2	Tab, White, A/SF/2	Nitroglycerin 2 mg	Nitrogard SR by Astra	Canadian	Vasodilator
ASI1	Tab, White, A/SI/1	Nitroglycerin 1 mg	Nitrogard SR by Astra	Canadian	Vasodilator
ASN3	Tab, White, A/SN/3	Nitroglycerin 3 mg	Nitrogard SR by Astra	Canadian	Vasodilator
ASPIRIN <> 44157	Tab, White, Round, Film Coated, Aspirin <> 44 over 157	Aspirin 325 mg	Aspirin by UDL	51079-0005	Analgesic

ID FRONT <> BACK	DESCRIPTION FRONT <> BACK	INGREDIENT & STRENGTH	BRAND (OR EQUIV.) & FIRM	NDC#	CLASS; SCH.
ASPIRIN44157	Tab, White, Round, Aspirin/44/157	Aspirin 325 mg	by LNK		Analgesic
AST10	Tab	Astemizole 10 mg	Hismanal by Pharmedix	53002-0642	Antihistamine
AST10 <> JANSSEN	Tab, AST Over 10	Astemizole 10 mg	Hismanal by Johnson & Johnson	59604-0510	Antihistamine
AST10 <> JANSSEN	Tab	Astemizole 10 mg	Hismanal by PDRX	55289-0527	Antihistamine
AST10 <> JANSSEN	Tab, AST over 10 <> Janssen	Astemizole 10 mg	Hismanal by Direct Dispensing	57866-6480	Antihistamine
AST10 <> JANSSEN	Tab, Debossed, AST Over 10	Astemizole 10 mg	Hismanal by St Marys Med	60760-0510	Antihistamine
AST10 <> JANSSEN	Tab, AST over 10	Astemizole 10 mg	Hismanal by Quality Care	60346-0568	Antihistamine
AST10 <> JANSSEN	Tab, Debossed	Astemizole 10 mg	Hismanal by Amerisource	62584-0510	Antihistamine
AST10 <> JANSSEN	Tab, AST over 10 <> Janssen	Astemizole 10 mg	Hismanal by Ortho	00062-0510	Antihistamine
AST10 <> JANSSEN	Tab, AST/10	Astemizole 10 mg	Hismanal by Kaiser	00179-1234	Antihistamine
AST10 <> JANSSEN	Tab, AST over 10 <> Janssen	Astemizole 10 mg	Hismanal by Janssen	50458-0510	Antihistamine
AST10 <> JANSSEN	Tab, AST/10	Astemizole 10 mg	Hismanal by Allscripts	54569-2467	Antihistamine
AST5	Tab, White, A/ST/5	Nitroglycerin 5 mg	Nitrogard SR by Astra	Canadian	Vasodilator
AT	Tab, Round, Abbott Logo	Pipobroman 25 mg	Vercyte by Abbott		Antineoplastic
AT05056	Tab, White, Round, AT 0.5/056	Lorazepam 0.5 mg	Ativan by ATI		Sedative/Hypnotic; C IV
AT053	Cap, White	Clorazepate Dipotassium 30.75 mg	Tranxene by ATI		Antianxiety; C IV
AT054	Cap, Orange	Clorazepate Dipotassium 7.5 mg	Tranxene by ATI		Antianxiety; C IV
AT055	Cap, Red	Clorazepate Dipotassium 15 mg	Tranxene by ATI		Antianxiety; C IV
AT083	Cap, Orange	Danazol 200 mg	Danocrine by ATI		Steroid
AT096	Tab, Green, Hexagonal	Chlorzoxazone 250 mg, Acetaminophen 300 mg	Parafon Forte by ATI		Muscle Relaxant
AT098	Tab, Yellow, Oblong	Theranatal Plus One	by ATI		Vitamin
AT100	Tab, Golden Yellow, Oblong	Therapeutic Vitamin Plus	Berocca Plus by ATI		Vitamin
AT10058	Tab, White, Round, AT 1.0/058	Lorazepam 1 mg	Ativan by ATI		Sedative/Hypnotic; C IV
AT101	Cap, Orange	Meclofenamate Sodium 50 mg	Meclomen by ATI		NSAID
AT102	Cap, Orange	Meclofenamate Sodium 100 mg	Meclomen by ATI		NSAID
AT109	Cap, Clear & Pink, AT-109	Oxazepam 10 mg	Serax by ATI		Sedative/Hypnotic; C IV
AT110	Cap, Clear & Orange, AT-110	Oxazepam 15 mg	Serax by ATI		Sedative/Hypnotic; C IV
AT113	Cap, Clear & White, AT-113	Oxazepam 30 mg	Serax by ATI		Sedative/Hypnotic; C IV
AT121	Tab, White, Round	Trazodone HCl 50 mg	Desyrel by ATI		Antidepressant
AT125	Tab, White, Round	Trazodone HCl 100 mg	Desyrel by ATI		Antidepressant
AT133	Tab, Yellow, Oblong	Therapeutic Vitamin	Berocca by ATI		Vitamin
AT135	Tab, White, Round	Methocarbamol 500 mg	Robaxin by ATI		Muscle Relaxant
AT137	Tab, White, Oblong	Methocarbamol 750 mg	Robaxin by ATI		Muscle Relaxant
AT141	Tab, White, Round	Prednisone 5 mg	Deltasone by ATI		Steroid
AT142	Tab, White, Round	Prednisone 10 mg	Deltasone by ATI		Steroid
AT143	Tab, White, Round	Prednisone 20 mg	Deltasone by ATI		Steroid
AT145	Tab, White, Round	Quinine Sulfate 260 mg	Quinamm by ATI		Antimalarial
AT146	Tab, White, Round	Quinine Sulfate 325 mg	by ATI		Antimalarial
AT147	Tab, Peach, Oblong	Fenoprofen Calcium 600 mg	Nalfon by ATI		NSAID
AT148	Tab, Orange, Round	Clonidine HCl 0.1 mg	Catapres by ATI		Antihypertensive
AT149	Tab, White, Round	Clonidine HCl 0.2 mg	Catapres by ATI		Antihypertensive
AT150	Tab, White, Round	Clonidine HCl 0.3 mg	Catapres by ATI		Antihypertensive
AT151	Cap, Orange & Yellow	Thiothixene 1 mg	Navane by ATI		Antipsychotic
AT152	Cap, Green & Yellow	Thiothixene 2 mg	Navane by ATI		Antipsychotic
AT153	Cap, Orange & White	Thiothixene 5 mg	Navane by ATI		Antipsychotic
AT154	Cap, Green & White	Thiothixene 10 mg	Navane by ATI		Antipsychotic
AT155	Cap, Blue & White	Thiothixene 20 mg	Navane by ATI		Antipsychotic
AT156	Tab, Blue, Round	Clorazepate Dipotassium 30.75 mg	Tranxene by ATI		Antianxiety; C IV
AT157	Tab, Peach, Round	Clorazepate Dipotassium 7.5 mg	Tranxene by ATI		Antianxiety; C IV
AT158	Tab, Pink, Round	Clorazepate Dipotassium 15 mg	Tranxene by ATI		Antianxiety; C IV
AT164	Tab, Yellow, Round, AT-164	Triamterene 75 mg, Hydrochlorothiazide 50 mg	Maxzide by ATI		Diuretic
AT165	Tab, White, Round	Metaproterenol Sulfate 10 mg	Alupent by ATI		Antiasthmatic

ID FRONT <> BACK	DESCRIPTION FRONT <> BACK	INGREDIENT & STRENGTH	BRAND (OR EQUIV.) & FIRM	NDC#	CLASS; SCH.
AT166	Tab, White, Round	Metaproterenol Sulfate 20 mg	Alupent by ATI		Antiasthmatic
AT167	Tab, Orange, Round	Maprotiline 25 mg	Ludiomil by ATI		Antidepressant
AT168	Tab, Orange, Round	Maprotiline 50 mg	Ludiomil by ATI		Antidepressant
AT169	Tab, White, Round	Maprotiline 75 mg	Ludiomil by ATI		Antidepressant
AT172	Tab, White, Round	Albuterol Sulfate 2 mg	Proventil by ATI		Antiasthmatic
AT174	Tab, Green, Oblong	Chlorzoxazone 500 mg	Parafon by ATI		Muscle Relaxant
AT177	Tab, White, Round	Albuterol Sulfate 4 mg	Proventil by ATI		Antiasthmatic
AT178	Cap, Light Brown	Fenoprofen Calcium 200 mg	Nalfon by ATI		NSAID
AT182	Cap, White	Prazosin HCl 1 mg	Minipress by ATI		Antihypertensive
AT184	Cap, Pink	Prazosin HCl 2 mg	Minipress by ATI		Antihypertensive
AT187	Cap, Blue	Prazosin HCl 5 mg	Minipress by ATI		Antihypertensive
AT190	Cap, Yellow	Fenoprofen Calcium 300 mg	Nalfon by ATI		NSAID
AT20060	Tab, White, Round, AT 2.0/060	Lorazepam 2 mg	Ativan by ATI		Sedative/Hypnotic; C IV
AT2012	Tab, White, Round, AT 201/2	Acetaminophen 300 mg, Codeine Phosphate 15 mg	Tylenol # 2 by ATI		Analgesic; C III
AT2023	Tab, White, Round, AT 202/3	Acetaminophen 300 mg, Codeine Phosphate 30 mg	Tylenol # 3 by ATI		Analgesic; C III
AT2034	Tab, White, Round, AT 203/4	Acetaminophen 300 mg, Codeine Phosphate 60 mg	Tylenol #4 by ATI		Analgesic; C III
AT211	Tab, White, Oval	Theralins RX	Natalin RX by ATI		Vitamin
AT4312	Tab, Orange & Pink & Purple, Round, AT-4312	Poly Vitamins, Fluoride 0.5 mg	Poly-Vi-Flor by ATI		Vitamin
ATA <> GEIGY	Tab, Brownish-Red, Round, Sugar Coated	Imipramine HCl 75 mg	Tofranil by Novartis	Canadian DIN# 00306487	Antidepressant
ATARAX10	Tab, Orange, Triangle Shaped, Sugar Coated	Hydroxyzine HCl 10 mg	Atarax by Roerig	00049-5600	Antihistamine
ATARAX25	Tab, Dark Green, Triangle Shaped, Sugar Coated	Hydroxyzine HCl 25 mg	Atarax by Roerig	00049-5610	Antihistamine
ATARAX25	Tab, Sugar Coated	Hydroxyzine HCl 25 mg	Atarax by Urgent Care Ctr	50716-0516	Antihistamine
ATASOL	Tab, White, Round	Acetaminophen 325 mg	Atasol by Horner	Canadian	Antipyretic
ATC	Tab, Light Tan, Round, A/TC	Levothyroxine 9.5 mcg, Liothyronine 2.25 mcg	Armour Thyroid 1/4 by Forest	00456-0457	Antithyroid
ATC	Tab, A Over Mortar & Pestle with TC Beneath	Levothyroxine 9.5 mcg, Liothyronine 2.25 mcg	Armour Thyroid by Allscripts	54569-3101	Antithyroid
ATD	Tab, Light Tan, Round, A/TD	Levothyroxine 19 mcg, Liothyronine 4.5 mcg	Armour Thyroid 1/2 by Forest	00456-0458	Antithyroid
ATD	Tab, A Over Mortar & Pestle with TD Beneath	Levothyroxine 19 mcg, Liothyronine 4.5 mcg	Armour Thyroid by Wal Mart	49035-0180	Antithyroid
ATE	Tab, Light Tan, Round, A/TE	Levothyroxine 38 mcg, Liothyronine 9 mcg	Armour Thyroid 1 by Forest	00456-0459	Antithyroid
ATE	Tab, A Over Mortar & Pestle with TE Beneath	Levothyroxine 38 mcg, Liothyronine 9 mcg	Armour Thyroid by Wal Mart	49035-0181	Antithyroid
ATE	Tab, A Over Mortar & Pestle with TE Beneath	Levothyroxine 38 mcg, Liothyronine 9 mcg	Armour Thyroid by Murfreesboro	51129-1635	Antithyroid
ATE	Tab, A, Armour Logo	Levothyroxine 38 mcg, Liothyronine 9 mcg	Armour Thyroid by Amerisource	62584-0459	Antithyroid
ATF	Tab, A Over Mortar & Pestle with TF Beneath	Levothyroxine 76 mcg, Liothyronine 18 mcg	Armour Thyroid by Wal Mart	49035-0182	Antithyroid
ATF	Tab, Light Tan, Round, A/TF	Levothyroxine 76 mcg, Liothyronine 18 mcg	Armour Thyroid 2 by Forest	00456-0461	Antithyroid
ATG	Tab, Light Tan, Round, Scored, A/TG	Levothyroxine 114 mcg, Liothyronine 27 mcg	Armour Thyroid 3 by Forest	00456-0462	Antithyroid
ATG	Tab, A Over Mortar & Pestle with TG Beneath	Levothyroxine 114 mcg, Liothyronine 27 mcg	Armour Thyroid by Wal Mart	49035-0183	Antithyroid
ATH	Tab, Light Tan, Round, A/TH	Levothyroxine 152 mcg, Liothyronine 36 mcg	Armour Thyroid 4 by Forest	00456-0463	Antithyroid
ATI	Tab, Light Tan, Round, Scored, A/TI	Levothyroxine 190 mcg, Liothyronine 45 mcg	Armour Thyroid 5 by Forest	00456-0464	Antithyroid
ATI076	Cap, White	Chlordiazepoxide HCl 5 mg, Clidinium Bromide 2.5 mg	Librax by ATI		Gastrointestinal; C IV
ATJ	Tab, Light Tan, Round, A/TJ	Levothyroxine 57 mcg, Liothyronine 13.5 mcg	Armour Thyroid 1 1/2 by Forest	00456-0460	Antithyroid
ATJ	Tab, Light Tan, Round	Levothyroxine 57 mcg, Liothyronine 13.5 mcg	Armour Thyroid by Allscripts	54569-4471	Antithyroid
ATJ	Tab, Light Tan, Round, A/TJ	Levothyroxine Sodium 57mcg, Liothyronine Sodium 13.5mcg	Armour Thyroid by Forest	00456-0460	Antithyroid
ATRAL <> 250MG	Cap, 250 mg	Tetracycline HCl 250 mg	by Quality Care	60346-0609	Antibiotic
ATRAL <> 500MG	Cap, 500 mg	Tetracycline HCl 500 mg	by Quality Care	60346-0435	Antibiotic
ATRAL250MG	Cap, Pink	Amoxicillin 250 mg	Amoxil by Lab A		Antibiotic
ATRAL250MG	Cap, Light Green	Cephalexin 250 mg	Keflex by Lab A		Antibiotic
ATRAL250MG	Cap, Warner Chilcott	Tetracycline HCl 250 mg	by Pharmedix	53002-0225	Antibiotic
ATRAL500MG	Cap, Pink	Amoxicillin 500 mg	Amoxil by Lab A		Antibiotic
ATRAL500MG	Cap, Gray & Orange	Cephalexin 500 mg	Keflex by Lab A		Antibiotic
ATRIANGLE <> ZOVIRAX	Tab, Shield Shaped	Acyclovir 400 mg	Zovirax by DRX	55045-2293	Antiviral

ID FRONT <> BACK	DESCRIPTION FRONT <> BACK	INGREDIENT & STRENGTH	BRAND (OR EQUIV.) & FIRM	NDC#	CLASS; SCH.
ATT	Tab, Yellow, Round	Tocainide HCl 400 mg	Tonocard by Astra	Canadian	Antiarrhythmic
AUF	Tab, White, Round, Schering Logo AUF	Griseofulvin 250 mg	Fulvicin UF by Schering	00085-0948	Antifungal
AUG	Tab, White, Round, Schering Logo	Griseofulvin 500 mg	Fulvicin-U/F by Schering	00085-0496	Antifungal
AUGMENTIN <> 250125	Tab, White, Oval	Amoxicillin Trihydrate 500 mg; Clavulanate Potassium 125 mg	Augmentin by Southwood Pharms	58016-0107	Antibiotic
AUGMENTIN <> 250125	Tab, Film Coated	Amoxicillin Trihydrate, Clavulanate Potassium	Augmentin by Casa De Amigos	62138-6075	Antibiotic
AUGMENTIN <> 250125	Tab, White, Oval, Film Coated, Augmentin <> 250 over 125	Amoxicillin 250 mg, Clavulanate Potassium 125 mg	Augmentin by Bayer	00280-1001	Antibiotic
AUGMENTIN <> 250125	Tab, White, Oval, Augmentin <> 250/125	Amoxicillin 250 mg, Clavulanic Acid 125 mg	Augmentin by SKB	00029-6075	Antibiotic
AUGMENTIN <> 250125	Tab, Film Coated	Amoxicillin Trihydrate, Clavulanate Potassium	Augmentin by Pharmedix	53002-0250	Antibiotic
AUGMENTIN <> 250MG	Tab, Film Coated, Tan in Silver Foil Wrap <> 250 MG	Amoxicillin Trihydrate, Clavulanate Potassium	Augmentin by Quality Care	60346-0074	Antibiotic
AUGMENTIN <> 500125	Tab, White, Oval, Film Coated, Augmentin <> 500/125	Amoxicillin 500 mg, Clavulanate Potassium Chewable 125 mg	Augmentin by Bayer	00280-1011	Antibiotic
AUGMENTIN <> 500125	Tab, White, Oval, Film Coated	Amoxicillin Trihydrate 500 mg; Clavulanate Potassium 125 mg	Augmentin by PDRX Pharms	55289-0296	Antibiotic
AUGMENTIN <> 500125	Tab, Film Coated, 500/125	Amoxicillin Trihydrate, Clavulanate Potassium	Augmentin by Amerisource	62584-0312	Antibiotic
AUGMENTIN <> 500125	Tab, Film Coated	Amoxicillin Trihydrate, Clavulanate Potassium	Augmentin by Casa De Amigos	62138-6080	Antibiotic
AUGMENTIN <> 500125	Tab, White, Oval, Film Coated, Augmentin <> 500/125	Amoxicillin Trihydrate, Clavulanate Potassium	Augmentin by SKB	00029-6080	Antibiotic
AUGMENTIN <> 500125	Tab, Film Coated	Amoxicillin Trihydrate, Clavulanate Potassium	Augmentin by Pharmedix	53002-0239	Antibiotic
AUGMENTIN <> 500125	Tab, Film Coated, 500/125	Amoxicillin Trihydrate, Clavulanate Potassium	Augmentin by HJ Harkins Co	52959-0021	Antibiotic
AUGMENTIN <> 500MG	Tab, Film Coated	Amoxicillin Trihydrate, Clavulanate Potassium	Augmentin by Quality Care	60346-0364	Antibiotic
AUGMENTIN200	Tab, Pink, Round	Amoxicillin 200 mg	Augmentin by SKB	00029-6071	Antibiotic
AUGMENTIN400	Tab, Pink, Round	Amoxicillin 400 mg	Augmentin by SKB	00029-6072	Antibiotic
AUGMENTIN875 <> SB	Tab, White, Cap Shaped, Coated	Amoxicillin Trihydrate, Clavulanate Potassium	Augmentin by SKB	00029-6086	Antibiotic
AUGMENTIN875 <> SB	Tab, White, Oblong	Amoxicillin Trihydrate, Clavulanate Potassium	Augmentin by Bayer	00280-1091	Antibiotic
AUGMENTIN875 <> SB	Tab, Coated	Amoxicillin Trihydrate, Clavulanate Potassium	Augmentin by HJ Harkins Co	52959-0478	Antibiotic
AUGMENTIN875 <> SB	Tab, White, Oblong, Scored	Clavulamate Potassium, Amoxicillin Trihydrate	Augmentin 875 by Copley	38245-0133	Antibiotic
AWYETH64	Tab, White, Pentagonal, A/Wyeth 64	Lorazepam 1 mg	Ativan by Wyeth		Sedative/Hypnotic; C IV
AWYETH65	Tab, White, Pentagonal, A/Wyeth 65	Lorazepam 2 mg	Ativan by Wyeth		Sedative/Hypnotic; C IV
AWYETH81	Tab, White, Pentagonal, A/Wyeth 81	Lorazepam 0.5 mg	Ativan by Wyeth		Sedative/Hypnotic; C IV
AX <> 3438	Tab, White, Round, Mottled, Apotex Logo	Selegiline HCl 5 mg	Selegiline HCl USP by SB	59742-3160	Antiparkinson
AX3438	Tab, White, Round	Selegiline HCl 5 mg	Eldepryl by Caraco		Antiparkinson
AXID150MG <> 3144	Cap, Axid 150 mg <> Symbol/3144	Nizatidine 150 mg	Axid by Nat Pharmpak Serv	55154-1803	Gastrointestinal
AXID150MG <> LILLY3144	Cap, Yellow	Nizatidine 150 mg	Axid by Promex Medcl	62301-0047	Gastrointestinal
AXID150MG <> LILLY3144	Cap	Nizatidine 150 mg	Axid by Eli Lilly	00002-3144	Gastrointestinal
AXID150MG <> LILLY3144	Cap, Dark Yellow & Pale Yellow	Nizatidine 150 mg	Axid by Murfreesboro	51129-3144	Gastrointestinal
AXID150MG <>	Cap, Dark Yellow & Pale Yellow	Nizatidine 150 mg	Axid by Allscripts	54569-2605	Gastrointestinal
AXID150MG <> LILLY3144	Cap	Nizatidine 150 mg	Axid by Pharmedix	53002-1041	Gastrointestinal
AXID150MG <> LILLY3144	Cap, Dark Yellow & Pale Yellow, Lilly 3144	Nizatidine 150 mg	Nizatidine by Med Pro	53978-2079	Gastrointestinal
AXID150MG <> LILLY3144	Cap, Dark Yellow & Pale Yellow	Nizatidine 150 mg	Axid by Quality Care	60346-0585	Gastrointestinal
AXID150MG <> LILLY3144	Cap, Dark Yellow & Pale Yellow	Nizatidine 150 mg	Axid by Promex Med	62301-0020	Gastrointestinal
AXID300MG <> LILLY3145	Cap	Nizatidine 300 mg	Axid by Eli Lilly	00002-3145	Gastrointestinal
AYC	Tab, Violet & White, Round, A/YC	Levothyroxine 12.5 mcg, Liothyronine Sodium 3.1 mcg	Thyrolar 1/4 by Forest	00456-0040	Antithyroid
AYD	Tab, Peach & White, Round, A/YD	Levothyroxine 25 mcg, Liothyronine Sodium 6.25 mcg	Thyrolar 1/2 by Forest	00456-0045	Antithyroid
AYE	Tab, Pink & White, Round, A/YE	Levothyroxine 50 mcg, Liothyronine Sodium 12.5 mcg	Thyrolar 1 by Forest	00456-0050	Antithyroid
AYE	Tab	Levothyroxine Sodium 50 mcg, Liothyronine Sodium 12.5 mcg	Thyrolar 1 by Allscripts	54569-3639	Antithyroid
AYERST	Cap, Green & White	Aspirin 325 mg, Phenobarbital 16.2 mg, Codeine Phosphate 64.8 mg	Phenaphen by Wyeth-Ayerst	Canadian	Analgesic

ID FRONT <> BACK	DESCRIPTION FRONT <> BACK	INGREDIENT & STRENGTH	BRAND (OR EQUIV.) & FIRM	NDC#	CLASS; SCH.
AYERST	Cap, Black & Green	Aspirin 325 mg, Pheonbarbital 16.2 mg, Codeine Phosphate 32.4 mg	Phenaphen by Wyeth-Ayerst	Canadian	Analgesic
AYERST	Tab, Orange, Oblong	B Complex Vitamin	Beminal by Whitehall-Robbins		Vitamin
AYERST	Cap, Red	Clofibrate 1g	by Wyeth-Ayerst	Canadian	Antihyperlipidemic
AYERST	Cap, Orange	Clofibrate 500 mg	Atromid-S by Wyeth-Ayerst	Canadian	Antihyperlipidemic
AYERST	Tab, White, Round, Scored	Dapsone 100 mg	by Wyeth-Ayerst	Canadian	Antimycobacterial
AYERST	Tab, Orange	Fenfluramine HCl 20 mg	Pondimin by Wyeth-Ayerst	Canadian	Anorexiant
AYERST	Tab, Pink	Glycopyrrolate 1 mg	Robinul by Wyeth-Ayerst	Canadian	Gastrointestinal
AYERST	Tab, Pink	Glycopyrrolate 2 mg	Robinul Forte by Wyeth-Ayerst	Canadian	Gastrointestinal
AYERST	Tab, White, Round	Magaldrate 480 mg	Riopan by Whitehall-Robbins		Gastrointestinal
AYERST	Tab, Blue	Metoclopramide 10 mg	Reglan by Wyeth-Ayerst	Canadian	Gastrointestinal
AYERST	Tab, White, Round	Primidone 250 mg	by Wyeth-Ayerst	Canadian	Anticonvulsant
AYERST250	Cap, Caramel & Red	Amoxicillin 250 mg	Amoxil by Ayerst		Antibiotic
AYERST252	Cap, Black	Vitamin Combination	Mediatric by Ayerst		Vitamin
AYERST500	Cap, Caramel & Red	Amoxicillin 500 mg	Amoxil by Ayerst		Antibiotic
AYERST5REGLAN	Tab, Blue, Oblong, Ayerst 5/Reglan	Metoclopramide 5 mg	Reglan by Wyeth-Ayerst	Canadian	Gastrointestinal
AYERST752	Tab, Orange, Oblong	Vitamin Combination	Mediatric by Ayerst		Vitamin
AYERST783	Tab, Yellow, Round	Sulfamethizole 500 mg, Phenazopyridine 50 mg	Thiosulfil-A Forte by Ayerst		Antibiotic; Urinary Analgesic
AYERST784	Tab, Red, Round	Sulfamethizole 250 mg, Phenazopyridine 50 mg	Thiosulfil-A by Ayerst		Antibiotic; Urinary Analgesic
AYERST786	Tab, White, Oval	Sulfamethizole 500 mg	Thiosulfil Forte by Ayerst		Antibiotic
AYERST878	Tab, Maroon, Round	Conjugated Estrogens 0.625 mg, Methyltestosterone 5 mg	Premarin w Methyltes by Ayerst		Estrogen
AYERST879	Tab, Yellow, Round	Conjugated Estrogens 1.25 mg, Methyltestosterone 10 mg	Premarin w Methyltes by Ayerst		Estrogen
AYERST880	Tab, Green, Oblong	Conjugated Estrogens 0.45 mg, Meprobamate 200 mg	PMB 200 by Ayerst		Estrogen
AYERST881	Tab, Pink, Oblong	Conjugated Estrogens 0.45 mg, Meprobamate 400 mg	PMB 400 by Ayerst		Estrogen
AYERSTMICROK	Cap, Orange, Ayerst/Micro-K	Potassium Chloride 600 mg	by Key	Canadian	Electrolytes
AYERSTMICROK10	Cap, Orange & White, Ayerst/Micro-K-10	Potassium Chloride 750 mg	by Key	Canadian	Electrolytes
AYF	Tab, Green & White, Round, A/YF	Levothyroxine 100 mcg, Liothyronine Sodium 25 mcg	Thyrolar 2 by Forest	00456-0055	Antithyroid
AYGESTIN	Tab, White, Oval	Norethindrone Acetate 5 mg	by ESI Lederle		Oral Contraceptive
AYH	Tab, White & Yellow, Round, A/YH	Levothyroxine 150 mcg, Liothyronine Sodium 37.5 mcg	Thyrolar 3 by Forest	00456-0060	Antithyroid
AZ	Tab, Yellow, Round, Scored	Azathioprine 50 mg	by Genpharm	55567-0084	Immunosuppressant
B	Tab, Beveled Edge, Debossed	Isosorbide Dinitrate 2.5 mg	by Barr	00555-0172	Antianginal
B <> 11	Tab, Light Green, Film Coated	Inert	Tri-Levlen 28 by Berlex	50419-0111	Placebo
B <> 21	Tab, Light Orange	Ethinyl Estradiol 0.03 mg, Levonorgestrel 0.15 mg	Levlen 28 by Berlex	50419-0021	Oral Contraceptive
B <> 22	Tab, Round, Sugar Coated	Ethinyl Estradiol 0.02 mg, Levonorgestrel 0.1 mg	Levlite 28 by Berlex	50419-0408	Oral Contraceptive
B <> 22	Tab, Round, Sugar Coated	Ethinyl Estradiol 0.02 mg, Levonorgestrel 0.1 mg	Levlite 21 by Berlex	50419-0406	Oral Contraceptive
B <> 22	Tab, Sugar Coated	Ethinyl Estradiol 0.02 mg, Levonorgestrel 0.1 mg	Levlite by Schering	12866-1163	Oral Contraceptive
B <> 22	Tab, Pink, Round	Levonorgestrel 0.1 mg, Ethinyl Estradiol 0.02 mg	Levlite by Schering Productions	64259-1165	Oral Contraceptive
B <> 252	Tab, Film Coated, Barr Logo	Dipyridamole 25 mg	by Quality Care	60346-0789	Antiplatelet
B <> 252	Tab, Film Coated	Dipyridamole 25 mg	by Heartland	61392-0549	Antiplatelet
B <> 252	Tab, Film Coated, Schein Logo	Dipyridamole 25 mg	by Schein	00364-2491	Antiplatelet
B <> 252	Tab, Film Coated, Barr Logo <> 252	Dipyridamole 25 mg	by Barr	00555-0252	Antiplatelet
B <> 252	Tab, Film Coated, Barr Logo	Dipyridamole 25 mg	by Geneva	00781-1890	Antiplatelet
B <> 252	Tab, White, Round, Film Coated	Dipyridamole 25 mg	Persantine by UDL	51079-0068	Antiplatelet
B <> 252	Tab, White, Round, Film Coated, Genpharm Logo	Dipyridamole 25 mg	by Genpharm	55567-0088	Antiplatelet
B <> 28	Tab, Pink	Ethinyl Estradiol 0.03 mg, Levonorgestrel 0.15 mg; See 50419-0021	Levlen 21 by Berlex	50419-0410	Oral Contraceptive
B <> 28	Tab, Pink	Inert	Levlen 21 by Berlex	50419-0028	Placebo
B <> 285	Tab, Film Coated	Dipyridamole 50 mg	by Heartland	61392-0552	Antiplatelet
B <> 285	Tab, Film Coated	Dipyridamole 50 mg	by Amerisource	62584-0370	Antianginal
B <> 285	Tab, Film Coated, Barr Logo	Dipyridamole 50 mg	by Geneva	00781-1678	Antiplatelet
B <> 285	Tab, Film Coated	Dipyridamole 50 mg	by Barr	00555-0285	Antiplatelet
B <> 285	Tab, White, Round, Film Coated	Dipyridamole 50 mg	Persantine by UDL	51079-0069	Antiplatelet

ID FRONT <> BACK	DESCRIPTION FRONT <> BACK	INGREDIENT & STRENGTH	BRAND (OR EQUIV.) & FIRM	NDC#	CLASS; SCH.
B <> 285	Tab, Film Coated	Dipyridamole 50 mg	by Allscripts	54569-0468	Antiplatelet
B <> 29	Tab, Round, Sugar Coated	Ethinyl Estradiol 0.02 mg, Levonorgestrel 0.1 mg	Levlite 28 by Berlex	50419-0408	Oral Contraceptive
B <> 484	Tab, White, Round, B <> 484	Leucovorin Calcium	Wellcovoring by UDL	51079-0581	Antineoplastic
B <> 484	Tab, Debossed	Leucovorin Calcium	by Rugby	00536-4148	Antineoplastic
B <> 484	Tab, Debossed	Leucovorin Calcium	by Barr	00555-0484	Antineoplastic
B <> 484	Tab, b <> 484	Leucovorin Calcium	by Supergen	62701-0900	Antineoplastic
B <> 484	Tab, Deboosed	Leucovorin Calcium	by Major	00904-2315	Antineoplastic
B <> 485	Tab, Pale Green, Round, B <> 485	Leucovorin Calcium	by Qualitest	00603-4183	Antineoplastic
B <> 485	Tab, Debossed	Leucovorin Calcium	Wellcovoring by UDL	51079-0582	Antineoplastic
B <> 485	Tab, Debossed	Leucovorin Calcium	by Barr	00555-0485	Antineoplastic
B <> 485	Tab, Debossed	Leucovorin Calcium	by Supergen	62701-0901	Antineoplastic
B <> 50902	Tab, Barr Logo <> 50/902	Naltrexone HCl 50 mg	by Qualitest	00603-4184	Antineoplastic
B <> 555606	Tab, White, Round, Scored, B <> 555 Over 606	Megestrol Acetate 20 mg	Naltrexone Hydrochloride by Barr	00555-0902	Opiod Antagonist
B <> 555606	Tab	Megestrol Acetate 20 mg	Megace by UDL	51079-0434	Progestin
B <> 555606	Tab, Debossed	Megestrol Acetate 20 mg	by Barr	00555-0606	Progestin
B <> 555607	Tab, Debossed as 555/607	Megestrol Acetate 20 mg	by Major	00904-3570	Progestin
B <> 555607	Tab, White, Round, Scored, B <> 555 Over 607	Megestrol Acetate 40 mg	by Supergen	62701-0920	Progestin
B <> 555779	Tab, Debossed	Medroxyprogesterone Acetate 10 mg	Megace by UDL	51079-0435	Progestin
B <> 555779	Tab, Debossed	Medroxyprogesterone Acetate 10 mg	by Major	00904-2690	Progestin
B <> 555779	Tab, Coated	Medroxyprogesterone Acetate 10 mg	by Qualitest	00603-4367	Progestin
B <> 555779	Tab, Debossed	Medroxyprogesterone Acetate 10 mg	by Barr	00555-0779	Progestin
B <> 555872	Tab, White, Round, Scored	Medroxyprogesterone Acetate 2.5 mg	by United Res	00677-1619	Progestin
B <> 555872	Tab, Coated, Debossed, 555/872	Medroxyprogesterone Acetate 2.5 mg	by Murfreesboro Ph	51129-1373	Progestin
B <> 555872	Tab, Coated	Medroxyprogesterone Acetate 2.5 mg	by Qualitest	00603-4365	Progestin
B <> 555873	Tab, Coated	Medroxyprogesterone Acetate 5 mg	by United Res	00677-1617	Progestin
B <> 555873	Tab, Coated, Debossed	Medroxyprogesterone Acetate 5 mg	by Barr	00555-0873	Progestin
B <> 555873	Tab, Coated	Medroxyprogesterone Acetate 5 mg	by United Res	00677-1618	Progestin
B <> 572	Tab, Coated	Methotrexate 2.5 mg	by Qualitest	00603-4366	Progestin
B <> 8861	Tab, Purple, Oval, Scored	Estradiol 1 mg	by Qualitest	00603-4499	Antineoplastic
B <> 95	Tab	Ethinyl Estradiol 0.03 mg, Ethinyl Estradiol 0.04 mg, Ethinyl Estradiol 0.03 mg, Levonorgestrel 0.05 mg, Levonorgestrel 0.125 mg, Levonorgestrel 0.075 mg	by DRX Pharm Consults	55045-2739	Hormone
B <> 95	Tab, Brown, Six	Ethinyl Estradiol 0.03 mg, Ethinyl Estradiol 0.04 mg, Ethinyl Estradiol 0.03 mg, Levonorgestrel 0.05 mg, Levonorgestrel 0.125 mg, Levonorgestrel 0.075 mg	Tri Levlen 28 by Nat Pharmpak Serv	55154-0304	Oral Contraceptive
B <> 95	Tab, Brown, Film Coated	Ethinyl Estradiol 0.03 mg, Ethinyl Estradiol 0.04 mg, Ethinyl Estradiol 0.03 mg, Levonorgestrel 0.05 mg, Levonorgestrel 0.125 mg, Levonorgestrel 0.050 mg	Tri Levlen 28 by Pharm Utilization	60491-0653	Oral Contraceptive
B <> 95	Tab, Brown, Film Coated	Ethinyl Estradiol 0.03 mg, Ethinyl Estradiol 0.04 mg, Ethinyl Estradiol 0.03 mg, Levonorgestrel 0.05 mg, Levonorgestrel 0.125 mg, Levonorgestrel 0.050 mg	Tri Levlen 21 by Berlex	50419-0195	Oral Contraceptive
B <> 96	Tab, Off-White to White, Five	Ethinyl Estradiol 0.03 mg, Ethinyl Estradiol 0.04 mg, Ethinyl Estradiol 0.03 mg, Levonorgestrel 0.05 mg, Levonorgestrel 0.125 mg, Levonorgestrel 0.075 mg	Tri-Levlen 28 by Berlex	50419-0195	Oral Contraceptive
B <> 96	Tab, Off-White to White, Film Coated	Ethinyl Estradiol 0.04 mg, Ethinyl Estradiol 0.04 mg, Ethinyl Estradiol 0.03 mg, Levonorgestrel 0.05 mg, Levonorgestrel 0.125 mg, Levonorgestrel 0.075 mg	Tri Levlen 28 by Pharm Utilization	60491-0653	Oral Contraceptive
B <> 96	Tab, Off-White to White, Film Coated	Ethinyl Estradiol 0.04 mg, Ethinyl Estradiol 0.04 mg, Ethinyl Estradiol 0.03 mg, Levonorgestrel 0.05 mg, Levonorgestrel 0.125 mg, Levonorgestrel 0.075 mg	Tri Levlen 21 by Berlex	50419-0196	Oral Contraceptive
B <> 97	Tab, Light Yellow, Ten	Ethinyl Estradiol 0.03 mg, Ethinyl Estradiol 0.04 mg, Ethinyl Estradiol 0.03 mg, Levonorgestrel 0.05 mg, Levonorgestrel 0.125 mg, Levonorgestrel 0.075 mg	Tri-Levlen 28 by Berlex	50419-0196	Oral Contraceptive
B <> 97	Tab, Light Yellow, Film Coated	Ethinyl Estradiol 0.03 mg, Ethinyl Estradiol 0.04 mg, Ethinyl Estradiol 0.03 mg, Levonorgestrel 0.05 mg, Levonorgestrel 0.125 mg, Levonorgestrel 0.075 mg	Tri Levlen 28 by Pharm Utilization	60491-0653	Oral Contraceptive
B <> 97	Tab, Light Yellow, Film Coated	Ethinyl Estradiol 0.03 mg, Ethinyl Estradiol 0.04 mg, Ethinyl Estradiol 0.03 mg, Levonorgestrel 0.05 mg, Levonorgestrel 0.125 mg, Levonorgestrel 0.125 mg	Tri-Levlen 28 by Berlex	50419-0197	Oral Contraceptive
B <> KERLONE20	Tab, White, Round, Coated, Greek Letter Beta <> Kerlone 20	Ethinyl Estradiol 0.03 mg, Ethinyl Estradiol 0.04 mg, Ethinyl Estradiol 0.03 mg, Levonorgestrel 0.05 mg, Levonorgestrel 0.125 mg, Levonorgestrel 0.125 mg	Tri Levlen 21 by Berlex	50419-0197	Oral Contraceptive
B003	Tab, Pink, Round, White Specks	Betaxolol HCl 20 mg	Kerlone by GD Searle	00025-5201	Antihypertensive
		Acetaminophen Chewable 80 mg	Tylenol Chewable by Biopharmaceutics		Antipyretic

ID FRONT <> BACK	DESCRIPTION FRONT <> BACK	INGREDIENT & STRENGTH	BRAND (OR EQUIV.) & FIRM	NDC#	CLASS; SCH.
B01	Tab, Yellow, Round	Bisacodyl 5 mg	Dulcolax by Upsher		Gastrointestinal
B01	Tab, Yellow, Round	Bisacodyl 5 mg	Dulcolax by BI		Gastrointestinal
B027	Tab, Blue, Round, B-027	Methenamine 40.8 mg, Phenyl Salicylcate 18.1 mg, Methylene Blue 5.4 mg, Benzoic Acid 4.5 mg	Urised by Breckenridge	51991-0027	Antibiotic; Urinary Tract
B035	Tab, Light Green, Oblong, B-035	Phenylephrine HCl 25 mg, Phenylpropanolamine HCl 50 mg, Chlorpheniramine Maleate 8 mg	Rutuss by Breckenridge	51991-0250	Cold Remedy
B042	Cap, White, B-042	Phenylpropanolamine HCl 25 mg	Polyhistine D pediatric by Breckenridge	51991-0042	Decongestant; Appetite Suppressant
B042	Cap, Opaque White, B-042	Phenylpropanolamine HCl 25 mg, Phenylotoloxamine Citrate 8 mg, Pheniramine Maleate 8 mg, Pyrilamine Maleate 8 mg	PPAH PTC PNM PRM PD by Prepackage Spec	58864-0029	Cold Remedy
B060	Tab, Violet, Oval, B-060	Arbinoxamine Maleate 8 mg, Pseudoephedrine HCl 120 mg	Coldec TR by Breckenridge	51991-0060	Cold Remedy
B080	Cap, Reddish Brown, Oval, Gelatin, B-080	Chloral Hydrate 500 mg	Noctec by Breckenridge	51991-0080	Sedative/Hypnotic; C IV
B1	Tab, Pink, Scored	Bisoprolol Fumarate 5 mg	Zebeta by Wyeth Pharms	52903-3816	Antihypertensive
B1 <> LL	Tab, Pink, Scored	Bisoprolol Fumarate 5 mg	Zebeta by Ayerst Lab (Div Wyeth)	00046-3816	Antihypertensive
B12 <> LL	Tab, Film Coated, B Above 12 <> Engraved within Heart Shape	Bisoprolol Fumarate 2.5 mg, Hydrochlorothiazide 6.25 mg	Ziac by Quality Care	60346-0775	Antihypertensive; Diuretic
B12 <> LL	Tab, Yellow, Round	Bisoprolol Fumarate 2.5 mg; Hydrochlorothiazide 6.25 mg	Ziac by Ayerst Lab (Div Wyeth)	00046-3238	Antihypertensive; Diuretic
B13 <> LL	Tab, Film Coated, A B over 13 <> LL Heart	Bisoprolol Fumarate 5 mg, Hydrochlorothiazide 6.25 mg	Ziac by Caremark	00339-6006	Antihypertensive; Diuretic
B130	Tab	Hyoscyamine Sulfate 0.125 mg	by Zenith Goldline	00182-1607	Gastrointestinal
B14 <> LL	Tab, White, Round	Bisoprolol Fumarate 10 mg; Hydrochlorothiazide 6.25 mg	Ziac by Ayerst Lab (Div Wyeth)	00046-3235	Antihypertensive; Diuretic
B14 <> LL	Tab, White, Round	Bisoprolol Fumarate 10 mg; Hydrochlorothiazide 6.25 mg	Ziac by Stevens Dee Fd	45868-4179	Antihypertensive; Diuretic
B145	Tab, Yellow, Round, Scored	Digoxin 0.125 mg	Digitek by Bertek Pharms	62794-0145	Cardiac Agent
B145	Tab, Yellow, Round, Scored, B over 145	Digitek 0.125 mg	Lanoxin by UDL	51079-0945	Cardiac Agent
B146	Tab, White, Round, Scored, B over 146	Digitek 0.25 mg	Lanoxin by UDL	51079-0946	Cardiac Agent
B146	Tab, Sugar Coated, B-146	Phenazopyridine HCl 100 mg	by Lini	58215-0313	Urinary Analgesic
B147	Tab, Sugar Coated, B-146	Phenazopyridine HCl 200 mg	by Lini	58215-0314	Urinary Analgesic
B147	Tab, Sugar Coated	Phenazopyridine HCl 200 mg	by Breckenridge	51991-0525	Urinary Analgesic
B147	Tab, Sugar Coated	Phenazopyridine HCl 200 mg	by Apotheca	12634-0189	Urinary Analgesic
B154	Tab, White, Oval, B-154	Elemental Iron 90 mg, Calcium 200 mg, Zinc 25 mg, Vitamin A 2700 IU, Vitamin D3 400 IU, Vitamin E 30 IU, Vitamin C 120 mg, Vitamin B6 20 mg, Docusate Sodium 50 mg	Prenate Ultra by Breckenridge	51991-0154	Vitamin/Mineral
B156	Tab, Sugar Coated	Dexchlorpheniramine Maleate 4 mg	by Lini	58215-0311	Antihistamine
B156	Tab, Sugar Coated	Dexchlorpheniramine Maleate 4 mg	by Breckenridge	51991-0470	Antihistamine
B157	Tab, Sugar Coated	Dexchlorpheniramine Maleate 6 mg	by United Res	00677-0669	Antihistamine
B157	Tab, Sugar Coated	Dexchlorpheniramine Maleate 6 mg	by Lini	58215-0312	Antihistamine
B158	Tab, White, Oval, B-158	Vitamin A 4000 IU, Vitamin C 80 mg, Vitamin D 400 IU, Vitamin E 15 IU, Niacin 17 mg, Calcium 200 mg, Iron 54 mg, Magnesium 100 mg, Zinc 25 mg, Copper 3 mg	Natalins Rx by Breckenridge	51991-0158	Vitamin
B158 <> FLOMAXO4MG	Cap, Green & Orange	Tamsulosin HCl 0.4 mg	Flomax by Caremark	00339-5560	Antiadrenergic
B15G	Tab, White, Round, B/1.5/G	Bromazepam 1.5 mg	by Genpharm	Canadian	Sedative
B167	Tab, Ex Release, B on One Side of Bisect and 167 on Other Side	Chlorpheniramine Maleate 8 mg, Methscopolamine Nitrate 2.5 mg, Phenylephrine HCl 20 mg	Guaivent DA by Lini	58215-0327	Cold Remedy
B168	Tab, Delayed Release, B-168	Atropine Sulfate 0.04 mg, Chlorpheniramine Maleate 8 mg, Hyoscyamine Sulfate 0.19 mg, Phenylephrine HCl 25 mg, Phenylpropanolamine HCl 50 mg, Scopolamine Hydrobromide 0.01 mg	Atrohist Plus by Lini	58215-0326	Cold Remedy
B17	Tab, Orange, Oval, Scored	Clonidine HCl 0.2 mg	Catapres by Phy Total Care	54868-0931	Antihypertensive
B172	Tab, Yellow, Round	Isosorbide Dinitrate Sublingual 2.5 mg	Isordil by Barr		Antianginal
B173	Tab, Pink, Round	Isosorbide Dinitrate Sublingual 5.0 mg	Isordil by Barr		Antianginal

ID FRONT <> BACK	DESCRIPTION FRONT <> BACK	INGREDIENT & STRENGTH	BRAND (OR EQUIV.) & FIRM	NDC#	CLASS; SCH.
B198	Cap, Maroon, Opaque, B-198	Polysaccharide Iron Complex 150 mg, Folic Acid 1 mg, Vitamine B12 25mcg	Niferex 150 Forte by Breckenridge	51991-0198	Vitamin
B2	Tab, B2	Ergotamine Tartrate 2 mg	Ergomar Sublingual by Lotus Biochemical Corp	59417-0120	Analgesic
B200	Tab, White, Round	Ibuprofen 200 mg	Advil by Barr		NSAID
B200	Tab, Blue, Oval, Film Coated	Polysaccharide Iron Complex 60 mg, Folic Acid 1 mg, Ascorbic Acid 1 mg, Vitamin B12 3mcg, Vitamin A 4000 IU, Vitamin D 400 IU, Thiamine 3 mg, Riboflavin 3 mg, Vitamin B6 2 mg, Niacinamide 10 mg, Calcium 125 mg, Zinc 18 mg	Niferex PC by Breckenridge	51991-0200	Vitamin
B202	Tab, White, Oval, B-202	Olysaccharide Iron Complex 60 mg, Folic Acid 1 mg, Vitamin B12 12mcg, Vitamin A 5000 IU, Vitamin D 400 IU, Thiamine 3 mg, Riboflavin 3.4 mg, Vitamin B6 4 mg, Niacinamide 20 mg, Calcium 250 mg, Zinc 25 mg, Vitamin C 80 mcg, Vitamin E 30 IU, Iodine 0.2 mg, Magnesium 10 mg, Copper 2 mg	Niferex PC Forte by Breckenridge	51991-0202	Vitamin
B203	Cap, Brown & Red, B-203	Polysaccharide Iron Complex 150 mg	Niferex 150 by Breckenridge	51991-0203	Vitamin
B237	Tab, Pink, Triangle	Perphenazine 2 mg, Amitriptyline 25 mg	Triavil by Barr		Antipsychotic; Antidepressant
B238	Tab, Light Green, Round	Perphenazine 4 mg, Amitriptyline 25 mg	Triavil by Barr		Antipsychotic; Antidepressant
B245	Tab, White, Triangle	Perphenazine 2 mg, Amitriptyline 10 mg	Triavil by Barr		Antipsychotic; Antidepressant
B246	Tab, Salmon, Triangle	Perphenazine 4 mg, Amitriptyline 10 mg	Triavil by Barr		Antipsychotic; Antidepressant
B252	Tab, Film Coated	Dipyridamole 25 mg	by Zenith Goldline	00182-1568	Antiplatelet
B252	Tab, Film Coated, Barr 252	Dipyridamole 25 mg	by Rugby	00536-3570	Antiplatelet
B252	Tab, Sugar Coated, B/252	Dipyridamole 25 mg	by Qualitest	00603-3383	Antiplatelet
B260	Tab, Beige, Round	Thioridazine HCl 10 mg	Mellaril by Barr		Antipsychotic
B261	Tab, Yellow, Round	Thioridazine HCl 25 mg	Mellaril by Barr		Antipsychotic
B277	Tab, White, Round	Isosorbide Dinitrate Sublingual 10 mg	Isordil by Barr		Antianginal
B285	Tab, Film Coated	Dipyridamole 50 mg	by Zenith Goldline	00182-1569	Antiplatelet
B285	Tab, Film Coated	Dipyridamole 50 mg	by Rugby	00536-3619	Antiplatelet
B285	Tab, Sugar Coated, B/285	Dipyridamole 50 mg	by Qualitest	00603-3384	Antiplatelet
B2C	Cap	Digoxin 0.1 mg	Lanoxicaps by Catalytica	63552-0272	Cardiac Agent
B2C	Cap, Yellow	Digoxin 0.1 mg	Lanoxicaps by Glaxo	53873-0272	Cardiac Agent
B2C	Cap, Yellow	Digoxin 0.1 mg	Lanoxicaps by Glaxo	00173-0272	Cardiac Agent
B2C	Cap, Clear & Yellow	Digoxin 0.1 mg	Lanoxicaps by Murfreesboro	51129-1246	Cardiac Agent
B2C <> B2C	Cap, Clear & Yellow	Digoxin 0.1 mg	Lanoxicaps by RP Scherer	11014-0748	Cardiac Agent
B3	Tab, Red, Round	Ferrous Sulfate 324 mg	by Paddock		Mineral
B3 <> LL	Tab, White, Scored	Bisoprolol Fumarate 10 mg	Zebeta by Ayerst Lab (Div Wyeth)	00046-3817	Antihypertensive
B3 <> LL	Tab, White, Scored	Bisoprolol Fumarate 10 mg	Zebeta by Wyeth Pharms	52903-3817	Antihypertensive
B329	Tab, Blue, Round	Thioridazine HCl 15 mg	Mellaril by Barr		Antipsychotic
B381	Tab, White, Round	Meperidine HCl 50 mg	Demerol by Barr		Analgesic; C II
B396	Cap, Blue	Phenylbutazone 100 mg	Butazolidin by Barr		Anti-Inflammatory
B397	Tab, Yellow, Round	Clonidine 0.1 mg	Catapres by Barr		Antihypertensive
B398	Tab, White, Round	Clonidine 0.2 mg	Catapres by Barr		Antihypertensive
B399	Tab, Green, Round	Clonidine 0.3 mg	Catapres by Barr		Antihypertensive
B3G	Tab, Pink, Round, B/3/G	Bromazepam 3 mg	by Genpharm	Canadian	Sedative
B477	Tab, White, Round	Haloperidol 0.5 mg	Haldol by Barr		Antipsychotic
B478	Tab, Yellow, Round	Haloperidol 1 mg	Haldol by Barr		Antipsychotic
B479	Tab, White, Round	Haloperidol 2 mg	Haldol by Barr		Antipsychotic
B480	Tab, Green, Round	Haloperidol 5 mg	Haldol by Barr		Antipsychotic
B484	Tab	Leucovorin Calcium	by Zenith Goldline	00182-1869	Antineoplastic
B485	Tab	Leucovorin Calcium	by Zenith Goldline	00182-1870	Antineoplastic
B52	Cap, Red	Vitamin A 50,000 Units	Alphalin by Lilly		Vitamin
B527	Tab, Off-White, Round	Doxycycline Hyclate 100 mg	Vibra-Tab by Martec		Antibiotic

ID FRONT <> BACK	DESCRIPTION FRONT <> BACK	INGREDIENT & STRENGTH	BRAND (OR EQUIV.) & FIRM	NDC#	CLASS; SCH.
B572	Tab, Coated	Methotrexate 2.5 mg	by Zenith Goldline	00182-1539	Antineoplastic
B572	Tab, Coated, B/572	Methotrexate 2.5 mg	by Barr	00555-0572	Antineoplastic
B572	Tab, Coated, Debossed B/572	Methotrexate 2.5 mg	by Supergen	62701-0940	Antineoplastic
B572	Tab, Coated, Debossed	Methotrexate 2.5 mg	by Major	00904-1749	Antineoplastic
B572	Tab, Coated, Debossed	Methotrexate 2.5 mg	by Geneva	00781-1076	Antineoplastic
B572	Tab, Coated, B/572	Methotrexate 2.5 mg	by HL Moore	00839-7905	Antineoplastic
B60	Cap, Brown	Ergocalciterol 50,000 Units	Deltalin by Lilly		Vitamin
B6G	Tab, Green, Round, B/6/G	Bromazepam 6 mg	by Genpharm	Canadian	Sedative
B700	Cap, Ex Release	Chlorpheniramine Maleate 4 mg, Methscopolamine Nitrate 1.25 mg, Phenylephrine HCl 10 mg	Extendryl Jr by Lini	58215-0325	Cold Remedy
B701	Tab	Dexbrompheniramine Maleate 6 mg, Pseudoephedrine Sulfate 120 mg	Drixoral Type by Lini	58215-0111	Cold Remedy
B701	Tab	Dexbrompheniramine Maleate 6 mg, Pseudoephedrine Sulfate 120 mg	Pharmadrine by Breckenridge	51991-0175	Cold Remedy
B8861	Tab, Light Purple, Oval, B 886/1	Estradiol 1 mg	Estrace by Barr		Hormone
B8872	Tab, Green, Oval, B 887/2	Estradiol 2 mg	Estrace by Barr		Hormone
B89912	Tab, White, Oval, B 899 1/2	Estradiol 0.5 mg	Estrace by Barr		Hormone
BAC10	Tab, BAC over 10	Baclofen 10 mg	by Rosemont	00832-1024	Muscle Relaxant
BAC10832	Tab, White, Round, Scored, BAC over 10/832	Baclofen 10 mg	Lioresal by Martec	52555-0695	Muscle Relaxant
BACTRIMDS <> ROCHE	Tab, Bactrim DS	Sulfamethoxazole 800 mg, Trimethoprim 160 mg	Bactrim DS by Hoffmann La Roche	00004-0117	Antibiotic
BACTRIMDS <> ROCHE	Tab	Sulfamethoxazole 800 mg, Trimethoprim 160 mg	Bactrim DS by DRX	55045-2291	Antibiotic
BACTRIMDS <> ROCHE	Tab, White, Oblong, Bactrim-DS	Sulfamethoxazole 800 mg, Trimethoprim 160 mg	Bactrim DS by St. Marys Med	60760-0102	Antibiotic
BACTRIMDS <> ROCHE	Tab, Bactrim DS	Sulfamethoxazole 800 mg, Trimethoprim 160 mg	Bactrim DS by Thrift Drug	59198-0258	Antibiotic
BACTRIMDS <> ROCHE	Tab	Sulfamethoxazole 800 mg, Trimethoprim 160 mg	Bactrim DS by Amerisource	62584-0117	Antibiotic
BACTRIMDS <> ROCHE	Tab, Bactrim DS	Sulfamethoxazole 800 mg, Trimethoprim 160 mg	Bactrim DS by Nat Pharmpak Serv	55154-3101	Antibiotic
BACTRIMDS <> ROCHE	Tab, White, Oblong	Trimethoprim 160 mg, Sulfamethoxazole 800 mg	Bactrim DS by Rightpak	65240-0612	Antibiotic
BACTRIMDS <> ROCHE	Tab, White, Oblong	Trimethoprim 160 mg, Sulfamethoxazole 800 mg	Bactrim DS by Med-Pro	53978-3380	Antibiotic
BAND0499 <> DYNACIN75MG	Cap, Gray, Dynacin 75 mg Band	Minocycline HCl 75 mg	Dynacin by Neuman Distr	64579-0307	Antibiotic
BAR011	Cap	Tetracycline HCl 500 mg	by Med Pro	53978-5048	Antibiotic
BAR159	Cap, Black Print, White Powder	Chlordiazepoxide HCl 25 mg	by Major	00904-0092	Antianxiety; C IV
BARR <> 8335	Tab, Peach, Oval, Scored	Warfarin Sodium 5 mg	by UDL	51079-0913	Anticoagulant
BARR <> 033	Cap, Black & Green	Chlordiazepoxide HCl 10 mg	Librium by UDL	51079-0375	Antianxiety; C IV
BARR <> 033	Cap	Chlordiazepoxide HCl 10 mg	by Med Pro	53978-3175	Antianxiety; C IV
BARR <> 033	Cap, Barr Logo	Chlordiazepoxide HCl 10 mg	by Geneva	00781-2082	Antianxiety; C IV
BARR <> 059	Cap, Pink	Diphenhydramine HCl 50 mg	Benadryl by UDL	51079-0066	Antihistamine
BARR <> 158	Cap, Green & Yellow	Chlordiazepoxide HCl 5 mg	Librium by UDL	51079-0374	Antianxiety; C IV
BARR <> 158	Cap, Barr Logo	Chlordiazepoxide HCl 5 mg	by Geneva	00781-2080	Antianxiety; C IV
BARR <> 158	Cap, Qualitest Logo	Chlordiazepoxide HCl 5 mg	by Qualitest	00603-2666	Antianxiety; C IV
BARR <> 158	Cap	Chlordiazepoxide HCl 5 mg	by Physicians Total Care	54868-2463	Antianxiety; C IV
BARR <> 159	Cap, Green & White	Chlordiazepoxide HCl 25 mg	Librium by UDL	51079-0141	Antianxiety; C IV
BARR <> 159	Cap, Green & White	Chlordiazepoxide HCl 25 mg	by PDRX	55289-0126	Antianxiety; C IV
BARR <> 259	Tab, Coated	Erythromycin Ethylsuccinate	by Barr	00555-0259	Antibiotic
BARR <> 262	Tab, Coated, Debossed	Thioridazine HCl 50 mg	by Barr	00555-0262	Antipsychotic
BARR <> 263	Tab, Coated, Debossed	Thioridazine HCl 100 mg	by Barr	00555-0263	Antipsychotic
BARR <> 285	Tab, White, Round, Film Coated	Dipyridamole 50 mg	by Allscripts	54569-0468	Antiplatelet
BARR <> 286	Tab, White, Round, Film	Dipyridamole 75 mg	by Genpharm	55567-0091	Antiplatelet
BARR <> 286	Tab, Film Coated	Dipyridamole 75 mg	by Nat Pharmpak Serv	55154-5817	Antiplatelet
BARR <> 286	Tab, Film Coated, Debossed	Dipyridamole 75 mg	by Heartland	61392-0553	Antiplatelet
BARR <> 286	Tab, Film Coated	Dipyridamole 75 mg	by Heartland	61392-0142	Antiplatelet
BARR <> 286	Tab, Film Coated	Dipyridamole 75 mg	by Quality Care	60346-0790	Antiplatelet
BARR <> 286	Tab, White, Round, Film Coated	Dipyridamole 75 mg	by Natl Pharmpak	55154-9304	Antiplatelet
BARR <> 286	Tab, White, Round, Film	Dipyridamole 75 mg	by Glaxo Wellcome	00173-0662	Antiplatelet
BARR <> 286	Tab, Film Coated	Dipyridamole 75 mg	by Zenith Goldline	00182-1570	Antiplatelet

ID FRONT <> BACK	DESCRIPTION FRONT <> BACK	INGREDIENT & STRENGTH	BRAND (OR EQUIV.) & FIRM	NDC#	CLASS; SCH.
BARR <> 286	Tab, Sugar Coated	Dipyridamole 75 mg	by Qualitest	00603-3385	Antiplatelet
BARR <> 286	Tab, Film Coated	Dipyridamole 75 mg	by Geneva	00781-1478	Antiplatelet
BARR <> 286	Tab, Film Coated	Dipyridamole 75 mg	by Schein	00364-2493	Antiplatelet
BARR <> 286	Tab, Film Coated	Dipyridamole 75 mg	by Barr	00555-0286	Antiplatelet
BARR <> 286	Tab, White, Round, Film Coated	Dipyridamole 75 mg	Persantine by UDL	51079-0070	Antiplatelet
BARR <> 286	Tab, Film Coated	Dipyridamole 75 mg	by Allscripts	54569-0470	Antiplatelet
BARR <> 286	Tab, Film Coated	Dipyridamole 75 mg	by Major	00904-1088	Antiplatelet
BARR <> 382	Tab, Debossed	Meperidine HCl 100 mg	by Barr	00555-0382	Analgesic; C II
BARR <> 446	Tab	Tamoxifen Citrate 10 mg	by Zeneca	00310-0446	Antiestrogen
BARR <> 446	Tab	Tamoxifen Citrate 10 mg	by Haines	59564-0144	Antiestrogen
BARR <> 545	Cap	Cephalexin Monohydrate	by Warner Chilcott	00047-0938	Antibiotic
BARR <> 555013	Tab, Coated	Erythromycin Stearate 250 mg	by Barr	00555-0013	Antibiotic
BARR <> 555163	Tab, White, Round, Scored	Diazepam 2 mg	by Southwood Pharms	58016-0274	Antianxiety; C IV
BARR <> 555163	Tab, Barr <> 555/163	Diazepam 2 mg	by Barr	00555-0163	Antianxiety; C IV
BARR <> 555164	Tab, 555/164	Diazepam 10 mg	by Quality Care	60346-0033	Antianxiety; C IV
BARR <> 555164	Tab, Blue, Round, Scored	Diazepam 10 mg	by Southwood Pharms	58016-0273	Antianxiety; C IV
BARR <> 555164	Tab, Barr <> 555/164	Diazepam 10 mg	by Barr	00555-0164	Antianxiety; C IV
BARR <> 555271	Tab, 555/271 Debossed	Sulfinpyrazone 100 mg	by Barr	00555-0271	Uricosuric
BARR <> 555363	Tab, 555/363	Diazepam 5 mg	by Quality Care	60346-0478	Antianxiety; C IV
BARR <> 555363	Tab, Yellow, Round, Scored	Diazepam 5 mg	by Southwood Pharms	58016-0275	Antianxiety; C IV
BARR <> 555363	Tab, 555/363	Diazepam 5 mg	by Barr	00555-0363	Antianxiety; C IV
BARR <> 555427	Tab, 555/427 Debossed	Hydrochlorothiazide 25 mg, Propranolol HCl 40 mg	by Barr	00555-0427	Diuretic; Antihypertensive
BARR <> 555428	Tab, 555/428 Debossed	Hydrochlorothiazide 25 mg, Propranolol HCl 80 mg	by Barr	00555-0428	Diuretic; Antihypertensive
BARR <> 555444	Tab, Debossed <> 555/444	Hydrochlorothiazide 50 mg, Triamterene 75 mg	by Rugby	00536-4927	Diuretic
BARR <> 555444	Tab, 555/444 Debossed	Hydrochlorothiazide 50 mg, Triamterene 75 mg	by Barr	00555-0444	Diuretic
BARR <> 555444	Tab	Hydrochlorothiazide 50 mg, Triamterene 75 mg	by PDRX	55289-0488	Diuretic
BARR <> 555444	Tab, 555/444	Hydrochlorothiazide 50 mg, Triamterene 75 mg	by Quality Care	60346-0704	Diuretic
BARR <> 555444	Tab, Company Logo Debossed <> 555/444 Debossed	Hydrochlorothiazide 50 mg, Triamterene 75 mg	by Major	00904-1965	Diuretic
BARR <> 555483	Tab, Light Yellow, Barr <> 555/483	Amiloride HCl 5 mg, Hydrochlorothiazide 50 mg	by Barr	00555-0483	Diuretic
BARR <> 555489	Tab, White, Round, Scored, Barr <> 555 over 489	Trazodone HCl 50 mg	by UDL	51079-0427	Antidepressant
BARR <> 555489	Tab, 555/489 Debossed	Trazodone HCl 50 mg	by Barr	00555-0489	Antidepressant
BARR <> 555489	Tab, Debossed 555/489	Trazodone HCl 50 mg	by Rugby	00536-4715	Antidepressant
BARR <> 555489	Tab, Film Coated, 555/489	Trazodone HCl 50 mg	by Nat Pharmpak Serv	55154-1406	Antidepressant
BARR <> 555490	Tab, Debossed 555/490	Trazodone HCl 100 mg	by Rugby	00536-4688	Antidepressant
BARR <> 555490	Tab, 555/490 Debossed	Trazodone HCl 100 mg	by Barr	00555-0490	Antidepressant
BARR <> 555490	Tab, White, Round, Scored, Barr <> 555 over 490	Trazodone HCl 100 mg	Desyrel by UDL	51079-0428	Antidepressant
BARR <> 555490	Tab, B Printed As Small B with 6-Sided Ring Inside of Circle <> 555 Over 490	Trazodone HCl 100 mg	by Murfreesboro	51129-1131	Antidepressant
BARR <> 555490	Tab, Film Coated, 555/490	Trazodone HCl 100 mg	by Quality Care	60346-0014	Antidepressant
BARR <> 555585	Tab, Stylized Barr	Chlorzoxazone 500 mg	by PDRX	55289-0633	Muscle Relaxant
BARR <> 555585	Tab, Light Green, 555/585	Chlorzoxazone 500 mg	by Quality Care	60346-0663	Muscle Relaxant
BARR <> 555585	Tab, Green, Round, Scored	Chlorzoxazone 500 mg	by Direct Dispensing	57866-3444	Muscle Relaxant
BARR <> 555585	Tab, Light Green, Round, Scored, Barr <> 555 over 585	Chlorzoxazone 500 mg	Parafon Forte by UDL	51079-0476	Muscle Relaxant
BARR <> 555585	Tab, 555/585	Chlorzoxazone 500 mg	by Barr	00555-0585	Muscle Relaxant
BARR <> 555607	Tab, Debossed, Barr <> 555/607	Megestrol Acetate 40 mg	by Warner Chilcott	00047-0108	Progestin
BARR <> 555607	Tab, 555/607 Debossed	Megestrol Acetate 40 mg	by Rugby	00536-4822	Progestin
BARR <> 555607	Tab, 555/607 Debossed	Megestrol Acetate 40 mg	by Barr	00555-0607	Progestin
BARR <> 555607	Tab, Debossed	Megestrol Acetate 40 mg	by CVS	51316-0239	Progestin
BARR <> 555607	Tab, 555/607 Beveled	Megestrol Acetate 40 mg	by Major	00904-3571	Progestin
BARR <> 555607	Tab, 555 Over 607	Megestrol Acetate 40 mg	by CVS Revco	00894-6651	Progestin

ID FRONT <> BACK	DESCRIPTION FRONT <> BACK	INGREDIENT & STRENGTH	BRAND (OR EQUIV.) & FIRM	NDC#	CLASS; SCH.
BARR <> 555607	Tab, 555/607	Megestrol Acetate 40 mg	by Qualitest	00603-4392	Progestin
BARR <> 555643	Tab, Barr Logo <> 555/643 Debossed	Hydrochlorothiazide 25 mg, Triamterene 37.5 mg	by Barr	00555-0643	Diuretic
BARR <> 555727	Tab, Yellow, Round, Flat, Scored, 555/727	Estropipate 0.75 mg	Estropipate USP by Heartland	61392-0617	Hormone
BARR <> 555728	Tab, Peach, Round, Flat, Scored, 555/728	Estropipate 1.5 mg	Estropipate USP by Heartland	61392-0707	Hormone
BARR <> 555729	Tab, Blue, Round, Flat, Scored, 555/729	Estropipate 3 mg	Estropipate USP by Heartland	61392-0715	Hormone
BARR <> 555831	Tab, in Lower Case <> 555/831, Beveled Edge	Warfarin Sodium 1 mg	by Barr	00555-0831	Anticoagulant
BARR <> 555832	Tab, in Lower Case <> 555/832, Beveled Edge	Warfarin Sodium 2.5 mg	by Barr	00555-0832	Anticoagulant
BARR <> 555833	Tab, 555/833	Warfarin Sodium 5 mg	by Barr	00555-0833	Anticoagulant
BARR <> 555834	Tab, 555/834	Warfarin Sodium 7.5 mg	by Barr	00555-0834	Anticoagulant
BARR <> 555835	Tab, 555/835	Warfarin Sodium 10 mg	by Barr	00555-0835	Anticoagulant
BARR <> 555869	Tab, Lavender, in Lower Case, Beveled Edge <> 555/869	Warfarin Sodium 2 mg	by Barr	00555-0869	Anticoagulant
BARR <> 555874	Tab, 555/874	Warfarin Sodium 4 mg	by Barr	00555-0874	Anticoagulant
BARR <> 584	Cap, Clear & Green	Erythromycin 250 mg	by Murfreesboro Ph	51129-1392	Antibiotic
BARR <> 8311	Tab, Pink, Oval, Scored	Warfarin Sodium 1 mg	by UDL	51079-0908	Anticoagulant
BARR <> 834712	Tab, Yellow, Oval, Scored	Warfarin Sodium 7.5 mg	by UDL	51079-0915	Anticoagulant
BARR <> 83510	Tab, White, Oval, Scored	Warfarin Sodium 10 mg	by UDL	51079-0916	Anticoagulant
BARR <> 8692	Tab, Purple, Oval, Scored	Warfarin Sodium 2 mg	by UDL	51079-0909	Anticoagulant
BARR <> 8744	Tab, Blue, Oval, Scored	Warfarin Sodium 4 mg	by UDL	51079-0912	Anticoagulant
BARR <> 904	Tab, Debossed	Tamoxifen Citrate 20 mg	by Zeneca	00310-0904	Antiestrogen
BARR <> 904	Tab	Tamoxifen Citrate 20 mg	by Barr	00555-0904	Antiestrogen
BARR <> 9253	Tab, Tan, Oval, Scored	Warfarin Sodium 3 mg	by UDL	51079-0911	Anticoagulant
BARR <> EBASE333MG	Tab, Barr <> E-Base 333 mg	Erythromycin 333 mg	E Base by Barr	00555-0495	Antibiotic
BARR <> EBASE333MG	Tab, Barr <> E-Base 333 mg	Erythromycin 333 mg	E Base by Barr	00555-0532	Antibiotic
BARR <> EBASE500MG	Tab, Barr <> E-Base 500 mg	Erythromycin 500 mg	E Base by Barr	00555-0533	Antibiotic
BARR010	Cap, Black & Yellow	Tetracycline HCl 500 mg	by HJ Harkins	52959-0336	Antibiotic
BARR010	Cap, Imprint in White Ink	Tetracycline HCl 500 mg	by Barr	00555-0010	Antibiotic
BARR010	Cap, Barr	Tetracycline HCl 500 mg	by Pharmedix	53002-0217	Antibiotic
BARR011	Orange	Tetracycline HCl 250 mg	by Southwood Pharms	58016-0101	Antibiotic
BARR011	Cap, Barr 011 in Black Ink	Tetracycline HCl 250 mg	by Barr	00555-0011	Antibiotic
BARR011	Cap	Tetracycline HCl 250 mg	by Pharmedix	53002-0225	Antibiotic
BARR011	Cap, Barr 011 in Black Ink	Tetracycline HCl 250 mg	by Major	00904-2416	Antibiotic
BARR011	Black & Yellow, Oblong	Tetracycline HCl 500 mg	by Southwood Pharms	58016-0102	Antibiotic
BARR033	Cap, Barr over 033	Chlordiazepoxide HCl 10 mg	by Quality Care	60346-0052	Antianxiety; C IV
BARR033	Cap	Chlordiazepoxide HCl 10 mg	by Zenith Goldline	00182-0978	Antianxiety; C IV
BARR033	Cap, White Print	Chlordiazepoxide HCl 10 mg	by Barr	00555-0033	Antianxiety; C IV
BARR033	Cap	Chlordiazepoxide HCl 10 mg	by Qualitest	00603-2667	Antianxiety; C IV
BARR033	Cap, White Print	Chlordiazepoxide HCl 10 mg	by Major	00904-0091	Antianxiety; C IV
BARR058	Cap, Clear & Pink	Diphenhydramine HCl 25 mg	by Barr	00555-0058	Antihistamine
BARR058 <> BARR058	Cap, Pink	Diphenhydramine HCl 50 mg	by Southwood Pharms	58016-0409	Antihistamine
BARR059	Cap	Diphenhydramine HCl 50 mg	by Nat Pharmpak Serv	55154-5530	Antihistamine
BARR059	Cap, Clear & Pink	Diphenhydramine HCl 50 mg	by Barr	00555-0059	Antihistamine
BARR059	Cap	Diphenhydramine HCl 50 mg	by Nat Pharmpak Serv	55154-5230	Antihistamine
BARR059	Cap	Diphenhydramine HCl 50 mg	by Med Pro	53978-0013	Antihistamine
BARR066 <> 100	Tab, Barr/066 <> Debossed	Isoniazid 100 mg	Isoniazid by Rugby	00536-5901	Antimycobacterial
BARR066 <> 100	Tab, Barr/066	Isoniazid 100 mg	Isoniazid by Barr	00555-0066	Antimycobacterial
BARR066 <> 100	Tab, White, Round, Flat, Barr/066	Isoniazid 100 mg	by Murfreesboro	51129-1562	Antimycobacterial
BARR066 <> 100	Tab, White, Round, Flat, Scored, Barr Over 066	Isoniazid 100 mg	by Murfreesboro	51129-1560	Antimycobacterial
BARR066 <> 100	Tab	Isoniazid 100 mg	Isoniazid by Quality Care	60346-0203	Antimycobacterial
BARR066 <> 100	Tab, Barr/066	Isoniazid 100 mg	Isoniazid by Medirex	57480-0495	Antimycobacterial
BARR066 <> 100	Tab, Debossed	Isoniazid 100 mg	Isoniazid by Prepackage Spec	58864-0298	Antimycobacterial
BARR066 <> 100	Tab, White, Round, Scored, Barr Over 066 <> 100	Isoniazid 100 mg	INH by UDL	51079-0082	Antimycobacterial
BARR066100	Tab, Barr 066 100	Isoniazid 100 mg	Isoniazid by Allscripts	54569-2942	Antimycobacterial

ID FRONT ⬦ BACK	DESCRIPTION FRONT ⬦ BACK	INGREDIENT & STRENGTH	BRAND (OR EQUIV.) & FIRM	NDC#	CLASS; SCH.
BARR071 ⬦ 300	Tab, Barr/071	Isoniazid 300 mg	Isoniazid by Barr	00555-0071	Antimycobacterial
BARR071 ⬦ 300	Tab, Barr/071 Debossed	Isoniazid 300 mg	Isoniazid by Rugby	00536-3941	Antimycobacterial
BARR071 ⬦ 300	Tab, Debossed, Barr/071 ⬦ 300	Isoniazid 300 mg	Isoniazid by Schein	00364-0151	Antimycobacterial
BARR071 ⬦ 300	Tab	Isoniazid 300 mg	Isoniazid by Quality Care	60346-0483	Antimycobacterial
BARR071 ⬦ 300	Tab, White, Round, Scored, Barr Over 071 ⬦ 300	Isoniazid 300 mg	INH by UDL	51079-0083	Antimycobacterial
BARR100324	Cap	Hydroxyzine Pamoate	by Zenith Goldline	00182-1991	Antihistamine
BARR115	Tab, Salmon, Round	Reserpine 0.1 mg, Hydralazine HCl 25 mg, Hydrochlorothiazide 15 mg	Serapes by Barr		Antihypertensive
BARR128	Cap, White Print	Decyclomine HCl 10 mg	by Barr	00555-0128	Gastrointestinal
BARR158	Cap	Chlordiazepoxide HCl 5 mg	by Zenith Goldline	00182-0977	Antianxiety; C IV
BARR158	Cap, Black Print	Chlordiazepoxide HCl 5 mg	by Barr	00555-0158	Antianxiety; C IV
BARR158	Cap	Chlordiazepoxide HCl 5 mg	by HL Moore	00839-1130	Antianxiety; C IV
BARR158	Cap, Black Print	Chlordiazepoxide HCl 5 mg	by Major	00904-0090	Antianxiety; C IV
BARR158	Cap, Green & Yellow	Chlordiazepoxide 5 mg	Librium by Geneva		Antianxiety; C IV
BARR159	Cap	Chlordiazepoxide HCl 25 mg	by Zenith Goldline	00182-0979	Antianxiety; C IV
BARR159	Cap, Black Print	Chlordiazepoxide HCl 25 mg	by Barr	00555-0159	Antianxiety; C IV
BARR159	Cap	Chlordiazepoxide HCl 25 mg	by Geneva	00781-2084	Antianxiety; C IV
BARR159	Cap, Barr over 159	Chlordiazepoxide HCl 25 mg	by Quality Care	60346-0260	Antianxiety; C IV
BARR170	Tab, White, Oval	Furosemide 20 mg	Lasix by Barr		Diuretic
BARR198 ⬦ 3	Tab, Barr/198 ⬦ 3	Acetaminophen 300 mg, Codeine Phosphate 30 mg	by Barr	00555-0198	Analgesic; C III
BARR198 ⬦ 3	Tab	Acetaminophen 300 mg, Codeine Phosphate 30 mg	by Pharmedix	53002-0101	Analgesic; C III
BARR214	Cap, Green & White	Chlordiazepoxide HCl 5 mg, Clidinium Bromide 2.5 mg	Librax by Barr		Gastrointestinal; C IV
BARR2172	Tab, White, Round, Barr 217/2	Acetaminophen 300 mg, Codeine 15 mg	Tylenol #2 by Barr		Analgesic; C III
BARR219	Tab, Pink, Oblong	Erythromycin Stearate 500 mg	Erythrocin by Barr		Antibiotic
BARR229 ⬦ 4	Tab	Acetaminophen 300 mg, Codeine Phosphate 60 mg	by Pharmedix	53002-0103	Analgesic; C III
BARR230 ⬦ BARR230	Cap, Reddish Orange, Barr over 230	Erythromycin Estolate	by Barr	00555-0230	Antibiotic
BARR243	Tab, White, Round	Chlordiazepoxide HCl 10 mg, Amitriptyline 25 mg	Limbitrol by Barr		Antianxiety; C IV
BARR244	Tab, Peach, Round	Chlordiazepoxide HCl 5 mg, Amitriptyline 12.5 mg	Limbitrol by Barr		Antianxiety; C IV
BARR248	Tab, White, Round, Barr/248	Methyldopa 500 mg	Aldomet by Barr		Antihypertensive
BARR259	Tab, Coated	Erythromycin Ethylsuccinate	by Pharmedix	53002-0206	Antibiotic
BARR260	Tab, Coated	Thioridazine HCl 10 mg	by Pharmedix	53002-1065	Antipsychotic
BARR2643	Tab, White, Round, Barr 264/3	Aspirin 325 mg, Codeine 30 mg	Empirin #3 by Barr		Analgesic; C III
BARR267	Tab, Yellow, Round	Chlorthalidone 25 mg	Hygroton by Barr		Diuretic
BARR268	Tab, Green, Round	Chlorthalidone 50 mg	Hygroton by Barr		Diuretic
BARR272	Cap, Barr 272 in Black Ink	Sulfinpyrazone 200 mg	by Barr	00555-0272	Uricosuric
BARR276	Tab, White, Round, Barr/276	Chlorpropamide 250 mg	Diabinese by Barr		Antidiabetic
BARR2804	Tab, White, Round	Aspirin 325 mg, Codeine 60 mg	Empirin #4 by Barr		Analgesic; C III
BARR286	Tab, Film Coated	Dipyridamole 75 mg	by Zenith Goldline	00182-1570	Antiplatelet
BARR288	Tab, Yellow, Round	Isosorbide Dinitrate 40 mg	Isordil by Barr		Antianginal
BARR2942	Tab, White, Round, Barr 294/2	Aspirin 325 mg, Codeine 15 mg	Empirin #2 by Barr		Analgesic; C III
BARR295 ⬦ DOXYTAB	Tab, Coated, Barr 295 ⬦ Doxy-Tab	Doxycycline Hyclate	by Barr	00555-0295	Antibiotic
BARR296 ⬦ DOXYCAP	Tab, Coated, Barr 296 ⬦ Doxy-Cap	Doxycycline Hyclate	by Barr	00555-0296	Antibiotic
BARR297 ⬦ DOXYCAP	Tab, Coated, Barr 297 ⬦ Doxy-Cap	Doxycycline Hyclate	by Barr	00555-0297	Antibiotic
BARR302	Cap, Red & Yellow, Opaque, Barr Underlined Over 302	Hydroxyzine Pamoate 50 mg	by Murfreesboro	51129-1483	Antihistamine
BARR30250	Cap, Ivory & Maroon, Barr 302/50	Hydroxyzine Pamoate 50 mg	Vistaril by Barr		Antihistamine
BARR321	Tab, White, Oblong, Barr/321	Sulfamethoxazole 400 mg, Trimethoprim 80 mg	Septra by Barr		Antibiotic
BARR322	Tab, White, Oval, Barr/322	Sulfamethoxazole 800 mg, Trimethoprim 160 mg	Septra by Barr		Antibiotic
BARR323 ⬦ 25	Cap, in Black Ink Barr Over 323	Hydroxyzine Pamoate 42.61 mg	by Barr	00555-0323	Antihistamine
BARR323 ⬦ 25	Cap, in Black Ink Barr Over 323	Hydroxyzine Pamoate 42.61 mg	by Qualitest	00603-3994	Antihistamine
BARR324 ⬦ 100	Cap, in Black Ink	Hydroxyzine Pamoate	by Barr	00555-0324	Antihistamine
BARR324100	Cap, Barr 324/100	Hydroxyzine Pamoate	by Rugby	00536-3896	Antihistamine
BARR325	Tab	Acetaminophen 500 mg, Hydrocodone Bitartrate 5 mg	by Pharmedix	53002-0119	Analgesic; C III
BARR327	Tab, Green, Round	Thioridazine HCl 150 mg	Mellaril by Barr		Antipsychotic

ID FRONT <> BACK	DESCRIPTION FRONT <> BACK	INGREDIENT & STRENGTH	BRAND (OR EQUIV.) & FIRM	NDC#	CLASS; SCH.
BARR328	Tab, Orange, Round	Thioridazine HCl 200 mg	Mellaril by Barr		Antipsychotic
BARR331	Cap, Blue & Red	Disopyramide Phosphate 100 mg	Norpace by Barr		Antiarrhythmic
BARR332	Cap, Ivory & Red	Disopyramide Phosphate 150 mg	Norpace by Barr		Antiarrhythmic
BARR336	Cap, Green & Green, Barr/336	Indomethacin 25 mg	Indocin by Barr		NSAID
BARR337	Cap, Green & Green, Barr/337	Indomethacin 50 mg	Indocin by Barr		NSAID
BARR349	Tab, Blue, Round	Chlorpropamide 100 mg	Diabinese by Barr		Antidiabetic
BARR350	Tab, Blue, Round	Chlorpropamide 250 mg	Diabinese by Barr		Antidiabetic
BARR357	Tab, White, Round	Methyldopa 125 mg	Aldomet by Barr		Antihypertensive
BARR358	Tab, White, Round	Methyldopa 250 mg	Aldomet by Barr		Antihypertensive
BARR374	Cap, White	Oxazepam 10 mg	Serax by Barr		Sedative/Hypnotic; C IV
BARR375	Cap, Red	Oxazepam 15 mg	Serax by Barr		Sedative/Hypnotic; C IV
BARR376	Cap, Maroon	Oxazepam 30 mg	Serax by Barr		Sedative/Hypnotic; C IV
BARR377	Cap, Blue & White, Barr/377	Flurazepam HCl 15 mg	Dalmane by Barr		Hypnotic; C IV
BARR378	Cap, Blue, Barr/378	Flurazepam HCl 30 mg	Dalmane by Barr		Hypnotic; C IV
BARR383	Tab, White, Round	Ergoloid Mesylates 1 mg	Hydergine by Barr		Ergot
BARR388	Tab, Orange, Round	Hydralazine HCl 10 mg	Apresoline by Barr		Antihypertensive
BARR389	Tab, Orange, Round, Barr/389	Hydralazine HCl 100 mg	Apresoline by Barr		Antihypertensive
BARR395	Tab, Orange & Red, Round	Phenylbutazone 100 mg	Butazolidin by Barr		Anti-Inflammatory
BARR396	Cap, Green & White	Phenylbutazone 100 mg	Butazolidin by Barr		Anti-Inflammatory
BARR404	Cap, Ivory	Doxepin HCl 25 mg	Sinequan by Barr		Antidepressant
BARR405	Cap, Ivory	Doxepin HCl 50 mg	Sinequan by Barr		Antidepressant
BARR406	Cap, Green	Doxepin HCl 75 mg	Sinequan by Barr		Antidepressant
BARR407	Cap, Green & White	Doxepin HCl 100 mg	Sinequan by Barr		Antidepressant
BARR415	Tab, White, Round	Tolazamide 100 mg	Tolinase by Barr		Antidiabetic
BARR416	Tab, White, Round	Tolazamide 250 mg	Tolinase by Barr		Antidiabetic
BARR417	Tab, White, Oval	Tolazamide 500 mg	Tolinase by Barr		Antidiabetic
BARR419	Tab, Coated	Ibuprofen 400 mg	by Pharmedix	53002-0337	NSAID
BARR420	Tab, Film Coated	Ibuprofen 600 mg	by Pharmedix	53002-0301	NSAID
BARR425	Tab, Beige, Round, Barr/425	Verapamil HCl 80 mg	Isoptin,Calan by Barr		Antihypertensive
BARR442	Tab	Acetohexamide 250 mg	by Barr	00555-0442	Antidiabetic
BARR443	Tab, White, Oblong, Scored	Acetohexamide 500 mg	by Amerisource	62584-0049	Antidiabetic
BARR443	Tab	Acetohexamide 500 mg	by Barr	00555-0443	Antidiabetic
BARR486	Tab, Blue, Round	Chlorthalidone 50 mg	Hygroton by Barr		Diuretic
BARR487	Cap, Green & White, Barr/487	Temazepam 15 mg	Restoril by Barr		Sedative/Hypnotic; C IV
BARR488	Cap, White, Barr/488	Temazepam 30 mg	Restoril by Barr		Sedative/Hypnotic; C IV
BARR499	Tab, Coated	Ibuprofen 800 mg	by Pharmedix	53002-0398	NSAID
BARR50 <> 302	Cap, in Black Ink	Hydroxyzine Pamoate 85.22 mg	by Barr	00555-0302	Antihistamine
BARR50 <> 302	Cap, in Black Ink	Hydroxyzine Pamoate 85.22 mg	by Qualitest	00603-3995	Antihistamine
BARR514	Cap, Black Print	Cephalexin Monohydrate	by Warner Chilcott	00047-0938	Antibiotic
BARR514	Cap, Black Print	Cephalexin Monohydrate	by Rugby	00536-0120	Antibiotic
BARR514	Cap, Black Print	Cephalexin Monohydrate	by Barr	00555-0514	Antibiotic
BARR514	Cap, Red & Tan w/ Black Print	Cephalexin Monohydrate 250 mg	by ESI Lederle	59911-5933	Antibiotic
BARR515	Cap, Black Print	Cephalexin Monohydrate	by Warner Chilcott	00047-0939	Antibiotic
BARR515	Cap, Black Print	Cephalexin Monohydrate	by Rugby	00536-0130	Antibiotic
BARR515	Cap, Black Print	Cephalexin Monohydrate	by Barr	00555-0515	Antibiotic
BARR515	Cap, Red	Cephalexin Monohydrate 500 mg	by ESI Lederle	59911-5934	Antibiotic
BARR546	Tab, Orange, Oblong	Cephalexin 500 mg	Keflex by Barr		Antibiotic
BARR550	Cap, Green & Pink	Cephradine 250 mg	Velosef by Barr		Antibiotic
BARR551	Cap, Green & Green	Cephradine 500 mg	Velosef by Barr		Antibiotic
BARR554	Cap, Maroon & Pink	Meclofenamate Sodium 50 mg	Meclomen by Barr		NSAID
BARR555	Cap, Maroon & White	Meclofenamate Sodium 100 mg	Meclomen by Barr		NSAID
BARR555196	Tab, White, Round, Barr 555/196	Furosemide 80 mg	Lasix by Barr		Diuretic

ID FRONT <> BACK	DESCRIPTION FRONT <> BACK	INGREDIENT & STRENGTH	BRAND (OR EQUIV.) & FIRM	NDC#	CLASS; SCH.
BARR555363	Tab	Diazepam 5 mg	by Pharmedix	53002-0334	Antianxiety; C IV
BARR555483	Tab	Amiloride HCl 5 mg, Hydrochlorothiazide 50 mg	by Zenith Goldline	00182-1877	Diuretic
BARR555483	Tab, Barr/455/483	Amiloride HCl 5 mg, Hydrochlorothiazide 50 mg	by Qualitest	00603-2188	Diuretic
BARR582	Cap, Brown & White, Opaque	Cefadroxil 500 mg	Cefadroxil USP by Caremark	00339-6154	Antibiotic
BARR582	Cap, Brown & White	Cefadroxil Hemihydrate 525 mg	by Ranbaxy Pharms	63304-0582	Antibiotic
BARR584	Cap, Delayed Release, White Pellets Imprinted in Gray	Erythromycin 250 mg	by Quality Care	60346-0017	Antibiotic
BARR584	Cap	Erythromycin 250 mg	by Pharmedix	53002-0252	Antibiotic
BARR584	Cap, Stylized Barr	Erythromycin 276.32 mg	by PDRX	55289-0645	Antibiotic
BARR584	Cap, Clear & Dark Green	Erythromycin 276.32 mg	by Barr	00555-0584	Antibiotic
BARR584	Cap, Gray Print, White Beads	Erythromycin 276.32 mg	by Rugby	00536-0354	Antibiotic
BARR584	Cap, Barr/584	Erythromycin 276.32 mg	by UDL	51079-0671	Antibiotic
BARR584	Cap, Gray Print, White Beads	Erythromycin 276.32 mg	by DRX	55045-2076	Antibiotic
BARR584	Cap, Gray Print	Erythromycin 276.32 mg	by Major	00904-2465	Antibiotic
BARR633	Cap, Barr Logo	Danazol 50 mg	by Barr	00555-0633	Steroid
BARR634	Cap, Barr Logo 634	Danazol 100 mg	by Barr	00555-0634	Steroid
BARR635	Cap	Danazol 200 mg	by Zenith Goldline	00182-1880	Steroid
BARR635	Cap	Danazol 200 mg	by Barr	00555-0635	Steroid
BARR732 <> 505050	Tab, White, Oval, Flat, Scored, 50 50 50	Trazodone HCl 150 mg	Trazodone HCl USP by Teva	00480-0290	Antidepressant
BARR733 <> 100100100	Tab, White, Oval, Flat, Scored, Middle 100 Perpendicular to the Others	Trazodone HCl 300 mg	Trazodone HCl USP by Teva	00480-0292	Antidepressant
BARR875	Cap, Barr 875, Barr Logo, in Black Ink	Hydrochlorothiazide 25 mg, Triamterene 37.5 mg	by Barr	00555-0875	Diuretic
BARR882	Cap, Pink & Purple	Hydroxyurea 500 mg	by Barr		Antineoplastic
BARR882	Cap, Pink & Purple	Hydroxyurea 500 mg	by Barr	00555-0882	Antineoplastic
BARR932	Cap, Brown & Olive	Minocycline HCl 50 mg	Minocin by Barr		Antibiotic
BARR933	Cap, Olive & White	Minocycline HCl 100 mg	Minocin by Barr		Antibiotic
BAYER	Cap, White, Oblong, Scored	Acetaminophen 325 mg	by Bayer	Canadian	Antipyretic
BAYER	Cap, Green	Aspirin 500 mg, Methocarbamol 500~400 mg	by Bayer	Canadian	Analgesic
BAYER <> LG	Tab, White with Orange Tinge, Coated, Triple Score	Praziquantel 600 mg	Biltricide by Bayer	00026-2521	Antihelmintic
BAYER <> M400	Tab, Red, Oblong, Film Coated	Moxifloxacin HCl 400 mg	Avelox by Bayer	00026-8581	Antibiotic
BAYER <> M400	Tab, Red, Oblong, Film Coated	Moxifloxacin HCl 400 mg	by Bayer (GM)	12527-8581	Antibiotic
BAYER 325	Cap, Yellow	Acetaminophen 325 mg	by Bayer		Antipyretic
BAYER 500	Cap, Yellow	Acetaminophen 500 mg	by Bayer	Canadian	Antipyretic
BAYER 855	Cap, Ivory	Nimodipine 30 mg	Nimotop by Bayer	Canadian	Antihypertensive
BAYER PLUS	Tab, White	Aspirin 325 mg, Calcium Carb 160 mg, Magnesium Carb 34 mg, Magnes. Oxide 63 mg	by Bayer	Canadian	Analgesic
BAYER10	Tab, Dusty Rose, Round, Bayer/10	Nifedipine 10 mg	Adalat PA by Bayer	Canadian	Antihypertensive
BAYER20	Tab, Dusty Rose, Round, Bayer/20	Nifedipine 20 mg	Adalat PA by Bayer	Canadian	Antihypertensive
BAYER855	Cap, Bayer/855	Nimodipine 30 mg	Nimotop by Bayer	00026-2855	Antihypertensive
BAYER855	Cap, Bayer/855	Nimodipine 30 mg	Nimotop by Nat Pharmpak Serv	55154-4804	Antihypertensive
BAYERCROSS	Tab, Peach, Scored	Acetaminophen 325 mg	by Bayer	Canadian	Antipyretic
BAYERCROSS	Tab, White, Bayer Logo	Acetaminophen 325 mg	by Bayer	Canadian	Antipyretic
BAYERCROSS	Tab, White	Aspirin 500 mg	by Bayer	Canadian	Analgesic
BAYERCROSS ASPRIRIN	Tab, Peach, Bayer Cross/Aspririn	Acetaminophen 80 mg	by Bayer	Canadian	Antipyretic
BAYERLG	Tab, White, Oblong, Bayer/LG	Praziquantel 600 mg	Biltricide by Bayer	Canadian	Antihelmintic
BB455	Tab, Orange, Oval, B/B 455	Verapamil HCl 120 mg	Isoptin,Calan by Barr		Antihypertensive
BBA	Tab, Salmon, Round, Schering Logo BBA	Acetophenazine Maleate 20 mg	Tindal by Schering		Antipsychotic
BC <> AMOX500	Cap	Amoxicillin 500 mg, Amoxicillin Trihydrate 574 mg	by Biochemie	43858-0355	Antibiotic
BC <> AMPI250	Cap	Ampicillin Trihydrate 288.7 mg	by Biochemie	43858-0282	Antibiotic
BC <> AMPI500	Cap	Ampicillin Trihydrate	by Biochemie	43858-0285	Antibiotic
BC <> SANDOZ	Tab, Ivory, Round, Sugar Coated	Pizotifen 0.5 mg	Sandomigran by Novartis	Canadian DIN# 00329320	Antimigraine

ID FRONT ⟺ BACK	DESCRIPTION FRONT ⟺ BACK	INGREDIENT & STRENGTH	BRAND (OR EQUIV.) & FIRM	NDC#	CLASS; SCH.
BC20832	Tab, White, Round, Scored, BC over 20/832	Baclofen 20 mg	Lioresal by Martec	52555-0696	Muscle Relaxant
BCI	Cap, Yellow	Doxercalciferol 2.5 mg	Hectorol by Bone Care	64894-0825	Calcium Metabolism
BCI	Cap, Yellow	Doxercalciferol 2.5 mg	Hectorol by Scherer Rp North	11014-1235	Calcium Metabolism
BCT212	Tab, BCT 2 1/2	Bromocriptine 2.5 mg	by Lek	48866-0105	Antiparkinson
BCT212	Tab, BCT 2 1/2	Bromocriptine 2.5 mg	by Rosemont	00832-0105	Antiparkinson
BDA	Tab, Pink, Round, Schering Logo BDA	Betamethasone 0.6 mg	Celestone by Schering	00085-0011	Steroid
BE	Tab, Lavender, Oval, Schering Logo BE	Methyltestosterone Buccal 10 mg	Oreton Buccal by Schering		Hormone; C III
BEACH ⟺ 1114	Tab, Film Coated	Methenamine Mandelate 500 mg, Sodium Phosphate, Monobasic, Monohydrate 500 mg	Uroqid Acid No 2 by Pharm Assoc	00121-0352	Antibiotic; Urinary Tract
BEACH ⟺ 1114	Tab, Film Coated	Methenamine Mandelate 500 mg, Sodium Phosphate, Monobasic, Monohydrate 500 mg	Uroqid Acid No 2 by Beach	00486-1114	Antibiotic; Urinary Tract
BEACH ⟺ 1114	Tab, Yellow, Oblong, Film	Methenamine Mandelate 500 mg, Sodium Phosphate, Monobasic 500 mg	Uroqid Acid No 2 by Neogen	59051-0090	Antibiotic; Urinary Tract
BEACH ⟺ 1114	Tab, Yellow, Oblong, Film Coated	Methenamine Mandelate 500 mg, Sodium Phosphate, Monobasic 500 mg	Uroqid by WestWard Pharm	00143-9023	Antibiotic; Urinary Tract
BEACH ⟺ 1125	Tab, Film Coated	Potassium Phosphate, Monobasic 155 mg, Sodium Phosphate, Dibasic, Anhydrous 852 mg, Sodium Phosphate, Monobasic, Monohydrate 130 mg	K Phos by Pharm Assoc	00121-0349	Electrolytes
BEACH ⟺ 1125	Tab, Film Coated	Potassium Phosphate, Monobasic 155 mg, Sodium Phosphate, Dibasic, Anhydrous 852 mg, Sodium Phosphate, Monobasic, Monohydrate 130 mg	K-Phos Neutral by Beach	00486-1125	Electrolytes
BEACH ⟺ 1134	Tab, White, Coated	Potassium Phosphate, Monobasic 305 mg, Sodium Phosphate, Monobasic 700 mg	K-Phos No 2 by Beach	00486-1134	Electrolytes
BEACH ⟺ 1134	Tab, Coated	Potassium Phosphate, Monobasic 305 mg, Sodium Phosphate, Monobasic 700 mg	K Phos No 2 by Pharm Assoc	00121-0386	Electrolytes
BEACH ⟺ 1134	Tab	Potassium Phosphate, Monobasic 500 mg	K Phos Original by Pharm Assoc	00121-0382	Electrolytes
BEACH ⟺ 1134	Tab, White, Oblong, Film Coated, Scored	Sodium Phosphate, Dibasic, Anhydrous 852 mg, Potassium Phosphate, Tribasic 155 mg; Sodium Phosphate, Monobasic, Monohydrate 130 mg	K Phos by WestWard Pharm	00143-9024	Electrolytes
BEACH ⟺ 1134	Tab, White, Oblong, Scored, Film	Sodium Phosphate, Dibasic, Anhydrous, Potassium Phosphate, Tribasic, Monobasic, Monohydrate	K Phos Neutral		Electrolytes
BEACH ⟺ 1135	Tab	Potassium Phosphate, Monobasic 155 mg, Sodium Phosphate, Monobasic 350 mg	K Phos M F by Pharm Assoc	00486-1135	Electrolytes
BEACH ⟺ 1136	Tab	Potassium Citrate Anhydrous 50 mg, Sodium Citrate, Anhydrous 950 mg	Citrolith by Pharm Assoc	00121-0374	Electrolytes
BEACH ⟺ 1136	Tab	Potassium Citrate Anhydrous 50 mg, Sodium Citrate, Anhydrous 950 mg	Citrolith by Beach	00486-1136	Electrolytes
BEACH ⟺ 1136	Tab, 11/36	Potassium Citrate Anhydrous 50 mg, Sodium Citrate, Anhydrous 950 mg	Citrolith by		Electrolytes
BEACH1111	Tab	Potassium Phosphate, Monobasic 500 mg	K-Phos Original by West Ward	00143-9001	Electrolytes
BEACH1111	Tab, White	Potassium Phosphate, Monobasic 500 mg	K Phos Original by Beach	00486-1111	Electrolytes
BEACH1112	Tab, Yellow, Round	Methenamine Mandelate 350 mg, Sodium Acid Phosphate 200 mg	Uroquid-Acid by Beach		Antibiotic; Urinary Tract
BEACH1115	Tab, Green, Oblong	Methenamine Mandelate 500 mg, Potassium Acid Phosphate 250 mg	Thiacide by Beach		Antibiotic; Urinary Tract
BEACH1132	Tab, Yellow, Round	Magnesium 600 mg, Vitamin B-6 25 mg	Beelith by Beach	00486-1132	Mineral; Vitamin
BEACH1135	Tab	Potassium Phosphate, Monobasic 155 mg, Sodium Phosphate, Monobasic 350 mg	K Phos MF by West Ward	00143-9002	Electrolytes
BEACH1135	Tab, White	Potassium Phosphate, Monobasic 155 mg, Sodium Phosphate, Monobasic 350 mg	K-Phos MF by Beach	00486-1135	Electrolytes
BEB ⟺ CG	Tab, Light Red, Round, Film Coated	Oxprenolol HCl 80 mg	Slow Trasicor by Novartis	Canadian DIN# 00534579	Antihypertensive
BEECHAM ⟺ 185	Tab	Penicillin V Potassium	by Quality Care	60346-0414	Antibiotic
BEECHAM ⟺ FASTIN	Cap, Blue & White Beads	Phentermine HCl 30 mg	Fastin by HJ Harkins Co	52959-0430	Anorexiant; C IV
BEECHAM ⟺ FASTIN	Cap, Blue & White Beads	Phentermine HCl 30 mg	Fastin by King	60793-0836	Anorexiant; C IV
BEECHAM ⟺ FASTIN	Cap, Beecham in White Ink ⟺ R Inside Circle to Right of Fastin in Red Ink	Phentermine HCl 30 mg	Fastin by SKB	00029-2205	Anorexiant; C IV
BEECHAM ⟺ FASTIN	Cap, Blue & Clear, Blue & White Beads	Phentermine HCl 30 mg	Fastin by PDRX	55289-0180	Anorexiant; C IV
BEECHAM186	Tab, White, Oval	Penicillin V Potassium 500 mg	Beepen-VK by SmithKline SKB		Antibiotic
BEMINAL	Tab, Brown, Oval	B Complex Vitamin	Beminal by Whitehall-Robbins		Vitamin
BEMINALC	Cap, Brown & Yellow	B Complex Vitamin	Beminal by Whitehall-Robbins		Vitamin
BENADRYL	Cap, Light Green	Diphenhydramine 12.5 mg, Pseudoephedrine 30 mg, Acetaminophen 500 mg	by Warner-Lambert	Canadian	Cold Remedy
BENTYL10	Cap, Bentyl over 10	Decyclomine HCl 10 mg	Bentyl by Quality Care	60346-0749	Gastrointestinal
BENTYL10	Cap, Blue	Decyclomine HCl 10 mg	Bentyl by Hoechst Marion Roussel	00088-0120	Gastrointestinal
BENTYL20	Tab, Light Blue	Decyclomine HCl 20 mg	Bentyl by Hoechst Marion Roussel	00088-0123	Gastrointestinal
BENTYL20	Tab	Decyclomine HCl 20 mg	Bentyl by Allscripts	54569-0418	Gastrointestinal

ID FRONT <> BACK	DESCRIPTION FRONT <> BACK	INGREDIENT & STRENGTH	BRAND (OR EQUIV.) & FIRM	NDC#	CLASS; SCH.
BENTYL20	Tab, Blue, Round	Dicyclomine HCl 20 mg	Bentyl by HJ Harkins	52959-0390	Gastrointestinal
BENYLIN	Cap, Green	Dextromethorphan 15 mg, Pseudoephedrine 30 mg, Guaifenesin 100 mg, Aceta 500 mg	by Warner Lambert	Canadian	Cold Remedy
BERLEX	Tab, White, Oblong, Scored	Sotalol HCl 80 mg	Betapace by Promex Medcl	62301-0051	Antiarrhythmic
BERLEX120	Tab, White, Capsule Shaped, Scored	Sotalol HCl 120 mg	Betapace AF/tm by Berlex	50419-11906	Antiarrhythmic
BERLEX120	Tab, White, Capsule Shaped, Scored	Sotalol HCl 120 mg	Betapace AF/tm by Berlex	50419-11911	Antiarrhythmic
BERLEX160	Tab, White, Capsule Shaped, Scored	Sotalol HCl 160 mg	Betapace AF/tm by Berlex	50419-11611	Antiarrhythmic
BERLEX160	Tab, White, Capsule Shaped, Scored	Sotalol HCl 160 mg	Betapace AF/tm by Berlex	50419-11606	Antiarrhythmic
BERLEX181	Cap, Blue & Yellow	Chlorpheniramine Maleate 8 mg, Pseudoephedrine HCl 120 mg	Deconamine SR by Berlex		Cold Remedy
BERLEX184	Tab, White, Round	Chlorpheniramine Maleate 4 mg, Pseudoephedrine HCl 60 mg	Deconamine by Berlex		Cold Remedy
BERLEX80	Tab, White, Capsule Shaped, Scored	Sotalol HCl 80 mg	Betapace Af/tm by Berlex	50419-11506	Antiarrhythmic
BERLEX80	Tab. White, Capsule Shaped, Scored	Sotalol HCl 80 mg	Betapace AF/tm by Berlex;	50419-11511	Antiarrhythmic
BERTEK 560	Cap, Light Lavender & White	Phenytoin Sodium 100 mg	by Mylan	00378-1560	Anticonvulsant
BERTEK560	Tab, Light Lavender & White, Cap Shaped, Bertek over 560	Extended Phenytoin Sodium 100 mg	Dilantin Kapseals	51079-0905	Anticonvulsant
BERTEK560	Cap, Purple & White	Phenytoin Sodium 100 mg	by Phy Total Care	54868-0040	Anticonvulsant
BERTEX560	Cap, Opaque & Purple, Bertex Over 560	Phenytoin Sodium 100 mg	by Prepackage Spec	58864-0397	Anticonvulsant
BETAPACE <> 80MG	Tab, Light Blue	Sotalol HCl 80 mg	by Caremark	00339-6051	Antiarrhythmic
BETAPACE <> 80MG	Tab, Light Blue, Betapace <> 80/mg	Sotalol HCl 80 mg	by Nat Pharmpak Serv	55154-0305	Antiarrhythmic
BGL	Tab, White, Round, BGL/Logo	Clobazam 10 mg	Frisium by Hoechst-Roussel	Canadian	Anticonvulsant
BHIOM	Tab	Acetic Acid 6 X, Aranea Diadema 8 X, Arsenic Trioxide 6 X, Asafoetida 6 X,	Migraine by Heel	50114-2236	Homeopathic
BHIOM	Tab	Aconite 5 X, Calcium Sulfide 10 X, Capsicum 6 X, Chamomile 4 X, Ferric Phosphate 10 X, Plantain 4 X, Potassium Chlorate 6 X, Pulsatilla 4 X	by Heel	50114-2279	Homeopathic
BI <> 18	Tab, Sugar Coated	Dipyridamole 50 mg	Persantine by Nat Pharmpak Serv	55154-0402	Antiplatelet
BI <> 18	Tab, Reddish Orange, Sugar Coated	Dipyridamole 50 mg	Persantine-50 by Boehringer Ingelheim	00597-0018	Antiplatelet
BI <> 19	Tab, Sugar Coated	Dipyridamole 75 mg	Persantine 75 by Boehringer Ingelheim	00597-0019	Antiplatelet
BI <> 64	Cap, Celery	Phendimetrazine Tartrate 105 mg	Prelu 2 by Quality Care	60346-0621	Anorexiant; C III
BI10	Tab	Chlorthalidone 15 mg, Clonidine HCl 0.3 mg	Combipres by Boehringer Ingelheim	00597-0010	Diuretic; Antihypertensive
BI10	Tab, Coated	Mesoridazine Besylate 10 mg	Serentil by Boehringer Ingelheim	00597-0020	Antipsychotic
BI100	Tab, Coated	Mesoridazine Besylate 100 mg	Serentil by Boehringer Ingelheim	00597-0023	Antipsychotic
BI11	Tab	Clonidine HCl 0.3 mg	Catapres by Boehringer Ingelheim	00597-0011	Antihypertensive
BI11	Tab, Peach, Oval, Scored	Clonidine HCl 0.3 mg	Catapres by DHHS Prog	11819-0111	Antihypertensive
BI12	Tab, Yellow, Round, BI/12	Bisacodyl 5 mg	Dulcolax by BI		Gastrointestinal
BI17	Tab, Orange, Round, BI/17	Dipyridamole 25 mg	Persantine by Genpharm	55567-0092	Antiplatelet
BI17	Tab, Orange, Round, BI/17	Dipyridamole 25 mg	Persantine by Glaxo Wellcome		Antiplatelet
BI17	Tab, Sugar Coated	Dipyridamole 25 mg	Persantine by Boehringer Ingelheim	00597-0017	Antiplatelet
BI18	Tab, Sugar Coated, BI Over 18	Dipyridamole 50 mg	Persantine by Amerisource	62584-0018	Antiplatelet
BI18	Tab, Orange, Round, BI/18	Dipyridamole 50 mg	Persantine by Glaxo Wellcome		Antiplatelet
BI19	Tab, Sugar Coated, BI Over 19	Dipyridamole 75 mg	Persantine by Leiner	59606-0718	Antiplatelet
BI19	Tab, Sugar Coated, BI/19	Dipyridamole 75 mg	Persantine by Pharm Utilization	60491-0507	Antiplatelet
BI19	Tab, Orange, Round, BI/19	Dipyridamole 75 mg	Persantine by Glaxo Wellcome	00173-0661	Antiplatelet
BI25	Tab, Coated	Mesoridazine Besylate 25 mg	Serentil by Boehringer Ingelheim	00597-0021	Antipsychotic
BI28	Tab, Yellow, Round, BI/28	Thiethylperazine Maleate 10 mg	Torecan by BI		Antiemetic
BI48	Tab, White, Round, BI/48	Theophylline SR 250 mg	Respbid by BI		Antiasthmatic
BI49	Tab, White, Oblong, BI/49	Theophylline SR 500 mg	Respbid by BI		Antiasthmatic
BI50	Tab, Coated	Mesoridazine Besylate 50 mg	Serentil by Boehringer Ingelheim	00597-0022	Antipsychotic
BI58 <> FLOMAX04MG	Cap, Olive Green, Gelatin Coated, BI 58 <> Flomax Over 0.4 mg	Tamsulosin HCl 0.4 mg	Flomax by Boehringer Ingelheim	00597-0058	Antiadrenergic
BI58 <> FLOMAX04MG	Cap, Gelatin Coated, BI 58 <> Flomax 0.4 mg	Tamsulosin HCl 0.4 mg	Flomax by Shaklee Tech	51248-0058	Antiadrenergic
BI58 <> FLOMAX4MG	Cap, Gelatin Coated, Flomax 0.4 mg	Tamsulosin HCl 0.4 mg	by Yamanouchi	12838-0058	Antiadrenergic
BI6	Tab, Tan, Oval	Clonidine HCl 0.1 mg	Catapres by Boehringer Ingelheim	00597-0006	Antihypertensive
BI6	Tab, Tan, Oval, Scored	Clonidine HCl 0.1 mg	Catapres by DHHS Prog	11819-0101	Antihypertensive

ID FRONT <> BACK	DESCRIPTION FRONT <> BACK	INGREDIENT & STRENGTH	BRAND (OR EQUIV.) & FIRM	NDC#	CLASS; SCH.
BI62	Tab, Pink, Round, BI/62	Phenmetrazine HCl 75 mg	Preludin Endurets by BI		Appetite Suppressant
BI64	Cap, Green	Phendimetrazine Tartrate 105 mg	Prelu-2 by Allscripts	54569-0395	Anorexiant; C III
BI66	Cap, Brown & Red	Mexiletine HCl 150 mg	by Roxane	00054-0066	Antiarrhythmic
BI66	Cap, Caramel	Mexiletine HCl 150 mg	Mexitil by Boehringer Ingelheim	00597-0066	Antiarrhythmic
BI67	Cap	Mexiletine HCl 200 mg	Mexitil by Boehringer Ingelheim	00597-0067	Antiarrhythmic
BI67	Cap, Red, BI/67	Mexiletine HCl 200 mg	by Roxane	00054-0067	Antiarrhythmic
BI68	Cap, Aqua Green & Red, BI/68	Mexiletine HCl 250 mg	by Roxane	00054-0068	Antiarrhythmic
BI68	Cap, Aqua Green	Mexiletine HCl 250 mg	Mexitil by Boehringer Ingelheim	00597-0068	Antiarrhythmic
BI7	Tab, Orange, Oval	Clonidine HCl 0.2 mg	Catapres by Boehringer Ingelheim	00597-0007	Antihypertensive
BI7	Tab, Orange, Oval, Scored	Clonidine HCl 0.2 mg	Catapres by DHHS Prog	11819-0102	Antihypertensive
BI72	Tab	Metaproterenol Sulfate 20 mg	Alupent by Boehringer Ingelheim	00597-0072	Antiasthmatic
BI74	Tab	Metaproterenol Sulfate 10 mg	Alupent by Boehringer Ingelheim	00597-0074	Antiasthmatic
BI76	Tab, White, Kidney Shaped, BI/76	Chlorthalidone 25 mg	Thalitone by BI		Diuretic
BI77	Tab, White, Kidney Shaped, BI/77	Chlorthalidone 15 mg	Thalitone by BI		Diuretic
BI8	Tab, Pink, Oval	Chlorthalidone 15 mg, Clonidine HCl 0.1 mg	Combipres by Boehringer Ingelheim	00597-0008	Diuretic; Antihypertensive
BI9	Tab, Blue, Oval	Chlorthalidone 15 mg, Clonidine HCl 0.2 mg	Combipres by Boehringer Ingelheim	00597-0009	Diuretic; Antihypertensive
BICRAFT149	Cap, Blue & Red, Biocraft over 149	Clindamycin HCl 150 mg	by Teva	00093-3171	Antibiotic
BIOCRAF02	Cap, Green & Light Green	Dicloxacillin Sodium 250 mg	Dynapen by Biocraft		Antibiotic
BIOCRAFT <> 01	Cap, Buff & Caramel	Amoxicillin 250 mg	by Quality Care	60346-0655	Antibiotic
BIOCRAFT <> 05	Cap, Scarlet	Ampicillin Trihydrate	by Schein	00364-2001	Antibiotic
BIOCRAFT <> 05	Cap, Scarlet	Ampicillin Trihydrate	by Quality Care	60346-0082	Antibiotic
BIOCRAFT <> 06	Cap, Scarlet	Ampicillin Trihydrate	by Quality Care	60346-0593	Antibiotic
BIOCRAFT <> 105	Tab, White, Oblong, Scored	Sucralfate 1 gm	by SKB	60351-4153	Gastrointestinal
BIOCRAFT <> 105	Tab, White, Oblong, Scored	Sucralfate 1 gm	by SKB	60351-4896	Gastrointestinal
BIOCRAFT <> 105	Tab	Sucralfate 1 gm	by Vangard	00615-4517	Gastrointestinal
BIOCRAFT <> 105	Tab, White, Oblong, Scored	Sucralfate 1 gm	by Allscripts	54569-4446	Gastrointestinal
BIOCRAFT <> 105	Tab, White, Oblong, Scored, Uncoated	Sucralfate 1 gm	by Sigma Tau	54482-0053	Gastrointestinal
BIOCRAFT <> 105	Tab, White, Oblong, Scored	Sucralfate 1 gm	by SKB	60351-5046	Gastrointestinal
BIOCRAFT <> 105	Tab	Sucralfate 1 gm	by Golden State	60429-0706	Gastrointestinal
BIOCRAFT <> 105105	Tab, White, Oblong, Scored	Sucralfate 1 gm	by Murfreesboro Ph	51129-1266	Gastrointestinal
BIOCRAFT <> 105105	Tab, White, Oblong, Scored, Biocraft <> 105/105	Sucralfate 1 gm	by Teva	00093-2210	Gastrointestinal
BIOCRAFT <> 105105	Tab, White, Oval Shaped, Scored, Biocraft <> 105/105	Sucralfate 1 gm	Carafate by UDL	51079-0871	Gastrointestinal
BIOCRAFT <> 112	Cap, Green & Opaque & Pink	Cephradine 250 mg	by Carlsbad	61442-0103	Antibiotic
BIOCRAFT <> 112	Cap, Light Green	Cephradine Monohydrate 250 mg	by Quality Care	60346-0040	Antibiotic
BIOCRAFT <> 113	Cap, Light Green	Cephradine 500 mg	by Schein	00364-2142	Antibiotic
BIOCRAFT <> 113	Cap, Light Green	Cephradine Monohydrate 500 mg	by Quality Care	60346-0041	Antibiotic
BIOCRAFT <> 115	Cap, Gray & Orange	Cephalexin 250 mg	by Caremark	00339-6167	Antibiotic
BIOCRAFT <> 117	Cap, Biocraft Labs	Cephalexin Monohydrate	by Quality Care	60346-0055	Antibiotic
BIOCRAFT <> 149	Cap	Clindamycin HCl	by Quality Care	60346-0018	Antibiotic
BIOCRAFT <> 16	Tab, White, Oval	Penicillin V Potassium 250 mg	by Teva	00093-1172	Antibiotic
BIOCRAFT <> 16	Tab	Penicillin V Potassium	by Quality Care	60346-0414	Antibiotic
BIOCRAFT <> 3	Tab	Sulfamethoxazole 800 mg, Trimethoprim 160 mg	by Zenith Goldline	00182-8844	Antibiotic
BIOCRAFT <> 3	Tab	Sulfamethoxazole 800 mg, Trimethoprim 160 mg	by Nat Pharmpak Serv	55154-5805	Antibiotic
BIOCRAFT <> 33	Tab	Sulfamethoxazole 800 mg, Trimethoprim 160 mg	SMX TMP by Vangard	00615-0170	Antibiotic
BIOCRAFT <> 33	Tab	Sulfamethoxazole 800 mg, Trimethoprim 160 mg	SMZ TMP DS by Quality Care	60346-0087	Antibiotic
BIOCRAFT <> 34	Tab, White, Round, Scored, Biocraft <> 3 over 4	Trimethoprim 100 mg	by Teva	00093-2158	Antibiotic
BIOCRAFT <> 34	Tab	Trimethoprim 100 mg	by Murfreesboro	51129-1204	Antibiotic
BIOCRAFT <> 49	Tab, Film Coated	Penicillin V Potassium	by Quality Care	60346-0095	Antibiotic
BIOCRAFT <> 49	Tab, White, Oval, Scored, Biocraft <> 4/9	Penicillin V Potassium 500 mg	by Teva	00093-1174	Antibiotic
BIOCRAFT <> 0101	Cap	Amoxicillin Trihydrate	by Urgent Care Ctr	50716-0606	Antibiotic

ID FRONT <> BACK	DESCRIPTION FRONT <> BACK	INGREDIENT & STRENGTH	BRAND (OR EQUIV.) & FIRM	NDC#	CLASS; SCH.
BIOCRAFT 185	Cap, White	Ketoprofen 25 mg	Orudis by Biocraft		NSAID
BIOCRAFT01	Cap, Buff & Caramel	Amoxicillin 250 mg	Amoxil by Biocraft		Antibiotic
BIOCRAFT01	Cap, Buff & Caramel	Amoxicillin Trihydrate	by Zenith Goldline	00182-1070	Antibiotic
BIOCRAFT01	Cap	Amoxicillin Trihydrate	by Qualitest	00603-2266	Antibiotic
BIOCRAFT01	Cap	Amoxicillin Trihydrate	by HL Moore	00839-6037	Antibiotic
BIOCRAFT01	Cap, Buff & Caramel	Amoxicillin Trihydrate	by Allscripts	54569-1746	Antibiotic
BIOCRAFT01	Cap	Amoxicillin Trihydrate	by Pharmedix	53002-0208	Antibiotic
BIOCRAFT01	Cap	Amoxicillin Trihydrate	by Med Pro	53978-5002	Antibiotic
BIOCRAFT01	Cap, Tan	Amoxicillin Trihydrate 250 mg	by Allscripts	54569-3876	Antibiotic
BIOCRAFT01	Cap, Beige & Brown	Amoxicillin Trihydrate 250 mg	by Allscripts	54569-3986	Antibiotic
BIOCRAFT01	Cap, Buff & Caramel, Biocraft over 01	Amoxicillin Trihydrate 250 mg	by Teva	00093-3107	Antibiotic
BIOCRAFT01	Cap, Buff or Caramel	Amoxicillin 250 mg	by Teva	17372-0613	Antibiotic
BIOCRAFT02	Cap	Amoxicillin Trihydrate	by Qualitest	00603-2267	Antibiotic
BIOCRAFT02	Cap	Dicloxacillin Sodium	by Prescription Dispensing	61807-0038	Antibiotic
BIOCRAFT02	Cap	Dicloxacillin Sodium	by Warner Chilcott	00047-0945	Antibiotic
BIOCRAFT02	Cap	Dicloxacillin Sodium	by Rugby	00536-1180	Antibiotic
BIOCRAFT02	Cap, Dark Green & Light Green	Dicloxacillin Sodium	by Pharmedix	53002-0220	Antibiotic
BIOCRAFT02	Cap	Dicloxacillin Sodium	by Apotheca	12634-0439	Antibiotic
BIOCRAFT02	Cap, Light Green & Medium Green	Dicloxacillin Sodium 250 mg	by Quality Care	60346-0480	Antibiotic
BIOCRAFT02	Cap, Light Green, Biocraft over 02	Dicloxacillin Sodium 250 mg	by Teva	00093-3123	Antibiotic
BIOCRAFT02	Cap	Dicloxacillin Sodium 250 mg	by Zenith Goldline	00182-1506	Antibiotic
BIOCRAFT02	Cap	Dicloxacillin Sodium 250 mg	by HJ Harkins Co	52959-0048	Antibiotic
BIOCRAFT02	Cap, Light Green	Dicloxacillin Sodium 250 mg	by Allscripts	54569-0384	Antibiotic
BIOCRAFT02	Cap, Light Green, Biocraft/02	Dicloxacillin Sodium	by Kaiser	00179-1048	Antibiotic
BIOCRAFT02	Cap	Dicloxacillin Sodium	by Urgent Care Ctr	50716-0222	Antibiotic
BIOCRAFT02	Cap, Light Green, Biocraft/02	Dicloxacillin Sodium	by UDL	51079-0610	Antibiotic
BIOCRAFT03	Cap, Buff	Amoxicillin Trihydrate	by Zenith Goldline	00182-1071	Antibiotic
BIOCRAFT03	Cap	Amoxicillin Trihydrate	by HL Moore	00839-6038	Antibiotic
BIOCRAFT03	Cap, Buff	Amoxicillin Trihydrate	by Allscripts	54569-1861	Antibiotic
BIOCRAFT03	Cap	Amoxicillin Trihydrate	by Med Pro	53978-5003	Antibiotic
BIOCRAFT03	Cap	Amoxicillin Trihydrate	by Pharmedix	53002-0216	Antibiotic
BIOCRAFT03	Cap, Buff	Amoxicillin Trihydrate 500 mg	by Allscripts	54569-3335	Antibiotic
BIOCRAFT03	Cap, Buff, Biocraft over 03	Amoxicillin Trihydrate 500 mg	by Teva	00093-3109	Antibiotic
BIOCRAFT03	Cap	Amoxicillin 500 mg	by Diversified Hlthcare Serv	55887-0982	Antibiotic
BIOCRAFT03	Cap, Buff or Caramel, Teva Logo	Amoxicillin 500 mg	by Quality Care	60346-0634	Antibiotic
BIOCRAFT03	Cap, Buff	Amoxicillin 500 mg	Amoxil by Biocraft		Antibiotic
BIOCRAFT03	Cap	Amoxicillin Trihydrate	by Urgent Care Ctr	50716-0607	Antibiotic
BIOCRAFT04	Cap, Light Green	Dicloxacillin Sodium	by Quality Care	60346-0229	Antibiotic
BIOCRAFT04	Cap	Dicloxacillin Sodium	by Warner Chilcott	00047-0946	Antibiotic
BIOCRAFT04	Cap	Dicloxacillin Sodium	by Zenith Goldline	00182-1507	Antibiotic
BIOCRAFT04	Cap, Light Green, Biocraft over 04	Dicloxacillin Sodium 500 mg	by Teva	00093-3125	Antibiotic
BIOCRAFT04	Cap	Dicloxacillin Sodium 500 mg	by Allscripts	54569-1889	Antibiotic
BIOCRAFT04	Cap	Dicloxacillin Sodium 500 mg	by HJ Harkins Co	52959-0049	Antibiotic
BIOCRAFT04	Cap	Dicloxacillin Sodium 500 mg	by HL Moore	00839-6614	Antibiotic
BIOCRAFT04	Cap, Biocraft/04	Dicloxacillin Sodium 500 mg	by UDL	51079-0611	Antibiotic
BIOCRAFT05	Cap	Ampicillin Trihydrate	by Signal Health	62125-0415	Antibiotic
BIOCRAFT05	Cap	Ampicillin Trihydrate	by Zenith Goldline	00182-0163	Antibiotic
BIOCRAFT05	Cap	Ampicillin Trihydrate	by HL Moore	00839-5087	Antibiotic
BIOCRAFT05	Cap	Ampicillin Trihydrate	by Qualitest	00603-2290	Antibiotic
BIOCRAFT05	Cap	Ampicillin Trihydrate	by Pharmedix	53002-0230	Antibiotic
BIOCRAFT05	Cap	Ampicillin Trihydrate	by Allscripts	54569-1719	Antibiotic
BIOCRAFT05	Cap	Ampicillin Trihydrate	by Apotheca	12634-0417	Antibiotic

ID FRONT <> BACK	DESCRIPTION FRONT <> BACK	INGREDIENT & STRENGTH	BRAND (OR EQUIV.) & FIRM	NDC#	CLASS; SCH.
BIOCRAFT05	Cap	Ampicillin Trihydrate	by Geneva	00781-2555	Antibiotic
BIOCRAFT05	Cap, Gray	Ampicillin Trihydrate 250 mg	by Southwood Pharms	58016-0148	Antibiotic
BIOCRAFT05	Cap, Gray & Scarlet, Biocraft over 05	Ampicillin Trihydrate 250 mg	by Teva	00093-3111	Antibiotic
BIOCRAFT05	Cap, Dark <> Light	Dicloxacillin Sodium	by Pharmedix	53002-0228	Antibiotic
BIOCRAFT05	Cap, Scarlet, Biocraft/05	Ampicillin Trihydrate	by Kaiser	00179-0085	Antibiotic
BIOCRAFT05	Cap, Scarlet, Biocraft/05	Ampicillin Trihydrate	by UDL	51079-0602	Antibiotic
BIOCRAFT06	Cap	Ampicillin Trihydrate	by Zenith Goldline	00182-0641	Antibiotic
BIOCRAFT06	Cap	Ampicillin Trihydrate	by Qualitest	00603-2291	Antibiotic
BIOCRAFT06	Cap	Ampicillin Trihydrate	by Med Pro	53978-5019	Antibiotic
BIOCRAFT06	Cap	Ampicillin Trihydrate	by Allscripts	54569-2411	Antibiotic
BIOCRAFT06	Cap	Ampicillin Trihydrate	by HJ Harkins Co	52959-0389	Antibiotic
BIOCRAFT06	Cap	Ampicillin Trihydrate	by Geneva	00781-2999	Antibiotic
BIOCRAFT06	Cap	Ampicillin Trihydrate	by Major	00904-2073	Antibiotic
BIOCRAFT06	Cap, Gray & Scarlet	Ampicillin Trihydrate 500 mg	by PDRX	55289-0024	Antibiotic
BIOCRAFT06	Cap, Gray & Scarlet, Biocraft over 06	Ampicillin Trihydrate 500 mg	by Teva	00093-3113	Antibiotic
BIOCRAFT06	Cap	Ampicillin Trihydrate 500 mg	by Apotheca	12634-0168	Antibiotic
BIOCRAFT112	Cap, Light Green	Cephradine 250 mg	by Schein	00364-2141	Antibiotic
BIOCRAFT112	Cap, Light Green & Pink, Opaque, Biocraft over 112	Cephradine 250 mg	by Teva	00093-3153	Antibiotic
BIOCRAFT112	Cap	Cephradine 250 mg	by Allscripts	54569-0325	Antibiotic
BIOCRAFT112	Cap	Cephradine Monohydrate 250 mg	by Prescription Dispensing	61807-0048	Antibiotic
BIOCRAFT112	Cap	Cephradine Monohydrate 250 mg	by Zenith Goldline	00182-1253	Antibiotic
BIOCRAFT112	Cap	Cephradine Monohydrate 250 mg	by Pharmedix	53002-0248	Antibiotic
BIOCRAFT112	Cap, Biocraft/112	Cephradine 250 mg	by UDL	51079-0606	Antibiotic
BIOCRAFT113	Cap, Light Green, Opaque, Biocraft over 113	Cephradine 500 mg	by Teva	00093-3155	Antibiotic
BIOCRAFT113	Cap	Cephradine 500 mg	by HJ Harkins Co	52959-0032	Antibiotic
BIOCRAFT113	Cap	Cephradine 500 mg	by Allscripts	54569-0326	Antibiotic
BIOCRAFT113	Cap	Cephradine Monohydrate 500 mg	by PDRX	55289-0597	Antibiotic
BIOCRAFT113	Cap	Cephradine Monohydrate 500 mg	by Zenith Goldline	00182-1254	Antibiotic
BIOCRAFT113	Cap	Cephradine Monohydrate 500 mg	by Pharmedix	53002-0249	Antibiotic
BIOCRAFT113	Cap, Biocraft/113	Cephradine 500 mg	by UDL	51079-0607	Antibiotic
BIOCRAFT114	Cap, Yellow	Cefadroxil 500 mg	Duricef by Biocraft		Antibiotic
BIOCRAFT115	Cap	Cephalexin 250 mg	by Darby Group	66467-0120	Antibiotic
BIOCRAFT115	Cap, Gray & Orange, Biocraft over 115	Cephalexin 250 mg	by Teva	00093-3145	Antibiotic
BIOCRAFT115	Cap	Cephalexin 250 mg	by Allscripts	54569-0304	Antibiotic
BIOCRAFT115	Cap, Biocraft over 115	Cephalexin Monohydrate	by Quality Care	60346-0441	Antibiotic
BIOCRAFT115	Cap, Swedish Orange	Cephalexin Monohydrate	by PDRX	55289-0057	Antibiotic
BIOCRAFT115	Cap	Cephalexin Monohydrate	by Signal Health	62125-0318	Antibiotic
BIOCRAFT115	Cap	Cephalexin Monohydrate	by Signal Health	62125-0317	Antibiotic
BIOCRAFT115	Cap	Cephalexin Monohydrate	by Zenith Goldline	00182-1278	Antibiotic
BIOCRAFT115	Cap	Cephalexin Monohydrate	by Rugby	00536-0120	Antibiotic
BIOCRAFT115	Cap	Cephalexin Monohydrate	by Qualitest	00603-2595	Antibiotic
BIOCRAFT115	Cap	Cephalexin Monohydrate	by Pharmedix	53002-0226	Antibiotic
BIOCRAFT115	Cap	Cephalexin Monohydrate	by Med Pro	53978-5020	Antibiotic
BIOCRAFT115	Cap	Cephalexin Monohydrate	by HL Moore	00839-7311	Antibiotic
BIOCRAFT115	Cap	Cephalexin Monohydrate	by Talbert Med	44514-0490	Antibiotic
BIOCRAFT115	Cap	Cephalexin Monohydrate	by Apotheca	12634-0433	Antibiotic
BIOCRAFT117	Cap, Orange, Biocraft over 117	Cephalexin 500 mg	by Teva	00093-3147	Antibiotic
BIOCRAFT117	Cap	Cephalexin 500 mg	by Nat Pharmpak Serv	55154-5522	Antibiotic
BIOCRAFT117	Cap	Cephalexin Monohydrate	by PDRX	55289-0057	Antibiotic
BIOCRAFT117	Cap	Cephalexin Monohydrate	by Signal Health	62125-0320	Antibiotic
BIOCRAFT117	Cap	Cephalexin Monohydrate	by Signal Health	62125-0319	Antibiotic
BIOCRAFT117	Cap	Cephalexin Monohydrate	by Zenith Goldline	00182-1279	Antibiotic

ID FRONT <> BACK	DESCRIPTION FRONT <> BACK	INGREDIENT & STRENGTH	BRAND (OR EQUIV.) & FIRM	NDC#	CLASS; SCH.
BIOCRAFT117	Cap	Cephalexin Monohydrate	by Rugby	00536-0130	Antibiotic
BIOCRAFT117	Cap	Cephalexin Monohydrate	by Allscripts	54569-0305	Antibiotic
BIOCRAFT117	Cap	Cephalexin Monohydrate	by Pharmedix	53002-0218	Antibiotic
BIOCRAFT117	Cap, Coated	Cephalexin Monohydrate	by Med Pro	53978-5021	Antibiotic
BIOCRAFT117	Cap	Cephalexin Monohydrate	by Apotheca	12634-0434	Antibiotic
BIOCRAFT117	Cap	Cephalexin Monohydrate	by Talbert Med	44514-0491	Antibiotic
BIOCRAFT117	Cap, Orange	Cephalexin Monohydrate 500 mg	by Allscripts	54569-3324	Antibiotic
BIOCRAFT117	Cap	Cephalexin 500 mg	by HL Moore	00839-7312	Antibiotic
BIOCRAFT117	Cap	Cephalexin 500 mg	by Darby Group	66467-0130	Antibiotic
BIOCRAFT117	Cap	Cephalexin Monohydrate	by Urgent Care Ctr	50716-0144	Antibiotic
BIOCRAFT117	Cap, Biocraft/117	Cephalexin Monohydrate	by UDL	51079-0605	Antibiotic
BIOCRAFT117	Cap, Biocraft/117	Cephalexin Monohydrate 541 mg	by Amerisource	62584-0328	Antibiotic
BIOCRAFT117	Cap	Cephalexin Monohydrate 541 mg	by Qualitest	00603-2596	Antibiotic
BIOCRAFT12	Cap, Blue & Opaque	Oxacillin 250 mg	Prostaphlin by Biocraft		Antibiotic
BIOCRAFT12	Cap, Blue, Opaque, Biocraft over 12	Oxacillin Sodium Monohydrate 250 mg	by Teva	00093-3115	Antibiotic
BIOCRAFT134	Cap	Minocycline HCl	by Rugby	00536-1482	Antibiotic
BIOCRAFT134	Cap	Minocycline HCl	by Zenith Goldline	00182-1102	Antibiotic
BIOCRAFT134	Cap	Minocycline HCl	by United Res	00677-1435	Antibiotic
BIOCRAFT134	Cap	Minocycline HCl	by Qualitest	00603-4678	Antibiotic
BIOCRAFT134	Cap	Minocycline HCl 50 mg	by Quality Care	60346-0830	Antibiotic
BIOCRAFT134	Cap, Pink, Biocraft over 134	Minocycline HCl 50 mg	by Teva	00093-3165	Antibiotic
BIOCRAFT135	Cap	Minocycline HCl	by Rugby	00536-1492	Antibiotic
BIOCRAFT135	Cap	Minocycline HCl	by Zenith Goldline	00182-1103	Antibiotic
BIOCRAFT135	Cap	Minocycline HCl	by Quality Care	60346-0831	Antibiotic
BIOCRAFT135	Cap	Minocycline HCl	by Major	00904-7683	Antibiotic
BIOCRAFT135	Cap	Minocycline HCl	by Qualitest	00603-4679	Antibiotic
BIOCRAFT135	Cap, Maroon & Pink, Biocraft over 135	Minocycline HCl 100 mg	by Teva	00093-3167	Antibiotic
BIOCRAFT14	Cap	Oxacillin Sodium	by Zenith Goldline	00182-1341	Antibiotic
BIOCRAFT14	Cap	Oxacillin Sodium	by Qualitest	00603-4928	Antibiotic
BIOCRAFT14	Cap, Blue, Opaque, Biocraft over 14	Oxacillin Sodium Monohydrate 500 mg	by Teva	00093-3117	Antibiotic
BIOCRAFT148	Cap, Red	Clindamycin HCl 75 mg	Cleocin by Biocraft		Antibiotic
BIOCRAFT148	Cap, Red, Biocraft over 148	Clindamycin HCl 75 mg	by Teva	00093-3169	Antibiotic
BIOCRAFT149	Cap	Ampicillin Trihydrate	by Pharmedix	53002-0231	Antibiotic
BIOCRAFT149	Cap	Clindamycin HCl	by Nat Pharmpak Serv	55154-5546	Antibiotic
BIOCRAFT149	Cap	Clindamycin HCl	by Zenith Goldline	00182-1202	Antibiotic
BIOCRAFT149	Cap	Clindamycin HCl	by Pharmedix	53002-0232	Antibiotic
BIOCRAFT149	Cap	Clindamycin HCl	by Allscripts	54569-3456	Antibiotic
BIOCRAFT149	Cap	Clindamycin HCl	by Major	00904-3838	Antibiotic
BIOCRAFT149	Cap	Clindamycin HCl	by Apotheca	12634-0092	Antibiotic
BIOCRAFT16	Tab	Penicillin V Potassium	by Major	00904-2450	Antibiotic
BIOCRAFT16	Tab	Penicillin V Potassium	by Qualitest	00603-5067	Antibiotic
BIOCRAFT16	Tab	Penicillin V Potassium	by Apotheca	12634-0468	Antibiotic
BIOCRAFT16	Tab	Penicillin V Potassium	by HL Moore	00839-5188	Antibiotic
BIOCRAFT16	Tab, White, Oval	Penicillin V Potassium 250 mg	by Southwood Pharms	58016-0146	Antibiotic
BIOCRAFT163	Cap, Blue & Yellow	Cinoxacin 250 mg	Cinobac by Biocraft		Antibiotic
BIOCRAFT164	Cap, Blue & Yellow	Cinoxacin 500 mg	Cinobac by Biocraft		Antibiotic
BIOCRAFT177	Cap	Potassium Chloride 600 mg	by Teva	00093-3189	Electrolytes
BIOCRAFT178	Cap	Potassium Chloride 750 mg	by Teva	00093-3190	Electrolytes
BIOCRAFT187	Cap	Ketoprofen 50 mg	Ketoprofen by Zenith Goldline	00182-1959	NSAID
BIOCRAFT187	Cap, Blue & Light Blue, Biocraft over 187	Ketoprofen 50 mg	by Teva	00093-3193	NSAID
BIOCRAFT187	Cap	Ketoprofen 50 mg	Ketoprofen by Pharmedix	53002-0588	NSAID
BIOCRAFT187	Cap, Light Blue	Ketoprofen 50 mg	Ketoprofen by Quality Care	60346-0856	NSAID

ID FRONT <> BACK	DESCRIPTION FRONT <> BACK	INGREDIENT & STRENGTH	BRAND (OR EQUIV.) & FIRM	NDC#	CLASS; SCH.
BIOCRAFT187	Cap, Light Blue	Ketoprofen 50 mg	Ketoprofen by Qualitest	00603-4177	NSAID
BIOCRAFT192	Cap	Ketoprofen 75 mg	Ketoprofen by Zenith Goldline	00182-1960	NSAID
BIOCRAFT192	Cap, Blue & White, Biocraft over 192	Ketoprofen 75 mg	by Teva	00093-3195	NSAID
BIOCRAFT192	Cap	Ketoprofen 75 mg	Ketoprofen by Allscripts	54569-3688	NSAID
BIOCRAFT192	Cap	Ketoprofen 75 mg	Ketoprofen by Pharmedix	53002-0531	NSAID
BIOCRAFT192	Cap	Ketoprofen 75 mg	Ketoprofen by Med Pro	53978-2082	NSAID
BIOCRAFT192	Cap	Ketoprofen 75 mg	Ketoprofen by Quality Care	60346-0667	NSAID
BIOCRAFT192	Cap	Ketoprofen 75 mg	Ketoprofen by Qualitest	00603-4178	NSAID
BIOCRAFT192	Cap	Ketoprofen 75 mg	Ketoprofen by Murfreesboro	51129-1103	NSAID
BIOCRAFT223	Cap, Gray & White	Cefaclor 250 mg	Ceclor by Biocraft		Antibiotic
BIOCRAFT224	Cap, Red & White	Cefaclor 500 mg	Ceclor by Biocraft		Antibiotic
BIOCRAFT28	Cap, Dark Green & Scarlet	Cloxacillin Sodium	by Quality Care	60346-0345	Antibiotic
BIOCRAFT28	Cap	Cloxacillin Sodium Monohydrate	by Zenith Goldline	00182-1358	Antibiotic
BIOCRAFT28	Cap	Cloxacillin Sodium Monohydrate	by Qualitest	00603-3029	Antibiotic
BIOCRAFT28	Cap, Green & Red	Cloxacillin Sodium Monohydrate 250 mg	by HJ Harkins	52959-0468	Antibiotic
BIOCRAFT28	Cap, Dark Green & Scarlet, Biocraft over 28	Cloxacillin Sodium Monohydrate 250 mg	by Teva	00093-3119	Antibiotic
BIOCRAFT3 <> 3	Tab	Sulfamethoxazole 800 mg, Trimethoprim 160 mg	by Allscripts	54569-0075	Antibiotic
BIOCRAFT30	Cap	Cloxacillin Sodium	by Zenith Goldline	00182-1359	Antibiotic
BIOCRAFT30	Cap, Dark Green & Scarlet, Biocraft over 30	Cloxacillin Sodium 500 mg	by Teva	00093-3121	Antibiotic
BIOCRAFT313	Tab	Sulfamethoxazole 800 mg, Trimethoprim 160 mg	by Apotheca	12634-0177	Antibiotic
BIOCRAFT33	Tab	Sulfamethoxazole 800 mg, Trimethoprim 160 mg	by Zenith Goldline	00182-1408	Antibiotic
BIOCRAFT33	Tab	Sulfamethoxazole 800 mg, Trimethoprim 160 mg	by Rugby	00536-4693	Antibiotic
BIOCRAFT33	Tab	Sulfamethoxazole 800 mg, Trimethoprim 160 mg	by United Res	00677-0784	Antibiotic
BIOCRAFT34	Tab	Trimethoprim 100 mg	by Rugby	00536-4686	Antibiotic
BIOCRAFT34	Tab	Trimethoprim 100 mg	by Zenith Goldline	00182-1536	Antibiotic
BIOCRAFT34	Tab	Trimethoprim 100 mg	by DRX	55045-2302	Antibiotic
BIOCRAFT34	Tab, Biocraft/34	Trimethoprim 100 mg	by Allscripts	54569-3153	Antibiotic
BIOCRAFT34	Tab, Biocraft/34	Trimethoprim 100 mg	by HL Moore	00839-7284	Antibiotic
BIOCRAFT34	Tab, Biocraft/34	Trimethoprim 100 mg	by Major	00904-1646	Antibiotic
BIOCRAFT40	Cap, Blue & Scarlet, Biocraft over 40	Disopyramide Phosphate 100 mg	by Teva	00093-3127	Antiarrhythmic
BIOCRAFT40	Cap	Disopyramide Phosphate 100 mg	by Zenith Goldline	00182-1743	Antiarrhythmic
BIOCRAFT41	Cap	Disopyramide 150 mg	by Zenith Goldline	00182-1744	Antiarrhythmic
BIOCRAFT41	Cap, Buff & Scarlet, Biocraft over 41	Disopyramide Phosphate 150 mg	by Teva	00093-3129	Antiarrhythmic
BIOCRAFT49	Tab	Penicillin V Potassium	by Zenith Goldline	00182-1537	Antibiotic
BIOCRAFT49	Tab	Penicillin V Potassium	by Prescription Dispensing	61807-0004	Antibiotic
BIOCRAFT49	Tab	Penicillin V Potassium	by Apotheca	12634-0422	Antibiotic
BIOCRAFT94	Tab, White, Oblong, Biocraft/94	Cyclacillin 250 mg	Cylcapen by Biocraft		Antibiotic
BIOCRAFT95	Tab, White, Oblong, Biocraft/95	Cyclacillin 500 mg	Cylcapen by Biocraft		Antibiotic
BIOCRAFTO149	Cap, Blue & Red, Biocrafto/149	Clindamycin HCL, 150 mg	Cleocin by UDL	51079-0598	Antibiotic
BIOHIST	Tab, White, Elliptical, Scored	Chlorpheniramine Maleate 12 mg, Pseudoephedrine HCl 120 mg	Biohist LA by Wakefield	59310-0112	Cold Remedy
BIOHIST	Tab, White, Oblong, Scored	Chlorpheniramine Maleate 12 mg; Pseudoephedrine HCl 120 mg	Biohist by Sovereign Pharms	58716-0662	Cold Remedy
BL <> 130	Tab, White, Round, Scored	Albuterol 2 mg	by Teva	00093-2226	Antiasthmatic
BL <> 130	Tab	Albuterol Sulfate	by UDL	51079-0657	Antiasthmatic
BL <> 131	Tab, White, Round, Scored	Albuterol 4 mg	by Teva	00093-2228	Antiasthmatic
BL <> 131	Tab	Albuterol Sulfate	by UDL	51079-0658	Antiasthmatic
BL <> 132	Tab, White, Round, Scored	Metaproterenol Sulfate 10 mg	by Nat Pharmpak Serv	55154-5586	Antiasthmatic
BL <> 133	Tab, Buff, Round, Scored	Metaproterenol Sulfate 20 mg	by Teva	00093-2232	Antiasthmatic
BL <> 136	Tab, White, Oblong, Scored, B/L <> 136	Cephalexin 250 mg	by Teva	00093-2238	Antibiotic
BL <> 137	Tab, White, Oblong, Scored, B/L <> 137	Cephalexin 500 mg	by Teva	00093-2240	Antibiotic
BL <> 15	Tab, White, Round, Scored, BL <> 1 over 5	Penicillin V Potassium 250 mg	by Teva	00093-1171	Antibiotic
BL <> 15	Tab, White, Round, Scored	Penicillin V Potassium 250 mg	Pen*Vee K by UDL	51079-0615	Antibiotic
BL <> 15	Tab	Penicillin V Potassium	by Quality Care	60346-0414	Antibiotic

ID FRONT <> BACK	DESCRIPTION FRONT <> BACK	INGREDIENT & STRENGTH	BRAND (OR EQUIV.) & FIRM	NDC#	CLASS; SCH.
BL <> 17	Tab	Penicillin V 500 mg	by Talbert Med	44514-0645	Antibiotic
BL <> 17	Tab, Film Coated	Penicillin V Potassium	by Quality Care	60346-0095	Antibiotic
BL <> 17	Tab, White, Round, Scored, BL <> 1 over 7	Penicillin V Potassium 500 mg	by Teva	00093-1173	Antibiotic
BL <> 18	Tab, Off-White, Round	Neomycin Sulfate 500 mg	by Teva	00093-1177	Antibiotic
BL <> 19	Tab, Yellow, Round	Imipramine HCl 10 mg	by Teva	00093-2111	Antidepressant
BL <> 20	Tab, Salmon, Round	Imipramine HCl 25 mg	by Teva	00093-2113	Antidepressant
BL <> 20	Tab, Salmon, Coated	Imipramine HCl 25 mg	by Schein	00364-0406	Antidepressant
BL <> 20	Tab, Salmon	Imipramine HCl 25 mg	by Allscripts	54569-0194	Antidepressant
BL <> 20	Tab, Salmon	Imipramine HCl 25 mg	by UDL	51079-0080	Antidepressant
BL <> 21	Tab, Green, Round	Imipramine HCl 50 mg	by Teva	00093-2117	Antidepressant
BL <> 21	Tab	Imipramine HCl 50 mg	by UDL	51079-0081	Antidepressant
BL <> 22	Tab, Pink, Round, Coated	Amitriptyline HCl 10 mg	by Teva	00093-2120	Antidepressant
BL <> 221	Tab, White to Off-White, Oblong, Chewable	Amoxicillin 125 mg	by Teva	00093-2267	Antibiotic
BL <> 221	Tab, White, Oblong, Scored, B/L <> 221	Amoxicillin 125 mg	by Barr	00555-0886	Antibiotic
BL <> 221	Tab, Chewable	Amoxicillin Trihydrate	by HL Moore	00839-7776	Antibiotic
BL <> 222	Tab, Chew, B/L	Amoxicillin Trihydrate	by St Marys Med	60760-0268	Antibiotic
BL <> 222	Tab, Chewable	Amoxicillin Trihydrate	by Quality Care	60346-0113	Antibiotic
BL <> 222	Tab, Chewable, Debossed	Amoxicillin Trihydrate	by Casa De Amigos	62138-6005	Antibiotic
BL <> 222	Tab, Chewable, B over L <> 222	Amoxicillin Trihydrate	by Allscripts	54569-3689	Antibiotic
BL <> 222	Tab, Chewable, B/L <> 222	Amoxicillin Trihydrate	by DRX	55045-2004	Antibiotic
BL <> 222	Tab, White to Off-White, Oblong, Scored, Chewable, B/L <> 222	Amoxicillin Trihydrate 250 mg	by Teva	00093-2268	Antibiotic
BL <> 23	Tab, Light Green, Round, Coated	Amitriptyline HCl 25 mg	by Teva	00093-2122	Antidepressant
BL <> 24	Tab, Brown, Round, Coated	Amitriptyline HCl 50 mg	by Teva	00093-2124	Antidepressant
BL <> 25	Tab, Lavender, Round, Coated	Amitriptyline HCl 75 mg	by Teva	00093-2126	Antidepressant
BL <> 26	Tab, Orange, Round, Coated, Scored	Amitriptyline HCl 100 mg	by Teva	00093-2128	Antidepressant
BL <> 32	Tab	Sulfamethoxazole 400 mg, Trimethoprim 80 mg	SMX TMP SS by PDRX	55289-0457	Antibiotic
BL <> 35	Tab, White, Round, Scored	Trimethoprim 200 mg	by Teva	00093-2159	Antibiotic
BL <> 92	Tab, White, Round, Scored	Metoclopramide HCl 5 mg	by Teva	00093-2204	Gastrointestinal
BL <> 92	Tab, White, Round	Metoclopramide HCl 5 mg	Reglan by UDL	51079-0629	Gastrointestinal
BL <> 92	Tab, Debossed	Metoclopramide HCl	by Rugby	00536-4038	Gastrointestinal
BL <> 92	Tab, White, Round	Metoclopramide HCl 5 mg	by Murfreesboro Ph	51129-1683	Gastrointestinal
BL <> 93	Tab, White, Round, Scored	Metoclopramide HCl 10 mg	by Teva	00093-2203	Gastrointestinal
BL <> L1	Tab	Mitotane 500 mg	Lysodren by Anabolic	00722-5240	Antineoplastic
BL <> V1	Tab	Penicillin V Potassium	by Quality Care	60346-0414	Antibiotic
BL 512	Tab, Yellow, Rectangular	Theophylline Anhydrous 300 mg	Quibron T by BMS		Antiasthmatic
BL 519	Tab, White, Rectangular	Theophylline Anhydrous SR 300 mg	Quibron T SR by BMS		Antiasthmatic
BL<> 17	Tab, White, Round, Scored	Penicillian-VK 500 mg	Pen*Vee K	51079-0616	Antibiotic
BL07	Tab, White, Round, BL/07	Penicillin G Potassium 200,000 Units	Pentids by Biocraft		Antibiotic
BL09	Tab, White, Round, BL/09	Penicillin G Potassium 250,000 Units	Pentids by Biocraft		Antibiotic
BL10	Tab, White, Round, BL/10	Penicillin G Potassium 400,000 Units	Pentids by Biocraft		Antibiotic
BL131	Tab, Coated, BL 131	Albuterol Sulfate 4.8 mg	by Quality Care	60346-0285	Antiasthmatic
BL131	Tab	Albuterol Sulfate 4.8 mg	by Zenith Goldline	00182-1012	Antiasthmatic
BL132	Tab	Metaproterenol Sulfate 10 mg	by Qualitest	00603-4464	Antiasthmatic
BL132	Tab, BL/132	Metaproterenol Sulfate 10 mg	by HL Moore	00839-7485	Antiasthmatic
BL132	Tab, BL/132	Metaproterenol Sulfate 10 mg	by Major	00904-2878	Antiasthmatic
BL132	Tab, White, Round, BL/132	Metaproterenol Sulfate 10 mg	by Teva	00093-2230	Antiasthmatic
BL132	Tab, BL/132 Debossed	Metaproterenol Sulfate 10 mg	by Quality Care	60346-0723	Antiasthmatic
BL133	Tab, BL/132	Metaproterenol Sulfate 20 mg	by Quality Care	60346-0141	Antiasthmatic
BL133	Tab	Metaproterenol Sulfate 20 mg	by Qualitest	00603-4465	Antiasthmatic
BL133	Tab, BL/132	Metaproterenol Sulfate 20 mg	by HL Moore	00839-7486	Antiasthmatic
BL136	Tab, Coated, BL/136	Cephalexin Monohydrate	by Diversified Hlthcare Serv	55887-0991	Antibiotic
BL136	Cap	Cephalexin 250 mg	by Darby Group	66467-0120	Antibiotic

ID FRONT <> BACK	DESCRIPTION FRONT <> BACK	INGREDIENT & STRENGTH	BRAND (OR EQUIV.) & FIRM	NDC#	CLASS; SCH.
BL136	Cap	Cephalexin 250 mg	by IDE Inter	00814-1605	Antibiotic
BL137	Tab, Coated	Cephalexin Monohydrate	by Zenith Goldline	00182-1887	Antibiotic
BL137	Tab, Coated	Cephalexin Monohydrate	by Pharmedix	53002-0298	Antibiotic
BL14	Cap	Oxacillin Sodium	by United Res	00677-0933	Antibiotic
BL141	Tab, White, Round, Scored, BL over 141	Baclofen 10 mg	by Teva	00093-2234	Muscle Relaxant
BL141	Tab	Baclofen 10 mg	by Vangard	00615-3541	Muscle Relaxant
BL142	Tab, White, Round, Scored, BL over 142	Baclofen 20 mg	by Teva	00093-2236	Muscle Relaxant
BL142	Tab	Baclofen 20 mg	by Vangard	00615-3542	Muscle Relaxant
BL142	Tab, BL over 142	Baclofen 20 mg	by UDL	51079-0669	Muscle Relaxant
BL15	Tab	Penicillin V Potassium	by PDRX	55289-0206	Antibiotic
BL15	Tab	Penicillin V Potassium	by Pharmedix	53002-0201	Antibiotic
BL15	Tab	Penicillin V Potassium	by Diversified Hlthcare Serv	55887-0980	Antibiotic
BL15	Tab, White, Round, BL/15	Penicillin V Potassium 250 mg	V-Cillin K by Biocraft		Antibiotic
BL15 <> BL15	Tab, White, Round, Scored	Penicillin V Potassium 250 mg	by Southwood Pharms	58016-0146	Antibiotic
BL17	Tab	Penicillin V 500 mg	by HL Moore	00839-1766	Antibiotic
BL17	Tab	Penicillin V Potassium	by Pharmedix	53002-0202	Antibiotic
BL17	Tab	Penicillin V Potassium	by St Marys Med	60760-0174	Antibiotic
BL17	Tab	Penicillin V Potassium	by Qualitest	00603-5068	Antibiotic
BL17	Tab, White, Round, BL/17	Penicillin V Potassium 500 mg	V-Cillin K by Biocraft		Antibiotic
BL17	Tab, White, Round, BL and 17	Penicillin V Potassium 500 mg	by Pharmafab	62542-0724	Antibiotic
BL170	Tab, White, Round	Amoxicillin Veterinary 50 mg	Biomox by Biocraft		Antibiotic
BL171	Tab, White, Round	Amoxicillin Veterinary 100 mg	Biomox by Biocraft		Antibiotic
BL172	Tab, White, Round	Amoxicillin Veterinary 200 mg	Biomox by Biocraft		Antibiotic
BL173	Tab, White, Round	Amoxicillin Veterinary 400 mg	Biomox by Biocraft		Antibiotic
BL18	Tab, White, Round, BL/18	Neomycin Sulfate 500 mg	Mycifradin by Biocraft		Antibiotic
BL18	Tab	Neomycin Sulfate 500 mg	by Rugby	00536-4064	Antibiotic
BL18	Tab	Neomycin Sulfate 500 mg	by Zenith Goldline	00182-0673	Antibiotic
BL19	Tab, Yellow, Round, BL/19	Imipramine HCl 10 mg	Tofranil by Biocraft		Antidepressant
BL19	Tab, Coated, BL/19	Imipramine HCl 10 mg	by Schein	00364-0443	Antidepressant
BL19	Tab, Coated, BL/19	Imipramine HCl 10 mg	by PDRX	55289-0149	Antidepressant
BL19	Tab, Coated, BL/19	Imipramine HCl 10 mg	by Allscripts	54569-2726	Antidepressant
BL19	Tab	Imipramine HCl 10 mg	by Heartland	61392-0025	Antidepressant
BL19	Tab, Sugar Coated, BL/19	Imipramine HCl 10 mg	by Quality Care	60346-0718	Antidepressant
BL19	Tab, Film Coated	Imipramine HCl 10 mg	by Qualitest	00603-4043	Antidepressant
BL19	Tab, BL/19	Imipramine HCl 10 mg	by HL Moore	00839-1370	Antidepressant
BL20	Tab, Salmon, Round, BL/20	Imipramine HCl 25 mg	Tofranil by Biocraft		Antidepressant
BL20	Tab	Imipramine HCl 25 mg	by Quality Care	60346-0460	Antidepressant
BL20	Tab, Salmon	Imipramine HCl 25 mg	by Heartland	61392-0026	Antidepressant
BL20	Tab, Coated, BL/20	Imipramine HCl 25 mg	by Kaiser	62224-3440	Antidepressant
BL20	Tab, Rust, Film Coated	Imipramine HCl 25 mg	by Qualitest	00603-4044	Antidepressant
BL207	Tab, Blue, Round, Scored	Nadolol 40 mg	Corgard by Thrift Services	59198-0375	Antihypertensive
BL207 <> CORGARD40	Tab, BL Over 207 <> Corgard 40	Nadolol 40 mg	Corgard by ER Squibb	00003-0207	Antihypertensive
BL207 <> CORGARD40	Tab	Nadolol 40 mg	Corgard by Repack Co of Amer	55306-0207	Antihypertensive
BL207 <> CORGARD40	Tab	Nadolol 40 mg	Corgard by Nat Pharmpak Serv	55154-0605	Antihypertensive
BL208 <> CORGARD120MG	Tab, Light Blue	Nadolol 120 mg	Corgard by ER Squibb	00003-0208	Antihypertensive
BL21	Tab, Green, Round, BL/21	Imipramine HCl 50 mg	Tofranil by Biocraft		Antidepressant
BL21	Tab, BL/21	Imipramine HCl 50 mg	by Schein	00364-0435	Antidepressant
BL21	Tab, Coated	Imipramine HCl 50 mg	by Med Pro	53978-0073	Antidepressant
BL21	Tab, Coated	Imipramine HCl 50 mg	by Pharmedix	53002-1066	Antidepressant
BL21	Tab, Sugar Coated	Imipramine HCl 50 mg	by Quality Care	60346-0709	Antidepressant
BL21	Tab, Coated, BL/21	Imipramine HCl 50 mg	by Kaiser	62224-3444	Antidepressant

ID FRONT <> BACK	DESCRIPTION FRONT <> BACK	INGREDIENT & STRENGTH	BRAND (OR EQUIV.) & FIRM	NDC#	CLASS; SCH.
BL21	Tab	Imipramine HCl 50 mg	by Heartland	61392-0027	Antidepressant
BL21	Tab, Film Coated	Imipramine HCl 50 mg	by Qualitest	00603-4045	Antidepressant
BL21	Tab, Coated, BL/21	Imipramine HCl 50 mg	by HL Moore	00839-1372	Antidepressant
BL22	Tab, Pink, Round, BL/22	Amitriptyline HCl 10 mg	Elavil by Biocraft		Antidepressant
BL22	Tab, Coated	Amitriptyline HCl 10 mg	by Pharmedix	53002-0491	Antidepressant
BL222	Tab, Chewalbe	Amoxicillin Trihydrate	by Zenith Goldline	00182-1962	Antibiotic
BL222	Tab, Chewable	Amoxicillin Trihydrate	by Med Pro	53978-1257	Antibiotic
BL23	Tab, Light Green, Coated, BL/23	Amitriptyline HCl 25 mg	by Quality Care	60346-0027	Antidepressant
BL23	Tab, Green, Round, BL/23	Amitriptyline HCl 25 mg	Elavil by Biocraft		Antidepressant
BL232 <> CORGARD20	Tab, BL Over 232 <> Corgard 20	Nadolol 20 mg	Corgard by ER Squibb	00003-0232	Antihypertensive
BL24	Tab, Film Coated, BL/24 Debossed	Amitriptyline HCl 50 mg	by Quality Care	60346-0673	Antidepressant
BL24	Tab, Brown, Round, BL/24	Amitriptyline HCl 50 mg	Elavil by Biocraft		Antidepressant
BL241 <> CORGARD80	Tab, BL/241 <> Corgard 80	Nadolol 80 mg	Corgard by Nat Pharmpak Serv	55154-0604	Antihypertensive
BL241 <> CORGARD80	Tab, Light Blue, BL Over 241	Nadolol 80 mg	Corgard by ER Squibb	00003-0241	Antihypertensive
BL246 <> CORGARD160MG	Tab, Dark Blue	Nadolol 160 mg	Corgard by ER Squibb	00003-0246	Antihypertensive
BL25	Tab, Lavender, Round, BL/25	Amitriptyline HCl 75 mg	Elavil by Biocraft		Antidepressant
BL26	Tab, Orange, Round	Amitriptyline HCl 100 mg	Elavil by Biocraft		Antidepressant
BL283 <> CORZIDE405	Tab, Bluish White to White, Dark Blue Specks, BL over 283 <> Corzide 40/5	Bendroflumethiazide 5 mg, Nadolol 40 mg	Corzide 40 5 by ER Squibb	00003-0283	Diuretic; Antihypertensive
BL284 <> CORZIDE805	Tab, Bluish White to White, Dark Blue Specks, BL over 284 <> Corzide 80/5	Bendroflumethiazide 5 mg, Nadolol 80 mg	Corzide 80 5 by ER Squibb	00003-0284	Diuretic; Antihypertensive
BL32	Tab	Sulfamethoxazole 400 mg, Trimethoprim 80 mg	by Zenith Goldline	00182-1478	Antibiotic
BL32	Tab	Sulfamethoxazole 400 mg, Trimethoprim 80 mg	by United Res	00677-0783	Antibiotic
BL35	Tab, BL/35 Biocraft	Trimethoprim 200 mg	by Rugby	00536-4683	Antibiotic
BL35	Tab	Trimethoprim 200 mg	by Pharmedix	53002-0291	Antibiotic
BL35	Tab	Trimethoprim 200 mg	by Quality Care	60346-0978	Antibiotic
BL35	Tab	Trimethoprim 200 mg	by Qualitest	00603-6265	Antibiotic
BL35	Tab, BL/35	Trimethoprim 200 mg	by HL Moore	00839-7433	Antibiotic
BL38	Tab, White, Round	Chloroquine 250 mg	Aralen Phosphate by Biocraft		Antimalarial
BL42	Tab, Green, Oval, BL/42	Thioridazine HCl 10 mg	Mellaril by Biocraft		Antipsychotic
BL46	Tab, Light Green, Oval, BL/46	Thioridazine HCl 100 mg	Mellaril by Biocraft		Antipsychotic
BL52	Tab, Yellow, Round, BL/52	Amiloride HCl 5 mg, Hydrochlorothiazide 50 mg	Moduretic by Biocraft		Diuretic
BL53	Tab, White, Oblong, BL/53	Furosemide (Veterinary) 12.5 mg	by Biocraft		Veterinary
BL54	Tab, White, Oblong, BL/54	Furosemide (Veterinary) 50 mg	by Biocraft		Veterinary
BL71	Tab, Brown, Round, BL/71	Clonidine 0.1 mg	Catapres by Biocraft		Antihypertensive
BL72	Tab, Purple, Round, BL/72	Clonidine 0.2 mg	Catapres by Biocraft		Antihypertensive
BL73	Tab, Pink, Round, BL/73	Clonidine 0.3 mg	Catapres by Biocraft		Antihypertensive
BL92	Tab, BL/92	Metoclopramide HCl 5 mg	by Quality Care	60346-0880	Gastrointestinal
BL92	Tab, Compressed, Debossed	Metoclopramide HCl 5.91 mg	by Allscripts	54569-3851	Gastrointestinal
BL92	Tab	Metoclopramide HCl 5.91 mg	by Nat Pharmpak Serv	55154-5226	Gastrointestinal
BL92	Tab, BL/92	Metoclopramide HCl	by Duramed	51285-0834	Gastrointestinal
BL92	Tab	Metoclopramide HCl	by Nat Pharmpak Serv	55154-5526	Gastrointestinal
BL92	Tab, BL/92	Metoclopramide HCl	by Major	00904-1069	Gastrointestinal
BL92	Tab, White, Round, BL/92	Metoclopramide HCl 5 mg	by Neuman Distr	64579-0047	Gastrointestinal
BL93	Tab, White, Round, BL/93	Metoclopramide HCl	by Duramed	51285-0805	Gastrointestinal
BL93	Tab, BL/93	Metoclopramide HCl	by Allscripts	54569-0434	Gastrointestinal
BL93	Tab, BL Over 93	Metoclopramide HCl	by Quality Care	60346-0802	Gastrointestinal
BL93	Tab, BL/93 Debossed	Metoclopramide HCl	by HL Moore	00839-7127	Gastrointestinal
BL93	Tab, White, Round, Scored, BL/93	Metoclopramide HCl 10 mg	by Neuman Distr	64579-0051	Gastrointestinal
BL93	Tab, White, Round, BL/93	Metoclopramide HCl 10 mg	Reglan by Biocraft		Gastrointestinal
BL93	Tab, White, Round, Scored	Metoclopramide HCl 10 mg	by Vangard Labs	00615-2536	Gastrointestinal

ID FRONT <> BACK	DESCRIPTION FRONT <> BACK	INGREDIENT & STRENGTH	BRAND (OR EQUIV.) & FIRM	NDC#	CLASS; SCH.
BLAINE	Tab, White	Magnesium Oxide 400 mg	Mag-Ox 400 by Blaine	00165-0022	Mineral
BLAINE0054	Cap, White	Magnesium Oxide 140 mg	Uro-Mag by Central		Mineral
BLAINE0054	Cap	Magnesium Oxide 140 mg	Uro-Mag by Blaine		Mineral
BLANSETT <> 30	Cap, Ex Release, Printed in Red Ink	Guaifenesin 250 mg, Pseudoephedrine HCl 120 mg	Nalex by Sovereign	58716-0010	Cold Remedy
BLANSETT33 <> NALEXJR	Cap, Ex Release, Blansett 33 Green Ink <> Nalex JR White Ink	Guaifenesin 300 mg, Pseudoephedrine HCl 60 mg	Nalex Jr by Sovereign	58716-0006	Cold Remedy
BLC1	Tab, Yellow, Oblong	Cefadroxil 1 GM	Ultracef by BMS		Antibiotic
BLKLOTRIX10MEQ770	Tab, Orange, Round, BL Klotrix 10mEq 770	Potassium Chloride ER 10 mEq	Klotrix by Apothecon		Electrolytes
BLL1	Tab, Engraved, BL Over L1	Mitotane 500 mg	Lysodren by Mead Johnson	00015-3080	Antineoplastic
BLLLD9	Cap, Coral, BL-LL-D9	Demeclocycline HCl 150 mg	Declomycin by Lederle		Antibiotic
BLN1 <> NALDECON	Tab, White, Red Specks, BL over N1 <> Naldecon around Perimeter	Chlorpheniramine Maleate 5 mg, Phenylephrine HCl 10 mg, Phenylpropanolamine HCl 40 mg, Phenyltoloxamine Citrate 15 mg	Naldecon by Mead Johnson	00015-5600	Cold Remedy
BLNI	Tab, Pink, Round	Phenylprop., Phenyleph., Phenyltolox., Chlorphenir.	Naldecon by Bristol		Cold Remedy
BLOCADREN <> MSD 136	Tab, Light Blue, Cap-Shaped	Timolol Maleate 10 mg	Blocadren by Merck	00006-0136	Antihypertensive
BLS1	Tab, Green, Round	Hydroflumethiazide 50 mg, Reserpine 0.125 mg	Salutensin by BMS		Diuretic; Antihypertensive
BLS2	Tab, White, Round	Hydroflumethiazide 50 mg	Saluron by BMS		Diuretic
BLS3	Tab, Yellow, Round	Hydroflumethiazide 25 mg, Reserpine 0.125 mg	Salutensin Demi by BMS		Diuretic; Antihypertensive
BLV1	Tab, Film Coated	Penicillin V Potassium	Veetids by ER Squibb	00003-0115	Antibiotic
BLV1	Tab	Penicillin V Potassium	by Patient	57575-0013	Antibiotic
BLV1	Tab, Film Coated	Penicillin V Potassium	by Talbert Med	44514-0643	Antibiotic
BLV1	Tab, White, Round	Penicillin V Potassium 250 mg	by Allscripts	54569-2702	Antibiotic
BLV2	Tab, White, Round	Penicillin V Potassium 500 mg	by Allscripts	54569-3503	Antibiotic
BLV2	Tab	Penicillin V 500 mg	by Patient	57575-0014	Antibiotic
BLV2	Tab, Film Coated	Penicillin V Potassium	Veetids by ER Squibb	00003-0116	Antibiotic
BLV2	Tab, Film Coated, BL/V2	Penicillin V Potassium	by Allscripts	54569-2710	Antibiotic
BLV2	Tab, Film Coated	Penicillin V Potassium	by Med Pro	53978-5055	Antibiotic
BLV2	Tab, Film Coated	Penicillin V Potassium	by Quality Care	60346-0095	Antibiotic
BLV2	Tab, White, Round	Penicillin V Potassium 500 mg	Betapen VK by BMS		Antibiotic
BLVI	Tab	Penicillin V Potassium	by Med Pro	53978-5042	Antibiotic
BM <> RGP	Cap	Acetaminophen 300 mg, Phenyltoloxamine Citrate 20 mg, Salicylamide 200 mg	by Pharmakon	55422-0411	Analgesic
BM <> RGP	Cap	Acetaminophen 300 mg, Phenyltoloxamine Citrate 20 mg, Salicylamide 200 mg	by Seatrace	00551-0411	Analgesic
BM102	Tab, Off-White to White, BM Logo/102	Torsemide 5 mg	Demadex by Boehringer Mannheim	53169-0102	Diuretic
BM103	Tab, Off-White to White, BM Logo/103	Torsemide 10 mg	Demadex by Boehringer Mannheim	53169-0103	Diuretic
BM103 <> BM103	Tab, BM Logo	Torsemide 10 mg	Demadex by Boehringer Mannheim	12871-3775	Diuretic
BM104	Tab, Off-White to White, BM Logo/104	Torsemide 20 mg	Demadex by Boehringer Mannheim	53169-0104	Diuretic
BM104 <> BM104	Tab, BM Logo	Torsemide 20 mg	Demadex by Boehringer Mannheim	12871-6507	Diuretic
BM105	Tab, Off-White to White, Beveled Edge, BM Logo/105	Torsemide 100 mg	Demadex by Boehringer Mannheim	53169-0105	Diuretic
BM105 <> BM105	Tab, BM Logo	Torsemide 100 mg	Demadex by Boehringer Mannheim	12871-6531	Diuretic
BM8 <> MAXZIDE	Tab, B on the Left and M8 on the Right of Score	Hydrochlorothiazide 50 mg, Triamterene 75 mg	Maxzide by Mylan	00378-7550	Diuretic
BM8 <> MAXZIDE	Tab, B on Left, M8 on Right of Score <> Beveled Edge	Hydrochlorothiazide 50 mg, Triamterene 75 mg	Maxzide by Bertek	62794-0460	Diuretic
BM9 <> MAXZIDE	Tab, B/M9	Hydrochlorothiazide 25 mg, Triamterene 37.5 mg	Maxzide by Caremark	00339-6094	Diuretic
BM9 <> MAXZIDE	Tab, B on Left of Score M9 on Right <> Beveled	Hydrochlorothiazide 25 mg, Triamterene 37.5 mg	Maxide 25 by Direct Dispensing	57866-6801	Diuretic
BM9 <> MAXZIDE	Tab, B on Left, M9 on Right of Score <> Beveled Edge	Hydrochlorothiazide 25 mg, Triamterene 37.5 mg	Maxide 25 by Bertek	62794-0464	Diuretic
BMD9	Tab, White, Round, BM/D9	Bezafibrate 400 mg	Bezalip SR by Roche	Canadian	Antihyperlipidemic
BMEU	Tab, White, Oblong, BM/EU	Glyburide 5 mg	by Boehringer Mannheim	Canadian	Antidiabetic
BMG6	Tab, White, Round, BM/G6	Bezafibrate 200 mg	Bezalip by Roche	Canadian	Antihyperlipidemic
BMP <> 140	Cap	Ampicillin Trihydrate	by Quality Care	60346-0082	Antibiotic
BMP <> 203	Tab, Pink, Round	Amoxicillin Trihydrate 200 mg	Amoxi-Tabs by Pfizer		Antibiotic
BMP 125	Tab, Yellow, Oblong	Esterified Estrogens 0.3 mg	Menest by Monarch	61570-0072	Hormone

ID FRONT <> BACK	DESCRIPTION FRONT <> BACK	INGREDIENT & STRENGTH	BRAND (OR EQUIV.) & FIRM	NDC#	CLASS; SCH.
BMP 126	Tab, Orange, Oblong	Esterified Estrogens 0.625 mg	Menest by Monarch	61570-0073	Hormone
BMP 127	Tab, Green, Oblong	Esterified Estrogens 1.25 mg	Menest by Monarch	61570-0074	Hormone
BMP112	Cap, Yellow	Atropine 0.13, Aspirin 130, Caffeine 8, Ipecac 3, Camphor 15	Dasin by SKB		Gastrointestinal
BMP121	Cap, Pink	Multivitamin Combination	Livitamin by SKB		Vitamin
BMP122	Cap, Green	Multivitamin Combination	Livitamin with IF by SKB		Vitamin
BMP123	Tab, Orange	Multivitamin	Livitamin Chewable by SKB		Vitamin
BMP125	Tab, Yellow, Oblong	Esterified Estrogens 0.3 mg	Menest by SmithKline SKB		Hormone
BMP126	Tab, Film Coated	Estrogens, Esterified 0.625 mg	Menest by SKB	00029-2810	Hormone
BMP127	Tab, Coated	Estrogens, Esterified 1.25 mg	Menest by SKB	00029-2820	Hormone
BMP128	Tab, Coated	Estrogens, Esterified 2.5 mg	Menest by King	60793-0840	Hormone
BMP128	Tab, Coated	Estrogens, Esterified 2.5 mg	Menest by SKB	00029-2830	Hormone
BMP141	Cap, Brown & Orange	Ampicillin 500 mg	Totacillin by SmithKline SKB		Antibiotic
BMP143	Cap, Brown & Yellow	Oxacillin Sodium 250 mg	Bactocill by SmithKline SKB		Antibiotic
BMP144	Cap, Brown & Yellow	Oxacillin Sodium 500 mg	Bactocill by SmithKline SKB		Antibiotic
BMP145	Tab, White, Round	Oxyphencyclimine HCl 10 mg	Daricon by SKB		Antispasmodic
BMP165	Cap, Blue & Cream	Dicloxacillin Sodium 250 mg	Dycill by SmithKline SKB		Antibiotic
BMP166	Cap, Blue & Cream	Dicloxacillin Sodium 500 mg	Dycill by SmithKline SKB		Antibiotic
BMP169	Cap, Beige & Lime	Cloxacillin Sodium 250 mg	Cloxapen by SKB		Antibiotic
BMP170	Cap, Beige & Lime	Cloxacillin Sodium 500 mg	Cloxapen by SKB		Antibiotic
BMP182	Cap	Codeine Phosphate 20 mg, Pseudoephedrine HCl 60 mg	Nucofed by King	60793-0852	Cold Remedy; C III
BMP182	Cap, Clear & Green	Codeine Phosphate 20 mg, Pseudoephedrine HCl 60 mg	Nucofed by Monarch	61570-0018	Cold Remedy; C III
BMP188	Tab, BMP/188	Acetaminophen 650 mg, Hydrocodone Bitartrate 7.5 mg	Anexsia by Nat Pharmpak Serv	55154-7101	Analgesic; C III
BMP189	Tab, Chewable	Amoxicillin 125 mg, Clavulanic Acid 31.25 mg	Augmentin by HJ Harkins Co	52959-0470	Antibiotic
BMP190	Tab, Mottled Yellow, Round	Amoxicillin Trihydrate 250 mg, Clavulanate Potassium 62.5 mg	Augmentin Chewable by Bayer	00280-1070	Antibiotic
BMP190	Tab, Chew	Amoxicillin Trihydrate, Clavulanate Potassium	Augmentin by Quality Care	60346-0590	Antibiotic
BMP190	Tab, Yellow, Round, Chewable	Amoxicillin Trihydrate, Clavulanate Potassium	Augmentin by SKB	00029-6047	Antibiotic
BMP192	Tab, Blue, Round	Metoclopramide 10 mg	Maxolon by SKB		Gastrointestinal
BMP207	Tab, White, Round	Hydrocodone Bitartrate 5 mg, Acetaminophen 500 mg	Anexsia by SKB		Analgesic; C III
BMP210	Tab, White, Oblong	Phenylephrine 10 mg, Guaifenesin 100 mg, DM 15 mg, Acetaminophen 300 mg	Conar-A by SKB		Cold Remedy
BMS	Tab, White, Hexagon	Nefazodone HCl 100 mg	Serzone by Va Cmop	65243-0102	Antidepressant
BMS <> 5040	Tab	Atenolol 50 mg	by Quality Care	60346-0719	Antihypertensive
BMS <> 5250	Tab, Coated	Diltiazem HCl 30 mg	by Quality Care	60346-0960	Antihypertensive
BMS <> 5250	Tab, Coated, Mottled	Diltiazem HCl 30 mg	by ER Squibb	00003-5250	Antihypertensive
BMS <> 5550	Tab, Coated, Slightly Mottled	Diltiazem HCl 30 mg	by Golden State	60429-0061	Antihypertensive
BMS <> 5550	Tab, Coated, Mottled	Diltiazem HCl 60 mg	by ER Squibb	00003-5550	Antihypertensive
BMS <> 5550	Tab, Coated, Scored	Diltiazem HCl 60 mg	by Golden State	60429-0062	Antihypertensive
BMS <> 5550	Tab, Mottled Clear, Film Coated, Scored	Diltiazem HCl 60 mg	by Med Pro	53978-1235	Antihypertensive
BMS <> 5770	Tab, Coated, Mottled	Diltiazem HCl 90 mg	by ER Squibb	00003-5770	Antihypertensive
BMS <> 5850	Tab, Coated, Mottled	Diltiazem HCl 120 mg	by ER Squibb	00003-5850	Antihypertensive
BMS <> 6060500	Tab, White, Round, Film Coated	Metformin HCl 500 mg	by Allscripts	54569-4202	Antidiabetic
BMS <> 6072	Tab, Pale Yellow, Cap Shaped, Film Coated	Glyburide 1.25 mg, Metformin HCl 250 mg	Glucovance by Bristol-Myers	00087-6072	Antidiabetic
BMS <> 6072	Tab, Yellow	Glyburide 1.25 mg; Metformin HCl 250 mg	Glucovance by Bristol Myers Squibb	12783-0072	Antidiabetic
BMS <> 6073	Tab, Orange	Glyburide 2.5 mg; Metformin HCl 500 mg	Glucovance by Bristol Myers Squibb	12783-0073	Antidiabetic
BMS <> 6073	Tab, Pale Orange, Cap Shaped, Film Coated	Glyburide 2.50 mg, Metformin HCl 500 mg	Glucovande by Bristol-Myers	00087-6073	Antidiabetic
BMS <> 6074	Tab, Yellow, Cap Shaped, Film Coated	Glyburide 5 mg, Metformin HCL 500 mg	Glucovance by Bistol-Myers	00087-6074	Antidiabetic
BMS <> MONOPRIL10	Tab, Off-White	Fosinopril Sodium 10 mg	Monopril by Direct Dispensing	57866-3800	Antihypertensive
BMS <> MONOPRIL10	Tab, Off-White, Diamond Shaped	Fosinopril Sodium 10 mg	by Allscripts	54569-3808	Antihypertensive
BMS <> MONOPRIL10	Tab, White, Diamond	Fosinopril Sodium 10 mg	Monopril by Va Cmop	65243-0092	Antihypertensive
BMS <> MONOPRIL10	Tab, Off-White, Diamond Shaped	Fosinopril Sodium 10 mg	Monopril by Bristol Myers	00087-0158	Antihypertensive
BMS <> MONOPRIL10	Tab, Off-White, Scored	Fosinopril Sodium 10 mg	Monopril by Caremark	00339-5745	Antihypertensive
BMS <> MONOPRIL20	Tab	Fosinopril Sodium 20 mg	Monopril by Direct Dispensing	57866-3803	Antihypertensive
BMS <> MONOPRIL20	Tab, White, Oval	Fosinopril Sodium 20 mg	Monopril by Va Cmop	65243-0093	Antihypertensive

ID FRONT <> BACK	DESCRIPTION FRONT <> BACK	INGREDIENT & STRENGTH	BRAND (OR EQUIV.) & FIRM	NDC#	CLASS; SCH.
BMS <> MONOPRIL20	Tab, White to Off-White, Oval	Fosinopril Sodium 20 mg	by Allscripts	54569-3809	Antihypertensive
BMS <> MONOPRIL20	Tab, Off-White, Oval	Fosinopril Sodium 20 mg	Monopril by Bristol Myers Squibb	00087-0609	Antihypertensive
BMS <> MONOPRIL20	Tab	Fosinopril Sodium 20 mg	Monopril by Bristol Myers	15548-0609	Antihypertensive
BMS <> MONOPRIL20	Tab, White, Oval	Fosinopril Sodium 20 mg	Monopril by JB	51111-0471	Antihypertensive
BMS <> MONOPRIL40	Tab, White, Hexagon	Fosinopril Sodium 40 mg	Monopril by Va Cmop	65243-0094	Antihypertensive
BMS <> MONOPRIL40	Tab, Off-White, Hexagonal	Fosinopril Sodium 40 mg	Monopril by Bristol Myers Squibb	00087-1202	Antihypertensive
BMS <> MONOPRIL40	Tab	Fosinopril Sodium 40 mg	Monopril by Bristol Myers	15548-0202	Antihypertensive
BMS <> TEQUIN200	Tab, White, Almond Shaped, Film Coated	Gatifloxacin 200 mg	by Bristol Myers Squibb	00015-1117	Antibiotic
BMS <> TEQUIN200	Tab, White, Film Coated	Gatifloxacin 200 mg	Tequin by Squibb Mfg	12783-0117	Antibiotic
BMS <> TEQUIN400	Tab, White, Film Coated	Gatifloxacin 400 mg	Tequin by Squibb Mfg	12783-0177	Antibiotic
BMS <> TEQUIN400	Tab, White, Film Coated	Gatifloxacin 400 mg	by Bristol Myers Squibb	00015-1177	Antibiotic
BMS <> W921	Tab, Film Coated	Metoprolol Tartrate 50 mg	by Quality Care	60346-0523	Antihypertensive
BMS <> W921	Tab	Metoprolol Tartrate 50 mg	by Apothecon	59772-3692	Antihypertensive
BMS <> W933	Tab	Metoprolol Tartrate 100 mg	by Apothecon	59772-3693	Antihypertensive
BMS <> W933	Tab	Metoprolol Tartrate 100 mg	by Quality Care	60346-0514	Antihypertensive
BMS 37	Tab, Pink, Round	Amoxicillin 125 mg	by Apothecon	59772-0037	Antibiotic
BMS 38	Tab, Pink, Round	Amoxicillin 250 mg	by Apothecon	59772-0038	Antibiotic
BMS 5040	Tab, Off-White, Round	Atenolol 50 mg	by ER Squibb	00003-5040	Antihypertensive
BMS 5240	Tab, Off-White, Round	Atenolol 100 mg	by ER Squibb	00003-5240	Antihypertensive
BMS100	Tab	Nefazodone HCl 50 mg	Serzone by Bristol Myers Squibb	00087-0057	Antidepressant
BMS100 <> 31	Tab	Nefazodone HCl 100 mg	Serzone by Kaiser	00179-1241	Antidepressant
BMS100 <> 32	Tab, White, Engraved	Nefazodone HCl 100 mg	Serzone by Bristol Myers Squibb	00087-0032	Antidepressant
BMS100 <> 32	Tab	Nefazodone HCl 100 mg	Serzone by Quality Care	60346-0172	Antidepressant
BMS100 <> 32	Tab	Nefazodone HCl 100 mg	Serzone by Bristol Myers	15548-0032	Antidepressant
BMS10032	Tab, White, Hexagonal, BMS 100/32	Nefazodone HCl 100 mg	Serzone by Bristol-Myers	Canadian	Antidepressant
BMS100MG	Tab, White, Hexagon, Scored	Nefazodone HCl 100 mg	Serzone by Direct Dispensing	57866-0912	Antidepressant
BMS150	Tab	Nefazodone HCl 50 mg	Serzone by Bristol Myers Squibb	00087-0057	Antidepressant
BMS150 <> 39	Tab, Peach, Engraved	Nefazodone HCl 150 mg	Serzone by Bristol Myers Squibb	00087-0039	Antidepressant
BMS150 <> 39	Tab	Nefazodone HCl 150 mg	Serzone by Kaiser	00179-1242	Antidepressant
BMS150 <> 39	Tab, BMS 150	Nefazodone HCl 150 mg	Serzone by Allscripts	54569-4127	Antidepressant
BMS150 <> 39	Tab, Peach, Hexagonal, Scored	Nefazodone HCl 150 mg	Serzone by Par	49884-0569	Antidepressant
BMS150 <> 39	Tab	Nefazodone HCl 150 mg	Serzone by Bristol Myers	15548-0039	Antidepressant
BMS15039	Tab, Peach, Hexagonal, BMS 150/39	Nefazodone HCl 150 mg	Serzone by Bristol-Myers	Canadian	Antidepressant
BMS1964 <> 15	Cap, Dark Red & Light Yellow, Black Print, BMS over 1964 <> 15	Stavudine 15 mg	Zerit by Bristol Myers	00003-1964	Antiviral
BMS196415	Cap, Red & Yellow, BMS 1964/15	Stavudine 15 mg	Zerit by Bristol-Myers	Canadian	Antiviral
BMS1965 <> 20	Cap, Brown	Stavudine 20 mg	Zerit by Murfreesboro Ph	51129-1396	Antiviral
BMS1965 <> 20	Cap, Light Brown, Black Print, BMS over 1965 <> 20	Stavudine 20 mg	Zerit by Bristol Myers	00003-1965	Antiviral
BMS196520	Cap, Light Brown, BMS 1965/20	Stavudine 20 mg	Zerit by Bristol-Myers	Canadian	Antiviral
BMS1966 <> 30	Cap, Dark Orange & Light Orange, Black Print, BMS over 1966 <> 30	Stavudine 30 mg	Zerit by Bristol Myers	00003-1966	Antiviral
BMS196630	Cap, Light Orange, BMS 1966/30	Stavudine 30 mg	Zerit by Bristol-Myers	Canadian	Antiviral
BMS1967 <> 40	Cap, Dark Orange, Black Print, BMS over 1967 <> 40	Stavudine 40 mg	Zerit by Bristol Myers	00003-1967	Antiviral
BMS1967 <> 40	Cap, Orange	Stavudine 40 mg	Zerit by Squibb Mfg	12783-0967	Antiviral
BMS196740	Tab, Orange, BMS 1967/40	Stavudine 40 mg	Zerit by Bristol-Myers	Canadian	Antiviral
BMS200 <> 33	Tab, Light Yellow	Nefazodone HCl 200 mg	Serzone by Bristol Myers Squibb	00087-0033	Antidepressant
BMS200 <> 33	Tab	Nefazodone HCl 200 mg	Serzone by Kaiser	00179-1243	Antidepressant
BMS200 <> 33	Tab, Light Yellow	Nefazodone HCl 200 mg	Serzone by Quality Care	60346-0175	Antidepressant
BMS200 <> 33	Tab	Nefazodone HCl 200 mg	Serzone by Bristol Myers	15548-0033	Antidepressant
BMS20033	Tab, Light Yellow, Hexagonal, BMS 200/33	Nefazodone HCl 200 mg	Serzone by Bristol-Myers	Canadian	Antidepressant
BMS250	Tab, White, Hexagon	Nefazodone HCl 250 mg	Serzone by Par	49884-0574	Antidepressant
BMS250 <> 41	Tab, White	Nefazodone HCl 250 mg	Serzone by Bristol Myers Squibb	00087-0041	Antidepressant
BMS250 <> 41	Tab	Nefazodone HCl 250 mg	Serzone by Kaiser	00179-1244	Antidepressant

ID FRONT <> BACK	DESCRIPTION FRONT <> BACK	INGREDIENT & STRENGTH	BRAND (OR EQUIV.) & FIRM	NDC#	CLASS; SCH.
BMS250 <> 41	Tab	Nefazodone HCl 250 mg	Serzone by Bristol Myers	15548-0041	Antidepressant
BMS30034	Tab, Peach, Hexagonal, BMS 300/34	Nefazodone HCl 300 mg	Serzone by Bristol-Myers	Canadian	Antidepressant
BMS32	Tab, White, Hexagonal	Serzone 100 mg	by Bristol-Myers		Antidepressant
BMS37	Tab, Chewable	Amoxicillin Trihydrate	by Bristol Myers Barcelaneta	55961-0035	Antibiotic
BMS38	Tab, Chewable	Amoxicillin Trihydrate	by Golden State	60429-0238	Antibiotic
BMS38	Tab, Chewable	Amoxicillin Trihydrate	by Bristol Myers Barcelaneta	55961-0036	Antibiotic
BMS50	Tab	Nefazodone HCl 50 mg	Serzone by Bristol Myers Squibb	00087-0057	Antidepressant
BMS50	Tab, Light Pink	Nefazodone HCl 50 mg	Serzone by Bristol Myers	15548-0031	Antidepressant
BMS50 <> 31	Tab	Nefazodone HCl 50 mg	Serzone by Murfreesboro	51129-1106	Antidepressant
BMS50 <> 31	Tab, Light Pink	Nefazodone HCl 50 mg	Serzone by Bristol Myers Squibb	00087-0031	Antidepressant
BMS5031	Tab, Pink, Hexagonal, BMS 50/31	Nefazodone HCl 50 mg	Serzone by Bristol-Myers	Canadian	Antidepressant
BMS50MG	Tab, Pink, Hexagon	Nefazodone HCl 50 mg	Serzone by Direct Dispensing	57866-0911	Antidepressant
BMS5240	Tab, White, Round	Atenolol 100 mg	Tenormin by BMS		Antihypertensive
BMS5250	Tab, Coated	Diltiazem HCl 30 mg	by Med Pro	53978-2064	Antihypertensive
BMS5550	Tab, Film Coated	Diltiazem HCl 60 mg	by Med Pro	53978-1235	Antihypertensive
BMS6060 <> 500	Tab, White to Off-White, Round, Film Coated	Metformin HCl 500 mg	Glucophage by Bristol Myers Squibb	00087-6060	Antidiabetic
BMS6060 <> 500	Tab, Film Coated, BMS 6060 Around the Outside	Metformin HCl 500 mg	Glucophage by PDRX	55289-0211	Antidiabetic
BMS6060 <> 500	Tab, Coated	Metformin HCl 500 mg	Glucophage by Heartland	61392-0717	Antidiabetic
BMS6060 <> 500	Tab, White, Round, Film	Metformin 500 mg	Glucophage by Purdue Pharma	59011-0103	Antidiabetic
BMS6063 <> 500	Tab, White to Off-White, Cap Shaped	Metformin HCl 500 mg	Glucophage XR by Bristol Myers	00087-6063	Antidiabetic
BMS6070	Tab, White, Round, Scored	Metformin HCl 850 mg	Glucophage by Va Cmop	65243-0047	Antidiabetic
BMS6070 <> 850	Tab, White, Round	Metformin HCl 850 mg	Glucophage by Kaiser Fdn	00179-1378	Antidiabetic
BMS6070 <> 850	Tab, White, Round	Metformin HCl 850 mg	Glucophage by Direct Dispensing	57866-9058	Antidiabetic
BMS6070 <> 850	Tab, White to Off-White, Round, Film Coated	Metformin HCl 850 mg	Glucophage by Bristol Myers Squibb	00087-6070	Antidiabetic
BMS6070 <> 850	Tab, Film Coated	Metformin HCl 850 mg	Glucophage by Caremark	00339-6085	Antidiabetic
BMS6070 <> 850	Tab, Round, Film Coated	Metformin HCl 850 mg	by Nat Pharmpak Serv	55154-5825	Antidiabetic
BMS6070 <> 850	Tab, White, Round, Film Coated	Metformin HCl 850 mg	Glucophage by Nat Pharmpak Serv	55154-5824	Antidiabetic
BMS6070 <> 850	Tab, White, Round, Film Coated	Metformin HCl 850 mg	Glucophage by Squibb Mfg	12783-0070	Antidiabetic
BMS6071 <> 1000	Tab, White, Oval	Metformin HCl 1000 mg	Glucophage by Direct Dispensing	57866-9057	Antidiabetic
BMS6071 <> 1000	Tab, White to Off-White, Oval, Scored, Film Coated	Metformin HCl 1000 mg	Glucophage by Bristol Myers Squibb	00087-6071	Antidiabetic
BMS6071 <> 1000	Tab, White, Oval, Film Coated	Metformin HCl 1000 mg	Glucophage by Caremark	00339-6173	Antidiabetic
BMS7491250	Cap, Blue & White, BMS 7491/250	Cefaclor 250 mg	Ceclor by BMS		Antibiotic
BMS7494500	Cap, Blue & Gray, BMS 7494/500	Cefaclor 500 mg	Ceclor by BMS		Antibiotic
BMS7720250	Tab, Film Coated	Cefprozil 250 mg	Cefzil by Quality Care	60346-0906	Antibiotic
BMS7720250	Tab, Film Coated	Cefprozil 250 mg	Cefzil by Bristol Myers Barcelaneta	55961-0720	Antibiotic
BMS7721500	Tab, Film Coated	Cefprozil 500 mg	Cefzil by Bristol Myers Barcelaneta	55961-0721	Antibiotic
BMS97	Tab, Pink, Round	Amoxicyllin 125 mg	by Apothecon		Antibiotic
BMSMONOPRIL10	Tab, White, Diamond Shaped, BMS/Monopril 10	Fosinopril Sodium 10 mg	by Bristol-Myers	Canadian	Antihypertensive
BMSMONOPRIL20	Tab, White, Oval, BMS/Monopril 20	Fosinopril Sodium 20 mg	by Bristol-Myers	Canadian	Antihypertensive
BN10G	Tab, White, BN/10/G	Baclofen 10 mg	by BDH	Canadian	Muscle Relaxant
BN20G	Tab, White, BN/20/G	Baclofen 20 mg	by BDH	Canadian	Muscle Relaxant
BNB <> CG	Tab, White, Round, Film Coated	Oxprenolol HCl 160 mg	Slow Trasicor by Novartis	Canadian DIN# 00534587	Antihypertensive
BNP6000	Cap, Clear & Orange	Diazoxide 50 mg	Proglycem by Baker		Diuretic
BNP7400	Cap, Orange	Tolmetin Sodium 400 mg	Tolectin DS by Baker		NSAID
BNP7600	Cap, Opaque & White	Pentosan Polysulfate Sodium 100 mg	Elmiron by Baker Cummins	Canadian	Analgesic
BNP7600	Cap	Pentosan Polysulfate Sodium 100 mg	Elmiron by Baker Norton	00575-7600	Analgesic
BNP7600	Cap, White, Gelatin Coated	Pentosan Polysulfate Sodium 100 mg	Elmiron by Alza	17314-9300	Analgesic
BOCK <> BOCK	Cap, ER, in Black Ink with White Beads	Pheniramine Maleate 16 mg, Phenylpropanolamine HCl 50 mg, Phenyltoloxamine Citrate 16 mg, Pyrilamine Maleate 16 mg	Poly Histine D by Sanofi	00024-1656	Cold Remedy

ID FRONT <> BACK	DESCRIPTION FRONT <> BACK	INGREDIENT & STRENGTH	BRAND (OR EQUIV.) & FIRM	NDC#	CLASS; SCH.
BOCK <> BOCK	Cap, Black Ink with White Beads	Pheniramine Maleate 8 mg, Phenylpropanolamine HCl 25 mg, Phenyltoloxamine Citrate 8 mg, Pyrilamine Maleate 8 mg	Poly Histine D by Sanofi	00024-1658	Cold Remedy
BOCK <> PN90	Tab, PN/90	Ascorbic Acid 120 mg, Calcium 250 mg, Cholecalciferol 10 mcg, Copper 2 mg, Cyanocobalamin 12 mcg, Docusate Sodium 50 mg, Folic Acid 1 mg, Iodine 150 mcg, Iron 90 mg, Niacinamide 20 mg, Pyridoxine HCl 20 mg, Riboflavin 3.4 mg, Thiamine Mononitrate 3 mg, Vitamin A Acetate 1.2 mg, Vitamin E Acetate 30 mg, Zinc 25 mg	Prenate 90 by Physicians Total Care	54868-2703	Vitamin
BOCK <> ZLA	Tab, Z/LA	Guaifenesin 600 mg, Pseudoephedrine HCl 120 mg	Zephrex LA by		Cold Remedy
BOCK <> ZLA	Tab, Film Coated	Guaifenesin 600 mg, Pseudoephedrine HCl 120 mg	Zephrex LA by Sanofi	00024-2627	Cold Remedy
BOCK330	Tab, Beige, Round	Ferrous Fumarate 110 mg, Docusate Na 20 mg, Vitamin C 200 mg	Hemaspan by Sanofi		Mineral
BOCK460	Tab, Bock over 460	Guaifenesin 400 mg, Pseudoephedrine HCl 60 mg	Zephrex by Sanofi	00024-2624	Cold Remedy
BOCK460	Tab, Blue, Oval, Scored	Guaifenesin 400 mg; Pseudoephedrine HCl 60 mg	Zephrex by Midland Pharms	45255-2070	Cold Remedy
BOCKHS33	Tab, Tan, Oblong	Ferrous Fumarate 335 mg, Vitamin C 200 mg, Docusate Na 20 mg	Hemaspan by KV		Mineral
BOCKPN	Tab, White, Oval	Prenatal Vitamin	Prenate Ultra by Sanofi		Vitamin
BOCKZLA	Tab, Orange, Oval, Bock Z/LA	Pseudoephedrine HCl 120 mg, Guaifenesin 600 mg	Zephrex LA by Sanofi		Cold Remedy
BOLAR227	Cap, Maroon	Triamterene 50 mg, Hydrochlorothiazide 25 mg	Dyazide by Bolar		Diuretic
BOLAR277	Cap, Red	Triamterene 50 mg, Hydrochlorothiazide 25 mg	Dyazide by Bolar		Diuretic
BOOTS0051	Tab, White, Round	Allopurinol 100 mg	Lopurin by Boots		Antigout
BOOTS0052	Tab, Orange, Round	Allopurinol 300 mg	Lopurin by Boots		Antigout
BP0004	Tab, White, Round	Primidone 250 mg	Mysoline by Bolar		Anticonvulsant
BP0005	Tab, White, Round	Methocarbamol 500 mg	Robaxin by Bolar		Muscle Relaxant
BP0007	Tab, White, Round	Trihexyphenidyl HCl 2 mg	Artane by Bolar		Antiparkinson
BP0011	Tab, Yellow, Round	Furosemide (Veterinary) 12.5 mg	Lasix by Bolar		Veterinary
BP0012	Tab, Yellow, Oblong	Furosemide (Veterinary) 50 mg	Lasix by Bolar		Veterinary
BP0017	Tab, Green, Round	Pentaerythritol Tetranitrate SR 80 mg	Peritrate SA by Bolar		Antianginal
BP0024	Tab, White, Round	Trihexyphenidyl HCl 5 mg	Artane by Bolar		Antiparkinson
BP0026	Tab, Green, Round	Isosorbide Dinitrate SA 40 mg	Isordil Tembid by Bolar		Antianginal
BP0036	Tab, White, Round	Chlorothiazide 250 mg	Diuril by Bolar		Diuretic
BP0037	Tab, White, Round	Orphenadrine Citrate SR 100 mg	Norflex by Bolar		Muscle Relaxant
BP0045	Tab, Pink, Round	Warfarin Sodium 5 mg	Coumadin by Bolar		Anticoagulant
BP0049	Tab, Green, Round	Isosorbide Dinitrate Oral 20 mg	Isordil by Bolar		Antianginal
BP0052	Tab, White, Round	Ergoloid Mesylates Sublingual 0.5 mg	Hydergine by Bolar		Ergot
BP0058	Tab, Orange, Round	Hydrochlorothiazide 100 mg	Hydrodiuril by Bolar		Diuretic
BP0059	Tab, Brownish Yellow, Round	Sulfasalazine 500 mg	Azulfidine by Bolar		Gastrointestinal
BP0065	Cap, White	Hydralazine HCl 25 mg, Hydrochlorothiazide 25 mg	Apresazide by Bolar		Antihypertensive
BP0066	Cap, Black & White	Hydralazine HCl 50 mg, Hydrochlorothiazide 50 mg	Apresazide by Bolar		Antihypertensive
BP0069	Tab, White, Oval	Ergoloid Mesylates Sublingual 1 mg	Hydergine by Bolar		Vasodilator
BP0073	Tab, White, Round	Bethanechol Chloride 5 mg	Urecholine by Bolar		Urinary Tract
BP0074	Tab, Pink, Round	Bethanechol Chloride 10 mg	Urecholine by Bolar		Urinary Tract
BP0075	Tab, Yellow, Round	Bethanechol Chloride 25 mg	Urecholine by Bolar		Urinary Tract
BP0083	Tab, Orange, Round	Hydralazine HCl 25 mg, Hydrochlorothiazide 15 mg	Apresoline/Esidrix by Bolar		Antihypertensive
BP0084	Cap, White	Phenytoin Sodium ER 100 mg	Dilantin by Bolar		Anticonvulsant
BP0093	Tab, Chartreuse, Round	Prochlorperazine 10 mg	Compazine by Bolar		Antiemetic
BP0094	Tab, White, Round	Carisoprodol 350 mg	Soma by Bolar		Muscle Relaxant
BP0111	Tab, Chartreuse, Round	Prochlorperazine 5 mg	Compazine by Bolar		Antiemetic
BP0129	Tab, White, Round	Spironolactone 25 mg, Hydrochlorothiazide 25 mg	Aldactazide by Bolar		Diuretic
BP0139	Tab, Green, Round	Fluoxymesterone 10 mg	Halotestin by Bolar		Steroid; C III
BP0149	Tab, White, Round	Acepromazine Maleate (Veterinary) 10 mg	by Bolar		Veterinary
BP0150	Tab, Yellow, Round	Acepromazine Maleate (Veterinary) 25 mg	by Bolar		Veterinary
BP0187	Tab, Pink, Oblong	Procainamide HCl SR 1000 mg	Procan SR by Bolar		Antiarrhythmic
BP0211	Tab, Blue, Round	Maprotiline HCl 25 mg	Ludiomil by Bolar		Antidepressant
BP0212	Tab, Yellow, Round	Maprotiline HCl 50 mg	Ludiomil by Bolar		Antidepressant
BP0213	Tab, White, Round	Maprotiline HCl 75 mg	Ludiomil by Bolar		Antidepressant

ID FRONT <> BACK	DESCRIPTION FRONT <> BACK	INGREDIENT & STRENGTH	BRAND (OR EQUIV.) & FIRM	NDC#	CLASS; SCH.
BP095	Tab, Lavender & White, Round	Carisoprodol 200 mg, Aspirin 325 mg	Soma Compound by Bolar		Muscle Relaxant
BP1	Tab, Green, Oblong	Thioridazine HCl 10 mg	Mellaril by Bolar		Antipsychotic
BP100	Cap, Green	Hydroxyzine Pamoate 25 mg	Vistaril by Bolar		Antihistamine
BP1007	Tab, White, Round	Trazodone HCl 50 mg	Desyrel by Bolar		Antidepressant
BP1008	Tab, White, Round	Trazodone HCl 100 mg	Desyrel by Bolar		Antidepressant
BP101	Cap, Green & White	Hydroxyzine Pamoate 50 mg	Vistaril by Bolar		Antihistamine
BP1015	Cap, Yellow	Nitrofurantoin 100 mg	Macrodantin by Bolar		Antibiotic
BP1016	Cap, White & Yellow	Nitrofurantoin 50 mg	Macrodantin by Bolar		Antibiotic
BP102	Cap, Gray & Green	Hydroxyzine Pamoate 100 mg	Vistaril by Bolar		Antihistamine
BP1027	Cap, Pink	Amantadine HCl 100 mg	Symmetrel by Bolar		Antiviral
BP111	Tab, Chartreuse, Round	Prochlorperazine 5 mg	Compazine by Bolar		Antiemetic
BP112	Tab, Chartreuse, Round	Prochlorperazine 25 mg	Compazine by Bolar		Antiemetic
BP117	Tab, Red, Round	Trifluoperazine HCl 5 mg	Stelazine by Bolar		Antipsychotic
BP118	Tab, Buff, Oblong	Thioridazine HCl 25 mg	Mellaril by Bolar		Antipsychotic
BP119	Tab, White, Oblong	Thioridazine HCl 50 mg	Mellaril by Bolar		Antipsychotic
BP120	Tab, Yellow, Oblong	Thioridazine HCl 100 mg	Mellaril by Bolar		Antipsychotic
BP121	Tab, Yellow, Oblong	Thioridazine HCl 150 mg	Mellaril by Bolar		Antipsychotic
BP122	Tab, Pink, Oblong	Thioridazine HCl 200 mg	Mellaril by Bolar		Antipsychotic
BP123	Tab, Peach, Round	Propranolol HCl 10 mg	Inderal by Bolar		Antihypertensive
BP124	Tab, Blue, Round	Propranolol HCl 20 mg	Inderal by Bolar		Antihypertensive
BP125	Tab, Green, Round	Propranolol HCl 40 mg	Inderal by Bolar		Antihypertensive
BP126	Tab, Yellow, Round	Propranolol HCl 80 mg	Inderal by Bolar		Antihypertensive
BP127	Tab, Yellow, Round	Hydroflumethiazide 25 mg, Reserpine 0.125 mg	Salutensin-Demi by Bolar		Diuretic; Antihypertensive
BP128	Tab, Green, Round	Hydroflumethiazide 50 mg, Reserpine 0.125 mg	Salutensin by Bolar		Diuretic; Antihypertensive
BP13	Tab, White, Round	Chlorothiazide 500 mg	Diuril by Bolar		Diuretic
BP131	Tab, Brownish Orange, Round	Sulfasalazine 500 mg	Azulfidine EN-tabs by Bolar		Gastrointestinal
BP132	Tab, Pink, Round	Chlorothiazide 500 mg, Reserpine 0.125 mg	Diupres by Bolar		Diuretic; Antihypertensive
BP133	Tab, White, Round	Allopurinol 100 mg	Zyloprim by Bolar		Antigout
BP134	Tab, Peach, Round	Allopurinol 300 mg	Zyloprim by Bolar		Antigout
BP135	Tab, Orange, Round	Guanethidine Monosulfate 10 mg	Ismelin by Bolar		Antihypertensive
BP136	Tab, White, Round	Guanethidine Monosulfate 25 mg	Ismelin by Bolar		Antihypertensive
BP137	Tab, Peach, Round	Fluoxymesterone 2 mg	Halotestin by Bolar		Steroid; C III
BP138	Tab, Green, Round	Fluoxymesterone 5 mg	Halotestin by Bolar		Steroid; C III
BP144	Tab, Lavender & White, Round	Carisoprodol 200 mg, Aspirin 325 mg	Soma Compound by Bolar		Muscle Relaxant
BP145	Cap, Green	Indomethacin 25 mg	Indocin by Bolar		NSAID
BP146	Cap, Green	Indomethacin 50 mg	Indocin by Bolar		NSAID
BP151	Tab, Red, Round	Trifluoperazine HCl 10 mg	Stelazine by Bolar		Antipsychotic
BP152	Tab, Blue, Oval	Procainamide HCl SR 250 mg	Procan SR by Bolar		Antiarrhythmic
BP153	Tab, Pink, Oval	Procainamide HCl SR 500 mg	Procan SR by Bolar		Antiarrhythmic
BP154	Tab, Buff, Oval	Procainamide HCl SR 750 mg	Procan SR by Bolar		Antiarrhythmic
BP157	Tab, Gray, Round	Methyclothiazide 5 mg, Deserpidine 0.5 mg	Enduronyl Forte by Bolar		Diuretic; Antihypertensive
BP158	Tab, Yellow, Round	Methyclothiazide 5 mg, Deserpidine 0.25 mg	Enduronyl by Bolar		Diuretic; Antihypertensive
BP163	Tab, White, Round	Fluphenazine HCl 1 mg	Prolixin by Bolar		Antipsychotic
BP164	Tab, Beige, Round	Fluphenazine HCl 2.5 mg	Prolixin by Bolar		Antipsychotic
BP165	Tab, Blue, Round	Fluphenazine HCl 5 mg	Prolixin by Bolar		Antipsychotic
BP166	Tab, Red, Round	Fluphenazine HCl 10 mg	Prolixin by Bolar		Antipsychotic
BP167	Tab, Blue, Round	Chlorpropamide 100 mg	Diabinese by Bolar		Antidiabetic

ID FRONT <> BACK	DESCRIPTION FRONT <> BACK	INGREDIENT & STRENGTH	BRAND (OR EQUIV.) & FIRM	NDC#	CLASS; SCH.
BP168	Tab, Blue, Round	Chlorpropamide 250 mg	Diabinese by Bolar		Antidiabetic
BP171	Tab, Red, Round	Trifluoperazine HCl 1 mg	Stelazine by Bolar		Antipsychotic
BP172	Tab, Red, Round	Trifluoperazine HCl 2 mg	Stelazine by Bolar		Antipsychotic
BP181	Tab, White, Round	Lorazepam 1 mg	Ativan by Bolar		Sedative/Hypnotic; C IV
BP182	Tab, White, Round	Lorazepam 2 mg	Ativan by Bolar		Sedative/Hypnotic; C IV
BP187	Tab, Pink, Oblong	Procainamide HCl SR 1000 mg	Procan SR by Bolar		Antiarrhythmic
BP2	Tab, White, Round	Lorazepam 0.5 mg	Ativan by Bolar		Sedative/Hypnotic; C IV
BP2005	Cap, Orange & White	Disopyramide Phosphate 100 mg	Norpace by Bolar		Antiarrhythmic
BP2006	Cap, Brown & Orange	Disopyramide Phosphate 150 mg	Norpace by Bolar		Antiarrhythmic
BP2014	Tab, White, Round	Methyldopa 125 mg	Aldomet by Bolar		Antihypertensive
BP2015	Tab, White, Round	Methyldopa 250 mg	Aldomet by Bolar		Antihypertensive
BP2016	Tab, White, Round	Methyldopa 500 mg	Aldomet by Bolar		Antihypertensive
BP2023	Cap, Blue	Decyclomine HCl 10 mg	Bentyl by Bolar		Gastrointestinal
BP2024	Cap, Maroon & Pink	Meclofenamate Sodium 50 mg	Meclomen by Bolar		NSAID
BP2025	Cap, Maroon & White	Meclofenamate Sodium 100 mg	Meclomen by Bolar		NSAID
BP2026	Tab, Blue, Round	Decyclomine HCl 20 mg	Bentyl by Bolar		Gastrointestinal
BP2027	Tab, White, Round	Metoclopramide HCl 10 mg	Reglan by Bolar		Gastrointestinal
BP2036	Tab, Chartreuse, Round	Methyldopa 250 mg, Hydrochlorothiazide 15 mg	Aldoril by Bolar		Antihypertensive
BP2037	Tab, Pink, Round	Methyldopa 250 mg, Hydrochlorothiazide 25 mg	Aldoril by Bolar		Antihypertensive
BP2038	Tab, Chartreuse, Oval	Methyldopa 500 mg, Hydrochlorothiazide 30 mg	Aldoril by Bolar		Antihypertensive
BP2039	Tab, Pink, Oval	Methyldopa 500 mg, Hydrochlorothiazide 50 mg	Aldoril by Bolar		Antihypertensive
BP2042	Tab, White, Round	Verapamil HCl 80 mg	Isoptin by Bolar		Antihypertensive
BP2043	Tab, White, Round	Verapamil HCl 120 mg	Isoptin by Bolar		Antihypertensive
BP2047	Tab, Green, Round	Hydrochlorothiazide 25 mg, Reserpine 0.125 mg	Hydropres by Bolar		Diuretic; Antihypertensive
BP2048	Tab, Green, Round	Hydrochlorothiazide 50 mg, Reserpine 0.125 mg	Hydropres by Bolar		Diuretic; Antihypertensive
BP2049	Tab, White, Round	Hydrochlorothiazide 15 mg, Reserpine 0.1 mg, Hydralazine 25 mg	Ser- by Bolar		Diuretic; Antihypertensive
BP2053	Tab, Orange, Round	Perphenazine 2 mg, Amitriptyline 25 mg	Triavil by Bolar		Antipsychotic; Antidepressant
BP2054	Tab, Yellow, Round	Perphenazine 4 mg, Amitriptyline 25 mg	Triavil by Bolar		Antipsychotic; Antidepressant
BP2055	Tab, Orange, Round	Perphenazine 4 mg, Amitriptyline 50 mg	Triavil by Bolar		Antipsychotic; Antidepressant
BP2056	Tab, Blue, Round	Perphenazine 2 mg, Amitriptyline 10 mg	Triavil by Bolar		Antipsychotic; Antidepressant
BP2057	Tab, Salmon, Round	Perphenazine 4 mg, Amitriptyline 10 mg	Triavil by Bolar		Antipsychotic; Antidepressant
BP2060	Tab, Pink, Round	Propranolol HCl 60 mg	Inderal by Bolar		Antihypertensive
BP2062	Tab, White, Round	Tolbutamide 250 mg	Orinase by Bolar		Antidiabetic
BP2063	Tab, White, Round	Tolbutamide 500 mg	Orinase by Bolar		Antidiabetic
BP2064	Tab, Green, Round	Pentaerythritol Tetranitrate 10 mg	Peritrate by Bolar		Antianginal
BP2066	Cap, Pink & White	Lithium Carbonate 300 mg	Eskalith by Bolar		Antipsychotic
BP2067	Tab, Green, Round	Pentaerythritol Tetranitrate 20 mg	Peritrate by Bolar		Antianginal
BP2068	Tab, White, Round	Tolazamide 100 mg	Tolinase by Bolar		Antidiabetic
BP2069	Tab, White, Round	Tolazamide 250 mg	Tolinase by Bolar		Antidiabetic
BP2070	Tab, White, Round	Tolazamide 500 mg	Tolinase by Bolar		Antidiabetic
BP2074	Tab, White, Oblong	Probenecid 0.5 GM, Colchicine 0.5 mg	ColBenemid by Bolar		Antigout
BP2075	Tab, Yellow, Round	Nitrofurantoin 50 mg	Furadantin by Bolar		Antibiotic
BP2076	Cap, Yellow	Procainamide HCl 250 mg	Pronestyl by Bolar		Antiarrhythmic
BP2078	Cap, Orange & Yellow	Procainamide HCl 500 mg	Pronestyl by Bolar		Antiarrhythmic

ID FRONT <> BACK	DESCRIPTION FRONT <> BACK	INGREDIENT & STRENGTH	BRAND (OR EQUIV.) & FIRM	NDC#	CLASS; SCH.
BP2080	Tab, Yellow, Round	Nitrofurantoin 100 mg	Furadantin by Bolar		Antibiotic
BP2081	Cap, Green & White	Flurazepam HCl 15 mg	Dalmane by Bolar		Hypnotic; C IV
BP2082	Cap, Green & White	Flurazepam HCl 30 mg	Dalmane by Bolar		Hypnotic; C IV
BP2085	Tab, Pink, Oblong	Propoxyphene Napsylate 50 mg, Acetaminophen 325 mg	Darvocet N by Bolar		Analgesic; C IV
BP2086	Tab, Pink, Oblong	Propoxyphene Napsylate 100 mg, Acetaminophen 650 mg	Darvocet N by Bolar		Analgesic; C IV
BP2087	Cap, Pink	Temazepam 15 mg	Restoril by Bolar		Sedative/Hypnotic; C IV
BP2088	Cap, Pink & Yellow	Temazepam 30 mg	Restoril by Bolar		Sedative/Hypnotic; C IV
BP2092	Tab, Lavender, Round	Trichlormethiazide 4 mg, Reserpine 0.1 mg	Naquival by Bolar		Diuretic; Antihypertensive
BP2093	Tab, Orange, Round	Hydrochlorothiazide 25 mg	Hydrodiuril by Bolar		Diuretic
BP2094	Tab, Orange, Round	Hydrochlorothiazide 50 mg	Hydrodiuril by Bolar		Diuretic
BP211	Tab, Blue, Round	Maprotiline HCl 25 mg	Ludiomil by Bolar		Antidepressant
BP2118	Cap, Purple & Yellow	Disopyramide Phosphate CR 100 mg	Norpace CR by Bolar		Antiarrhythmic
BP2119	Cap, Orange & Purple	Disopyramide Phosphate CR 150 mg	Norpace CR by Bolar		Antiarrhythmic
BP212	Tab, Yellow, Round	Maprotiline HCl 50 mg	Ludiomil by Bolar		Antidepressant
BP2126	Cap, White	Potassium Chloride 750 mg	Micro K 10 by Bolar		Electrolytes
BP213	Tab, White, Round	Maprotiline HCl 75 mg	Ludiomil by Bolar		Antidepressant
BP2150	Tab, White, Round	Isoniazid 100 mg	by Bolar		Antimycobacterial
BP2155	Tab, White, Round	Isoniazid 300 mg	by Bolar		Antimycobacterial
BP28	Tab, Brown, Round	Imipramine HCl 25 mg	Tofranil by Bolar		Antidepressant
BP3000	Tab, White, Round	Quinidine Gluconate SR 324 mg	Quinaglute Duratabs by Bolar		Antiarrhythmic
BP3020	Tab, Blue, Round	Trichlormethiazide 4 mg	Naqua by Bolar		Diuretic
BP31	Tab, Pink, Oblong	Thioridazine HCl 15 mg	Mellaril by Bolar		Antipsychotic
BP32	Tab, Blue, Pentagon	Dexamethasone 0.75 mg	Decadron by Bolar		Steroid
BP33	Tab, Peach, Round	Chlorthalidone 25 mg	Hygroton by Bolar		Diuretic
BP34	Tab, Blue, Round	Chlorthalidone 50 mg	Hygroton by Bolar		Diuretic
BP35	Tab, White, Round	Chlorthalidone 100 mg	Hygroton by Bolar		Diuretic
BP39	Tab, Yellow, Triangular	Imipramine HCl 10 mg	Tofranil by Bolar		Antidepressant
BP40	Tab, Green, Round	Imipramine HCl 50 mg	Tofranil by Bolar		Antidepressant
BP41	Tab, White, Round	Ergoloid Mesylates Oral 1 mg	Hydergine by Bolar		Ergot
BP42	Tab, White, Round	Acetazolamide 250 mg	Diamox by Bolar		Diuretic
BP44	Tab, Orange, Round	Warfarin Sodium 2.5 mg	Coumadin by Bolar		Anticoagulant
BP46	Tab, Yellow, Round	Warfarin Sodium 7.5 mg	Coumadin by Bolar		Anticoagulant
BP47	Tab, White, Round	Warfarin Sodium 10 mg	Coumadin by Bolar		Anticoagulant
BP50	Tab, Lavender, Round	Warfarin Sodium 2 mg	Coumadin by Bolar		Anticoagulant
BP5000	Tab, White, Round	Spironolactone 25 mg	Aldactone by Bolar		Diuretic
BP5010	Tab, Yellow, Round	Bethanechol Chloride 50 mg	Urecholine by Bolar		Urinary Tract
BP56	Tab, Pink, Round	Chlorothiazide 250 mg, Reserpine 0.125 mg	Diupres by Bolar		Diuretic; Antihypertensive
BP6	Tab, White, Oblong	Methocarbamol 750 mg	Robaxin by Bolar		Muscle Relaxant
BP60	Tab, White, Round	Liothyronine Sodium 25 mcg	Cytomel by Bolar		Antithyroid
BP62	Tab, Orange, Round	Methyclothiazide 2.5 mg	Enduron by Bolar		Diuretic
BP63	Tab, Reddish Orange, Round	Methyclothiazide 5 mg	Enduron by Bolar		Diuretic
BP64	Cap, Blue	Hydralazine HCl 100 mg, Hydrochlorothiazide 50 mg	Apresazide by Bolar		Antihypertensive
BP72	Tab, White, Round	Hydroflumethiazide 50 mg	Saluron by Bolar		Diuretic
BP76	Tab, Red, Round	Oxtriphylline 100 mg	Choledyl by Bolar		Antiasthmatic
BP77	Tab, Yellow, Round	Oxtriphylline 200 mg	Choledyl by Bolar		Antiasthmatic
BP78	Tab, White, Round	Cyproheptadine HCl 4 mg	Periactin by Bolar		Antihistamine
BP79	Tab, White, Round	Clonidine HCl 0.1 mg	Catapres by Bolar		Antihypertensive
BP80	Tab, Orange, Round	Clonidine HCl 0.2 mg	Catapres by Bolar		Antihypertensive
BP81	Tab, Peach, Round	Clonidine HCl 0.3 mg	Catapres by Bolar		Antihypertensive
BP87	Tab, Green, Round	Sulfamethoxazole 500 mg	Gantanol by Bolar		Antibiotic

ID FRONT ⟷ BACK	DESCRIPTION FRONT ⟷ BACK	INGREDIENT & STRENGTH	BRAND (OR EQUIV.) & FIRM	NDC#	CLASS; SCH.
BP88	Tab, White, Round	Primidone (Veterinary) 250 mg	by Bolar		Veterinary
BP9000	Tab, White, Round	Quinine Sulfate 260 mg	Quinamm by Bolar		Antimalarial
BP93	Tab, Chartreuse, Round	Prochlorperazine 10 mg	Compazine by Bolar		Antiemetic
BP956	Tab, White, Oblong	Methyltestosterone Buccal 5 mg	Android 5 by Heather		Hormone; C III
BP958	Tab, Green, Square	Methyltestosterone 10 mg	Android 10 by Heather		Hormone; C III
BP996	Tab, Orange, Square	Methyltestosterone 25 mg	Android 25 by Heather		Hormone; C III
BP998	Tab, White, Round	Fluoxymesterone 10 mg	Android F by Heather		Steroid; C III
BPI2	Tab, White, Round	AcetAminophen 300 mg, Codeine Phosphate 15 mg	Tylenol #2 by Noramco		Analgesic; C III
BPM ⟷ PSE	Cap, Clear & Green, in Black	Brompheniramine Maleate 12 mg, Pseudoephedrine HCl 120 mg	BPM PSEH 08 by Bryant	63629-4488	Cold Remedy
BPM189	Tab, Yellow, Round	Amoxicillin 125 mg, Clavulanate Potassium Chewable 31.25 mg	Augmentin by SKB	00029-6073	Antibiotic
BPM190	Tab, Yellow, Round	Amoxicillin 250 mg, Clavulanate Potassium Chewable 62.5 mg	Augmentin by SKB	00029-6047	Antibiotic
BRA200	Tab	Calcium Acetate 667 mg	Phoslo by Braintree	52268-0200	Vitamin/Mineral
BREON100	Cap, Brown & White	Theophylline Anhydrous 100 mg	Bronkodyl by Sanofi		Antiasthmatic
BREON200	Cap, Red	Guaifenesin 200 mg	Breonesin by Sanofi		Expectorant
BREON200	Cap, Green & White	Theophylline Anhydrous 200 mg	Bronkodyl by Sanofi		Antiasthmatic
BREONT100	Tab, Peach, Oblong	Chlormezanone 100 mg	Trancopal by Sanofi		Antihistamine
BREONT200	Tab, Green, Oblong	Chlormezanone 200 mg	Trancopal by Sanofi		Antihistamine
BRISTOL	Cap	Amoxicillin Trihydrate	by Talbert Med	44514-0077	Antibiotic
BRISTOL ⟷ 278	Cap, Burgundy & Salmon	Amoxicillin 250 mg	by Quality Care	60346-0655	Antibiotic
BRISTOL ⟷ 7279	Cap, Burgundy & Salmon	Amoxicillin 500 mg	by Quality Care	60346-0634	Antibiotic
BRISTOL ⟷ 7992	Cap	Ampicillin Trihydrate	by Quality Care	60346-0082	Antibiotic
BRISTOL ⟷ 7993	Cap	Ampicillin Trihydrate	by Quality Care	60346-0593	Antibiotic
BRISTOL1257892	Cap, Light Blue & White	Dicloxacillin Sodium 125 mg	by Apothecon		Antibiotic
BRISTOL3030 ⟷ 10MG	Cap, Bristol Over 3030 ⟷ 10 mg	Lomustine 10 mg	Ceenu by Mead Johnson	00015-3030	Antineoplastic
BRISTOL303010MG	Cap	Lomustine 10 mg	by Bristol	Canadian	Antineoplastic
BRISTOL3031 ⟷ 40MG	Cap, Moss Green, Bristol over 3031 ⟷ 40 mg	Lomustine 40 mg	Ceenu by Mead Johnson	00015-3031	Antineoplastic
BRISTOL303140MG	Cap	Lomustine 40 mg	by Bristol	Canadian	Antineoplastic
BRISTOL3032 ⟷ 100MG	Cap, Bristol Over 3032 ⟷ 100 mg	Lomustine 100 mg	Ceenu by Mead Johnson	00015-3032	Antineoplastic
BRISTOL3032100MG	Cap	Lomustine 100 mg	by Bristol	Canadian	Antineoplastic
BRISTOL3091	Cap, Black Print, Bristol over 3091	Etoposide 50 mg	Vepesid by Mead Johnson	00015-3091	Antineoplastic
BRISTOL3506	Cap	Kanamycin Sulfate	Kantrex by Mead Johnson	00015-3506	Anthelmintic
BRISTOL515	Cap, White & Yellow	Theophylline 300 mg, Guaifenesin 180 mg	Quibron 300 by Bristol		Antiasthmatic
BRISTOL516	Cap, Yellow	Theophylline 150 mg, Guaifenesin 90 mg	Quibron by Bristol		Antiasthmatic
BRISTOL7271	Cap, Black & Blue, White Print	Cefadroxil Hemihydrate	by Quality Care	60346-0022	Antibiotic
BRISTOL7271	Cap	Cefadroxil Monohydrate	by Prescription Dispensing	61807-0123	Antibiotic
BRISTOL7271	Cap, White Print	Cefadroxil Monohydrate	by DRX	55045-2426	Antibiotic
BRISTOL7271	Cap, Black & Blue	Cefadroxil Monohydrate 500 mg	by Natl Pharmpak	55154-7604	Antibiotic
BRISTOL7271	Cap, White Ink	Cefadroxil 500 mg	by Apothecon	59772-7271	Antibiotic
BRISTOL7271500	Cap, Black	Cefadroxil 500 mg	Ultracef by BMS		Antibiotic
BRISTOL7278	Cap, Flesh, Black Print	Amoxicillin Trihydrate	Trimox by ER Squibb	00003-0101	Antibiotic
BRISTOL7279	Cap	Amoxicillin Trihydrate	by Med Pro	53978-5003	Antibiotic
BRISTOL7279	Cap, Flesh, Black Print	Amoxicillin Trihydrate	Trimox by ER Squibb	00003-0109	Antibiotic
BRISTOL732 ⟷ ENKAID25MG	Cap, Bristol 732 ⟷ Enkaid 25 mg	Encainide HCl 25 mg	Enkaid by Bristol Myers Squibb	00087-0732	Antiarrhythmic
BRISTOL734 ⟷ ENKAID35MG	Cap, Bristol 734 ⟷ Enkaid 35 mg	Encainide HCl 35 mg	Enkaid by Bristol Myers Squibb	00087-0734	Antiarrhythmic
BRISTOL7375	Cap, Blue & Purple	Cephalexin Monohydrate 250 mg	Cefanex by BMS		Antibiotic
BRISTOL7376 ⟷ 500MG	Cap, Bristol over 7376 ⟷ 500 mg	Cephalexin Monohydrate	by Quality Care	60346-0055	Antibiotic
BRISTOL7496	Cap, Black & Orange	Cloxacillin 500 mg	Tegopen by BMS		Antibiotic
BRISTOL7578	Cap	Amoxicillin Trihydrate	by Med Pro	53978-5002	Antibiotic

ID FRONT <> BACK	DESCRIPTION FRONT <> BACK	INGREDIENT & STRENGTH	BRAND (OR EQUIV.) & FIRM	NDC#	CLASS; SCH.
BRISTOL7658500	Cap, Blue & White, Bristol 7658/500	Dicloxacillin Sodium 500 mg	Dynapen by BMS		Antibiotic
BRISTOL7892125	Cap, Blue & White, Bristol 7892/125	Dicloxacillin Sodium 125 mg	Dynapen by BMS		Antibiotic
BRISTOL7893250	Cap, Blue & White, Bristol 7893/250	Dicloxacillin Sodium 250 mg	Dynapen by BMS		Antibiotic
BRISTOL7922	Cap, Gray & Scarlet	Ampicillin 250 mg	Principen by BMS		Antibiotic
BRISTOL7923	Cap, Gray & Scarlet	Ampicillin 500 mg	Principen by BMS		Antibiotic
BRISTOL7935	Cap, Black & Orange	Cloxacillin 250 mg	Tegopen by Bristol		Antibiotic
BRISTOL7936	Cap, Black & Orange	Cloxacillin Sodium 250 mg	Tegopen by BMS		Antibiotic
BRISTOL7977	Cap, Pink	Oxacillin Sodium 250 mg	Prostaphlin by BMS		Antibiotic
BRISTOL7982	Cap, Pink	Oxacillin Sodium 500 mg	Prostaphlin by BMS		Antibiotic
BRISTOL7992	Cap	Ampicillin Trihydrate 250 mg	by Med Pro	53978-5018	Antibiotic
BRISTOL7992	Cap, Black Print	Ampicillin Trihydrate	Principen by ER Squibb	00003-0122	Antibiotic
BRISTOL7993	Cap	Ampicillin Trihydrate	by Med Pro	53978-5019	Antibiotic
BRISTOL7993	Cap, Black Print	Ampicillin Trihydrate	Principen by ER Squibb	00003-0134	Antibiotic
BRISTOL7993	Cap, Gray & Red, Black Print	Ampicillin 500 mg	by Bayer	00280-1092	Antibiotic
BRL <> 1127	Tab, Blue, Oblong, Scored	Sucralfate 1 gm	by Blue Ridge	59273-0001	Gastrointestinal
BRL <> 1127	Tab, Blue, Oblong	Sucralfate 1 gm	by Solvay	00032-1101	Gastrointestinal
BRL <> 1127	Tab, Blue, Oblong	Sucralfate 1 gm	Carafate by SKB	00135-0176	Gastrointestinal
BRL <> 1127	Tab	Sucralfate 1 gm	by Hoechst Roussel	00088-1127	Gastrointestinal
BRL <> 1127	Tab, Embossed	Sucralfate 1 gm	by Rugby	00536-1127	Gastrointestinal
BRL120 <> 3104	Tab, White, Oblong	Diltiazem HCl 120 mg	by Endo		Antihypertensive
BRL120 <> 3104	Tab, White, Oblong, Scored	Diltiazem HCl 120 mg	by Blue Ridge	59273-0005	Antihypertensive
BRL120 <> 3104	Tab, White	Diltiazem HCl 120 mg	Cardizem by Rugby	52544-0778	Antihypertensive
BRL1203104	Tab, Coated	Diltiazem HCl 120 mg	by Rugby	00536-3104	Antihypertensive
BRL30 <> 3101	Tab, Blue, Round, BRL 30	Diltiazem HCl 30 mg	by Elan Hold	60274-0884	Antihypertensive
BRL30 <> 3101	Tab, Blue, Round, Scored	Diltiazem HCl 30 mg	by Blue Ridge	59273-0002	Antihypertensive
BRL30 <> 3101	Tab, Blue, Round	Diltiazem HCl 30 mg	Cardizem by Rugby	52544-0775	Antihypertensive
BRL30301	Tab, Coated	Diltiazem HCl 30 mg	by Rugby	00536-3101	Antihypertensive
BRL4777	Tab, Blue, Round	Oxybutynin Chloride 5 mg	Ditropan by Rugby		Urinary
BRL4777	Tab	Oxybutynin Chloride 5 mg	by Rugby	00536-5672	Urinary
BRL60 <> 3102	Tab, White, Round, Scored	Diltiazem HCl 60 mg	by Fielding	00421-0158	Antihypertensive
BRL60 <> 3102	Tab, White, Round, Scored, BRL 60	Diltiazem HCl 60 mg	by Endo	60951-0675	Antihypertensive
BRL60 <> 3102	Tab, White, Round, Scored	Diltiazem HCl 60 mg	by Blue Ridge	59273-0003	Antihypertensive
BRL603102	Tab, Coated	Diltiazem HCl 60 mg	by Rugby	00536-3102	Antihypertensive
BRL90 <> 3103	Tab, Blue, Oblong, Scored, BRL 90	Diltiazem HCl 90 mg	by Endo	63481-0653	Antihypertensive
BRL90 <> 3103	Tab, Blue, Oblong, Scored	Diltiazem HCl 90 mg	by Blue Ridge	59273-0004	Antihypertensive
BRL90 <> 3103	Tab, Blue, Oblong, Scored	Diltiazem HCl 90 mg	by Fielding	00421-0748	Antihypertensive
BRL903103	Tab, Coated	Diltiazem HCl 90 mg	by Rugby	00536-3103	Antihypertensive
BROMFED <> MURO12120	Cap, Light Green, Ex Release, <> Muro 12-120	Brompheniramine Maleate 12 mg, Pseudoephedrine HCl 120 mg	Bromfed by Thrift Drug	59198-0190	Cold Remedy
BROMFED <> MURO12120	Cap, Bromfed <> Muro 12-120	Brompheniramine Maleate 12 mg, Pseudoephedrine HCl 120 mg	Bromfed by Muro	00451-4000	Cold Remedy
BROMFEDMURO12120	Cap, Clear & Green, Bromfed Muro 12-120	Brompheniramine Maleate 12 mg, Pseudoephedrine HCl 120 mg	BPM PSEH 07 by Bryant	63629-2200	Cold Remedy
BROMFEDPD <> MURO660	Cap, Bromfed-PD <> Muro 6-60	Brompheniramine Maleate 6 mg, Pseudoephedrine HCl 60 mg	Bromfed-PD by Muro	00451-4001	Cold Remedy
BROMFEDPD <> MURO660	Cap, Bromfed-PD <> Muro 6-60	Brompheniramine Maleate 6 mg, Pseudoephedrine HCl 60 mg	Bromfed PD by Nat Pharmpak Serv	55154-4301	Cold Remedy
BROMFEDPD <> MURO660	Cap, Dark Green, Ex Release, Bromfed-PD <> Muro 6-60	Brompheniramine Maleate 6 mg, Pseudoephedrine HCl 60 mg	Bromfed PD by Thrift Drug	59198-0189	Cold Remedy
BROMFEDPD <> MURO660	Cap, Clear & Green, Bromfed-PD <> Muro 6 60, Contains White Beads	Brompheniramine Maleate 6 mg, Pseudoephedrine HCl 60 mg	Bromfed PD by Capellon	64543-0111	Cold Remedy
BROMFEDPDMUR660	Cap, Clear & Green, Bromfed-PD Muro 6-60 in Blue	Brompheniramine Maleate 6 mg, Pseudoephedrine HCl 60 mg	BPM PSEH PD 08 by Capellon	64543-0089	Cold Remedy
BRONTEX	Tab, Red, Oblong	Codeine Phosphate 10 mg, Guaifenensin 300 mg	Brontex by Dixon	17236-0375	Analgesic; C III

ID FRONT <> BACK	DESCRIPTION FRONT <> BACK	INGREDIENT & STRENGTH	BRAND (OR EQUIV.) & FIRM	NDC#	CLASS; SCH.
BRONTEX	Tab, Coated	Codeine Phosphate 10 mg, Guaifenesin 300 mg	Brontex by Quality Care	60346-0304	Cold Remedy; C III
BRONTEX	Tab, Coated	Codeine Phosphate 10 mg, Guaifenesin 300 mg	Brontex by Procter & Gamble	00149-0440	Cold Remedy; C III
BROWN <> MYLAN3205	Cap	Prazosin HCl 5 mg	by Allscripts	54569-2584	Antihypertensive
BTG11	Tab, White, Oval	Oxandrolone 2.5 mg	Oxandrin by BTG		Steroid
BU10 <> NU	Tab, White, Rectangular, Scored	Buspirone 10 mg	by Nu Pharm	Canadian DIN# 02207672	Antianxiety
BU10APO	Tab, White, Pillow, BU 10/APO	Buspirone 10 mg	Buspirone by Apotex	Canadian	Antianxiety
BU5APO	Tab, White, Pillow, BU 5/APO	Buspirone 5 mg	by Apotex	Canadian	Antianxiety
BUCETUAD307	Cap, White, Opaque, Bucet/UAD 307	Acetaminophen 650 mg, Butalbital 50 mg	Bucet by Forest	00785-2307	Analgesic
BULL	Tab, White, Novo Nordisk Bull Logo	Repaglinide 0.5 mg	Prandin by Novo Nordisk	00169-0081	Antidiabetic
BULL	Tab, Yellow, Novo Nordisk Bull Logo	Repaglinide 1 mg	Prandin by Novo Nordisk	00169-0082	Antidiabetic
BULL	Tab, Red, Novo Nordisk Bull Logo	Repaglinide 2 mg	Prandin by Novo Nordisk	00169-0084	Antidiabetic
BUMEX <> ROCHE	Tab	Bumetanide 2 mg	Bumex by Med Pro	53978-2035	Diuretic
BUMEX05 <> ROCHE	Tab, Bumex 0.5 <> Roche	Bumetanide 0.5 mg	Bumex by Nat Pharmpak Serv	55154-3103	Diuretic
BUMEX05 <> ROCHE	Tab, Light Green, Bumex 0.5	Bumetanide 0.5 mg	Bumex by Thrift Drug	59198-0257	Diuretic
BUMEX05 <> ROCHE	Tab, Green, Oval, Bumex over 0.5 <> Roche	Bumetanide 0.5 mg	Bumex by Capellon	64543-0141	Diuretic
BUMEX05 <> ROCHE	Tab, Bumex 0.5 <> Roche	Bumetanide 0.5 mg	Bumex by Hoffmann La Roche	00004-0125	Diuretic
BUMEX1	Tab, Yellow, Oval, Bumex over 1	Bumetanide 1 mg	Bumex by Capellon	64543-0131	Diuretic
BUMEX1 <> ROCHE	Tab	Bumetanide 1 mg	Bumex by Thrift Drug	59198-0256	Diuretic
BUMEX1 <> ROCHE	Tab	Bumetanide 1 mg	Bumex by Nat Pharmpak Serv	55154-3104	Diuretic
BUMEX1 <> ROCHE	Tab	Bumetanide 1 mg	Bumex by Hoffmann La Roche	00004-0121	Diuretic
BUMEX1 <> ROCHE	Tab, Bumex/1 <> Roche	Bumetanide 1 mg	Bumex by Med Pro	53978-0241	Diuretic
BUMEX2 <> ROCHE	Tab	Bumetanide 2 mg	Bumex by Thrift Drug	59198-0101	Diuretic
BUMEX2 <> ROCHE	Tab	Bumetanide 2 mg	Bumex by Nat Pharmpak Serv	55154-3105	Diuretic
BUMEX2 <> ROCHE	Tab	Bumetanide 2 mg	Bumex by Quality Care	60346-0310	Diuretic
BUMEX2 <> ROCHE	Tab	Bumetanide 2 mg	Bumex by Amerisource	62584-0162	Diuretic
BUMEX2 <> ROCHE	Tab	Bumetanide 2 mg	Bumex by Hoffmann La Roche	00004-0162	Diuretic
BUSPAR	Tab, MJ Logo	Buspirone HCl 10 mg	Buspar by Amerisource	62584-0819	Antianxiety
BUSPAR	Tab, MJ Logo	Buspirone HCl 10 mg	Buspar by Drug Distr	52985-0156	Antianxiety
BUSPAR	Tab, MJ Logo	Buspirone HCl 5 mg	Buspar by Amerisource	62584-0818	Antianxiety
BUSPAR	Tab, MJ Logo	Buspirone HCl 5 mg	Buspar by Drug Distr	52985-0155	Antianxiety
BUSPAR <> 10MG	Tab, MJ Logo	Buspirone HCl 10 mg	by Med Pro	53978-3024	Antianxiety
BUSPAR <> 10MJ	Tab, Buspar <> 10 over MJ	Buspirone HCl 10 mg	Buspar by Nat Pharmpak Serv	55154-2010	Antianxiety
BUSPAR <> MJ10	Tab, Mead Johnson Logo 10	Buspirone HCl 10 mg	Buspar by Quality Care	60346-0162	Antianxiety
BUSPAR <> MJ10	Tab, MJ Logo	Buspirone HCl 10 mg	Buspar by Heartland	61392-0602	Antianxiety
BUSPAR <> MJ10	Tab, White, Ovoid-Rectangular, Scored	Buspirone HCl 10 mg	Buspar by Bristol Myers Squibb	00087-0819	Antianxiety
BUSPAR <> MJ10	Tab	Buspirone HCl 10 mg	Buspar by Pharmedix	53002-1017	Antianxiety
BUSPAR <> MJ10	Tab	Buspirone HCl 10 mg	Buspar by CVS Revco	00894-5215	Antianxiety
BUSPAR <> MJ5	Tab, Ovoid Rectangular, <> MJ Logo Then 5	Buspirone HCl 5 mg	Buspar by Heartland	61392-0601	Antianxiety
BUSPAR <> MJ5	Tab, White, Ovoid-Rectangular, Scored	Buspirone HCl 5 mg	Buspar by Bristol Myers Squibb	00087-0818	Antianxiety
BUSPARBL	Tab, White, Pillow, Buspar/BL Bristol Logo	Buspirone 10 mg	by Bristol	Canadian	Antianxiety
BUSPIRONEPMS10MG	Cap, White, Buspirone/pms/10 mg	Buspirone 10 mg	by Pharmascience	Canadian	Antianxiety
BUTEXFORTE <> 070	Cap, White, Opaque	Acetaminophen 650 mg, Butalbital 50 mg	Butex Forte by Alphapharm	57315-0013	Analgesic
BUTIBEL <> 37046	Tab, Red, Round, Butibel <> 37 over 046	Belladonna Extract 15 mg, Butabarbital Sodium 15 mg	Butibel by Wallace	00037-0046	Gastrointestinal; C IV
BUTISOLSODIUM <> 37112	Tab, Lavender, Scored, Butisol Sodium <> 37 over 112	Butabarbital Sodium 15 mg	Butisol Sodium by Wallace	00037-0112	Sedative; C III
BUTISOLSODIUM <> 37113	Tab, Green, Scored, Butisol Sodium <> 37 over 113	Butabarbital Sodium 30 mg	Butisol Sodium by Wallace	00037-0113	Sedative; C III
BUTISOLSODIUM <> 37114	Tab, Orange, Scored, Butisol Sodium <> 37 over 114	Butabarbital Sodium 50 mg	Butisol Sodium by Wallace	00037-0114	Sedative; C III
BV	Tab, Round	Cyproterone Acetate 50 mg	Androcur by Berlex Canada	Canadian	Antiandrogen

ID FRONT <> BACK	DESCRIPTION FRONT <> BACK	INGREDIENT & STRENGTH	BRAND (OR EQUIV.) & FIRM	NDC#	CLASS; SCH.
BVF <> 0117	Tab, White, Oblong	Pentoxifylline 400 mg	Pentoxifylline ER by Pharmafab	62542-0725	Anticoagulent
BVF <> 117	Tab, White, Oblong	Pentoxifylline 400 mg	by Vangard Labs	00615-4523	Anticoagulent
BVF120	Cap, Lavender	Diltiazem 120 mg	by Crystaal	Canadian	Antihypertensive
BVF180	Cap, Blue-Green & White	Diltiazem 180 mg	by Crystaal	Canadian	Antihypertensive
BVF240	Cap, Bluish-Green & Lavender	Diltiazem 240 mg	by Crystaal	Canadian	Antihypertensive
BVF300	Cap, Lavender & White	Diltiazem 300 mg	by Crystaal	Canadian	Antihypertensive
BVF300	Cap, Ivory	Diltiazem HCl 300 mg	by Biovail	62660-0010	Antihypertensive
BVF360	Cap, Blue & Green	Diltiazem 360 mg	by Crystaal	Canadian	Antihypertensive
BX <> SEARLE	Tab, Blue, Round	Norethindrone, Ethinyl Estradiol	Synphasic 28 day by Pharmacia	Canadian DIN# 02187116	Oral Contraceptive
BX <> SEARLE	Tab, Blue, Round	Norethindrone, Ethinyl Estradiol	Synphasic 21 day by Pharmacia	Canadian DIN# 02187108	Oral Contraceptive
BX <> SEARLE	Tab, White, Round	Norethindrone, Ethinyl Estradiol	Synphasic 28 day by Pharmacia	Canadian DIN# 02187116	Oral Contraceptive
BX <> SEARLE	Tab, White, Round	Norethindrone, Ethinyl Estradiol	Synphasic 21 day by Pharmacia	Canadian DIN# 02187108	Oral Contraceptive
BX <> SEARLE	Tab, Blue, Round	Norethindrone, Ethinyl Estradiol 0.5, 35	Brevicon .5/35 21 day by Pharmacia	Canadian DIN# 02187068	Oral Contraceptive
BX <> SEARLE	Tab, Blue, Round	Norethindrone, Ethinyl Estradiol 0.5/35	Brevicon .5/35 28 day by Pharmacia	Canadian DIN# 02187094	Oral Contraceptive
BX <> SEARLE	Tab, White, Round	Norethindrone, Ethinyl Estradiol 1/35	Select 1/35 21 day by Pharmacia	Canadian DIN# 02197502	Oral Contraceptive
BX <> SEARLE	Tab, White, Round	Norethindrone, Ethinyl Estradiol 1/35	Brevicon 1/35 28 day by Pharmacia	Canadian DIN# 02189062	Oral Contraceptive
BX <> SEARLE	Tab, White, Round	Norethindrone, Ethinyl Estradiol 1/35	Select 1/35 28 day by Pharmacia	Canadian DIN# 02199297	Oral Contraceptive
BX <> SEARLE	Tab, White, Round	Norethindrone, Ethinyl Estradiol 1/35	Brevicon 1/35 21 day by Pharmacia	Canadian DIN# 02189054	Oral Contraceptive
C	Tab, White, Round	Atenolol 25 mg	Tenomin by IPR		Antihypertensive
C	Tab, White, Oval, Film, C in Black Ink	Phenylpropanolamine HCl 75 mg	Acutrim Complete by Physicians Total Care	54868-4107	Decongestant; Appetite Suppressant
C	Tab, White, Oblong, Scored, Caplet	Pseudoephedrine HCl 60 mg, Guaifenesin 400 mg	Congestac by B F Ascher	00225-0580	Cold Remedy
C	Tab, White, Round, C Inside Flask <> Clock Design	Quinidine Gluconate 324 mg	Quinaglute Duratabs by RX PAK	65084-0127	Antiarrhythmic
C	Tab, White, Round	Quinidine Gluconate 324 mg	Quinaglute by Rightpac	65240-0727	Antiarrhythmic
C	Tab, ER, C in A Flask Embossed <> Clock-Like Design	Quinidine Gluconate 324 mg	Quinaglute by Caremark	00339-5327	Antiarrhythmic
C	Tab, ER, C Inside Flask Design <> Clock Like Design	Quinidine Gluconate 324 mg	by Med Pro	53978-0739	Antiarrhythmic
C	Tab, ER, C in A Flask <> Clock Like Design	Quinidine Gluconate 324 mg	Quinaglute Dura by CVS	51316-0024	Antiarrhythmic
C	Tab, White, ER, C in Flask <> Clock Design, w/Bone Specks, Imprint 4 Triangles in Square Around 2 Clocks	Quinidine Gluconate 324 mg	Quinaglute Dura by Amerisource	62584-0101	Antiarrhythmic
C	Tab, ER, C in Flask Design <> Clock Design	Quinidine Gluconate 324 mg	Quinaglute Dura by Nat Pharmpak Serv	55154-0303	Antiarrhythmic
C	Tab, White, Round, C in Flask Design <> Clock Design	Quinidine Gluconate 324 mg	Quinaglute Dura by Berlex	50419-0101	Antiarrhythmic
C <> 200	Tab, Pink, Round	Amiodarone HCl 200 mg	Cordorone by Wyeth Pharms	52903-4188	Antiarrhythmic

ID FRONT ⟷ BACK	DESCRIPTION FRONT ⟷ BACK	INGREDIENT & STRENGTH	BRAND (OR EQUIV.) & FIRM	NDC#	CLASS; SCH.
C ⟷ 317	Tab, Mottled White, Oblong	Guaifenesin 300 mg, Phenylpropanolamine HCl 20 mg	Miraphen PE by Martec		Cold Remedy
C ⟷ 355	Tab, Green, Oblong	Guaifenesin 600 mg; Dextromethorphan Hydrobromide 30 mg	by Caraco Pharm	57664-0355	Cold Remedy
C ⟷ 51	Tab	Atenolol 50 mg, Chlorthalidone 25 mg	by IPR	54921-0115	Antihypertensive; Diuretic
C ⟷ 71	Tab	Atenolol 100 mg, Chlorthalidone 25 mg	by IPR	54921-0117	Antihypertensive; Diuretic
C ⟷ 8648	Tab, Layered	Phendimetrazine Tartrate 35 mg	Bontril PDM by Carnrick	00086-0048	Anorexiant; C III
C ⟷ 8650	Cap, Opaque & Purple	Acetaminophen 325 mg, Butalbital 50 mg	Phrenilin by Quality Care	60346-0915	Analgesic
C ⟷ 8650	Tab	Acetaminophen 325 mg, Butalbital 50 mg	Phrenilin by Carnrick	00086-0050	Analgesic
C ⟷ 8650	Cap, Opaque & Purple	Acetaminophen 650 mg, Butalbital 50 mg	Phrenilin Forte by American Pharm	58605-0514	Analgesic
C ⟷ 8650	Tab, Purple, Oblong, Scored	Acetaminophen 325 mg; Butalbital 50 mg	Phrenilin by Thrift Services	59198-0364	Analgesic
C ⟷ 8656	Tab, Purple, Round, Scored	Acetaminophen 325 mg, Butalbital 50 mg	Phrenilin by Able		Analgesic
C ⟷ 8656	Cap	Acetaminophen 650 mg, Butalbital 50 mg	Phrenilin Forte by Carnrick	00086-0056	Analgesic
C ⟷ 8656	Cap, Purple	Butalbital 50 mg; Acetaminophen 650 mg	Phrenilin Forte by Thrift Services	59198-0365	Analgesic
C ⟷ 8657	Cap	Acetaminophen 500 mg, Hydrocodone Bitartrate 5 mg	Hydrocet by Carnrick	00086-0057	Analgesic; C III
C ⟷ 8662	Tab, Pink, Oblong, Scored	Metaxalone 400 mg	Skelaxin by Thrift Services	59198-0367	Muscle Relaxant
C ⟷ 8662	Tab, Pink, Scored	Metaxalone 400 mg	Skelaxin by HJ Harkins	52959-0410	Muscle Relaxant
C ⟷ 8662	Tab, Pink, Oblong, Scored	Metaxalone 400 mg	Skelaxin by Rx Pac	65084-0167	Muscle Relaxant
C ⟷ 8662	Tab, Lavender, C with Dot on Top Tip, ⟷ 86 Over 62	Metaxalone 400 mg	Skelaxin by Carnrick	00086-0062	Muscle Relaxant
C ⟷ 8662	Tab	Metaxalone 400 mg	Skelaxin by Drug Distr	52985-0226	Muscle Relaxant
C ⟷ 8662	Tab, Pale Rose	Metaxalone 400 mg	Skelaxin by Allscripts	54569-0855	Muscle Relaxant
C ⟷ 8662	Tab	Metaxalone 400 mg	Skelaxin by CVS	51316-0231	Muscle Relaxant
C ⟷ 8662	Tab	Metaxalone 400 mg	Skelaxin by Direct Dispensing	57866-4637	Muscle Relaxant
C ⟷ 8662	Tab, Pale Rose	Metaxalone 400 mg	Skelaxin by Amerisource	62584-0033	Muscle Relaxant
C ⟷ 8662	Tab, Pale Rose	Metaxalone 400 mg	Skelaxin by Quality Care	60346-0057	Muscle Relaxant
C ⟷ 8673	Tab, White with Blue Specks	Guaifenesin 400 mg, Phenylpropanolamine HCl 75 mg	Exgest LA by Carnrick	00086-0063	Cold Remedy
C ⟷ 8673	Tab, White, Oval, Scored	Phenylpropanolamine HCl 75 mg, Guaifenesin 400 mg	Exgest by Eckerd	19458-0832	Cold Remedy
C ⟷ 8674	Tab	Atropine 0.025 mg, Difenoxin HCl 1 mg	Motofen by Physicians Total Care	54868-3510	Antidiarrheal; C IV
C ⟷ 8674	Tab, White, Scored	Difenoxin HCl 1 mg; Atropine Sulfate 0.025 mg	Motofen by West Ward Pharm	00143-9031	Antidiarrheal; C IV
C ⟷ AMEN	Tab	Medroxyprogesterone Acetate 10 mg	Amen by Eckerd Drug	19458-0831	Progestin
C ⟷ CLOCK	Tab, White, Round	Quinidine Gluconate SR 324 mg	Quinaglute Duratabs by RX PAK	65084-0132	Antiarrhythmic
C ⟷ CYCRIN	Tab, Peach, Oval, Scored	Medroxyprogesterone Acetate 10 mg	by Southwood Pharms	58016-0926	Progestin
C ⟷ CYCRIN	Tab, Purple, Oval, Scored	Medroxyprogesterone Acetate 5 mg	by Kaiser Fdn Health	62224-4334	Progestin
C ⟷ SCORED	Tab	Estrogens, Conjugated 0.625 mg, Medroxyprogesterone Acetate 2.5 mg	Prempro by Pharm Utilization	60491-0904	Hormone
C1	Tab, Coated	Bendroflumethiazide 4 mg, Rauwolfia Serpentina 50 mg	by Rugby	00536-4502	Diuretic; Antihypertensive
C1	Cap, Pink	Choline Magnesium Trisalicylate 1000 mg	Trilisate by Amide	51285-0904	NSAID
C1	Tab, Blue, Round	Rauwolfia Serpentina 50 mg, Bendroflumethiazide 100 mg	Rauzide by Econlab		Antihypertensive
C1	Tab, Film Coated	Salicylate 1000 mg	by Rugby	00536-3470	NSAID
C1	Tab, Pink, Cap-Shaped, Film Coated	Salicylate 1000 mg	by Amide	52152-0086	NSAID
C10	Cap, Black & Green	Chlordiazepoxide 10 mg	Librium by Geneva		Antianxiety; C IV
C1000J	Tab, White, C 1000/J	Sulfadiazine 820 mg, Trimethoprim 180 mg	Coptin by Jouveinal	Canadian	Antibiotic
C100G	Tab, White, Oval, C 100/G	Captopril 100 mg	by Genpharm	Canadian	Antihypertensive
C103	Tab, Blue, Round, Coated, C/103	Salsalate 500 mg	by Duramed	51285-0296	NSAID
C105	Tab, Blue, Cap-Shaped, Coated, C/105	Salsalate 750 mg	by Duramed	51285-0297	NSAID
C11 ⟷ M	Tab, Green, Round, Scored	Clozapine 100 mg	by UDL	51079-0922	Antipsychotic
C110	Tab, Blue, Round, Scored	Clonazepam 1 mg	Ceberclon by Cebert	64019-0110	Anticonvulsant; C IV
C110	Tab, Blue, Round, Scored	Clonazepam 1 mg	Ceberclon by EON Labs Mfg	00185-2110	Anticonvulsant; C IV
C111	Cap, Yellow	Clofibrate 500 mg	Atromid-S by Rosemont		Antihyperlipidemic
C122	Cap, Yellow, Gelatin, C-122	Amantadine HCl 100 mg	by UDL	51079-0481	Antiviral
C122	Cap, Gelatin, Coated, C-122	Amantadine HCl 100 mg	by Rosemont	00832-1015	Antiviral
C122	Cap, Gelatin	Amantadine HCl 100 mg	by United Res	00677-1128	Antiviral

ID FRONT <> BACK	DESCRIPTION FRONT <> BACK	INGREDIENT & STRENGTH	BRAND (OR EQUIV.) & FIRM	NDC#	CLASS; SCH.
C122	Cap, Gelatin, C-122	Amantadine HCl 100 mg	by Rugby	00536-3043	Antiviral
C122	Cap, Yellow, Gelatin Coated, C-122	Amantadine HCl 100 mg	by Duramed	51285-0839	Antiviral
C122	Cap, C-122	Amantadine HCl 100 mg	by Allscripts	54569-0084	Antiviral
C122	Cap, Gelatin	Amantadine HCl 100 mg	by HJ Harkins Co	52959-0007	Antiviral
C122	Cap, Gelatin, C-122	Amantadine HCl 100 mg	by Banner Pharmacaps	10888-3185	Antiviral
C122	Cap, Yellow, Gelatin	Amantadine HCl 100 mg	by Dixon Shane	17236-0849	Antiviral
C122	Cap, Yellow, C-122	Amantadine HCl 100 mg	by Apotheca	12634-0536	Antiviral
C122	Cap, C-122	Amantadine HCl 100 mg	by Direct Dispensing	57866-3090	Antiviral
C122	Cap, Yellow, Gelatin, C-122	Amantadine HCl 100 mg	Symmetrel by Martec	52555-0675	Antiviral
C125SYC	Tab, White, Oblong, C 12.5/Syc	Captopril 12.5 mg	by Altimed	Canadian DIN# 00851639	Antihypertensive
C13 <> M	Tab, Yellow, Round, Scored, C over 13 <> M	Clonazepam 0.5 mg	Klonopin by UDL	51079-0881	Anticonvulsant; C IV
C133	Cap, Yellow, Soft Gelatin, C-133	Valproic Acid 250 mg	Depakene	51079-0298	Anticonvulsant
C133	Cap, Gelatin	Valproic Acid 250 mg	by Banner	00832-1007	Anticonvulsant
C133	Cap, Yellow	Valproic Acid 250 mg	Depakene by Rosemont		Anticonvulsant
C133	Cap, Yellow, Gelatin, C-133	Valproic Acid 250 mg	Depakene by Martec	52555-0688	Anticonvulsant
C135	Tab, White, Oval	Doxylamine Succinate 25 mg	by Perrigo	00113-0403	Sleep Aid
C14 <> M	Tab, Light Green, Round, Scored, C over 14 <> M	Clonazepam 1 mg	Klonopin by UDL	51079-0882	Anticonvulsant; C IV
C15 <> M	Tab, White, Round, Scored, C over 15 <> M	Clonazepam 2 mg	Klonopin by UDL	51079-0883	Anticonvulsant; C IV
C177	Tab, Blue, Round, C-177	Bromatapp E.R.	Dimetapp by Copley		Cold Remedy
C177	Tab, Blue, Round	Phenylpropanolamine 75 mg, Brompheniramine 12 mg	by Perrigo	00113-0451	Cold Remedy
C1M	Tab, M to the Right of the Score and C1 to the Left of the Score	Captopril 12.5 mg	by Heartland	61392-0604	Antihypertensive
C200	Tab, Pink, Round, C/200	Amiodarone HCl 200 mg	Cordarone by Wyeth-Ayerst	Canadian	Antiarrhythmic
C200 <> WYETH4188	Tab	Amiodarone HCl 200 mg	Cordarone by Amerisource	62584-0345	Antiarrhythmic
C200 <> WYETH4188	Tab, Pink, Round, Convex, Scored, Raised C and Marked 200 <> Wyeth 4188	Amiodarone HCl 200 mg	Cordarone by Apothecon	59772-0363	Antiarrhythmic
C200 <> WYETH4188	Tab, C/200 <> Wyeth/4188	Amiodarone HCl 200 mg	Cordarone by Wyeth Labs	00008-4188	Antiarrhythmic
C200 <> WYETH4188	Tab, C 200 <> Wyeth/4188	Amiodarone HCl 200 mg	Cordarone by Caremark	00339-6082	Antiarrhythmic
C200 <> WYETH4188	Tab	Amiodarone HCl 200 mg	Cordarone by Nat Pharmpak Serv	55154-4202	Antiarrhythmic
C200 <> WYETH4188	Tab	Amiodarone HCl 200 mg	by Med Pro	53978-2092	Antiarrhythmic
C21	Tab, White, Oval, with Pink Specks	Hydrocodone Bitartrate 5 mg, Aspirin 500 mg	Azdone by Schwarz Pharma		Analgesic; C III
C229	Tab, Green, ROUnd	Dexbrompheniramine 6 mg, Pseudoephedrine 120 mg	by Perrigo		Cold Remedy
C229	Tab, Blue, Round	Pseudoephedrine 120 mg, Dexbrompheniramine 6 mg	Drixoral by Granutec		Cold Remedy
C25	Tab, White, Square	Captopril 25 mg	by Genpharm	Canadian	Antihypertensive
C25	Cap, Green & White	Chlordiazepoxide 25 mg	Librium by Geneva		Antianxiety; C IV
C25SYC	Tab, White, Square, C 25/Syc	Captopril 25 mg	by Altimed	Canadian DIN# 00851833	Antihypertensive
C27	Cap, Clear & Red, C-27	Docusate Sodium 100 mg	Colace by Chase		Laxative
C27	Cap, Orange & Red	Docusate Sodium 100 mg	Colace by Chase		Laxative
C275 <> PF	Tab, Bone	Quinidine Polygalacturonate 275 mg	Cardioquin by Purdue Frederick	00034-5470	Antiarrhythmic
C275PF	Tab, White, Round, C/275/PF	Quinidine Polygalacturonate 275 mg	Cardioquim by Purdue Frederick	Canadian	Antiarrhythmic
C29	Cap, Clear & Orange, C-29	Docusate Sodium 250 mg	Colace by Chase		Laxative
C29	Cap, Red	Docusate Sodium 250 mg	by Chase		Laxative
C29	Cap, Orange & Red	Docusate Sodium 250 mg	Colace by Chase		Laxative
C2C	Cap	Digoxin 0.2 mg	Lanoxicaps by Catalytica	63552-0274	Cardiac Agent
C2C	Cap, Green	Digoxin 0.2 mg	Lanoxicaps by Glaxo (CA)	53873-0274	Cardiac Agent
C2C	Cap, Green	Digoxin 0.2 mg	Lanoxicaps by Glaxo	00173-0274	Cardiac Agent
C2C <> C2C	Cap, Clear & Light Green	Digoxin 0.2 mg	Lanoxicaps by RP Scherer	11014-0749	Cardiac Agent
C31	Tab, Orange, Round	Clonazepam 0.5 mg	by ICN	Canadian	Anticonvulsant
C3148	Cap, Yellow	Clofibrate 500 mg	Atromid S by Chase		Antihyperlipidemic

ID FRONT <> BACK	DESCRIPTION FRONT <> BACK	INGREDIENT & STRENGTH	BRAND (OR EQUIV.) & FIRM	NDC#	CLASS; SCH.
C32	Tab, Green, Round	Clonazepam 1 mg	by ICN	Canadian	Anticonvulsant
C3227	Cap, White, C-3227	Nifedipine 10 mg	Procardia by Chase		Antihypertensive
C33	Tab, White, Round	Clonazepam 2 mg	by ICN	Canadian	Anticonvulsant
C33 <> LL	Tab	Leucovorin Calcium 5 mg	by Immunex	58406-0624	Antineoplastic
C34 <> LL	Tab	Leucovorin Calcium 16.2 mg	by Immunex	58406-0626	Antineoplastic
C3453	Cap, White, C-3453	Nifedipine 20 mg	Procardia by Chase		Antihypertensive
C3543	Cap, White, C-3543	Nifedipine 20 mg	Procardia by Chase		Antihypertensive
C360LL	Tab, Orange, Oblong, C/360-LL	Calcium, Vitamin D	Caltrate Jr w/D by Lederle		Vitamin/Mineral
C39	Cap, Red	Docusate Sodium 100 mg, Casanthranol 30 mg	Peri-Colace by Chase		Laxative
C40LL	Tab, Brown, Oblong, C/40 LL	Calcium 600 mg, Vitamin D	Caltrate 600 w/D by Lederle		Vitamin/Mineral
C42	Tab, Powder Blue, Round, C/42	Colnidine HCl 0.1 mg	by Lederle		Antihypertensive
C428	Tab, White	Isosorbide Dinitrate 20 mg	Coradur by Glaxo	Canadian	Antianginal
C45	Tab, White, Round	Atenolol 50 mg	Tenormin by IPR		Antihypertensive
C45LL	Tab, Red, Oblong, C/45 LL	Calcium 600 mg, Iron	Caltrate 600 w/Fe by Lederle		Vitamin/Mineral
C5	Cap, Green & Yellow	Chlordiazepoxide 5 mg	Librium by Geneva		Antianxiety; C IV
C500J	Tab, White, C 500/J	Sulfadiazine 410 mg, Trimethoprim 90 mg	Coptin by Jouveinal	Canadian	Antibiotic
C50G	Tab, White, Oval, C 50/G	Captopril 50 mg	by Genpharm	Canadian	Antihypertensive
C54	Cap, Blue & Pink	Cefaclor 250 mg	Ceclor by Lederle		Antibiotic
C58	Cap, Blue & Lavender	Cefaclor 500 mg	Ceclor by Lederle		Antibiotic
C600LL	Tab, White, Oblong, C/600-LL	Calcium 600 mg	Caltrate 600 by Lederle		Vitamin/Mineral
C62 <> LEDERLE	Cap, Light Green	Cephradine Monohydrate 500 mg	by Quality Care	60346-0041	Antibiotic
C66 <> SKF	Tab, Yellow-Green, Coated	Prochlorperazine Maleate 8.1 mg	Compazine by Allscripts	54569-0352	Antiemetic
C66 <> SKF	Tab, Coated	Prochlorperazine Maleate 8.1 mg	Compazine by Quality Care	60346-0271	Antiemetic
C67 <> SKF	Tab, Yellow-Green, Coated	Prochlorperazine Maleate 16.2 mg	Compazine by Quality Care	60346-0860	Antiemetic
C6BVP	Tab, Off-White, Round, C6 B/VP	Cefadroxil 100 mg	Cef-Tab by Bristol Myers		Antibiotic
C7 <> M	Tab, Peach, Round, Scored, C/7 <> M	Clozapine 25 mg	by UDL	51079-0921	Antipsychotic
C86120	Cap, Red, with Pink Band, C/86120	Acetaminophen 325 mg, Chloralantipyrine 100 mg, Isometheptene Mucate 65 mg	Midrin by Allscripts	54569-0343	Analgesic
C86120	Cap, Pink Band	Acetaminophen 325 mg, Dichloralantipyrine 100 mg, Isometheptene Mucate 65 mg	Midrin by Carnrick	00086-0120	Cold Remedy
C86120	Cap, Purple Band	Acetaminophen 325 mg, Dichloralantipyrine 100 mg, Isometheptene Mucate 65 mg	Midrin by Pharmedix	53002-0545	Cold Remedy
C86204	Tab, Pink, Round	Phenindamine 24 mg, Chlorpheniramine 4 mg, Phenylpropanolamine 50 mg	Nolamine by Carnrick		Cold Remedy
C8647	Cap, Clear Yellow	Phendimetrazine Tartrate 105 mg	Bontril by Carnrick	00086-0047	Anorexiant; C III
C8647	Cap	Phendimetrazine Tartrate 105 mg	Bontril by Quality Care	62682-1034	Anorexiant; C III
C8647	Cap	Phendimetrazine Tartrate 105 mg	Bontril Sr by D M Graham	00756-0250	Anorexiant; C III
C8652	Tab, White, Oblong	Phenindamine Tartrate 25 mg	Nolahist by Carnrick		Antihistamine
C8655	Cap, Amethyst & White	Butalbital 50 mg, Acetaminophen 650 mg, Codeine 30 mg	Phrenilin #3 by Carnrick		Analgesic; C III
C8662	Tab	Metaxalone 400 mg	Skelaxin by Pharmedix	53002-0459	Muscle Relaxant
C8666	Tab, Peach, Round	Acetaminophen 650 mg, Chlorpheniramine 4 mg, Phenylpropanolamine 25 mg	Sinulin by Carnrick		Cold Remedy
C8671	Tab, White, Round	Salsalate 500 mg	Salflex by Carnrick		NSAID
C8672	Tab, White, Oval	Salsalate 750 mg	Salflex by Carnrick		NSAID
C8674	Tab, White, Pentagonal	Difenoxin HCl 1 mg, Atropine Sulfate 0.25 mg	Motofen by Carnrick		Antidiarrheal; C IV
C90	Tab, White, Round	Atenolol 100 mg	Tenormin by IPR		Antihypertensive
C9BZYLOPRIM	Tab, Peach, Round, C9B/Zyloprim	Allopurinol 300 mg	by Glaxo	Canadian	Antigout
CAFERGOT	Tab, Mottled Yellowish White, Round	Caffeine 100 mg, Ergotamine Tartrate 1 mg	by Novartis	Canadian DIN# 00176095	Analgesic
CAFERGOT	Tab, Beige, Round, Sugar Coated	Ergotamine Tartrate 1 mg, Caffeine 100 mg	Cafergot by Novartis	00078-0349	Antimigraine
CAFFEINE <> GPI30	Cap, Pink & White	Caffeine 200 mg	Keep Alert by Caremark	00339-5410	Stimulant
CAFFEINEGPI30	Cap, Pink & White, Bullet Shaped, Caffeine/GPI 30	Caffeine 200 mg	Keep Alert by Reese	10956-0661	Stimulant
CALAN <> 40	Tab, Pink, Round, Coated	Verapamil HCl 40 mg	Calan by GD Searle	00025-1771	Antihypertensive
CALAN <> 80	Tab, Film Coated	Verapamil HCl 80 mg	Calan by Nat Pharmpak Serv	55154-3603	Antihypertensive
CALAN <> 80	Tab, Peach, Oval, Scored	Verapamil HCl 80 mg	Calan by Rightpak	65240-0619	Antihypertensive
CALAN <> 80	Tab, Peach, Oval, Scored	Verapamil HCl 80 mg	Calan by Med-Pro	53978-3398	Antihypertensive

ID FRONT <> BACK	DESCRIPTION FRONT <> BACK	INGREDIENT & STRENGTH	BRAND (OR EQUIV.) & FIRM	NDC#	CLASS; SCH.
CALAN <> 80	Tab, Peach, Oval, Film Coated	Verapamil HCl 80 mg	Calan by GD Searle	00025-1851	Antihypertensive
CALAN <> 80	Tab, Film Coated	Verapamil HCl 80 mg	Calan by Amerisource	62584-0852	Antihypertensive
CALAN <> 80	Tab, Film Coated, Debossed	Verapamil HCl 80 mg	Calan by Thrift Drug	59198-0015	Antihypertensive
CALAN <> SR120	Tab, Light Violet, Film Coated	Verapamil HCl 120 mg	Calan Sr by Quality Care	60346-0298	Antihypertensive
CALAN <> SR120	Tab, Light Violet, Oval	Verapamil HCl 120 mg	Calan Sr by GD Searle	00025-1901	Antihypertensive
CALAN <> SR180	Cap, Light Pink, Oval, Film Coated	Calan SR 180 mg	by Allscripts	54569-8555	Vitamin
CALAN <> SR180	Tab, Light Pink, Oval	Verapamil HCl 180 mg	Calan Sr by GD Searle	00025-1911	Antihypertensive
CALAN <> SR180	Tab	Verapamil HCl 180 mg	Calan Sr by Nat Pharmpak Serv	55154-3616	Antihypertensive
CALAN <> SR180	Tab	Verapamil HCl 180 mg	Calan Sr by Allscripts	54569-3802	Antihypertensive
CALAN <> SR240	Tab, Green, Oblong, Film Coated, Scored	Verapamil HCl 240 mg	Calan SR by Rx Pac	65084-0141	Antihypertensive
CALAN <> SR240	Tab, Film Coated, SR/240	Verapamil HCl 240 mg	Calan Sr by GD Searle	00014-1891	Antihypertensive
CALAN <> SR240	Tab, Green, Oblong, Scored, Film Coated	Verapamil HCl 240 mg	Calan SR Sustained Release by Teva	00480-0788	Antihypertensive
CALAN <> SR240	Tab, Light Green, Film Coated, Debossed, <> SR 240	Verapamil HCl 240 mg	Calan Sr by Nat Pharmpak Serv	55154-3615	Antihypertensive
CALAN <> SR240	Tab, Film Coated, SR/240	Verapamil HCl 240 mg	by Med Pro	53978-0588	Antihypertensive
CALAN <> SR240	Tab, Light Green, Cap-Shaped	Verapamil 240 mg	Calan Sr by GD Searle	00025-1891	Antihypertensive
CALAN120	Tab, Film Coated	Verapamil HCl 120 mg	Calan by Amerisource	62584-0861	Antihypertensive
CALAN120	Tab, Brown, Oval, Film Coated	Verapamil HCl 120 mg	Calan by GD Searle	00025-1861	Antihypertensive
CAPOTEN <> 125	Tab, Mottled White, Round, Capoten <> 12.5	Captopril 12.5 mg	Capoten by ER Squibb	00003-0450	Antihypertensive
CAPOTEN <> 125	Tab, Capoten <> 12.5	Captopril 12.5 mg	Capoten by Nat Pharmpak Serv	55154-3706	Antihypertensive
CAPOTEN <> 25	Tab, Mottled	Captopril 25 mg	Capoten by ER Squibb	00003-0452	Antihypertensive
CAPOTEN <> 25	Tab	Captopril 25 mg	Capoten by Nat Pharmpak Serv	55154-3707	Antihypertensive
CAPOTEN <> 50	Tab	Captopril 50 mg	Capoten by Nat Pharmpak Serv	55154-3708	Antihypertensive
CAPOTEN <> 50	Tab, Mottled	Captopril 50 mg	Capoten by ER Squibb	00003-0482	Antihypertensive
CAPOTEN 100	Tab, White, Oval	Captopril 100 mg	by Squibb	Canadian	Antihypertensive
CAPOTEN 25	Tab, White, Square	Captopril 25 mg	by Squibb	Canadian	Antihypertensive
CAPOTEN 50	Tab, White, Oval	Captopril 50 mg	by Squibb	Canadian	Antihypertensive
CAPOTEN100	Tab, Mottled, Oval	Captopril 100 mg	Capoten by ER Squibb	00003-0485	Antihypertensive
CAPOTEN125	Tab, Capoten 12.5	Captopril 12.5 mg	Capoten by Allscripts	54569-0522	Antihypertensive
CAPOTEN25	Tab	Captopril 25 mg	Capoten by Allscripts	54569-0523	Antihypertensive
CAPOTEN25	Tab	Captopril 25 mg	by Med Pro	53978-0236	Antihypertensive
CAPOZIDE2515	Tab, White to Off-White, Orange Specks, Capozide 25/15	Captopril 25 mg, Hydrochlorothiazide 15 mg	Capozide 25/15 by ER Squibb	00003-0338	Antihypertensive; Diuretic
CAPOZIDE2525	Tab, Mottled, Capozide over 25/25	Captopril 25 mg, Hydrochlorothiazide 25 mg	Capozide 25/25 by ER Squibb	00003-0349	Antihypertensive; Diuretic
CAPOZIDE5015	Tab, White to Off-White, Mottled Orange, Capozide over 50/15	Captopril 50 mg, Hydrochlorothiazide 15 mg	Capozide 50/15 by ER Squibb	00003-0384	Antihypertensive; Diuretic
CAPOZIDE5025	Tab, Mottled, Capozide over 50/25	Captopril 50 mg, Hydrochlorothiazide 25 mg	Capozide 50/25 by ER Squibb	00003-0390	Antihypertensive; Diuretic
CARACO <> 105105	Tab, Film Coated, Caraco <> 105/105	Salsalate 750 mg	by Allscripts	54569-1712	NSAID
CARACO <> 152	Tab	Guaifenesin 600 mg	by Caraco	57664-0152	Expectorant
CARACO <> 152	Tab, Green, Oblong, Scored	Guaifenesin LA 600 mg	by Med Pro	53978-3361	Expectorant
CARACO <> 157	Tab	Guaifenesin 400 mg, Phenylpropanolamine HCl 75 mg	Miraphen LA by Caraco	57664-0157	Cold Remedy
CARACO <> 872	Cap, RP Scherer Logo 872	Nifedipine 10 mg	by Quality Care	60346-0803	Antihypertensive
CARACO166	Tab, White, Oblong	Metoprolol Tartrate 50 mg	Lopressor by Caraco		Antihypertensive
CARACO167	Tab, White, Oblong	Metoprolol Tartrate 100 mg	Lopressor by Caraco		Antihypertensive
CARACO199	Tab, White, Round	Yohimbine HCl 5.4 mg	Yocon by Caraco		Impotence Agent
CARACO872	Cap	Nifedipine 10 mg	by Qualitest	00603-4759	Antihypertensive
CARACO872	Cap, Caraco/872	Nifedipine 10 mg	by RP Scherer	11014-0956	Antihypertensive
CARACO873	Cap	Nifedipine 20 mg	by Qualitest	00603-4760	Antihypertensive
CARACO873	Cap, Reddish Brown	Nifedipine 20 mg	by RP Scherer	11014-0966	Antihypertensive
CARAFATE <> 1712	Tab	Sucralfate 1 gm	Carafate by Heartland	61392-0606	Gastrointestinal
CARAFATE <> 1712	Tab	Sucralfate 1 gm	Carafate by Amerisource	62584-0712	Gastrointestinal

ID FRONT <> BACK	DESCRIPTION FRONT <> BACK	INGREDIENT & STRENGTH	BRAND (OR EQUIV.) & FIRM	NDC#	CLASS; SCH.
CARAFATE <> 1712	Tab, Light Pink, Carafate <> 17 Over 12	Sucralfate 1 gm	Carafate by Quality Care	60346-0922	Gastrointestinal
CARAFATE <> 1712	Tab	Sucralfate 1 gm	Carafate by Giant Food	11146-0041	Gastrointestinal
CARAFATE <> 1712	Tab	Sucralfate 1 gm	Carafate by Murfreesboro	51129-1166	Gastrointestinal
CARAFATE <> 1712	Tab, Pink, Oblong, Scored	Sucralfate 1 gm	Carafate by SKB	00007-4896	Gastrointestinal
CARAFATE <> 1712	Tab, Light Pink	Sucralfate 1 gm	Carafate by Hoechst Roussel	00088-1712	Gastrointestinal
CARAFATE <> 1712	Tab, Light Pink	Sucralfate 1 gm	Carafate by HJ Harkins Co	52959-0052	Gastrointestinal
CARAFATE <> 1712	Tab	Sucralfate 1 gm	Carafate by Allscripts	54569-0422	Gastrointestinal
CARAFATE <> 1712	Tab	Sucralfate 1 gm	by Med Pro	53978-3070	Gastrointestinal
CARAFATE <> 1712	Tab	Sucralfate 1 gm	Carafate by Nat Pharmpak Serv	55154-2207	Gastrointestinal
CARAFATE1712 <> 1MG	Tab	Sucralfate 1 gm	Carafate by Med Pro	53978-0305	Gastrointestinal
CARBEX	Tab, Coated	Selegiline HCl 5 mg	Carbex by Dupont Pharma	00056-0408	Antiparkinson
CARBEX	Tab, White, Oval	Selegiline HCl 5 mg	Carbex by Endo Labs	63481-0408	Antiparkinson
CARDENE <> ROCHE	Cap, Blue	Nicardipine HCl 30 mg	Cardene by ICN Dutch Holdings	64158-0437	Antihypertensive
CARDENE20 <> ROCHE	Cap, Blue Band	Nicardipine HCl 20 mg	Cardene by Repack Co of Amer	55306-2437	Antihypertensive
CARDENE20MG <> ROCHE	Cap, with Blue Band	Nicardipine HCl 20 mg	Cardene by Murfreesboro	51129-1125	Antihypertensive
CARDENE20MG <> ROCHE	Cap, with Brillant Blue Band	Nicardipine HCl 20 mg	Cardene by Hoffmann La Roche	00004-0183	Antihypertensive
CARDENE20MG <> ROCHE	Cap, Opaque & White, Hard Gel	Nicardipine HCl 20 mg	Cardene by Par	49884-0589	Antihypertensive
CARDENE20MG <> ROCHE	Cap	Nicardipine HCl 20 mg	Cardene by Syntex	18393-0437	Antihypertensive
CARDENE30MG <> ROCHE	Cap, with Brillant Blue Band	Nicardipine HCl 30 mg	Cardene by Hoffmann La Roche	00004-0184	Antihypertensive
CARDENE30MG <> ROCHE	Cap, Blue Band	Nicardipine HCl 30 mg	Cardene by Repack Co	55306-2438	Antihypertensive
CARDENE30MG <> ROCHE	Cap, with Brillant Blue Band	Nicardipine HCl 30 mg	Cardene by Murfreesboro	51129-1206	Antihypertensive
CARDENE30MG <> ROCHE	Cap, Gelatin Coated	Nicardipine HCl 30 mg	Cardene by Syntex	18393-0438	Antihypertensive
CARDENE30MG <> SYNTEX2438	Cap, Blue & Opaque	Nicardipine HCl 30 mg	Cardene by Par	49884-0579	Antihypertensive
CARDENESR30MG <> ROCHE	Cap	Nicardipine HCl 30 mg	Cardene SR by Hoffmann La Roche	00004-0180	Antihypertensive
CARDENESR30MG <> SYNTEX2440	Cap	Nicardipine HCl 30 mg	Cardene Sr by Physicians Total Care	54868-3817	Antihypertensive
CARDENESR45MG <> ROCHE	Cap	Nicardipine HCl 45 mg	Cardene SR by Hoffmann La Roche	00004-0181	Antihypertensive
CARDENESR60MG <> ROCHE	Cap	Nicardipine HCl 60 mg	Cardene SR by Hoffmann La Roche	00004-0182	Antihypertensive
CARDIZEM <> CARDIZEMSR60	Cap, Brown	Diltiazem HCl 60 mg	Cardizem SR by Eckerd Drug	19458-0905	Antihypertensive
CARDIZEM <> CARDIZEMSR90	Cap, Brown	Diltiazem HCl 90 mg	Cardizem SR by Eckerd Drug	19458-0906	Antihypertensive
CARDIZEM <> CARDIZEMSR90MG	Cap, Gold, Cardizem Logo <> Cardizem SR 90 mg	Diltiazem HCl 90 mg	Cardizem Sr by Elan	56125-0006	Antihypertensive
CARDIZEM240MG	Cap, Blue	Diltiazem HCl 240 mg	Cardizen CD by Elan Hold	60274-0300	Antihypertensive
CARDIZEM300MG	Cap, Blue & Light Gray, Cardizem 300 mg <> Hoechst Logo	Diltiazem HCl 300 mg	Cardizem CD by Hoechst Roussel	00088-1798	Antihypertensive
CARDIZEMCD <> 180MG	Tab, Blue, Oblong	Diltiazem HCl 180 mg	by Egis	48581-5112	Antihypertensive
CARDIZEMCD <> 300MG	Cap, Blue & Gray	Diltiazem 300 mg	Cardizem CD by Eckerd Drug	19458-0895	Antihypertensive

ID FRONT <> BACK	DESCRIPTION FRONT <> BACK	INGREDIENT & STRENGTH	BRAND (OR EQUIV.) & FIRM	NDC#	CLASS; SCH.
CARDIZEMCD120MG	Cap, Blue	Diltiazem HCl 120 mg	Cardizem CD by Elan	56125-0065	Antihypertensive
CARDIZEMCD120MG	Cap, Light Turquoise Blue, Cardizem CD/120 mg <> Hoechst Logo	Diltiazem HCl 120 mg	Cardizem CD by Hoechst Roussel	00088-1795	Antihypertensive
CARDIZEMCD120MG	Cap, MMD Logo	Diltiazem HCl 120 mg	Cardizem CD by Nat Pharmpak Serv	55154-2212	Antihypertensive
CARDIZEMCD12OMG	Cap, Blue	Diltiazem HCl 120 mg	Cardizem CD by Elan Hold	60274-0100	Antihypertensive
CARDIZEMCD180	Cap, Ex Release, MMD Logo	Diltiazem HCl 180 mg	Cardizem CD by Pharm Utilization	60491-0120	Antihypertensive
CARDIZEMCD180	Cap, Blue	Diltiazem HCl 180 mg	Cardizem CD by Rightpak	65240-0607	Antihypertensive
CARDIZEMCD180	Cap, Blue	Diltiazem HCl 180 mg	Cardizem CD by Rx Pac	65084-0114	Antihypertensive
CARDIZEMCD180	Cap, Blue	Diltiazem HCl 180 mg	Cardizem CD by Wal Mart	49035-0187	Antihypertensive
CARDIZEMCD180MG	Cap, Blue	Diltiazem HCl 180 mg	Cardizem CD by Eckerd Drug	19458-0899	Antihypertensive
CARDIZEMCD180MG	Cap, Blue, Cardizem CD 180 mg	Diltiazem HCl 180 mg	Cardizem CD by Elan Hold	60274-0200	Antihypertensive
CARDIZEMCD180MG	Cap, Ex Release, MMD Logo	Diltiazem HCl 180 mg	Cardizem CD by Amerisource	62584-0796	Antihypertensive
CARDIZEMCD180MG	Cap, Dark Blue & Light Blue, Cardizem CD/180 mg <> Hoechst Logo	Diltiazem HCl 180 mg	Cardizem CD by Hoechst Roussel	00088-1796	Antihypertensive
CARDIZEMCD180MG	Cap, Light Turquoise, MMD Logo	Diltiazem HCl 180 mg	Cardizem CD by Allscripts	54569-3803	Antihypertensive
CARDIZEMCD180MG	Cap, Dark Blue & Light Blue, MMD Logo	Diltiazem HCl 180 mg	Cardizem CD by Nat Pharmpak Serv	55154-2208	Antihypertensive
CARDIZEMCD240MG	Cap, Dark Blue, Cardizem CD/240 mg <> Hoechst Logo	Diltiazem HCl 240 mg	Cardizem CD by Hoechst Roussel	00088-1797	Antihypertensive
CARDIZEMCD240MG	Cap, MMD Logo	Diltiazem HCl 240 mg	Cardizem CD by Nat Pharmpak Serv	55154-2210	Antihypertensive
CARDIZEMCD240MG	Cap, MMD Logo	Diltiazem HCl 240 mg	Cardizem CD by Allscripts	54569-3804	Antihypertensive
CARDIZEMCD240MG	Cap, MMD Logo	Diltiazem HCl 240 mg	by Med Pro	53978-3062	Antihypertensive
CARDIZEMCD300MG	Cap, MMD Logo	Diltiazem HCl 300 mg	Cardizem CD by Nat Pharmpak Serv	55154-2211	Antihypertensive
CARDIZEMCD300MG	Cap, Cardizem CD/300 mg	Diltiazem HCl 300 mg	Cardizem CD by Murfreesboro	51129-9732	Antihypertensive
CARDIZEMSR120	Cap, Brown	Diltiazem HCl 120 mg	Cardizem SR by Egis	48581-5111	Antihypertensive
CARDIZEMSR120MG	Cap, Light Turquoise	Diltiazem 120 mg	by Hoechst Marion Roussel	Canadian	Antihypertensive
CARDIZEMSR120MG	Cap, Brown & Caramel	Diltiazem HCl 120 mg	Cardizem SR by Hoechst Marion Roussel	00088-1779	Antihypertensive
CARDIZEMSR180MG	Cap, Blue & Turquoise	Diltiazem 180 mg	by Hoechst Marion Roussel	Canadian	Antihypertensive
CARDIZEMSR240MG	Cap, Light Blue	Diltiazem 240 mg	by Hoechst Marion Roussel	Canadian	Antihypertensive
CARDIZEMSR300MG	Cap, Light Blue & Light Gray	Diltiazem 300 mg	by Hoechst Marion Roussel	Canadian	Antihypertensive
CARDIZEMSR60MG	Cap, Brown & Ivory	Diltiazem HCl 60 mg	Cardizem SR by Hoechst Marion Roussel	00088-1777	Antihypertensive
CARDIZEMSR60MG	Cap, Brown & Ivory	Diltiazem 60 mg	by Hoechst Marion Roussel	Canadian	Antihypertensive
CARDIZEMSR90MG	Cap, Brown & Gold	Diltiazem 90 mg	by Hoechst Marion Roussel	Canadian	Antihypertensive
CARDIZEMSR90MG	Cap, Brown & Gold	Diltiazem HCl 90 mg	Cardizem SR by Hoechst Marion Roussel	00088-1778	Antihypertensive
CARDIZEMSR90MG	Cap, Cardizem Logo	Diltiazem HCl 90 mg	Cardizem Sr by Allscripts	54569-2912	Antihypertensive
CARDIZEMSR90MG <> CARDIZEM	Cap, Gold, Cardizem SR 90 mg <> Cardizem Logo	Diltiazem HCl 90 mg	Cardizem Sr by Elan	56125-0006	Antihypertensive
CARDUA	Tab	Doxazosin Mesylate 8 mg	Cardura by Pharm Utilization	60491-0123	Antihypertensive
CARDURA	Tab, Yellow, Oblong, Scored	Doxazosin 2 mg	CarDura by H J Harkins Co	52959-0003	Antihypertensive
CARDURA	Tab, White, Round, Scored	Doxazosin Mesylate 1 mg	Cardura by Allscripts	54569-4864	Antihypertensive
CARDURA	Tab, Yellow, Round, Scored	Doxazosin Mesylate 2 mg	Cardura by Allscripts	54569-4865	Antihypertensive
CARDURA <> 1MG	Tab, White, Oblong, Cardura <> 1/mg	Doxazosin Mesylate 1 mg	Cardura by Roerig	00049-2750	Antihypertensive
CARDURA <> 4MG	Tab	Doxazosin Mesylate 4 mg	Cardura by Nat Pharmpak Serv	55154-3216	Antihypertensive
CARDURA <> 4MG	Tab, Orange, Oblong, Cardura <> 4/mg	Doxazosin Mesylate 4 mg	Cardura by Roerig	00049-2770	Antihypertensive
CARDURA1ASTRA	Tab, White, Round, Cardura 1/Astra	Doxazosin 1 mg	Cardura by Astra	Canadian	Antihypertensive
CARDURA1ASTRA	Tab, White, Diamond, Cardura 1/Astra	Doxazosin 4 mg	Cardura by Astra	Canadian	Antihypertensive
CARDURA2ASTRA	Tab, White, Oval, Cardura 2/Astra	Doxazosin 2 mg	Cardura by Astra	Canadian	Antihypertensive
CARDURA2MG	Tab	Doxazosin Mesylate 2 mg	by Med Pro	53978-3071	Antihypertensive
CARDURA4MG	Tab	Doxazosin Mesylate 4 mg	Cardura by Allscripts	54569-3250	Antihypertensive
CARNITORST	Tab, White	Levocarnitine 330 mg	by Sigma	Canadian	Carnitine Replem
CATAFLAM <> 50	Tab, Coated	Diclofenac Potassium 50 mg	Cataflam by PDRX	55289-0818	NSAID

ID FRONT <> BACK	DESCRIPTION FRONT <> BACK	INGREDIENT & STRENGTH	BRAND (OR EQUIV.) & FIRM	NDC#	CLASS; SCH.
CATAFLAM <> 50	Tab, Coated	Diclofenac Potassium 50 mg	Cataflam by Quality Care	60346-0975	NSAID
CATAFLAM <> 50	Tab, Coated	Diclofenac Potassium 50 mg	Cataflam by Direct Dispensing	57866-1182	NSAID
CATAFLAM <> 50	Tab, Brown, Round	Diclofenac Potassium 50 mg	Cataflam by HJ Harkins	52959-0344	NSAID
CATAFLAM <> 50	Tab, Light Brown, Round	Diclofenac Potassium 50 mg	Cataflam by Novartis	00028-0151	NSAID
CATAFLAM <> 50	Tab, Coated	Diclofenac Potassium 50 mg	Cataflam by DRX	55045-2225	NSAID
CATAFLAM <> 50	Tab, Coated	Diclofenac Potassium 50 mg	Cataflam by Allscripts	54569-3823	NSAID
CATAFLAM <> 50	Tab, Coated	Diclofenac Potassium 50 mg	Cataflam by Novartis	17088-0151	NSAID
CB300	Tab, Pale, Film Coated	Cimetidine 300 mg	by Penn	58437-0001	Gastrointestinal
CB400	Tab, Pale, Film Coated	Cimetidine 400 mg	by Penn	58437-0002	Gastrointestinal
CB400	Tab, Film Coated	Cimetidine 400 mg	by Allscripts	54569-3838	Gastrointestinal
CB800	Tab, Pale, Film Coated	Cimetidine 800 mg	by Penn	58437-0003	Gastrointestinal
CBF	Tab, Sugar Coated	Ascorbic Acid 120 mg, Beta-Carotene 4000 Units, Calcium 200 mg, Cyanocobalamin 8 mcg, Folic Acid 1 mg, Iodine 150 mcg, Iron 50 mg, Niacin 20 mg, Pyridoxine HCl 3 mg, Riboflavin 3 mg, Thiamine HCl 3 mg, Vitamin D 400 Units, Vitamin E 30 Units, Zinc 15 mg	Nestabs Cbf by Fielding	00421-1997	Vitamin
CBF	Tab, Sugar Coated	Ascorbic Acid 120 mg, Beta-Carotene 4000 Units, Calcium 200 mg, Cyanocobalamin 8 mcg, Folic Acid 1 mg, Iodine 150 mcg, Iron 50 mg, Niacin 20 mg, Pyridoxine HCl 3 mg, Riboflavin 3 mg, Thiamine HCl 3 mg, Vitamin D 400 Units, Vitamin E 30 Units, Zinc 15 mg	Nestabs Cbf by JB	51111-0004	Vitamin
CC	Tab, Gray & Green, Round, C/C	Chlorophyllin Copper Complex Sodium 14 mg	Chloresium by Rystan		Gastrointestinal
CC <> 0147	Cap, C-C in a Box	Phentermine HCl 30 mg	T Diet by Jones	52604-0010	Anorexiant; C IV
CC <> 105	Tab, Blue, Cap-Shaped, Film Coated, Scored	Salsalate 750 mg	by Allscripts	54569-1712	NSAID
CC <> 1875	Cap, CC <> 18.75	Phentermine HCl 18.75 mg	by Quality Care	60346-0102	Anorexiant; C IV
CC0147	Cap	Phentermine HCl 30 mg	by DRX	55045-1264	Anorexiant; C IV
CC0147	Cap	Phentermine HCl 30 mg	by DRX	55045-2231	Anorexiant; C IV
CC0147	Cap	Phentermine HCl 30 mg	by Quality Care	62682-7025	Anorexiant; C IV
CC0147	Cap, C-C/0147	Phentermine HCl 30 mg	by Qualitest	00603-5190	Anorexiant; C IV
CC0147	Cap, Black	Phentermine HCl	by Allscripts	54569-3248	Anorexiant; C IV
CC0147	Cap, C-C/0147 in a Box	Phentermine HCl 30 mg	Phnt 30 Phentride 30 by JMI Canton	00252-9151	Anorexiant; C IV
CC0147	Cap, C-C/0147 in a Box	Phentermine HCl 30 mg	Pty 30 Phentride 30 by JMI Canton	00252-9152	Anorexiant; C IV
CC0147	Cap, C-C/0147 in a Box	Phentermine HCl 30 mg	Phentride by Jones	52604-9151	Anorexiant; C IV
CC0147	Cap, C-C/0147 in a Box	Phentermine HCl 30 mg	Phentride by Jones	52604-9152	Anorexiant; C IV
CC0147	Cap, C-C/0147 in a Box	Phentermine HCl 30 mg	by Jones	52604-9153	Anorexiant; C IV
CC101	Tab, Yellow, Oval	Meclizine HCl 25 mg	Antivert by Camall		Antiemetic
CC102	Tab	Phentermine HCl 8 mg	by Zenith Goldline	00182-0204	Anorexiant; C IV
CC102	Tab	Phentermine HCl 8 mg	by Allscripts	54569-2753	Anorexiant; C IV
CC102	Tab	Phentermine HCl 8 mg	by DRX	55045-1688	Anorexiant; C IV
CC102	Tab, C-C/102, C-C is in a Box	Phentermine HCl 8 mg	Phentride Phntg by Jones	52604-9161	Anorexiant; C IV
CC102	Tab, Green, Round, Flat, Scored	Phentermine HCl 8 mg	by Physicians Total Care	54868-4067	Anorexiant; C IV
CC102	Tab, Green, Round, Flat, Scored	Phentermine HCl 8 mg	by Physicians Total Care	54868-4076	Anorexiant; C IV
CC102	Tab	Phentermine HCl 8 mg	by PDRX	55289-0803	Anorexiant; C IV
CC102	Tab	Phentermine HCl 8 mg	Raphtre by Macnary	55982-0003	Anorexiant; C IV
CC102	Tab	Phentermine HCl 8 mg	by Ems Disp	62792-0102	Anorexiant; C IV
CC102	Tab	Phentermine HCl 8 mg	by Quality Care	60346-0215	Anorexiant; C IV
CC105	Tab, White, Round, Double Scored	Phendimetrazine Tartrate 35 mg	by PDRX Pharms	55289-0300	Anorexiant; C III
CC105	Tab, Gray, Round, Double Scored	Phendimetrazine Tartrate 35 mg	by PDRX Pharms	55289-0285	Anorexiant; C III
CC105	Tab, Gray, Round	Phendimetrazine Tartrate 35 mg	Plegine by Camall		Anorexiant; C III
CC105	Tab, White, Round	Phendimetrazine Tartrate 35 mg	Plegine by Camall		Anorexiant; C III
CC105	Tab, Yellow, Round	Phendimetrazine Tartrate 35 mg	Plegine by Camall		Anorexiant; C III
CC105	Tab, Pink, Round	Phendimetrazine Tartrate 35 mg	Plegine by Camall		Anorexiant; C III
CC105	Tab, Pink, Round, Scored	Phendimetrazine Tartrate 35 mg	by Physicians Total Care	54868-1341	Anorexiant; C III
CC105	Tab, C-C in a Box 105	Phendimetrazine Tartrate 35 mg	by Jones	52604-9143	Anorexiant; C III

ID FRONT <> BACK	DESCRIPTION FRONT <> BACK	INGREDIENT & STRENGTH	BRAND (OR EQUIV.) & FIRM	NDC#	CLASS; SCH.
CC107	Tab, C-C in a Box/107	Phendimetrazine Tartrate 35 mg	Oby Obezine by JMI Canton	00252-9145	Anorexiant; C III
CC107	Tab	Phendimetrazine Tartrate 35 mg	by Allscripts	54569-2668	Anorexiant; C III
CC107	Tab, Yellow, Round, Scored	Phendimetrazine Tartrate 35 mg	by Physicians Total Care	54868-1288	Anorexiant; C III
CC107	Tab, C-C/107, C-C is in a Box	Phendimetrazine Tartrate 35 mg	Obezine by Jones	52604-9145	Anorexiant; C III
CC107	Tab, Yellow, Round, Scored	Phendimetrazine Tartrate 35 mg	by Physicians Total Care	54868-1502	Anorexiant; C III
CC107	Tab	Phendimetrazine Tartrate 35 mg	by DRX	55045-2010	Anorexiant; C III
CC107	Tab, Compressed, CC 107	Phendimetrazine Tartrate 35 mg	Rapdone by Macnary	55982-0001	Anorexiant; C III
CC107	Tab	Phendimetrazine Tartrate 35 mg	by Quality Care	62682-7035	Anorexiant; C III
CC107	Tab, [C-C] Over 107	Phendimetrazine Tartrate 35 mg	by Quality Care	60346-0562	Anorexiant; C III
CC107	Tab	Phendimetrazine Tartrate 35 mg	by United Res	00677-1499	Anorexiant; C III
CC108	Tab	Hydrochlorothiazide 50 mg	by Geneva	00781-1481	Diuretic
CC108	Tab	Hydrochlorothiazide 50 mg	by Qualitest	00603-3859	Diuretic
CC109	Tab	Diethylpropion HCl 25 mg	Radtue by Macnary	55982-0002	Antianorexiant; C IV
CC109	Tab	Diethylpropion HCl 25 mg	by PDRX	55289-0794	Antianorexiant; C IV
CC109	Tab, CC Over 109	Diethylpropion HCl 25 mg	by Quality Care	60346-0060	Antianorexiant; C IV
CC109	Tab, CC 109	Diethylpropion HCl 25 mg	by Quality Care	62682-7044	Antianorexiant; C IV
CC109	Tab	Diethylpropion HCl 25 mg	by Zenith Goldline	00182-1436	Antianorexiant; C IV
CC109	Tab, Blue, Round	Diethylpropion HCl 25 mg	by Dupont Pharma	00056-0627	Antianorexiant; C IV
CC109	Tab, White, Round	Diethylpropion HCl 25 mg	by Dupont Pharma	00056-0623	Antianorexiant; C IV
CC109	Tab, C-C/109, C-C is in a Box	Diethylpropion HCl 25 mg	by JMI Canton	00252-9159	Antianorexiant; C IV
CC109	Tab	Diethylpropion HCl 25 mg	by Allscripts	54569-2059	Antianorexiant; C IV
CC109	Tab, C-C/109	Diethylpropion HCl 25 mg	by Jones	52604-9159	Antianorexiant; C IV
CC109	Tab, Blue, Round	Diethylpropion HCl 25 mg	by Southwood Pharms	58016-0835	Antianorexiant; C IV
CC116	Tab, Imprinting Logo	Hydrochlorothiazide 25 mg	by Camall	00147-0116	Diuretic
CC116	Tab	Hydrochlorothiazide 25 mg	Hctz by Quality Care	60346-0184	Diuretic
CC116	Tab	Hydrochlorothiazide 25 mg	by Heartland	61392-0011	Diuretic
CC116	Tab	Hydrochlorothiazide 25 mg	by Qualitest	00603-3858	Diuretic
CC116	Tab, Imprinting Logo	Hydrochlorothiazide 25 mg	by United Res	00677-0346	Diuretic
CC116	Tab	Hydrochlorothiazide 25 mg	by Geneva	00781-1480	Diuretic
CC116	Tab	Hydrochlorothiazide 25 mg	by Talbert Med	44514-0410	Diuretic
CC116	Tab	Hydrochlorothiazide 25 mg	by Apotheca	12634-0445	Diuretic
CC123	Tab	Hydrochlorothiazide 25 mg	by United Res	00677-0346	Diuretic
CC124	Tab, Pink, Round, CC Inside Rectangle and 124	Hydralazine HCl 25 mg, Hydrochlorothiazide 15 mg, Reserpine 0.1 mg	Uniserp by Rx Pak	65084-0184	Antihypertensive; Diuretic
CC124	Tab, Salmon	Hydralazine HCl 25 mg, Hydrochlorothiazide 15 mg, Reserpine 0.1 mg	by Zenith Goldline	00182-1820	Antihypertensive; Diuretic
CC124	Tab	Hydralazine HCl 25 mg, Hydrochlorothiazide 15 mg, Reserpine 0.1 mg	Uni Serp by United Res	00677-0415	Antihypertensive; Diuretic
CC124	Tab	Hydralazine HCl 25 mg, Hydrochlorothiazide 15 mg, Reserpine 0.1 mg	Tri Hydroserpine by Rugby	00536-4909	Antihypertensive; Diuretic
CC124	Tab, CC-124	Hydralazine HCl 25 mg, Hydrochlorothiazide 15 mg, Reserpine 0.1 mg	by Qualitest	00603-3807	Antihypertensive; Diuretic
CC125	Tab, Green, Round	Hydrochlorothiazide 50 mg, Reserpine 0.125 mg	Serpasil-Esidrix by Camall		Diuretic; Antihypertensive
CC135	Tab, Green & White, Oblong, Double Scored	Phendimetrazine Tartrate 35 mg	by PDRX Pharms	55289-0294	Anorexiant; C III
CC135	Tab, White, with Green Specks	Phendimetrazine Tartrate 35 mg	Obezine Obgw by Jones	52604-9142	Anorexiant; C III
CC136	Tab	Phentermine HCl 8 mg	by DRX	55045-2274	Anorexiant; C IV
CC136	Tab	Phentermine HCl 8 mg	by PDRX	55289-0801	Anorexiant; C IV
CC136	Tab	Phentermine HCl 8 mg	by Quality Care	60346-0215	Anorexiant; C IV
CC137	Tab, Blue, Oval	Meclizine HCl 12.5 mg	Antivert by Camall		Antiemetic
CC143	Tab, Aqua, Round	Trichlormethiazide 4 mg	Metahydrin by Camall		Diuretic
CC143	Tab	Trichlormethiazide 4 mg	by Zenith Goldline	00182-0517	Diuretic

ID FRONT <> BACK	DESCRIPTION FRONT <> BACK	INGREDIENT & STRENGTH	BRAND (OR EQUIV.) & FIRM	NDC#	CLASS; SCH.
CC143	Tab	Trichlormethiazide 4 mg	by PDRX	55289-0795	Diuretic
CC166	Tab, Green, Round	Phendimetrazine Tartrate 35 mg	Plegine by Camall		Anorexiant; C III
CC1875	Cap, Gray & Yellow, CC 18.75	Phentermine HCl 18.75 mg	by Camall		Anorexiant; C IV
CC1875	Cap, CC 18.75	Phentermine HCl 18.75 mg	by Camall	00147-0249	Anorexiant; C IV
CC1875	Cap	Phentermine HCl 18.75 mg	by Allscripts	54569-2669	Anorexiant; C IV
CC1875	Cap, CC 18.75	Phentermine HCl 18.75 mg	by Ems Disp	62792-0249	Anorexiant; C IV
CC1875	Cap, Logo CC 18.75	Phentermine HCl 18.75 mg	by Apotheca	12634-0517	Anorexiant; C IV
CC227	Tab, Tan, Round	Thyroid 3 gr	by Camall		Thyroid
CC232	Tab, White, with Blue Specks	Phentermine HCl 37.5 mg	Pbw Phentride by JMI Canton	00252-9156	Anorexiant; C IV
CC232	Tab	Phentermine HCl 37.5 mg	by Zenith Goldline	00182-0205	Anorexiant; C IV
CC232	Tab, Blue Specks	Phentermine HCl 37.5 mg	by Camall	00147-0248	Anorexiant; C IV
CC232	Tab, White, with Blue Specks	Phentermine HCl 37.5 mg	Phentride by Jones	52604-9156	Anorexiant; C IV
CC232	Tab	Phentermine HCl 37.5 mg	by Allscripts	54569-2504	Anorexiant; C IV
CC232	Tab, White, with Blue Specks	Phentermine HCl 37.5 mg	by Physicians Total Care	54868-4091	Anorexiant; C IV
CC232	Tab, Blue Specks	Phentermine HCl 37.5 mg	by PDRX	55289-0701	Anorexiant; C IV
CC232	Tab	Phentermine HCl 37.5 mg	by Quality Care	60346-0084	Anorexiant; C IV
CC232	Tab	Phentermine HCl 37.5 mg	by PDRX	55289-0865	Anorexiant; C IV
CC232	Tab	Phentermine HCl 37.5 mg	by Quality Care	62682-7038	Anorexiant; C IV
CC232	Tab, Yellow, Oblong, Scored	Phentermine HCl 37.5 mg	by Compumed	00403-5312	Anorexiant; C IV
CC232	Tab, Blue Specks	Phentermine HCl 37.5 mg	by Qualitest	00603-5191	Anorexiant; C IV
CC232	Tab, White, w/ Blue Specks	Phentermine HCl 37.5 mg	by Allscripts	54569-3203	Anorexiant; C IV
CC236	Tab, White, Round	Cyproheptadine HCl 4 mg	Periactin by Camall		Antihistamine
CC238	Tab, White, Round	Potassium Gluconate 500 mg	Potassium Gluconate by Camall		Electrolytes
CC242	Tab, Tan, Round	Thyroid 0.5 gr	by Camall		Thryoid
CC243	Tab, Tan, Round	Thyroid 1 gr	by Camall		Thyroid
CC244	Tab, Tan, Round	Thyroid 2 gr	by Camall		Thyroid
CC245	Tab, Pink, Oval	Chromium Picolinate 200 mcg	Pichrome by Camall		Supplement
CC250	Tab, White, Oblong	Vitamin Combination	by Camall		Vitamin
CC255	Tab, Orange, Round	Hydralazine HCl 10 mg	Apresoline by Camall		Antihypertensive
CC255	Tab, Orange, Round	Hydralazine HCl 10 mg	by Camall	00147-0255	Antihypertensive
CC256	Tab, Orange, Round	Hydralazane HCl 25 mg	by Camall	00147-0256	Antihypertensive
CC256	Tab, Orange, Round	Hydralazine HCl 25 mg	Apresoline by Camall		Antihypertensive
CC257	Tab, Orange, Round	Hydralazane HCl 50 mg	by Camall	00147-0257	Antihypertensive
CC257	Tab, Orange, Round	Hydralazine HCl 50 mg	Apresoline by Camall		Antihypertensive
CC258	Tab, Orange, Round	Hydralazane HCl 100 mg	by Camall	00147-0258	Antihypertensive
CC258	Tab, Orange, Round	Hydralazine HCl 100 mg	Apresoline by Camall		Antihypertensive
CC270	Tab, Yellow, Oval	Phenylpropanolamine HCl 37.5 mg	by Camall		Decongestant; Appetite Suppressant
CC270	Tab, Gray, Oval	Phenylpropanolamine HCl 37.5 mg	by Camall		Decongestant; Appetite Suppressant
CC270	Tab, Pink, Oval	Phenylpropanolamine HCl 37.5 mg	by Camall		Decongestant; Appetite Suppressant
CC270	Tab, Blue, Oval	Phenylpropanolamine HCl 37.5 mg	by Camall		Decongestant; Appetite Suppressant
CC270	Tab, Green, Oval	Phenylpropanolamine HCl 37.5 mg	by Camall		Decongestant; Appetite Suppressant
CC270	Tab, Peach, Oval	Phenylpropanolamine HCl 37.5 mg	by Camall		Decongestant; Appetite Suppressant
CC270	Tab, White, Oval	Phenylpropanolamine HCl 37.5 mg	by Camall		Decongestant; Appetite Suppressant
CC375	Cap, Black & Red, CC 37.5	Phentermine HCl 37.5 mg	by Camall		Anorexiant; C IV
CC375	Cap, Yellow, CC 37.5	Phentermine HCl 37.5 mg	by Camall		Anorexiant; C IV

ID FRONT <> BACK	DESCRIPTION FRONT <> BACK	INGREDIENT & STRENGTH	BRAND (OR EQUIV.) & FIRM	NDC#	CLASS; SCH.
CC375	Cap, Clear & Green, CC 37.5	Phentermine HCl 37.5 mg	by Camall		Anorexiant; C IV
CC375	Cap, Brown & Clear, CC 37.5	Phentermine HCl 37.5 mg	by Camall		Anorexiant; C IV
CC375	Cap, Black, CC 37.5	Phentermine HCl 37.5 mg	by Camall		Anorexiant; C IV
CC375	Cap, Black & Yellow, CC 37.5	Phentermine HCl 37.5 mg	by Camall		Anorexiant; C IV
CC375	Cap, Clear, with Orange & White Beads, CC 37.5	Phentermine HCl 37.5 mg	Pbc Phentride by JMI Canton	00252-9155	Anorexiant; C IV
CC375	Cap, Logo CC 37.5	Phentermine HCl 37.5 mg	by DRX	55045-2294	Anorexiant; C IV
CC375	Cap, Orange & White Beads, CC 37.5	Phentermine HCl 37.5 mg	by DRX	55045-2289	Anorexiant; C IV
CC375	Cap, Clear, with Orange & White Beads, CC 37.5	Phentermine HCl 37.5 mg	Phentride by Jones	52604-9155	Anorexiant; C IV
CC375	Cap, Clear & Green, CC 37.5	Phentermine 37.5 mg	by Physicians Total Care	54868-4059	Anorexiant; C IV
CC375	Tab, CC 37.5	Phentermine HCl 37.5 mg	by Ems Disp	62792-0231	Anorexiant; C IV
CC375	Cap, CC 37.5	Phentermine HCl 37.5 mg	by Quality Care	60346-0426	Anorexiant; C IV
CC375	Cap, CC 37.5	Phentermine HCl 37.5 mg	by Quality Care	62682-7043	Anorexiant; C IV
CC375	Cap, CC 37.5	Phentermine HCl 37.5 mg	by Apotheca	12634-0515	Anorexiant; C IV
CC375P	Tab, Pink, Round, CC 37.5P	Phenylpropanolamine 37.5 mg	by Camall		Decongestant; Appetite Suppressant
CC375P	Tab, Peach, Round, CC 37.5P	Phenylpropanolamine 37.5 mg	by Camall		Decongestant; Appetite Suppressant
CC375P	Tab, Gray, Round, CC 37.5P	Phenylpropanolamine 37.5 mg	by Camall		Decongestant; Appetite Suppressant
CC375P	Tab, White, Round, CC 37.5P	Phenylpropanolamine 37.5 mg	by Camall		Decongestant; Appetite Suppressant
CC375P	Tab, White, Round, Green Specks, CC 37.5P	Phenylpropanolamine 37.5 mg	by Camall		Decongestant; Appetite Suppressant
CC375P	Tab, Yellow, Round, CC 37.5P	Phenylpropanolamine 37.5 mg	by Camall		Decongestant; Appetite Suppressant
CC375P	Tab, Green, Round, CC 37.5P	Phenylpropanolamine 37.5 mg	by Camall		Decongestant; Appetite Suppressant
CC525	Tab, Purple, Oval	Zinc 15 mg, Chromium 200 mcg	by Camall		Mineral Supplement
CC75P	Cap, Blue & Clear	Phenylpropanolamine 75 mg	by Camall		Decongestant; Appetite Suppressant
CC75P	Cap, Black	Phenylpropanolamine 75 mg	by Camall		Decongestant; Appetite Suppressant
CC75P	Cap, Black & Yellow	Phenylpropanolamine 75 mg	by Camall		Decongestant; Appetite Suppressant
CC75P	Cap, Yellow	Phenylpropanolamine 75 mg	by Camall		Decongestant; Appetite Suppressant
CDAY	Cap, Yellow, C-Day	Acetaminophen 650 mg, Pseudoephedrine 60 mg, Dextromethorphan 30 mg	by SmithKline SKB	Canadian	Cold Remedy
CDAY	Tab, Yellow, Oblong, C-Day	Acetaminophen 650 mg, Pseudophed 60 mg, Dextromethorphan 30 mg	Contact by SmithKline SKB	Canadian	Cold Remedy
CDC <> GEIGY	Tab, Light Yellow, Round, Film Coated	Metoprolol Tartrate 200 mg	Lopresor SR by Novartis	Canadian DIN# 00534560	Antihypertensive
CDC322	Tab, CDC/322	Yohimbine HCl 5.4 mg	Thybine Blue by JMI Canton	00252-3223	Impotence Agent
CDX50	Tab, Film Coated, Casodex Logo	Bicalutamide 50 mg	Casodex by Zeneca	62311-0705	Antiandrogen
CDX50	Tab, White, CDX50/Zeneca Logo	Bicalutamide 50 mg	by Zeneca	Canadian	Antiandrogen
CDX50	Tab, White, Film Coated, Casodex Logo	Bicalutamide 50 mg	Casodex by AstraZeneca	00310-0705	Antiandrogen
CECLOR 250 <> LILLY3061	Cap, Ceclor over 250 <> Lilly over 3061	Cefaclor 250 mg	Ceclor by Quality Care	60346-0104	Antibiotic
CECLOR 250 MG <> LILLY3061	Cap	Cefaclor Anhydrous 250 mg	Ceclor by Eli Lilly	00002-3061	Antibiotic
CECLOR 500 MG <> LILLY3062	Cap, Ceclor 500 mg <> Lilly over 3062	Cefaclor 500 mg	Ceclor by Quality Care	60346-0640	Antibiotic

ID FRONT <> BACK	DESCRIPTION FRONT <> BACK	INGREDIENT & STRENGTH	BRAND (OR EQUIV.) & FIRM	NDC#	CLASS; SCH.
CECLOR 500 MG <> LILLY3062	Cap	Cefaclor Monohydrate 500 mg	Ceclor by Eli Lilly	00002-3062	Antibiotic
CECLOR250 <> LILLY3061	Cap	Cefaclor 250 mg	by Pharmedix	53002-0211	Antibiotic
CECLOR250MG <> LILLY3061	Cap, Purple & White	Cefaclor Anhydrous 250 mg	Ceclor by HJ Harkins	52959-0027	Antibiotic
CECLOR500MG <> LILLY3062	Cap	Cefaclor 500 mg	by Pharmedix	53002-0244	Antibiotic
CECLORCD375MG	Tab	Cefaclor 375 mg	Ceclor CD by Dura	51479-0036	Antibiotic
CECLORCD500LILL	Tab	Cefaclor 500 mg	Ceclor CD by Allscripts	54569-4463	Antibiotic
CECLORCD500MG	Tab	Cefaclor 500 mg	Ceclor CD by Dura	51479-0035	Antibiotic
CEDAX400	Cap, White	Ceftibuten Dihydrate 400 mg	Cedax by Schering	00085-0691	Antibiotic
CEFACLO R250 <> LEDERLEC54	Cap, in Black Ink	Cefaclor Monohydrate 250 mg	by Quality Care	60346-0202	Antibiotic
CEFACLOR 250 MG <> LEDERLEC54	Cap	Cefaclor Monohydrate	by UDL	51079-0617	Antibiotic
CEFACLOR 500 MG <> LEDERLEC58	Cap, Lavender	Cefaclor Monohydrate	by UDL	51079-0618	Antibiotic
CEFACLOR250 <> ZENITH4760	Cap	Cefaclor Monohydrate 250 mg	by PDRX	55289-0749	Antibiotic
CEFACLOR250 MG <> 2614SCHEIN	Cap, Purple	Cefaclor 250 mg	by Schein	00364-2614	Antibiotic
CEFACLOR500 MG <> 2615SCHEIN	Cap, Purple & Yellow	Cefaclor 500 mg	by Schein	00364-2615	Antibiotic
CELGENE	Cap, White, Hard Gel	Thalidomide 50 mg	Thalomid by Celgene	59572-0105	Immunomodulator
CELGENE	Cap, White	Thalidomide 50 mg	Thalomid by Penn Pharms	63069-0630	Immunomodulator
CELGENE	Cap, Opaque & White	Thalidomide 50 mg	Thalomid by Takeda	64764-0151	Immunomodulator
CELLCEPT250	Cap, Blue & Brown	Mycophenolate Mofetil 250 mg	CellCept by Roche	Canadian	Immunosuppressant
CELLCEPT250 <> ROCHE	Cap, Printed in Black	Mycophenolate Mofetil 250 mg	Cellcept by Syntex	18393-0259	Immunosuppressant
CELLCEPT250 <> ROCHE	Cap, Blue & Brown, Hard Gel	Mycophenolate Mofetil 250 mg	Cellcept by Murfreesboro Ph	51129-1358	Immunosuppressant
CELLCEPT250 <> ROCHE	Cap	Mycophenolate Mofetil 250 mg	Cellcept by Hoffmann La Roche	00004-0259	Immunosuppressant
CELLCEPT500	Tab, Lavender, Cap-Shaped	Mycophenolate Mofetil 500 mg	CellCept by Roche	Canadian	Immunosuppressant
CELLCEPT500 <> ROCHE	Tab, Lavender, Coated, in Black Ink	Mycophenolate Mofetil 500 mg	Cellcept by Hoffmann La Roche	00004-0260	Immunosuppressant
CELLCEPT500 <> ROCHE	Tab, Purple, Oblong, Film	Mycophenolate Mofetil 500 mg	Cellcept by Novartis	00078-0327	Immunosuppressant
CELLCEPT500 <> ROCHE	Tab, Coated	Mycophenolate Mofetil 500 mg	Cellcept by Syntex	18393-0923	Immunosuppressant
CENTRAL130MG	Cap, Clear	Theophylline Anhydrous 130 mg	Theoclear LA-130 by Schwarz Pharma		Antiasthmatic
CENTRAL13105	Tab, Blue, Oval, Central 131/05	Vitamin Combination	Niferex-PN by Schwarz Pharma		Vitamin
CENTRAL13107	Tab, Red, Round, Central 131/07	Prednisone 5 mg	Prednicen-M by Schwarz Pharma		Steroid
CENTRAL20	Tab, Lavender, Round	Vitamin, Mineral Supplement	Niferex by Schwarz Pharma		Vitamin
CENTRAL2200	Tab, Brown, Round	Vitamin, Mineral Supplement	Niferex by Schwarz Pharma		Vitamin
CENTRAL260MG	Cap, Clear	Theophylline Anhydrous 260 mg	Theoclear LA-260 by Schwarz Pharma		Antiasthmatic
CENTRAL40	Cap, Clear & Red	Chlorpheniramine 8 mg, Pseudoephedrine 120 mg	Codimal LA by Schwarz Pharma		Cold Remedy
CENTRAL4220	Cap, Clear & Orange	Vitamin Combination	Niferex-150 by Schwarz Pharma		Vitamin
CENTRAL4330	Cap, Clear & Red	Vitamin Combination	Niferex-150 Forte by Schwarz Pharma		Vitamin
CENTRAL44	Cap, Brown & Red	Vitamin Combination	Niferex-150 Forte by Schwarz Pharma		Vitamin
CENTRAL5005	Tab, White, Oval, Central 500/5	Hydrocodone 5 mg, Acetaminophen 500 mg	Co-Gesic by Schwarz Pharma		Analgesic; C III

ID FRONT <> BACK	DESCRIPTION FRONT <> BACK	INGREDIENT & STRENGTH	BRAND (OR EQUIV.) & FIRM	NDC#	CLASS; SCH.
CENTRAL500MG	Tab, Pink, Round	Salsalate 500 mg	Mono-Gesic by Schwarz Pharma		NSAID
CENTRAL604	Cap, Clear, Central 60/4	Chlorpheniramine Maleate 4 mg, Pseudoephedrine 60 mg	Codimal LA Half by Schwarz Pharma		Cold Remedy
CENTRAL750MG	Tab, Pink, Oval	Salsalate 750 mg	Mono-Gesic by Schwarz Pharma		NSAID
CENTRALC	Cap, Red & White	Chlorpheniramine 2 mg, Pseudoephedrine 30 mg, Acetaminophen 325 mg	Codimal by Schwarz Pharma		Cold Remedy
CENTURY PHARMACEUTICALS LOGO	Tab, White, Round	Simethicone 40 mg	D-Gas by Century	00436-0989	Antiflatulent
CF	Cap, Clear & Orange, CF over Abbott Logo	Pentobarbital Sodium 50 mg	Nembutal by Abbott	00074-3150	Sedative/Hypnotic; C II
CG <> BEB	Tab, Light Red, Round, Film Coated	Oxprenolol HCl 80 mg	Slow Trasicor by Novartis	Canadian DIN# 00534579	Antihypertensive
CG <> BNB	Tab, White, Round, Film Coated	Oxprenolol HCl 160 mg	Slow Trasicor by Novartis	Canadian DIN# 00534587	Antihypertensive
CG <> CG	Tab, Light Yellow, Round, Film Coated, Scored	Oxprenolol HCl 80 mg	Trasicor by Novartis	Canadian DIN# 00402583	Antihypertensive
CG <> FV	Tab, Dark Yellow, Round	Letrozole 2.5 mg	Femara by Novartis	Canadian DIN# 02231384	Antineoplastic
CG <> FV	Tab, Dark Yellow, Round, Film Coated	Letrozole 2.5 mg	Femara by Novartis	00078-0249	Antineoplastic
CG <> HC	Tab, Beige & Orange, Oval, Scored	Carbamazepine 200 mg	Tegretol CR by Novartis	Canadian DIN# 00773611	Anticonvulsant
CG <> HGH	Tab, Light Orange	Hydrochlorothiazide 12.5 mg, Valsartan 80 mg	Diovan HCT by Novartis	00078-0314	Diuretic; Antihypertensive
CG <> HGH	Tab, Light Orange, Oval, Film Coated	Hydrochlorothiazide 12.5 mg, Valsartan 80 mg	Diovan HCT by Novartis	Canadian DIN# 02241900	Diuretic; Antihypertensive
CG <> HGH	Tab, Orange, Oblong	Valsartan 80 mg, Hydrochlorothiazide 12.5 mg	Diovan by Allscripts	54569-4766	Antihypertensive
CG <> HHH	Tab, Dark Red	Hydrochlorothiazide 12.5 mg, Valsartan 160 mg	Diovan HCT by Novartis	00078-0315	Diuretic; Antihypertensive
CG <> HHH	Tab, Dark Red, Oval, Film Coated	Hydrochlorothiazide 12.5 mg, Valsartan 160 mg	Diovan HCT by Novartis	Canadian DIN# 02241901	Diuretic; Antihypertensive
CG <> HO	Tab, Dark Yellow, Cap Shaped, Film Coated	Benazepril HCl 10 mg	Lotensin by Novartis	Canadian DIN# 00885843	Antihypertensive
CG <> HP	Tab, Reddish-Orange, Cap Shaped, Film Coated	Benazepril HCl 20 mg	Lotensin by Novartis	Canadian DIN# 00885851	Antihypertensive
CG <> LV	Tab, Light Yellow, Cap Shaped, Film Coated	Benazepril HCl 5 mg	Lotensin by Geigy	Canadian DIN# 00885835	Antihypertensive
CG <> TD	Tab, Yellow, Oval, Film Coated, Scored	Oxcarbazepine 150 mg	Trileptal FCT by Novartis Pharm AG	17088-0010	Anticonvulsant
CG <> TD	Tab, Yellow, Oval, Film Coated, Scored, C/G <> T/D	Oxcarbazepine 150 mg	Tripetal by Novartis Pharms	00078-0336	Anticonvulsant
CG 503	Tab, White	Ferrous Sulfate 160 mg	by Novartis	Canadian	Mineral
CG622	White, Oblong	Terazosin HCl 1 mg	by Kaiser Fdn	00179-1359	Antihypertensive
CGCG <> ENEENE	Tab, Brownish-Orange, Oval, Scored	Carbamazepine 400 mg	Tegretol by Geigy	Canadian DIN# 00755583	Anticonvulsant

ID FRONT <> BACK	DESCRIPTION FRONT <> BACK	INGREDIENT & STRENGTH	BRAND (OR EQUIV.) & FIRM	NDC#	CLASS; SCH.
CGCG <> TETE	Tab, Yellow, Oval, Film Coated, Scored	Oxcarbazepine 300 mg	Trileptal FCT by Novartis Pharm AG	17088-0011	Anticonvulsant
CGCG <> TETE	Tab, Yellow, Oval, Film Coated, Scored, CG/CG <> TE/TE	Oxcarbazepine 300 mg	Tripeptal by Novartis Pharms	00078-0337	Anticonvulsant
CGCG <> TFTF	Tab, Yellow, Oval, Film Coated, Scored	Oxcarbazepine 600 mg	Trileptal FCT by Novartis Pharm AG	17088-0012	Anticonvulsant
CGCG <> TFTF	Tab, Yellow, Oval, Film Coated, Scored, CG/CG <> TF/TF	Oxcarbazepine 600 mg	Tripeptal by Novartis Pharms	00078-0338	Anticonvulsant
CGCGTFTF	Tab, Yellow, Oval, Slightly Biconvex, Film Coated, Scored on both, TF/TF <> CG/CG	Oxcarbazepine 600 mg	Trileptal by Novartis	00078-0339	Anticonvulsant
CGCS	Cap, Brown & Red, CG/CS	Rifampin 300 mg	by Novartis	Canadian	Antibiotic
CGFXF	Cap, Clear, Gelatin w/ White Powder	Fomoterol Fumarate 12 mg	Foradil by Novartis	Canadian DIN# 02230898	Antiasthmatic
CGFZF	Cap, Flesh & Light Gray, Opaque	Valsartan 80 mg	Diovan by Novartis	Canadian DIN# 02236808	Antihypertensive
CGFZF	Cap, Light Gray & Light Pink, Opaque, CG FZF	Valsartan 80 mg	Diovan by Novartis	00083-4000	Antihypertensive
CGGOG	Cap, Flesh & Dark Gray, Opaque	Valsartan 160 mg	Diovan by Novartis	Canadian DIN# 02236809	Antihypertensive
CGGOG	Cap, Dark Gray & Light Pink, Opaque, CG GOG	Valsartan 160 mg	Diovan by Novartis	00083-4001	Antihypertensive
CGJZ	Cap, Brown & Red, CG/JZ	Rifampin 150 mg	by Novartis	Canadian	Antibiotic
CGLV	Tab, Light Yellow, Oblong, CG/LV	Benazepril HCl 5 mg	Lotensin by Novartis	Canadian	Antihypertensive
CH	Cap, Yellow, CH over Abbott Logo	Pentobarbital Sodium 100 mg	Nembutal by Abbott	00074-3114	Sedative/Hypnotic; C II
CHEMET100	Cap	Succimer 100 mg	Chemet by Sanofi	00024-0333	Chelating Agent
CHEMET100	Cap, Filled with White Beads	Succimer 100 mg	Chemet by Sanofi	00024-0333	Chelating Agent
CHEW <> DURA	Tab, Chewable	Chlorpheniramine Maleate 2 mg, Methscopolamine Nitrate 1.25 mg, Phenylephrine HCl 10 mg	D A by Anabolic	00722-6219	Cold Remedy
CHEWEZ	Tab, Chew, Chew over EZ <> Abbott Logo	Erythromycin Ethylsuccinate	Eryped by Quality Care	60346-0032	Antibiotic
CHLORAFED <> ROBERTS136	Cap, Black Print, White Beads	Chlorpheniramine Maleate 8 mg, Pseudoephedrine HCl 120 mg	Chlorafed	00131-4513	Cold Remedy
CHLORAFEDHS <> ROBERTS135	Cap, White Beads, Black Print	Chlorpheniramine Maleate 4 mg, Pseudoephedrine HCl 60 mg	Chlorafed		Cold Remedy
CI10G	Tab, Yellow, Triangular, CI/10/G	Clomipramine 10 mg	Gen Clomipramine by Genpharm	Canadian	OCD
CI25G	Tab, Yellow, Biconvex, CI/25/G	Clomipramine 25 mg	Gen Clomipramine by Genpharm	Canadian	OCD
CI50G	Tab, White, Biconvex, CI/50/G	Clomipramine 50 mg	Gen Clomipramine by Genpharm	Canadian	OCD
CIBA <> 154	Cap, Caramel & Scarlet	Rifampin 300 mg	by Geneva	00781-2018	Antibiotic
CIBA <> 16	Tab, White, Round, Film Coated	Methylphenidate HCl 20 mg	Ritalin by Novartis	Canadian DIN# 00632775	Stimulant
CIBA <> A	Tab, White, Round, Film Coated, Scored	Oxprenolol HCl 40 mg	Trasicor by Novartis	Canadian DIN# 00402575	Antihypertensive
CIBA <> AB	Tab, Pale Blue, Round, Scored	Methylphenidate HCl 10 mg	Ritalin by Novartis	Canadian DIN# 00005606	Stimulant
CIBA <> CO	Tab, Cream, Round, Film Coated	Maprotiline 10 mg	Ludiomil by Ciba	Canadian DIN# 00641855	Antidepressant
CIBA <> DP	Tab, Brownish-Orange, Round, Film Coated	Maprotiline 25 mg	Ludiomil by Ciba	Canadian DIN# 00360481	Antidepressant
CIBA <> ER	Tab, Brownish-Yellow, Round, Film Coated	Maprotiline HCl 50 mg	Ludiomil by Novartis	Canadian DIN# 00360503	Antidepressant

ID FRONT <> BACK	DESCRIPTION FRONT <> BACK	INGREDIENT & STRENGTH	BRAND (OR EQUIV.) & FIRM	NDC#	CLASS; SCH.
CIBA <> FA	Tab, White, Scored	Hydralazine HCl 10 mg	Apresoline by Novartis	Canadian DIN# 00005525	Antihypertensive
CIBA <> GF	Tab, Blue, Round, Coated	Hydralazine HCl 25 mg	Apresoline by Novartis	Canadian DIN# 00005533	Antihypertensive
CIBA <> HG	Tab, Pink, Round, Coated	Hydralazine HCl 50 mg	Apresoline by Novartis	Canadian DIN# 00005541	Antihypertensive
CIBA <> PN	Tab, Pale Yellow, Round, Scored	Methylphenidate HCl 20 mg	Ritalin by Novartis	Canadian DIN# 00005614	Stimulant
CIBA101	Tab, Peach, Round	Hydralazine HCl 100 mg	Apresoline by Ciba		Antihypertensive
CIBA103	Tab, White, Round	Guanethidine Monosulfate 25 mg	Isimil by Ciba		Antihypertensive
CIBA104	Tab, Yellow, Round	Reserpine 0.2 mg, Hydralazine HCl 50 mg	Serpasil-Apresoline2 by Ciba		Antihypertensive
CIBA110	Tab, Orange, Oval	Maprotiline HCl 25 mg	Ludiomil by Ciba		Antidepressant
CIBA129	Tab, Orange, Round	Hydralazine HCl 25 mg, Hydrochlorothiazide 15 mg	Apresoline-Esidrix by Ciba		Antihypertensive
CIBA13	Tab, Orange, Round	Reserpine 0.1 mg, Hydrochlorothiazide 25 mg	Serpasil-Esidrix #1 by Ciba		Antihypertensive
CIBA130	Tab, White, Round, Ciba/130	Metyrapone 250 mg	Metopirone by Ciba	Canadian	Diagnostic
CIBA130	Tab, White, Round	Metyrapone 250 mg	Metopirone by Ciba		Diagnostic
CIBA135	Tab, White, Oval	Maprotiline HCl 75 mg	Ludiomil by Ciba		Antidepressant
CIBA154	Cap	Rifampin 300 mg	Rimactane by Ciba Geigy	14656-0154	Antibiotic
CIBA154	Cap	Rifampin 300 mg	Rimactane by Novartis	17088-7189	Antibiotic
CIBA16	Tab	Methylphenidate HCl 20 mg	Ritalin Sr by Caremark	00339-4084	Stimulant; C II
CIBA16	Tab, White, Round, Coated	Methylphenidate HCl 20 mg	Ritalin SR by Novartis	00083-0016	Stimulant; C II
CIBA165	Tab, Orange, Round	Potassium Chloride 600 mg (8 mEq)	Slow K by Ciba		Electrolytes
CIBA192	Tab, Blue, Round	Hydrochlorothiazide 100 mg	Esidrix by Ciba		Diuretic
CIBA22	Tab	Hydrochlorothiazide 25 mg	Esidrix by Ciba Geigy	14656-0022	Diuretic
CIBA24	Tab, White, Round, Scored	Aminoglutethimide 250 mg	Cytadren by Novartis Pharms (Ca)	61615-0103	Sedative; C II
CIBA24	Tab, White, Round	Aminoglutethimide 250 mg	Cytadren by Ciba		Sedative; C II
CIBA26	Tab, Orange, Round	Maprotiline HCl 50 mg	Ludiomil by Ciba		Antidepressant
CIBA3	Tab, Green, Round	Methylphenidate HCl 10 mg	Ritalin by Ciba		Stimulant; C II
CIBA3	Tab, Pale Green, Round, Scored	Methylphenidate HCl 10 mg	Ritalin by Novartis	00083-0003	Stimulant; C II
CIBA3	Tab, Pale Green	Methylphenidate HCl 10 mg	Ritalin by Caremark	00339-4083	Stimulant; C II
CIBA30	Tab, White, Round	Methyltestosterone 10 mg	Metandren by Ciba		Hormone; C III
CIBA32	Tab, Yellow, Round	Methyltestosterone 25 mg	Metandren by Ciba		Hormone; C III
CIBA34	Tab, Yellow, Round	Methylphenidate HCl 20 mg	Ritalin by Phy Total Care	54868-2762	Stimulant; C II
CIBA34	Tab, Pale Yellow	Methylphenidate HCl 20 mg	Ritalin HCl by Caremark	00339-4085	Stimulant; C II
CIBA34	Tab, Pale Yellow, Round, Scored	Methylphenidate HCl 20 mg	Ritalin by Novartis	00083-0034	Stimulant; C II
CIBA34	Tab, Yellow, Round, Scored	Methylphenidate HCl 20 mg	Ritalin by Phy Total Care	54868-2418	Stimulant; C II
CIBA35	Tab, White, Round	Reserpine 0.1 mg	Serpasil by Ciba		Antihypertensive
CIBA36	Tab, White, Round	Reserpine 0.25 mg	Serpasil by Ciba		Antihypertensive
CIBA37	Tab, Yellow, Round	Hydralazine HCl 10 mg	Apresoline by Ciba		Antihypertensive
CIBA39	Tab, Blue, Round	Hydralazine HCl 25 mg	Apresoline by Ciba		Antihypertensive
CIBA40	Tab, Yellow, Round	Reserpine 0.1 mg, Hydralazine HCl 25 mg	Serpasil-Apresoline1 by Ciba		Antihypertensive
CIBA41	Tab, White, Round	Sulfinpyrazone 100 mg	Anturane by Ciba		Uricosuric
CIBA46	Tab	Hydrochlorothiazide 50 mg	Esidrix by Ciba Geigy	14656-0046	Diuretic
CIBA47	Tab, White, Round	Guanethidine Monosulfate 10 mg, Hydrochlorothiazide 25 mg	Esimil by Ciba		Antihypertensive
CIBA49	Tab, Yellow, Round	Guanethidine Monosulfate 10 mg	Esimil by Ciba		Antihypertensive
CIBA51	Tab, White, Oval	Methyltestosterone Sublingual 5 mg	Metandren Linguets by Ciba		Hormone; C III
CIBA64	Tab, Yellow, Oval	Methyltestosterone Sublingual 10 mg	Metandren Linguets by Ciba		Hormone; C III
CIBA65	Tab, Peach, Round	Lithium Carbonate 300 mg	Lithobid by Ciba		Antipsychotic

ID FRONT <> BACK	DESCRIPTION FRONT <> BACK	INGREDIENT & STRENGTH	BRAND (OR EQUIV.) & FIRM	NDC#	CLASS; SCH.
CIBA7	Tab, Yellow, Round	Methylphenidate HCl 5 mg	Ritalin by Novartis	00083-0007	Stimulant; C II
CIBA7	Tab, Yellow, Round	Methylphenidate HCl 5 mg	Ritalin HCl by Caremark	00339-4082	Stimulant; C II
CIBA71	Tab, Pink, Round	Reserpine 0.1 mg, Hydralazine HCl 25 mg, Hydrochlorothiazide 15 mg	Ser- by Ciba		Antihypertensive
CIBA73	Tab, Blue, Round	Hydralazine HCl 50 mg	Apresoline by Ciba		Antihypertensive
CIBA97	Tab, Orange, Round	Reserpine 0.1 mg, Hydrochlorothiazide 50 mg	Serpasil-Esidrix #2 by Ciba		Antihypertensive
CIBAAC	Tab, Pink, Round, Ciba/AC	Reserpine 0.1 mg, Hydralazine 25 mg, Hydrochlorothiazide 15 mg	by Novartis	Canadian	Antihypertensive
CIBAAC	Tab, Pink, Round, Ciba/AC	Reserpine Hydralazine HCl 15 mg	Ser-Ap-Es by Novartis	Canadian	Antihypertensive
CIBAAI	Tab, White, Round, Ciba/AI	Oxprenolol HCl 40 mg	Trasicor by Ciba	Canadian	Antihypertensive
CIBABNB	Tab, White, Round, Ciba/BNB	Oxprenolol 160 mg	Slow-Trasicor by Ciba	Canadian	Antihypertensive
CIBACG	Tab, Light Yellow, Round, Ciba/CG	Oxprenolol HCl 80 mg	Trasicor by Ciba	Canadian	Antihypertensive
CIBACO	Tab, Cream, Round, Ciba/CO	Maprotiline HCl 10 mg	Ludiomil by Novartis	Canadian	Antidepressant
CIBADP	Tab, Brown & Yellow, Round, Ciba/DP	Maprotiline HCl 25 mg	Ludiomil by Novartis	Canadian	Antidepressant
CIBAFS	Tab, Brown & Red, Round, Ciba/FS	Maprotiline HCl 75 mg	Ludiomil by Novartis	Canadian	Antidepressant
CIBAGG	Tab, White, Round, Ciba/GG	Aminoglutethimide 250 mg	Cytadren by Ciba	Canadian	Sedative
CIBAJL	Tab, White, Round, Ciba/JL	Methyltestosterone 10 mg	Metandren by Novartis	Canadian	Hormone; C III
CIBAKM	Tab, White, Round, Ciba/KM	Methyltestosterone 25 mg	Metandren by Novartis	Canadian	Hormone; C III
CIBALJ	Tab, Blue, Round, Ciba/LJ	Tripelennamine HCl 50 mg	by Novartis	Canadian	Antihistamine
CIBASP	Tab, White, Round, Ciba/SP	Reserpine 0.25 mg	Serapsil by Ciba	Canadian	Antihypertensive
CIBATP	Tab, Yellow, Ciba/TP	Ferrous Sulfate 160 mg, Folic Acid 400 mcg	Slow-Fe Folic by Ciba	Canadian	Mineral
CIBATRASICOR20	Tab, White, Round, Ciba/Trasicor/20	Oxprenolol HCl 20 mg	Trasicor by Novartis	Canadian	Antihypertensive
CIBATRASICOR20	Tab, White, Round, Ciba/Trasicor 20	Oxprenolol HCl 20 mg	Trasicor by Ciba	Canadian	Antihypertensive
CIL 5	Tab, Reddish Brown, Oval	Cilazapril 5 mg	Inhibace by Roche	Canadian	Antihypertensive
CIL1	Tab, Yellow, Oval	Cilazapril 1 mg	Inhibace by Roche	Canadian	Antihypertensive
CIL25	Tab, Tabish Brown & Pink, Oval, Cil 2.5	Cilazapril 2.5 mg	Inhibace by Roche	Canadian	Antihypertensive
CINOBAC250MG <> OCL55	Cap, Cinobac 250 mg <> OCL 55	Cinoxacin 250 mg	Cinobac by Eli Lilly	00002-3055	Antibiotic
CINOBAC250MG <> OCL55	Cap, Cinobac 250 mg <> OCL 55	Cinoxacin 250 mg	Cinobac by Eli Lilly	00002-0055	Antibiotic
CINOBAC25OMG <> OCL55	Cap	Cinoxacin 250 mg	Cinobac by Oclassen	55515-0055	Antibiotic
CINOBAC500MG <> OCL56	Cap	Cinoxacin 500 mg	Cinobac by Oclassen	55515-0056	Antibiotic
CINOBAC500MG <> OCL56	Cap, Cinobac 500 mg <> OCL 56	Cinoxacin 500 mg	Cinobac by Eli Lilly	00002-0056	Antibiotic
CIPRO <> 100	Tab, Yellow, Round, Film Coated	Ciprofloxacin HCl 100 mg	Cipro Cystitis Pack by Compumed	00403-2558	Antibiotic
CIPRO <> 100	Tab, Film Coated	Ciprofloxacin HCl 116.4 mg	Ciprobay by Bayer	00026-8511	Antibiotic
CIPRO <> 250	Tab, Slightly Yellowish, Film Coated	Ciprofloxacin HCl	Cipro by HJ Harkins Co	52959-0171	Antibiotic
CIPRO <> 250	Tab, Yellow, Oblong	Ciprofloxacin HCl 250 mg	Cipro by Direct Dispensing	57866-6250	Antibiotic
CIPRO <> 250	Tab, Yellow, Round, Film Coated	Ciprofloxacin HCl 250 mg	Cipro by Compumed	00403-4258	Antibiotic
CIPRO <> 250	Tab, Pale Yellow, Film Coated	Ciprofloxacin HCl 291.5 mg	Cipro by Quality Care	60346-0433	Antibiotic
CIPRO <> 250	Tab, Film Coated	Ciprofloxacin HCl 291.5 mg	Cipro by Amerisource	62584-0335	Antibiotic
CIPRO <> 250	Tab, Film Coated	Ciprofloxacin HCl 291.5 mg	Ciprobay by Bayer	00026-8512	Antibiotic
CIPRO <> 250	Tab, Film Coated	Ciprofloxacin HCl 291.5 mg	Cipro by Nat Pharmpak Serv	55154-4806	Antibiotic
CIPRO <> 250	Tab, Film Coated	Ciprofloxacin HCl 291.5 mg	Cipro by Apotheca	12634-0423	Antibiotic
CIPRO <> 500	Tab, Film Coated	Ciprofloxacin HCl	Cipro by HJ Harkins Co	52959-0037	Antibiotic
CIPRO <> 500	Tab, Yellow, Oblong, Film Coated	Ciprofloxacin HCl 500 mg	Cipro by Allscripts	54569-4820	Antibiotic
CIPRO <> 500	Tab, Yellow, Oblong, Film Coated	Ciprofloxacin HCl 500 mg	Cipro by Compumed	00403-4522	Antibiotic
CIPRO <> 500	Tab, Film Coated	Ciprofloxacin HCl 583 mg	Cipro by Amerisource	62584-0336	Antibiotic
CIPRO <> 500	Tab, Film Coated	Ciprofloxacin HCl 583 mg	Cipro by Prescription Dispensing	61807-0035	Antibiotic
CIPRO <> 500	Tab, Pale Yellow, Film Coated	Ciprofloxacin HCl 583 mg	Cipro by Quality Care	60346-0031	Antibiotic
CIPRO <> 500	Tab, Film Coated	Ciprofloxacin HCl 583 mg	Ciprobay by Bayer	00026-8513	Antibiotic
CIPRO <> 500	Tab, Film Coated	Ciprofloxacin HCl 583 mg	Cipro by PDRX	55289-0371	Antibiotic

ID FRONT <> BACK	DESCRIPTION FRONT <> BACK	INGREDIENT & STRENGTH	BRAND (OR EQUIV.) & FIRM	NDC#	CLASS; SCH.
CIPRO <> 500	Tab, Coated	Ciprofloxacin HCl 583 mg	Cipro by Physicians Total Care	54868-0939	Antibiotic
CIPRO <> 500	Tab, Coated	Ciprofloxacin HCl 583 mg	Cipro by HJ Harkins Co	52959-0036	Antibiotic
CIPRO <> 500	Tab, Slightly Yellowish, Film Coated	Ciprofloxacin HCl 583 mg	by Med Pro	53978-3075	Antibiotic
CIPRO <> 500	Tab, Film Coated	Ciprofloxacin HCl 583 mg	Cipro by Nat Pharmpak Serv	55154-4801	Antibiotic
CIPRO <> 750	Tab, Film Coated	Ciprofloxacin HCl	Cipro by Nat Pharmpak Serv	55154-4807	Antibiotic
CIPRO <> 750	Tab, Yellow, Oblong, Film, Coated	Ciprofloxacin HCl 750 mg	Cipro by Compumed	00403-4650	Antibiotic
CIPRO <> 750	Tab, Film Coated	Ciprofloxacin HCl 874.5 mg	Ciprobay by Bayer	00026-8514	Antibiotic
CIPRO <> 750	Tab, Film Coated	Ciprofloxacin HCl 874.5 mg	Cipro by Physicians Total Care	54868-1184	Antibiotic
CIPRO100	Tab, White, Round, Cipro/100	Ciprofloxacin HCl 100 mg	Cipro by Bayer	Canadian	Antibiotic
CIPRO250	Tab, White, Round, Cipro/250	Ciprofloxacin HCl 250 mg	Cipro by Bayer	Canadian	Antibiotic
CIPRO250	Tab, Film Coated	Ciprofloxacin HCl 291.5 mg	Cipro by Pharmedix	53002-0279	Antibiotic
CIPRO250	Tab, Film Coated, Cipro/250	Ciprofloxacin HCl 291.5 mg	Cipro by Allscripts	54569-1648	Antibiotic
CIPRO500	Tab, White, Oblong, Cipro/500	Ciprofloxacin HCl 500 mg	Cipro by Bayer	Canadian	Antibiotic
CIPRO500	Tab, Film Coated	Ciprofloxacin HCl 583 mg	Cipro by Allscripts	54569-1723	Antibiotic
CIPRO750	Tab, White, Oblong, Cipro/750	Ciprofloxacin HCl 750 mg	Cipro by Bayer	Canadian	Antibiotic
CIPRO750	Tab, Film Coated	Ciprofloxacin HCl 874.5 mg	Cipro by Allscripts	54569-2488	Antibiotic
CIPRO750	Tab, Film Coated	Ciprofloxacin HCl 874.5 mg	Cipro by Pharmedix	53002-0268	Antibiotic
CIR 3MG	Cap, Light Gray & Pink	Budesonide 3 mg	Entocort by Astra	Canadian	Steroid
CIS20JANSSEN	Tab, Beige & White, Circular, CIS/20/Janssen	Cisapride 20 mg	Prepulsid by Janssen	Canadian	Gastrointestinal
CIS5JANSSEN	Tab, Beige & White, Circular, CIS/5/Janssen	Cisapride 5 mg	Prepulsid by Janssen	Canadian	Gastrointestinal
CL	Tab, Green & Light Green	Pentaerythritol Tetranitrate 80 mg	Peritrate by Parke-Davis	Canadian	Antianginal
CL	Tab, Green	Pentaerythritol Tetranitrate 80 mg	Peritrate by Parke-Davis	Canadian	Antianginal
CL 209	Tab, Brown, Round	Senna Concentrate 187 mg	Senna-Gen by Concord Labs		Gastrointestinal
CL 600	Tab, White	Gemfibrozil 600 mg	by Altimed	Canadian	Antihyperlipidemic
CL1	Tab, Yellow, Round, CL/1	Isosorbide Dinitrate SL 2.5 mg	Isordil by Geneva		Antianginal
CL15	Tab, White, Round	Nylidrin 12 mg	Arlidin by Geneva		Vasodilator
CL201	Tab, White, Round	Furosemide 40 mg	Lasix by Geneva		Diuretic
CL219	Tab, White, Round, CL 219 <> +	Gualfenesin 200 mg, Ephedrine 25 mg	by Concord		Cold Remedy
CL284	Tab, White, Round	Isoxsuprine 20 mg	Vasodilan by Geneva		Vasodilator
CL300	Cap, Maroon & White	Gemfibrozil 300 mg	by Altimed	Canadian	Antihyperlipidemic
CL400	Tab, Beige, Round	Caffeine 100 mg, Ergotamine Tartrate 1 mg	Cafergot by Geneva	00781-1995	Analgesic
CL400	Tab, Beige, Round	Ergotamine Tartrate 1 mg; Caffeine 100 mg	Ercaf by Allscripts	54569-1996	Antimigraine
CL512	Cap, Green & Yellow	Nitroglycerin SR 9 mg	Nitrobid by Geneva		Vasodilator
CL555	Tab, Lavender, Round, CL55/5	Trifluoperazine HCl 5 mg	Stelazine by Cord		Antipsychotic
CLARITIN10 <> 458	Tab, White	Loratadine 10 mg	Claritin by Patient 1st	57575-0100	Antihistamine
CLARITIN10 <> 458	Tab, White, Round	Loratadine 10 mg	Claritin by Neuman Distbtrs	64579-0251	Antihistamine
CLARITIN10 <> 458	Tab, White, Round	Loratadine 10 mg	Claritin by Natl Pharmpak	55154-3513	Antihistamine
CLARITIN10 <> 458	Tab, White, Oblong	Loratadine 10 mg	Claritin by Southwood Pharms	58016-0560	Antihistamine
CLARITIN10 <> 458	Tab, White, Round, Claritin 10	Loratadine 10 mg	Claritin by Mylan	00378-3358	Antihistamine
CLARITIN10 <> 458	Tab	Loratadine 10 mg	Claritin by HJ Harkins Co	52959-0452	Antihistamine
CLARITIN10 <> 458	Tab, Off-White	Loratadine 10 mg	Claritin by Urgent Care Ctr	50716-0267	Antihistamine
CLARITIN10 <> 458	Tab	Loratadine 10 mg	Claritin by Allscripts	54569-3738	Antihistamine
CLARITIN10 <> 458	Tab	Loratadine 10 mg	Claritin by Direct Dispensing	57866-3500	Antihistamine
CLARITIN10 <> 458	Tab	Loratadine 10 mg	Claritin by Amerisource	62584-0458	Antihistamine
CLARITIN10 <> 458	Tab	Loratadine 10 mg	Claritin by Quality Care	60346-0941	Antihistamine
CLARITIN10 <> 458	Tab	Loratadine 10 mg	Claritin DR by Schering	00085-0458	Antihistamine
CLARITIN10 <> 458	Tab, White, Round	Loratadine 10 mg	Claritin by Compumed	00403-4369	Antihistamine
CLARITIND	Tab, White, Claritin-D	Loratadine 5 mg, Pseudoephedrine Sulfate 120 mg	Claritin D by Schering	00085-0635	Cold Remedy
CLARITIND	Tab, ER, Branded in Green	Loratadine 5 mg, Pseudoephedrine Sulfate 120 mg	Claritin-D by Allscripts	54569-4094	Cold Remedy
CLARITIND	Tab, ER, Branded in Green	Loratadine 5 mg, Pseudoephedrine Sulfate 120 mg	Claritin D by DRX	55045-2263	Cold Remedy
CLARITIND	Tab, ER, Branded in Green	Loratadine 5 mg, Pseudoephedrine Sulfate 120 mg	Claritin D by HJ Harkins Co	52959-0443	Cold Remedy
CLARITIND	Tab, Green Print	Loratadine 5 mg, Pseudoephedrine Sulfate 120 mg	Claritin D by Direct Dispensing	57866-3401	Cold Remedy

ID FRONT <> BACK	DESCRIPTION FRONT <> BACK	INGREDIENT & STRENGTH	BRAND (OR EQUIV.) & FIRM	NDC#	CLASS; SCH.
CLARITIND	Tab, White	Loratadine 5 mg; Pseudoephedrine Sulfate 120 mg	Claritin D by Compumed	00403-5323	Cold Remedy
CLARITIND <> CLARITIND	Tab, Film Coated, Branded in Green	Loratadine 5 mg, Pseudoephedrine Sulfate 120 mg	Claritin D 12 Hr by Caremark	00339-6021	Cold Remedy
CLARITIND24HOUR	Tab, Off-White, Oval, Film Coated, Branded in Black	Loratadine 10 mg, Pseudoephedrine 240 mg	Claritin D 24 Hour by Murfreesboro	51129-1555	Cold Remedy
CLARITIND24HOUR	Tab, Off-White, Oval, Film Coated, Branded in Black	Loratadine 10 mg, Pseudoephedrine Sulfate 240 mg	Claritin D 24 Hr by Schering	00085-1233	Cold Remedy
CLARITIND24HOUR	Tab, Film Coated, Branded in Black	Loratadine 10 mg, Pseudoephedrine Sulfate 240 mg	Claritin D 24 Hr by Caremark	00339-6110	Cold Remedy
CLARITIND24HOUR	Tab, Film Coated, Branded in Black	Loratadine 10 mg, Pseudoephedrine Sulfate 240 mg	Claritin D 24 Hr by Allscripts	54569-4382	Cold Remedy
CLARITIND24HOUR	Tab, White, Round, Film Coated	Loratadine 10 mg; Pseudoephedrine Sulfate 240 mg	Claritin D by Compumed	00403-0915	Cold Remedy
CLEAR <> 59743060	Cap	Brompheniramine Maleate 12 mg, Pseudoephedrine HCl 120 mg	by Qualitest	00603-2505	Cold Remedy
CLEOCIN300MG <> CLEOCIN300MG	Cap	Clindamycin HCl	Cleocin HCl by Pharmacia & Upjohn	00009-0395	Antibiotic
CLEOCIN300MG <> CLEOCIN300MG	Cap	Clindamycin HCl	Cleocin by Nat Pharmpak Serv	55154-3923	Antibiotic
CLINORIL <> MSD942	Tab	Sulindac 150 mg	Clinoril by Merck Sharp and Dohme	62904-0941	NSAID
CLINORIL <> MSD942	Tab, Bright Yellow, Hexagon-Shaped	Sulindac 200 mg	Clinoril by Merck	00006-0942	NSAID
CLINORIL <> MSD942	Tab	Sulindac 200 mg	Clinoril by Allscripts	54569-0268	NSAID
CLINORIL <> MSD942	Tab	Sulindac 200 mg	Clinoril by Merck Sharp and Dohme	62904-0942	NSAID
CLOMID50	Tab, White, Round	Clomiphene Citrate 50 mg	Clomid by Hoechst Marion Roussel	00068-0226	Infertility
CLONAZEPAM	Tab, Blue, Cylindrical	Clonazepam 0.25 mg	by Pharmascience	Canadian	Anticonvulsant
CLONAZEPAMPMS05	Tab, Orange, Cylindrical, Clonazepam/pms/0.5	Clonazepam 0.5 mg	by Pharmascience	Canadian	Anticonvulsant
CLONAZEPAMPMS10	Tab, Pink, Round, Clonazepam/pms/1.0	Clonazepam 1 mg	by Pharmascience	Canadian	Anticonvulsant
CLONAZEPAMPMS20	Tab, White, Cylindrical, Clonazepam/pms/2.0	Clonazepam 2 mg	by Pharmascience	Canadian	Anticonvulsant
CLORAZIL25	Tab, Yellow, Round, Clorazil/25	Clozapine 25 mg	Clozaril by Novartis	Canadian	Antipsychotic
CLOZARIL <> 100	Tab, Pale Yellow, Round, Scored	Clozapine 100 mg	Clozaril by Novartis	00078-0127	Antipsychotic
CLOZARIL <> 100	Tab	Clozapine 100 mg	Clozaril by Physicians Total Care	54868-3576	Antipsychotic
CLOZARIL <> 100	Tab, Yellow, Round, Scored	Clozapine 100 mg	by DHHS Prog	11819-0166	Antipsychotic
CLOZARIL <> 100	Tab, Yellow, Round, Scored	Clozapine 100 mg	Clozaril by Dixon	17236-0303	Antipsychotic
CLOZARIL <> 100MG	Tab, Pale Yellow, Round, Scored	Clozapine 100 mg	Clozaril by Novartis	Canadian DIN# 00894745	Antipsychotic
CLOZARIL <> 25	Tab, Yellow, Round, Scored	Clozapine 25 mg	Clozaril by Direct Dispensing	57866-4421	Antipsychotic
CLOZARIL <> 25	Tab, Yellow, Round, Scored	Clozapine 25 mg	Clozaril by Natl Pharmpak	55154-3412	Antipsychotic
CLOZARIL <> 25	Tab, Pale Yellow, Round, Scored	Clozapine 25 mg	Clozaril by Novartis	00078-0126	Antipsychotic
CLOZARIL <> 25	Tab, Yellow, Round	Clozapine 25 mg	Clozaril by Dista Prod	00777-3107	Antipsychotic
CLOZARIL <> 25	Tab, Yellow, Round, Scored	Clozapine 25 mg	by DHHS Prog	11819-0165	Antipsychotic
CLOZARIL <> 25MG	Tab, Pale Yellow, Round, Scored	Clozapine 25 mg	Clozaril by Novartis	Canadian DIN# 00894737	Antipsychotic
CN05 <> G	Tab, CN over 0.5 <> G	Clonazepam 0.5 mg	by Alphapharm	57315-0017	Anticonvulsant; C IV
CN05 <> G	Tab, Yellow, Round, Scored, CN/0.5 <> G	Clonazepam 0.5 mg	by D M Graham	00756-0269	Anticonvulsant; C IV
CN1 <> G	Tab, CN over 1 <> G	Clonazepam 1 mg	by Alphapharm	57315-0018	Anticonvulsant; C IV
CN1 <> G	Tab, Yellow, Round, Scored, CN/1	Clonazepam 1 mg	by Danbury	61955-2628	Anticonvulsant; C IV
CN2 <> G	Tab, CN over 2 <> G	Clonazepam 2 mg	by Alphapharm	57315-0019	Anticonvulsant; C IV
CN2 <> G	Tab, White, Round, Scored, CN/2	Clonazepam 2 mg	by Danbury	61955-2629	Anticonvulsant; C IV
CNIGHT	Tab, Blue, C-Night	Acetaminophen 650 mg, Pseudoephedrine 60 mg, Diphenhydramine 50 mg	by SmithKline SKB	Canadian	Cold Remedy
CO <> CIBA	Tab, Cream, Round, Film Coated	Maprotiline 10 mg	Ludiomil by Ciba	Canadian DIN# 00641855	Antidepressant
COGENTIN <> MSD60	Tab, White, Round	Benztropine Mesylate 2 mg	Cogentin by Merck	00006-0060	Antiparkinson
COGENTIN <> MSD635	Tab, White, Oval	Benztropine Mesylate 1 mg	Cogentin by Merck	00006-0635	Antiparkinson
COGNEX10	Cap, Dark Green	Tacrine HCl 10 mg	Cognex by Parke Davis	00071-0096	Antialzheimers
COGNEX20	Cap, Light Blue & Yellow	Tacrine HCl 20 mg	Cognex by Parke Davis	00071-0097	Antialzheimers

ID FRONT <> BACK	DESCRIPTION FRONT <> BACK	INGREDIENT & STRENGTH	BRAND (OR EQUIV.) & FIRM	NDC#	CLASS; SCH.
COGNEX30	Cap, Orange & Yellow	Tacrine HCl 30 mg	Cognex by Parke Davis	00071-0095	Antialzheimers
COGNEX40	Cap, Lavender & Yellow,	Tacrine HCl 40 mg	Cognex by Parke Davis	00071-0098	Antialzheimers
COMHIST <> RPC066	Tab	Chlorpheniramine Maleate 2 mg, Phenylephrine HCl 10 mg, Phenyltoloxamine Citrate 25 mg	Comhist by Roberts	54092-0066	Cold Remedy
COMHISTLA <> ROBERTS	Cap	Chlorpheniramine Maleate 4 mg, Phenylephrine HCl 20 mg, Phenyltoloxamine Citrate 50 mg	Comhist LA by Roberts	54092-0065	Cold Remedy; C III
COMPOZ	Tab, White, Oblong	Dyphenhydramine HCl 50 mg	Compoz by Medtech		Antihistamine
COMTAN	Tab, Orange, Oval, Film	Entacapone 200 mg	Comtan by Halsey Drug	00904-5171	Antiparkinson
COMTAN	Tab, Orange, Oval, Film	Entacapone 200 mg	Comtan by Haines	59564-0197	Antiparkinson
COMTAN	Tab, Brownish-Orange, Oval	Entacapone 200 mg	Comtan by Novartis	00078-0003	Antiparkinson
COMTAN	Tab, Brownish Orange, Oval, Film Coated	Entacapone 200 mg	Comtan by Novartis	00078-0327	Antiparkinson
COMTRIMDS <> 9393	Tab	Sulfamethoxazole 800 mg, Trimethoprim 160 mg	SMZ TMP DS by Quality Care	60346-0087	Antibiotic
CONTACT	Cap, Gray & Red	Chlorpheniramine Maleate 12 mg, Phenylpropanolamine 75 mg	by SmithKline SKB	Canadian	Cold Remedy
CONTACTC	Cap, Gray & White, Contact-C	Pseudoephedrine HCl 120 mg	by SmithKline SKB	Canadian	Decongestant
COP <> 014	Tab, Chewable	Sodium Fluoride 1.1 mg	Luride Half Strength by Colgate Oral	00126-0014	Element
COP <> 186	Tab, Chewable	Fluoride Ion 0.25 mg, Sodium Fluoride 0.55 mg	Luride Vanilla by Colgate Oral	00126-0186	Mineral
COP006	Tab, Pink, Round	Sodium Fluoride 1 mg	Luride by Colgate Oral PH.		Element
COPEY <> 150	Tab	Naproxen 500 mg	by Qualitest	00603-4732	NSAID
COPEY <> 443	Tab	Naproxen 375 mg	by Qualitest	00603-4731	NSAID
COPLEY	Tab, Film Coated	Procainamide HCl 750 mg	by Zenith Goldline	00182-1709	Antiarrhythmic
COPLEY <> 111	Tab, Yellowish Tan, Coated	Ascorbic Acid 120 mg, Beta-Carotene 4.2 mg, Calcium Carbonate 490.76 mg, Cholecalciferol 0.49 mg, Cupric Oxide 2.5 mg, Cyanocobalamin 12 mcg, Ferrous Fumarate 197.75 mg, Folic Acid 1 mg, Niacinamide 21 mg, Pyridoxine HCl 10.5 mg, Riboflavin 3.15 mg, Thiamine Mononitrate 1.575 mg, Vitamin A Acetate 8.4 mg, Vitamin E Acetate 44 mg, Zinc Oxide 31.12 mg	Prenatal One Mg Plus Iron by Copley	38245-0111	Vitamin
COPLEY <> 113	Tab, Buff	Chlorpheniramine Tannate 8 mg, Phenylephrine Tannate 25 mg, Pyrilamine Tannate 25 mg	R-Tannate by Schein	00364-2196	Cold Remedy
COPLEY <> 114	Tab, Film Coated	Procainamide HCl 750 mg	by Murfreesboro	51129-1174	Antiarrhythmic
COPLEY <> 114	Tab, Film Coated	Procainamide HCl 750 mg	by HL Moore	00839-7029	Antiarrhythmic
COPLEY <> 114	Tab, Film Coated	Procainamide HCl 750 mg	by Copley	38245-0114	Antiarrhythmic
COPLEY <> 1166	Tab, Orange, Pink & Purple, Chewable	Ascorbic Acid 34.5 mg, Cyanocobalamin 4.9 mcg, Folic Acid 0.35 mg, Niacinamide 14.17 mg, Pyridoxine HCl 1.1 mg, Riboflavin 1.26 mg, Sodium Ascorbate 32.2 mg, Sodium Fluoride 2.21 mg, Thiamine Mononitrate 1.15 mg, Vitamin A Palmitate 5.5 mg, Vitamin D 0.194 mg, Vitamin E Acetate 15.75 mg	Polyvitamin by Schein	00364-1075	Vitamin
COPLEY <> 136	Tab	Metoprolol Tartrate 50 mg	by Copley	38245-0136	Antihypertensive
COPLEY <> 146	Tab, Off-White	Naproxen 250 mg	by Quality Care	60346-0816	NSAID
COPLEY <> 150	Tab, Film Coated	Naproxen Sodium 550 mg	by Prescription Dispensing	61807-0021	NSAID
COPLEY <> 150	Tab, White, Oblong	Naproxen 500 mg	by Southwood Pharms	58016-0289	NSAID
COPLEY <> 150	Tab, Off-White	Naproxen 500 mg	by Quality Care	60346-0815	NSAID
COPLEY <> 150	Tab, Off-White	Naproxen 500 mg	by Copley	38245-0150	NSAID
COPLEY <> 150	Tab, White, Oblong	Naproxen 500 mg	by Nutramax	38206-0400	NSAID
COPLEY <> 152	Tab, Film Coated	Ascorbic Acid 200 mg, Biotin 0.15 mg, Calcium Pantothenate 27.17 mg, Chromic Chloride 0.51 mg, Cupric Oxide 3.75 mg, Cyanocobalamin 50 mcg, Ferrous Fumarate 82.2 mg, Folic Acid 0.8 mg, Magnesium Oxide 82.89 mg, Manganese 50 mg, Manganese Sulfate 15.5 mg, Niacinamide Ascorbate 400 mg, Pyridoxine HCl 30.25 mg, Riboflavin 20 mg, Thiamine Mononitrate 20 mg, Vitamin A Acetate 10.75 mg, Vitamin E Acetate 30 mg, Zinc Oxide 27.99 mg	Berplex Plus by Schein	00364-0814	Vitamin

ID FRONT <> BACK	DESCRIPTION FRONT <> BACK	INGREDIENT & STRENGTH	BRAND (OR EQUIV.) & FIRM	NDC#	CLASS; SCH.
COPLEY <> 152	Tab, Golden Yellow, Film Coated	Ascorbic Acid 200 mg, Biotin 0.15 mg, Calcium Pantothenate 27.17 mg, Chromic Chloride 0.51 mg, Cupric Oxide 3.75 mg, Cyanocobalamin 50 mcg, Ferrous Fumarate 82.2 mg, Folic Acid 0.8 mg, Magnesium Oxide 82.89 mg, Manganese 50 mg, Manganese Sulfate 15.5 mg, Niacinamide Ascorbate 400 mg, Pyridoxine HCl 30.25 mg, Riboflavin 20 mg, Thiamine Mononitrate 20 mg, Vitamin A Acetate 10.75 mg, Vitamin E Acetate 30 mg, Zinc Oxide 27.99 mg	B Complex Vit Plus by Copley	38245-0152	Vitamin
COPLEY <> 158	Tab, Chewable	Ascorbic Acid 34.5 mg, Cyanocobalamin 4.9 mcg, Folic Acid 0.35 mg, Niacinamide 14.16 mg, Pyridoxine HCl 1.1 mg, Riboflavin 1.2 mg, Sodium Ascorbate 32.2 mg, Sodium Fluoride 1.1 mg, Thiamine Mononitrate 1.15 mg, Vitamin A Acetate 5.5 mg, Vitamin D 0.194 mg, Vitamin E Acetate 15.75 mg	Polyvitamin by Schein	00364-1157	Vitamin
COPLEY <> 159	Tab, Chewable	Cholecalciferol 0.194 mg, Cupric Oxide 1.25 mg, Cyanocobalamin 4.9 mcg, Ferrous Fumarate 36.5 mg, Folic Acid 0.35 mg, Niacinamide 14.17 mg, Pyridoxine HCl 1.1 mg, Riboflavin 1.26 mg, Sodium Ascorbate 32.2 mg, Sodium Fluoride 2.21 mg, Thiamine Mononitrate 1.15 mg, Vitamin A Acetate 5.5 mg, Vitamin E 15.75 mg, Zinc Oxide 12.5 mg	Polyvitamin by Schein	00364-0770	Vitamin
COPLEY <> 165	Tab, Film Coated	Ascorbic Acid 17.53 mg, Beta-Carotene 0.56 mg, Calcium Carbonate 249.41 mg, Calcium Pantothenate 4.18 mg, Cholecalciferol 0.25 mg, Cupric Oxide 2.02 mg, Ferrous Fumarate 82.15 mg, Magnesium Oxide 82.93 mg, Niacinamide Ascorbate 8.54 mg, Pyridoxine HCl 2.43 mg, Riboflavin 0.84 mg, Thiamine Mononitrate 1 mg, Vitamin A Acetate 2680 Units, Zinc Oxide 15.56 mg	Prenatal Rx by Copley	38245-0165	Vitamin
COPLEY <> 188	Tab	Procainamide HCl 500 mg	by Zenith Goldline	00182-1708	Antiarrhythmic
COPLEY <> 188	Tab, Pink, Oblong, Film	Procainamide HCl 500 mg	by Quality Care	62682-1014	Antiarrhythmic
COPLEY <> 188	Cap	Procainamide HCl 500 mg	by Qualitest	00603-5411	Antiarrhythmic
COPLEY <> 188	Tab, Ex Release	Procainamide HCl 500 mg	by Copley	38245-0188	Antiarrhythmic
COPLEY <> 188	Tab	Procainamide HCl 500 mg	by HL Moore	00839-7028	Antiarrhythmic
COPLEY <> 197	Tab, Dark Red, Chewable	Ascorbic Acid 34.47 mg, Cholecalciferol 0.194 mg, Cupric Oxide 1.25 mg, Cyanocobalamin 4.9 mcg, Ferrous Fumarate 36.48 mg, Folic Acid 0.35 mg, Niacinamide 14.16 mg, Pyridoxine HCl 1.1 mg, Riboflavin 1.258 mg, Sodium Fluoride 1.1 mg, Thiamine Mononitrate 1.15 mg, Vitamin A Acetate 5.5 mg, Vitamin E Acetate 15.75 mg, Zinc Oxide 12.5 mg	Polyvitamin by Schein	00364-2506	Vitamin
COPLEY <> 225	Tab, Film Coated	Potassium Chloride 600 mg	by Schein	00364-0861	Electrolytes
COPLEY <> 381 381	Tab, Light Green, Rounded Hexagon	Glyburide 3 mg	Micronized by Copley	38245-0381	Antidiabetic
COPLEY <> 381381	Tab, Green, Hexagon, Scored	Glyburide 1.5 mg	by Blue Ridge	59273-0016	Antidiabetic
COPLEY <> 381381	Tab, Green, Hexagon, Scored	Glyburide 3 mg	by Blue Ridge	59273-0017	Antidiabetic
COPLEY <> 381381	Tab, Green, Hexagon, Scored	Glyburide 3 mg	by Kaiser	00179-1336	Antidiabetic
COPLEY <> 381381	Tab	Glyburide 3 mg	Micronized by DRX	55045-2267	Antidiabetic
COPLEY <> 381381	Tab, Green, Hexagon, Scored	Micronized Glyburide	by Neuman Distr	64579-0187	Antidiabetic
COPLEY <> 381381	Tab, Green, Hexagon, Scored	Micronized Glyburide 3 mg	by Neuman Distr	64579-0222	Antidiabetic
COPLEY <> 381381	Tab, Green, Hexagon, Scored	Micronized Glyburide 3 mg	by Neuman Distr	64579-0223	Antidiabetic
COPLEY <> 411	Tab, Shallow Concave	Methazolamide 25 mg	by Copley	38245-0411	Diuretic
COPLEY <> 417	Tab, Light Blue	Metoprolol Tartrate 100 mg	by Copley	38245-0417	Antihypertensive
COPLEY <> 443	Tab, Off-White	Naproxen 375 mg	by Quality Care	60346-0817	NSAID
COPLEY <> 443	Tab, White, Oblong	Naproxen 375 mg	by Nutramax	38206-0201	NSAID
COPLEY <> 443	Tab, Off-White	Naproxen 375 mg	by Copley	38245-0443	NSAID
COPLEY <> 443	Tab, White, Oblong	Naproxen 375 mg	by Southwood Pharms	58016-0267	NSAID
COPLEY <> 643	Tab, Debossed	Prochlorperazine 5 mg	by Qualitest	00603-5418	Antiemetic
COPLEY <> 643	Tab, Film Coated, Debossed	Prochlorperazine Maleate	by UDL	51079-0541	Antiemetic
COPLEY <> 643	Tab, Film Coated	Prochlorperazine Maleate 8.26 mg	by HJ Harkins Co	52959-0511	Antiemetic
COPLEY <> 643	Tab, Film Coated	Prochlorperazine Maleate 8.26 mg	by Quality Care	62682-7046	Antiemetic
COPLEY <> 643	Tab, Film Coated	Prochlorperazine Maleate 8.26 mg	by Copley	38245-0643	Antiemetic
COPLEY <> 652	Tab, Debossed	Prochlorperazine 10 mg	by Qualitest	00603-5419	Antiemetic
COPLEY <> 652	Tab, Film Coated, Debossed	Prochlorperazine Maleate	by UDL	51079-0542	Antiemetic

ID FRONT <> BACK	DESCRIPTION FRONT <> BACK	INGREDIENT & STRENGTH	BRAND (OR EQUIV.) & FIRM	NDC#	CLASS; SCH.
COPLEY <> 652	Tab, Yellow, Round, Film	Prochlorperazine Maleate 10 mg	by Ranbaxy	63304-0655	Antiemetic
COPLEY <> 652	Tab, Yellow, Round, Film Coated	Prochlorperazine Maleate 10 mg	by Phy Total Care	54868-1082	Antiemetic
COPLEY <> 652	Tab, Film Coated	Prochlorperazine Maleate 16.53 mg	by HJ Harkins Co	52959-0476	Antiemetic
COPLEY <> 652	Tab, Film Coated	Prochlorperazine Maleate 16.53 mg	by Copley	38245-0652	Antiemetic
COPLEY <> 712	Tab	Atenolol 50 mg	by Copley	38245-0712	Antihypertensive
COPLEY <> 713	Tab	Atenolol 100 mg	by Copley	38245-0713	Antihypertensive
COPLEY <> 725725	Tab, Pink, Hexagon, Scored	Glyburide 1.5 mg	by Blue Ridge	59273-0016	Antidiabetic
COPLEY <> 725725	Tab, Rounded Hexagon	Glyburide 1.5 mg	Micronized by Merrell	00068-3203	Antidiabetic
COPLEY <> 725725	Tab, Rounded Hexagon	Glyburide 1.5 mg	Micronized by Copley	38245-0725	Antidiabetic
COPLEY <> 725725	Tab, Pink, Hexagon, Scored	Micronized Glyburide	by Neuman Distr	64579-0206	Antidiabetic
COPLEY <> 741	Tab, Light Blue, Film Coated	Naproxen Sodium 275 mg	by Copley	38245-0741	NSAID
COPLEY <> 744	Tab, Film Coated, Debossed	Naproxen Sodium 550 mg	by St Marys Med	60760-0744	NSAID
COPLEY <> 744	Tab, Film Coated	Naproxen Sodium 550 mg	by Copley	38245-0744	NSAID
COPLEY 177	Tab, Blue, Round	Phenylpropanolamine, Brompheniramine, Phenylepherine	Dimetapp by Copley		Cold Remedy
COPLEY0159	Tab, Chewable	Cholecalciferol 0.194 mg, Cupric Oxide 1.25 mg, Cyanocobalamin 4.9 mcg, Ferrous Fumarate 36.5 mg, Folic Acid 0.35 mg, Niacinamide 14.17 mg, Pyridoxine HCl 1.1 mg, Riboflavin 1.26 mg, Sodium Ascorbate 32.2 mg, Sodium Fluoride 2.21 mg, Thiamine Mononitrate 1.15 mg, Vitamin A Acetate 5.5 mg, Vitamin E 15.75 mg, Zinc Oxide 12.5 mg	Multivitamins by Copley	38245-0159	Vitamin
COPLEY0519	Tab, Square	Vitamin 1 mg, Fluoride (Chewable) 1 mg	Poly-Vi-Flor by Copley		Vitamin
COPLEY107	Tab, Peach, Round	Mebendazole 100 mg	by Allscripts	54569-4962	Anthelmintic
COPLEY107	Tab, Peach, Round	Mebendazole 100 mg	by DRX Pharm Consults	55045-2742	Anthelmintic
COPLEY107	Tab, Chew, Debossed	Mebendazole 100 mg	by Physicians Total Care	54868-3732	Anthelmintic
COPLEY107	Tab, Bevel Edge, Chew	Mebendazole 100 mg	by Copley	38245-0107	Anthelmintic
COPLEY111	Tab, Coated	Ascorbic Acid 120 mg, Beta-Carotene 4.2 mg, Calcium Carbonate 490.76 mg, Cholecalciferol 0.49 mg, Cupric Oxide 2.5 mg, Cyanocobalamin 12 mcg, Ferrous Fumarate 197.75 mg, Folic Acid 1 mg, Niacinamide 21 mg, Pyridoxine HCl 10.5 mg, Riboflavin 3.15 mg, Thiamine Mononitrate 1.575 mg, Vitamin A Acetate 8.4 mg, Vitamin E Acetate 44 mg, Zinc Oxide 31.12 mg	Prenatal 1 Mg Plus Iron by Zenith Goldline	00182-4463	Vitamin
COPLEY113	Tab	Chlorpheniramine Tannate 8 mg, Phenylephrine Tannate 25 mg, Pyrilamine Tannate 25 mg	R Tannate by Pharmedix	53002-0480	Cold Remedy
COPLEY113	Tab, Buff	Chlorpheniramine Tannate 8 mg, Phenylephrine Tannate 25 mg, Pyrilamine Tannate 25 mg	R Tannate by Copley	38245-0113	Cold Remedy
COPLEY114	Tab, Buff, Film Coated	Procainamide HCl 750 mg	by Qualitest	00603-5412	Antiarrhythmic
COPLEY114	Tab, Film Coated	Procainamide HCl 750 mg	by United Res	00677-0988	Antiarrhythmic
COPLEY117	Tab, Ex Release	Procainamide HCl 1000 mg	by Copley	38245-0117	Antiarrhythmic
COPLEY123	Tab, Purple, Round	Sodium Fluoride 0.5 mg	Luride by Copley		Element
COPLEY126	Tab, Pink, Oblong	Multivitamin, Folic Acid 500	Iberet Folic 500 by Copley		Vitamin
COPLEY131	Tab, Pink, Round	Sodium Fluoride 2.2 mg	by		Element
COPLEY131	Tab, Chew, Copley over 131	Sodium Fluoride 2.2 mg	by Quality Care	60346-0263	Element
COPLEY131	Tab, Chew	Sodium Fluoride 2.2 mg	by Copley	38245-0131	Element
COPLEY133	Tab, Pink, Round, Scored, Copley over 133	Amiodarone HCl 200 mg	by UDL	51079-0906	Antiarrhythmic
COPLEY133	Tab, Pink, Round, Scored	Amiodarone HCl 200 mg	Amiodarone HCl by Apotheca	12634-0552	Antiarrhythmic
COPLEY133	Tab, Pink, Round, Scored	Amiodarone HCl 200 mg	by Teva	55953-9133	Antiarrhythmic
COPLEY143	Tab, Aqua, Oblong	Salsalate 500 mg	Disalcid by Copley		NSAID
COPLEY144	Tab, Aqua, Oblong	Salsalate 750 mg	Disalcid by Copley		NSAID
COPLEY146	Tab, White, Round	Naproxen 250 mg	by Southwood Pharms	58016-0314	NSAID
COPLEY146	Tab, Off-White	Naproxen 250 mg	by Copley	38245-0146	NSAID
COPLEY146	Tab	Naproxen 250 mg	by Qualitest	00603-4730	NSAID
COPLEY151	Tab, Green	B Complex Vitamins	Berocca by Copley		Vitamin

ID FRONT <> BACK	DESCRIPTION FRONT <> BACK	INGREDIENT & STRENGTH	BRAND (OR EQUIV.) & FIRM	NDC#	CLASS; SCH.
COPLEY158	Tab, Orange, Pink & Purple, Chewable	Ascorbic Acid 34.5 mg, Cyanocobalamin 4.9 mcg, Folic Acid 0.35 mg, Niacinamide 14.16 mg, Pyridoxine HCl 1.1 mg, Riboflavin 1.2 mg, Sodium Ascorbate 32.2 mg, Sodium Fluoride 1.1 mg, Thiamine Mononitrate 1.15 mg, Vitamin A Acetate 5.5 mg, Vitamin D 0.194 mg, Vitamin E Acetate 15.75 mg	Multivitamins by Copley	38245-0158	Vitamin
COPLEY166	Tab, Orange, Pink & Purple, Chewable	Ascorbic Acid 34.5 mg, Cyanocobalamin 4.9 mcg, Folic Acid 0.35 mg, Niacinamide 14.17 mg, Pyridoxine HCl 1.1 mg, Riboflavin 1.26 mg, Sodium Ascorbate 32.2 mg, Sodium Fluoride 2.21 mg, Thiamine Mononitrate 1.15 mg, Vitamin A Palmitate 5.5 mg, Vitamin D 0.194 mg, Vitamin E Acetate 15.75 mg	Multiple Vitamins by Copley	38245-0166	Vitamin
COPLEY169	Tab, White, Oval	Prenatal Vitamin RX	Natalins RX by Copley		Vitamin
COPLEY170	Tab, Blue, Oblong	Prenatal Vitamin, Folic Acid	Pramet FA by Copley		Vitamin
COPLEY175	Tab, Film Coated	Quinidine Sulfate 300 mg	by Copley	38245-0175	Antiarrhythmic
COPLEY176	Tab, Orange & Pink & Purple, Pillow	Triple Vitamins 1 mg, Fluoride 1 mg	Tri-Vi-Flor by Copley		Vitamin
COPLEY188	Tab, Ex Release	Procainamide HCl 500 mg	by United Res	00677-0987	Antiarrhythmic
COPLEY192	Tab, Blue, Oblong	Prenatal Vitamins, Zinc	Zenate by Copley		Vitamin
COPLEY197	Tab, Chewable	Ascorbic Acid 34.47 mg, Cholecalciferol 0.194 mg, Cupric Oxide 1.25 mg, Cyanocobalamin 4.9 mcg, Ferrous Fumarate 36.48 mg, Folic Acid 0.35 mg, Niacinamide 14.16 mg, Pyridoxine HCl 1.1 mg, Riboflavin 1.258 mg, Sodium Fluoride 1.1 mg, Thiamine Mononitrate 1.15 mg, Vitamin A Acetate 5.5 mg, Vitamin E Acetate 15.75 mg, Zinc Oxide 12.5 mg	Multivitamin by DRX	55045-1949	Vitamin
COPLEY197	Tab, Chewable	Ascorbic Acid 34.47 mg, Cholecalciferol 0.194 mg, Cupric Oxide 1.25 mg, Cyanocobalamin 4.9 mcg, Ferrous Fumarate 36.48 mg, Folic Acid 0.35 mg, Niacinamide 14.16 mg, Pyridoxine HCl 1.1 mg, Riboflavin 1.258 mg, Sodium Fluoride 1.1 mg, Thiamine Mononitrate 1.15 mg, Vitamin A Acetate 5.5 mg, Vitamin E Acetate 15.75 mg, Zinc Oxide 12.5 mg	Multivitamins by Copley	38245-0197	Vitamin
COPLEY206	Tab, Blue, Round	Amitriptyline HCl 10 mg	Elavil by Copley		Antidepressant
COPLEY207	Tab, Yellow, Round	Amitriptyline HCl 25 mg	Elavil by Copley		Antidepressant
COPLEY208	Tab, Beige, Round	Amitriptyline HCl 50 mg	Elavil by Copley		Antidepressant
COPLEY209	Tab, Orange, Round	Amitriptyline HCl 75 mg	Elavil by Copley		Antidepressant
COPLEY210	Tab, Pink, Round	Amitriptyline HCl 100 mg	Elavil by Copley		Antidepressant
COPLEY211	Tab, Blue, Oblong	Amitriptyline HCl 150 mg	Elavil by Copley		Antidepressant
COPLEY225	Tab, Film Coated	Potassium Chloride 600 mg	by Geneva	00781-1516	Electrolytes
COPLEY225	Tab, Film Coated	Potassium Chloride 600 mg	by Murfreesboro	51129-8245	Electrolytes
COPLEY225	Tab, Orange, Round, Film Coated, Copley over 225	Potassium Chloride 600 mg	Slow-K by UDL	51079-0744	Electrolytes
COPLEY225	Tab, Film Coated	Potassium Chloride 600 mg	by Pharmedix	53002-1039	Electrolytes
COPLEY225	Tab, Film Coated	Potassium Chloride 600 mg	by Quality Care	60346-0453	Electrolytes
COPLEY225	Tab, Film Coated	Potassium Chloride 600 mg	by Copley	38245-0225	Electrolytes
COPLEY225	Tab, Film Coated	Potassium Chloride 600 mg	by United Res	00677-1096	Electrolytes
COPLEY231	Tab, Peach, Oblong	Choline Magnesium Trisalicylate 500 mg	Trilisate by Copley		NSAID
COPLEY233	Tab, White, Oblong	Choline Magnesium Trisalicylate 750 mg	Trilisate by Copley		NSAID
COPLEY299 <> ACYCLOVIR200	Cap	Acyclovir 200 mg	by Copley	38245-0299	Antiviral
COPLEY312	Tab	Captopril 50 mg	by Copley	38245-0312	Antihypertensive
COPLEY380 <> URSODIOL300MG	Cap, Red & White	Ursodiol 300 mg	Ursodiol by Copley Pharm	38245-0380	Gastrointestinal
COPLEY381	Tab, Green, Hexagonal	Glyburide (Micronized) 3 mg	Glynase by Copley		Antidiabetic
COPLEY411	Tab	Methazolamide 25 mg	by Qualitest	00603-4470	Diuretic
COPLEY424	Tab	Methazolamide 50 mg	by Qualitest	00603-4471	Diuretic
COPLEY424	Tab	Methazolamide 50 mg	by Copley	38245-0424	Diuretic
COPLEY427	Tab	Diclofenac Sodium 75 mg	by Copley	38245-0427	NSAID
COPLEY431	Tab	Diclofenac Sodium 25 mg	by Copley	38245-0431	NSAID
COPLEY447	Tab, Orange, Round	Iodinated Glycerol 30 mg	Organidin by Copley		Expectorant
COPLEY457	Tab, Orange, Oblong	Magnesium Gluconate	by Copley		Mineral

ID FRONT <> BACK	DESCRIPTION FRONT <> BACK	INGREDIENT & STRENGTH	BRAND (OR EQUIV.) & FIRM	NDC#	CLASS; SCH.
COPLEY471	Tab	Captopril 25 mg	by Copley	38245-0471	Antihypertensive
COPLEY472	Tab, Peach, Round, Scored	Pemoline 75 mg	Pemoline by Pharmafab	62542-0410	Stimulant; C IV
COPLEY474	Tab, Pink, Round	Diclofenac Sodium 50 mg	Lodine by HJ Harkins	52959-0436	NSAID
COPLEY474	Tab	Diclofenac Sodium 50 mg	by Copley	38245-0474	NSAID
COPLEY524	Tab, White, Round, Scored	Pemoline 37.5 mg	Pemoline by Pharmafab	62542-0453	Stimulant; C IV
COPLEY524	Tab, White, Round	Pemoline 37.5 mg	by Copley Pharm	38245-0577	Stimulant; C IV
COPLEY541	Tab, Peach, Round, Scored	Pemoline 18.75 mg	by Copley Pharm	38245-0541	Stimulant; C IV
COPLEY631	Tab	Diltiazem HCl 30 mg	by Medirex	57480-0489	Antihypertensive
COPLEY631	Tab	Diltiazem HCl 30 mg	by Geneva	00781-1158	Antihypertensive
COPLEY631	Tab, Film Coated	Diltiazem HCl 30 mg	by Qualitest	00603-3319	Antihypertensive
COPLEY631	Tab	Diltiazem HCl 30 mg	by Copley	38245-0631	Antihypertensive
COPLEY653	Tab	Captopril 100 mg	by Copley	38245-0653	Antihypertensive
COPLEY662	Tab, Film Coated, Copley 662	Diltiazem HCl 60 mg	by Qualitest	00603-3320	Antihypertensive
COPLEY662	Tab	Diltiazem HCl 60 mg	by Medirex	57480-0490	Antihypertensive
COPLEY662	Tab	Diltiazem HCl 60 mg	by Geneva	00781-1159	Antihypertensive
COPLEY662	Tab, Film Coated	Diltiazem HCl 60 mg	by Med Pro	53978-1235	Antihypertensive
COPLEY662	Tab	Diltiazem HCl 60 mg	by Copley	38245-0662	Antihypertensive
COPLEY691	Tab	Diltiazem HCl 90 mg	by Medirex	57480-0491	Antihypertensive
COPLEY691	Tab	Diltiazem HCl 90 mg	by Geneva	00781-1174	Antihypertensive
COPLEY691	Tab, Pale Blue	Diltiazem HCl 90 mg	by Copley	38245-0691	Antihypertensive
COPLEY711 <> 8	Tab	Guanabenz Acetate 10.28 mg	by Copley	38245-0711	Antihypertensive
COPLEY717 <> 4	Tab	Guanabenz Acetate 5.14 mg	by Copley	38245-0717	Antihypertensive
COPLEY720	Tab	Diltiazem HCl 120 mg	by Medirex	57480-0492	Antihypertensive
COPLEY720	Tab, Film Coated, Copley 720	Diltiazem HCl 120 mg	by Qualitest	00603-3322	Antihypertensive
COPLEY720	Tab	Diltiazem HCl 120 mg	by Geneva	00781-1175	Antihypertensive
COPLEY720	Tab	Diltiazem HCl 120 mg	by Copley	38245-0720	Antihypertensive
COPLEY724	Tab	Nadolol 80 mg	Nadolol by Copley	38245-0724	Antihypertensive
COPLEY725	Tab, Pink, Hexagonal	Glyburide (Micronized) 1.5 mg	Glynase by Copley		Antidiabetic
COPLEY727	Tab	Nadolol 120 mg	Nadolol by Copley	38245-0727	Antihypertensive
COPLEY731	Tab	Nadolol 160 mg	Nadolol by Copley	38245-0731	Antihypertensive
COPLEY743	Tab	Captopril 12.5 mg	by Copley	38245-0743	Antihypertensive
COPLEY774	Tab, White, Oblong, Film	Hydroxychloroquine Sulfate 200 mg	by Murfreesboro	51129-1468	Antimalarial
COPLEY774	Tab, Film Coated, Debossed	Hydroxychloroquine Sulfate 200 mg	by Physicians Total Care	54868-3821	Antimalarial
COPLEY774	Tab, Film Coated	Hydroxychloroquine Sulfate 200 mg	by Copley	38245-0774	Antimalarial
COPLEY774	Tab, Coated	Hydroxychloroquine Sulfate 201 mg	by HL Moore	00839-7963	Antimalarial
CORGARD120MG <> BL208	Tab, Light Blue	Nadolol 120 mg	Corgard by ER Squibb	00003-0208	Antihypertensive
CORGARD160MG <> BL246	Tab, Dark Blue	Nadolol 160 mg	Corgard by ER Squibb	00003-0246	Antihypertensive
CORGARD160SQUIBB	Tab, Blue, Oblong, Corgard 160/Squibb	Nadolol 160 mg	Corgard by Squibb	Canadian	Antihypertensive
CORGARD20 <> BL232	Tab, Corgard 20 <> BL Over 232	Nadolol 20 mg	Corgard by ER Squibb	00003-0232	Antihypertensive
CORGARD40	Tab, White, Round	Nadolol 40 mg	Corgard by Squibb	Canadian	Antihypertensive
CORGARD40 <> BL207	Tab, Corgard 40 <> BL Over 207	Nadolol 40 mg	Corgard by ER Squibb	00003-0207	Antihypertensive
CORGARD40 <> BL207	Tab	Nadolol 40 mg	Corgard by Repack Co of Amer	55306-0207	Antihypertensive
CORGARD40 <> BL207	Tab	Nadolol 40 mg	Corgard by Nat Pharmpak Serv	55154-0605	Antihypertensive
CORGARD40 <> PPP207	Tab	Nadolol 40 mg	Nadolol by Pharmedix	53002-1018	Antihypertensive
CORGARD80 <> BL241	Tab, Corgard 80 <> BL/241	Nadolol 80 mg	Corgard by Nat Pharmpak Serv	55154-0604	Antihypertensive
CORGARD80 <> BL241	Tab, Light Blue	Nadolol 80 mg	Corgard by ER Squibb	00003-0241	Antihypertensive
CORGARD80SQUIBB	Tab, White, Round, Corgard 80/Squibb	Nadolol 80 mg	Corgard by Squibb	Canadian	Antihypertensive

ID FRONT <> BACK	DESCRIPTION FRONT <> BACK	INGREDIENT & STRENGTH	BRAND (OR EQUIV.) & FIRM	NDC#	CLASS; SCH.
CORTEF10	Tab, White, Round, Scored	Hydrocortisone 10 mg	Cortef by Upjohn	Canadian DIN# 00030910	Steroid
CORTEF20	Tab, White, Round, Scored	Hydrocortisone 20 mg	Cortef by Upjohn	Canadian DIN# 00030929	Steroid
CORTEF20	Tab	Hydrocortisone 20 mg	Cortef by Murfreesboro	51129-9004	Steroid
CORTEF5	Tab	Hydrocortisone 5 mg	Cortef by Physicians Total Care	54868-3924	Steroid
CORTONE <> MSD219	Tab	Cortisone Acetate 25 mg	by Merck	00006-0219	Steroid
CORZIDE405 <> BL283	Tab, Bluish White to White, Dark Blue Specks, Corzide 40/5 <> BL over 283	Bendroflumethiazide 5 mg, Nadolol 40 mg	Corzide 40 5 by ER Squibb	00003-0283	Diuretic; Antihypertensive
CORZIDE805 <> BL284	Tab, Bluish White to White, Dark Blue Specks, Corzide 80/5 <> BL over 284	Bendroflumethiazide 5 mg, Nadolol 80 mg	Corzide 80 5 by ER Squibb	00003-0284	Diuretic; Antihypertensive
COTAZYMECS20	Cap, Orange, Gelatin w/ Dark Blue Print, Organon Logo Cotazym ECS 20	Amylase 55,000 USP, Lipase 20,000 USP, Proteasse 55,000 USP	Cotazym ECS 20 by Organon	Canadian DIN# 00821373	Gastrointestinal
COTAZYMECS4	Cap, Clear & Pink, Gelatin w/ Dark Blue Print, Organon Logo Cotazym ECS 4	Amylase 11,000 USP, Lipase 4,000 USP, Proteasse 11,000 USP	Cotazym ECS 4 by Organon	Canadian DIN# 02181215	Gastrointestinal
COTAZYMECS8	Cap, Clear, Gelatin w/ Dark Blue Print, Organon Logo Cotazym ECS 8	Amylase 30,000 USP, Lipase 8,000 USP, Proteasse 30,000 USP	Cotazym ECS 8 by Organon	Canadian DIN# 00502790	Gastrointestinal
COTRIM <> 9393	Tab, 93 on Left, 93 on Right	Sulfamethoxazole 400 mg, Trimethoprim 80 mg	SMZ TMP by Quality Care	60346-0559	Antibiotic
COTRIM <> 9393	Tab, White, Round, Scored, Cotrim <> 93 over 93	Sulfamethoxazole 400 mg, Trimethorprim 80 mg	Cotrim by Teva	00093-0188	Antibiotic
COTRIMDS <> 9393	Tab, Cotrim DS <> 93 on Left, 93 on Right	Sulfamethoxazole 800 mg, Trimethoprim 160 mg	SMZ TMP DS by Quality Care	60346-0087	Antibiotic
COTRIMDS <> 9393	Tab, White, Oblong, Scored, Cotrim DS <> 93/93	Sulfamethoxazole 800 mg, Trimethorprim 160 mg	Cotrim DS by Teva	00093-0189	Antibiotic
COUMADIN1	Tab	Warfarin Sodium 1 mg	Coumadin by Caremark	00339-5088	Anticoagulant
COUMADIN1 <> DUPONT	Tab	Warfarin Sodium 1 mg	Coumadin by Nat Pharmpak Serv	55154-7701	Anticoagulant
COUMADIN1 <> DUPONT	Tab, Pink, Round, Scored	Warfarin Sodium 1 mg	Coumadin by Eckerd	19458-0907	Anticoagulant
COUMADIN1 <> DUPONT	Tab, Pink, Round, Scored	Warfarin Sodium 1 mg	Coumadin by Du Pont Pharma	00056-0169	Anticoagulant
COUMADIN1 <> DUPONT	Tab	Warfarin Sodium 1 mg	by Med Pro	53978-3302	Anticoagulant
COUMADIN10 <> DUPONT	Tab, White, Round, Scored	Warfarin Sodium 10 mg	Coumadin by Dupont Pharma	00056-0174	Anticoagulant
COUMADIN10 <> DUPONT	Tab	Warfarin Sodium 10 mg	Coumadin by Nat Pharmpak Serv	55154-7707	Anticoagulant
COUMADIN10DUPONT	Tab, White, Coumadin/10/Dupont	Warfarin Sodium 10 mg	Coumadin by Dupont	Canadian	Anticoagulant
COUMADIN1DUPONT	Tab, Pink, Coumadin/1/Dupont	Warfarin Sodium 1 mg	Coumadin by Dupont	Canadian	Anticoagulant
COUMADIN2 <> DUPONT	Tab, Lavender, Round, Scored	Warfarin Sodium 2 mg	Coumadin by Dupont Pharma	00056-0170	Anticoagulant
COUMADIN2 <> DUPONT	Tab, Lavender, on One Face, the Number is Superimposed	Warfarin Sodium 2 mg	Coumadin by PDRX	55289-0143	Anticoagulant
COUMADIN2 <> DUPONT	Tab, Purple, Round, Scored, Coumadin on Top of Line and 2 on Line	Warfarin Sodium 2 mg	Coumadin by Thrift Drug	59198-0346	Anticoagulant
COUMADIN2 <> DUPONT	Tab, Lavender, Coumadin/2 <> Dupont	Warfarin Sodium 2 mg	Coumadin by Amerisource	62584-0348	Anticoagulant
COUMADIN2 <> DUPONT	Tab, Lavender	Warfarin Sodium 2 mg	Coumadin by Nat Pharmpak Serv	55154-7702	Anticoagulant

ID FRONT <> BACK	DESCRIPTION FRONT <> BACK	INGREDIENT & STRENGTH	BRAND (OR EQUIV.) & FIRM	NDC#	CLASS; SCH.
COUMADIN2 <> DUPONT	Tab, Purple, Round, Scored	Warfarin Sodium 2 mg	Coumadin by Eckerd	19458-0908	Anticoagulant
COUMADIN212 <> DUPONT	Tab, Coumadin over 2 1/2	Warfarin Sodium 2.5 mg	Coumadin by Quality Care	60346-0918	Anticoagulant
COUMADIN212 <> DUPONT	Tab, Green	Warfarin Sodium 2.5 mg	Coumadin by Dupont	Canadian	Anticoagulant
COUMADIN212 <> DUPONT	Tab, Green, Round, Scored, Coumadin 2 1/2 <> Dupont	Warfarin Sodium 2.5 mg	Coumadin by Dupont Pharma	00056-0176	Anticoagulant
COUMADIN212 <> DUPONT	Tab, Coumadin Inscribed with 2 1/2 Superimposed <> Inscribed	Warfarin Sodium 2.5 mg	Coumadin by Caremark	00339-5087	Anticoagulant
COUMADIN212 <> DUPONT	Tab, Coumadin 2 1/2	Warfarin Sodium 2.5 mg	by Med Pro	53978-3301	Anticoagulant
COUMADIN212 <> DUPONT	Tab, Coumadin 2 1/2	Warfarin Sodium 2.5 mg	Coumadin by Nat Pharmpak Serv	55154-7703	Anticoagulant
COUMADIN212DUPO	Tab, Coumadin 2 1/2 Dupont	Warfarin Sodium 2.5 mg	Coumadin by Allscripts	54569-0212	Anticoagulant
COUMADIN25 <> DUPONT	Tab, Green, Round, 2.5, Scored	Warfarin Sodium 2.5 mg	Coumadin by Eckerd	19458-0909	Anticoagulant
COUMADIN2DUPONT	Tab, Lavender, Coumadin/2/Dupont	Warfarin Sodium 2 mg	Coumadin by Dupont	Canadian	Anticoagulant
COUMADIN3 <> DUPONT	Tab, Tan, Round, Scored	Warfarin Sodium 3 mg	Coumadin by Dupont Pharma	00056-0188	Anticoagulant
COUMADIN3 <> DUPONT	Tab, Tan, Round, Scored	Warfarin Sodium 3 mg	Coumadin by Eckerd	19458-0910	Anticoagulant
COUMADIN4 <> DUPONT	Tab, Blue, Round, Scored	Warfarin Sodium 4 mg	Coumadin by Du Pont Pharma	00056-0168	Anticoagulant
COUMADIN4 <> DUPONT	Tab, Blue, Round, Scored	Warfarin Sodium 4 mg	Coumadin by Eckerd	19458-0911	Anticoagulant
COUMADIN4DUPONT	Tab, Blue, Coumadin/4/Dupont	Warfarin Sodium 4 mg	Coumadin by Dupont	Canadian	Anticoagulant
COUMADIN5 <> DUPONT	Tab, Peach, Round, Scored	Warfarin Sodium 5 mg	Coumadin by Dupont Pharma	00056-0172	Anticoagulant
COUMADIN5 <> DUPONT	Tab, Coumadin Inscribed, 5 Superimposed	Warfarin Sodium 5 mg	Coumadin by Caremark	00339-5089	Anticoagulant
COUMADIN5 <> DUPONT	Tab	Warfarin Sodium 5 mg	Coumadin by Allscripts	54569-0159	Anticoagulant
COUMADIN5 <> DUPONT	Tab, 5 Superimposed	Warfarin Sodium 5 mg	by Med Pro	53978-0314	Anticoagulant
COUMADIN5 <> DUPONT	Tab, Superimposed	Warfarin Sodium 5 mg	Coumadin by Amerisource	62584-0172	Anticoagulant
COUMADIN5 <> DUPONT	Tab, Peach, Round, Scored, Coumadin on Top of Line and 5 on Line	Warfarin Sodium 5 mg	Coumadin by Thrift Drug	59198-0347	Anticoagulant
COUMADIN5 <> DUPONT	Tab, 5 Superimposed	Warfarin Sodium 5 mg	Coumadin by Nat Pharmpak Serv	55154-7704	Anticoagulant
COUMADIN5 <> DUPONT	Tab, Peach, Round, Scored	Warfarin Sodium 5 mg	Coumadin by Eckerd	19458-0912	Anticoagulant
COUMADIN5DUPONT	Tab, Peach, Coumadin/5/Dupont	Warfarin Sodium 5 mg	Coumadin by Dupont	Canadian	Anticoagulant
COUMADIN6 <> DUPONT	Tab, Teal, Round, Coated	Warfarin Sodium 6 mg	Coumadin by Dupont Pharma	00056-0189	Anticoagulant
COUMADIN712 <> DUPONT	Tab, Yellow, Round, Scored, Coumadin 7 1/2 <> Dupont	Warfarin Sodium 7.5 mg	Coumadin by Dupont Pharma	00056-0173	Anticoagulant
COUMADIN712 <> DUPONT	Tab, Coumadin 7 1/2	Warfarin Sodium 7.5 mg	Coumadin by Nat Pharmpak Serv	55154-7706	Anticoagulant
COVERAHS2011	Tab, Lavender, Round, Film Coated, Covera-HS 2011	Verapamil HCl 180 mg	Covera HS by GD Searle	00025-2011	Antihypertensive
COVERAHS2021	Tab, Pale Yellow, Round, Film Coated, Covera-HS 2021	Verapamil HCl 240 mg	Covera HS by GD Searle	00025-2021	Antihypertensive

ID FRONT <> BACK	DESCRIPTION FRONT <> BACK	INGREDIENT & STRENGTH	BRAND (OR EQUIV.) & FIRM	NDC#	CLASS; SCH.
COVERAHS2021	Tab, Film Coated, Covera-HS 2021	Verapamil HCl 240 mg	Covera HS by Caremark	00339-5884	Antihypertensive
COZAAR <> MRK952	Tab, Green, Oval, Film Coated	Losartan Potassium 50 mg	Cozaar by Phy Total Care	54868-3726	Antihypertensive
COZAAR <> MRK952	Tab, Teardrop, Film Coated	Losartan Potassium 50 mg	Cozaar by Nat Pharmpak Serv	55154-5016	Antihypertensive
CP <> 266	Tab, Coated, Imprinted in Black Ink	Thioridazine HCl 25 mg	by Heartland	61392-0463	Antipsychotic
CP <> 270	Tab, Coated	Thioridazine HCl 200 mg	by Creighton Prod	50752-0270	Antipsychotic
CP <> 275	Tab, Creighton	Acetaminophen 325 mg, Butalbital 50 mg, Caffeine 40 mg	by Quality Care	60346-0703	Analgesic
CP <> 275	Tab	Acetaminophen 325 mg, Butalbital 50 mg, Caffeine 40 mg	Fiorpap by Creighton Prod	50752-0275	Analgesic
CP250 <> NORTRIPTYLINE10	Cap	Nortriptyline 10 mg	by Creighton Prod	50752-0250	Antidepressant
CP251 <> NORTRIPTYLINE25	Cap, Green & White, Opaque	Nortriptyline HCl	by Quality Care	60346-0757	Antidepressant
CP252	Cap, Green & Yellow	Nortriptyline HCl 50 mg	Pamelor by Creighton		Antidepressant
CP253	Cap, Green	Nortriptyline HCl 75 mg	Aventyl HCl by Novartis		Antidepressant
CP253	Cap, Green	Nortriptyline HCl 75 mg	Pamelor by Geneva	00781-2633	Antidepressant
CP262	Tab, White, Round	Bromocriptine 2.5 mg	Parlodel by Novartis		Antiparkinson
CP264	Tab, Yellow Green, Round	Thioridazine 10 mg	Mellaril by Creighton		Antipsychotic
CP265	Tab, White, Round	Thioridazine 15 mg	Mellaril by Creighton		Antipsychotic
CP267	Tab, White, Round	Thioridazine 50 mg	Mellaril by Creighton		Antipsychotic
CP268	Tab, Coated	Thioridazine HCl 100 mg	by Creighton Prod	50752-0268	Antipsychotic
CP269	Tab, Yellow, Round	Thioridazine 150 mg	Mellaril by Creighton		Antipsychotic
CP271	Cap, Pink & White	Temazepam 7.5 mg	Restoril by Creighton		Sedative/Hypnotic; C IV
CP271	Cap, Pink & White	Temazepam 7.5 mg	Restoril by Geneva	00781-2209	Sedative/Hypnotic; C IV
CP272	Cap, Aqua & White	Temazepam 15 mg	Restoril by Creighton		Sedative/Hypnotic; C IV
CP273	Cap, Aqua	Temazepam 30 mg	Restoril by Creighton		Sedative/Hypnotic; C IV
CP277	Tab, White, Round	Butalbital 50 mg, Aspirin 325 mg, Caffeine 40 mg	Fiorinal by Creighton		Analgesic
CP278	Cap, Green & Lime Green	Butalbital 50 mg, Aspirin 325 mg, Caffeine 40 mg	Fiorinal by Geneva	00781-2120	Analgesic
CP278	Cap, Green	Butalbital 50 mg, Aspirin 325 mg, Caffeine 40 mg	Fiorinal by Novartis		Analgesic
CP279	Cap, Blue & Yellow	Aspirin 325 mg, Butalbital 50 mg, Caffeine 40 mg, Codeine Phosphate 30 mg	by Quality Care	60346-0738	Analgesic; C III
CP279	Cap, Blue & Yellow	Codeine 30 mg, Butalbital 50 mg, Caffeine 40 mg, Aspirin 325 mg	Fiorinal with Codeine by Geneva	00781-2221	Analgesic; C III
CP279	Cap, Blue & Yellow	Codeine 30 mg, Butalbital 50 mg, Caffeine 40 mg, Aspirin 325 mg	Fiorinal with Codeine by Novartis		Analgesic; C III
CP800	Cap	Ampicillin Trihydrate	by Medpharm	62780-0657	Antibiotic
CP800	Cap, Gray & Red, Opaque	Ampicillin 250 mg	by Bayer	12527-2885	Antibiotic
CP800	Cap, Scarlet	Ampicillin Trihydrate	by Consolidated Pharmaceutical Group	61423-0800	Antibiotic
CP805	Cap, Scarlet	Ampicillin Trihydrate 500 mg	by Consolidated Pharmaceutical Group	61423-0805	Antibiotic
CP805	Cap, Gray & Red, Opaque	Ampicillin 500 mg	by Bertek	62794-0001	Antibiotic
CP820	Cap, Buff and Caramel	Amoxicillin Trihydrate	by Consolidated Pharmaceutical Group	61423-0820	Antibiotic
CP820	Cap, Beige & Caramel	Amoxicillin Trihydrate	by Medpharm	62780-0658	Antibiotic
CP820	Cap	Amoxicillin Trihydrate	by Qualitest	00603-2266	Antibiotic
CP820	Cap	Amoxicillin Trihydrate	by Richmond	54738-0108	Antibiotic
CP820	Cap, Beige & Brown	Amoxicillin 250 mg	by Barr	00555-0728	Antibiotic
CP825	Cap, Buff	Amoxicillin Trihydrate	by Consolidated Pharmaceutical Group	61423-0825	Antibiotic
CP825	Cap, Buff	Amoxicillin Trihydrate	by Qualitest	00603-2267	Antibiotic
CP825	Cap, Buff	Amoxicillin Trihydrate	by Richmond	54738-0110	Antibiotic
CP825	Cap, Beige	Amoxicillin 500 mg	by Barr	00555-0729	Antibiotic
CP840	Tab, White, Oval	Penicillin V Potassium 250 mg	by Pharmafab	62542-0691	Antibiotic
CP840	Tab	Penicillin V Potassium	by Richmond	54738-0122	Antibiotic
CP840	Tab	Penicillin V Potassium	by Medpharm	62780-0659	Antibiotic
CP840	Tab	Penicillin V Potassium	by Consolidated Pharmaceutical Group	61423-0840	Antibiotic
CP845	Tab	Penicillin V Potassium	by Richmond	54738-0123	Antibiotic
CP845	Tab	Penicillin V Potassium	by Consolidated Pharmaceutical Group	61423-0845	Antibiotic
CP845	Tab, White, Oval	Penicillin V Potassium 500 mg	by Pharmafab	62542-0704	Antibiotic

ID FRONT <> BACK	DESCRIPTION FRONT <> BACK	INGREDIENT & STRENGTH	BRAND (OR EQUIV.) & FIRM	NDC#	CLASS; SCH.
CPC1121	Tab, White, Oval, CPC 11/21	Elemental Iron 90 mg, Calcium 200 mg, Zinc 25 mg, Vitamin A 4000 IU, Vitamin D3 400 IU, Vitamin E 30 IU, Vitamin C 120 mg, Docusate Sodium 50 mg	Prenate 90 by Breckenridge	51991-0152	Vitamin/Mineral
CPC1125	Tab, White	Prenatal Vitamins	Vernate Advanced by Rugby		Vitamin
CPC1167	Tab, Brown, Round	Phenazopyridine HCl 95 mg	UTI Relief by Consumers Choice Systems	61814-9505	Urinary Analgesic
CPC120	Tab, Yellow, Round	Folic Acid 1 mg	by Contract Pharmacal		Vitamin
CPC120	Cap, Clear & Coral	Hyoscyamine Sulfate 0.375 mg	Levsinex by Pecos Pharmaceuticals		Gastrointestinal
CPC1620	Cap	Hyoscyamine Sulfate 0.375 mg	by Mutual	53489-0240	Gastrointestinal
CPC1620	Tab	Hyoscyamine Sulfate 0.375 mg	by Zenith Goldline	00182-1993	Gastrointestinal
CPC1620	Cap	Hyoscyamine Sulfate 0.375 mg	by Rugby	00536-5592	Gastrointestinal
CPC1620	Cap	Hyoscyamine Sulfate 0.375 mg	by Lini	58215-0305	Gastrointestinal
CPC1620	Cap, Brown & White Beads	Hyoscyamine Sulfate 0.375 mg	by United Res	00677-1507	Gastrointestinal
CPC1620	Cap	Hyoscyamine Sulfate 0.375 mg	by Pecos	59879-0109	Gastrointestinal
CPC1620	Cap, Brown & White Beads	Hyoscyamine Sulfate 0.375 mg	by Major	00904-7833	Gastrointestinal
CPC1667	Tab, Red, Round	Phenazopyridine 97 mg	Re-Azo by Reese	10956-0551	Urinary Analgesic
CPC1724	Tab, Blue, Round, Film Coated	Methenamine 40.8 mg, Benzoic Acid 4.5 mg, Phenyl Salicylate 18.1 mg; Methylene Blue 5.4 mg; Hyoscyamine Sulfate 0.03 mg, Atropine Sulfate 0.03 mg	by Contract Pharma	10267-1724	Antibiotic; Urinary Tract
CPC1991	Tab, Beige, Oval	Vitamin A 5000 IU, Vitamin D3 400 IU, Vitamin E 30 IU, Vitamin C 120 mg, Calcium 200 mg	Materna by Breckenridge	51991-0155	Vitamin
CPC365	Cap, Orange & Yellow	Acetaminophen 325 mg, Phenylpropanolamine 12.5 mg, Chlorpheniramine 2 mg, Dextromethorphan 10 mg	Multi Symptom Cold Relief by Contract		Cold Remedy
CPC3712	Cap, White, CPC 37 1/2	Phenylpropanolamine HCl 37.5 mg	Phenylpropanolamine by Quality Care		Decongestant; Appetite Suppressant
CPC464	Cap, Brown & Red	Liver Stomach Concentrate 240 mg, Vitamin B12 15 mcg, Iron 110 mg, Asorbic Acid 75 mg, Folic Acid 0.5 mg	Ferocon by Breckenridge	51991-0635	Vitamin
CPC464	Cap, Brown & Red	Multivitamin, Mineral	Trinsicon by Moore		Vitamin
CPC465	Cap, Orange	Phenylpropanolamine HCl (Timed Release) 75 mg	Just-One-Per-Day by Reese	10956-0603	Decongestant; Appetite Suppressant
CPC836	Cap, Pink	Diphenhydramine 50 mg	Benadryl		Antihistamine
CPC860	Tab, Red, Cap Shaped	Phenazopyridine HCl 200 mg	Pyridium by Breckenridge	51991-0525	Urinary Analgesic
CPC860	Cap, Red	Phenazopyridine HCl 200 mg	by Breckenridge	51991-0525	Urinary Analgesic
CPI	Tab, CPI Logo	Aprobarbital 25 mg, Butabarbital Sodium 50 mg, Phenobarbital 25 mg	Triple Barbital by Century	00436-0198	Sedative; C IV
CPI	Tab, CPI Logo	Phenobarbital 7.5 mg	by Century	00436-0864	Sedative/Hypnotic; C IV
CPI <> 2	Tab, CPI Logo	Phenobarbital 30 mg	by Century	00436-0869	Sedative/Hypnotic; C IV
CPI <> 2	Tab, CPI Logo	Phenobarbital 30 mg	by Century	00436-0129	Sedative/Hypnotic; C IV
CPI <> 2	Tab, CPI Logo	Phenobarbital 30 mg	by Century	00436-0870	Sedative/Hypnotic; C IV
CPI <> 4	Tab, CPI Logo	Phenobarbital 16.2 mg	by Century	00436-0867	Sedative/Hypnotic; C IV
CPI <> 4	Tab, CPI Logo	Phenobarbital 16.2 mg	by Century	00436-0866	Sedative/Hypnotic; C IV
CPI107	Tab, Peach, Round	Mebendazole 100 mg	Vermox by Copley		Antihelmintic
CPI111	Tab, Yellow, Oval	Prenatal Vitamin + Iron 1 mg	Stuartnatal Plus by Copley		Vitamin
CPI113	Tab, Off-White, Oblong	Phenylephrine 25 mg, Chlorpheniramine 8 mg, Pyrilamine 25 mg	Rynatan by Copley		Cold Remedy
CPI114	Tab, Orange, Oblong	Procainamide HCl ER 750 mg	Procan SR by Copley		Antiarrhythmic
CPI117	Tab, Red, Oblong	Procainamide HCl ER 1000 mg	Procan SR by Copley		Antiarrhythmic
CPI131	Tab, Pink, Round	Sodium Fluoride 2.2 mg	Luride by Copley		Element
CPI135	Tab, White, Oval	Doxylamine Succinate 25 mg	Unisom by Copley		Sleep Aid
CPI146	Tab, Off-White, Round	Naproxen 250 mg	Naprosyn by Copley		NSAID
CPI150	Tab, Off-White, Oblong	Naproxen 500 mg	Naprosyn by Copley		NSAID
CPI152	Tab, Yellow, Oval	B Complex Vitamin Plus	Berocca Plus by Copley		Vitamin
CPI158	Tab, Orange or Pink or Purple, Square	Multivitamins, Fluoride 0.5 mg	Poly-Vi-Flor 0.5mg by Copley		Vitamin
CPI159	Tab, Purple, Square	Multivitamins 1 mg, Fluoride + Iron 1 mg	Poly-Vi-Flor w Iron by Copley		Vitamin
CPI166	Tab, Orange or Pink or Purple, Square	Multivitamins 1 mg, Fluoride 1 mg	Poly-Vi-Flor 1mg by Copley		Vitamin
CPI169	Tab, White, Oval	Prenatal Vitamin RX	Natalins RX by Copley		Vitamin

ID FRONT <> BACK	DESCRIPTION FRONT <> BACK	INGREDIENT & STRENGTH	BRAND (OR EQUIV.) & FIRM	NDC#	CLASS; SCH.
CPI175	Tab, White, Round	Quinidine Sulfate ER 300 mg	Quinidex by Copley		Antiarrhythmic
CPI177	Tab, Blue, Round	Bromatapp E.R.	Dimetapp by Copley		Cold Remedy
CPI188	Tab, Orange, Oblong	Procainamide HCl ER 500 mg	Procan SR by Copley		Antiarrhythmic
CPI197	Tab, Pink, Square	Multivitamin, Fluoride + Iron 0.5 mg	Poly-Vi-Flor w Iron by Copley		Vitamin
CPI225	Tab, Orange, Round	Potassium Chloride ER 600 mg (8 mEq)	Slow K by Copley		Electrolytes
CPI312	White	Captopril 50 mg	Capoten by Copley		Antihypertensive
CPI381	Tab, Green, Hexagonal	Glyburide (Micronized) 3 mg	Glynase by Copley		Antidiabetic
CPI411	Tab, White, Square	Methazolamide 25 mg	Neptazane by Copley		Diuretic
CPI424	Tab, White, Round	Methazolamide 50 mg	Neptazane by Copley		Diuretic
CPI443	Tab, Off-White, Oblong	Naproxen 375 mg	Naprosyn by Copley		NSAID
CPI471	Tab, White, Round	Captopril 25 mg	Capoten by Copley		Antihypertensive
CPI514	Tab, White, Oval	Prenatal Vitamin, Zinc	Zenate by Copley		Vitamin
CPI631	Tab, Blue, Round	Diltiazem HCl 30 mg	Cardizem by Copley		Antihypertensive
CPI643	Tab, Yellow, Round	Prochlorperazine 5 mg	Compazine by Copley		Antiemetic
CPI652	Tab, Yellow, Round	Prochlorperazine 10 mg	Compazine by Copley		Antiemetic
CPI653	White	Captopril 100 mg	Capoten by Copley		Antihypertensive
CPI662	Tab, White, Round	Diltiazem HCl 60 mg	Cardizem by Copley		Antihypertensive
CPI691	Tab, Blue, Oblong	Diltiazem HCl 90 mg	Cardizem by Copley		Antihypertensive
CPI711	Tab, Peach, Square	Guanabenz Acetate 8 mg	Wytensin by Copley		Antihypertensive
CPI717	Tab, Peach, Square	Guanabenz Acetate 4 mg	Wytensin by Copley		Antihypertensive
CPI720	Tab, White, Oblong	Diltiazem HCl 120 mg	Cardizem by Copley		Antihypertensive
CPI724	Tab, Blue, Round	Nadolol 80 mg	Corgard by Copley		Antihypertensive
CPI725	Tab, Pink, Hexagonal	Glyburide (Micronized) 1.5 mg	Glynase by Copley		Antidiabetic
CPI727	Tab, Blue, Oblong	Nadolol 120 mg	Corgard by Copley		Antihypertensive
CPI731	Tab, Blue, Oblong	Nadolol 160 mg	Corgard by Copley		Antihypertensive
CPI743	Tab, White, Round	Captopril 12.5 mg	Capoten by Copley		Antihypertensive
CPI774	Tab, White, Oblong	Hydroxychloroquine Sulfate 200 mg	Plaquenil by Copley		Antimalarial
CPL	Tab, Blue & Green, Round, CPL Logo	Chlorpheniramine Maleate 2 mg, Phenylephrine HCl 5 mg	Hista Tab Plus by Century	00436-0633	Cold Remedy
CPM <> PSE	Cap, Blue & Clear	Chlorpheniramine Maleate 8 mg, Pseudoephedrine HCl 120 mg	CPM PSEH 08 by Compumed	00403-0010	Cold Remedy
CPMPSE	Cap, Blue & Clear	Chlorpheniramine Maleate 8 mg, Pseudoephedrine HCl 120 mg	by Allscripts	54569-4122	Cold Remedy
CPMPSE	Cap, Blue, CPM over PSE	Chlorpheniramine Maleate 8 mg; Pseudoephedrine HCl 120 mg	by Pfab	62542-0260	Cold Remedy
CPW5088	Cap, Blue & Clear, Blue & White Beads, CPW 50-88	Caffeine 200 mg	Fastlene by BDI		Stimulant
CPW50888	Cap, Black, CPW 50-888	Caffeine 200 mg	Dextrophin by Clifton Pharm.		Stimulant
CPW50888	Cap, Black, CPW 50-888	Caffeine 250 mg	Dextrophin by Clifton Pharm.		Stimulant
CPW50888	Cap, Black, CPW 50-888	Caffeine 350 mg	Dextrophin by Clifton Pharm.		Stimulant
CRIXIVAN200MG	Cap, Opaque & White	Indinavir 200 mg	by MSD	Canadian	Antiviral
CRIXIVAN200MG	Cap	Indinavir Sulfate 200 mg	Crixivan by Merck	00006-0571	Antiviral
CRIXIVAN400	Cap, White	Indinavir Sulfate 400 mg	Crixivan by Murfreesboro	51129-1546	Antiviral
CRIXIVAN400MG	Cap, Opaque & White	Indinavir 400 mg	by MSD	Canadian	Antiviral
CRIXIVAN400MG	Cap, White	Indinavir Sulfate 400 mg	Crixivan by Murfreesboro Ph	51129-1651	Antiviral
CRIXIVAN400MG	Cap	Indinavir Sulfate 400 mg	Crixivan by Merck	00006-0573	Antiviral
CRIXIVAN400MG	Cap, White, in Green Ink	Indinavir Sulfate 400 mg	Crixivan by Murfreesboro	51129-1547	Antiviral
CRIXIVAN400MG	Cap, White, in Green Ink	Indinavir Sulfate 400 mg	Crixivan by Murfreesboro	51129-1544	Antiviral
CS11SILVER	Tab, Gray, Oblong, CS 11-Silver	Multivitamin, Minerals	Centrum Silver by Lederle		Vitamin
CSCOTT <> 110	Tab, Sugar Coated, C Scott	Thyroid 1 gr	by JMI Canton	00252-7007	Thyroid
CT937	Tab, White, Round	Calcium Lactate 10 gr	by Fresh		Vitamin/Mineral
CTI101	Tab, White, Round	Diclofenac Sodium 25 mg	Diclofenac Sodium DR by DRX	55045-2681	NSAID
CTI102	Tab, White, Round	Diclofenac Sodium 50 mg	Diclofenac Sodium DR by DRX	55045-2682	NSAID
CTI103	Tab, White, Round	Diclofenac Sodium 75 mg	Diclofenac Sodium DR by DRX	55045-2685	NSAID
CTI112	Tab, White, Oval	Acyclovir 400 mg	Acyclovir USP by Amerisource	62584-0798	Antiviral
CTI113	Tab, White, Oval	Acyclovir 800 mg	Acyclovir by Amerisource	62584-0816	Antiviral
CTX088	Tab, Peach & White, Oblong, Scored, Film Coated	Acetaminophen 500 mg, Phenylephrine HCl 40 mg, Chlorpheniramine Maleate 8 mg	Histex SR by Alphapharm	57315-0012	Cold Remedy

ID FRONT <> BACK	DESCRIPTION FRONT <> BACK	INGREDIENT & STRENGTH	BRAND (OR EQUIV.) & FIRM	NDC#	CLASS; SCH.
CY	Tab, White, Cap Shaped, Film Coated, CY engraved in arcs	Tranexamic Acid 500 mg	by Pharmacia	Canadian DIN# 02064405	Hemostatic
CY	Tab, White, Round	Tranexamic Acid 500 mg	Cyklokapron by Pharmacia		Hemostatic
CY250	Cap, Green, CY250/Syntex Logo	Ganciclovir Sodium 250 mg	Cytovene by Roche	Canadian	Antiviral
CY4	Tab, White	Cyproheptadine HCl 4 mg	by Pharmascience	Canadian	Antihistamine
CYCRIN	Tab, Peach, Oval	Medroxyprogesterone Acetate 10 mg	Cycrin by ESI Lederle		Progestin
CYCRIN <> C	Tab, Light Purple, Oval	Medroxyprogesterone Acetate 5 mg	Cycrin by ESI Lederle	59911-5897	Progestin
CYCRIN <> C	Tab, Peach, Oval, Scored	Medroxyprogesterone Acetate 10 mg	by Southwood Pharms	58016-0926	Progestin
CYCRIN <> C	Tab, Purple, Oval, Scored	Medroxyprogesterone Acetate 5 mg	by Kaiser Fdn Health	62224-4334	Progestin
CYCRIN <> C	Tab, Purple, Oval, Opposing C	MedroxyproGesterone Acetate 5 mg	by Nat Pharmpak Serv	55154-5577	Progestin
CYCRIN <> OPPOSINGCS	Tab, Debossed, Cycrin <> Opposing C's	Medroxyprogesterone Acetate 10 mg	by Kaiser	62224-4331	Progestin
CYSTA50 <> MYLAN	Cap, Cysta over 50	Cysteamine Bitartrate	Cystagon by Mylan	00378-9040	Nephropathic Cystimosis
CYSTAGON150 <> MYLAN	Cap, Cystagon over 150	Cysteamine Bitartrate	Cystagon by Mylan	00378-9045	Nephropathic Cystimosis
CYTOVENE250 <> ROCHE	Cap, Gelatin Coated	Ganciclovir 250 mg	Cytovene by Hoffmann La Roche	00004-0269	Antiviral
CYTOVENE250 <> ROCHE	Cap	Ganciclovir 250 mg	Cytovene by Syntex	18393-0269	Antiviral
CYTOVENE50 <> ROCHE	Cap, Dark Blue Print, 2 Blue Bands	Ganciclovir 500 mg	Cytovene by Syntex	18393-0914	Antiviral
CYTOVENE500 <> ROCHE	Cap	Ganciclovir 500 mg	Cytovene by Hoffmann La Roche	00004-0278	Antiviral
D	Tab, Pink, Round, Schering Logo/D	Amitriptyline HCl 2 mg, Perphenazine 25 mg	Etrafon by Bayer	Canadian	Antipsychotic
D	Tab, Green, Round	Chlorophyllin Copper Complex Sodium 100 mg	Derifil by Rystan		Gastrointestinal
D	Tab, White, Round	Lactose Enzyme 3000 FCC	by Blistex		Gastrointestinal
D	Tab, Pink, Logo/D	Perphenazine 2 mg, Amitriptyline 25 mg	by Schering	Canadian	Antipsychotic; Antidepressant
D14 <> JMI	Tab, White, Scored	Liothyronine Sodium	Cytomel by Jones	52604-3414	Antithyroid
D147	Cap	Phentermine HCl 30 mg	by United Res	00677-0460	Anorexiant; C IV
D150	Tab	Desogestrel 0.15 mg, Ethinyl Estradiol 0.03 mg	Orthocept 28 Day by Dept Health Central Pharm	53808-0042	Oral Contraceptive
D150 <> ORTHO	Tab, Orange	Desogestrel 150 mcg, Ethinyl Estradiol 3 mcg	Ortho Cept 28 by Ortho	00062-1796	Oral Contraceptive
D150 <> ORTHO	Tab, Peach, Round	Desogestrel 150 mcg, Ethinyl Estradiol 3 mcg	Ortho Cept 21 by Ortho	00062-1795	Oral Contraceptive
D3 <> DIAMOX	Cap	Acetazolamide 500 mg	Diamox ER Sequels by Lederle	00005-4465	Diuretic
D31	Tab, Pink, Round	Meperidine HCl 50 mg, Acetaminophen 300 mg	Demerol APAP by Sanofi		Analgesic; C II
D35 <> W	Tab, D/35	Meperidine HCl 50 mg	Demerol Hydrochloride by Sanofi	00024-0335	Analgesic; C II
D35 <> W	Tab, Coated, D/35	Meperidine HCl 50 mg	Demerol by Bayer	00280-0335	Analgesic; C II
D37 <> W	Tab, D/37	Meperidine HCl 100 mg	Demerol Hydrochloride by Sanofi	00024-0337	Analgesic; C II
D37 <> W	Tab, Coated, D/37	Meperidine HCl 100 mg	Demerol by Bayer	00280-0337	Analgesic; C II
D3V	Cap, Reddish Brown, Oval, Soft Gelatin	Testosterone Undecanoate 40 mg	Andriol by Organon	Canadian	Hormone
D44 <> LL	Tab	Dipyridamole 25 mg	by PDRX	55289-0748	Antiplatelet
D44 <> LL	Tab, D over 44	Dipyridamole 25 mg	by Lederle	00005-3743	Antiplatelet
D44 <> LL	Tab, Film Coated, D over 44	Dipyridamole 25 mg	by UDL	51079-0068	Antiplatelet
D45	Tab, Coated	Dipyridamole 50 mg	by Nat Pharmpak Serv	55154-5506	Antiplatelet
D45	Tab, Film Coated, UDL Logo	Dipyridamole 50 mg	by UDL	51079-0069	Antiplatelet
D45 <> LL	Tab, Purple, Round	Dipyridamole 50 mg	by Caremark	00339-5107	Antiplatelet
D46	Tab, Coated	Dipyridamole 75 mg	by Nat Pharmpak Serv	55154-5507	Antiplatelet
D46	Tab, Film Coated, UDL Logo	Dipyridamole 75 mg	by UDL	51079-0070	Antiplatelet
D46 <> LL	Tab, Purple, Round	Dipyridamole 75 mg	by Caremark	00339-5109	Antiplatelet

ID FRONT <> BACK	DESCRIPTION FRONT <> BACK	INGREDIENT & STRENGTH	BRAND (OR EQUIV.) & FIRM	NDC#	CLASS; SCH.
D46 <> LL	Tab, Coated, D over 46	Dipyridamole 75 mg	by Lederle	00005-3791	Antiplatelet
D50	Tab, Brown, Round	Dipyridamole 50 mg	Dipyridamone by Apotex	Canadian	Antiplatelet
D500 <> NU	Tab, Orange, Cap Shaped, Film Coated	Diflusinal 500 mg	by Nu Pharm	Canadian DIN# 02058413	NSAID
D51 <> LL	Tab	Diazepam 2 mg	by Allscripts	54569-0947	Antianxiety; C IV
D51 <> LL	Tab, D over 51 <> LL	Diazepam 2 mg	by UDL	51079-0284	Antianxiety; C IV
D51 <> LL	Tab, D over 51 <> LL	Diazepam 2 mg	by Lederle	50053-3128	Antianxiety; C IV
D52 <> LL	Tab, Scored, D over 52 <> LL	Diazepam 5 mg	by Nat Pharmpak Serv	55154-5554	Antianxiety; C IV
D52 <> LL	Tab, D Above, 52 Below	Diazepam 5 mg	by Quality Care	60346-0478	Antianxiety; C IV
D52 <> LL	Tab, Tan & White, Round, Scored	Diazepam 5 mg	by Southwood Pharms	58016-0275	Antianxiety; C IV
D52 <> LL	Tab, D over 52 <> LL	Diazepam 5 mg	by UDL	51079-0285	Antianxiety; C IV
D52 <> LL	Tab, D over 52 <> LL	Diazepam 5 mg	by Lederle	50053-3129	Antianxiety; C IV
D53 <> LL	Tab, D over 53 <> LL	Diazepam 10 mg	by Lederle	50053-3130	Antianxiety; C IV
D53 <> LL	Tab	Diazepam 10 mg	by Allscripts	54569-0936	Antianxiety; C IV
D53 <> LL	Tab, Green, Round, Scored	Diazepam 10 mg	by Southwood Pharms	58016-0273	Antianxiety; C IV
D53 <> LL	Tab, D over 53 <> LL	Diazepam 10 mg	by UDL	51079-0286	Antianxiety; C IV
D71	Tab, Film Coated	Diltiazem HCl 30 mg	by Nat Pharmpak Serv	55154-5504	Antihypertensive
D71 <> LL	Tab, Film Coated	Diltiazem HCl 30 mg	by Amerisource	62584-0366	Antihypertensive
D71 <> LL	Tab, Convex, Film Coated	Diltiazem HCl 30 mg	by UDL	51079-0745	Antihypertensive
D72 <> LL	Tab, Light Blue, Film Coated	Diltiazem HCl 60 mg	by Lederle	00005-3334	Antihypertensive
D72 <> LL	Tab, Film Coated, D over 72 <> LL	Diltiazem HCl 60 mg	by UDL	51079-0746	Antihypertensive
D75	Tab, Red, Round	Dipyridamole 75 mg	Dipyridamone by Apotex	Canadian	Antiplatelet
D75 <> LL	Tab, Coated	Diltiazem HCl 90 mg	by PDRX	55289-0893	Antihypertensive
D75 <> LL	Tab, Coated	Diltiazem HCl 90 mg	by Quality Care	60346-0503	Antihypertensive
D75 <> LL	Tab, Film Coated, D/75	Diltiazem HCl 90 mg	by UDL	51079-0747	Antihypertensive
D92 <> W	Cap, White Print, D92 <> W in circle	Ergocalciferol 1.25 mg	Drisdol by Sanofi	00024-0392	Vitamin
D92 <> W	Cap, White Print, W in a Circle	Ergocalciferol 1.25 mg	Drisdol by Bayer	00280-0392	Vitamin
DA <> DURA	Tab, D/A <> DU/RA	Chlorpheniramine Maleate 8 mg, Methscopolamine Nitrate 2.5 mg, Phenylephrine HCl 20 mg	Dura Vent by Anabolic	00722-6072	Cold Remedy
DAII <> DURA	Tab	Chlorpheniramine Maleate 4 mg, Methscopolamine Nitrate 1.25 mg, Phenylephrine HCl 10 mg	Da II by Anabolic	00722-6354	Cold Remedy
DALLERGY	Tab, Off-White	Chlorpheniramine Maleate 8 mg, Methscopolamine Nitrate 2.5 mg, Phenylephrine HCl 20 mg	Dallergy by Anabolic	00722-6273	Cold Remedy
DALLERGY	Tab	Mivacurium Chloride 8 mg, Methscopolamine Nitrate 2.5 mg, Phenylephrine HCl 20 mg	Dallergy IR by Anabolic CA	00722-6457	Cold Remedy
DALLERGY <> 12H	Tab, White, Cap Shaped, Scored	Chlorpheniramine Maleate 8 mg, Methscopolamine Nitrate 2.5 mg, Phenylephrine HCl 20 mg	Dallergy ER by Laser	00277-0180	Cold Remedy
DALLERGY <> LASER	Tab, White, Round, Scored	Chlorpheniramine Maleate 4 mg, Methscopolamine Nitrate 1.25 mg, Phenylephrine HCl 10 mg	Dallergy by Laser	00277-0160	Cold Remedy
DALLERGYJR <> LASER176	Cap, Ex Release, Dallergy JR <> Laser over 176	Brompheniramine Maleate 6 mg, Pseudoephedrine HCl 60 mg	Dallergy Jr by Sovereign	58716-0028	Cold Remedy
DALLERGYJR <> LASER176	Cap, Maize, Opaque	Brompheniramine Maleate 6 mg, Pseudoephedrine HCl 60 mg	Dallergy JR by Laser	00277-0176	Cold Remedy
DALMANE15ROCHE	Cap, Orange, Dalmane/15 Roche	Flurazepam HCl 15 mg	Dalmane by Roche	Canadian	Hypnotic
DALMANE30ROCHE	Cap, Ivory & Red, Dalmane/30 Roche	Flurazepam HCl 30 mg	Dalmane by Roche	Canadian	Hypnotic
DAN <> 100P	Tab, White, Round, Scored	Phenobarbital 100 mg	by Schein	00364-0206	Sedative/Hypnotic; C IV
DAN <> 15P	Tab, White, Round, Scored	Phenobarbital 15 mg	by Schein	00364-2444	Sedative/Hypnotic; C IV
DAN <> 30P	Tab, White, Round, Scored	Phenobarbital 30 mg	by Schein	00364-0203	Sedative/Hypnotic; C IV
DAN <> 5050	Tab, Orange, Round, Film Coated	Hydralazine HCl 25 mg	by Schein	00364-0144	Antihypertensive
DAN <> 5052	Tab	Prednisone 5 mg	by Nat Pharmpak Serv	55154-5208	Steroid
DAN <> 5055	Tab, Orange, Round, Film Coated	Hydralazine HCl 50 mg	by Schein	00364-0145	Antihypertensive

ID FRONT <> BACK	DESCRIPTION FRONT <> BACK	INGREDIENT & STRENGTH	BRAND (OR EQUIV.) & FIRM	NDC#	CLASS; SCH.
DAN <> 5319	Tab, White, Round	Promethazine HCl 50 mg	by Schein	00364-0345	Antiemetic; Antihistamine
DAN <> 5319	Tab	Promethazine HCl 50 mg	by Danbury	00591-5319	Antiemetic; Antihistamine
DAN <> 5373	Tab	Isosorbide Dinitrate 10 mg	by Danbury	00591-5373	Antianginal
DAN <> 5385	Tab	Isosorbide Dinitrate 5 mg	by Danbury	00591-5385	Antianginal
DAN <> 5385	Tab, White, Round	Isosorbide Dinitrate 5 mg	by Schein	00364-0368	Antianginal
DAN <> 5387	Tab	Isosorbide Dinitrate 2.5 mg	by Danbury	00591-5387	Antianginal
DAN <> 5387	Tab, Yellow, Round	Isosorbide Dinitrate 2.5 mg	by Schein	00364-0367	Antianginal
DAN <> 5428	Tab, Light Yellow, Round	Reserpine 0.1 mg, Hydralazine HCl 25 mg, Hydrochlorothiazide 15 mg	by Schein	00364-0361	Antihypertensive
DAN <> 5444	Tab, White, Round, Scored	Chlorothiazide 250 mg	by Schein	00364-0389	Diuretic
DAN <> 5501	Tab, White, Oval, Sublingual	Ergoloid Mesylates 1 mg	by Schein	00364-0446	Ergot
DAN <> 5502	Tab, White, Round, Sublingual	Ergoloid Mesylates 0.5 mg	by Schein	00364-0415	Ergot
DAN <> 5503	Tab, Amber-Yellow, Round	Sulfasalazine 500 mg	by Schein	00364-0444	Gastrointestinal
DAN <> 5504	Tab, White, Round	Ergoloid Mesylates 1 mg	by Schein	00364-0622	Ergot
DAN <> 5507	Tab, Yellow, Round	Chlorthalidone 25 mg	by Schein	00364-0564	Diuretic
DAN <> 5507	Tab, Orange, Round	Chlorthalidone 25 mg	by Schein	00364-0592	Diuretic
DAN <> 5513	Tab, White, Round	Carisoprodol 350 mg	by Kaiser Fdn	00179-1349	Muscle Relaxant
DAN <> 5513	Tab, White, Round	Carisoprodol 350 mg	by Schein	00364-0475	Muscle Relaxant
DAN <> 5513	Tab	Carisoprodol 350 mg	by Danbury	00591-5513	Muscle Relaxant
DAN <> 5513	Tab	Carisoprodol 350 mg	by Urgent Care Ctr	50716-0202	Muscle Relaxant
DAN <> 5513	Tab	Carisoprodol 350 mg	by Allscripts	54569-1709	Muscle Relaxant
DAN <> 5513	Tab	Carisoprodol 350 mg	by Allscripts	54569-3403	Muscle Relaxant
DAN <> 5513	Tab	Carisoprodol 350 mg	by Quality Care	60346-0635	Muscle Relaxant
DAN <> 5516	Tab, White, Round	Quinine Sulfate 260 mg	by Schein	00364-0560	Antimalarial
DAN <> 5518	Tab, Light Green, Round	Chlorthalidone 50 mg	by Schein	00364-0528	Diuretic
DAN <> 5518	Tab, Light Blue, Round	Chlorthalidone 50 mg	by Schein	00364-0593	Diuretic
DAN <> 5522	Tab, Coated	Hydroxyzine HCl 10 mg	by Danbury	00591-5522	Antihistamine
DAN <> 5522	Tab, Orange, Round, Film Coated	Hydroxyzine HCl 10 mg	by Schein	00364-0494	Antihistamine
DAN <> 5522	Tab, Coated	Hydroxyzine HCl 10 mg	by Heartland	61392-0012	Antihistamine
DAN <> 5523	Tab, Film Coated	Hydroxyzine HCl 25 mg	by Heartland	61392-0013	Antihistamine
DAN <> 5523	Tab, Green, Round, Film Coated	Hydroxyzine HCl 25 mg	by Schein	00364-0495	Antihistamine
DAN <> 5523	Tab, Film Coated	Hydroxyzine HCl 25 mg	by Danbury	00591-5523	Antihistamine
DAN <> 5523	Tab, Film Coated	Hydroxyzine HCl 25 mg	by Vangard	00615-1526	Antihistamine
DAN <> 5523	Tab, Film Coated	Hydroxyzine HCl 25 mg	by Quality Care	60346-0086	Antihistamine
DAN <> 5538	Tab, ER	Quinidine Gluconate 324 mg	by Danbury	00591-5538	Antiarrhythmic
DAN <> 5538	Tab, Off-White, Round, Ex Release	Quinidine Gluconate 324 mg	by Schein	00364-0604	Antiarrhythmic
DAN <> 5540	Tab	Metronidazole 250 mg	by Danbury	00591-5540	Antibiotic
DAN <> 5540	Tab, Off-White to White, Round	Metronidazole 250 mg	by Schein	00364-0595	Antibiotic
DAN <> 5540	Tab	Metronidazole 250 mg	by Nat Pharmpak Serv	55154-5212	Antibiotic
DAN <> 5540	Tab	Metronidazole 250 mg	by Allscripts	54569-0965	Antibiotic
DAN <> 5547	Tab, White, Oval, Scored	Sulfamethoxazole 800 mg, Trimethoprim 160 mg	by Va Cmop	65243-0067	Antibiotic
DAN <> 5549	Tab, White, Round, Film Coated	Chloroquine Phosphate 500 mg	by Schein	00364-2431	Antimalarial
DAN <> 5552	Tab	Metronidazole 500 mg	by Nat Pharmpak Serv	55154-5234	Antibiotic
DAN <> 5553	Tab, Light Orange, Round, Film Coated	Doxycycline Hyclate 100 mg	by Schein	00364-2063	Antibiotic
DAN <> 5553	Tab, Orange, Round, Film Coated	Doxycycline Hyclate	by Murfreesboro Ph	51129-1357	Antibiotic
DAN <> 5553	Tab, Film Coated	Doxycycline Hyclate	by Danbury	00591-5553	Antibiotic
DAN <> 5562	Tab, White, Oval, Film Coated, Ex Release	Procainamide HCl 250 mg	by Schein	00364-0715	Antiarrhythmic
DAN <> 5562	Tab, Film Coated	Procainamide HCl 250 mg	by Danbury	00591-5562	Antiarrhythmic
DAN <> 5565	Tab, Yellow, Round, Film Coated	Hydroxyzine HCl 50 mg	by Schein	00364-0496	Antihistamine
DAN <> 5565	Tab, Sugar Coated	Hydroxyzine HCl 50 mg	by Allscripts	54569-0409	Antihistamine
DAN <> 5565	Tab, Coated	Hydroxyzine HCl 50 mg	by Med Pro	53978-3186	Antihistamine

ID FRONT <> BACK	DESCRIPTION FRONT <> BACK	INGREDIENT & STRENGTH	BRAND (OR EQUIV.) & FIRM	NDC#	CLASS; SCH.
DAN <> 5565	Tab, Coated	Hydroxyzine HCl 50 mg	by Quality Care	60346-0796	Antihistamine
DAN <> 5565	Tab, Coated	Hydroxyzine HCl 50 mg	by Danbury	00591-5565	Antihistamine
DAN <> 5569	Tab, Orange, Round, Film Coated	Thioridazine HCl 100 mg	by Schein	00364-0670	Antipsychotic
DAN <> 5572	Tab, White, Round, Film Coated	Thioridazine HCl 15 mg	by Schein	00364-0669	Antipsychotic
DAN <> 5576	Tab, White, Round	Furosemide 20 mg	by Schein	00364-0568	Diuretic
DAN <> 5580	Tab, Orange, Round, Film Coated	Thioridazine HCl 150 mg	by Schein	00364-0723	Antipsychotic
DAN <> 5581	Tab, Orange, Round, Film Coated	Thioridazine HCl 200 mg	by Schein	00364-0724	Antipsychotic
DAN <> 5584	Tab, White, Round, Film Coated	Ibuprofen 400 mg	by Schein	00364-0765	NSAID
DAN <> 5585	Tab, White, Round, Film Coated	Ibuprofen 200 mg	by Schein	00364-2145	NSAID
DAN <> 5586	Tab, White, Oval, Film Coated	Ibuprofen 600 mg	by Schein	00364-0766	NSAID
DAN <> 5587	Tab, White, Round, Film Coated	Methyldopa 500 mg	by Schein	00364-0708	Antihypertensive
DAN <> 5588	Tab, White, Round, Film Coated	Methyldopa 250 mg	by Schein	00364-0707	Antihypertensive
DAN <> 5600	Tab, Film Coated	Trazodone HCl 50 mg	by Allscripts	54569-1470	Antidepressant
DAN <> 5601	Tab, Film Coated	Verapamil HCl 80 mg	by Nat Pharmpak Serv	55154-5227	Antihypertensive
DAN <> 5637	Cap, Coral	Meclofenamate Sodium	by Quality Care	60346-0350	NSAID
DAN <> 5644	Tab, White, Oval, Film Coated	Ibuprofen 800 mg	by Schein	00364-2137	NSAID
DAN <> 5658	Tab, Film Coated	Cyclobenzaprine HCl 10 mg	by Danbury	00591-5658	Muscle Relaxant
DAN <> 5658	Tab, Film Coated	Cyclobenzaprine HCl 10 mg	by Vangard	00615-3520	Muscle Relaxant
DAN <> 5658	Tab, White, Round, Film Coated	Cyclobenzaprine HCl 10 mg	by Schein	00364-2348	Muscle Relaxant
DAN <> 5658	Tab, Film Coated	Cyclobenzaprine HCl 10 mg	by Nat Pharmpak Serv	55154-5217	Muscle Relaxant
DAN <> 5658	Tab, Film Coated	Cyclobenzaprine HCl 10 mg	by Heartland	61392-0830	Muscle Relaxant
DAN <> 5658	Tab, Film Coated	Cyclobenzaprine HCl 10 mg	by Heartland	61392-0098	Muscle Relaxant
DAN <> 5658	Tab, Film Coated	Cyclobenzaprine HCl 10 mg	by Amerisource	62584-0354	Muscle Relaxant
DAN <> 5658	Tab, Film Coated	Cyclobenzaprine HCl 10 mg	by PDRX	55289-0567	Muscle Relaxant
DAN <> 5658	Tab, Film Coated	Cyclobenzaprine HCl 10 mg	by Quality Care	60346-0581	Muscle Relaxant
DAN <> 5658	Tab, White, Round	Cyclobenzaprine HCl 10 mg	by Southwood Pharms	58016-0234	Muscle Relaxant
DAN <> 5661	Tab	Sulindac 150 mg	by Danbury	00591-5661	NSAID
DAN <> 5661	Tab, Yellow, Round	Sulindac 150 mg	by Schein	00364-2441	NSAID
DAN <> 5661	Tab	Sulindac 150 mg	by Quality Care	60346-0044	NSAID
DAN <> 5661	Tab	Sulindac 150 mg	by Direct Dispensing	57866-4621	NSAID
DAN <> 5661	Tab, Yellow, Round	Sulindac 150 mg	by St. Marys Med	60760-0290	NSAID
DAN <> 5662	Tab, Off-White, Oval, Scored	Nalidixic Acid 1 gm	by Schein	00364-2325	Antibiotic
DAN <> 5678	Tab, White, Round, Film Coated	Chlordiazepoxide 10 mg, Amitriptyline 25 mg	by Schein	00364-2158	Antianxiety; C IV
DAN <> 5679	Tab, Light Green, Round, Film Coated	Chlordiazepoxide 5 mg, Amitriptyline 12.5 mg	by Schein	00364-2157	Antianxiety; C IV
DAN <> 5682	Tab, Yellow, Round, Scored	Triamterene 75 mg, Hydrochlorothiazide 50 mg	by Schein	00364-2242	Diuretic
DAN <> 5726	Cap, Dark Green & Light Green	Hydroxyzine Pamoate 25 mg	by Schein	00364-0483	Antihistamine
DAN <> 5726	Cap, Dark Green & Light Green	Hydroxyzine Pamoate 43 mg	by Quality Care	60346-0208	Antihistamine
DAN <> 5782	Tab, White, Round, Scored	Atenolol 50 mg, Chlorthalidone 25 mg	by Schein	00364-2527	Antihypertensive; Diuretic
DAN <> 5783	Tab, White, Round	Atenolol 100 mg, Chlorthalidone 25 mg	by Schein	00364-2528	Antihypertensive; Diuretic
DAN <> 5912	Tab, Blue, Oval, Scored	Captopril 50 mg, Hydrochlorothiazide 25 mg	by Schein	00364-2640	Antihypertensive; Diuretic
DAN <> 60P	Tab, White, Round, Scored	Phenobarbital 60 mg	by Schein	00364-0697	Sedative/Hypnotic; C IV
DAN <> 944	Tab	Colchicine 0.6 mg	by Heartland	61392-0174	Antigout
DAN <> 944	Tab, White, Round	Colchicine 0.6 mg	by Schein	00364-0074	Antigout
DAN <> 944	Tab	Colchicine 0.6 mg	by Danbury	00591-0944	Antigout
DAN <> 944	Tab	Colchicine 0.6 mg	by Allscripts	54569-0236	Antigout
DAN <> A22	Tab, Yellow, Round, Film Coated	Ranitidine HCl 150 mg	by Schein	00364-2633	Gastrointestinal
DAN <> A23	Tab, Yellow, Cap-Shaped, Film Coated	Ranitidine HCl 300 mg	by Schein	00364-2634	Gastrointestinal
DAN01 <> 5609	Tab, White, Pentagonal, Scored, Dan 0.1 <> 5609	Clonidine HCl 0.1 mg	by Schein	00364-0820	Antihypertensive
DAN02 <> 5612	Tab, Light Yellow, Pentagonal, Scored, Dan 0.2 <> 5612	Clonidine HCl 0.2 mg	by Schein	00364-0821	Antihypertensive

ID FRONT <> BACK	DESCRIPTION FRONT <> BACK	INGREDIENT & STRENGTH	BRAND (OR EQUIV.) & FIRM	NDC#	CLASS; SCH.
DAN025 <> 5449	Tab, Orange, Pentagonal, Scored, Dan 0.25 <> 5449	Dexamethasone 0.25 mg	by Schein	00364-0397	Steroid
DAN03 <> 5613	Tab, Light Blue, Pentagonal, Scored, Dan 0.3 <> 5613	Clonidine HCl 0.3 mg	by Schein	00364-0824	Antihypertensive
DAN05 <> 5605	Tab, White, Round, Scored, Dan 0.5 <> 5605	Haloperidol 0.5 mg	by Schein	00364-2204	Antipsychotic
DAN05 <> 5625	Tab, White, Round, Scored, Dan 0.5 <> 5625	Lorazepam 0.5 mg	by Schein	00364-0793	Sedative/Hypnotic; C IV
DAN050 <> 5450	Tab, Yellow, Pentagonal, Scored, Dan 0.50 <> 5450	Dexamethasone 0.5 mg	by Schein	00364-0398	Steroid
DAN075 <> 5361	Tab, Light Blue, Dan 0.75 <> 5361	Dexamethasone 0.75 mg	by Quality Care	60346-0550	Steroid
DAN075 <> 5361	Tab, Light Blue, Round, Scored, Dan 0.75 <> 5361	Dexamethasone 0.75 mg	by Schein	00364-0098	Steroid
DAN1 <> 5604	Tab, Peach, Round, Scored	Haloperidol 1 mg	by Schein	00364-2205	Antipsychotic
DAN1 <> 5624	Tab, White, Round, Scored	Lorazepam 1 mg	by Schein	00364-0794	Sedative/Hypnotic; C IV
DAN10 <> 5554	Tab, Orange, Round, Scored	Propranolol HCl 10 mg	by Schein	00364-0756	Antihypertensive
DAN10 <> 5566	Tab, Yellow-Green, Triangular	Thioridazine HCl 10 mg	by Schein	00364-2317	Antipsychotic
DAN10 <> 5620	Tab, Light Blue, Round, Scored	Diazepam 10 mg	by Schein	00364-0776	Antianxiety; C IV
DAN10 <> 5643	Tab, White, Round, Scored	Minoxidil 10 mg	by Schein	00364-2173	Antihypertensive
DAN10 <> 5724	Tab, White, Round, Scored	Metaproterenol Sulfate 10 mg	by Schein	00364-2283	Antiasthmatic
DAN10 <> 5730	Tab, White, Round, Scored	Baclofen 10 mg	by Schein	00364-2312	Muscle Relaxant
DAN10 <> 5737	Tab, White, Round, Scored	Timolol Maleate 10 mg	by Schein	00364-2358	Antihypertensive
DAN10 <> 5883	Tab, Green, Round, Scored	Methylphenidate HCl 10 mg	by Danbury	00591-5883	Stimulant; C II
DAN10 <> 5883	Tab, Green, Round, Scored	Methylphenidate HCl 10 mg	by Schein	00364-0479	Stimulant; C II
DAN100	Tab	Atenolol 100 mg	by Danbury	00591-5778	Antihypertensive
DAN100 <> 5715	Tab, Blue, Round, Scored	Amoxapine 100 mg	by Schein	00364-2434	Antidepressant
DAN100 <> 5715	Tab	Amoxapine 100 mg	by Danbury	00591-5715	Antidepressant
DAN100 <> 5778	Tab, White, Round	Atenolol 100 mg	by Schein	00364-2514	Antihypertensive
DAN100 <> 5859	Tab, White, Round, Quadrisected	Captopril 100 mg	by Schein	00364-2631	Antihypertensive
DAN1005778	Tab, Coated, Dan/100/5778	Atenolol 100 mg	by Duramed	51285-0838	Antihypertensive
DAN1005859	Tab, White, Round, Scored	Captopril 100 mg	Captopril USP by Caremark	00339-5851	Antihypertensive
DAN105724	Tab, White, Round	Metaproterenol Sulfate 10 mg	Alupent by Danbury		Antiasthmatic
DAN105730	Tab, White, Round, Dan-10, 5730	Baclofen 10 mg	Lioresal by Danbury		Muscle Relaxant
DAN10MG <> NORTRIPTYLINE	Cap, Green & White	Nortriptyline HCl 10 mg	by Allscripts	54569-4146	Antidepressant
DAN10MG <> NORTRIPTYLINE	Cap, Deep Green	Nortriptyline HCl	by Danbury	00591-5786	Antidepressant
DAN10MG <> NORTRIPTYLINE	Cap	Nortriptyline HCl	by Heartland	61392-0361	Antidepressant
DAN10MG <> NORTRIPTYLINE	Cap, Deep Green	Nortriptyline HCl	by Danbury	61955-2508	Antidepressant
DAN1153	Tab, White, Round	Carisoprodol 350 mg	Soma by Danbury		Muscle Relaxant
DAN1255856	Tab, White, Round, Scored, Dan 12.5 5856	Captopril 12.5 mg	Captopril USP by Caremark	00339-5781	Antihypertensive
DAN15 <> 5451	Tab, White, Pentagonal, Scored, Dan 1.5 <> 5451	Dexamethasone 1.5 mg	by Schein	00364-0399	Steroid
DAN15 <> 5607	Tab, White, Round, Film Coated	Methyldopa 250 mg, Hydrochlorothiazide 15 mg	by Schein	00364-0827	Antihypertensive
DAN150 <> 5716	Tab	Amoxapine 150 mg	by Danbury	00591-5716	Antidepressant
DAN150 <> 5716	Tab, Orange, Round, Scored	Amoxapine 150 mg	by Schein	00364-2435	Antidepressant
DAN2 <> 5603	Tab, Yellow, Round, Scored	Haloperidol 2 mg	by Schein	00364-2206	Antipsychotic
DAN2 <> 5621	Tab, White, Round, Scored	Diazepam 2 mg	by Schein	00364-0774	Antianxiety; C IV
DAN2 <> 5622	Tab, White, Round, Scored	Lorazepam 2 mg	by Schein	00364-0795	Sedative/Hypnotic; C IV
DAN2 <> 5710	Tab, White, Round, Scored	Albuterol 2 mg	by Schein	00364-2438	Antiasthmatic
DAN20 <> 5555	Tab, Blue, Round, Scored	Propranolol HCl 20 mg	by Schein	00364-0757	Antihypertensive
DAN20 <> 5725	Tab, White, Round, Scored	Metaproterenol Sulfate 20 mg	by Schein	00364-2284	Antiasthmatic
DAN20 <> 5731	Tab, White, Round, Scored	Baclofen 20 mg	by Schein	00364-2313	Muscle Relaxant
DAN20 <> 5738	Tab, White, Cap Shaped, Scored	Timolol Maleate 20 mg	by Schein	00364-2359	Antihypertensive
DAN20 <> 5884	Tab, Peach, Round, Scored	Methylphenidate HCl 20 mg	by Schein	00364-0562	Stimulant; C II
DAN20 <> 5884	Tab, Peach, Round, Scored	Methylphenidate HCl 20 mg	by Danbury	00591-5884	Stimulant; C II
DAN205725	Tab, White, Round	Metaproterenol Sulfate 20 mg	Alupent by Danbury		Antiasthmatic

ID FRONT <> BACK	DESCRIPTION FRONT <> BACK	INGREDIENT & STRENGTH	BRAND (OR EQUIV.) & FIRM	NDC#	CLASS; SCH.
DAN205731	Tab, White, Round, Dan-20, 5731	Baclofen 20 mg	Lioresal by Danbury		Muscle Relaxant
DAN205738	Tab, White, Oblong, Dan/20 5738	Timolol Maleate 20 mg	Blocadren by Danbury		Antihypertensive
DAN25 <> 5542	Tab, Beige, Triangular, Film Coated	Thioridazine HCl 25 mg	by Schein	00364-0662	Antipsychotic
DAN25 <> 5608	Tab, White, Round, Film Coated	Methyldopa 250 mg, Hydrochlorothiazide 25 mg	by Schein	00364-0828	Antihypertensive
DAN25 <> 5642	Tab, White, Round, Scored, Dan 2.5 <> 5642	Minoxidil 2.5 mg	by Schein	00364-2172	Antihypertensive
DAN25 <> 5713	Tab, White, Round, Scored	Amoxapine 25 mg	by Schein	00364-2432	Antidepressant
DAN25 <> 5713	Tab	Amoxapine 25 mg	by Danbury	00591-5713	Antidepressant
DAN25 <> A7	Tab, White, Round, Scored	Captopril 25 mg	by Schein	00364-2629	Antihypertensive
DAN25 <> NORTRIPTYLINE	Cap	Nortriptyline HCl	by Nat Pharmpak Serv	55154-5220	Antidepressant
DAN250 <> 5816	Cap, Light Green, Round	Naproxen 250 mg	by Schein	00364-2562	NSAID
DAN250 <> 5816	Tab, Green, Round	Naproxen 250 mg	by Danbury Pharma	00591-5816	NSAID
DAN25MG <> NORTRIPTYLINE	Cap, Deep Green & White	Nortriptyline HCl	by Quality Care	60346-0757	Antidepressant
DAN25MG <> NORTRIPTYLINE	Cap	Nortriptyline HCl	by Heartland	61392-0364	Antidepressant
DAN25MG <> NORTRIPTYLINE	Cap, Deep Green	Nortriptyline HCl	by Danbury	00591-5787	Antidepressant
DAN25MG <> NORTRIPTYLINE	Cap	Nortriptyline HCl	by Danbury	61955-2509	Antidepressant
DAN30 <> 5611	Tab, White, Round, Film Coated	Methyldopa 500 mg, Hydrochlorothiazide 30 mg	by Schein	00364-2400	Antihypertensive
DAN375 <> 5817	Tab, Purple, Oblong	Naproxen 375 mg	by Danbury Pharma	00591-5817	NSAID
DAN375 <> 5817	Tab, Lavender, Cap Shaped	Naproxen 375 mg	by Schein	00364-2563	NSAID
DAN4 <> 5711	Tab, White, Round, Scored	Albuterol 4 mg	by Schein	00364-2439	Antiasthmatic
DAN40 <> 5556	Tab, Green, Round, Scored	Propranolol HCl 40 mg	by Schein	00364-0758	Antihypertensive
DAN5 <> 5606	Tab, Blue, Round, Scored	Haloperidol 5 mg	by Schein	00364-2207	Antipsychotic
DAN5 <> 5619	Tab, Yellow, Round, Scored	Diazepam 5 mg	by Schein	00364-0775	Antianxiety; C IV
DAN5 <> 5736	Tab, White, Round	Timolol Maleate 5 mg	by Schein	00364-2357	Antihypertensive
DAN5 <> 5882	Tab, Purple, Round	Methylphenidate HCl 5 mg	by Schein	00364-0561	Stimulant; C II
DAN5 <> 5882	Tab, Purple, Round	Methylphenidate HCl 5 mg	by Danbury	00591-5882	Stimulant; C II
DAN50 <> 5568	Tab, White, Triangular, Film Coated	Thioridazine HCl 50 mg	by Schein	00364-2318	Antipsychotic
DAN50 <> 5610	Tab, White, Round, Film Coated, Scored	Methyldopa 500 mg, Hydrochlorothiazide 50 mg	by Schein	00364-2401	Antihypertensive
DAN50 <> 5714	Tab, Orange, Round, Scored	Amoxapine 50 mg	by Schein	00364-2433	Antidepressant
DAN50 <> 5714	Tab	Amoxapine 50 mg	by Danbury	00591-5714	Antidepressant
DAN50 <> 5777	Tab	Atenolol 50 mg	by Danbury	61955-2513	Antihypertensive
DAN50 <> 5777	Tab	Atenolol 50 mg	by Danbury	00591-5777	Antihypertensive
DAN50 <> 5777	Tab, White, Round, Scored	Atenolol 50 mg	by Schein	00364-2513	Antihypertensive
DAN50 <> 5858	Tab, White, Round, Scored	Captopril 50 mg	by Schein	00364-2630	Antihypertensive
DAN500 <> 5706	Tab, Light Green, Round, Scored	Chlorzoxazone 500 mg	by Schein	00364-2255	Muscle Relaxant
DAN500 <> 5818	Tab, Green, Oblong	Naproxen 500 mg	by Danbury Pharma	00591-5818	NSAID
DAN500 <> 5818	Tab, Light Green, Cap Shaped	Naproxen 500 mg	by Schein	00364-2564	NSAID
DAN5002	Cap, Clear & Pink	Diphenhydramine HCl 25 mg	Benadryl by Danbury		Antihistamine
DAN5003	Cap, Pink	Diphenhydramine HCl 50 mg	Benadryl by Danbury		Antihistamine
DAN5005706	Tab, Green, Round, Dan-500, 5706	Chlorzoxazone 500 mg	Parafon Forte DSC by Danbury		Muscle Relaxant
DAN5026 <> DAN5026	Cap	Procainamide HCl 250 mg	by Danbury	00591-5026	Antiarrhythmic
DAN5028	Cap, Clear	Quinine 5 gr	by Danbury		Antimalarial
DAN5050	Tab, Orange, Round	Hydralazine HCl 25 mg	Apresoline by Danbury		Antihypertensive
DAN5055	Tab, Orange, Round	Hydralazine HCl 50 mg	Apresoline by Danbury		Antihypertensive
DAN505777	Tab, White, Round, Dan/50/5777	Atenolol 50 mg	by Duramed	51285-0837	Antihypertensive
DAN5058	Tab, Bluish Green, Round, Dan/5058	Tripelennamine HCl 50 mg	PBZ by Danbury		Antihistamine
DAN505858	Tab, White, Round, Scored	Captopril 50 mg	Captopril by Caremark	00339-5840	Antihypertensive
DAN5059	Tab, Peach, Round	Prednisolone 5 mg	by Danbury		Steroid

ID FRONT <> BACK	DESCRIPTION FRONT <> BACK	INGREDIENT & STRENGTH	BRAND (OR EQUIV.) & FIRM	NDC#	CLASS; SCH.
DAN50MG <> NORTRIPTYLINE	Cap	Nortriptyline HCl	by Danbury	61955-2510	Antidepressant
DAN50MG <> NORTRIPTYLINE	Cap	Nortriptyline HCl	by Danbury	00591-5788	Antidepressant
DAN50MG <> NORTRIPTYLINE	Cap	Nortriptyline HCl	by Heartland	61392-0367	Antidepressant
DAN5162	Cap	Tetracycline HCl 250 mg	by Talbert Med	44514-0884	Antibiotic
DAN5162	Cap	Tetracycline HCl 500 mg	by Med Pro	53978-5048	Antibiotic
DAN5183	Tab, White, Round	Hydrocortisone 20 mg	Cortone by Danbury		Steroid
DAN5196	Cap, Brown & Clear	Papaverine HCl 150 mg	Pavabid by Danbury		Vasodilator
DAN5204	Tab, White, Round	Pseudoephedrine HCl 60 mg	Sudafed by Danbury		Decongestant
DAN5216	Tab, Yellow, Round, Dan/5216	Folic Acid 1 mg	Folvite by Danbury		Vitamin
DAN526	Tab, White, Round	Isoniazid 300 mg	by Danbury		Antimycobacterial
DAN5304	Tab, Gray, Round	Promethazine HCl 12.5 mg	Phenergan by Danbury		Antiemetic; Antihistamine
DAN5307	Tab, White, Round	Promethazine HCl 25 mg	Phenergan by Danbury		Antiemetic; Antihistamine
DAN5316	Tab, White, Round	Phenylbutazone (Veterinary) 100 mg	Butazolidin by Danbury		Veterinary
DAN5321	Tab, White, Round, Dan/5321	Primidone 250 mg	Mysoline by Danbury		Anticonvulsant
DAN5325	Tab, White, Oblong	Colchicine 0.5 mg, Probenecid 500 mg	ColBenemid by Danbury		Antigout
DAN5326	Tab, White, Oblong	Probenecid 500 mg, Colchicine 0.5 mg	ColBenemid by Danbury		Antigout
DAN5333 <> DAN5333	Cap	Procainamide HCl 500 mg	by Danbury	00591-5333	Antiarrhythmic
DAN5335	Tab, White, Round, Dan/5335	Trihexyphenidyl 2 mg	Artane by Danbury		Antiparkinson
DAN5337	Tab, White, Round, Dan/5337	Trihexyphenidyl 5 mg	Artane by Danbury		Antiparkinson
DAN5342	Tab, White, Round	Nylidrin HCl 6 mg	Arlidin by Danbury		Vasodilator
DAN5345	Tab, Peach, Round	Hydrochlorothiazide 50 mg	Esidrix by Danbury		Diuretic
DAN5347	Tab	Probenecid 500 mg	by Pharmedix	53002-0397	Antigout
DAN5350 <> DAN5350	Cap	Procainamide HCl 375 mg	by Danbury	00591-5350	Antiarrhythmic
DAN5361075	Tab, Blue, Round, Dan 5361 0.75	Dexamethasone 0.75 mg	Decadron by Danbury		Steroid
DAN5368	Tab, White, Round, Dan/5368	Disulfiram 500 mg	Antabuse by Danbury		Antialcoholism
DAN5369	Tab, White, Round, Dan/5369	Bethanechol 10 mg	Urecholine by Danbury		Urinary Tract
DAN5374	Tab, Pink, Round	Isosorbide Dinitrate 5 mg	Isordil by Danbury		Antianginal
DAN5374	Tab, White, Round	Isosorbide Dinitrate 5 mg	Isordil by Danbury		Antianginal
DAN5376	Tab, White, Round, Dan/5376	Disulfiram 250 mg	Antabuse by Danbury		Antialcoholism
DAN5381	Tab	Methocarbamol 500 mg	by Pharmedix	53002-0304	Muscle Relaxant
DAN5388	Tab, White, Oblong, Dan/5388	Triamcinolone 4 mg	Aristocort by Danbury		Steroid
DAN5390	Tab, White, Round	Nylidrin HCl 12 mg	Arlidin by Danbury		Vasodilator
DAN5402	Tab, Yellow, Round, Dan/5402	Bethanechol 25 mg	Urecholine by Danbury		Urinary Tract
DAN5406	Tab, Green, Round, Dan/5406	Hydrochlorothiazide 25 mg, Reserpine 0.125 mg	Hydropres by Danbury		Diuretic; Antihypertensive
DAN5407	Tab, Green, Round, Dan/5407	Hydrochlorothiazide 50 mg, Reserpine 0.125 mg	Hydropres by Danbury		Diuretic; Antihypertensive
DAN5428	Tab, Yellow, Round	Hydrochlorothiazide 15 mg, Hydralazine HCl 25 mg, Reserpine 0.1 mg	Ser-Ap-Es by Danbury		Diuretic; Antihypertensive
DAN5434	Tab, White, Round	Triprolidine HCl 2.5 mg, Pseudoephedrine HCl 60 mg	Actifed by Danbury		Cold Remedy
DAN5438	Tab, White, Round	Quinidine Sulfate 200 mg	by Danbury		Antiarrhythmic
DAN5440	Tab, Blue, Oblong	Doxycycline Hyclate 100 mg	by H J Harkins Co	52959-0467	Antibiotic
DAN5440	Cap	Doxycycline Hyclate	by Allscripts	54569-1840	Antibiotic
DAN5440	Cap	Doxycycline Hyclate	by Pharmedix	53002-0212	Antibiotic
DAN5440	Cap, Blue	Doxycycline Hyclate 100 mg	by Danbury Pr	61955-2033	Antibiotic
DAN5440 <> DAN5440	Cap	Doxycycline Hyclate	by Danbury	00591-5440	Antibiotic
DAN5442	Tab, White, Round, Dan/5442	Prednisone 10 mg	Deltasone by Geneva		Steroid

ID FRONT <> BACK	DESCRIPTION FRONT <> BACK	INGREDIENT & STRENGTH	BRAND (OR EQUIV.) & FIRM	NDC#	CLASS; SCH.
DAN5443	Tab, Peach, Round	Prednisone 20 mg	Deltasone by Danbury		Steroid
DAN5444	Tab, White, Round	Chlorothiazide 250 mg	Diuril by Danbury		Diuretic
DAN5449025	Tab, Orange, Pentagonal, Dan 5449 0.25	Dexamethasone 0.25 mg	Decadron by Danbury		Steroid
DAN545005	Tab, Yellow, Pentagonal, Dan 5450 0.5	Dexamethasone 0.5 mg	Decadron by Danbury		Steroid
DAN545115	Tab, White, Pentagonal, Dan 5451 1.5	Dexamethasone 1.5 mg	Decadron by Danbury		Steroid
DAN5453	Tab, White, Round	Quinidine Sulfate 100 mg	by Danbury		Antiarrhythmic
DAN5454	Tab, White, Round, Dan/5454	Quinidine Sulfate 300 mg	by Danbury		Antiarrhythmic
DAN5455	Tab, Blue, Round	Chlorpropamide 250 mg	Diabinese by Danbury		Antidiabetic
DAN5479	Cap, Ivory & Orange, Dan/5479	Erythromycin Estolate 250 mg	Ilosone by Danbury		Antibiotic
DAN5484	Tab, White, Round	Cyproheptadine HCl 4 mg	Periactin by Danbury		Antihistamine
DAN5490	Tab, White, Round	Prednisone 50 mg	Deltasone by Danbury		Steroid
DAN5495	Tab, Peach, Round	Chlorzoxazone 250 mg	Parafon by Danbury		Muscle Relaxant
DAN5496	Tab, Buff, Round	Spironolactone 25 mg, Hydrochlorothiazide 25 mg	Aldactazide by Danbury		Diuretic
DAN5501	Tab, White, Round	Ergoloid Mesylates S.L. 1 mg	Hydergine by Danbury		Ergot
DAN5502	Tab, White, Round	Ergoloid Mesylates S.L. 0.5 mg	Hydergine by Danbury		Ergot
DAN5503	Tab, Butterscotch, Round, Dan/5503	Sulfasalazine 500 mg	Azulfidine by Danbury		Gastrointestinal
DAN5504	Tab, White, Round	Ergoloid Mesylates Oral 1 mg	Hydergine by Danbury		Ergot
DAN5506	Tab, Red, Round	Pseudoephedrine HCl 30 mg	Sudafed by Danbury		Decongestant
DAN5507	Tab, Yellow, Round	Chlorthalidone 25 mg	Hygroton by Danbury		Diuretic
DAN5508	Tab, White, Round	Tolbutamide 500 mg	Orinase by Danbury		Antidiabetic
DAN5510	Tab, White, Round	Dipyridamole 25 mg	Persantine by Danbury		Antiplatelet
DAN5511	Tab, White, Round	Dipyridamole 50 mg	Persantine by Danbury		Antiplatelet
DAN5512	Tab, White, Round	Dipyridamole 75 mg	Persantine by Danbury		Antiplatelet
DAN5513	Tab	Carisoprodol 350 mg	by Pharmedix	53002-0356	Muscle Relaxant
DAN5514	Tab, White, Round	Sulfinpyrazone 100 mg	Azulfidine by Danbury		Uricosuric
DAN5515	Tab, Yellow, Round	Bethanechol Chloride 50 mg	Urecholine by Danbury		Urinary Tract
DAN5516	Tab, White, Round	Quinine Sulfate 260 mg	Quinamm by Danbury		Antimalarial
DAN5518	Tab, Green, Round	Chlorthalidone 50 mg	Hygroton by Danbury		Diuretic
DAN5520	Cap, Black & Yellow	Tetracylcine HCl 500 mg	Achromycin V by Danbury		Antibiotic
DAN5522	Tab, Sugar Coated	Hydroxyzine HCl 10 mg	by Allscripts	54569-0406	Antihistamine
DAN5523	Tab, Sugar Coated	Hydroxyzine HCl 25 mg	by Allscripts	54569-0413	Antihistamine
DAN5523	Tab, Sugar Coated	Hydroxyzine HCl 25 mg	by Med Pro	53978-3066	Antihistamine
DAN5523	Tab, Film Coated	Hydroxyzine HCl 25 mg	by Nat Pharmpak Serv	55154-5203	Antihistamine
DAN5532	Tab, Film Coated	Hydroxyzine HCl 25 mg	by Direct Dispensing	57866-3874	Antihistamine
DAN5535	Cap	Doxycycline Hyclate	by Allscripts	54569-0147	Antibiotic
DAN5535	Cap, Blue & White	Doxycycline Hyclate 50 mg	by Danbury Pr	61955-2032	Antibiotic
DAN5535 <> DAN5535	Cap	Doxycycline Hyclate	by Danbury	00591-5535	Antibiotic
DAN5540	Tab	Metronidazole 250 mg	by Med Pro	53978-0215	Antibiotic
DAN5543	Tab, White, Round	Allopurinol 100 mg	Zyloprim by Danbury		Antigout
DAN5544	Tab, Orange, Round	Allopurinol 300 mg	Zyloprim by Danbury		Antigout
DAN5546	Tab, White, Round, Dan/5546	Sulfamethoxazole 400 mg, Trimethoprim 80 mg	Bactrim by Danbury		Antibiotic
DAN5547	Tab, White, Oval, Dan/5547	Sulfamethoxazole 800 mg, Trimethoprim 160 mg	Bactrim DS by Danbury		Antibiotic
DAN5548	Tab, White, Round, Dan/5548	Chloroquine Phosphate 250 mg	Aralen by Danbury		Antimalarial
DAN5549	Tab, White, Round	Chloroquine Phosphate 500 mg	Aralen by Danbury		Antimalarial
DAN5553	Tab, Film Coated	Doxycycline Hyclate	by Med Pro	53978-3028	Antibiotic
DAN5553	Tab, Film Coated	Doxycycline Hyclate	by Pharmedix	53002-0271	Antibiotic
DAN5554 <> 10	Tab	Propranolol HCl 10 mg	by Danbury	00591-5554	Antihypertensive
DAN555410	Tab	Propranolol HCl 10 mg	by Med Pro	53978-0034	Antihypertensive
DAN5555 <> 20	Tab	Propranolol HCl 20 mg	by Quality Care	60346-0598	Antihypertensive
DAN5555 <> 20	Tab, Blue, Round, Scored	Propranolol HCl 20 mg	by RX PAK	65084-0101	Antihypertensive
DAN5555 <> 20	Tab, Blue, Round, Scored	Propranolol HCl 20 mg	by Vangard Labs	00615-2562	Antihypertensive
DAN5555 <> 20	Tab	Propranolol HCl 20 mg	by Danbury	00591-5555	Antihypertensive

ID FRONT <> BACK	DESCRIPTION FRONT <> BACK	INGREDIENT & STRENGTH	BRAND (OR EQUIV.) & FIRM	NDC#	CLASS; SCH.
DAN5556 <> 40	Tab, Green, Round, Scored	Propranolol HCl 40 mg	by RX PAK	65084-0102	Antihypertensive
DAN5556 <> 40	Tab, Green, Round, Scored	Propranolol HCl 40 mg	by Vangard Labs	00615-2563	Antihypertensive
DAN5556 <> 40	Tab	Propranolol HCl 40 mg	by Danbury	00591-5556	Antihypertensive
DAN5557 <> 80	Tab	Propranolol HCl 80 mg	by Danbury	00591-5557	Antihypertensive
DAN5560 <> DAN5560	Cap	Disopyramide Phosphate	by Danbury	00591-5560	Antiarrhythmic
DAN5561 <> DAN5561	Cap	Disopyramide Phosphate	by Danbury	00591-5561	Antiarrhythmic
DAN5569	Tab, Orange, Round	Thioridazine HCl 100 mg	Mellaril by Danbury		Antipsychotic
DAN5571	Tab, White, Round	Trimethoprim 100 mg	Trimpex by Danbury		Antibiotic
DAN5572	Tab, White, Round	Thioridazine HCl 15 mg	Mellaril by Danbury		Antipsychotic
DAN5575	Tab, White, Round	Furosemide 40 mg	Lasix by Danbury		Diuretic
DAN5576	Tab, White, Round	Furosemide 20 mg	Lasix by Danbury		Diuretic
DAN5579	Tab, Blue, Round	Chlorpropamide 100 mg	Diabinese by Danbury		Antidiabetic
DAN5580	Tab, Orange, Round	Thioridazine HCl 150 mg	Mellaril by Danbury		Antipsychotic
DAN5581	Tab, Orange, Round, Dan/5581	Thioridazine 200 mg	Mellaril by Danbury		Antipsychotic
DAN5582	Tab, White, Round	Tolazamide 250 mg	Tolinase by Danbury		Antidiabetic
DAN5584	Tab, White, Round	Ibuprofen 400 mg	Motrin by Danbury		NSAID
DAN5585	Tab, White, Round	Ibuprofen 200 mg	Advil by Danbury		NSAID
DAN5586	Tab, White, Oval	Ibuprofen 600 mg	Motrin by Danbury		NSAID
DAN5587	Tab, Round, White, Dan-5587	Methyldopa 500 mg	Aldomet by Danbury		Antihypertensive
DAN5588	Tab, Round, White, Dan-5588	Methyldopa 250 mg	Aldomet by Danbury		Antihypertensive
DAN5589	Tab, White, Round	Metoclopramide HCl 10 mg	Reglan by Danbury		Gastrointestinal
DAN5590	Tab, White, Round	Tolazamide 500 mg	Tolinase by Danbury		Antidiabetic
DAN5591	Tab, White, Round	Tolazamide 100 mg	Tolinase by Danbury		Antidiabetic
DAN5592	Cap	Thiothixene 2 mg	by Quality Care	60346-0841	Antipsychotic
DAN5592 <> DAN5592	Cap	Thiothixene 2 mg	by Danbury	00591-5592	Antipsychotic
DAN5593 <> DAN5593	Cap	Thiothixene 1 mg	by Danbury	00591-5593	Antipsychotic
DAN5594 <> DAN5594	Cap	Thiothixene 10 mg	by Danbury	00591-5594	Antipsychotic
DAN5595	Cap, Opaque & Orange	Thiothixene 5 mg	by Taro	52549-4032	Antipsychotic
DAN5595 <> DAN5595	Cap, Green & Opaque	Thiothixene 2 mg	by Taro	52549-4033	Antipsychotic
DAN5595 <> DAN5595	Cap	Thiothixene 5 mg	by Danbury	00591-5595	Antipsychotic
DAN5599	Tab, White, Round	Trazodone 100 mg	Desyrel by Danbury		Antidepressant
DAN5601	Tab, Film Coated	Verapamil HCl 80 mg	by Pharmedix	53002-1027	Antihypertensive
DAN5602	Tab, Coated	Verapamil HCl 120 mg	by Pharmedix	53002-1074	Antihypertensive
DAN56032	Tab, Yellow, Round, Dan 5603/2	Haloperidol 2 mg	Haldol by Danbury		Antipsychotic
DAN56041	Tab, Peach, Round, Dan 5604/1	Haloperidol 1 mg	Haldol by Danbury		Antipsychotic
DAN560505	Tab, White, Round, Dan 5605 0.5	Haloperidol 0.5 mg	Haldol by Danbury		Antipsychotic
DAN56065	Tab, Blue, Round, Dan 5606/5	Haloperidol 5 mg	Haldol by Danbury		Antipsychotic
DAN560715	Tab, White, Round	Methyldopa 250 mg, Hydrochlorothiazide 15 mg	Aldoril 15 by Danbury		Antihypertensive
DAN560825	Tab, White, Round	Methyldopa 250 mg, Hydrochlorothiazide 25 mg	Aldoril 25 by Danbury		Antihypertensive
DAN5609 <> 01	Tab, Dan 5609 <> 0.1	Clonidine HCl 0.1 mg	by Quality Care	60346-0786	Antihypertensive
DAN5609 <> 01	Tab, Dan 5609 <> 0.1	Clonidine HCl 0.1 mg	by Danbury	00591-5609	Antihypertensive
DAN560901	Tab, White, Pentagonal, Dan 5609/0.1	Clonidine 0.1 mg	Catapres by Danbury		Antihypertensive
DAN561050	Tab, White, Round	Methyldopa 500 mg, Hydrochlorothiazide 50 mg	Aldoril D50 by Danbury		Antihypertensive
DAN561130	Tab, White, Round	Methyldopa 500 mg, Hydrochlorothiazide 30 mg	Aldoril D30 by Danbury		Antihypertensive
DAN5612 <> 02	Tab, Dan 5612 <> 0.2	Clonidine HCl 0.2 mg	by Danbury	00591-5612	Antihypertensive
DAN561202	Tab, Yellow, Pentagonal, Dan 5612/0.2	Clonidine 0.2 mg	Catapres by Danbury		Antihypertensive
DAN5613 <> 03	Tab, Dan 5613 <> 0.3	Clonidine HCl 0.3 mg	by Danbury	00591-5613	Antihypertensive
DAN5613 <> 03	Tab	Clonidine HCl 0.3 mg	by Allscripts	54569-2801	Antihypertensive
DAN561303	Tab, Blue, Pentagonal, Dan 5613/0.3	Clonidine 0.3 mg	Catapres by Danbury		Antihypertensive
DAN5614	Cap, Blue & White	Flurazepam HCl 15 mg	Dalmane by Danbury		Hypnotic; C IV
DAN5615	Cap	Flurazepam HCl 30 mg	by Quality Care	60346-0762	Hypnotic; C IV
DAN5616	Cap, Red	Oxazepam 15 mg	Serax by Danbury		Sedative/Hypnotic; C IV

ID FRONT <> BACK	DESCRIPTION FRONT <> BACK	INGREDIENT & STRENGTH	BRAND (OR EQUIV.) & FIRM	NDC#	CLASS; SCH.
DAN5617	Cap, White	Oxazepam 10 mg	Serax by Danbury		Sedative/Hypnotic; C IV
DAN5618	Cap, Maroon	Oxazepam 30 mg	Serax by Danbury		Sedative/Hypnotic; C IV
DAN5619 <> 5	Tab	Diazepam 5 mg	by St Marys Med	60760-0775	Antianxiety; C IV
DAN5619 <> 5	Tab, Yellow, Round, Scored	Diazepam 5 mg	by DRX	55045-2656	Antianxiety; C IV
DAN5619 <> 5	Tab, Dan over 5619	Diazepam 5 mg	by Quality Care	60346-0478	Antianxiety; C IV
DAN5619 <> 5	Tab	Diazepam 5 mg	by Danbury	00591-5619	Antianxiety; C IV
DAN5619 <> 5	Tab, Yellow, Round, Scored	Diazepam 5 mg	by Vangard Labs	00615-1533	Antianxiety; C IV
DAN5620 <> 10	Tab	Diazepam 10 mg	by St Marys Med	60760-0776	Antianxiety; C IV
DAN5620 <> 10	Tab, Light Blue	Diazepam 10 mg	by Quality Care	60346-0033	Antianxiety; C IV
DAN5620 <> 10	Tab	Diazepam 10 mg	by Danbury	00591-5620	Antianxiety; C IV
DAN5621 <> 2	Tab, White, Round, Scored	Diazepam 2 mg	by Vangard Labs	00615-1532	Antianxiety; C IV
DAN5621 <> 2	Tab, Dan over 5621	Diazepam 2 mg	by Quality Care	60346-0579	Antianxiety; C IV
DAN5621 <> 2	Tab, White, Round, Scored	Diazepam 2 mg	by DRX	55045-2652	Antianxiety; C IV
DAN5621 <> 2	Tab, White, Round, Scored	Diazepam 2 mg	by Murfreesboro Ph	51129-1302	Antianxiety; C IV
DAN5621 <> 2	Tab	Diazepam 2 mg	by Danbury	00591-5621	Antianxiety; C IV
DAN56222	Tab, White, Round, Dan 5622/2	Lorazepam 2 mg	Ativan by Danbury		Sedative/Hypnotic; C IV
DAN562360	Tab, Red, Round, Dan 5623/60	Propranolol HCl 60 mg	Inderal by Danbury		Antihypertensive
DAN56241	Tab, White, Round, Dan 5624/1	Lorazepam 1 mg	Ativan by Danbury		Sedative/Hypnotic; C IV
DAN562505	Tab, White, Round, Dan 5625/0.5	Lorazepam 0.5 mg	Ativan by Danbury		Sedative/Hypnotic; C IV
DAN5629	Cap, Beige	Doxepin HCl 10 mg	by Heartland Healthcare	61392-0120	Antidepressant
DAN5629	Cap, Tan, Opaque	Doxepin HCl 10 mg	by H J Harkins Co	52959-0246	Antidepressant
DAN5629	Cap, Beige, Opaque	Doxepin HCl 10 mg	by H J Harkins Co	52959-0366	Antidepressant
DAN5629	Cap, Green & Opaque	Doxepin HCl 10 mg	by H J Harkins Co	52959-0369	Antidepressant
DAN5629 <> DAN5629	Cap	Doxepin HCl	by Danbury	00591-5629	Antidepressant
DAN5630	Cap, Dan over 5630	Doxepin HCl	by Quality Care	60346-0553	Antidepressant
DAN5630 <> DAN5630	Cap	Doxepin HCl	by Danbury	00591-5630	Antidepressant
DAN5630 <> DAN5630	Cap, Ivory & White, Opaque	Doxepin HCl 25 mg	by H J Harkins Co	52959-0377	Antidepressant
DAN5631	Cap, Ivory, Opaque	Doxepin HCl 50 mg	by H J Harkins Co	52959-0012	Antidepressant
DAN5631	Cap, Cap	Doxepin HCl 50 mg	by H J Harkins Co	52959-0391	Antidepressant
DAN5631 <> DAN5631	Cap	Doxepin HCl	by Danbury	00591-5631	Antidepressant
DAN5632	Cap, Green	Doxepin HCl 75 mg	by Heartland Healthcare	61392-0933	Antidepressant
DAN5632 <> DAN5632	Cap	Doxepin HCl	by Danbury	00591-5632	Antidepressant
DAN5633 <> DAN5633	Cap, Light Green	Doxepin HCl	by Danbury	00591-5633	Antidepressant
DAN563590	Tab, Lavender, Round, Dan 5635/90	Propranolol HCl 90 mg	Inderal by Danbury		Antihypertensive
DAN5636 <> DAN5636	Cap	Meclofenamate Sodium	by Danbury	00591-5636	NSAID
DAN5637	Cap	Meclofenamate Sodium	by Pharmedix	53002-0400	NSAID
DAN5637 <> DAN5637	Cap	Meclofenamate Sodium	by Danbury	00591-5637	NSAID
DAN5642 <> 25	Tab, Dan 5642 <> 2.5	Minoxidil 2.5 mg	by Danbury	00591-5642	Antihypertensive
DAN564225	Tab, White, Round, Dan 5642/2.5	Minoxidil 2.5 mg	Loniten by Danbury		Antihypertensive
DAN5643 <> 10	Tab	Minoxidil 10 mg	by Danbury	00591-5643	Antihypertensive
DAN5644	Tab, White, Oval	Ibuprofen 800 mg	Motrin by Danbury		NSAID
DAN5658	Tab, Film Coated	Cyclobenzaprine HCl 10 mg	by Pharmedix	53002-0308	Muscle Relaxant
DAN5658	Tab, Film Coated	Cyclobenzaprine HCl 10 mg	by Danbury	61955-2348	Muscle Relaxant
DAN5658	Tab, White, Round, Film Coated	Cyclobenzaprine HCl 10 mg	by DJ Pharma	64455-0013	Muscle Relaxant
DAN5659	Tab, White, Round	Furosemide 80 mg	Lasix by Danbury		Diuretic
DAN5660	Tab	Sulindac 200 mg	by Pharmedix	53002-0388	NSAID
DAN5662	Tab, Off-White, Oval, Dan/5662	Nalidixic Acid 1 gm	NegGram by Danbury		Antibiotic
DAN5677	Tab, Off-White, Round, Dan/5677	Nalidixic Acid 500 mg	NegGram by Danbury		Antibiotic
DAN5678	Tab, White, Round	Chlordiazepoxide 10 mg, Amitriptyline HCl 25 mg	Limbitrol by Danbury		Antianxiety; C IV
DAN5679	Tab, Green, Round	Chlordiazepoxide 5 mg, Amitriptyline HCl 12.5 mg	Limbitrol by Danbury		Antianxiety; C IV
DAN5682	Cap	Hydrochlorothiazide 25 mg, Triamterene 50 mg	by Med Pro	53978-5009	Diuretic
DAN5682	Tab, Flat-faced and Bevel-edged, Compressed Powder, Dan/5682	Hydrochlorothiazide 50 mg, Triamterene 75 mg	by Kaiser	00179-1132	Diuretic

ID FRONT <> BACK	DESCRIPTION FRONT <> BACK	INGREDIENT & STRENGTH	BRAND (OR EQUIV.) & FIRM	NDC#	CLASS; SCH.
DAN5682	Tab	Hydrochlorothiazide 50 mg, Triamterene 75 mg	by Danbury	00591-5682	Diuretic
DAN5682	Tab	Hydrochlorothiazide 50 mg, Triamterene 75 mg	by Quality Care	60346-0704	Diuretic
DAN5682	Tab, Yellow, Round, Scored	Hydrochlorothiazide 50 mg, Triamterene 75 mg	by Heartland Hlthcare	61392-0965	Diuretic
DAN5693	Cap, Orange	Prazosin HCl 5 mg	Minipress by Danbury		Antihypertensive
DAN5694 <> MINOCYCLINE100	Cap, Dark Gray	Minocycline HCl	by Danbury	00591-5695	Antibiotic
DAN5694 <> MINOCYCLINE50	Cap	Minocycline HCl	by Danbury	00591-5694	Antibiotic
DAN5694 <> MINOCYCLINE50	Cap	Minocycline HCl	by Danbury	61955-2497	Antibiotic
DAN5695 <> MINOCYCLINE100	Cap	Minocycline HCl	by Danbury	61955-2498	Antibiotic
DAN5696	Cap, Gray	Prazosin HCl 2 mg	Minipress by Danbury		Antihypertensive
DAN5697	Cap	Prazosin HCl	by Pharmedix	53002-0499	Antihypertensive
DAN5708	Cap	Clindamycin HCl	by St Marys Med	60760-0337	Antibiotic
DAN5708 <> DAN5708	Cap	Clindamycin HCl	by Quality Care	60346-0018	Antibiotic
DAN5708 <> DAN5708	Cap	Clindamycin HCl	by Danbury	00591-5708	Antibiotic
DAN57102	Tab, White, Round, Dan-5710, 2	Albuterol Sulfate 2 mg	Ventolin by Danbury		Antiasthmatic
DAN57114	Tab, White, Round, Dan-5711, 4	Albuterol Sulfate 4 mg	Ventolin by Danbury		Antiasthmatic
DAN571325	Tab, White, Round	Amoxapine 25 mg	Asendin by Danbury		Antidepressant
DAN571450	Tab, Orange, Round	Amoxapine 50 mg	Asendin by Danbury		Antidepressant
DAN5715100	Tab, Blue, Round	Amoxapine 100 mg	Asendin by Danbury		Antidepressant
DAN5716150	Tab, Orange, Round	Amoxapine 150 mg	Asendin by Danbury		Antidepressant
DAN5726	Cap, Green	Hydroxyzine Pamoate 25 mg	by Heartland Hlthcare	61392-0801	Antihistamine
DAN5726 <> DAN5726	Cap, Dark Green & Light Green	Hydroxyzine Pamoate	by Danbury	00591-5726	Antihistamine
DAN5730 <> 10	Tab	Baclofen 10 mg	by Heartland	61392-0706	Muscle Relaxant
DAN5730 <> 10	Tab, White, Round, Scored	Baclofen 10 mg	by Heartland Hlthcare	61392-0090	Muscle Relaxant
DAN5730 <> 10	Tab	Baclofen 10 mg	by Amerisource	62584-0623	Muscle Relaxant
DAN5730 <> 10	Tab	Baclofen 10 mg	by Danbury	00591-5730	Muscle Relaxant
DAN5731 <> 20	Tab	Baclofen 20 mg	by Amerisource	62584-0624	Muscle Relaxant
DAN5731 <> 20	Tab	Baclofen 20 mg	by Danbury	00591-5731	Muscle Relaxant
DAN57365	Tab, White, Round	Timolol Maleate 5 mg	Blocadren by Danbury		Antihypertensive
DAN573710	Tab, White, Round	Timolol Maleate 10 mg	Blocadren by Danbury		Antihypertensive
DAN577750	Tab, White, Round, Dan-5777, 50	Atenolol 50 mg	Tenormin by Danbury		Antihypertensive
DAN5778100	Tab, White, Round, Dan-5778, 100	Atenolol 100 mg	Tenormin by Danbury		Antihypertensive
DAN5782	Tab	Atenolol 50 mg, Chlorthalidone 25 mg	by Danbury	00591-5782	Antihypertensive; Diuretic
DAN5783	Tab	Atenolol 100 mg, Chlorthalidone 25 mg	by Danbury	00591-5783	Antihypertensive; Diuretic
DAN5912	Tab	Captopril 50 mg, Hydrochlorothiazide 25 mg	by Danbury	00591-5912	Antihypertensive; Diuretic
DAN75MG <> NORTRIPTYLINE	Cap	Nortriptyline HCl	by Danbury	61955-2511	Antidepressant
DAN75MG <> NORTRIPTYLINE	Cap	Nortriptyline HCl	by Danbury	00591-5789	Antidepressant
DAN75MG <> NORTRIPTYLINE	Cap	Nortriptyline HCl	by Heartland	61392-0370	Antidepressant
DAN80 <> 5557	Tab, Yellow, Round, Scored	Propranolol HCl 80 mg	by Schein	00364-0760	Antihypertensive
DAN937	Tab, White, Round	Papaverine HCl 60 mg	by Danbury		Vasodilator
DAN938	Tab, White, Round	Papaverine HCl 100 mg	by Danbury		Vasodilator
DAN944	Tab	Colchicine 0.6 mg	by Pharmedix	53002-0444	Antigout
DANA22	Tab, Yellow, Round, Film Coated	Ranitidine HCl 150 mg	by Dixon Shane	17236-0741	Gastrointestinal

ID FRONT <> BACK	DESCRIPTION FRONT <> BACK	INGREDIENT & STRENGTH	BRAND (OR EQUIV.) & FIRM	NDC#	CLASS; SCH.
DANA22	Tab, Film Coated	Ranitidine HCl 167.5 mg	by Ranbaxy	63304-0745	Gastrointestinal
DANA22	Tab, Film Coated	Ranitidine HCl 167.5 mg	by Danbury	00591-8013	Gastrointestinal
DANA23	Tab, Coated	Ranitidine HCl 336 mg	by Ranbaxy	63304-0746	Gastrointestinal
DANA23	Tab, Yellow	Ranitidine HCl 336 mg	by Apotheca	12634-0560	Gastrointestinal
DANA23	Tab, Coated	Ranitidine HCl 336 mg	by Danbury	00591-8014	Gastrointestinal
DANAND5538	Tab, White, Round	Quinidine Gluconate 324 mg	by Heartland Healthcare	61392-0952	Antiarrhythmic
DANBURY5373	Tab	Isosorbide Dinitrate 10 mg	by Pharmedix	53002-0451	Antianginal
DANDAN <> 5052	Tab, White, Round, Scored	Prednisone 5 mg	by Schein	00364-0218	Steroid
DANDAN <> 5052	Tab	Prednisone 5 mg	by Danbury	00591-5052	Steroid
DANDAN <> 5052	Tab, White, Round, Scored	Prednisone 10 mg	by Southwood Pharms	58016-0216	Steroid
DANDAN <> 5052	Tab	Prednisone 10 mg	by Vangard	00615-3593	Steroid
DANDAN <> 5052	Tab	Prednisone 5 mg	by Vangard	00615-0536	Steroid
DANDAN <> 5052	Tab	Prednisone 5 mg	by Vedco	50989-0601	Steroid
DANDAN <> 5052	Tab	Prednisone 5 mg	by Quality Care	60346-0515	Steroid
DANDAN <> 5052	Tab	Prednisone 5 mg	by Heartland	61392-0408	Steroid
DANDAN <> 5052	Tab	Prednisone 5 mg	by Danbury	61955-0218	Steroid
DANDAN <> 5052	Tab	Prednisone 5 mg	by WA Butler	11695-1801	Steroid
DANDAN <> 5058	Tab, Blue-Green, Round, Scored	Tripelennamine HCl 50 mg	by Schein	00364-0281	Antihistamine
DANDAN <> 5059	Tab	Prednisolone 5 mg	by Darby Group	66467-4346	Steroid
DANDAN <> 5059	Tab, Peach, Round, Scored	Prednisolone 5 mg	by Schein	00364-0217	Steroid
DANDAN <> 5216	Tab	Folic Acid 1 mg	by Quality Care	60346-0697	Vitamin
DANDAN <> 5216	Tab	Folic Acid 1 mg	by Vangard	00615-0664	Vitamin
DANDAN <> 5216	Tab, Yellow, Round, Scored	Folic Acid 1 mg	by Schein	00364-0137	Vitamin
DANDAN <> 5216	Tab	Folic Acid 1 mg	by Danbury	00591-5216	Vitamin
DANDAN <> 526	Tab, White, Round, Scored	Isoniazid 300 mg	by Schein	00364-0151	Antimycobacterial
DANDAN <> 5307	Tab, White, Round, Scored	Promethazine HCl 25 mg	by Ranbaxy	63304-0690	Antiemetic; Antihistamine
DANDAN <> 5307	Tab, White, Round, Scored	Promethazine HCl 25 mg	by Schein	00364-0222	Antiemetic; Antihistamine
DANDAN <> 5307	Tab	Promethazine HCl 25 mg	by Danbury	00591-5307	Antiemetic; Antihistamine
DANDAN <> 5307	Tab	Promethazine HCl 25 mg	by Allscripts	54569-1754	Antiemetic; Antihistamine
DANDAN <> 5307	Tab	Promethazine HCl 25 mg	by Quality Care	60346-0085	Antiemetic; Antihistamine
DANDAN <> 5321	Tab	Primidone 250 mg	by Danbury	00591-5321	Anticonvulsant
DANDAN <> 5321	Tab, White, Round, Scored	Primidone 250 mg	by Schein	00364-0366	Anticonvulsant
DANDAN <> 5321	Tab, White, Round, Scored	Primidone 250 mg	by Quality Care	60346-0367	Anticonvulsant
DANDAN <> 5321	Tab	Primidone 250 mg	by Vangard	00615-2521	Anticonvulsant
DANDAN <> 5325	Tab, White, Cap Shaped, Scored	Colchicine 0.5 mg, Probenecid 500 mg	by Schein	00364-0315	Antigout
DANDAN <> 5325	Tab	Colchicine 0.5 mg, Probenecid 500 mg	Col Probenecid by Danbury	00591-5325	Antigout
DANDAN <> 5335	Tab, White, Round, Scored	Trihexyphenidyl HCl 2 mg	by Heartland Healthcare	61392-0634	Antiparkinson
DANDAN <> 5335	Tab	Trihexyphenidyl HCl 2 mg	by Danbury	00591-5335	Antiparkinson
DANDAN <> 5335	Tab, White, Round, Scored	Trihexyphenidyl HCl 2 mg	by Schein	00364-0408	Antiparkinson
DANDAN <> 5335	Tab	Trihexyphenidyl HCl 2 mg	by Vangard	00615-0675	Antiparkinson
DANDAN <> 5335	Tab	Trihexyphenidyl HCl 2 mg	by Quality Care	60346-0844	Antiparkinson
DANDAN <> 5335	Tab	Trihexyphenidyl HCl 2 mg	by Amerisource	62584-0886	Antiparkinson
DANDAN <> 5335	Tab	Trihexyphenidyl HCl 2 mg	by Danbury	61955-0408	Antiparkinson
DANDAN <> 5335	Tab	Trihexyphenidyl HCl 2 mg	by Octofoil	63467-0301	Antiparkinson
DANDAN <> 5337	Tab, White, Round, Scored	Trihexyphenidyl HCl 5 mg	by Schein	00364-0409	Antiparkinson
DANDAN <> 5337	Tab	Trihexyphenidyl HCl 5 mg	by Danbury	00591-5337	Antiparkinson
DANDAN <> 5337	Tab	Trihexyphenidyl HCl 5 mg	by Danbury	61955-0409	Antiparkinson

ID FRONT <> BACK	DESCRIPTION FRONT <> BACK	INGREDIENT & STRENGTH	BRAND (OR EQUIV.) & FIRM	NDC#	CLASS; SCH.
DANDAN <> 5337	Tab	Trihexyphenidyl HCl 5 mg	by Amerisource	62584-0887	Antiparkinson
DANDAN <> 5342	Tab, White, Round, Scored	Nylidrin 6 mg	by Schein	00364-0391	Vasodilator
DANDAN <> 5345	Tab	Hydrochlorothiazide 50 mg	by Talbert Med	44514-0411	Diuretic
DANDAN <> 5345	Tab, Peach, Round, Scored	Hydrochlorothiazide 50 mg	by Schein	00364-0328	Diuretic
DANDAN <> 5347	Tab, Yellow, Cap-Shaped, Film Coated, Scored	Probenecid 500 mg	by Schein	00364-0314	Antigout
DANDAN <> 5347	Tab	Probenecid 500 mg	by Danbury	00591-5347	Antigout
DANDAN <> 5368	Tab, Off-White, Round, Scored	Disulfiram 500 mg	by Schein	00364-0337	Antialcoholism
DANDAN <> 5369	Tab, White, Round, Scored	Bethanechol Chloride 10 mg	by Bryant	63629-1164	Urinary Tract
DANDAN <> 5369	Tab, White, Round, Scored	Bethanechol Chloride 10 mg	by Schein	00364-0349	Urinary Tract
DANDAN <> 5369	Tab	Bethanechol Chloride 10 mg	by Danbury	00591-5369	Urinary Tract
DANDAN <> 5373	Tab, White, Round, Scored	Isosorbide Dinitrate 10 mg	by Schein	00364-0341	Antianginal
DANDAN <> 5373	Tab	Isosorbide Dinitrate 10 mg	by Quality Care	60346-0577	Antianginal
DANDAN <> 5374	Tab, White, Round, Scored	Isosorbide Dinitrate 5 mg	by Schein	00364-0340	Antianginal
DANDAN <> 5374	Tab	Isosorbide Dinitrate 5 mg	by Danbury	00591-5374	Antianginal
DANDAN <> 5381	Tab	Methocarbamol 500 mg	by Danbury	00591-5381	Muscle Relaxant
DANDAN <> 5381	Tab	Methocarbamol 500 mg	by Kaiser	00179-0446	Muscle Relaxant
DANDAN <> 5381	Tab, White, Round, Scored	Methocarbamol 500 mg	by Schein	00364-0346	Muscle Relaxant
DANDAN <> 5381	Tab	Methocarbamol 500 mg	by Quality Care	60346-0080	Muscle Relaxant
DANDAN <> 5381	Tab	Methocarbamol 500 mg	by Talbert Med	44514-0557	Muscle Relaxant
DANDAN <> 5382	Tab	Methocarbamol 750 mg	by Kaiser	00179-0447	Muscle Relaxant
DANDAN <> 5382	Tab	Methocarbamol 750 mg	by Danbury	00591-5382	Muscle Relaxant
DANDAN <> 5382	Tab, White, Cap-Shaped, Scored	Methocarbamol 750 mg	by Schein	00364-0347	Muscle Relaxant
DANDAN <> 5382	Tab	Methocarbamol 750 mg	by Allscripts	54569-0843	Muscle Relaxant
DANDAN <> 5382	Tab	Methocarbamol 750 mg	by Talbert Med	44514-0558	Muscle Relaxant
DANDAN <> 5388	Tab, White, Cap-Shaped, Scored	Triamcinolone 4 mg	by Schein	00364-0352	Steroid
DANDAN <> 5390	Tab, White, Round, Scored	Nylidrin 12 mg	by Schein	00364-0392	Vasodilator
DANDAN <> 5402	Tab, Yellow, Round, Scored	Bethanechol Chloride 25 mg	by Schein	00364-0410	Urinary Tract
DANDAN <> 5402	Tab	Bethanechol Chloride 25 mg	by Danbury	00591-5402	Urinary Tract
DANDAN <> 5406	Tab, Green, Round, Scored	Reserpine 0.125 mg, Hydrochlorothiazide 25 mg	by Schein	00364-0354	Antihypertensive
DANDAN <> 5407	Tab, Green, Round, Scored	Reserpine 0.125 mg, Hydrochlorothiazide 50 mg	by Schein	00364-0355	Antihypertensive
DANDAN <> 5430	Tab, White, Round, Scored	Acetazolamide 250 mg	by Amerisource	62584-0043	Diuretic
DANDAN <> 5430	Tab	Acetazolamide 250 mg	by Quality Care	60346-0734	Diuretic
DANDAN <> 5430	Tab, White, Round, Scored	Acetazolamide 250 mg	by Schein	00364-0400	Diuretic
DANDAN <> 5430	Tab	Acetazolamide 250 mg	by Danbury	00591-5430	Diuretic
DANDAN <> 5438	Tab	Quinidine Sulfate 200 mg	by Danbury	00591-5438	Antiarrhythmic
DANDAN <> 5438	Tab, White, Round, Scored	Quinidine Sulfate 200 mg	by Schein	00364-0229	Antiarrhythmic
DANDAN <> 5442	Tab, White, Round, Scored	Prednisone 10 mg	by Schein	00364-0461	Steroid
DANDAN <> 5442	Tab	Prednisone 10 mg	by Danbury	00591-5442	Steroid
DANDAN <> 5442	Tab	Prednisone 10 mg	by Med Pro	53978-3037	Steroid
DANDAN <> 5442	Tab	Prednisone 10 mg	by Allscripts	54569-0331	Steroid
DANDAN <> 5442	Tab	Prednisone 10 mg	by Allscripts	54569-3302	Steroid
DANDAN <> 5442	Tab	Prednisone 10 mg	by Nat Pharmpak Serv	55154-5215	Steroid
DANDAN <> 5442	Tab	Prednisone 10 mg	by Quality Care	60346-0058	Steroid
DANDAN <> 5442	Tab	Prednisone 10 mg	by Danbury	61955-0461	Steroid
DANDAN <> 5442	Tab	Prednisone 10 mg	by Heartland	61392-0417	Steroid
DANDAN <> 5443	Tab	Prednisone 20 mg	by Danbury	61955-0442	Steroid
DANDAN <> 5443	Tab	Prednisone 20 mg	by Quality Care	60346-0094	Steroid
DANDAN <> 5443	Tab, Peach, Round, Scored	Prednisone 20 mg	by Qualitest	00603-2551	Steroid
DANDAN <> 5443	Tab	Prednisone 20 mg	by WA Butler	11695-1802	Steroid
DANDAN <> 5443	Tab	Prednisone 20 mg	by Vangard	00615-1542	Steroid
DANDAN <> 5443	Tab	Prednisone 20 mg	by Danbury	00591-5443	Steroid
DANDAN <> 5443	Tab, Peach, Round, Scored	Prednisone 20 mg	by Schein	00364-0442	Steroid

ID FRONT <> BACK	DESCRIPTION FRONT <> BACK	INGREDIENT & STRENGTH	BRAND (OR EQUIV.) & FIRM	NDC#	CLASS; SCH.
DANDAN <> 5443	Tab	Prednisone 20 mg	by HJ Harkins Co	52959-0127	Steroid
DANDAN <> 5443	Tab	Prednisone 20 mg	by Allscripts	54569-0332	Steroid
DANDAN <> 5443	Tab	Prednisone 20 mg	by Vedco	50989-0602	Steroid
DANDAN <> 5443	Tab, Peach, Round, Scored	Prednisone 20 mg	by Allscripts	54569-3043	Steroid
DANDAN <> 5454	Tab	Quinidine Sulfate 300 mg	by Danbury	00591-5454	Antiarrhythmic
DANDAN <> 5454	Tab, White, Round, Scored	Quinidine Sulfate 300 mg	by Schein	00364-0582	Antiarrhythmic
DANDAN <> 5455	Tab, Blue, Tab, Blue, Round, Scored	Chlorpropamide 250 mg	by Schein	00364-0510	Antidiabetic
DANDAN <> 5496	Tab, Buff, Round, Scored	Spironolactone 25 mg, Hydrochlorothiazide 25 mg	by Schein	00364-0513	Diuretic
DANDAN <> 5508	Tab, White, Round, Scored	Tolbutamide 500 mg	by Schein	00364-0477	Antidiabetic
DANDAN <> 5515	Tab	Bethanechol Chloride 50 mg	by Danbury	00591-5515	Urinary Tract
DANDAN <> 5515	Tab, Yellow, Round, Scored	Bethanechol Chloride 50 mg	by Schein	00364-0590	Urinary Tract
DANDAN <> 5543	Tab	Allopurinol 100 mg	by Danbury	61955-0632	Antigout
DANDAN <> 5543	Tab	Allopurinol 100 mg	by Quality Care	60346-0774	Antigout
DANDAN <> 5543	Tab, White, Round, Scored	Allopurinol 100 mg	by Natl Pharmpak	55154-5239	Antigout
DANDAN <> 5543	Tab	Allopurinol 100 mg	by Danbury	00591-5543	Antigout
DANDAN <> 5543	Tab, White, Round, Scored	Allopurinol 100 mg	by Schein	00364-0632	Antigout
DANDAN <> 5544	Tab	Allopurinol 300 mg	by Danbury	61955-0633	Antigout
DANDAN <> 5544	Tab, Orange, Round, Scored	Allopurinol 300 mg	by Schein	00364-0633	Antigout
DANDAN <> 5544	Tab	Allopurinol 300 mg	by Danbury	00591-5544	Antigout
DANDAN <> 5544	Tab, Orange, Round, Scored	Allopurinol 300 mg	by Apotheca	12634-0498	Antigout
DANDAN <> 5546	Tab, White, Round, Scored	Sulfamethoxazole 400 mg, Trimethoprim 80 mg	by Schein	00364-2068	Antibiotic
DANDAN <> 5546	Tab	Sulfamethoxazole 400 mg, Trimethoprim 80 mg	by Danbury	00591-5546	Antibiotic
DANDAN <> 5546	Tab	Sulfamethoxazole 400 mg, Trimethoprim 80 mg	by Allscripts	54569-0269	Antibiotic
DANDAN <> 5546	Tab, White, Round, Scored	Sulfamethoxazole 400 mg, Trimethoprim 80 mg	by St. Marys Med	60760-0004	Antibiotic
DANDAN <> 5547	Tab	Sulfamethoxazole 800 mg, Trimethoprim 160 mg	by Danbury	00591-5547	Antibiotic
DANDAN <> 5547	Tab, White, Oval, Scored	Sulfamethoxazole 800 mg, Trimethoprim 160 mg	by Schein	00364-2069	Antibiotic
DANDAN <> 5547	Tab	Sulfamethoxazole 800 mg, Trimethoprim 160 mg	Trimeth Sulfa DS by Pharmedix	53002-0210	Antibiotic
DANDAN <> 5548	Tab, White, Round, Scored	Chloroquine Phosphate 250 mg	by Schein	00364-0470	Antimalarial
DANDAN <> 5552	Tab, Off-White to White, Round	Metronidazole 500 mg	by Schein	00364-0687	Antibiotic
DANDAN <> 5552	Tab	Metronidazole 500 mg	by Danbury	00591-5552	Antibiotic
DANDAN <> 5563	Tab, White, Oval, Film Coated, Scored, Ex Release	Procainamide HCl 500 mg	by Schein	00364-0716	Antiarrhythmic
DANDAN <> 5564	Tab, White, Oval, Film Coated, Scored, Ex Release	Procainamide HCl 750 mg	by Schein	00364-0717	Antiarrhythmic
DANDAN <> 5571	Tab, White, Oval, Scored	Trimethoprim 100 mg	by Schein	00364-0649	Antibiotic
DANDAN <> 5571	Tab	Trimethoprim 100 mg	by Danbury	00591-5571	Antibiotic
DANDAN <> 5575	Tab, White, Round, Scored	Furosemide 40 mg	by Schein	00364-0514	Diuretic
DANDAN <> 5579	Tab, Blue, Round, Scored	Chlorpropamide 100 mg	by Schein	00364-0699	Antidiabetic
DANDAN <> 5582	Tab, White, Round, Scored	Tolazamide 250 mg	by Schein	00364-0720	Antidiabetic
DANDAN <> 5589	Tab	Metoclopramide HCl	by Quality Care	60346-0802	Gastrointestinal
DANDAN <> 5589	Tab	Metoclopramide HCl	by Danbury	00591-5589	Gastrointestinal
DANDAN <> 5589	Tab, White, Round, Scored	Metoclopramide HCl 10 mg	by Schein	00364-0769	Gastrointestinal
DANDAN <> 5590	Tab, White, Round, Scored	Tolazamide 500 mg	by Schein	00364-0722	Antidiabetic
DANDAN <> 5591	Tab, White, Round, Scored	Tolazamide 100 mg	by Schein	00364-0721	Antidiabetic
DANDAN <> 5597	Tab, White, Cap Shaped, Scored	Acetohexamide 500 mg	by Schein	00364-2233	Antidiabetic
DANDAN <> 5597	Tab	Acetohexamide 500 mg	by Danbury	00591-5597	Antidiabetic
DANDAN <> 5598	Tab, White, Cap Shaped, Scored	Acetohexamide 250 mg	by Schein	00364-2232	Antidiabetic
DANDAN <> 5598	Tab	Acetohexamide 250 mg	by Danbury	00591-5598	Antidiabetic
DANDAN <> 5599	Tab, White, Round, Film Coated, Scored	Trazodone HCl 100 mg	by Schein	00364-2110	Antidepressant
DANDAN <> 5599	Tab, Coated	Trazodone HCl 100 mg	by Danbury	00591-5599	Antidepressant
DANDAN <> 5600	Tab, Coated	Trazodone HCl 50 mg	by Danbury	00591-5600	Antidepressant
DANDAN <> 5600	Tab, White, Round, Film Coated, Scored	Trazodone HCl 50 mg	by Schein	00364-2109	Antidepressant
DANDAN <> 5600	Tab, Coated	Trazodone HCl 50 mg	by Quality Care	60346-0620	Antidepressant
DANDAN <> 5601	Tab, White, Round, Film Coated, Scored	Verapamil HCl 80 mg	by Schein	00364-2111	Antihypertensive

ID FRONT <> BACK	DESCRIPTION FRONT <> BACK	INGREDIENT & STRENGTH	BRAND (OR EQUIV.) & FIRM	NDC#	CLASS; SCH.
DANDAN <> 5601	Tab, Film Coated	Verapamil HCl 80 mg	by Danbury	00591-5601	Antihypertensive
DANDAN <> 5601	Tab, Film Coated	Verapamil HCl 80 mg	by Amerisource	62584-0888	Antihypertensive
DANDAN <> 5602	Tab, Dan/Dan <> 5602	Clonidine HCl 0.2 mg	by Nat Pharmpak Serv	55154-5229	Antihypertensive
DANDAN <> 5602	Tab, Coated	Verapamil HCl 120 mg	by Amerisource	62584-0889	Antihypertensive
DANDAN <> 5602	Tab, White, Round, Scored, Film	Verapamil HCl 120 mg	by Ther Rx	64011-0024	Antihypertensive
DANDAN <> 5602	Tab, Coated	Verapamil HCl 120 mg	by Danbury	00591-5602	Antihypertensive
DANDAN <> 5602	Tab, White, Round, Coated, Scored	Verapamil HCl 120 mg	by Schein	00364-2112	Antihypertensive
DANDAN <> 5659	Tab, White, Round, Scored	Furosemide 80 mg	by Schein	00364-0700	Diuretic
DANDAN <> 5660	Tab, Yellow, Round, Scored	Sulindac 200 mg	by Schein	00364-2442	NSAID
DANDAN <> 5660	Tab	Sulindac 200 mg	by Danbury	00591-5660	NSAID
DANDAN <> 5660	Tab	Sulindac 200 mg	by HJ Harkins Co	52959-0195	NSAID
DANDAN <> 5660	Tab	Sulindac 200 mg	by Allscripts	54569-4032	NSAID
DANDAN <> 5660	Tab, Dan Dan <> 56/60	Sulindac 200 mg	by Quality Care	60346-0686	NSAID
DANDAN <> 5660	Tab	Sulindac 200 mg	by St Marys Med	60760-0424	NSAID
DANDAN <> 5660	Tab	Sulindac 200 mg	by PDRX	55289-0930	NSAID
DANDAN <> 5677	Tab, Off-White, Round, Scored	Nalidixic Acid 500 mg	by Schein	00364-2324	Antibiotic
DANDAN <> 5704	Tab, White, Cap Shaped, Film Coated, Scored	Fenoprofen Calcium 600 mg	by Schein	00364-2316	NSAID
DANDAN5059	Tab	Prednisolone 5 mg	by Danbury	00591-5059	Steroid
DANDAN5059	Tab	Prednisolone 5 mg	by Vedco	50989-0600	Steroid
DANDAN5059	Tab	Prednisolone 5 mg	by WA Butler	11695-1800	Steroid
DANDAN5216	Tab	Folic Acid 1 mg	by Amerisource	62584-0708	Vitamin
DANDAN5216	Tab, Yellow, Round, Scored	Folic Acid 1 mg	by JB	51111-0087	Vitamin
DANDAN5381	Tab	Methocarbamol 500 mg	by Allscripts	54569-0852	Muscle Relaxant
DANDAN5430	Tab, White, Round	Acetazolamide 250 mg	by Compumed	00403-0058	Diuretic
DANDAN5438	Tab, White, Round, Scored	Quinidine Sulfate 200 mg	by Heartland Healthcare	61392-0953	Antiarrhythmic
DANDAN5442	Tab	Prednisone 10 mg	by Amerisource	62584-0833	Steroid
DANDAN5443	Tab	Prednisone 20 mg	by Amerisource	62584-0834	Steroid
DANDAN5543	Tab	Allopurinol 100 mg	by Allscripts	54569-0233	Antigout
DANDAN5544	Tab	Allopurinol 300 mg	by Allscripts	54569-0235	Antigout
DANDAN5547	Tab	Sulfamethoxazole 800 mg, Trimethoprim 160 mg	by Nat Pharmpak Serv	55154-5205	Antibiotic
DANDAN5547	Tab, White, Oval, Scored	Sulfamethoxazole 800 mg, Trimethoprim 160 mg	by Amerisource Health	62584-0399	Antibiotic
DANDAN5547	Tab, White, Oval, Scored	Trimethoprim 160 mg, Sulfamethoxazole 800 mg	SMZ/TMP DS by Southwood Pharms	58016-0109	Antibiotic
DANDAN5562	Tab, White, Oval, Dan/Dan 5562	Procainamide HCl SR 250 mg	Procan SR by Danbury		Antiarrhythmic
DANDAN5563	Tab, White, Oval, Dan/Dan 5563	Procainamide HCl SR 500 mg	Procan SR by Danbury		Antiarrhythmic
DANDAN5564	Tab, White, Oval, Dan/Dan 5564	Procainamide HCl SR 750 mg	Procan SR by Danbury		Antiarrhythmic
DANDAN5589	Tab	Metoclopramide HCl	by Nat Pharmpak Serv	55154-5202	Gastrointestinal
DANDAN5589	Tab	Metoclopramide HCl 10 mg	by Med Pro	53978-5011	Gastrointestinal
DANDAN5704	Tab, White, Dan/Dan 5704	Fenoprofen Calcium 600 mg	Nalfon by Danbury		NSAID
DANP100	Tab, White, Round, Dan-P 100	Phenobarbital 100 mg	by Danbury		Sedative/Hypnotic; C IV
DANP15	Tab, White, Round, Dan-P 15	Phenobarbital 15 mg	by Danbury		Sedative/Hypnotic; C IV
DANP30	Tab, White, Round, Dan-P 30	Phenobarbital 30 mg	by Danbury		Sedative/Hypnotic; C IV
DANP60	Tab, White, Round, Dan-P 60	Phenobarbital 60 mg	by Danbury		Sedative/Hypnotic; C IV
DANTRIUM	Cap, Orange & Tan	Dantrolene Sodium 100 mg	Dantrium by Procter & Gamble	00149-0033	Muscle Relaxant
DANTRIUM100MG 01490033	Cap, Brown to Tan & Orange, Opaque w/ Three Black Bands, Dantrium 100 mg 0149 0033	Dantrolene Sodium 100 mg	Dantrium Caps by Procter & Gamble	Canadian DIN# 01997602	Muscle Relaxant
DANTRIUM25MG <> 01490030	Cap, Beige & Orange, Opaque, Dantrium 25 mg <> 0149-0030	Dantrolene Sodium 25 mg	Dantrium by Drug Distr	52985-0231	Muscle Relaxant
DANTRIUM25MG <> 014930	Cap, Orange & Tan	Dantrolene Sodium 25 mg	Dantrium by Procter & Gamble	00149-0030	Muscle Relaxant

ID FRONT <> BACK	DESCRIPTION FRONT <> BACK	INGREDIENT & STRENGTH	BRAND (OR EQUIV.) & FIRM	NDC#	CLASS; SCH.
DANTRIUM25MG 01490030	Cap, Brown to Tan & Orange, Opaque w/ One Black Band, Dantrium 25 mg 0149 0030	Dantrolene Sodium 25 mg	Dantrium th Procter & Gamble	Canadian DIN# 01997602	Muscle Relaxant
DANTRIUM50MG <> 014931	Cap, Orange & Tan	Dantrolene Sodium 50 mg	Dantrium by Procter & Gamble	00149-0031	Muscle Relaxant
DARAPRIM <> A3A	Tab	Pyrimethamine 25 mg	Daraprim by Catalytica	63552-0201	Antiprotozoal
DARAPRIM <> A3A	Tab	Pyrimethamine 25 mg	Daraprim by Glaxo	00173-0201	Antiprotozoal
DARAPRIMA3A	Tab, White, Biconvex	Pyrimethamine 25 mg	Daraprim by B.W. Inc	Canadian	Antiprotozoal
DARVOCETN100	Tab, Film Coated, Darvocet-N 100	Acetaminophen 650 mg, Propoxyphene Napsylate 100 mg	Darvocet N 100 by Caremark	00339-4045	Analgesic; C IV
DARVOCETN100	Tab, Film Coated, Darvocet-N 100	Acetaminophen 650 mg, Propoxyphene Napsylate 100 mg	Darvocet N by Quality Care	60346-0685	Analgesic; C IV
DARVOCETN100 <> LILLY	Tab, Dark Orange, Film Coated, Darvocet-N 100 <> Lilly	Acetaminophen 650 mg, Propoxyphene Napsylate 100 mg	Darvocet N 100 by Eli Lilly	00002-0363	Analgesic; C IV
DARVOCETN100 <> LILLY	Tab, Film Coated	Acetaminophen 650 mg, Propoxyphene Napsylate 100 mg	Darvocet N 100 by Med Pro	53978-3084	Analgesic; C IV
DARVOCETN100 <> LILLY	Tab, Film Coated	Acetaminophen 650 mg, Propoxyphene Napsylate 100 mg	Darvocet N by Nat Pharmpak Serv	55154-1807	Analgesic; C IV
DARVOCETN100 <> LILLY	Tab, Film Coated, Darvocet-N 100	Acetaminophen 650 mg, Propoxyphene Napsylate 100 mg	Darvocet N 100 by Allscripts	54569-0007	Analgesic; C IV
DARVON <> LILLYH03 LILLY	Cap, Pink, with Dark Pink Band	Propoxyphene HCl 65 mg	Darvon by Eli Lilly	00002-0803	Analgesic; C IV
DARVONCOMP65 <> LILLY3111	Cap	Aspirin 389 mg, Caffeine 32.4 mg, Propoxyphene HCl 65 mg	Darvon Compound 65 by Med Pro	53978-3083	Analgesic; C IV
DARVONCOMP65 <> LILLY3111	Cap, Darvon Comp 65 <> Lilly 3111	Aspirin 389 mg, Caffeine 32.4 mg, Propoxyphene HCl 65 mg	Darvon Compound 65 by Eli Lilly	00002-3111	Analgesic; C IV
DARVONN100 <> LILLY	Tab, Buff, Darvon-N 100 <> Lilly	Propoxyphene Napsylate 100 mg	Darvon N by Eli Lilly	00002-0353	Analgesic; C IV
DARVONN100 <> LILLY	Tab, Buff, Darvon-N 100 <> Lilly	Propoxyphene Napsylate 100 mg	Darvon N by Med Pro	53978-3082	Analgesic; C IV
DAYPRO <> 1381	Cap, White, Scored, Film	Oxaprozin 600 mg	by PF	48692-0013	NSAID
DAYPRO <> 1381	Tab, Film Coated, Daypro <> 13/81	Oxaprozin 600 mg	Daypro by GD Searle	00014-1381	NSAID
DAYPRO <> 1381	Tab, Film Coated	Oxaprozin 600 mg	Daypro by GD Searle	00025-1381	NSAID
DAYPRO <> 1381	Tab, White, Oblong, Scored, Film	Oxaprozin 600 mg	Daypro by Perrigo	00113-0995	NSAID
DAYPRO <> 1381	Tab, Film Coated	Oxaprozin 600 mg	Daypro by Caremark	00339-5881	NSAID
DAYPRO <> 1381	Tab, Film Coated, Daypro <> 13/81	Oxaprozin 600 mg	Daypro by DRX	55045-2120	NSAID
DAYPRO <> 1381	Tab, Film Coated	Oxaprozin 600 mg	Daypro by Allscripts	54569-3702	NSAID
DAYPRO <> 1381	Tab, Film Coated	Oxaprozin 600 mg	Daypro by HJ Harkins Co	52959-0252	NSAID
DAYPRO <> 1381	Tab, Film Coated	Oxaprozin 600 mg	Daypro by Quality Care	60346-0722	NSAID
DAYPRO <> 1381	Tab, Film Coated, Debossed	Oxaprozin 600 mg	Daypro by Amerisource	62584-0381	NSAID
DAYPRO <> 1381	Tab, Film Coated	Oxaprozin 600 mg	Daypro by Prescription Dispensing	61807-0079	NSAID
DAYPRO <> 1381	Tab, Film Coated	Oxaprozin 600 mg	Daypro by St Marys Med	60760-0381	NSAID
DAYPRO <> 1381	Cap, White, Scored, Film Coated	Oxaprozin 600 mg	by Pharmacia	Canadian DIN# 02027860	NSAID
DAYPRO1381	Tab, White, Oblong, Daypro/1381	Oxaprozin 600 mg	by Searle	Canadian	NSAID
DBETHEX <> 260	Tab, Coated, Scored	Ascorbic Acid 100 mg, Biotin 30 mcg, Calcium Carbonate, Precipitated 250 mg, Chromic Chloride 25 mcg, Cupric Oxide 2 mg, Cyanocobalamin 12 mcg, Ferrous Fumarate 60 mg, Folic Acid 1 mg, Magnesium Oxide 25 mg, Manganese Sulfate 5 mg, Niacinamide 20 mg, Pantothenic Acid 10 mg, Potassium Iodide 150 mcg, Pyridoxine HCl 10 mg, Riboflavin 3.4 mg, Sodium Molybdate 25 mcg, Thiamine HCl 3 mg, Vitamin A 5000 Units, Vitamin D 400 Units, Vitamin E 30 Units, Zinc Oxide 25 mg	Prenatal Mtr by KV	10609-1351	Vitamin
DCI <> PANCRECARBMS4	Cap, Delayed Release, Blue Ink	Amylase 25000 Units, Lipase 4000 Units, Protease 25000 Units	Pancrecarb Ms-4 by Digestive Care	59767-0002	Gastrointestinal

ID FRONT <> BACK	DESCRIPTION FRONT <> BACK	INGREDIENT & STRENGTH	BRAND (OR EQUIV.) & FIRM	NDC#	CLASS; SCH.
DCI <> PANCRECARBMS8	Cap, Delayed Release	Amylase 40000 Units, Lipase 8000 Units, Protease 45000 Units	Pancrecarb Ms-8 by Digestive Care	59767-0001	Gastrointestinal
DDAVP01 <> RPR	Tab, White, Oblong, DDAVP 0.1 <> RPR	Desmopressin Acetate 0.1 mg	DDAVP by RPR	00075-0016	Antidiuretic
DDAVP02 <> RPR	Tab, DDAVP Over 0.2 <> RPR	Desmopressin Acetate 0.2 mg	DDAVP by Promex Med	62301-0030	Antidiuretic
DDAVP02 <> RPR	Tab, White, Oblong, DDAVP 0.2 <> RPR Logo	Desmopressin Acetate 0.2 mg	DDAVP by RPR	00075-0026	Antidiuretic
DE	Cap, Black, D & E	Caffeine 325 mg	by D & E		Stimulant
DE	Tab, White, Oblong	Lactose Enzyme 3000 FCC	by Blistex		Gastrointestinal
DE200	Tab, Pink, Heart Shaped	Caffeine 200 mg	by DNE Pharm		Stimulant
DECADRON <> MSD63	Tab, Bluish-Green	Dexamethasone 0.75 mg	Decadron by Merck	00006-0063	Steroid
DEES25	Cap, Yellow, Gray Print, D & E ES25	Ephedrine Sulphate 25 mg	Ephedrine Sulphate by D & E Pharma		Supplement
DEFEN	Tab	Guaifenesin 600 mg, Pseudoephedrine HCl 60 mg	Defen LA by Anabolic	00722-6298	Cold Remedy
DELTASONE	Tab	Prednisone 5 mg	by Urgent Care Ctr	50716-0305	Steroid
DELTASONE <> 10	Tab	Prednisone 10 mg	Deltasone by Quality Care	60346-0721	Steroid
DELTASONE10	Tab	Prednisone 10 mg	Deltasone by Pharmacia & Upjohn	00009-0193	Steroid
DELTASONE20	Tab	Prednisone 20 mg	Deltasone by Pharmacia & Upjohn	00009-0165	Steroid
DELTASONE20	Tab	Prednisone 20 mg	Deltasone by Allscripts	54569-4017	Steroid
DELTASONE5	Tab	Prednisone 5 mg	Deltasone by Pharmacia & Upjohn	00009-0045	Steroid
DELTASONE5	Tab, White, Round, Scored	Prednisone 5 mg	Deltasone by Qualitest	00603-2542	Steroid
DELTASONE5	Tab	Prednisone 5 mg	by DHHS Prog	11819-0051	Steroid
DEPAKENE	Cap, Orange, Gelatin	Valproic Acid 250 mg	Depakene by Abbott	00074-5681	Anticonvulsant
DEPAKOTESPRINKLE 125MG	Cap, Blue & White, Opaque, This Side/End Up on Top Half	Divalproex Sodium	Depakote by Abbott	00074-6114	Anticonvulsant
DESPECSR <> 44	Tab, Green, Oblong, Scored	Guaifenesin 600 mg, Phenylpropanolamine HCl 75 mg	GFN PPAH 01 by Med Pro	53978-3315	Cold Remedy
DESYREL <> MJ775	Tab, Orange, Round, Scored	Trazodone HCl 50 mg	Desyrel by Rx Pac	65084-0233	Antidepressant
DESYREL <> MJ775	Tab, Film Coated	Trazodone HCl 50 mg	Desyrel by Leiner	59606-0629	Antidepressant
DESYREL <> MJ775	Tab, Film Coated	Trazodone HCl 50 mg	Desyrel by Amerisource	62584-0775	Antidepressant
DESYREL <> MJ776	Tab, White, Round, Scored, Film	Trazodone HCl 100 mg	Desyrel by Teva	00480-0536	Antidepressant
DESYREL <> MJ776	Tab, Film Coated	Trazodone HCl 100 mg	Desyrel by Amerisource	62584-0776	Antidepressant
DESYRELMJ <> 775	Tab, Film Coated	Trazodone HCl 50 mg	Desyrel by Quality Care	60346-0504	Antidepressant
DESYRELMJ775	Tab, Orange, Round	Trazodone HCl 50 mg	Desyrel by Rightpak	65240-0629	Antidepressant
DESYRELMJ775	Tab, Film Coated	Trazodone HCl 50 mg	Desyrel by Bristol Myers Squibb	00087-0775	Antidepressant
DESYRELMJ775	Tab, Film Coated	Trazodone HCl 50 mg	Desyrel by Nat Pharmpak Serv	55154-2001	Antidepressant
DESYRELMJ776	Tab, Off-White to White, Film Coated	Trazodone HCl 100 mg	Desyrel by Bristol Myers Squibb	00087-0776	Antidepressant
DESYRELMJ776	Tab, White, Round, Scored	Trazodone HCl 100 mg	Desyrel by Rightpak	65240-0630	Antidepressant
DF	Tab, White, Round	Terazosin HCl 1 mg	Hytrin by Abbott	00074-3322	Antihypertensive
DH	Tab, Orange, Round	Terazosin HCl 2 mg	Hytrin by Abbott	00074-3323	Antihypertensive
DH	Tab, Peach, Round	Terazosin HCl 2 mg	Hytrin by Abbott	00074-3323	Antihypertensive
DI	Tab, Green, Round	Terazosin HCl 10 mg	Hytrin by Abbott	00074-3322	Antihypertensive
DIAB	Tab, DIA/B	Glyburide 5 mg	by Coventry	61372-0578	Antidiabetic
DIAB <> HOECHST	Tab	Glyburide 5 mg	Diabeta by Rite Aid	11822-5186	Antidiabetic
DIAB <> HOECHST	Tab, Peach, Oblong	Glyburide 1.25 mg	Diabeta by Hoechst Roussel	00039-0053	Antidiabetic
DIAB <> HOECHST	Tab	Glyburide 1.25 mg	Diabeta by Merrell	00068-1210	Antidiabetic
DIAB <> HOECHST	Tab	Glyburide 2.5 mg	Diabeta by Thrift Drug	59198-0022	Antidiabetic
DIAB <> HOECHST	Tab, Diab <> Hoechst	Glyburide 2.5 mg	Diabeta by Quality Care	60346-0890	Antidiabetic
DIAB <> HOECHST	Tab, Diab <> Hoechst	Glyburide 2.5 mg	Diabeta by Amerisource	62584-0361	Antidiabetic
DIAB <> HOECHST	Tab, Pink, Oblong, Scored	Glyburide 2.5 mg	Diabeta by Natl Pharmpak	55154-1206	Antidiabetic
DIAB <> HOECHST	Tab, Greek Letter Beta	Glyburide 2.5 mg	Diabeta by Merrell	00068-1211	Antidiabetic
DIAB <> HOECHST	Tab, Light Pink, Oblong	Glyburide 2.5 mg	Diabeta by Hoechst Roussel	00039-0051	Antidiabetic
DIAB <> HOECHST	Tab, Light Green, DIA B	Glyburide 5 mg	Diabeta by Quality Care	60346-0730	Antidiabetic
DIAB <> HOECHST	Tab, Light Green	Glyburide 5 mg	Diabeta by Thrift Drug	59198-0023	Antidiabetic
DIAB <> HOECHST	Tab	Glyburide 5 mg	Diabeta by Merrell	00068-1212	Antidiabetic
DIAB <> HOECHST	Tab, Light Green, Oblong	Glyburide 5 mg	Diabeta by Hoechst Roussel	00039-0052	Antidiabetic

ID FRONT <> BACK	DESCRIPTION FRONT <> BACK	INGREDIENT & STRENGTH	BRAND (OR EQUIV.) & FIRM	NDC#	CLASS; SCH.
DIAB <> HOECHST	Tab, DIA/B <> Hoechst	Glyburide 5 mg	Diabeta by Nat Pharmpak Serv	55154-1201	Antidiabetic
DIABHOECHST	Tab, DIA-B Hoechst	Glyburide 5 mg	Diabeta by Allscripts	54569-0200	Antidiabetic
DIAMOX <> D3	Cap	Acetazolamide 500 mg	Diamox ER Sequels by Lederle	00005-4465	Diuretic
DIAMOX D3	Cap, Orange	Acetazolamide 500 mg	by Storz	Canadian	Diuretic
DIAMOX250 <> LLD2	Tab, Diamox 250 <> LL in Upper Right Quad, D2 in Lower Left Quadrant	Acetazolamide 250 mg	Diamox by Thrift Drug	59198-0186	Diuretic
DIAMOX250 <> LLD2	Tab	Acetazolamide 250 mg	Diamox by Storz Ophtha	57706-0755	Diuretic
DIAMOXD3	Cap, Diamox over D3	Acetazolamide 500 mg	Diamox Sequels by Haines	59564-0142	Diuretic
DIAZEPAM10 <> PAR192	Tab	Diazepam 10 mg	by Par	49884-0192	Antianxiety; C IV
DIAZEPAM2 <> PAR190	Tab	Diazepam 2 mg	by Par	49884-0190	Antianxiety; C IV
DIAZEPAM5 <> PAR191	Tab	Diazepam 5 mg	by Par	49884-0191	Antianxiety; C IV
DIDREX50	Tab, Coated	Benzphetamine HCl 50 mg	Didrex by Quality Care	60346-0678	Sympathomimetic; C III
DIDREX50	Tab, Coated	Benzphetamine HCl 50 mg	Didrex by Compumed	00403-0059	Sympathomimetic; C III
DIDREX50	Tab, Coated	Benzphetamine HCl 50 mg	Didrex by Allscripts	54569-0389	Sympathomimetic; C III
DIDREX50	Tab, Coated	Benzphetamine HCl 50 mg	Didrex by Allscripts	54569-2949	Sympathomimetic; C III
DIFLUCAN100 <> PFIZER	Tab, Pink, Trapezoid	Fluconazole 100 mg	Diflucan by Pfizer	Canadian DIN# 00891819	Antifungal
DIFLUCAN100 <> ROERIG	Tab, Coated, Diflucan/100 <> Roerig	Fluconazole 100 mg	Diflucan by Nat Pharmpak Serv	55154-3214	Antifungal
DIFLUCAN100 <> ROERIG	Tab, Coated	Fluconazole 100 mg	Diflucan by Amerisource	62584-0362	Antifungal
DIFLUCAN100 <> ROERIG	Tab, Pink, Trapezoidal, Coated, Diflucan/100 <> Roerig	Fluconazole 100 mg	Diflucan by Roerig	00049-3420	Antifungal
DIFLUCAN100 <> ROERIG	Tab, Coated	Fluconazole 100 mg	Diflucan by Allscripts	54569-3926	Antifungal
DIFLUCAN100 <> ROERIG	Tab, Coated	Fluconazole 100 mg	by Med Pro	53978-3012	Antifungal
DIFLUCAN200 <> ROERIG	Tab, Coated	Fluconazole 200 mg	Diflucan by Nat Pharmpak Serv	55154-3215	Antifungal
DIFLUCAN200 <> ROERIG	Tab, Coated	Fluconazole 200 mg	Diflucan by Amerisource	62584-0363	Antifungal
DIFLUCAN200 <> ROERIG	Tab, Pink, Trapezoidal, Coated, Diflucan/200 <> Roerig	Fluconazole 200 mg	Diflucan by Roerig	00049-3430	Antifungal
DIFLUCAN200 <> ROERIG	Tab, Coated	Fluconazole 200 mg	by Med Pro	53978-3105	Antifungal
DIFLUCAN200 <> ROERIG	Tab	Fluconazole 200 mg	Diflucan by Allscripts	54569-3269	Antifungal
DIFLUCAN50 <> PFIZER	Tab, Pink, Trapezoid	Fluconazole 50 mg	Diflucan by Pfizer	Canadian DIN# 00891800	Antifungal
DIFLUGAN50 <> ROERIG	Tab, Coated	Fluconazole 50 mg	Diflucan by Pharm Utilization	60491-0194	Antifungal
DILACOR240	Cap, White	Diltiazem HCl 240 mg	Dilacor XR by Rx Pac	65084-0242	Antihypertensive
DILACORXR <> 180MG	Cap, Ex Release	Diltiazem HCl 180 mg	by Kaiser	62224-9339	Antihypertensive
DILACORXR120MG	Cap, Gold, Ex Release, RPR Logo in 3/4 Circle over Dilacor XR <> Old Imprint, RPR over 0250 over 120 mg	Diltiazem HCl 120 mg	Dilacor XR by Leiner	59606-0776	Antihypertensive
DILACORXR120MG	Cap, Gold, Ex Release	Diltiazem HCl 120 mg	Dilacor XR by Amerisource	62584-0250	Antihypertensive
DILACORXR120MG	Cap, Gold, RPR Logo over Dilacor XR over 120 mg	Diltiazem HCl 120 mg	Dilacor XR by RPR	00075-0250	Antihypertensive
DILACORXR120MG	Cap, Gold, Ex Release	Diltiazem HCl 120 mg	Dilacor XR by Drug Distr	52985-0223	Antihypertensive
DILACORXR120MG	Cap, Dilacor XR/120 mg <> Logo	Diltiazem HCl 120 mg	Dilacor XR by Nat Pharmpak Serv	55154-4020	Antihypertensive

ID FRONT <> BACK	DESCRIPTION FRONT <> BACK	INGREDIENT & STRENGTH	BRAND (OR EQUIV.) & FIRM	NDC#	CLASS; SCH.
DILACORXR120MG <> RPR	Cap, Gold	Diltiazem HCl 120 mg	Dilacor XR by Thrift Drug	59198-0259	Antihypertensive
DILACORXR180	Cap, Peach & Purple	Diltiazem HCl 180 mg	Dilacor XR by Rx Pac	65084-0240	Antihypertensive
DILACORXR180MG	Cap, Ex Release	Diltiazem HCl 180 mg	Dilacor XR by Leiner	59606-0736	Antihypertensive
DILACORXR180MG	Cap, Orange & White	Diltiazem HCl 180 mg	Dilacor XR by Amerisource	62584-0251	Antihypertensive
DILACORXR180MG	Cap	Diltiazem HCl 180 mg	Dilacor XR by RPR	00075-0251	Antihypertensive
DILACORXR180MG	Cap, Orange & White	Diltiazem HCl 180 mg	Dilacor XR by Nat Pharmpak Serv	55154-4021	Antihypertensive
DILACORXR180MG <> RPR	Cap, Ex Release	Diltiazem HCl 180 mg	Dilacor XR by Thrift Drug	59198-0260	Antihypertensive
DILACORXR240MG	Cap, Ex Release	Diltiazem HCl 240 mg	Dilacor XR by Leiner	59606-0639	Antihypertensive
DILACORXR240MG	Cap, Ex Release	Diltiazem HCl 240 mg	Dilacor XR by Amerisource	62584-0252	Antihypertensive
DILACORXR240MG	Cap	Diltiazem HCl 240 mg	Dilacor XR by Caremark	00339-5903	Antihypertensive
DILACORXR240MG	Cap, Dilacor XR/240 mg <> Lines/Logo	Diltiazem HCl 240 mg	Dilacor XR by Nat Pharmpak Serv	55154-4022	Antihypertensive
DILEXG	Tab, White, Round	Dyphylline 200 mg; Guaifenesin 200 mg	Dilex-G by Poly Pharms	50991-0400	Antiasthmatic
DIOVOL	Cap, Blue	Aluminum Hydroxide 200 mg	by Horner	Canadian	Gastrointestinal
DIOVOL EX	Tab, White, Round	Aluminum Hydroxide 600 mg	by Horner	Canadian	Gastrointestinal
DIPENTUM250MG	Cap, Beige	Olsalazine Sodium 250 mg	Dipentum by Pharmacia & Upjohn	00013-0105	Gastrointestinal
DIPENTUM250MG	Cap	Olsalazine Sodium 250 mg	Dipentum by Pharmacia & Upjohn	59632-0105	Gastrointestinal
DIPENTUM250MG	Cap, Beige, Opaque, Gelatin	Olsalazine Sodium 250 mg	by Pharmacia	Canadian DIN# 02063808	Gastrointestinal
DISALCID <> 3M	Tab, Aqua, Round, Bisected, Film Coated	Salsalate 500 mg	Disalcid by 3M	00089-0149	NSAID
DISALCID <> 3M	Cap, Aqua & White	Salsalate 500 mg	Disalcid by 3M	00089-0148	NSAID
DISALCID750 <> 3M	Tab, Aqua, Oblong, Scored, Film Coated	Salsalate 750 mg	Disalcid by RX PAK	65084-0216	NSAID
DISALCID750 <> 3M	Tab, Blue, Oblong, Film Coated, Bisected	Salsalate 750 mg	Disalcid by Rx Pac	65084-0212	NSAID
DISALCID750 <> 3M	Tab, Aqua, Cap-Shaped, Bisected, Film Coated	Salsalate 750 mg	Disalcid by 3M	00089-0151	NSAID
DISALCID750 <> 3M	Tab, Film Coated	Salsalate 750 mg	Disalcid by Nat Pharmpak Serv	55154-2902	NSAID
DISALCID750 <> 3M	Tab, Film Coated	Salsalate 750 mg	Disalcid by Thrift Drug	59198-0121	NSAID
DISALCID750 <> 3M	Tab, Film Coated, Embossed	Salsalate 750 mg	Disalcid by Amerisource	62584-0151	NSAID
DISALCID750 <> 3M	Tab, Film Coated	Salsalate 750 mg	Disalcid by Leiner	59606-0635	NSAID
DISTA3104 <> PROZAC10	Cap	Fluoxetine HCl 10 mg	Prozac by Quality Care	60346-0971	Antidepressant
DISTA3104 <> PROZAC10	Cap	Fluoxetine HCl 10 mg	Prozac by Kaiser	00179-1252	Antidepressant
DISTA3104 <> PROZAC10MG	Cap	Fluoxetine HCl 10 mg	Prozac by Kaiser	62224-1115	Antidepressant
DISTA3104 <> PROZAC10MG	Cap, Green	Fluoxetine HCl 10 mg	Prozac by Eli Lilly	00002-3104	Antidepressant
DISTA3104 <> PROZAC10MG	Cap	Fluoxetine HCl 10 mg	Prozac by Dista Prod	00777-3104	Antidepressant
DISTA3104 <> PROZAC10MG	Cap	Fluoxetine HCl 10 mg	Prozac by Allscripts	54569-4129	Antidepressant
DISTA3104 <> PROZAC10MG	Cap, Green, Opaque	Fluoxetine HCl 10 mg	Prozac by Invamed	52189-0310	Antidepressant
DISTA3105 <> PROZAC20	Cap, Beige & Green	Fluoxetine 20 mg	Prozac by Southwood Pharms	58016-0828	Antidepressant
DISTA3105 <> PROZAC20MG	Cap, Gelatin Coated	Fluoxetine 20 mg	Prozac by Heartland	61392-0235	Antidepressant
DISTA3105 <> PROZAC20MG	Cap, Gelatin Coated	Fluoxetine 20 mg	Prozac by Promex Med	62301-0008	Antidepressant
DISTA3105 <> PROZAC20MG	Cap, Off-White, Gelatin Coated	Fluoxetine 20 mg	Prozac by Quality Care	60346-0004	Antidepressant

ID FRONT <> BACK	DESCRIPTION FRONT <> BACK	INGREDIENT & STRENGTH	BRAND (OR EQUIV.) & FIRM	NDC#	CLASS; SCH.
DISTA3105 <> PROZAC20MG	Cap, Green & White	Fluoxetine 20 mg	Prozac by Va Cmop	65243-0031	Antidepressant
DISTA3105 <> PROZAC20MG	Cap, Green & White	Fluoxetine 20 mg	Prozac by Eli Lilly	00002-3105	Antidepressant
DISTA3105 <> PROZAC20MG	Cap, Green & Yellow, Gelatin	Fluoxetine 20 mg	Prozac by Dista Prod	00777-3105	Antidepressant
DISTA3105 <> PROZAC20MG	Cap, Gelatin	Fluoxetine 20 mg	Prozac by Pharmedix	53002-1016	Antidepressant
DISTA3105 <> PROZAC20MG	Cap, Gelatin Coated	Fluoxetine 20 mg	Prozac by Allscripts	54569-1732	Antidepressant
DISTA3105 <> PROZAC20MG	Cap, Gelatin	Fluoxetine 20 mg	by Med Pro	53978-1033	Antidepressant
DISTA3105 <> PROZAC20MG	Cap, Green & White, Opaque	Fluoxetine HCl 20 mg	Prozac by Invamed	52189-0262	Antidepressant
DISTA3106 <> PROZAC20MG	Cap, Green & Opaque & Orange	Fluoxetine 20 mg	Prozac by Kaiser	00179-1159	Antidepressant
DISTA3107 <> PROZAC40MG	Cap, Green & Orange, Opaque	Fluoxetine 40 mg	Prozac by Dista Prod	00777-3107	Antidepressant
DISTA3107 <> PROZAC40MG	Cap, Green & Orange, Opaque	Fluoxetine HCl 40 mg	Prozac by Invamed	52189-0309	Antidepressant
DISTA3123	Cap, Green & Yellow, Oval	Chlorpheniramine Maleate 4 mg, Pseudoephedrine HCl 60 mg	Co-Pyronil 2 by Lilly		Cold Remedy
DISTAH09 <> ILOSONE250MG	Cap	Erythromycin 250 mg	Ilosone by Dista Prod	00777-0809	Antibiotic
DISTAH69 <> KEFLEX250	Cap	Cephalexin Monohydrate	Keflex by Quality Care	60346-0649	Antibiotic
DISTAH69 <> KEFLEX250	Cap	Cephalexin Monohydrate 250 mg	Keflex by Lilly	00110-0869	Antibiotic
DISTAH69 <> KEFLEX250	Cap	Cephalexin Monohydrate 250 mg	Keflex by Dista Prod	00777-0869	Antibiotic
DISTAH71 <> KEFLEX500	Cap, Dark Green & Light Green	Cephalexin Monohydrate 500 mg	Keflex by Carlsbad	61442-0102	Antibiotic
DISTAH74	Cap, Blue	Ethinamate 500 mg	Valmid by Dista Prod		Hypnotic
DISTAH77 <> NALFON	Cap	Fenoprofen Calcium 324 mg	Nalfon by Dista Prod	00777-0877	NSAID
DISTAH77 <> NALFON	Cap	Fenoprofen Calcium 324 mg	Nalfon by Physicians Total Care	54868-0856	NSAID
DISTANALFON	Yellow, Oblong, Dista/Nalfon	Fenoprofen Calcium 600 mg	Nalfon by Lilly		NSAID
DISTAU26	Tab, Coated	Erythromycin Estolate	Ilosone by Dista Prod	00777-2126	Antibiotic
DITROPAN <> 1375	Tab, Ditropan <> 13/75	Oxybutynin Chloride 5 mg	Ditropan by Hoechst Roussel	00088-1375	Urinary
DITROPAN <> 1375	Tab, Ditropan <> 13/75	Oxybutynin Chloride 5 mg	Ditropan by Nat Pharmpak Serv	55154-2209	Urinary
DITROPAN <> 9200	Tab, Blue, Ditropan <> 92-00	Oxybutynin Chloride 5 mg	Ditropan by Alza	17314-9200	Urinary
DIUPRES <> MSD 405	Tab	Chlorothiazide 500 mg, Reserpine 0.125 mg	Diupres-500 by Merck	00006-0405	Diuretic; Antihypertensive
DJ	Tab, Tan, Round	Terazosin HCl 5 mg	Hytrin by Abbott	00074-3324	Antihypertensive
DJ	Tab, Salmon, Round	Terazosin HCl 5 mg	Hytrin by Abbott	00074-3324	Antihypertensive
DL430	Tab	Metoclopramide HCl	by Qualitest	00603-4617	Gastrointestinal
DL517	Tab	Metoclopramide HCl	by Qualitest	00603-4616	Gastrointestinal
DLANOXINX3A	Tab	Digoxin 0.25 mg	Lanoxin by Med Pro	53978-0177	Cardiac Agent
DMSP <> 272	Tab	Carbidopa 25 mg, Levodopa 100 mg	by Murfreesboro	51129-1127	Antiparkinson
DMSP019	Tab, White, Oval	Cimetidine 200 mg	Tagamet by Dupont		Gastrointestinal
DMSP050	Tab, White, Oval	Cimetidine 300 mg	Tagamet by Dupont		Gastrointestinal
DMSP087	Tab, White, Oval	Cimetidine 400 mg	Tagamet by Dupont		Gastrointestinal
DMSP088	Tab, White, Oval	Cimetidine 800 mg	Tagamet by Dupont		Gastrointestinal
DMSP251	Tab, Dapple Blue, Oval	Carbidopa 25 mg, Levodopa 250 mg	Sinemet by Dupont		Antiparkinson

ID FRONT <> BACK	DESCRIPTION FRONT <> BACK	INGREDIENT & STRENGTH	BRAND (OR EQUIV.) & FIRM	NDC#	CLASS; SCH.
DMSP271	Tab, Dapple Blue, Oval	Carbidopa 10 mg, Levodopa 100 mg	Sinemet by Dupont		Antiparkinson
DMSP272	Tab, Yellow, Oval	Carbidopa 25 mg, Levodopa 100 mg	Sinemet by Dupont		Antiparkinson
DOLACET <> ROBERTS138	Cap	Acetaminophen 500 mg, Hydrocodone Bitartrate 5 mg	Dolacet by Roberts	54092-0138	Analgesic; C III
DOLACET <> ROBERTS138	Cap	Acetaminophen 500 mg, Hydrocodone Bitartrate 5 mg	by Mikart	46672-0247	Analgesic; C III
DOLOBID	Tab, Peach, Oblong	Diflunisal 250 mg	by Frosst	Canadian	NSAID
DOLOBID	Tab, Orange, Oblong	Diflunisal 500 mg	by Frosst	Canadian	NSAID
DOLOBID <> MSD675	Tab, Peach, Cap Shaped, Film Coated	Diflunisal 250 mg	Dolobid by Merck	00006-0675	NSAID
DOLOBID <> MSD697	Tab, Film Coated	Diflunisal 500 mg	Dolobid by Quality Care	60346-0940	NSAID
DOLOBID <> MSD697	Tab, Orange, Oblong, Film Coated	Diflunisal 500 mg	Dolobid by Dura		NSAID
DOLOBID <> MSD697	Tab, Film Coated	Diflunisal 500 mg	Dolobid by Allscripts	54569-0296	NSAID
DONNATAL <> AHR	Tab, Film Coated	Atropine Sulfate 0.0582 mg, Hyoscyamine Sulfate 0.3111 mg, Phenobarbital 48.6 mg, Scopolamine Hydrobromide 0.0195 mg	Antispasmotic by Pharmedix	53002-0449	Gastrointestinal; C IV
DONNATALEXTENTA <> AHR	Tab, Pale Green, Film Coated	Atropine Sulfate 0.0582 mg, Hyoscyamine Sulfate 0.3111 mg, Phenobarbital 48.6 mg, Scopolamine Hydrobromide 0.0195 mg	Donnatal by Thrift Drug	59198-0233	Gastrointestinal; C IV
DORAL <>15	Tab, Light Orange w/ White Speckles, Capsule-shaped, Doral <> 15	Quazepam 15 mg	Doral by Wallace	00037-9002	Sedative Hypnotic; CIV
DORAL <> 75	Tab, Light Orange w/ White Specks, Cap Shaped, Doral <> 7.5	Quazepam 7.5 mg	Doral by Wallace	00037-9000	Sedative/Hypnotic; C IV
DORAL <> 75	Tab, Slightly White Specks, Impressed with 7.5	Quazepam 7.5 mg	Doral by Quality Care	60346-0865	Sedative/Hypnotic; C IV
DORMIN25MG	Cap, Pink	Diphenhydramine HCl 25 mg	Dormin by Randob		Antihistamine
DORYX	Cap, White Print	Doxycycline Hyclate	Doryx by Pharm Utilization	60491-0215	Antibiotic
DORYX	Cap, Clear	Doxycycline Hyclate	Doryx by Physicians Total Care	54868-1491	Antibiotic
DORYX <> DORYX	Cap, White Print	Doxycycline Hyclate	Doryx by Warner Chilcott	00430-0838	Antibiotic
DORYX <> DORYX	Cap, White Print	Doxycycline Hyclate	Doryx by Faulding	50546-0400	Antibiotic
DORYX PD	Cap, Yellow	Doxycycline Hyclate 100 mg	by Parke-Davis	Canadian	Antibiotic
DORYXPD	Cap	Doxycycline Hyclate	Doryx by Parke Davis	00071-0838	Antibiotic
DOXYCAP <> BARR296	Cap, Doxy-Cap <> Barr over 296	Doxycycline Hyclate	by Barr	00555-0296	Antibiotic
DOXYCAP <> BARR297	Cap, Doxy-Cap <> Barr over 297	Doxycycline Hyclate	by Barr	00555-0297	Antibiotic
DOXYCIN 100	Tab, Orange	Doxycycline Hyclate 100 mg	Doxycin by Riva	Canadian	Antibiotic
DOXYTAB <> BARR295	Tab, Coated, Doxy-Tab <> Barr 295	Doxycycline Hyclate	by Barr	00555-0295	Antibiotic
DOXYTEC100	Tab, Light Orange, Round, Film Coated, Scored, Doxytec over 100	Doxycycline Hyclate 100 mg	by Altimed	Canadian DIN# 02091232	Antibiotic
DP <> 200	Tab	Levothyroxine Sodium 200 mcg	Levoxyl by Jones	52604-1112	Antithyroid
DP <> 301	Tab, Duramed Logo	Methylprednisolone 4 mg	by Quality Care	60346-0608	Steroid
DP <> 417	Tab, Green, Oblong, Scored, Film Coated, Duramed Logo	Guaifenesin 600 mg	by Lilly	00110-4117	Expectorant
DP <> 501	Tab, Lavender, Round, Duramed Logo	Estradiol 0.5 mg	by Duramed	51285-0501	Hormone
DP <> 502	Tab, Rose, Round, Duramed Logo	Estradiol 1 mg	by Duramed	51285-0502	Hormone
DP <> 504	Tab, Duramed Logo	Estradiol 2 mg	by Duramed	51285-0504	Hormone
DP <> 521	Tab, Orange, Round	Prochlorperazine 5 mg	by Duramed Pharms	51285-0521	Antiemetic
DP <> 570	Tab, White, Round	Desogestrel 0.15 mg; Ethinyl Estradiol 0.03 mg	Apri by Allscripts	54569-4878	Oral Contraceptive
DP <> 575	Tab, Pink, Round	Desogestrel 0.15 mg; Ethinyl Estradiol 0.03 mg	Apri by Allscripts	54569-4878	Oral Contraceptive
DP <> CIBA	Tab, Brownish-Orange, Round, Film Coated	Maprotiline 25 mg	Ludiomil by Ciba	Canadian DIN# 00360481	Antidepressant
DP <> M	Tab, Mottled Pink, D-P	Aspirin 500 mg, Hydrocodone Bitartrate 5 mg	Damason P by Quality Care	60346-0748	Analgesic; C III
DP <> M	Tab	Aspirin 500 mg, Hydrocodone Bitartrate 5 mg	Damason P by Mason Pharmaceuticals	12758-0057	Analgesic; C III

ID FRONT <> BACK	DESCRIPTION FRONT <> BACK	INGREDIENT & STRENGTH	BRAND (OR EQUIV.) & FIRM	NDC#	CLASS; SCH.
DP <> TOUROCC	Tab, White, Oblong	Guaifenesin 575 mg; Pseudoephedrine HCl 60 mg; Dextromethorphan Hydrobromide 30 mg	by Pfab	62542-0770	Cold Remedy
DP01	Tab, Tan, Round	Clonidine HCl 0.1 mg	Catapres by Duramed		Antihypertensive
DP02	Tab, Orange, Round	Clonidine HCl 0.2 mg	Catapres by Duramed		Antihypertensive
DP03	Tab, Peach, Round	Clonidine HCl 0.3 mg	Catapres by Duramed		Antihypertensive
DP082 <> TUSSIGON	Tab, DP/082	Homatropine Methylbromide 1.5 mg, Hydrocodone Bitartrate 5 mg	Tussigon by Quality Care	60346-0947	Cold Remedy; C III
DP082 <> TUSSIGON	Tab, Blue, Round, Scored, dp/082 <> Tussigon	Homatropine Methylbromide 1.5 mg, Hydrocodone Bitartrate 5 mg	Tussigon by JMI Daniels	00689-0082	Cold Remedy; C III
DP10	Tab, Peach, Round	Propranolol 10 mg	Inderal by Duramed		Antihypertensive
DP100 <> LEVOXYL	Tab	Levothyroxine Sodium 100 mcg	Levoxyl by Jones	52604-1110	Antithyroid
DP100 <> LEVOXYL	Tab, Yellow, Oval, Scored	Levothyroxine Sodium 100 mcg	Levoxyl by JMI Daniels	00689-1110	Antithyroid
DP11	Tab, Lavender, Round	Trifluoperazine HCl 1 mg	Stelazine by Duramed		Antipsychotic
DP112 <> LEVOXYL	Tab	Levothyroxine Sodium 112 mcg	Levoxyl by Jones	52604-1130	Antithyroid
DP112 <> LEVOXYL	Tab, Rose, Oval, Scored, dp/112 <> Levoxyl	Levothyroxine Sodium 112 mcg	Levoxyl by JMI Daniels	00689-1130	Antithyroid
DP12	Tab, Lavender, Round	Trifluoperazine HCl 2 mg	Stelazine by Duramed		Antipsychotic
DP125	Tab	Levothyroxine Sodium 125 mcg	Levoxyl by Jones	52604-1120	Antithyroid
DP125 <> LEVOXYL	Tab, Brown, Oval, Scored, dp/125 <> Levoxyl	Levothyroxine Sodium 125 mcg	Levoxyl by JMI Daniels	00689-1120	Antithyroid
DP13	Tab, Lavender, Round	Trifluoperazine HCl 5 mg	Stelazine by Duramed		Antipsychotic
DP137	Tab	Levothyroxine Sodium 137 mcg	Levoxyl by Jones	52604-1135	Antithyroid
DP137 <> LEVOXYL	Tab, Dark Blue, Oval, Scored, dp/137 <> Levoxyl	Levothyroxine Sodium 137 mcg	Levoxyl by JMI Daniels	00689-1135	Antithyroid
DP14	Tab, Lavender, Round	Trifluoperazine HCl 10 mg	Stelazine by Duramed		Antipsychotic
DP150	Tab, Light Blue	Levothyroxine Sodium 150 mcg	Levoxyl by Jones	52604-1111	Antithyroid
DP150 <> LEVOXYL	Tab, Blue, Oval, Scored	Levothyroxine Sodium 150 mcg	Levoxyl by JMI Daniels	00689-1111	Antithyroid
DP1625	Tab	Estropipate 0.75 mg	by United Res	00677-1508	Hormone
DP175 <> LEVOXYL	Tab, Turquoise	Levothyroxine Sodium 175 mcg	Levoxyl by Jones	52604-1122	Antithyroid
DP175 <> LEVOXYL	Tab, Turquoise, Oval, Scored, dp/175 <> Levoxyl	Levothyroxine Sodium 175 mcg	Levoxyl by JMI Daniels	00689-1122	Antithyroid
DP20	Tab, Blue, Round	Propranolol 20 mg	Inderal by Duramed		Antihypertensive
DP200 <> LEVOXYL	Tab, Pink, Oval, Scored	Levothyroxine Sodium 200 mcg	Levoxyl by JMI Daniels	00689-1112	Antithyroid
DP223	Tab, White, Round	Aminophylline 100 mg	Aminophyllin by Duramed		Antiasthmatic
DP224	Tab, White, Round	Aminophylline 200 mg	Aminophyllin by Duramed		Antiasthmatic
DP225	Tab, White, Round	Haloperidol 0.5 mg	Haldol by Duramed		Antipsychotic
DP226	Tab, Yellow, Round	Haloperidol 1 mg	Haldol by Duramed		Antipsychotic
DP227	Tab, Lavender, Round	Haloperidol 2 mg	Haldol by Duramed		Antipsychotic
DP228	Tab, Green, Round	Haloperidol 5 mg	Haldol by Duramed		Antipsychotic
DP229	Tab, Aqua, Round	Haloperidol 10 mg	Haldol by Duramed		Antipsychotic
DP230	Tab, Salmon, Round	Haloperidol 20 mg	Haldol by Duramed		Antipsychotic
DP241	Tab, Yellow, Oval	Choline Magnesium Trisalate 500 mg	Trilisate by Duramed		NSAID
DP242	Tab, Blue, Oval	Choline Magnesium Trisalate 750 mg	Trilisate by Duramed		NSAID
DP246	Tab, White, Round	Cyproheptadine HCl 4 mg	Periactin by Duramed		Antihistamine
DP25 <> LEVOXYL	Tab, dp/25	Levothyroxine Sodium 25 mcg	Levoxyl by Jones	52604-1117	Antithyroid
DP25 <> LEVOXYL	Tab, Orange, Oval, Scored, dp/25 <> Levoxyl	Levothyroxine Sodium 25 mcg	Levoxyl by JMI Daniels	00689-1117	Antithyroid
DP251	Tab, Blue, Round	Chlorpropamide 250 mg	Diabinese by Duramed		Antidiabetic
DP252	Tab, Blue, Round, dp-252	Chlorpropamide 100 mg	Diabinese by Duramed		Antidiabetic
DP265	Cap, Green, Oblong	Hydroxyzine Pamoate 25 mg	Vistaril by Duramed		Antihistamine
DP266	Cap, Green & White, Oblong	Hydroxyzine Pamoate 50 mg	Vistaril by Duramed		Antihistamine
DP267	Cap, Gray & Green, Oblong	Hydroxyzine Pamoate 100 mg	Vistaril by Duramed		Antihistamine
DP274	Tab, White, Round	Isoniazid 100 mg	INH by Duramed		Antimycobacterial
DP275	Cap, Green, Oblong	Indomethacin 25 mg	Indocin by Duramed		NSAID
DP276	Cap, Green	Indomethacin 50 mg	Indocin by Duramed		NSAID
DP277	Tab	Isoniazid 300 mg	Isoniazid by Zenith Goldline	00182-1356	Antimycobacterial
DP277	Tab, White, Round	Isoniazid 300 mg	Isoniazid by Duramed	51285-0277	Antimycobacterial
DP277	Tab	Isoniazid 300 mg	Isoniazid by Allscripts	54569-2509	Antimycobacterial
DP293	Cap	Guaifenesin 200 mg, Phenylephrine HCl 5 mg, Phenylpropanolamine HCl 45 mg	Quintex by Qualitest	00603-5665	Cold Remedy

ID FRONT <> BACK	DESCRIPTION FRONT <> BACK	INGREDIENT & STRENGTH	BRAND (OR EQUIV.) & FIRM	NDC#	CLASS; SCH.
DP293	Cap, Beige & Orange	Guaifenesin 200 mg, Phenylephrine HCl 5 mg, Phenylpropanolamine HCl 45 mg	Duratex by Duramed	51285-0293	Cold Remedy
DP293	Cap	Guaifenesin 200 mg, Phenylephrine HCl 5 mg, Phenylpropanolamine HCl 45 mg	Guiatex by Rugby	00536-4459	Cold Remedy
DP294	Tab, Ex Release, Duramed Logo 294	Guaifenesin 400 mg, Phenylpropanolamine HCl 75 mg	Enomine LA by Quality Care	60346-0339	Cold Remedy
DP295	Tab, Ex Release, Duramed Logo 295	Guaifenesin 400 mg, Phenylpropanolamine HCl 75 mg	Enomine LA by Quality Care	60346-0339	Cold Remedy
DP295	Tab	Guaifenesin 400 mg, Phenylpropanolamine HCl 75 mg	by Pharmedix	53002-0323	Cold Remedy
DP295	Tab, Blue, Oval	Guaifenesin 400 mg, Phenylpropanolamine HCl 75 mg	by Duramed	51285-0295	Cold Remedy
DP296	Tab, Blue, Round	Salsalate 500 mg	Disalcid by Amide		NSAID
DP296	Tab, Yellow, Cap Shaped, Coated	Salsalate 500 mg	by Duramed	51285-0858	NSAID
DP297	Tab, Yellow, Oblong	Salsalate 750 mg	Disalcid by Amide		NSAID
DP297	Tab, Yellow, Cap Shaped	Salsalate 750 mg	by Duramed	51285-0859	NSAID
DP298	Tab, Yellow, Round	Salsalate 500 mg	Disalcid by Duramed		NSAID
DP299	Tab, Yellow, Oblong	Salsalate 750 mg	Disalcid by Duramed		NSAID
DP3	Tab	Acetaminophen 300 mg, Codeine 30 mg	by Major	00904-0175	Analgesic; C III
DP30	Tab, White, Round	Conjugated Estrogens 0.3 mg	Premarin by Duramed		Estrogen
DP300 <> LEVOXYL	Tab, Green, Oval, Scored, dp/300 <> Levoxyl	Levothyroxine Sodium 300 mcg	Levoxyl by JMI Daniels	00689-1121	Antithyroid
DP301	Tab, White, Oval, Scored	Methylprednisolone 4 mg	by Neuman Distr	64579-0039	Steroid
DP301	Tab, Film Coated	Methylprednisolone 4 mg	by Schein	00364-0467	Steroid
DP301	Tab	Methylprednisolone 4 mg	by Zenith Goldline	00182-1050	Steroid
DP301	Tab, White, Oval, Duramed Logo	Methylprednisolone 4 mg	by Duramed	51285-0301	Steroid
DP301	Tab	Methylprednisolone 4 mg	by Pharmedix	53002-0312	Steroid
DP301	Tab	Methylprednisolone 4 mg	by United Res	00677-0565	Steroid
DP301	Tab	Methylprednisolone 4 mg	by HL Moore	00839-6224	Steroid
DP301	Tab	Methylprednisolone 4 mg	by Qualitest	00603-4593	Steroid
DP31	Tab, White, Round	Conjugated Estrogens 0.625 mg	Premarin by Duramed		Estrogen
DP311 <> TOURODM	Cap, Blue	Dextromethorphan 30 mg, Guaifensin 575 mg	Touro DM by Dartmouth	58869-0411	Cold Remedy
DP311 <> TOURODM	Tab, DP 311 <> Touro DM	Dextromethorphan Hydrobromide 30 mg, Guaifenesin 600 mg	Touro DM by Anabolic	00722-6297	Cold Remedy
DP311 <> TOURODM	Tab, Blue, Oblong, Scored, DP over 311	Guaifenesin 575 mg, Dextromethorphan Hydriodide 30 mg	by Martec		Cold Remedy
DP312	Tab, White, Round	Prednisone 10 mg	Deltasone by Duramed		Steroid
DP313	Tab, Orange, Round	Prednisone 20 mg	Deltasone by Duramed		Steroid
DP314	Tab, Yellow, Round	Prochlorperazine 5 mg	Compazine by Duramed		Antiemetic
DP315	Tab, Yellow, Round	Prochlorperazine 10 mg	Compazine by Duramed		Antiemetic
DP316	Tab, Yellow, Round	Prochlorperazine 25 mg	Compazine by Duramed		Antiemetic
DP32	Tab, White, Round	Conjugated Estrogens 1.25 mg	Premarin by Duramed		Estrogen
DP321 <> TOUROEX	Tab, White, Ex Release, DP/321 <> Touro EX	Guaifenesin 575 mg	Touro EX by Dartmouth	58869-0421	Expectorant
DP321 <> TOUROEX	Tab, DP/321 <> Touro EX	Guaifenesin 575 mg	Touro EX by Anabolic	00722-6394	Expectorant
DP321 <> TOUROEX	Tab, DP/321 <> Touro EX	Guaifenesin 600 mg	Touro EX by Anabolic	00722-6282	Expectorant
DP325	Tab, White, Round	Tolazamide 100 mg	Tolinase by Duramed		Antidiabetic
DP327	Tab, White, Round	Tolazamide 500 mg	Tolinase by Duramed		Antidiabetic
DP332	Tab, Yellow, Round	Propranolol 40 mg, Hydrochlorothiazide 25 mg	Inderide by Duramed		Antihypertensive
DP333	Tab, Yellow, Round	Propranolol 80 mg, Hydrochlorothiazide 25 mg	Inderide by Duramed		Antihypertensive
DP34	Tab, White, Round	Conjugated Estrogens 2.5 mg	Premarin by Duramed		Estrogen
DP364	Cap, Scarlet & White	Isometheptene Mucate 65 mg, Dichloralphenazone 100 mg, Acetaminophen 325 mg	Midrin by Amide		Analgesic
DP371	Tab, White, Round	Methyldopa 250 mg	Aldomet by Duramed		Antihypertensive
DP372	Tab, White, Round	Methyldopa 500 mg	Aldomet by Duramed		Antihypertensive
DP40	Tab	Propranolol HCl 40 mg	by Pharmedix	53002-0495	Antihypertensive
DP401	Tab, Yellow, Cap Shaped, Film Coated	Guaifenesin 600 mg, Pseudoephedrine HCl 120 mg	by Duramed	51285-0401	Cold Remedy
DP417	Tab, Green, Cap Shaped, Film Coated	Guaifenesin 600 mg	by Duramed	51285-0417	Expectorant
DP42	Tab, Red, Round, Duramed Logo and 42	Synthetic Conjugated Estrogens 0.625 mg	by Duramed	51285-0442	Hormone
DP420	Tab, Film Coated, DP Logo	Dextromethorphan Hydrobromide 30 mg, Guaifenesin 600 mg	by Quality Care	60346-0182	Cold Remedy
DP420	Tab, White, Cap Shaped	Dextromethorphan Hydrobromide 30 mg, Guaifenesin 600 mg	by Duramed	51285-0420	Cold Remedy
DP421 <> TOUROEX	Tab, White, Oblong, Scored	Guaifenesin 575 mg	by Pfab	62542-0705	Expectorant
DP43	Tab, White, Round, Duramed Logo 43	Synthetic Conjugated Estrogens 0.9 mg	by Duramed	51285-0443	Hormone

ID FRONT <> BACK	DESCRIPTION FRONT <> BACK	INGREDIENT & STRENGTH	BRAND (OR EQUIV.) & FIRM	NDC#	CLASS; SCH.
DP436 <> TOUROLA	Tab, DP/436 <> Touro LA	Guaifenesin 500 mg, Pseudoephedrine HCl 120 mg	Touro LA by Anabolic	00722-6284	Cold Remedy
DP480	Tab, Light Pink, Cap Shaped	Verapamil HCl SR 120 mg	Isoptin SR by Duramed	51285-0480	Antihypertensive
DP482	Tab, Light Pink, Cap Shaped	Verapamil HCl SR 240 mg	Isoptin SR by Duramed	51285-0482	Antihypertensive
DP50 <> LEVOXYL	Tab, dp/50 <> Levoxyl	Levothyroxine Sodium 50 mcg	Levoxyl by Jones	52604-1118	Antithyroid
DP50 <> LEVOXYL	Tab, White, Oval, Scored, dp/50 <> Levoxyl	Levothyroxine Sodium 50 mcg	Levoxyl by JMI Daniels	00689-1118	Antithyroid
DP501	Tab, Purple, Round, Scored, D Over P 501	Estradiol 0.5 mg	by Heartland	61392-0176	Hormone
DP504	Tab, Blue, Round, Scored, D Over P 504	Estradiol 2 mg	by Heartland	61392-0121	Hormone
DP509	Tab, Yellow, Oval, Scored	Methotrexate 2.5 mg	by Kiel	59063-0114	Antineoplastic
DP509	Tab, Yellow, Round	Methotrexate Sodium 2.5 mg	Methotrexate by Kiel	51285-0509	Antineoplastic
DP548	Cap, Buff & Dark Green	Hydroxyurea 500 mg	Hydrea by Duramed	51285-0548	Antineoplastic
DP575	Tab, Medium Rose, Round	Desogestrel 0.15 mg, Ethinyl Estradiol 0.03 mg	Desogen/Otho-Cept by Organon & RW Johnson	51285-0576	Oral Contraceptive
DP60	Tab, Pink, Round	Propranolol 60 mg	Inderal by Duramed		Antihypertensive
DP610	Tab, Off-White, Round	Oxycodone 5 mg, Acetaminophen 325 mg	Percocet by Duramed	51285-0610	Analgesic; C II
DP622	Tab, Yellow, Round	Diazepam 5 mg	Valium by Duramed		Antianxiety; C IV
DP623	Tab, Blue, Round	Diazepam 10 mg	Valium by Duramed		Antianxiety; C IV
DP636 <> TOURLA	Tab, White, Oblong, Scored	Guaifenesin 525 mg; Pseudoephedrine HCl 120 mg	by Pfab	62542-0755	Cold Remedy
DP636 <> TOURLA	Tab, White, Oblong	Guaifenesin 525 mg; Pseudoephedrine HCl 120 mg	Touro LA by Dartmouth Pharms	58869-0636	Cold Remedy
DP651	Cap, Blue & Clear	Phentermine HCl 30 mg	Fastin by Duramed		Anorexiant; C IV
DP660	Cap, Green & White	Temazepam 15 mg	Restoril by Duramed		Sedative/Hypnotic; C IV
DP661	Cap, White	Temazepam 30 mg	Restoril by Duramed		Sedative/Hypnotic; C IV
DP70	Yellow, Scored	Digoxin 0.125 mg	by Eckerd Drug	19458-0892	Cardiac Agent
DP75 <> LEVOXYL	Tab	Levothyroxine Sodium 75 mcg	Levoxyl by Jones	52604-1119	Antithyroid
DP75 <> LEVOXYL	Tab, Purple, Oval, Scored, dp/75 <> Levoxyl	Levothyroxine Sodium 75 mcg	Levoxyl by JMI Daniels	00689-1119	Antithyroid
DP80	Tab, Yellow, Round, dp/80	Propranolol 80 mg	Inderal by Duramed		Antihypertensive
DP825	Tab, Beige, Cap Shaped	Chlorpheniramine Tannate 8 mg, Phenylephrine Tannate 25 mg, Pyrilamine Tannate 25 mg	Triotann by Duramed	51285-0825	Cold Remedy
DP832	Tab, Pale Pink, Cap Shaped	Choline Magnesium Trisalicylate 500 mg	Trilisate by Amide	51285-0902	NSAID
DP833	Tab, White, Cap Shaped, Film Coated	Salicylate 750 mg	Choline Magnesium Trisalicylate by Duramed	51285-0903	NSAID
DP849	Tab, White, Cap Shaped	Butalbital 50 mg, Acetaminophen 325 mg, Caffeine 40 mg	Fioricet by Mikart		Analgesic
DP877	Tab, White, Round	Yohimbine HCl 5.4 mg	Yocon by Mikart		Impotence Agent
DP877	Tab, White, Round	Yohimbine HCl 5.4 mg	by Duramed	51285-0877	Impotence Agent
DP88 <> LEVOXYL	Tab	Levothyroxine Sodium 88 mcg	Levoxyl by Jones	52604-1132	Antithyroid
DP88 <> LEVOXYL	Tab, Olive, Oval, Scored, dp/88 <> Levoxyl	Levothyroxine Sodium 88 mcg	Levoxyl by JMI Daniels	00689-1132	Antithyroid
DP896	Tab, Blue, Cap Shaped	Durasal II 5,45,200 mg	Deconsal II by Sovereign	51285-0293	Cold Remedy
DP90	Tab, Lavender, Round	Propranolol 90 mg	Inderal by Duramed		Antihypertensive
DP914	Tab, White, Round	Digoxin 0.125 mg	Lanoxin by Jerome Stevens	51285-0914	Cardiac Agent
DP915	Tab, White, Round	Digoxin 0.25 mg	by Duramed		Cardiac Agent
DP915	Tab, White, Round	Digoxin 0.25 mg	Lanoxin by Jerome Stevens	51285-0915	Cardiac Agent
DP932	Tab, White, Round	Hyoscyamine Sulfate 0.125 mg	Levsin by Rugby		Gastrointestinal
DP932	Tab, White, Round	Hyoscyamine Sulfate 0.125 mg	Levsin by Amide	51285-0932	Gastrointestinal
DP933	Tab, Orange, Cap-Shaped, Ex Release	Hyoscyamine Sulfate 0.375 mg	by Duramed	51285-0933	Gastrointestinal
DP933	Tab, White, Oblong, Scored	Hyoscyamine Sulfate 0.375 mg	by Duramed Pharms	51285-0937	Gastrointestinal
DP935	Tab, Blue, Round	Hyoscyamine Sulfate SL 0.125 mg	Levsin SL by Amide	51285-0935	Gastrointestinal
DP935	Tab, White, Round	Hyoscyamine Sulfate 0.125 mg	Levsin SL by Rugby		Gastrointestinal
DP970	Tab, Yellow, Round	Digoxin 0.125 mg	by Duramed	51285-0970	Cardiac Agent
DP971	Tab, White, Round	Digoxin 0.25 mg	by Duramed	51285-0971	Cardiac Agent
DP972	Tab, Green, Round	Digoxin 0.5 mg	Lanoxin by Amide	51285-0972	Cardiac Agent
DPI <> 3	Tab	Acetaminophen 300 mg, Codeine Phosphate 30 mg	by Quality Care	60346-0059	Analgesic; C III
DPI <> 364	Cap, Scarlet, Black Print	Acetaminophen 325 mg, Dichloralantipyrine 100 mg, Isometheptene Mucate 65 mg	Duradrin by Kaiser	00179-1222	Cold Remedy
DPI <> 364	Cap, Scarlet, DPI or DP	Acetaminophen 325 mg, Dichloralantipyrine 100 mg, Isometheptene Mucate 65 mg	Midchlor by Schein	00364-2342	Cold Remedy

ID FRONT <> BACK	DESCRIPTION FRONT <> BACK	INGREDIENT & STRENGTH	BRAND (OR EQUIV.) & FIRM	NDC#	CLASS; SCH.
DPI <> 4	Tab	Acetaminophen 300 mg, Codeine Phosphate 60 mg	by Quality Care	60346-0632	Analgesic; C III
DPI <> 488	Cap, Opaque & White	Triamterene 37.5 mg, Hydrochlorothiazide 25 mg	Dyazide by Duramed	51285-0488	Diuretic
DPI <> 644	Cap	Acetaminophen 500 mg, Oxycodone HCl 5 mg	by Schein	00364-2395	Analgesic; C II
DPI 364	Cap, Scarlet & White	Duradrin 325,100,65 mg	Midrin by Duramed	51285-0364	Analgesic
DPI125	Tab, White, Diamond Shaped	Estropipate 1.5 mg	by Duramed	51285-0876	Hormone
DPI2	Tab	Acetaminophen 300 mg, Codeine 15 mg	by Elge	58298-0954	Analgesic; C III
DPI2	Tab	Acetaminophen 300 mg, Codeine 15 mg	by Zenith Goldline	00182-1268	Analgesic; C III
DPI2	Tab	Acetaminophen 300 mg, Codeine 15 mg	by McNeil	52021-0600	Analgesic; C III
DPI2	Tab	Acetaminophen 300 mg, Codeine 15 mg	by Major	00904-0571	Analgesic; C III
DPI2	Tab, White, Round	Acetaminophen 300 mg, Codeine Phosphate 15 mg	by Duramed	51285-0600	Analgesic; C III
DPI2 <> DPI2	Tab	Acetaminophen 300 mg, Codeine 15 mg	by United Res	00677-0611	Analgesic; C III
DPI3	Tab	Acetaminophen 300 mg, Codeine 30 mg	by Elge	58298-0953	Analgesic; C III
DPI3	Tab	Acetaminophen 300 mg, Codeine 30 mg	by Zenith Goldline	00182-0948	Analgesic; C III
DPI3	Tab	Acetaminophen 300 mg, Codeine 30 mg	by United Res	00677-0612	Analgesic; C III
DPI3	Tab	Acetaminophen 300 mg, Codeine 30 mg	by McNeil	52021-0601	Analgesic; C III
DPI3	Tab, White, Round	Acetaminophen 300 mg, Codeine Phosphate 30 mg	Tylenol #3 by Noramco		Analgesic; C III
DPI3	Tab, White, Round	Acetaminophen 300 mg, Codeine Phosphate 30 mg	by Duramed	51285-0601	Analgesic; C III
DPI364	Cap, Scarlet	Acetaminophen 325 mg, Dichloralantipyrine 100 mg, Isometheptene Mucate 65 mg	Duradrin by Duramed	51285-0364	Cold Remedy
DPI4	Tab	Acetaminophen 300 mg, Codeine 60 mg	by Elge	58298-0951	Analgesic; C III
DPI4	Tab	Acetaminophen 300 mg, Codeine 60 mg	by Zenith Goldline	00182-1338	Analgesic; C III
DPI4	Tab	Acetaminophen 300 mg, Codeine 60 mg	by United Res	00677-0632	Analgesic; C III
DPI4	Tab	Acetaminophen 300 mg, Codeine 60 mg	by McNeil	52021-0602	Analgesic; C III
DPI4	Tab	Acetaminophen 300 mg, Codeine 60 mg	by Major	00904-3916	Analgesic; C III
DPI4	Tab, White, Round	Acetaminophen 300 mg, Codeine Phosphate 60 mg	by Prepackage Spec	58864-0005	Analgesic; C III
DPI4	Tab, White, Round	Acetaminophen 300 mg, Codeine Phosphate 60 mg	Tylenol #4 by Noramco		Analgesic; C III
DPI4	Tab, White, Round	Acetaminophen 300 mg, Codeine Phosphate 60 mg	by Duramed	51285-0602	Analgesic; C III
DPI625	Tab, Light Orange, Diamond Shaped	Estropipate 0.75 mg	by Duramed	51285-0875	Hormone
DPI644	Cap	Acetaminophen 500 mg, Oxycodone HCl 5 mg	by Zenith Goldline	00182-9175	Analgesic; C II
DPI644	Cap, Red & White	Acetaminophen 500 mg, Oxycodone HCl 5 mg	by Duramed	51285-0644	Analgesic; C II
DPI644	Cap, Red & White	Acetaminophen 500 mg, Oxycodone HCl 5 mg	by McNeil	52021-0644	Analgesic; C II
DPI658	Cap, Red & White	Oxycodone 5 mg, Acetaminophen 500 mg	Tylox by Duramed	51285-0658	Analgesic; C II
DPI855	Cap, Clear & White	Guaifenesin 250 mg, Pseudoephedrine HCl 120 mg	by Duramed	51285-0855	Cold Remedy
DPI856	Cap, Blue & Clear	Guaifenesin 300 mg, Pseudoephedrine HCl 60 mg	by Duramed	51285-0856	Cold Remedy
DPI894	Cap, White	Guaifenesin 250 mg; Pseudoephedrine HCl 120 mg	by Pfab	62542-0454	Cold Remedy
DPI895	Cap, Blue	Guaifenesin 300 mg; Pseudoephedrine HCl 60 mg	by Pfab	62542-0406	Cold Remedy
DRISTANNDESEF	Cap, Yellow	Acetaminophen 500 mg, D-Pseudoephedrine HCl 30 mg	Dristan by Whitehall-Robbins		Cold Remedy
DRISTANSINUS1	Cap, White, Oval	Ibuprofen 200 mg, Pseudoephedrine HCl 30 mg	Dristan by Whitehall-Robbins		Cold Remedy
DRIXORAL	Tab, Green, Sphere, Schering Logo	Dexbrompheniramine Maleate 6 mg, Pseudoephed Sulfate 120 mg	Drixoral by Schering	Canadian	Cold Remedy
DRIXORALND	Tab, Yellow, Round, Drixoral N. D.	Pseudoephedrine Sulfate 120 mg	Drixoral N.D. by Schering	Canadian	Decongestant
DROXIA6335	Cap, Blue-Green, Hard Gel, Black Print	Hydroxyurea 200 mg	Droxia by ER Squibb	00003-6335	Antineoplastic
DROXIA6336	Cap, Purple, Black Print	Hydroxyurea 300 mg	Droxia by ER Squibb	00003-6336	Antineoplastic
DROXIA6337	Cap, Orange, Hard Gel, Black Print	Hydroxyurea 400 mg	Droxia by ER Squibb	00003-6337	Antineoplastic
DS	Cap, White, Gelatin, DS over Abbott Logo	Ritonavir 100 mg	Norvir by Abbott	00074-6633	Antiviral
DT	Tab, White, Round, Biconvex, Film Coated, with Arcs Above and Below the Letters DT	Tolterodine 2 mg	Detrol by Pharmacia & Upjohn	00009-4544	Urinary Tract
DT	Tab, White, Round, Film Coated	Tolterodine 2 mg	by Pharmacia	Canadian DIN# 02239065	Urinary Tract
DT	Tab, White, Round	Tolterodine Tartrate 2 mg	Detrol by Phy Total Care	54868-2824	Urinary Tract
DT	Tab, White, Round	Tolterodine Tartrate 2 mg	Detrol by Pharmacia Upjohn (It)	10829-4544	Urinary Tract
DT30G	Tab, Green, Round, DT 30/G	Diltiazem 30 mg	by Genpharm	Canadian	Antihypertensive
DT60	Tab, Yellow, Round	Diltiazem HCl 60 mg	by Genpharm	Canadian	Antihypertensive

ID FRONT <> BACK	DESCRIPTION FRONT <> BACK	INGREDIENT & STRENGTH	BRAND (OR EQUIV.) & FIRM	NDC#	CLASS; SCH.
DUNHALL0805	Cap, Red	Doxycycline Hyclate 100 mg	Doxy-D by Dunhall		Antibiotic
DUNHALL2811	Cap, Orange & White	Acetaminophen 325 mg, Butalbital 50 mg	Triaprin by Dunhall		Analgesic
DUNHALL2829	Cap, Red & Yellow	Carbetapentane 20 mg, Phenyleph. 10 mg, Phenylprop. 10 mg, Pot.Guaiacol 45 mg	Cophene-X by Dunhall		Cold Remedy
DUPHAR 313	Tab, White, Oval	Fluvoxamine Maleate 100 mg	Luvox by Solvay Kingswood	Canadian	OCD
DUPONT <> 11	Tab, Pale Yellow, Cap-Shaped, Coated	Naltrexone HCl 50 mg	Revia by Du Pont Pharma	00056-0011	Opiod Antagonist
DUPONT <> COUMADIN1	Tab, Pink, Round, Scored	Warfarin Sodium 1 mg	Coumadin by Eckerd	19458-0907	Anticoagulant
DUPONT <> COUMADIN1	Tab, Pink, Round, Scored	Warfarin Sodium 1 mg	Coumadin by Dupont Pharma	00056-0169	Anticoagulant
DUPONT <> COUMADIN1	Tab	Warfarin Sodium 1 mg	by Med Pro	53978-3302	Anticoagulant
DUPONT <> COUMADIN1	Tab	Warfarin Sodium 1 mg	Coumadin by Nat Pharmpak Serv	55154-7701	Anticoagulant
DUPONT <> COUMADIN10	Tab, White, Round, Scored	Warfarin Sodium 10 mg	Coumadin by Dupont Pharma	00056-0174	Anticoagulant
DUPONT <> COUMADIN10	Tab	Warfarin Sodium 10 mg	Coumadin by Nat Pharmpak Serv	55154-7707	Anticoagulant
DUPONT <> COUMADIN2	Tab, Lavender, Round, Scored	Warfarin Sodium 2 mg	Coumadin by Du Pont Pharma	00056-0170	Anticoagulant
DUPONT <> COUMADIN2	Tab, Lavender, <> On One Face, the Number is Superimposed	Warfarin Sodium 2 mg	Coumadin by PDRX	55289-0143	Anticoagulant
DUPONT <> COUMADIN2	Tab, Lavender	Warfarin Sodium 2 mg	Coumadin by Nat Pharmpak Serv	55154-7702	Anticoagulant
DUPONT <> COUMADIN2	Tab, Lavender, Dupont <> Coumadin/2	Warfarin Sodium 2 mg	Coumadin by Amerisource	62584-0348	Anticoagulant
DUPONT <> COUMADIN2	Tab, Purple, Round, Scored	Warfarin Sodium 2 mg	Coumadin by Eckerd	19458-0908	Anticoagulant
DUPONT <> COUMADIN212	Tab, Dupont <> Coumadin 2 1/2	Warfarin Sodium 2.5 mg	Coumadin by Nat Pharmpak Serv	55154-7703	Anticoagulant
DUPONT <> COUMADIN212	Tab, Dupont <> Coumadin over 2 1/2	Warfarin Sodium 2.5 mg	Coumadin by Quality Care	60346-0918	Anticoagulant
DUPONT <> COUMADIN212	Tab, Green, Round, Scored, Dupont <> Coumadin 2 1/2	Warfarin Sodium 2.5 mg	Coumadin by Dupont Pharma	00056-0176	Anticoagulant
DUPONT <> COUMADIN212	Tab, Dupont <> Coumadin 2 1/2	Warfarin Sodium 2.5 mg	Coumadin by Caremark	00339-5087	Anticoagulant
DUPONT <> COUMADIN212	Tab, Dupont <> Coumadin 2 1/2	Warfarin Sodium 2.5 mg	by Med Pro	53978-3301	Anticoagulant
DUPONT <> COUMADIN25	Tab, Green, Round, Scored, Dupont <> Coumadin 2.5	Warfarin Sodium 2.5 mg	Coumadin by Eckerd	19458-0909	Anticoagulant
DUPONT <> COUMADIN3	Tab, Tan, Round, Scored	Warfarin Sodium 3 mg	Coumadin by Dupont Pharma	00056-0188	Anticoagulant
DUPONT <> COUMADIN3	Tab, Tan, Round, Scored	Warfarin Sodium 3 mg	Coumadin by Eckerd	19458-0910	Anticoagulant
DUPONT <> COUMADIN4	Tab, Blue, Round, Scored	Warfarin Sodium 4 mg	Coumadin by Du Pont Pharma	00056-0168	Anticoagulant
DUPONT <> COUMADIN4	Tab, Blue, Round, Scored	Warfarin Sodium 4 mg	Coumadin by Eckerd	19458-0911	Anticoagulant
DUPONT <> COUMADIN5	Tab, Peach, Round, Scored	Warfarin Sodium 5 mg	Coumadin by Dupont Pharma	00056-0172	Anticoagulant
DUPONT <> COUMADIN5	Tab	Warfarin Sodium 5 mg	Coumadin by Caremark	00339-5089	Anticoagulant

ID FRONT <> BACK	DESCRIPTION FRONT <> BACK	INGREDIENT & STRENGTH	BRAND (OR EQUIV.) & FIRM	NDC#	CLASS; SCH.
DUPONT <> COUMADIN5	Tab	Warfarin Sodium 5 mg	Coumadin by Allscripts	54569-0159	Anticoagulant
DUPONT <> COUMADIN5	Tab	Warfarin Sodium 5 mg	by Med Pro	53978-0314	Anticoagulant
DUPONT <> COUMADIN5	Tab	Warfarin Sodium 5 mg	Coumadin by Amerisource	62584-0172	Anticoagulant
DUPONT <> COUMADIN5	Tab	Warfarin Sodium 5 mg	Coumadin by Nat Pharmpak Serv	55154-7704	Anticoagulant
DUPONT <> COUMADIN5	Tab, Peach, Round, Scored	Warfarin Sodium 5 mg	Coumadin by Eckerd	19458-0912	Anticoagulant
DUPONT <> COUMADIN6	Tab, Teal, Round, Coated	Warfarin Sodium 6 mg	Coumadin by Dupont Pharma	00056-0189	Anticoagulant
DUPONT <> COUMADIN712	Tab, Yellow, Round, Scored, Dupont <> Coumadin 7 1/2	Warfarin Sodium 7.5 mg	Coumadin by Dupont Pharma	00056-0173	Anticoagulant
DUPONT <> COUMADIN712	Tab, Dupont <> Coumadin 7 1/2	Warfarin Sodium 7.5 mg	Coumadin by Nat Pharmpak Serv	55154-7706	Anticoagulant
DUPONT <> HYCODAN	Tab, White, Round, Scored	Hydrocodone Bitartrate 5 mg, Homatropine Methylbromide 1.5 mg	Hycodan by DRX Pharm Consults	55045-2728	Analgesic; C III
DUPONT <> PERCOCET	Tab	Acetaminophen 325 mg, Oxycodone HCl 5 mg	Percocet by Dupont	00590-0127	Analgesic; C II
DUPONT <> PERCODANDEMI	Tab, Dupont <> Perdocan-Demi	Aspirin 325 mg, Oxycodone HCl 2.25 mg, Oxycodone Terephthalate 0.19 mg	Percodan Demi by Dupont	00590-0166	Analgesic; C II
DUPONT <> TREXAN	Tab, Debossed	Naltrexone HCl 50 mg	Trexan by Du Pont Pharma	00056-0080	Opiod Antagonist
DUPONT11	Tab, Yellow, Oblong, Dupont/11	Naltrexone 50 mg	Revia by DuPont Pharma	Canadian	Opiod Antagonist
DUPONTCOUMADIN2	Tab	Warfarin Sodium 2 mg	Coumadin by Allscripts	54569-0158	Anticoagulant
DUPONTHYCODAN	Tab	Homatropine Methylbromide 1.5 mg, Hydrocodone Bitartrate 5 mg	Hycodan by Du Pont Pharma	00056-0042	Cold Remedy; C III
DUPONTHYCOMINE	Tab, Coral, Dupont/Hycomine	Acetaminophen 250 mg, Caffeine 30 mg, Chlorpheniramine Maleate 2 mg, Hydrocodone Bitartrate 5 mg, Phenylephrine HCl 10 mg	Hycomine Compound by Du Pont Pharma	00056-0048	Cold Remedy; C III
DUPONTPHARMA <> SYMMETREL	Cap	Amantadine HCl 100 mg	by Dupont Pharma	00056-0315	Antiviral
DUPONTZYDONE	Cap, White, Red Band, Red Print	Acetaminophen 500 mg, Hydrocodone Bitartrate 5 mg	Zydone by Du Pont Pharma	00056-0091	Analgesic; C III
DURA <> 009	Tab, Light Blue, DU-RA	Guaifenesin 600 mg	Fenesin by Anabolic	00722-6139	Expectorant
DURA <> 009	Tab, Blue, Oblong, Scored	Guaifenesin 600 mg	Fenesin by Med Pro	53978-3363	Expectorant
DURA <> 15	Tab, White, Scored	Guaifenesin 600 mg; Pseudoephedrine HCl 120 mg	by DJ Pharma	64455-0015	Cold Remedy
DURA <> 15	Tab, White, Oblong	Guaifenesin 600 mg; Pseudoephedrine HCl 120 mg	Guai Vent PSE by Anabolic Ca	00722-6310	Cold Remedy
DURA <> 7575	Tab, Dura <> 7.5/7.5	Guaifenesin 600 mg, Phenylpropanolamine HCl 75 mg	Dura Vent by Anabolic	00722-6051	Cold Remedy
DURA <> 7575	Tab, Dura <> 7.5/7.5	Guaifenesin 600 mg, Phenylpropanolamine HCl 75 mg	by DHHS Prog	11819-0049	Cold Remedy
DURA <> 7575	Tab, White, Oblong, Scored, Dura <> 7.5/7.5	Guaifenesin 600 mg, Phenylpropanolamine HCl 75 mg	Dura Vent by Med Pro	53978-3334	Cold Remedy
DURA <> 7575	Tab, Dura <> 7.5/7.5	Guaifenesin 600 mg, Phenylpropanolamine HCl 75 mg	Dura Vent by CVS	51316-0242	Cold Remedy
DURA <> CHEW	Tab, Chewable	Chlorpheniramine Maleate 2 mg, Methscopolamine Nitrate 1.25 mg, Phenylephrine HCl 10 mg	D A by Anabolic	00722-6219	Cold Remedy
DURA <> CHEW	Tab, Orange, Scored	Methscopolamine Nitrate 1.25 mg, Phenylephrine HCl 10 mg, Dextromethorphan Hydrobromide 25 mg	DA Chewable by Neuman Distr	64579-0015	Cold Remedy
DURA <> DA	Tab, DU/RA <> D/A	Chlorpheniramine Maleate 8 mg, Methscopolamine Nitrate 2.5 mg, Phenylephrine HCl 20 mg	Dura Vent by Anabolic	00722-6072	Cold Remedy
DURA <> DA	Tab, Brown, Oblong, Scored	Methscopolamine Nitrate 2.5 mg, Phenylephrine HCl 20 mg, Chlorpheniramine Maleate 8 mg	Dura Vent DA by Neuman Distr	64579-0016	Cold Remedy
DURA <> DAII	Tab	Chlorpheniramine Maleate 4 mg, Methscopolamine Nitrate 1.25 mg, Phenylephrine HCl 10 mg	Da II by Anabolic	00722-6354	Cold Remedy
DURA <> DAII	Tab, White, Oblong	Methscopolamine Nitrate 1.25 mg, Phenylephrine HCl 10 mg, Chlorpheniramine Maleate 4 mg	DA II by Neuman Distr	64579-0014	Cold Remedy
DURA <> FDM014	Tab, Film Coated	Dextromethorphan Hydrobromide 30 mg, Guaifenesin 600 mg	by PDRX	55289-0625	Cold Remedy

ID FRONT <> BACK	DESCRIPTION FRONT <> BACK	INGREDIENT & STRENGTH	BRAND (OR EQUIV.) & FIRM	NDC#	CLASS; SCH.
DURA <> FDM014	Tab, DU/RA <> FDM 014	Dextromethorphan Hydrobromide 30 mg, Guaifenesin 600 mg	Fenesin DM by Anabolic	00722-6275	Cold Remedy
DURA015	Tab, White, Oblong	Guaifenesin 600 mg, Pseudoephedrine 120 mg	Guai-Vent/PSE by Dura		Cold Remedy
DURA017	Tab, Pink, Oval	Brompheniramine Maleate 4 mg, Pseudoephedrine 60 mg	Rondec Chewable by Dura		Cold Remedy
DURADAJR	Tab, Orange	Chlorpheniramine 2 mg, Phenylephrine 10 mg, Methscopolamine 1.25 mg	Dura- by Dura		Cold Remedy
DURADAJR	Tab, Orange	Chlorpheniramine 2 mg, Phenylephrine 10 mg, Methscopolamine 1.25 mg	Dura-Vent DA Chew by Dura		Cold Remedy
DURAGEST <> 51479005	Cap, Gray & White, Dura-Gest <> 51479005	Guaifenesin 200 mg, Phenylephrine HCl 5 mg, Phenylpropanolamine HCl 45 mg	Dura Gest by Mallinckrodt Hobart	00406-1124	Cold Remedy
DURAGEST <> 51479005	Cap, Dura-Gest	Guaifenesin 200 mg, Phenylephrine HCl 5 mg, Phenylpropanolamine HCl 45 mg	Enomine by Quality Care	60346-0725	Cold Remedy
DURICEF500 <> APP784	Cap	Cefadroxil 500 mg	Duricef by Pharmedix	53002-0284	Antibiotic
DURICEF500 <> PPP784	Cap, Duricef over 500 <> PPP over 784	Cefadroxil 500 mg	Duricef by Nat Pharmpak Serv	55154-2009	Antibiotic
DURICEF500MG <> PPP784	Cap	Cefadroxil 500 mg	Duricef by Bristol Myers Barcelaneta	55961-0784	Antibiotic
DURICEF500MG <> PPP784	Cap	Cefadroxil 500 mg	Duricef by Prestige Packaging	58056-0348	Antibiotic
DURICEF500MG <> PPP784	Cap, Duricef 500 mg <> PPP 784	Cefadroxil 500 mg	Duricef by Bristol Myers Squibb	00087-0784	Antibiotic
DURICEF500MG <> PPP784	Cap	Cefadroxil 500 mg	Duricef by Allscripts	54569-0108	Antibiotic
DURICEF500MG <> PPP784	Cap, Duricef over 500 mg <> PPP784	Cefadroxil Monohydrate	Duricef by Quality Care	60346-0641	Antibiotic
DYAZIDE <> SB	Cap	Hydrochlorothiazide 25 mg, Triamterene 37.5 mg	Dyazide by Allscripts	54569-3824	Diuretic
DYAZIDE <> SB	Cap, Opaque	Hydrochlorothiazide 25 mg, Triamterene 37.5 mg	Dyazide by Amerisource	62584-0365	Diuretic
DYAZIDESB	Cap	Hydrochlorothiazide 25 mg, Triamterene 37.5 mg	Dyazide by Wal Mart	49035-0170	Diuretic
DYAZIDESB	Cap	Hydrochlorothiazide 25 mg, Triamterene 37.5 mg	Dyazide by Physicians Total Care	54868-3366	Diuretic
DYAZIDESB	Cap	Hydrochlorothiazide 25 mg, Triamterene 37.5 mg	Dyazide by Repack	55306-3650	Diuretic
DYAZIDESB	Cap, Opaque & Red & White	Triamterene 37.5 mg, Hydrochlorothiazide 25 mg	Dyazide by Teva	00480-0733	Diuretic
DYAZIDESB	Cap	Hydrochlorothiazide 25 mg, Triamterene 37.5 mg	Dyazide by SKB	00007-3650	Diuretic
DYAZIDESB	Cap, Opaque & Red & White, Dyazide over SB	Hydrochlorothiazide 25 mg, Triamterene 37.5 mg	Dyazide by Murfreesboro	51129-1385	Diuretic
DYFLEXG	Tab, Dyflex/G	Dyphylline 200 mg, Guaifenesin 200 mg	Dyflex G by EMREX Econo	38130-0012	Antiasthmatic
DYNABAC <> VC5364	Tab, Delayed Release	Dirithromycin 250 mg	Dynabac by Quality Care	60346-0601	Antibiotic
DYNABAC<> UC5364	Tab, White, Oval, Coated	Dirithromycin 250 mg	Dynabac by Eli Lilly	00002-0490	Antibiotic
DYNABACUC5364	Tab, Coated	Dirithromycin 250 mg	Dynabac by Sanofi	00024-0490	Antibiotic
DYNABACUC5364	Tab, White, Enteric Coated	Dirithromycin 250 mg	Dynabac by Muro Pharm	00451-0490	Antibiotic
DYNACIN <> 498	Cap, Gray & White	Minocycline HCl 100 mg	Dynacin by Natl Pharmpak	55154-9101	Antibiotic
DYNACIN100MG <> 498	Cap, Gray & White	Minocycline HCl 100 mg	Dynacin by WalMart	49035-0186	Antibiotic
DYNACIN50MG <> 497	Cap, White	Minocycline HCl 50 mg	Dynacin by Natl Pharmpak	55154-9102	Antibiotic
DYNACIN75MG <> 499	Cap, Gray	Minocycline HCl 75 mg	Dynacin by Rx Pac	65084-0236	Antibiotic
DYNACIN75MG <> 499	Cap, Gray	Minocycline HCl 75 mg	Dynacin by Eckerd	19458-0914	Antibiotic
DYNACIRC <> 25	Cap, Dynacirc <> 2.5 Sandoz Logo	Isradipine 2.5 mg	Dynacirc by Caremark	00339-5719	Antihypertensive
DYNACIRC <> 25S	Tab, White, Oblong, Dynacirc <> 2.5 S	Isradipine 2.5 mg	Dynacirc by Murfreesboro	51129-1588	Antihypertensive
DYNACIRC <> 5S	Cap, Pink	Isradipine 5 mg	Dynacirc by Murfreesboro	51129-1589	Antihypertensive
DYNACIRCCR10	Tab, DR, in Red Ink	Isradipine 10 mg	Dynacirc CR by Novartis	00078-0236	Antihypertensive
DYNACIRCCR5	Tab, DR, in Red Ink	Isradipine 5 mg	Dynacirc CR by Novartis	00078-0235	Antihypertensive
DYNACN0499	Cap, Gray	Minocycline HCl 75 mg	Dynacin by Wal Mart	49035-0195	Antibiotic
DYRENIUMSKF100MG	Cap, Red, Dyrenium/SKF/100 mg	Triamterene 100 mg	Dyrenium by SKB		Diuretic
DYRENIUMSKF50MG	Cap, Red, Dyrenium/SKF/50 mg	Triamterene 50 mg	Dyrenium by SKB		Diuretic
E	Tab, White, Round	I-Isomer Selegilline HCl 5 mg	Eldepryl by Draxis	Canadian	Antiparkinson
E	Tab, White	Seleniline HCl 5 mg	Eldepryl by Draxis	Canadian	Antiparkinson

ID FRONT ⬦ BACK	DESCRIPTION FRONT ⬦ BACK	INGREDIENT & STRENGTH	BRAND (OR EQUIV.) & FIRM	NDC#	CLASS; SCH.
E ⬦ 10	Tab, Red, Octagonal	Acetaminophen 400 mg, Hydrocodone Bitartrate 10 mg	Zydone by Endo Labs	63481-0698	Analgesic; C III
E ⬦ 10	Tab, Red, Octagonal	Acetaminophen 400 mg, Hydrocodone Bitartrate 10 mg	Zydone by Allscripts	54569-4732	Analgesic; C III
E ⬦ 10	Tab, Red, Octagonal	Acetaminophen 400 mg; Hydrocodone Bitartrate 10 mg	Zydone by West Pharm	52967-0275	Analgesic; C III
E ⬦ 10	Tab, Red, Octagon, Convex	Hydrocodone Bitartrate 10 mg, Acetaminophen 400 mg	Zydone by Murfreesboro	51129-1442	Analgesic; C III
E ⬦ 10	Tab, Red, Octagon, Convex	Hydrocodone Bitartrate 5 mg, Acetaminophen 400 mg	Zydone by Murfreesboro	51129-1450	Analgesic; C III
E ⬦ 10	Tab, Red, Octagon, Convex	Hydrocodone Bitatrate 10 mg, Acetaminophen 400 mg	Zydone by Murfreesboro	51129-1460	Analgesic; C III
E ⬦ 134	Tab	Reserpine 0.25 mg	by Allscripts	54569-0597	Antihypertensive
E ⬦ 2	Tab, Blue, Coated	Hydromorphone HCl 2 mg	Dilaudid by Ethex	58177-0298	Analgesic; C II
E ⬦ 2	Tab, Coated	Hydromorphone HCl 2 mg	by KV	10609-1366	Analgesic; C II
E ⬦ 4	Tab, Tan, Coated	Hydromorphone HCl 4 mg	Dilaudid by Ethex	58177-0299	Analgesic; C II
E ⬦ 4	Tab, Coated	Hydromorphone HCl 4 mg	by KV	10609-1367	Analgesic; C II
E ⬦ 5	Tab, Yellow, Octagonal	Acetaminophen 400 mg; Hydrocodone Bitartrate 5 mg	Zydone by West Pharm	52967-0273	Analgesic; C III
E ⬦ 5	Tab, Yellow, Octagonal	Acetaminophen 500 mg, Hydrocodone Bitartrate 5 mg	Zydone by Endo Labs	63481-0668	Analgesic; C III
E ⬦ 5	Tab, Yellow, Oblong, Convex	Hydrocodone Bitartrate 10 mg, Acetaminophen 400 mg	Zydone by Murfreesboro	51129-1443	Analgesic; C III
E ⬦ 5	Tab, Yellow, Oblong, Convex	Hydrocodone Bitartrate 5 mg, Acetaminophen 400 mg	Zydone by Murfreesboro	51129-1446	Analgesic; C III
E ⬦ 5	Tab	Hydrocodone Bitatrate 5 mg, Acetaminophen 400 mg	Zydone by Murfreesboro	51129-1461	Analgesic; C III
E ⬦ 75	Tab, White, E ⬦ 7.5	Lisinopril 2.5 mg	Prinivil by Allscripts	54569-4721	Antihypertensive
E ⬦ 75	Tab, Blue, Octagonal, E ⬦ 7.5	Acyclovir 800 mg	Zydone by Allscripts	54569-4724	Antiviral
E ⬦ 75	Tab, Blue, Octagonal, E ⬦ 7.5	Acetaminophen 400 mg, Hydrocodone Bitartrate 7.5 mg	Zydone by Endo Labs	63481-0669	Analgesic; C III
E ⬦ 75	Tab, Blue, Octagon, Convex, E ⬦ 7.5	Acetaminophen 400 mg; Hydrocodone Bitartrate 7.5 mg	Zydone by West Pharm	52967-0274	Analgesic; C III
E ⬦ 75	Tab, Blue, Octagon, Convex, E ⬦ 7.5	Hydrocodone Bitartrate 7.5 mg, Acetaminophen 400 mg	Zydone by Murfreesboro	51129-1454	Analgesic; C III
E ⬦ HYDROGESIC	Cap, Edwards Logo	Hydrocodone Bitatrate 7.5 mg, Acetaminophen 400 mg	Zydone by Murfreesboro	51129-1462	Analgesic; C III
E0019	Tab, Blue, Round	Acetaminophen 500 mg, Hydrocodone Bitartrate 5 mg	Hydrogesic by Edwards	00485-0050	Analgesic; C III
E1 ⬦ 511	Tab, White, Round	Desipramine HCl 25 mg	Norpramin by Eon		Antidepressant
E1 ⬦ 511	Tab, White, Round, Scored	Estradiol 0.5 mg	by ESI Lederle	59911-5879	Hormone
E10	Tab, White, Round, Scored, Film-Coated, E over 10	Estradiol 0.5 mg	by Ayerst Lab (Div Wyeth)	00046-5879	Hormone
E10	Tab, White, Round	Labetalol HCl 100 mg	Trandate by UDL	51079-0928	Antihypertensive
E10	Tab, White, Round, Film Coated	Labetalol HCl 100 mg	by Eon	00185-0010	Antihypertensive
E112	Tab, Eon Logo	Labetalol HCl 100 mg	by Caremark	00339-6186	Antihypertensive
E112	Tab, White, Oval	Sulfamethoxazole 800 mg, Trimethoprim 160 mg	by Rugby	00536-4693	Antibiotic
E112	Tab	Sulfamethoxazole 800 mg, Trimethoprim 160 mg	Bactrim DS by Eon	00185-0112	Antibiotic
E112	Tab, Eon Logo	Sulfamethoxazole 800 mg, Trimethoprim 160 mg	by Kaiser	00179-0372	Antibiotic
E112	Tab, E on Left, 112 on Right	Sulfamethoxazole 800 mg, Trimethoprim 160 mg	by Darby Group	66467-4693	Antibiotic
E112	Tab, White, Oval, Scored	Sulfamethoxazole 800 mg, Trimethoprim 160 mg	SMZ TMP DS by Quality Care	60346-0087	Antibiotic
E114	Tab, Yellow, Round	Trimethoprim 160 mg, Sulfamethoxazole 800 mg	by Haines Pharms	59564-0199	Antibiotic
E115	Tab, Off-White, Oval	Enalapril Maleate 2.5 mg	by Eon	00185-0114	Antihypertensive
E117	Tab, White, Round, Scored, Film-Coated, E over 117	Ticlopidine HCl 250 mg	by Eon	00185-0115	Anticoagulant
E117	Tab, White, Round	Labetalol HCl 200 mg	Trandate by UDL	51079-0929	Antihypertensive
E117	Tab, White, Round, Film Coated	Labetalol HCl 200 mg	by Eon	00185-0117	Antihypertensive
E118	Tab, White, Round	Labetalol HCl 200 mg	by Caremark	00339-6187	Antihypertensive
E12 ⬦ SKF	Cap	Labetalol HCl 300 mg	by Eon	00185-0118	Antihypertensive
E120	Tab, White, Oval, Film Coated	Dextroamphetamine Sulfate 5 mg	Dexedrine by Physicians Total Care	54868-3402	Stimulant; C II
E120	Tab, White, Oval, Film Coated	Isosorbide Mononitrate 120 mg	by Ethex	58177-0201	Antianginal
E121	Tab, White, Round, Scored	Isosorbide Mononitrate 120 mg	by KV Pharm	10609-1368	Antianginal
E121	Tab, White, Round, Scored	Captopril 12.5 mg	Captopril by Caremark	00339-5918	Antihypertensive
E1217	Cap, Green & Yellow	Captopril 12.5 mg	Captopril USP by Caremark	00339-5948	Antihypertensive
E1217	Cap, ER	Nitroglycerin 9 mg	Nitrobid ER by Eon	00185-1217	Vasodilator
E122	Tab, White, Round, Scored	Nitroglycerin 9 mg	by Major	00904-0647	Vasodilator
E122	Tab, White, Round, Scored	Captopril 25 mg	Captopril USP by Caremark	00339-6112	Antihypertensive
E123	Tab, White, Round, Scored	Captopril 25 mg	Captopril by Caremark	00339-5920	Antihypertensive
E1235	Cap, Blue & Yellow	Captopril 50 mg	Captopril by Caremark	00339-5944	Antihypertensive
		Nitroglycerin 6.5 mg	Nitrobid ER by Eon	00185-1235	Vasodilator

ID FRONT <> BACK	DESCRIPTION FRONT <> BACK	INGREDIENT & STRENGTH	BRAND (OR EQUIV.) & FIRM	NDC#	CLASS; SCH.
E1235	Cap, ER	Nitroglycerin 6.5 mg	by Rugby	00536-4084	Vasodilator
E1235	Cap, ER	Nitroglycerin 6.5 mg	by Major	00904-0644	Vasodilator
E1235 <> E1235	Tab, Blue & Clear, Oval	Nitroglycerin 6.5 mg	by PDRX	55289-0310	Vasodilator
E124	Tab, White, Round, Scored	Captopril 100 mg	Captopril USP by Caremark	00339-6127	Antihypertensive
E124	Tab, White, Round, Scored	Captopril 100 mg	Captopril by Caremark	00339-5946	Antihypertensive
E127	Tab, White, Round	Enalapril Maleate 5 mg	by Eon	00185-0127	Antihypertensive
E128	Tab, Green, Round, Scored, Eon Logo 128	Bumetanide 0.5 mg	by Caraco	57664-0221	Diuretic
E128	Tab, Green, Round, Scored, E over 128	Bumetanide 0.5 mg	Bumex by UDL	51079-0891	Diuretic
E128	Tab, Green, Round, Eon Logo	Bumetanide 0.5 mg	Bumex by Eon	00185-0128	Diuretic
E128	Tab	Bumetanide 0.5 mg	by Geneva	00781-1821	Diuretic
E128	Tab	Bumetanide 0.5 mg	by Major	00904-5102	Diuretic
E129	Tab, Yellow, Round, Scored	Bumetanide 1 mg	by Caraco	57664-0315	Diuretic
E129	Tab, Yellow, Round, Scored, E over 129	Bumetanide 1 mg	by UDL	51079-0892	Diuretic
E129	Tab	Bumetanide 1 mg	by Geneva	00781-1822	Diuretic
E129	Tab, Yellow, Round, Eon Logo	Bumetanide 1 mg	Bumex by Eon	00185-0129	Diuretic
E129	Tab	Bumetanide 1 mg	by Major	00904-5103	Diuretic
E129	Tab, Yellow, Round	Bumetanide 1 mg	by Caremark	00339-6185	Diuretic
E13	Tab, Green	Ferrous Sulfate 325 mg	by Eon	00185-0013	Mineral
E130	Tab, Beige to Light Brown, Round, Scored, E over 130	Bumetanide 2 mg	Bumex by UDL	51079-0893	Diuretic
E130	Tab, Light Brown, Round, Eon Logo	Bumetanide 2 mg	Bumex by Eon	00185-0130	Diuretic
E130	Tab, Eon Logo 130	Bumetanide 2 mg	by Major	00904-5104	Diuretic
E1303	Cap, Clear	Quinine Sulfate 325 mg	by Eon		Antimalarial
E1303	Cap, Clear	Quinine Sulfate 325 mg	by Eon		Antimalarial
E1304	Cap, Dark Blue & Clear	Chlorpheniramine Maleate 8 mg, Pseudoephedrine HCl 120 mg	Deconamine SR by Eon	00185-1304	Cold Remedy
E1304	Cap, Eon Logo 1304	Chlorpheniramine Maleate 8 mg, Pseudoephedrine HCl 120 mg	by DHHS Prog	11819-0055	Cold Remedy
E1304	Cap, Dark Blue	Chlorpheniramine Maleate 8 mg, Pseudoephedrine HCl 120 mg	Pseudo Chlor by Allscripts	54569-4122	Cold Remedy
E1304	Cap, Blue & Clear	Chlorpheniramine Maleate 8 mg, Pseudoephedrine HCl 120 mg	Deconamine SR by Geneva	00781-2915	Cold Remedy
E1304	Cap, Eon Logo 1304	Chlorpheniramine Maleate 8 mg, Pseudoephedrine HCl 120 mg	Pseudo Chlor Caps by Major	00904-7777	Cold Remedy
E1304	Cap, Blue & Clear	Chlorpheniramine Maleate 8 mg; Pseudoephedrine HCl 120 mg	Sanfed A by C J Sant Pharm	60527-0304	Cold Remedy
E131	Tab, White, Round	Methadone HCl 10 mg	by Eon	00185-0131	Analgesic; C II
E131	Tab, White, Round, Eon Logo over 131	Methadone HCl 10 mg	by Nat Pharmpak Serv	55154-6905	Analgesic; C II
E132	Tab, White, Quadrasected	Methadone HCl 40 mg	by Eon	00185-0132	Analgesic; C II
E132	Tab, White, Scored, E over 132	Methadone HCl 40 mg	by Nat Pharmpak Serv	55154-5826	Analgesic; C II
E134	Tab, White, Round	Reserpine 0.25 mg	Serpasil by Eon	00185-0134	Antihypertensive
E134	Tab	Reserpine 0.25 mg	by United Res	00677-0126	Antihypertensive
E139	Tab, White, Oval	Etodolac 500 mg	by Eon	00185-0139	NSAID
E14	Tab, Yellow	Chlorpheniramine Maleate 4 mg	by Eon	00185-1064	Antihistamine
E140	Tab, Film Coated, E-40	Etodolac 400 mg	by Mylan	00378-2237	NSAID
E140	Tab, White, Oval, Film Coated, E-140	Etodolac 400 mg	Lodine by Eon	00185-0140	NSAID
E140	Tab, White, Oval, Film Coated, E-140	Etodolac 400 mg	by Heartland	61392-0828	NSAID
E140	Tab, White, Oval, Film Coated	Etodolac 400 mg	by HJ Harkins	52959-0471	NSAID
E144	Tab, Yellow, Round	Amiodarone HCl 200 mg	by Eon	00185-0144	Antiarrhythmic
E147	Tab, Salmon, Round	Enalapril Maleate 10 mg	by Eon	00185-0147	Antihypertensive
E157	Tab, Beige, Round	Fluvoxamine Maleate 100 mg	by Eon	00185-0157	OCD
E17	Tab, Off-White, Round	Fluvoxamine Maleate 25 mg	by Eon	00185-0017	OCD
E170	Tab, Light Blue, Cap Shaped	Sotalol 120 mg	by Eon	00185-0170	Antiarrhythmic
E171	Tab, Light Blue, Cap Shaped	Sotalol 80 mg	by Eon	00185-0171	Antiarrhythmic
E174	Tab, Light Blue, Cap Shaped	Sotalol 240 mg	by Eon	00185-0174	Antiarrhythmic
E175	Tab, Orange, Round	Bupropion HCl 75 mg	by Eon	00185-0175	Antidepressant
E176	Tab, Red, Round	Bupropion HCl 100 mg	by Eon	00185-0176	Antidepressant
E177	Tab, Light Blue, Cap Shaped	Sotalol 160 mg	by Eon	00185-0177	Antiarrhythmic
E19	Tab, Light Blue, Round, Film Coated, E over 19	Desipramine HCl 25 mg	Norpramin by UDL	51079-0489	Antidepressant

ID FRONT <> BACK	DESCRIPTION FRONT <> BACK	INGREDIENT & STRENGTH	BRAND (OR EQUIV.) & FIRM	NDC#	CLASS; SCH.
E19	Tab, Blue, Round, Film Coated	Desipramine HCl 25 mg	by DRX		Antidepressant
E19	Tab, Light Blue, Round, Film Coated	Desipramine HCl 25 mg	Norpramin by Eon	00185-0019	Antidepressant
E19	Tab, Coated	Desipramine HCl 25 mg	by Major	00904-1570	Antidepressant
E19	Tab, Coated	Desipramine HCl 25 mg	by Prescription Dispensing	61807-0130	Antidepressant
E19 <> SKF	Tab	Dextroamphetamine Sulfate 5 mg	Dexedrine by Abbott	00074-3241	Stimulant; C II
E21	Tab, White, Round	Methadone HCl 5 mg	by Eon	00185-0021	Analgesic; C II
E21	Tab, White, Round, Eon Logo over 21	Methadone HCl 5 mg	by Nat Pharmpak Serv	55154-6904	Analgesic; C II
E214	Tab, Peach, Round	Enalapril Maleate 20 mg	by Eon	00185-0214	Antihypertensive
E217	Tab, Light Yellow, Oval	Amiodarone HCl 400 mg	by Eon	00185-0217	Antiarrhythmic
E22	Tab, White, Round	Orphenadrine Citrate ER 100 mg	by Eon	00185-0022	Muscle Relaxant
E220	Tab, Sugar Coated, Stylized E	Atropine Sulfate 0.03 mg, Benzoic Acid 4.5 mg, Hyoscyamine 0.03 mg, Methenamine 40.8 mg, Methylene Blue 5.4 mg, Phenyl Salicylate 18.1 mg	Urinary Antiseptic by PDRX	55289-0518	Antiseptic
E220	Tab, Dark Blue, Sugar Coated, Eon Logo 220	Atropine Sulfate 0.03 mg, Benzoic Acid 4.5 mg, Hyoscyamine 0.03 mg, Methenamine 40.8 mg, Methylene Blue 5.4 mg, Phenyl Salicylate 18.1 mg	Urinary Antiseptic No. 2 by Quality Care	60346-0124	Antiseptic
E230	Tab, Blue, Round	Urinary Antiseptic #2	Hexalol by Eon		Urinary Tract
E24	Tab, White, Round	Diphenoxylate HCl 2.5 mg, Atropine Sulfate 0.025 mg	by Eon	00185-0024	Antidiarrheal; C V
E243	Tab, Yellow, Round	Rabeprazole Sodium 20 mg	Aciphex by RX PAK	65084-0145	Gastrointestinal
E243	Tab, Yellow, Round	Rabeprazole Sodium 20 mg	Aciphex by RX PAK	65084-0147	Gastrointestinal
E245 <> 5	Tab, Film Coated	Donepezil HCl 5 mg	Aricept by Eisai	62856-0245	Antialzheimers
E246 <> 10	Tab, Film Coated	Donepezil HCl 10 mg	Aricept by Eisai	62856-0246	Antialzheimers
E26	Cap, Red, E-26	Docusate Calcium 240 mg	Surfak by Chase		Laxative
E27	Cap, Orange & Red, E-27	Docusate Sodium 100 mg	Colace by Chase		Laxative
E27	Tab, Yellow, Round	Fluvoxamine Maleate 50 mg	by Eon	00185-0027	OCD
E29	Tab, White, Round, Coated, Eon Logo	Desipramine HCl 10 mg	by Eon	00185-0029	Antidepressant
E29	Tab, Eon Logo	Desipramine HCl 10 mg	by Zenith Goldline	00182-2652	Antidepressant
E29	Cap, Orange & Red, E-29	Docusate Sodium 250 mg	Colace by Chase		Laxative
E3 <> M	Tab, White, Round, Flat, Scored, Uncoated	Estradiol 0.5 mg	Estradiol by Heartland	61392-0122	Hormone
E30	Tab, Red, Oval, Film Coated, Scored	Isosorbide Mononitrate 30 mg	by Ethex	58177-0222	Antianginal
E30	Tab, Red, Oval, Film Coated	Isosorbide Mononitrate 30 mg	by KV Pharm	10609-1396	Antianginal
E30	Tab, Red, Oval, Scored	Isosorbide Mononitrate 60 mg	by Ethex	58177-0238	Antianginal
E31	Tab, White, Round, Eon Logo	Captopril 12.5 mg	Captopril by Eon	00185-0031	Antihypertensive
E32	Tab, White, Round	Reserpine 0.1 mg	Serpasil by Eon	00185-0032	Antihypertensive
E32	Tab, Eon Logo 32	Reserpine 0.1 mg	by Quality Care	60346-0837	Antihypertensive
E32	Tab, Eon Logo 32	Reserpine 0.1 mg	by Apotheca	12634-0442	Antihypertensive
E33 <> SKF	Cap, Red	Phenoxybenzamine HCl 10 mg	Dibenzyline by Wellspring Pharm	65197-0001	Antihypertensive
E345	Cap, Ex Release, with Beads	Caramiphen Edisylate 40 mg, Phenylpropanolamine HCl 75 mg	Tusso Gest ER by Quality Care	60346-0476	Cold Remedy
E345	Cap, Clear & White	Caramiphen Edisylate 40 mg, Phenylpropanolamine HCl 75 mg	Ordrine AT by Eon	00185-0345	Cold Remedy
E39	Tab, White to Off-White, Cap Shaped	Naltrexone HCl 50 mg	by Eon	00185-0039	Opiod Antagonist
E4	Tab, Blue, Round	Hydromorphone HCl 4 mg	Dilaudid by KV		Analgesic; C II
E4 <> M	Tab, Pink, Round, Flat, Scored, Uncoated	Estradiol 1 mg	Estradiol by Heartland	61392-0149	Hormone
E435	Tab	Isoniazid 100 mg	Isoniazid by Med Pro	53978-3065	Antimycobacterial
E4350	Tab, White, Round, Scored	Isoniazid 300 mg	by HJ Harkins	52959-0419	Antimycobacterial
E4350	Tab, White, Round	Isoniazid 300 mg	Isoniazid by Eon	00185-4350	Antimycobacterial
E4350	Tab	Isoniazid 300 mg	Isoniazid by Rugby	00536-3941	Antimycobacterial
E4350	Tab	Isoniazid 300 mg	Isoniazid by Med Pro	53978-1305	Antimycobacterial
E4350	Tab	Isoniazid 300 mg	Isoniazid by Major	00904-2096	Antimycobacterial
E4351	Tab, White, Round	Isoniazid 100 mg	INH by Eon		Antimycobacterial
E4351	Tab, White, Round	Isoniazid 100 mg	INH by Eon		Antimycobacterial
E4354	Tab, White, Round, Scored	Amoxicillin Trihydrate 250 mg; Clavulanate Potassium 125 mg	Augmentin by Southwood Pharms	58016-0106	Antibiotic
E4354	Tab, White, Round, E over 4354	Isoniazid 100 mg	Isoniazid by Eon	00185-4351	Antimycobacterial
E4354	Tab	Isoniazid 100 mg	Isoniazid by Quality Care	60346-0203	Antimycobacterial
E4354	Tab	Isoniazid 100 mg	Isoniazid by Major	00904-2095	Antimycobacterial

ID FRONT <> BACK	DESCRIPTION FRONT <> BACK	INGREDIENT & STRENGTH	BRAND (OR EQUIV.) & FIRM	NDC#	CLASS; SCH.
E471	Tab, Round, Eon Logo	Captopril 50 mg	by Eon	00185-0471	Antihypertensive
E474	Tab	Acetaminophen 500 mg, Hydrocodone Bitartrate 5 mg	by Eon	00185-0474	Analgesic; C III
E475	Tab	Acetaminophen 750 mg, Hydrocodone Bitartrate 7.5 mg	by Eon	00185-0475	Analgesic; C III
E491	Tab, White, Round	Captopril 100 mg	Capoten by Eon		Antihypertensive
E5 <> M	Tab, Blue, Round, Flat, Scored, Uncoated	Estradiol 2 mg	Estradiol by Heartland	61392-0175	Hormone
E5 <> M	Tab, Blue, Round	Estradiol 2 mg	by Mylan Pharms	00378-1458	Hormone
E5000	Cap, Blue & White Pellets	Phentermine HCl 30 mg	by HJ Harkins Co	52959-0440	Anorexiant; C IV
E5000	Cap	Phentermine HCl 30 mg	by Allscripts	54569-3069	Anorexiant; C IV
E5000	Cap	Phentermine HCl 30 mg	by Golden State	60429-0523	Anorexiant; C IV
E5000	Cap, Blue & Clear	Phentermine HCl 30 mg	by Compumed	00403-0874	Anorexiant; C IV
E5000	Cap	Phentermine HCl 30 mg	by Major	00904-0614	Anorexiant; C IV
E5000	Cap	Phentermine HCl 30 mg	by Apotheca	12634-0516	Anorexiant; C IV
E5000	Cap	Phentermine HCl 30 mg	by Zenith Goldline	00182-1026	Anorexiant; C IV
E5000	Cap, Blue & Clear w/ White Beads	Phentermine HCl 30 mg	Fastin by Eon	00185-5000	Anorexiant; C IV
E51	Tab, White, Round	Doxazosin 1 mg	by Eon	00185-0051	Antihypertensive
E511	Tab, White, Round, Scored	Quinidine Sulfate 200 mg	by Murfreesboro Ph	51129-1364	Antiarrhythmic
E511	Tab, Compressed, E/511	Quinidine Sulfate 200 mg	by Kaiser	00179-0639	Antiarrhythmic
E511	Tab, White, Round	Quinidine Sulfate 200 mg	by Eon	00185-4346	Antiarrhythmic
E511	Tab	Quinidine Sulfate 200 mg	by Zenith Goldline	00182-0144	Antiarrhythmic
E511	Tab	Quinidine Sulfate 200 mg	by United Res	00677-0122	Antiarrhythmic
E512	Tab, White, Round	Quinidine Sulfate 300 mg	by Eon	00185-1047	Antiarrhythmic
E512	Tab, Eon Logo	Quinidine Sulfate 300 mg	by Rugby	00536-4429	Antiarrhythmic
E512	Tab, Eon Logo	Quinidine Sulfate 300 mg	by United Res	00677-1209	Antiarrhythmic
E5156	Cap, ER	Papaverine HCl 150 mg	by Zenith Goldline	00182-0181	Vasodilator
E5156	Cap, Brown & Clear	Papaverine HCl 150 mg	Pavabid SR by Eon	00185-5156	Vasodilator
E5156	Cap, ER	Papaverine HCl 150 mg	by Geneva	00781-2000	Vasodilator
E5174	Cap, Amethyst & Clear	Nitroglycerin 2.5 mg	Nitrobid SR by Eon	00185-5174	Vasodilator
E5174	Cap, Lavender, Ex Release	Nitroglycerin 2.5 mg	by Rugby	00536-4083	Vasodilator
E5174	Cap, ER	Nitroglycerin 2.5 mg	by Major	00904-0643	Vasodilator
E5174 <> E5174	Tab, Purple, Oval	Nitroglycerin 2.5 mg	by PDRX	55289-0319	Vasodilator
E52	Tab, Yellow, Round	Doxazosin 2 mg	by Eon	00185-0052	Antihypertensive
E5254	Cap, Brown & Clear	Phendimetrazine Tartrate 105 mg	by Eon	00185-5254	Anorexiant; C III
E530 <> 10	Tab, White, Round	Isoxsuprine HCl 10 mg	Vasodilan by Eon	00185-0530	Vasodilator
E531 <> 20	Tab, White, Round	Isoxsuprine HCl 20 mg	Vasodilan by Eon	00185-0531	Vasodilator
E535	Tab, White, Round	Tolbutamide 500 mg	Orinase by Eon		Antidiabetic
E5380	Cap, Red & Scarlet, Opaque	Ascorbic Acid 75 mg, Cyanocobalamin 15 mcg, Ferrous Fumarate 110 mg, Folic Acid 0.5 mg, Liver With Stomach 240 mg	Foltrin by Eon	00185-5380	Vitamin
E5380	Cap	Ascorbic Acid 75 mg, Cyanocobalamin 15 mcg, Ferrous Fumarate 110 mg, Folic Acid 0.5 mg, Liver With Stomach 240 mg	Contrin by Geneva	00781-2025	Vitamin
E5380	Cap, Maroon & Red	Ascorbic Acid 75 mg, Cyanocobalamin 15 mcg, Ferrous Fumarate 110 mg, Folic Acid 0.5 mg, Liver With Stomach 240 mg	Trinsicon by Geneva	00781-2025	Vitamin
E5385	Cap, Clear & Red	Ferrous Sulfate SR 250 mg	by Eon		Mineral
E551	Tab, Compressed, Eon Logo	Metronidazole 250 mg	by Quality Care	60346-0592	Antibiotic
E555	Tab, Compressed, Eon Logo	Metronidazole 500 mg	by Quality Care	60346-0507	Antibiotic
E58	Tab, Orange, Round	Doxazosin 4 mg	by Eon	00185-0058	Antihypertensive
E59	Tab, Green, Round	Doxazosin 8 mg	by Eon	00185-0059	Antihypertensive
E591	Tab, Round, Eon Logo	Captopril 100 mg	by Eon	00185-0591	Antihypertensive
E60	Tab, Yellow, Oval, Film Coated, Scored	Isosorbide Mononitrate 60 mg	by KV Pharm	10609-1395	Antianginal
E61	Tab, White, Round, Eon Logo	Captopril 25 mg	Captopril by Eon	00185-0061	Antihypertensive
E613	Cap, Green	Hydroxyzine Pamoate 25 mg	by Vangard Labs	00615-0331	Antihistamine
E613	Cap, Dark Green & Light Green	Hydroxyzine Pamoate 25 mg	Vistaril by Eon	00185-0613	Antihistamine
E613	Cap, Green & Light Green	Hydroxyzine Pamoate 25 mg	Vistaril by Geneva	00781-2252	Antihistamine

ID FRONT <> BACK	DESCRIPTION FRONT <> BACK	INGREDIENT & STRENGTH	BRAND (OR EQUIV.) & FIRM	NDC#	CLASS; SCH.
E613	Cap, Dark Green & Light Green	Hydroxyzine Pamoate 43 mg	by Major	00904-0362	Antihistamine
E613	Cap	Hydroxyzine Pamoate 43 mg	by HL Moore	00839-6270	Antihistamine
E613	Cap, URL	Hydroxyzine Pamoate 43 mg	by United Res	00677-0596	Antihistamine
E613	Cap, Dark Green & Light Green	Hydroxyzine Pamoate 85 mg	by Physicians Total Care	54868-1854	Antihistamine
E615	Cap, Clear & Dark Blue	Decyclomine HCl 10 mg	by Chelsea	46193-0105	Gastrointestinal
E615	Cap	Hydroxyzine Pamoate	by Rugby	00536-3894	Antihistamine
E615	Cap, Dark Green	Hydroxyzine Pamoate	by Quality Care	60346-0797	Antihistamine
E615	Cap, Dark Green & White	Hydroxyzine Pamoate 50 mg	Vistaril by Eon	00185-0615	Antihistamine
E615	Cap, Green & White, E 615	Hydroxyzine Pamoate 50 mg	Viataril by Geneva	00781-2254	Antihistamine
E615	Cap	Hydroxyzine Pamoate 85 mg	by Major	00904-0363	Antihistamine
E615	Cap	Hydroxyzine Pamoate 85 mg	by HL Moore	00839-6271	Antihistamine
E615 <> E615	Cap, Dark Blue	Decyclomine HCl 10 mg	by Endo	60951-0615	Gastrointestinal
E615 <> E615	Cap, Dark Green	Hydroxyzine Pamoate 43 mg	by Mova	55370-0877	Antihistamine
E615 <> E615	Cap	Hydroxyzine Pamoate 85 mg	by Mova	55370-0878	Antihistamine
E616	Tab, Blue, Round	Decyclomine HCl 20 mg	by Endo	60951-0616	Gastrointestinal
E616	Tab	Decyclomine HCl 20 mg	by Chelsea	46193-0115	Gastrointestinal
E617	Cap, White	Chlordiazepoxide HCl 5 mg, Clidinium Bromide 2.5 mg	Librax by Eon	00185-0617	Gastrointestinal; C IV
E620	Tab, Coated	Seleginine HCl 5 mg	Carbex by Endo	63481-0408	Antiparkinson
E63	Tab, Yellow, Round, Convex, Scored, E Over 63	Clonazepam 0.5 mg	by Danbury	61955-2631	Anticonvulsant; C IV
E63	Tab, Yellow, Round, Convex, Scored, E Over 63	Clonazepam 0.5 mg	by Danbury	61955-8856	Anticonvulsant; C IV
E63	Tab, Yellow, Round, Scored	Clonazepam 0.5 mg	by Southwood Pharms	58016-0183	Anticonvulsant; C IV
E63	Tab, Light Yellow, Round, E over 63	Clonazepam 0.5 mg	Klonopin by Eon	00185-0063	Anticonvulsant; C IV
E63	Tab, Yellow, Round, Scored, E over 63	Clonazepam 0.5 mg	by DHHS Prog	11819-0088	Anticonvulsant; C IV
E64	Tab, Light Blue, Round, E over 64	Clonazepam 1 mg	Klonopin by Eon	00185-0064	Anticonvulsant; C IV
E64	Tab, Blue, Round, Scored, E over 64	Clonazepam 1 mg	by DHHS Prog	11819-0015	Anticonvulsant; C IV
E64	Tab, Blue, Round, Convex, Scored, E Over 64	Clonazepam 1 mg	by Danbury	61955-2630	Anticonvulsant; C IV
E64	Tab, Blue, Round, Scored	Clonazepam 1 mg	by Compumed	00403-2660	Anticonvulsant; C IV
E640	Cap, Black	Phentermine HCl 30 mg	by Eon	00185-0640	Anorexiant; C IV
E640	Cap, Black	Phentermine HCl 37.5 mg	by Compumed	00403-0468	Anorexiant; C IV
E644	Cap, Gray & Yellow	Phentermine HCl 15 mg	Ionamin by Eon		Anorexiant; C IV
E647	Cap	Phentermine HCl 30 mg	by Allscripts	54569-0392	Anorexiant; C IV
E647	Cap, E over 647	Phentermine HCl 30 mg	by Quality Care	60346-0763	Anorexiant; C IV
E647	Cap	Phentermine HCl 30 mg	by Major	00904-3921	Anorexiant; C IV
E647	Cap, Yellow	Phentermine HCl 30 mg	by Compumed	00403-5074	Anorexiant; C IV
E647	Cap, Yellow	Phentermine HCl 30 mg	by HJ Harkins	52959-0432	Anorexiant; C IV
E647	Cap, Yellow	Phentermine HCl 30 mg	by Eon	00185-0647	Anorexiant; C IV
E648	Cap, E Over 648	Diphenhydramine HCl 25 mg	by Quality Care	60346-0589	Antihistamine
E648	Cap, Clear & Pink	Diphenhydramine HCl 25 mg	by Eon	00185-0648	Antihistamine
E649	Cap, Pink	Diphenhydramine HCl 50 mg	Benadryl by Eon	00185-0649	Antihistamine
E65	Tab, White, Round, E over 65	Clonazepam 2 mg	Klonopin by Eon	00185-0065	Anticonvulsant; C IV
E652 <> 15	Tab, Blue, Round	Morphine Sulfate 15 mg	Morphine Sulfate by Novartis	00043-0149	Analgesic; C II
E652 <> 15	Tab, Blue, Round	Morphine Sulfate 15 mg	Morphine Sulfate ER by Novartis	00067-0143	Analgesic; C II
E652 <> 15	Tab, Blue, Round	Morphine Sulfate 15 mg	by Endo Labs	60951-0652	Analgesic; C II
E652 <> 15	Tab, Blue, Round	Morphine Sulfate 15 mg	by Dupont Pharma	00056-0652	Analgesic; C II
E653 <> 30	Tab, Green, Round	Morphine Sulfate 30 mg	Morphine Sulfate ER by Novartis	00067-0148	Analgesic; C II
E653 <> 30	Tab, Green, Round	Morphine Sulfate 30 mg	Morphine Sulfate ER by Novartis	00067-0140	Analgesic; C II
E653 <> 30	Tab, Green, Round	Morphine Sulfate 30 mg	by Dupont Pharma	00056-0653	Analgesic; C II
E653 <> 30	Tab, Green, Round	Morphine Sulfate 30 mg	by Endo Labs	60951-0653	Analgesic; C II
E654	Tab, White to Off-White w/ Blue Speckles, Cap Shaped	Phentermine HCl 30 mg	by Eon	00185-0654	Anorexiant; C IV
E655 <> 60	Tab, Orange, Round	Morphine Sulfate 60 mg	by Endo Pharms	60951-0655	Analgesic; C II
E655 <> 60	Tab, Orange, Oblong	Morphine Sulfate 60 mg	by Dupont Pharma	00056-0655	Analgesic; C II
E660	Cap, Orange	Acetaminophen 500 mg; Oxycodone 5 mg	by Dupont Pharma	00056-0660	Analgesic; C II

ID FRONT <> BACK	DESCRIPTION FRONT <> BACK	INGREDIENT & STRENGTH	BRAND (OR EQUIV.) & FIRM	NDC#	CLASS; SCH.
E660 <> E660	Cap, Orangish Red	Acetaminophen 500 mg; Oxycodone 5 mg	by Endo Pharms	60951-0660	Analgesic; C II
E670	Cap, Orange & Yellow	Tetracycline HCl 250 mg	Sumycin by Eon		Antibiotic
E675 <> E675	Cap, Blue & Yellow	Aspirin 325 mg, Butalbital 50 mg, Caffeine 40 mg, Codeine Phosphate 30 mg	by Endo Labs	60951-0675	Analgesic; C III
E675 <> E675	Tab, Blue & Yellow, Oblong, Red Axial Print	Aspirin 325 mg, Butalital 50 mg, Caffeine 40 mg, Codeine Phosphate 30 mg	by Caremark	00339-5299	Analgesic; C III
E693	Tab, Coated	Salsalate 500 mg	by Major	00904-5072	NSAID
E694	Tab, Coated	Salsalate 750 mg	by Major	00904-5073	NSAID
E7	Tab, Tan, Oblong	Chlorpheniramine 8 mg, Phenylephrine 25 mg, Pyrilamine 25 mg	Rynatann by Eon		Cold Remedy
E7	Tab, White, Round, Scored	Estradiol 1 mg	by Ayerst Lab (Div Wyeth)	00046-5880	Hormone
E7 <> 511	Tab, White, Round	Estradiol 1 mg	by ESI Lederle	59911-5880	Hormone
E701	Tab, Orange, Round	Bisoprolol Fumarate 2.5 mg, Hydrochlorothiazide 6.25 mg	by Eon	00185-0701	Antihypertensive; Diuretic
E704	Tab, Red, Round	Bisoprolol Fumarate 5 mg, Hydrochlorothiazide 6.25 mg	by Eon	00185-0704	Antihypertensive; Diuretic
E707	Tab, White, Round	Bisoprolol Fumarate 10 mg, Hydrochlorothiazide 6.25 mg	by Eon	00185-0707	Antihypertensive; Diuretic
E713	Tab, Green & White, Round, Eon Logo	Aspirin 385 mg, Caffeine 30 mg, Orphenadrine Citrate 25 mg	Norgesic by Eon	00185-0713	Analgesic; Muscle Relaxant
E713	Tab, Eon Logo 713	Aspirin 385 mg, Caffeine 30 mg, Orphenadrine Citrate 25 mg	by Major	00904-5238	Analgesic; Muscle Relaxant
E714	Tab, Green & White, Cap Shaped, Eon Logo	Aspirin 770 mg, Caffeine 60 mg, Orphenadrine Citrate 50 mg	Norgesic Forteby Eon	00185-0714	Analgesic
E716	Tab, White, Round, Eon Logo-716	Meprobamate 200 mg	Miltown by Eon	00185-0716	Sedative/Hypnotic; C IV
E716	Tab	Meprobamate 200 mg	by Major	00904-0044	Sedative/Hypnotic; C IV
E716	Tab, Eon Logo-716	Meprobamate 200 mg	by United Res	00677-0232	Sedative/Hypnotic; C IV
E717	Tab	Meprobamate 200 mg	by Darby Group	66467-4006	Sedative/Hypnotic; C IV
E717	Tab, White, Round	Meprobamate 400 mg	Miltown by Eon	00185-0717	Sedative/Hypnotic; C IV
E717	Tab	Meprobamate 400 mg	by Zenith Goldline	00182-0294	Sedative/Hypnotic; C IV
E717	Tab	Meprobamate 400 mg	by United Res	00677-0233	Sedative/Hypnotic; C IV
E720	Cap, Clear & Green	Indomethacin 75 mg	Indocin SR by Eon	00185-0720	NSAID
E720 <> E720	Cap, Clear & Green	Indomethacin 75 mg	by Endo Pharms	60951-0738	NSAID
E721	Tab, Blue, Round, Coated, E over 721	Desipramine HCl 50 mg	Norpramin by Eon	00185-0721	Antidepressant
E721	Tab, Coated	Desipramine HCl 50 mg	by Major	00904-1571	Antidepressant
E721	Tab, Blue, Round, Film Coated, E over 721	Desipramine HCL 50 mg	Norpramin by UDL	51079-0490	Antidepressant
E722	Tab, Light Blue, Round, Film Coated, E over 722	Desipramine HCl 75 mg	Norpramin by UDL	51079-0491	Antidepressant
E722	Tab, Light Blue, Round, Coated	Desipramine HCl 75 mg	Norpramin by Eon	00185-0722	Antidepressant
E722	Tab, Coated	Desipramine HCl 75 mg	by Major	00904-1572	Antidepressant
E724	Tab, Eon Logo 724	Aspirin 325 mg, Carisoprodol 200 mg	by Zenith Goldline	00182-1821	Analgesic; Muscle Relaxant
E724	Tab, Lavender & White	Aspirin 325 mg, Carisoprodol 200 mg	by Rugby	00536-3429	Analgesic; Muscle Relaxant
E724	Tab, Lavender & White, Round, Eon Logo	Aspirin 325 mg, Carisoprodol 200 mg	Soma Compound by Eon	00185-0724	Analgesic; Muscle Relaxant
E724	Tab, Lavender & White	Aspirin 325 mg, Carisoprodol 200 mg	by United Res	00677-1068	Analgesic; Muscle Relaxant
E724	Tab	Aspirin 325 mg, Carisoprodol 200 mg	by Major	00904-0356	Analgesic; Muscle Relaxant
E736	Tab, Coated	Desipramine HCl 100 mg	by Zenith Goldline	00182-1316	Antidepressant
E736	Tab, Blue, Round, Coated	Desipramine HCl 100 mg	Norpramin by Eon	00185-0736	Antidepressant
E736	Tab, Coated	Desipramine HCl 100 mg	by Major	00904-1573	Antidepressant
E745	Tab, Eon Logo	Guaifenesin 400 mg, Phenylpropanolamine HCl 75 mg	by Golden State	60429-0233	Cold Remedy
E745	Tab, Light Blue, Ex Release, EON Labs Logo 745	Guaifenesin 400 mg, Phenylpropanolamine HCl 75 mg	Enomine LA by Quality Care	60346-0339	Cold Remedy
E745	Tab, Light Blue, E/745	Guaifenesin 400 mg, Phenylpropanolamine HCl 75 mg	Guaifen PPA by Kaiser	00179-1137	Cold Remedy
E745	Tab, Light Blue, E/745	Guaifenesin 400 mg, Phenylpropanolamine HCl 75 mg	by UDL	51079-0859	Cold Remedy

ID FRONT <> BACK	DESCRIPTION FRONT <> BACK	INGREDIENT & STRENGTH	BRAND (OR EQUIV.) & FIRM	NDC#	CLASS; SCH.
E745	Tab	Guaifenesin 400 mg, Phenylpropanolamine HCl 75 mg	by Med Pro	53978-5012	Cold Remedy
E745	Tab, Blue, Round, Scored	Guaifenesin 400 mg; Phenylpropanolamine HCl 75 mg	Santex LA by C J Sant Pharm	60527-0745	Cold Remedy
E745	Tab, Light Blue, Oval	Phenylpropanolamine HCl 75 mg, Guaifenesin 400 mg	Guaipax SR by Eon	00185-0745	Cold Remedy
E749	Tab	Aspirin 325 mg, Carisoprodol 200 mg, Codeine Phosphate 16 mg	by Rugby	00536-5753	Analgesic; C III
E749	Tab, White & Yellow, Round, Eon Logo	Aspirin 325 mg, Carisoprodol 200 mg, Codeine Phosphate 16 mg	Soma Comp. With Cod. by Eon	00185-0749	Analgesic; C III
E749	Tab	Aspirin 325 mg, Carisoprodol 200 mg, Codeine Phosphate 16 mg	by Qualitest	00603-2584	Analgesic; C III
E749	Tab, White & Yellow, Round	Carisoprodol 200 mg; Aspirin 325 mg; Codeine Phosphate 16 mg	by DRX Pharm Consults	55045-2779	Analgesic; C III
E75	Tab, Oblong, Scored	Phendimetrazine Tartrate 35 mg	by PDRX Pharms	55289-0295	Anorexiant; C III
E75	Tab, Pink, Oblong	Phendimetrazine Tartrate 35 mg	by Southwood Pharms	58016-0854	Anorexiant; C III
E75	Tab, Blue, Pink & White, Cap Shaped	Phendimetrazine Tartrate 35 mg	by Eon	00185-4055	Anorexiant; C III
E750	Tab, Brown, Round	Nystatin 500,000 Units	Mycostatin by Eon		Antifungal
E750	Tab, Brown, Round	Nystatin 500,000 units	Mycostatin by Eon		Antifungal
E757	Tab, White, Oblong	Sulfadiazine 500 mg	by Solvay	00032-1103	Antibiotic
E757	Tab, White, Cap Shaped	Sulfadiazine 500 mg	Microsulfon by Eon	00185-0757	Antibiotic
E757	Tab	Sulfadiazine 500 mg	by UDL	51079-0840	Antibiotic
E757	Tab, White, Oblong	Sulfadiazine 500 mg	by Sovereign	58716-0057	Antibiotic
E76	Tab, Yellow, Round, Scored	Phendimetrazine Tartrate 35 mg	by Allscripts	54569-4336	Anorexiant; C III
E76	Tab, Light Yellow, Round	Phendimetrazine Tartrate 35 mg	by Eon	00185-4057	Anorexiant; C III
E76	Tab, Yellow, Round, Scored	Phendimetrazine Tartrate 35 mg	by Physicians Total Care	54868-2277	Anorexiant; C III
E76	Tab, Eon Logo 76	Phendimetrazine Tartrate 35 mg	by Quality Care	62682-7035	Anorexiant; C III
E76	Tab, E over 76	Phendimetrazine Tartrate 35 mg	by Quality Care	60346-0562	Anorexiant; C III
E76	Tab	Phendimetrazine Tartrate 35 mg	by HL Moore	00839-5108	Anorexiant; C III
E760	Tab, Coated, Eon Logo	Desipramine HCl 150 mg	by Zenith Goldline	00182-2653	Antidepressant
E760	Tab, White, Round, Coated, Eon Logo	Desipramine HCl 150 mg	Norpramin by Eon	00185-0760	Antidepressant
E760	Tab, Coated	Desipramine HCl 150 mg	by Major	00904-5190	Antidepressant
E761	Tab, Yellow, Oblong	Salsalate 500 mg	Disalcid by Eon		NSAID
E762	Tab, Yellow, Oblong	Salsalate 750 mg	Disalcid by Eon		NSAID
E77	Tab, Pink, Cap Shaped	Phendimetrazine Tartrate 35 mg	by Eon	00185-4093	Anorexiant; C III
E77 <> 511	Tab, White, Round	Estradiol 2 mg	by ESI Lederle	59911-5882	Hormone
E77 <> 511	Tab, White, Round, Scored	Estradiol 2 mg	by Ayerst Lab (Div Wyeth)	00046-5882	Hormone
E77 <> 511	Tab, White, Round	Estrogen	Etradiol Tab by Ayerst Lab		Hormone
E771	Tab, Pink, Round	Bisoprolol Fumarate 5 mg	by Eon	00185-0771	Antihypertensive
E771	Tab	Meprobamate 400 mg	by Major	00904-0045	Sedative/Hypnotic; C IV
E771	Tab	Meprobamate 400 mg	by Qualitest	00603-4440	Sedative/Hypnotic; C IV
E771	Tab	Meprobamate 400 mg	by HL Moore	00839-5004	Sedative/Hypnotic; C IV
E774	Tab, White, Round	Bisoprolol Fumarate 10 mg	by Eon	00185-0774	Antihypertensive
E784	Tab, Ex Release, Eon Logo 784	Guaifenesin 600 mg, Pseudoephedrine HCl 120 mg	Enomine PSE by Quality Care	60346-0933	Cold Remedy
E784	Tab, White, Oval	Guaifenesin 600 mg, Pseudoephedrine HCl 120 mg	Guaipax PSE by Eon	00185-0784	Cold Remedy
E799	Cap, Red	Rifampin 300 mg	by RX PAK	65084-0185	Antibiotic
E799	Cap, Red	Rifampin 300 mg	Rimactane by Eon	00185-0799	Antibiotic
E799	Cap, Red	Rifampin 300 mg	Rifadin by UDL	51079-0890	Antibiotic
E799 <> E799	Cap, Red	Rifampin 300 mg	by Murfreesboro Ph	51129-1402	Antibiotic
E801	Cap, Orange	Rifampin 150 mg	Rimactane by Eon	00185-0801	Antibiotic
E805	Cap, Yellow	Doxycycline 50 mg	by Eon	00185-0805	Antibiotic
E810	Cap, Brown	Doxycycline 100 mg	by Eon	00185-0810	Antibiotic
E839	Cap, Red, E-839	Docusate Sodium 100 mg, Casanthranol 30 mg	Peri-Colace by Chase		Laxative
E856	Tab, Blue, Oblong	Salsalate 500 mg	Disalcid by Eon		NSAID
E857	Tab, Blue, Oblong	Salsalate 750 mg	Disalcid by Eon		NSAID
E882	Cap, Gray & Yellow	Phentermine 15 mg	by Physicians Total Care	54868-4048	Anorexiant; C IV
E882	Cap, Gray & Yellow, Scored	Phentermine HCl 15 mg	by HJ Harkins	52959-0426	Anorexiant; C IV
E882	Cap, Gray & Yellow	Phentermine HCl 15 mg	by Eon	00185-0644	Anorexiant; C IV
E882	Cap, Gray & Yellow	Phentermine HCl 15 mg	by Physicians Total Care	54868-4073	Anorexiant; C IV

ID FRONT <> BACK	DESCRIPTION FRONT <> BACK	INGREDIENT & STRENGTH	BRAND (OR EQUIV.) & FIRM	NDC#	CLASS; SCH.
E882	Cap	Phentermine HCl 15 mg	by Allscripts	54569-4143	Anorexiant; C IV
E882	Cap, Eon Logo	Phentermine HCl 15 mg	by Physicians Total Care	54868-0283	Anorexiant; C IV
E882	Cap, Eon Logo 882	Phentermine HCl 15 mg	by Quality Care	60346-0133	Anorexiant; C IV
E882	Cap	Phentermine HCl 15 mg	by PDRX	55289-0791	Anorexiant; C IV
E882	Cap, Gray & Yellow	Phentermine HCl 18.75 mg	by Physicians Total Care	54868-4092	Anorexiant; C IV
E932	Cap, Clear, Oblong, Gelatin w/ Yellowish Oily Liquid	Cyclosporine 25 mg	by Eon	00185-0932	Immunosuppressant
E933	Cap, Clear, Oblong, Gelatin w/ Yellowish Oily Liquid	Cyclosporine 100 mg	by Eon	00185-0933	Immunosuppressant
E968	Cap, Light Green	Chlordiazepoxide HCl 5 mg, Clidinium Bromide 2.5 mg	by Eon	00185-0968	Gastrointestinal; C IV
E968 <> E968	Cap, Light Green, Black Print	Chlordiazepoxide HCl 5 mg, Clidinium Bromide 2.5 mg	by Kaiser	00179-0170	Gastrointestinal; C IV
E988	Tab, White, Round	Quinine Sulfate 260 mg	Quinamm by Eon		Antimalarial
E998	Tab, White, Round	Yohimbine HCl 5.4 mg	Yocon by Eon	00185-0998	Impotence Agent
EA	Tab, Film Coated, Logo	Erythromycin 500 mg	by Quality Care	60346-0077	Antibiotic
EA	Tab, Pink, Cap Shaped, EA <> Abbott Logo	Erythromycin 500 mg	Erythromycin Base by Abbott	00074-6227	Antibiotic
EA	Tab, Film Coated, Abbott Logo	Erythromycin 500 mg	by Allscripts	54569-2502	Antibiotic
EA	Tab, Film Coated, Abbott Logo	Erythromycin 500 mg	by Apotheca	12634-0507	Antibiotic
EA	Tab, Pink, Oval, Film, Abbott Logo	ErythroMycin 500 mg	by Halsey Drug	00904-5392	Antibiotic
EATON036	Tab, Yellow, Round	Nitrofurantoin 50 mg	Furadantin by Norwich		Antibiotic
EATON037	Tab, Yellow, Round	Nitrofurantoin 100 mg	Furadantin by Norwich		Antibiotic
EATON072	Tab, Brown, Round	Furazolidone 100 mg	Furoxone by Norwich		Antibiotic
EB	Tab, Coated, Logo	Erythromycin 250 mg	by Quality Care	60346-0037	Antibiotic
EB	Tab, Pink, Cap Shaped, Film Coated, EB over Abbott Logo	Erythromycin 250 mg	Erythromycin Base by Abbott	00074-6326	Antibiotic
EB <> A	Tab, Film Coated, Abbott Logo	Erythromycin Stearate	by Apotheca	12634-0163	Antibiotic
EBASE333MG <> BARR	Tab, E-Base 333 mg <> Barr	Erythromycin 333 mg	E Base by Barr	00555-0532	Antibiotic
EBASE333MG <> BARR	Tab, E-Base 333 mg <> Barr	Erythromycin 333 mg	E Base by Barr	00555-0495	Antibiotic
EBASE500MG <> BARR	Tab, E-Base 500 mg <> Barr	Erythromycin 500 mg	E Base by Barr	00555-0533	Antibiotic
EC	Tab, Abbott Logo	Erythromycin 250 mg	Ery Tab by Nat Pharmpak Serv	55154-0107	Antibiotic
EC	Tab, Delayed Release, Logo	Erythromycin 250 mg	Ery-Tab by Quality Care	60346-0108	Antibiotic
EC	Tab, Delayed Release, Abbott Labs Symbol	Erythromycin 250 mg	Ery Tab by Amerisource	62584-0372	Antibiotic
EC	Tab, Black Print, Abbott Logo	Erythromycin 250 mg	by Kaiser	00179-1055	Antibiotic
EC	Tab, Abbott Logo	Erythromycin 250 mg	Ery Tab by Allscripts	54569-3563	Antibiotic
EC	Tab, Abbott Logo	Erythromycin 250 mg	Ery Tab by Pharmedix	53002-0203	Antibiotic
EC	Tab, White, Oval, Enteric Coated, EC <> Abbott Logo	Erythromycin Delayed Release 250 mg	Ery-Tab by Abbott	00074-6304	Antibiotic
ECNAPROSYN	Tab, DR, Syntex	Naproxen 500 mg	EC Naprosyn by PDRX	55289-0693	NSAID
ECNAPROSYN <> 375	Tab, DR	Naproxen 375 mg	Naprosyn by Syntex	18393-0255	NSAID
ECNAPROSYN <> 375	Tab, DR	Naproxen 375 mg	E C Naprosyn by PDRX	55289-0267	NSAID
ECNAPROSYN <> 375	Tab, DR	Naproxen 375 mg	EC Naprosyn by Allscripts	54569-3981	NSAID
ECNAPROSYN <> 375	Tab, DR, Syntex	Naproxen 375 mg	EC Naprosyn by DRX	55045-2425	NSAID
ECNAPROSYN <> 375	Tab, White, Oblong	Naxproxen 375 mg	EC Naprosyn Delayed Release by Par	49884-0567	NSAID
ECNAPROSYN <> 500	Tab, DR	Naproxen 500 mg	EC Naprosyn by Allscripts	54569-3982	NSAID
ECNAPROSYN <> 500	Tab, DR	Naproxen 500 mg	Naprosyn EC by HJ Harkins Co	52959-0456	NSAID
ECNAPROSYN <> 500	Tab, DR	Naproxen 500 mg	EC Naprosyn by DRX	55045-2441	NSAID
ECNAPROSYN <> 500	Tab, DR	Naproxen 500 mg	EC Naprosyn by Quality Care	60346-0334	NSAID
ECNAPROSYN <> 500	Tab, White, Oblong	Naproxen 500 mg	Naprosyn EC by Compumed	00403-0717	NSAID
ECNAPROSYN <> 500	Tab, DR	Naproxen 500 mg	Naprosyn by Syntex	18393-0256	NSAID
ECNAPROSYN <> 500	Tab, White, Oblong	Naxproxen 500 mg	EC Naprosyn Delayed Release by Par	49884-0568	NSAID
ECR0141	Tab, ECR/0141	Acetaminophen 500 mg, Hydrocodone Bitartrate 5 mg	Panacet 5 500 by		Analgesic; C III
ECR25	Tab, White, Cap Shaped, Scored, ECR 2.5	Hydrocodone 2.5 mg, Guaifenesin 300 mg	Pneumotussin by ECR	00095-0066	Analgesic; C III; Expectorant
ECR600	Tab, Ex Release, ECR/600	Guaifenesin 600 mg	Pneumomist by Sovereign	58716-0603	Expectorant
ECR6006	Cap, Clear	Pseudoephedrine 60 mg, Brompheniarmine 6 mg	Lodrane LD by ECR	00095-6006	Cold Remedy
ECR6006 <> ECR6006	Cap, Ex Release, ECR Over 6006	Brompheniramine Maleate 6 mg, Pseudoephedrine HCl 60 mg	Lodrane LD by Sovereign	58716-0027	Cold Remedy
ED	Tab, Light Brown, E/D	Chlorpheniramine Maleate 8 mg, Phenylephrine HCl 20 mg	Ed A Hist by Anabolic	00722-6287	Cold Remedy

ID FRONT <> BACK	DESCRIPTION FRONT <> BACK	INGREDIENT & STRENGTH	BRAND (OR EQUIV.) & FIRM	NDC#	CLASS; SCH.
ED	Tab, Delayed Release, Logo	Erythromycin 500 mg	Ery-Tab by Quality Care	60346-0644	Antibiotic
ED	Tab, Abbott Logo	Erythromycin 500 mg	by Kaiser	00179-1056	Antibiotic
ED	Tab, Abbott Logo	Erythromycin 500 mg	Ery Tab by Pharmedix	53002-0205	Antibiotic
ED	Tab, Abbott Logo	Erythromycin 500 mg	Ery Tab by Allscripts	54569-2508	Antibiotic
ED	Tab, White, Oval, Enteric Coated, ED <> Abbott Logo	Erythromycin Delayed Release 500 mg	Ery-Tab by Abbott	00074-6321	Antibiotic
EDEPRYL5MG	Cap, Blue, Somer Logo/ Edepryl 5 mg	Selegiline HCl 5 mg	by Somerset		Antiparkinson
EDFLEX	Cap, ED-Flex	Acetaminophen 300 mg, Phenyltoloxamine Citrate 20 mg, Salicylamide 200 mg	Ed Flex by Edwards	00485-0066	Analgesic
EDFLEX	Cap, ED-Flex	Acetaminophen 300 mg, Phenyltoloxamine Citrate 20 mg, Salicylamide 200 mg	Ed Flex by Seatrace	00551-0066	Analgesic
EE	Tab, Coated, Abbott Logo	Erythromycin Ethylsuccinate	EES Tablets by Nat Pharmpak Serv	55154-0101	Antibiotic
EE	Tab, Coated, Logo Over EE	Erythromycin Ethylsuccinate	EES Tablets by Quality Care	60346-0617	Antibiotic
EE	Tab, Coated, Abbott Logo	Erythromycin Ethylsuccinate	by Kaiser	00179-1014	Antibiotic
EE	Tab, Cotaed, Abbott Logo	Erythromycin Ethylsuccinate	E E S by Pharmedix	53002-0295	Antibiotic
EE	Tab, Pink, Oval	Erythromycin Ethylsuccinate 400 mg	EES 400 by Murfreesboro Ph	51129-1421	Antibiotic
EE	Tab, Pink	Erythromycin Ethylsuccinate 400 mg	EES by Rightpak	65240-0636	Antibiotic
EE	Tab, Pink, Oval, Film Coated, EE over Abbott Logo	Erythromycin Ethylsuccinate 400 mg	EES 400 by Abbott	00074-5729	Antibiotic
EF	Tab, White, Round, Abbott Logo	Erythromycin Ethylsuccinate 200 mg	EES Chewable by Abbott		Antibiotic
EFF <> 20	Tab, White, Round, Debossed	Methazolamide 50 mg	by Duramed	51285-0969	Diuretic
EFF <> 20	Tab, White, Round, Scored	Methazolamide 50 mg	Neptazane by Lederle Labs	55806-0020	Diuretic
EFF <> 20	Tab	Methazolamide 50 mg	by Mikart	46672-0109	Diuretic
EFF <> 21	Tab, White, Round, Debossed	Methazolamide 25 mg	by Duramed	51285-0968	Diuretic
EFF <> 21	Tab, White, Round	Methazolamide 25 mg	Neptazane by Lederle Labs	55806-0021	Diuretic
EFF20	Tab	Methazolamide 50 mg	by Zenith Goldline	00182-1076	Diuretic
EFF20	Tab, Mikart	Methazolamide 50 mg	by Rugby	00536-5616	Diuretic
EFF21	Tab	Methazolamide 25 mg	by Zenith Goldline	00182-1075	Diuretic
EGIS111 <> PIROXICAM	Cap, Blue & Red	Piroxicam 10 mg	Piroxicam USP by Prestige	58056-0344	NSAID
EGIS111 <> PIROXICAM10MG	Cap, Blue & Red	Piroxicam 10 mg	by Prestige	58056-0347	NSAID
EGIS112 <> PIROXICAM20MG	Cap, Red	Piroxicam 20 mg	Piroxicam USP by Prestige	58056-0345	NSAID
EGIS112 <> PIROXICAM20MG	Cap, Red	Piroxicam 20 mg	by Promeco SA	64674-0006	NSAID
EH	Tab, Delayed Release, Logo	Erythromycin 333 mg	by Quality Care	60346-0098	Antibiotic
EH	Tab	Erythromycin 333 mg	Ery Tab by Med Pro	53978-0089	Antibiotic
EH	Tab, Abbott Logo	Erythromycin 333 mg	Ery Tab by Pharmedix	53002-0204	Antibiotic
EH	Tab, Abbott Logo	Erythromycin 333 mg	Ery Tab by Allscripts	54569-2199	Antibiotic
EH	Tab, White, Oval, Enteric Coated, EH <> Abbott Logo	Erythromycin Delayed Release 333 mg	Ery-Tab by Abbott	00074-6320	Antibiotic
EI <> KTAB	Tab, K-Tab, Film Coated	Potassium Chloride 750 mg	K Tab ER by Heartland	61392-0900	Electrolytes
EK	Tab, White, Oval, EK over Abbott Logo	Erythromycin 500 mg	PCE by Abbott	00074-3389	Antibiotic
EK <> A	Tab, Delayed Release, Abbott Symbol	Erythromycin 500 mg	PCE by Quality Care	60346-0445	Antibiotic
EK25	Tab, Lime	Potassium 977.5 mg (25 mEq)	Effer-K by Nomax	51801-0002	Electrolytes
EK25	Tab, Orange	Potassium 977.5 mg (25 mEq)	Effer-K by Nomax	51801-0001	Electrolytes
EL <> 130	Tab	Hyoscyamine Sulfate 0.125 mg	by Anabolic	00722-6294	Gastrointestinal
EL <> 740	Cap, Ex Release	Chlorpheniramine Maleate 8 mg, Pseudoephedrine HCl 120 mg	Colfed A by Pharmafab	62542-0253	Cold Remedy
EL <> 740	Cap	Chlorpheniramine Maleate 8 mg, Pseudoephedrine HCl 120 mg	N D Clear by Seatrace	00551-0147	Cold Remedy
EL <> 860	Cap	Guaifenesin 250 mg, Pseudoephedrine HCl 120 mg	Guaibid D by Econolab	55053-0860	Cold Remedy
EL <> 860	Cap	Guaifenesin 250 mg, Pseudoephedrine HCl 120 mg	by United Res	00677-1503	Cold Remedy
EL <> 870	Cap, Ex Release	Guaifenesin 300 mg, Pseudoephedrine HCl 60 mg	Guaibid D Ped by Pharmafab	62542-0401	Cold Remedy
EL040	Tab	Guaifenesin 600 mg	by Zenith Goldline	00182-1188	Expectorant
EL040	Tab, Light Green, Ex Release, EL/040	Guaifenesin 600 mg	Mucobid LA by Theraids	59037-6159	Expectorant
EL040	Tab, Light Green, Delayed Release, EL 040	Guaifenesin 600 mg	by Quality Care	60346-0863	Expectorant
EL069	Tab, Blue, Round	Rauwolfia Serpentina 50 mg, Bendroflumethiazide 4 mg	Rauzide by Econolab		Antihypertensive

ID FRONT <> BACK	DESCRIPTION FRONT <> BACK	INGREDIENT & STRENGTH	BRAND (OR EQUIV.) & FIRM	NDC#	CLASS; SCH.
EL073	Tab, Green, Oval	Phenyleph 25 mg, Phenylpro 50 mg, Chlorphen 8 mg, Hyosc 0.19 mg, Atro 0.04 mg, Scop 0.01 mg	Ru-tuss by Econolab		Cold Remedy
EL077	Tab, Violet, Oval	Carbinoxamine Maleate 8 mg, Pseudoephedrine 120 mg	Rondec TR by Economed		Cold Remedy
EL082	Tab, White, Oval	Carbinoxamine Maleate 4 mg, Pseudoephedrine 60 mg	Rondec by Economed		Cold Remedy
EL090	Tab, Green	Guaifenesin 600 mg, Dextromethorphan Hydrobromide 60 mg	by Econolab		Cold Remedy
EL111	Tab, Blue, Round	Hyoscyamine 0.15 mg	Cystospaz by Econolab		Gastrointestinal
EL122	Tab, Pink, Oval	Carbetapentane 60 mg, Chlorpheniramine 5 mg, Ephedrine 10 mg, PhenEph. 10 mg	Rynatuss by Econolab		Cold Remedy
EL124	Tab	Belladonna Alkaloids 0.2 mg, Ergotamine Tartrate 0.6 mg, Phenobarbital 40 mg	Bellamine by Quality Care	60346-0639	Gastrointestinal; C IV
EL124	Tab, Blue	Belladonna Alkaloids 0.2 mg, Ergotamine Tartrate 0.6 mg, Phenobarbital 40 mg	Spastrin by Anabolic	00722-6307	Gastrointestinal; C IV
EL124	Tab, Blue, Round, Cross Scored	Phenobarbital 40 mg, Ergotamine Tartrate 0.6 mg, Belladonna Alkaloids 0.2 mg	Bel Tabs by United Res	00677-1660	Antimigraine; C IV
EL125	Cap, Blue & Clear	Bromopheniramine Maleate 6 mg, Pseudoephedrine 60 mg	Bromfed PD by Econolab		Cold Remedy
EL140	Tab, Blue	Guaifenesin 600 mg, Pseudoephedrine 60 mg	Deconsal II by Econolab		Cold Remedy
EL158	Tab, Beige, OTC, EL 158	Polycarbophil 625 mg	Fibercon by Breckenridge	51991-0007	Gastrointestinal
EL175	Tab, Pink, Round	Meprobamate 400 mg, Benactyzine HCl 1 mg	Deprol by Econolab		Sedative/Hypnotic; C IV
EL191	Tab, Beige, Oval	Phenylephrine 25 mg, Chlorpheniramine 8 mg, Pyrilamine 25 mg	Rynatan by Econolab		Cold Remedy
EL222 <> EL222	Cap, Ex Release, EL-222	Brompheniramine Maleate 6 mg, Pseudoephedrine HCl 60 mg	Nalfed PD by Sovereign	58716-0031	Cold Remedy
EL270	Tab, Pink, Round	Guaifenesin 200 mg	Organidin NR by Econolab		Expectorant
EL310	Cap, ER, EL-310	Hyoscyamine Sulfate 0.375 mg	by Major	00904-7833	Gastrointestinal
EL310	Cap, ER, EL-310	Hyoscyamine Sulfate 0.375 mg	by Pharmafab	62542-0310	Gastrointestinal
EL320	Tab, EL/320	Amylase 30000 Units, Lipase 8000 Units, Protease 30000 Units	Pancrelipase by Anabolic	00722-6089	Gastrointestinal
EL320	Tab, Cream, Round, Scored	Lipase 8000 Unt, Protease 30000 Unt, Amylase 30000 Unt	Pancrelipase by Murfreesboro Ph	51129-1428	Gastrointestinal
EL320	Tab, Off-White, Round, EL 320	Lipase 8000, Amylase 30000, Protease 30000	Viokase by Breckenridge	51991-0520	Gastrointestinal
EL323	Cap, Clear & White	Lipase, Amylase, Protease	Pancrease by Econolab		Gastrointestinal
EL323	Cap	Pancreatic Enzyme	Pancrease by Anabolic		Gastrointestinal
EL410	Tab, Orange, Oblong, Scored	Hyoscyamine Sulfate 0.375 mg	by Murfreesboro	51129-1488	Gastrointestinal
EL410	Tab, ER	Hyoscyamine Sulfate 0.375 mg	by Pegasus	55246-0970	Gastrointestinal
EL410	Tab, ER	Hyoscyamine Sulfate 0.375 mg	by Econolab	55053-0410	Gastrointestinal
EL44	Cap	Trimethobenzamide HCl 250 mg	by Zenith Goldline	00182-1396	Antiemetic
EL444	Cap, Anabolic	Trimethobenzamide HCl 250 mg	by Rugby	00536-4727	Antiemetic
EL444	Cap, Light Blue	Trimethobenzamide HCl 250 mg	Tigan by Breckenridge	51991-0625	Antiemetic
EL444	Cap, Dark Blue & Light Blue, EL 444	Trimethobenzamide HCl 250 mg	by Anabolic	00722-6149	Antiemetic
EL444	Cap	Trimethobenzamide HCl 250 mg	by United Res	00677-1383	Antiemetic
EL514	Tab	Aspirin 800 mg	by Rugby	00536-3320	Analgesic
EL518	Tab, Pink, Oval	Pseudoephedrine 60 mg, Chlorpheniramine 4 mg, Acetaminophen 650 mg	by Econolab		Cold Remedy
EL522	Tab	Dyphylline 200 mg, Guaifenesin 200 mg	by Econolab	55053-0522	Antiasthmatic
EL522	Tab	Dyphylline 200 mg, Guaifenesin 200 mg	by Pegasus	55246-0953	Antiasthmatic
EL522	Tab, White, Round, Scored	Dyphylline 200 mg, Guaifenesin 200 mg	Dyphylline GG by H J Harkins Co	52959-0482	Antiasthmatic
EL524	Cap, Clear & Yellow	Chlorphen 4 mg, Phenyltolox 20 mg, Phenylephrine 50 mg	Comhist LA by Econolab		Cold Remedy
EL525	Tab, Coated, EL/525	Belladonna Alkaloid Malate 125 mcg, Caffeine 100 mg, Ergotamine Tartrate 1 mg, Pentobarbital Sodium 30 mg	Micomp PB by Anabolic	00722-6090	Gastrointestinal; C IV
EL717	Tab	Hyoscyamine Sulfate 0.125 mg	by United Res	00677-1536	Gastrointestinal
EL717	Tab, Light Blue Green	Hyoscyamine Sulfate 0.125 mg	Hyosol SL by Econolab	55053-0717	Gastrointestinal
EL717 <> RUGBY5575	Tab	Hyoscyamine Sulfate 0.125 mg	Hyosol SL by Pegasus	55246-0949	Gastrointestinal
EL730	Tab, EL-730	Yohimbine HCl 5.4 mg	by Major	00904-3255	Impotence Agent
EL730 <> RUGBY4989	Tab	Yohimbine HCl 5.4 mg	by Pegasus	55246-0947	Impotence Agent
EL740	Cap	Chlorpheniramine 8 mg, Pseudoephedrine HCl 120 mg	by Zenith Goldline	00182-1151	Cold Remedy
EL740	Cap, Black Print, White Beads	Chlorpheniramine Maleate 8 mg, Pseudoephedrine HCl 120 mg	Colfed A by Econolab	55053-0740	Cold Remedy
EL740	Cap, Black Print, White Beads	Chlorpheniramine Maleate 8 mg, Pseudoephedrine HCl 120 mg	by HL Moore	00839-7178	Cold Remedy
EL800	Cap, Ex Release	Chlorpheniramine Maleate 4 mg, Pseudoephedrine HCl 60 mg	Dynafed by Pharmafab	62542-0201	Cold Remedy
EL800	Cap, Clear, Red Beads, EL-800	Chlorpheniramine Maleate 4 mg, Pseudoephedrine HCl 60 mg	Dynahist ER by Breckenridge	51991-0217	Cold Remedy

ID FRONT <> BACK	DESCRIPTION FRONT <> BACK	INGREDIENT & STRENGTH	BRAND (OR EQUIV.) & FIRM	NDC#	CLASS; SCH.
EL840	Tab, Coated	Ascorbic Acid 120 mg, Calcium 250 mg, Copper 2 mg, Cyanocobalamin 12 mcg, Docusate Sodium 50 mg, Folic Acid 1 mg, Iodine 0.15 mg, Iron 90 mg, Niacinamide 20 mg, Pyridoxine HCl 20 mg, Riboflavin 3.4 mg, Thiamine Mononitrate 3 mg, Vitamin A Acetate 4000 Units, Vitamin D 400 Units, Vitamin E 30 Units, Zinc 25 mg	Obnate 90 by Intertech	60917-0001	Vitamin
EL860	Cap, Ex Release	Guaifenesin 250 mg, Pseudoephedrine HCl 120 mg	Guaibid D by Pharmafab	62542-0452	Cold Remedy
EL870	Cap, Black Print, White Beads	Guaifenesin 300 mg, Pseudoephedrine HCl 60 mg	Guaibid D Ped by Econolab	55053-0870	Cold Remedy
EL880	Cap, Clear & White	Lipase, Protease, Amylase	Creon-10 by Econolab		Gastrointestinal
EL890	Tab, Coated	Ascorbic Acid 100 mg, Biotin 30 mcg, Calcium 250 mg, Chromium 25 mcg, Copper 2 mg, Cyanocobalamin 12 mcg, Folic Acid 1 mg, Iodine 150 mcg, Iron 60 mg, Magnesium 25 mg, Manganese 5 mg, Molybdenum 25 mcg, Niacinamide 20 mg, Pantothenic Acid 10 mg, Pyridoxine HCl 10 mg, Riboflavin 3.4 mg, Thiamine Mononitrate 3 mg, Vitamin A Acetate 5000 Units, Vitamin D 400 Units, Vitamin E Acetate 30 Units, Zinc 25 mg	Preterna by Intertech	60917-0002	Vitamin
EL950	Tab, Film Coated	Ascorbic Acid 70 mg, Calcium 200 mg, Cyanocobalamin 2.2 mcg, Folic Acid 1 mg, Iodine 175 mcg, Iron 65 mg, Magnesium 100 mg, Niacin 17 mg, Pyridoxine HCl 2.2 mg, Riboflavin 1.6 mg, Selenium 65 mcg, Thiamine Mononitrate 1.5 mg, Vitamin A 4000 Units, Vitamin D 400 Units, Vitamin E 10 Units, Zinc 15 mg	Zitamin by Intertech	60917-0003	Vitamin
ELAVIL <> 40	Tab, Blue, Round, Film Coated	Amitriptyline HCl 10 mg	Elavil by HJ Harkins	52959-0396	Antidepressant
ELAVIL <> 40	Tab, Coated	Amitriptyline HCl 10 mg	Elavil by Zeneca	00310-0040	Antidepressant
ELAVIL <> 41	Tab, Film Coated	Amitriptyline HCl 50 mg	Elavil by Zeneca	00310-0041	Antidepressant
ELAVIL <> 42	Tab, Film Coated	Amitriptyline HCl 75 mg	Elavil by Zeneca	00310-0042	Antidepressant
ELAVIL <> 43	Tab, Film Coated	Amitriptyline HCl 100 mg	Elavil by Zeneca	00310-0043	Antidepressant
ELAVIL <> 43	Tab, Film Coated	Amitriptyline HCl 100 mg	Elavil by Merck	00006-0435	Antidepressant
ELAVIL <> 45	Tab, Yellow, Round, Film Coated	Amitriptyline HCl 25 mg	by Allscripts	54569-0174	Antidepressant
ELAVIL <> 45	Tab, Yellow, Round	Amitriptyline HCl 25 mg	Elavil by Rightpak	65240-0637	Antidepressant
ELAVIL <> 45	Tab, Film Coated	Amitriptyline HCl 25 mg	Elavil by Zeneca	00310-0045	Antidepressant
ELAVIL <> 45	Tab, Film Coated	Amitriptyline HCl 25 mg	Elavil by Physicians Total Care	54868-0409	Antidepressant
ELAVIL <> 47	Tab, Film Coated	Amitriptyline HCl 150 mg	Elavil by Zeneca	00310-0047	Antidepressant
ELAVILSTUART45	Tab, Film Coated	Amitriptyline HCl 25 mg	Elavil by Allscripts	54569-0174	Antidepressant
ELDEPRYL5MG	Cap, Aqua Blue Opaque, Eldepryl/5 mg <> Somerset Logo	Eldepryl 5 mg (Selegiline HCL)	by UDL	51079-0887	Antiparkinson
ELDEPRYL5MG	Cap, Somerset Logo Imprinted	Selegiline HCl 5 mg	Eldepryl by Somerset	39506-0022	Antiparkinson
ELDER600	Cap, Salmon	Methoxsalen 10 mg	8-MOP by ICN		Dermatologic
ELDERCAPS <> MP	Cap	Ascorbic Acid 200 mg, Calcium Pantothenate 10 mg, Cholecalciferol 400 Units, Folic Acid 1 mg, Magnesium Sulfate, Manganese Sulfate, Niacinamide 25 mg, Pyridoxine HCl 2 mg, Riboflavin 5 mg, Thiamine Mononitrate 10 mg, Vitamin A 4000 Units, Vitamin E 25 Units, Zinc Sulfate	Eldercaps by Merz	00259-0393	Vitamin
ELDERCAPS <> MP	Cap	Ascorbic Acid 200 mg, Calcium Pantothenate 10 mg, Cholecalciferol 400 Units, Folic Acid 1 mg, Magnesium Sulfate, Manganese Sulfate, Niacinamide 25 mg, Pyridoxine HCl 2 mg, Riboflavin 5 mg, Thiamine Mononitrate 10 mg, Vitamin A 4000 Units, Vitamin E 25 Units, Zinc Sulfate	Eldercaps by Anabolic	00722-6386	Vitamin
ELN30	Tab, Brownish-Red, Round, Film Coated, ELN over 30	Nifedipine 30 mg	by Teva Pharms	00093-1021	Antihypertensive
ELP10	Tab, Brown, Round	Enalapril Maleate 10 mg	by Mova Pharms	55370-0924	Antihypertensive
ELP10	Tab, Pink, Round	Enalapril Maleate 10 mg	by LEK Pharm	48866-0303	Antihypertensive
ELP20	Tab, Gray, Round	Enalapril Maleate 20 mg	by Mova Pharms	55370-0925	Antihypertensive
ELP20	Tab, Gray & Purple, Round	Enalapril Maleate 20 mg	by LEK Pharm	48866-0304	Antihypertensive
ELP212	Tab, Yellow, Round, Scored	Enalapril Maleate 2.5 mg	by Mova Pharms	55370-0922	Antihypertensive
ELP212	Tab, Yellow, Round	Enalapril Maleate 2.5 mg	by LEK Pharm	48866-0301	Antihypertensive
ELP5	Tab, Pink, Round, Scored	Enalapril Maleate 5 mg	by Mova Pharms	55370-0923	Antihypertensive
ELP5	Tab, Pink, Round, Scored	Enalapril Maleate 5 mg	by LEK Pharm	48866-0302	Antihypertensive
EM	Tab, White, Round	Dyphylline 200 mg	Dyflex by Lemmon		Antiasthmatic
EM	Tab, Pink, Round, Schering Logo EM	Ethinyl Estradiol 0.05 mg	Estinyl by Schering		Oral Contraceptive
EM10	Tab, White, Round, Scored	Methimazole 10 mg	by Par Pharm	49884-0641	Antithyroid

| --- | --- | --- | --- | --- | --- |
EM5	Tab, White, Round, Scored	Methimazole 5 mg	by Par Pharm	49884-0640	Antithyroid
EMBEL320	Tab	Amylase 30000 Units, Lipase 8000 Units, Protease 30000 Units	Pancrelipase by Zenith Goldline	00182-1741	Gastrointestinal
EMCYT140MG <> PHARMACIA	Cap	Estramustine Phosphate Sodium	Emcyt by Pharmacia & Upjohn	00013-0132	Antineoplastic
EMPRACET 30 K9B	Tab, Peach, Round	Acetaminophen 300 mg, Codeine Phosphate 30 mg	by Glaxo	Canadian	Analgesic
EMPRACET 60 L9B	Tab, Peach, Round	Acetaminophen 300 mg, Codeine Phosphate 60 mg	by Glaxo	Canadian	Analgesic
EMTEC30	Tab, Peach, Round, Scored, Emtec-30	Acetaminophen 300 mg, Codeine Phosphate 30 mg	by Altimed	Canadian DIN# 00608882	Analgesic
EMYCIN <> 250MG	Tab, Delayed Release, E-Mycin <> 250 mg	Erythromycin 250 mg	by Quality Care	60346-0630	Antibiotic
EMYCIN250MG	Tab, Delayed Release, Printed in Black	Erythromycin 250 mg	by Casa De Amigos	62138-6304	Antibiotic
EMYCIN250MG	Tab, E-Mycin 250 mg	Erythromycin 250 mg	by PDRX	55289-0120	Antibiotic
EMYCIN250MG	Tab	Erythromycin 250 mg	by Allscripts	54569-0123	Antibiotic
EMYCIN333	Tab, Orange	Erythromycin 333 mg	by Urgent Care Ctr	50716-0376	Antibiotic
EMYCIN333MG	Tab, Orange Print	Erythromycin 333 mg	by Prestige Packaging	58056-0194	Antibiotic
EMYCIN333MG	Tab, Orange Print	Erythromycin 333 mg	by Nat Pharmpak Serv	55154-0504	Antibiotic
EMYCIN333MG	Tab, White, Round	Erythromycin 333 mg	E Mycin by Rightpak	65240-0645	Antibiotic
EMYCIN333MG	Tab, White, Round	Erythromycin 333 mg	E Mycin by Rx Pac	65084-0223	Antibiotic
EMYCIN333MG	Tab, Orange Print	Erythromycin 333 mg	by Drug Distr	52985-0180	Antibiotic
EMYCIN333MG	Tab, E-Mycin 333 mg	Erythromycin 333 mg	by Allscripts	54569-0129	Antibiotic
EMYCIN333MG	Tab, White, Round, Convex, Enterick E-Mycin 333 mg in Orange	Levothyroxine Sodium 333 mg	E Mycin by Murfreesboro	51129-1647	Antithyroid
EMYCIN33MG	Tab, Delayed Release, Printed in Orange	Erythromycin 333 mg	by Amerisource	62584-0208	Antibiotic
ENDO	Tab, White	Oxycodone 5 mg, Acetaminophen 325 mg	Percocet by Dupont	Canadian	Analgesic; C II
ENDO	Tab, Yellow	Oxycodone 5 mg, Acetylsalicylic 325 mg	Percodan by Dupont	Canadian	Analgesic; C II
ENDO	Tab	Selegiline HCl 5 mg	by Dupont Pharma	00056-0620	Antiparkinson
ENDO	Tab, White, Oval	Selegiline HCl 5 mg	by Endo	60951-0620	Antiparkinson
ENDO <> 631	Tab, Film Coated	Cimetidine 300 mg	by Quality Care	60346-0944	Gastrointestinal
ENDO <> 721	Tab, Coated	Captopril 12.5 mg	by Dupont Pharma	00056-0721	Antihypertensive
ENDO10010	Tab, Blue, Oval, Endo/100/10	Levodopa 100 mg, Carbidopa 10 mg	by Endo	Canadian	Antiparkinson
ENDO10025	Tab, Yellow, Oval, Endo/100/25	Levodopa 100 mg, Carbidopa 25 mg	by Endo	Canadian	Antiparkinson
ENDO25025	Tab, Light Blue, Oval, Endo/250/25	Levodopa 250 mg, Carbidopa 25 mg	by Endo	Canadian	Antiparkinson
ENDO602	Tab, White, Round, Scored	Acetaminophen 325 mg, Oxycodone HCl 5 mg	Endocet by Endo	60951-0602	Analgesic; C II
ENDO602	Tab, Endo 602	Acetaminophen 325 mg, Oxycodone HCl 5 mg	Endocet by Dupont	00590-0602	Analgesic; C II
ENDO603	Tab, Dark Blue, Oval, Scored	Carbidopa, Dl- 10 mg, Levodopa 100 mg	by Endo	60951-0603	Antiparkinson
ENDO605	Tab, Yellow, Oval	Carbidopa 25 mg, Levodopa 100 mg	Sinemet by Endo		Antiparkinson
ENDO605	Tab, Yellow, Oval, Scored	Carbidopa, Dl- 25 mg, Levodopa 100 mg	by Endo	60951-0605	Antiparkinson
ENDO607	Tab, Blue, Oval	Carbidopa 25 mg, Levodopa 250 mg	Sinemet by Endo		Antiparkinson
ENDO607	Tab, Light Blue, Oval, Scored	Carbidopa, Dl- 25 mg, Levodopa 250 mg	by Endo	60951-0607	Antiparkinson
ENDO610	Tab, Yellow, Round, Scored	Aspirin 325 mg, Oxycodone HCl 4.5 mg, Oxycodone Terephthalate 0.38 mg	Endodan by Endo	60951-0610	Analgesic; C II
ENDO610	Tab	Aspirin 325 mg, Oxycodone HCl 4.5 mg, Oxycodone Terephthalate 0.38 mg	Endodan by Dupont	00590-0610	Analgesic; C II
ENDO630	Tab, White, Oval	Cimetidine 200 mg	by Endo	60951-0630	Gastrointestinal
ENDO631	Tab, White, Oval, Film Coated	Cimetidine 300 mg	by Endo	60951-0631	Gastrointestinal
ENDO631	Tab, Film Coated, Debossed	Cimetidine 300 mg	by Amerisource	62584-0631	Gastrointestinal
ENDO631	Tab, Film Coated	Cimetidine 300 mg	by Dupont Pharma	00056-0631	Gastrointestinal
ENDO632	Tab, White, Oval, Scored, Film Coated	Cimetidine 400 mg	by Endo	60951-0632	Gastrointestinal
ENDO632	Tab, Film Coated, Debossed	Cimetidine 400 mg	by Amerisource	62584-0632	Gastrointestinal
ENDO632	Tab, Film Coated	Cimetidine 400 mg	by Dupont Pharma	00056-0632	Gastrointestinal
ENDO632	Tab, Film Coated	Cimetidine 400 mg	by Med Pro	53978-2009	Gastrointestinal
ENDO633	Tab, White, Oval, Scored, Film Coated	Cimetidine 800 mg	by Endo	60951-0633	Gastrointestinal
ENDO688 <> ENDO688	Cap, Gelatin Coated	Etodolac 200 mg	by Endo	60951-0688	NSAID
ENDO688 <> ENDO688	Cap, Gelatin	Etodolac 200 mg	by Dupont Pharma	00056-0688	NSAID
ENDO689	Cap, Gelatin Coated, Imprinted in Red	Etodolac 300 mg	by Endo	60951-0689	NSAID

ID FRONT <> BACK	DESCRIPTION FRONT <> BACK	INGREDIENT & STRENGTH	BRAND (OR EQUIV.) & FIRM	NDC#	CLASS; SCH.
ENDO689 <> ENDO689	Cap, Gelatin	Etodolac 300 mg	by Dupont Pharma	00056-0689	NSAID
ENDO711	Tab	Glipizide 5 mg	by Rugby	00536-5702	Antidiabetic
ENDO711	Tab	Glipizide 5 mg	by Quality Care	62682-5002	Antidiabetic
ENDO711	Tab, White, Round	Glipizide 5 mg	by Endo	60951-0711	Antidiabetic
ENDO714	Tab, White, Round	Glipizide 10 mg	by Endo	60951-0714	Antidiabetic
ENDO714	Tab	Glipizide 10 mg	by Dupont Pharma	00056-0714	Antidiabetic
ENDO714	Tab	Glipizide 10 mg	by Rugby	00536-5703	Antidiabetic
ENDO721	Tab, Coated	Captopril 12.5 mg	by Endo	60951-0721	Antihypertensive
ENDO722	Tab	Captopril 25 mg	by Direct Dispensing	57866-6106	Antihypertensive
ENDO722	Tab, Coated	Captopril 25 mg	by Endo	60951-0722	Antihypertensive
ENDO722	Tab, Coated	Captopril 25 mg	by Dupont Pharma	00056-0722	Antihypertensive
ENDO724	Tab, Coated	Captopril 50 mg	by Endo	60951-0724	Antihypertensive
ENDO724	Tab, Coated	Captopril 50 mg	by Dupont Pharma	00056-0724	Antihypertensive
ENDO727	Tab, Coated	Captopril 100 mg	by Endo	60951-0727	Antihypertensive
ENDO727	Tab, Coated	Captopril 100 mg	by Dupont Pharma	00056-0727	Antihypertensive
ENDO731	Tab, Peach, Round, Scored	Captopril 50 mg, Hydrochlorothiazide 25 mg	by Endo	60951-0731	Antihypertensive; Diuretic
ENDO731	Tab	Captopril 50 mg, Hydrochlorothiazide 25 mg	by Dupont Pharma	00056-0731	Antihypertensive; Diuretic
ENDO733	Tab, White, Round, Scored	Captopril 25 mg, Hydrochlorothiazide 15 mg	by Endo	60951-0733	Antihypertensive; Diuretic
ENDO733	Tab	Captopril 25 mg, Hydrochlorothiazide 15 mg	by Dupont Pharma	00056-0733	Antihypertensive; Diuretic
ENDO739	Tab, White, Round, Scored	Captopril 50 mg, Hydrochlorothiazide 15 mg	by Endo	60951-0739	Antihypertensive; Diuretic
ENDO739	Tab	Captopril 50 mg, Hydrochlorothiazide 15 mg	by Dupont Pharma	00056-0739	Antihypertensive; Diuretic
ENDO741	Tab, Peach, Round, Scored	Captopril 25 mg, Hydrochlorothiazide 25 mg	by Endo	60951-0741	Antihypertensive; Diuretic
ENDO741	Tab	Captopril 25 mg, Hydrochlorothiazide 25 mg	by Dupont Pharma	00056-0741	Antihypertensive; Diuretic
ENDO744	Tab	Etodolac 400 mg	by Endo	60951-0744	NSAID
ENDO744	Tab	Etodolac 400 mg	by Dupont Pharma	00056-0744	NSAID
ENDURON	Tab, Orange, Square, Scored, Enduron over Abbott Logo	Methyclothiazide 2.5 mg	Enduron by Abbott	00074-6827	Diuretic
ENDURON	Tab, Salmon, Square, Scored, Enduron over Abbott Logo	Methyclothiazide 5 mg	Enduron by Abbott	00074-6812	Diuretic
ENEENE <> CGCG	Tab, Brownish-Orange, Oval, Scored	Carbamazepine 400 mg	Tegretol by Geigy	Canadian DIN# 00755583	Anticonvulsant
ENKAID25MG <> BRISTOL732	Cap, Enkaid 25 mg <> Bristol 732	Encainide HCl 25 mg	Enkaid by Bristol Myers Squibb	00087-0732	Antiarrhythmic
ENKAID35MG <> BRISTOL734	Cap, Enkaid 25 mg <> Bristol 734	Encainide HCl 35 mg	Enkaid by Bristol Myers Squibb	00087-0734	Antiarrhythmic
ENT	Tab, Ex Release	Brompheniramine Maleate 12 mg, Phenylpropanolamine HCl 75 mg	E N T by Sovereign	58716-0641	Cold Remedy
ENTEX <> 01490412	Cap	Guaifenesin 200 mg, Phenylephrine HCl 5 mg, Phenylpropanolamine HCl 45 mg	Entex by Amerisource	62584-0412	Cold Remedy
ENTEX <> 51479030	Tab	Guaifenesin 200 mg, Phenylephrine HCl 5 mg, Phenylpropanolamine HCl 45 mg	Entex by Welpharm	63375-6378	Cold Remedy
ENTEX LA <> 01490436	Tab, Ex Release	Guaifenesin 400 mg, Phenylpropanolamine HCl 75 mg	Entex LA by Leiner	59606-0641	Cold Remedy
ENTEX51479030	Cap, Orange & White	Guaifenesin 200 mg, Phenylephrine HCl 5 mg, Phenylpropanolamine HCl 45 mg	Entex by Dura	51479-0030	Cold Remedy
ENTEXLA <> 01490436	Tab	Guaifenesin 400 mg, Phenylpropanolamine HCl 75 mg	Entex LA by Amerisource	62584-0436	Cold Remedy
ENTEXLA <> 01490436	Tab	Guaifenesin 400 mg, Phenylpropanolamine HCl 75 mg	Entex LA by Quality Care	60346-0336	Cold Remedy
ENTEXLA <> 01490436	Tab	Guaifenesin 400 mg, Phenylpropanolamine HCl 75 mg	Entex LA by Caremark	00339-5128	Cold Remedy
ENTEXLA <> 01490436	Tab	Guaifenesin 400 mg, Phenylpropanolamine HCl 75 mg	Entex LA by Urgent Care Ctr	50716-0436	Cold Remedy
ENTEXLA <> 01490436	Tab	Guaifenesin 400 mg, Phenylpropanolamine HCl 75 mg	Entex LA by Nat Pharmpak Serv	55154-2303	Cold Remedy

ID FRONT <> BACK	DESCRIPTION FRONT <> BACK	INGREDIENT & STRENGTH	BRAND (OR EQUIV.) & FIRM	NDC#	CLASS; SCH.
ENTEXLA <> 033033	Tab, Film Coated	Guaifenesin 400 mg, Phenylpropanolamine HCl 75 mg	Entex LA by Welpharm	63375-6377	Cold Remedy
ENTEXLA <> 033033	Tab, Orange, Oblong, Scored	Guaifenesin 400 mg, Phenylpropanolamine HCl 75 mg	Entex LA by Martec		Cold Remedy
ENTEXLA <> 033033	Tab, Orange, Scored	Guaifenesin 400 mg, Phenylpropanolamine HCl 75 mg	Entex LA by Dura	51479-0033	Cold Remedy
ENTEXPSE <> 032032	Tab, Yellow, Scored, Film Coated	Guaifenesin 600 mg, Pseudoephedrine HCl 120 mg	Entex PSE by Dura	51479-0032	Cold Remedy
ENTEXPSE <> 032032	Tab, Film Coated, Entex PSE <> 032 over 032	Guaifenesin 600 mg, Pseudoephedrine HCl 120 mg	Entex PSE by Welpharm	63375-6376	Cold Remedy
ENTROPHEN 975MG	Tab, Yellow, Oval	Acetaminophen 975 mg	by Johnson & Johnson	Canadian	Antipyretic
ENTROPHEN325MG	Cap, Yellow, Film Coated	Acetaminophen 325 mg	Entrophen by Johnson & Johnson	Canadian DIN# 02050161	Antipyretic
ENTROPHEN325MG	Tab, Brown, Round, Film Coated	Acetaminophen 325 mg	Entrophen by Johnson & Johnson	Canadian DIN# 0010332	Antipyretic
ENTROPHEN500MG	Tab, Pink, Oval, Film Coated	Acetaminophen 500 mg	Entrophen by Johnson & Johnson	Canadian DIN# 00852015	Antipyretic
ENTROPHEN650MG	Cap, Orange, Film Coated	Acetaminophen 650 mg	Entrophen by Johnson & Johnson	Canadian DIN# 01905392	Antipyretic
ENTROPHEN650MG	Tab, Orange, Oval, Film Coated	Acetaminophen 650 mg	Entrophen by Johnson & Johnson	Canadian DIN# 00010340	Antipyretic
EON720	Cap, Green & Clear, Eon Logo 720	Indomethacin ER 75 mg	by Allscripts	54569-1518	NSAID
EP	Tab, Peach, Round, Schering Logo EP	Ethinyl Estradiol 0.5 mg	Estinyl by Schering		Hormone
EP103	Tab, White, Round, Scored	Pseudoephedrine HCl 60 mg	by RX PAK	65084-0107	Decongestant
EP103	Tab, White, Round, Scored	Pseudoephedrine HCl 60 mg	by RX PAK	65084-0108	Decongestant
EP104	Tab, White, Round, EP 104	Colchicine 0.6 mg	by DJ Pharma	64455-0005	Antigout
EP104	Tab, White, Round	Colchicine 0.6 mg	by Dixon	17236-0655	Antigout
EP105	Tab, Green, Oval	Magnesium Salicylate 600 mg, Phenyltolaxamine 25 mg	by Nat Pharmpak Serv	55154-5237	Analgesic
EP105	Tab, Green, Oblong, Bisected	Magnesium Salicylate 600 mg, Phenyltolaxamine 25 mg	by Nat Pharmpak Serv	55154-5241	Analgesic
EP105	Tab, Green, Oblong, Bisected	Phenyltoloxamine Citrate 25 mg, Magnesium Salicylate Tetrahydrate Citrate 600 mg	Mag Phen by Physicians Total Care	54868-2469	Cold Remedy
EP915	Tab, White, Round	Phenobarbital 15 mg	by United Res	00677-1731	Sedative/Hypnotic; C IV
EP915	Tab, White, Round	Phenobarbital 15 mg	by Excellium	64125-0915	Sedative/Hypnotic; C IV
EPH3252243850	Cap, Crimson, EPH 325 224/3850	Ephedra 325 mg	Ephedra 325 by NVE Pharm		Supplement
EPI101	Cap, Red & White	Dichloralantipyrine 100 mg; Acetaminophen 325 mg; Isometheptene Mucate 65 mg	Migraine by Excellium	64125-0101	Antimigraine
EPI132 <> 5	Tab, EPI Over 132	Oxycodone HCl 5 mg	Percolone by Du Pont Pharma	00056-0132	Analgesic; C II
EPI132 <> 5	Tab, White, Round, Scored, EPI Over 132 <> 5	Oxycodone HCl 5 mg	Percolone by Endo	63481-0132	Analgesic; C II
EPITOL <> 9393	Tab, White, Round, Scored, Epitol <> 93 over 93	Carbamazepine 200 mg	Epitol by Teva	00093-0090	Anticonvulsant
EPITOL <> 9393	Tab, White, Round, Scored	Carbamazepine 200 mg	Epitol by Caremark	00339-6132	Anticonvulsant
EQUAGESIC	Tab, White & Yellow, Equa-Gesic	Meprobamate 200 mg, Aspirin 75 mg, Ethoheptazine 250 mg	Equagesic by Wyeth-Ayerst	Canadian	Sedative/Hypnotic
EQUANIL400	Tab, White	Meprobamate 400 mg	Equanil by Wyeth-Ayerst	Canadian	Sedative/Hypnotic
ER	Tab, Beige, Round, Schering Logo ER	Ethinyl Estradiol 0.02 mg	Estinyl by Schering		Hormone
ER	Cap, Clear & Maroon, Opaque, w/ Pink & Yellow Beads, ER over Abbott Logo	Erythromycin Delayed Release 250 mg	by Abbott	00074-6301	Antibiotic
ER <> CIBA	Tab, Brownish-Yellow, Round, Film Coated	Maprotiline HCl 50 mg	Ludiomil by Novartis	Canadian DIN# 00360503	Antidepressant
ERCIBA	Tab, Brown & Yellow, Round, ER/Ciba	Maprotiline 50 mg	Ludiomil by Ciba	Canadian	Antidepressant
EREX	Tab	Yohimbine HCl 5.4 mg	Erex by Sovereign	58716-0613	Impotence Agent
ERVA54	Tab, White, Round, Erva 5.4	Yohimbine HCl 5.4 mg	Yocon by Royce		Impotence Agent
ERVA54	Tab, Erva 5.4	Yohimbine HCl 5.4 mg	by Royce	51875-0361	Impotence Agent

ID FRONT <> BACK	DESCRIPTION FRONT <> BACK	INGREDIENT & STRENGTH	BRAND (OR EQUIV.) & FIRM	NDC#	CLASS; SCH.
ERYC <> PD696	Cap, Clear & Orange, Opaque	Erythromycin 250 mg	Eryc by Parke-Davis	Canadian DIN# 00607142	Antibiotic
ERYC <> PD696	Cap, Clear & Orange	Erythromycin 250 mg	Eryc by Murfreesboro Ph	51129-1422	Antibiotic
ERYC <> PD696	Cap, P-D 696	Erythromycin 250 mg	Eryc by Parke Davis	00071-0696	Antibiotic
ERYC <> PD696	Cap, P-D 696	Erythromycin 250 mg	Eryc by Allscripts	54569-0131	Antibiotic
ERYC333MG	Cap, Clear & Yellow, Eryc/333 mg	Erythromycin 333 mg	by Frosst	Canadian	Antibiotic
ES	Tab, Film Coated, Logo	Erythromycin Stearate	by Quality Care	60346-0580	Antibiotic
ES	Tab, Film Coated, Abbott Logo	Erythromycin Stearate	by Allscripts	54569-0124	Antibiotic
ES	Tab, Film Coated, Abbott Logo	Erythromycin Stearate	by Pharmedix	53002-0270	Antibiotic
ES	Tab, Pink, Round, Film Coated, ES <> Abbott Logo	Erythromycin Stearate 250 mg	Erythrocin by Abbott	00074-6346	Antibiotic
ESGICPLUS <> FOREST0372	Cap, White Print	Acetaminophen 500 mg, Butalbital 50 mg, Caffeine 40 mg	Esgic Plus by Eckerd Drug	19458-0844	Analgesic
ESGICPLUS <> FOREST0372	Cap	Acetaminophen 500 mg, Butalbital 50 mg, Caffeine 40 mg	by Mikart	46672-0273	Analgesic
ESGICPLUS <> FOREST0372	Cap, Red	Acetaminophen 500 mg, Butalbital 50 mg, Caffeine 40 mg	by Allscripts	54569-3441	Analgesic
ESGICPLUS <> FOREST0372	Cap, Red, White Print	Acetaminophen 500 mg, Butalbital 50 mg, Caffeine 40 mg	Esgic Plus by Forest	00456-0679	Analgesic
ESGICPLUS <> FOREST0372	Cap, Red & White	Acetaminophen 500 mg; Butalbital 50 mg; Caffeine 40 mg	Esgic Plus by Med-Pro	53978-3396	Analgesic
ESGICPLUS <> FOREST0372	Cap, Red	Butalbital 50 mg; Acetaminophen 500 mg; Caffeine 40 mg	Esgic Plus by Thrift Services	59198-0332	Analgesic
ESKALITH <> SB	Cap, Gray & Yellow	Lithium Carbonate 300 mg	Eskalith by Mylan	00378-0423	Antipsychotic
ESKALITHSB	Cap, Gray & Yellow, Eskalith/SB	Lithium Carbonate 300 mg	Eskalith by SKB	00007-4007	Antipsychotic
ESMAALOXPLUS	Tab, Pink, Round	Magnesium Hydroxide 350 mg	by Novartis	Canadian	Mineral
ESTAC <> 500	Cap, Blue, Film Coated	Acetaminophen 500 mg, Chlorzoxazone 250 mg	Extra Strength Tylenol Aches & Strains by McNeil	Canadian DIN# 02155214	Analgesic; Muscle Relaxant
ET	Tab, Coated, Abbott Logo	Erythromycin Stearate	by Allscripts	54569-0125	Antibiotic
ET	Tab, Coated, Abbott Logo	Erythromycin Stearate	by Pharmedix	53002-0269	Antibiotic
ET	Tab, Pink, Oval, Film Coated, ET <> Abbott Logo	Erythromycin Stearate 500 mg	Erythrocin by Abbott	00074-6316	Antibiotic
ET500 <> G	Tab, Blue, Oval, Film Coated	Etodolac 500 mg	by Genpharm	55567-0032	NSAID
ET7	Tab	Chlorpheniramine Tannate 8 mg, Phenylephrine Tannate 25 mg, Pyrilamine Tannate 25 mg	Tritan by Eon	00185-0700	Cold Remedy
ETH <> 15	Tab, White, Partially Bisected	Morphine Sulfate 15 mg	MSIR by Ethex	58177-0313	Analgesic; C II
ETH <> 15	Tab, Partially Bisect	Morphine Sulfate 15 mg	by KV	10609-1405	Analgesic; C II
ETH <> 274	Tab, Coated	Hyoscyamine Sulfate 0.125 mg	by KV	10609-1352	Gastrointestinal
ETH <> 274	Tab, White, Oval, Coated	Hyoscyamine Sulfate 0.125 mg	Levsin by Ethex	58177-0274	Gastrointestinal
ETH <> 315	Tab, Orange & Rust, Beveled Edge, Partially Bisect	Oxycodone HCl 5 mg	Roxicodone by Ethex	58177-0315	Analgesic; C II
ETH <> 315	Tab, Beveled Edge, Partially Bisect	Oxycodone HCl 5 mg	by KV	10609-1419	Analgesic; C II
ETH 301	Tab, White, Round	Ketorolac 10 mg	Toradol by Syntex		NSAID
ETH042	Cap, Maroon	Ascorbic Acid 250 mg; Ferrous Fumarate 200 mg; Cyanocobalamin 10 mcg	Anemagen by Accucaps Inds	61474-4070	Vitamin
ETH255	Tab, ETH/255	Hyoscyamine Sulfate 0.125 mg	by KV	10609-1347	Gastrointestinal
ETH255	Tab, White	Hyoscyamine Sulfate 0.125 mg	Levsin/SL by Ethex	58177-0255	Gastrointestinal
ETH266 <> 1MG	Tab, Light Purple, Oblong	Doxazosin Mesylate 1 mg	Cardura by Pfizer	58177-0266	Antihypertensive
ETH267 <> 2MG	Tab, Yellow, Oblong	Doxazosin Mesylate 2 mg	Cardura by Pfizer	58177-0267	Antihypertensive
ETH268 <> 4MG	Tab, Pink, Oblong, Scored	Doxazosin Mesylate 4 mg	Cardura by Pfizer	58177-0268	Antihypertensive
ETH269 <> 8MG	Tab, Blue, Oblong	Doxazosin Mesylate 8 mg	Cardura by Pfizer	58177-0269	Antihypertensive
ETH30	Cap, Brown, ETH/30	Morphine Sulfate IR 30 mg	by KV Pharm.		Analgesic; C II
ETHEX <> 001	Cap, ER, in Red	Potassium Chloride 750 mg	Micro-K 10 by Ethex	58177-0001	Electrolytes
ETHEX <> 001	Cap, ER	Potassium Chloride 750 mg	by Heartland	61392-0402	Electrolytes

ID FRONT <> BACK	DESCRIPTION FRONT <> BACK	INGREDIENT & STRENGTH	BRAND (OR EQUIV.) & FIRM	NDC#	CLASS; SCH.
ETHEX <> 002	Cap, Orange & Purple	Disopyramide Phosphate	Norpace by Ethex	58177-0002	Antiarrhythmic
ETHEX <> 004	Cap, Lavender, Ex Release, in Black Ink	Nitroglycerin 2.5 mg	Nitrobid by Ethex	58177-0004	Vasodilator
ETHEX <> 005	Cap, Blue & Orange, Ex Release, in Black Ink	Nitroglycerin 6.5 mg	Nitrobid by Ethex	58177-0005	Vasodilator
ETHEX <> 006	Cap, Clear, Ex Release, in Black Ink	Nitroglycerin 9 mg	Nitrobid by Ethex	58177-0006	Vasodilator
ETHEX <> 024	Cap, Opaque & Orange	Cyanocobalamin 25 mcg, Folic Acid 1 mg, Iron 150 mg	FE Tinic 150 by DJ Pharma	64455-0009	Vitamin
ETHEX <> 025	Cap, Gelatin, White Print	Cyanocobalamin 25 mcg, Folic Acid 1 mg, Iron 150 mg	Fe Tinic 150 by KV	10609-1365	Vitamin
ETHEX <> 025	Cap, Maroon, Gelatin Coated	Cyanocobalamin 25 mcg, Folic Acid 1 mg, Iron 150 mg	Fe Tinic 150 by Ethex	58177-0025	Vitamin
ETHEX <> 027	Cap, Maroon	Meperidine HCl 50 mg, Promethazine HCl 25 mg	Mepergan by Ethex	58177-0027	Analgesic; C II
ETHEX <> 027	Cap, White Ink	Meperidine HCl 50 mg, Promethazine HCl 25 mg	by KV	10609-1398	Analgesic; C II
ETHEX <> 037	Cap, Green	Trimethobenzamide HCl 250 mg	Tigan by Ethex	58177-0037	Antiemetic
ETHEX <> 037	Cap	Trimethobenzamide HCl 250 mg	by KV	10609-1401	Antiemetic
ETHEX <> 041	Cap, Beige & Opaque & White, in Black Ink	Oxycodone HCl 5 mg	by Pharmafab	62542-0257	Analgesic; C II
ETHEX <> 1	Cap, Clear, Hard Gel	Potassium Chloride 750 mg	by Eckerd	19458-0877	Electrolytes
ETHEX <> 15	Cap, Blue & Clear	Guaifenesin 300 mg; Pseudoephedrine HCl 60 mg	Pseudovent by Ethex	58177-0046	Cold Remedy
ETHEX <> 16	Cap, White	Guaifenesin 250 mg; Pseudoephedrine HCl 120 mg	Pseudovent by Ethex	58177-0045	Cold Remedy
ETHEX <> 208	Tab, White, Oblong, Scored	Guaifenesin 600 mg; Pseudoephedrine HCl 120 mg	by Murfreesboro Ph	51129-1390	Cold Remedy
ETHEX <> 213	Tab, Green, Oblong, Scored	Dextromethorphan Hydrobromide 30 mg, Guaifenesin 600 mg	Guaifenex DM ER by DRX	55045-2623	Cold Remedy
ETHEX <> 216	Tab, White, Oval, Coated	Ascorbic Acid 80 mg, Beta-Carotene 0.4 mg, Biotin 30 mcg, Calcium 200 mg, Copper 3 mg, Cyanocobalamin 2.5 mcg, Folic Acid 1 mg, Iron 60 mg, Magnesium 100 mg, Niacinamide 17 mg, Pantothenic Acid 7 mg, Pyridoxine HCl 4.86 mg, Riboflavin 1.6 mg, Thiamine 1.5 mg, Vitamin A 0.8 mg, Vitamin D 10 mcg, Vitamin E 10 mg, Zinc 25 mg	Prenatal Rx by Ethex	58177-0216	Vitamin
ETHEX <> 225	Tab, Pink, Oval, Scored	Ascorbic Acid 120 mg, Calcium 200 mg, Copper 2 mg, Cyanocobalamin 12 mcg, Folic Acid 1 mg, Iron 27 mg, Niacinamide 20 mg, Pyridoxine HCl 10 mg, Riboflavin 3 mg, Thiamine HCl 1.84 mg, Vitamin A 4000 Units, Vitamin D 400 Units, Vitamin E 22 mg, Zinc 25 mg	Natalcare Plus by Ethex	58177-0225	Vitamin
ETHEX <> 225	Tab, Scored	Ascorbic Acid 120 mg, Calcium 200 mg, Copper 2 mg, Cyanocobalamin 12 mcg, Folic Acid 1 mg, Iron 27 mg, Niacinamide 20 mg, Pyridoxine HCl 10 mg, Riboflavin 3 mg, Thiamine HCl 1.84 mg, Vitamin A 4000 Units, Vitamin D 400 Units, Vitamin E 22 mg, Zinc 25 mg	Natalcare Plus by KV	10609-1382	Vitamin
ETHEX <> 232	Tab, Peach, Film Coated	Ascorbic Acid 50 mg, Calcium 250 mg, Copper 2 mg, Folic Acid 1 mg, Iron 40 mg, Magnesium 50 mg, Pyridoxine HCl 2 mg, Vitamin D 6 mcg, Vitamin E 3.5 mg, Zinc 15 mg	Natalcare by Ethex	58177-0232	Vitamin
ETHEX <> 234	Tab, Buff, Cap-Shaped	Phenylephrine Tannate 25 mg	R-Tannate by Ethex	58177-0234	Decongestant
ETHEX <> 275	Tab, White, Film Coated	Ascorbic Acid 70 mg, Calcium 200 mg, Cyanocobalamin 2.2 mcg, Folic Acid 1 mg, Iodine 175 mcg, Iron 65 mg, Magnesium 100 mg, Niacin 17 mg, Pyridoxine HCl 2.2 mg, Riboflavin 1.6 mg, Thiamine HCl 1.5 mg, Vitamin A 3000 Units, Vitamin D 400 Units, Vitamin E 10 Units, Zinc 15 mg	Prenatal Z by Ethex	58177-0275	Vitamin
ETHEX <> 275	Tab, Film Coated	Ascorbic Acid 70 mg, Calcium 200 mg, Cyanocobalamin 2.2 mcg, Folic Acid 1 mg, Iodine 175 mcg, Iron 65 mg, Magnesium 100 mg, Niacin 17 mg, Pyridoxine HCl 2.2 mg, Riboflavin 1.6 mg, Thiamine HCl 1.5 mg, Vitamin A 3000 Units, Vitamin D 400 Units, Vitamin E 10 Units, Zinc 15 mg	Prenatal Z by KV	10609-1360	Vitamin
ETHEX <> 292	Tab, Beige, Oval, Film Coated	Ascorbic Acid 120 mg, Calcium 200 mg, Cholecalciferol 400 Units, Copper 2 mg, Cyanocobalamin 12 mcg, Docusate Sodium 50 mg, Folic Acid 1 mg, Iodine 150 mcg, Iron 90 mg, Niacinamide 20 mg, Pyridoxine HCl 20 mg, Riboflavin 3.4 mg, Thiamine HCl 3 mg, Vitamin A 2700 Units, Vitamin E 30 Units, Zinc 25 mg	Ultra Natalcare by Ethex	58177-0292	Vitamin
ETHEX <> 292	Tab, Film Coated, Scored	Ascorbic Acid 120 mg, Calcium 200 mg, Cholecalciferol 400 Units, Copper 2 mg, Cyanocobalamin 12 mcg, Docusate Sodium 50 mg, Folic Acid 1 mg, Iodine 150 mcg, Iron 90 mg, Niacinamide 20 mg, Pyridoxine HCl 20 mg, Riboflavin 3.4 mg, Thiamine HCl 3 mg, Vitamin A 2700 Units, Vitamin E 30 Units, Zinc 25 mg	Ultra Natalcare by KV	10609-1358	Vitamin
ETHEX <> 30	Tab, White, Partially Bisected	Morphine Sulfate 30 mg	MSIR by Ethex	58177-0314	Analgesic; C II
ETHEX <> 30	Tab, Partially Bisected	Morphine Sulfate 30 mg	by KV	10609-1406	Analgesic; C II

ID FRONT <> BACK	DESCRIPTION FRONT <> BACK	INGREDIENT & STRENGTH	BRAND (OR EQUIV.) & FIRM	NDC#	CLASS; SCH.
ETHEX <> 301	Tab, White, Round, Film Coated	Ketorolac Tromethamine 10 mg	by Murfreesboro Ph	51129-1437	NSAID
ETHEX <> 301	Tab, Film Coated, Red Ink	Ketorolac Tromethamine 10 mg	by Allscripts	54569-4494	NSAID
ETHEX <> 301	Tab, White, Film Coated, in Red Ink	Ketorolac Tromethamine 10 mg	Toradol by Ethex	58177-0301	NSAID
ETHEX <> 301	Tab, White, Round, Film Coated	Ketorolac Tromethamine 10 mg	by Compumed	00403-4136	NSAID
ETHEX <> 301	Tab, Film Coated, Red-Printed	Ketorolac Tromethamine 10 mg	by Syntex	18393-0301	NSAID
ETHEX <> 302	Tab, DR	Naproxen 375 mg	by Syntex	18393-0257	NSAID
ETHEX <> 302	Tab, DR	Naproxen 375 mg	by Allscripts	54569-4523	NSAID
ETHEX <> 303	Tab	Naproxen 500 mg	by Allscripts	54569-4520	NSAID
ETHEX <> 303	Tab, DR	Naproxen 500 mg	by PDRX	55289-0307	NSAID
ETHEX <> 303	Tab, DR	Naproxen 500 mg	by Syntex	18393-0258	NSAID
ETHEX <> 308	Tab, White, Film Coated, Scored	Guaifenesin 1200 mg	Guaifenex G by Ethex	58177-0308	Expectorant
ETHEX <> 308	Tab, Film Coated, Scored	Guaifenesin 1200 mg	Guaifenex G by KV	10609-1397	Expectorant
ETHEX <> 316	Tab, Tan, Oval, Film Coated, Scored	Ascorbic Acid 120 mg, Biotin 30 mcg, Calcium 200 mg, Chromium 25 mcg, Copper 2 mg, Cyanocobalamin 12 mcg, Folic Acid 1 mg, Iodine 150 mcg, Iron 27 mg, Magnesium 25 mg, Manganese 5 mg, Molybdenum 25 mcg, Niacinamide 20 mg, Pantothenic Acid 10 mg, Pyridoxine HCl 10 mg, Riboflavin 3.4 mg, Selenium 20 mcg, Thiamine HCl 3 mg, Vitamin A 5000 Units, Vitamin D 400 Units, Vitamin E 30 mg, Zinc 25 mg	Prenatal Mtr by Ethex	58177-0316	Vitamin
ETHEX <> 316	Tab, Film Coated, Scored	Ascorbic Acid 120 mg, Biotin 30 mcg, Calcium 200 mg, Chromium 25 mcg, Copper 2 mg, Cyanocobalamin 12 mcg, Folic Acid 1 mg, Iodine 150 mcg, Iron 27 mg, Magnesium 25 mg, Manganese 5 mg, Molybdenum 25 mcg, Niacinamide 20 mg, Pantothenic Acid 10 mg, Pyridoxine HCl 10 mg, Riboflavin 3.4 mg, Selenium 20 mcg, Thiamine HCl 3 mg, Vitamin A 5000 Units, Vitamin D 400 Units, Vitamin E 30 mg, Zinc 25 mg	Prenatal Mtr by KV	10609-1412	Vitamin
ETHEX <> 317	Tab, White, Oval	Prenatal Multivitamin	Enfamil Natalins by Ethex	58177-0317	Vitamin
ETHEX <> 322	Tab, Orange	Prenatal Multivitamin	NataFort by Ethex	58177-0322	Vitamin
ETHEX <> 322	Tab, Orange, Oval, Film	Vitamin A 1000 Units, Ascorbic Acid 120 mg, Iron 60 mg, Cholecalsifecol, Vitamin E, Thiamine 2 mg, Riboflavin 3 mg, Niacinamide 20 mg, Pyridoxine HCl 10 mg, Folic Acid 1 mg, Cyanocobalomin 12 mcg	Natalcare CFE 60 by Thrift Drug	59198-0320	Vitamin
ETHEX <> 328	Tab, White, Oval	Prenatal Multivitamin	Nestabs CBF by Ethex	58177-0328	Vitamin
ETHEX <> 329	Tab, Purple, Oval	Prenatal Multivitamin	Nestabs FA by Ethex	58177-0329	Vitamin
ETHEX <> 350	Tab, White, Oval	Vitamin A 2700 unt; Ascorbic Acid 120 mg; Calcium 200 mg; Iron 90 mg; Vitamin D 400 unt; Thiamine HCl 3 mg; Riboflavin 3.4 mg; Niacinamide 20 mg; Pyridoxine HCl 20 mg; Folic Acid 1 mg; Cyanocobalamin 12 mcg; Zinc 25 mg; Copper 2 mg; Magnesium 30 mg	Advanced Natalcare Prenatal Vitamins by Ethex	58177-0350	Vitamin
ETHEX <> 350	Tab, White, Oval	Vitamin A 2700 unt, Ascorbic Acid 120 mg, Calcium 200 mg, Iron 90 mg; Vitamin D 400 unt; Thiamine HCl 3 mg; Riboflavin 3.4 mg; Niacinamide 20 mg; Pyridoxine HCl 20 mg; Folic Acid 1 mg; Cyanocobalamin 12 mcg; Zinc 25 mg, Copper 2 mg, Magnesium 30 mg	Advanced Natalcare Prenatal Vitamins by KV Pharm	10609-1463	Vitamin
ETHEX 015	Cap, Blue & Clear	Guaifenesin 300 mg, Pseudoephedrine 60 mg	Guaifed PD by KV		Cold Remedy
ETHEX 277	Tab, Blue, Oval	AM Guaifensin 600 mg, Pseudoephedrine 60 mg, PM Guaif 600 mg, Dextrom 30 mg	Syn RX DM by Ethex	58177-0277	Cold Remedy
ETHEX001	Cap, Clear	Potassium Chloride 10 mEq	by Purdue Pharma	59011-0100	Electrolytes
ETHEX001	Cap	Potassium Chloride 750 mg	by Med Pro	53978-5044	Electrolytes
ETHEX001	Cap, Clear, Hard Gel	Potassium Chloride 750 mg	by Promeco SA	64674-0018	Electrolytes
ETHEX001	Cap, Clear, Ex Release, with White Beads	Potassium Chloride 750 mg	by Quality Care	60346-0112	Electrolytes
ETHEX001	Cap, Clear, Hard Gel	Potassium Chloride 750 mg	by Vangard Labs	00615-1318	Electrolytes
ETHEX003	Cap, Purple & Yellow	Disopyramide Phosphate ER 100 mg	Norpace CR by KV		Antiarrhythmic
ETHEX005	Cap, ER	Nitroglycerin 6.5 mg	by Physicians Total Care	54868-0689	Vasodilator
ETHEX005	Cap, ER	Nitroglycerin 6.5 mg	by KV	10609-0635	Vasodilator
ETHEX015	Cap, Blue & Clear, Ethex/015	Phenylpropanolamine HCl 60 mg, Guaifenesin 300 mg	Guaifed-PD by Ethex	58177-0015	Cold Remedy
ETHEX016	Cap, Clear & White	Guaifenesin 250 mg, Pseudoephedrine 120 mg	Guaifed by KV		Cold Remedy
ETHEX016	Cap, Clear & White, Ethex/016	Phenylpropanolamine HCl 120 mg, Guaifenesin 250 mg	Guaifed by Ethex	58177-0016	Cold Remedy

ID FRONT <> BACK	DESCRIPTION FRONT <> BACK	INGREDIENT & STRENGTH	BRAND (OR EQUIV.) & FIRM	NDC#	CLASS; SCH.
ETHEX017	Cap, Clear	Hyoscyamine Sulfate 0.375 mg	Levsinex by KV		Gastrointestinal
ETHEX017	Cap, Clear, Ethex/017	Hyoscyamine 0.375 mg	Levsinex by Ethex	58177-0017	Gastrointestinal
ETHEX019	Cap, Clear & Green, Ex Release, with Beads, in Black Ink	Brompheniramine Maleate 12 mg, Pseudoephedrine HCl 120 mg	Nasal Decongestant by Quality Care	60346-0929	Cold Remedy
ETHEX019	Cap, Clear & Green, Ethex/019	Pseudoephedrine 120 mg	Bromfed by Ethex	58177-0019	Decongestant
ETHEX020	Cap, Clear & Green	Bromopheniramine 6 mg, Pseuodephedrine 60 mg	Bromfed PD by KV		Cold Remedy
ETHEX020	Cap, Clear & Green, Ethex/020	Pseudoephedrine 60 mg	Bromfed PD by Ethex	58177-0020	Decongestant
ETHEX022	Cap, Pink & White	Phenylprop. 50 mg, Phenyltol. 16 mg, Pyrilamine 16 mg, Pheniramine 16 mg	Poly-Histine D by KV		Cold Remedy
ETHEX022	Cap, Pink & White, Ethex/022	Phenylpropanolamine HCl 50 mg, Phenyltoloxamine Citrate 16 mg, Pyrilamine Maleate 16 mg, Pheniramine Maleate 16 mg	Poly-Histine-D by Ethex	58177-0022	Cold Remedy
ETHEX023	Cap, White	Phenylprop. 25 mg, Phenyltol. 8 mg, Pyrilamine 8 mg, Pheniramine 8 mg	Poly-Histine D Ped by KV		Cold Remedy
ETHEX023	Cap, White, Ethex/023	Phenylpropanolamine HCl 25 mg, Phenyltoloxamine Citrate 8 mg, Pyrilamine Maleate 8 mg, Pheniramine Maleate 8 mg	Poly-Histine-D Ped by Ethex	58177-0023	Cold Remedy
ETHEX024	Cap, Orange	Iron 150 mg	Fe-Tinic by KV		Mineral
ETHEX024	Cap, Orange	Iron 150 mg	Niferex by Ethex	58177-0024	Mineral
ETHEX027	Cap, Maroon, Ethex/027	Merperidine HCl 50 mg, Promethazine HCl 25 mg	Mepergan Fortis by Ethex	58177-0027	Analgesic
ETHEX041	Cap, Peach & White	Oxycodone HCl 5 mg	OXYIR by Ethex	58177-0041	Analgesic; C II
ETHEX042	Cap, Maroon	Ferrous Fum 200 mg~10 mcg, Ascorbic 250 mg, Cyanocob 10 mcg	Chromagen by Ethex	58177-0042	Mineral
ETHEX043	Cap, Brown & Green, Gelatin, Ethex/043	Ferrous Fumarate 200 mg, Ascoribic Acid 250 mg	Chromagen FA by Ethex	58177-0043	Mineral
ETHEX044	Cap, Brown	Liver Concentrate 240 mg, Ascorbic Acid 75 mg, Cyanocobalamin 15 mcg; Iron 110 mg; Folic Acid 0.5 mg	Conison by Ethex	58177-0044	Deficiency Anemias
ETHEX044	Cap, Brown	Liver Concentrate 240 mg, Ascorbic Acid 75 mg, Cyanocobalamin 15 mcg; Iron 110 mg, Folic Acid 0.5 mg	Conison by KV Pharm	10609-1458	Deficiency Anemias
ETHEX048	Cap, Blue & Clear	Lipase 12000 unt, Amylase 39000 unt, Protease 39000 unt	Pangestyme UL 12 by Ethex	58177-0048	Gastrointestinal
ETHEX048	Cap, Blue & Clear	Lipase 12000 unt, Amylase 39000 unt, Protease 39000 unt	Pangestyme UL 12 by KV Pharm	10609-1468	Gastrointestinal
ETHEX049	Cap, Blue	Lipase 18000 unt, Amylase 58500 unt, Protease 58500 unt	Pangestyme UL 18 by Ethex	58177-0049	Gastrointestinal
ETHEX050	Cap, Clear & Green	Lipase 20000 unt, Amylase 65000 unt, Protease 65000 unt	Pangestyme UL 20 by Ethex	58177-0050	Gastrointestinal
ETHEX050	Cap, Clear & Green	Lipase 20000 unt, Amylase 65000 unt, Protease 65000 unt	Pangestyme UL 20 by KV Pharm	10609-1470	Gastrointestinal
ETHEX204	Tab, White, Oval	Guaifenesin 600 mg, Phenylpropanolamine HCl 75 mg	Dura-Vent by Ethex	58177-0204	Cold Remedy
ETHEX204	Tab, White, Oval	Phenylpropanolamine 75 mg, Guaifenesin 600 mg	Dura-Vent by KV		Cold Remedy
ETHEX205	Tab, White, Oval	Guaifenesin 600 mg	Humibid LA by Ethex	58177-0205	Expectorant
ETHEX205	Tab, Ethex/205	Guaifenesin 600 mg, Pseudoephedrine HCl 60 mg	Guaifenex Rx by KV	10609-1362	Cold Remedy
ETHEX208	Tab, White, Oval	Guaifenesin 600 mg, Phenylpropanolamine HCl 120 mg	Guaifenex PSE 120 by Ethex	58177-0208	Cold Remedy
ETHEX208	Tab, Yellow, Oval	Pseudoephedrine HCl 120 mg, Guaifenesin 600 mg	Entex PSE by KV		Cold Remedy
ETHEX212	Tab, Pink, Oval, Film Coated, Ethex/212	Ascorbic Acid 120 mg, Calcium 250 mg, Copper 2 mg, Cyanocobalamin 12 mcg, Docusate Sodium 50 mg, Folic Acid 1 mg, Iodine 0.15 mg, Iron 90 mg, Niacinamide 20 mg, Pyridoxine HCl 20 mg, Riboflavin 3.4 mg, Thiamine Mononitrate 3 mg, Vitamin A 4000 Units, Vitamin D 400 Units, Vitamin E 30 Units, Zinc 25 mg	Prenatal Mr 90 by Ethex	58177-0212	Vitamin
ETHEX213	Tab, Green, Ethex/213	Dextromethorphan Hydrobromide 30 mg, Guaifenesin 600 mg, Pseudoephedrine HCl 60 mg	Guaifenex Rx DM by Ethex	58177-0277	Cold Remedy
ETHEX213	Tab, Ethex/213	Dextromethorphan Hydrobromide 30 mg, Guaifenesin 600 mg, Pseudoephedrine HCl 60 mg	Guaifenex Rx DM by KV	10609-1363	Cold Remedy
ETHEX213	Tab, Green, Oval, Ethex/213	Dextromethorphan Hydrobromide 30 mg, Guaifenesin 600 mg	Guaifenex DM by Ethex	58177-0213	Cold Remedy
ETHEX213	Tab, Blue, Ethex/213	Guaifenesin 600 mg, Pseudoephedrine HCl 60 mg	Guaifenex Rx by Ethex	58177-0276	Cold Remedy
ETHEX214	Tab, Blue, Ethex/214	Dextromethorphan Hydrobromide 30 mg, Guaifenesin 600 mg, Pseudoephedrine HCl 60 mg	Guaifenex Rx DM by Ethex	58177-0277	Cold Remedy
ETHEX214	Tab, Ethex/214	Dextromethorphan Hydrobromide 30 mg, Guaifenesin 600 mg, Pseudoephedrine HCl 60 mg	Guaifenex Rx DM by KV	10609-1363	Cold Remedy
ETHEX214	Tab, Blue, Ethex/213	Guaifenesin 600 mg, Pseudoephedrine HCl 60 mg	Guaifenex Rx by Ethex	58177-0276	Cold Remedy
ETHEX214	Tab, Blue, Oval, Ethex/214	Guaifenesin 600 mg, Pseudoephedrine HCl 60 mg	Guaifenex PSE 60 by Ethex	58177-0214	Cold Remedy
ETHEX214	Tab, Ethex/214	Guaifenesin 600 mg, Pseudoephedrine HCl 60 mg	Guaifenex PSE 60 by KV	10609-1312	Cold Remedy
ETHEX214	Tab, Ethex/214	Guaifenesin 600 mg, Pseudoephedrine HCl 60 mg	Guaifenex Rx by KV	10609-1362	Cold Remedy
ETHEX217	Tab, Tan, Oblong	Prenatal Vitamin	Materna by KV		Vitamin

ID FRONT <> BACK	DESCRIPTION FRONT <> BACK	INGREDIENT & STRENGTH	BRAND (OR EQUIV.) & FIRM	NDC#	CLASS; SCH.
ETHEX218	Tab, Blue, Oblong	Prenatal Vitamin	Zenate by KV		Vitamin
ETHEX223	Tab, Coated	Codeine Phosphate 10 mg, Guaifenesin 300 mg	by Quality Care	62682-8003	Cold Remedy; C III
ETHEX223	Tab, Red, Oval, Ethex/223	Guaifenesin 300 mg, Codeine Phsphate 10 mg	Guaifenesin by Ethex	58177-0223	Analgesic; C III
ETHEX224	Tab, White, Cap-Shaped	Prenatal Multivitamin	Zenate by KV		Vitamin
ETHEX227	Tab, Film Coated, Ethex/227	Chlorpheniramine Maleate 8 mg, Methscopolamine Nitrate 2.5 mg, Phenylephrine HCl 20 mg	Hista Vent DA by KV	10609-1332	Cold Remedy
ETHEX227	Cap, Brown, Ethex/227	Chlorpheniramine Maleate 8 mg, Phenylephrine HCl 20 mg, Methscopolamine Nitrate 2.5 mg	Dura-Vent by Ethex	58177-0227	Cold Remedy
ETHEX234	Tab, Buff, Oblong	Phenylephrine 25 mg, Chlorpheniramine 8 mg, Pyrilamine 25 mg	Rynatan by Carter-Wallace		Cold Remedy
ETHEX236	Tab, Orange & White, Round	Carisoprodol Compound (Aspirin 325 mg, Carisoprodol 200 mg)	Soma Compound by Carter-Wallace		Muscle Relaxant
ETHEX237	Tab, Peach, Ethex/237	Hyoscyamine Sulfate 0.375 mg	Levbid by Ethex	58177-0237	Gastrointestinal
ETHEX237	Tab, Ex Release, Ethex/237	Hyoscyamine Sulfate 0.375 mg	by KV	10609-1345	Gastrointestinal
ETHEX256	Tab, Yellow, Caplet	Multivitamin	Nephro-Vite by KV		Vitamin
ETHEX257	Tab, Blue, Oval, Film Coated	Ascorbic Acid 50 mg, Calcium 125 mg, Cyanocobalamin 3 mcg, Folic Acid 1 mg, Iron 60 mg, Niacinamide 10 mg, Pyridoxine HCl 2 mg, Riboflavin 3 mg, Thiamine Mononitrate 3 mg, Vitamin A 4000 Units, Vitamin D 400 Units, Zinc 18 mg	Natalcare Pic by Ethex	58177-0257	Vitamin
ETHEX257	Tab, Film Coated	Ascorbic Acid 50 mg, Calcium 125 mg, Cyanocobalamin 3 mcg, Folic Acid 1 mg, Iron 60 mg, Niacinamide 10 mg, Pyridoxine HCl 2 mg, Riboflavin 3 mg, Thiamine Mononitrate 3 mg, Vitamin A 4000 Units, Vitamin D 400 Units, Zinc 18 mg	Natalcare Pic by KV	10609-1374	Vitamin
ETHEX258	Tab, White, Oval, Film Coated	Ascorbic Acid 80 mg, Calcium 250 mg, Copper 2 mg, Cyanocobalamin 12 mcg, Folic Acid 1 mg, Iodine 0.2 mg, Iron 60 mg, Magnesium 10 mg, Niacinamide 20 mg, Pyridoxine HCl 4 mg, Riboflavin 3.4 mg, Thiamine 3 mg, Vitamin A Acetate 5000 Units, Vitamin D 400 Units, Vitamin E 30 Units, Zinc 25 mg	Natalcare Pic Forte by Ethex	58177-0258	Vitamin
ETHEX258	Tab, Film Coated, Ethex/258	Ascorbic Acid 80 mg, Calcium 250 mg, Copper 2 mg, Cyanocobalamin 12 mcg, Folic Acid 1 mg, Iodine 0.2 mg, Iron 60 mg, Magnesium 10 mg, Niacinamide 20 mg, Pyridoxine HCl 4 mg, Riboflavin 3.4 mg, Thiamine 3 mg, Vitamin A Acetate 5000 Units, Vitamin D 400 Units, Vitamin E 30 Units, Zinc 25 mg	Natalcare Pic Forte by KV	10609-1369	Vitamin
ETHEX260	Tab, Tan, Ovaloid	Prenatal Vitamin, Beta Carotene	Materna/Beta Caroten by KV		Vitamin
ETHEX276	Tab, Blue, Oval	Guaifenesin 600 mg, Phenylpropanolamine 60 mg, HCl 600 mg	Syn RX by Ethex	58177-0276	Cold Remedy
ETHEX302	Tab, White, Ethex/302	Enteric Naproxen 375 mg	EC Naprosyn by Ethex	58177-0302	NSAID
ETHEX303	Tab, White, Ethex/303	Enteric Naproxen 500 mg	EC Naprosyn by Ethex	58177-0303	NSAID
ETHMOZINE200 <> ROBERTS	Tab, Film Coated	Moricizine HCl 200 mg	by Roberts	54092-0046	Antiarrhythmic
ETHMOZINE250 <> ROBERTS	Tab, Film Coated	Moricizine HCl 250 mg	by Roberts	54092-0047	Antiarrhythmic
ETHMOZINE300 <> ROBERTS	Tab, Film Coated	Moricizine HCl 300 mg	by Roberts	54092-0048	Antiarrhythmic
ETO200	Cap, Black & Pink	Etodolac 200 mg	by Taro Pharm (IS)	52549-4016	NSAID
ETO200	Cap, Black & Pink	Etodolac 200 mg	by Taro Pharms (US)	51672-4016	NSAID
ETO300	Cap, Black & Pink	Etodolac 300 mg	by Taro Pharms (US)	51672-4017	NSAID
ETO300	Cap, Black & Pink	Etodolac 300 mg	by Taro Pharm (IS)	52549-4017	NSAID
EUFLEX	Tab, Yellow, Round	Flutamide 250 mg	Euflex by Schering	Canadian	Antiandrogen
EV0072	Tab, Film Coated	Ascorbic Acid 60 mg, Calcium 125 mg, Cyanocobalamin 5 mcg, Folic Acid 1 mg, Iron 65 mg, Niacin 15 mg, Pyridoxine HCl 2.5 mg, Riboflavin 1.8 mg, Thiamine Mononitrate 1.1 mg, Vitamin A 6000 Units, Vitamin D 400 Units, Vitamin E 30 Units	Vitafol by Lini	58215-0301	Vitamin
EV0078	Tab, Film Coated	Ascorbic Acid 60 mg, Calcium 125 mg, Cyanocobalamin 5 mcg, Folic Acid 1 mg, Iron 65 mg, Magnesium 25 mg, Niacin 15 mg, Pyridoxine HCl 2.5 mg, Riboflavin 1.8 mg, Selenium 65 mcg, Thiamine HCl 1.6 mg, Vitamin A 4000 Units, Vitamin D 400 Units, Vitamin E 30 Units, Zinc 15 mg	Vitafol PN by Lini	58215-0121	Vitamin

ID FRONT <> BACK	DESCRIPTION FRONT <> BACK	INGREDIENT & STRENGTH	BRAND (OR EQUIV.) & FIRM	NDC#	CLASS; SCH.
EV0078	Tab, Film Coated	Ascorbic Acid 60 mg, Calcium 125 mg, Cyanocobalamin 5 mcg, Folic Acid 1 mg, Iron 65 mg, Magnesium 25 mg, Niacin 15 mg, Pyridoxine HCl 2.5 mg, Riboflavin 1.8 mg, Thiamine HCl 1.6 mg, Vitamin A 4000 Units, Vitamin D 400 Units, Vitamin E 30 Units, Zinc 15 mg	Vitafol PN by Lini	58215-0134	Vitamin
EV0078	Tab, Blue, Film Coated	Ascorbic Acid 60 mg, Calcium 125 mg, Cyanocobalamin 5 mcg, Folic Acid 1 mg, Iron 65 mg, Magnesium 25 mg, Niacin 15 mg, Pyridoxine HCl 2.5 mg, Riboflavin 1.8 mg, Thiamine HCl 1.6 mg, Vitamin A 4000 Units, Vitamin D 400 Units, Vitamin E 30 Units, Zinc 15 mg	Vitafol PN by Everett	00642-0078	Vitamin
EV0204	Tab, Film Coated	Ascorbic Acid 500 mg, Biotin 0.15 mg, Chromium 0.1 mg, Copper 3 mg, Cyanocobalamin 50 mcg, Folic Acid 0.8 mg, Iron 10 mg, Magnesium 50 mg, Molybdenum 25 mcg, Niacin 100 mg, Pantothenic Acid 25 mg, Pyridoxine HCl 25 mg, Riboflavin 20 mg, Selenium 50 mcg, Thiamine HCl 20 mg, Vitamin A 4000 Units, Vitamin E 60 Units, Zinc 15 mg	Strovite Forte by Lini	58215-0328	Vitamin
EV0204	Tab, Green, Film Coated	Ascorbic Acid 500 mg, Biotin 0.15 mg, Chromium 0.1 mg, Copper 3 mg, Cyanocobalamin 50 mcg, Folic Acid 0.8 mg, Iron 10 mg, Magnesium 50 mg, Molybdenum 25 mcg, Niacin 100 mg, Pantothenic Acid 25 mg, Pyridoxine HCl 25 mg, Riboflavin 20 mg, Selenium 50 mcg, Thiamine HCl 20 mg, Vitamin A 4000 Units, Vitamin E 60 Units, Zinc 15 mg	Strovite Forte by Everett	00642-0204	Vitamin
EV0300	Cap, White, Film Coated	Biotin 300 mcg, Chromium 200 mcg, Folic Acid 2.5 mg, Niacin 20 mg, Pantothenic Acid 10 mg, Selenium 70 mcg, Vitamin B1 3 mg, Vitamin B2 2 mg, Vitamin B6 15 mg, Vitamin B12 12 mg, Vitamin C 50 mg, Vitamin E 35 IU, Zinc 20 mg	Renax by Everett	00642-0300	Vitamin
EV0650	Tab, White, Oblong, Scored	Guaifenesin 600 mg; Pseudoephedrine HCl 60 mg; Dextromethorphan Hydrobromide 30 mg	by Pfab	62542-0771	Cold Remedy
EV201	Tab, Film Coated	Ascorbic Acid 500 mg, Biotin 0.15 mg, Chromium 0.1 mg, Copper 3 mg, Cyanocobalamin 50 mcg, Folic Acid 0.8 mg, Iron 27 mg, Magnesium 50 mg, Manganese 5 mg, Niacin 100 mg, Pantothenic Acid 25 mg, Pyridoxine HCl 25 mg, Riboflavin 20 mg, Thiamine HCl 20 mg, Vitamin A 5000 Units, Vitamin E 30 Units, Zinc 22.5 mg	Strovite Plus by Lini	58215-0330	Vitamin
EV201	Tab, Film Coated	Ascorbic Acid 500 mg, Biotin 0.15 mg, Chromium 0.1 mg, Copper 3 mg, Cyanocobalamin 50 mcg, Folic Acid 0.8 mg, Iron 27 mg, Magnesium 50 mg, Manganese 5 mg, Niacin 100 mg, Pantothenic Acid 25 mg, Pyridoxine HCl 25 mg, Riboflavin 20 mg, Thiamine Mononitrate 20 mg, Vitamin A 5000 Units, Vitamin E 30 Units, Zinc 22.5 mg	Bacmin by Marnel	00682-3000	Vitamin
EV201	Tab, Dark Red, Film Coated	Ascorbic Acid 500 mg, Biotin 0.15 mg, Chromium 0.1 mg, Copper 3 mg, Cyanocobalamin 50 mcg, Folic Acid 0.8 mg, Iron 27 mg, Magnesium 50 mg, Manganese 5 mg, Niacin 100 mg, Pantothenic Acid 25 mg, Pyridoxine HCl 25 mg, Riboflavin 20 mg, Thiamine HCl 20 mg, Vitamin A 5000 Units, Vitamin E 30 Units, Zinc 22.5 mg	Strovite Plus by Everett	00642-0201	Vitamin
EV201	Tab, Dark Red, Film Coated	Ascorbic Acid 500 mg, Biotin 0.15 mg, Chromium 0.1 mg, Copper 3 mg, Cyanocobalamin 50 mcg, Folic Acid 0.8 mg, Iron 27 mg, Magnesium 50 mg, Manganese 5 mg, Niacin 100 mg, Pantothenic Acid 25 mg, Pyridoxine HCl 25 mg, Riboflavin 20 mg, Thiamine Mononitrate 20 mg, Vitamin A 5000 Units, Vitamin E 30 Units, Zinc 22.5 mg	Bacmin by Lini	58215-0316	Vitamin
EVERETT0072	Tab, Maroon, Oblong	Multivitamin, Iron, Folic Acid	Vitafol by Everett		Vitamin
EVERETT0078	Tab, Blue, Oblong	Prenatal Vitamin	by Everett		Vitamin
EVERETT0201	Tab, Pink, Oblong	Multivitamin, Minerals	Strovite Plus by Everett		Vitamin
EVERETT0204	Tab, Green, Oblong	Multivitamin, Minerals	Strovite Forte by Everett		Vitamin
EVERETT162	Tab, White, Round	Butalbital 50 mg, Caffeine 40 mg, Acetaminophen 325 mg	Repan by Everett		Analgesic
EVERETT164	Cap, White	Butalbital 50 mg, Caffeine 40 mg, Acetaminophen 325 mg	Repan by Everett		Analgesic
EVERETT166	Tab, Blue	Butalbital 50 mg, Acetaminophen 650 mg	Repan CF by Everett		Analgesic

ID FRONT <> BACK	DESCRIPTION FRONT <> BACK	INGREDIENT & STRENGTH	BRAND (OR EQUIV.) & FIRM	NDC#	CLASS; SCH.
EVOO78	Cap, Blue, Scored	Magnesium Oxide, Zinc Gluconate, Cyanocobalamin, Folic Acid, Thiamine Mononitrate, Pyridoxine HCl, Riboflavin, Calcium Carbonate, Tocopheryl Acetate, Beta-Carotene, Niacinamide, Ascorbic Acid, Ferrous Fumarate	Vitafol PN by Nat Pharmpak Serv	55154-4921	Mineral
EWGEIGY	Tab, Peach, Round, EW/Geigy	Desipramine HCl 25 mg	Pertofrane by Geigy	Canadian	Antidepressant
EXELO45MG	Cap, Red, Exelon 4.5 mg in White Ink	Rivastigmine Tartrate 4.5 mg	Exelon by Novartis Pharms	00078-0325	Antialzheimers
EXELON15MG	Cap, Yellow, Gelatin, Exelon 1.5 mg	Rivastigmine 1.5 mg	Exelon by Novartis Pharm AG	Canadian DIN# 02242115	Antialzheimers
EXELON15MG	Cap, Yellow, Exelon 1.5 mg in Red Ink	Rivastigmine Tartrate 1.5 mg	Exelon by Novartis Pharms	00078-0323	Antialzheimers
EXELON15MG	Cap, Yellow	Rivastigmine Tartrate 1.5 mg	Exelon by Novartis Pharm AG	17088-0018	Antialzheimers
EXELON3MG	Cap, Orange, Gelatin	Rivastigmine 3 mg	Exelon by Novartis Pharm AG	Canadian DIN# 02242116	Antialzheimers
EXELON3MG	Cap, Orange	Rivastigmine Tartrate 3 mg	Exelon by Novartis Pharm AG	17088-0019	Antialzheimers
EXELON3MG	Cap, Orange, Exelon 3 mg in Red Ink	Rivastigmine Tartrate 3 mg	Exelon by Novartis Pharms	00078-0324	Antialzheimers
EXELON45MG	Cap, Red, Gelatin, Exelon 4.5 mg	Rivastigmine 4.5 mg	Exelon by Novartis Pharm AG	Canadian DIN# 02242117	Antialzheimers
EXELON45MG	Cap, Red	Rivastigmine Tartrate 4.5 mg	Exelon by Novartis Pharm AG	17088-0020	Antialzheimers
EXELON6MG	Cap, Orange & Red, Gelatin	Rivastigmine 6 mg	Exelon by Novartis Pharm AG	Canadian DIN# 02242118	Antialzheimers
EXELON6MG	Cap, Orange & Red, Exelon 6 mg in red ink	Rivastigmine Tartrate 6 mg	Exelon by Novartis Pharms	00078-0326	Antialzheimers
EXELON6MG	Cap, Orange	Rivastigmine Tartrate 6 mg	Exelon by Novartis Pharm AG	17088-0021	Antialzheimers
EZCHEW	Tab, White, Round, Chewable	Erythromycin Chewable 200 mg	EryPed Chewable by Abbott	00074-6314	Antibiotic
EZOL <> EZOL	Cap, Green Print	Acetaminophen 325 mg, Butalbital 50 mg, Caffeine 40 mg	Ezol by Stewart Jackson	45985-0578	Analgesic
F	Tab, Pink, Round, Schering Logo/F	Amitriptyline HCl 4 mg, Perphenazine 25 mg	Etrafon by Bayer	Canadian	Antipsychotic
F	Cap	Ascorbic Acid 100 mg, Biotin 150 mcg, Cyanocobalamin 6 mcg, Folic Acid 1 mg, Niacin 20 mg, Pantothenic Acid 5 mg, Pyridoxine HCl 10 mg, Riboflavin 1.7 mg, Thiamine Mononitrate 1.5 mg	Nephrocaps Vit by Fleming	00256-0185	Vitamin
F	Cap, F Within a Triangle	Ascorbic Acid 100 mg, Biotin 150 mcg, Cyanocobalamin 6 mcg, Folic Acid 1 mg, Niacin 20 mg, Pantothenic Acid 5 mg, Pyridoxine HCl 10 mg, Riboflavin 1.7 mg, Thiamine 1.5 mg	Nephrocaps by Quality Care	62682-9000	Vitamin
F	Tab, Red, Logo/F	Perphenazine 4 mg, Amitriptyline 25 mg	by Schering	Canadian	Antipsychotic; Antidepressant
F	Tab, Scored	Propoxyphene HCl 65 mg	by Frosst	Canadian	Analgesic
F	Tab, Salmon, Oval, Scored	Propoxyphene HCl 65 mg, Aspirin 375 mg, Caffeine 30 mg	by Frosst	Canadian	Analgesic
F <> A1	Tab, Yellow, Oblong	Triamcinolone 1 mg	Aristocort by Fujisawa	00469-5121	Steroid
F <> A4	Tab	Triamcinolone 4 mg	Aristocort by Lederle	00005-4419	Steroid
F <> A4	Tab	Triamcinolone 4 mg	Aristocort by Fujisawa	00469-5124	Steroid
F01CPI	Tab, Yellow, Round, F01/CPI	Folic Acid 1 mg	Folvite by Charlotte/Phoe		Vitamin
F04	Cap, Gray & Red	Cycloserine 250 mg	Seromycin by Lilly		Antibiotic
F05	Tab, Chewable, F over 0.5	Fluoride Ion	Fluoritab by Fluoritab	00288-5509	Mineral
F05	Tab, Chewable, F over 0.5	Fluoride Ion	Fluoritab by Fluoritab	00288-5511	Mineral
F05	Tab, Chewable, F over 0.5	Fluoride Ion	Fluoritab by Fluoritab	00288-5510	Mineral
F05	Tab, Chewable, F over 0.5	Fluoride Ion	Fluoritab by Century	00436-0776	Mineral
F05	Tab, Chewable, F over 0.5	Fluoride Ion	Fluoritab by Century	00436-0778	Mineral
F05	Tab, Chewable, F over 0.5	Fluoride Ion	Fluoritab by Century	00436-0777	Mineral
F1	Tab, Chewable, F/1	Fluoride Ion	Fluoritab by Fluoritab	00288-1108	Mineral
F1	Tab, Chewable, F/1	Fluoride Ion	Fluoritab by Century	00436-0774	Mineral
F1	Tab, Chew, F/1	Sodium Fluoride 1.1 mg	Fluoritab by Fluoritab	00288-1106	Element
F1	Tab, Chew, F/1	Sodium Fluoride 1.1 mg	Fluoritab by Century	00436-0772	Element

ID FRONT <> BACK	DESCRIPTION FRONT <> BACK	INGREDIENT & STRENGTH	BRAND (OR EQUIV.) & FIRM	NDC#	CLASS; SCH.
F1	Tab, Chew, F Over 1	Sodium Fluoride 1.1 mg	Fluoritab by Century	00436-0770	Element
F100	Tab, White	Flurbiprofen 100 mg	by Knoll	Canadian	NSAID
F11 <> LL	Tab	Furosemide 20 mg	by Quality Care	60346-0761	Diuretic
F11 <> LL	Tab	Furosemide 20 mg	by UDL	51079-0072	Diuretic
F12 <> LL	Tab, F over 12 <> LL	Furosemide 40 mg	by UDL	51079-0073	Diuretic
F13 <> LL	Tab, F over 13 <> LL	Furosemide 80 mg	by UDL	51079-0527	Diuretic
F14	Cap, Yellow	Ephedrine Sulfate 25 mg, Amobarbital 50 mg	Ephedrine & Amytal by Lilly		Antiasthmatic
F15	Cap, Red	Comb. Liver Stomach Conc., Iron, B Vitamins	Lextron by Lilly		Digestant
F16	Cap, Red	Comb. Liver Stomach Conc., Iron, B Vitamins	Lextron Ferrous by Lilly		Digestant
F19	Cap, Brown	Liver Stomach Concentrate	Extralin by Lilly		Hematinic
F2	Tab, Chewable, F/2	Fluoride Ion	Fluoritab by Fluoritab	00288-2203	Mineral
F2	Tab, Chewable, F over 2	Fluoride Ion	Fluoritab by Fluoritab	00288-2204	Mineral
F2	Tab, Chewable, F over 2	Fluoride Ion	Fluoritab by Century	00436-0775	Mineral
F2	Tab, Chewable, F/2	Fluoride Ion	Fluoritab by Century	00436-0773	Mineral
F2	Tab, Chew, F/2	Sodium Fluoride 2.2 mg	Fluoritab by Century	00436-0771	Element
F22 <> LL	Tab, Film Coated, F/22	Fenoprofen Calcium	by UDL	51079-0477	NSAID
F22 <> LL	Tab, Film Coated	Fenoprofen Calcium 691.8 mg	by Quality Care	60346-0233	NSAID
F23	Cap, Blue	Amobarbital Sodium 60 mg	Amytal Sodium by Lilly		Sedative/Hypnotic; C II
F25	Cap, Pink	Ephedrine Sulfate 50 mg	by Lilly		Antiasthmatic
F2F	Cap, White	Triprolidine HCl 2.5 mg, Pseudoephedrene 60 mg, Acetaminophen 500 mg	Actifed Plus ES by Warner Wellcome	Canadian	Cold Remedy
F33	Cap, Blue	Amobarbital Sodium 200 mg	Amytal Sodium by Lilly		Sedative/Hypnotic; C II
F34	Cap, Pink	Arsenic Extract 250 mg	Carbarsone by Lilly		Poison
F36	Cap, Clear	Papaverine 15 mg, Codeine 15 mg	Copavin by Lilly		Analgesic
F39	Cap, Pink	Quinidine Sulfate 200 mg	by Lilly		Antiarrhythmic
F40	Cap, Orange	Secobarbital Sodium 100 mg	Seconal by Lilly		Sedative/Hypnotic; C II
F42	Cap, Orange	Secobarbital Sodium 50 mg	Seconal by Lilly		Sedative/Hypnotic; C II
F5	Tab, White, Round, F/5	Warfarin Sodium 5 mg	by Frosst	Canadian	Anticoagulant
F50	Tab, White	Flurbiprofen 50 mg	by Knoll	Canadian	NSAID
F6171MG	Cap, White	Tacrolimus 1 mg	Prograf by Fujisawa	00469-0617	Immunosuppressant
F64	Cap, Blue & Orange	Amobarbital Sodium 25 mg, Secobarbital Sodium 25 mg	Tuinal by Lilly		Sedative/Hypnotic; C II
F65	Cap, Blue & Orange	Amobarbital Sodium 50 mg, Secobarbital Sodium 50 mg	Tuinal by Lilly		Sedative/Hypnotic; C II
F6575MG	Cap, Pink	Tacrolimus 5 mg	Prograf by Fujisawa	00469-0657	Immunosuppressant
F66	Cap, Blue & Orange	Amobarbital Sodium 100 mg, Secobarbital Sodium 100 mg	Tuinal by Lilly		Sedative/Hypnotic; C II
F66LL	Tab, Beige, Oblong, F/66-LL	Fibercon	Fibercon by Lederle		Laxative
F74	Cap, Red	Vitamin Combination	Tycopan by Lilly		Vitamin
F96	Cap, Brown	Liver Stomach Concentrate, Vitamin Comb.	Reticulex by Lilly		Hematinic
F9BZYLOPRIM	Tab, White, Round, F9B/Zyloprim	Allopurinol 200 mg	by Glaxo	Canadian	Antigout
FA	Tab, Yellow, Oval	Beta-Carotene 4000 Unt; Ascorbic Acid 120 mg; Thiamine HCl 3 mg; Riboflavin 3 mg; Pyridoxine HCl 3 mg; Cyanocobalamin 8 mcg; Niacin 20 mg; Vitamin D 400 Unt; Vitamin E 30 Unt; Folic Acid 1 mg; Calcium 200 mg; Iodine 150 mcg; Iron 29 mg; Zinc 15 mg	Nestabs FA by JB Labs	51111-0008	Vitamin/Mineral
FA <> CIBA	Tab, White, Scored	Hydralazine HCl 10 mg	Apresoline by Novartis	Canadian DIN# 00005525	Antihypertensive
FA2	Tab, Pink, Oblong	Triamcinolone 2 mg	Aristocort by Fujisawa		Steroid
FA8	Tab, Yellow, Oblong	Triamcinolone 8 mg	Aristocort by Fujisawa		Steroid
FAMVIR <> 125	Tab, Film Coated	Famciclovir 125 mg	Famvir by SKB	60351-4115	Antiviral
FAMVIR <> 125	Tab, White, Round, Film Coated	Famciclovir 125 mg	Famvir by Phy Total Care	54868-3882	Antiviral
FAMVIR <> 125	Tab, White, Round, Film Coated	Famciclovir 125 mg	by SmithKline SKB	Canadian DIN# 02229110	Antiviral
FAMVIR <> 125	Tab, White, Film Coated	Famciclovir 125 mg	Famvir by SKB	00007-4115	Antiviral

ID FRONT <> BACK	DESCRIPTION FRONT <> BACK	INGREDIENT & STRENGTH	BRAND (OR EQUIV.) & FIRM	NDC#	CLASS; SCH.
FAMVIR <> 125	Tab, White, Round, Film Coated	Famciclovir 125 mg	Famvir by Novartis	00078-0366	Antiviral
FAMVIR <> 125	Tab, Film Coated	Famciclovir 125 mg	Famvir by Allscripts	54569-4533	Antiviral
FAMVIR <> 125	Tab, Film Coated	Famciclovir 125 mg	Famvir by Apotheca	12634-0508	Antiviral
FAMVIR <> 250	Tab, Film Coated	Famciclovir 250 mg	Famvir by SKB	60351-4116	Antiviral
FAMVIR <> 250	Tab, White, Round, Film Coated	Famciclovir 250 mg	by SmithKline SKB	Canadian DIN# 02229129	Antiviral
FAMVIR <> 250	Tab, White, Round, Film Coated	Famciclovir 250 mg	Famvir by SKB	00007-4116	Antiviral
FAMVIR <> 250	Tab, White, Round, Film Coated	Famciclovir 250 mg	Famvir by Novartis	00078-0367	Antiviral
FAMVIR <> 250	Tab, Film Coated	Famciclovir 250 mg	Famvir by Physicians Total Care	54868-3969	Antiviral
FAMVIR <> 500	Tab, Film Coated	Famciclovir 500 mg	Famvir by SKB	60351-4117	Antiviral
FAMVIR <> 500	Tab, White, Oval, Film Coated	Famciclovir 500 mg	by SmithKline SKB	Canadian DIN# 02177102	Antiviral
FAMVIR <> 500	Tab, White, Round, Film Coated	Famciclovir 500 mg	Famvir by SKB	00007-4117	Antiviral
FAMVIR <> 500	Tab, White, Round, Film Coated	Famciclovir 500 mg	Famvir by Novartis	00078-0368	Antiviral
FAMVIR <> 500	Tab, Film Coated	Famciclovir 500 mg	Famvir by Allscripts	54569-4534	Antiviral
FANSIDARROCHE	Tab	Pyrimethamine 25 mg, Sulfadoxine 500 mg	Fansidar by F Hoffmann La Roche	12806-0161	Antimalarial
FASTIN <> BEECHAM	Cap, Blue & Clear	Phentermine HCl 30 mg	Fastin by PDRX	55289-0180	Anorexiant; C IV
FASTIN <> BEECHAM	Cap, Blue & White Beads	Phentermine HCl 30 mg	Fastin by HJ Harkins Co	52959-0430	Anorexiant; C IV
FASTIN <> BEECHAM	Cap, Blue & White Beads	Phentermine HCl 30 mg	Fastin by King	60793-0836	Anorexiant; C IV
FASTIN <> BEECHAM	Cap, R inside Circle to Right of Fastin in Red Ink <> Beecham in White Ink	Phentermine HCl 30 mg	Fastin by SKB	00029-2205	Anorexiant; C IV
FC	Tab, White, Oval, Abbott Logo	Temafloxacin HCl 400 mg	Omniflox by Abbott		Antibiotic
FC <> SANDOZ78107	Cap, Sandoz Logo F-C <> Sandoz 78-107	Aspirin 325 mg, Butalbital 50 mg, Caffeine 40 mg, Codeine Phosphate 30 mg	Fiorinal w Codeine #3 by Allscripts	54569-0341	Analgesic; C III
FC1SANDOZ78105	Cap, Red & Yellow, F-C #1 Sandoz 78-105	Codeine 7.5 mg, Butalbital 50 mg, Caffeine 40 mg, Aspirin 325 mg	Fiorinal #1 by Sandoz		Analgesic; C III
FC2SANDOZ78106	Cap, Gray & Yellow, F-C #2 Sandoz 78-106	Codeine 15 mg, Butalbital 50 mg, Caffeine 40 mg, Aspirin 325 mg	Fiorinal #2 by Sandoz		Analgesic; C III
FC3SANDOZ78107	Cap, Blue & Yellow, F-C #3 Sandoz 78-107	Codeine 30 mg, Butalbital 50 mg, Caffeine 40 mg, Aspirin 325 mg	Fiorinal #3 by Sandoz		Analgesic; C III
FDM014 <> DURA	Tab, Film Coated	Dextromethorphan Hydrobromide 30 mg, Guaifenesin 600 mg	by PDRX	55289-0625	Cold Remedy
FDM014 <> DURA	Tab, Blue, Oblong, Scored	Dextromethorphan Hydrobromide 30 mg, Guaifenesin 600 mg	Fenesin DM by DRX	55045-2621	Cold Remedy
FDM014 <> DURA	Tab, FDM 014 <> DU/RA	Dextromethorphan Hydrobromide 30 mg, Guaifenesin 600 mg	Fenesin DM by Anabolic	00722-6275	Cold Remedy
FE	Tab, Red, Round	Ferrous Sulfate 300 mg	Feratab by Upsher	00245-0053	Mineral
FE	Tab, Green, Round	Ferrous Gluconate 300 mg	Fergon by Upsher	00245-0061	Mineral
FELDENE <> PFIZER323	Cap, Maroon	Piroxicam 20 mg	Feldene by Pfizer	00069-3230	NSAID
FELDENE <> PFIZER323	Cap	Piroxicam 20 mg	by Pharmedix	53002-0389	NSAID
FELDENE <> PFIZER323	Cap	Piroxicam 20 mg	Feldene by Allscripts	54569-0272	NSAID
FELDENE <> PFIZER323	Cap	Piroxicam 20 mg	Feldene by Nat Pharmpak Serv	55154-2702	NSAID
FELDENE <> PFIZER323	Cap	Piroxicam 20 mg	Feldene by Quality Care	60346-0241	NSAID
FELDENE <> PFIZER323	Cap	Piroxicam 20 mg	Feldene by Amerisource	62584-0230	NSAID
FELDENE <> PFIZER323	Cap, Maroon, Hard Gel	Piroxicam 20 mg	Feldene by Prestige	58056-0340	NSAID
FELDENEPFIZER	Cap, Blue & Maroon, Opaque, Gelatin	Piroxicam 10 mg	Feldene by Pfizer	Canadian DIN# 00525596	NSAID

ID FRONT <> BACK	DESCRIPTION FRONT <> BACK	INGREDIENT & STRENGTH	BRAND (OR EQUIV.) & FIRM	NDC#	CLASS; SCH.
FELDENEPFIZER	Cap, Maroon, Opaque, Gelatin	Piroxicam 20 mg	Feldene by Pfizer	Canadian DIN# 00525618	NSAID
FH <> GEIGY	Tab, Cream, Round, Sugar Coated	Clomipramine HCl 25 mg	Anafranil by Novartis	Canadian DIN# 00324019	OCD
FIII	Cap, ER, White Beads in Capsule	Theophylline 65 mg	Aerolate III by Fleming	00256-0150	Antiasthmatic
FIORICET	Tab, Sandoz Logo <> Three Head Profile	Acetaminophen 325 mg, Butalbital 50 mg, Caffeine 40 mg	Floricet by Repack	55306-0084	Analgesic
FIORICET	Tab, Logo of Triangle with an S <> Three Headed Profile Logo	Acetaminophen 325 mg, Butalbital 50 mg, Caffeine 40 mg	Fioricet by Leiner	59606-0649	Analgesic
FIORICET	Tab, Light Blue, Fioricet Logo <> Three Head Profile	Acetaminophen 325 mg, Butalbital 50 mg, Caffeine 40 mg	Fioricet by Amerisource	62584-0084	Analgesic
FIORICET	Tab, S in a Triangle Fioricet <> 3 Faces	Acetaminophen 325 mg, Butalbital 50 mg, Caffeine 40 mg	Fioricet by Novartis	00078-0084	Analgesic
FIORICET	Tab, Blue, Round, S in a triangle and Fioricet <> Three Head Profile	Acetaminophen 325 mg, Butalbital 50 mg, Caffeine 40 mg	Fioricet by Able		Analgesic
FIORICET	Tab, Blue, Round, Fioricet and Logo <> Three Head Profile	Acetaminophen 325 mg, Butalbital 50 mg, Caffeine 40 mg	Fioricet by Able		Analgesic
FIORICET	Tab, Sandoz Logo	Acetaminophen 325 mg, Butalbital 50 mg, Caffeine 40 mg	Fioricet by Allscripts	54569-0013	Analgesic
FIORICET	Tab, Light Blue, Fioricet S in triangle <> Three Heads Profile	Acetaminophen 325 mg, Butalbital 50 mg, Caffeine 40 mg	Fioricet by CVS Revco	00894-6131	Analgesic
FIORICETCODEINE	Cap, Dark Blue & Gray, Opaque, Red Print, Four-Head Profile	Codeine Phosphate 30 mg, Butalbital 50 mg, Caffeine 40 mg, Acetaminophen 325 mg	Fioricet with Codeine by Novartis	00078-0243	Analgesic; C III
FIORICETS	Tab, Fio-Ricet, S in a Triangle <> 3 Head Profile	Acetaminophen 325 mg, Butalbital 50 mg, Caffeine 40 mg	Fioricet by Prestige Packaging	58056-0349	Analgesic
FIORICETS	Tab, Blue	Caffeine 40 mg; Butalbital 50 mg; Acetaminophen 325 mg	Fioricet by Rightpak	65240-0649	Antimigraine/Other Headaches
FIORINAL <> S	Tab, White, Round, Fiorinal <> S in a triangle	Butalbital 50 mg, Caffeine 40 mg, Aspirin 330 mg	by Novartis	Canadian DIN# 00275328	Analgesic
FIORINAL78103 <> FIORINAL78103	Cap, Dark Green & Light Green, Fiorinal 78-103 <> Fiorinal 78-103	Aspirin 325 mg, Butalbital 50 mg, Caffeine 40 mg	Fiorinal by Novartis	00078-0103	Analgesic; C III
FIORINAL78103 <> FIORINAL78103	Cap, Green	Butalbital 50 mg; Caffeine 40 mg; Aspirin 325 mg	Fiorinal by Med-Pro	53978-3395	Analgesic
FIORINALC12S	Cap, Blue & Light Blue, Gelatin, Fiorinal C 1/2 S in a triangle	Butalbital 50 mg, Caffeine 40 mg, Aspirin 330 mg	by Novartis	Canadian DIN# 00176206	Analgesic
FIORINALC14S	Cap, Blue & White, Gelatin, Fiorinal C 1/4 S in a triangle	Butalbital 50 mg, Caffeine 40 mg, Aspirin 330 mg	by Novartis	Canadian DIN# 00176192	Analgesic
FIORINALS	Cap, Blue & Purple, Gelatin, Fiorinal w/ S inside a triangle	Butalbital 50 mg, Caffeine 40 mg, Aspirin 330 mg	by Novartis	Canadian DIN# 00226327	Analgesic
FISONS101	Cap, Clear	Sodium Cromoglycate 100 mg	by Rhone-Poulenc Rorer	Canadian	Antiasthmatic
FISONSINTALP	Cap, Clear & Yellow, Fisons/Intal-p	Sodium Cromogryclate 20 mg	by Rhone-Poulenc Rorer	Canadian	Antiasthmatic
FJ	Tab, Orange-Peach, Round, FJ <> Abbott Logo	Tiagabine HCl 2 mg	Gabitril by Abbott	00074-3963	Anticonvulsant
FJR	Cap, Clear & Red, F in Triangle Logo JR	Anhydrous Theophylline 130 mg	Aerolate JR by Fleming		Antiasthmatic
FJR	Cap, White Beads	Chlorpheniramine Maleate 4 mg, Methscopolamine Nitrate 1.25 mg, Phenylephrine HCl 10 mg	Extendryl Jr by Fleming	00256-0177	Cold Remedy
FJR	Cap, Green & Red, F in Triangle Logo JR	Chlorpheniramine 4 mg, Phenylephrine 10 mg, Methscopolamine 1.25 mg	Extendryl JR by Fleming		Cold Remedy
FJR	Cap, Blue & Clear, F in triangle JR	Guaifenesin 125 mg, Pseudoephedrine 60 mg	Congess JR by Fleming		Cold Remedy
FJR	Cap, White Beads	Guaifenesin 125 mg, Pseudoephedrine HCl 60 mg	Congess Jr by Fleming	00256-0174	Cold Remedy
FJR	Cap, Clear & Red, Ex Release, with White Beads, F in Triangle Symbol	Theophylline 130 mg	Aerolate Jr by Fleming	00256-0114	Antiasthmatic
FJR <> FJR	Cap, Ex Release, Logo F and JR	Guaifenesin 125 mg, Pseudoephedrine HCl 60 mg	Congess Jr by Pharmafab	62542-0420	Cold Remedy
FK	Tab, Yellow, Round, Film Coated	Tiagabine HCl 4 mg	Gabitril by Abbott Hlth	60692-3904	Anticonvulsant
FK	Tab, Yellow, Round, FK <> Abbott Logo	Tiagabine HCl 4 mg	Gabitril by Abbott	00074-3904	Anticonvulsant
FL	Cap, Ex Release, Printed in Red Ink <> Symbols of 2 Hearts in Red Ink	Chlorpheniramine Maleate 4 mg, Pseudoephedrine HCl 60 mg	Kronofed A Jr by Sovereign	58716-0043	Cold Remedy

ID FRONT <> BACK	DESCRIPTION FRONT <> BACK	INGREDIENT & STRENGTH	BRAND (OR EQUIV.) & FIRM	NDC#	CLASS; SCH.
FL	Cap, Two Red Hearts	Chlorpheniramine Maleate 4 mg, Pseudoephedrine HCl 60 mg	Kronofed A Jr by Ferndale	00496-0434	Cold Remedy
FL	Cap, Two Hearts	Chlorpheniramine Maleate 8 mg, Pseudoephedrine HCl 120 mg	Kronofed A by DRX	55045-2454	Cold Remedy
FL	Cap, Ex Release, Symbols of 2 Hearts	Chlorpheniramine Maleate 8 mg, Pseudoephedrine HCl 120 mg	Kronofed A by Sovereign	58716-0042	Cold Remedy
FL	Cap, Two Black Hearts	Chlorpheniramine Maleate 8 mg, Pseudoephedrine HCl 120 mg	Kronofed A by Ferndale	00496-0382	Cold Remedy
FL	Cap, Two Hearts	Chlorpheniramine Maleate 8 mg, Pseudoephedrine HCl 120 mg	by United Res	00677-1086	Cold Remedy
FL	Cap, 2 Heart Figures	Chlorpheniramine Maleate 8 mg, Pseudoephedrine HCl 120 mg	Decongestamine Sr by Pharmedix	53002-0465	Cold Remedy
FL	Tab, Green, Oval, Film Coated	Tiagabine HCl 12 mg	Gabitril by Abbott Hlth	60692-3910	Anticonvulsant
FL	Tab, Green, Ovaloid, FL <> Abbott Logo	Tiagabine HCl 12 mg	Gabitril by Abbott	00074-3910	Anticonvulsant
FL <> 100	Tab, Logo FL <> Compressed Tab	Levothyroxine Sodium 100 mcg	by Kaiser	00179-0458	Antithyroid
FL <> 125	Tab, Logo <> Compressed Tab	Levothyroxine Sodium 125 mcg	by Kaiser	00179-1210	Antithyroid
FL <> 150	Tab, Logo FL <> Compressed Tab	Levothyroxine Sodium 150 mcg	by Kaiser	00179-0459	Antithyroid
FL <> 200	Tab, Logo FL <> Compressed Tab	Levothyroxine Sodium 200 mcg	by Kaiser	00179-0460	Antithyroid
FL <> 50	Tab, Logo FL <> Compressed Tab	Levothyroxine Sodium 50 mcg	by Kaiser	00179-0457	Antithyroid
FL1033	Tab	Belladonna Alkaloids 0.2 mg, Ergotamine Tartrate 0.6 mg, Phenobarbital 40 mg	by Zenith Goldline	00182-1990	Gastrointestinal; C IV
FL112	Tab, Rose, Round	Levothyroxine Sodium 112 mcg	Levothroid by Forest	00456-0330	Antithyroid
FL125	Tab, Purple, Round	Levothyroxine Sodium 125 mcg	Levothroid by Forest	00456-0324	Antithyroid
FL137	Tab, Blue, Round	Levothyroxine Sodium 137 mcg	Levothroid by Forest	00456-0331	Antithyroid
FL175	Tab, Turquoise, Round	Levothyroxine Sodium 175 mcg	Levothroid by Forest	00456-0326	Antithyroid
FL25	Tab, Orange, Round	Levothyroxine Sodium 25 mcg	Levothroid by Forest	00456-0320	Antithyroid
FL300	Tab, Green, Round	Levothyroxine Sodium 300 mcg	Levothroid by Forest	00456-0328	Antithyroid
FL75	Tab, Gray, Round	Levothyroxine Sodium 75 mcg	Levothroid by Forest	00456-0322	Antithyroid
FL88	Tab, Blue, Round	Levothyroxine Sodium 88 mcg	Levothroid by Forest		Antithyroid
FL99	Cap, White	Chlorpheniramine Maleate 4 mg, Pseudoephedrine HCl 60 mg	Kronofed A JR by Collagenex	64682-0007	Cold Remedy
FLAGYL <> 375	Cap	Metronidazole 375 mg	Flagyl by GD Searle	00025-1942	Antibiotic
FLAGYL <> 375	Cap, Light Green	Metronidazole 375 mg	Flagyl by Physicians Total Care	54868-3786	Antibiotic
FLAGYL <> 500	Tab, Film Coated	Metronidazole 500 mg	Flagyl by GD Searle	00025-1821	Antibiotic
FLAGYL <> 500	Tab, Film Coated, Debossed	Metronidazole 500 mg	Flagyl by Thrift Drug	59198-0030	Antibiotic
FLAGYL <> 500	Tab, Blue, Oblong, Film	Metronidazole 500 mg	Flagyl by Neuman Distr	64579-0118	Antibiotic
FLAGYL250 <> SEARLE1831	Tab, Film Coated	Metronidazole 250 mg	Flagyl by GD Searle	00025-1831	Antibiotic
FLAGYL250 <> SEARLE1831	Tab, Film Coated	Metronidazole 250 mg	Flagyl by Thrift Drug	59198-0311	Antibiotic
FLAGYL250 <> SEARLE1831	Tab, Film Coated, Debossed	Metronidazole 250 mg	Flagyl by Amerisource	62584-0831	Antibiotic
FLAGYLER <> SEARLE1961	Tab, Blue, Oval, Film Coated	Metronidazole 750 mg	Flagyl by Mova Pharms	55370-0562	Antibiotic
FLAGYLER <> SEARLE1961	Tab, Film Coated	Metronidazole 750 mg	Flagyl ER by GD Searle	00025-1961	Antibiotic
FLEXERIL <> MSD931	Tab, Butterscotch Yellow, D-Shaped, Film Coated	Cyclobenzaprine HCl 10 mg	Flexeril by Merck	00006-0931	Muscle Relaxant
FLEXERIL <> MSD931	Tab, Film Coated	Cyclobenzaprine HCl 10 mg	Flexeril by Nat Pharmpak Serv	55154-5007	Muscle Relaxant
FLEXERIL <> MSD931	Tab, D-Shaped, Film Coated	Cyclobenzaprine HCl 10 mg	Flexeril by Allscripts	54569-0835	Muscle Relaxant
FLEXERIL <> MSD931	Tab, D-Shaped, Film Coated	Cyclobenzaprine HCl 10 mg	Flexeril by Allscripts	54569-4008	Muscle Relaxant
FLEXERIL <> MSD931	Tab, Butterscotch Yellow, D-Shaped, Film Coated	Cyclobenzaprine HCl 10 mg	Flexeril by Quality Care	60346-0471	Muscle Relaxant
FLING <> 150	Tab, Blue, Round, Scored	Levothyroxine Sodium 0.15 mg	Synthroid by Rx Pac	65084-0182	Antithyroid
FLINT	Tab, Orange, Round, Scored	Levothyroxine Sodium 0.025 mg	Synthroid by Rx Pac	65084-0174	Antithyroid
FLINT <> 100	Tab	Levothyroxine Sodium 0.1 mg	Synthroid by Nat Pharmpak Serv	55154-0906	Antithyroid
FLINT <> 100	Tab	Levothyroxine Sodium 0.1 mg	Synthroid by Giant Food	11146-0305	Antithyroid
FLINT <> 100	Tab	Levothyroxine Sodium 0.1 mg	Synthroid by Rite Aid	11822-5193	Antithyroid
FLINT <> 100	Tab, BASF <> 100 is Debossed	Levothyroxine Sodium 0.1 mg	Synthroid by Allscripts	54569-0909	Antithyroid
FLINT <> 100	Tab, Yellow, Round, Scored	Levothyroxine Sodium 100 mcg	Synthroid by Knoll	00048-1070	Antithyroid
FLINT <> 100MCG	Tab, Debossed	Levothyroxine Sodium 0.1 mg	Synthroid by Amerisource	62584-0070	Antithyroid
FLINT <> 100MCG	Tab, Yellow, Round, Scored	Levothyroxine Sodium 0.1 mg	Synthroid by Wal Mart	49035-0194	Antithyroid

ID FRONT <> BACK	DESCRIPTION FRONT <> BACK	INGREDIENT & STRENGTH	BRAND (OR EQUIV.) & FIRM	NDC#	CLASS; SCH.
FLINT <> 100MCG	Tab, Yellow, Round, Scored	Levothyroxine Sodium 0.1 mg	Synthroid by Rightpac	65240-0742	Antithyroid
FLINT <> 112	Tab, Pink, Round, Scored, 112 on Bisect	Levothyroxine Sodium 0.112 mg	Synthroid by Murfreesboro	51129-1646	Antithyroid
FLINT <> 112	Tab	Levothyroxine Sodium 0.112 mg	Synthroid by Nat Pharmpak Serv	55154-0911	Antithyroid
FLINT <> 112	Tab, Rose, Round, Scored	Levothyroxine Sodium 112 mcg	Synthroid by Knoll	00048-1080	Antithyroid
FLINT <> 112	Tab, Pink, Round, Scored, 112 on Bisect	Levothyroxine Sodium 112 mcg	Synthroid by Murfreesboro	51129-1664	Antithyroid
FLINT <> 112MCG	Tab, Round, Scored	Levothyroxine Sodium 0.112 mg	Synthroid by Rightpac	65240-0743	Antithyroid
FLINT <> 112MCG	Tab, Debossed	Levothyroxine Sodium 0.112 mg	Synthroid by Amerisource	62584-0080	Antithyroid
FLINT <> 125	Tab	Levothyroxine Sodium 0.125 mg	Synthroid by Nat Pharmpak Serv	55154-0909	Antithyroid
FLINT <> 125	Tab	Levothyroxine Sodium 0.125 mg	Synthroid by Rite Aid	11822-5285	Antithyroid
FLINT <> 125	Tab	Levothyroxine Sodium 0.125 mg	Synthroid by Giant Food	11146-0303	Antithyroid
FLINT <> 125	Tab, Brown, Round, Scored	Levothyroxine Sodium 125 mcg	Synthroid by Knoll	00048-1130	Antithyroid
FLINT <> 125MCG	Tab, Brown, Round, Scored	Levothyroxine Sodium 0.125 mg	Synthroid by Rightpac	65240-0744	Antithyroid
FLINT <> 125MCG	Tab, Debossed	Levothyroxine Sodium 0.125 mg	Synthroid by Amerisource	62584-0130	Antithyroid
FLINT <> 150	Tab	Levothyroxine Sodium 0.15 mg	Synthroid by Nat Pharmpak Serv	55154-0905	Antithyroid
FLINT <> 150	Tab	Levothyroxine Sodium 0.15 mg	Synthroid by Giant Food	11146-0304	Antithyroid
FLINT <> 150	Tab	Levothyroxine Sodium 0.15 mg	Synthroid by Rite Aid	11822-5210	Antithyroid
FLINT <> 150	Tab, Blue, Round, Scored	Levothyroxine Sodium 150 mcg	Synthroid by Knoll	00048-1090	Antithyroid
FLINT <> 150MCG	Tab, Blue, Round, Scored	Levothyroxine Sodium 0.15 mg	Synthroid by Wal Mart	49035-0193	Antithyroid
FLINT <> 150MCG	Tab, Debossed	Levothyroxine Sodium 0.15 mg	Synthroid by Amerisource	62584-0090	Antithyroid
FLINT <> 175	Tab, Purple, Round, Scored	Levothyroxine Sodium 0.175 mg	Synthroid by Murfreesboro	51129-1648	Antithyroid
FLINT <> 175	Tab, Lilac, Round, Scored	Levothyroxine Sodium 175 mcg	Synthroid by Knoll	00048-1100	Antithyroid
FLINT <> 175MCG	Tab, Purple, Round, Scored	Levothyroxine Sodium 0.175 mg	Synthroid by Rightpac	65240-0758	Antithyroid
FLINT <> 200	Tab	Levothyroxine Sodium 0.2 mg	Synthroid by Rite Aid	11822-5194	Antithyroid
FLINT <> 200	Tab	Levothyroxine Sodium 0.2 mg	Synthroid by Giant Food	11146-0306	Antithyroid
FLINT <> 200	Tab, Pink, Round, Scored	Levothyroxine Sodium 0.2 mg	Synthroid by Rx Pac	65084-0160	Antithyroid
FLINT <> 200	Tab	Levothyroxine Sodium 0.2 mg	Synthroid by Wal Mart	49035-0172	Antithyroid
FLINT <> 200	Tab	Levothyroxine Sodium 0.2 mg	Synthroid by Nat Pharmpak Serv	55154-0907	Antithyroid
FLINT <> 200	Tab, Pink, Round, Scored	Levothyroxine Sodium 200 mcg	Synthroid by Knoll	00048-1140	Antithyroid
FLINT <> 200MCG	Tab, Debossed	Levothyroxine Sodium 0.2 mg	Synthroid by Amerisource	62584-0140	Antithyroid
FLINT <> 25	Tab	Levothyroxine Sodium 0.025 mg	Synthroid by Rite Aid	11822-5287	Antithyroid
FLINT <> 25	Tab, Orange, Round, Scord	Levothyroxine Sodium 25 mcg	Synthroid by Knoll	00048-1020	Antithyroid
FLINT <> 25MCG	Tab, Orange, Round, Scored	Levothyroxine Sodium 0.025 mg	Synthroid by Rightpac	65240-0739	Antithyroid
FLINT <> 25MCG	Tab, Debossed	Levothyroxine Sodium 0.025 mg	Synthroid by Amerisource	62584-0020	Antithyroid
FLINT <> 300	Tab, Debossed	Levothyroxine Sodium 0.3 mg	Synthroid by CVS	51316-0246	Antithyroid
FLINT <> 300	Tab, Debossed, Score is Vertical with 300 Running Horizontal Thru Break in Score	Levothyroxine Sodium 0.3 mg	Synthroid by Thrift Drug	59198-0298	Antithyroid
FLINT <> 300	Tab, Debossed	Levothyroxine Sodium 0.3 mg	Synthroid by Amerisource	62584-0170	Antithyroid
FLINT <> 300	Tab, Green, Round, Scored	Levothyroxine Sodium 300 mcg	Synthroid by Knoll	00048-1170	Antithyroid
FLINT <> 50	Tab	Levothyroxine Sodium 0.05 mg	Synthroid by Physicians Total Care	54868-1011	Antithyroid
FLINT <> 50	Tab	Levothyroxine Sodium 0.05 mg	Synthroid by Knoll BV	55445-0104	Antithyroid
FLINT <> 50	Tab	Levothyroxine Sodium 0.05 mg	Synthroid by Giant Food	11146-0301	Antithyroid
FLINT <> 50	Tab, White, Round, Scored	Levothyroxine Sodium 50 mcg	Synthroid by Knoll	00048-1040	Antithyroid
FLINT <> 50MCG	Tab, Debossed	Levothyroxine Sodium 0.05 mg	Synthroid by Amerisource	62584-0040	Antithyroid
FLINT <> 50MCG	Tab, White, Round, Scored	Levothyroxine Sodium 0.05 mg	Synthroid by Rightpac	65240-0740	Antithyroid
FLINT <> 50MCG	Tab, White, Round, Scored	Levothyroxine Sodium 50 mcg	Synthroid by Murfreesboro	51129-1659	Antithyroid
FLINT <> 75	Tab, Purple, Round, Scored 75 on Bisect	Levothyroxine Sodium 0.075 mg	Synthroid by Murfreesboro	51129-1656	Antithyroid
FLINT <> 75	Tab	Levothyroxine Sodium 0.075 mg	Synthroid by Nat Pharmpak Serv	55154-0904	Antithyroid
FLINT <> 75	Tab	Levothyroxine Sodium 0.075 mg	Synthroid by Rite Aid	11822-5286	Antithyroid
FLINT <> 75	Tab	Levothyroxine Sodium 0.075 mg	Synthroid by Giant Food	11146-0302	Antithyroid
FLINT <> 75	Tab, Violet, Round, Scored	Levothyroxine Sodium 75 mcg	Synthroid by Knoll	00048-1050	Antithyroid
FLINT <> 75	Tab, Purple, Round, Scored	Levothyroxine Sodium 75 mcg	by Murfreesboro	51129-1658	Antithyroid
FLINT <> 75MCG	Tab, Debossed	Levothyroxine Sodium 0.075 mg	Synthroid by Amerisource	62584-0050	Antithyroid

ID FRONT <> BACK	DESCRIPTION FRONT <> BACK	INGREDIENT & STRENGTH	BRAND (OR EQUIV.) & FIRM	NDC#	CLASS; SCH.
FLINT <> 88	Tab, Green, Round, Scored	Levothyroxine Sodium 0.088 mg	Synthroid by Phy Total Care	54868-2705	Antithyroid
FLINT <> 88	Tab, Green, Round, Scored	Levothyroxine Sodium 0.088 mg	Synthroid by Murfreesboro	51129-1645	Antithyroid
FLINT <> 88	Tab, Olive, Round, Scored	Levothyroxine Sodium 88 mcg	Synthroid by Knoll	00048-1060	Antithyroid
FLINT <> 88MCG	Tab, Olive, Round, Scored	Levothyroxine Sodium 0.088 mg	Synthroid by Rightpac	65240-0757	Antithyroid
FLINT100	Tab	Levothyroxine Sodium 0.1 mg	Synthroid by Quality Care	60346-0850	Antithyroid
FLINT100	Tab, Flint 100	Levothyroxine Sodium 0.1 mg	Synthroid by Med Pro	53978-1038	Antithyroid
FLINT100	Tab	Levothyroxine Sodium 0.1 mg	Synthroid by Pharmedix	53002-1056	Antithyroid
FLINT100MCG	Tab, Yellow, Round, Scored	Levothyroxine Sodium 100 mcg	Synthroid by Murfreesboro	51129-1660	Antithyroid
FLINT112	Tab	Levothyroxine Sodium 0.112 mg	Synthroid by CVS	51316-0201	Antithyroid
FLINT112	Tab, Debossed	Levothyroxine Sodium 0.112 mg	Synthroid by Repack Co of Amer	55306-1080	Antithyroid
FLINT112MCG	Tab, Rose	Levothyroxine Sodium 0.112 mg	Synthroid by Thrift Drug	59198-0303	Antithyroid
FLINT125MCG	Tab, Brown, Round, Scored	Levothyroxine Sodium 125 mcg	Synthroid by Murfreesboro	51129-1662	Antithyroid
FLINT150	Tab	Levothyroxine Sodium 0.15 mg	Synthroid by Med Pro	53978-0999	Antithyroid
FLINT175MCG	Tab, Purple, Round, Scored	Levothyroxine Sodium 175 mcg	Synthroid by Murfreesboro	51129-1639	Antithyroid
FLINT175MCG	Tab, Blue, Round, Scored	Levothyroxine Sodium 0.175 mg	Synthroid by Rx Pac	65084-0196	Antithyroid
FLINT200	Tab	Levothyroxine Sodium 0.2 mg	Synthroid by Med Pro	53978-0856	Antithyroid
FLINT25	Tab	Levothyroxine Sodium 0.025 mg	Synthroid by Haines	59564-0115	Antithyroid
FLINT25MCG	Tab, Orange, Round, Scored	Levothyroxine Sodium 0.025 mg	Synthroid by Thrift Services	59198-0337	Antithyroid
FLINT300MCG	Tab, Green, Round, Scored	Levothyroxine Sodium 300 mcg	Synthroid by Murfreesboro	51129-1663	Antithyroid
FLINT3P1093	Tab, Blue, Round, Scored	Levothyroxine Sodium 0.15 mg	Synthroid by Rightpac	65240-0745	Antithyroid
FLINT3P1143	Tab, Pink, Round, Scored	Levothyroxine Sodium 0.2 mg	Synthroid by Rightpac	65240-0746	Antithyroid
FLINT3P1173	Tab, Green, Round, Scored	Levothyroxine Sodium 0.3 mg	Synthroid by Rightpac	65240-0747	Antithyroid
FLINT50	Tab	Levothyroxine Sodium 0.05 mg	Synthroid by Med Pro	53978-0589	Antithyroid
FLINT75MCG	Tab, Purple, Round	Levothyroxine Sodium 0.075 mg	Synthroid by Phy Total Care	54868-2005	Antithyroid
FLINT75MCG	Tab, Purple, Round, Scored	Levothyroxine Sodium 75 mcg	Synthroid by Murfreesboro	51129-1661	Antithyroid
FLINT88MCG	Tab, Green, Round, Scored	Levothyroxine Sodium 0.088 mg	Synthroid by Rx Pac	65084-0222	Antithyroid
FLINT88MCG	Tab, Green, Round, Scored	Levothyroxine Sodium 88 mcg	Synthroid by Murfreesboro	51129-1667	Antithyroid
FLINT88MCG	Tab, Green, Round, Scored	Levothyroxine Sodium 88 mcg	Synthroid by Murfreesboro	51129-1641	Antithyroid
FLLA	Tab, Mint Green, Round	Levothyroxine Sodium 88 mcg	Levothroid by Forest	00456-0329	Antithyroid
FLLC	Tab, Blue, Round	Levothyroxine Sodium 137 mcg	Levothroid by Forest	00456-0331	Antithyroid
FLLJ	Tab, Rose, Round	Levothyroxine Sodium 112 mcg	Levothroid by Forest	00456-0330	Antithyroid
FLOMAX04MG <> BI58	Cap, Olive Green, Gelatin Coated, Flomax over 0.4 mg <> BI 58	Tamsulosin HCl 0.4 mg	Flomax by Boehringer Ingelheim	00597-0058	Antiadrenergic
FLOMAX04MG <> BI58	Cap, Gelatin Coated, Flomax 0.4 mg <> BI 58	Tamsulosin HCl 0.4 mg	Flomax by Shaklee Tech	51248-0058	Antiadrenergic
FLOMAX04MG <> BI58	Cap, Green & Orange	Tamsulosin HCl 0.4 mg	Flomax by Caremark	00339-5560	Antiadrenergic
FLOMAX04MG <> BI58	Cap, Gelatin Coated, Flomax 0.4 mg	Tamsulosin HCl 0.4 mg	by Yamanouchi	12838-0058	Antiadrenergic
FLORICETS	Tab, Floricets <> 3 Head Profile	Acetaminophen 325 mg, Butalbital 50 mg, Caffeine 40 mg	Fioricet by Nat Pharmpak Serv	55154-3416	Analgesic
FLOXIN <> 200	Tab, Yellow, Film	Ofloxacin 200 mg	Floxin by Bristol Myers Squibb	64747-0429	Antibiotic
FLOXIN <> 200MG	Tab, Light Yellow, Film Coated	Ofloxacin 200 mg	Floxin by Quality Care	60346-0647	Antibiotic
FLOXIN <> 300	Tab, White, Film	Ofloxacin 300 mg	Floxin by Boca Pharmacal	64376-0503	Antibiotic
FLOXIN <> 300MG	Tab, Film Coated	Ofloxacin 300 mg	Ofloxacin by Med Pro	53978-3018	Antibiotic
FLOXIN <> 300MG	Tab, Film Coated	Ofloxacin 300 mg	Floxin by Quality Care	60346-0716	Antibiotic
FLOXIN <> 400	Tab, Pale Gold, Film Coated	Ofloxacin 400 mg	Floxin by Quality Care	60346-0400	Antibiotic
FLOXIN200	Tab, Light Yellow, Floxin/200	Ofloxacin 200 mg	Floxin by Ortho	Canadian	Antibiotic
FLOXIN200	Tab, Light Yellow, Film Coated	Ofloxacin 200 mg	Floxin by McNeil	00045-1540	Antibiotic
FLOXIN200	Tab, Light Yellow, Film Coated	Ofloxacin 200 mg	Floxin by Ortho	00062-1540	Antibiotic
FLOXIN200	Tab, Film Coated	Ofloxacin 200 mg	Floxin by McNeil	52021-0540	Antibiotic
FLOXIN200	Tab, Coated	Ofloxacin 200 mg	Floxin by Allscripts	54569-3268	Antibiotic
FLOXIN200	Tab, Film Coated	Ofloxacin 200 mg	Floxin by Physicians Total Care	54868-2641	Antibiotic
FLOXIN200MG	Tab, Film Coated	Ofloxacin 200 mg	Ofloxacin by Med Pro	53978-3014	Antibiotic
FLOXIN300	Tab, White, Floxin/300	Ofloxacin 300 mg	Floxin by Ortho	Canadian	Antibiotic
FLOXIN300	Tab, White, Film Coated	Ofloxacin 300 mg	Floxin by Ortho	00062-1541	Antibiotic
FLOXIN300	Tab, Film Coated	Ofloxacin 300 mg	Floxin by McNeil	00045-1541	Antibiotic

ID FRONT <> BACK	DESCRIPTION FRONT <> BACK	INGREDIENT & STRENGTH	BRAND (OR EQUIV.) & FIRM	NDC#	CLASS; SCH.
FLOXIN300	Tab, Coated	Ofloxacin 300 mg	Floxin by Allscripts	54569-3872	Antibiotic
FLOXIN300	Tab, Film Coated	Ofloxacin 300 mg	Floxin by McNeil	52021-0541	Antibiotic
FLOXIN400	Tab, Gold, Floxin/400	Ofloxacin 400 mg	Floxin by Ortho	Canadian	Antibiotic
FLOXIN400	Tab, Yellow, Round, Film Coated	Ofloxacin 400 mg	Floxin by Natl Pharmpak	55154-0551	Antibiotic
FLOXIN400	Tab, Gold, Film Coated	Ofloxacin 400 mg	Floxin by McNeil	00045-1542	Antibiotic
FLOXIN400	Tab, Pale Gold, Film Coated	Ofloxacin 400 mg	Floxin by Ortho	00062-1542	Antibiotic
FLOXIN400	Tab, Gold, Film Coated	Ofloxacin 400 mg	Floxin by McNeil	52021-0542	Antibiotic
FLOXIN400	Tab, Film Coated	Ofloxacin 400 mg	Floxin by Allscripts	54569-3293	Antibiotic
FLOXIN400MG	Tab, Yellow, Film	Ofloxacin 400 mg	Floxin by PDRX	55289-0406	Antibiotic
FLUMADINE100 <> FOREST	Tab, Orange, Oval, Film Coated	Rimantadine HCl 100 mg	Flumadine by HJ Harkins	52959-0490	Antiviral
FLUMADINE100 <> FOREST	Tab, Film Coated	Rimantadine HCl 100 mg	Flumadine by Allscripts	54569-3773	Antiviral
FLUMADINE100 <> FOREST	Tab, Film Coated	Rimantadine HCl 100 mg	Flumadine by DRX	55045-2085	Antiviral
FLUMADINE100 <> FOREST	Tab, Film Coated	Rimantadine HCl 100 mg	Flumadine by Quality Care	60346-0903	Antiviral
FLUMADINE100 FOREST	Tab, Orange, Oval, Film Coated, Flumadine 100/Forest	Rimantadine HCl 100 mg	Flumadine by Forest	00456-0521	Antiviral
FLUORIDE1MG	Tab, Off-White	Ascorbic Acid 60 mg, Sodium Fluoride 2.2 mg, Vitamin A 3000 Units, Vitamin D 400 U	Flor-Dac by IVC Ind	00417-1899	Vitamin
FLUORIDE1MG	Tab	Sodium Fluoride 2.2 mg	Fluorabon by IVC Ind	00417-1699	Element
FLUORIDE1MG	Tab	Sodium Fluoride 2.2 mg	Fluorabon by IVC Ind	00417-1599	Element
FLUORIDE1MG	Tab, Chewable	Sodium Fluoride 2.21 mg	Fluoro by IVC Ind	00417-0672	Element
FLUORIDE1MG	Tab, Chewable	Sodium Fluoride 2.21 mg	by IVC Ind	00417-0318	Element
FLUORIDE1MG	Tab, Chewable	Sodium Fluoride 2.21 mg	by IVC Ind	00417-0317	Element
FLUORIDE1MG	Tab, Chewable	Sodium Fluoride 2.21 mg	Fluorabon by IVC Ind	00417-0229	Element
FLURAZEPAM15 <> WESTWARD	Cap Black Print	Flurazepam HCl 15 mg	by Kaiser	00179-1098	Hypnotic; C IV
FLURAZEPAM15 <> WESTWARD	Tab, Blue & White, Oblong	Flurazepam HCl 15 mg	by Southwood Pharms	58016-0811	Hypnotic; C IV
FLURAZEPAM30 <> WESTWARD	Tab, Blue, Oblong	Flurazepam HCl 30 mg	by Southwood Pharms	58016-0812	Hypnotic; C IV
FLURAZEPAM30 <> WESTWARD	Cap, Black Print	Flurazepam HCl 30 mg	by Kaiser	00179-1099	Hypnotic; C IV
FM	Tab, Blue, Oval, Film Coated	Tiagabine HCl 16 mg	Gabitril by Abbott Hlth	60692-3960	Anticonvulsant
FM	Tab, Blue, Ovaloid, FM <> Abbott Logo	Tiagabine HCl 16 mg	Gabitril by Abbott	00074-3960	Anticonvulsant
FM20G	Tab, Beige, D-Shaped, FM 20/G	Famotidine 20 mg	by Genpharm	Canadian	Gastrointestinal
FM40G	Tab, Light Brown, D-Shaped, FM 40/G	Famotidine 40 mg	by Genpharm	Canadian	Gastrointestinal
FN	Tab, Pink, Oval, Film Coated	Tiagabine HCl 20 mg	Gabitril by Abbott Hlth	60692-3982	Anticonvulsant
FN	Tab, Pink, Ovaloid, FN <> Abbott Logo	Tiagabine HCl 20 mg	Gabitril by Abbott	00074-3982	Anticonvulsant
FO1CPI	Tab, Yellow, Round, FO1/CPI	Folic Acid 1 mg	Folvite by Charlotte/Phoe		Vitamin
FOREST	Cap	Acetaminophen 500 mg, Hydrocodone Bitartrate 5 mg	Bancap HC by Pharmedix	53002-0120	Analgesic; C III
FOREST <> 355	Cap, Blue & Pink	Racemethionine 200 mg	Pedameth by Forest	00456-0355	Urinary
FOREST <> 678	Tab	Acetaminophen 500 mg, Butalbital 50 mg, Caffeine 40 mg	Esgic-Plus by Quality Care	60346-0957	Analgesic
FOREST <> 678	Tab	Acetaminophen 500 mg, Butalbital 50 mg, Caffeine 40 mg	Esgic Plus by PDRX	55289-0264	Analgesic
FOREST <> 678	Tab	Acetaminophen 500 mg, Butalbital 50 mg, Caffeine 40 mg	Esgic Plus by Nat Pharmpak Serv	55154-4602	Analgesic
FOREST <> 678	Tab, White, Oblong, Scored	Acetaminophen 500 mg; Butalbital 50 mg; Caffeine 40 mg	Esgic Plus by Rx Pac	65084-0195	Analgesic
FOREST <> 678	Tab, White, Oblong, Scored	Acetaminophen 500 mg; Butalbital 50 mg; Caffeine 40 mg	Esgic Plus by Rightpak	65240-0644	Analgesic
FOREST <> FLUMADINE100	Tab, Orange, Oval, Film Coated	Rimantadine HCl 100 mg	Flumadine by HJ Harkins	52959-0490	Antiviral
FOREST <> FLUMADINE100	Tab, Film Coated	Rimantadine HCl 100 mg	Flumadine by Allscripts	54569-3773	Antiviral

ID FRONT <> BACK	DESCRIPTION FRONT <> BACK	INGREDIENT & STRENGTH	BRAND (OR EQUIV.) & FIRM	NDC#	CLASS; SCH.
FOREST <> FLUMADINE100	Tab, Film Coated	Rimantadine HCl 100 mg	Flumadine by DRX	55045-2085	Antiviral
FOREST <> FLUMADINE100	Tab, Film Coated	Rimantadine HCl 100 mg	Flumadine by Quality Care	60346-0903	Antiviral
FOREST 295	Tab, Pink, Sugar Coated	Potassium Iodide 135 mg, Niacinamide Hydroiodide 25 mg	Iodo-Niacin by Forest	00456-0295	Expectorant
FOREST0372 <> ESGICPLUS	Cap, Red	Acetaminophen 500 mg, Butalbital 50 mg, Caffeine 40 mg	Esgic Plus by Allscripts	54569-4740	Analgesic
FOREST0372 <> ESGICPLUS	Cap, White Print	Acetaminophen 500 mg, Butalbital 50 mg, Caffeine 40 mg	Esgic Plus by Eckerd Drug	19458-0844	Analgesic
FOREST0372 <> ESGICPLUS	Cap	Acetaminophen 500 mg, Butalbital 50 mg, Caffeine 40 mg	by Mikart	46672-0273	Analgesic
FOREST0372 <> ESGICPLUS	Cap, Red	Acetaminophen 500 mg, Butalbital 50 mg, Caffeine 40 mg	by Allscripts	54569-3441	Analgesic
FOREST0372 <> ESGICPLUS	Cap, Red, White Print	Acetaminophen 500 mg, Butalbital 50 mg, Caffeine 40 mg	Esgic Plus by Forest	00456-0679	Analgesic
FOREST0372 <> ESGICPLUS	Cap, Red & White	Acetaminophen 500 mg; Butalbital 50 mg; Caffeine 40 mg	Esgic Plus by Med-Pro	53978-3396	Analgesic
FOREST0372 <> ESGICPLUS	Cap, Red	Butalbital 50 mg; Acetaminophen 500 mg; Caffeine 40 mg	Esgic Plus by Thrift Services	59198-0332	Analgesic
FOREST100	Tab, White, Round	Theophylline SR 100 mg	Duraphyl by Forest		Antiasthmatic
FOREST1054	Cap, Blue & Pink	Racemethionine 200 mg	Pedameth by Forest		Urinary
FOREST150	Tab, Burgundy, Round	Guaifenesin 200 mg	Amonidrin by Forest		Expectorant
FOREST161	Tab, White, Round	Powdered Opium 1.23 mg, Bismuth Subcarbonate 125 mg, Calcium Carb. 125 mg	Diabismul by Forest		Gastrointestinal
FOREST200	Tab, White, Oblong	Theophylline SR 200 mg	Duraphyl by Forest		Antiasthmatic
FOREST245	Tab, Green, Round	Aminoacetic Acid 150 mg, Calcium Carbonate 300 mg	Glycate by Forest		Bladder Irrigation
FOREST251	Tab, Blue, Oblong	Sulfamethazole 500 mg	Proklar by Forest		Antibiotic
FOREST281	Tab, Green, Round	Dehydrochloric Acid 125 mg, Pb 8 mg, Homatropine Methylbromide 2.5 mg	G.B.S. by Forest		Gastrointestinal; C IV
FOREST300	Tab, White, Oblong	Theophylline SR 300 mg	Duraphyl by Forest		Antiasthmatic
FOREST346	Tab, Blue, Round	Rauwolfia Serpentina 50 mg	Rauverid by Forest		Antihypertensive
FOREST372	Tab, Brown	Ferrous Fumarate 100 mg (33 mg elemental iron)	Feostat by Forest	00456-0372	Mineral
FOREST372	Tab, Brown, Round	Ferrous Fumarate 33.3 mg (Fe)	Feostat by Forest		Mineral
FOREST416	Tab, Green, Round	Hydrocodone 5 mg, Acetaminophen 300 mg	Vicodin by Forest		Analgesic; C III
FOREST416	Tab, Green	Hydrocodone Bitartrate 5 mg, Acetaminophen 500 mg	by Forest Pharma	00456-0416	Analgesic; C III
FOREST416	Tab, Green, Round	Hydrocodone Bitartrate 5 mg, Acetaminophen 500 mg	by Forest Pharma	00456-0641	Analgesic; C III
FOREST429	Tab, White, Round	Phenobarbital 16 mg, Sodium Nitrate 65 mg	Soniphen by Forest		Sedative/Hypnotic; C IV
FOREST452	Cap, Orange & Yellow	Tetracycline HCl 250 mg	by Forest		Antibiotic
FOREST4910	Cap, Black & Blue, Forest/4910	Butalbital 50 mg, Caffeine 40 mg, Acetaminophen 500 mg, Codeine 30 mg	by Forest		Analgesic; C III
FOREST4922	Cap, Blue & White, Forest/4922	Butalbital 50 mg, Caffeine 40 mg, Acetaminophen 500 mg, Codeine 7.5 mg	by Forest		Analgesic; C III
FOREST4924	Cap, Blue & White, Forest/4924	Butalbital 50 mg, Caffeine 40 mg, Acetaminophen 500 mg, Codeine 10 mg	by Forest		Analgesic; C III
FOREST4930	Cap, Red & White, Forest/4930	Caffeine 30 mg, Acetaminophen 356.4 mg, Hydrocodone 5 mg	by Forest		Analgesic; C III
FOREST516	Tab, Green, Round	Phendimetrazine 35 mg	Metra by Forest		Anorexiant; C III
FOREST536	Tab, Orange, Round	Rauwolfia Serpentina 100 mg	Wolfina 100 by Forest		Antihypertensive
FOREST546	Cap, Red & White	Butalbital 50 mg, Acetaminophen 325 mg	Bancap by Forest	00456-0546	Analgesic
FOREST573	Cap, Brown & Red	Opium 3 mg, Bismuth Subcarbonate 60 mg, Kaolin 350 mg	KBP/O by Forest		Gastrointestinal
FOREST591	Tab, Orange, Round	Dextromethorphan Hydrobromide 15 mg, Guaifenesin 100 mg	Queltuss by Forest		Cold Remedy
FOREST606	Cap, Black	Phentermine HCl 30 mg	Obermine by Forest		Anorexiant; C IV
FOREST610	Cap, Orange & Yellow	Hydrocodone 5 mg, Acetaminophen 500 mg	Bancap HC by Forest	00456-0546	Analgesic; C III
FOREST610	Cap, Black & Red	Hydrocodone Bitartrate 5 mg, Acetaminophen 500 mg	by Forest Pharma	00456-0610	Analgesic; C III
FOREST610A	Cap, Orange & Yellow	Acetaminophen 500 mg, Hydrocodone Bitartrate 5 mg	Bancap HC by Forest	00456-0601	Analgesic; C III
FOREST617	Cap, Clearish Red	Chlorpheniramine Maleate 4 mg, Acetaminophen 325 mg, Phenylpropanolamine HCl 25 mg, Powdered Opium 2 mg	Hista-Derfule by Forest	00456-0617	Anlagesic
FOREST621	Tab, White, Oblong	Hyoscyamine Sulfate 0.125 mg	Neoquess by Forest		Gastrointestinal

ID FRONT <> BACK	DESCRIPTION FRONT <> BACK	INGREDIENT & STRENGTH	BRAND (OR EQUIV.) & FIRM	NDC#	CLASS; SCH.
FOREST624	Tab, Green, Oblong	Phenylpropanolamine 25 mg, Chlorpheniramine 4 mg, Acetaminophen 325 mg	Conex by Forest		Cold Remedy
FOREST627	Tab, Chartreuse, Round	Phenylpropanolamine 37.5 mg, Chlorpheniramine 4 mg	Conex DA by Forest		Cold Remedy
FOREST628	Cap, Clear & Orange	Chlorpheniramine Maleate 8 mg, Phenylpropanolamine HCl 75 mg	Dehist by Forest	00456-0628	Cold Remedy
FOREST630	Tab, White, Round	Acetaminophen 325 mg, Caffeine 40 mg, Butalbital 50 mg	Esgic by Forest	00456-0629	Analgesic
FOREST631	Cap, White, Opaque	Acetaminophen 325 mg, Butalbital 50 mg, Caffeine 40 mg	Esgic by Forest	00535-0012	Analgesic
FOREST631	Cap, White, Opaque	Butalbital 50 mg, Acetaminophen 325 mg, Anhydrous Caffeine 40 mg	Esgic by Forest	0535-0012	Analgesic
FOREST641	Tab, Green, Round	Hydrocodone 5 mg, Acetaminophen 500 mg	Anodynos DHC by Forest		Analgesic; C III
FOREST642	Cap, White, Soft-Gel	Theophylline Anhydrous, 100 mg	Elixophyllin DF by Forest	00456-0642	Antiasthmatic
FOREST643	Cap, White, Soft-Gel	Theophylline Anhydrous, 200 mg	Elixophyllin DF by Forest	00456-0643	Antiasthmatic
FOREST646	Cap, Clear, with White Nonpareils	Theophylline Anhydrous, 125 mg	Elixophyllin SR by Forest	00456-0646	Antiasthmatic
FOREST647	Cap, Clear, with White Nonpareils	Theophylline Anhydrous, 250 mg	Elixophyllin SR by Forest	00456-0647	Antiasthmatic
FOREST674	Tab, White, Round	Butalbital 50 mg, Acetaminophen 325 mg	Esgic CF by Forest	00456-0674	Analgesic
FOREST677	Cap, Black & Blue	Butalbital 50 mg, Acetaminophen 325 mg, Anhydrous caffeine 40 mg, Codeine Phosphate 30 mg	Esgic with Codeine by Forest	00456-0677	Analgesic; C III
FOREST678	Tab, Scored, Forest over 678	Acetaminophen 500 mg, Butalbital 50 mg, Caffeine 40 mg	Esgic Plus by Amerisource	62584-0678	Analgesic
FOREST678	Tab, White, Cap Shaped, Scored	acetaminophen 500 mg, Butalbital 50 mg, Caffeine 40 mg	by Allscripts	54569-3441	Analgesic
FOREST678	Tab, White, Cap Shaped, Scored	Acetaminophen 500 mg, Butalbital 50 mg, Caffeine 40 mg	Esgic Plus by Forest	00456-0678	Analgesic
FOREST678	Tab	Acetaminophen 500 mg, Butalbital 50 mg, Caffeine 40 mg	Esgic Plus by CVS	51316-0228	Analgesic
FOREST678	Tab, White, Oblong, Scored	Acetaminophen 500 mg; Butalbital 50 mg; Caffeine 40 mg	Esgic Plus by Thrift Services	59198-0333	Analgesic
FOREST678	Tab, White, Oblong, Scored	Butabital 50 mg, Acetaminophen 500 mg, Caffeine 40 mg	Esgic Plus by Caremark	00339-4111	Analgesic
FOREST707	Cap, Blue & Clear	Sucrose 75%, Starch 25%	Cebocap 1 by Forest	00456-0707	Placebo
FOREST707	Cap, Clear & Green, Old	Sucrose 75%, Starch 25%	Cebocap 2 by Forest Pharma	00456-0708	Placebo
FOREST707	Cap, Clear & Orange, Old	Sucrose 75%, Starch 25%	Cebocap 3 by Forest Pharma	00456-0709	Placebo
FOREST708	Cap, Clear & Green, New	Sucrose 75%, Starch 25%	Cebocap 2 by Forest	00456-0708	Placebo
FOREST709	Cap, Clear & Orange, New	Sucrose 75%, Starch 25%	Cebocap 3 by Forest	00456-0709	Placebo
FOREST766	Cap, Yellow	Phentermine HCl 30 mg	Obermine by Forest		Anorexiant; C IV
FORSLEEP <> RESTORIL15MG	Cap, For Sleep over For Sleep <> Restoril 15 mg over Restoril 15 mg	Temazepam 15 mg	Restoril by Novartis	00078-0098	Sedative/Hypnotic; C IV
FORSLEEP <> RESTORIL15MG	Cap, For Sleep over For Sleep <> Restoril 15 mg over Restoril 15 mg	Temazepam 15 mg	Restoril by Med Pro	53978-3080	Sedative/Hypnotic; C IV
FORSLEEP <> RESTORIL30MG	Cap, For Sleep over For Sleep <> Restoril 30 mg over Restoril 30 mg	Temazepam 30 mg	Restoril by Novartis	00078-0099	Sedative/Hypnotic; C IV
FORSLEEP <> RESTORIL30MG	Cap, For Sleep over For Sleep <> Restoril 30 mg over Restoril 30 mg	Temazepam 30 mg	Restoril by Med Pro	53978-3081	Sedative/Hypnotic; C IV
FOSAMAX <> MRK936	Tab, Fosamax Bone Image <> MRK 936 Bone Image	Alendronate Sodium 13.05 mg	Fosamax by Physicians Total Care	54868-3857	Antiosteoporosis
FOSAMAX <> MRK936	Tab, White, Round	Alendronate Sodium 10 mg	Fosamax by Heartland Hlthcare	61392-0854	Antiosteoporosis
FOSAMAX <> MRK936	Tab, White, Round, Bone Image	Alendronate Sodium 10 mg	Fosamax by Merck	00006-0936	Antiosteoporosis
FOSOMAX <> MRK212	Tab, White, Triangular, Bone Print	Alendronate Sodium 40 mg	Fosamax by Merck	00006-0212	Antiosteoporosis
FP <> 20MG	Tab, Pink, Oval, Scored, Film Coated	Citalopharm Hydrobromide 20 mg	Celexa by Compumed	00403-4894	Antidepressant
FP <> 20MG	Tab, Pink, Oval, Film Coated, Scored	Citalopram Hydrobromide 20 mg	Celexa by Forest	00456-4020	Antidepressant
FP <> 20MG	Tab, Film Coated, F/P	Citalopram Hydrobromide 24.98 mg	Celexa by Forest	63711-0120	Antidepressant
FP <> 40MG	Tab, White, Oval, Film Coated, Scored	Citalopram Hydrobromide 40 mg	Celexa by Forest	00456-4040	Antidepressant
FP <> 40MG	Tab, Film Coated, F/P	Citalopram Hydrobromide 49.96 mg	Celexa by Forest	63711-0140	Antidepressant
FR	Cap, Abbott Logo	Fenofibrate 67 mg	Tricor by Fournier Pharma	63924-0001	Antihyperlipidemic
FR	Cap, Yellow, FR over Abbott Logo	Fenofibrate Micronized 67 mg	Tri-Cor by Abbott	00074-4342	Antihyperlipidemic
FR1	Tab, White, Round	Acetaminophen 500 mg	Tylenol by Ultratab		Antipyretic
FROSST	Tab, Light Blue, Oblong	Timolol Maleate 20 mg	Blocadren by Frosst	Canadian	Antihypertensive
FROSST	Tab, White	Timolol Maleate 5 mg	Blocadren by Frosst	Canadian	Antihypertensive
FROSST 412	Tab, White, Doscoid	Bethanechol Chloride 10 mg	Urecholine by Frosst	Canadian	Urinary Tract
FROSST222AFR	Tab, White, Round, Frosst/222AF-R	Acetaminophen 325 mg	by Frosst	Canadian	Antipyretic
FROSST222AFX	Tab, White, Round, Frosst/222AF-X	Acetaminophen 500 mg	by Frosst	Canadian	Antipyretic
FROSST67	Tab, Light Blue, Hexagonal	Timolol Maleate 10 mg	Timolide by Frosst	Canadian	Antihypertensive

ID FRONT <> BACK	DESCRIPTION FRONT <> BACK	INGREDIENT & STRENGTH	BRAND (OR EQUIV.) & FIRM	NDC#	CLASS; SCH.
FROSST893	Tab, White, Round, Frosst/893	Acetaminophen 300 mg, Codeine Phosphate 30 mg, Caffeine Citrate 8 mg	Exdol by Frosst	Canadian	Analgesic
FROSST894	Tab, White, Round, Frosst/894	Acetaminophen 300 mg, Codeine Phosphate 30 mg, Caffeine Citrate 15 mg	Exdol by Frosst	Canadian	Analgesic
FROSST895	Tab, White, Round, Frosst/895	Acetaminophen 300 mg, Codeine Phosphate 30 mg, Caffeine Citrate 30 mg	Exdol by Frosst	Canadian	Analgesic
FS	Tab, White, Oval, Abb. Logo	Temafloxacin HCl 600 mg	Omniflox by Abbott		Antibiotic
FSCIBA	Tab, Reddish-Brown, Round, FS/Ciba	Maprotiline 75 mg	Ludiomil by Ciba	Canadian	Antidepressant
FSR	Cap, Clear & Red, F in Triangle Logo SR	Anhydrous Theophylline 260 mg	Aerolate SR by Fleming		Antiasthmatic
FSR	Cap, Green & Red, F in Triangle Logo SR	Chlorpheniramine 8 mg, Phenylephrine 20 mg, Methscopolamine 2.5 mg	Extendryl SR by Fleming		Cold Remedy
FSR	Cap, F in triangle	Chlorpheniramine Maleate 8 mg, Methscopolamine Nitrate 2.5 mg, Phenylephrine HCl 20 mg	Extendryl Sr by Fleming	00256-0111	Cold Remedy
FSR	Cap, Yellow	Flurbiprofen 200 mg	by Knoll	Canadian	NSAID
FSR	Cap, Blue & Clear, F in triangle SR	Guaifenesin 250 mg, Pseudoephedrine 120 mg	Congess SR by Fleming		Cold Remedy
FSR	Cap	Guaifenesin 250 mg, Pseudoephedrine HCl 120 mg	Congess Sr by Fleming	00256-0173	Cold Remedy
FSR	Cap, Green & Red	Phenylephrine HCl 20 mg, Methscopolamine Nitrate 2.5 mg, Chlorpheniramine Maleate 8 mg	Extendryl SR by DRX Pharm Consults	55045-2601	Cold Remedy
FSR	Cap, Clear & Red, Ex Release, with White Beads, F in Triangle	Theophylline 260 mg	Aerolate Sr by Fleming	00256-0115	Antiasthmatic
FULVICINPG	Tab, White, Oval, Fulvicin P/G	Griseofulvin Ultramicrosize 165 mg	Fulvicin P/G by Schering		Antifungal
FULVICINPG <> 352	Tab, Off White, Fulvicin P/G	Griseofulvin, Ultramicrocrystalline 330 mg	Fulvicin P G 330 by Pharm Utilization	60491-0275	Antifungal
FV <> CG	Tab, Dark Yellow, Round, Film Coated	Letrozole 2.5 mg	Femara by Novartis	00078-0249	Antineoplastic
FV <> CG	Tab, Dark Yellow, Round	Letrozole 2.5 mg	Femara by Novartis	Canadian DIN# 02231384	Antineoplastic
FVCG	Tab, Yellow, Round, FV/CG	Letrozole 2.5 mg	Femara by Novartis	Canadian	Antineoplastic
FWH 600	Tab, Blue, Ellipsoid	Cimetidine 600 mg	Peptol by Horner	Canadian	Gastrointestinal
FWH 800	Tab, Peach, Ellipsoid	Cimetidine 800 mg	Peptol by Horner	Canadian	Gastrointestinal
FWH200	Tab, Light Yellow, Round, FWH/200	Cimetidine 200 mg	Peptol by Horner	Canadian	Gastrointestinal
FWH300	Tab, Blue, Round, FWH/300	Cimetidine 300 mg	Peptol by Horner	Canadian	Gastrointestinal
FWH400	Tab, Peach, Round, FWH/400	Cimetidine 400 mg	Peptol by Horner	Canadian	Gastrointestinal
G <> 0030	Tab, Off-White, Film Coated, G <> 00 Over 30	Ranitidine HCl 168 mg	by Genpharm	55567-0030	Gastrointestinal
G <> 0030	Tab, White	Ranitidine 150 mg	by Mylan		Gastrointestinal
G <> 0031	Tab, White	Ranitidine 300 mg	by Mylan		Gastrointestinal
G <> 0031	Tab, Film Coated	Ranitidine HCl 336 mg	by Genpharm	55567-0031	Gastrointestinal
G <> 0034	Cap	Acyclovir 200 mg	by Genpharm	55567-0034	Antiviral
G <> 0034	Cap, Blue & Opaque	Acyclovir 200 mg	by Amerisource	62584-0736	Antiviral
G <> 0037	Tab	Acyclovir 800 mg	by Genpharm	55567-0037	Antiviral
G <> 0037	Tab, Blue, Oval	Acyclovir 800 mg	by Amerisource	62584-0783	Antiviral
G <> 0041	Cap	Nicardipine HCl 20 mg	by Genpharm	55567-0041	Antihypertensive
G <> 0041	Cap, Blue & Opaque & White, Hard Gel	Nicardipine HCl 20 mg	by Par	49884-0596	Antihypertensive
G <> 0042	Cap	Nicardipine HCl 30 mg	by Genpharm	55567-0042	Antihypertensive
G <> 0042	Cap, Blue & Opaque, Hard Gel	Nicardipine HCl 30 mg	by Par	49884-0599	Antihypertensive
G <> 026	Cap	Piroxicam 10 mg	by Par	49884-0440	NSAID
G <> 026	Cap, Dark Green & Olive	Piroxicam 10 mg	by Genpharm	55567-0026	NSAID
G <> 027	Cap	Piroxicam 20 mg	by Par	49884-0441	NSAID
G <> 027	Cap, 027	Piroxicam 20 mg	by Genpharm	55567-0027	NSAID
G <> 05	Tab, White, Oval, Scored, G <> 0.5	Estradiol 0.51 mg	by Teva	00093-1057	Hormone
G <> 05	Tab, G <> 0.5	Estradiol 0.51 mg	by AAI	27280-0004	Hormone
G <> 1	Tab, White, Hexagon, Scored	Estradiol 1 mg	by Teva	00093-1058	Hormone
G <> 1	Tab	Estradiol 1 mg	by AAI	27280-0005	Hormone
G <> 100	Tab	Atenolol 100 mg	by Par	49884-0457	Antihypertensive
G <> 1189500	Tab	Chlorzoxazone 500 mg	by Royce	51875-0239	Muscle Relaxant
G <> 180605	Tab, G <> 1806 0.5	Lorazepam 0.51 mg	by Royce	51875-0240	Sedative/Hypnotic; C IV
G <> 18071	Tab, G <> 1807 1	Lorazepam 1 mg	by Royce	51875-0241	Sedative/Hypnotic; C IV
G <> 18082	Tab, G <> 1808 2	Lorazepam 2 mg	by Royce	51875-0242	Sedative/Hypnotic; C IV

ID FRONT <> BACK	DESCRIPTION FRONT <> BACK	INGREDIENT & STRENGTH	BRAND (OR EQUIV.) & FIRM	NDC#	CLASS; SCH.
G <> 2	Tab, White, Round, Scored	Estradiol 2 mg	by Teva	00093-1059	Hormone
G <> 2	Tab	Estradiol 2 mg	by AAI	27280-0006	Hormone
G <> 2011	Tab, White, Round	Orphenadrine Citrate 100 mg	by Global Pharms (Ca)	00115-2011	Muscle Relaxant
G <> 30	Tab, White, Round, Film Coated	Ranitidine HCl 150 mg	by Mylan Pharms	00378-3252	Gastrointestinal
G <> 31	Tab, White, Oblong, Film Coated	Ranitidine HCl 300 mg	by Mylan Pharms	00378-3254	Gastrointestinal
G <> 38	Cap, Gray	Etodolac 200 mg	by Genpharm	55567-0038	NSAID
G <> 39	Cap, Gray	Etodolac 300 mg	by Genpharm	55567-0039	NSAID
G <> 40	Tab, Orange, Oval, Film Coated	Etodolac 400 mg	by Genpharm	55567-0040	NSAID
G <> 50	Tab	Atenolol 50 mg	by Par	49884-0456	Antihypertensive
G <> 53511	Tab, Gilbert Logo	Acetaminophen 325 mg, Butalbital 50 mg, Caffeine 40 mg	Esgic by Nat Pharmpak Serv	55154-4601	Analgesic
G <> 600	Tab, Film Coated	Ibuprofen 600 mg	by Quality Care	60346-0556	NSAID
G <> 800	Tab, Film Coated	Ibuprofen 400 mg	by Quality Care	60346-0030	NSAID
G <> 891		Levonorgestrel 0.25 mg, Ethinyl Estradiol 0.05 mg	Preven Emergency Contraceptive by Gynetics	63955-0020	Oral Contraceptive
G <> 891	Tab	Levonorgestrel 0.25 mg, Ethinyl Estradiol 0.05 mg	by Barr	00555-0891	Oral Contraceptive
G <> A100	Tab, A Over 100	Atenolol 100 mg	by Amerisource	62584-0621	Antihypertensive
G <> A50	Tab	Atenolol 50 mg	by Quality Care	60346-0719	Antihypertensive
G <> A50	Tab, A Over 50	Atenolol 50 mg	by Amerisource	62584-0620	Antihypertensive
G <> AC 400	Cap, Orange & Purple	Acebutolol HCl 400 mg	by Par Pharm	49884-0588	Antihypertensive
G <> AC200	Cap, Orange & Purple	Acebutolol HCl 200 mg	by Alphapharm	57315-0025	Antihypertensive
G <> AC200	Cap, Orange & Purple	Acebutolol HCl 200 mg	by Par Pharm	49884-0587	Antihypertensive
G <> AC200	Cap, Orange & Purple	Acebutolol HCl 200 mg	by Genpharm	55567-0089	Antihypertensive
G <> AC400	Cap, Orange & Purple	Acebutolol HCl 400 mg	by Alphapharm	57315-0026	Antihypertensive
G <> AC400	Cap, Orange & Purple	Acebutolol HCl 400 mg	by Genpharm	55567-0090	Antihypertensive
G <> AL025	Tab, Light Yellow, Coated, <> AL/0.25	Alprazolam 0.25 mg	by Quality Care	60346-0876	Antianxiety; C IV
G <> AL025	Tab	Alprazolam 0.25 mg	by Par	49884-0448	Antianxiety; C IV
G <> AL05	Tab	Alprazolam 0.5 mg	by Par	49884-0449	Antianxiety; C IV
G <> AL10	Tab	Alprazolam 1 mg	by Par	49884-0450	Antianxiety; C IV
G <> AL10	Tab, G <> AL 1.0	Alprazolam 1 mg	by Alphapharm	57315-0008	Antianxiety; C IV
G <> AL10	Tab, G <> AL 1.0	Alprazolam 1 mg	by Direct Dispensing	57866-4636	Antianxiety; C IV
G <> CN05	Tab, G <> CN over 0.5	Clonazepam 0.5 mg	by Alphapharm	57315-0017	Anticonvulsant; C IV
G <> CN1	Tab, G <> CN over 1	Clonazepam 1 mg	by Alphapharm	57315-0018	Anticonvulsant; C IV
G <> CN2	Tab, G <> CN over 2	Clonazepam 2 mg	by Alphapharm	57315-0019	Anticonvulsant; C IV
G <> ET500	Tab, Blue, Oval, Convex, Film	Etodolac 500 mg	by Heartland	61392-0916	NSAID
G <> ET500	Tab, Blue, Oval, Film Coated	Etodolac 500 mg	by Genpharm	55567-0032	NSAID
G <> GP10	Tab	Glipizide 10 mg	by Par	49884-0452	Antidiabetic
G <> GP5	Tab	Glipizide 5 mg	by Par	49884-0451	Antidiabetic
G <> GU1	Tab, White, Oval	Guanfacine HCl 1 mg	by Par Pharm	49884-0572	Antihypertensive
G <> GU1	Tab, White, Oval	Guanfacine HCl 1 mg	by Genpharm	55567-0051	Antihypertensive
G <> GU2	Tab, White, Oval	Guanfacine HCl 2 mg	by Par Pharm	49884-0573	Antihypertensive
G <> GU2	Tab, White, Oval	Guanfacine HCl 2 mg	by Genpharm	55567-0052	Antihypertensive
G <> IE125	Tab, Film Coated, G <> IE Over 1.25	Indapamide 1.25 mg	by Alphapharm	57315-0027	Diuretic
G <> IE25	Tab, Film Coated, G <> IE Over 2.5	Indapamide 2.5 mg	by Alphapharm	57315-0028	Diuretic
G <> P10	Tab	Pindolol 10 mg	by Par	49884-0443	Antihypertensive
G <> P10	Tab	Pindolol 10 mg	by Genpharm	55567-0016	Antihypertensive
G <> P10	Tab	Pindolol 10 mg	by United Res	00677-1458	Antihypertensive
G <> P5	Tab	Pindolol 5 mg	by Par	49884-0442	Antihypertensive
G <> P5	Tab	Pindolol 5 mg	by Genpharm	55567-0015	Antihypertensive
G <> P5	Tab	Pindolol 5 mg	by United Res	00677-1457	Antihypertensive
G <> S	Tab, White, Oblong, Scored	Sotalol HCl 80 mg	by Par Pharm	49884-0582	Antiarrhythmic
G <> S120	Tab, White, Oblong	Sotalol HCl 120 mg	by Genpharm	55567-0076	Antiarrhythmic
G <> S120	Tab, White, Oblong	Sotalol HCl 120 mg	by Par Pharm	49884-0583	Antiarrhythmic

ID FRONT <> BACK	DESCRIPTION FRONT <> BACK	INGREDIENT & STRENGTH	BRAND (OR EQUIV.) & FIRM	NDC#	CLASS; SCH.
G <> S160	Tab, White, Oblong	Sotalol HCl 160 mg	by Par Pharm	49884-0584	Antiarrhythmic
G <> S240	Tab, White, Oblong	Sotalol HCl 240 mg	by Par Pharm	49884-0585	Antiarrhythmic
G <> S240	Tab, White, Oblong	Sotalol HCl 240 mg	by Genpharm	55567-0059	Antiarrhythmic
G <> S5E	Tab, White, Round	Selegiline HCl 5 mg	by Par Pharm	49884-0610	Antiparkinson
G <> SE5	Tab, White, Round, Convex, G <> SE over 5	Selegiline HCl 5 mg	Selegiline HCl by Schein	00364-2830	Antiparkinson
G <> SR	Cap, Orange, Abbott Logo	Fenofibrate 200 mg	Tricor Micronized by Integrity	64731-0187	Antihyperlipidemic
G <> T250	Tab, White, Oval, Convex, Film	Ticlopidine HCl 250 mg	Ticlopidine HCl by Teva	00093-0154	Anticoagulant
G <> T250	Tab, White, Oval, Convex, Film	Ticlopidine HCl 250 mg	by Teva	00093-0290	Anticoagulant
G <> TR125	Tab	Triazolam 0.125 mg	by Par	49884-0453	Sedative/Hypnotic; C IV
G <> TR125	Tab, TR/125	Triazolam 0.125 mg	by Qualitest	00603-6186	Sedative/Hypnotic; C IV
G <> TR250	Tab	Triazolam 0.25 mg	by Par	49884-0454	Sedative/Hypnotic; C IV
G <> TR250	Tab, TR/250	Triazolam 0.25 mg	by Quality Care	60346-0886	Sedative/Hypnotic; C IV
G <> TR250	Tab, TR/250	Triazolam 0.25 mg	by Qualitest	00603-6187	Sedative/Hypnotic; C IV
G 3723	Tab, White, Oval	Flurbiprofen 50 mg	Ansaid by Greenstone		NSAID
G0036	Tab, G over 0036	Acyclovir 400 mg	by Genpharm	55567-0036	Antiviral
G0036	Tab, White, Pentagon, G Over 0036	Acyclovir 400 mg	by Amerisource	62584-0749	Antiviral
G004	Tab, Red, Oval	Docusate Sodium 100 mg	by Group Health	58087-0110	Laxative
G0104	Cap, Black & Purple, G-0104	Phenylpropanolamine HCl 75 mg, Caramiphen Edisylate 40 mg	Tuss- by Pioneer		Cold Remedy
G0112 <> Z2416	Cap, Orange & Yellow	Tetracycline HCl 250 mg	Tetrex by Zenith Goldline	00172-2416	Antibiotic
G0131	Cap, Clear	Quinine Sulfate 325 mg	by Nutro Laboratories		Antimalarial
G03	Tab	Hydralazine HCl 25 mg	by Zenith Goldline	00182-0554	Antihypertensive
G04	Tab	Hydralazine HCl 10 mg	by Zenith Goldline	00182-0905	Antihypertensive
G05	Tab	Hydralazine HCl 50 mg	by Zenith Goldline	00182-0555	Antihypertensive
G0506	Tab, White, Round, G-0506	Reserpine 0.1 mg, Hydralazine HCl 25 mg, Hydrochlorothiazide 15 mg	Ser- by Zenith		Antihypertensive
G0507	Tab, Yellow, Round	Folic Acid 1 mg	Folvite by West-ward		Vitamin
G0556	Tab	Hydrochlorothiazide 25 mg	by Zenith Goldline	00182-0556	Diuretic
G0557	Tab	Hydrochlorothiazide 50 mg	by Zenith Goldline	00182-0557	Diuretic
G06	Tab	Hydralazine HCl 100 mg	by Zenith Goldline	00182-1553	Antihypertensive
G0679 <> Z2407	Cap	Tetracycline HCl 500 mg	by Zenith Goldline	00182-0679	Antibiotic
G0679 <> Z2407	Cap, Black & Yellow	Tetracycline HCl 500 mg	Tetrex by Zenith Goldline	00172-2407	Antibiotic
G07	Tab, Sugar Coated	Hydroxyzine HCl 10 mg	by Zenith Goldline	00182-1492	Antihistamine
G08	Tab, Sugar Coated	Hydroxyzine HCl 25 mg	by Zenith Goldline	00182-1493	Antihistamine
G09	Tab, Sugar Coated	Hydroxyzine HCl 50 mg	by Zenith Goldline	00182-1494	Antihistamine
G10	Tab, White, Oval	Medroxyprogesterone Acetate 10 mg	by Genpharm	Canadian	Progestin
G100BAYERCROSS	Tab, Off-White, Round, G100/Bayer Cross	Acarbose 100 mg	Prandase by Bayer	Canadian	Antidiabetic
G1043	Tab	Amoxapine 25 mg	by Zenith Goldline	00182-1043	Antidepressant
G1044	Tab, Salmon, Round	Amoxapine 50 mg	Asendin by Watson		Antidepressant
G1094	Tab, Red, Round	Phenylprop. 40 mg, Phenyleph. 10 mg, Phenyltoxlox. 15 mg, Chlorphenir. 5 mg	Naldecon by Rosemont		Cold Remedy
G1098	Cap, Light Green	Hydroxyzine Pamoate 25 mg	Vistaril by Zenith Goldline	00182-1098	Antihistamine
G1098 <> Z2911	Cap, Dark Green & Light Green	Hydroxyzine Pamoate 25 mg	Vistaril by Zenith Goldline	00172-2911	Antihistamine
G1099 <> Z2909	Cap, Green & White	Hydroxyzine Pamoate 50 mg	Vistaril by Zenith Goldline	00172-2909	Antihistamine
G1140	Tab, Flesh, Oblong	Amitriptyline HCl 150 mg	Elavil by MD		Antidepressant
G1161	Tab, White, Round	Furosemide 40 mg	Lasix by Watson		Diuretic
G1170	Tab	Furosemide 20 mg	by Med Pro	53978-5031	Diuretic
G1189	Tab	Chlorzoxazone 500 mg	by Zenith Goldline	00182-1189	Muscle Relaxant
G1234	Cap	Acetaminophen 325 mg, Dichloralantipyrine 100 mg, Isomethepene Mucate (1:1) 65 mg	Ida by Zenith Goldline	00182-1234	Cold Remedy
G1300	Tab, White, Round	Verapamil HCl 80 mg	Isoptin by Watson		Antihypertensive
G1301	Tab, White, Round	Verapamil HCl 120 mg	Isoptin by Watson		Antihypertensive
G1330 <> Z2971	Tab, White, Round	Metronidazole 250 mg	Flagyl by Zenith Goldline	00172-2971	Antibiotic
G135	Tab, White, Round	Doxylamine Succinate 25 mg	Unisom by Granutec		Sleep Aid

| --- | --- | --- | --- | --- | --- |
G14	Tab, Green, Oblong	Acetaminophen 500 mg, Pseudophed HCl 60 mg, Dexbrophen Mal 2 mg	Super Sina Care by Apothecary Products		Cold Remedy
G1410	Tab, White, Round	Acetaminophen 325 mg	Tylenol by Granutec		Antipyretic
G1457	Tab, White, Round	Acetaminophen 500 mg	Tylenol Ex-Strength by Granutec		Antipyretic
G150	Tab, White, Round, G/150	Ranitidine 150 mg	by Genpharm	Canadian	Gastrointestinal
G150MG <> 3328	Cap, G 150 MG	Clindamycin HCl	by Quality Care	60346-0018	Antibiotic
G150MG3328	Cap, Light Blue & Green	Clindamycin HCl	by Allscripts	54569-3456	Antibiotic
G17	Tab, Light Blue, Oval	Naproxen Sodium 220 mg	by Novopharm		NSAID
G17 <> LL	Tab, Film Coated	Gemfibrozil 600 mg	by Vangard	00615-3559	Antihyperlipidemic
G1724	Tab, White, Round	Quinidine Sulfate 300 mg	by Eon		Antiarrhythmic
G1736	Tab	Furosemide 80 mg	by Zenith Goldline	00182-1736	Diuretic
G1789	Tab	Metoclopramide HCl 10 mg	by Med Pro	53978-5011	Gastrointestinal
G1802	Tab, Yellow, Round	Salsalate 500 mg	Disalcid by Rosemont Pharmaceutical		NSAID
G1803	Tab, Yellow, Oblong	Salsalate 750 mg	Disalcid by Rosemont Pharmaceutical		NSAID
G180605	Tab, White, Round, G 1806/0.5	Lorazepam 0.5 mg	Ativan by Royce		Sedative/Hypnotic; C IV
G1808	Tab	Lorazepam 2 mg	by Zenith Goldline	00182-1808	Sedative/Hypnotic; C IV
G1839	Tab, Film Coated	Potassium Chloride 600 mg	by Zenith Goldline	00182-1839	Electrolytes
G1840	Tab, Film Coated	Potassium Chloride 750 mg	by Zenith Goldline	00182-1840	Electrolytes
G1872	Tab, Yellow, Round	Triamterene 75 mg, Hydrochlorothiazide 50 mg	Maxzide by Watson		Diuretic
G1919	Tab, Film Coated	Cyclobenzaprine HCl 10 mg	by Invamed	52189-0252	Muscle Relaxant
G1LL	Tab, Brown, Oblong, G1-LL	Vitamin, Mineral	Gevral by Lederle		Vitamin
G2	Tab, White, Round, G-2	Triprolidine HCl 2.5 mg, Psuedoephedrine 60 mg	Actifed by K.C.		Cold Remedy
G2 <> AL	Tab, White, Oblong, Scored	Alprazolam 2 mg	by Par Pharm	49884-0400	Antianxiety; C IV
G2 <> MYLAN	Tab, White, Round, Scored	Glipizide 10 mg	by Kaiser	00179-1316	Antidiabetic
G21	Tab, Film Coated	Amitriptyline HCl 10 mg	by Zenith Goldline	00182-1018	Antidepressant
G2152	Tab, White, Oblong	Acetaminophen 500 mg	Tylenol Ex-Strength by Baker		Antipyretic
G22	Tab, Coated, G-22	Amitriptyline HCl 25 mg	by Quality Care	60346-0027	Antidepressant
G22	Tab, Film Coated	Amitriptyline HCl 25 mg	by Zenith Goldline	00182-1019	Antidepressant
G23	Tab, Film Coated	Amitriptyline HCl 50 mg	by Zenith Goldline	00182-1020	Antidepressant
G237	Cap, Green	Chloral Hydrate 500 mg	Noctec by R. P. Scherer		Sedative/Hypnotic; C IV
G24	Tab, Film Coated	Amitriptyline HCl 75 mg	by Zenith Goldline	00182-1021	Antidepressant
G25	Tab, Film Coated	Amitriptyline HCl 100 mg	by Zenith Goldline	00182-1063	Antidepressant
G25	Tab	Atenolol 25 mg	by Genpharm	55567-0025	Antihypertensive
G25	Tab, Peach, Oval, G 2.5	Medroxyprogesterone Acetate 2.5 mg	by Genpharm	Canadian	Progestin
G283	Cap, Natural & Pink	Diphenhydramine HCl 25 mg	by PFI		Antihistamine
G284	Cap, Blue	Pseudoephedrine 60 mg, Diphenhydramine 25 mg	by PFI		Cold Remedy
G29	Tab	Chlorpropamide 250 mg	by Zenith Goldline	00182-1852	Antidiabetic
G297	Cap	Chloral Hydrate 500 mg	by United Res	00677-0225	Sedative/Hypnotic; C IV
G297	Cap, Clear & Light Green	Chloral Hydrate 500 mg	by RP Scherer	11014-0918	Sedative/Hypnotic; C IV
G2LL	Tab, Maroon, Oblong, G2-LL	Vitamin, Mineral	Gevral T by Lederle		Vitamin
G30	Tab	Chlorthalidone 25 mg	by Zenith Goldline	00182-1434	Diuretic
G300	Tab, White, Oblong, G/300	Ranitidine 300 mg	by Genpharm	Canadian	Gastrointestinal
G324	Cap, Red	Chloral Hydrate 500 mg	Noctec by R. P. Scherer		Sedative/Hypnotic; C IV
G3327 <> 4	Tab, White, Oval, Scored	Methylprednisolone 4 mg	by Pharmacia & Upjohn	00009-3327	Steroid
G33274	Tab, White, Oval, G 3327/4	Methylprednisolone 4 mg	Medrol by Greenstone		Steroid
G33274	Tab, White, Elliptical, G 3327/4	Methylprednisone Acetate 4 mg	Medrol by Upjohn		Steroid
G3328	Cap, Blue & Green	Clindamycin HCl 150 mg	Cleocin by Greenstone		Antibiotic
G359 <> 832	Tab	Fluoxymesterone 10 mg	by Qualitest	00603-3645	Steroid; C III
G3717	Tab, White	Triazolam 0.125 mg	by HJ Harkins	52959-0401	Sedative/Hypnotic; C IV
G3717	Tab, White	Triazolam 0.125 mg	by DRX Pharm Consults	55045-2550	Sedative/Hypnotic; C IV
G3717	Tab	Triazolam 0.125 mg	by St Marys Med	60760-0717	Sedative/Hypnotic; C IV
G3717	Tab, White, Scored	Triazolam 0.125 mg	by Pharmacia & Upjohn	00009-3717	Sedative/Hypnotic; C IV

ID FRONT <> BACK	DESCRIPTION FRONT <> BACK	INGREDIENT & STRENGTH	BRAND (OR EQUIV.) & FIRM	NDC#	CLASS; SCH.
G3718	Tab, Blue, Scored	Triazolam 0.25 mg	by HJ Harkins	52959-0402	Sedative/Hypnotic; C IV
G3718	Tab, Blue, Oval, Scored	Triazolam 0.25 mg	by Allscripts	54569-3966	Sedative/Hypnotic; C IV
G3718	Tab	Triazolam 0.25 mg	by Quality Care	60346-0886	Sedative/Hypnotic; C IV
G3718	Tab, Blue, Scored	Triazolam 0.25 mg	by Pharmacia & Upjohn	00009-3718	Sedative/Hypnotic; C IV
G3719	Tab, Coated, G 3719	Alprazolam 0.25 mg	by Quality Care	60346-0876	Antianxiety; C IV
G3719	Tab, Coated	Alprazolam 0.25 mg	by Pharmacia & Upjohn	00009-3719	Antianxiety; C IV
G3720	Tab, Peach, Oval, Scored	Alprazolam 0.5 mg	by HJ Harkins	52959-0457	Antianxiety; C IV
G3720	Tab, Peach, Elliptical	Alprazolam 0.5 mg	Xanax by Greenstone		Antianxiety; C IV
G3720	Tab, Peach, Oval, Scored	Alprazolam 0.5 mg	by Pharmacia & Upjohn	00009-3720	Antianxiety; C IV
G3721	Tab, Coated	Alprazolam 1 mg	by Physicians Total Care	54868-3005	Antianxiety; C IV
G3721	Tab, Coated, G 3721	Alprazolam 1 mg	by Quality Care	60346-0932	Antianxiety; C IV
G3721	Tab, Coated	Alprazolam 1 mg	by Golden State	60429-0504	Antianxiety; C IV
G3721	Tab, Coated	Alprazolam 1 mg	by Pharmacia & Upjohn	00009-3721	Antianxiety; C IV
G3722	Tab, Coated, Multi Scored	Alprazolam 2 mg	by Golden State	60429-0505	Antianxiety; C IV
G3722	Tab, White, Oblong	Alprazolam 2 mg	by Allscripts	54569-4900	Antianxiety; C IV
G3722	Tab, Coated, Scored	Alprazolam 2 mg	by Pharmacia & Upjohn	00009-3722	Antianxiety; C IV
G3724	Tab, Coated	Flurbiprofen 100 mg	by Pharmacia & Upjohn	00009-3724	NSAID
G3724	Tab, Coated	Flurbiprofen 100 mg	by Repack Co of Amer	55306-3724	NSAID
G3725	Tab, White, Round	Glyburide 1.25 mg	Diabeta by Greenstone		Antidiabetic
G3726	Tab	Glyburide 2.5 mg	by Direct Dispensing	57866-6408	Antidiabetic
G3726	Tab	Glyburide 2.5 mg	by Caremark	00339-5912	Antidiabetic
G3726	Tab	Glyburide 2.5 mg	by DRX	55045-2322	Antidiabetic
G3726	Tab, Pink, Round, Scored	Glyburide 2.5 mg	by Pharmacia & Upjohn	00009-3726	Antidiabetic
G3727	Tab, Blue, Round, Scored	Glyburide 5 mg	by Pharmacia & Upjohn	00009-3727	Antidiabetic
G3727	Tab	Glyburide 5 mg	by Direct Dispensing	57866-6409	Antidiabetic
G3727	Tab, Blue, Round, Scored	Glyburide 5 mg	by HJ Harkins	52959-0449	Antidiabetic
G3727	Tab	Glyburide 5 mg	by Caremark	00339-5914	Antidiabetic
G3727	Tab	Glyburide 5 mg	by DRX	55045-2138	Antidiabetic
G3727	Tab, Blue, Round, Scored	Glyburide 5 mg	by KV	10609-1438	Antidiabetic
G3740	Tab	Medroxyprogesterone Acetate 2.5 mg	by Pharmacia & Upjohn	00009-3740	Progestin
G3740	Tab, Compressed	Medroxyprogesterone Acetate 2.5 mg	by Kaiser	00179-1201	Progestin
G3740	Tab	Medroxyprogesterone Acetate 2.5 mg	by Quality Care	60346-0213	Progestin
G3740	Tab	Medroxyprogesterone Acetate 2.5 mg	by Apotheca	12634-0432	Progestin
G3741	Tab	Medroxyprogesterone Acetate 5 mg	by Pharmacia & Upjohn	00009-3741	Progestin
G3741	Tab, Compressed	Medroxyprogesterone Acetate 5 mg	by Kaiser	00179-1202	Progestin
G3741	Tab	Medroxyprogesterone Acetate 5 mg	by PDRX	55289-0908	Progestin
G3742	Tab, White, Round, Scored	Medroxyprogesterone Acetate 10 mg	by Nat Pharmpak Serv	55154-5568	Progestin
G3742	Tab	Medroxyprogesterone Acetate 10 mg	by Pharmacia & Upjohn	00009-3742	Progestin
G3742	Tab, Compressed	Medroxyprogesterone Acetate 10 mg	by Kaiser	00179-1117	Progestin
G3783	Tab, Yellow, Ovoid, Scored	Glyburide 6 mg	Micronized Glyburide by Kaiser	00179-1325	Antidiabetic
G3783	Tab, Yellow, Oval, Scored	Glyburide Micronized 6 mg	by Lederle	59911-3606	Antidiabetic
G3783	Tab, Yellow, Oval	Glyburide Micronized 6 mg	by Greenstone		Antidiabetic
G383	Cap, Red	Guaifenesin	Robitussin Gelcaps by Granutec		Expectorant
G4 <> M	Tab	Guanfacine HCl	by Mylan	00378-1160	Antihypertensive
G400	Tab, Film Coated	Ibuprofen 400 mg	by Apotheca	12634-0171	NSAID
G400	Tab, Coated	Ibuprofen 400 mg	by Pharmacia & Upjohn	00009-7378	NSAID
G400	Tab, Film Coated	Ibuprofen 400 mg	by Caremark	00339-6076	NSAID
G400	Tab, Film Coated	Ibuprofen 400 mg	by Allscripts	54569-0285	NSAID
G400	Tab, Film Coated	Ibuprofen 400 mg	by Quality Care	60346-0430	NSAID
G400	Tab, Coated	Ibuprofen 400 mg	by Prescription Dispensing	61807-0027	NSAID
G403 <> G403	Cap, White with Blue Print, Gelatin	Sevelamer HCl 403 mg	Renagel by Genzyme/GelTex	58468-4709	Phosphate Binder
G42	Cap, Clear & Red	Docusate 100 mg	Colace by Goldcaps		Laxative

ID FRONT <> BACK	DESCRIPTION FRONT <> BACK	INGREDIENT & STRENGTH	BRAND (OR EQUIV.) & FIRM	NDC#	CLASS; SCH.
G43	Cap, Red	Docusate 100 mg, Casanthrol 30 mg	Peri-Colace by Goldcaps		Laxative
G463 <> 832	Tab	Medroxyprogesterone Acetate 10 mg	by Quality Care	60346-0571	Progestin
G463 <> 832	Tab	Medroxyprogesterone Acetate 10 mg	by Qualitest	00603-4368	Progestin
G465832	Tab, White, Round, G 465/832	Megesterol Acetate 20 mg	Megace by Rosemont		Progestin
G466832	Tab, White, Round, G 466/832	Megesterol Acetate 40 mg	Megace by Rosemont		Progestin
G5	Tab, Red & Yellow, Oblong	Acetaminophen 500 mg	Tylenol by Granutec		Antipyretic
G5	Tab, Blue, Oval	Medroxyprogesterone Acetate 5 mg	by Genpharm	Canadian	Progestin
G5 <> M	Tab	Guanfacine HCl	by Mylan	00378-1190	Antihypertensive
G500 <> G500	Tab, Yellow, Round, Scored	Sulfasalazine 500 mg	by St. Marys Med	60760-0138	Gastrointestinal
G500 <> G500	Tab, Yellow, Round, Scored	Sulfasalazine 500 mg	Azulfidine by St. Marys Med	60760-0237	Gastrointestinal
G50BAYERCROSS	Tab, Off-White, Round, G50/Bayer Cross	Acarbose 50 mg	Prandase by Bayer	Canadian	Antidiabetic
G52 <> G52	Tab, Pink, Round	Ranitidine HCl 75 mg	Ranitidine HCl by RX PAK	65084-0173	Gastrointestinal
G600	Tab	Ibuprofen 600 mg	by Pharmacia & Upjohn	00009-7379	NSAID
G600	Tab	Ibuprofen 600 mg	by Caremark	00339-6077	NSAID
G600	Tab, Coated	Ibuprofen 600 mg	by Allscripts	54569-0287	NSAID
G600	Tab, Film Coated	Ibuprofen 600 mg	by Med Pro	53978-5006	NSAID
G600	Tab, Coated	Ibuprofen 600 mg	by Apotheca	12634-0191	NSAID
G600 <> TTC	Tab	Guaifenesin 600 mg	by United Res	00677-1475	Expectorant
G600 <> TTC	Tab, Light Green, Delayed Release, G 600	Guaifenesin 600 mg	by Quality Care	60346-0863	Expectorant
G800	Tab, Coated	Ibuprofen 800 mg	by Pharmacia & Upjohn	00009-7380	NSAID
G800	Tab, Coated	Ibuprofen 800 mg	by Caremark	00339-6078	NSAID
G800	Tab	Ibuprofen 800 mg	by Allscripts	54569-3332	NSAID
G800	Tab, Coated	Ibuprofen 800 mg	by Allscripts	54569-0289	NSAID
G800	Tab, Film Coated	Ibuprofen 800 mg	by Med Pro	53978-5007	NSAID
GA100	Tab, Coated	Atenolol 100 mg	by Zenith Goldline	00182-1005	Antihypertensive
GA50	Tab	Atenolol 50 mg	by Zenith Goldline	00182-1004	Antihypertensive
GA50	Tab	Atenolol 50 mg	by Med Pro	53978-1199	Antihypertensive
GANTACID	Tab, White, Round, G/Antacid	Calcium Carbonate 585 mg, Magensium Hydro 120 mg, Simethicone 30 mg	Gastrozepin by Boehringer Ingelheim	Canadian	Vitamin/Mineral
GAT100	Tab, White, Round, G/AT/100	Atenolol 100 mg	Gen Atenolol by Genpharm	Canadian	Antihypertensive
GAT100	Tab, White, Round, G/AT/100	Atenolol 100 mg	by Genpharm	Canadian	Antihypertensive
GAT50	Tab, White, Round, G/AT/50	Atenolol 50 mg	Gen Atenolol by Genpharm	Canadian	Antihypertensive
GAT60	Tab, White, Round, G/AT/60	Atenolol 60 mg	by Genpharm	Canadian	Antihypertensive
GATE <> MOBAN10	Tab	Molindone HCl 10 mg	Moban by Gate	57844-0915	Antipsychotic
GATE <> MOBAN100	Tab	Molindone HCl 100 mg	Moban by Gate	57844-0918	Antipsychotic
GATE <> MOBAN25	Tab	Molindone HCl 25 mg	Moban by Gate	57844-0916	Antipsychotic
GATE <> MOBAN5	Tab	Molindone HCl 5 mg	Moban by Gate	57844-0914	Antipsychotic
GATE <> MOBAN510	Tab	Molindone HCl 50 mg	Moban by Gate	57844-0917	Antipsychotic
GAVISCONEXTRA	Tab, White, Round, Gaviscon/Extra	Alginic Acid 400 mg	Gaviscon by SmithKline SKB	Canadian	Gastrointestinal
GBN10	Tab, White, Round, G BN/10	Baclofen 10 mg	Lioresal by Genpharm		Muscle Relaxant
GBN20	Tab, White, Round, G BN/20	Baclofen 20 mg	Lioresal by Genpharm		Muscle Relaxant
GC125	Tab, White, Oblong, G/C 12.5	Captopril 12.5 mg	by Genpharm	Canadian	Antihypertensive
GDC103	Tab, White, Round	Simethicone 80 mg	Mylicon-80 by Guardian		Antiflatulent
GDC127	Tab, Multi-Colored, Round	Calcium Carbonate 750 mg	Tums E-X by Guardian		Vitamin/Mineral
GE5GG	Tab, White, Oblong, GE/5/G/G	Glyburide 5 mg	Gen Glybe by Genpharm	Canadian	Antidiabetic
GEIGEY136	Tab, Orange, Round	Imipramine HCl 50 mg	Tofranil by Novartis Pharms (Ca)	61615-0106	Antidepressant
GEIGEY32	Tab, Orange, Triangle	Imipramine HCl 10 mg	Tofranil by Novartis Pharms (Ca)	61615-0104	Antidepressant
GEIGY	Tab, White, Round, Scored	Carbamazepine 200 mg	Tegretol by Novartis	Canadian DIN# 00010405	Anticonvulsant
GEIGY	Cap	Clofazimine 50 mg	Lamprene by Novartis	17088-0108	Antileprosy

ID FRONT <> BACK	DESCRIPTION FRONT <> BACK	INGREDIENT & STRENGTH	BRAND (OR EQUIV.) & FIRM	NDC#	CLASS; SCH.
GEIGY	Tab, White, Round, Scored	Nicoumalone 4 mg	Sintrom by Geigy	Canadian DIN# 00010391	Anticoagulant
GEIGY <> 3535	Tab	Hydrochlorothiazide 25 mg, Metoprolol Tartrate 50 mg	Lopressor HCT by Novartis	00028-0035	Diuretic; Antihypertensive
GEIGY <> 5151	Tab, Coated	Metoprolol Tartrate 50 mg	Lopressor by Novartis	00028-0051	Antihypertensive
GEIGY <> 5151	Tab, Coated	Metoprolol Tartrate 50 mg	Lopressor by Caremark	00339-5213	Antihypertensive
GEIGY <> 5151	Tab, Coated, Geigy <> 51/51	Metoprolol Tartrate 50 mg	Lopressor by Wal Mart	49035-0179	Antihypertensive
GEIGY <> 5151	Tab, Coated	Metoprolol Tartrate 50 mg	Lopressor by Nat Pharmpak Serv	55154-1009	Antihypertensive
GEIGY <> 5151	Tab, Light Red, Cap Shaped, Film Coated, Scored	Metoprolol Tartrate 50 mg	Lopresor by Novartis	Canadian DIN# 00397423	Antihypertensive
GEIGY <> 5353	Tab,	Hydrochlorothiazide 25 mg, Metoprolol Tartrate 100 mg	Lopressor HCT by Novartis	00028-0053	Diuretic; Antihypertensive
GEIGY <> 5353	Tab, Pink & White	Hydrochlorothiazide 25 mg, Metoprolol Tartrate 100 mg	Lopressor HCT by Pharm Utilization	60491-0371	Diuretic; Antihypertensive
GEIGY <> 7171	Tab, Light Blue, Cap Shaped, Film Coated, Scored	Metoprolol Tartrate 100 mg	Lopresor by Novartis	Canadian DIN# 00397431	Antihypertensive
GEIGY <> 7171	Tab, Film Coated	Metoprolol Tartrate 100 mg	Lopressor by Novartis	00028-0071	Antihypertensive
GEIGY <> 7373	Tab	Hydrochlorothiazide 50 mg, Metoprolol Tartrate 100 mg	Lopressor HCT by Novartis	00028-0073	Diuretic; Antihypertensive
GEIGY <> ATA	Tab, Brownish-Red, Round, Sugar Coated	Imipramine HCl 75 mg	Tofranil by Novartis	Canadian DIN# 00306487	Antidepressant
GEIGY <> CDC	Tab, Light Yellow, Round, Film Coated	Metoprolol Tartrate 200 mg	Lopresor SR by Novartis	Canadian DIN# 00534560	Antihypertensive
GEIGY <> FH	Tab, Cream, Round, Sugar Coated	Clomipramine HCl 25 mg	Anafranil by Novartis	Canadian DIN# 00324019	OCD
GEIGY <> GW	Tab, White to Off-White, Cap Shaped, Scored	Baclofen 20 mg	Lioresal by Geigy	Canadian DIN# 00636576	Muscle Relaxant
GEIGY <> KJ	Tab, White to Off-White, Oval, Scored	Baclofen 10 mg	Lioresal by Geigy	Canadian DIN# 00455881	Muscle Relaxant
GEIGY <> KR100	Tab, Brownish-Orange, Round, Film Coated	Metoprolol Tartrate 100 mg	Lopresor SR by Novartis	Canadian DIN# 00658855	Antihypertensive
GEIGY <> LB	Tab, Brownish-Red, Round, Sugar Coated	Imipramine HCl 50 mg	Tofranil by Novartis	Canadian DIN# 00010480	Antidepressant
GEIGY <> LP	Tab, White, Round, Film Coated	Clomipramine HCl 50 mg	Anafranil by Novartis	Canadian DIN# 00402591	OCD
GEIGY <> MR	Tab, White w/ Red Specks, Round, Scored	Carbamazepine 100 mg	Tegretol Chewtabs by Novartis	Canadian DIN# 00369810	Anticonvulsant
GEIGY <> PU	Tab, White w/ Red Specks, Oval, Scored	Carbamazepine 200 mg	Tegretol Chewtabs by Novartis	Canadian DIN# 00665088	Anticonvulsant

ID FRONT <> BACK	DESCRIPTION FRONT <> BACK	INGREDIENT & STRENGTH	BRAND (OR EQUIV.) & FIRM	NDC#	CLASS; SCH.
GEIGY105	Tab, White, Round, Scored	Terbutaline Sulfate 5 mg	Brethine by Rightpak	65240-0614	Antiasthmatic
GEIGY105	Tab	Terbutaline Sulfate 5 mg	Brethine by Novartis	00028-0105	Antiasthmatic
GEIGY105	Tab	Terbutaline Sulfate 5 mg	Brethine by Physicians Total Care	54868-1240	Antiasthmatic
GEIGY105	Tab	Terbutaline Sulfate 5 mg	Brethine by Drug Distr	52985-0114	Antiasthmatic
GEIGY105	Tab	Terbutaline Sulfate 5 mg	Brethine by Amerisource	62584-0105	Antiasthmatic
GEIGY105	Tab	Terbutaline Sulfate 5 mg	Brethine by Thrift Drug	59198-0012	Antiasthmatic
GEIGY105	Tab	Terbutaline Sulfate 5 mg	Brethine by Nat Pharmpak Serv	55154-1002	Antiasthmatic
GEIGY105	Tab, White, Round, Scored	Terbutaline Sulfate 5 mg	Brethine by Syntex	18393-0150	Antiasthmatic
GEIGY108	Cap, Brown	Clofazimine 50 mg	Lamprene by Geigy		Antileprosy
GEIGY109	Cap, Brown	Clofazimine 100 mg	Lamprene by Geigy		Antileprosy
GEIGY111	Tab, White, Round	Tripelennamine HCl 25 mg	PBZ by Geigy		Antihistamine
GEIGY117	Tab	Tripelennamine HCl 50 mg	PBZ by Novartis	00028-0117	Antihistamine
GEIGY136	Tab, Coral, Round	Imipramine HCl 50 mg	Tofranil by Geigy		Antidepressant
GEIGY14	Tab, Red, Round	Phenylbutazone 100 mg	Butazolidin by Geigy		Anti-Inflammatory
GEIGY140	Tab, Coral, Round	Imipramine HCl 25 mg	Tofranil by Geigy		Antidepressant
GEIGY140	Tab, Orange, Round	Imipramine HCl 25 mg	Tofranil by Novartis Pharms (Ca)	61615-0105	Antidepressant
GEIGY20	Cap, Coral	Imipramine Pamoate	Tofranil-Pm by Novartis	00028-0020	Antidepressant
GEIGY22	Cap, Coral, in Black Ink	Imipramine Pamoate 150 mg	Tofranil Pm by Novartis	00028-0022	Antidepressant
GEIGY23	Tab, White, Oval	Baclofen 10 mg	Lioresal by Geigy		Muscle Relaxant
GEIGY32	Tab, Coral, Round	Imipramine HCl 10 mg	Tofranil by Geigy		Antidepressant
GEIGY33	Tab, White, Oblong	Baclofen 20 mg	Lioresal by Geigy		Muscle Relaxant
GEIGY40	Cap, Coral & Dark Yellow	Imipramine Pamoate 100 mg	Tofranil Pm by Novartis	00028-0040	Antidepressant
GEIGY42	Tab, Pink, Oval	Theophylline Anhydrous 200 mg	Constant-T by Geigy		Antiasthmatic
GEIGY45	Cap, Coral & Ivory	Imipramine Pamoate 125 mg	Tofranil Pm by Novartis	00028-0045	Antidepressant
GEIGY47	Tab, White, Round, Red Specks	Carbamazepine Chewable 100 mg	Tegretol by Geigy		Anticonvulsant
GEIGY48	Tab, Lavender, Round	Tripelennamine HCl SR 100 mg	PBZ-SR by Geigy		Antihistamine
GEIGY51	Tab, Film Coated	Metoprolol Tartrate 50 mg	by Med Pro	53978-2058	Antihypertensive
GEIGY52	Tab, White, Round, Red Specks	Carbamazepine Chewable 100 mg	Tegretol by Geigy		Anticonvulsant
GEIGY57	Tab, Blue, Oval	Theophylline Anhydrous 300 mg	Constant-T by Geigy		Antiasthmatic
GEIGY72	Tab, White, Oval	Terbutaline Sulfate 2.5 mg	Brethine by Rightpak	65240-0613	Antiasthmatic
GEIGY72	Tab	Terbutaline Sulfate 2.5 mg	Brethine by Novartis	00028-0072	Antiasthmatic
GEIGY72	Tab	Terbutaline Sulfate 2.5 mg	Brethine by Drug Distr	52985-0113	Antiasthmatic
GEIGY72	Tab	Terbutaline Sulfate 2.5 mg	Brethine by Thrift Drug	59198-0134	Antiasthmatic
GEIGY72	Tab	Terbutaline Sulfate 2.5 mg	Brethine by Nat Pharmpak Serv	55154-1001	Antiasthmatic
GEIGY72	Tab	Terbutaline Sulfate 2.5 mg	Brethine by Rite Aid	11822-5296	Antiasthmatic
GEIGY72	Tab, White, Oval, Scored	Terbutaline Sulfate 2.5 mg	Brethine by Syntex	18393-0149	Antiasthmatic
GEIGYANTURAN	Tab, White, Round, Geigy/Anturan	Sulfinpyrazone 200 mg	Anturan by Novartis	Canadian	Uricosuric
GEIGYDK	Tab, Cream, Triangular, Geigy/DK	Clomipramine HCl 10 mg	Anafranil by Novartis	Canadian	OCD
GEIGYDK	Tab, Cream, Triangular	Clomipramine HCl 10 mg	Anafranil by Geigy		OCD
GEIGYFH	Tab, Cream, Round	Clomipramine HCl 25 mg	Anafranil by Geigy		OCD
GEIGYFK	Tab, White, Round, Geigy/FK	Sulfinpyrazone 100 mg	Anturan by Novartis	Canadian	Uricosuric
GEIGYFP	Tab, White, Round	Phenylbutazone 100 mg	Alka Butazolidin by Geigy		Anti-Inflammatory
GEIGYFT	Tab, Brown & Red, Triangle, Geigy/FT	Imipramine HCl 10 mg	Tofranil by Geigy	Canadian	Antidepressant
GEIGYFT	Tab, Brown & Red, Triangular, Geigy/FT	Imipramine HCl 10 mg	Tofranil by Novartis	Canadian	Antidepressant
GEIGYKJ	Tab, White, Oval, Geigy/KJ	Baclofen 10 mg	by Novartis	Canadian	Muscle Relaxant
GEIGYLP	Tab, Cream, Round	Clomipramine HCl 50 mg	Anafranil by Geigy		OCD
GEIGYPU	Tab, White, Oval, Geigy/P/U	Carbamazepine 200 mg	Tegretol by Geigy	Canadian	Anticonvulsant
GEIGYZA	Tab, Beige & Yellow, Round, Geigy/ZA	Chlorthalidone 50 mg	Hygroton by Novartis	Canadian	Diuretic
GF <> CIBA	Tab, Blue, Round, Coated	Hydralazine HCl 25 mg	Apresoline by Novartis	Canadian DIN# 00005533	Antihypertensive
GF1200	Tab, White, Oblong, Scored	Guaifenesin 1200 mg	by Pfab	62542-0711	Expectorant

ID FRONT <> BACK	DESCRIPTION FRONT <> BACK	INGREDIENT & STRENGTH	BRAND (OR EQUIV.) & FIRM	NDC#	CLASS; SCH.
GF1200	Tab, White, Oblong, Scored	Guaifenesin 1200 mg	GFN 1200 by Eli Lilly	00002-1095	Expectorant
GF1200	Tab, White, Oblong, Scored	Guaifenesin 1200 mg	by Lilly	00110-4116	Expectorant
GF200	Tab, Pink, Oblong, Scored	Guaifenesin 200 mg	by Lilly	00110-3105	Expectorant
GF200	Tab, Pink, Oblong, Scored	Guaifenesin 200 mg	GFN 200 01 by Lex	49523-0124	Expectorant
GF600	Tab, Green, Oblong, Scored	Guaifenesin 600 mg	GFN 600 04 by Eli Lilly	00002-1094	Expectorant
GF600	Tab, Green, Oblong, Scored	Guaifenesin 600 mg	by Lilly	00110-3107	Expectorant
GFDM	Tab, Green, Oblong, Scored, GF over DM	Guaifenesin 600 mg, Dextromethorphan Hydriodide 30 mg	GFN DTMH 03 by McNeil	52021-0645	Cold Remedy
GFDM	Tab, Green, Oblong, Scored	Guaifenesin 600 mg, Pseudoephedrine 30 mg	by Med Pro	53978-3341	Cold Remedy
GFN <> PSE	Cap, Blue & Clear, Opaque	Guaifenesin 300 mg, Pseudoephedrine 60 mg	by Martec		Cold Remedy
GFN <> PSE	Cap, Blue & Clear, Black Print	Guaifenesin 300 mg, Pseudoephedrine HCl 60 mg	GFN PSEH PD 05 by Martec		Cold Remedy
GFP120	Tab, Yellow, Oblong, Scored	Guaifenesin 600 mg, Pseudoephedrine HCl 120 mg	GFN 700 PSEH 120 01 by Med Pro	53978-3350	Cold Remedy
GFP120	Cap, Yellow, Scored	Guaifenesin 600 mg, Pseudoephedrine 120 mg	Guiatex PSE CapTABS by Med Pro	53978-3344	Cold Remedy
GFP60	Tab, Blue, Oblong, Scored	Guaifenesin 600 mg, Pseudoephedrine 60 mg	Guiatex II SR by Med Pro	53978-3342	Cold Remedy
GFP60	Tab, Blue, Oblong, Scored	Guaifenesin 600 mg, Pseudoephedrine HCl 60 mg	GFN 600 PSEH 60 03 by Med Pro	53978-3345	Cold Remedy
GFP60	Tab, Blue, Oblong, Scored	Guaifenesin 600 mg; Pseudoephedrine HCl 60 mg	by Pfab	62542-0745	Cold Remedy
GFPP	Tab, White, Oblong, Scored	Guaifenesin 600 mg, Phenylpropanolamine HCl 75 mg	GFN PPAH 03 by Med Pro	53978-3317	Cold Remedy
GFPP	Tab, White, Oblong, Scored	Guaifenesin 600 mg, Phenylpropanolamine HCl 75 mg	by Med Pro	53978-3319	Cold Remedy
GG	Tab	Acetaminophen 300 mg, Codeine Phosphate 30 mg	by Patient	57575-0026	Analgesic; C III
GG	Cap	Cephalexin 500 mg	by Patient	57575-0082	Antibiotic
GG	Tab	Meclizine HCl 25 mg	by Patient	57575-0065	Antiemetic
GG <> 101	Tab, White, Compressed	Methocarbamol 750 mg	Robaxin by Geneva	00781-1750	Muscle Relaxant
GG <> 105	Tab, White, Round, Scored	Haloperidol 0.5 mg	by Natl Pharmpak	55154-5412	Antipsychotic
GG <> 105	Tab	Haloperidol 0.5 mg	by Med Pro	53978-3043	Antipsychotic
GG <> 105	Tab	Haloperidol 0.5 mg	by PDRX	55289-0157	Antipsychotic
GG <> 123	Tab, Debossed	Haloperidol 1 mg	by Golden State	60429-0087	Antipsychotic
GG <> 123	Tab, Yellow, Round, Scored	Haloperidol 1 mg	by Natl Pharmpak	55154-5413	Antipsychotic
GG <> 123	Tab	Haloperidol 1 mg	by Med Pro	53978-3004	Antipsychotic
GG <> 124	Tab, Pink, Round, Scored	Haloperidol 2 mg	Haloperidol by Geneva	00781-1393	Antipsychotic
GG <> 126	Tab, Light Green, Round, Scored	Haloperidol 10 mg	Haloperidol by Geneva	00781-1397	Antipsychotic
GG <> 134	Tab, Coral, Round, Scored	Haloperidol 20 mg	Haloperidol by Geneva	00781-1398	Antipsychotic
GG <> 172	Tab, Yellow, Round, Scored, Compressed	Hydrochlorothiazide 50 mg, Triamterene 75 mg	Maxzide by Geneva	00781-1008	Diuretic
GG <> 190	Tab, White, Round, Scored, Compressed	Methocarbamol 500 mg	Robaxin by Geneva	00781-1760	Muscle Relaxant
GG <> 191	Tab, Blue, Round	Amoxapine 100 mg	Asendin by Geneva	00781-1846	Antidepressant
GG <> 201	Tab, White, Round, Scored	Furosemide 40 mg	Lasix by Geneva	00781-1966	Diuretic
GG <> 225	Tab, White, Round, Compressed	Promethazine HCl 25 mg	Phenergan by Geneva	00781-1830	Antiemetic; Antihistamine
GG <> 227	Tab, Green, Round, Scored, Compressed	Isosorbide Dinitrate 20 mg	Isordil by Geneva	00781-1695	Antianginal
GG <> 259	Tab, Pink, Round, Scored, Compressed	Isosorbide Dinitrate 5 mg	Isordil by Geneva	00781-1635	Antianginal
GG <> 26	Tab, White, Round, Scored, Compressed	Isosorbide Dinitrate 10 mg	Isordil by Geneva	00781-1556	Antianginal
GG <> 274	Tab, White, Round, Scored, Compressed	Isoxsuprine HCl 10 mg	Vasodilan by Geneva	00781-1840	Vasodilator
GG <> 284	Tab, White, Round, Scored, Compressed	Isoxsuprine HCl 20 mg	Vasodilan by Geneva	00781-1842	Vasodilator
GG <> 38	Tab, Lavender, Film Coated	Hydroxyzine HCl 25 mg	by Quality Care	60346-0086	Antihistamine
GG <> 4	Tab	Atropine Sulfate 0.025 mg, Diphenoxylate HCl 2.5 mg	Lonox by Quality Care	60346-0437	Antidiarrheal; C V
GG <> 42	Tab	Imipramine HCl 50 mg	by Allscripts	54569-0196	Antidepressant
GG <> 42	Tab, Green, Round, Film	Imipramine HCl 50 mg	by Murfreesboro	51129-1533	Antidepressant
GG <> 42	Tab, Coated, Debossed	Imipramine HCl 50 mg	by Golden State	60429-0097	Antidepressant
GG <> 429	Tab, Green, Cap Shaped, Film Coated	Cimetidine 400 mg	Tagamet by Geneva	00781-1449	Gastrointestinal
GG <> 430	Tab, Green, Cap Shaped	Cimetidine 800 mg	Tagamet by Geneva	00781-1444	Gastrointestinal
GG <> 438	Tab, White, Round, Scored, Compressed	Pindolol 5 mg	Visken by Geneva	00781-1168	Antihypertensive
GG <> 439	Tab, White, Round, Scored, Compressed	Pindolol 10 mg	Visken by Geneva	00781-1169	Antihypertensive
GG <> 445	Tab, Yellow, Round, Scored	Enalapril 2.5 mg	Vasotec by Geneva	00781-1229	Antihypertensive
GG <> 47	Tab, Beige, Round, Film, Debossed	Imipramine HCl 25 mg	by Murfreesboro	51129-1532	Antidepressant

ID FRONT <> BACK	DESCRIPTION FRONT <> BACK	INGREDIENT & STRENGTH	BRAND (OR EQUIV.) & FIRM	NDC#	CLASS; SCH.
GG <> 47	Tab, Film Coated	Imipramine HCl 25 mg	by Direct Dispensing	57866-3930	Antidepressant
GG <> 47	Tab, Film Coated, Debossed	Imipramine HCl 25 mg	by Golden State	60429-0096	Antidepressant
GG <> 482	Tab, White, Round, Scored	Enalapril 5 mg	Vasotec by Geneva	00781-1231	Antihypertensive
GG <> 517	Cap, Light Green	Indomethacin 25 mg	by Quality Care	60346-0684	NSAID
GG <> 531	Cap, Green & White	Temazepam 15 mg	Temazepam by St. Marys Med	60760-0552	Sedative/Hypnotic; C IV
GG <> 535	Cap	Nitrofurantoin 50 mg	by Quality Care	60346-0616	Antibiotic
GG <> 536	Cap	Nitrofurantoin 100 mg	by Quality Care	60346-0008	Antibiotic
GG <> 724	Tab	Naproxen 250 mg	by Quality Care	60346-0816	NSAID
GG <> 739	Tab, Delayed Release	Diclofenac Sodium 75 mg	by Quality Care	60346-0463	NSAID
GG <> 76	Tab, Coated	Flurbiprofen 100 mg	by Quality Care	60346-0968	NSAID
GG <> 780	Tab, White, Round, Film Coated	Methylphenidate HCl 20 mg	by Caremark	00339-4103	Stimulant; C II
GG <> 783	Tab, Yellow, Round	Methylphenidate HCl 5 mg	by Caremark	00339-4100	Stimulant; C II
GG <> 789	Tab, Green, Round, Scored	Methylphenidate HCl 10 mg	by Caremark	00339-4101	Stimulant; C II
GG <> 91	Tab, White, Round	Lorazepam 0.5 mg	by Heartland Healthcare	61392-0455	Sedative/Hypnotic; C IV
GG <> 91	Tab, White, Round	Lorazepam 0.5 mg	by Allscripts	54569-2687	Sedative/Hypnotic; C IV
GG <> 92	Tab, White, Round, Scored	Lorazepam 1 mg	by Allscripts	54569-1585	Sedative/Hypnotic; C IV
GG 100	Tab, Film Coated	Acetaminophen 650 mg, Propoxyphene Napsylate 100 mg	by Golden State	60429-0518	Analgesic; C IV
GG 220 <> 3	Tab	Acetaminophen 300 mg, Codeine Phosphate 30 mg	by Golden State	60429-0500	Analgesic; C III
GG 60	Tab, Scored	Allopurinol 300 mg	by Golden State	60429-0014	Antigout
GG03	Tab	Captopril 12.5 mg	by Med Pro	53978-0939	Antihypertensive
GG1	Tab, Yellow, Round	Isosorbide Dinitrate SL 2.5 mg	Isordil by Geneva		Antianginal
GG100	Tab, Coated	Acetaminophen 650 mg, Propoxyphene Napsylate 100 mg	by Geneva	00781-1720	Analgesic; C IV
GG100	Tab, Coated, Geneva Logo	Acetaminophen 650 mg, Propoxyphene Napsylate 100 mg	Propoxy N APAP by Quality Care	60346-0610	Analgesic; C IV
GG100	Tab, Coated	Acetaminophen 650 mg, Propoxyphene Napsylate 100 mg	by Med Pro	53978-5013	Analgesic; C IV
GG101	Tab	Methocarbamol 750 mg	by Urgent Care Ctr	50716-0750	Muscle Relaxant
GG101	Tab, Debossed	Methocarbamol 750 mg	by Nat Pharmpak Serv	55154-5410	Muscle Relaxant
GG101	Tab, Debossed	Methocarbamol 750 mg	by Golden State	60429-0119	Muscle Relaxant
GG103	Tab, Film Coated	Metronidazole 250 mg	by Urgent Care Ctr	50716-0263	Antibiotic
GG103	Tab	Metronidazole 250 mg	by Golden State	60429-0128	Antibiotic
GG103	Tab, Film Coated	Metronidazole 250 mg	by Geneva	00781-1742	Antibiotic
GG104	Tab, White, Round	Methyldopa 125 mg	Aldomet by Geneva		Antihypertensive
GG105	Tab, White, Round, Scored	Haloperidol 0.5 mg	by Geneva	00781-1391	Antipsychotic
GG106	Tab	Amiloride HCl 5 mg, Hydrochlorothiazide 50 mg	by Geneva	00781-1119	Diuretic
GG106	Tab, GG 106	Amiloride HCl 5 mg, Hydrochlorothiazide 50 mg	by Physicians Total Care	54868-0667	Diuretic
GG107	Tab, White, Round, Film Coated	Perphenazine 4 mg	by Pharmafab	62542-0791	Antipsychotic
GG107	Tab, Film Coated	Perphenazine 4 mg	by Quality Care	60346-0835	Antipsychotic
GG107	Tab, Film Coated, Debossed	Perphenazine 4 mg	by Golden State	60429-0153	Antipsychotic
GG107	Tab, White, Round, Film Coated	Perphenazine 4 mg	Trilafon by Geneva	00781-1047	Antipsychotic
GG107	Tab, Film Coated	Perphenazine 4 mg	by Vangard	00615-3585	Antipsychotic
GG108	Tab, Film Coated, Debossed	Perphenazine 8 mg	by Golden State	60429-0154	Antipsychotic
GG108	Tab, White, Round, Film Coated	Perphenazine 8 mg	Trilafon by Geneva	00781-1048	Antipsychotic
GG108	Tab, Film Coated	Perphenazine 8 mg	by Vangard	00615-4511	Antipsychotic
GG108	Tab, White, Round, Film Coated	Perphenazine 8 mg	by Heartland Healthcare	61392-0084	Antipsychotic
GG109	Tab, White, Round, Film Coated	Perphenazine 16 mg	Trilafon by Geneva	00781-1049	Antipsychotic
GG109	Tab, Coated	Perphenazine 16 mg	by Vangard	00615-4512	Antipsychotic
GG11	Tab, Coated	Chlorthalidone 25 mg	by Geneva	00781-1726	Diuretic
GG110	Tab, Green, Round	Chlorzoxazone 250 mg, Acetaminophen 300 mg	Parafon Forte by Geneva		Muscle Relaxant
GG111	Tab, Coated	Methyldopa 250 mg	by Geneva	00781-1320	Antihypertensive
GG112	Tab	Acetaminophen 650 mg, Propoxyphene HCl 65 mg	by Quality Care	60346-0909	Analgesic; C IV
GG112	Tab, Coated	Acetaminophen 650 mg, Propoxyphene HCl 65 mg	by Geneva	00781-1378	Analgesic; C IV
GG113	Tab	Metoclopramide HCl	by Geneva	00781-1301	Gastrointestinal
GG114	Tab, White, Round	Ergoloid Mesylates 1 mg	Hydergine by Danbury		Ergot

ID FRONT <> BACK	DESCRIPTION FRONT <> BACK	INGREDIENT & STRENGTH	BRAND (OR EQUIV.) & FIRM	NDC#	CLASS; SCH.
GG115	Tab, White, Oval	Ergoloid Mesylates SL 1 mg	Hydergine by Danbury		Ergot
GG116	Tab, White, Round	Ergoloid Mesylates SL 0.5 mg	Hydergine by Danbury		Ergot
GG118	Tab	Chlorpheniramine Maleate 5 mg, Phenylephrine HCl 10 mg, Phenylpropanolamine HCl 40 mg, Phenyltoloxamine Citrate 15 mg	by Geneva	00781-1576	Cold Remedy
GG118	Tab, White, Round, Blue Specks	Decongestant SR	Naldecon by Geneva		Cold Remedy
GG119	Tab, White, Round	Butalbital 50 mg, Aspirin 40 mg, Caffeine 325 mg	Fiorinal by Geneva		Analgesic
GG12	Tab, White, Round	Medroxyprogesterone Acetate 10 mg	Provera by Solvay		Progestin
GG1214	Tab, White, Round, GG 121/4	Acetaminophen 300 mg, Codeine 60 mg	Tylenol w/Codeine by Geneva		Analgesic; C III
GG122	Tab, Brownish Yellow	Sulfasalazine 500 mg	Azulfidine by Bolar		Gastrointestinal
GG123	Tab, Yellow, Round, Scored	Haloperidol 1 mg	by Geneva	00781-1392	Antipsychotic
GG124	Tab, Debossed	Haloperidol 2 mg	by Golden State	60429-0088	Antipsychotic
GG124	Tab	Haloperidol 2 mg	by Med Pro	53978-3006	Antipsychotic
GG125	Tab, Debossed	Haloperidol 5 mg	by Golden State	60429-0089	Antipsychotic
GG125	Tab, Green, Round	Haloperidol 5 mg	Haloperidol by Geneva	00781-1396	Antipsychotic
GG125	Tab	Haloperidol 5 mg	by Med Pro	53978-3003	Antipsychotic
GG126	Tab, Light Green, Debossed	Haloperidol 10 mg	by Golden State	60429-0090	Antipsychotic
GG127	Tab, White, Round	Quinine Sulfate 260 mg	by Geneva		Antimalarial
GG13	Tab	Captopril 12.5 mg	by Geneva	00781-1828	Antihypertensive
GG13	Tab, Blue-Green, Coated	Chlorthalidone 50 mg	by Geneva	00781-1728	Diuretic
GG130	Tab	Aminophylline 100 mg	by Geneva	00781-1214	Antiasthmatic
GG132	Tab, White, Round	Verapamil 80 mg	Isoptin by Geneva		Antihypertensive
GG132	Tab, Film Coated	Verapamil HCl 80 mg	by Med Pro	53978-7001	Antihypertensive
GG132	Tab, Film Coated	Verapamil HCl 80 mg	by Golden State	60429-0196	Antihypertensive
GG132	Tab, Partial Score, Film Coated	Verapamil HCl 80 mg	by Murfreesboro	51129-1187	Antihypertensive
GG132	Tab, White, Round, Scored, Film Coated, GG/132	Verapamil HCl 80 mg	Isoptin by Geneva	00781-1016	Antihypertensive
GG133	Tab, Film Coated	Verapamil HCl 120 mg	by Med Pro	53978-7002	Antihypertensive
GG133	Tab, White, Round, Scored, Film Coated	Verapamil HCl 120 mg	Isoptin by Geneva	00781-1017	Antihypertensive
GG134	Tab	Haloperidol 20 mg	by Physicians Total Care	54868-2569	Antipsychotic
GG1343	Tab, White, Round	Reserpine 0.1 mg, Hydralazine 25 mg, Hydrochlorothiazide 15 mg	Ser-Ap-Es by Danbury		Antihypertensive
GG14	Tab, Peach, Round	Prednisolone 5 mg	Delta Cortef by Geneva		Steroid
GG141	Tab, Blue & White, Two Layered	Meclizine HCl 12.5 mg	by Kaiser	00179-1115	Antiemetic
GG141	Tab, Blue & White, 2 Layered	Meclizine HCl 12.5 mg	by Caremark	00339-5222	Antiemetic
GG141	Tab	Meclizine HCl 12.5 mg	by Quality Care	60346-0056	Antiemetic
GG141	Tab, Blue & White, Oval, Scored	Meclizine HCl 12.5 mg	Antivert by Geneva	00781-1542	Antiemetic
GG141	Tab, Blue, Oval	Meclizine HCl 12.5 mg	Antivert by Geneva	00781-1345	Antiemetic
GG142	Tab, White, Round	Tolbutamide 500 mg	Orinase by Geneva		Antidiabetic
GG144	Tab	Chlorpropamide 250 mg	by Pharmedix	53002-0347	Antidiabetic
GG145	Tab, Yellow, Round	Dimenhydrinate 50 mg	Dramamine by Geneva		Antiemetic
GG15	Tab, White, Round	Nylidrin 12 mg	Arlidin by Geneva		Vasodilator
GG150	Tab	Meprobamate 400 mg	by DRX	55045-1753	Sedative/Hypnotic; C IV
GG150	Tab	Meprobamate 400 mg	by Quality Care	62682-7032	Sedative/Hypnotic; C IV
GG1513	Tab	Aspirin 325 mg, Codeine Phosphate 30 mg	by Geneva	00781-1660	Analgesic; C III
GG153	Tab	Hydrochlorothiazide 25 mg, Propranolol HCl 40 mg	by Geneva	00781-1431	Diuretic; Antihypertensive
GG154	Tab	Hydrochlorothiazide 25 mg, Propranolol HCl 80 mg	by Geneva	00781-1432	Diuretic; Antihypertensive
GG155	Tab, Peach, Round	Prednisone 20 mg	Deltasone by Geneva		Steroid
GG156	Tab, White, Round	Prednisone 10 mg	Deltasone by Geneva		Steroid
GG157	Tab, White, Round	Prednisone 50 mg	Deltasone by Geneva		Steroid
GG158	Tab, White, Round	Sulfisoxazole 500 mg	Gantrisin by Geneva		Antibiotic
GG159	Tab, White, Oblong	Clemastine Fumarate 1.34 mg	Tavist by Geneva		Antihistamine
GG159	Tab, White	Clemastine Fumarate 1.34 mg	Tavist by Geneva	00781-1358	Antihistamine

ID FRONT <> BACK	DESCRIPTION FRONT <> BACK	INGREDIENT & STRENGTH	BRAND (OR EQUIV.) & FIRM	NDC#	CLASS; SCH.
GG160	Tab, White, Round	Clemastine Fumarate 2.68 mg	Tavist by Geneva	00781-1359	Antihistamine
GG1614	Tab	Aspirin 325 mg, Codeine Phosphate 60 mg	by Geneva	00781-1875	Analgesic; C III
GG162	Tab, White	Triazolam 0.125 mg	Halcion by Upjohn		Sedative/Hypnotic; C IV
GG162	Tab, White, Scored	Triazolam 0.125 mg	Halcion by Geneva	00781-1441	Sedative/Hypnotic; C IV
GG163	Tab, Powder Blue	Triazolam 0.25 mg	by Allscripts	54569-3966	Sedative/Hypnotic; C IV
GG163	Tab, Blue, Scored	Triazolam 0.25 mg	Halcion by Geneva	00781-1442	Sedative/Hypnotic; C IV
GG165	Tab	Hydrochlorothiazide 25 mg, Triamterene 37.5 mg	by Physicians Total Care	54868-2679	Diuretic
GG165	Tab, Debossed	Hydrochlorothiazide 25 mg, Triamterene 37.5 mg	by PDRX	55289-0090	Diuretic
GG165	Tab, Debossed	Hydrochlorothiazide 25 mg, Triamterene 37.5 mg	by Golden State	60429-0232	Diuretic
GG165	Tab	Hydrochlorothiazide 25 mg, Triamterene 37.5 mg	by Heartland	61392-0829	Diuretic
GG165	Tab, Green, Round	Hydrochlorothiazide 25 mg, Triamterene 37.5 mg	Maxzide-25 by Geneva	00781-1123	Diuretic
GG165	Tab, Green, Round, Scored	Triamterene 37.5 mg, Hydrochlorothiazide 25 mg	by Teva	00480-0637	Diuretic
GG166	Tab, White, Round, Film Coated	Desipramine HCl 75 mg	Norpramin by Geneva	00781-1974	Antidepressant
GG166	Tab, Film Coated	Desipramine HCl 75 mg	by Murfreesboro	51129-1208	Antidepressant
GG167	Tab, White, Round, Coated	Desipramine HCl 100 mg	Norpramin by Geneva		Antidepressant
GG167	Tab, White, Round, Film Coated	Desipramine HCl 100 mg	Norpramin by Geneva	00781-1975	Antidepressant
GG168	Tab, White, Round, Film Coated	Desipramine HCl 150 mg	Norpramin by Geneva	00781-1976	Antidepressant
GG169	Tab, White, Round, Film	Verapamil HCl 40 mg	by Thrift Drug	59198-0309	Antihypertensive
GG169	Tab, White, Round, Film Coated	Verapamil HCl 40 mg	Isoptin by Geneva	00781-1014	Antihypertensive
GG172	Cap	Hydrochlorothiazide 25 mg, Triamterene 50 mg	by Med Pro	53978-5009	Diuretic
GG172	Tab	Hydrochlorothiazide 50 mg, Triamterene 75 mg	by Quality Care	60346-0704	Diuretic
GG172	Tab	Hydrochlorothiazide 50 mg, Triamterene 75 mg	by Diversified Healthcare Serv	55887-0996	Diuretic
GG172	Tab	Hydrochlorothiazide 50 mg, Triamterene 75 mg	by Golden State	60429-0191	Diuretic
GG172	Tab, Yellow, Round, Scored	Triamterene 75 mg, Hydrochlorothiazide 50 mg	by Teva	00480-0752	Diuretic
GG174	Tab, White, Round	Sulfamethoxazole 400 mg, Trimethoprim 80 mg	Bactrim by Geneva		Antibiotic
GG175	Tab, White, Oval	Sulfamethoxazole 800 mg, Trimethoprim 160 mg	Bactrim DS by Geneva		Antibiotic
GG177	Tab	Captopril 25 mg	by Golden State	60429-0030	Antihypertensive
GG177	Tab	Captopril 25 mg	by Geneva	00781-1829	Antihypertensive
GG177	Tab	Captopril 25 mg	by Med Pro	53978-0236	Antihypertensive
GG178	Tab	Captopril 50 mg	by Geneva	00781-1838	Antihypertensive
GG178	Tab	Captopril 50 mg	by Med Pro	53978-0517	Antihypertensive
GG178	Tab	Captopril 50 mg	by Golden State	60429-0031	Antihypertensive
GG178	Tab, White, Round, Scored	Captopril 50 mg	by Haines Pharms	59564-0128	Antihypertensive
GG179	Tab	Captopril 100 mg	by Geneva	00781-1839	Antihypertensive
GG18	Tab, Coated	Perphenazine 2 mg	by Heartland	61392-0082	Antipsychotic
GG18	Tab, Coated	Perphenazine 2 mg	by Golden State	60429-0152	Antipsychotic
GG18	Tab, White, Round, Film Coated	Perphenazine 2 mg	Trilafon by Geneva	00781-1046	Antipsychotic
GG18	Tab, Coated	Perphenazine 2 mg	by Vangard	00615-3584	Antipsychotic
GG180	Tab, White, Round	Aminophylline 200 mg	Aminophyllin by Geneva		Antiasthmatic
GG181	Tab, White, Round, Scored	Methazolamide 50 mg	by Allscripts	54569-3864	Diuretic
GG181	Tab, White, Round, Scored	Methazolamide 50 mg	by Nat Pharmpak Serv	55154-8705	Diuretic
GG181	Tab, Debossed	Methazolamide 50 mg	by Quality Care	60346-0412	Diuretic
GG181	Tab, White, Round, Scored	Methazolamide 50 mg	Neptazane by Geneva	00781-1071	Diuretic
GG182	Tab	Timolol Maleate 10 mg	by Geneva	00781-1127	Antihypertensive
GG183	Tab	Timolol Maleate 20 mg	by Geneva	00781-1128	Antihypertensive
GG185	Tab, White, Round	Glutethimide 500 mg	Doriden by Geneva		Hypnotic
GG190	Tab	Methocarbamol 500 mg	by Quality Care	60346-0080	Muscle Relaxant
GG190	Tab, Debossed	Methocarbamol 500 mg	by Golden State	60429-0118	Muscle Relaxant
GG191	Tab, Blue, Round	Amoxapine 100 mg	Asendin by Geneva		Antidepressant
GG192	Tab, Light Orange, Round, Scored	Amoxapine 150 mg	Asendin by Geneva	00781-1847	Antidepressant
GG195	Tab, Debossed	Metronidazole 500 mg	by Golden State	60429-0129	Antibiotic
GG195	Tab, Film Coated	Metronidazole 500 mg	by Geneva	00781-1747	Antibiotic

ID FRONT <> BACK	DESCRIPTION FRONT <> BACK	INGREDIENT & STRENGTH	BRAND (OR EQUIV.) & FIRM	NDC#	CLASS; SCH.
GG196	Tab, Yellow, Round	Chlorpheniramine Maleate 4 mg	Chlor-trimeton by Geneva		Antihistamine
GG197	Tab, White, Oval	Acetohexamide 250 mg	Dymelor by Rosemont		Antidiabetic
GG198	Tab, White, Oblong	Acetohexamide. 500 mg	Dymelor by Rosemont		Antidiabetic
GG199	Tab, White, Round	Acetaminophen 325 mg	Tylenol by Geneva		Antipyretic
GG2	Tab	Isosorbide Dinitrate 5 mg	by Geneva	00781-1565	Antianginal
GG2	Tab, Pink, Round, GG/2	Isosorbide Dinitrate SL 5 mg	Isordil by Geneva		Antianginal
GG200	Tab, Pink, Oblong	Propoxyphene Napsylate 100 mg, Acetaminophen 650 mg	Darvocet N by Bolar		Analgesic; C IV
GG201	Tab	Furosemide 40 mg	by Med Pro	53978-5032	Diuretic
GG201	Tab, White, Round, Scored	Furosemide 40 mg	by JB	51111-0472	Diuretic
GG201	Tab, White, Round, Scored	Furosemide 40 mg	by Vangard Labs	00615-0446	Diuretic
GG201	Tab	Furosemide 40 mg	by Murfreesboro	51129-1281	Diuretic
GG21	Tab, White, Round, Scored	Furosemide 20 mg	Lasix by Geneva	00781-1818	Diuretic
GG21	Tab, White, Round, Scored	Furosemide 20 mg	by Vangard Labs	00615-1569	Diuretic
GG21	Tab, White, Round, Scored	Furosemide 20 mg	by JB	51111-0475	Diuretic
GG210	Tab, Yellow, Round, Scored	Azathioprine 50 mg	Imuran by Geneva		Immunosuppressant
GG210	Tab, Yellow, Oblong, Scored	Azathioprine 50 mg	by Caremark	00339-6181	Immunosuppressant
GG210	Tab, Yellow, Cap Shaped, Scored	Azathioprine 50 mg	Imuran by Geneva	00781-1059	Immunosuppressant
GG211	Tab, White, Round, Scored	Bromocriptine 2.5 mg	Parlodel by Geneva		Sedative
GG211	Tab, White, Round	Bromocriptine 2.5 mg	Parlodel by Geneva	00781-1817	Antiparkinson
GG213	Tab, Blue, Round, Film Coated	Amitriptyline HCl 10 mg, Perphenazine 2 mg	Triavil by Geneva	00781-1265	Antipsychotic
GG214	Tab, Orange, Round	Perphenazine 2 mg, Amitriptyline 25 mg	Triavil by Geneva		Antipsychotic; Antidepressant
GG214	Tab, Orange, Round, Film Coated	Perphenazine 2 mg, Amitriptyline 25 mg	Triavil by Geneva	00781-1273	Antipsychotic; Antidepressant
GG215	Tab, Coated	Amitriptyline HCl 10 mg, Perphenazine 4 mg	by Geneva	00781-1266	Antipsychotic
GG216	Tab, Yellow, Round	Perphenazine 4 mg, Amitriptyline 25 mg	Triavil by Geneva	00781-1267	Antipsychotic; Antidepressant
GG217	Tab, Orange, Round, Film Coated	Amitriptyline HCl 50 mg, Perphenazine 4 mg	Triavil by Geneva	00781-1268	Antipsychotic
GG217	Tab, Film Coated	Amitriptyline HCl 50 mg, Perphenazine 4 mg	by Physicians Total Care	54868-3927	Antipsychotic
GG2182	Tab, White, Round, GG 218/2	Acetaminophen 300 mg, Codeine 15 mg	Tylenol w/Codeine by KV		Analgesic; C III
GG219	Tab, Film Coated	Hydrochlorothiazide 15 mg, Methyldopa 250 mg	by Geneva	00781-1809	Diuretic; Antihypertensive
GG22	Tab, White, Round, Scored	Pseudoephedrine 60 mg	Sudafed by Geneva	00781-1535	Decongestant
GG22	Tab, White, Round	Pseudoephedrine 60 mg	Sudafed by Geneva		Decongestant
GG220	Tab	Acetaminophen 300 mg, Codeine Phosphate 30 mg	by Geneva	00781-1752	Analgesic; C III
GG220	Tab, Pink, Oblong	Propoxyphene Napsylate 100 mg, Acetaminophen 650 mg	Darvocet N by Bolar		Analgesic; C IV
GG220 <> 13	Tab	Acetaminophen 300 mg, Codeine Phosphate 30 mg	by Med Pro	53978-2086	Analgesic; C III
GG220 <> 3	Tab	Acetaminophen 300 mg, Codeine Phosphate 30 mg	by Quality Care	60346-0059	Analgesic; C III
GG224	Tab, White, Oblong	Phenylpropanolamine HCl 75 mg, Guaifenesin 400 mg	Entex LA by Amide		Cold Remedy
GG225	Tab, White, Round, Scored	Promethazine HCl 25 mg	by Allscripts	54569-1754	Antiemetic; Antihistamine
GG225	Tab, Geneva	Promethazine HCl 25 mg	by Pharmedix	53002-0402	Antiemetic; Antihistamine
GG225	Tab	Promethazine HCl 25 mg	by Quality Care	60346-0085	Antiemetic; Antihistamine
GG227	Tab	Isosorbide Dinitrate 20 mg	by Med Pro	53978-5039	Antianginal
GG227	Tab	Isosorbide Dinitrate 20 mg	by Nat Pharmpak Serv	55154-5407	Antianginal
GG227	Tab	Isosorbide Dinitrate 20 mg	by Golden State	60429-0102	Antianginal
GG229	Tab, Yellow, Round	Isosorbide Dinitrate ER 40 mg	Isordil by Geneva		Antianginal
GG232	Tab, White, Oblong	Hydrocodone 5 mg, Acetaminophen 500 mg	Vicodin by Rosemont		Analgesic; C III
GG234	Tab, White, Oval	Methylprednisolone 4 mg	Medrol by Duramed		Steroid

ID FRONT <> BACK	DESCRIPTION FRONT <> BACK	INGREDIENT & STRENGTH	BRAND (OR EQUIV.) & FIRM	NDC#	CLASS; SCH.
GG235	Tab	Promethazine HCl 50 mg	by Physicians Total Care	54868-2844	Antiemetic; Antihistamine
GG235	Tab, Debossed	Promethazine HCl 50 mg	by St Marys Med	60760-0832	Antiemetic; Antihistamine
GG235	Tab, Pink, Round	Promethazine HCl 50 mg	Phenergan by Geneva	00781-1832	Antiemetic; Antihistamine
GG236	Tab, Yellow, Round, Scored	Sulindac 150 mg	Clinoril by Geneva	00781-1811	NSAID
GG237	Tab, Yellow, Round, Scored	Sulindac 200 mg	by Murfreesboro Ph	51129-1685	NSAID
GG237	Tab, Yellow, Round	Sulindac 200 mg	by Va Cmop	65243-0066	NSAID
GG237	Tab, Coated	Sulindac 200 mg	by Golden State	60429-0172	NSAID
GG237	Tab, Yellow, Round, Scored	Sulindac 200 mg	Clinoril by Geneva	00781-1812	NSAID
GG238	Tab, White, Round	Glyburide 1.25 mg	Diabeta by Greenstone		Antidiabetic
GG238	Tab, White, Round, Scored	Glyburide 1.25 mg	by Pharmacia & Upjohn	00009-3725	Antidiabetic
GG239	Tab	Glyburide 2.5 mg	by Golden State	60429-0084	Antidiabetic
GG239	Tab, Dark Pink, Round, Scored	Glyburide 2.5 mg	Micronase R.N. by Geneva	00781-1456	Antidiabetic
GG24	Tab, White, Round	Theophylline 130 mg, Ephedrine Sulfate 25 mg, Hydroxyzine HCl 10 mg	Marax by Geneva		Antiasthmatic
GG240	Tab	Glyburide 5 mg	by Quality Care	60346-0938	Antidiabetic
GG240	Tab	Glyburide 5 mg	by Golden State	60429-0085	Antidiabetic
GG240	Tab	Glyburide 5 mg	by Med Pro	53978-0694	Antidiabetic
GG240	Tab, Blue, Round, Scored	Glyburide 5 mg	by KV	10609-1447	Antidiabetic
GG242	Tab	Methyclothiazide 5 mg	by Geneva	00781-1810	Diuretic
GG243	Tab, Film Coated	Hydrochlorothiazide 30 mg, Methyldopa 500 mg	by Geneva	00781-1843	Diuretic; Antihypertensive
GG244	Tab	Methyclothiazide 2.5 mg	by Geneva	00781-1803	Diuretic
GG245	Tab, White, Round	Minoxidil 10 mg	Loniten by Quantum		Antihypertensive
GG249	Tab, White, Rectangular	Alprazolam 2 mg	by PDRX Pharms	55289-0523	Antianxiety; C IV
GG249	Tab, White, Rectangular, Scored, Coated	Alprazolam 2 mg	Xanax by Geneva	00781-1089	Antianxiety; C IV
GG25	Tab, White, Round	Triprolidine HCl 2.5 mg, Pseudoephedrine HCl 60 mg	Actifed by Geneva		Cold Remedy
GG250	Tab	Quinidine Gluconate 324 mg	by Med Pro	53978-2085	Antiarrhythmic
GG250	Tab, Ex Release	Quinidine Gluconate 324 mg	by Geneva	00781-1804	Antiarrhythmic
GG250	Tab, Ex Release	Quinidine Gluconate 324 mg	by Golden State	60429-0167	Antiarrhythmic
GG251	Tab	Carbidopa 10 mg, Levodopa 100 mg	by Geneva	00781-1626	Antiparkinson
GG252	Tab	Carbidopa 25 mg, Levodopa 100 mg	by Geneva	00781-1627	Antiparkinson
GG254	Tab	Fenoprofen Calcium 600 mg	by Geneva	00781-1863	NSAID
GG255	Tab, White, Round, Coated	Dexbrompheniramine Maleate 6 mg, Pseudoephedrine Sulfate 120 mg	Drixoral by Geneva	00781-1600	Cold Remedy
GG256	Tab, White, Oval, Scored	Alprazolam 0.25 mg	Xanax by Geneva	00781-1061	Antianxiety; C IV
GG256	Tab, Coated	Alprazolam 0.25 mg	by Murfreesboro	51129-1341	Antianxiety; C IV
GG256	Tab	Alprazolam 0.25 mg	by Murfreesboro	51129-1345	Antianxiety; C IV
GG256	Tab, Coated	Alprazolam 0.25 mg	by Med Pro	53978-1300	Antianxiety; C IV
GG256	Tab, White, Oval, Scored	Alprazolam 0.25 mg	Xanax by Geneva	00781-1326	Antianxiety; C IV
GG256	Tab, White, Oval, Scored	Alprazolam 0.25 mg	by Apotheca	12634-0529	Antianxiety; C IV
GG257	Tab, Peach, Oval, Scored	Alprazolam 0.5 mg	Xanax by Geneva	00781-1077	Antianxiety; C IV
GG258	Tab, Blue, Oval	Alprazolam 1 mg	by Compumed	00403-4578	Antianxiety; C IV
GG258	Tab, Blue, Oval, Scored	Alprazolam 1 mg	by Apotheca	12634-0530	Antianxiety; C IV
GG258	Tab, Blue, Oval, Scored	Alprazolam 1 mg	Xanax R.N. by Geneva	00781-1328	Antianxiety; C IV
GG258	Tab, Blue, Oval, Scored	Alprazolam 1 mg	Xanax by Geneva	00781-1079	Antianxiety; C IV
GG26	Tab	Isosorbide Dinitrate 10 mg	by Med Pro	53978-5038	Antianginal
GG26	Tab	Isosorbide Dinitrate 10 mg	by Nat Pharmpak Serv	55154-5406	Antianginal
GG26	Tab	Isosorbide Dinitrate 10 mg	by Golden State	60429-0101	Antianginal
GG26	Tab, Debossed	Isosorbide Dinitrate 10 mg	by Quality Care	60346-0577	Antianginal
GG260	Tab, White, Round, Film Coated, Scored	Hydroxychloroquine Sulfate 200 mg	by Murfreesboro Ph	51129-1369	Antimalarial
GG260	Tab, Film Coated	Hydroxychloroquine Sulfate 200 mg	by Golden State	60429-0700	Antimalarial

ID FRONT <> BACK	DESCRIPTION FRONT <> BACK	INGREDIENT & STRENGTH	BRAND (OR EQUIV.) & FIRM	NDC#	CLASS; SCH.
GG260	Tab, White, Round, Film Coated	Hydroxychloroquine Sulfate 200 mg	Plaquenil by Geneva	00781-1407	Antimalarial
GG261	Tab, Football Shaped	Meclizine HCl 25 mg	by Kaiser	00179-1116	Antiemetic
GG261	Tab	Meclizine HCl 25 mg	by Quality Care	60346-0694	Antiemetic
GG261	Tab, Yellow, Oval, Scored	Meclizine HCl 25 mg	Antivert by Geneva	00781-1375	Antiemetic
GG261	Tab, White & Yellow, Oval, Scored	Meclizine HCl 25 mg	Antivert by Geneva	00781-1544	Antiemetic
GG263	Tab	Atenolol 50 mg	by Golden State	60429-0025	Antihypertensive
GG263	Tab, White, Round, Scored	Atenolol 50 mg	by Haines Pharms	59564-0126	Antihypertensive
GG263	Tab, White, Round, Scored	Atenolol 50 mg	by Natl Pharmpak	55154-5411	Antihypertensive
GG263	Tab, White, Round, Scored	Atenolol 50 mg	by Allscripts	54569-3432	Antihypertensive
GG263	Tab, White, Round, Scored	Atenolol 50 mg	by Va Cmop	65243-0014	Antihypertensive
GG263	Tab	Atenolol 50 mg	by Zenith Goldline	00182-1004	Antihypertensive
GG263	Tab, White, Round, Scored	Atenolol 50 mg	Tenormin by Geneva	00781-1506	Antihypertensive
GG263	Tab, White, Round	Atenolol 50 mg	by Duramed	51285-0837	Antihypertensive
GG263	Tab	Atenolol 50 mg	by Med Pro	53978-1199	Antihypertensive
GG263	Tab, White, Round, Scored	Atenolol 50 mg	by Compumed	00403-4582	Antihypertensive
GG264	Tab, Coated	Atenolol 100 mg	by Golden State	60429-0026	Antihypertensive
GG264	Tab	Atenolol 100 mg	by Direct Dispensing	57866-3331	Antihypertensive
GG264	Tab, White, Round	Atenolol 100 mg	by Southwood Pharms	58016-0771	Antihypertensive
GG264	Tab	Atenolol 100 mg	by Quality Care		Antihypertensive
GG264	Tab, Coated	Atenolol 100 mg	by Zenith Goldline	00182-1005	Antihypertensive
GG264	Tab, White, Round	Atenolol 100 mg	Tenormin by Geneva	00781-1507	Antihypertensive
GG264	Tab, White, Round, Coated	Atenolol 100 mg	by Duramed	51285-0838	Antihypertensive
GG264	Tab, Coated	Atenolol 100 mg	by Med Pro	53978-2027	Antihypertensive
GG265	Tab, Film Coated	Hydrochlorothiazide 25 mg, Methyldopa 250 mg	by Geneva	00781-1819	Diuretic; Antihypertensive
GG27	Tab, Peach, Round	Hydrochlorothiazide 50 mg	Hydrodiuril by Geneva		Diuretic
GG270	Tab	Tolazamide 100 mg	by Geneva	00781-1922	Antidiabetic
GG271	Tab	Tolazamide 250 mg	by Geneva	00781-1932	Antidiabetic
GG272	Tab	Tolazamide 500 mg	by Geneva	00781-1942	Antidiabetic
GG28	Tab, Peach, Round	Hydrochlorothiazide 25 mg	Hydrodiuril by Geneva		Diuretic
GG284	Tab, Debossed	Isoxsuprine HCl 20 mg	by Physicians Total Care	54868-1464	Vasodilator
GG285	Tab	Quinidine Sulfate 200 mg	by Geneva	00781-1900	Antiarrhythmic
GG286	Tab	Quinidine Sulfate 300 mg	by Geneva	00781-1902	Antiarrhythmic
GG288	Tab, Butterscotch Yellow, Round, Film Coated	Cyclobenzaprine HCl 10 mg	Flexeril by Geneva	00781-1324	Muscle Relaxant
GG288	Tab, Butterscotch Yellow, Coated	Cyclobenzaprine HCl 10 mg	by Med Pro	53978-1035	Muscle Relaxant
GG288	Tab, Coated	Cyclobenzaprine HCl 10 mg	by Golden State	60429-0052	Muscle Relaxant
GG289	Tab, Film Coated	Hydrochlorothiazide 50 mg, Methyldopa 500 mg	by Geneva	00781-1853	Diuretic; Antihypertensive
GG291	Tab, White, Round	Ibuprofen 400 mg	Motrin by Ciba		NSAID
GG292	Tab, White, Oval	Ibuprofen 600 mg	Motrin by Interpharm		NSAID
GG293	Tab, White, Round	Ibuprofen 200 mg	Nuprin by Geneva		NSAID
GG294	Tab, White, Oblong	Ibuprofen 800 mg	Motrin by Geneva		NSAID
GG295	Tab, White, Round	Albuterol 4 mg	Proventil by Geneva		Antiasthmatic
GG295	Tab, White, Round, Scored	Albuterol Sulfate 4 mg	Proventil by Geneva	00781-1672	Antiasthmatic
GG30	Tab, Coated	Thioridazine HCl 10 mg	by Heartland	61392-0462	Antipsychotic
GG30	Tab, Orange, Film Coated	Thioridazine HCl 10 mg	Mellaril by Geneva	00781-1604	Antipsychotic
GG300	Cap, Maroon & White, G/G 300	Gemfibrozil 300 mg	by Genpharm	Canadian	Antihyperlipidemic
GG31 <> 15	Tab, Orange, Round, Film Coated	Thioridazine HCl 15 mg	by Heartland Healthcare	61392-0464	Antipsychotic
GG31 <> 15	Tab, Film Coated	Thioridazine HCl 15 mg	by Murfreesboro	51129-1110	Antipsychotic
GG31 <> 15	Tab, Film Coated	Thioridazine HCl 15 mg	by Vangard	00615-2505	Antipsychotic
GG31 <> 15	Tab, Orange, Round, Film Coated	Thioridazine HCl 15 mg	Mellaril by Geneva	00781-1614	Antipsychotic
GG32 <> 25	Tab, Coated	Thioridazine HCl 25 mg	by Heartland	61392-0463	Antipsychotic

ID FRONT ⬦ BACK	DESCRIPTION FRONT ⬦ BACK	INGREDIENT & STRENGTH	BRAND (OR EQUIV.) & FIRM	NDC#	CLASS; SCH.
GG32 ⬦ 25	Tab, Orange, Round, Film Coated	Thioridazine HCl 25 mg	Mellaril by Geneva	00781-1624	Antipsychotic
GG32 ⬦ 25	Tab, Orange, Round	Thioridazine HCl 25 mg	by Direct Dispensing	57866-4642	Antipsychotic
GG33 ⬦ 50	Tab, Film Coated	Thioridazine HCl 50 mg	by Heartland	61392-0819	Antipsychotic
GG33 ⬦ 50	Tab, Orange, Round, Film Coated	Thioridazine HCl 50 mg	Mellaril by Geneva	00781-1634	Antipsychotic
GG34 ⬦ 100	Tab, Film Coated	Thioridazine HCl 100 mg	by Heartland	61392-0144	Antipsychotic
GG34 ⬦ 100	Tab, Orange, Round, Film Coated	Thioridazine HCl 100 mg	Mellaril by Geneva	00781-1644	Antipsychotic
GG34100	Tab, Film Coated	Thioridazine HCl 100 mg	by Med Pro	53978-2007	Antipsychotic
GG35	Tab, Orange, Round, Film Coated	Thioridazine HCl 150 mg	Mellaril by Geneva	00781-1664	Antipsychotic
GG35	Tab, Film Coated	Thioridazine HCl 150 mg	by Vangard	00615-2509	Antipsychotic
GG36	Tab, White, Round, Scored	Methazolamide 50 mg	by Heartland Healthcare	61392-0890	Diuretic
GG36	Tab, Orange, Round, Film Coated	Thioridazine HCl 200 mg	by Heartland Healthcare	61392-0465	Antipsychotic
GG36	Tab, Film Coated	Thioridazine HCl 200 mg	by Vangard	00615-2510	Antipsychotic
GG36	Tab, Orange, Round, Film Coated	Thioridazine HCl 200 mg	Mellaril by Geneva	00781-1674	Antipsychotic
GG37	Tab, Lavender, Round	Hydroxyzine HCl 10 mg	Atarax by Geneva		Antihistamine
GG39	Tab, Purple, Round	Hydroxyzine HCl 50 mg	Atarax by Geneva		Antihistamine
GG4	Tab, White, Round	Atropine Sulfate 0.025 mg, Diphenoxylate HCl 2.5 mg	by Allscripts	54569-0222	Antidiarrheal; C V
GG4	Tab, White, Round	Atropine Sulfate 0.025 mg, Diphenoxylate HCl 2.5 mg	Lomotil by Geneva	00781-1262	Antidiarrheal; C V
GG4	Tab	Atropine Sulfate 0.025 mg, Diphenoxylate HCl 2.5 mg	by HJ Harkins Co	52959-0157	Antidiarrheal; C V
GG4	Tab, White, Round	Diphenoxylate HCl 2.5 mg, Atropine Sulfate 0.025 mg	by Genpharm	55567-0054	Antidiarrheal; C V
GG40	Tab, Coated, GG Over 40	Amitriptyline HCl 10 mg	by Quality Care	60346-0354	Antidepressant
GG40	Tab, Pink, Round, Film Coated	Amitriptyline HCl 10 mg	Elavil by Geneva	00781-1486	Antidepressant
GG405	Tab, White, Round	Acetaminophen 500 mg	Tylenol by Geneva		Antipyretic
GG407 ⬦ 50	Tab, Butterscotch, Film Coated, Debossed	Chlorpromazine HCl 50 mg	by Golden State	60429-0042	Antipsychotic
GG407 ⬦ 50	Tab, Yellow, Round, Film Coated	Chlorpromazine HCl 50 mg	by Murfreesboro Ph	51129-1361	Antipsychotic
GG407 ⬦ 50	Tab, Yellow, Round, Film Coated	Chlorpromazine HCl 50 mg	by Haines Pharms	59564-0130	Antipsychotic
GG407 ⬦ 50	Tab, Butterscotch Yellow, Round, Film Coated	Chlorpromazine HCl 50 mg	Thorazine by Geneva	00781-1717	Antipsychotic
GG41	Tab, Yellow, Round, Film Coated	Imipramine HCl 10 mg	Tofranil by Geneva	00781-1762	Antidepressant
GG411	Tab, White, Round	Carisoprodol 350 mg	by Caremark	00339-6147	Muscle Relaxant
GG411	Tab, White, Round	Carisoprodol 350 mg	Soma by Geneva	00781-1050	Muscle Relaxant
GG414	Tab, White, Round, Film Coated, Scored	Metoprolol Tartrate 50 mg	by Murfreesboro Ph	51129-1419	Antihypertensive
GG414	Tab, Film Coated	Metoprolol Tartrate 50 mg	by Nat Pharmpak Serv	55154-5405	Antihypertensive
GG414	Tab, Film Coated	Metoprolol Tartrate 50 mg	by Med Pro	53978-2058	Antihypertensive
GG414	Tab, Film Coated	Metoprolol Tartrate 50 mg	by Quality Care	60346-0523	Antihypertensive
GG414	Tab, Film Coated	Metoprolol Tartrate 50 mg	by Golden State	60429-0126	Antihypertensive
GG414	Tab, Coated	Metoprolol Tartrate 50 mg	by Direct Dispensing	57866-6578	Antihypertensive
GG414	Tab, White, Round, Film Coated	Metoprolol Tartrate 50 mg	Lopressor by Geneva	00781-1223	Antihypertensive
GG414	Tab, Film Coated	Metoprolol Tartrate 50 mg	by Geneva	00781-1371	Antihypertensive
GG414	Tab, White, Round, Scored, Film	Metoprolol Tartrate 50 mg	by Neuman Distr	64579-0093	Antihypertensive
GG415	Tab, White, Round, Scored, Film	Metoprolol Tartrate 100 mg	by Neuman Distr	64579-0094	Antihypertensive
GG415	Tab, Film Coated	Metoprolol Tartrate 100 mg	by Nat Pharmpak Serv	55154-5409	Antihypertensive
GG415	Tab, Film Coated	Metoprolol Tartrate 100 mg	by Golden State	60429-0127	Antihypertensive
GG415	Tab, White, Round, Film Coated	Metoprolol Tartrate 100 mg	Lopressor by Geneva	00781-1228	Antihypertensive
GG415	Tab, Film Coated	Metoprolol Tartrate 100 mg	by Geneva	00781-1372	Antihypertensive
GG416	Tab, Green, Round	Hydralazine HCl 50 mg	Apresoline by Geneva		Antihypertensive
GG417	Tab, Film Coated	Naproxen Sodium 275 mg	by Murfreesboro	51129-1318	NSAID
GG417	Tab, Film Coated	Naproxen Sodium 275 mg	by Quality Care	60346-0875	NSAID
GG417	Tab, Yellow, Oval, Film Coated	Naproxen Sodium 275 mg	Anaprox by Geneva	00781-1187	NSAID
GG418	Tab, White, Oval, Film Coated	Naproxen Sodium 550 mg	Anaprox by Geneva	00781-1188	NSAID
GG418	Tab, Film Coated	Naproxen Sodium 550 mg	by St Marys Med	60760-0188	NSAID
GG418	Tab, Film Coated	Naproxen Sodium 550 mg	by Quality Care	60346-0826	NSAID
GG419	Tab, Film Coated	Trazodone HCl 50 mg	by Med Pro	53978-0495	Antidepressant
GG419	Tab, Film Coated, Debossed	Trazodone HCl 50 mg	by Amerisource	62584-0882	Antidepressant

ID FRONT <> BACK	DESCRIPTION FRONT <> BACK	INGREDIENT & STRENGTH	BRAND (OR EQUIV.) & FIRM	NDC#	CLASS; SCH.
GG419	Tab, Scored, Film Coated	Trazodone HCl 50 mg	by Golden State	60429-0187	Antidepressant
GG419	Tab, White, Round, Scored, Film Coated	Trazodone HCl 50 mg	Desyrel by Geneva	00781-1807	Antidepressant
GG42	Tab, Sugar Coated, GG over 42	Imipramine HCl 50 mg	by Quality Care	60346-0709	Antidepressant
GG42	Tab, Green, Round, Film Coated	Imipramine HCl 50 mg	Tofranil by Geneva	00781-1766	Antidepressant
GG420	Tab, Film Coated	Trazodone HCl 100 mg	by Med Pro	53978-0563	Antidepressant
GG420	Tab, Film Coated	Trazodone HCl 100 mg	by Golden State	60429-0188	Antidepressant
GG420	Tab, White, Round, Scored, Film Coated	Trazodone HCl 100 mg	Desyrel by Geneva	00781-1808	Antidepressant
GG421	Tab	Chlorzoxazone 250 mg	by Geneva	00781-1303	Muscle Relaxant
GG422	Tab	Chlorzoxazone 500 mg	by Geneva	00781-1304	Muscle Relaxant
GG427	Tab, Green, Round, Film Coated	Cimetidine 200 mg	Tagamet by Geneva	00781-1447	Gastrointestinal
GG428	Tab, Green, Round, Film Coated	Cimetidine 300 mg	Tagamet by Geneva	00781-1448	Gastrointestinal
GG429	Tab, Film Coated	Cimetidine 400 mg	by Quality Care	60346-0945	Gastrointestinal
GG429	Tab, Green, Oblong, Film Coated, Scored	Cimetidine 400 mg	by Murfreesboro Ph	51129-1347	Gastrointestinal
GG429	Tab, Green, Oblong, Scored, Film Coated	Cimetidine 400 mg	by Compumed	00403-2021	Gastrointestinal
GG430	Tab, Film Coated	Cimetidine 800 mg	by HJ Harkins Co	52959-0376	Gastrointestinal
GG431	Tab, Coated, Debossed	Amitriptyline HCl 50 mg	by Golden State	60429-0017	Antidepressant
GG431	Tab, Brown, Round, Film Coated	Amitriptyline HCl 50 mg	Elavil by Geneva	00781-1488	Antidepressant
GG432	Tab, White, Round	Conjugated Estrogens 0.3 mg	Premarin by Duramed		Estrogen
GG433	Tab, White, Round	Conjugated Estrogens 0.625 mg	Premarin by Duramed		Estrogen
GG434	Tab, White, Round	Conjugated Estrogens 1.25 mg	Premarin by Duramed		Estrogen
GG435	Tab, White, Round	Conjugated Estrogens 2.5 mg	Premarin by Duramed		Estrogen
GG436	Tab, Brown, Round	Nystatin Oral 500,000 Units	Mycostatin by Eon		Antifungal
GG437 <> 100	Tab, Coated	Chlorpromazine HCl 100 mg	by Haines	59564-0131	Antipsychotic
GG437 <> 100	Tab, Butterscotch, Coated, Debossed	Chlorpromazine HCl 100 mg	by Golden State	60429-0043	Antipsychotic
GG437 <> 100	Tab, Yellow, Round, Film	Chlorpromazine HCl 100 mg	by Compumed		Antipsychotic
GG437 <> 100	Tab, Butterscotch Yellow, Round, Film Coated	Chlorpromazine HCl 100 mg	Thorazine by Geneva	00781-1718	Antipsychotic
GG44	Tab, Coated	Amitriptyline HCl 25 mg	by Quality Care	60346-0027	Antidepressant
GG44	Tab, Coated, Debossed	Amitriptyline HCl 25 mg	by Golden State	60429-0016	Antidepressant
GG44	Tab, Green, Round	Amitriptyline HCl 25 mg	by Va Cmop	65243-0006	Antidepressant
GG44	Tab, Green, Round, Film	Amitriptyline HCl 25 mg	by Astra Zeneca	00186-0451	Antidepressant
GG44	Tab, Light Green, Round, Film Coated	Amitriptyline HCl 25 mg	Elavil by Geneva	00781-1487	Antidepressant
GG441	Tab, Debossed	Carisoprodol 350 mg	by Golden State	60429-0035	Muscle Relaxant
GG441	Tab, Cream & Orange Specks, Round	Chewable Vitamin, Fluoride 0.5 mg	Poly-Vi-Flor by Amide		Vitamin
GG444	Tab, White, Round	Pseudoephedrine 120 mg, Dexbrompheniramine SA 6 mg	Drixoral by Geneva		Cold Remedy
GG447	Tab, Blue, Round	Phenylpropanolamine HCl 75 mg, Brompheniramine Sulfate 12 mg	Dimetapp Ext. by Geneva		Cold Remedy
GG45	Tab, White, Round	Dipyridamole 50 mg	Persantine by Geneva		Antiplatelet
GG450	Tab, Light Green, Round, Film Coated	Amitriptyline HCl 150 mg	Elavil by Geneva	00781-1491	Antidepressant
GG451	Tab, Purple, Round, Film Coated	Amitriptyline HCl 75 mg	Elavil by Geneva	00781-1489	Antidepressant
GG455 <> 10	Tab, Yellow, Round, Film Coated	Chlorpromazine HCl 10 mg	by Heartland Hlthcare	61392-0880	Antipsychotic
GG455 <> 10	Tab, Butterscotch Yellow, Round, Film Coated	Chlorpromazine HCl 10 mg	Thorazine by Geneva	00781-1715	Antipsychotic
GG457 <> 200	Tab, Yellow, Round, Film Coated	Chlorpomazine HCl 200 mg	by Murfreesboro Ph	51129-1370	Antipsychotic
GG457 <> 200	Tab, Butterscotch Yellow, Round, Film Coated	Chlorpromazine HCl 200 mg	Thorazine by Geneva	00781-1719	Antipsychotic
GG457 <> 200	Tab, Butterscotch Yellow, Film Coated	Chlorpromazine HCl 200 mg	by Physicians Total Care	54868-2465	Antipsychotic
GG458	Tab, White, Oblong	Acetaminophen 500 mg	Tylenol by Geneva		Antipyretic
GG459	Tab, White, Oblong	Acetaminophen 325 mg	Tylenol by Geneva		Antipyretic
GG461	Tab, Orange, Round, Film Coated	Amitriptyline HCl 100 mg	Elavil by Geneva	00781-1490	Antidepressant
GG464	Tab, Film Coated	Dipyridamole 75 mg	by Geneva	00781-1478	Antiplatelet
GG47	Tab, Beige, Round, Film Coated	Imipramine HCl 25 mg	Tofranil by Geneva	00781-1764	Antidepressant
GG471	Tab, Film Coated	Methyldopa 500 mg	Methyldopa by Geneva	00781-1322	Antihypertensive
GG472	Tab, White, Oblong	Procainamide HCl SR 250 mg	Procan SR by Geneva		Antiarrhythmic
GG473	Tab, White, Oblong	Procainamide HCl SR 500 mg	Procan SR by Geneva		Antiarrhythmic
GG474	Tab, White, Oblong	Procainamide HCl SR 750 mg	Procan SR by Danbury		Antiarrhythmic

ID FRONT <> BACK	DESCRIPTION FRONT <> BACK	INGREDIENT & STRENGTH	BRAND (OR EQUIV.) & FIRM	NDC#	CLASS; SCH.
GG475	Tab, White, Round	Hydralazine HCl 10 mg	Apresoline by Geneva		Antihypertensive
GG476 <> 25	Tab, Butterscotch, Coated	Chlorpromazine HCl 25 mg	by Heartland	61392-0040	Antipsychotic
GG476 <> 25	Tab, Butterscotch, Coated	Chlorpromazine HCl 25 mg	by Quality Care	62682-7045	Antipsychotic
GG476 <> 25	Tab, Butterscotch Yelllow, Round, Film Coated	Chlorpromazine HCl 25 mg	Thorazine by Geneva	00781-1716	Antipsychotic
GG477	Tab, Blue, Round	Brompheniramine 12 mg, Phenylephrine 15 mg, Phenylpropanolamine 15 mg	Dimetapp by Geneva		Cold Remedy
GG48	Tab, Red, Round	Pseudoephedrine 30 mg	Sudafed by Geneva		Decongestant
GG48	Tab, Red, Round, Film Coated	Pseudoephedrine 30 mg	Sudafed by Geneva	00781-1533	Decongestant
GG480	Tab, White, Oblong	Prenatal Vitamins, Zinc	Stuart 1+1 Zinc by Amide		Vitamin
GG481	Tab, Tan, Oblong	Prenatal Vitamin, Zinc Improved	Stuart 1+1 by Amide		Vitamin
GG483	Tab, Salmon, Round	Enalapril 10 mg	Vasotec by Geneva	00781-1232	Antihypertensive
GG484	Tab, Peach, Round	Enalapril 20 mg	Vasotec by Geneva	00781-1233	Antihypertensive
GG485	Tab, Green, Round	Hydralazine HCl 25 mg	Apresoline by Geneva		Antihypertensive
GG487	Tab, White, Oblong	Probenecid 500 mg, Colchicine 0.5 mg	ColBenemid by Danbury		Antigout
GG488	Tab, Beige, Round, Film Coated	Fluphenazine HCl 2.5 mg	Prolixin by Geneva	00781-1437	Antipsychotic
GG489	Tab, Orange, Round	Fluphenazine HCl 5 mg	by Direct Dispensing	57866-4405	Antipsychotic
GG489	Tab, Light Rust, Round, Film Coated	Fluphenazine HCl 5 mg	Prolixin by Geneva	00781-1438	Antipsychotic
GG489	Tab, Coated	Fluphenazine HCl 5 mg	by Murfreesboro	51129-1258	Antipsychotic
GG49	Tab, Film Coated	Dipyridamole 25 mg	by Geneva	00781-1890	Antiplatelet
GG490	Tab, Rust, Film Coated	Fluphenazine HCl 10 mg	by Golden State	60429-0075	Antipsychotic
GG490	Tab, Rust, Round, Film Coated	Fluphenazine HCl 10 mg	Prolixin by Geneva	00781-1439	Antipsychotic
GG501	Cap, Blue & Yellow	Nitroglycerin SR 6.5 mg	Nitrobid by Geneva		Vasodilator
GG502	Cap	Chlorpheniramine Maleate 12 mg, Phenylpropanolamine HCl 75 mg	by Geneva	00781-2427	Cold Remedy
GG502 <> GG502	Cap, Blue & Clear	Phenylpropanolamine HCl 75 mg, Chlorpheniramine Maleate 12 mg	Propade by Mallinckrodt Hobart	00406-0421	Cold Remedy
GG502 <> GG502	Cap, Blue & Clear	Phenylpropanolamine HCl 75 mg, Chlorpheniramine Maleate 12 mg	by Geneva Pharms	00781-2424	Cold Remedy
GG503	Cap, Brown & Clear	Papaverine TD 150 mg	Pavabid by Geneva		Vasodilator
GG505	Cap, White, Black & Pink Bands, Opaque	Oxazepam 10 mg	Serax by Geneva	00781-2809	Sedative/Hypnotic; C IV
GG506	Cap, White, Black & Red Bands, Opaque	Oxazepam 15 mg	Serax by Geneva	00781-2810	Sedative/Hypnotic; C IV
GG506 <> GG506	Cap, White, GG 506 in Red Ink <> GG 506 in Black Ink	Oxazepam 15 mg	by Pharmacia & Upjohn	00009-5012	Sedative/Hypnotic; C IV
GG507	Cap, White, Black & Maroon Bands, Opaque	Oxazepam 30 mg	Serax by Geneva	00781-2811	Sedative/Hypnotic; C IV
GG51	Tab, Lavender, Round, Film Coated	Trifluoperazine HCl 1 mg	Stelazine by Geneva	00781-1030	Antipsychotic
GG51 <> 1	Tab, Purple, Round	Trifluoperazine HCl 1 mg	by Apotheca	12634-0678	Antipsychotic
GG511	Tab, Film Coated	Trifluoperazine HCl 1 mg	by Geneva	00781-1030	Antipsychotic
GG512	Cap, Green & Yellow	Nitroglycerin SR 9 mg	Nitrobid by Geneva		Vasodilator
GG515	Cap, Clear	Quinine Sulfate 5 gr	by Geneva		Antimalarial
GG517	Cap	Indomethacin 25 mg	by Golden State	60429-0098	NSAID
GG517	Cap	Indomethacin 25 mg	by Geneva	00781-2325	NSAID
GG518	Cap	Indomethacin 50 mg	by Geneva	00781-2350	NSAID
GG52	Tab, Yellow, Round	Levothyroxine 0.1 mg	Synthroid by Rosemont		Antithyroid
GG52 <> 2	Tab, Lavender, Round, Film Coated	Trifluoperazine HCl 2 mg	Stelazine by Geneva	00781-1032	Antipsychotic
GG522	Cap, Blue & White	Flurazepam 15 mg	Dalmane by Par		Hypnotic; C IV
GG523	Cap, Blue	Flurazepam 30 mg	Dalmane by Par		Hypnotic; C IV
GG524	Cap	Meclofenamate Sodium	by Geneva	00781-2702	NSAID
GG525	Cap	Meclofenamate Sodium	by Geneva	00781-2703	NSAID
GG526	Cap, White Bands	Clorazepate 30.75 mg	Tranxene by Geneva		Antianxiety; C IV
GG527	Cap, White Bands	Clorazepate 7.5 mg	Tranxene by Geneva		Antianxiety; C IV
GG527	Tab, White, Round	Prednisone 50 mg	Deltasone by Geneva		Steroid
GG528	Cap, White Bands	Clorazepate 15 mg	Tranxene by Geneva		Antianxiety; C IV
GG53 <> 2	Tab, Coated, Debossed	Trifluoperazine HCl 2 mg	by Med Pro	53978-2090	Antipsychotic
GG53 <> 2	Tab, Coated, Debossed	Trifluoperazine HCl 2 mg	by Heartland	61392-0822	Antipsychotic
GG53 <> 2	Tab, Lavender, Coated, Debossed	Trifluoperazine HCl 2 mg	by Golden State	60429-0192	Antipsychotic
GG53 <> 2	Tab, Coated	Trifluoperazine HCl 2 mg	by Vangard	00615-3598	Antipsychotic
GG530	Cap, White, with Green Bands	Loperamide HCl 2 mg	Imodium by Geneva	00781-2761	Antidiarrheal

ID FRONT <> BACK	DESCRIPTION FRONT <> BACK	INGREDIENT & STRENGTH	BRAND (OR EQUIV.) & FIRM	NDC#	CLASS; SCH.
GG531	Cap, Dark Green & White	Temazepam 15 mg	Restoril by Geneva	00781-2201	Sedative/Hypnotic; C IV
GG531 <> GG531	Cap, Green & White	Temazepam 15 mg	by St. Marys Med	60760-0711	Sedative/Hypnotic; C IV
GG532	Cap, White	Temazepam 30 mg	Restoril by Geneva	00781-2202	Sedative/Hypnotic; C IV
GG533	Cap, GG over 533	Diphenhydramine HCl 25 mg	by Quality Care	60346-0589	Antihistamine
GG533	Cap	Diphenhydramine HCl 25 mg	by Geneva	00781-2458	Antihistamine
GG535	Cap, Opaque & White & Yellow	Nitrofurantoin 50 mg	by Parmed	00349-8279	Antibiotic
GG535	Cap	Nitrofurantoin 50 mg	by Procter & Gamble	00149-2502	Antibiotic
GG535	Cap, White & Yellow	Nitrofurantoin 50 mg	Macrodantin by Geneva	00781-2502	Antibiotic
GG535	Cap, White & Yellow	Nitrofurantoin Macrocrystalline 50 mg	by Compumed	00403-1528	Antibiotic
GG536	Cap, Yellow	Nitrofurantoin 100 mg	by Southwood Pharms	58016-0141	Antibiotic
GG536	Cap, Yellow	Nitrofurantoin 100 mg	Macrodantin by Geneva	00781-2503	Antibiotic
GG536	Cap, Opaque	Nitrofurantoin 100 mg	by Procter & Gamble	00149-2503	Antibiotic
GG536	Cap, Opaque	Nitrofurantoin 100 mg	by Quality Care	60346-0008	Antibiotic
GG537	Cap, Caramel & White	Bromocriptine 5 mg	Parlodel by Geneva		Antiparkinson
GG537	Cap, Caramel & White	Bromocriptine 5 mg	Parlodel by Geneva	00781-2819	Antiparkinson
GG538	Cap	Nitrofurantoin 25 mg	by Procter & Gamble	00149-2501	Antibiotic
GG538	Cap	Nitrofurantoin 25 mg	by Geneva	00781-2501	Antibiotic
GG54	Tab, White, Round	Levothyroxine 0.2 mg	Synthroid by Rosemont		Antithyroid
GG541	Cap, GG Over 541	Diphenhydramine HCl 50 mg	by Quality Care	60346-0045	Antihistamine
GG541	Cap	Diphenhydramine HCl 50 mg	by Geneva	00781-2498	Antihistamine
GG55 <> 5	Tab, Coated, Debossed	Trifluoperazine HCl 5 mg	by Med Pro	53978-2089	Antipsychotic
GG55 <> 5	Tab, Coated	Trifluoperazine HCl 5 mg	by Quality Care	62682-7031	Antipsychotic
GG55 <> 5	Tab, Lavender, Coated, Debossed	Trifluoperazine HCl 5 mg	by Golden State	60429-0193	Antipsychotic
GG55 <> 5	Tab, Lavender, Round, Film Coated	Trifluoperazine HCl 5 mg	Stelazine by Geneva	00781-1034	Antipsychotic
GG551	Cap, Yellow	Procainamide HCl 250 mg	Pronestyl by Geneva		Antiarrhythmic
GG552	Cap, Orange & White	Procainamide HCl 375 mg	Pronestyl by Geneva		Antiarrhythmic
GG553	Cap	Diphenhydramine HCl 25 mg	by PDRX	55289-0479	Antihistamine
GG553	Cap, Orange & Yellow	Procainamide HCl 500 mg	Pronestyl by Geneva		Antiarrhythmic
GG554	Cap, Black & Clear	Niacin SR 125 mg	Nicobid by Eon		Vitamin
GG556	Cap, Gray & Orange	Cephalexin 250 mg	Keflex by Novopharm		Antibiotic
GG558	Cap, Black, Gold & White	Fenoprofen Calcium 200 mg	Nalfon by Geneva		NSAID
GG559	Cap, Gold Bands	Fenoprofen Calcium 345.9 mg	by DRX	55045-2450	NSAID
GG559	Cap	Fenoprofen Calcium 345.9 mg	by Geneva	00781-2862	NSAID
GG56	Cap	Disopyramide Phosphate	by Geneva	00781-2110	Antiarrhythmic
GG564	Cap, Clear & Green	Niacin SR 250 mg	Nicobid by Eon		Vitamin
GG565	Cap, White, Black and Orange Bands	Nortriptyline HCl 10 mg	Pamelor by Geneva	00781-2630	Antidepressant
GG565	Cap	Nortriptyline HCl	by Vangard	00615-1306	Antidepressant
GG565	Cap, Black & Orange Bands	Nortriptyline HCl	by Caremark	00339-5804	Antidepressant
GG566	Cap, White	Nortriptyline HCl 25 mg	by Compumed	00403-1594	Antidepressant
GG566	Cap, White	Nortriptyline HCl 25 mg	by Apotheca	12634-0680	Antidepressant
GG566	Cap, White, Black & Orange Bands	Nortriptyline HCl 25 mg	Pamelor by Geneva	00781-2631	Antidepressant
GG566	Cap, Black and Orange Bands	Nortriptyline HCl	by Caremark	00339-5768	Antidepressant
GG566	Cap	Nortriptyline HCl	by Vangard	00615-1307	Antidepressant
GG567	Cap, White, Black Bands	Nortriptyline HCl 50 mg	Pamelor by Geneva	00781-2632	Antidepressant
GG567	Cap	Nortriptyline HCl	by Caremark	00339-5770	Antidepressant
GG567	Cap	Nortriptyline HCl	by Vangard	00615-1315	Antidepressant
GG567 <> GG567	Cap, Black Bands	Nortriptyline HCl	by Murfreesboro	51129-1259	Antidepressant
GG568	Cap, Orange Ink Bands	Nortriptyline HCl 75 mg	by Geneva	00781-2633	Antidepressant
GG57	Cap	Disopyramide Phosphate	by Geneva	00781-2115	Antiarrhythmic
GG570	Cap, Clear & Green	Chlorpheniramine Maleate TD 8 mg	Teldrin by Geneva		Antihistamine
GG571	Cap, White	Chlordiazepoxide HCl 5 mg, Clidinium Bromide 2.5 mg	Librax by Geneva		Gastrointestinal; C IV
GG572	Cap	Doxepin HCl	by Geneva	00781-2801	Antidepressant

ID FRONT <> BACK	DESCRIPTION FRONT <> BACK	INGREDIENT & STRENGTH	BRAND (OR EQUIV.) & FIRM	NDC#	CLASS; SCH.
GG573	Cap	Doxepin HCl	by Geneva	00781-2802	Antidepressant
GG574	Cap	Doxepin HCl	by Geneva	00781-2803	Antidepressant
GG576	Cap, Red and Gold Ink Bands	Doxepin HCl	by Quality Care	60346-0793	Antidepressant
GG576	Cap	Doxepin HCl	by Geneva	00781-2800	Antidepressant
GG577	Cap, White, Blue & Green Band	Doxepin HCl 100 mg	Sinequan by Geneva		Antidepressant
GG58 <> 10	Tab, Purple, Round, Film Coated	Trifluoperazine HCl 10 mg	by Teva	00480-0753	Antipsychotic
GG58 <> 10	Tab, Lavender, Round, Film Coated	Trifluoperazine HCl 10mg	Stelazine by Geneva	00781-1036	Antipsychotic
GG580	Cap	Hydrochlorothiazide 25 mg, Triamterene 50 mg	by Caremark	00339-5619	Diuretic
GG580	Cap	Hydrochlorothiazide 25 mg, Triamterene 50 mg	by Med Pro	53978-0835	Diuretic
GG580	Cap	Hydrochlorothiazide 25 mg, Triamterene 50 mg	by Med Pro	53978-5009	Diuretic
GG580	Cap	Hydrochlorothiazide 25 mg, Triamterene 50 mg	by Golden State	60429-0190	Diuretic
GG580	Cap	Hydrochlorothiazide 25 mg, Triamterene 50 mg	by Quality Care	60346-0771	Diuretic
GG580	Cap	Hydrochlorothiazide 25 mg, Triamterene 50 mg	by Qualitest	00603-6181	Diuretic
GG580	Cap	Hydrochlorothiazide 25 mg, Triamterene 50 mg	by Geneva	00781-2540	Diuretic
GG580	Cap	Hydrochlorothiazide 25 mg, Triamterene 50 mg	by Geneva	00781-2715	Diuretic
GG580 <> GG580	Cap	Hydrochlorothiazide 25 mg, Triamterene 50 mg	by Murfreesboro	51129-1319	Diuretic
GG581	Cap	Aspirin 389 mg, Caffeine 32.4 mg, Propoxyphene HCl 65 mg	by Geneva	00781-2367	Analgesic; C IV
GG5810	Tab, Lavender, Round, GG58/10	Trifluoperazine HCl 10 mg	Stelazine by Geneva		Antipsychotic
GG582	Cap, Green	Hydroxyzine Pamoate 25 mg	Vistaril by Eon		Antihistamine
GG583	Cap, Green & White	Hydroxyzine Pamoate 50 mg	Vistaril by Eon		Antihistamine
GG584	Cap, Dark Green	Hydroxyzine Pamoate 100 mg	Vistaril by Geneva		Antihistamine
GG589	Cap, White, Gold & Orange Bands	Thiothixene 1 mg	Navane by Geneva	00781-2226	Antipsychotic
GG59	Tab	Allopurinol 100 mg	by Geneva	00781-1080	Antigout
GG590	Cap, Clear & Green	Chlorpheniramine Maleate TD 12 mg	Chlor-trimeton by Geneva		Antihistamine
GG591	Cap	Propoxyphene HCl 65 mg	by Geneva	00781-2140	Analgesic; C IV
GG592	Cap, Black & White bands	Prazosin 1 mg	Minipress by Geneva		Antihypertensive
GG593	Cap, Black & Pink & White Bd	Prazosin 2 mg	Minipress by Geneva		Antihypertensive
GG594	Cap, Black & Pink & White Bd	Prazosin 5 mg	Minipress by Geneva		Antihypertensive
GG596	Cap, White, Blue & Gold Bands	Thiothixene 2 mg	Navane by Geneva	00781-2227	Antipsychotic
GG597	Cap	Thiothixene 5 mg	by Golden State	60429-0185	Antipsychotic
GG597	Cap	Thiothixene 5 mg	by Quality Care	60346-0842	Antipsychotic
GG597	Cap, White, Opaque, Black & Orange Bands	Thiothixene 5 mg	Navane by Geneva	00781-2228	Antipsychotic
GG598	Cap	Thiothixene 10 mg	by Golden State	60429-0186	Antipsychotic
GG598	Cap, White, Black & Blue Bands	Thiothixene 10 mg	Navane by Geneva	00781-2229	Antipsychotic
GG60	Tab	Allopurinol 300 mg	by Geneva	00781-1082	Antigout
GG60	Tab	Allopurinol 300 mg	by Med Pro	53978-5001	Antigout
GG600	Cap, White	Hydrochlorothiazide 25 mg, Triamterene 37.5 mg	Dyazide by SKB		Diuretic
GG606	Cap, White	Hydrochlorothiazide 25 mg, Triamterene 37.5 mg	by Murfreesboro	51129-1391	Diuretic
GG606	Cap	Hydrochlorothiazide 25 mg, Triamterene 37.5 mg	by Allscripts	54569-3967	Diuretic
GG606	Cap, White, Printed in Black Ink	Hydrochlorothiazide 25 mg, Triamterene 37.5 mg	by Murfreesboro	51129-1411	Diuretic
GG606	Cap	Hydrochlorothiazide 25 mg, Triamterene 37.5 mg	by Geneva	00781-2056	Diuretic
GG606	Cap, White, Opaque, Black & Yellow Bands, Black Print	Hydrochlorothiazide 25 mg, Triamterene 37.5 mg	Dyazide (Lite) by Geneva	00781-2074	Diuretic
GG606	Cap, White, Black Print	Triamterene 37.5 mg, Hydrochlorothiazide 25 mg	Digoxin HCTZ by Teva	00480-0638	Diuretic
GG606	Cap, White	Triamterene 37.5 mg; Hydrochlorothiazide 25 mg	by Vangard Labs	00615-1333	Diuretic
GG606 <> GG606	Cap, White	Triamterene 75 mg; Hydrochlorothiazide 50 mg	by Southwood Pharms	58016-0520	Diuretic
GG61	Tab, White, Round	Chlorpropamide 100 mg	Diabinese by Geneva		Antidiabetic
GG614	Cap, Caramel with Off-White Powder, Opaque	Ranitidine HCl 150 mg	Zantac by Geneva	00781-2855	Gastrointestinal
GG615	Cap, Caramel with Off-White Powder, Opaque	Ranitidine HCl 300 mg	Zantac by Geneva	00781-2865	Gastrointestinal
GG62	Tab, Pink, Round	Sodium Fluoride 2.2 mg	Luride by Trinity		Element
GG621	Cap, White, Opaque, with Black & White Imprint	Terazosin 1 mg	Hytrin by Geneva	00781-2051	Antihypertensive
GG621	Cap, White	Terazosin HCl 1 mg	by Heartland Healthcare	61392-0943	Antihypertensive
GG621 <> GG621	Cap, White	Terazosin HCl 1 mg	Terazosin HCl by St. Marys Med	60760-0884	Antihypertensive

ID FRONT <> BACK	DESCRIPTION FRONT <> BACK	INGREDIENT & STRENGTH	BRAND (OR EQUIV.) & FIRM	NDC#	CLASS; SCH.
GG622	Cap, YellowBlack Print	Terazosin HCl 2 mg	by Syntex	18393-0148	Antihypertensive
GG622	Cap, Yellow, Opaque, with Black & White Imprint	Terazosin 2 mg	Hytrin by Geneva	00781-2052	Antihypertensive
GG622	Cap, Yellow	Terazosin HCl 2 mg	by Heartland Healthcare	61392-0944	Antihypertensive
GG622	Cap, Yellow	Terazosin HCl 2 mg	by Allscripts	54569-4874	Antihypertensive
GG622 <> GG622	Cap, Yellow	Terazosin HCl 2 mg	Terazosin HCl by Stason	60763-2041	Antihypertensive
GG623	Cap, Pink, Opaque, with Black & White Imprint	Terazosin 5 mg	Hytrin by Geneva	00781-2053	Antihypertensive
GG623	Cap, Pink	Terazosin HCl 5 mg	by Heartland Healthcare	61392-0945	Antihypertensive
GG623	Cap, Pink	Terazosin HCl 5 mg	by Allscripts	54569-4875	Antihypertensive
GG623 <> GG623	Tab, Pink, Oblong	Terazosin HCl 5 mg	Terazosin HCl by St. Marys Med	60760-0789	Antihypertensive
GG624	Cap, Blue	Terazosin HCl 10 mg	by Allscripts	54569-4876	Antihypertensive
GG624	Cap, Auqa, Opaque, with Black & White Imprint	Terazosin 10 mg	Hytrin by Geneva	00781-2054	Antihypertensive
GG624	Cap, Blue	Terazosin HCl 10 mg	by Heartland Healthcare	61392-0946	Antihypertensive
GG624 <> GG624	Cap, Aqua	Terazosin HCl 10 mg	Terazosin HCl by Stason	60793-0883	Antihypertensive
GG63	Tab, White, Round, Film Coated	Desipramine HCl 10 mg	Norpramin by Geneva	00781-1971	Antidepressant
GG64	Tab, White, Round, Coated	Desipramine HCl 25 mg	Norpramin by Geneva		Antidepressant
GG64	Tab, White, Round, Film Coated	Desipramine HCl 25 mg	Norpramin by Geneva	00781-1972	Antidepressant
GG64	Tab, Sugar Coated	Desipramine HCl 25 mg	by Allscripts	54569-0404	Antidepressant
GG64	Tab, White, Round	Desipramine HCl 25 mg	by Southwood Pharms	58016-0853	Antidepressant
GG65	Tab, Coated, GG Over 65	Desipramine HCl 50 mg	by Quality Care	60346-0732	Antidepressant
GG65	Tab, White, Round, Film Coated	Desipramine HCl 50 mg	Norpramin by Geneva	00781-1973	Antidepressant
GG66	Tab	Diazepam 2 mg	by Geneva	00781-1482	Antianxiety; C IV
GG67	Tab	Diazepam 5 mg	by Geneva	00781-1483	Antianxiety; C IV
GG68	Tab	Diazepam 10 mg	by Geneva	00781-1484	Antianxiety; C IV
GG705	Tab, Pink & White, Round, Film Coated	Ranitidine 150 mg	by Murfreesboro Ph	51129-1417	Gastrointestinal
GG705	Tab, Pink, Round, Film Coated	Ranitidine 150 mg	by RX PAK	65084-0150	Gastrointestinal
GG705	Tab, White, Round, Film Coated	Ranitidine 150 mg	by RX PAK	65084-0159	Gastrointestinal
GG705	Tab, White, Round	Ranitidine 150 mg	by Direct Dispensing	57866-6930	Gastrointestinal
GG705	Tab, Pink, Round	Ranitidine 150 mg	by Va Cmop	65243-0060	Gastrointestinal
GG705	Tab, Film Coated	Ranitidine 150 mg	by Caremark	00339-5332	Gastrointestinal
GG705	Tab, Pink, Film Coated	Ranitidine 150 mg	by Haines	59564-0200	Gastrointestinal
GG705	Tab, Pink, Round, Film Coated	Ranitidine 150 mg	Zantac by Geneva	00781-1883	Gastrointestinal
GG705	Tab, Pink, Round, Film Coated	Ranitidine 150 mg	by Compumed	00403-2342	Gastrointestinal
GG705	Tab, Off White & Pink, Film Coated	Ranitidine 150 mg	by Vangard	00615-4513	Gastrointestinal
GG706	Tab, Orange, Round, Film Coated	Ranitidine 300 mg	Zantac by Geneva	00781-1884	Gastrointestinal
GG71	Tab, Peach, Round	Propranolol 10 mg	Inderal by Geneva		Antihypertensive
GG72	Tab, Blue, Round	Propranolol 20 mg	Inderal by Geneva		Antihypertensive
GG721	Tab, White, Round	Terazosin 1 mg	Hytrin by Geneva	00781-1551	Antihypertensive
GG722	Tab, Orange, Round	Terazosin 2 mg	Hytrin by Geneva	00781-1561	Antihypertensive
GG723	Tab, Tan, Round	Terazosin 5 mg	Hytrin by Geneva	00781-1571	Antihypertensive
GG724	Tab	Naproxen 250 mg	by Golden State	60429-0133	NSAID
GG724	Tab, Yellow, Round	Naproxen 250 mg	by Geneva	00781-1163	NSAID
GG724	Tab	Naproxen 250 mg	by Talbert Med	44514-0601	NSAID
GG725	Tab	Naproxen 375 mg	by Haines	59564-0137	NSAID
GG725	Tab	Naproxen 375 mg	by Quality Care	60346-0817	NSAID
GG725	Tab, Debossed	Naproxen 375 mg	by Golden State	60429-0134	NSAID
GG725	Tab, Orange, Oblong	Naproxen 375 mg	by Nutramax	38206-0101	NSAID
GG725	Tab, Orange, Cap-Shaped	Naproxen 375 mg	by Geneva	00781-1164	NSAID
GG726	Tab	Naproxen 500 mg	by Med Pro	53978-2083	NSAID
GG726	Tab, Yellow, Oblong	Naproxen 500 mg	by Opti Med	63369-0321	NSAID
GG726	Tab	Naproxen 500 mg	by Haines	59564-0138	NSAID
GG726	Tab	Naproxen 500 mg	by Quality Care	60346-0815	NSAID
GG726	Tab	Naproxen 500 mg	by Golden State	60429-0135	NSAID

ID FRONT <> BACK	DESCRIPTION FRONT <> BACK	INGREDIENT & STRENGTH	BRAND (OR EQUIV.) & FIRM	NDC#	CLASS; SCH.
GG726	Tab, Yellow, Cap-Shaped	Naproxen 500 mg	by Geneva	00781-1165	NSAID
GG73	Tab, Green, Round	Propranolol 40 mg	Inderal by Geneva		Antihypertensive
GG733	Tab, Green, Round	Salsalate 500 mg	Disalcid by Geneva		NSAID
GG734	Tab, Green, Oblong	Salsalate 750 mg	Disalcid by Geneva		NSAID
GG735	Tab, White, Oval	Flurbiprofen 50 mg	Ansaid by Greenstone		NSAID
GG736	Tab, Blue, Round, Film Coated	Flurbiprofen 100 mg	Ansaid by Geneva	00781-1129	NSAID
GG737	Tab, Yellow, Round, Enteric Coated	Diclofenac Sodium 25 mg	by DRX	55045-2696	NSAID
GG737	Tab, Yellow, Round, Film Coated	Diclofenac Sodium 25 mg	Voltaren by Geneva	00781-1785	NSAID
GG737 <> GG737	Tab	Diclofenac Sodium 25 mg	by Geneva	00781-1285	NSAID
GG738	Tab	Diclofenac Sodium 50 mg	by Direct Dispensing	57866-6923	NSAID
GG738	Tab, Delayed Release	Diclofenac Sodium 50 mg	by Quality Care	60346-0238	NSAID
GG738	Tab	Diclofenac Sodium 50 mg	by Vangard	00615-4506	NSAID
GG738	Tab	Diclofenac Sodium 50 mg	by Geneva	00781-1287	NSAID
GG738	Tab, Brown, Round, Film Coated	Diclofenac Sodium 50 mg	Voltaren by Geneva	00781-1787	NSAID
GG738	Tab	Diclofenac Sodium 50 mg	by Physicians Total Care	54868-3659	NSAID
GG738	Tab	Diclofenac Sodium 50 mg	by Allscripts	54569-4165	NSAID
GG738	Tab, Delayed Release	Diclofenac Sodium 50 mg	by DRX	55045-2275	NSAID
GG738	Tab, Coated	Diclofenac Sodium 50 mg	by Novartis	17088-1029	NSAID
GG739	Tab, Pink, Round, Film Coated	Diclofenac Sodium 75 mg	Voltaren by Geneva	00781-1789	NSAID
GG739	Tab	Diclofenac Sodium 75 mg	by Vangard	00615-4507	NSAID
GG739	Tab	Diclofenac Sodium 75 mg	by DRX	55045-2247	NSAID
GG739	Tab	Diclofenac Sodium 75 mg	by Allscripts	54569-4166	NSAID
GG739	Tab, Pink, Round, Enteric Coated	Diclofenac Sodium 75 mg	by Compumed	00403-2904	NSAID
GG739	Tab	Diclofenac Sodium 75 mg	by Direct Dispensing	57866-6924	NSAID
GG739	Tab, Pink, Round, Enteric Coated	Diclofenac Sodium 75 mg	by DRX	55045-2689	NSAID
GG739	Tab, Pink, Triangular	Diclofenac Sodium 75 mg	by Phy Total Care	54868-3837	NSAID
GG739	Tab, Pink, Round, Enteric Coated	Diclofenac Sodium DR 75 mg	by DRX	55045-2699	NSAID
GG739 <> GG739	Tab	Diclofenac Sodium 75 mg	by Geneva	00781-1289	NSAID
GG74	Tab, Salmon, Round	Propranolol 60 mg	Inderal by Geneva		Antihypertensive
GG75	Tab, Yellow, Round	Propranolol 80 mg	Inderal by Geneva		Antihypertensive
GG759	Tab, Brown, Round	Diclofenac Potassium 50 mg	Cataflam by DRX	55045-2675	NSAID
GG759	Tab, Light Brown, Round	Diclofenac Potassium 50 mg	Cataflam by Geneva		NSAID
GG759	Tab, Light Brown, Round, Sugar Coated	Diclofenac Potassium 50 mg	Cataflam IR by Geneva	00781-1297	NSAID
GG76	Tab, Green, Round	Levothyroxine 0.3 mg	Synthroid by Rosemont		Antithyroid
GG77	Tab, Blue, Round	Levothyroxine 0.15 mg	Synthroid by Rosemont		Antithyroid
GG771	Tab, White, Round, Scored	Glipizide 5 mg	by Kaiser	00179-1303	Antidiabetic
GG771	Tab	Glipizide 5 mg	by Vangard	00615-3595	Antidiabetic
GG771	Tab, White, Round, Scored	Glipizide 5 mg	Glucotrol by Geneva	00781-1452	Antidiabetic
GG771	Tab	Glipizide 5 mg	by Nat Pharmpak Serv	55154-5408	Antidiabetic
GG771	Tab	Glipizide 5 mg	by Med Pro	53978-2013	Antidiabetic
GG771	Tab	Glipizide 5 mg	by Quality Care	62682-5002	Antidiabetic
GG771	Tab	Glipizide 5 mg	by Golden State	60429-0082	Antidiabetic
GG771	Tab	Glipizide 5 mg	by Direct Dispensing	57866-6463	Antidiabetic
GG771	Tab, White, Round, Scored	Glipizide 5 mg	by Allscripts	54569-3841	Antidiabetic
GG772	Tab	Glipizide 10 mg	by Direct Dispensing	57866-6462	Antidiabetic
GG772	Tab	Glipizide 10 mg	by Golden State	60429-0083	Antidiabetic
GG772	Tab, White, Round, Scored	Glipizide 10 mg	by Allscripts	54569-3842	Antidiabetic
GG772	Tab, White, Round, Scored	Glipizide 10 mg	by Kaiser	00179-1305	Antidiabetic
GG772	Tab	Glipizide 10 mg	by Vangard	00615-3596	Antidiabetic
GG772	Tab, White, Round, Scored	Glipizide 10 mg	Glucotrol by Geneva	00781-1453	Antidiabetic
GG772	Tab	Glipizide 10 mg	by Med Pro	53978-2014	Antidiabetic
GG774	Tab, Film Coated	Etodolac 400 mg	by Geneva	00781-1234	NSAID

ID FRONT <> BACK	DESCRIPTION FRONT <> BACK	INGREDIENT & STRENGTH	BRAND (OR EQUIV.) & FIRM	NDC#	CLASS; SCH.
GG78	Tab	Methazolamide 25 mg	by Quality Care	60346-0602	Diuretic
GG78	Tab, White, Round	Methazolamide 25 mg	by Nat Pharmpak Serv	55154-7206	Diuretic
GG78	Tab, White, Round	Methazolamide 25 mg	Neptazane by Geneva	00781-1072	Diuretic
GG780	Tab, White, Round	Methylphenidate 20 mg	by Geneva		Stimulant; C II
GG780	Tab, White, Round, Scored	Methylphenidate HCl 20 mg	Ritalin SR by Geneva	00781-1754	Stimulant; C II
GG783	Tab, Yellow, Round, Scored	Methylphenidate HCl 5 mg	Ritalin by Geneva	00781-1748	Stimulant; C II
GG789	Tab, Pale Green, Round, Scored	Methylphenidate HCl 10 mg	Ritalin by Geneva	00781-1749	Stimulant; C II
GG79	Tab, White, Round	Prednisone 5 mg	Meticorten by Geneva		Steroid
GG790	Tab, Light Yellow, Round, Scored	Methylphenidate HCl 20 mg	Ritalin by Geneva	00781-1753	Stimulant; C II
GG8	Tab, White, Round	Nylidrin 6 mg	Arlidin by Geneva		Vasodilator
GG80	Tab, White, Round, Scored	Furosemide 80 mg	by Geneva	00781-1446	Diuretic
GG80	Tab, White, Round, Scored	Furosemide 80 mg	by Vangard Labs	00615-1571	Diuretic
GG80	Tab, White, Round, Scored	Furosemide 80 mg	by JB	51111-0478	Diuretic
GG801	Cap, Light Green, Dark Green Bands	Ketoprofen 75 mg	Ketoprofen by Quality Care	60346-0667	NSAID
GG801	Cap	Ketoprofen 75 mg	Ketoprofen by Geneva	00781-2411	NSAID
GG802	Cap, White	Ketoprofen 50 mg	Orudis by Geneva		NSAID
GG802	Cap	Ketoprofen 50 mg	Ketoprofen by Geneva	00781-2410	NSAID
GG807	Cap, Orange, Oblong	Phenylpropanolamine 45 mg, PE 5 mg, Guaifenesin 200 mg	Entex by Amide		Cold Remedy
GG81	Tab	Clonidine HCl 0.1 mg	by Quality Care	60346-0786	Antihypertensive
GG81	Tab	Clonidine HCl 0.1 mg	by Geneva	00781-1471	Antihypertensive
GG82	Tab	Clonidine HCl 0.2 mg	by Geneva	00781-1472	Antihypertensive
GG822	Cap, White, Orange & Yellow Bands	Clomipramine HCl 25 mg	Anafranil by Geneva	00781-2027	OCD
GG822	Cap, Orange	Clomipramine HCl 25 mg	by D M Graham	00756-0205	OCD
GG823	Cap, White	Clomipramine HCl 50 mg	by CTEX	62022-0070	OCD
GG823	Cap, White	Clomipramine HCl 50 mg	by Copley	38245-0472	OCD
GG823	Cap, White, Opaque, Blue & Yellow Bands	Clomipramine HCl 50 mg	Anafranil by Geneva	00781-2037	OCD
GG823	Cap, White, Blue & Yellow Bands	Clomipramine HCl 50 mg	by Copley	38245-0524	OCD
GG824	Cap, White, Dark Yellow & Yellow Bands	Clomipramine HCl 75 mg	Anafranil by Geneva	00781-2047	OCD
GG825	Cap, Caramel & Red Bands	Mexiletine HCl 150 mg	by Vangard	00615-1326	Antiarrhythmic
GG825	Cap, White, Caramel & Red Bands	Mexiletine HCl 150 mg	Mexitil by Geneva	00781-2130	Antiarrhythmic
GG826	Cap, White, Red Bands	Mexiletine HCl 200 mg	Mexitil by Geneva	00781-2131	Antiarrhythmic
GG827	Cap, White, Aqua and Red Bands	Mexiletine HCl 250 mg	Mexitil by Geneva	00781-2132	Antiarrhythmic
GG83	Tab	Clonidine HCl 0.3 mg	by Geneva	00781-1473	Antihypertensive
GG832	Cap, Gray & Black Bands, White Powder	Etodolac 200 mg	by Geneva	00781-2012	NSAID
GG84	Tab	Timolol Maleate 5 mg	by Geneva	00781-1126	Antihypertensive
GG85	Tab, GG 85	Spironolactone 25 mg	by Quality Care	60346-0810	Diuretic
GG85	Tab	Spironolactone 25 mg	by Golden State	60429-0229	Diuretic
GG85	Tab, White, Round, Film Coated	Spironolactone 25 mg	Aldactone by Geneva	00781-1599	Diuretic
GG89	Tab, White, Round, Scored	Amoxapine 25 mg	Asendin by Geneva	00781-1844	Antidepressant
GG90	Tab, Orange, Round, Scored	Amoxapine 50 mg	Asendin by Geneva	00781-1845	Antidepressant
GG904	Tab, Pink, Round, Film Coated	Diclofenac Sodium 100 mg	Voltaren by DRX	55045-2698	NSAID
GG904	Tab, Light Pink, Round, Sugar Coated	Diclofenac Sodium 100 mg	Voltaren SR by Geneva	00781-1381	NSAID
GG91	Tab, White, Round, Scored	Lorazepam 0.5 mg	Ativan by Geneva	00781-1403	Sedative/Hypnotic; C IV
GG92	Tab	Lorazepam 1 mg	by Med Pro	53978-5008	Sedative/Hypnotic; C IV
GG92	Tab, White, Round, Scored	Lorazepam 1 mg	by Nat Pharmpak Serv	55154-1501	Sedative/Hypnotic; C IV
GG92	Tab, White, Round, Scored	Lorazepam 1 mg	by Nat Pharmpak Serv	55154-0215	Sedative/Hypnotic; C IV
GG92	Tab	Lorazepam 1 mg	by Golden State	60429-0512	Sedative/Hypnotic; C IV
GG92	Tab	Lorazepam 1 mg	by Quality Care	60346-0047	Sedative/Hypnotic; C IV
GG92	Tab, White, Round, Scored	Lorazepam 1 mg	Ativan by Geneva	00781-1404	Sedative/Hypnotic; C IV
GG92	Tab, White, Round, Scored	Lorazepam 1 mg	by Heartland Healthcare	61392-0449	Sedative/Hypnotic; C IV
GG92	Tab, White, Round, Scored	Lorazepam 1 mg	by Direct Dispensing	57866-9653	Sedative/Hypnotic; C IV
GG92	Tab, White, Round, Scored	Lorazepam 1 mg	by Apotheca	12634-0681	Sedative/Hypnotic; C IV

ID FRONT <> BACK	DESCRIPTION FRONT <> BACK	INGREDIENT & STRENGTH	BRAND (OR EQUIV.) & FIRM	NDC#	CLASS; SCH.
GG929	Tab, Purple, Round, Film Coated	Bupropion HCl 75 mg	by Invamed	52189-0361	Antidepressant
GG93	Tab, White, Round, Scored	Lorazepam 2 mg	by Heartland Healthcare	61392-0452	Sedative/Hypnotic; C IV
GG93	Tab	Lorazepam 2 mg	by Med Pro	53978-0608	Sedative/Hypnotic; C IV
GG93	Tab, White, Round, Scored	Lorazepam 2 mg	by Nat Pharmpak Serv	55154-0709	Sedative/Hypnotic; C IV
GG93	Tab	Lorazepam 2 mg	by Golden State	60429-0513	Sedative/Hypnotic; C IV
GG93	Tab, White, Round, Scored	Lorazepam 2 mg	by Compumed	00403-0012	Sedative/Hypnotic; C IV
GG93	Tab, White, Round, Scored	Lorazepam 2 mg	Ativan by Geneva	00781-1405	Sedative/Hypnotic; C IV
GG93	Tab, White, Round, Scored	Lorazepam 2 mg	by Allscripts	54569-2173	Sedative/Hypnotic; C IV
GG930	Tab, Lavender, Round, Film Coated	Bupropion HCl 100 mg	Wellbutrin by Geneva	00781-1064	Antidepressant
GG930	Tab, Lavender, Round	Bupropion HCl 75 mg	by Geneva Pharms	00781-1053	Antidepressant
GG931	Tab, White, Round	Orphenadrine Citrate 100 mg	by Geneva Pharms	00781-1649	Muscle Relaxant
GG932	Tab, White, Round, Scored	Pemoline 18.75 mg	by Geneva Pharms	00781-1731	Stimulant; C IV
GG933	Tab, White, Round, Scored	Pemoline 37.5 mg	Cylert by Geneva	00781-1741	Stimulant; C IV
GG934	Tab, White, Round, Scored	Pemoline 75 mg	by Geneva Pharms	00781-1751	Stimulant; C IV
GG935	Tab, White, Cap-Shaped	Naproxen DR 375 mg	EC Naprosyn by Geneva	00781-1646	NSAID
GG936	Tab, White, Cap-Shaped, Film Coated	Naproxen 500 mg	By Allscripts	54569-4520	NSAID
GG936	Tab, White, Cap-Shaped	Naproxen DR 500 mg	EC naprosyn by Geneva	00781-1653	NSAID
GG94	Tab, White, Round, Scored	Albuterol Sulfate 2 mg	Proventil by Geneva	00781-1671	Antiasthmatic
GG95	Tab, White, Round	Spironolactone 25 mg, Hydrochlorothiazide 25 mg	Aldactazide by Geneva		Diuretic
GG97	Tab, Orange, Round, Film Coated	Fluphenazine HCl 1 mg	by Invamed	52189-0313	Antipsychotic
GG97	Tab, Rust, Round, Film Coated	Fluphenazine HCl 1 mg	Prolixin by Geneva	00781-1436	Antipsychotic
GGAVISCON	Tab, White, Round, G/Gaviscon	Alginic Acid 200 mg	Gaviscon by SmithKline SKB	Canadian	Gastrointestinal
GGC1	Tab, Light Green, Round	Terazosin 10 mg	Hytrin by Geneva	00781-1541	Antihypertensive
GGC3	Tab	Captopril 12.5 mg	by Golden State	60429-0029	Antihypertensive
GGC3	Tab, White, Round	Captopril 12.5 mg	Capoten by Geneva		Antihypertensive
GGG5	Cap, Orange, Red & Yellow	Acetaminophen 500 mg	Tylenol by Granutec		Antipyretic
GGL7	Tab	Atenolol 25 mg	by Haines	59564-0125	Antihypertensive
GGL7	Tab	Atenolol 25 mg	by Golden State	60429-0211	Antihypertensive
GGL7	Tab, White, Round	Atenolol 25 mg	By Heartland Healthcare	61392-0542	Antihypertensive
GGL7	Tab, White, Round	Atenolol 25 mg	by Direct Dispensing	57866-3332	Antihypertensive
GGL7	Tab, White, Round	Atenolol 25 mg	Tenormin by Geneva		Antihypertensive
GGL7	Tab	Atenolol 25 mg	by Zenith Goldline	00182-1001	Antihypertensive
GGL7	Tab	Atenolol 25 mg	by Vangard	00615-3544	Antihypertensive
GGL7	Tab, White, Round	Atenolol 25 mg	Tenormin by Geneva	00781-1078	Antihypertensive
GGL7	Tab, White, Round	Atenolol 25 mg	by Duramed	51285-0836	Antihypertensive
GGL7	Tab	Atenolol 25 mg	by Allscripts	54569-3885	Antihypertensive
GGM	Cap, Brown	Clofazimine 100 mg	Lamprene by Geigy		Antileprosy
GIL307	Tab, Scored	Phenylephrine HCl 10 mg	Gilchew by Gil Pharm	58552-0307	Decongestant
GIL307	Tab, Scored	Phenylephrine HCl 10 mg	Gilchew IR by Nadin	14836-0307	Decongestant
GILGIL <> 303303	Tab, White, Oval, Scored	Guaifenesin 600 mg; Dextromethorphan Hydrobromide 30 mg; Phenylephrine HCl 20 mg	Giltuss by Sovereign Pharms	58716-0646	Cold Remedy
GILGIL <> 303303	Tab, White, Oval	Guaifenesin 600 mg; Dextromethorphan Hydrobromide 30 mg; Phenylephrine HCl 20 mg	Giltuss by Gil Pharm	58552-0303	Cold Remedy
GL <> 500	Tab, Coated	Metformin HCl 500 mg	Glucophage by Allscripts	54569-4202	Antidiabetic
GL <> 53511	Tab, Gilbert Logo G with Overlayed L <> 535-11	Acetaminophen 325 mg, Butalbital 50 mg, Caffeine 40 mg	Esgic by Prestige Packaging	58056-0354	Analgesic
GL <> 53511	Tab, White, Oblong, Scored	Butalbital 50 mg; Acetaminophen 325 mg; Caffeine 40 mg	Esgic by Rx Pac	65084-0126	Analgesic
GL500 <> GL500	Tab, Coated	Metformin HCl 500 mg	Glucophage by Caremark	00339-6022	Antidiabetic
GL53511	Tab, White, Cap Shaped, Scored, GL 535-11	Acetaminophen 325 mg, Butalbital 50 mg, Caffeine 40 mg	Esgic by Gilbert	00535-0011	Analgesic
GL53511	Tab, White, Round, GL 535-11	Butalbital 50 mg, Acetaminophen 325 mg, Caffeine 40 mg	by Forest Pharma	0535-0011	Analgesic
GL53512	Cap, White, Opaque, GL 535-12	Acetaminophen 325 mg, Butalbital 50 mg, Caffeine 40 mg	Esgic by Gilbert	00535-0012	Analgesic
GL53512	Cap, White, Opaque, GL 535-12	Butalbital 50 mg, Acetaminophen 325 mg, Anhydrous Caffeine 40 mg	by Forest Pharma	0535-0012	Analgesic
GL850	Tab, White, Oblong	Metformin 850 mg	Glucophage by BMS		Antidiabetic

ID FRONT <> BACK	DESCRIPTION FRONT <> BACK	INGREDIENT & STRENGTH	BRAND (OR EQUIV.) & FIRM	NDC#	CLASS; SCH.
GLAXCO <> ZANTAC150	Tab, Film Coated	Ranitidine HCl	by Med Pro	53978-2075	Gastrointestinal
GLAXO <> 250	Tab, White, Oblong	Cefuroxime Axetil 250 mg	Ceftin by Glaxo Wellcome	00173-7004	Antibiotic
GLAXO <> 387	Tab, Film Coated	Cefuroxime Axetil	Ceftin by Amerisource	62584-0325	Antibiotic
GLAXO <> 387	Tab, Film Coated	Cefuroxime Axetil	Ceftin by Glaxo	00173-0387	Antibiotic
GLAXO <> 387	Tab, Film Coated	Cefuroxime Axetil	Ceftin by Nat Pharmpak Serv	55154-1109	Antibiotic
GLAXO <> 387	Tab, Film Coated	Cefuroxime Axetil	Ceftin by Glaxo	51952-1347	Antibiotic
GLAXO <> 387	Tab, Light Blue, Film Coated	Cefuroxime Axetil	by Med Pro	53978-2088	Antibiotic
GLAXO <> 387	Tab, Light Blue, Film Coated	Cefuroxime Axetil 250 mg	Ceftin by Quality Care	60346-0369	Antibiotic
GLAXO <> 387	Tab, Film Coated	Cefuroxime Axetil 250 mg	Ceftin by Glaxo	51947-8121	Antibiotic
GLAXO <> 394	Tab, Film Coated	Cefuroxime Axetil	Ceftin by Glaxo	00173-0394	Antibiotic
GLAXO <> 394	Tab, Film Coated	Cefuroxime Axetil	Ceftin by Nat Pharmpak Serv	55154-1111	Antibiotic
GLAXO <> 395	Tab, Film Coated	Cefuroxime Axetil	Ceftin by Glaxo	00173-0395	Antibiotic
GLAXO <> 4	Tab, White, Oval, Film Coated	Ondansetron HCl	Zofran by Glaxo Wellcome	00173-0446	Antiemetic
GLAXO <> 500	Tab, White, Oblong	Cefuroxime Axetil 500 mg	Ceftin by Glaxo Wellcome	00173-7005	Antibiotic
GLAXO <> 8	Tab, Yellow, Oval	Ondansetron HCl 8 mg	Zofran by Glaxo Wellcome	00173-0447	Antiemetic
GLAXO <> ZANTAC150	Tab, Film Coated	Ranitidine HCl 150 mg	Zantac by Allscripts	54569-0445	Gastrointestinal
GLAXO <> ZANTAC150	Tab, Film Coated	Ranitidine HCl 150 mg	Zantac by Pharmedix	53002-0552	Gastrointestinal
GLAXO <> ZANTAC150	Tab, Film Coated	Ranitidine HCl 150 mg	Zantac by Kaiser	00179-1079	Gastrointestinal
GLAXO <> ZANTAC150	Tab, Film Coated	Ranitidine HCl 150 mg	Zantac by Glaxo	00173-0344	Gastrointestinal
GLAXO <> ZANTAC150	Cap, Imprinted in Blue	Ranitidine HCl 150 mg	by Nat Pharmpak Serv	55154-1110	Gastrointestinal
GLAXO <> ZANTAC150	Tab, Film Coated	Ranitidine HCl 150 mg	Zantac by Quality Care	60346-0729	Gastrointestinal
GLAXO <> ZANTAC150	Tab, Film Coated	Ranitidine HCl 150 mg	Zantac by Amerisource	62584-0488	Gastrointestinal
GLAXO <> ZANTAC150	Tab, Film Coated	Ranitidine HCl 150 mg	Zantac by Prescription Dispensing	61807-0054	Gastrointestinal
GLAXO <> ZANTAC150	Tab, Film Coated	Ranitidine HCl 150 mg	Zantac by Nat Pharmpak Serv	55154-1107	Gastrointestinal
GLAXO <> ZANTAC300	Tab, Film Coated	Ranitidine HCl 300 mg	Zantac by Kaiser	00179-1211	Gastrointestinal
GLAXO <> ZANTAC300	Tab	Ranitidine HCl 336 mg	Zantac by Pharmedix	53002-1028	Gastrointestinal
GLAXO <> ZANTAC300	Tab	Ranitidine HCl 336 mg	Zantac by Allscripts	54569-0444	Gastrointestinal
GLAXO <> ZANTAC300	Tab, Embossed	Ranitidine HCl 336 mg	Zantac by Amerisource	62584-0393	Gastrointestinal
GLAXO <>387	Tab, Blue, Oblong	Cefuroxime Axetil 250 mg	Ceftin by Allscripts	54569-1792	Antibiotic
GLAXO268	Tab, Blue & Clear	Theophylline SR 260 mg	Theobid Duracap by Glaxo Wellcome		Antiasthmatic
GLAXO281	Tab, Yellow, Oval	Ethaverine HCl 100 mg	Ethatab by Glaxo Wellcome		Vasodilator
GLAXO295	Cap, Blue & Clear	Theophylline SR 130 mg	Theobid Jr Duracap by Glaxo Wellcome		Antiasthmatic
GLAXO309	Cap, Clear & Pink	Phenylpropanolamine 75 mg, Chlorpheniramine 8 mg	Histabid Duracaps by Glaxo Wellcome		Cold Remedy
GLAXO316	Cap, Black & Orange	Vitamin Combination	Vicon Forte by Glaxo Wellcome		Vitamin
GLAXO371	Tab, Peach, Oval	Labetalol HCl 100 mg, Hydrochlorothiazide 25 mg	Trandate HCT by Glaxo Wellcome		Antihypertensive
GLAXO372	Tab, White, Oval	Labetalol HCl 200 mg, Hydrochlorothiazide 25 mg	Trandate HCT by Glaxo Wellcome		Antihypertensive
GLAXO373	Tab, Peach, Oval	Labetalol HCl 300 mg, Hydrochlorothiazide 25 mg	Trandate HCT by Glaxo Wellcome		Antihypertensive
GLAXO387	Tab, Coated	Cefuroxime Axetil 250 mg	Ceftin by Pharmedix	53002-0275	Antibiotic
GLAXO394	Tab, Coated	Cefuroxime Axetil 500 mg	Ceftin by Pharmedix	53002-0267	Antibiotic
GLAXO4	Tab, White, Oval, Glaxo/4	Ondansetron HCl 4 mg	Zofran by Glaxo Wellcome		Antiemetic
GLAXO4	Tab, Yellow, Oval, Glaxo/4	Ondansetron HCl Dihydrate 4 mg	Zofran by Glaxo Wellcome	Canadian	Antiemetic
GLAXOGLAXO <> VENTOLIN2	Tab, Glaxo over Glaxo <> Ventolin over 2	Albuterol Sulfate	Ventolin by Glaxo	00173-0341	Antiasthmatic
GLAXOGLAXO <> VENTOLIN4	Tab, Glaxo over Glaxo <> Ventolin over 4	Albuterol Sulfate	Ventolin by Glaxo	00173-0342	Antiasthmatic
GLAXOWELLCOME <> ZANTAC150	Cap, Blue Ink	Ranitidine HCl 150 mg	Zantac Geldose by Glaxo	00173-0428	Gastrointestinal
GLAXOWELLCOME <> ZANTAC150	Cap, Blue Ink	Ranitidine HCl 150 mg	Zantac Geldose by Glaxo	00173-0481	Gastrointestinal
GLAXOWELLCOME <> ZANTAC300	Cap, Blue Ink	Ranitidine HCl 300 mg	Zantac Geldose by Glaxo	00173-0429	Gastrointestinal

ID FRONT <> BACK	DESCRIPTION FRONT <> BACK	INGREDIENT & STRENGTH	BRAND (OR EQUIV.) & FIRM	NDC#	CLASS; SCH.
GLAXOWELLCOME <> ZANTAC300	Tab	Ranitidine HCl 336 mg	Zantac by Glaxo	00173-0393	Gastrointestinal
GLAXOZANTAC150	Tab, White, Round, Glaxo/Zantac/150	Ranitidine HCl 150 mg	Zantac by Glaxo	Canadian	Gastrointestinal
GLAXOZANTAC300	Tab, White, Oblong, Glaxo/Zantac 300	Ranitidine HCl 300 mg	Zantac by Glaxo	Canadian	Gastrointestinal
GLUCOTROLXL10	Tab	Glipizide 10 mg	Glucotrol XL by Allscripts	54569-3938	Antidiabetic
GLUCOTROLXL5	Tab	Glipizide 5 mg	Glucotrol XL by Allscripts	54569-3937	Antidiabetic
GLY	Tab, White, Round, Gly/Logo	Glyburide 2.5 mg	Albert Glyburide by Albert Pharma	Canadian	Antidiabetic
GLYBUR <> 364364	Tab	Glyburide 5 mg	by Copley	38245-0364	Antidiabetic
GLYBUR <> 364364	Tab	Glyburide 5 mg	by PDRX	55289-0892	Antidiabetic
GLYBUR <> 364364	Tab, 364 364	Glyburide 5 mg	by Quality Care	60346-0938	Antidiabetic
GLYBUR <> 364364	Tab, Blue, Oblong, Scored	Glyburide 5 mg	by Blue Ridge	59273-0015	Antidiabetic
GLYBUR <> 364364	Tab	Glyburide 5 mg	by Merrell	00068-3202	Antidiabetic
GLYBUR <> 364364	Tab, Blue, Oblong, Scored	Glyburide 5 mg	by KV	10609-1416	Antidiabetic
GLYBUR <> 364364	Tab	Glyburide 5 mg	by Allscripts	54569-3831	Antidiabetic
GLYBUR <> 433433	Tab	Glyburide 2.5 mg	by Coventry	61372-0577	Antidiabetic
GLYBUR <> 433433	Tab, Pink, Oblong, Scored	Glyburide 2.5 mg	by Blue Ridge	59273-0014	Antidiabetic
GLYBUR <> 433433	Tab	Glyburide 2.5 mg	by Merrell	00068-3201	Antidiabetic
GLYBUR <> 433433	Tab, Pink, Oblong, Scored	Glyburide 2.5 mg	by KV	10609-1415	Antidiabetic
GLYBUR <> 433433	Tab	Glyburide 2.5 mg	by Allscripts	54569-3830	Antidiabetic
GLYBUR <> 433433	Tab	Glyburide 2.5 mg	by Copley	38245-0433	Antidiabetic
GLYBUR <> 433433	Tab, Pink, Oblong, Scored	Glyburide 5 mg	by Blue Ridge	59273-0015	Antidiabetic
GLYBUR <> 433433	Tab, Pink, Oblong, Scored	Glyburide 5 mg	by KV	10609-1420	Antidiabetic
GLYBUR <> 477477	Tab, White, Oblong, Scored	Glyburide 5 mg	by KV	10609-1421	Antidiabetic
GLYBUR <> 477477	Tab	Glyburide 1.25 mg	by Coventry	61372-0576	Antidiabetic
GLYBUR <> 477477	Tab, White, Oblong, Scored	Glyburide 1.25 mg	by Blue Ridge	59273-0013	Antidiabetic
GLYBUR <> 477477	Tab, Glybur <> 477/477	Glyburide 1.25 mg	by Merrell	00068-3200	Antidiabetic
GLYBUR <> 477477	Tab, White, Oblong, Scored	Glyburide 1.25 mg	by KV	10609-1407	Antidiabetic
GLYBUR <> 477477	Tab, Glybur <> 477/477	Glyburide 1.25 mg	by Copley	38245-0477	Antidiabetic
GLYBUR <> 477477	Tab, White, Oblong, Scored	Glyburide 5 mg	by Blue Ridge	59273-0015	Antidiabetic
GLYBUR364	Tab, Blue, Oblong	Glyburide 5 mg	Diabeta by Copley		Antidiabetic
GLYBUR433	Tab, Pink, Oblong	Glyburide 2.5 mg	Diabeta by Copley		Antidiabetic
GLYBUR477	Tab, White, Oblong	Glyburide 1.25 mg	Diabeta by Copley		Antidiabetic
GLYGLY <> ALBERT	Tab, White, Round, Scored, Gly over Gly <> Albert Logo	Glyburide 2.5 mg	by Altimed	Canadian DIN# 01900927	Antidiabetic
GLYNASE1PT	Tab, Blue, Scored	Glyburide 3 mg	Glynase by Med-Pro	53978-3383	Antidiabetic
GLYNASE3 <> PT	Tab, Coated	Glyburide 3 mg	Glynase Prestab by Thrift Drug	59198-0171	Antidiabetic
GLYNASE3 <> PTPT	Tab, Coated, PT Score PT	Glyburide 3 mg	Glynase Prestab by Amerisource	62584-0352	Antidiabetic
GLYNASE3 <> PTPT	Tab, Coated, Glynase/3 <> PT/PT	Glyburide 3 mg	Glynase Prestab by Nat Pharmpak Serv	55154-3909	Antidiabetic
GLYNASE3 <> PTPT	Tab, Coated	Glyburide 3 mg	Glynase Prestab by Pharmacia & Upjohn	00009-0352	Antidiabetic
GLYNASE3 <> PTPT	Tab, Coated, Scored	Glyburide 3 mg	Glynase by Physicians Total Care	54868-3017	Antidiabetic
GLYNASE3PT	Tab, Blue, Oblong, Scored, Glynase 3/PT	Glyburide 3 mg	Glynase Prestab by Kiel	59063-0111	Antidiabetic
GLYNASE3PT	Tab, Coated, Glynase 3/PT	Glyburide 3 mg	Glynase by Drug Distr	52985-0224	Antidiabetic
GLYNASE3PT <> PT	Tab, Coated, Glynase 3/PT <> PT	Glyburide 3 mg	Glynase by Allscripts	54569-3690	Antidiabetic
GLYNASE6	Tab, Yellow, Oval, Scored	Glyburide 6 mg	Glynase Prestab by Kaiser	62224-7447	Antidiabetic
GLYNASE6 <> PTPT	Tab, Coated, Glynase 6 <> PT/PT	Glyburide 6 mg	Glynase Prestabs by Thrift Drug	59198-0003	Antidiabetic
GLYNASE6 <> PTPT	Tab, Yellow, Oblong, Scored	Glyburide 6 mg	by Allscripts	54569-4695	Antidiabetic
GLYNASE6 <> PTPT	Tab, Coated	Glyburide 6 mg	Glynase Prestab by Pharmacia & Upjohn	00009-3449	Antidiabetic

ID FRONT <> BACK	DESCRIPTION FRONT <> BACK	INGREDIENT & STRENGTH	BRAND (OR EQUIV.) & FIRM	NDC#	CLASS; SCH.
GLYNASE6 <> PTPT	Tab, Coated	Glyburide 6 mg	Glynase Prestabs by Nat Pharmpak Serv	55154-3917	Antidiabetic
GLYNASE6 <> PTPT	Tab, Coated, Glynase over 6 <> PT PT	Glyburide 6 mg	Glynase Prestab by Physicians Total Care	54868-3711	Antidiabetic
GLYNASE6PT	Tab, Coated, Glynase 6/PT	Glyburide 6 mg	Glynase Prestab by Amerisource	62584-0449	Antidiabetic
GLYNASE6PT	Tab, Yellow, Oblong, Scored	Glyburide 6 mg	Glynase Prestab by Kaiser	00179-1332	Antidiabetic
GLYNASE6PT	Tab, Coated, Glynase 6/PT	Glyburide 6 mg	Glynase by Drug Distr	52985-0225	Antidiabetic
GLYNASE6PT	Tab, Coated, Glynase 6/PT	Glyburide 6 mg	Glynase Prestab by DRX	55045-2338	Antidiabetic
GLYNASE6PT	Tab, Coated	Glyburide 6 mg	Glynase Prestab by Repack Co	55306-3449	Antidiabetic
GLYNASE6PT	Tab, Yellow, Oblong, Scored	Glyburide 6 mg	Glynase Prestab by Compumed	00403-4629	Antidiabetic
GLYNASE6PT	Tab, Yellow, Oval, Scored, Glynase 6/PT	Glyburide 6 mg	Glynase Prestab by KV	10609-1325	Antidiabetic
GLYNASE6PT	Tab, Coated, Glynase 6/PT	Glyburide 6 mg	Glynase by Leiner	59606-0723	Antidiabetic
GLYNASE6PT <> PT	Tab, Yellow, Scored	Glyburide 6 mg	Glynase by Rightpac	65240-0723	Antidiabetic
GLYSET <> 100	Tab, White, Round, Film	Miglitol 100 mg	Glyset by Neuman Distr	64579-0243	Antidiabetic
GLYSET <> 25	Tab, White, Round, Film	Miglitol 25 mg	Glyset by Neuman Distr	64579-0240	Antidiabetic
GLYSET <> 25	Tab, White, Round, Film	Miglitol 25 mg	Glyset by Neuman Distr	64579-0224	Antidiabetic
GLYSET <> 25	Tab, White, Round, Film	Miglitol 25 mg	Glyset by Neuman Distr	64579-0249	Antidiabetic
GLYSET <> 50	Tab, White, Round, Film	Miglitol 50 mg	Glyset by Neuman Distr	64579-0226	Antidiabetic
GLYSET <> 50	Tab, White, Round, Film	Miglitol 50 mg	Glyset by Neuman Distr	64579-0242	Antidiabetic
GOG <> CG	Cap	Valsartan 160 mg	Diovan by Novartis	17088-4001	Antihypertensive
GP10	Tab, White, Round, G/P 10	Pindolol 10 mg	Visken by Par		Antihypertensive
GP10 <> G	Tab	Glipizide 10 mg	by Par	49884-0452	Antidiabetic
GP10G	Tab, White, Oval	Glipizide 10 mg	Glucotrol by Par		Antidiabetic
GP147	Tab, Yellow, Oval	Bisoprolol Fumarate 2.5 mg, Hydrochlorothiazide 6.25 mg	Ziac by Geneva	00781-1841	Antihypertensive; Diuretic
GP148	Tab, Tan, Oval	Bisoprolol Fumarate 5 mg, Hydrochlorothiazide 6.25 mg	Ziac by Geneva	00781-1824	Antihypertensive; Diuretic
GP149	Tab, White, Oval	Bisoprolol Fumarate 10 mg, Hydrochlorothiazide 6.25 mg	Ziac by Geneva	00781-1833	Antihypertensive; Diuretic
GP151	Tab, White, Round	Doxazosin Mesylate 1 mg	Cardura by Geneva	00781-5001	Antihypertensive
GP152	Tab, Yellow, Round	Doxazosin Mesylate 2 mg	Cardura by Geneva	00781-5002	Antihypertensive
GP153	Tab, Beige, Round	Doxazosin Mesylate 4 mg	Cardura by Geneva	00781-5003	Antihypertensive
GP154	Tab, Light Green, Round	Doxazosin Mesylate 8 mg	Cardura by Geneva	00781-5004	Antihypertensive
GP300	Cap, Maroon	Vitamin, Iron	Ferrogen by Tishcon		Vitamin
GP5	Tab, White, Round G/P 5	Pindolol 5 mg	Gen Pindolol by Genpharm	Canadian	Antihypertensive
GP5	Tab, White, Round, G/P 5	Pindolol 5 mg	Visken by Par		Antihypertensive
GP5 <> G	Tab,	Glipizide 5 mg	by Par	49884-0451	Antidiabetic
GP5G	Tab, White, Oval	Glipizide 5 mg	Glucotrol by Par		Antidiabetic
GPCM200	Tab, Green, Round, G/p CM 200	Cimetidine 200 mg	by Genpharm	Canadian	Gastrointestinal
GPCM300	Tab, Green, Round, G/p CM 300	Cimetidine 300 mg	by Genpharm	Canadian	Gastrointestinal
GPCM400	Tab, Green, Ellipsoid, G/p CM 400	Cimetidine 400 mg	by Genpharm	Canadian	Gastrointestinal
GPCM600	Tab, Green, Ellipsoid, G/p CM 600	Cimetidine 600 mg	by Genpharm	Canadian	Gastrointestinal
GPCM800	Tab, Green, Ellipsoid, G/p CM 800	Cimetidine 800 mg	by Genpharm	Canadian	Gastrointestinal
GPI <> S1	Tab, White with Green Specks	Acetaminophen 325 mg, Phenylephrine HCl 5 mg, Chlorpheniramine Maleate 2 mg	Super Cold Tabs by Reese	10956-0771	Cold Remedy
GRISACTIN <> 330	Tab	Griseofulvin, Ultramicrosize 330 mg	Grisactin Ultra by Pharm Utilization	60491-0290	Antifungal
GRISACTIN250	Cap	Griseofulvin, Microcrystalline 250 mg	Grisactin by Pharmedix	53002-0277	Antifungal
GRISACTINULTRA	Tab	Griseofulvin, Ultramicrosize 250 mg	Grisactin Ultra by Allscripts	54569-1472	Antifungal
GRISPEG <> 125	Tab, Film Coated	Griseofulvin, Ultramicrosize 125 mg	Gris Peg by Novartis	00043-0800	Antifungal
GRISPEG <> 250	Tab, Film Coated, Gris-Peg <> 250	Griseofulvin 250 mg	Gris Peg by Quality Care	60346-0953	Antifungal
GRISPEG <> 250	Tab, Film Coated, Gris-Peg <> 250	Griseofulvin 250 mg	Gris Peg by Leiner	59606-0654	Antifungal
GRISPEG <> 250	Tab, Film Coated	Griseofulvin 250 mg	Gris Peg by Amerisource	62584-0773	Antifungal
GRISPEG <> 250	Tab, Film Coated	Griseofulvin 250 mg	Gris Peg by Novartis	00043-0801	Antifungal

ID FRONT <> BACK	DESCRIPTION FRONT <> BACK	INGREDIENT & STRENGTH	BRAND (OR EQUIV.) & FIRM	NDC#	CLASS; SCH.
GRISPEG <> 250	Tab, Film Coated	Griseofulvin 250 mg	Gris-Peg by Allergan	00023-0773	Antifungal
GS	Tab	Metronidazole 500 mg	by Patient	57575-0089	Antibiotic
GS <> S160	Tab, White, Oblong	Sotalol HCl 160 mg	by Genpharm	55567-0058	Antiarrhythmic
GS160	Tab, Blue, Oblong, G/S/160	Sotalol HCl 160 mg	by Genpharm	Canadian	Antiarrhythmic
GS240	Tab, Blue, Oblong, G/S/240	Sotalol HCl 240 mg	by Genpharm	Canadian	Antiarrhythmic
GS80	Tab, Blue, Oblong, G/S/80	Sotalol HCl 80 mg	by Genpharm	Canadian	Antiarrhythmic
GTN10	Tab, White, Round, G TN/10	Tamoxifen Citrate 10 mg	Nolvadex by Genpharm		Antiestrogen
GTN20	Tab, White, Octagonal, G TN/20	Tamoxifen Citrate 20 mg	by Genpharm		Antiestrogen
GU1 <> G	Tab, White, Oval	Guanfacine HCl 1 mg	by Par Pharm	49884-0572	Antihypertensive
GU1 <> G	Tab, White, Oval	Guanfacine HCl 1 mg	by Genpharm	55567-0051	Antihypertensive
GU2 <> G	Tab, White, Oval	Guanfacine HCl 2 mg	by Par Pharm	49884-0573	Antihypertensive
GU2 <> G	Tab, White, Oval	Guanfacine HCl 2 mg	by Genpharm	55567-0052	Antihypertensive
GUAIFED <> MURO120250	Cap, Ex Release, Muro 120-250	Guaifenesin 250 mg, Pseudoephedrine HCl 120 mg	Guaifed by Thrift Drug	59198-0192	Cold Remedy
GUAIFED <> MURO120250	Cap, Guaifed <> Muro 120-250	Guaifenesin 250 mg, Pseudoephedrine HCl 120 mg	Guaifed by Muro	00451-4002	Cold Remedy
GUAIFED <> MURO120250	Cap, Clear & Opaque & White, Guaifed <> Muro 120-250	Guaifenesin 250 mg, Pseudoephedrine HCl 120 mg	by Martec	52555-0159	Cold Remedy
GUAIFED <> MURO120250	Cap, Guaifed <> Muro 120-250	Guaifenesin 250 mg, Pseudoephedrine HCl 120 mg	Guaifed by Nat Pharmpak Serv	55154-4302	Cold Remedy
GUAIFEDMURO1202	Cap, Clear & White	Guaifenesin 250 mg; Pseudoephedrine HCl 120 mg	Guaifed by Rx Pac	65084-0213	Cold Remedy
GUAIFEDPD <> MURO60300	Cap, Ex Release, Guaifed PD <> Muro 60-300	Guaifenesin 300 mg, Pseudoephedrine HCl 60 mg	Guaifed PD by Thrift Drug	59198-0191	Cold Remedy
GUAIFEDPD <> MURO60300	Cap, Guaifed PD <> Muro 60-300	Guaifenesin 300 mg, Pseudoephedrine HCl 60 mg	Guaifed PD by Muro	00451-4003	Cold Remedy
GUAIFEDPD <> MURO60300	Cap, Blue & Clear & Opaque, Guaifed-PD <> Muro 60-300	Guaifenesin 300 mg, Pseudoephedrine HCl 60 mg	GFN PSEH PD 04 by Martec		Cold Remedy
GUAIFEDPD <> MURO60300	Cap	Guaifenesin 300 mg, Pseudoephedrine HCl 60 mg	by Pharmedix	53002-0623	Cold Remedy
GUAIFEDPD <> MURO60300	Cap, Blue & Clear, Oblong	Guaifenesin 300 mg, Pseudoephedrine HCl 60 mg	Guaifed PD by Martec		Cold Remedy
GUAIFEDPD <> MURO60300	Cap, Guaifed PD <> Muro 60-300	Guaifenesin 300 mg, Pseudoephedrine HCl 60 mg	Guaifed PD by Nat Pharmpak Serv	55154-4303	Cold Remedy
GUAIMAXD <> SP2055	Tab, White to Off-White, Scored	Guaifenesin 600 mg, Pseudoephedrine HCl 120 mg	Guaimax-D by Schwarz Pharma	00131-2055	Cold Remedy
GUAIMAXD <> SP2055	Tab, White, Round, Guaimax-D <> SP 2055	Pseudoephedrine HCl 120 mg, Guaifenesin 600 mg	Guaimax-D by Schwarz		Cold Remedy
GW <> GEIGY	Tab, White to Off-White, Cap Shaped, Scored	Baclofen 20 mg	Lioresal by Geigy	Canadian DIN# 00636576	Muscle Relaxant
GX623	Tab, Yellow, Oblong, Convex, Film Coated	Abacavir Sulfate 300 mg	Ziagen by Abbott	60692-3870	Antiviral
GX623	Tab, Yellow, Oblong, Convex, Film Coated	Abacavir Sulfate 300 mg	Ziagen by Abbott	60692-3869	Antiviral
GXCC1	Cap, White, Opaque	Amprenavir 50 mg	Agenerase by Block	10158-0428	Antiviral
GXCC2	Cap, Opaque & White	Amprenavir 150 mg	Agenerase by Biovail	62660-0025	Antiviral
GXCE3	Tab, Film Coated	Naratriptan HCl 1 mg	Amerge by Glaxo	00173-0561	Antimigraine
GXCE3	Tab, D Shaped, Film Coated	Naratriptan HCl 1 mg	Amerge by Glaxo	51947-8291	Antimigraine
GXCE5	Tab, Film Coated	Naratriptan HCl 2.5 mg	Amerge by Glaxo	00173-0562	Antimigraine
GXCE5	Tab, Film Coated	Naratriptan HCl 2.5 mg	Amerge by Glaxo	51947-8290	Antimigraine
GXCF7 <> 24	Tab, Pink, Oval	Ondansetron HCl 24 mg	Zofran by Glaxo Wellcome	00173-0680	Antiemetic
GXCG5	Tab, Tan, Oblong, Film Coated	Lamivudine 100 mg	Epivir by Glaxo	53873-0662	Antiviral
GXCG5	Tab, Yellow, Oblong, Convex, Film	Lamivudine 100 mg	Epivir HBV by Murfreesboro	51129-1623	Antiviral
GXCG5	Tab, Yellow, Oblong, Convex, Film	Lamivudine 100 mg	Epivir HBV by Murfreesboro	51129-1621	Antiviral
GXCG7	Tab, Pink, Round	Atovaquone 62.5 mg; Proguanil HCl 25 mg	Malarone by Glaxo Wellcome	00173-0676	Antiprotazoal
GXCG7	Tab, Pink, Round	Atovaquone 62.5 mg; Proguanil HCl 25 mg	Malarone by Glaxo	53873-0676	Antiprotazoal

ID FRONT <> BACK	DESCRIPTION FRONT <> BACK	INGREDIENT & STRENGTH	BRAND (OR EQUIV.) & FIRM	NDC#	CLASS; SCH.
GXCJ7	Tab, White, Diamond	Lamivudine 150 mg	by Glaxo	Canadian	Antiviral
GXCJ7 <> 150	Tab, Film Coated	Lamivudine 150 mg	Epivir by Glaxo	00173-0470	Antiviral
GXCJ7 <> 150	Tab, Film Coated	Lamivudine 150 mg	Epivir by Allscripts	54569-4221	Antiviral
GXCJ7 <> 150	Tab, White, Diamond, Film Coated	Lamivudine 150 mg	Epivir by Murfreesboro	51129-1624	Antiviral
GXCJ7 <> 150	Tab, Film Coated	Lamivudine 150 mg	Epivir by Physicians Total Care	54868-3693	Antiviral
GXCJ7 <> 150	Tab, Film Coated	Lamivudine 150 mg	Epivir by Quality Care	62682-1016	Antiviral
GXCJ7 <> 150	Tab, Film Coated	Lamivudine 150 mg	Epivir by St Marys Med	60760-0470	Antiviral
GXCJ7 <> 150	Tab, White, Diamond, Film Coated	Lamivudine 150 mg	Epivir by Compumed	00403-4977	Antiviral
GXCK3	Tab, White & Yellow, Round	Grepafloxacin HCl 200 mg	by Glaxo	Canadian	Antibiotic
GXCK3	Tab, Film Coated	Grepafloxacin HCl 200 mg	Raxar by Glaxo	00173-0566	Antibiotic
GXCK3	Tab, Film Coated	Grepafloxacin HCl 200 mg	Raxar by Otsuka	46602-0003	Antibiotic
GXCK5	Tab, Pale Yellow to White, Film Coated	Grepafloxacin HCl	Raxar by Glaxo	00173-0657	Antibiotic
GXCK5	Tab, Pale Yellow to White, Film Coated	Grepafloxacin HCl	Itmd Raxar Aqfc by Glaxo	51947-8295	Antibiotic
GXCK7	Tab, Pale Yellow to White, Film Coated	Grepafloxacin HCl	Raxar by Glaxo	00173-0658	Antibiotic
GXCK7	Tab, Film Coated	Grepafloxacin HCl	Itmd Raxar Aqfc by Glaxo	51947-8296	Antibiotic
GXCL2	Tab, White, Elliptical-Shaped, Chewable	Lamotrigine 5 mg	Lamictal by Glaxo Wellcome	00173-0527	Anticonvulsant
GXCL5	Tab, White, Cap-Shaped, Chewable	Lamotrigine 25 mg	Lamictal by Glaxo Wellcome	00173-0526	Anticonvulsant
GXCM3	Tab, Pink, Round	Atovaquone 250 mg; Proguanil HCl 100 mg	Malarone by Glaxo Wellcome	00173-0675	Antiprotazoal
GXCM3	Tab, Pink, Round	Atovaquone 250 mg; Proguanil HCl 100 mg	Malarone by Glaxo	53873-0675	Antiprotazoal
GXCT1	Tab, Blue, Oval, Film Coated	Alosetron 1 mg	Lotronex by Glaxo Wellcome	00173-0690	Gastrointestinal
GXCW3 <> 300	Tab, Film Coated	Zidovudine 300 mg	Retrovir by Catalytica	63552-0501	Antiviral
GXCW3 <> 300	Tab, White, Round, Film Coated	Zidovudine 300 mg	Retrovir by Glaxo	00173-0501	Antiviral
GXCW3 <> 300	Tab, Film Coated	Zidovudine 300 mg	Retrovir by DRX	55045-2488	Antiviral
GXFC3	Tab, Film Coated	Lamivudine 150 mg, Zidovudine 300 mg	Combivir by Glaxo	00173-0595	Antiviral
H	Tab, Coated	Ascorbic Acid 100 mg, Biotin, D- 300 mcg, Cyanocobalamin 6 mcg, Folic Acid 1000 mcg, Niacinamide 20 mg, Pantothenic Acid 10 mg, Pyridoxine HCl 10 mg, Riboflavin 1.7 mg, Thiamine Mononitrate 1.5 mg	Dailyvite Multi Vit by Hillestad	10542-0010	Vitamin
H <> HALDOL10MCNEIL	Tab, Aqua, H <> Haldol 10 McNeil	Haloperidol 10 mg	Haldol by McNeil	00045-0246	Antipsychotic
H <> HALDOL12MCNEIL	Tab, White, H <> Haldol 1/2 McNeil	Haloperidol 0.5 mg	Haldol by McNeil	00045-0240	Antipsychotic
H <> HALDOL1MCNEIL	Tab, Yellow, H <> Haldol 1 McNeil	Haloperidol 1 mg	Haldol by McNeil	00045-0241	Antipsychotic
H <> HALDOL20MCNEIL	Tab, Salmon, H <> Haldol 20 McNeil	Haloperidol 20 mg	Haldol by McNeil	00045-0248	Antipsychotic
H <> HALDOL2MCNEIL	Tab, Pink, H <> Haldol 2 McNeil	Haloperidol 2 mg	Haldol by McNeil	00045-0242	Antipsychotic
H <> HALDOL5MCNEIL	Tab, Green, H <> Haldol 5 McNeil	Haloperidol 5 mg	Haldol by McNeil	00045-0245	Antipsychotic
H04	Tab, White, Round	Meperidine HCl 50 mg	Pethadol by Halsey		Analgesic; C II
H05	Tab, White, Round	Meperidine HCl 100 mg	Pethadol by Halsey		Analgesic; C II
H09	Cap, Brown & Orange	Erythromycin Estolate 250 mg	Ilosone by Lilly		Antibiotic
H1	Tab, White, Round	Captopril 12.5 mg	Capoten by Hallmark		Antihypertensive
H1	Tab, White, Round	Captopril 12.5 mg	Capoten by Duramed	51285-0950	Antihypertensive
H1	Tab, White, Cap-Shaped	Naproxen 275 mg	Anaprox by Mova	55370-0918	NSAID
H1	Tab, Film Coated	Naproxen Sodium 275 mg	by AL Hikma	59115-0002	NSAID
H1	Tab, White, Oblong, Film Coated	Naproxen Sodium 275 mg	by WestWard Pharm	00143-9916	NSAID
H10	Cap, Blue & Pink	Vitamin Combination	En-cebrin F by Lilly		Vitamin
H11	Tab, White, Round	Captopril 25 mg	Capoten by Hallmark		Antihypertensive
H11	Tab, White, Round	Captopril 25 mg	Capoten by Duramed	51285-0951	Antihypertensive
H11 <> LL	Tab, Film Coated	Hydralazine HCl 25 mg	by Amerisource	62584-0733	Antihypertensive
H11 <> LL	Tab, Film Coated	Hydralazine HCl 25 mg	by Caremark	00339-5145	Antihypertensive
H11 <> LL	Tab, Film Coated	Hydralazine HCl 25 mg	by Med Pro	53978-3051	Antihypertensive
H11 <> LL	Tab, Film Coated	Hydralazine HCl 25 mg	by UDL	51079-0075	Antihypertensive
H11 <> LL	Tab, Film Coated	Hydralazine HCl 25 mg	by PDRX	55289-0133	Antihypertensive

ID FRONT <> BACK	DESCRIPTION FRONT <> BACK	INGREDIENT & STRENGTH	BRAND (OR EQUIV.) & FIRM	NDC#	CLASS; SCH.
H111	Tab, White, Round	Captopril 50 mg	Capoten by Duramed	51285-0952	Antihypertensive
H111	Tab, Light Blue, H Over 111	Hyoscyamine 0.15 mg	Hyospaz by Econolab	55053-0111	Gastrointestinal
H112	Tab, White, Round	Captopril 100 mg	Capoten by Hallmark		Antihypertensive
H114	Tab, White, Round	Glipizide 5 mg	by Duramed	51285-0598	Antidiabetic
H115	Tab, White, Round	Glipizide 10 mg	by Duramed	51285-0599	Antidiabetic
H12	Tab, White, Round	Captopril 100 mg	Capoten by Duramed	51285-0953	Antihypertensive
H12 <> LL	Tab, Coated	Hydralazine HCl 50 mg	by UDL	51079-0076	Antihypertensive
H124	Tab, Peach, Round	Hydrochlorothiazide 50 mg	Hydrodiuril by Heather		Diuretic
H12PF	Cap, Orange, H12/PF	Hydromorphone HCl 12 mg	by Purdue Frederick	Canadian	Analgesic
H14 <> LL	Tab, Peach, Round, Scored	Hydrochlorothiazide 25 mg	by Natl Pharmpak	55154-5574	Diuretic
H14 <> LL	Tab, H Over 14	Hydrochlorothiazide 25 mg	by Lederle	00005-3752	Diuretic
H14 <> LL	Tab, Peach, Round, Scored, H Over 14 <> LL	Hydrochlorothiazide 25 mg	HydroDiuril UDL	51079-0049	Diuretic
H14 <> LL	Tab, Peach, Round, Scored	Hydrochlorothiazide 25 mg	by Murfreesboro	51129-1201	Diuretic
H15	Loz, Orange	Benzocaine 15 mg	Bi-Zets by Reese	10956-0713	Topical Anesthetic
H15	Loz, Cherry	Benzocaine 15 mg, Dextromethorphan HBr 10 mg	Tetra-Formula by Reese	10956-0749	Topical Anesthetic
H15 <> LL	Tab, H Over 15	Hydrochlorothiazide 50 mg	by Lederle	00005-3753	Diuretic
H15 <> LL	Tab, Peach, Round, Scored, H Over 15 <> LL	Hydrochlorothiazide 50 mg	HydroDiuril by UDL	51079-0111	Diuretic
H15 <> LL	Tab	Hydrochlorothiazide 50 mg	by Amerisource	62584-0737	Diuretic
H17	Cap, White & Yellow	Nortriptyline HCl 10 mg	by Lilly	Canadian	Antidepressant
H17	Cap, White & Yellow	Nortriptyline HCl 10 mg	Aventyl HCl by Lilly		Antidepressant
H187	Tab, Salmon, Round	Prednisolone 5 mg	Sterane by Heather		Steroid
H19	Cap, White & Yellow	Nortriptyline HCl 25 mg	by Lilly	Canadian	Antidepressant
H19	Cap, White & Yellow	Nortriptyline HCl 25 mg	Aventyl HCl by Lilly		Antidepressant
H193	Tab, White, Round	Methocarbamol 500 mg	Robaxin by Heather		Muscle Relaxant
H196	Tab, Brown, Oblong	Methenamine Mandelate 500 mg	Mandelamine by Heather		Antibiotic; Urinary Tract
H2	Tab, Film Coated	Naproxen Sodium 550 mg	by AL Hikma	59115-0001	NSAID
H2	Tab, White, Cap-Shaped, Film Coated	Naproxen Sodium 550 mg	Anaprox DS by West Ward	00143-9908	NSAID
H202	Tab, White, Round	Sulfisoxazole 500 mg	Gantrisin by Heather		Antibiotic
H203	Cap, Black & Yellow	Tetracycline HCl 500 mg	Achromycin V by Heather		Antibiotic
H214	Cap, Blue & Yellow	Tetracycline HCl 250 mg	Achromycin V by Heather		Antibiotic
H214	Cap, Orange & Yellow	Tetracycline HCl 250 mg	Achromycin V by Heather		Antibiotic
H24PF	Cap, Gray, H24/PF	Hydromorphone HCl 24 mg	by Purdue Frederick	Canadian	Analgesic
H303 <> 3	Tab, White, Round, H/303 <> 3	Acetaminophen 300 mg, Codeine#3 30 mg	Tylenal w/Codeine by Duramed	51285-0303	Analgesic; C III
H30PF	Cap, Red, H30/PF	Hydromorphone HCl 30 mg	by Purdue Frederick	Canadian	Analgesic
H33	Tab, Chew	Nickel Sulfate 1 X, Potassium Bromate 1 X, Zinc Bromide 4 X	Psorizide Ultra by Loma Lux	61480-0124	Supplement
H373	Tab, Film Coated, H 373	Guaifenesin 400 mg, Phenylpropanolamine HCl 75 mg	Stamoist LA by Huckaby	58407-0374	Cold Remedy
H3PF	Cap, Green, H3/PF	Hydromorphone HCl 3 mg	Hydromor Contin by Purdue Frederick	Canadian	Analgesic
H403	Tab, Green, Round	Sulfamethoxazole 500 mg	Gantanol by Heather		Antibiotic
H501	Tab, White, Oblong	Methocarbamol 750 mg	Robaxin by Heather		Muscle Relaxant
H503	Tab, Purple, Oval	Methenamine Mandelate 1 gm	Mandelamine by Heather		Antibiotic; Urinary Tract
H510	Tab, White, Oval	Methylprednisolone 4 mg	Medrol by Heather		Steroid
H513	Tab, White, Round	Cortisone Acetate 25 mg	Cortone Acetate by Heather		Steroid
H527	Tab, White, Round	Prednisone 50 mg	Deltasone by Heather		Steroid
H539	Cap, Aqua	Doxycycline Hyclate 100 mg	Doxycin by Riva	Canadian	Antibiotic
H64	Cap, Pink	Propoxyphene Napsylate 100 mg	by Lilly	Canadian	Analgesic
H69	Cap, Green & White	Cephalexin 250 mg	Keflex by Lilly		Antibiotic
H6PF	Cap, Pink, H6/PF	Hydromorphone HCl 6 mg	by Purdue Frederick	Canadian	Analgesic
H71	Cap, Green	Cephalexin 500 mg	Keflex by Lilly		Antibiotic
H72	Cap, Black	Vitamin Combination	Theracebrin by Lilly		Vitamin
H74	Cap, Blue	Ethinamate 500 mg	Valmid by Lilly		Hypnotic
H76	Cap, White & Yellow	Fenoprofen Calcium 200 mg	Nalfon by Lilly		NSAID
H77	Cap, Yellow	Fenoprofen Calcium 300 mg	Nalfon by Lilly		NSAID

ID FRONT <> BACK	DESCRIPTION FRONT <> BACK	INGREDIENT & STRENGTH	BRAND (OR EQUIV.) & FIRM	NDC#	CLASS; SCH.
HALCION0125	Tab, Coated	Triazolam 0.125 mg	by Pharmedix	53002-0634	Sedative/Hypnotic; C IV
HALCION025	Tab	Triazolam 0.25 mg	by Pharmedix	53002-0380	Sedative/Hypnotic; C IV
HALCION025	Tab, Halcion 0.25	Triazolam 0.25 mg	Halcion by Quality Care	60346-0588	Sedative/Hypnotic; C IV
HALCON025	Tab	Triazolam 0.25 mg	Halcion by PDRX	55289-0128	Sedative/Hypnotic; C IV
HALDOL10MCNEIL <> H	Tab, Haldol 10 McNeil <> H	Haloperidol 10 mg	Haldol by McNeil	00045-0246	Antipsychotic
HALDOL12MCNEIL <> H	Tab, Haldol 1/2 McNeil <> H	Haloperidol 0.5 mg	Haldol by McNeil	00045-0240	Antipsychotic
HALDOL1MCNEIL <> H	Tab, Haldol 1 McNeil <> H	Haloperidol 1 mg	Haldol by McNeil	00045-0241	Antipsychotic
HALDOL20MCNEIL <> H	Tab, Salmon, Haldol 20 McNeil<> H	Haloperidol 20 mg	Haldol by McNeil	00045-0248	Antipsychotic
HALDOL2MCNEIL <> H	Tab, Haldol 2 McNeil <> H	Haloperidol 2 mg	Haldol by McNeil	00045-0242	Antipsychotic
HALDOL5MCNEIL <> H	Tab, Haldol 5 McNeil <> H	Haloperidol 5 mg	Haldol by McNeil	00045-0245	Antipsychotic
HALFAN	Tab, White, Oblong	Halofantrine 250 mg	by SmithKline SKB	Canadian	Antimalarial
HALFAN	Tab, Coated	Halofantrine HCl 250 mg	Halfan by King	60793-0880	Antimalarial
HAUCK053	Cap, Maroon & Pink, Hauck Logo 053	Phendimetrazine Tartrate 35 mg	Wehless by W.E.Hauck		Anorexiant; C III
HAUCK087	Tab, Orange	Hydrocodone Bitartrate 5 mg, Guaifenesin 300 mg	Entuss by W.E.Hauck		Analgesic; C III
HAUCK202BESTA	Cap, Orange	Vitamin Combination	Besta by W.E.Hauck		Vitamin
HAUCK258	Tab, White	Hydrocodone Bitartrate 5 mg, Guaifenesin 300 mg, Pseudoephedrine 30 mg	Entuss-D by W.E.Hauck		Analgesic; C III
HAW301	Tab, White, Oblong, Scored	Guaifenesin 600 mg, Pseudoephedrine HCl 90 mg .	GFN 600 PSEH 90 by Med Pro	53978-3354	Cold Remedy
HAW301	Tab, Oblong, Scored	Pseudoephedrine HCl 90 mg, Guaifenesin 600 mg	H 9600 SR by RX PAK	65084-0111	Cold Remedy
HB93614	Tab, Green, Round	Phenobarbital 16.2 mg, Belladonna Extract 10.8 mg	Belap by Lemmon		Gastrointestinal; C IV
HC	Tab, Gray, HC over Abbott Logo	Divalproex Sodium	Depakote ER by Abbott	00074-7126	Anticonvulsant
HC <> CG	Tab, Beige & Orange, Oval, Scored	Carbamazepine 200 mg	Tegretol CR by Novartis	Canadian DIN# 00773611	Anticonvulsant
HD <> 512	Tab	Acetaminophen 325 mg, Oxycodone HCl 5 mg	by Schein	00364-0605	Analgesic; C II
HD <> 567	Tab	Acetaminophen 325 mg, Butalbital 50 mg, Caffeine 40 mg	by Schein	00364-2297	Analgesic
HD <> 725	Cap	Doxycycline Hyclate	by Quality Care	60346-0449	Antibiotic
HD004	Tab, White, Round	Meperidine HCl 50 mg	Demerol by Halsey		Analgesic; C II
HD005	Tab, White, Round	Meperidine HCl 100 mg	Demerol by Halsey		Analgesic; C II
HD0656	Cap, Green	Chlordiazepoxide HCl 5 mg, Clidinium Bromide 2.5 mg	Clinoxide by Halsey		Gastrointestinal; C IV
HD157	Cap, Clear	Quinine Sulfate 325 mg	by Halsey		Antimalarial
HD4	Tab, White, Round	Meperidine HCl 50 mg	Pethadol by Halsey		Analgesic; C II
HD5	Tab, White, Round	Meperidine HCl 100 mg	Pethadol by Halsey		Analgesic; C II
HD512	Tab	Acetaminophen 325 mg, Oxycodone HCl 5 mg	by Qualitest	00603-4998	Analgesic; C II
HD532 <> HD532	Cap	Acetaminophen 500 mg, Oxycodone HCl 5 mg	by Superior	00144-0630	Analgesic; C II
HD532 <> HD532	Cap	Acetaminophen 500 mg, Oxycodone HCl 5 mg	by Rugby	00536-3219	Analgesic; C II
HD532 <> HD532	Cap	Acetaminophen 500 mg, Oxycodone HCl 5 mg	by Zenith Goldline	00182-9175	Analgesic; C II
HD532 <> HD532	Cap, Buff & Scarlet	Acetaminophen 500 mg, Oxycodone HCl 5 mg	by Qualitest	00603-4997	Analgesic; C II
HD532 <> HD532	Cap	Acetaminophen 500 mg, Oxycodone HCl 5 mg	by Parmed	00349-8659	Analgesic; C II
HD532 <> HD532	Cap	Acetaminophen 500 mg, Oxycodone HCl 5 mg	by Mallinckrodt Hobart	00406-0532	Analgesic; C II
HD532 <> HD532	Cap	Acetaminophen 500 mg, Oxycodone HCl 5 mg	by Halsey Drug	00879-0532	Analgesic; C II
HD567	Tab, Debossed	Acetaminophen 325 mg, Butalbital 50 mg, Caffeine 40 mg	by Quality Care	60346-0703	Analgesic
HD567	Tab	Acetaminophen 325 mg, Butalbital 50 mg, Caffeine 40 mg	by Kaiser	00179-1278	Analgesic
HD567	Tab	Acetaminophen 325 mg, Butalbital 50 mg, Caffeine 40 mg	by Warner Chilcott	00047-0106	Analgesic
HD567	Tab	Acetaminophen 325 mg, Butalbital 50 mg, Caffeine 40 mg	by United Res	00677-1242	Analgesic
HD567	Tab	Acetaminophen 325 mg, Butalbital 50 mg, Caffeine 40 mg	by Murfreesboro	51129-7401	Analgesic
HD567	Tab	Acetaminophen 325 mg, Butalbital 50 mg, Caffeine 40 mg	by DRX	55045-1582	Analgesic

ID FRONT <> BACK	DESCRIPTION FRONT <> BACK	INGREDIENT & STRENGTH	BRAND (OR EQUIV.) & FIRM	NDC#	CLASS; SCH.
HD567	Tab, White, Round	Acetaminophen 325 mg, Caffeine 40 mg, Butalbital 50 mg	by Adams	53014-0003	Analgesic
HD567	Tab, White, Round	Butalbital 50 mg, Acetaminophen 325 mg, Caffeine 40 mg	Fioricet by Watson	52544-0485	Analgesic
HD711	Tab, White	Propoxyphene 100 mg, Acetaminophen 650 mg	Darvocet N 100 by Halsey		Analgesic; C IV
HD7152	Tab, White, Round, HD 715/#2	Hydromorphone HCl 2 mg	Dilaudid by Halsey		Analgesic; C II
HD7174	Tab, White, Round, HD 717/#4	Hydromorphone HCl 4 mg	Dilaudid by Halsey		Analgesic; C II
HD724	Tab, Beige, Round	Doxycycline Hyclate 50 mg	Vibra-Tab by Halsey		Antibiotic
HD725	Tab, Yellow Interior, Film Coated	Doxycycline Hyclate	by Kaiser	00179-1170	Antibiotic
HD765	Tab	Acetaminophen 500 mg, Hydrocodone Bitartrate 5 mg	by Halsey Drug	00879-0765	Analgesic; C III
HD765	Tab, White, Oval, Scored	Acetaminophen 500 mg; Hydrocodone Bitartrate 5 mg	by UDL	51079-0933	Analgesic; C III
HD778	Tab	Acetaminophen 650 mg, Hydrocodone Bitartrate 10 mg	by Halsey Drug	00879-0778	Analgesic; C III
HD779	Tab	Acetaminophen 750 mg, Hydrocodone Bitartrate 7.5 mg	by Halsey Drug	00879-0779	Analgesic; C III
HD780	Tab	Acetaminophen 650 mg, Hydrocodone Bitartrate 7.5 mg	by Halsey Drug	00879-0780	Analgesic; C III
HEART <> 2771	Tab, Off-White, Oval, Biconvex	Irbesartan 75 mg	Avapro by BMS	00087-2771	Antihypertensive
HEART <> 2772	Tab, Off-White, Oval, Biconvex	Irbesartan 150 mg	Avapro by BMS	00087-2772	Antihypertensive
HEART <> 2773	Tab, Off-White, Oval, Biconvex	Irbesartan 300 mg	Avapro by BMS	00087-2773	Antihypertensive
HEART <> 2775	Tab, Peach, Oval, Biconvex	Irbesartan 150 mg, Hydrochlorothiazide 12.5 mg	Avalide by BMS	00087-2775	Antihypertensive
HEART <> 2776	Tab, Peach, Oval, Biconvex	Irbesartan 300 mg, Hydrochlorothiazide 12.5 mg	Avalide by BMS	00087-2776	Antihypertensive
HEEL	Tab	Ambra Grisea 6 X, Cocculus Indicus 4 X, Conium 3 X, Petroleum 8 X	Vertigoheel by Heel	50114-6155	Homeopathic
HEXALEN50MG <> USB001	Cap, Clear	Altretamine 50 mg	Hexalen by US Bioscience	58178-0001	Antineoplastic
HEXALEN50MG <> USB001	Cap	Altretamine 50 mg	Hexalen by AAI	27280-0001	Antineoplastic
HFC	Tab, Brown & Red, Circular, H/FC	Felodipine 10 mg	Renedil by Hoechst-Roussel	Canadian	Antihypertensive
HFC	Tab, Pink, Circular, H/FC	Felodipine 5 mg	Renedil by Hoechst-Roussel	Canadian	Antihypertensive
HFF	Tab, Yellow, Circular, H/FF	Felodipine 2.5 mg	Renedil by Hoechst-Roussel	Canadian	Antihypertensive
HG <> CIBA	Tab, Pink, Round, Coated	Hydralazine HCl 50 mg	Apresoline by Novartis	Canadian DIN# 00005541	Antihypertensive
HGH <> CG	Tab, Light Orange	Hydrochlorothiazide 12.5 mg, Valsartan 80 mg	Diovan HCT by Novartis	00078-0314	Diuretic; Antihypertensive
HGH <> CG	Tab	Hydrochlorothiazide 12.5 mg, Valsartan 80 mg	Diovan HCT by Novartis	17088-3932	Diuretic; Antihypertensive
HGH <> CG	Tab, Light Orange, Oval, Film Coated	Hydrochlorothiazide 12.5 mg, Valsartan 80 mg	Diovan HCT by Novartis	Canadian DIN# 02241900	Diuretic; Antihypertensive
HGH <> CG	Tab, Orange, Oblong	Valsartan 80 mg, Hydrochlorothiazide 12.5 mg	Diovan by Allscripts	54569-4766	Antihypertensive
HH	Cap, H H <> Abbott Logo	Terazosin HCl 1 mg	Hytrin by Allscripts	54569-4196	Antihypertensive
HH	Cap, Abbott Logo	Terazosin HCl 1 mg	Hytrin by Nat Pharmpak Serv	55154-0115	Antihypertensive
HH	Cap, Gray, HH <> Abbott Logo	Terazosin HCl 1 mg	Hytrin by Abbott	00074-3805	Antihypertensive
HH	Cap, Gray	Terazosin HCl 1 mg	Hytrin by Va Cmop	65243-0088	Antihypertensive
HH	Cap, Abbott Logo HH	Terazosin HCl	Hytrin by Quality Care	60346-0438	Antihypertensive
HH	Cap, Orange, Gelatin	Valproic Acid 250 mg	Depakene by Abbott	00074-5681	Anticonvulsant
HH	Cap, Orange, Gelatin	Valproic Acid 250 mg	Depakene by Abbott	00074-5681	Anticonvulsant
HHA <> HHA	Cap, Warm Gray, HH-A <> HH-A	Terazosin HCl 1 mg	Terazosin by RP Scherer	11014-1031	Antihypertensive
HHDP	Cap, Clear, Imprinted in Black	Phenyltoloxamine Citrate 8 mg, Pheniramine Maleate 8 mg, Pyrilamine Maleate 8 mg, Phenylpropanolamine HCl 25 mg	Highland Histine D PED by Prepackage Spec	58864-0359	Cold Remedy
HHH <> CG	Tab, Dark Red	Hydrochlorothiazide 12.5 mg, Valsartan 160 mg	Diovan HCT by Novartis	00078-0315	Diuretic; Antihypertensive
HHH <> CG	Tab	Hydrochlorothiazide 12.5 mg, Valsartan 160 mg	Diovan HCT by Novartis	17088-3933	Diuretic; Antihypertensive

ID FRONT <> BACK	DESCRIPTION FRONT <> BACK	INGREDIENT & STRENGTH	BRAND (OR EQUIV.) & FIRM	NDC#	CLASS; SCH.
HHH <> CG	Tab, Dark Red, Oval, Film Coated	Hydrochlorothiazide 12.5 mg, Valsartan 160 mg	Diovan HCT by Novartis	Canadian DIN# 02241901	Diuretic; Antihypertensive
HIGHLAND	Cap, Clear & Red, in Black	Phenyltoloxamine Citrate 16 mg, Pheniramine Maleate 16 mg, Pyrilamine Maleate 16 mg, Phenylpropanolamine HCl 50 mg	Highland Histine D by Prepackage Spec	58864-0149	Cold Remedy
HIVID0375 <> ROCHE	Tab, Film Coated, Hivid 0.375 <> Roche	Zalcitabine 0.375 mg	Hivid by Hoffmann La Roche	00004-0220	Antiviral
HIVID0375 <> ROCHE	Tab, Film Coated, Hivid 0.375 <> Roche	Zalcitabine 0.375 mg	Hivid by Pharm Utilization	60491-0296	Antiviral
HIVID0375 <> ROCHE	Tab, Beige, Oval, Film, Hivid 0.375 <> Roche	Zalcitabine 0.375 mg	Hivid by United Res	00677-1683	Antiviral
HIVID0375ROCHE	Tab, Beige, Oval, Hivid 0.375/Roche	Zalcitabine 0.375 mg	Hivid by Roche	Canadian	Antiviral
HIVID0750 <> ROCHE	Tab, Coated, Hivid 0.375 <> Roche	Zalcitabine 0.75 mg	Hivid by Allscripts	54569-3877	Antiviral
HIVID0750 <> ROCHE	Tab, Coated, Hivid 0.375 <> Roche	Zalcitabine 0.75 mg	Hivid by Pharm Utilization	60491-0297	Antiviral
HIVID0750ROCHE	Tab, Gray, Oval, Hivid 0.750/Roche	Zalcitabine 0.750 mg	Hivid by Roche	Canadian	Antiviral
HK	Cap, Abbott Logo HK	Terazosin HCl 5 mg	Hytrin by Allscripts	54569-4062	Antihypertensive
HK	Cap, Abbott Logo	Terazosin HCl 5 mg	Hytrin by PDRX	55289-0070	Antihypertensive
HK	Cap, Red, HK <> Abbott Logo	Terazosin HCl 5 mg	Hytrin by Abbott	00074-3807	Antihypertensive
HK	Cap, Red	Terazosin HCl 5 mg	Hytrin by Va Cmop	65243-0069	Antihypertensive
HK	Cap, HK <> Abbott Logo	Terazosin HCl	Hytrin by Quality Care	60346-0370	Antihypertensive
HKA <> HKA	Cap, HK-A	Terazosin HCl 5 mg	Terazosin by RP Scherer	11014-1033	Antihypertensive
HL	Tab, Green, Round	Herbal Laxative 486 mg	by PFI		Laxative
HLT41	Tab, Gray, Round	Trimeprazine Tartrate 2.5 mg	Temaril by Forest		Antipruritic
HLT50	Cap, Gray & Natural	Trimeprazine Tartrate 5 mg	Temaril Spansule by Forest		Antipruritic
HN	Cap, Blue, HN <> Abbott Logo	Terazosin HCl 10 mg	Hytrin by Abbott	00074-3808	Antihypertensive
HN	Cap, Abbott Logo HN	Terazosin HCl 10 mg	Hytrin by Allscripts	54569-4051	Antihypertensive
HN	Cap, Blue	Terazosin HCl 10 mg	Hytrin by Va Cmop	65243-0089	Antihypertensive
HN	Cap, HN <> Abbott Logo	Terazosin HCl	Hytrin by Quality Care	60346-0436	Antihypertensive
HNA <> NHA	Cap, HN-A	Terazosin HCl 10 mg	Terazosin by RP Scherer	11014-1034	Antihypertensive
HO <> CG	Tab, Dark Yellow, Cap Shaped, Film Coated	Benazepril HCl 10 mg	Lotensin by Novartis	Canadian DIN# 00885843	Antihypertensive
HOECHST <> DIAB	Tab, Pink, Oblong, Scored	Glyburide 2.5 mg	Diabeta by Natl Pharmpak	55154-1206	Antidiabetic
HOECHST	Tab	Glyburide 2.5 mg	Diabeta by Drug Distr	52985-0221	Antidiabetic
HOECHST <> ALTACE10MG	Cap, Blue, Hard Gel	Ramipril 10 mg	Altace by Monarch Pharms	61570-0120	Antihypertensive
HOECHST <> ALTACE10MG	Cap, Blue, Gelatin Coated	Ramipril 10 mg	Altace by Hoechst Roussel	00039-0106	Antihypertensive
HOECHST <> ALTACE10MG	Cap, ER, Altace over 10 mg	Ramipril 10 mg	Altace by Caremark	00339-6047	Antihypertensive
HOECHST <> ALTACE10MG	Cap, Gelatin Coated	Ramipril 10 mg	Altace by Hoechst Roussel	00088-0106	Antihypertensive
HOECHST <> ALTACE10MG	Cap, ER	Ramipril 10 mg	Altace by Physicians Total Care	54868-3846	Antihypertensive
HOECHST <> ALTACE125MG	Cap, Yellow, Gelatin, Altace 1.25 mg <> Hoechst	Ramipril 1.25 mg	Altace by Monarch Pharms	61570-0110	Antihypertensive
HOECHST <> ALTACE125MG	Cap, Gelatin Coated, Hoechst <> Altace 1.25 mg	Ramipril 1.25 mg	Altace by Hoechst Roussel	00088-0103	Antihypertensive
HOECHST <> ALTACE25MG	Cap, Orange	Ramipril 2.5 mg	Altace by Rx Pac	65084-0234	Antihypertensive
HOECHST <> ALTACE25MG	Cap, Orange, Gelatin Coated, Hoechst <> Altace 2.5 mg	Ramipril 2.5 mg	Altace by Hoechst Roussel	00039-0104	Antihypertensive
HOECHST <> ALTACE25MG	Cap, Gelatin Coated, Hoechst <> Altace 2.5 mg	Ramipril 2.5 mg	Altace by Hoechst Roussel	00088-0104	Antihypertensive

ID FRONT <> BACK	DESCRIPTION FRONT <> BACK	INGREDIENT & STRENGTH	BRAND (OR EQUIV.) & FIRM	NDC#	CLASS; SCH.
HOECHST <> ALTACE25MG	Cap, ER, Hoechst <> Altace 2.5 mg	Ramipril 2.5 mg	Altace by Allscripts	54569-3713	Antihypertensive
HOECHST <> ALTACE5MG	Cap, Red	Ramipril 5 mg	Altace by Rx Pac	65084-0235	Antihypertensive
HOECHST <> ALTACE5MG	Cap, Gelatin Coated	Ramipril 5 mg	Altace by Hoechst Roussel	00039-0105	Antihypertensive
HOECHST <> ALTACE5MG	Cap, Gelatin Coated, Hoechst <> Altace 5 mg	Ramipril 5 mg	Altace by Hoechst Roussel	00088-0105	Antihypertensive
HOECHST <> ALTACE5MG	Cap	Ramipril 5 mg	Altace by Allscripts	54569-3714	Antihypertensive
HOECHST <> ALTACE5MG	Cap, ER	Ramipril 5 mg	Altace by Quality Care	60346-0618	Antihypertensive
HOECHST <> ALTACETM	Cap, Gelatin Coated, TM Appears in Superscripts	Ramipril 5 mg	Altace by Hoechst Roussel	00039-0105	Antihypertensive
HOECHST <> DIAB	Tab	Glyburide 5 mg	Diabeta by Rite Aid	11822-5186	Antidiabetic
HOECHST <> DIAB	Tab	Glyburide 1.25 mg	Diabeta by Merrell	00068-1210	Antidiabetic
HOECHST <> DIAB	Tab	Glyburide 2.5 mg	Diabeta by Thrift Drug	59198-0022	Antidiabetic
HOECHST <> DIAB	Tab	Glyburide 2.5 mg	Diabeta by Quality Care	60346-0890	Antidiabetic
HOECHST <> DIAB	Tab	Glyburide 2.5 mg	Diabeta by Amerisource	62584-0361	Antidiabetic
HOECHST <> DIAB	Tab, Greek Letter Beta	Glyburide 2.5 mg	Diabeta by Merrell	00068-1211	Antidiabetic
HOECHST <> DIAB	Tab, Light Green, Hoechst <> DIA/B	Glyburide 5 mg	Diabeta by Quality Care	60346-0730	Antidiabetic
HOECHST <> DIAB	Tab, Light Green	Glyburide 5 mg	Diabeta by Thrift Drug	59198-0023	Antidiabetic
HOECHST <> DIAB	Tab	Glyburide 5 mg	Diabeta by Merrell	00068-1212	Antidiabetic
HOECHST <> DIAB	Tab, Hoechst <> DIA/B	Glyburide 5 mg	Diabeta by Nat Pharmpak Serv	55154-1201	Antidiabetic
HOECHST <> LASIX	Tab	Furosemide 20 mg	Lasix by Thrift Drug	59198-0224	Diuretic
HOECHST <> LASIX	Tab	Furosemide 20 mg	Lasix by Leiner	59606-0679	Diuretic
HOECHST <> LASIX	Tab	Furosemide 20 mg	Lasix by Pharm Utilization	60491-0359	Diuretic
HOECHST <> LASIX	Tab	Furosemide 20 mg	Lasix by Amerisource	62584-0067	Diuretic
HOECHST <> LASIX	Tab	Furosemide 20 mg	Lasix by Caremark	00339-5203	Diuretic
HOECHST <> LASIX	Tab	Furosemide 20 mg	Lasix by Drug Distr	52985-0072	Diuretic
HOECHST <> LASIX	Tab	Furosemide 20 mg	Lasix by Thrift Drug	59198-0068	Diuretic
HOECHST <> LASIX40	Tab, Hoechst Logo <> Lasix 40	Furosemide 40 mg	Lasix by Wal Mart	49035-0156	Diuretic
HOECHST <> LASIX40	Tab	Furosemide 40 mg	Lasix by Allscripts	54569-0573	Diuretic
HOECHST <> LASIX40	Tab	Furosemide 40 mg	Lasix by Thrift Drug	59198-0024	Diuretic
HOECHST <> LASIX80	Tab, Facetted Edged	Furosemide 80 mg	Lasix by Merrell	00068-1215	Diuretic
HOECHST <> LASIXR	Tab, Lasix Logo	Furosemide 20 mg	Lasix by Hoechst Roussel	00039-0067	Diuretic
HOECHST <> LASIXR	Tab, White, Oval, Hoechst <> Lasix (R)	Furosemide 20 mg	Lasix by Hoechst Roussel	00039-0060	Diuretic
HOECHST <> LASIXR40	Tab, White, Round, Hoechst <> Lasix (R) 40	Furosemide 40 mg			
HOECHST <> TRENTAL	Tab, Film Coated	Pentoxifylline 400 mg	Trental by Allscripts	54569-0668	Anticoagulent
HOECHST <> TRENTAL	Tab, Film Coated	Pentoxifylline 400 mg	Trental by Pharmedix	53002-1040	Anticoagulent
HOESCHT72	Tab, White, Round	Digestive Enzymes	Festal II by Hoechst		Digestant
HOESCHT73	Tab, Orange, Round	Digestive Enzymes, Atropine Methyl Nitrate	Festalan by Hoechst		Digestant
HOLD <> HOLD	Tab, Red, Round	Dextromethorphan HBr 5 mg	Hold by B F Ascher	00225-0630	Antitussive
HOLD <> HOLD	Tab, Amber, Round	Dextromethorphan HBr 5 mg	Hold by B F Ascher	00225-0640	Antitussive
HOLD <> HOLD	Tab, Yellow, Round	Dextromethorphan HBr 5 mg	Hold by B F Ascher	00225-0620	Antitussive
HOPE <> 301	Tab, White, Round, Uncoated	Scopolamine Hydrobromide 0.4 mg	by Sanofi	00024-0133	Antiemetic
HOPE <> 301	Tab, White, Round	Scopolamine Hydrobromide 0.4 mg	Scopace by Sanofi	00024-0140	Antiemetic
HOPE <> 301	Tab	Scopolamine Hydrobromide 0.4 mg	Scopace by Hope	60267-0301	Antiemetic
HOPE <> 301	Tab	Scopolamine Hydrobromide 0.4 mg	by Anabolic	00722-6383	Antiemetic
HOPE <> 742	Tab	Atropine Sulfate 0.4 mg	by Anabolic	00722-6685	Gastrointestinal
HORIZON205	Tab, White, Round, Scored	Glycopyrrolate 2 mg	Robinul Forte by Horizon Pharm	59630-0205	Gastrointestinal
HORNER	Tab, Salmon, Shield	Tolbutamide 500 mg	Mobenol by Horner	Canadian	Antidiabetic
HORNER15MG	Tab, White, Oval, Horner/15/mg	Flurazepam MonoHCl 15 mg	Somnol by Horner	Canadian	Hypnotic

ID FRONT <> BACK	DESCRIPTION FRONT <> BACK	INGREDIENT & STRENGTH	BRAND (OR EQUIV.) & FIRM	NDC#	CLASS; SCH.
HORNER200MG	Cap, White	Ibuprofen 200 mg	Amersol by Horner		NSAID
HORNER300MG	Cap, Yellow	Ibuprofen 300 mg	Amersol by Horner		NSAID
HORNER30MG	Tab, Light Blue, Oval, Horner/30/mg	Flurazepam MonoHCl 30 mg	Somnol by Horner	Canadian	Hypnotic
HORNER400MG	Cap, Scarlet	Ibuprofen 400 mg	Amersol by Horner		NSAID
HOYT <> 006	Tab, Pink, Round, Chew	Sodium Fluoride 2.2 mg	Luride Cherry by Colgate Oral	00126-0006	Element
HOYT007	Tab, White, Round	Sodium Fluoride 1 mg	Luride SF by Colgate	00126-0007	Element
HOYT013	Tab, Blue, Round	Sodium Fluoride 0.5 mg	Luride by Colgate	00126-0013	Element
HOYT014	Tab, Purple, Round	Sodium Fluoride 0.5 mg	Luride by Colgate	00126-0014	Element
HOYT140	Tab, Green, Round	Sodium Fluoride 1 mg	Luride by Colgate	00126-0140	Element
HOYT141	Tab, Yellow, Round	Sodium Fluoride 1 mg	Luride by Colgate	00126-0141	Element
HOYT142	Tab, Orange, Round	Sodium Fluoride 1 mg	Luride by Colgate	00126-0142	Element
HOYT186	Tab, Beige, Round	Sodium Fluoride 0.25 mg	Luride by Colgate	00126-0186	Element
HP <> CG	Tab, Reddish-Orange, Cap Shaped, Film Coated	Benazepril HCl 20 mg	Lotensin by Novartis	Canadian DIN# 00885851	Antihypertensive
HP15	Tab, Film Coated	Chlorpheniramine Maleate 8 mg, Methscopolamine Nitrate 2.5 mg, Pseudoephedrine HCl 120 mg	Mescolor by Horizon	59630-0150	Cold Remedy
HP15	Tab, Film Coated, HP/15	Chlorpheniramine Maleate 8 mg, Methscopolamine Nitrate 2.5 mg, Pseudoephedrine HCl 120 mg	Mescolor LA TR by Anabolic	00722-6293	Cold Remedy
HPC200	Tab, White, Round, Scored	Glycopyrrolate 1 mg	Robinul by Horizon Pharm	59630-0200	Gastrointestinal
HPS	Tab	Ergonovine Maleate 0.2 mg	by Pharmafab	62542-0902	Ergot
HPS	Tab	Ergonovine Maleate 0.2 mg	by Home Prescription	63704-0001	Ergot
HPS	Tab, White, Round	Ergonovine Maleate 0.2 mg	by Halsey Drug	00904-5387	Ergot
HPS	Tab, White, Round	Ergonovine Maleate 0.2 mg	Ergonovine by Halsey Drug	00904-5386	Ergot
HR	Tab, White, Round, Scored	Caffeine 200 mg	Overtime by BDI		Stimulant
HR	Tab, Pink, Heart Shaped	Caffine 200 mg	Valentine by BDI		Stimulant
HR	Tab, Blue, Round, Scored	Diphenhydramine	Snooze Fast by BDI		Antihistamine
HR	Tab, Brown, Round, Scored	Ginkgo Biloba Extract	Ginkgo Biloba by BDI		Supplement
HR	Tab, Yellow, Round, Scored	Melatonin 3 mg	Melatonin by BDI		Supplement
HR2020	Tab, White, Cap Shaped, Blue, Pink & Yellow Specks, HR/20/20	Caffine 200 mg	20/20 by BDI		Stimulant
HR225MINI	Tab, White, Round, HR 225/Mini	Ephedrine HCl 25 mg, Guaifenesin 200 mg	Mini Two-Way Action by BDI		Antiasthmatic
HS33	Tab, Beige, Round	Ferrous Fumarate 110 mg, Docusate Na 20 mg, Vitamin C 200 mg	Hemaspan by Sanofi		Mineral
HT15	Loz, Cherry	Benzocaine 15 mg, Dextromethorphan HBr 7.5 mg	Tetra-Formula by Reese	10956-0714	Topical Anesthetic
HTI76	Tab, White, Kidney Shape, <> HTI Over 76	Chlorthalidone 25 mg	Thalitone by Monarch	61570-0023	Diuretic
HTI77	Tab, White, Kidney, HTI/77	Chlorthalidone 15 mg	Thalitone by Monarch	61570-0024	Diuretic
HY	Cap, Yellow, HY <> Abbott Logo	Terazosin HCl 2 mg	Hytrin by Abbott	00074-3806	Antihypertensive
HY	Cap, Abbott Logo	Terazosin HCl 2 mg	Hytrin by Physicians Total Care	54868-3842	Antihypertensive
HY	Cap, Abbott Logo	Terazosin HCl 2 mg	Hytrin by Allscripts	54569-4111	Antihypertensive
HY	Cap, Yellow	Terazosin HCl 2 mg	Hytrin by Va Cmop	65243-0068	Antihypertensive
HY	Cap, Abbott Logo	Terazosin HCl	Hytrin by Quality Care	60346-0330	Antihypertensive
HYA <> HYA	Cap, HY-A	Terazosin HCl 2 mg	Terazosin by RP Scherer	11014-1032	Antihypertensive
HYCODAN	Tab, White, Round	Hydrocodone Bitartrate 5 mg, Homatropine 1.5 mg	Hycodan by Endo		Analgesic; C III
HYCODAN	Tab, White, Round, Scored	Hydrocodone Bitartrate 5 mg, Homatropine Methylbromide 1.5 mg	Hycodan by Endo Labs	63481-0042	Analgesic; C III
HYCODAN <> DUPONT	Tab, White, Round, Scored	Hydrocodone Bitartrate 5 mg, Homatropine Methylbromide 1.5 mg	Hycodan by DRX Pharm Consults	55045-2728	Analgesic; C III
HYCOMINE	Tab, Coral Pink, Round, Scored	Acetaminophen 250 mg, Caffeine 30 mg, Chlorpheniramine Maleate 2 mg, Hydrocodone Bitartrate 5 mg, Phenylephrine HCl 10 mg	Hycomine Compound by Endo Labs	63481-0048	Cold Remedy; C III
HYCOMINE	Tab, Red, Round	Hydrocodone Bitartrate, Chlorpheniramine Maleate	Hycomine by Endo		Analgesic; C III
HYDERGINE <> S	Tab, White, Round	Ergoloid Mesylates 1 mg	Hydergine by Novartis Pharms (Ca)	61615-0102	Ergot
HYDREA830	Cap	Hydroxyurea 500 mg	Hydrea by ER Squibb	00003-0830	Antineoplastic
HYDRODIURIL <> MSD 105	Tab, Peach, Round, MSD on Left, 105 on Right	Hydrochlorothiazide 50 mg	Hydrodiuril by Merck	00006-0105	Diuretic
HYDROGESIC <> E	Cap, Edwards Logo	Acetaminophen 500 mg, Hydrocodone Bitartrate 5 mg	Hydrogesic by Edwards	00485-0050	Analgesic; C III

ID FRONT <> BACK	DESCRIPTION FRONT <> BACK	INGREDIENT & STRENGTH	BRAND (OR EQUIV.) & FIRM	NDC#	CLASS; SCH.
HYDROXY <> CUT	Cap, White, with Red Ink	Hydroxagen 2000 mg, MaHuang extract 334 mg, Guarana extract 910 mg, Willow Bark extract 100 mg, L-Carnitine 100 mg, Chromium Picolinate 300 mcg	Hydroxy-Cut by Muscletech	OTC	Supplement
HYLOREL10	Tab	Guanadrel Sulfate 10 mg	Hylorel by Medeva	53014-0787	Antihypertensive
HYLOREL25	Tab, White, Oval	Guanadrel Sulfate 25 mg	Hylorel by Medeva	53014-0788	Antihypertensive
HYZAAR <> MRK 717	Tab, Yellow, Teardrop Shape, Film Coated	Hydrochlorothiazide 12.5 mg, Losartan Potassium 50 mg	Hyzaar by Merck	00006-0717	Diuretic; Antihypertensive
HYZAAR <> MRK717	Tab, Yellow, Oval, Film Coated	Losartan Potassium 50 mg; Hydrochlorothiazide 12.5 mg	Hyzaar by Allscripts	54569-4722	Antihypertensive
I	Cap, Yellow	Benzonatate 100 mg	Tessalon by Inwood		Antitussive
I	Cap	Benzonatate 100 mg	by Zenith Goldline	00182-1080	Antitussive
I <> 25	Tab, Coated	Sumatriptan Succinate 25 mg	Imitrex by Glaxo	00173-0460	Antimigraine
I <> 25	Tab, Coated	Sumatriptan Succinate 25 mg	Imitrex by Physicians Total Care	54868-3777	Antimigraine
I <> INDERAL10	Tab	Propranolol HCl 10 mg	Inderal by Ayerst	00046-0421	Antihypertensive
I <> INDERAL10	Tab	Propranolol HCl 10 mg	Inderal by Thrift Drug	59198-0038	Antihypertensive
I <> INDERAL10	Tab	Propranolol HCl 10 mg	Inderal by Amerisource	62584-0421	Antihypertensive
I <> INDERAL20	Tab, Powder Blue, Raised I <> Inderal over 20	Propranolol HCl 20 mg	Inderal by Ayerst	00046-0422	Antihypertensive
I <> INDERAL20	Tab	Propranolol HCl 10 mg	Inderal by Nat Pharmpak Serv	55154-0204	Antihypertensive
I <> INDERAL20	Tab	Propranolol HCl 20 mg	Inderal by Thrift Drug	59198-0039	Antihypertensive
I <> INDERAL20	Tab	Propranolol HCl 20 mg	Inderal by PDRX	55289-0131	Antihypertensive
I <> INDERAL20	Tab	Propranolol HCl 20 mg	Inderal by Amerisource	62584-0422	Antihypertensive
I <> INDERAL20	Tab, Embossed <> Imprinted	Propranolol HCl 20 mg	Inderal by Nat Pharmpak Serv	55154-0205	Antihypertensive
I <> INDERAL40	Tab, Green, Hexagon, Scored	Propranolol 40 mg	Inderal by Respa	60575-0087	Antihypertensive
I <> INDERAL40	Tab, Mint Green	Propranolol HCl 40 mg	Inderal by Ayerst	00046-0424	Antihypertensive
I <> INDERAL40	Tab	Propranolol HCl 40 mg	Inderal by Thrift Drug	59198-0040	Antihypertensive
I <> INDERAL40	Tab	Propranolol HCl 40 mg	Inderal by Amerisource	62584-0424	Antihypertensive
I <> INDERAL60	Tab, Raised I <> Inderal over 60	Propranolol HCl 60 mg	Inderal by Ayerst	00046-0426	Antihypertensive
I <> INDERAL80	Tab	Propranolol HCl 80 mg	Inderal by Ayerst	00046-0428	Antihypertensive
I <> INDERAL80	Tab	Propranolol HCl 80 mg	Inderal by Thrift Drug	59198-0041	Antihypertensive
I <> INDERAL80	Cap	Propranolol HCl 80 mg	Inderal LA by Murfreesboro	51129-1304	Antihypertensive
I <> INDERAL80	Tab, Coated, Embossed	Propranolol HCl 80 mg	Inderal by Pharm Utilization	60491-0319	Antihypertensive
I <> INDERAL80	Tab, Coated	Propranolol HCl 80 mg	Inderal by Amerisource	62584-0428	Antihypertensive
I <> INDERAL80	Tab, Coated	Propranolol HCl 80 mg	Inderal by Nat Pharmpak Serv	55154-0208	Antihypertensive
I <> INDERIDE4025	Tab, Raised I <> Inderide 40 Over 25	Hydrochlorothiazide 25 mg, Propranolol HCl 40 mg	Inderide by Ayerst	00046-0484	Diuretic; Antihypertensive
I <> SMP	Tab, Coated	Sumatriptan Succinate 25 mg	Imitrex by Glaxo	00173-0460	Antimigraine
I2	Tab, White, Round	Ibuprofen 200 mg	Advil by Perrigo	00113-0628	NSAID
I2	Tab, Brown, Round, Film, I-2	Ibuprofen 200 mg	by Murfreesboro	51129-1508	NSAID
I67	Tab, Film Coated	Carbinoxamine Maleate 8 mg, Pseudoephedrine HCl 120 mg	Cardec by Zenith Goldline	00182-1130	Cold Remedy
IA	Tab, Gray, Round, Film Coated, IA over Abbott Logo	Carteolol HCl 2.5 mg	Cartrol by Abbott	00074-1664	Antihypertensive
IB2	Tab, White, Round	Ibuprofen 200 mg	Advil by Par		NSAID
IB2	Tab, White, Oblong	Ibuprofen 200 mg	Advil by Par		NSAID
IB2	Tab, Brown, Round	Ibuprofen 200 mg	Advil by Perrigo	00113-0488	NSAID
IBU <> 400	Tab, Film Coated	Ibuprofen 400 mg	by Quality Care	60346-0430	NSAID
IBU400	Tab, Film Coated	Ibuprofen 400 mg	by Geneva	00781-1352	NSAID
IBU400	Tab, Film Coated	Ibuprofen 400 mg	by Baker Cummins	63171-1809	NSAID
IBU400	Tab, White, Round	Ibuprofen 400 mg	by Vangard Labs	00615-2525	NSAID
IBU400	Tab, White, Oblong, Film	Ibuprofen 400 mg	by Murfreesboro	51129-1519	NSAID
IBU400	Tab, Film Coated	Ibuprofen 400 mg	by Quality Care	60346-0430	NSAID
IBU400	Tab, Coated, Printed in Black	Ibuprofen 400 mg	by Golden State	60429-0092	NSAID
IBU400	Tab, Film Coated	Ibuprofen 400 mg	IBU by BASF	10117-0467	NSAID
IBU400	Tab	Ibuprofen 400 mg	by Talbert Med	44514-0574	NSAID
IBU600	Tab, Film Coated	Ibuprofen 600 mg	by Baker Cummins	63171-1810	NSAID
IBU600	Tab, White, Round	Ibuprofen 600 mg	by Vangard Labs	00615-2526	NSAID

ID FRONT <> BACK	DESCRIPTION FRONT <> BACK	INGREDIENT & STRENGTH	BRAND (OR EQUIV.) & FIRM	NDC#	CLASS; SCH.
IBU600	Tab, White, Oblong, Film	Ibuprofen 600 mg	by Murfreesboro	51129-1518	NSAID
IBU600	Tab, Film Coated	Ibuprofen 600 mg	IBU by Par	49884-0468	NSAID
IBU600	Tab, Film Coated	Ibuprofen 600 mg	by Quality Care	60346-0556	NSAID
IBU600	Tab, Coated	Ibuprofen 600 mg	by Golden State	60429-0093	NSAID
IBU600	Tab, Film Coated	Ibuprofen 600 mg	by Amerisource	62584-0747	NSAID
IBU600	Tab, Film Coated	Ibuprofen 600 mg	IBU by BASF	10117-0468	NSAID
IBU600	Tab, Film Coated	Ibuprofen 600 mg	by Geneva	00781-1362	NSAID
IBU800	Tab, Film Coated	Ibuprofen 800 mg	by Warner Chilcott	00047-0914	NSAID
IBU800	Tab, Film Coated	Ibuprofen 800 mg	by Schein	00364-2137	NSAID
IBU800	Tab, Film Coated	Ibuprofen 800 mg	by Zenith Goldline	00172-3648	NSAID
IBU800	Tab, Film Coated	Ibuprofen 800 mg	by Med Pro	53978-5007	NSAID
IBU800	Tab, White, Oblong, Film Coated	Ibuprofen 800 mg	by Murfreesboro	51129-1520	NSAID
IBU800	Tab, Film Coated	Ibuprofen 800 mg	IBU Ibuprofen by Par	49884-0469	NSAID
IBU800	Tab, Film Coated	Ibuprofen 800 mg	by Quality Care	60346-0030	NSAID
IBU800	Tab, Film Coated	Ibuprofen 800 mg	by Golden State	60429-0094	NSAID
IBU800	Tab, Coated, Printed in Black	Ibuprofen 800 mg	by HL Moore	00839-7236	NSAID
IBU800	Tab, Film Coated	Ibuprofen 800 mg	by IDE Inter	00814-3816	NSAID
IBU800	Tab, Film Coated	Ibuprofen 800 mg	IBU by BASF	10117-0173	NSAID
IBU800	Tab, Film Coated	Ibuprofen 800 mg	by Major	00904-1760	NSAID
IBU800	Tab, White, Cap-Shaped, Film Coated	Ibuprofen 800 mg	Motrin by Geneva	00781-1363	NSAID
IBU800	Tab, Film Coated	Ibuprofen 800 mg	by HL Moore	00839-7239	NSAID
IBU800	Tab, White, Round	Ibuprofen 800 mg	by Vangard Labs	00615-2528	NSAID
IC	Tab, White, Round, Film Coated, IC over Abbott Logo	Carteolol HCl 5 mg	Cartrol by Abbott	00074-1665	Antihypertensive
ICAPS	Tab, Off-White, Cap-Shaped	Ascorbic Acid, Zinc Acetate, Vitamin E Acetate, Manganese Hydrolyzed Vegetable Protein Chelate, Copper Hydrolyzed Vegetable Protein Chelate, Riboflavin, Beta Carotene, Selenium Hydrolyzed Vegetable Protein Chelate	ICAPS by Alcon	Canadian	Vitamin
ICAPS	Tab, Yellow, Cap-Shaped	Ascorbic Acid, Zinc Acetate, Vitamin E Acetate, Manganese Hydrolyzed vegetable Protein Chelate, Copper Hydrolyzed Vegetable Protein Chelate, Riboflavin, Beta Carotene, Selenium Hydrolyzed Vegetable Protein Chelate	ICAPS by Alcon	Canadian	Vitamin
ICI <> 105	Tab, White, Round	Atenolol 50 mg	Tenormin by AstraZeneca	00310-0105	Antihypertensive
ICI101	Tab, White, Round	Atenolol 100 mg	Tenormin by AstraZeneca	00310-0101	Antihypertensive
ICI115	Tab, White, Round	Atenolol 50 mg, Chlorthalidone 25 mg	Tenoretic 50 by AstraZeneca	00310-0115	Antihypertensive; Diuretic
ICI117	Tab, White, Round	Atenolol 100 mg, Chlorthalidone 25 mg	Tenoretic 100 by AstraZeneca	00310-0117	Antihypertensive; Diuretic
ICN	Cap	Methoxsalen 10 mg	Oxsoralen Ultra by Pharm Utilization	60491-0826	Dermatologic
ICN <> 650	Cap, Gelatin Coated	Methoxsalen 10 mg	Oxsoralen Ultra by RP Scherer	11014-1123	Dermatologic
ICN <> 650	Cap	Methoxsalen 10 mg	Oxsoralen Ultra by Banner Pharmacaps	10888-4554	Dermatologic
ICN D12	Tab, Blue, Oval	Dexamethasone 750 mcg	by ICN	Canadian	Steroid
ICN E12	Tab, Blue	Ethambutol HCl 400 mg	Etibi by ICN	Canadian	Antituberculosis
ICN N11	Tab, White	Aminosalicylate Sodium 500 mg	by ICN	Canadian	Antimycobacterial
ICN021	Tab, Blue, Round	Oxybutynin Chloride 5 mg	by ICN	Canadian	Urinary
ICN0901	Cap, Red	Methyltestosterone 10 mg	Testred by ICN		Hormone; C III
ICN122	Tab, White	Isoniazid 300 mg	by ICN	Canadian	Antimycobacterial
ICN303	Tab, White, Round, ICN/303	Trioxsalen 5 mg	by ICN	Canadian	Psoralen
ICN303	Tab, White, Round	Trioxsalen 5 mg	Trisoralen by ICN		Psoralen
ICN3100	Tab, White, Round	Neostigmine Bromide 15 mg	Prostigmin by Hoffman LaRoche		Muscle Stimulant
ICN311	Tab, White, Round	Methyltestosterone 10 mg	Android 10 by Schering		Hormone; C III
ICN499	Tab, Peach, Round	Methyltestosterone 25 mg	Android 25 by Schering		Hormone; C III
ICN60	Tab, White, Round	Pyridostigmine Bromide 60 mg	Mestinon by Hoffman LaRoche		Muscle Stimulant
ICN600	Cap, Light Pink	Methoxsalen 10 mg	by ICN	Canadian	Dermatologic
ICN650	Cap, Green, ICN/650	Methoxsalen 10 mg	by ICN	Canadian	Dermatologic

ID FRONT <> BACK	DESCRIPTION FRONT <> BACK	INGREDIENT & STRENGTH	BRAND (OR EQUIV.) & FIRM	NDC#	CLASS; SCH.
ICNA17	Cap, Blue & Pink	Diphenhydramine HCl 25 mg	Allerdryl by ICN		Antihistamine
ICNA17	Cap, Light Blue & Pink	Diphenhydramine HCl 25 mg	Allerdryl by ICN	Canadian	Antihistamine
ICNA18	Cap, Pink & White	Diphenhydramine 50 mg	by ICN	Canadian	Antihistamine
ICNA18	Cap, Pink & White	Diphenhydramine HCl 50 mg	Allerdryl by ICN		Antihistamine
ICNA21	Tab, White, Round	Allopurinol 100 mg	Zyloprim by ICN		Antigout
ICNA22	Tab, Orange, Rectangular	Allopurinol 200 mg	Alloprin by ICN		Antigout
ICNA23	Tab, Orange, Round	Allopurinol 300 mg	Zyloprim by ICN		Antigout
ICNB11	Tab, White, Round	Probenecid 500 mg	Benuryl by ICN	Canadian	Antigout
ICNC11	Cap, Orange & White	Lithium Carbonate 150 mg	by ICN	Canadian	Antipsychotic
ICNC12	Cap, Flesh	Lithium Carbonate 300 mg	by ICN	Canadian	Antipsychotic
ICNC13	Cap, Blue & Opaque	Lithium Carbonate 600 mg	by ICN	Canadian	Antipsychotic
ICNC23	Tab, White	Cortisone Acetate 25 mg	Cortisone Ace ICN by ICN	Canadian	Steroid
ICND11	Tab, Yellow, Oval	Dexamethasone 500 mcg	by ICN	Canadian	Steroid
ICND13	Tab, Green, Oval	Dexamethasone 4 mg	by ICN	Canadian	Steroid
ICNF11	Cap, Blue	Decyclomine HCl 10 mg	Formulex by ICN	Canadian	Gastrointestinal
ICNM180	Cap, Straw	Pyridostigmine 180 mg	by ICN	Canadian	Muscle Stimulant
ICNM180	Tab, Yellow, Oblong	Pyridostigmine Bromide 180 mg	Mestinon Timespan by Hoffman LaRoche		Muscle Stimulant
ICNN31	Cap, White & Yellow	Nortriptyline HCl 10 mg	by ICN	Canadian	Antidepressant
ICNN32	Cap, White & Yellow	Nortriptyline HCl 25 mg	by ICN	Canadian	Antidepressant
ICNP17	Tab, Maroon	Phenazopyridine HCl 100 mg	Phenazo by ICN	Canadian	Urinary Analgesic
ICNP18	Tab, Maroon	Phenazopyridine HCl 200 mg	Phenazo by ICN	Canadian	Urinary Analgesic
ICNP6	Tab, White	Procyclidine HCl 5 mg	Procyclid by ICN	Canadian	Antiparkinson
ICNP8	Tab, Peach, Round	Propantheline Bromide 15 mg	Propanthel by ICN	Canadian	Gastrointestinal
ICNR11	Cap, Opaque & Scarlet	Rifampin 150 mg	Rofact by ICN	Canadian	Antibiotic
ICNR12	Cap, Brown & Scarlet	Rifampin 300 mg	Rofact by ICN	Canadian	Antibiotic
ICNS11	Tab, Brown & Yellow, Round	Sulfasalazine 500 mg	SAS by ICN	Canadian	Gastrointestinal
ICNS14	Tab, Brown & Yellow, Oval	Sulfasalazine 500 mg	SAS by ICN	Canadian	Gastrointestinal
ICNS31	Tab, Light Blue, Oblong	Sotalol HCl 80 mg	by ICN	Canadian	Antiarrhythmic
ICNS32	Tab, Light Blue, Oblong	Sotalol HCl 160 mg	by ICN	Canadian	Antiarrhythmic
ICNS33	Tab, Light Blue, Oblong	Sotalol HCl 240 mg	by ICN	Canadian	Antiarrhythmic
ICNT11	Tab, White	Pyrazinamide 500 mg	Tebrazid by ICN	Canadian	Antibiotic
ICNT17	Cap, White	L-Tryptophan 500 mg	by ICN	Canadian DIN# 02240334	Supplement
ICNT21	Tab, Orange	Trazodone HCl 50 mg	by ICN	Canadian	Antidepressant
ICNT22	Tab, White	Trazodone HCl 100 mg	by ICN	Canadian	Antidepressant
ICNT23	Tab, Orange	Trazodone HCl 150 mg	by ICN	Canadian	Antidepressant
ICNW1	Tab, White	Prednisone 1 mg	by ICN	Canadian	Steroid
ID <> 300	Cap, Ex Release	Chlorpheniramine Maleate 8 mg, Pseudoephedrine HCl 120 mg	Deconomed Sr by Sovereign	58716-0044	Cold Remedy
ID <> 301	Cap, Ex Release	Brompheniramine Maleate 12 mg, Pseudoephedrine HCl 120 mg	Iofed by Sovereign	58716-0045	Cold Remedy
ID <> 301	Cap	Brompheniramine Maleate 12 mg, Pseudoephedrine HCl 120 mg	Iofed by Physicians Total Care	54868-3989	Cold Remedy
ID <> 302	Cap, Ex Release	Brompheniramine Maleate 6 mg, Pseudoephedrine HCl 60 mg	Iofed PD by Sovereign	58716-0046	Cold Remedy
ID <> 308	Cap	Trimethobenzamide HCl 250 mg	by Sovereign	58716-0055	Antiemetic
ID <> 311	Cap, Ex Release	Chlorpheniramine Maleate 8 mg	by Sovereign	58716-0051	Antihistamine
ID <> 312	Cap, Ex Release	Chlorpheniramine Maleate 12 mg	by Sovereign	58716-0049	Antihistamine
ID111	Tab, Coated, ID/111	Yohimbine HCl 5.4 mg	by Sovereign	58716-0653	Impotence Agent
ID112	Tab, Ex Release, Embossed, ID 112	Dextromethorphan Hydrobromide 30 mg, Guaifenesin 600 mg, Pseudoephedrine HCl 60 mg	Med Rx DM by Iomed	61646-0701	Cold Remedy
ID112	Tab, Ex Release, ID/112	Dextromethorphan Hydrobromide 30 mg, Guaifenesin 600 mg	Iobid DM by Sovereign	58716-0654	Cold Remedy
ID121	Tab, Yellow, Oblong, Scored	Guaifenesin 600 mg, Pseudoephedrine 120 mg	Entex PSE by Martec	52555-0635	Cold Remedy
ID121	Tab, Ex Release, ID/121	Guaifenesin 600 mg, Pseudoephedrine HCl 120 mg	Iotex PSE by Sovereign	58716-0657	Cold Remedy

ID FRONT <> BACK	DESCRIPTION FRONT <> BACK	INGREDIENT & STRENGTH	BRAND (OR EQUIV.) & FIRM	NDC#	CLASS; SCH.
ID122	Tab, Ex Release, Embossed, ID 122	Dextromethorphan Hydrobromide 30 mg, Guaifenesin 600 mg, Pseudoephedrine HCl 60 mg	Med Rx DM by Iomed	61646-0701	Cold Remedy
ID122	Tab, Ex Release, Embossed, ID 122	Guaifenesin 600 mg, Pseudoephedrine HCl 60 mg	Med Rx by Iomed	61646-0700	Cold Remedy
ID122	Tab, Ex Release, ID/122	Guaifenesin 600 mg, Pseudoephedrine HCl 60 mg	Iosal II by Sovereign	58716-0655	Cold Remedy
ID122	Tab	Guaifenesin 600 mg, Pseudoephedrine HCl 60 mg	Decongest II by Qualitest	00603-3116	Cold Remedy
ID125	Tab, White, Oblong, Scored	Guaifenesin 600 mg	Humibid LA by Martec	52555-0628	Expectorant
ID125	Tab, Ex Release, Embossed, ID 125	Guaifenesin 600 mg, Pseudoephedrine HCl 60 mg	Med Rx by Iomed	61646-0700	Cold Remedy
ID125	Tab, Ex Release, ID/125	Guaifenesin 600 mg	by Sovereign	58716-0656	Expectorant
ID152	Tab, Film Coated	Dexbrompheniramine Maleate 6 mg, Pseudoephedrine Sulfate 120 mg	Drexophed Sr by Qualitest	00603-3505	Cold Remedy
ID155	Tab, ID/155	Hyoscyamine Sulfate 0.375 mg	by Sovereign	58716-0673	Gastrointestinal
ID155	Tab	Hyoscyamine Sulfate 0.375 mg	by Iomed	61646-0155	Gastrointestinal
ID155	Tab, ER	Hyoscyamine Sulfate 0.375 mg	by United Res	00677-1611	Gastrointestinal
ID156	Tab	Hyoscyamine Sulfate 0.125 mg	by Sovereign	58716-0651	Gastrointestinal
ID156	Tab	Hyoscyamine Sulfate 0.125 mg	by Iomed	61646-0156	Gastrointestinal
ID156	Tab, ID/156	Hyoscyamine Sulfate 0.125 mg	by Sovereign	58716-0675	Gastrointestinal
ID172	Tab, White, Oblong, Scored, ID/172	Guaifenesin 1200 mg	by Lotus Biochem	59417-0403	Expectorant
ID172	Tab, White, Oblong, Scored	Guaifenesin 1200 mg	by Iopharm Labs	61646-0172	Expectorant
ID301	Cap	Brompheniramine Maleate 12 mg, Pseudoephedrine HCl 120 mg	by Qualitest	00603-2505	Cold Remedy
ID302	Cap, Dark Green	Brompheniramine Maleate 6 mg, Pseudoephedrine HCl 60 mg	by Qualitest	00603-2506	Cold Remedy
IE125 <> G	Tab, Orange, Round, Convex, Film	Indapamide 1.25 mg	by Murfreesboro	51129-1540	Diuretic
IE125 <> G	Tab, Film Coated, IE Over 1.25 <> G	Indapamide 1.25 mg	by Alphapharm	57315-0027	Diuretic
IE25 <> G	Tab, White, Round, Convex, Film	Indapamide 2.5 mg	by Murfreesboro	51129-1543	Diuretic
IE25 <> G	Tab, Film Coated, IE over 2.5 <> G	Indapamide 2.5 mg	by Alphapharm	57315-0028	Diuretic
IE25G	Tab, Pink, Round, IE 2.5/G	Indapamide Hemihydrate 2.5 mg	by Genpharm	Canadian	Diuretic
II	Tab, White, Abbott Logo	Phenacemide 500 mg	Phenurone by Abbott		Anticonvulsant
IINDERAL10	Tab, Orange, Hexagon, Scored	Propranolol HCl 10 mg	Inderal by RP Scherer SA	64566-0001	Antihypertensive
IINDERAL20	Tab, Blue, Hexagon, Scored	Propranolol HCl 20 mg	Inderal by RP Scherer SA	64566-0002	Antihypertensive
IKA11	Tab, White, Round	Clomiphene Citrate 50 mg	Serophene by Serono	44087-8090	Infertility
IL	Tab, Yellow, Round, IL in White	Benzonatate 100 mg	by Boca Pharmacal	64376-0502	Antitussive
IL	Cap, Yellow	Benzonatate 100 mg	by HJ Harkins	52959-0411	Antitussive
IL	Cap, Clear & Yellow, Gelatin, Round Perle	Benzonatate 100 mg	by Inwood	00258-3654	Antitussive
IL	Cap, Clear Yellow, Gelatin	Benzonatate 100 mg	by Teva	00093-0060	Antitussive
IL	Cap	Benzonatate 100 mg	Tessalon by RP Scherer	11014-1200	Antitussive
IL	Cap	Benzonatate 100 mg	Tessalon Perles by RP Scherer	11014-0732	Antitussive
IL <> 3581	Tab, ER	Theophylline 300 mg	by Schein	00364-0660	Antiasthmatic
IL <> 3583	Tab, Ex Release	Theophylline 200 mg	by Schein	00364-0681	Antiasthmatic
IL <> 3607	Cap, Lavender, Ex Release	Indomethacin 75 mg	by Schein	00364-2211	NSAID
IL <> 3607	Cap, Clear & Lavender, Ex Release	Indomethacin 75 mg	by Quality Care	60346-0687	NSAID
IL <> 3607	Cap, Lavender, Ex Release	Indomethacin 75 mg	by Qualitest	00603-4070	NSAID
IL <> 3609	Cap, ER	Propranolol HCl 60 mg	by Qualitest	00603-5497	Antihypertensive
IL <> 3610	Cap, ER	Propranolol HCl 80 mg	by Qualitest	00603-5498	Antihypertensive
IL <> 3611	Cap, ER	Propranolol HCl 120 mg	by Qualitest	00603-5499	Antihypertensive
IL <> 3613	Tab, Peach, Round, Scored	Isosorbide Dinitrate 40 mg	by Allscripts	54569-0454	Antianginal
IL3531	Tab	Theophylline Anhydrous 300 mg	by Med Pro	53978-0320	Antiasthmatic
IL3549	Tab, Peach, Round, Scored	Isosorbide Dinirtate 40 mg	by Inwood	00258-3613	Antianginal
IL3549	Tab, Ex Release, IL/3459	Isosorbide Dinitrate 40 mg	by Inwood	00258-3549	Antianginal
IL3549	Tab, ER	Isosorbide Dinitrate 40 mg	by Zenith Goldline	00182-0879	Antianginal
IL3549	Tab, IL/3459	Isosorbide Dinitrate 40 mg	by Allscripts	54569-0454	Antianginal
IL3549	Tab, Diamond Shaped, Ex Release	Isosorbide Dinitrate 40 mg	by Murfreesboro	51129-1315	Antianginal
IL3549	Tab, Ex Release, IL/3459	Isosorbide Dinitrate 40 mg	by Quality Care	60346-0280	Antianginal
IL3549	Tab, Ex Release, IL/3459	Isosorbide Dinitrate 40 mg	by Major	00904-2149	Antianginal
IL3549	Tab, ER	Isosorbide Dinitrate 40 mg	by Geneva	00781-1417	Antianginal

ID FRONT <> BACK	DESCRIPTION FRONT <> BACK	INGREDIENT & STRENGTH	BRAND (OR EQUIV.) & FIRM	NDC#	CLASS; SCH.
IL3549	Tab, ER	Isosorbide Dinitrate 40 mg	by United Res	00677-0473	Antianginal
IL3575	Cap, Clear & White	Isosorbide Dinitrate 40 mg	by Inwood		Antianginal
IL3575	Cap, Clear & White, IL/3575	Isosorbide Dinitrate C.R. 40 mg	Isordil by Inwood		Antianginal
IL3577	Cap, Clear & White, IL/3577	Pentaerythritol Tetranitrate C.R. 80 mg	Peritrate by Inwood		Antianginal
IL3581	Tab, White, Oblong, IL/3581	Theophylline 300 mg	Theochron by Astra	Canadian	Antiasthmatic
IL3581	Tab, Ex Release, IL/3581	Theophylline 300 mg	by Baker Cummins	63171-1400	Antiasthmatic
IL3581	Tab, White, Cap Shaped, Scored	Theophylline 300 mg	by Inwood	00258-3581	Antiasthmatic
IL3581	Tab, ER	Theophylline 300 mg	by Rugby	00536-4652	Antiasthmatic
IL3581	Tab, White, Cap Shaped, Scored	Theophylline 300 mg	Theochron by Forest	00456-4330	Antiasthmatic
IL3581	Tab, ER	Theophylline 300 mg	by Zenith Goldline	00182-1400	Antiasthmatic
IL3581	Tab, ER	Theophylline 300 mg	by Teva	00093-0589	Antiasthmatic
IL3581	Tab, ER	Theophylline 300 mg	by Pharmedix	53002-0335	Antiasthmatic
IL3581	Tab, Ex Release, IL/3581	Theophylline 300 mg	by Quality Care	60346-0596	Antiasthmatic
IL3581	Tab, Ex Release, IL/3581	Theophylline 300 mg	by United Res	00677-0817	Antiasthmatic
IL3581	Tab, White, Oblong, Scored	Theophylline 300 mg	by Dixon Shane	17236-0325	Antiasthmatic
IL3581	Tab, ER	Theophylline 300 mg	by HL Moore	00839-6693	Antiasthmatic
IL3581	Tab, ER	Theophylline 300 mg	Theochron ER by Forest	10418-0064	Antiasthmatic
IL3581	Tab, ER	Theophylline 300 mg	by Major	00904-1612	Antiasthmatic
IL3581	Tab, White, Oblong	Theophylline 300 mg CR	by Allscripts	54569-2483	Antiasthmatic
IL3581	Tab	Theophylline 200 mg	by Baker Cummins	63171-1590	Antiasthmatic
IL3583	Tab, White, Oval, Scored	Theophylline 200 mg	Theochron by Forest	00456-4320	Antiasthmatic
IL3583	Tab, Ex Release	Theophylline 200 mg	by Teva	00093-0588	Antiasthmatic
IL3583	Tab, White, Oval, Scored	Theophylline 200 mg	by Inwood	00258-3583	Antiasthmatic
IL3583	Tab, Ex Release	Theophylline 200 mg	by Zenith Goldline	00182-1590	Antiasthmatic
IL3583	Tab, Ex Release	Theophylline 200 mg	by Rugby	00536-4651	Antiasthmatic
IL3583	Tab, ER	Theophylline 200 mg	by Pharmedix	53002-0330	Antiasthmatic
IL3583	Tab, ER	Theophylline 200 mg	by Allscripts	54569-2482	Antiasthmatic
IL3583	Tab	Theophylline 200 mg	by Med Pro	53978-0319	Antiasthmatic
IL3583	Tab, Ex Release, IL/3583	Theophylline 200 mg	by Quality Care	60346-0669	Antiasthmatic
IL3583	Tab, ER	Theophylline 200 mg	by Major	00904-1611	Antiasthmatic
IL3583	Tab	Theophylline 200 mg	by United Res	00677-0846	Antiasthmatic
IL3583	Tab, White, Oval, Scored	Theophylline 200 mg	by Dixon Shane	17236-0324	Antiasthmatic
IL3583	Tab, ER	Theophylline 200 mg	Theochron ER by Forest	10418-0109	Antiasthmatic
IL3584	Tab, Ex Release, IL/3584	Theophylline 100 mg	by Baker Cummins	63171-1589	Antiasthmatic
IL3584	Tab, White, Round, IL/3584	Theophylline 100 mg	Theochron by Astra	Canadian	Antiasthmatic
IL3584	Tab, Ex Release, IL/3584	Theophylline 100 mg	by Teva	00093-0599	Antiasthmatic
IL3584	Tab, ER	Theophylline 100 mg	by Rugby	00536-4650	Antiasthmatic
IL3584	Tab, White, Round, Scored	Theophylline 100 mg	by Inwood	00258-3584	Antiasthmatic
IL3584	Tab, White, Round, Scored	Theophylline 100 mg	Theochron by Forest	00456-4310	Antiasthmatic
IL3584	Tab, ER	Theophylline 100 mg	by Zenith Goldline	00182-1589	Antiasthmatic
IL3584	Tab, Ex Release	Theophylline 100 mg	by Major	00904-1610	Antiasthmatic
IL3584	Tab, Ex Release	Theophylline 100 mg	by HL Moore	00839-6730	Antiasthmatic
IL3584	Tab, Ex Release	Theophylline 100 mg	Theochron ER by Forest	10418-0110	Antiasthmatic
IL3584	Tab, White, Oval, IL/3584	Theophylline 200 mg	Theochron by Astra	Canadian	Antiasthmatic
IL3587	Tab, White, Round	Carbamazepine 200 mg	by Inwood	00258-3587	Anticonvulsant
IL3587	Tab, IL/3587	Carbamazepine 200 mg	by Qualitest	00603-2563	Anticonvulsant
IL3587	Tab	Carbamazepine 200 mg	by United Res	00677-1099	Anticonvulsant
IL3587	Tab	Carbamazepine 200 mg	by DRX	55045-1516	Anticonvulsant
IL3587	Tab, White, Round, Scored	Carbamazepine 200 mg	by Dixon Shane	17236-0352	Anticonvulsant
IL3587	Tab	Carbemazepine 200 mg	by Major	00904-3855	Anticonvulsant
IL3587	Tab, White, Round	Carbamazepine 200 mg	by Inwood	00258-3587	Anticonvulsant
IL3587	Tab	Carbamazepine 200 mg	by Quality Care	60346-0777	Anticonvulsant

ID FRONT <> BACK	DESCRIPTION FRONT <> BACK	INGREDIENT & STRENGTH	BRAND (OR EQUIV.) & FIRM	NDC#	CLASS; SCH.
IL3607	Cap, ER, Off-White Beads	Indomethacin 75 mg	by Warner Chilcott	00047-0875	NSAID
IL3607	Cap, ER	Indomethacin 75 mg	by Zenith Goldline	00182-1469	NSAID
IL3607	Cap, Clear & Lavender w/ White Beads	Indomethacin 75 mg	by Inwood	00258-3607	NSAID
IL3607	Cap, ER	Indomethacin 75 mg	by Rugby	00536-4939	NSAID
IL3607	Cap	Indomethacin 75 mg	by Pharmedix	53002-0399	NSAID
IL3607	Cap, ER	Indomethacin 75 mg	by Allscripts	54569-1518	NSAID
IL3607	Cap, ER, Off-White Beads	Indomethacin 75 mg	by HJ Harkins Co	52959-0082	NSAID
IL3607	Cap, ER, Off-White Beads	Indomethacin 75 mg	by Brightstone	62939-7012	NSAID
IL3607	Cap, ER	Indomethacin 75 mg	by Major	00904-1178	NSAID
IL3607	Cap, ER	Indomethacin 75 mg	by United Res	00677-1197	NSAID
IL3607	Cap, Purple, IL-3607	Indomethacin ER 75 mg	by Geneva	00781-2153	NSAID
IL3609	Cap, ER	Propranolol HCl 60 mg	by Murfreesboro	51129-1554	NSAID
IL3609	Cap, Brown & Clear, Opaque, IL over 3609	Propranolol HCl 60 mg	by Zenith Goldline	00182-1926	Antihypertensive
IL3609	Cap, Brown & Clear	Propranolol HCl 60 mg	by Teva	00093-0691	Antihypertensive
IL3609	Cap, ER	Propranolol HCl 60 mg	by Inwood	00258-3609	Antihypertensive
IL3609	Cap, ER, Off-White Beads, <> IL/3609	Propranolol HCl 60 mg	by Geneva	00781-2061	Antihypertensive
IL3609	Cap, ER, Off-White Beads, <> IL/3609	Propranolol HCl 60 mg	by United Res	00677-1363	Antihypertensive
IL3610	Cap, Blue & Clear	Propranolol HCl 80 mg	by Major	00904-0421	Antihypertensive
IL3610	Cap, ER	Propranolol HCl 80 mg	by Inwood	00258-3610	Antihypertensive
IL3610	Cap, Blue & Clear, Opaque, IL over 3610	Propranolol HCl 80 mg	by Zenith Goldline	00182-1927	Antihypertensive
IL3610	Cap, ER, Off-White Beads	Propranolol HCl 80 mg	by Teva	00093-0692	Antihypertensive
IL3610	Cap, Opaque Blue, Ex Release, Off-White Beads	Propranolol HCl 80 mg	by DRX	55045-2461	Antihypertensive
IL3610	Cap, ER	Propranolol HCl 80 mg	by Major	00904-0422	Antihypertensive
IL3611	Cap, Blue & Clear	Propranolol HCl 120 mg	by Geneva	00781-2062	Antihypertensive
IL3611	Cap, ER, Off-White Beads	Propranolol HCl 120 mg	by Inwood	00258-3611	Antihypertensive
IL3611	Cap, ER	Propranolol HCl 120 mg	by Major	00904-0423	Antihypertensive
IL3612	Cap, Blue & Clear	Propranolol HCl 160 mg	by Geneva	00781-2063	Antihypertensive
IL3612	Cap, Blue & Clear, Opaque, IL over 3612	Propranolol HCl 160 mg	by Inwood	00258-3612	Antihypertensive
IL3612	Cap, ER	Propranolol HCl 160 mg	by Teva	00093-0694	Antihypertensive
IL3612	Cap, ER, Off White Beads	Propranolol HCl 160 mg	by Zenith Goldline	00182-1929	Antihypertensive
IL3612	Cap, ER	Propranolol HCl 160 mg	by DRX	55045-2388	Antihypertensive
IL3612	Cap, ER, Off-White Beads, <> IL/3612	Propranolol HCl 160 mg	by Geneva	00781-2064	Antihypertensive
IL3612	Cap, ER	Propranolol HCl 160 mg	by United Res	00677-1366	Antihypertensive
IL3613	Tab, Peach, Round, Scored	Isosorbide Dinitrate 40 mg	by Qualitest	00603-5500	Antihypertensive
IL3613	Tab, Peach, Round	Isosorbide Dinitrate 40 mg	by Inwood	00258-3613	Antianginal
IL3614	Tab, White, Oblong	Theophylline ER 450 mg	by Murfreesboro	51129-1566	Antianginal
IL3614450	Cap, Off-White, Cap-Shaped, IL 3614/450	Theophylline 450 mg	Theodur by Inwood		Antiasthmatic
IL3614450	Tab, Off-White, Ex Release	Theophylline 450 mg	by Inwood	00258-3614	Antiasthmatic
IL3622	Tab, White, Cap Shaped, Scored	Acetaminophen 650 mg, Hydrocodone Bitartrate 7.5 mg	by Major	00904-1613	Antiasthmatic
IL3622	Tab	Acetaminophen 650 mg, Hydrocodone Bitartrate 7.5 mg	by Inwood	00258-3622	Analgesic; C III
IL3625	Cap, ER, Off White Beads	Theophylline Anhydrous 300 mg	by HL Moore	00839-8061	Analgesic; C III
IL3625	Cap, ER	Theophylline Anhydrous 300 mg	by Major	00904-7849	Antiasthmatic
IL3625	Cap, Clear & White w/ Off-White Beads	Theophylline Anhydrous 300 mg	by Qualitest	00603-5952	Antiasthmatic
IL3625	Cap, ER, Inwood	Theophylline Anhydrous 300 mg	by Inwood	00258-3625	Antiasthmatic
IL3625	Cap, Clear & White, Opaque	Theophylline Anhydrous 300 mg	by Rugby	00536-5634	Antiasthmatic
IL3634	Cap, ER, Off White Beads	Theophylline Anhydrous 300 mg	by Teva	00093-0940	Antiasthmatic
IL3634	Cap, ER	Theophylline Anhydrous 200 mg	by Major	00904-7848	Antiasthmatic
IL3634	Cap, Clear & White w/ Off-White Beads	Theophylline Anhydrous 200 mg	by Qualitest	00603-5951	Antiasthmatic
IL3634	Cap, Clear & White, Opaque	Theophylline 200 mg	by Inwood	00258-3634	Antiasthmatic
IL3637	Cap, Clear & White, Ex Release, with Off-White Beads	Theophylline Anhydrous 200 mg	by Teva	00093-0938	Antiasthmatic
IL3638	Cap, Clear & White, Ex Release, with Off-White Beads	Theophylline Anhydrous 100 mg	by Inwood	00258-3637	Antiasthmatic
		Theophylline Anhydrous 125 mg	by Inwood	00258-3638	Antiasthmatic

ID FRONT <> BACK	DESCRIPTION FRONT <> BACK	INGREDIENT & STRENGTH	BRAND (OR EQUIV.) & FIRM	NDC#	CLASS; SCH.
IL3638	Cap, ER	Theophylline Anhydrous 125 mg	by Qualitest	00603-5950	Antiasthmatic
IL3638	Cap, Clear	Theophylline Anhydrous 125 mg	by Teva	00093-0936	Antiasthmatic
IL3657	Cap, White	Acetaminophen 500 mg, Butalbital 50 mg, Caffeine 40 mg	by Inwood	00258-3657	Analgesic
IL3657	Tab, White, Oblong, Scored	Butalbital 50 mg, Acetaminophen 500 mg, Caffeine 40 mg	by Caremark	00339-5021	Analgesic
IL3657	Tab, White, Oblong, Scored	Choline Magnesium 500 mg	by Allscripts	54569-4733	NSAID
IL3658	Tab, Light Blue, Scored	Acetaminophen 650 mg, Hydrocodone 10 mg	by Inwood	00258-3658	Analgesic; C III
IL3658	Tab, Light Blue	Acetaminophen 650 mg, Hydrocodone Bitartrate 10 mg	by DRX	55045-2386	Analgesic; C III
IL3658	Tab, Light Blue	Acetaminophen 650 mg, Hydrocodone Bitartrate 10 mg	by Inwood	00258-3658	Analgesic; C III
IL3658	Tab	Acetaminophen 650 mg, Hydrocodone Bitartrate 10 mg	by HL Moore	00839-8048	Analgesic; C III
IL3658	Tab	Acetaminophen 650 mg, Hydrocodone Bitartrate 10 mg	by Major	00904-5127	Analgesic; C III
IL3660	Tab, White	Hydrocodone 7.5 mg, Acetaminophen 750 mg	by Inwood		Analgesic; C III
IL3660	Tab, White, IL-3660	Hydrocodone 7.5 mg, Acetaminophen 750 mg	by Forest		Analgesic; C III
IL3661	Tab, White, IL-3661	Hydrocodone 10 mg, Acetaminophen 660 mg	by Forest		Analgesic; C III
IL3661	Tab, White	Hydrocodone 10 mg, Acetaminophen 660 mg	by Inwood		Analgesic; C III
IL3662	Tab, White	Hydrocodone 7.5 mg, Acetaminophen 500 mg	by Inwood		Analgesic; C III
IL3662	Tab, White, IL-3662	Hydrocodone 7.5 mg, Acetaminophen 750 mg	by Forest		Analgesic; C III
IL3711	Tab, Orange, Oval, Film Coated	Rimantadine HCl 100 mg	by RX PAK	65084-0189	Antiviral
IL3853	Tab, Ex Release, Inwood	Theophylline 200 mg	by HL Moore	00839-6729	Antiasthmatic
ILOSONE250MG <> DISTAH09	Cap	Erythromycin 250 mg	Ilosone by DISTA Prod	00777-0809	Antibiotic
ILOSONE250MGH09	Cap, Ivory & Opaque, Ilosone 250 mg/H09	Erythromycin 250 mg	by Lilly	Canadian	Antibiotic
IMAX100	Cap, Red	Isometheptene Mucate 65 mg, Dichloralphenazone 100 mg, Acetaminophen 325 mg	Midrin by Breckenridge	51991-0395	Analgesic
IMDUR <> 120	Tab, White, Oval	Isosorbide Mononitrate 120 mg	Imdur by Schering	00085-1153	Antianginal
IMDUR <> 120	Tab	Isosorbide Mononitrate 120 mg	Imdur by Pharm Utilization	60491-0314	Antianginal
IMDUR <> 120MG	Tab, White	Isosorbide Mononitrate 120 mg	Imdur by Murfreesboro	51129-1574	Antianginal
IMDUR <> 30	Tab, Rose	Isosorbide Mononitrate 30 mg	Imdur ER by Schering	00085-3306	Antianginal
IMDUR <> 3030	Tab, Rose	Isosorbide Mononitrate 30 mg	Imdur by Caremark	00339-6002	Antianginal
IMDUR <> 3030	Tab, ER	Isosorbide Mononitrate 30 mg	Imdur by Astra AB	17228-3306	Antianginal
IMDUR <> 30MG	Tab, Red, Oval, Scored	Isosorbide Mononitrate 30 mg	Imdur by Murfreesboro	51129-1573	Antianginal
IMDUR <> 60	Tab, ER	Isosorbide Mononitrate 60 mg	Imdur by Caremark	00339-6004	Antianginal
IMDUR <> 60	Tab, Yellow	Isosorbide Mononitrate 60 mg	Imdur ER by Schering	00085-4110	Antianginal
IMDUR <> 60	Tab, ER	Isosorbide Mononitrate 60 mg	Imdur by Caremark	00339-6003	Antianginal
IMDUR <> 60	Tab, ER	Isosorbide Mononitrate 60 mg	Imdur by Nat Pharmpak Serv	55154-3512	Antianginal
IMDUR <> 60MG	Tab, Yellow, Scored	Isosorbide Mononitrate 60 mg	Imdur by Murfreesboro	51129-1575	Antianginal
IMITREX <> 50	Tab, Coated	Sumatriptan Succinate 50 mg	Imitrex by Physicians Total Care	54868-3852	Antimigraine
IMITREX <> 50	Tab, Coated	Sumatriptan Succinate 50 mg	Imitrex by Pharm Utilization	60491-0318	Antimigraine
IMITREX <> 50	Tab, Coated	Sumatriptan Succinate 50 mg	Imitrex by Glaxo	00173-0459	Antimigraine
IMODIUM <> JANSSEN	Cap, Dark Green & Light Green	Loperamide 2 mg	Imodium by Janssen	50458-0400	Antidiarrheal
IMODIUM <> JANSSEN	Cap, Dark Green & Light Green	Loperamide 2 mg	Imodium by Johnson & Johnson	59604-0400	Antidiarrheal
IMODIUM <> JANSSEN	Cap, Dark Green & Light Green	Loperamide 2 mg	Imodium by Quality Care	60346-0942	Antidiarrheal
IMODIUM <> JANSSEN	Cap, Light Green	Loperamide HCl 2 mg	Imodium by Allscripts	54569-0219	Antidiarrheal
IMODIUM2125	Tab, Green, Round, Scored, Chewable, Imodium 2/125	Loperamide 2 mg, Simethicone 125 mg	Imodium by McNeil	Canadian DIN# 02237297	Antidiarrheal
IMODIUMAD2MG	Cap, Light Green, Scored, Imodium A-D 2 mg	Loperamide 2 mg	Imodium by McNeil	Canadian DIN# 02183862	Antidiarrheal
IMOVANE	Tab, Blue, Oval, Logo	Zopiclone 7.5 mg	by Rhodiapharm	Canadian	Hypnotic
IMURAN <> 50	Tab, Off-White to Yellow, Overlapping Circle Shape	Azathioprine 50 mg	Imuran by Catalytica	63552-0597	Immunosuppressant
IMURAN 50	Tab, Yellow, Dumbbell	Azathioprine 50 mg	by Glaxo	Canadian	Immunosuppressant
IMURAN50	Tab	Azathioprine 50 mg	Imuran by Glaxo	00173-0597	Immunosuppressant
IMURAN50MG	Tab, Peanut Shaped	Azathioprine 50 mg	Imuran by Pharmedix	53002-0486	Immunosuppressant

ID FRONT <> BACK	DESCRIPTION FRONT <> BACK	INGREDIENT & STRENGTH	BRAND (OR EQUIV.) & FIRM	NDC#	CLASS; SCH.
IND25	Cap, Cream	Indomethacin 25 mg	Rhodacine by Rhodiapharm	Canadian	NSAID
IND50	Cap, Light Brown	Indomethacin 50 mg	Rhodacine by Rhodiapharm	Canadian	NSAID
INDERAL10	Tab	Propranolol HCl 10 mg	by Med Pro	53978-0034	Antihypertensive
INDERAL10	Tab, Embossed with an I	Propranolol HCl 10 mg	Inderal by Drug Distr	52985-0036	Antihypertensive
INDERAL10	Tab	Propranolol HCl 10 mg	Inderal by Nat Pharmpak Serv	55154-0204	Antihypertensive
INDERAL10	Tab, Embossed with an I	Propranolol HCl 10 mg	Inderal by Leiner	59606-0660	Antihypertensive
INDERAL10 <> I	Tab	Propranolol HCl 10 mg	Inderal by Ayerst	00046-0421	Antihypertensive
INDERAL10 <> I	Tab	Propranolol HCl 10 mg	Inderal by Amerisource	62584-0421	Antihypertensive
INDERAL10 <> I	Tab	Propranolol HCl 10 mg	Inderal by Thrift Drug	59198-0038	Antihypertensive
INDERAL20	Tab, Embossed with I <> Ayerst	Propranolol HCl 20 mg	Inderal by Caremark	00339-5167	Antihypertensive
INDERAL20	Tab, Embossed with an I	Propranolol HCl 20 mg	Inderal by Drug Distr	52985-0037	Antihypertensive
INDERAL20	Tab, Embossed with an I	Propranolol HCl 20 mg	Inderal by Leiner	59606-0661	Antihypertensive
INDERAL20 <> I	Tab, Powder Blue, Inderal over 20 <> Raised I	Propranolol HCl 20 mg	Inderal by Ayerst	00046-0422	Antihypertensive
INDERAL20 <> I	Tab, Imprinted <> Embossed	Propranolol HCl 10 mg	Inderal by Nat Pharmpak Serv	55154-0204	Antihypertensive
INDERAL20 <> I	Tab, Blue, Hexagon, Scored	Propranolol HCl 20 mg	Inderal by Right Pak	65240-0668	Antihypertensive
INDERAL20 <> I	Tab	Propranolol HCl 20 mg	Inderal by Thrift Drug	59198-0039	Antihypertensive
INDERAL20 <> I	Tab, Imprinted <> Embossed	Propranolol HCl 20 mg	Inderal by PDRX	55289-0131	Antihypertensive
INDERAL20 <> I	Tab	Propranolol HCl 20 mg	Inderal by Nat Pharmpak Serv	55154-0205	Antihypertensive
INDERAL40	Tab, Embossed with an I	Propranolol HCl 40 mg	Inderal by Amerisource	62584-0422	Antihypertensive
INDERAL40	Tab	Propranolol HCl 40 mg	Inderal by Drug Distr	52985-0019	Antihypertensive
INDERAL40	Tab, Embossed with an I	Propranolol HCl 40 mg	Inderal by Nat Pharmpak Serv	55154-0206	Antihypertensive
INDERAL40	Tab, Green, Hexagon, Scored	Propranolol HCl 40 mg	Inderal by Leiner	59606-0662	Antihypertensive
INDERAL40 <> I	Tab, Mint Green, Inderal over 40 <> Raised I	Propranolol HCl 40 mg	Inderal by Rightpak	65240-0662	Antihypertensive
INDERAL40 <> I	Tab	Propranolol HCl 40 mg	Inderal by Ayerst	00046-0424	Antihypertensive
INDERAL40 <> I	Tab	Propranolol HCl 40 mg	Inderal by Thrift Drug	59198-0040	Antihypertensive
INDERAL40 <> I	Tab, Green, Hexagon, Scored	Propranolol HCl 40 mg	Inderal by Amerisource	62584-0424	Antihypertensive
INDERAL60 <> I	Tab, Inderal over 60 <> Raised I	Propranolol HCl 60 mg	Inderal by Right Pak	65240-0741	Antihypertensive
INDERAL80	Tab, Embossed with an I	Propranolol HCl 80 mg	Inderal by Ayerst	00046-0426	Antihypertensive
INDERAL80 <> I	Tab	Propranolol HCl 80 mg	Inderal by Leiner	59606-0663	Antihypertensive
INDERAL80 <> I	Cap	Propranolol HCl 80 mg	Inderal by Ayerst	00046-0428	Antihypertensive
INDERAL80 <> I	Tab	Propranolol HCl 80 mg	Inderal LA by Murfreesboro	51129-1304	Antihypertensive
INDERAL80 <> I	Tab	Propranolol HCl 80 mg	Inderal by Thrift Drug	59198-0041	Antihypertensive
INDERAL80 <> I	Tab, Coated, Embossed	Propranolol HCl 80 mg	Inderal by Amerisource	62584-0428	Antihypertensive
INDERAL80 <> I	Tab, Coated, Embossed	Propranolol HCl 80 mg	Inderal by Nat Pharmpak Serv	55154-0208	Antihypertensive
INDERAL80	Tab	Propranolol HCl 80 mg	Inderal by Pharm Utilization	60491-0319	Antihypertensive
INDERALLA	Cap, ER, Printed on Wide White Band <> 3 Narrow White Band	Propranolol HCl 80 mg	Inderal by Caremark	00339-5171	Antihypertensive
INDERALLA120	Cap, Dark Blue & Light Blue, Inderal-LA 120	Propranolol HCl 120 mg	Inderal LA by Repack Co of Amer	55306-0080	Antihypertensive
INDERALLA120	Cap, Blue	Propranolol HCl 120 mg	by Wyeth-Ayerst	Canadian	Antihypertensive
INDERALLA120	Cap, Dark Blue & Light Blue, 3 White Bands	Propranolol HCl 120 mg	Inderal LA by Rightpak	65240-0666	Antihypertensive
INDERALLA120	Cap, Dark Blue & Light Blue, 3 Narrow Bands, 1 Wide Band	Propranolol HCl 120 mg	Inderal LA by Ayerst	00046-0473	Antihypertensive
INDERALLA120	Cap, Dark Blue & Light Blue, 3 Narrow Bands	Propranolol HCl 120 mg	Inderal LA by Physicians Total Care	54868-1442	Antihypertensive
INDERALLA120	Cap, ER, Inderal LA 120 <> Lines	Propranolol HCl 120 mg	Inderal LA by Thrift Drug	59198-0043	Antihypertensive
INDERALLA120	Cap, 3 Narrow Bands, 1 Wide Band	Propranolol HCl 120 mg	Inderal LA by Nat Pharmpak Serv	55154-0202	Antihypertensive
INDERALLA120	Cap, Blue, 3 Narrow Bands, 1 Wide Band	Propranolol HCl 120 mg	Inderal LA by Amerisource	62584-0473	Antihypertensive
INDERALLA160	Cap, Dark blue, Inderal-LA 160	Propranolol HCl 160 mg	Inderal LA by RX PAK	65084-0104	Antihypertensive
INDERALLA160	Cap, ER, Inderal LA 120 in White Letters <> 3 White Stripes	Propranolol HCl 160 mg	by Wyeth-Ayerst	Canadian	Antihypertensive
INDERALLA160	Cap, Dark Blue, Ex Release, Inderal LA 160 <> 3 Narrow Bands, 1 Wide Band	Propranolol HCl 160 mg	Inderal LA by Ayerst	00046-0479	Antihypertensive
INDERALLA160	Cap, ER, Inderal LA 160 <> Identified by 3 Bands, 1 Wide	Propranolol HCl 160 mg	Inderal LA by Thrift Drug	59198-0044	Antihypertensive
INDERALLA160	Cap, ER, Inderal LA 160 <> 3 Narrow Bands and 1 Wide band	Propranolol HCl 160 mg	Inderal LA by Amerisource	62584-0479	Antihypertensive
INDERALLA160	Cap, ER, Inderal LA 160 <> Lines	Propranolol HCl 160 mg	Inderal LA by Pharm Utilization	60491-0323	Antihypertensive
			Inderal LA by Nat Pharmpak Serv	55154-0203	Antihypertensive

ID FRONT <> BACK	DESCRIPTION FRONT <> BACK	INGREDIENT & STRENGTH	BRAND (OR EQUIV.) & FIRM	NDC#	CLASS; SCH.
INDERALLA60	Cap, Blue & White, 3 Narrow Bands and 1 Wide Band and Inderal LA 60	Lansoprazole 60 mg	Inderal LA by Murfreesboro	51129-1625	Gastrointestinal
INDERALLA60	Cap, Light Blue & White, Inderal-LA 60	Propranolol HCl 60 mg	by Wyeth-Ayerst	Canadian	Antihypertensive
INDERALLA60	Cap, White	Propranolol HCl 60 mg	Inderal LA by Rightpak	65240-0664	Antihypertensive
INDERALLA60	Cap, Blue & White, Ex Release, Inderal LA 60 <> 3 White Stripes	Propranolol HCl 60 mg	Inderal LA by Ayerst	00046-0470	Antihypertensive
INDERALLA60	Cap, Blue & White, Inderal LA 60, 3 Narrow Bands and 1 Wide Band	Propranolol HCl 60 mg	Inderal LA by RX PAK	65084-0105	Antihypertensive
INDERALLA60	Cap, Blue & White, Inderal LA 60 Within the Blue Band <> 3 Narrow Bands	Propranolol HCl 60 mg	Inderal LA by Respa	60575-0733	Antihypertensive
INDERALLA60	Cap, Light Blue, Ex Release, Inderal LA 60, 3 Narrow Bands, 1 Wide Band	Propranolol HCl 60 mg	Inderal LA by Thrift Drug	59198-0226	Antihypertensive
INDERALLA60	Cap, ER	Propranolol HCl 60 mg	Inderal LA by Leiner	59606-0664	Antihypertensive
INDERALLA80	Cap, Blue	Propranolol HCl 80 mg	Inderal LA by Rightpak	65240-0665	Antihypertensive
INDERALLA80	Cap, Light Blue, Inderal-LA 80	Propranolol HCl 80 mg	by Wyeth-Ayerst	Canadian	Antihypertensive
INDERALLA80	Cap, ER, Inderal LA 80 <>3 Narrow Bands, 1 Wide Band	Propranolol HCl 80 mg	Inderal LA by Physicians Total Care	54868-0680	Antihypertensive
INDERALLA80	Cap, Light Blue, Ex Release, Inderal LA 80 <> Three Narrow Bands on One End	Propranolol HCl 80 mg	Inderal LA by Thrift Drug	59198-0042	Antihypertensive
INDERALLA80	Cap, Blue, Inderal LA 80	Propranolol HCl 80 mg	Inderal LA by Rising Pharma	64980-0101	Antihypertensive
INDERALLA80	Cap, Blue, Inderal 80, 3 Narrow Bands and 1 Wide Band	Propranolol HCl 80 mg	Inderal LA by RX PAK	65084-0103	Antihypertensive
INDERALLA80	Cap, ER, Inderal LA 80 <> 3 Narrow Bands, 1 Wide Band	Propranolol HCl 80 mg	Inderal LA by Amerisource	62584-0471	Antihypertensive
INDERALLA80	Cap	Propranolol HCl 80 mg	Inderal LA by Nat Pharmpak Serv	55154-0201	Antihypertensive
INDERIDE4025 <> I	Tab, Inderide 40 Over 25 <> Raised I	Hydrochlorothiazide 25 mg, Propranolol HCl 40 mg	Inderide by Ayerst	00046-0484	Diuretic; Antihypertensive
INDERIDELA12050	Cap, ER, Inderide LA 120/50	Hydrochlorothiazide 50 mg, Propranolol HCl 120 mg	Inderide LA by Pharm Utilization	60491-0328	Diuretic; Antihypertensive
INDERIDELA16050	Cap, ER, Inderide LA 160/50	Hydrochlorothiazide 50 mg, Propranolol HCl 160 mg	Inderide LA by Pharm Utilization	60491-0329	Diuretic; Antihypertensive
INDERIDELA8050	Cap, ER, Inderide LA 80/50	Hydrochlorothiazide 50 mg, Propranolol HCl 80 mg	Inderide LA by Pharm Utilization	60491-0327	Diuretic; Antihypertensive
INDOCIN <> MSD25	Cap, Light Blue & White	Indomethacin 25 mg	Indocin by Merck	00006-0025	NSAID
INDOCINSR <> 695	Cap, Clear	Indomethacin 75 mg	Indocin SR by Murfreesboro	51129-1551	NSAID
INDOCINSR <> MSD693	Cap, Blue & Clear & Opaque, Indocin SR Containing Blue & White Pellets	Indomethacin 75 mg	Indocin SR by Murfreesboro	51129-1548	NSAID
INDOCINSR695	Cap, Clear, Blue & White Pellets, Indocin SR over 695	Indomethacin 75 mg	by Allscripts	54569-0279	NSAID
INDOCINSR695	Cap, Clear, Indocin SR Over 695, Black Ink	Indomethacin 75 mg	Indocin SR by Murfreesboro	51129-1550	NSAID
INDOCINSRMSD693	Cap	Indomethacin 75 mg	Indocin Sr by Allscripts	54569-0279	NSAID
INDOTEC25TEC	Cap, Blue & White, Indotec 25/TEC	Indomethacin 25 mg	by Technilab	Canadian DIN# 02143364	NSAID
INDOTEC50TEC	Cap, Blue & White, Indotec 50/TEC	Indomethacin 50 mg	by Technilab	Canadian DIN# 02143372	NSAID
INGELHEIM TOWERLOGO	Tab, White, Round	Dipyridamole 100 mg	by Boehringer Ingelheim	Canadian	Antiplatelet
INGELHEIM TOWERLOGO	Tab, Orange, Round	Dipyridamole 25 mg	by Boehringer Ingelheim	Canadian	Antiplatelet
INGELHEIM TOWERLOGO	Tab, Red, Round	Dipyridamole 50 mg	by Boehringer Ingelheim	Canadian	Antiplatelet
INGELHEIM TOWERLOGO	Tab, Orange & Red, Round	Dipyridamole 75 mg	by Boehringer Ingelheim	Canadian	Antiplatelet
INOR	Tab, White, Round	Levonorgestrel 0.75 mg	Plan B by Womens Capital	64836-0000	Oral Contraceptive

ID FRONT <> BACK	DESCRIPTION FRONT <> BACK	INGREDIENT & STRENGTH	BRAND (OR EQUIV.) & FIRM	NDC#	CLASS; SCH.
INOR	Tab, White, Round	Levonorgestrel 0.75 mg	by Chem Works Gedeon	45541-1223	Oral Contraceptive
INV <> 205	Tab, Film Coated	Hydrochlorothiazide 15 mg, Methyldopa 250 mg	by Qualitest	00603-4543	Diuretic; Antihypertensive
INV <> 206	Tab, Film Coated	Hydrochlorothiazide 25 mg, Methyldopa 250 mg	by Qualitest	00603-4544	Diuretic; Antihypertensive
INV <> 211	Cap	Amantadine HCl 100 mg	by Caremark	00339-5780	Antiviral
INV <> 211	Cap, Red	Amantadine HCl 100 mg	by Apotheca	12634-0539	Antiviral
INV <> 250	Tab, White, Oblong, Film Coated	Hydroxychloroquine Sulfate 200 mg	by Murfreesboro Ph	51129-1426	Antimalarial
INV <> 250	Tab, White, Oblong, Film Coated	Hydroxychloroquine Sulfate 200 mg	by DRX Pharm Consults	55045-2766	Antimalarial
INV <> 250	Tab, Film Coated	Hydroxychloroquine Sulfate 200 mg	by Invamed	52189-0250	Antimalarial
INV <> 252	Tab, Film Coated	Cyclobenzaprine HCl 10 mg	by Physicians Total Care	54868-1110	Muscle Relaxant
INV <> 259	Tab	Atenolol 25 mg	by Apothecon	62269-0259	Antihypertensive
INV <> 259	Tab	Atenolol 25 mg	by Invamed	52189-0259	Antihypertensive
INV <> 261	Tab, White, Round	Methazolamide 25 mg	by Apothecon	62269-0261	Diuretic
INV <> 261	Tab, White, Round	Methazolamide 25 mg	by Invamed	52189-0261	Diuretic
INV <> 271	Tab, Scored	Captopril 12.5 mg	by Schein	00364-2628	Antihypertensive
INV <> 271	Tab, Scored	Captopril 12.5 mg	by Invamed	52189-0271	Antihypertensive
INV <> 278	Tab, Purple, Round, Film Coated	Trifluoperazine HCl 1 mg	by Apothecon	62269-0278	Antipsychotic
INV <> 278	Tab, Purple, Round, Film Coated	Trifluoperazine HCl 1 mg	by Invamed	52189-0278	Antipsychotic
INV100274	Tab, White, Oval	Captopril 100 mg	Capoten by Invamed		Antihypertensive
INV101	Tab, White, Round	Valu-Foam	Gaviscon by Duramed		GERD
INV208	Tab, White, Round	Benztropine Mesylate 0.5 mg	by Apothecon	62269-0208	Antiparkinson
INV208	Tab	Benztropine Mesylate 0.5 mg	by Heartland	61392-0167	Antiparkinson
INV208	Tab, Scored, INV over 208	Benztropine Mesylate 0.5 mg	by Invamed	52189-0208	Antiparkinson
INV209	Tab	Benztropine Mesylate 1 mg	by Heartland	61392-0170	Antiparkinson
INV209	Tab	Benztropine Mesylate 1 mg	by Golden State	60429-0027	Antiparkinson
INV209	Tab, Identification Logo INV and 209	Benztropine Mesylate 1 mg	by Quality Care	60346-0776	Antiparkinson
INV209	Tab, White, Oval	Benztropine Mesylate 1 mg	by Apothecon	62269-0209	Antiparkinson
INV209	Tab, Scored, INV over 209	Benztropine Mesylate 1 mg	by Invamed	52189-0209	Antiparkinson
INV210	Tab	Benztropine Mesylate 2 mg	by Quality Care	60346-0699	Antiparkinson
INV210	Tab, White, Orund	Benztropine Mesylate 2 mg	by Apothecon	62269-0210	Antiparkinson
INV210	Tab	Benztropine Mesylate 2 mg	by Golden State	60429-0028	Antiparkinson
INV210	Tab	Benztropine Mesylate 2 mg	by Geneva	00781-1367	Antiparkinson
INV210	Tab, Scored, INV over 210	Benztropine Mesylate 2 mg	by Invamed	52189-0210	Antiparkinson
INV210	Tab	Benztropine Mesylate 2 mg	by Med Pro	53978-2093	Antiparkinson
INV211	Cap	Amantadine HCl 100 mg	by Qualitest	00603-2164	Antiviral
INV211	Cap, INV Over 211	Amantadine HCl 100 mg	by Invamed	52189-0211	Antiviral
INV211	Cap	Amantadine HCl 100 mg	by Quality Care	60346-0079	Antiviral
INV211	Cap, Red	Amantadine HCl 100 mg	by Apothecon	62269-0211	Antiviral
INV211 <> INV211	Cap, Red	Amantadine HCl 100 mg	by Apotheca	12634-0538	Antiviral
INV220	Tab, Yellow, Round	Aspirin Delayed Release (E.C.) 15 gr	Easprin by Duramed		Analgesic
INV221	Tab, White, Round	Ibuprofen 200 mg	Advil by Invamed		NSAID
INV221	Tab, White, Round, Film Coated, INV 221	Ibuprofen 200 mg	Nuprin by Geneva	00781-1349	NSAID
INV227	Tab	Metoclopramide 5 mg	by Zenith Goldline	00182-1898	Gastrointestinal
INV228	Tab, Film Coated, INV over 228	Cimetidine 200 mg	by Invamed	52189-0228	Gastrointestinal
INV228	Tab, Film Coated, INV Over 228	Cimetidine 200 mg	by Apothecon	62269-0228	Gastrointestinal
INV229	Tab, Film Coated, INV Over 229	Cimetidine 300 mg	by Apothecon	62269-0229	Gastrointestinal
INV229	Tab, Film Coated, INV over 229	Cimetidine 300 mg	by Invamed	52189-0229	Gastrointestinal
INV230	Tab, Film Coated, INV/230	Cimetidine 400 mg	by Apothecon	62269-0230	Gastrointestinal
INV230	Tab, Film Coated, Scored	Cimetidine 400 mg	by Invamed	52189-0230	Gastrointestinal
INV231	Tab, Film Coated, INV/231	Cimetidine 800 mg	by Apothecon	62269-0231	Gastrointestinal
INV231	Tab, Film Coated, Scored	Cimetidine 800 mg	by Invamed	52189-0231	Gastrointestinal

ID FRONT <> BACK	DESCRIPTION FRONT <> BACK	INGREDIENT & STRENGTH	BRAND (OR EQUIV.) & FIRM	NDC#	CLASS; SCH.
INV232	Tab, White, Oblong	Aspirin SR 800 mg	ZORprin by Duramed		Analgesic
INV234	Tab	Chlorpheniramine Tannate 8 mg, Phenylephrine Tannate 25 mg, Pyrilamine Tannate 25 mg	R Tannamine by Qualitest	00603-5687	Cold Remedy
INV234	Tab	Chlorpheniramine Tannate 8 mg, Phenylephrine Tannate 25 mg, Pyrilamine Tannate 25 mg	R Tannamine by Physicians Total Care	54868-2189	Cold Remedy
INV236 <> 20	Tab	Nadolol 20 mg	Nadolol by Schein	00364-2652	Antihypertensive
INV236 <> 20	Tab, Engraved INV Above and 236 Below the Bisect	Nadolol 20 mg	Nadolol by Invamed	52189-0236	Antihypertensive
INV236 <> 20	Tab	Nadolol 20 mg	Nadolol by Major	00904-5069	Antihypertensive
INV236 <> 20	Tab, INV/236 <> 20	Nadolol 20 mg	Nadolol by Geneva	00781-1181	Antihypertensive
INV236 <> 20	Tab	Nadolol 20 mg	Nadolol by HL Moore	00839-7869	Antihypertensive
INV237 <> 40	Tab	Nadolol 40 mg	Nadolol by Schein	00364-2653	Antihypertensive
INV237 <> 40	Tab, Engraved INV Above and 237 Below the Bisect	Nadolol 40 mg	Nadolol by Invamed	52189-0237	Antihypertensive
INV237 <> 40	Tab	Nadolol 40 mg	Nadolol by Major	00904-5070	Antihypertensive
INV237 <> 40	Tab	Nadolol 40 mg	Nadolol by Geneva	00781-1182	Antihypertensive
INV237 <> 40	Tab	Nadolol 40 mg	Nadolol by HL Moore	00839-7870	Antihypertensive
INV238 <> 80	Tab, Engraved INV Above and 238 Below the Bisect	Nadolol 80 mg	Nadolol by Invamed	52189-0238	Antihypertensive
INV238 <> 80	Tab	Nadolol 80 mg	Nadolol by Geneva	00781-1183	Antihypertensive
INV238 <> 80	Tab	Nadolol 80 mg	Nadolol by Major	00904-5071	Antihypertensive
INV238 <> 80	Tab	Nadolol 80 mg	Nadolol by HL Moore	00839-7871	Antihypertensive
INV238 <> 80	Tab	Nadolol 80 mg	Nadolol by Schein	00364-2654	Antihypertensive
INV241	Tab, White, Oval	Choline Magnesium Trisalate 500 mg	Trilisate by Duramed		NSAID
INV241	Tab, Yellow, Oblong	Choline Magnesium Trisalicylate 500 mg	Trilisate by Invamed		NSAID
INV242	Tab, White, Oval	Choline Magnesium Trisalate 750 mg	Trilisate by Duramed		NSAID
INV242	Cap, Blue, INV/242	Choline Magnesium Trisalicylate 750 mg	Trilisate by Invamed		NSAID
INV244	Tab, Coated, INV and 244	Salsalate 750 mg	by Quality Care	60346-0034	NSAID
INV246	Tab, Film Coated, Engraved INV Above 246	Indapamide 1.25 mg	by Invamed	52189-0246	Diuretic
INV246	Tab, Film Coated, Engraved INV Above 246	Indapamide 1.25 mg	by Apothecon	62269-0246	Diuretic
INV247	Tab, Film Coated, INV Above 247	Indapamide 2.5 mg	by Invamed	52189-0247	Diuretic
INV247	Tab, Film Coated, INV Above 247	Indapamide 2.5 mg	by Apothecon	62269-0247	Diuretic
INV250	Tab, Film Coated	Hydroxychloroquine Sulfate 200 mg	by Apothecon	62269-0250	Antimalarial
INV252	Tab, Film Coated, INV over 252	Cyclobenzaprine HCl 10 mg	by Invamed	52189-0252	Muscle Relaxant
INV252	Tab, Film Coated	Cyclobenzaprine HCl 10 mg	by Urgent Care Ctr	50716-0932	Muscle Relaxant
INV252	Tab, Film Coated, INV over 252	Cyclobenzaprine HCl 10 mg	by Apothecon	62269-0252	Muscle Relaxant
INV252	Tab, Film Coated, INV over 252	Cyclobenzaprine HCl 10 mg	by Quality Care	60346-0581	Muscle Relaxant
INV25272	Tab, White, Round	Captopril 25 mg	Capoten by Invamed		Antihypertensive
INV256	Tab, Invamed Logo	Atenolol 50 mg	by Quality Care	60346-0719	Antihypertensive
INV256	Tab, INV over 256	Atenolol 50 mg	by Apothecon	62269-0256	Antihypertensive
INV256	Tab, Scored, INV over 256	Atenolol 50 mg	by Invamed	52189-0256	Antihypertensive
INV256	Tab	Atenolol 50 mg	by Med Pro	53978-1199	Antihypertensive
INV257	Tab, INV over 257	Atenolol 100 mg	by Apothecon	62269-0257	Antihypertensive
INV257	Tab, INV over 257	Atenolol 100 mg	by Invamed	52189-0257	Antihypertensive
INV260	Tab, White, Round, Scored	Methazolamide 50 mg	by Invamed	52189-0260	Diuretic
INV260	Tab, White, Round, Scored	Methazolamide 50 mg	by Apothecon	62269-0260	Diuretic
INV260	Tab, White, Round	Methazolamide 50 mg	Neptazane by Invamed		Diuretic
INV261	Tab, White, Round	Methazolamide 25 mg	Neptazane by Invamed		Diuretic
INV262	Tab, Brown, Oblong, Film	Ibuprofen 200 mg	by Murfreesboro	51129-1517	NSAID
INV263	Tab, INV Over 263	Metoclopramide 5 mg	by Zenith Goldline	00182-1898	Gastrointestinal
INV263	Tab, INV Over 263	Metoclopramide 5 mg	by Invamed	52189-0263	Gastrointestinal
INV263	Tab, INV Over 263	Metoclopramide 5 mg	by Apothecon	62269-0263	Gastrointestinal
INV263	Tab, INV Over 263	Metoclopramide 5 mg	by United Res	00677-1323	Gastrointestinal
INV264	Tab, INV Above and 264 Below Bisect	Metoclopramide 10 mg	by Invamed	52189-0264	Gastrointestinal
INV264	Tab, INV Above and 264 Below Bisect	Metoclopramide 10 mg	by Apothecon	62269-0264	Gastrointestinal

ID FRONT <> BACK	DESCRIPTION FRONT <> BACK	INGREDIENT & STRENGTH	BRAND (OR EQUIV.) & FIRM	NDC#	CLASS; SCH.
INV265	Tab, Green & White, Round	Orphenadrine 25 mg, Aspirin 325 mg, Caffeine 30 mg	Norgesic by Invamed		Muscle Relaxant
INV265	Tab, Green & White, Round	Orphenadrine Citrate 25 mg, Aspirin 385 mg, Caffeine 30 mg	by Apothecon	62269-0265	Muscle Relaxant
INV265	Tab, Green & White, Round	Orphenadrine Citrate 25 mg; Aspirin 428 mg; Caffeine 30 mg	Invagesic by Invamed	52189-0265	Muscle Relaxant
INV266	Tab, Green & White, Oblong	Orphenadrine 50 mg, Aspirin 770 mg, Caffeine 60 mg	Norgesic Forte by Invamed		Muscle Relaxant
INV266	Tab, Green & White, Cap-Shaped	Orphenadrine Citrate 50 mg, Aspirin 750 mg, Caffeine 60 mg	by Apothecon	62269-0266	Muscle Relaxant
INV266	Tab, Green & White, Oblong, Scored	Orphenadrine Citrate 50 mg; Aspirin 856 mg; Caffeine 60 mg	Invagesic Forte by Invamed	52189-0266	Muscle Relaxant
INV266	Tab, Green & White, Oblong, Scored	Orphenadrine Citrate 50 mg, Caffeine 60 mg, Aspirin 856 mg	by DRX Pharm Consults	55045-2777	Muscle Relaxant
INV272 <> 25	Tab, INV over 272	Captopril 25 mg	by Schein	00364-2629	Antihypertensive
INV272 <> 25	Tab, Quadrisected, INV over 272 <> 25	Captopril 25 mg	by Invamed	52189-0272	Antihypertensive
INV273 <> 50	Tab, Scored	Captopril 50 mg	by Invamed	52189-0273	Antihypertensive
INV274 <> 100	Tab, Scored	Captopril 100 mg	by Invamed	52189-0274	Antihypertensive
INV275 <> 5	Tab, Pale Yellow, Round	Prochlorperazine 10 mg	by Apothecon	62269-0275	Antiemetic
INV275 <> 5	Tab, Yellow, Round, Film Coated	Prochlorperazine Maleate 5 mg	by Murfreesboro Ph	51129-1427	Antiemetic
INV275 <> 5	Tab, Yellow, Round, Film Coated	Prochlorperazine Maleate 5 mg	by Invamed	52189-0275	Antiemetic
INV2755	Tab, Pale Yellow, Round	Prochlorperazine 5 mg	Compazine by Invamed		Antiemetic
INV276 <> 10	Tab, Pale Yellow, Round	Prochlorperazine 10 mg	by Apothecon	62269-0276	Antiemetic
INV276 <> 10	Tab, Yellow, Round, Film Coated	Prochlorperazine Maleate 10 mg	by Invamed	52189-0276	Antiemetic
INV276 <> 10	Tab, Yellow, Round, Film Coated	Prochlorperazine Maleate 10 mg	by Apotheca	12634-0676	Antiemetic
INV27610	Tab, Yellow, Round	Prochlorperazine 10 mg	Compazine by Invamed		Antiemetic
INV277 <> 25	Tab, Yellow, Round, Film Coated	Prochlorperazine Maleate 25 mg	by Invamed	52189-0277	Antiemetic
INV27725	Tab, Yellow, Round	Prochlorperazine 25 mg	Compazine by Invamed	52152-0188	Antiemetic
INV278	Tab, Lavender, Round	Trifluoperazine HCl 1 mg	Stelazine by Invamed		Antipsychotic
INV279	Tab, Lavender, Round	Trifluoperazine HCl 2 mg	Stelazine by Invamed		Antipsychotic
INV279	Tab, Purple, Round, Film Coated	Trifluoperazine HCl 2 mg	by Apothecon	62269-0279	Antipsychotic
INV279 <> 2	Tab, Purple, Round, Film Coated	Trifluoperazine HCl 2 mg	by Invamed	52189-0279	Antipsychotic
INV280	Tab, Purple, Round, Film Coated	Trifluoperazine HCl 10 mg	by Apothecon	62269-0281	Antipsychotic
INV280	Tab, Lavender, Round	Trifluoperazine HCl 5 mg	Stelazine by Invamed		Antipsychotic
INV280 <> 5	Tab, Purple, Round, Film Coated	Trifluoperazine HCl 5 mg	by Invamed	52189-0280	Antipsychotic
INV280 <> 5	Tab, Purple, Round, Film Coated	Trifluoperazine HCl 5 mg	by Apothecon	62269-0280	Antipsychotic
INV281	Tab, Lavender, Round	Trifluoperazine HCl 10 mg	Stelazine by Invamed		Antipsychotic
INV281 <> 10	Tab, Purple, Round, Film Coated	Trifluoperazine HCl 10 mg	by Invamed	52189-0281	Antipsychotic
INV286	Tab, Coated	Naproxen Sodium 275 mg	by Zenith Goldline	00182-1974	NSAID
INV286	Tab, Coated	Naproxen Sodium 275 mg	by Invamed	52189-0286	NSAID
INV286	Tab, Coated	Naproxen Sodium 275 mg	by Apothecon	62269-0286	NSAID
INV286	Tab, Light Blue, Coated	Naproxen Sodium 275 mg	by Qualitest	00603-4733	NSAID
INV287	Tab, White, Oval	Naproxen Sodium 550 mg	by Apothecon	62269-0287	NSAID
INV287	Tab, Film Coated, INV Over 287	Naproxen Sodium 550 mg	by Quality Care	60346-0826	NSAID
INV287	Tab, White, Oval, Film, Debossed INV 287	Naproxen Sodium 550 mg	by Par	49884-0499	NSAID
INV287	Tab, Coated	Naproxen Sodium 550 mg	by Invamed	52189-0287	NSAID
INV287	Tab, Light Blue, Film Coated	Naproxen Sodium 550 mg	by Qualitest	00603-4734	NSAID
INV289	Tab, White, Oblong, Film Coated	Naproxen 375 mg	by Apothecon	62269-0289	NSAID
INV289	Tab, White, Oblong, Film Coated	Naproxen 375 mg	by Invamed	52189-0289	NSAID
INV289	Tab, White, Oblong	Naproxen 375 mg	EC Naprosyn by Invamed		NSAID
INV289	Tab, White, Oblong	Naproxen Sodium 375 mg	by Bristol-Myers		NSAID
INV290	Tab, White, Oblong, Film Coated	Naproxen 500 mg	by Invamed	52189-0290	NSAID
INV290	Tab, White, Oblong, Film Coated	Naproxen 500 mg	by Apothecon	62269-0290	NSAID
INV290	Tab, White, Oblong	Naproxen 500 mg	EC Naprosyn by Invamed		NSAID
INV290	Tab, White, Oblong	Naproxen Sodium 500 mg	by Bristol-Myers		NSAID
INV291	Tab, Scored	Glipizide 5 mg	by Invamed	52189-0291	Antidiabetic
INV291	Tab	Glipizide 5 mg	by Quality Care	62682-5002	Antidiabetic
INV291	Tab	Glipizide 5 mg	by Apothecon	62269-0291	Antidiabetic
INV292	Tab, INV/292	Glipizide 10 mg	by Apothecon	62269-0292	Antidiabetic

ID FRONT <> BACK	DESCRIPTION FRONT <> BACK	INGREDIENT & STRENGTH	BRAND (OR EQUIV.) & FIRM	NDC#	CLASS; SCH.
INV292	Tab, Scored	Glipizide 10 mg	by Invamed	52189-0292	Antidiabetic
INV293	Tab, White, Round, Scored	Glyburide 1.5 mg	by Apothecon	62269-0293	Antidiabetic
INV293	Tab, White, Round, Scored	Glyburide 1.5 mg	by Invamed	52189-0293	Antidiabetic
INV293	Tab, White, Round	Glyburide 1.5 mg	by Bristol-Myers		Antidiabetic
INV293	Tab, White, Round	Glyburide 1.5 mg	Glynase by Invamed		Antidiabetic
INV294	Tab, Blue, Round, Scored	Glyburide 3 mg	by Invamed	52189-0294	Antidiabetic
INV294	Tab, Blue, Round, Scored	Glyburide 3 mg	by Apothecon	62269-0294	Antidiabetic
INV294	Tab, Blue, Round	Glyburide 3 mg	Glynase by Invamed		Antidiabetic
INV294	Tab, Blue, Round	Glyburide 3 mg	by Bristol-Myers		Antidiabetic
INV296	Tab, Blue, Round	Salsalate 500 mg	Disalcid by Duramed		NSAID
INV297	Tab, Blue, Oblong	Salsalate 750 mg	Disalcid by Duramed		NSAID
INV309	Tab, Pink, Square	Warfarin Sodium 1 mg	Coumadin by Invamed		Anticoagulant
INV309 <> 1	Tab, Pink, Square, Scored, INV Above 309 Below Bisect	Warfarin Sodium 1 mg	by Torpharm	62318-0027	Anticoagulant
INV309 <> 1	Tab, Pink, Square, Scored, INV Bisect 309	Warfarin Sodium 1 mg	Warfarin Sodium by UDL	51079-0900	Anticoagulant
INV310	Tab, Lavender, Square	Warfarin Sodium 2 mg	Coumadin by Invamed		Anticoagulant
INV310 <> 2	Tab, Purple, Square, INV Above and 310 Below Bisect	Warfarin Sodium 2 mg	by Torpharm	62318-0033	Anticoagulant
INV310 <> 2	Tab, Purple, Square, Scored, INV Bisect 310	Warfarin Sodium 2 mg	Warfarin Sodium by UDL	51079-0901	Anticoagulant
INV3102	Tab, Lavender, Square, INV 310/2	Warfarin Sodium 2 mg	by Bristol-Myers		Anticoagulant
INV311	Tab, Green, Square	Warfarin Sodium 2.5 mg	Coumadin by Invamed		Anticoagulant
INV311 <> 25	Tab, Green, Square, Scored, INV over 311 <> 2.5	Warfarin Sodium 2.5 mg	by Torpharm	62318-0055	Anticoagulant
INV311 <> 25	Tab, Green, Square, Scored, INV over 311 <> 2.5	Warfarin Sodium 2.5 mg	Warfarin Sodium by UDL	51079-0902	Anticoagulant
INV31125	Tab, Green, Square, INV 311/2.5	Warfarin Sodium 2.5 mg	by Bristol-Myers		Anticoagulant
INV312	Tab, Blue, Square	Warfarin Sodium 4 mg	Coumadin by Invamed		Anticoagulant
INV312 <> 4	Tab, Blue, Square, INV Above and 312 Below Bisect	Warfarin Sodium 4 mg	by Torpharm	62318-3438	Anticoagulant
INV312 <> 4	Tab, Blue, Square, Scored, INV Bisect 312	Warfarin Sodium 4 mg	Warfarin Sodium by UDL	51079-0903	Anticoagulant
INV3124	Tab, Blue, Square, INV 312/4	Warfarin Sodium 4 mg	by Bristol-Myers		Anticoagulant
INV313	Tab, Peach, Square	Warfarin Sodium 5 mg	Coumadin by Invamed		Anticoagulant
INV313 <> 5	Tab, Peach, Square, INV Bisect 313	Warfarin Sodium 5 mg	by Trigen	59746-0113	Anticoagulant
INV313 <> 5	Tab, Peach, Square, INV Bisect 313	Warfarin Sodium 5 mg	Warfarin Sodium by UDL	51079-0905	Anticoagulant
INV3135	Tab, Peach, Square, INV 313/5	Warfarin Sodium 5 mg	by Bristol-Myers		Anticoagulant
INV314	Tab, Yellow, Square	Warfarin Sodium 7.5 mg	Coumadin by Invamed		Anticoagulant
INV314 <> 75	Tab, Yellow, Square, Scored, INV 314 <> 7.5	Warfarin Sodium 7.5 mg	Warfarin Sodium by Unimed	00051-5044	Anticoagulant
INV314 <> 75	Tab, Yellow, Square, INV over 314 <> 7.5	Warfarin Sodium 7.5 mg	by Trigen	59746-0115	Anticoagulant
INV31475	Tab, Yellow, Square, INV 314/7.5	Warfarin Sodium 7.5 mg	by Bristol-Myers		Anticoagulant
INV315	Tab, White, Square	Warfarin Sodium 10 mg	Coumadin by Invamed		Anticoagulant
INV315 <> 10	Tab, White, Square, Scored, INV Over 315	Warfarin Sodium 10 mg	Warfarin Sodium by Unimed	00051-5046	Anticoagulant
INV315 <> 10	Tab, White, Square, Scored, INV Above and 315 Below	Warfarin Sodium 10 mg	by Truett	11312-0127	Anticoagulant
INV31510	Tab, White, Square, INV 315/10	Warfarin Sodium 10 mg	by Bristol-Myers		Anticoagulant
INV320	Tab, Film Coated, Scored	Gemfibrozil 600 mg	by Apothecon	62269-0320	Antihyperlipidemic
INV320	Tab, Film Coated, INV to Left, 320 to Right of Score	Gemfibrozil 600 mg	by Golden State	60429-0081	Antihyperlipidemic
INV320	Tab, White, Oval, Scored, Film Coated	Gemfibrozil 600 mg	by Kaiser	00179-1292	Antihyperlipidemic
INV320	Tab, Film Coated, Scored	Gemfibrozil 600 mg	by Invamed	52189-0320	Antihyperlipidemic
INV321	Cap, Orange & White	Clomipramine HCl 25 mg	Anafranil by Invamed		OCD
INV321 <> INV321	Cap, White & Yellow, Gelatin	Clomipramine HCl 25 mg	by Invamed	52189-0321	OCD
INV321 <> INV321	Cap, White & Yellow, Hard Gel	Clomipramine HCl 25 mg	by Apothecon	62269-0321	OCD
INV322	Cap, Blue	Clomipramine HCl 50 mg	Anafranil by Invamed		OCD
INV322 <> INV322	Cap, Blue & White, Gelatin	Clomipramine HCl 50 mg	by Invamed	52189-0322	OCD
INV322 <> INV322	Cap, Blue & White	Clomipramine HCl 50 mg	by Apothecon	62269-0322	OCD
INV323	Cap, Yellow	Clomipramine HCl 75 mg	Anafranil by Invamed		OCD
INV323 <> INV323	Cap, White & Yellow	Clomipramine HCl 75 mg	by Invamed	52189-0323	OCD
INV323 <> INV323	Cap, White & Yellow	Clomipramine HCl 75 mg	by Apothecon	62269-0323	OCD
INV328	Cap, Green & White	Nortriptyline 10 mg	Pamelor by Invamed		Antidepressant

ID FRONT <> BACK	DESCRIPTION FRONT <> BACK	INGREDIENT & STRENGTH	BRAND (OR EQUIV.) & FIRM	NDC#	CLASS; SCH.
INV329	Cap, Green & White	Nortriptyline 25 mg	Pamelor by Invamed		Antidepressant
INV330	Cap, White	Nortriptyline 50 mg	Pamelor by Invamed		Antidepressant
INV331	Cap, Green	Nortriptyline 75 mg	Pamelor by Invamed		Antidepressant
INV336	Tab, White, Round	Orphenadrine Citrate 100 mg	by Invamed	52189-0336	Muscle Relaxant
INV336	Tab, White, Round	Orphenadrine Citrate 100 mg	by Bristol-Myers		Muscle Relaxant
INV336	Tab, White, Round	Orphenadrine Citrate 100 mg	Norflex by Invamed		Muscle Relaxant
INV336	Tab, White, Round	Orphenadrine Citrate 100 mg	Orphenadrine Citrate by Perrigo	00113-0203	Muscle Relaxant
INV350	Tab, Yellow, Oval, Film Coated	Etodolac 400 mg	by Phy Total Care	54868-3955	NSAID
INV350	Tab, Yellow, Oval, Film Coated	Etodolac 400 mg	by Apothecon	62269-0350	NSAID
INV350	Tab, Yellow, Oval, Film Coated	Etodolac 400 mg	by Invamed	52189-0350	NSAID
INV350	Tab, Yellow, Oval	Etodolac 400 mg	Lodine by Invamed		NSAID
INV351	Tab, White, Oval	Methylprednisolone 4 mg	by Bristol-Myers		Steroid
INV351	Tab, White, Oval, Scored	Methylprednisolone 4 mg	by Invamed	52189-0351	Steroid
INV351	Tab, White, Round, Scored	Methylprednisolone 4 mg	by Apothecon	62269-0351	Steroid
INV351	Tab, White, Oval, Scored, INV Above 351	Methylprednisolone 4 mg	MethylpRednisolone by Neuman Distr	64579-0037	Steroid
INV351	Tab, White, Oval	Methylprednisolone 4 mg	Medrol by Invamed		Steroid
INV353	Tab, Yellow, Round, Scored	Clonazepam 0.5 mg	by Invamed	52189-0353	Anticonvulsant; C IV
INV353	Tab, Yellow, Round, Scored	Clonazepam 0.5 mg	by Apothecon	62269-0353	Anticonvulsant; C IV
INV353	Tab, Yellow, Round	Clonazepam 0.5 mg	Klonopin by Invamed		Anticonvulsant; C IV
INV353	Tab, Yellow, Round, Scored	Clonazepam 0.5 mg	by DHHS Prog	11819-0083	Anticonvulsant; C IV
INV354	Tab, Green, Round	Clonazepam 1 mg	Klonopin by Invamed		Anticonvulsant; C IV
INV354	Tab, Green, Round	Clonazepam 1 mg	by Bristol-Myers		Anticonvulsant; C IV
INV354	Tab, Green, Round, Scored	Clonazepam 1 mg	by Apothecon	62269-0354	Anticonvulsant; C IV
INV354	Tab, Green, Round, Scored	Clonazepam 1 mg	by Invamed	52189-0354	Anticonvulsant; C IV
INV354	Tab, Green, Round, Scored	Clonazepam 1 mg	by DHHS Prog	11819-0081	Anticonvulsant; C IV
INV355	Tab, White, Round, Scored	Clonazepam 2 mg	by Invamed	52189-0355	Anticonvulsant; C IV
INV355	Tab, White, Round, Scored	Clonazepam 2 mg	by Apothecon	62269-0355	Anticonvulsant; C IV
INV355	Tab, White, Round	Clonazepam 2 mg	Klonopin by Invamed		Anticonvulsant; C IV
INV355	Tab, White, Round	Clonazepam 2 mg	by Bristol-Myers		Anticonvulsant; C IV
INV355	Tab, White, Round, Scored	Clonazepam 2 mg	by DHHS Prog	11819-0087	Anticonvulsant; C IV
INV359	Cap, Gray & White	Etodolac 200 mg	by Apothecon	62269-0359	NSAID
INV359	Cap, Gray & White	Etodolac 200 mg	by Invamed	52189-0359	NSAID
INV359	Cap, Gray & White	Etodolac 200 mg	Lodine by Invamed		NSAID
INV360	Cap, Gray	Etodolac 300 mg	by Apothecon	62269-0360	NSAID
INV360	Cap, Gray	Etodolac 300 mg	by Invamed	52189-0360	NSAID
INV360	Cap, Gray	Etodolac 300 mg	by DRX Pharm Consults	55045-2592	NSAID
INV360	Cap, Gray	Etodolac 300 mg	by Bristol-Myers		NSAID
INV360	Cap, Gray	Etodolac 300 mg	Lodine by Invamed		NSAID
INV362	Tab, Purple, Round, Film Coated	Bupropion HCl 100 mg	by Invamed	52189-0362	Antidepressant
INV375	Tab, Orange, Round, Film, INV Over 375	Ticlopidine HCl 250 mg	by Taro	52549-4035	Anticoagulant
INV375	Tab, Light Orange, Round, Film Coated, INV 375	Ticlopidine HCl 250 mg	Ticlid by Geneva	00781-1514	Anticoagulant
INV375	Tab, Orange, Round, Film, INV Over 375	Ticlopidine HCl 250 mg	Ticlopidine HCl by Teva	00093-0280	Anticoagulant
INV383	Tab, White, Round, Film, INV over 383	Diclofenac Potassium 50 mg	Diclofenac Potassium by DRX	55045-2672	NSAID
INV391	Tab, White, Round, Scored	Pemoline 18.75 mg	by Invamed	52189-0391	Stimulant; C IV
INV391	Tab, White, Round, Scored	Pemoline 18.75 mg	by Apothecon	62269-0391	Stimulant; C IV
INV392	Tab, White, Round	Pemoline 37.5 mg	Pemoline by Pharmafab	62542-0460	Stimulant; C IV
INV393	Tab, White, Round, INV Above 393	Pemoline 75 mg	Pemoline by Pharmafab	62542-0690	Stimulant; C IV
INV394	Tab, Peach, Round, Scored, INV 394	Leucovorin Calcium 15 mg	Leucovorin Calcium by Murfreesboro	51129-1627	Antineoplastic
INV50273	Tab, White, Oval	Captopril 50 mg	Capoten by Invamed		Antihypertensive
INV535	Tab, Yellow, Round, INV/535	Clonazepam 0.5 mg	by Invamed		Anticonvulsant; C IV
INV75 <> NORTRIPTYLINE	Cap, Green	Nortriptyline HCl 75 mg	by Invamed	52189-0331	Antidepressant

ID FRONT <> BACK	DESCRIPTION FRONT <> BACK	INGREDIENT & STRENGTH	BRAND (OR EQUIV.) & FIRM	NDC#	CLASS; SCH.
INV75 <> NORTRIPTYLINEIN	Cap, Green	Nortriptyline HCl 75 mg	by Apothecon	62269-0331	Antidepressant
IONAMIN15	Cap	Phentermine Resin Complex	Ionamin by Quality Care	62682-7036	Anorexiant; C IV
IONAMIN15	Cap, ER	Phentermine Resin Complex	Ionamin by PDRX	55289-0987	Anorexiant; C IV
IONAMIN15	Cap, Gray & Yellow	Phentermine Resin Complex 15 mg	Ionamin by HJ Harkins	52959-0418	Anorexiant; C IV
IONAMIN15	Cap, Gray & Yellow	Phentermine Resin Complex 15 mg	Ionamin by Physicians Total Care		Anorexiant; C IV
IONAMIN15	Cap, Gray & Yellow, Ionamin 15	Phentermine Resin Complex 15 mg	Ionamin by Medeva	53014-0903	Anorexiant; C IV
IONAMIN15	Cap, ER	Phentermine Resin Complex	Ionamin by Allscripts	54569-2290	Anorexiant; C IV
IONAMIN30	Cap	Phentermine	Ionamin by Allscripts	54569-0393	Anorexiant; C IV
IONAMIN30	Cap	Phentermine	Ionamin by Nat Pharmpak Serv	55154-6302	Anorexiant; C IV
IONAMIN30	Cap, Yellow	Phentermine 30 mg	Ionamin by Compumed	00403-1069	Anorexiant; C IV
IONAMIN30	Cap, Yellow	Phentermine Resin 30 mg	Ionamin by Medeva	53014-0904	Anorexiant; C IV
IONAMIN30	Cap, ER	Phentermine Resin Complex	Ionamin by DRX	55045-2295	Anorexiant; C IV
IONAMIN30	Cap, ER, Ionamin 30	Phentermine Resin Complex	Ionamin by PDRX	55289-0731	Anorexiant; C IV
IONAMIN30	Cap, ER, Ionamin 30 <> Fisons	Phentermine Resin Complex	Ionamin by DRX	55045-2443	Anorexiant; C IV
IONAMIN30	Cap, ER	Phentermine Resin Complex	Ionamin by Quality Care	62682-7037	Anorexiant; C IV
IP001	Tab, White, Round	Acetaminophen 500 mg	Tylenol by Interpharm		Antipyretic
IP011	Tab, White, Round	Acetaminophen 325 mg	Tylenol by Interpharm		Antipyretic
IP018	Tab, White, Oblong	Acetaminophen 500 mg	Tylenol by Interpharm		Antipyretic
IP029	Tab	Aspirin 800 mg	by United Res	00677-1172	Analgesic
IP037	Tab, Yellow, Round	Chlorpheniramine Maleate 4 mg	Chlor-trimeton by Interpharm		Antihistamine
IP050	Tab, Pink, Round	Acetaminophen 325 mg, Pseudophedrine HCl 30 mg	Sinutab by Interpharm		Cold Remedy
IP064	Cap, Pink & White	Diphenhydramine 25 mg	Benadryl by Interpharm		Antihistamine
IP131	Tab, Coated	Ibuprofen 400 mg	by Qualitest	00603-4018	NSAID
IP131 <> 400	Tab, Coated	Ibuprofen 400 mg	by Prescription Dispensing	61807-0027	NSAID
IP131 <> 400	Tab, Film Coated	Ibuprofen 400 mg	by Quality Care	60346-0430	NSAID
IP131 <> 400	Tab, White, Round, Convex, Film	Ibuprofen 400 mg	Ibuprofen by Murfreesboro	51129-1523	NSAID
IP131 <> 400	Tab, White, Round, Convex, Film	Ibuprofen 400 mg	by Murfreesboro	51129-1525	NSAID
IP131 <> 400	Tab, Coated	Ibuprofen 400 mg	by Golden State	60429-0092	NSAID
IP131 <> 400	Tab, White, Round, Film Coated	Ibuprofen 400 mg	by Goldline Labs	00182-1809	NSAID
IP132	Tab, Coated	Ibuprofen 600 mg	by Qualitest	00603-4019	NSAID
IP132 <> 600	Tab, Film Coated	Ibuprofen 600 mg	by Urgent Care Ctr	50716-0743	NSAID
IP132 <> 600	Tab, White, Oval, Film	Ibuprofen 600 mg	by Murfreesboro	51129-1526	NSAID
IP132 <> 600	Tab, White, Round	Ibuprofen 600 mg	by Breckenridge	51991-0730	NSAID
IP132 <> 600	Tab, Film Coated	Ibuprofen 600 mg	by Quality Care	60346-0556	NSAID
IP132 <> 600	Tab, Coated	Ibuprofen 600 mg	by Golden State	60429-0093	NSAID
IP132 <> 600	Tab, Coated	Ibuprofen 600 mg	by Prescription Dispensing	61807-0011	NSAID
IP132 <> 600	Tab, White, Oval, Film Coated	Ibuprofen 600 mg	by Major Pharms	00904-5186	NSAID
IP135	Tab, White, Round	Ibuprofen 200 mg	Advil by Interpharm		NSAID
IP136	Cap, Red	Isometheptene Mucate 65 mg, Dichloralphenazone 100 mg, Acetaminophen 325 mg	Midrin by Interpharm		Analgesic
IP137	Tab, Coated	Ibuprofen 800 mg	by Qualitest	00603-4020	NSAID
IP137 <> 800	Tab, Film Coated	Ibuprofen 800 mg	by Urgent Care Ctr	50716-0726	NSAID
IP137 <> 800	Tab, White, Oblong, Film	Ibuprofen 800 mg	by Murfreesboro	51129-1528	NSAID
IP137 <> 800	Tab, White, Round	Ibuprofen 800 mg	by Breckenridge	51991-0740	NSAID
IP137 <> 800	Tab, Coated	Ibuprofen 800 mg	by Golden State	60429-0094	NSAID
IP137 <> 800	Tab, Film Coated	Ibuprofen 800 mg	by Quality Care	60346-0030	NSAID
IP137 <> 800	Tab, Coated	Ibuprofen 800 mg	by Prescription Dispensing	61807-0012	NSAID
IP137 <> 800	Tab, White, Film Coated	Ibuprofen 800 mg	by Major Pharms	00904-5187	NSAID
IP138 <> 400	Tab, White, Round	Ibuprofen 400 mg	by Breckenridge	51991-0720	NSAID
IP138200	Tab, White, Oblong, IP138/200	Ibuprofen 200 mg	Advil by Interpharm		NSAID
IP141	Cap, Red	Isometheptene Mucate 65 mg, Dichloralphenazone 100 mg, Acetaminophen 325 mg	Midrin by Interpharm		Analgesic

ID FRONT <> BACK	DESCRIPTION FRONT <> BACK	INGREDIENT & STRENGTH	BRAND (OR EQUIV.) & FIRM	NDC#	CLASS; SCH.
IP191	Tab, Film Coated	Ascorbic Acid 60 mg, Biotin 300 mcg, Cyanocobalamin 6 mcg, Folic Acid 1 mg, Niacinamide 20 mg, Pantothenic Acid 10 mg, Pyridoxine HCl 10 mg, Riboflavin 1.7 mg, Thiamine Mononitrate 1.5 mg	Nephro Vite Rx by Interpharm	53746-0191	Vitamin
IP211	Tab, Pink, Oblong	Pseudoephedrine 60 mg, Chlorpheniramine 4 mg, Acetaminophen 650 mg	Singlet by Interpharm		Cold Remedy
IP221	Tab, Compressed, IP/221	Pseudoephedrine HCl 60 mg	by Kaiser	00179-0659	Decongestant
IP251	Tab, White, Round	Quinine Sulfate 260 mg	Quinamm by Interpharm		Antimalarial
IP274	Tab, Pink, Round	Simethicone 80 mg	Mylicon by Interpharm		Antiflatulent
IP276	Tab, Blue, Round	Salsalate 500 mg	Disalcid by Interpharm		NSAID
IP277	Tab, Film Coated, Debossed	Salsalate 750 mg	by Golden State	60429-0207	NSAID
IP288	Tab, IP/288	Pseudoephedrine HCl 60 mg, Triprolidine HCl 2.5 mg	Triprolidine by Kaiser	00179-0820	Cold Remedy
IP94	Tab, White, Round	Guafenesin 1200 mg	Duravent by Breckenridge	51991-0049	Expectorant
IP94	Tab, White, Oblong	Phenylpropanolamine HCl 75 mg, Guaifenesin 600 mg	Duravent by Interpharm		Cold Remedy
IP95	Tab, White, Oblong	Guaifenesin 600 mg, Pseudoephedrine 120 mg	Duratuss by Interpharm		Cold Remedy
IP96	Tab, Blue, Oval, IP/96	Guaifenesin 400 mg, Phenylpropanolamine HCl 75 mg	by Martec		Cold Remedy
IP96	Tab	Guaifenesin 400 mg, Phenylpropanolamine HCl 75 mg	by Interpharm	53746-0096	Cold Remedy
IP96	Tab, Blue, Oval	Phenylpropanolamine HCl 75 mg, Guaifenesin LA 400 mg	Entex LA by Interpharm		Cold Remedy
IP97	Tab, Yellow, Oval	Guiadrine PSE	Entex PSE by Breckenridge	51991-0245	Cold Remedy
IP97	Tab	Guaifenesin 600 mg, Pseudoephedrine HCl 120 mg	Enomine PSE by Quality Care	60346-0933	Cold Remedy
IP97	Tab, Film Coated	Guaifenesin 600 mg, Pseudoephedrine HCl 120 mg	by Zenith Goldline	00182-1740	Cold Remedy
IP98	Tab	Guaifenesin 600 mg, Pseudoephedrine HCl 60 mg	by Zenith Goldline	00182-1037	Cold Remedy
IP99	Tab, Film Coated	Dextromethorphan Hydrobromide 30 mg, Guaifenesin 600 mg	by Zenith Goldline	00182-1042	Cold Remedy
IP99	Tab	Dextromethorphan Hydrobromide 30 mg, Guaifenesin 600 mg	by Rugby	00536-5591	Cold Remedy
IP99	Tab, Green, Cap Shaped	Guiadrine DM	Humibid DM by Breckenridge	51991-0285	Expectorant
IP99	Tab, Green, Oblong	Guaifenesin 600 mg, Dextromethorphan Hydrobromide 30 mg	Guaifenesin DM by Med Pro	53978-3183	Cold Remedy
ISMO20	Tab, Orange, Round, Scored	Isosorbide Mononitrate 20 mg	Ismo by Wyeth Labs	00008-0771	Antianginal
ISMO20	Tab, Film Coated	Isosorbide Mononitrate 20 mg	Ismo by A H Robins	00031-0771	Antianginal
ISMO20	Tab, Film Coated	Isosorbide Mononitrate 20 mg	Ismo by Nat Pharmpak Serv	55154-4206	Antianginal
ISMO20	Tab, Film Coated	Isosorbide Mononitrate 20 mg	Ismo by Physicians Total Care	54868-3001	Antianginal
ISMO20W	Tab, Orange, Biconvex, Ismo 20/W	Isosorbide 5-Mononitrate 20 mg	by Wyeth-Ayerst	Canadian	Antianginal
ISODRIL10	Tab, White	Isosorbide Dinitrate 10 mg	Isordil by Wyeth-Ayerst	Canadian	Antianginal
ISODRIL30	Tab, White	Isosorbide Dinitrate 30 mg	Isordil by Wyeth-Ayerst	Canadian	Antianginal
ISOPTIN120 <> KNOLL	Tab, Film Coated, Isoptin 120	Verapamil HCl 120 mg	Isoptin by Knoll	00044-1823	Antihypertensive
ISOPTIN80 <> KNOLL	Tab, Film Coated	Verapamil HCl 80 mg	by Med Pro	53978-7001	Antihypertensive
ISOPTIN80 <> KNOLL	Tab, Film Coated, Isoptin 80	Verapamil HCl 80 mg	Isoptin by Knoll	00044-1822	Antihypertensive
ISOPTIN80 <> KNOLL	Tab, Film Coated, Embossed	Verapamil HCl 80 mg	Isoptin by Amerisource	62584-0822	Antihypertensive
ISOPTINSR	Tab, Light Green, Film Coated, <> Embossed with Double Knoll Triangle	Verapamil HCl 240 mg	Isoptin Sr by PDRX	55289-0078	Antihypertensive
ISORDIL10	Tab, White	Isosorbide Dinitrate 10 mg	by Wyeth-Ayerst	Canadian	Antianginal
J	Tab, White	Trimebutine Maleate 100 mg	Modulon by Jouveinal	Canadian	Motility Regulator
J	Tab, White	Trimebutine Maleate 200 mg	Modulon by Jouveinal	Canadian	Motility Regulator
J02	Tab, White, Round	Atropine Sulfate 0.4 mg	by Lilly		Gastrointestinal
J09	Tab, White, Round	Codeine Sulfate 15 mg	by Lilly		Analgesic; C III
J10	Tab, White, Round	Codeine Sulfate 30 mg	by Lilly		Analgesic; C III
J11	Tab, White, Round	Codeine Sulfate 60 mg	by Lilly		Analgesic; C III
J13	Tab, White, Round	Colchicine 0.6 mg	by Lilly		Antigout
J2 <> LL	Tab, J Above & 2 Below Score <> LL —Lederle	Methazolamide 50 mg	by Allscripts	54569-3864	Diuretic
J20	Tab, White, Round	Quinidine Sulfate 200 mg	by Lilly		Antiarrhythmic
J25	Tab, Brown, Round	Thyroid 60 mg	by Lilly		Thyroid
J26	Tab, Brown, Round	Thyroid 120 mg	by Lilly		Thyroid
J29	Tab, Brown, Round	Thyroid 30 mg	by Lilly		Thyroid
J31	Tab, White, Round	Phenobarbital 15 mg	by Lilly		Sedative/Hypnotic; C IV
J32	Tab, White, Round	Phenobarbital 30 mg	by Lilly		Sedative/Hypnotic; C IV

ID FRONT <> BACK	DESCRIPTION FRONT <> BACK	INGREDIENT & STRENGTH	BRAND (OR EQUIV.) & FIRM	NDC#	CLASS; SCH.
J33	Tab, White, Round	Phenobarbital 100 mg	by Lilly		Sedative/Hypnotic; C IV
J36	Tab, White, Round	Ergonovine Maleate 0.2 mg	Ergotrate Maleate by Lilly		Antimigraine
J37	Tab, White, Round	Phenobarbital 60 mg	by Lilly		Sedative/Hypnotic; C IV
J52	Tab, White, Round	Diethylstilbestrol 1 mg	by Lilly		Hormone
J54	Tab, White, Round	Diethylstilbestrol 5 mg	by Lilly		Hormone
J60	Tab, Pink, Round	Digitoxin 0.1 mg	Crystodigin by Lilly		Cardiac Agent
J61	Tab, White, Round	Papaverine HCl 30 mg	by Lilly		Vasodilator
J62	Tab, White, Round	Papaverine HCl 60 mg	by Lilly		Vasodilator
J64	Tab, White, Round	Methadone HCl 5 mg	Dolophine by Lilly		Analgesic; C II
J69	Tab, White, Round	Propylthiouracil 50 mg	by Lilly		Antithyroid
J72	Tab, White, Round	Methadone HCl 10 mg	Dolophine by Lilly		Analgesic; C II
J73	Tab, White, Oblong	Methyltestosterone 10 mg	by Lilly		Hormone; C III
J74	Tab, White, Round	Methyltestosterone 25 mg	by Lilly		Hormone; C III
J75	Tab, Orange, Round	Digitoxin 0.05 mg	Crystodigin by Lilly		Cardiac Agent
J75	Tab, White, Round	Isoproterenol HCl 10 mg	Isuprel by Sanofi		Antiasthmatic
J76	Tab, Yellow, Round	Digitoxin 0.15 mg	Crystodigin by Lilly		Cardiac Agent
J77	Tab, White, Round	Isoproterenol HCl 15 mg	Isuprel by Sanofi		Antiasthmatic
J94	Tab, White, Round, Beveled, Scored	Methimazole 5 mg	Tapazole by Neuman Distr	64579-0001	Antithyroid
J94	Tab, White, Round, Scored	Methimazole 5 mg	by Jones	52604-1094	Antithyroid
J95	Tab, White, Round, Scored	Methimazole 10 mg	Tapazole by DRX Pharm Consults	55045-2749	Antithyroid
J95	Tab, White, Round, Scored	Methimazole 10 mg	by Jones	52604-1095	Antithyroid
J96	Tab, White, Round	Methyltestosterone 5 mg, Diethylstilbestrol 0.25 mg	Tylosterone by Lilly		Hormone; C III
JACOBUS <> 100101	Tab, Jacobus <> 100/101	Dapsone 100 mg	by Jacobus	49938-0101	Antimycobacterial
JACOBUS <> 100101	Tab, Scored, Jacobus <> 100 over 101	Dapsone 100 mg	by Physicians Total Care	54868-3801	Antimycobacterial
JACOBUS <> 25102	Tab, Jacobus <> 25/102	Dapsone 25 mg	by Jacobus	49938-0102	Antimycobacterial
JACOBUS <> 25102	Tab, Jacobus <> 25 over 102	Dapsone 25 mg	by PDRX	55289-0188	Antimycobacterial
JACOBUS0704	Tab, Tan, Jacobus 107-04	Aminosalicylic Acid Granules DR 4 GM	Paser(R) by Jacobus		Antimycobacterial
JANSSEN	Tab, Chew	Mebendazole 100 mg	by Dept Health Central Pharm	53808-0003	Anthelmintic
JANSSEN <> AST10	Tab	Astemizole 10 mg	Hismanal by PDRX	55289-0527	Antihistamine
JANSSEN <> AST10	Tab, AST Over 10	Astemizole 10 mg	Hismanal by Quality Care	60346-0568	Antihistamine
JANSSEN <> AST10	Tab, Janssen <> AST over 10	Astemizole 10 mg	Hismanal by Direct Dispensing	57866-6480	Antihistamine
JANSSEN <> AST10	Tab, Debossed <> Debossed, AST Over 10	Astemizole 10 mg	Hismanal by St Marys Med	60760-0510	Antihistamine
JANSSEN <> AST10	Tab, AST Over 10	Astemizole 10 mg	Hismanal by Johnson & Johnson	59604-0510	Antihistamine
JANSSEN <> AST10	Tab, Debossed	Astemizole 10 mg	Hismanal by Amerisource	62584-0510	Antihistamine
JANSSEN <> AST10	Tab, Janssen <> AST over 10	Astemizole 10 mg	Hismanal by Ortho	00062-0510	Antihistamine
JANSSEN <> AST10	Tab, AST over 10	Astemizole 10 mg	Hismanal by Kaiser	00179-1234	Antihistamine
JANSSEN <> AST10	Tab, AST over 10	Astemizole 10 mg	Hismanal by Allscripts	54569-2467	Antihistamine
JANSSEN <> AST10	Tab, Janssen <> AST over 10	Astemizole 10 mg	Hismanal by Janssen	50458-0510	Antihistamine
JANSSEN <> IMODIUM	Cap, Dark Green & Light Green	Loperamide 2 mg	Imodium by Janssen	50458-0400	Antidiarrheal
JANSSEN <> IMODIUM	Cap, Dark Green & Light Green	Loperamide 2 mg	Imodium by Quality Care	60346-0942	Antidiarrheal
JANSSEN <> IMODIUM	Cap, Dark Green & Light Green	Loperamide 2 mg	Imodium by Johnson & Johnson	59604-0400	Antidiarrheal
JANSSEN <> IMODIUM	Cap, Light Green	Loperamide HCl 2 mg	Imodium by Allscripts	54569-0219	Antidiarrheal
JANSSEN <> L50	Tab, Coated, L Over 50	Levamisole HCl 59 mg	Ergamisol by Janssen	50458-0270	Immunomodulator
JANSSEN <> NIZORAL	Tab, White, Scored	Ketoconazole 200 mg	Nizoral by HJ Harkins	52959-0197	Antifungal
JANSSEN <> NIZORAL	Tab	Ketoconazole 200 mg	Nizoral by Janssen	50458-0220	Antifungal
JANSSEN <> NIZORAL	Tab	Ketoconazole 200 mg	Nizoral by Johnson & Johnson	59604-0220	Antifungal
JANSSEN <> NIZORAL	Tab	Ketoconazole 200 mg	Nizoral by Quality Care	60346-0247	Antifungal
JANSSEN <> NIZORAL	Tab, Debossed	Ketoconazole 200 mg	Nizoral by Direct Dispensing	57866-6570	Antifungal
JANSSEN <> NIZORAL	Tab	Ketoconazole 200 mg	Nizoral by Pharm Utilization	60491-0454	Antifungal
JANSSEN <> P10	Tab, P/10	Cisapride 10 mg	Propulsid by Johnson & Johnson	59604-0430	Gastrointestinal
JANSSEN <> P10	Tab, Janssen <> P/10	Cisapride 10 mg	Propulsid by PDRX	55289-0105	Gastrointestinal
JANSSEN <> P10	Tab, P Over 10	Cisapride 10 mg	Propulsid by Quality Care	60346-0490	Gastrointestinal

369

ID FRONT <> BACK	DESCRIPTION FRONT <> BACK	INGREDIENT & STRENGTH	BRAND (OR EQUIV.) & FIRM	NDC#	CLASS; SCH.
JANSSEN <> P10	Tab, Janssen <> P over 10	Cisapride 10 mg	by Pharm Packaging Ctr	54383-0077	Gastrointestinal
JANSSEN <> P10	Tab, Janssen <> P/10	Cisapride 10 mg	Propulsid by Nat Pharmpak Serv	55154-1402	Gastrointestinal
JANSSEN <> P10	Tab, P/10	Cisapride Monohydrate	Propulsid by Allscripts	54569-4238	Gastrointestinal
JANSSEN <> P20	Tab, Also Comes in Blue, <> P/20	Cisapride 20 mg	Propulsid by Johnson & Johnson	59604-0440	Gastrointestinal
JANSSEN <> P20	Tab, Janssen <> P/20	Cisapride 20 mg	Propulsid by Janssen	50458-0440	Gastrointestinal
JANSSEN <> R1	Tab, White	Risperidone 1 mg	Risperdal by Va Cmop	65243-0061	Antipsychotic
JANSSEN <> R1	Tab, Coated, R/1	Risperidone 1 mg	Risperdal by Janssen	50458-0300	Antipsychotic
JANSSEN <> R1	Tab, Coated	Risperidone 1 mg	Risperdal by Johnson & Johnson	59604-0300	Antipsychotic
JANSSEN <> R2	Tab, Orange, Oblong, Coated	Risperidone 2 mg	Risperdal by Janssen	50458-0320	Antipsychotic
JANSSEN <> R2	Tab, Coated	Risperidone 2 mg	Risperdal by Johnson & Johnson	59604-0320	Antipsychotic
JANSSEN <> R3	Tab, Coated	Risperidone 3 mg	Risperdal by Janssen	50458-0330	Antipsychotic
JANSSEN <> R3	Tab, Coated	Risperidone 3 mg	Risperdal by Johnson & Johnson	59604-0330	Antipsychotic
JANSSEN <> R4	Tab, Coated	Risperidone 4 mg	Risperdal by Janssen	50458-0350	Antipsychotic
JANSSEN <> R4	Tab, Coated	Risperidone 4 mg	Risperdal by Johnson & Johnson	59604-0350	Antipsychotic
JANSSEN <> RIS	Tab, Yellow	Risperidone 0.25 mg	Risperdal by Janssen Cilag	62579-0301	Antipsychotic
JANSSEN <> RIS025	Tab, Yellow, Janssen <> RIS 0.25	Risperidone 0.25 mg	Risperdal by RX PAK	65084-0194	Antipsychotic
JANSSEN <> RIS025	Tab, Yellow, Janssen <> RIS 0.25	Risperidone 0.25 mg	Risperdal by RX PAK	65084-0190	Antipsychotic
JANSSEN <> RIS05	Tab, Red, Janssen <> RIS 0.5	Risperidone 0.5 mg	Risperdal by RX PAK	65084-0191	Antipsychotic
JANSSEN <> RIS05	Tab, Red, Janssen <> RIS 0.5	Risperidone 0.5 mg	Risperdal by RX PAK	65084-0197	Antipsychotic
JANSSEN <> SPORANOX100	Cap, Blue & Pink	Itraconazole 100 mg	Sporanox by Allscripts	54569-4869	Antifungal
JANSSEN <> SPORANOX100	Cap	Itraconazole 100 mg	Sporanox by Nat Pharmpak Serv	55154-1404	Antifungal
JANSSEN <> SPORANOX100	Cap	Itraconazole 100 mg	Sporanox by Physicians Total Care	54868-3706	Antifungal
JANSSEN <> SPORANOX100	Cap	Itraconazole 100 mg	Sporanox by Janssen	50458-0290	Antifungal
JANSSEN <> SPORANOX100	Cap	Itraconazole 100 mg	Sporanox by Johnson & Johnson	59604-0290	Antifungal
JANSSEN <> SPORANOX100	Cap	Itraconazole 100 mg	Sporanox by Janssen	12578-0290	Antifungal
JANSSEN <> VERMOX	Tab, Pink, Round	Mebendazole 100 mg	Vermox by HJ Harkins	52959-0160	Anthelmintic
JANSSEN <> VERMOX	Tab, Chew	Mebendazole 100 mg	Vermox by Janssen	50458-0110	Anthelmintic
JANSSEN <> VERMOX	Tab, Chew	Mebendazole 100 mg	Vermox C by Johnson & Johnson	59604-0110	Anthelmintic
JANSSEN1	Tab, White, Round	Risperidone 1 mg	by Apotheca	12634-0679	Antipsychotic
JANSSENAST10	Tab, White, Round	Astemizole 10 mg	Hismanal by Johnson & Johnson	Canadian	Antihistamine
JANSSENIMODIUM	Cap	Loperamide 2 mg	Imodium by Nat Pharmpak Serv	55154-1401	Antidiarrheal
JANSSENP <> 10	Tab, Janssen/P <> 10	Cisapride 10 mg	Propulsid by Janssen	50458-0430	Gastrointestinal
JANSSENP10	Tab, Janssen P/10	Cisapride 10 mg	Propulsid by Caremark	00339-5887	Gastrointestinal
JANSSENP10	Tab, White, Scored	Cisapride 10 mg	Propulsid by Compumed	00403-4662	Gastrointestinal
JANSSENP10	Tab	Cisapride 10 mg	by Med Pro	53978-2062	Gastrointestinal
JANSSENP20	Tab	Cisapride 20 mg	Propulsid by Caremark	00339-6024	Gastrointestinal
JANSSENR1	Tab, White, Scored	Risperidone 1 mg	Risperdal by RX PAK	65084-0198	Antipsychotic
JANSSENR1	Tab, Coated	Risperidone 1 mg	Risperdal by Nat Pharmpak Serv	55154-1405	Antipsychotic
JANSSENR4	Tab, Green, Oblong, Coated	Risperidone 4 mg	Risperdal by Physicians Total Care	54868-3515	Antipsychotic
JC <> SANOREX	Tab, Peach, Round, Scored	Mazindol 2 mg	Sanorex by Novartis	Canadian DIN# 00285544	Anorexiant
JD	Tab, White, Round, Sch. Logo JD	Methyltestosterone 10 mg	Oreton by Schering		Hormone; C III
JE	Tab, Peach, Round, Sch. Logo JE	Methyltestosterone 25 mg	Oreton by Schering		Hormone; C III
JIMINT1	Tab, Tan, Round, Jimi/NT 1	Thyroid 64.8 mg	Westhroid by Jones		Thyroid
JIMITH1	Tab, Blue, Round, Jimi TH-1	Thyroid 64.8 mg	Westhroid by Jones		Thyroid

ID FRONT <> BACK	DESCRIPTION FRONT <> BACK	INGREDIENT & STRENGTH	BRAND (OR EQUIV.) & FIRM	NDC#	CLASS; SCH.
JIMITH1	Tab, Pink, Round, Jimi TH-1	Thyroid 64.8 mg	Westhroid by Jones		Thyroid
JIMITH1	Tab, Red, Round, Jimi TH-1	Thyroid 64.8 mg	Westhroid by Jones		Thyroid
JIMITH1	Tab, Yellow, Round, Jimi TH-1	Thyroid 64.8 mg	Westhroid by Jones		Thyroid
JMI <> 6792	Tab	Atropine Sulfate 0.0194 mg, Hyoscyamine Sulfate 0.1037 mg, Phenobarbital 16.2 mg, Scopolamine Hydrobromide 0.0065 mg	Belladonna PB by Quality Care	60346-0042	Gastrointestinal; C IV
JMI <> APT	Tab, Sugar Coated	Thyroid 3 gr	Westhroid Apt 2 by JMI Canton	00252-7505	Thyroid
JMI <> APT	Tab, Sugar Coated	Thyroid 3 gr	Westhroid Apt 2 by Jones	52604-7505	Thyroid
JMI <> D14	Tab, Round, Scored	Liothyronine Sodium	Cytomel by Jones	52604-3414	Antithyroid
JMI <> NT112	Tab, NT Over 1 1/2	Thyroid 97.2 mg	Nature Thyroid by JMI Canton	00252-3304	Thyroid
JMI <> NT112	Tab, NT Over 1 1/2	Thyroid 97.2 mg	Nature Thyroid by Jones	52604-3304	Thyroid
JMI <> NT12	Tab, NT Over 1 1/2	Thyroid 32.4 mg	Nature Thyroid by JMI Canton	00252-3299	Thyroid
JMI <> NT12	Tab, NT Over 1 1/2	Thyroid 32.4 mg	Nature Thyroid by Jones	52604-3299	Thyroid
JMI <> NT3	Tab	Thyroid 3 gr	Nature Thyroid by Jones	52604-3312	Thyroid
JMI3166	Tab, Green & Pink & Yellow, JMI/3166	Phenobarbital 30 mg	by JMI Canton	00252-3166	Sedative/Hypnotic; C IV
JMI4450	Tab, Salmon, Round	Guaifenesin 200 mg	Organidin NR by Jones		Expectorant
JMI627	Tab, Sugar Coated, JMI/627	Thyroid 64.8 mg	by JMI Canton	00252-0627	Thyroid
JMI627	Tab, JMI/3166	Thyroid 64.8 mg	by Jones	52604-0627	Thyroid
JMI628	Tab, Sugar Coated, JMI/627	Thyroid 129.6 mg	by JMI Canton	00252-0628	Thyroid
JMI628	Tab, JMI/628	Thyroid 129.6 mg	by Jones	52604-0628	Thyroid
JMI629	Tab, Sugar Coated, JMI/627	Thyroid 194.4 mg	by JMI Canton	00252-0629	Thyroid
JMI629	Tab, Sugar Coated, JMI/629	Thyroid 194.4 mg	by Jones	52604-0629	Thyroid
JMI674	Tab, JMI/674	Thyroid 64.8 mg	by JMI Canton	00252-0674	Thyroid
JMI674	Tab, JMI/674	Thyroid 64.8 mg	by Jones	52604-0674	Thyroid
JMI675	Tab, JMI/675	Thyroid 129.6 mg	by JMI Canton	00252-0675	Thyroid
JMI675	Tab, JMI/675	Thyroid 129.6 mg	by Jones	52604-0675	Thyroid
JMI6792	Tab, JMI/6792	Atropine Sulfate 0.0194 mg, Hyoscyamine Sulfate 0.1037 mg, Phenobarbital 16.2 mg, Scopolamine Hydrobromide 0.0065 mg	Hyanatol Pb Belladonna by Jones	52604-6792	Gastrointestinal; C IV
JMI6792	Tab, Embossed, JMI/6792	Atropine Sulfate 0.0194 mg, Hyoscyamine Sulfate 0.1037 mg, Phenobarbital 16.2 mg, Scopolamine Hydrobromide 0.0065 mg	Donnaphen by Alphagen	59743-0027	Gastrointestinal; C IV
JMI6792	Tab, JMI/6792	Atropine Sulfate 0.0194 mg, Hyoscyamine Sulfate 0.1037 mg, Phenobarbital 16.2 mg, Scopolamine Hydrobromide 0.0065 mg	by JMI Canton	00252-6792	Gastrointestinal; C IV
JMI686	Tab, Sugar Coated, JMI/686	Thyroid 32.4 mg	by JMI Canton	00252-0626	Thyroid
JMI686	Tab, JMI/686	Thyroid 32.4 mg	by JMI Canton	00252-0686	Thyroid
JMI686	Tab, JMI/686	Thyroid 32.4 mg	by Jones	52604-0626	Thyroid
JMI686	Tab, JMI/686	Thyroid 32.4 mg	by Jones	52604-0686	Thyroid
JMI7070	Tab, JMI/7070	Thyroid 0.5 gr	Westhroid Th 1/2 by JMI Canton	00252-7070	Thyroid
JMI7070	Tab, JMI/7070	Thyroid 0.5 gr	Westhroid Th 1/2 by Jones	52604-7070	Thyroid
JMI7073	Tab, JMI/7073	Thyroid 1 gr	Westhroid Th 1 by JMI Canton	00252-7073	Thyroid
JMI7073	Tab, JMI/7073	Thyroid 1 gr	Westhroid Th 1 by Jones	52604-7073	Thyroid
JMI7080	Tab, JMI/7080	Thyroid 2 gr	Westhroid Th 2 by JMI Canton	00252-7080	Thyroid
JMI7080	Tab, JMI/7080	Thyroid 2 gr	Westhroid Th 2 by Jones	52604-7080	Thyroid
JMI7087	Tab, JMI/7087	Thyroid 3 gr	Westhroid Th 3 by JMI Canton	00252-7087	Thyroid
JMI7087	Tab, JMI/7087	Thyroid 3 gr	Westhroid Th 3 by Jones	52604-7087	Thyroid
JMI7090	Tab, Tan, with Green, Red, Yellow Specks, JMI/7090	Thyroid 3 gr	Westhroid Thv 3 by JMI Canton	00252-7090	Thyroid
JMI7092	Tab, JMI/7092	Thyroid 4 gr	Westhroid Th 4 by JMI Canton	00252-7092	Thyroid
JMI7092	Tab, JMI/7092	Thyroid 4 gr	Westhroid Th 4 by Jones	52604-7092	Thyroid
JMI7095	Tab, JMI/7095	Thyroid 5 gr	Westhroid Th 5 by JMI Canton	00252-7095	Thyroid
JMI7095	Tab, JMI/7095	Thyroid 5 gr	Westhroid Th 5 by Jones	52604-7095	Thyroid
JMI776	Tab, JMI/776	Thyroid 32.4 mg	by JMI Canton	00252-7004	Thyroid
JMI776	Tab, JMI/776	Thyroid 32.4 mg	by Jones	52604-0776	Thyroid
JMI776	Tab, JMI/776	Thyroid 32.4 mg	by Jones	52604-7004	Thyroid
JMI776	Tab	Thyroid 32.4 mg	by United Res	00677-0150	Thyroid

ID FRONT <> BACK	DESCRIPTION FRONT <> BACK	INGREDIENT & STRENGTH	BRAND (OR EQUIV.) & FIRM	NDC#	CLASS; SCH.
JMI777	Tab, JMI 777	Levothyroxine 38 mcg, Liothyronine 9 mcg	by Qualitest	00603-6046	Antithyroid
JMI777	Tab, JMI 777	Thyroid 64.8 mg	by JMI Canton	00252-0777	Thyroid
JMI777	Tab, JMI 777	Thyroid 64.8 mg	by JMI Canton	00252-7006	Thyroid
JMI777	Tab, JMI 777	Thyroid 64.8 mg	by Jones	52604-0777	Thyroid
JMI777	Tab, JMI 777	Thyroid 64.8 mg	by Quality Care	60346-0905	Thyroid
JMI777	Tab	Thyroid 64.8 mg	by United Res	00677-0151	Thyroid
JMI777	Tab, JMI 777	Thyroid 65 mg	Etwon by Macnary	55982-0013	Thyroid
JMI778	Tab, JMI 778	Levothyroxine 76 mcg, Liothyronine 18 mcg	by Qualitest	00603-6047	Antithyroid
JMI778	Tab, JMI 778	Thyroid 129.6 mg	by JMI Canton	00252-0778	Thyroid
JMI778	Tab	Thyroid 129.6 mg	by United Res	00677-0153	Thyroid
JMI778	Tab, JMI 778	Thyroid 194.4 mg	by Jones	52604-0778	Thyroid
JMI779	Tab, JMI 779	Levothyroxine 114 mcg, Liothyronine 27 mcg	by Qualitest	00603-6048	Antithyroid
JMI779	Tab, JMI 779	Thyroid 194.4 mg	by JMI Canton	00252-7023	
JMID14	Tab, White, Round	Liothyronine Sodium 5 mcg	Cytomel by Jones		Antithyroid
JMID16	Tab, White, Round, Scored, JMI over D16	Liothyronine Sodium	Cytomel by Jones	52604-3416	Antithyroid
JMID16	Tab, White, Round	Liothyronine Sodium 25 mcg	Cytomel by Jones		Antithyroid
JMID17	Tab, White, Round, Scored, JMI over D17	Liothyronine Sodium	Cytomel by Jones	52604-3417	Antithyroid
JMID17	Tab, White, Round	Liothyronine Sodium 50 mcg	Cytomel by Jones		Antithyroid
JMIK	Tab, Off-White, JMI/K	Potassium Bicarbonate 648 mg	Quic K by JMI Canton	00252-5745	Electrolytes
JMIK	Tab, Off-White, JMI/K	Potassium Bicarbonate 648 mg	Quic K by Jones	52604-5745	Electrolytes
JMINT1	Tab, JMI/NT1	Thyroid 1 gr	Nature Thyroid by JMI Canton	00252-3300	Thyroid
JMINT1	Tab, JMI Over NT1	Thyroid 1 gr	Nature Thyroid by Jones	52604-3300	Thyroid
JMINT2	Tab, JMI/NT2	Thyroid 2 gr	Parloid Thyroid Rn2 by JMI Canton	00252-3308	Thyroid
JMINT2	Tab, Tan, Round, JMI Over NT2	Thyroid 2 gr	Nature Thyroid by Jones	52604-3308	Thyroid
JMITH1	Tab, Sugar Coated, JMI/TH-1	Thyroid 1 gr	Westhroid Thp 11 by JMI Canton	00252-7077	Thyroid
JMITH1	Tab, Sugar Coated, JMI/TH-1	Thyroid 1 gr	Westhroid Thr 1 by JMI Canton	00252-7075	Thyroid
JMITH1	Tab, Sugar Coated, JMI/TH-1	Thyroid 1 gr	Westhroid Thy 1 by JMI Canton	00252-7076	Thyroid
JMITH1	Tab, Sugar Coated, JMI/TH-1	Thyroid 1 gr	Westhroid Thb 1 by JMI Canton	00252-7074	Thyroid
JMITH1	Tab, Sugar Coated, JMI/TH-1	Thyroid 1 gr	Westhroid Thb 1 by Jones	52604-7074	Thyroid
JMITH1	Tab, Sugar Coated, JMI/TH-1	Thyroid 1 gr	Westhroid Thr 1 by Jones	52604-7075	Thyroid
JMITH1	Tab, Sugar Coated, JMI/TH-1	Thyroid 1 gr	Westhroid Thp 11 by Jones	52604-7077	Thyroid
JMITH1	Tab, Sugar Coated, JMI/TH-1	Thyroid 1 gr	Westhroid Thy 1 by Jones	52604-7076	Thyroid
JMITH2	Tab, Sugar Coated, JMI/TH-2	Thyroid 2 gr	Westhroid Thp 21 by JMI Canton	00252-7084	Thyroid
JMITH2	Tab, Sugar Coated, JMI/TH-2	Thyroid 2 gr	Westhroid Thb 2 by JMI Canton	00252-7081	Thyroid
JMITH2	Tab, Sugar Coated, JMI/TH-2	Thyroid 2 gr	Westhroid Thy 2 by JMI Canton	00252-7083	Thyroid
JMITH2	Tab, Sugar Coated, JMI/TH-2	Thyroid 2 gr	Westhroid Thr 2 by JMI Canton	00252-7082	Thyroid
JMITH2	Tab, Blue, Round, Sugar Coated, JMI/TH-2	Thyroid 2 gr	Westhroid Thy 2 by Jones	52604-7083	Thyroid
JMITH2	Tab, Yellow, Round, Sugar Coated, JMI/TH-2	Thyroid 2 gr	Westhroid Thr 2 by Jones	52604-7082	Thyroid
JMITH2	Tab, Pink, Round, Sugar Coated, JMI/TH-2	Thyroid 2 gr	Westhroid Thb 2 by Jones	52604-7081	Thyroid
JMITH2	Tab, Red, Round, Sugar Coated, JMI/TH-2	Thyroid 2 gr	Westhroid Thp 21 by Jones	52604-7084	Thyroid
JMITH3	Tab, White, Round, JMI TH-3	Thyroid 194.4 mg	Nature Thyroid by Jones		Thyroid
JMITH3	Tab, Sugar Coated, JMI/TH-3	Thyroid 3 gr	Westhroid Thg 32 by JMI Canton	00252-7088	Thyroid
JMITH3	Tab, Sugar Coated, JMI/TH-3	Thyroid 3 gr	Westhroid Thb 33 by JMI Canton	00252-7089	Thyroid
JMITH3	Tab, Green, Round, Sugar Coated, JMI/TH-3	Thyroid 3 gr	Westhroid Thg 32 by Jones	52604-7088	Thyroid
JMITH3	Tab, Blue, Round, Sugar Coated, JMI/TH-3	Thyroid 3 gr	Westhroid Thb 33 by Jones	52604-7089	Thyroid
JMITH4	Tab, Fuchsia, Sugar Coated, JMI/TH-4	Thyroid 4 gr	Westhroid Thf 4 by JMI Canton	00252-7093	Thyroid
JMITH4	Tab, Fuchsia, Round, Sugar Coated, JMI/TH-4	Thyroid 4 gr	Westhroid Thf 4 by Jones	52604-7093	Thyroid
JMITH5	Tab, Sugar Coated, JMI/TH-5	Thyroid 5 gr	Westhroid Thb 5 by JMI Canton	00252-7097	Thyroid
JMITH5	Tab, Blue, Round, Sugar Coated, JMI/TH-5	Thyroid 5 gr	Westhroid Thb 5 by Jones	52604-7097	Thyroid
JMIY	Tab, White, JMI/Y	Yohimbine HCl 5.4 mg	Yocon by JMI Canton	00252-3245	Impotence Agent
JPI406	Tab, White, Oval, Scored, JPI/406	Chlorpheniramine Maleate 8 mg, Phenylephrine HCl 20 mg, Methscopolamine Nitrate 2.5 mg	Vanex Forte-D by Jones	52604-0127	Cold Remedy

ID FRONT <> BACK	DESCRIPTION FRONT <> BACK	INGREDIENT & STRENGTH	BRAND (OR EQUIV.) & FIRM	NDC#	CLASS; SCH.
JPI406	Tab, White, Oblong	Chlorpheniramine Maleate 8 mg; Methscopolamine Nitrate 2.5 mg; Phenylephrine HCl 20 mg	Vanex Forte D by Anabolic Ca	00722-6447	Cold Remedy
JPI406	Tab, White, Oval, Scored	Chlorpheniramine Maleate 8mb, Phenylephrine HCl 20 mg, Methimazole 10mg	Drize-R by Jones Pharma	52604-0406	Cold Remedy
JSP <> 513	Tab, Peach, Round, Scored	Levothyroxine Sodium 25 mg	Unithroid by Watson	52544-0902	Antithyroid
JSP <> 514	Tab, White, Round, Scored	Levothyroxine Sodium 50 mg	Unithroid by Watson	52544-0903	Antithyroid
JSP <> 515	Tab, Purple, Round, Scored	Levothyroxine Sodium 75 mg	Unithroid by Watson	52544-0904	Antithyroid
JSP <> 516	Tab	Levothyroxine Sodium 0.1 mg	by Jones	52604-7701	Antithyroid
JSP <> 516	Tab, Yellow, Round, Scored	Levothyroxine Sodium 100 mg	Unithroid by Watson	52544-0906	Antithyroid
JSP <> 519	Tab, Tan, Round, Scored	Levothyroxine Sodium 125 mg	Unithroid by Watson	52544-0908	Antithyroid
JSP <> 520	Tab	Levothyroxine Sodium 0.15 mg	by JMI Canton	00252-7700	Antithyroid
JSP <> 520	Tab, Debossed	Levothyroxine Sodium 0.15 mg	Estre by Macnary	55982-0015	Antithyroid
JSP <> 520	Tab, Blue, Round, Scored	Levothyroxine Sodium 150 mg	Unithroid by Watson	52544-0909	Antithyroid
JSP <> 522	Tab, Pink, Round, Scored	Levothyroxine Sodium 200 mg	Unithroid by Watson	52544-0911	Antithyroid
JSP <> 523	Tab, Green, Round, Scored	Levothyroxine Sodium 300 mg	Unithroid by Watson	52544-0912	Antithyroid
JSP <> 561	Tab, Olive, Round, Scored	Levothyroxine Sodium 88 mg	Unithroid by Watson	52544-0905	Antithyroid
JSP <> 562	Tab, Rose, Round, Scored	Levothyroxine Sodium 112 mg	Unithroid by Watson	52544-0907	Antithyroid
JSP <> 563	Tab, Lilac, Round, Scored	Levothyroxine Sodium 175 mg	Unithroid by Watson	52544-0910	Antithyroid
JSP125	Tab, Debossed, Color Coded	Levothyroxine Sodium 0.125 mg	by PDRX	55289-0858	Antithyroid
JSP485	Tab, Mustard Yellow, Coated, JSP-485	Ascorbic Acid 120 mg, Calcium Phosphate 64.4 mg, Calcium Sulfate 215 mg, Copper, Cyanocobalamin 12 mcg, Ergocalciferol, Folic Acid 1.21 mg, Iron 199 mg, Niacinamide 20 mg, Pyridoxine HCl 10 mg, Riboflavin 9 mg, Thiamine Mononitrate 4.5 mg, Vitamin A Acetate 8 mg, Vitamin E 22 mg, Zinc Oxide 31 mg	Prenatal 1+ Improved by Jerome Stevens	50564-0485	Vitamin
JSP485	Tab, Mustard, Oval	Prenatal 1+1 Improved	Stuartnatal 1+1 by Jerome Stevens		Vitamin
JSP490	Tab, Pink & White, Round	Methocarbamol 400 mg, Aspirin 325 mg	Robaxisal by Jerome Stevens		Muscle Relaxant
JSP507	Cap, Blue & Yellow	Butalbital 50 mg, Aspirin 325 mg, Caffeine 40 mg, Codeine 30 mg	Fiorinal #3 by Jerome Stevens		Analgesic; C III
JSP507	Tab, Blue & Yellow, Oblong	Codeine 30 mg, Butalbital 50 mg, Caffeine 40 mg, Aspirin 325 mg	by Dixon	17236-0358	Analgesic; C III
JSP507	Tab, Blue & Yellow, Oblong	Codeine 30 mg, Butalbital 50 mg, Caffeine 40 mg, Aspirin 325 mg	by Dixon	17236-0359	Analgesic; C III
JSP508	Cap	Acetaminophen 325 mg, Dichloralantipyrine 100 mg, Isometheptene Mucate 65 mg	by Jerome Stevens	50564-0508	Cold Remedy
JSP508	Cap	Acetaminophen 325 mg, Dichloralantipyrine 100 mg, Isometheptene Mucate 65 mg	by Physicians Total Care	54868-1514	Cold Remedy
JSP510	Cap	Chlorpheniramine 8 mg, Pseudoephedrine HCl 120 mg	by Zenith Goldline	00182-1151	Cold Remedy
JSP510	Cap, JSP-510	Chlorpheniramine 8 mg, Pseudoephedrine HCl 120 mg	Decongestant Sr by Jerome Stevens	50564-0510	Cold Remedy
JSP513	Tab	Levothyroxine Sodium 0.025 mg	by Zenith Goldline	00182-1529	Antithyroid
JSP513	Tab, JSP-513 Embossed	Levothyroxine Sodium 0.025 mg	by Jerome Stevens	50564-0513	Antithyroid
JSP514	Tab, JSP-514 Embossed	Levothyroxine Sodium 0.05 mg	by Jerome Stevens	50564-0514	Antithyroid
JSP515	Tab, JSP-515 Embossed	Levothyroxine Sodium 0.075 mg	by Jerome Stevens	50564-0515	Antithyroid
JSP515	Tab	Levothyroxine Sodium 0.075 mg	by Pharm Packaging Ctr	54383-0086	Antithyroid
JSP516	Tab, JSP-516 Embossed	Levothyroxine Sodium 0.1 mg	by Jerome Stevens	50564-0516	Antithyroid
JSP516	Tab	Levothyroxine Sodium 100 mcg	by United Res	00677-0078	Antithyroid
JSP519	Tab	Levothyroxine Sodium 0.1 mg	by Zenith Goldline	00182-1516	Antithyroid
JSP519	Tab, JSP-519 Embossed	Levothyroxine Sodium 0.125 mg	by Jerome Stevens	50564-0519	Antithyroid
JSP520	Tab	Levothyroxine Sodium 0.15 mg	by Zenith Goldline	00182-1117	Antithyroid
JSP520	Tab, JSP-520 Embossed	Levothyroxine Sodium 0.15 mg	by Jerome Stevens	50564-0520	Antithyroid
JSP520	Tab, Light Blue, JSP 520	Levothyroxine Sodium 150 mcg	by Quality Care	60346-0801	Antithyroid
JSP520	Tab	Levothyroxine Sodium 150 mcg	by United Res	00677-0992	Antithyroid
JSP522	Tab, JSP-522 Embossed	Levothyroxine Sodium 0.2 mg	by Jerome Stevens	50564-0522	Antithyroid
JSP522	Tab	Levothyroxine Sodium 200 mcg	by United Res	00677-0079	Antithyroid
JSP523	Tab	Levothyroxine Sodium 0.3 mg	by Zenith Goldline	00182-1119	Antithyroid
JSP523	Tab, JSP-523 Embossed	Levothyroxine Sodium 0.3 mg	by Jerome Stevens	50564-0523	Antithyroid
JSP523	Tab, Light Green, JSP <>	Levothyroxine Sodium 0.3 mg	by Quality Care	60346-0474	Antithyroid
JSP526	Cap, Dark Green, JSP-526	Brompheniramine Maleate 6 mg, Pseudoephedrine HCl 60 mg	Nasal Decongestant PD by Jerome Stevens	50564-0526	Cold Remedy

ID FRONT <> BACK	DESCRIPTION FRONT <> BACK	INGREDIENT & STRENGTH	BRAND (OR EQUIV.) & FIRM	NDC#	CLASS; SCH.
JSP526	Cap, Clear & Green, Ex Release, with White Beads, JSP 526	Brompheniramine Maleate 12 mg, Pseudoephedrine HCl 120 mg	Nasal Decongestant TR by Quality Care	60346-0929	Cold Remedy
JSP527	Cap, Light Green, JSP-527	Brompheniramine Maleate 12 mg, Pseudoephedrine HCl 120 mg	Nasal Decongestant by Jerome Stevens	50564-0527	Cold Remedy
JSP533	Tab, Ex Release, JSP-533 Embossed	Isosorbide Dinitrate 40 mg	by Jerome Stevens	50564-0533	Antianginal
JSP533	Tab, Ex Release, JSP-533	Isosorbide Dinitrate 40 mg	by Quality Care	60346-0280	Antianginal
JSP533	Tab, ER	Isosorbide Dinitrate 40 mg	by Qualitest	00603-4120	Antianginal
JSP539	Tab	Hyoscyamine Sulfate 0.125 mg	by Zenith Goldline	00182-1607	Gastrointestinal
JSP539	Tab, JSP-539 Embossed	Hyoscyamine Sulfate 0.125 mg	by Jerome Stevens	50564-0539	Gastrointestinal
JSP540	Tab, Film Coated, Jerome Stevens	Methenamine Mandelate 500 mg	by Rugby	00536-4022	Antibiotic; Urinary Tract
JSP540	Tab, Film Coated, JSP-540 Embossed	Methenamine Mandelate 500 mg	by Jerome Stevens	50564-0540	Antibiotic; Urinary Tract
JSP541	Tab, Film Coated, JSP-541 Embossed	Methenamine Mandelate 1000 mg	by Jerome Stevens	50564-0541	Antibiotic; Urinary Tract
JSP544	Tab, JSP-544	Digoxin 0.125 mg	by Jerome Stevens	50564-0544	Cardiac Agent
JSP545	Tab, JSP-545	Digoxin 0.25 mg	by Jerome Stevens	50564-0545	Cardiac Agent
JSP547	Tab, White, Round	Yohimbine HCl 5.4 mg	Yocon by Jerome Stevens		Impotence Agent
JSP548	Tab, JSP-548	Guaifenesin 600 mg	by Jerome Stevens	50564-0548	Expectorant
JSP551	Tab, Mustard, Oval	Prenatal Vitamin Plus	Stuartnatal Plus by Jerome Stevens		Vitamin
JSP552	Tab, Green, Round	Hyoscyamine Sulfate SL 0.125 mg	Levsin SL by Jerome Stevens		Gastrointestinal
JSP553	Tab	Codeine Phosphate 10 mg, Guaifenesin 300 mg	by Pecos	59879-0512	Cold Remedy; C III
JSP553	Tab, Coated	Codeine Phosphate 10 mg, Guaifenesin 300 mg	by Quality Care	62682-8003	Cold Remedy; C III
JSP553	Tab	Codeine Phosphate 10 mg, Guaifenesin 300 mg	by Zenith Goldline	00182-0151	Cold Remedy; C III
JSP553	Tab, JSP-553	Codeine Phosphate 10 mg, Guaifenesin 300 mg	by Jerome Stevens	50564-0553	Cold Remedy; C III
JU <> VISKEN15	Tab, White, Round, Scored	Pindolol 15 mg	Visken by Novartis	Canadian DIN# 00417289	Antihypertensive
JUL42 <> PAL	Tab, White, Scored	Pseudoephedrine HCl 80 mg, Guaifenesin 800 mg	Panmist LA by Sovereign Pharms	58716-0692	Cold Remedy
JUVISKEN15	Tab, White, JU/Visken 15	Pindolol 15 mg	Visken by Sandoz	Canadian	Antihypertensive
K	Tab, Pink w/ White Specks, Round	Attapulgite 300 mg	Kaopectate by Johnson & Johnson	Canadian DIN# 02229948	Antidiarrheal
K	Tab, Light Pink, Round, Chewable	Kaopectate 300 mg	by Upjohn		Antidiarrheal
K	Tab, Efferv	Potassium Bicarbonate 0.5 gm, Potassium Chloride 1.5 gm	Efferv Potassium Chloride by Qualitest	00603-3508	Electrolytes
K	Tab, Efferv	Potassium Bicarbonate 0.5 gm, Potassium Chloride 1.5 gm	Efferv Potassium Chloride by Tower	50201-1300	Electrolytes
K	Tab, Efferv	Potassium Bicarbonate 0.5 gm, Potassium Chloride 1.5 gm	Efferv Potassium Chloride by Bajamar Chem	44184-0025	Electrolytes
K	Tab, Orange, Round	Potassium Bicarbonate 2.5 g	Effervescent by Tower Labs.		Electrolytes
K	Cap, Orange	Valproic Acid 250 mg	by Altimed	Canadian DIN# 02140047	Anticonvulsant
K	Cap, Orange	Valproic Acid 250 mg	Kenral Valproic by Kenral	Canadian	Anticonvulsant
K	Tab, Pink, Round	Vitamin B Complex	Apatate by Kenwood		Vitamin
K 250	Tab, White	Erythromycin 250 mg	Erythromycin by Kenral	Canadian	Antibiotic
K0183	Tab, Chewable	Chlorpheniramine Maleate 1 mg, Pseudoephedrine HCl 15 mg	Deconamine Childrens by Kenwood	00482-0183	Cold Remedy
K0183	Tab, Chewable	Chlorpheniramine Maleate 1 mg, Pseudoephedrine HCl 15 mg	Deconamine by Lini	58215-0324	Cold Remedy
K0659	Tab, White, Oval	Ergoloid Mesylate SL 1 mg	Hydergine by KV		Ergot
K0849	Cap, Brown & Clear	Papaverine HCl SR 150 mg	Pavabid by KV		Vasodilator
K1	Tab, White, Triangular, Film Coated	Granisetron HCl 1.12 mg	Kytril by SKB	60351-4151	Antiemetic
K1	Tab, White, Triangular, Film Coated	Granisetron HCl 1.12 mg	Kytril by SKB	00029-4151	Antiemetic
K1	Tab, Green, Round	Hydromorphone HCl 1 mg	Dilaudid by Knoll		Analgesic; C II
K1	Tab, Blue, Round	Medroxyprogesterone Acetate 5 mg	by AltiMed	Canadian DIN# 02148560	Progestin

ID FRONT <> BACK	DESCRIPTION FRONT <> BACK	INGREDIENT & STRENGTH	BRAND (OR EQUIV.) & FIRM	NDC#	CLASS; SCH.
K10 <> ALRA	Tab, Film Coated, Debossed, K+10 <> Alra	Potassium Chloride 750 mg	by PDRX	55289-0359	Electrolytes
K10 <> ALRA	Tab, Film Coated, K+10 <> Alra	Potassium Chloride 750 mg	K Plus 10 by Quality Care	62682-6025	Electrolytes
K10 <> ALRA	Tab, Film Coated, K+19	Potassium Chloride 750 mg	by Golden State	60429-0215	Electrolytes
K100	Cap, Clear	Morphine Sulfate 100 mg	by Knoll	Canadian	Analgesic
K100	Tab, White, Oblong	Ranitidine 300 mg	by Altimed	Canadian	Gastrointestinal
K100	Tab, White, Oblong	Ranitidine HCl 336 mg	Ranitidine by Kenral	Canadian DIN# 00828688	Gastrointestinal
K101	Tab, White, Round	Ranitidine HCl 168 mg	Ranitidine by Kenral	Canadian DIN# 00828823	Gastrointestinal
K101	Tab, White, Round	Ranitidine 150 mg	by Altimed	Canadian	Gastrointestinal
K104	Tab, White, Elliptical	Flurbiprofen 50 mg	Flurbiprofen by Kenral	Canadian	NSAID
K104	Tab, White, Elliptical	Flurbiprofen 50 mg	by Altimed	Canadian DIN# 00675202	NSAID
K105	Tab, Blue, Elliptical	Flurbiprofen 100 mg	Flurbiprofen by Kenral	Canadian	NSAID
K105	Tab, Blue, Elliptical	Flurbiprofen 100 mg	by Altimed	Canadian DIN# 00675199	NSAID
K108	Tab, Yellow, Round	Desipramine 25 mg	by Altimed	Canadian DIN# 01948784	Antidepressant
K108	Tab, Yellow, Round	Desipramine 25 mg	Desipramine by Kenral	Canadian	Antidepressant
K109	Tab, Green, Round	Desipramine 50 mg	Desipramine by Kenral	Canadian	Antidepressant
K109	Tab, Green, Round	Desipramine 50 mg	by Altimed	Canadian DIN# 01948792	Antidepressant
K11	Tab, White, Triangle, Convex, Film Coated	Granisetron HCl 1 mg	Kytril by Lederle	59911-5552	Antiemetic
K110	Tab, Orange, Round	Desipramine 75 mg	by Altimed	Canadian DIN# 01948806	Antidepressant
K110	Tab, Orange, Round	Desipramine 75 mg	Desipramine by Kenral	Canadian	Antidepressant
K113	Tab, White	Domperidone 10 mg	by Altimed	Canadian DIN# 01912070	Gastrointestinal
K113	Tab, White	Domperidone Maleate 12.72 mg	Domperidone Mal by Kenral	Canadian	Gastrointestinal
K124	Tab, Orange	Doxycycline Hyclate 100 mg	by AltiMed	Canadian	Antibiotic
K17	Tab, Orange	Prazosin HCl 1 mg	by AltiMed	Canadian DIN# 02139979	Antihypertensive
K18	Tab, White, Round	Prazosin 2 mg	by Altimed	Canadian	Antihypertensive
K18	Tab, White, Round	Prazosin HCl 2 mg	by AltiMed	Canadian DIN# 02139987	Antihypertensive
K182	Tab, Coated, K Underlined	Guaifenesin 300 mg, Hydrocodone Bitartrate 5 mg, Pseudoephedrine HCl 30 mg	Deconamine CX by Kenwood	00482-0182	Cold Remedy; C III
K19	Tab, White, Diamond	Prazosin HCl 5 mg	by AltiMed	Canadian DIN# 02139995	Antihypertensive
K2	Tab, White, Triangle, Convex, Film	Granisetron HCl 2 mg	Kytril by Lederle	59911-5551	Antiemetic
K2	Tab, White, Triangle, Convex, Film	Granisetron HCl 2.0 mg	Kytril by Lederle	59911-5550	Antiemetic
K2	Tab, Orange, Round	Hydromorphone HCl 2 mg	Dilaudid by Knoll		Analgesic; C II

ID FRONT <> BACK	DESCRIPTION FRONT <> BACK	INGREDIENT & STRENGTH	BRAND (OR EQUIV.) & FIRM	NDC#	CLASS; SCH.
K20	Tab, Blue, Round	Desipramine 10 mg	by Altimed	Canadian DIN# 01948776	Antidepressant
K20	Tab, Blue, Round	Desipramine 10 mg	Desipramine by Kenral	Canadian	Antidepressant
K20	Cap, Clear	Morphine Sulfate 20 mg	by Knoll	Canadian	Analgesic
K21	Tab, Light Green, Oblong	Loperamide HCl 2 mg	Kenral Loperamide by Kenral	Canadian	Antidiarrheal
K211	Tab	Morphine Sulfate 30 mg	by King	60793-0211	Analgesic; C II
K212	Tab	Morphine Sulfate 15 mg	by King	60793-0212	Analgesic; C II
K250	Tab, White, Circular	Erythromycin 250 mg	by Altimed	Canadian	Antibiotic
K27	Tab, White, Round	Pseudoephedrine HCl 60 mg	by PDK Labs		Decongestant
K29	Tab, White, Oval, Scored	Alprazolam 0.25 mg	by Altimed	Canadian DIN# 00677485	Antianxiety
K2A <> MYLERAN	Tab	Busulfan 2 mg	Myleran by Catalytica	63552-0713	Antineoplastic
K2A <> MYLERAN	Tab	Busulfan 2 mg	Myleran by Glaxo	00173-0713	Antineoplastic
K3	Tab, Pink, Round	Hydromorphone HCl 3 mg	Dilaudid by Knoll		Analgesic; C II
K3	Tab, White, Round	Medroxyprogesterone Acetate 10 mg	by AltiMed	Canadian DIN# 02148579	Progestin
K30	Tab, White, Round	Codeine Sulfate 30 mg	by Knoll		Analgesic; C III
K300	Tab, White	Ibuprofen 300 mg	Ibuprofen by Kenral	Canadian	NSAID
K300	Tab, White, Circular	Ibuprofen 300 mg	by Altimed	Canadian	NSAID
K4	Tab, Yellow, Round	Hydromorphone HCl 4 mg	Dilaudid by Knoll		Analgesic; C II
K4	Tab, Powder Blue, Elliptical, K/4	Triazolam 0.25 mg	by Altimed	Canadian	Sedative/Hypnotic
K4	Tab, Blue, K/4	Triazolam 0.25 mg	Triazolam by Kenral	Canadian	Sedative/Hypnotic
K400	Tab, Orange, Circular	Ibuprofen 400 mg	by Altimed	Canadian	NSAID
K400	Tab, Orange	Ibuprofen 400 mg	Ibuprofen by Kenral	Canadian	NSAID
K5	Tab, White, Circular	Prednisone 5 mg	by Altimed	Canadian	Steroid
K5	Tab, White, Circular, Scored	Prednisone 5 mg	Prednisone by Kenral	Canadian	Steroid
K50	Cap, Clear	Morphine Sulfate 50 mg	by Knoll	Canadian	Analgesic
K55	Tab, Peach, Oval, Scored	Alprazolam 0.5 mg	by Altimed	Canadian DIN# 00677477	Antianxiety
K56	Tab, White, Round	Acetaminophen 250 mg, Aspirin 250 mg, Caffeine 64 mg	Pain Relief II by PDK Labs		Analgesic
K6	Tab, Orange, Round	Medroxyprogesterone Acetate 2.5 mg	by AltiMed	Canadian DIN# 02148552	Progestin
K60	Tab, White, Round	Codeine Sulfate 60 mg	by Knoll		Analgesic; C III
K600	Cap, Peach	Ibuprofen 600 mg	by Altimed	Canadian	NSAID
K600	Tab, Peach	Ibuprofen 600 mg	Ibuprofen by Kenral	Canadian	NSAID
K634	Cap, Clear & Lavender, K-634	Nitroglycerin TD 2.5 mg	Nitrobid by KV		Vasodilator
K635	Cap, Blue & Yellow, K-635	Nitroglycerin TD 6.5 mg	Nitrobid by KV		Vasodilator
K698	Cap, Clear	Nitroglycerin TD 9 mg	Nitrobid by KV		Antianginal
K713	Cap, Blue & Maroon	Piroxicam 10 mg	by Altimed	Canadian DIN# 02139952	NSAID
K713	Cap, Blue & Maroon	Piroxicam 10 mg	Kenral Piroxicam by Kenral	Canadian	NSAID
K714	Cap, Maroon & Opaque	Piroxicam 20 mg	by Altimed	Canadian DIN# 02139960	NSAID
K714	Cap, Maroon & Opaque	Piroxicam 20 mg	Kenral Piroxicam by Kenral	Canadian	NSAID

ID FRONT <> BACK	DESCRIPTION FRONT <> BACK	INGREDIENT & STRENGTH	BRAND (OR EQUIV.) & FIRM	NDC#	CLASS; SCH.
K715	Cap, Pink & Scarlet	Doxepin HCl 10 mg	by AltiMed	Canadian DIN# 02140071	Antidepressant
K716	Cap, Blue & Pink	Doxepin HCl 25 mg	by AltiMed	Canadian DIN# 02140098	Antidepressant
K717	Cap, Flesh & Pink	Doxepin HCl 50 mg	by AltiMed	Canadian DIN# 02140101	Antidepressant
K718	Cap, Flesh	Domperidone 75 mg	by Altimed	Canadian	Gastrointestinal
K718	Cap, Flesh	Doxepin HCl 75 mg	by AltiMed	Canadian DIN# 02140128	Antidepressant
K750	Cap, Blue	Doxycycline Hyclate 100 mg	by AltiMed	Canadian	Antibiotic
K8	Tab, Orange, Round	Potassium Chloride SA 600 mg	Slow K by Alra		Electrolytes
K8	Tab, Violet, K/8	Triazolam 0.125 mg	Triazolam by Kenral	Canadian	Sedative/Hypnotic
K8	Tab, Light Violet, Elliptical, K/8	Triazolam 0.125 mg	by Altimed	Canadian	Sedative/Hypnotic
K8 <> ALRA	Tab, Film Coated, K+8	Potassium Chloride 600 mg	by Golden State	60429-0158	Electrolytes
KADIAN <> 100MG	Cap	Morphine Sulfate 100 mg	Kadian ER by Purepac	00228-2055	Analgesic; C II
KADIAN <> 20MG	Cap	Morphine Sulfate 20 mg	Kadian ER by Purepac	00228-2043	Analgesic; C II
KADIAN <> 50MG	Cap	Morphine Sulfate 50 mg	Kadian ER by Purepac	00228-2045	Analgesic; C II
KADIAN100MG	Cap, Green, Opaque	Morphine Sulfate 100 mg	Kadian ER by Faulding	63857-0324	Analgesic; C II
KADIAN20MG	Cap, Yellow, Opaque	Morphine Sulfate 20 mg	Kadian ER by Faulding	63857-0322	Analgesic; C II
KADIAN50MG	Cap, Blue, Opaque	Morphine Sulfate 50 mg	Kadian ER by Faulding	63857-0323	Analgesic; C II
KAO600	Tab, White, Ellipsoidal	Attapulgite 600 mg	Kaopectate by Johnson & Johnson	Canadian DIN# 02229953	Antidiarrheal
KAO750	Tab, White, Cap Shaped	Attapulgite 750 mg	Kaopectate by Johnson & Johnson	Canadian DIN# 02229949	Antidiarrheal
KBI2	Tab, White, Round	Hydrocodone Bitartrate 7.5 mg, Acetaminophen 750 mg	by Heartland Hlthcare	61392-0921	Analgesic; C III
KCl10BOLARKV	Cap, Clear, KCl 10/Bolar/KV	Potassium Chloride 10 mEq	Micro K 10 by Bolar		Electrolytes
KDUR10	Tab, White, Oblong, K-DUR 10	Potassium Chloride 750 mg	K-Dur 10 ER by Schering	00085-0263	Electrolytes
KDUR10	Tab, ER	Potassium Chloride 750 mg	by Med Pro	53978-2060	Electrolytes
KDUR10	Tab, Ex Release, K-DUR 10	Potassium Chloride 750 mg	K Dur by Nat Pharmpak Serv	55154-1505	Electrolytes
KDUR10	Tab, Ex Release, K-DUR 10	Potassium Chloride 750 mg	K Dur by Amerisource	62584-0404	Electrolytes
KDUR20	Tab, Off-White, Oblong, K-DUR 20	Potassium Chloride 20 mEq	K-DUR by Schering	Canadian	Electrolytes
KDUR20	Tab, White, Oblong, Scored	Potassium Chloride 20 meq	K Dur 20 by Rightpak	65240-0675	Electrolytes
KDUR20	Tab, White, Oblong, K-DUR 20	Potassium Chloride 20 mEq	K Dur 20 ER by Schering	00085-0787	Electrolytes
KDUR20	Tab, ER	Potassium Chloride 20 mEq	K Dur Sr by Nat Pharmpak Serv	55154-1504	Electrolytes
KDUR20	Tab, Ex Release K DUR 20	Potassium Chloride 20 mEq	by Med Pro	53978-2061	Electrolytes
KDUR20	Tab, Ex Release K DUR 20	Potassium Chloride 20 mEq	K Dur by PDRX	55289-0079	Electrolytes
KDUR20	Tab, ER	Potassium Chloride 20 mEq	K Dur by Amerisource	62584-0787	Electrolytes
KEENE7788	Cap, Green Print, Keene/7788	Acetaminophen 325 mg, Butalbital 50 mg, Caffeine 40 mg	Endolor by Keene	00588-7788	Analgesic
KEFLEX250 <> DISTAH69	Cap	Cephalexin Monohydrate	Keflex by Quality Care	60346-0649	Antibiotic
KEFLEX250 <> DISTAH69	Cap	Cephalexin Monohydrate 250 mg	Keflex by Lilly	00110-0869	Antibiotic
KEFLEX250 <> DISTAH69	Cap	Cephalexin Monohydrate 250 mg	Keflex by DISTA Prod	00777-0869	Antibiotic
KEFTAB <> 500	Tab, Dark Green, Elliptical, Coated	Cephalexin HCl	Keftab by Quality Care	60346-0650	Antibiotic
KEFTAB500	Tab	Cephalexin HCl	Keftab by DISTA Prod	00777-4143	Antibiotic

ID FRONT <> BACK	DESCRIPTION FRONT <> BACK	INGREDIENT & STRENGTH	BRAND (OR EQUIV.) & FIRM	NDC#	CLASS; SCH.
KEFTAB500	Tab, Green, Oval	Cephalexin HCl 500 mg	Keftab by Carlsbad	61442-0101	Antibiotic
KEM	Tab, White, Round, Sch. Logo KEM	Prednisone 1 mg	Meticorten by Schering		Steroid
KEMADRIN <> S3A	Tab	Procyclidine HCl 5 mg	Kemadrin by Catalytica	63552-0604	Antiparkinson
KEMADRIN <> S3A	Tab, White, Round	Procyclidine HCl 5 mg	Kemadrin by Monarch	61570-0059	Antiparkinson
KEMADRINS3A	Tab, White, Round, Kemadrin/S3A	Procyclidine HCl 5 mg	by Glaxo	Canadian	Antiparkinson
KENWOOD <> ADEFLORM	Tab	Ascorbic Acid 100 mg, Calcium 250 mg, Calcium Pantothenate 10 mg, Cyanocobalamin 2 mcg, Fluorides 1 mg, Iron 30 mg, Niacinamide 20 mg, Pyridoxine HCl 10 mg, Riboflavin 2.5 mg, Thiamine Mononitrate 1.5 mg, Vitamin A 6000 Units, Vitamin D 400 Units	Adeflor M by Kenwood	00482-0115	Vitamin
KENWOOD181	Cap	Chlorpheniramine Maleate 8 mg, Pseudoephedrine HCl 120 mg	Deconamine Sr by Nat Pharmpak Serv	55154-6401	Cold Remedy
KENWOOD181	Cap	Chlorpheniramine Maleate 8 mg, Pseudoephedrine HCl 120 mg	Deconamine Sr by Thrift Drug	59198-0183	Cold Remedy
KENWOOD181	Cap	Chlorpheniramine Maleate 8 mg, Pseudoephedrine HCl 120 mg	Deconamine Sr by Kenwood	00482-0181	Cold Remedy
KENWOOD184	Tab	Chlorpheniramine Maleate 4 mg, Pseudoephedrine HCl 60 mg	Deconamine by Kenwood	00482-0184	Cold Remedy
KERLONE10	Tab, White, Round, Coated	Betaxolol HCl 10 mg	Kerlone by GD Searle	00025-5101	Antihypertensive
KERLONE20 <> B	Tab, White, Round, Coated, Kerlone 20 <> Greek Letter Beta	Betaxolol HCl 20 mg	Kerlone by GD Searle	00025-5201	Antihypertensive
KET10	Tab, White, Round	Ketorolac 10 mg	Toradol by Roche	Canadian	NSAID
KETOPROFEN	Cap, Green & Ivory, Logo	Ketoprofen 50 mg	by Pharmascience	Canadian	NSAID
KETOPROFENER 200MG <> SHN	Cap, Ketoprofen ER 200 MG	Ketoprofen 200 mg	Ketoprofen by Schein	00364-2667	NSAID
KETOPROFENER 200MG <> SHN	Cap, ER, Ketoprofen ER 200 MG	Ketoprofen 200 mg	Ketoprofen by Danbury	00591-8847	NSAID
KETOPROFENER 200MG <> SHN	Cap, Blue & Opaque & White, Ketoprofen ER 200 MG	Ketoprofen 200 mg	by Murfreesboro	51129-1596	NSAID
KETOPROFENER 200MG <> SHN	Cap, ER, Ketoprofen ER 200 MG	Ketoprofen 200 mg	Ketoprofen by Elan	56125-0102	NSAID
KH	Cap, Red	Ethchlorvynol 500 mg	Placidyl by Abbott	00074-6685	Hypnotic; C IV
KH2 <> ORGANON	Tab, Film Coated, KH over 2 <> Organon	Desogestrel 0.15 mg, Ethinyl Estradiol 0.02 mg, Ethinyl Estradiol 0.01 mg	Mircette by Organon	00052-0281	Oral Contraceptive
KH2 <> ORGANON	Tab, Film Coated, K H over 2 <> Organon	Desogestrel 0.15 mg, Ethinyl Estradiol 0.02 mg, Ethinyl Estradiol 0.01 mg	Mircette by NV Organon	12860-0281	Oral Contraceptive
KH2 <> ORGANON	Tab, KH Over 2	Desogestrel 0.15 mg, Ethinyl Estradiol 0.03 mg	Desogen by Organon	60889-0261	Oral Contraceptive
KH2 <> ORGANON	Tab, Film Coated, K H over 2 <> Organon	Desogestrel 0.15 mg, Ethinyl Estradiol 0.03 mg	Desogen by Organon	00052-0261	Oral Contraceptive .
KH2 <> ORGANON	Tab, Green, Round	Inate	Marvelon 28 by Organon	Canadian DIN# 02042479	Placebo
KJ	Tab, Yellow, Oval, Abbott Logo <> KJ	Clarithromycin 500 mg	Biaxin XL by Abbott	00074-3165	Antibiotic
KJ <> GEIGY	Tab, White to Off-White, Oval, Scored	Baclofen 10 mg	Lioresal by Geigy	Canadian DIN# 00455881	Muscle Relaxant
KL	Tab, Film Coated, Abbott Logo	Clarithromycin 500 mg	Biaxin by PDRX	55289-0021	Antibiotic
KL	Tab, Delayed Release, Abbott Labs Logo	Clarithromycin 500 mg	Biaxin by Quality Care	60346-0351	Antibiotic
KL	Tab, Film Coated, Abbott Logo in Blue	Clarithromycin 500 mg	Biaxin by Amerisource	62584-0317	Antibiotic
KL	Tab, Delayed Release, Imprinted in Blue with Abbott Logo	Clarithromycin 500 mg	Biaxin by Promex Med	62301-0001	Antibiotic
KL	Tab, Abbott Logo	Clarithromycin 500 mg	Biaxin by Nat Pharmpak Serv	55154-0109	Antibiotic
KL	Tab, Yellow, Oval, Blue Print, KL over Abbott Logo	Clarithromycin 500 mg	Biaxin by Abbott	00074-2586	Antibiotic
KL	Tab, Yellow, Oval, Abbott Logo <> KL	Clarithromycin 500 mg	Biaxin by Abbott	00074-2586	Antibiotic
KL	Tab, Abbott Logo	Clarithromycin 500 mg	by Med Pro	53978-3038	Antibiotic
KL	Tab, Film Coated, Abbott Logo	Clarithromycin 500 mg	Biaxin by Allscripts	54569-3439	Antibiotic
KL	Tab, Film Coated, Abbott Logo	Clarithromycin 500 mg	Biaxin by HJ Harkins Co	52959-0230	Antibiotic
KL	Tab, Film Coated, Abbott Logo	Clarithromycin 500 mg	Biaxin by DRX	55045-1865	Antibiotic
KL	Tab, Light Yellow, Film Coated, Abbott Logo	Clarithromycin 500 mg	Biaxin by Murfreesboro	51129-2586	Antibiotic
KL	Tab, K/L	Yohimbine HCl 5.4 mg	Yohimex by JMI Canton	00252-3230	Impotence Agent
KL <> A	Tab, Yellow, Oval, Film Coated	Clarithromycin 500 mg	Biaxin by Promex Medcl	62301-0037	Antibiotic
KL107	Tab, Delayed Release, KL 107	Guaifenesin 600 mg	by Quality Care	60346-0863	Expectorant

ID FRONT <> BACK	DESCRIPTION FRONT <> BACK	INGREDIENT & STRENGTH	BRAND (OR EQUIV.) & FIRM	NDC#	CLASS; SCH.
KL107	Tab, Ex Release, KL-107	Guaifenesin 600 mg	Humavent LA by WE	59196-0008	Expectorant
KL107	Tab, Ex Release	Guaifenesin 600 mg	Guaispan by Warner Kiel	62291-0102	Expectorant
KL107	Tab, Ex Release, KL-107	Guaifenesin 600 mg	by Kiel	59063-0107	Expectorant
KL109	Tab, Ex Release, KL-109	Guaifenesin 600 mg, Phenylpropanolamine HCl 75 mg	Sinuvent by WE	59196-0001	Cold Remedy
KL109	Tab, Ex Release, KL-109	Guaifenesin 600 mg, Phenylpropanolamine HCl 75 mg	Vental by Alphagen	59743-0049	Cold Remedy
KL109	Tab, Ex Release, KL-109	Guaifenesin 600 mg, Phenylpropanolamine HCl 75 mg	by Kiel	59063-0109	Cold Remedy
KL110	Tab, Light Blue, Cap Shaped	Dextromethorphan Hydrobromide 30 mg, Guaifenesin 600 mg	S Pack DM by Duramed	51285-0589	Cold Remedy
KL110	Tab, Light Blue, Cap Shaped, KL-110	Dextromethorphan Hydrobromide 30 mg, Guaifenesin 600 mg	Deconsal II by Kiel	51285-0565	Cold Remedy
KL110	Tab, Blue & Green, Cap Shaped, Film Coated	Guaifenesin 600 mg	S Pack Kit by Duramed	51285-0588	Expectorant
KL111	Tab, White, Round, Unscored, with KL 111	Orphenadrine Citrate 100 mg	Orphenadrine Citrate ER by Perrigo	00113-0368	Muscle Relaxant
KL112	Tab, KL-112	Carbinoxamine Maleate 8 mg, Pseudoephedrine HCl 120 mg	Carbodec by Rugby	00536-4453	Cold Remedy
KLONOPIN05ROCHE	Tab	Clonazepam 0.5 mg	Klonopin by Roche	59643-0068	Anticonvulsant; C IV
KLONOPIN05ROCHE	Tab, Klonopin 0.5 Roche	Clonazepam 0.5 mg	Klonopin by Hoffmann La Roche	00004-0068	Anticonvulsant; C IV
KLONOPIN1ROCHE	Tab	Clonazepam 1 mg	Klonopin by Roche	59643-0058	Anticonvulsant; C IV
KLONOPIN2ROCHE	Tab	Clonazepam 2 mg	Klonopin by Roche	59643-0098	Anticonvulsant; C IV
KLONOPINROCHE	Tab	Clonazepam 1 mg	Klonopin by Allscripts	54569-2727	Anticonvulsant; C IV
KLORCON10	Tab, Yellow, Round, Film, KLOR-CON 10	Potassium Chloride 750 mg	Klor-Con 10 by Purdue Frederick	00034-1201	Electrolytes
KLORCON10	Tab, Film Coated	Potassium Chloride 750 mg	Klor Con 10 by Caremark	00339-6011	Electrolytes
KLORCON8	Tab, Film Coated, KLOR-CON/8	Potassium Chloride 600 mg	by Kaiser	00179-1164	Electrolytes
KLORCON8	Tab, Blue, Round, Klor-Con 8	Potassium Chloride 8mEq	Klor-Con 8 by Upsher-Smith	00245-0040	Electrolytes
KLOTRIXBL770MEQ	Tab, ER, in Black Ink BL in Center with Klotrix 10 MEQ 770 Around Tab Face	Potassium Chloride 10 mEq	Klotrix by Bristol Myers Squibb	00087-0770	Electrolytes
KN	Cap, Green	Ethchlorvynol 750 mg	Placidyl by Abbott	00074-6630	Hypnotic; C IV
KNOLL <> 120SR	Tab, Purple, Oval, Film, 120 SR	Verapamil HCl 120 mg	Isoptin SR by Teva	00480-1006	Antihypertensive
KNOLL <> ISOPTIN120	Tab, Film Coated, Isoptin 120	Verapamil HCl 120 mg	Isoptin by Knoll	00044-1823	Antihypertensive
KNOLL <> ISOPTIN80	Tab, Film Coated	Verapamil HCl 80 mg	by Med Pro	53978-7001	Antihypertensive
KNOLL <> ISOPTIN80	Tab, Film Coated, Isoptin 80	Verapamil HCl 80 mg	Isoptin by Knoll	00044-1822	Antihypertensive
KNOLL <> ISOPTIN80	Tab, Film Coated, Embossed	Verapamil HCl 80 mg	Isoptin by Amerisource	62584-0822	Antihypertensive
KNOLL1	Tab, Pink, Round, Scored	Trandolapril 1 mg	Mavik by Murfreesboro Ph	51129-1400	Antihypertensive
KNOLL1	Tab, Salmon, Round	Trandolapril 1 mg	Mavik by Knoll	00048-5805	Antihypertensive
KNOLL120SR	Tab, Violet, Oval	Verapamil HCl SR 120 mg	Isoptin SR by Knoll		Antihypertensive
KNOLL2	Tab, Yellow, Round	Trandolapril 2 mg	Mavik by Knoll	00048-5806	Antihypertensive
KNOLL4	Tab, Rose, Round	Trandolapril 4 mg	Mavik by Knoll	00048-5807	Antihypertensive
KOK	Tab, White, Round, KO/K with Arrow	Acetaminophen 325 mg	APAP by PDK		Analgesic
KOLRCON10	Tab, Yellow, Round, Kolr-Con 10	Potassium Chloride 10 mEq	Klor-Con 10 y Upsher-Smith	00245-0041	Electrolytes
KOS	Tab, Ex Release, Printed 375, 500 or 750	Niacin 750 mg	Niaspan by KOS	60598-0004	Vitamin
KOS <> 1000	Tab, Ex Release, Debossed	Niacin 1000 mg	Niaspan by KOS	60598-0003	Vitamin
KOS <> 500	Tab, White, Oblong	Niacin 500 mg	Niaspan by DRX Pharm Consults	55045-2767	Vitamin
KOS <> 500	Tab, Ex Release, Debossed	Niacin 500 mg	Niaspan by KOS	60598-0001	Vitamin
KOS <> 750	Tab, Ex Release, Debossed	Niacin 750 mg	Niaspan by KOS	60598-0002	Vitamin
KP <> 101	Tab, Gold, Compressed, KP Logo	Sulfasalazine 500 mg	Azulfidine by Thrift Drug	59198-0010	Gastrointestinal
KP <> 102	Tab, Gold, Elliptical-Shaped, Film Coated	Sulfasalazine 500 mg	Azulfidine EN by Thrift Drug	59198-0230	Gastrointestinal
KP1026	Cap	Codeine Phosphate 20 mg, Pseudoephedrine HCl 60 mg	Kg Fed by King	60793-0026	Cold Remedy; C III
KPH <> 101	Tab	Sulfasalazine 500 mg	Azulfidine by Pharmacia & Upjohn	59632-0101	Gastrointestinal
KPH <> 101	Tab, Orangish Yellow, Round, KPh <> 101	Sulfasalazine 500 mg	by Pharmacia	Canadian DIN# 02064480	Gastrointestinal
KPH <> 101	Tab, Mustard	Sulfasalazine 500 mg	Azulfidine by Pharmacia & Upjohn	00013-0101	Gastrointestinal
KPH <> 102	Tab, Film Coated	Sulfasalazine 500 mg	Azulfidine EN Tabs by Pharmacia & Upjohn	59632-0102	Gastrointestinal

ID FRONT <> BACK	DESCRIPTION FRONT <> BACK	INGREDIENT & STRENGTH	BRAND (OR EQUIV.) & FIRM	NDC#	CLASS; SCH.
KPH <> 102	Tab, Orange, Elliptical, Enteric Coated, KPh <> 102	Sulfasalazine 500 mg	by Pharmacia	Canadian DIN# 02064472	Gastrointestinal
KPH <> 102	Tab, Yellow, Oval, Enteric Coated	Sulfasalazine 500 mg	Azulfidine by Natl Pharmpak	55154-2801	Gastrointestinal
KPH <> 102	Tab, Gold, Film Coated	Sulfasalazine 500 mg	Azulfidine EN Tabs by Wal Mart	49035-0167	Gastrointestinal
KPH <> 102	Tab, Yellow	Sulfasalazine 500 mg	Azulfidine by Rx Pac	65084-0171	Gastrointestinal
KPH <> 102	Tab, Mustard, Film Coated	Sulfasalazine 500 mg	Azulfidine EN Tabs by Pharmacia & Upjohn	00013-0102	Gastrointestinal
KPH101	Tab, Orange & Yellow, Round, Kph/101	Sulfasalazine 500 mg	by Pharmacia	Canadian	Gastrointestinal
KPH102	Tab, Orange, Elliptical, Kph/102	Sulfasalazine 500 mg	by Pharmacia	Canadian	Gastrointestinal
KPI <> 13	Tab, Light Green, Oval, Ex Release	Guaifenesin 600 mg	Monafed by Monarch	61570-0026	Expectorant
KPI1	Tab	Acetaminophen 500 mg, Hydrocodone Bitartrate 5 mg	by King	60793-0844	Analgesic; C III
KPI1	Tab, White, Round, KPI 1	Acetaminophen 500 mg, Hydrocodone Bitartrate 5 mg	Lortab by Endo	60951-0639	Analgesic; C III
KPI12	Tab	Acetaminophen 750 mg, Hydrocodone Bitartrate 7.5 mg	by Mallinckrodt Hobart	00406-0360	Analgesic; C III
KPI13	Tab, Light Green	Guaifenesin 600 mg	Monafed by King	60793-0850	Expectorant
KPI13	Tab, Ex Release	Guaifenesin 600 mg	by King	60793-0049	Expectorant
KPI14	Tab, Green, Oval, Ex Release	Dextromethorphan Hydrobromide 30 mg, Guaifenesin 600 mg	Monafed DM by Monarch	61570-0027	Cold Remedy
KPI14	Tab, Ex Release, Embossed	Dextromethorphan Hydrobromide 30 mg, Guaifenesin 600 mg	by King	60793-0050	Cold Remedy
KPI14	Tab, Ex Release, Embossed	Dextromethorphan Hydrobromide 30 mg, Guaifenesin 600 mg	Monafed DM by King	60793-0851	Cold Remedy
KPI2	Tab, White, Round	Acetaminophen 750 mg, Hydrocodone Bitartrate 7.5 mg	by Endo	60951-0641	Analgesic; C III
KPI2	Tab	Acetaminophen 750 mg, Hydrocodone Bitartrate 7.5 mg	by King	60793-0846	Analgesic; C III
KPI2	Tab, White, Round, Scored	Acetaminophen 750 mg, Hydrocodone Bitartrate 7.5 mg	by Allscripts	54569-3909	Analgesic; C III
KPI2	Tab, White, Round, Scored	Acetaminophen 750 mg, Hydrocodone Bitartrate 7.5 mg	Vicodin ES by Geneva	00781-1532	Analgesic; C III
KPI2	Tab, Light Blue, Round	Hydrocodone 7.5 mg, Acetaminophen 750 mg	Vicodin ES by King Pharmaceutical		Analgesic; C III
KPI33	Cap	Phentermine HCl 30 mg	by King	60793-0009	Anorexiant; C IV
KPI4	Tab, Debossed	Acetaminophen 650 mg, Hydrocodone Bitartrate 7.5 mg	by King	60793-0845	Analgesic; C III
KPI4	Tab, Debossed	Acetaminophen 650 mg, Hydrocodone Bitartrate 7.5 mg	by Endo	60951-0640	Analgesic; C III
KPI4	Tab	Acetaminophen 650 mg, Hydrocodone Bitartrate 7.5 mg	by Mallinckrodt Hobart	00406-0359	Analgesic; C III
KPI4	Tab, White, Cap Shaped, Scored	Acetaminophen 650 mg, Hydrocodone Bitartrate 7.5 mg	Lorcet Plus by Geneva	00781-1523	Analgesic; C III
KPI4	Tab	Acetaminophen 650 mg, Hydrocodone Bitartrate 7.5 mg	by Major	00904-3440	Analgesic; C III
KPI4	Tab, White, Oblong	Hydrocodone 7.5 mg, Acetaminophen 650 mg	Lorcet Plus by King Pharmaceutical		Analgesic; C III
KPI4	Tab, White, Oblong	Hydrocodone Bitartrate 7.5 mg, Acetaminophen 650 mg	by Heartland Hlthcare	61392-0922	Analgesic; C III
KR100 <> GEIGY	Tab, Brownish-Orange, Round, Film Coated	Metoprolol Tartrate 100 mg	Lopresor SR by Novartis	Canadian DIN# 00658855	Antihypertensive
KREMERSURBAN055	Cap, Clear	Pseudoephedrine HCl 120 mg, Chlorpheniramine 8 mg	Fedahist Timecaps by Schwarz Pharma		Cold remedy
KREMERSURBAN320	Cap, Clear & Violet, Kremers-Urban 320	Nitroglycerin SR 2.5 mg	Nitrocine Timecaps by Schwarz Pharma		Vasodilator
KREMERSURBAN330	Cap, Blue & Orange, Kremers-Urban 330	Nitroglycerin SR 6.5 mg	Nitrocine Timecaps by Schwarz Pharma		Vasodilator
KREMERSURBAN340	Cap, Clear, Kremers-Urban 340	Nitroglycerin SR 9 mg	Nitrocine Timecaps by Schwarz Pharma		Vasodilator
KREMERSURBAN475	Cap, Green & White	Enzyme Combination	Kutrase by Schwarz		Digestant
KREMERSURBAN505	Cap, Orange & White, Kremers Urban/505	Lactase 250 mg	by Rivex Pharma	Canadian	Gastrointestinal
KREMERSURBAN505	Cap, Orange & White, Kremers-Urban 505	Lactase Enzyme 250 mg	Lactrase by Schwarz		Gastrointestinal
KREMERSURBAN522	Cap, White & Yellow	Amylase 30 mg, Protease 6 mg, Lipase 75 mg, Cellulase 2 mg	Ku-Zyme by Schwarz		Gastrointestinal
KREMERSURBAN525	Cap, White	Pancrelipase	Ku-Zyme HP by Schwarz		Gastrointestinal
KREMERSURBAN537	Cap, Brown & Clear	Hyoscyamine Sulfate 0.375 mg	Levsinex Timecaps by Schwarz		Gastrointestinal
KREMERSURBAN539	Cap, Clear & Pink, Kremers-Urban 539	Hyoscyamine Sulfate 0.375 mg, Phenobarbital 45 mg	Levsinex Pb Timecaps by Schwarz Pharma		Gastrointestinal
KREMERSURBANE <> 537	Cap, ER	Hyoscyamine Sulfate 0.375 mg	Levsinex by Drug Distr	52985-0228	Gastrointestinal
KS2 <> ORGANON	Tab, Film Coated, KS over 2 <> Organon	Desogestrel 0.15 mg, Ethinyl Estradiol 0.02 mg, Ethinyl Estradiol 0.01 mg	Mircette by Organon	00052-0281	Oral Contraceptive
KS2 <> ORGANON	Tab, Film Coated, K S over 2 <> Organon	Desogestrel 0.15 mg, Ethinyl Estradiol 0.02 mg, Ethinyl Estradiol 0.01 mg	Mircette by NV Organon	12860-0281	Oral Contraceptive
KT	Tab, Yellow, Oval, Film Coated	Clarithromycin 250 mg	Biaxin by Natl Pharmpak	55154-0122	Antibiotic

ID FRONT <> BACK	DESCRIPTION FRONT <> BACK	INGREDIENT & STRENGTH	BRAND (OR EQUIV.) & FIRM	NDC#	CLASS; SCH.
KT	Tab, Yellow, Oval, Blue Print, KT over Abbott Logo	Clarithromycin 250 mg	Biaxin by Abbott	00074-3368	Antibiotic
KT	Tab, Abbott Logo	Clarithromycin 250 mg	Biaxin by Physicians Total Care	54868-3820	Antibiotic
KT	Tab, Film Coated, Abbott Logo	Clarithromycin 250 mg	Biaxin by Allscripts	54569-3556	Antibiotic
KT	Tab, Film Coated, Abbott Logo	Clarithromycin 250 mg	Biaxin by HJ Harkins Co	52959-0442	Antibiotic
KT	Tab, Film Coated, Abbott Logo	Clarithromycin 250 mg	Biaxin by DRX	55045-2165	Antibiotic
KT	Tab, Yellow, Oval, Film Coated, Abbott Logo	Clarithromycin 250 mg	Biaxin by Contract	10267-2155	Antibiotic
KT	Tab, Yellow, Oblong	Clarithromycin 250 mg	Biaxin by Compumed	00403-4625	Antibiotic
KTAB	Tab, Yellow, Ovaloid, Film Coated, K-TAB <> Abbott Logo	Potassium Chloride 750 mg	K-Tab ER by Abbott	00074-7804	Electrolytes
KTAB	Tab, Film Coated, K-Tab <> Symbol	Potassium Chloride 750 mg	K Tab by Nat Pharmpak Serv	55154-0106	Electrolytes
KTAB <> A	Tab, Yellow, Oval, Film Coated	Potassium Chloride 750 mg	K Tab by Abbott	00074-7804	Electrolytes
KTAB <> ABBOTT	Tab, Yellow, Oval, Film Coated, K-Tab	Potassium Chloride 750 mg	K Tab by Promex Med	62301-0036	Electrolytes
KTAB <> EI	Tab, Film Coated, K-Tab	Potassium Chloride 750 mg	K Tab ER by Heartland	61392-0900	Electrolytes
KU <> 101	Tab, White, Scored	Hyoscyamine Sulfate 0.125 mg	by Murfreesboro	51129-1501	Gastrointestinal
KU <> 101	Tab, White, Scored	Hyoscyamine Sulfate 0.125 mg	by Schwarz Pharma Mfg	00131-9101	Gastrointestinal
KU <> 101	Tab, White	Hyoscyamine Sulfate 0.125 mg	by Kremers Urban	62175-0101	Gastrointestinal
KU <> 102	Tab, Blue, Round, Flat, Beveled, Scored	Hyoscyamine Sulfate 0.125 mg	by Murfreesboro	51129-1503	Gastrointestinal
KU <> 102	Tab, White, Round	Hyoscyamine Sulfate 0.125 mg	by Schwarz Pharma Mfg	00131-9102	Gastrointestinal
KU <> 102	Tab, White, Round, Scored, Sublingual	Hyoscyamine Sulfate 0.125 mg	by Kremers Urban	62175-0102	Gastrointestinal
KU <> 103	Cap, Brown & Clear	Hyoscyamine Sulfate 0.375 mg	by Murfreesboro	51129-1505	Gastrointestinal
KU050	Tab, White, Oval	Pseudoephedrine HCl 60 mg, Chlorpheniramine Maleate 4 mg	Fedahist by Schwarz		Cold Remedy
KU1	Tab, Yellow, Oval	Ergocalciferol 1.25 mg	Calciferol by Schwarz Pharma		Vitamin
KU103	Cap, Brown & White	Hyoscyamine Sulfate 0.375 mg	by Schwarz Pharma Mfg	00131-9103	Gastrointestinal
KU103	Cap, Brown & White	Hyoscyamine Sulfate 0.375 mg	by Kremers Urban	62175-0103	Gastrointestinal
KU106 <> 10	Tab, White	Isosorbide Mononitrate 10 mg	by Kremers Urban	62175-0106	Antianginal
KU106 <> 10	Tab, White, Round, Scored	Isosorbide Mononitrate 10 mg	by Schwarz Pharma Mfg	00131-9106	Antianginal
KU107 <> 20	Tab, White	Isosorbide Mononitrate 20 mg	by Kremers Urban	62175-0107	Antianginal
KU107 <> 20	Tab, White, Round, Scored	Isosorbide Mononitrate 20 mg	by Schwarz Pharma Mfg	00131-9107	Antianginal
KU107 <> 20	Tab, KU 107	Isosorbide Mononitrate 20 mg	by Physicians Total Care	54868-3822	Antianginal
KU108	Tab, Light Orange, Oblong, Scored	Hyoscyamine Sulfate 0.375 mg	by Schwarz Pharma Mfg	00131-9108	Gastrointestinal
KU108	Tab, Orange, Scored	Hyoscyamine Sulfate ER 0.375 mg	by Murfreesboro	51129-1502	Gastrointestinal
KU108	Tab, Light Orange, Ex Release	Hyoscyamine Sulfate 0.375 mg	by Kremers Urban	62175-0108	Gastrointestinal
KU119	Tab, White, Cap Shaped, Scored	Isosorbide Mononitrate 60 mg	Imdur ER by Kremers Urban	62175-0119	Antianginal
KU119	Tab, White, Oblong, Scored	Isosorbide Mononitrate 60 mg	by Schwarz Pharma Mfg	00131-9119	Antianginal
KU120	Cap	Pseudoephedrine 120 mg, Chlorpheniramine 8 mg	GG-Cen by Kremers Urban		Cold Remedy
KU128	Tab, White, Cap Shaped, Scored	Isosorbide Mononitrate 30 mg	Imdur ER by Kremers Urban	62175-0128	Antianginal
KU128	Tab, White, Oblong, Scored	Isosorbide Mononitrate 30 mg	by Schwarz Pharma Mfg	00131-9128	Antianginal
KU129	Tab, White, Cap Shaped	Isosorbide Mononitrate 120 mg	Imdur ER by Kremers Urban	62175-0129	Antianginal
KU129	Tab, White, Oblong, Scored	Isosorbide Mononitrate 120 mg	by Schwarz Pharma Mfg	00131-9129	Antianginal
KU171	Tab, White, Oval	Aspirin 325 mg, Acetaminophen 325 mg	Gemnisyn by Schwarz		Analgesic
KU202	Tab, Gray, Round	Belladona Extract 15 mg, Phenobarbital 15 mg	Chardonna-2 by Schwarz		Gastrointestinal; C IV
KU531	Tab, White, K-U/531	Hyoscyamine 0.125 mg	by Rivex Pharma	Canadian	Gastrointestinal
KU531	Tab, White, Round, K-U 531	Hyoscyamine Sulfate 0.125 mg	Levsin by Schwarz		Gastrointestinal
KU534	Tab, Pink, Round, K-U 534	Hyoscyamine Sulfate 0.125 mg, Phenobarbital 15 mg	Levsin Pb by Schwarz		Gastrointestinal; C IV
L	Tab, Orange, Round	Iodinated Glycerol 30 mg	Organidin by LuChem		Expectorant
L	Tab, Off-White, Hexagonal	Propranolol HCl 40 mg, Hydrochlorothiazide 25 mg	by Wyeth-Ayerst	Canadian	Antihypertensive
L	Tab, Off-White, Hexagonal	Propranolol HCl 80 mg, Hydrochlorothiazide 25 mg	by Wyeth-Ayerst	Canadian	Antihypertensive
L <> N144500	Cap	Cephalexin Monohydrate 541 mg	by United Res	00677-1159	Antibiotic
L014	Tab, White	Acetaminophen 500 mg	Tylenol by Leiner		Antipyretic
L016	Tab, White, Round	Acetaminophen 500 mg	APAP by Leiner		Analgesic
L021	Tab, Yellow, Round	Chlorpheniramine 4 mg	by Leiner		Antihistamine
L030	Tab, Yellow, Oblong	Phenylpropanolamine 75 mg	by Leiher		Decongestant; Appetite Suppressant

ID FRONT ◇ BACK	DESCRIPTION FRONT ◇ BACK	INGREDIENT & STRENGTH	BRAND (OR EQUIV.) & FIRM	NDC#	CLASS; SCH.
L036	Cap, Light Blue	Diphenhydramine 25 mg	Ex Stre Non A PM by Leiner		Antihistamine
L039	Tab, Yellow, Round	Meclizine HCl 25 mg	Antivert by Perrigo		Antiemetic
L040	Tab, Blue, Round	Diphenhydramine 25 mg	Diphenhydramine by Leiner		Antihistamine
L042	Tab, Green, Oblong	Iron, Ferrous Fumarate	Ferro Sequel		Mineral
L052	Tab, White, Football Shaped, Black Specks	Calcium Polycaebophil 625 mg	by Leiner Health		Vitamin/Mineral
L077	Tab, Orange, Cap Shaped	Acetaminophen 500 mg, Pseudoephedine HCl 30 mg	Phed Sinus Cap by Leiner Health Products		Cold Remedy
L1	Tab, Green, Round	Ferrous Sulfate 65 mg	by Perrigo		Mineral
L1 ◇ BL	Tab	Mitotane 500 mg	Lysodren by Anabolic	00722-5240	Antineoplastic
L101	Cap, Green & White	Pseudoephedrine 30 mg, Acetaminophen 500 mg	Non-Aspirin Sinus by Perrigo		Cold Remedy
L110	Tab, Red	Yohimbine HCl 5.4 mg	by Zenith Goldline	00182-1625	Impotence Agent
L113	Tab, White, Oblong	Lactase Enzyme	by Perrigo		Gastrointestinal
L12	Tab, White, Oblong, Scored, L/12	Guaifenesin 1200 mg	Liquibid 1200 by Lederle	59911-5887	Expectorant
L12	Tab, White, Oblong, Scored	Guaifenesin 1200 mg	Liquibid by Sovereign Pharms	58716-0683	Expectorant
L12	Tab, White, Oblong, Scored	Guaifenesin 1200 mg	Liquibid by Eckerd	19458-0913	Expectorant
L126	Tab, White, Cap-Shaped	Pseudoephedrine 30 mg, Dextromethorphan 15 mg, Acetaminophen 325 mg	Non by Perrigo	00113-0126	Cold Remedy
L128	Cap, Blue & White	Calcium Carbonate 311 mg, Magnesium Carbonate 232 mg	by Perrigo		Vitamin/Mineral
L171	Cap, White, Blue Band	Acetaminophen 500 mg, Diphenhydramine HCl 25 mg	by Perrigo		Cold Remedy
L172	Tab, Pink, Round	Acetaminophen 160 mg	by Perrigo	00113-0172	Antipyretic
L173	Cap, Green & Yellow	Chlorphenamine 2 mg, Pseudoephedrine 30 mg, Acetaminophen 500 mg	by Perrigo		Cold Remedy
L179	Tab, Multi-colored, Round	Calcium Carbonate 750 mg	by Perrigo	00113-0179	Vitamin/Mineral
L187	Tab, Red & Yellow, Round	Acetaminophen 500 mg	Tylenol by Perrigo		Antipyretic
L193	Cap, Green	Pseudoeph 30, Doxylamine 6.25, Acetaminophen 250, Dextromethorphan 10	by Perrigo	00113-0193	Cold Remedy
L2	Tab, Green, Round	Ferrous Gluconate 36 mg	by Perrigo	00113-0554	Mineral
L2	Tab, Green, Oblong, L-2	Loperamide 2 mg	Imodium by Novopharm		Antidiarrheal
L216	Tab, Lavender, Round	Pseudoephedrine 7.5 mg, Acetaminophen 80 mg, Chlorpheniramine 0.5 mg	by Perrigo	00113-0216	Cold Remedy
L226	Cap, Red	Pseudoephedrine 30 mg, Dextromethorphan 10 mg, Guaifenesin 200 mg	by Perrigo	00113-0226	Cold Remedy
L235	Tab, White, Round	Dihydroxyaluminum Sodium Carbonate 300 mg	Rolaids by Perrigo		Gastrointestinal
L240	Tab, Beige, Round	Phenolphthalein 90 mg	by Perrigo	00113-0240	Gastrointestinal
L259	Tab, Round	Aspirin 81 mg	Aspirin Lo-Dose by Perrigo		Analgesic
L282	Tab, White, Oblong	Clemastine Fumarate 1.34 mg	by L Perrigo	00113-0282	Antihistamine
L299	Tab, White, Oblong	Acetaminophen 500 mg, Calcium Carbonate 250 mg	by Perrigo		Analgesic
L33	Tab, White, Round	Aspirin 325 mg, Codeine 30 mg	Empirin #3 by Lee		Analgesic; C III
L33	Tab, White, Round	Aspirin 325 mg, Codeine 60 mg	Empirin #4 by Lee		Analgesic; C III
L368	Tab, Blue, Oval	Naproxen Sodium 220 mg	Naproxen Sodium by Par	49884-0545	NSAID
L4	Tab, Green, Oblong	Prenatal Vitamin	by Perrigo		Vitamin
L403	Tab, White, Round	Acetaminophen 325 mg	by Perrigo	00113-0403	Antipyretic
L405	Tab, White, Round	Acetaminophen 500 mg	by Perrigo	00113-0405	Antipyretic
L406	Tab, Blue, Round	Diphenhydramine HCl 25 mg	by Perrigo	00113-0406	Antihistamine
L409	Tab, Yellow, Round	Caffeine 200 mg	by Perrigo	00113-0409	Stimulant
L410	Tab, Light Peach, Oblong	Acetaminophen 500 mg, Pseudoephedrine 30 mg	by Perrigo	00113-0410	Cold Remedy
L415	Tab, White, Round	Aspirin 400 mg, Caffeine 32 mg	by Perrigo	00113-0415	Analgesic
L419	Tab, White, Round	Phenylpropanolamine 15 mg, Diphenhydramine 38.33 mg, Aspirin 325 mg	by Perrigo		Cold Remedy
L420	Tab, Yellow, Round	Pseudoeph 30 mg, Dextometh 10 mg, Acetaminophen 325 mg, Chlorpheniramine 2 mg	by Perrigo		Cold Remedy
L421	Tab, White, Round	Aspirin 325 mg, Sodium Bicarbonate 1916 mg, Citric Acid 1000 mg	by Perrigo	00113-0421	Analgesic
L427	Tab, Yellow, Oblong	Chlorpheniramine 2 mg, Pseudoephedrine 30 mg, Acetaminophen 500 mg	by Perrigo	00113-0071	Cold Remedy
L429	Tab, Orange, Round	Aspirin 325 mg	Ecotrin by Perrigo		Analgesic
L430	Tab, White, Round	Aspirin 250 mg, Acetaminophen 250 mg, Caffeine 65 mg	by Perrigo	00113-0430	Analgesic
L432	Tab, Red, Round	Pseudoephedrine 30 mg	Sudafed by Perrigo	00113-0432	Decongestant
L434	Tab, White, Round	Triprolidine 2.5 mg, Pseudoephedrine 60 mg	Actifed by Perrigo		Cold Remedy
L437	Tab, Blue, Cap Shaped	Diphenhydramine 25 mg, Acetaminophen 500 mg	by Perrigo	00113-0437	Antihistamine

ID FRONT <> BACK	DESCRIPTION FRONT <> BACK	INGREDIENT & STRENGTH	BRAND (OR EQUIV.) & FIRM	NDC#	CLASS; SCH.
L438	Tab, Green, Caplet	Pseudoephedrine 30 mg, Acetaminophen 500 mg	by Perrigo	00113-0438	Cold Remedy
L447	Tab, Orange, Oval	Pseudoephedrine 30 mg, Acetaminophen 500 mg	by Perrigo	00113-0447	Cold Remedy
L449	Tab, Round	Acetaminophen 160 mg	by Perrigo	00113-0449	Antipyretic
L450	Tab, Lavender, Round	Pseudoephedrine 60 mg, Chlorpheniramine 4 mg	by Perrigo	00113-0450	Cold Remedy
L452	Tab, White, Round	Aspirin 325 mg, Aluminum Magnesium Hydrox 50 mg, Ca Carbonate 50 mg	by Perrigo	00113-0452	Analgesic
L453	Tab, White, Cap Shaped	Acetaminophen 325 mg	by Perrigo	00113-0453	Antipyretic
L458	Tab, Yellow, Oblong	Phenylpropanolamine 75 mg	by Perrigo	00113-0458	Decongestant; Appetite Suppressant
L459	Tab, Yellow, Oblong	Phenylpropanolamine 25 mg, Chlorpheniramine 4 mg	by Perrigo		Cold Remedy
L462	Cap, Clear & Pink, Red Band	Diphenhydramine 25 mg	by Perrigo	00113-0462	Antihistamine
L463	Tab, Yellow, Round	Chlorpheniramine 4 mg	by Perrigo	00113-0463	Antihistamine
L465PM	Tab, Blue & White, Round	Acetaminophen 500 mg, Diphenhydramine 25 mg	by Perrigo	00113-0465	Cold Remedy
L467	Tab, Orange, Round	Aspirin Children Chewable 81 mg	Bayer Child by Perrigo	00113-0259	Analgesic
L469	Tab, Pink, Round	Bismuth Subsalicylate 300 mg	by Perrigo	00113-0469	Gastrointestinal
L470	Cap, Yellow, with 1 Red Band	Acetaminophen 500 mg	Tylenol by Perrigo		Antipyretic
L478	Tab, Multi-colored, Round	Calcium Carbonate 500 mg	Tums by Perrigo	00113-0478	Vitamin/Mineral
L479	Tab, Pink, Oblong	Diphenhydramine 25 mg	by Perrigo	00113-0479	Antihistamine
L479	Tab, Pink, Oblong	Diphenhydramine HCl 25 mg	by Geneva	00781-2052	Antihistamine
L480	Tab, Yellow, Oval	Pseudoephedrine 30 mg, Chlorpheniramine 2 mg, Acetaminophen 500 mg	by Perrigo	00113-0480	Cold Remedy
L481	Tab, Lavender, Round	Acetaminophen 80 mg	by Perrigo	00113-0481	Antipyretic
L482	Cap, Clear	Phenylpropanolamine 75 mg, Chlorpheniramine 8 mg	Contac by Perrigo	00113-0482	Cold Remedy
L484	Tab, White, Cap Shaped	Acetaminophen 500 mg	Tylenol by Perrigo	00113-0484	Antipyretic
L485	Tab, White, Round	Calcium Carbonate 500 mg	by Perrigo	00113-0485	Vitamin/Mineral
L486	Cap, Red & White, Oval	Docusate Sodium 100 mg	by Perrigo	00113-0486	Laxative
L492	Tab, Pink, Round	Acetaminophen 80 mg	by Perrigo	00113-0492	Antipyretic
L494	Tab, White, Round	Phenylpropanolamine 15 mg, Chlorpheniramine 2 mg, Aspirin 325 mg	by Perrigo	00113-0494	Cold Remedy
L495	Cap, Red, Oval	Docusate Sodium 100 mg, Casanthranol 30 mg	by Perrigo	00113-0495	Laxative
L496	Tab, Blue, Round	Phenylpropanolamine 25 mg, Brompheniramine 4 mg	by Perrigo		Cold Remedy
L50 <> JANSSEN	Tab, Coated, L Over 50	Levamisole HCl 59 mg	Ergamisol by Janssen	50458-0270	Immunomodulator
L501	Tab, Blue, Oblong	Phenylpropan 12.5 mg, Dextrometh 15 mg, Acetaminophen 500 mg, Chlorpheniramine 2 mg	by Perrigo	00113-0501	Cold Remedy
L507	Tab, Purple, Round	Phenylpropanolamine 6.25 mg, Brompheniramine 1 mg	by Perrigo		Cold Remedy
L50JANSSEN	Tab, White, L50/Janssen	Levamisole 50 mg	by Janssen	Canadian	Immunomodulator
L524	Tab, White, Round	Pseudoephedrine 30 mg, Acetaminophen 325 mg	by Perrigo	00113-0524	Cold Remedy
L535	Tab, Yellow	Aspirin 81 mg	by Perrigo		Analgesic
L537	Cap, Green	Pseudoephedrine 30 mg, Guaifenesin 200 mg	by Perrigo	00113-0537	Cold Remedy
L556	Tab, White, Round	Brompheniramine 2 mg, Aspirin 500 mg, Dextrometh 10 mg, Phenylpropan 12.5 mg	by Perrigo		Cold Remedy
L562	Cap, Orange	Pseudoephedrine 30 mg, Guaifenesin 100 mg, Dextrometh 10 mg, Acetaminophen 250 mg	by Perrigo	00113-0080	Cold Remedy
L576	Cap, Orange & Yellow	Pseudoephedrine 30 mg, Dextromethorphan 15 mg, Acetaminophen 325 mg	Non by Perrigo		Cold Remedy
L582	Tab, White, Oblong	Aspirin 325 mg	by Perrigo	00113-0582	Analgesic
L596	Tab, White, Cap-Shaped	Pheudoephedrine 30 mg, Dextromethorphan 15 mg, Acetaminophen 500 mg	by Perrigo	00113-0596	Cold Remedy
L609	Tab, Green, Oblong	Phenyleph 25 mg, Phenylpro 50 mg, Chlorphen 8 mg, Hyosc 0.19 mg, Atro 0.04 mg, Scop 0.01 mg	Ru-tuss by Norton		Cold Remedy
L642	Tab, White, Round	Aspirin, Calcium Carbonate	by Perrigo	00113-0642	Analgesic
L643	Tab, White, Round	Pseudoephedrine 30 mg, Acetaminophen 500 mg	by Perrigo	00113-0642	Cold Remedy
L670	Tab, White, Round	Quinine Sulfate 260 mg	Quinamm by LuChem		Antimalarial
L685	Tab, Beige	Thyroid 32.5 mg	by Taro	52549-4034	Thyroid
L686	Tab	Thyroid 1 gr	by Pharmedix	53002-1029	Thyroid
L687	Tab, Tan, Round	Thyroid 120 mg	Thyroid by LuChem		Thyroid
L754	Tab, Green, Oblong	Phenylephrine 20 mg, Guaifenesin 300 mg	Endal by Norton		Cold Remedy
L837	Tab, Blue & White, Round	Acetaminophen 500 mg, Diphenhydramine 25 mg	Tylenol PM by Perrigo	00113-0837	Cold Remedy

383

ID FRONT <> BACK	DESCRIPTION FRONT <> BACK	INGREDIENT & STRENGTH	BRAND (OR EQUIV.) & FIRM	NDC#	CLASS; SCH.
L860	Tab, White, Round	Phenylpropanolamine 75 mg, Clemastine 1.34 mg	by Perrigo	00113-0860	Cold Remedy
L877	Tab, Orange & Yellow	Acetaminophen 500 mg	Tylenol by Perrigo	00113-0877	Antipyretic
L890	Tab, White, Round	Dimenhydrinate 50 mg	by Perrigo	00113-0890	Antiemetic
L995	Tab, White, Round	Ibuprofen 200 mg	Ibuprofen by Murfreesboro	51129-1521	NSAID
LACTAID	Tab, White, Cap Shaped, Chewable	Lactase 3000 units	Regular Strength Lactaid Tables By McNeil	Canadian DIN# 02230653	Gastrointestinal
LACTAID	Tab, White, Cap Shaped	Lactase 5000 units	Lactaid Ultra By McNeil	Canadian DIN# 02231507	Gastrointestinal
LACTAID	Tab, White, Round, Chewable	Lactase 9,000 units	by McNeil	Canadian DIN# 02239664	Gastrointestinal
LACTAID	Tab, White, Round, Chewable	Lactase 9000 units	Lactaid Ultra Chewable Tablets by McNeil	Canadian DIN# 02239548	Gastrointestinal
LACTAIDES	Tab, White, Cap Shaped, Chewable	Lactase 4500 Units	Lactaid by McNeil	Canadian DIN# 02230654	Gastrointestinal
LAFLI	Tab, Mint Green, Round, Compressed, Uncoated, Partly Convex, LA/FLI Logo	Levothyroxine Sodium 88 mcg	by Forest	00456-0329	Antithyroid
LAMICTAL <> 100	Tab, Peach, Hexagon, Scored	Lamotrigine 100 mg	Lamictal by Glaxo Wellcome	00173-0594	Anticonvulsant
LAMICTAL <> 25	Tab, White, Hexagon, Scored	Lamotrigine 25 mg	Lamictal by Glaxo Wellcome	00173-0594	Anticonvulsant
LAMICTAL100	Tab, Peach, Shield	Lamotrigine 100 mg	Lamictal by B.W. Inc	Canadian	Anticonvulsant
LAMICTAL100	Tab, Shield-Shaped	Lamotrigine 100 mg	Lamictal by Catalytica	63552-0642	Anticonvulsant
LAMICTAL100	Tab, Peach, Shield-Shaped	Lamotrigine 100 mg	Lamictal by Glaxo Wellcome	00173-0642	Anticonvulsant
LAMICTAL150	Tab	Lamotrigine 150 mg	Lamictal by Catalytica	63552-0643	Anticonvulsant
LAMICTAL150	Tab, Cream, Shield	Lamotrigine 150 mg	Lamictal by B.W. Inc	Canadian	Anticonvulsant
LAMICTAL150	Tab, Cream, Shield-Shaped	Lamotrigine 150 mg	Lamictal by Glaxo	00173-0643	Anticonvulsant
LAMICTAL200	Tab	Lamotrigine 200 mg	Lamictal by Catalytica	63552-0644	Anticonvulsant
LAMICTAL200	Tab, Blue, Shield-Shaped	Lamotrigine 200 mg	Lamictal by Glaxo Wellcome	00173-0644	Anticonvulsant
LAMICTAL25	Tab, White, Shield	Lamotrigine 25 mg	Lamictal by B.W. Inc	Canadian	Anticonvulsant
LAMICTAL25	Tab, Lamictal 25	Lamotrigine 25 mg	Lamictal by Catalytica	63552-0633	Anticonvulsant
LAMICTAL25	Tab, White, Shield-Shaped	Lamotrigine 25 mg	Lamictal by Glaxo Wellcome	00173-0633	Anticonvulsant
LAMISIL <> 250	Tab, White, Round	Terbinafine HCl 250 mg	Lamisil by Novartis Pharms (Ca)	61615-0101	Antifungal
LAMISIL <> 250	Tab, White to Yellow-Tinged White, Round	Terbinafine HCl 250 mg	Lamisil by Novartis	00078-0179	Antifungal
LAMISIL <> 250	Tab, Lamisil in Circular Form	Terbinafine HCl 250 mg	Lamisil by Novartis	17088-9586	Antifungal
LAMISIL <> 250	Tab, White to Off White, Round, Scored	Terbinafine HCl 250 mg	Lamisil by Novartis Pharms (CA)	61615-0100	Antifungal
LAMISIL125	Tab, White & Yellow, Round	Terbinafine HCl 125 mg	Lamisil by Sandoz	Canadian	Antifungal
LAMISIL250	Tab, Whitish-Yellow, Round, Scored	Terbinafine HCl 250 mg	Lamisil by Sandoz	Canadian DIN# 02031116	Antifungal
LAN	Cap, Blue	Dicyclomine 10 mg	Bentyl by Mova	55370-0854	Gastrointestinal
LAN <> 1231	Tab	Primidone 250 mg	by Qualitest	00603-5370	Anticonvulsant
LAN 0586	Cap	Decyclomine HCl 10 mg	by Kaiser	62224-9119	Gastrointestinal
LAN0586	Cap, Blue	Decyclomine HCl 10 mg	by DRX	55045-2729	Gastrointestinal
LAN0586	Cap, White Powder Fill	Decyclomine HCl 10 mg	by Quality Care	60346-0911	Gastrointestinal
LAN0586	Cap, Blue	Decyclomine HCl 10 mg	by Novopharm	55953-0555	Gastrointestinal
LAN0586	Cap	Decyclomine HCl 10 mg	by Zenith Goldline	00182-0519	Gastrointestinal
LAN0586	Cap	Decyclomine HCl 10 mg	by Qualitest	00603-3265	Gastrointestinal
LAN0586	Cap	Decyclomine HCl 10 mg	by Lannett	00527-0586	Gastrointestinal
LAN0586	Cap	Decyclomine HCl 10 mg	by United Res	00677-0341	Gastrointestinal

ID FRONT <> BACK	DESCRIPTION FRONT <> BACK	INGREDIENT & STRENGTH	BRAND (OR EQUIV.) & FIRM	NDC#	CLASS; SCH.
LAN0586	Cap, Blue	Decyclomine HCl 10 mg	by Duramed	51285-0929	Gastrointestinal
LAN0586	Cap, Blue	Dicyclomine 10 mg	Bentyl by MOVA	55370-0854	Gastrointestinal
LAN1050	Tab, White, Round	Acetazolamide 250 mg	Diamox by Lannett		Diuretic
LAN1109	Tab, White, Round	Isoniazide 300 mg	INH by Lannett		Antimycobacterial
LAN1149 <> LAN1149	Tab, Lan over 1149	Aminosalicylate Sodium 500 mg	by Lannett	00527-1149	Antimycobacterial
LAN1200	Tab	Prednisone 5 mg	by Lannett	00527-1200	Steroid
LAN1231	Tab, LAN Over 1231	Primidone 250 mg	by Lannett	00527-1231	Anticonvulsant
LAN1231	Tab, Lannet	Primidone 250 mg	by Rugby	00536-4373	Anticonvulsant
LAN1231	Tab, White, Round, Debossed LAN/1231	Primidone 250 mg	by Duramed	51285-0939	Anticonvulsant
LAN1231	Tab, White, Round, Scored	Primidone 250 mg	Mysoline by MOVA	55370-0888	Anticonvulsant
LAN1231	Tab, White, Round, Debossed LAN/1231	Primidone 250 mg	by Novopharm	55953-0527	Anticonvulsant
LAN1231	Tab, White, Round, Scored	Primidone 250 mg	by Dixon Shane	17236-0547	Anticonvulsant
LAN1231	Tab	Primidone 250 mg	by United Res	00677-0354	Anticonvulsant
LAN1262	Tab, LAN Over 1262	Prednisone 20 mg	by Lannett	00527-1262	Steriod
LAN1282	Tab, Blue, Round	Dicyclomine HCl 20 mg	by Lannett	00527-1282	Gastrointestinal
LANNETT <> 05271552	Cap, Dark Green & Light Green, Lannett <> 0527/1552	Aspirin 325 mg, Butalbital 50 mg, Caffeine 40 mg	by Novopharm	55953-0633	Analgesic; C III
LANNETT <> 05271552	Cap, Lannett <> 0527/1552	Aspirin 325 mg, Butalbital 50 mg, Caffeine 40 mg	by Lannett	00527-1552	Analgesic; C III
LANNETT05271552	Cap, Lannett 0527/1552	Aspirin 325 mg, Butalbital 50 mg, Caffeine 40 mg	by Qualitest	00603-2550	Analgesic; C III
LANOXIN <> X3A	Tab, White, Scored	Digoxin 0.25 mg	Lanoxin by Va Cmop	65243-0024	Cardiac Agent
LANOXIN <> X3A	Tab	Digoxin 0.25 mg	Lanoxin by Amerisource	62584-0249	Cardiac Agent
LANOXIN <> X3A	Tab	Digoxin 0.25 mg	Lanoxin by Catalytica	63552-0249	Cardiac Agent
LANOXIN <> X3A	Tab	Digoxin 0.25 mg	by Med Pro	53978-3060	Cardiac Agent
LANOXIN <> Y3B	Tab	Digoxin 0.125 mg	Lanoxin by Catalytica	63552-0242	Cardiac Agent
LANOXIN <> Y3B	Tab, Yellow, Scored	Digoxin 0.125 mg	Lanoxin by Va Cmop	65243-0023	Cardiac Agent
LANOXIN <> Y3B	Tab	Digoxin 0.125 mg	Lanoxin by Amerisource	62584-0242	Cardiac Agent
LANOXIN <> Y3B	Tab	Digoxin 0.125 mg	by Med Pro	53978-3061	Cardiac Agent
LANOXIN <> Y3B	Tab, Yellow, Scored	Digoxin 0.125 mg	Lanoxin by Eckerd Drug	19458-0880	Cardiac Agent
LANOXIN <> Y3B	Tab	Digoxin 0.125 mg	Lanoxin by Quality Care	60346-0396	Cardiac Agent
LANOXIN <> Y3B	Tab	Digoxin 125 mcg	Lanoxin by Thrift Drug	59198-0232	Cardiac Agent
LANOXIN <> Y3B	Tab, Yellow, Scored	Digoxin 125 mcg	Lanoxin by Eckerd Drug	19458-0889	Cardiac Agent
LANOXIN Y3B	Tab, Yellow, Round	Digoxin 0.125 mg	by Glaxo	Canadian	Cardiac Agent
LANOXINU3A	Tab, Peach, Round	Digoxin 0.0625 mg	by Glaxo	Canadian	Cardiac Agent
LANOXINX3A	Tab	Digoxin 0.25 mg	Lanoxin by Leiner	59606-0678	Cardiac Agent
LANOXINX3A	Tab	Digoxin 0.25 mg	by Kaiser	62224-9228	Cardiac Agent
LANOXINX3A	Tab	Digoxin 0.25 mg	Lanoxin by Nat Pharmpak Serv	55154-0702	Cardiac Agent
LANOXINX3A	Tab, White, Round	Digoxin 0.25 mg	by Glaxo	Canadian	Cardiac Agent
LANOXINX3A	Tab, Yellow, Round, Scored	Digoxin 0.25 mg	Lanoxin by Thrift Services	59198-0373	Cardiac Agent
LANOXINX3A	Tab, Lanoxin over X3A	Digoxin 0.25 mg	by Kaiser	00179-0404	Cardiac Agent
LANOXINX3A	Tab	Digoxin 0.25 mg	Lanoxin by Glaxo	00173-0249	Cardiac Agent
LANOXINX3A	Tab	Digoxin 0.25 mg	Lanoxin by Caremark	00339-5202	Cardiac Agent
LANOXINX3A	Tab, Lanoxin over X3A	Digoxin 0.25 mg	by Vangard	00615-0518	Cardiac Agent
LANOXINX3A	Tab, Lanoxin over X3A	Digoxin 0.25 mg	Lanoxin by CVS	51316-0245	Cardiac Agent
LANOXINX3A	Tab	Digoxin 0.25 mg	Lanoxin by Allscripts	54569-0484	Cardiac Agent
LANOXINX3A	Tab, Lanoxin over X3A	Digoxin 0.25 mg	Lanoxin by Murfreesboro	51129-1311	Cardiac Agent
LANOXINX3A	Tab	Digoxin 0.25 mg	Lanoxin by Pharmedix	53002-0366	Cardiac Agent
LANOXINX3A	Tab, White, Round, Scored	Digoxin 0.25 mg	Lanoxin by Eckerd Drug	19458-0887	Cardiac Agent
LANOXINX3A	Tab	Digoxin 0.25 mg	by Talbert Med	44514-0499	Cardiac Agent
LANOXINX3A	Tab, White, Round, Scored	Digoxin 250 mcg	Lanoxin by Eckerd Drug	19458-0891	Cardiac Agent
LANOXINY3B	Tab	Digoxin 0.125 mg	Lanoxin by Glaxo	00173-0242	Cardiac Agent
LANOXINY3B	Tab	Digoxin 0.125 mg	Lanoxin by Caremark	00339-5198	Cardiac Agent
LANOXINY3B	Tab, Lanoxin/Y3B	Digoxin 0.125 mg	by Vangard	00615-0547	Cardiac Agent
LANOXINY3B	Tab, Scored, Lanoxin over Y3B	Digoxin 0.125 mg	Lanoxin by DRX	55045-2130	Cardiac Agent

ID FRONT <> BACK	DESCRIPTION FRONT <> BACK	INGREDIENT & STRENGTH	BRAND (OR EQUIV.) & FIRM	NDC#	CLASS; SCH.
LANOXINY3B	Tab	Digoxin 0.125 mg	Lanoxin by Allscripts	54569-0483	Cardiac Agent
LANOXINY3B	Tab	Digoxin 0.125 mg	by Talbert Med	44514-0498	Cardiac Agent
LANOXINY3B	Tab, Yellow, Round, Scored	Digoxin 0.125 mg	Lanoxin by Eckerd Drug	19458-0885	Cardiac Agent
LANOXINY3B	Tab	Digoxin 0.125 mg	by Kaiser	62224-9226	Cardiac Agent
LANOXINY3B	Tab	Digoxin 0.125 mg	Lanoxin by Nat Pharmpak Serv	55154-0701	Cardiac Agent
LANOXINY3B	Tab	Digoxin 125 mcg	Lanoxin by Leiner	59606-0677	Cardiac Agent
LANOXINY3B	Tab, Lanoxin/Y3B	Digoxin 125 mcg	Lanoxin by Kaiser	00179-0377	Cardiac Agent
LANOXINY3B	Tab, Lanoxin/Y3B	Digoxin 125 mcg	Lanoxin by Med Pro	53978-0202	Cardiac Agent
LARIAM250ROCHE	Tab	Mefloquine HCl 250 mg	Lariam by PDRX	55289-0780	Antiprotozoal
LARIAM250ROCHE	Tab	Mefloquine HCl 250 mg	Lariam by DRX	55045-2459	Antiprotozoal
LARIAM250ROCHE	Tab	Mefloquine HCl 250 mg	Lariam by F Hoffmann La Roche	12806-7460	Antiprotozoal
LASER <> 0174	Cap, Clear & Green, Opaque	Guaifenesin 200 mg, Pseudoephedrine HCl 60 mg	GFN PSEH PD 10 by Marnel	00682-1445	Cold Remedy
LASER <> DALLERGY	Tab, White, Round, Scored	Chlorpheniramine Maleate 4 mg, Methscopolamine Nitrate 1.25 mg, Phenylephrine HCl 10 mg	Dallergy by Laser	00277-0160	Cold Remedy
LASER0169	Cap, Clear & Orange	Guaifenesin 250 mg, Pseudoephedrine HCl 120 mg	Respaire 120 SR by Laser	00277-0169	Cold Remedy
LASER0172	Cap, Orange & Red	Multihematinic	Fumatinic by Laser		Vitamin
LASER0174	Cap, Clear & Green	Guaifenesin 200 mg, Pseudoephedrine HCl 60 mg	Respaire 60 SR by Laser	00277-0174	Cold Remedy
LASER0181	Cap	Ascorbic Acid 60 mg, Cyanocobalamin 5 mcg, Ferrous Fumarate 200 mg	Fumatinic by Opti Med	63369-0181	Vitamin
LASER0181	Cap, Clear & Maroon	Ascorbic Acid 60 mg, Cyanocobalamin 5 mcg, Ferrous Fumarate 200 mg	Fumatinic by Laser	00277-0181	Vitamin
LASER0181	Cap, Clear & Maroon	Multihematinic, Vitamin B 12, Vitamin C	Fumatinic by Anabolic		Vitamin
LASER173	Tab, Film Coated	Ascorbic Acid 100 mg, Calcium Carbonate 200 mg, Cupric Sulfate, Anhydrous 2 mg, Cyanocobalamin 12 mcg, Ferrous Fumarate 65 mg, Folic Acid 1 mg, Magnesium Oxide 10 mg, Niacinamide 20 mg, Potassium Iodide 0.15 mg, Pyridoxine HCl 5 mg, Riboflavin 3.4 mg, Thiamine Mononitrate 3 mg, Vitamin A Acetate 4000 Units, Vitamin D 400 Units, Vitamin E 30 Units, Zinc Sulfate 15 mg	Lactocal F by Opti Med	63369-0179	Vitamin
LASER173	Tab, White, Oval, Film Coated	Ascorbic Acid 100 mg, Calcium Carbonate 200 mg, Cupric Sulfate, Anhydrous 2 mg, Cyanocobalamin 12 mcg, Ferrous Fumarate 65 mg, Folic Acid 1 mg, Magnesium Oxide 10 mg, Niacinamide 20 mg, Potassium Iodide 0.15 mg, Pyridoxine HCl 5 mg, Riboflavin 3.4 mg, Thiamine Mononitrate 3 mg, Vitamin A Acetate 4000 Units, Vitamin D 400 Units, Vitamin E 30 Units, Zinc Sulfate 15 mg	Lactocal F by Laser	00277-0179	Vitamin
LASER176 <> DALLERGYJR	Cap, Ex Release, Laser over 176 <> Dallergy JR	Brompheniramine Maleate 6 mg, Pseudoephedrine HCl 60 mg	Dallergy Jr by Sovereign	58716-0028	Cold Remedy
LASER176 <> DALLERGYJR	Cap, Maize, Opaque	Brompheniramine Maleate 6 mg; Pseudoephedrine HCl 60 mg	Dallergy JR by Laser	00277-0176	Cold Remedy
LASER35	Tab, Orange, Round	Phendimetrazine Tartrate 35 mg	Trimstat by Laser		Anorexiant; C III
LASIX <> HOECHST	Tab	Furosemide 20 mg	Lasix by Pharm Utilization	60491-0359	Diuretic
LASIX <> HOECHST	Tab	Furosemide 20 mg	Lasix by Leiner	59606-0679	Diuretic
LASIX <> HOECHST	Tab	Furosemide 20 mg	Lasix by Thrift Drug	59198-0224	Diuretic
LASIX <> HOECHST	Tab	Furosemide 20 mg	Lasix by Amerisource	62584-0067	Diuretic
LASIX <> HOECHST	Tab	Furosemide 20 mg	Lasix by Caremark	00339-5203	Diuretic
LASIX <> HOECHST	Tab	Furosemide 20 mg	Lasix by Drug Distr	52985-0072	Diuretic
LASIX40	Tab, Hoechst Logo	Furosemide 40 mg	Lasix by Amerisource	62584-0060	Diuretic
LASIX40	Tab, Hoechst Logo	Furosemide 40 mg	Lasix by Drug Distr	52985-0220	Diuretic
LASIX40 <> HOECHST	Tab	Furosemide 40 mg	Lasix by Allscripts	54569-0573	Diuretic
LASIX40 <> HOECHST	Tab	Furosemide 40 mg	Lasix by Wal Mart	49035-0156	Diuretic
LASIX40 <> HOECHST	Tab, Lasix 40 <> Hoechst Logo	Furosemide 40 mg	Lasix by Thrift Drug	59198-0068	Diuretic
LASIX80	Tab, Hoechst Logo on This Side	Furosemide 80 mg	Lasix by Pharm Utilization	60491-0361	Diuretic
LASIX80	Tab, Lasix 80 <> Hoechst Logo	Furosemide 80 mg	Lasix by Wal Mart	49035-0171	Diuretic
LASIX80	Tab, White, Round, Lasix 80 <> Hoechst Logo	Furosemide 80 mg	Lasix by Hoechst Roussel	00039-0066	Diuretic
LASIX80 <> HOECHST	Tab, Facetted Edged	Furosemide 80 mg	Lasix by Thrift Drug	59198-0024	Diuretic
LASIXR <> HOECHST	Tab, Lasix Logo	Furosemide 20 mg	Lasix by Merrell	00068-1215	Diuretic
LASIXR <> HOECHST	Tab, Lasix (R) <> Hoechst	Furosemide 20 mg	Lasix by Hoechst Roussel	00039-0067	Diuretic

ID FRONT <> BACK	DESCRIPTION FRONT <> BACK	INGREDIENT & STRENGTH	BRAND (OR EQUIV.) & FIRM	NDC#	CLASS; SCH.
LASIXR40	Tab, Lasix Logo 40 <> Hoechst Logo	Furosemide 40 mg	Lasix by Merrell	00068-1216	Diuretic
LASIXR40 <> HOECHST	Tab, Lasix (R) 40 <> Hoechst	Furosemide 40 mg	Lasix by Hoechst Roussel	00039-0060	Diuretic
LASIXR80	Tab, Lasix Logo 80 <> Hoechst Logo	Furosemide 80 mg	Lasix by Merrell	00068-1217	Diuretic
IATIVAN	Tab, White, Oblong, I/Ativan	Lorazepam 1 mg	by Wyeth-Ayerst	Canadian	Sedative/Hypnotic
LB <> GEIGY	Tab, Brownish-Red, Round, Sugar Coated	Imipramine HCl 50 mg	Tofranil by Novartis	Canadian DIN# 00010480	Antidepressant
LB <> VISKEN5	Tab, White, Round, Scored	Pindolol 5 mg	Visken by Sandoz	Canadian DIN# 00417270	Antihypertensive
LB2	Tab, Green, Round	Ergotamine Tartrate 2 mg	Ergomar Sublingual by Lotus Biochem	59417-0120	Analgesic
LB210	Tab, Blue, Triangular, LB/2-10	Perphenazine 2 mg, Amitriptyline HCl 10 mg	Triavil by Watson		Antipsychotic; Antidepressant
LB210	Tab, Blue, Triangular, LB 2-10	Perphenazine 2 mg, Amitriptyline HCl 10 mg	Triavil by Lotus BioChem	59417-0401	Antipsychotic; Antidepressant
LB225	Tab, Light Orange, Triangular, LB/2-25	Perphenazine 2 mg, Amitriptyline HCl 25 mg	Triavil by Watson		Antipsychotic; Antidepressant
LB225	Tab, Orange, Triangular, LB 2-25	Perphenazine 2 mg, Amitriptyline HCl 25 mg	Triavil by Lotus BioChem	59417-0402	Antipsychotic; Antidepressant
LB410	Tab, Beige, Triangular, LB/4-10	Perphenazine 4 mg, Amitriptyline HCl 10 mg	Triavil by Watson		Antipsychotic; Antidepressant
LB410	Tab, Beige, Triangle, Convex	Perphenazine 4 mg, Amitriptyline HCl 10 mg	Triavil by Pharmafab	62542-0915	Antipsychotic; Antidepressant
LB425	Tab, Yellow, Triangular, LB/4-25	Perphenazine 4 mg, Amitriptyline HCl 25 mg	Triavil by Watson		Antipsychotic; Antidepressant
LB425	Tab, Yellow, Triangular, LB 4-25	Perphenazine 4 mg, Amitriptyline HCl 25 mg	Triavil by Lotus BioChem	59417-0404	Antipsychotic; Antidepressant
LB975	Tab, White, Oval, Green Ink, LB-975	Aspirin 975 mg	Easprin by Lotus BioChem	59417-0975	Analgesic
LBS01	Tab, Yellow, Round	Mecamylamine HCl 2.5 mg	Inversine by Layton	65525-0626	Antihypertensive
LBSO1	Tab, Yellow, Round	Mecamylamine HCl 2.5 mg	Inversine by Oread	63015-0626	Antihypertensive
LBSO1 <> LBSO1	Tab, Yellow, Round	Mecamylmine HCl 2.5 mg	Inversine by Siegfried CMS	17205-0626	Antihypertensive
LBVISKEN5	Tab, White, Round, LB/Visken 5	Pindolol 5 mg	Visken by Novartis	Canadian	Antihypertensive
LC738	Tab, LC/738	Propranolol HCl 10 mg	Inderal by LC		Antihypertensive
LC739	Tab, LC/739	Propranolol HCl 20 mg	Inderal by LC		Antihypertensive
LC740	Tab, LC/740	Propranolol HCl 40 mg	Inderal by LC		Antihypertensive
LC741	Tab, LC/741	Propranolol HCl 80 mg	Inderal by LC		Antihypertensive
LC770	Cap, LC/770	Phenytoin Sodium Prompt 100 mg	by LC		Anticonvulsant
LCUSV	Tab, Blue, Round, LC/USV	Levothyroxine Sodium 137 mcg	by Forest	00456-0331	Antithyroid
LDM	Tab, Pink, Oblong, Scored	Dextromethorphan Hydrobromide 60 mg; Guaifenesin 1200 mg	Tussibid by Sovereign Pharms	58716-0694	Cold Remedy
LDY	Tab, White, Round	Glyburide 2.5 mg	Diabeta by Hoechst-Roussel	Canadian	Antidiabetic
LE	Tab, White, Square, Abbott Logo	Trimethadione 150 mg	Tridione Dulcet by Abbott	00074-3753	Anticonvulsant
LEDERLE <> C62	Cap, Light Green	Cephradine Monohydrate 500 mg	by Quality Care	60346-0041	Antibiotic
LEDERLE <> P69	Cap, Flesh	Prazosin HCl 1 mg	by Quality Care	60346-0572	Antihypertensive
LEDERLE <> P70	Cap	Prazosin HCl	by Quality Care	60346-0805	Antihypertensive
LEDERLE 4516	Tab, White, Round	Diethylcarbamazine Citrate 50 mg	Hetrazan by Wyeth-Ayerst	Canadian	Antiparasitic
LEDERLE C9	Cap, Green & Yellow	Chlordiazepoxide HCl 5 mg	Librium by Lederle		Antianxiety; C IV
LEDERLE100MG <> LEDERLEM46	Cap, Lederle over 100 mg <> Lederle over M46	Minocycline HCl 100 mg	Minocin by Allscripts	54569-2899	Antibiotic
LEDERLE119	Cap, Pink	Indomethacin 25 mg	by Southwood Pharms	58016-0235	NSAID
LEDERLE250A3	Cap, Blue & Yellow	Tetracycline HCl 250 mg	Achromycin V by Lederle		Antibiotic
LEDERLE250A31	Cap, Green & White	Ampicillin Trihydrate 250 mg	Principen by Lederle		Antibiotic

ID FRONT <> BACK	DESCRIPTION FRONT <> BACK	INGREDIENT & STRENGTH	BRAND (OR EQUIV.) & FIRM	NDC#	CLASS; SCH.
LEDERLE250MG <> LEDERLEA3	Cap, Dark Blue, Lederle 250 mg <> Lederle A-3	Tetracycline HCl 250 mg	Achromycin V by Lederle	00005-4880	Antibiotic
LEDERLE500A32	Cap, Green & White	Ampicillin Trihydrate 500 mg	Principen by Lederle		Antibiotic
LEDERLE500A5	Cap, Blue & Yellow	Tetracycline HCl 500 mg	Achromycin V by Lederle		Antibiotic
LEDERLE500MG <> LEDERLEA5	Cap, Lederle over 500 mg <> Lederle over A5	Tetracycline HCl 500 mg	by Quality Care	60346-0435	Antibiotic
LEDERLEA20	Cap, Blue, Lederle/A20	Acetaminophen 500 mg	Tylenol by Lederle		Antipyretic
LEDERLEA3 <> LEDERLE250MG	Cap, Dark Blue, Lederle A-3 <> Lederle 250 mg	Tetracycline HCl 250 mg	Achromycin V by Lederle	00005-4880	Antibiotic
LEDERLEA33	Cap, Gray & White	Amoxicillin 250 mg	Amoxil by Lederle		Antibiotic
LEDERLEA34	Cap	Amoxicillin 500 mg	Amoxil by Lederle		Antibiotic
LEDERLEC10	Cap, Black & Green	Chlordiazepoxide HCl 10 mg	Librium by Lederle		Antianxiety; C IV
LEDERLEC11	Cap, Green & White	Chlordiazepoxide HCl 25 mg	Librium by Lederle		Antianxiety; C IV
LEDERLEC17	Cap, Green & Natural	Chlorpheniramine Maleate TD 8 mg	Teldrin by Lederle		Antihistamine
LEDERLEC18	Cap, Green & Natural	Chlorpheniramine Maleate TD 12 mg	Teldrin by Lederle		Antihistamine
LEDERLEC54 <> CEFACLOR250	Cap, in Black Ink	Cefaclor Monohydrate 250 mg	by Quality Care	60346-0202	Antibiotic
LEDERLEC54 <> CEFACLOR250MG	Cap	Cefaclor Monohydrate	by UDL	51079-0617	Antibiotic
LEDERLEC55	Cap, Lavender & White	Clorazepate Dipotassium 30.75 mg	Tranxene by Lederle		Antianxiety; C IV
LEDERLEC56	Cap, Lavender & Maroon	Clorazepate Dipotassium 7.5 mg	Tranxene by Lederle		Antianxiety; C IV
LEDERLEC57	Cap, Lavender	Clorazepate Dipotassium 15 mg	Tranxene by Lederle		Antianxiety; C IV
LEDERLEC58 <> CEFACLOR500MG	Cap, Lavender	Cefaclor Monohydrate	by UDL	51079-0618	Antibiotic
LEDERLEC61	Cap, Green & Pink	Cephradine 250 mg	Velosef by Lederle		Antibiotic
LEDERLEC62	Cap, Green	Cephradine 500 mg	Velosef by Lederle		Antibiotic
LEDERLEC64	Cap, Gray & Red	Cephalexin 250 mg	Keflex by Lederle		Antibiotic
LEDERLEC65	Cap, Red	Cephalexin 500 mg	Keflex by Lederle		Antibiotic
LEDERLED16	Cap, Green	Dicloxacillin Sodium 250 mg	Dynapen by Lederle		Antibiotic
LEDERLED17	Cap, Green	Dicloxacillin Sodium 500 mg	Dynapen by Lederle		Antibiotic
LEDERLED22	Cap, Brown & Green	Doxycycline Hyclate 50 mg	Vibramycin by Lederle		Antibiotic
LEDERLED23	Cap, Blue	Decyclomine HCl 10 mg	Bentyl by Lederle		Gastrointestinal
LEDERLED25	Cap, Brown	Doxycycline Hyclate 100 mg	Vibramycin by Lederle		Antibiotic
LEDERLED3	Cap, Orange	Acetazolamide 500 mg	Diamox Sequels by Lederle		Diuretic
LEDERLED35	Tab, Pink, Oval	Propoxyphene HCl 65 mg, Acetaminophen 650 mg	Wygesic by Lederle		Analgesic; C IV
LEDERLED36	Cap, Pink	Propoxyphene HCl 65 mg	Darvon by Lederle		Analgesic; C IV
LEDERLED43	Cap, Buff & Red	Disopyramide 150 mg	Norpace by Lederle		Antiarrhythmic
LEDERLED47	Cap, Ivory & White	Doxepin 25 mg	Sinequan by Lederle		Antidepressant
LEDERLED48	Cap, Ivory	Doxepin 50 mg	Sinequan by Lederle		Antidepressant
LEDERLED49	Cap, Green	Doxepin 75 mg	Sinequan by Lederle		Antidepressant
LEDERLED50	Cap, Buff	Doxepin 10 mg	Sinequan by Lederle		Antidepressant
LEDERLED54	Cap, Green & White	Doxepin 100 mg	Sinequan by Lederle		Antidepressant
LEDERLED55	Cap, Gray & Orange	Doxepin 150 mg	Sinequan by Lederle		Antidepressant
LEDERLED62	Cap, Blue & Red	Disopyramide 100 mg	Norpace by Lederle		Antiarrhythmic
LEDERLEF15	Cap, Blue & White	Flurazepam 15 mg	Dalmane by Lederle		Hypnotic; C IV
LEDERLEF30	Cap, Blue	Flurazepam 30 mg	Dalmane by Lederle		Hypnotic; C IV
LEDERLEI19	Cap, Pink & White	Indomethacin 25 mg	by Caremark	00339-5471	NSAID
LEDERLEI20	Cap, Pink & White	Indomethacin 50 mg	by Caremark	00339-5473	NSAID
LEDERLEI20	Cap, Lederle over 120	Indomethacin 50 mg	by UDL	51079-0191	NSAID
LEDERLEK1	Cap, Green	Ketoprofen 25 mg	Orudis by Lederle		NSAID
LEDERLEK2	Cap	Ketoprofen 50 mg	Ketoprofen by Lederle	00005-3285	NSAID
LEDERLEK2	Cap	Ketoprofen 50 mg	Ketoprofen by Physicians Total Care	54868-2414	NSAID

ID FRONT <> BACK	DESCRIPTION FRONT <> BACK	INGREDIENT & STRENGTH	BRAND (OR EQUIV.) & FIRM	NDC#	CLASS; SCH.
LEDERLEK2	Cap	Ketoprofen 50 mg	Ketoprofen by PDRX	55289-0287	NSAID
LEDERLEK2	Cap	Ketoprofen 50 mg	Ketoprofen by Direct Dispensing	57866-4638	NSAID
LEDERLEK2	Cap, Light Green, Imprint is on Both Cap and Body	Ketoprofen 50 mg	Ketoprofen by Quality Care	60346-0856	NSAID
LEDERLEK3	Cap, White	Ketoprofen 75 mg	Orudis by Lederle		NSAID
LEDERLEK3	Cap	Ketoprofen 75 mg	Ketoprofen by Physicians Total Care	54868-2415	NSAID
LEDERLEK3	Cap	Ketoprofen 75 mg	Ketoprofen by Quality Care	60346-0667	NSAID
LEDERLEL1	Cap, Green, Lederle/L1	Loxapine Succinate 5 mg	Loxitane by Watson		Antipsychotic
LEDERLEL2	Cap, Green & Yellow, Lederle/L2	Loxapine Succinate 10 mg	Loxitane by Watson		Antipsychotic
LEDERLEL3	Cap, Green, Lederle/L3	Loxapine Succinate 25 mg	Loxitane by Watson		Antipsychotic
LEDERLEL4	Cap, Blue & Green, Lederle/L4	Loxapine Succinate 50 mg	Loxitane by Watson		Antipsychotic
LEDERLELLC81	Tab, White, Oval	Cephalexin 250 mg	Keflex by Lederle		Antibiotic
LEDERLELLC82	Tab, White, Oval	Cephalexin 500 mg	Keflex by Lederle		Antibiotic
LEDERLEM2MINOCIN	Cap, Orange & Purple, Lederle M2/Minocin	Minocycline HCl 100 mg	by Wyeth-Ayerst	Canadian	Antibiotic
LEDERLEM2MINOCIN	Cap, Orange, Lederle M2/Minocin	Minocycline HCl 50 mg	by Wyeth-Ayerst	Canadian	Antibiotic
LEDERLEM41	Cap, Coral	Meclofenamate Sodium 50 mg	Meclomen by Lederle		NSAID
LEDERLEM42	Cap, Coral & White	Meclofenamate Sodium 100 mg	Meclomen by Lederle		NSAID
LEDERLEM4550MG	Cap, Green & Yellow	Minocycline 50 mg	Minocin by Lederle		Antibiotic
LEDERLEM46 <> LEDERLE100MG	Cap, Lederle over M46 <> Lederle over 100 mg	Minocycline HCl 100 mg	Minocin by Allscripts	54569-2899	Antibiotic
LEDERLEM46 <> LEDERLE100MG	Cap, Green & Opaque, Lederle over M46 <> Lederle over 100 mg	Minocycline HCl 100 mg	Minocin by Neuman Distr	64579-0304	Antibiotic
LEDERLEM46100MG	Cap, Green	Minocycline 100 mg	Minocin by Lederle		Antibiotic
LEDERLEN20	Cap, Natural & Purple	Nitroglycerin SR 2.5 mg	Nitrobid by Lederle		Vasodilator
LEDERLEN21	Cap, Blue & Yellow	Nitroglycerin SR 6.5 mg	Nitrobid by Lederle		Vasodilator
LEDERLEN22	Cap, Amber & Green	Nitroglycerin SR 9 mg	Nitrobid by Lederle		Vasodilator
LEDERLEOI19	Cap, Lederle O/I19	Indomethacin 25 mg	by UDL	51079-0190	NSAID
LEDERLEP11	Cap, Brown & Natural	Papaverine HCl TD 150 mg	Pavabid by Lederle		Vasodilator
LEDERLEP29	Cap, Yellow	Procainamide HCl 250 mg	Pronestyl by Lederle		Antiarrhythmic
LEDERLEP30	Cap, Orange & White	Procainamide HCl 375 mg	Pronestyl by Lederle		Antiarrhythmic
LEDERLEP31	Cap, Orange & Yellow	Procainamide HCl 500 mg	Pronestyl by Lederle		Antiarrhythmic
LEDERLEP53	Cap, Transparent	Phenytoin Sodium ER 100 mg	Dilantin by Lederle		Anticonvulsant
LEDERLEP69	Cap, Flesh, Lederle over P69	Prazosin HCl	by UDL	51079-0630	Antihypertensive
LEDERLEP70	Cap, Lederle over P70	Prazosin HCl	by UDL	51079-0631	Antihypertensive
LEDERLEP71	Cap, Lederle/P71	Prazosin HCl	by UDL	51079-0632	Antihypertensive
LEDERLEQ15	Cap, Transparent	Quinine Sulfate 325 mg	by Lederle		Antimalarial
LEDERLES5	Cap, Brown	Vitamin, Mineral	Stresscaps by Lederle		Vitamin
LEDERLET32	Cap, Peach	Temazepam 15 mg	Restoril by Lederle		Sedative/Hypnotic; C IV
LEDERLET33	Cap, Yellow	Temazepam 30 mg	Restoril by Lederle		Sedative/Hypnotic; C IV
LEDERLEU21 CENTRUMJR	Cap, Orange, Pink & Purple, Oval, Lederle U21/Centrum Jr	12 Vitamins & Minerals	Centrum by Whitehall-Robbins		Vitamin
LEDERLEU22 CENTRUMJR	Cap, Orange & Pink, Oval, Lederle U22/Centrum Jr	17 Vitamins & Minerals	Centrum by Whitehall-Robbins		Vitamin
LEDERLEV6 <> VERELAN360	Cap, ER, Lederle over V6 on Left <> Verelan over 360 on Right	Verapamil HCl 360 mg	Verelan by Elan Hold	60274-0360	Antihypertensive
LEDERLEV7 <> VERELAN180	Cap, ER, Lederle over V7 on Left <> Verelan over 180 on Right	Verapamil HCl 180 mg	Verelan by Elan Hold	60274-0180	Antihypertensive
LEDERLEV8 <> VERELAN120	Cap, ER, Lederle over V8 on Left <> Verelan over 120 on Right	Verapamil HCl 120 mg	Verelan by Elan Hold	60274-0120	Antihypertensive
LEDERLEV9 <> VERELAN240	Cap, ER, Lederle over V9 on Left <> Verelan over 240 on Right	Verapamil HCl 240 mg	Verelan by Elan Hold	60274-0240	Antihypertensive
LEKCT4	Tab, Coated	Cimetidine 400 mg	by Lek	48866-0103	Gastrointestinal
LEKCT4	Tab, White, Cap Shaped, Coated	Cimetidine 400 mg	Tagamet by Rosemont	00832-0103	Gastrointestinal

ID FRONT <> BACK	DESCRIPTION FRONT <> BACK	INGREDIENT & STRENGTH	BRAND (OR EQUIV.) & FIRM	NDC#	CLASS; SCH.
LEKCT4	Tab, Coated	Cimetidine 400 mg	by United Res	00677-1529	Gastrointestinal
LEKCT4	Tab, Coated	Cimetidine 400 mg	by Schein	00364-2593	Gastrointestinal
LEKCT4	Tab, Coated	Cimetidine 400 mg	by Martec	52555-0710	Gastrointestinal
LEMMON	Tab, Yellow, Oblong	Hydralazine HCl 25 mg	Dralzine by Lemmon		Antihypertensive
LEMMON	Tab, Blue, Round	Promethazine HCl 25 mg	Phenergan by Lemmon		Antiemetic; Antihistamine
LEMMON <> 99	Tab, Blue & White, Oblong, Scored, Lemmon <> 9/9	Phentermine HCl 37.5 mg	Adipex P by Teva	00093-0009	Anorexiant; C IV
LEMMON <> 99	Tab, Mottled Blue & White	Phentermine HCl 37.5 mg	Adipex P by Allscripts	54569-1718	Anorexiant; C IV
LEMMON <> 99	Tab, Blue Speckled	Phentermine HCl 37.5 mg	Adipex P by Gate	57844-0009	Anorexiant; C IV
LEMMON <> LEMMON	Tab	Acetaminophen 300 mg, Codeine Phosphate 30 mg	by Kaiser	00179-0038	Analgesic; C III
LEMMON <> ORAP2	Tab, White, Oval, Scored, Lemmon <> Orap/2	Pimozide 2 mg	Orap by Teva	00093-0187	Antipsychotic
LEMMON <> ORAP2	Tab	Pimozide 2 mg	Orap by Gate	57844-0187	Antipsychotic
LEMMON110	Tab, White, Round	Acetaminophen 300 mg, Salicylamide 300 mg, Phenylpropanol 60 mg, Chlorpheniramine 4 mg	Rhinex D-Lay by Lemmon		Cold Remedy
LEMMON128	Tab, White, Round	Dyphylline 200 mg, Guaifenesin 200 mg	Neothylline-GG by Lemmon		Antiasthmatic
LEMMON133	Cap, Clear & Green	Dextroamphetamine Sulfate 15 mg	Dexampex by Lemmon		Stimulant; C II
LEMMON169	Tab, Yellow, Round	Opium, Bismuth Sulgal, Pectin, Kaolin, Zinc Phenolsulf	B.P.P. by Lemmon		Gastrointestinal
LEMMON178	Tab, Pink, Oblong	Methamphetamine HCl 10 mg	Methampex by Lemmon		Stimulant; C II
LEMMON179	Tab, Blue, Oblong	Dextroamphetamine Sulfate 5 mg	Dexampex by Lemmon		Stimulant; C II
LEMMON180	Tab, Pink, Oblong	Dextroamphetamine Sulfate 10 mg	Dexampex by Lemmon		Stimulant; C II
LEMMON277	Cap, Green & White	Phendimetrazine Tartrate 35 mg	Statobex by Lemmon		Anorexiant; C III
LEMMON30	Tab, White, Round	Dyphylline 200 mg	Neothylline by Lemmon		Antiasthmatic
LEMMON368	Cap, Blue	Pheniramine, Pyrilamine, Phenylpropan, Phenylephrine	Allerstat by Lemmon		Cold Remedy
LEMMON37	Tab, White, Oblong	Dyphylline 400 mg	Neothylline by Lemmon		Antiasthmatic
LEMMON71	Tab, Oblong, Green & White Specks	Phendimetrazine tartrate 35 mg	Statobex by Lemmon		Anorexiant; C III
LEMMON714	Tab, White, Round	Methaqualone HCl 300 mg	Quaalude by Lemmon		Hypnotic
LEMMON77	Tab, Green, Oblong	Phendimetrazine Tartrate 35 mg	Statobex-G by Lemmon		Anorexiant; C III
LEMMON86	Tab, White, Round	Secobarbital 50 mg, Butabarbital 30 mg, Phenobarbital 15 mg	S.B.P. by Lemmon		Sedative/Hypnotic; C IV
LEMMON9	Tab, Blue & White, Oblong	Phentermine HCl 37.5 mg	Adipex-P by Lemmon		Anorexiant; C IV
LEMMON93205	Tab, Pink, Round	Phenobarbital, Hyoscyamine, Atropine, Scopolamine	Donphen by Lemmon		Gastrointestinal; C IV
LEMMON9393	Tab, Blue & White	Phentermine HCl 37.5 mg	Adipex P by Quality Care	60346-0344	Anorexiant; C IV
LEMON99	Tab, Blue & White, Oblong, Scored	Phentermine HCl 37.5 mg	Adipex P by Physicians Total Care		Anorexiant; C IV
LEOPHARMALOGO	Tab, White, Round, Scored, Leo Pharma Logo=Assyrian Lion	Bumetanide 1 mg	Burinex by Novartis	Canadian DIN# 00728284	Diuretic
LEOPHARMALOGO	Tab, White, Round, Scored, Leo Pharma Logo=Assyrian Lion	Bumetanide 2 mg	Burinex by Novartis	Canadian DIN# 02176076	Diuretic
LEOPHARMALOGO	Tab, White, Oval, Film Coated, Leo Pharma Logo=Assyrian Lion	Pivampicillin 500 mg	Pondocillin by Leo Pharma	Canadian DIN# 00582247	Antibiotic
LEOPHARMALOGO	Tab, White, Film Coated, Leo Pharma Logo=Assyrian Lion	Pivmecillinam 200 mg	Selexid by Leo Pharma	Canadian DIN# 00657212	Antibiotic
LESCOL <> 20	Cap, Brown & Light Brown, Lescol Logo <> Triangle Logo 20	Fluvastatin Sodium 20 mg	Lescol by Novartis	00078-0176	Antihyperlipidemic
LESCOL <> 20	Cap, Sandoz Logo	Fluvastatin Sodium 20 mg	Lescol by Allscripts	54569-3821	Antihyperlipidemic
LESCOL <> 40	Cap, Brown & Gold, Lescol Logo <> Triangle Logo 40	Fluvastatin Sodium 40 mg	Lescol by Novartis	00078-0234	Antihyperlipidemic
LESCOL <> 4040	Cap, Brown & Gold, Lescol <> Logo 40 Logo 40	Acetaminophen 500 mg, Hydrocodone Bitartrate 7.5 mg	by Allscripts	54569-4761	Analgesic; C III
LESCOL <> S20	Cap, Lescol & Lescol Logo Printed Twice <> S in Triangle and 20 Printed Twice	Fluvastatin Sodium 20 mg	Lescol by Pharm Utilization	60491-0355	Antihyperlipidemic
LESCOL <> S20	Cap, Triangle with S Inside	Fluvastatin Sodium 20 mg	Lescol by Amerisource	62584-0176	Antihyperlipidemic
LESCOL <> S40	Cap, Gold, Lescol Logo Lescol Logo <> Sandoz Logo 40	Fluvastatin Sodium 40 mg	Lescol by DRX	55045-2369	Antihyperlipidemic

ID FRONT <> BACK	DESCRIPTION FRONT <> BACK	INGREDIENT & STRENGTH	BRAND (OR EQUIV.) & FIRM	NDC#	CLASS; SCH.
LESCOL <> S40	Cap, Lescol over Lescol Logo Twice <> S Inside Triangle and 40 Imprinted Twice	Fluvastatin Sodium 40 mg	Lescol by Pharm Utilization	60491-0356	Antihyperlipidemic
LESCOLLESCOL <> S2020	Cap, Light Brown & Brown, Gelatin, Lescol Logo Lescol Logo <> S in triangle 20 20	Fluvastatin Sodium 20 mg	Lescol by Novartis	Canadian DIN# 02061562	Antihyperlipidemic
LESCOLLESCOL <> S4040	Cap, Gold & Brown, Gelatin, Lescol Logo Lescol Logo <> S in triangle 40 40	Fluvastatin Sodium 40 mg	Lescol by Novartis	Canadian DIN# 02061570	Antihyperlipidemic
LESCOLXL <> 80	Tab, Yellow, Round, Film Coated	Fluvastatin Sodium 80 mg	Lescol XL by Novartis	00078-0354	Antihyperlipidemic
LEVAQUIN <> 250	Tab, Pink, Square	Levofloxacin 250 mg	Levaquin by Allscripts	54569-4915	Antibiotic
LEVAQUIN <> 250	Tab, Pink, Rectangle	Levofloxacin 250 mg	Levaquin by Phy Total Care	54868-4175	Antibiotic
LEVAQUIN <> 250	Tab, Pink, Rectangle, Film	Levofloxacin 250 mg	Levaquin by Murfreesboro	51129-1630	Antibiotic
LEVAQUIN <> 500	Tab, Peach, Rectangle	Levofloxacin 500 mg	Levaquin by Phy Total Care	54868-3923	Antibiotic
LEVAQUIN <> 500	Peach	Levofloxacin 500 mg	Levaquin by Murfreesboro	51129-1628	Antibiotic
LEVOT100M	Tab, Yellow, Round, Levo-T/100/M	Levothyroxine Sodium 100 mcg	by Pharmascience	Canadian	Antithyroid
LEVOT125M	Tab, Brown, Round, Levo-T/125/M	Levothyroxine Sodium 0.125 mg	by Pharmascience	Canadian	Antithyroid
LEVOT150M	Tab, Blue, Round, Levo-T/150/M	Levothyroxine Sodium 0.15 mg	by Pharmascience	Canadian	Antithyroid
LEVOT200M	Tab, Pink, Round, Levo-T/200/M	Levothyroxine Sodium 0.2 mg	by Pharmascience	Canadian	Antithyroid
LEVOT25M	Tab, Orange, Round, Levo-T/25/M	Levothyroxine Sodium 0.025 mg	by Pharmascience	Canadian	Antithyroid
LEVOT300M	Tab, Green, Round, Levo-T/300/M	Levothyroxine Sodium 0.3 mg	by Pharmascience	Canadian	Antithyroid
LEVOT50M	Tab, White, Round, Levo-T/50/M	Levothyroxine Sodium 0.05 mg	by Pharmascience	Canadian	Antithyroid
LEVOT75M	Tab, Violet, Round, Levo-T/75/M	Levothyroxine Sodium 0.075 mg	by Pharmascience	Canadian	Antithyroid
LEVOXYL <> DP100	Tab	Levothyroxine Sodium 100 mcg	Levoxyl by Jones	52604-1110	Antithyroid
LEVOXYL <> DP100	Tab, Yellow, Oval, Scored	Levothyroxine Sodium 100 mcg	Levoxyl by JMI Daniels	00689-1110	Antithyroid
LEVOXYL <> DP112	Tab	Levothyroxine Sodium 112 mcg	Levoxyl by Jones	52604-1130	Antithyroid
LEVOXYL <> DP112	Tab, Rose, Oval, Scored, Levoxyl <> dp/112	Levothyroxine Sodium 112 mcg	Levoxyl by JMI Daniels	00689-1130	Antithyroid
LEVOXYL <> DP125	Tab, Brown, Oval, Scored, Levoxyl <> dp/125	Levothyroxine Sodium 125 mcg	Levoxyl by JMI Daniels	00689-1120	Antithyroid
LEVOXYL <> DP137	Tab, Dark Blue, Oval, Scored, Levoxyl <> dp/137	Levothyroxine Sodium 137 mcg	Levoxyl by JMI Daniels	00689-1135	Antithyroid
LEVOXYL <> DP150	Tab, Blue, Oval, Scored	Levothyroxine Sodium 150 mcg	Levoxyl by JMI Daniels	00689-1111	Antithyroid
LEVOXYL <> DP175	Tab, Turquoise	Levothyroxine Sodium 175 mcg	Levoxyl by Jones	52604-1122	Antithyroid
LEVOXYL <> DP175	Tab, Turquoise, Oval, Scored, Levoxyl <> dp/175	Levothyroxine Sodium 175 mcg	Levoxyl by JMI Daniels	00689-1122	Antithyroid
LEVOXYL <> DP200	Tab, Pink, Oval, Scored	Levothyroxine Sodium 200 mcg	Levoxyl by JMI Daniels	00689-1112	Antithyroid
LEVOXYL <> DP25	Tab, DP/25	Levothyroxine Sodium 25 mcg	Levoxyl by Jones	52604-1117	Antithyroid
LEVOXYL <> DP25	Tab, Orange, Oval, Scored, Levoxyl <> dp/25	Levothyroxine Sodium 25 mcg	Levoxyl by JMI Daniels	00689-1117	Antithyroid
LEVOXYL <> DP300	Tab, Green, Oval, Scored, Levoxyl <> dp/300	Levothyroxine Sodium 300 mcg	Levoxyl by JMI Daniels	00689-1121	Antithyroid
LEVOXYL <> DP50	Tab, DP/50	Levothyroxine Sodium 50 mcg	Levoxyl by Jones	52604-1118	Antithyroid
LEVOXYL <> DP50	Tab, White, Oval, Scored, Levoxyl <> dp/50	Levothyroxine Sodium 50 mcg	Levoxyl by JMI Daniels	00689-1118	Antithyroid
LEVOXYL <> DP75	Tab	Levothyroxine Sodium 75 mcg	Levoxyl by Jones	52604-1119	Antithyroid
LEVOXYL <> DP75	Tab, Purple, Oval, Scored, Levoxyl <> dp/75	Levothyroxine Sodium 75 mcg	Levoxyl by JMI Daniels	00689-1119	Antithyroid
LEVOXYL <> DP88	Tab	Levothyroxine Sodium 88 mcg	Levoxyl by Jones	52604-1132	Antithyroid
LEVOXYL <> DP88	Tab, Olive, Oval, Scored, Levoxyl <> dp/88	Levothyroxine Sodium 88 mcg	Levoxyl by JMI Daniels	00689-1132	Antithyroid
LEXXEL155	Tab, Film Coated, MERCK	Enalapril Maleate 5 mg, Felodipine 5 mg	Lexxel by Promex Med	62301-0027	Antihypertensive
LEXXEL155	Tab, White, Round, Film Coated, Lexxel 1, 5-5	Enalapril Maleate 5 mg, Felodipine 5 mg	Lexxel by AstraZeneca	00186-0001	Antihypertensive
LEXXEL2525	Tab, White, Round, Film Coated, Lexxel 2, 5-2.5	Enalapril Maleate 5 mg, Felodipine 2.5 mg	Lexxel by AstraZeneca	00186-0002	Antihypertensive
LF	Tab, White, Round, Abb. Logo	Warfarin Sodium 10 mg	Panwarfin by Abbott		Anticoagulant
LG <> BAYER	Tab, White, Coated, with Orange Tinge <> Triple Score on Side 1	Praziquantel 600 mg	Biltricide by Bayer	00026-2521	Antihelmintic
LH	Cap	Chlorpheniramine Maleate 4 mg, Phenylephrine HCl 20 mg, Phenyltoloxamine Citrate 50 mg	Linhist LA by Pharmedix	53002-0355	Cold Remedy; C III
LH524	Cap	Chlorpheniramine Maleate 4 mg, Phenylephrine HCl 20 mg, Phenyltoloxamine Citrate 50 mg	by Zenith Goldline	00182-1574	Cold Remedy; C III
LHUSV	Tab, Purple, Round, LH/USV	Levothyroxine Sodium 125 mcg	Levothroid by Forest	00456-0324	Antithyroid
LI3611	Cap, ER	Propranolol HCl 120 mg	by Zenith Goldline	00182-1928	Antihypertensive

ID FRONT <> BACK	DESCRIPTION FRONT <> BACK	INGREDIENT & STRENGTH	BRAND (OR EQUIV.) & FIRM	NDC#	CLASS; SCH.
LIBRAXROCHE	Cap, Librax over Roche <> Librax over Roche	Chlordiazepoxide HCl 5 mg, Clidinium Bromide 2.5 mg	Librax by Roche	00140-0007	Gastrointestinal; C IV
LILLY <> 300490MG	Cap, Clear & Green, Opaque	Fluoxetine 90 mg	Prozac by Lilly	00002-3004	Antidepressant
LILLY <> 4115	Tab, White, Round	Olanzapine 5 mg	Zyprexa by Lilly Del Caribe	00110-4115	Antipsychotic
LILLY <> 4116	Tab, White, Round, Film, in Blue Ink	Olanzapine 7.5 mg	Zyprexa by PDRX		Antipsychotic
LILLY <> 4117	Tab, White, Round, Film, in Blue Ink	Olanzapine 10 mg	Zyprexa by PDRX		Antipsychotic
LILLY <> DARVOCETN100	Tab, Dark Orange, Film Coated, Lilly <> Darvocet-N 100	Acetaminophen 650 mg, Propoxyphene Napsylate 100 mg	Darvocet N 100 by Eli Lilly	00002-0363	Analgesic; C IV
LILLY <> DARVOCETN100	Tab, Film Coated	Acetaminophen 650 mg, Propoxyphene Napsylate 100 mg	Darvocet N 100 by Med Pro	53978-3084	Analgesic; C IV
LILLY <> DARVOCETN100	Tab, Film Coated	Acetaminophen 650 mg, Propoxyphene Napsylate 100 mg	Darvocet N by Nat Pharmpak Serv	55154-1807	Analgesic; C IV
LILLY <> DARVOCETN100	Tab, Film Coated, Darvocet-N 100	Acetaminophen 650 mg, Propoxyphene Napsylate 100 mg	Darvocet N 100 by Allscripts	54569-0007	Analgesic; C IV
LILLY <> DARVONN100	Tab, Buff, Lilly <> Darvon-N-100	Propoxyphene Napsylate 100 mg	Darvon N by Eli Lilly	00002-0353	Analgesic; C IV
LILLY <> DARVONN100	Tab, Buff, Lilly <> Darvon-N-100	Propoxyphene Napsylate 100 mg	Darvon N by Med Pro	53978-3082	Analgesic; C IV
LILLY3061 <> CECLOR250	Cap, Lilly over 3061 <> Ceclor over 250	Cefaclor 250 mg	Ceclor by Quality Care	60346-0104	Antibiotic
LILLY3061 <> CECLOR250	Cap	Cefaclor 250 mg	by Pharmedix	53002-0211	Antibiotic
LILLY3061 <> CECLOR250MG	Cap	Cefaclor 250 mg	Ceclor by Eli Lilly	00002-3061	Antibiotic
LILLY3061 <> CECLOR250MG	Cap, Purple & White	Cefaclor Anhydrous 250 mg	Ceclor by HJ Harkins	52959-0027	Antibiotic
LILLY3062 <> CECLOR500MG	Cap, Lilly over 3062 <> Ceclor 500 mg	Cefaclor 500 mg	Ceclor by Quality Care	60346-0640	Antibiotic
LILLY3062 <> CECLOR500MG	Cap	Cefaclor 500 mg	by Pharmedix	53002-0244	Antibiotic
LILLY3062 <> CECLOR500MG	Cap	Cefaclor Monohydrate 500 mg	Ceclor by Eli Lilly	00002-3062	Antibiotic
LILLY3104 PROZAC10MG	Cap, Gray & Green, Lilly 3104/Prozac 10 mg	Fluoxetine HCl 10 mg	Prozac by Lilly	Canadian	Antidepressant
LILLY3105 PROZAC20MG	Cap, Green & White, Lilly 3105/Prozac 20 mg	Fluoxetine HCl 20 mg	Prozac by Lilly	Canadian	Antidepressant
LILLY3111 <> DARVONCOMP65	Cap	Aspirin 389 mg, Caffeine 32.4 mg, Propoxyphene HCl 65 mg	Darvon Compound 65 by Med Pro	53978-3083	Analgesic; C IV
LILLY3111 <> DARVONCOMP65	Cap, Lilly 3111 <> Darvon Comp 65	Aspirin 389 mg, Caffeine 32.4 mg, Propoxyphene HCl 65 mg	Darvon Compound 65 by Eli Lilly	00002-3111	Analgesic; C IV
LILLY3125 <> VANCOCINHCL125	Cap, Also Imprinted mg After 125	Vancomycin HCl	by Nat Pharmpak Serv	55154-1805	Antibiotic
LILLY3144 <> AXID150MG	Cap, Yellow	Nizatidine 150 mg	Axid by Promex Medcl	62301-0047	Gastrointestinal
LILLY3144 <> AXID150MG	Cap	Nizatidine 150 mg	Axid by Eli Lilly	00002-3144	Gastrointestinal
LILLY3144 <> AXID150MG	Cap, Dark Yellow & Pale Yellow	Nizatidine 150 mg	Axid by Murfreesboro	51129-3144	Gastrointestinal
LILLY3144 <> AXID150MG	Cap, Dark Yellow & Pale Yellow	Nizatidine 150 mg	Nizatidine by Med Pro	53978-2079	Gastrointestinal
LILLY3144 <> AXID150MG	Cap, Dark Yellow & Pale Yellow, Pulvule Shaped, Gel Filled	Nizatidine 150 mg	Axid by Allscripts	54569-2605	Gastrointestinal

ID FRONT <> BACK	DESCRIPTION FRONT <> BACK	INGREDIENT & STRENGTH	BRAND (OR EQUIV.) & FIRM	NDC#	CLASS; SCH.
LILLY3144 <> AXID150MG	Cap, Opaque & Yellow	Nizatidine 150 mg	Axid by PDRX	55289-0348	Gastrointestinal
LILLY3144 <> AXID150MG	Cap	Nizatidine 150 mg	Axid by Pharmedix	53002-1041	Gastrointestinal
LILLY3144 <> AXID150MG	Cap, Dark Yellow & Pale Yellow, Lilly over 3144 <> Axid over 150 mg	Nizatidine 150 mg	Axid by Quality Care	60346-0585	Gastrointestinal
LILLY3144 <> AXID150MG	Cap, Dark Yellow & Pale Yellow	Nizatidine 150 mg	Axid by Promex Med	62301-0020	Gastrointestinal
LILLY3145 <> AXID300MG	Cap	Nizatidine 300 mg	Axid by Eli Lilly	00002-3145	Gastrointestinal
LILLY3170 <> LORABID200MG	Cap, Blue-Gray, Bullet Shaped	Loracarbef	Lorabid by Allscripts	54569-3659	Antibiotic
LILLY3170 <> LORABID200MG	Cap, Blue & Gray, Lilly 3170 <> Lorabid 200 mg	Loracarbef 200 mg	Lorabid by Eli Lilly	00002-3170	Antibiotic
LILLY3171 <> LORABID400MG	Cap, Blue & Pink, Lilly 3171 <> Lorabid 400 mg	Loracarbef 400 mg	Lorabid by Eli Lilly	00002-3171	Antibiotic
LILLY3171 <> LORABID400MG	Cap, Coated, Lilly 3171 <> Lorabid 400 mg	Loracarbef 400 mg	Lorabid by Allscripts	54569-4219	Antibiotic
LILLY3210	Cap, Pink & Purple	Fluoxetine 10 mg	Sarafem by Lilly	00002-3210	Antidepressant
LILLY3220 <> 20MG	Cap, Pink & Purple	Fluoxetine 20 mg	Sarafem by Lilly	00002-3220	Antidepressant
LILLY4112	Tab, White, Round, Film Coated	Olanzapine 2.5 mg	Zyprexa by Phcy Care	65070-0192	Antipsychotic
LILLY4112	Tab, Imprinted in Blue Ink	Olanzapine 2.5 mg	Zyprexa by Lilly	00110-4112	Antipsychotic
LILLY4112	Tab, White, Round, Coated, with Blue Print	Olanzapine 2.5 mg	Zyprexa by Eli Lilly	00002-4112	Antipsychotic
LILLY4115	Tab, White, Round, Lilly/4115	Olanzapine 5 mg	by Lilly	Canadian	Antipsycotic
LILLY4115	Tab, White, Round	Olanzapine 5 mg	by Med-Pro	53978-3371	Antipsychotic
LILLY4115	Tab, Soluble, Blue Ink	Olanzapine 5 mg	Zyprexa by Eli Lilly	00002-4115	Antipsychotic
LILLY4116	Tab, White, Round, Lilly/4116	Olanzapine 7.5 mg	by Lilly	Canadian	Antipsycotic
LILLY4116	Tab, Soluble	Olanzapine 7.5 mg	Zyprexa by Eli Lilly	00002-4116	Antipsychotic
LILLY4117	Tab, White, Round, Lilly/4117	Olanzapine 10 mg	by Lilly	Canadian	Antipsychotic
LILLY4117	Tab, Soluble, Imprinted with Blue Ink	Olanzapine 10 mg	Zyprexa by Eli Lilly	00002-4117	Antipsychotic
LILLY4131	Tab, Ivory, Rectangular	Pergolide Mesylate 0.05 mg	Permax by Lilly		Antiparkinson
LILLY4133	Tab, Pink, Rectangular	Pergolide Mesylate 0.25 mg	Permax by Lilly		Antiparkinson
LILLY4135	Tab, Pink, Rectangular	Pergolide Mesylate 1 mg	Permax by Lilly		Antiparkinson
LILLY4165	Tab, White, Oblong, Film	Raloxifene HCl 60 mg	Evista by RX PAK	65084-0149	Antiosteoporosis
LILLY4165	Tab, White, Oval, Film	Raloxifene HCl 60 mg	Evista by RX PAK	65084-0148	Antiosteoporosis
LILLY4165	Tab, White, Oblong	Raloxifene HCl 60 mg	Evista by Lilly		Antiosteoporosis
LILLY4165	Tab, White, Oval, Coated, with Blue Print	Raloxifene HCl 60 mg	Evista by Eli Lilly	00002-4165	Antiosteoporosis
LILLY4165	Tab, Film Coated	Raloxifene HCl 60 mg	Evista by Lilly	00110-4165	Antiosteoporosis
LILLY4415	Tab, Blue, Oval	Olanzapine 15 mg	Zyprexa by Eli Lilly	00002-4415	Antipsychotic
LILLY4420	Tab, Pink, Elliptical	Olanzapine 20 mg	Zyprexa by Lilly		Antipsychotic
LILLYDARVOCETN100	Tab, Orange, Oblong, Lilly/Darvocet-N 100	Propoxyphene Napsylate 100 mg, Acetaminophen 650 mg	Darvocet-N 100 by Lilly		Analgesic; C IV
LILLYDARVOCETN50	Tab, Coated, Lilly Darvocet N50	Acetaminophen 325 mg, Propoxyphene Napsylate 50 mg	Darvocet N 50 by Eli Lilly	00002-0351	Analgesic; C IV
LILLYDARVOCETN50	Tab, Orange, Oblong	Propoxyphene Napsylate 50 mg, Acetaminophen 325 mg	Darvocet N 50 by Lilly		Analgesic; C IV
LILLYDYNABAC4215	Tab	Dirithromycin 250 mg	Dynabac by Eli Lilly	00002-4215	Antibiotic
LILLYF40 <> LILLYF40	Cap	Secobarbital Sodium 100 mg	by Eli Lilly	00002-0640	Sedative/Hypnotic; C II
LILLYF47	Cap, Blue & Orange	Aminophylline 130 mg, Ephedrine 25 mg, Amobarbital 25 mg	Amesec by Lilly		Antiasthmatic
LILLYF65 <> LILLYF65	Cap, Lilly F65	Amobarbital Sodium 50 mg, Secobarbital Sodium 50 mg	Tuinal by Eli Lilly	00002-0665	Sedative/Hypnotic; C II
LILLYH02	Cap, Pink	Propoxyphene HCl 32 mg	Darvon by Lilly		Analgesic; C IV
LILLYH03 <> DARVON	Cap, Pink, with Dark Pink Band <> in Edible Black Ink	Propoxyphene HCl 65 mg	Darvon by Eli Lilly	00002-0803	Analgesic; C IV
LILLYH17 <> LILLYH17	Cap, White & Yellow	Nortriptyline HCl	Aventyl Hydrochloride by Eli Lilly	00002-0817	Antidepressant
LILLYH19 <> LILLYH19	Cap, White & Yellow	Nortriptyline HCl 25 mg	Aventyl Hydrochloride by Eli Lilly	00002-0819	Antidepressant
LILLYJ31	Tab	Phenobarbital 15 mg	by Eli Lilly	00002-1031	Sedative/Hypnotic; C IV

ID FRONT <> BACK	DESCRIPTION FRONT <> BACK	INGREDIENT & STRENGTH	BRAND (OR EQUIV.) & FIRM	NDC#	CLASS; SCH.
LILLYJ32	Tab	Phenobarbital 30 mg	by Eli Lilly	00002-1032	Sedative/Hypnotic; C IV
LILLYJ33	Tab	Phenobarbital 100 mg	by Eli Lilly	00002-1033	Sedative/Hypnotic; C IV
LILLYJ37	Tab	Phenobarbital 60 mg	by Eli Lilly	00002-1037	Sedative/Hypnotic; C IV
LILLYJ64	Tab	Methadone HCl 5 mg	Dolophine Hydrochloride by Eli Lilly	00002-1064	Analgesic; C II
LILLYJ72	Tab	Methadone 10 mg	Dolophine Hydrochloride by Eli Lilly	00002-1072	Analgesic; C II
LILLYJ94	Tab, White, Round, Beveled, Scored	Methimazole 5 mg	Tapazole by Neuman Distr	64579-0002	Antithyroid
LILLYJ95	Tab, White, Round, Beveled, Scored	Methimazole 10 mg	Tapazole by Neuman Distr	64579-0003	Antithyroid
LILLYNALFON	Tab, Yellow, Oblong, Lilly/Nalfon	Fenoprofen Calcium 600 mg	Naflon by Lilly	Canadian	NSAID
LILLYT24	Tab, White, Round	Sodium Chloride 1 GM	by Lilly		Electrolyte
LILLYT29	Tab, White, Round	Sodium Bicarbonate 10 gr	by Lilly		Vitamin
LILLYU03	Tab, Lilly U03	Acetohexamide 250 mg	Dymelor by Eli Lilly	00002-2103	Antidiabetic
LILLYU53	Tab	Methadone HCl 40 mg	by Eli Lilly	00002-2153	Analgesic; C II
LINES <> DILACORXR240MG	Cap, Lines/Logo <> Dilacor XR/240 mg	Diltiazem HCl 240 mg	Dilacor XR by Nat Pharmpak Serv	55154-4022	Antihypertensive
LINES <> INDERALLA80	Cap	Propranolol HCl 80 mg	Inderal LA by Ayerst	00046-0471	Antihypertensive
LINES <> INDERALLA80	Cap	Propranolol HCl 80 mg	Inderal LA by Nat Pharmpak Serv	55154-0201	Antihypertensive
LINES01490008 <> MACRODANTIN50MG	Cap, Lines/01490008 <> Macrodantin 50 mg	Nitrofurantoin 50 mg	Macrodantin by Nat Pharmpak Serv	55154-2301	Antibiotic
LIPIDIL 100MG	Cap, Orange	Fenofibrate 100 mg	by Fournier Pharma	Canadian	Antihyperlipidemic
LIPIDIL MICRO	Cap, Orange	Fenofibrate, micronized 200 mg	Lipidil Micro by Fournier Pharma	Canadian	Antihyperlipidemic
LIPIDIL MICRO	Cap, Yellow	Fenofibrate, micronized 67 mg	Lipidil Micro Dou by Fournier Pharma	Canadian	Antihyperlipidemic
LIQUIBID	Tab, White, Oblong, Scored, Liqu/Ibid	Guaifenesin 600 mg	Liquibid Sustained Release by Lederle	59911-5888	Expectorant
LIQUIBID	Tab, Ex Release, Liqu/Ibid	Guaifenesin 600 mg	Liquibid by Sovereign	58716-0604	Expectorant
LIQUIBID	Tab	Guaifenesin 600 mg	Liquibid by ION	11808-0300	Expectorant
LIQUIBID	Tab, White, Oblong, Scored	Guaifenesin 600 mg	Liquibid by Eckerd	19458-0834	Expectorant
LIQUIBIDD	Tab, Ex Release, Liquibid-D	Guaifenesin 600 mg, Phenylephrine HCl 40 mg	Liquibid D by Sovereign	58716-0648	Cold Remedy
LIQUIBIDD	Tab, White, Oval, Scored	Guaifenesin 600 mg, Phenylephrine HCl 40 mg	Liquibid D SR by Med Pro	53978-3313	Cold Remedy
LITHIZINE150	Cap, Aqua & Green	Lithium Carbonate 150 mg	Lithizine by Technilab	Canadian	Antipsychotic
LITHIZINE300	Cap, Aqua & Green	Lithium Carbonate 300 mg	Lithizine by Technilab	Canadian	Antipsychotic
LJUSV	Tab, Rose, Round, LJ/USV	Levothyroxine Sodium 112 mcg	Levothroid by Forest	00456-0330	Antithyroid
LK	Tab, Salmon, Round, Abbott Logo	Deserpidine 0.25 mg	Harmonyl by Abbott		Antihypertensive
LKUSV	Tab, Orange, Round, LK/USV	Levothyroxine Sodium 25 mcg	Levothroid by Forest	00456-0320	Antithyroid
LL	Tab, Gray, Round, Abb. Logo	Hydrochlorothiazide 25 mg, Deserpidine 0.25 mg	Oreticyl Forte by Abbott		Diuretic; Antihypertensive
LL <> A10	Tab, LL <> A/10	Aminocaproic Acid 500 mg	Amicar by Immunex	58406-0612	Hemostatic
LL <> A49	Tab, Lederle Logo <> A/49	Atenolol 50 mg	by Quality Care	60346-0719	Antihypertensive
LL <> A49	Tab	Atenolol 50 mg	by Kaiser	62224-7224	Antihypertensive
LL <> A49	Tab	Atenolol 50 mg	by Baker Cummins	63171-1004	Antihypertensive
LL <> A49	Tab, Kaiser Logo	Atenolol 50 mg	by Kaiser	00179-1165	Antihypertensive
LL <> A49	Tab	Atenolol 50 mg	by Vangard	00615-3532	Antihypertensive
LL <> A49	Tab	Atenolol 50 mg	by UDL	51079-0684	Antihypertensive
LL <> A51	Tab	Alprazolam 0.25 mg	by Nat Pharmpak Serv	55154-5553	Antianxiety; C IV
LL <> A51	Tab, Coated, Lederle Logo <> A 51	Alprazolam 0.25 mg	by Quality Care	60346-0876	Antianxiety; C IV
LL <> A51	Tab	Alprazolam 0.25 mg	by Vangard	00615-0426	Antianxiety; C IV
LL <> A51	Tab, A/51	Alprazolam 0.25 mg	by UDL	51079-0788	Antianxiety; C IV
LL <> A52	Tab	Alprazolam 0.5 mg	by Vangard	00615-0401	Antianxiety; C IV
LL <> A52	Tab	Alprazolam 0.5 mg	by Caremark	00339-4057	Antianxiety; C IV
LL <> A52	Tab, A/52	Alprazolam 0.5 mg	by UDL	51079-0789	Antianxiety; C IV
LL <> A53	Tab, A/53	Alprazolam 1 mg	by UDL	51079-0790	Antianxiety; C IV
LL <> A53	Tab	Alprazolam 1 mg	by Caremark	00339-4054	Antianxiety; C IV

ID FRONT <> BACK	DESCRIPTION FRONT <> BACK	INGREDIENT & STRENGTH	BRAND (OR EQUIV.) & FIRM	NDC#	CLASS; SCH.
LL <> A7	Tab	Atenolol 25 mg	by Nat Pharmpak Serv	55154-5511	Antihypertensive
LL <> A7	Tab, White, Round	Atenolol 25 mg	Tenormin by Lederle	00005-3218	Antihypertensive
LL <> A7	Tab	Atenolol 25 mg	by Med Pro	53978-3055	Antihypertensive
LL <> A71	Tab, Lederle Logo	Atenolol 100 mg	by Quality Care	60346-0914	Antihypertensive
LL <> A71	Tab	Atenolol 100 mg	by Kaiser	62224-7331	Antihypertensive
LL <> A71	Tab, Kaiser Logo	Atenolol 100 mg	by Kaiser	00179-1166	Antihypertensive
LL <> A71	Tab, LL <> A over 71	Atenolol 100 mg	by UDL	51079-0685	Antihypertensive
LL <> B1	Tab, Pink, Scored	Bisoprolol Fumarate 5 mg	Zebeta by Ayerst Lab (Div Wyeth)	00046-3816	Antihypertensive
LL <> B12	Tab, Film Coated, Engraved Within Heart Shape <> B Above 12	Bisoprolol Fumarate 2.5 mg, Hydrochlorothiazide 6.25 mg	Ziac by Quality Care	60346-0775	Antihypertensive; Diuretic
LL <> B12	Tab, Yellow, Round	Bisoprolol Fumarate 2.5 mg; Hydrochlorothiazide 6.25 mg	Ziac by Ayerst Lab (Div Wyeth)	00046-3238	Antihypertensive; Diuretic
LL <> B13	Tab, Film Coated, LL Heart <> A B over 13	Bisoprolol Fumarate 5 mg, Hydrochlorothiazide 6.25 mg	Ziac by Caremark	00339-6006	Antihypertensive; Diuretic
LL <> B14	Tab, White, Round	Bisoprolol Fumarate 10 mg; Hydrochlorothiazide 6.25 mg	Ziac by Ayerst Lab (Div Wyeth)	00046-3235	Antihypertensive; Diuretic
LL <> B14	Tab, White, Round	Bisoprolol Fumarate 10 mg; Hydrochlorothiazide 6.25 mg	Ziac by Stevens Dee Fd	45868-4179	Antihypertensive; Diuretic
LL <> B3	Tab, White, Scored	Bisoprolol Fumarate 10 mg	Zebeta by Wyeth Pharms	52903-3817	Antihypertensive
LL <> B3	Tab, White, Scored	Bisoprolol Fumarate 10 mg	Zebeta by Ayerst Lab (Div Wyeth)	00046-3817	Antihypertensive
LL <> C33	Tab	Leucovorin Calcium 5 mg	by Immunex	58406-0624	Antineoplastic
LL <> C34	Tab	Leucovorin Calcium 16.2 mg	by Immunex	58406-0626	Antineoplastic
LL <> D44	Tab	Dipyridamole 25 mg	by PDRX	55289-0748	Antiplatelet
LL <> D44	Tab, D over 44	Dipyridamole 25 mg	by Lederle	00005-3743	Antiplatelet
LL <> D44	Tab, Film Coated, D over 44	Dipyridamole 25 mg	by UDL	51079-0068	Antiplatelet
LL <> D45	Tab, Purple, Round	Dipyridamole 50 mg	by Caremark	00339-5107	Antiplatelet
LL <> D46	Tab, Purple, Round	Dipyridamole 75 mg	by Caremark	00339-5109	Antianginal
LL <> D46	Tab, Coated, D over 46	Dipyridamole 75 mg	by Lederle	00005-3791	Antiplatelet
LL <> D51	Tab, LL <> D over 51	Diazepam 2 mg	by UDL	51079-0284	Antianxiety; C IV
LL <> D51	Tab	Diazepam 2 mg	by Allscripts	54569-0947	Antianxiety; C IV
LL <> D51	Tab, LL <> D over 51	Diazepam 2 mg	by Lederle	50053-3128	Antianxiety; C IV
LL <> D52	Tab, D Above, 52 Below	Diazepam 5 mg	by Quality Care	60346-0478	Antianxiety; C IV
LL <> D52	Tab, Scored, LL <> D over 52	Diazepam 5 mg	by Nat Pharmpak Serv	55154-5554	Antianxiety; C IV
LL <> D52	Tab, Tan & White, Round, Scored	Diazepam 5 mg	by Southwood Pharms	58016-0275	Antianxiety; C IV
LL <> D52	Tab, LL <> D over 52	Diazepam 5 mg	by UDL	51079-0285	Antianxiety; C IV
LL <> D52	Tab, LL <> D over 52	Diazepam 5 mg	by Lederle	50053-3129	Antianxiety; C IV
LL <> D53	Tab	Diazepam 10 mg	by Allscripts	54569-0936	Antianxiety; C IV
LL <> D53	Tab, LL <> D over 53	Diazepam 10 mg	by Lederle	50053-3130	Antianxiety; C IV
LL <> D53	Tab, Green, Round, Scored	Diazepam 10 mg	by Southwood Pharms	58016-0273	Antianxiety; C IV
LL <> D53	Tab, LL <> D over 53	Diazepam 10 mg	by UDL	51079-0286	Antianxiety; C IV
LL <> D71	Tab, Film Coated	Diltiazem HCl 30 mg	by Amerisource	62584-0366	Antihypertensive
LL <> D71	Tab, Convex, Film Coated	Diltiazem HCl 30 mg	by UDL	51079-0745	Antihypertensive
LL <> D72	Tab, Light Blue, Film Coated	Diltiazem HCl 60 mg	by Lederle	00005-3334	Antihypertensive
LL <> D72	Tab, Blue, Round, Scored, Film, Mottled	Diltiazem HCl 60 mg	by Excellium	64125-0105	Antihypertensive
LL <> D72	Tab, Film Coated, LL <> D over 72	Diltiazem HCl 60 mg	by UDL	51079-0746	Antihypertensive
LL <> D75	Tab, Coated	Diltiazem HCl 90 mg	by PDRX	55289-0893	Antihypertensive
LL <> D75	Tab, Coated	Diltiazem HCl 90 mg	by Quality Care	60346-0503	Antihypertensive
LL <> D75	Tab, Film Coated, D/75	Diltiazem HCl 90 mg	by UDL	51079-0747	Antihypertensive
LL <> D75	Tab, Mottled Blue, Oblong, Scored, Film Coated	Diltiazem HCl 90 mg	by Eckerd Drug	19458-0896	Antihypertensive
LL <> F11	Tab, Lederle	Furosemide 20 mg	by Quality Care	60346-0761	Diuretic
LL <> F11	Tab	Furosemide 20 mg	by UDL	51079-0072	Diuretic
LL <> F12	Tab, LL <> F over 12	Furosemide 40 mg	by UDL	51079-0073	Diuretic

396

ID FRONT <> BACK	DESCRIPTION FRONT <> BACK	INGREDIENT & STRENGTH	BRAND (OR EQUIV.) & FIRM	NDC#	CLASS; SCH.
LL <> F13	Tab, LL <> F over 13	Furosemide 80 mg	by UDL	51079-0527	Diuretic
LL <> F22	Tab, Film Coated, F/22	Fenoprofen Calcium	by UDL	51079-0477	NSAID
LL <> F22	Tab, Film Coated	Fenoprofen Calcium 691.8 mg	by Quality Care	60346-0233	NSAID
LL <> G17	Tab, Film Coated	Gemfibrozil 600 mg	by Vangard	00615-3559	Antihyperlipidemic
LL <> H11	Tab, Film Coated	Hydralazine HCl 25 mg	by Amerisource	62584-0733	Antihypertensive
LL <> H11	Tab, Film Coated	Hydralazine HCl 25 mg	by Caremark	00339-5145	Antihypertensive
LL <> H11	Tab, Film Coated	Hydralazine HCl 25 mg	by Med Pro	53978-3051	Antihypertensive
LL <> H11	Tab, Film Coated	Hydralazine HCl 25 mg	by PDRX	55289-0133	Antihypertensive
LL <> H12	Tab, Coated	Hydralazine HCl 50 mg	by UDL	51079-0075	Antihypertensive
LL <> H14	Tab, Peach, Round, Scored	Hydrochlorothiazide 25 mg	by Natl Pharmpak	55154-5574	Diuretic
LL <> H14	Tab, H Over 14	Hydrochlorothiazide 25 mg	by Lederle	00005-3752	Diuretic
LL <> H14	Tab, Peach, Round, Scored, LL <> H Over 14	Hydrochlorothiazide 25 mg	HydroDiuril UDL	51079-0049	Diuretic
LL <> H15	Tab, H Over 15	Hydrochlorothiazide 50 mg	by Lederle	00005-3753	Diuretic
LL <> H15	Tab, Peach, Round, Scored, LL <> H Over 15	Hydrochlorothiazide 50 mg	HydroDiuril By UDL	51079-0111	Diuretic
LL <> H15	Tab	Hydrochlorothiazide 50 mg	by Amerisource	62584-0737	Diuretic
LL <> J2	Tab,—Lederle <> J Above & 2 Below Score	Methazolamide 50 mg	by Allscripts	54569-3864	Diuretic
LL <> M19	Tab	Methocarbamol 500 mg	by Lederle	00005-3562	Muscle Relaxant
LL <> M19	Tab, Lederle Logo	Methocarbamol 500 mg	by Quality Care	60346-0080	Muscle Relaxant
LL <> M19	Tab	Methocarbamol 500 mg	by Nat Pharmpak Serv	55154-5541	Muscle Relaxant
LL <> M19	Tab, M Over 19	Methocarbamol 500 mg	by UDL	51079-0091	Muscle Relaxant
LL <> M20	Tab, M/20	Methocarbamol 750 mg	by UDL	51079-0092	Muscle Relaxant
LL <> M22	Tab, Coated	Methyldopa 250 mg	by UDL	51079-0200	Antihypertensive
LL <> M22	Tab, Peach, Round, Convex	Methyldopa 250 mg	by Neuman Dist	64579-0018	Antihypertensive
LL <> M22	Tab, Coated	Methyldopa 250 mg	by Lederle	00005-3850	Antihypertensive
LL <> M23	Tab, Peach, Round, Convex	Methyldopa 500 mg	by Neuman Dist	64579-0019	Antihypertensive
LL <> M23	Tab, Coated	Methyldopa 500 mg	by UDL	51079-0201	Antihypertensive
LL <> M23	Tab, Coated	Methyldopa 500 mg	by Lederle	00005-3851	Antihypertensive
LL <> M23	Tab, Coated	Methyldopa 500 mg	by Caremark	00339-5231	Antihypertensive
LL <> M6	Tab, White, Round, Film Coated	Myambutol HCl 100 mg	Myambutol by Dura	51479-0046	Antituberculosis
LL <> M6	Tab, White, Round	Myambutol HCl 100 mg	Myambutol by Lederle Pharm	00005-5015	Antituberculosis
LL <> M6	Tab, White, Round	Ethambutol HCl 100 mg	Myambutol by Lederle	00005-0046	Antituberculosis
LL <> M7	Tab, White, Round, Film Coated, Scored	Ethambutol HCl 400 mg	Myambutol by DRX Pharm Consults	55045-2763	Antituberculosis
LL <> M7	Tab	Ethambutol HCl 400 mg	Myambutol by Allscripts	54569-3070	Antituberculosis
LL <> M7	Tab, White, Round, Scored, Film	Ethambutol HCl 400 mg	Myambutol by Heartland	61392-0725	Antituberculosis
LL <> M7	Tab, White, Round, Scored, Film	Ethambutol HCl 400 mg	Myambutol by Heartland	61392-0724	Antituberculosis
LL <> N11	Tab, N Over 11	Naproxen 250 mg	by UDL	51079-0793	NSAID
LL <> N17	Tab, Lavender, N 17	Naproxen 375 mg	by UDL	51079-0794	NSAID
LL <> N17	Tab	Naproxen 375 mg	by Physicians Total Care	54868-2965	NSAID
LL <> N77	Tab	Naproxen 500 mg	by UDL	51079-0795	NSAID
LL <> N77	Tab	Naproxen 500 mg	by St Marys Med	60760-0452	NSAID
LL <> P33	Tab	Propylthiouracil 50 mg	by Physicians Total Care	54868-1752	Antithyroid
LL <> P36	Tab	Pyrazinamide 500 mg	by Lederle	00005-5093	Antibiotic
LL <> P36	Tab	Pyrazinamide 500 mg	by Allscripts	54569-3950	Antibiotic
LL <> P36	Tab	Pyrazinamide 500 mg	by PDRX	55289-0283	Antibiotic
LL <> P36	Tab, White, Round, Scored, LL <> P over 36	Pyrazinamide 500 mg	Lederle by UDL	51079-0691	Antibiotic
LL <> P36	Tab	Pyrazinamide 500 mg	by Amerisource	62584-0848	Antibiotic
LL <> Q11	Tab, Q' Over 11	Quinidine Sulfate 200 mg	by UDL	51079-0031	Antiarrhythmic
LL <> S11	Tab, White, Round, Scored	Selegiline HCl 5 mg	by Lederle Pharm	00005-3254	Antiparkinson
LL <> S11	Tab, White, Round	Selegiline HCl 5 mg	by ESI Lederle	59911-3254	Antiparkinson
LL <> S16	Tab	Sulindac 150 mg	by Lederle	00005-3550	NSAID
LL <> S16	Tab	Sulindac 150 mg	by Caremark	00339-5696	NSAID

ID FRONT ◇ BACK	DESCRIPTION FRONT ◇ BACK	INGREDIENT & STRENGTH	BRAND (OR EQUIV.) & FIRM	NDC#	CLASS; SCH.
LL ◇ S16	Tab, S Over 16	Sulindac 150 mg	by UDL	51079-0666	NSAID
LL ◇ S16	Tab	Sulindac 150 mg	by Quality Care	60346-0044	NSAID
LL ◇ S17	Tab	Sulindac 200 mg	by Quality Care	60346-0686	NSAID
LL ◇ T1	Tab, Dark Red, Coated	Ascorbic Acid 600 mg, Cobalamin Concentrate 25 mcg, Docusate Sodium 50 mg, Ferrous Fumarate 350 mg, Folic Acid 1 mg, Intrinsic Factor 75 mg, Tocopheryl Succinate 30 Units	Trihemic 600 by Lederle	00005-4590	Vitamin
LL N6	Tab, Yellow, Oval	Nystatin Vaginal 100,000 Units	Nilstat by Lederle		Antifungal
LL077	Tab, Blue, Round	Diltiazem HCl 120 mg	Cardizem by Lederle		Antihypertensive
LL100	Tab, Yellow, Round	Levothyroxine Sodium 100 mcg	Levo-T by Lederle		Antithyroid
LL100A17	Tab, Blue, Heptagonal, LL100/A17	Amoxapine 100 mg	by Wyeth-Ayerst	Canadian	Antidepressant
LL10X2	Tab, Light Green, Round, LL/10/x/2	Loxapine 10 mg	by Wyeth-Ayerst	Canadian	Antipsychotic
LL112	Tab, LL 1/12	Furosemide 40 mg	by Med Pro	53978-5032	Diuretic
LL125	Tab, Beige, Round	Levothyroxine Sodium 125 mcg	Levo-T by Lederle		Antithyroid
LL150	Tab, Blue, Round	Levothyroxine Sodium 150 mcg	Levo-T by Lederle		Antithyroid
LL15C35	Tab, Yellow, Oval, LL15/C35	Leucovorin 15 mg	Leucovorin by Immunex		Antineoplastic
LL15C35	Tab, Yellow, Oval	Leucovorin Calcium 15 mg	Leucovorin by Lederle		Antineoplastic
LL200	Tab, Pink, Round	Levothyroxine Sodium 200 mcg	Levo-T by Lederle		Antithyroid
LL200 ◇ SUPRAX	Tab, Film Coated, Divided Break Line	Cefixime 200 mg	Suprax by Quality Care	60346-0220	Antibiotic
LL25	Tab, Peach, Round	Levothyroxine Sodium 25 mcg	Levo-T by Lederle		Antithyroid
LL25A13	Tab, White, Heptagonal, LL25/A13	Amoxapine 25 mg	by Wyeth-Ayerst	Canadian	Antidepressant
LL25X3	Tab, Pink, Round, LL/25/x/3	Loxapine 25 mg	by Wyeth-Ayerst	Canadian	Antipsychotic
LL300	Tab, Green, Round	Levothyroxine Sodium 300 mcg	Levo-T by Lederle		Antithyroid
LL400 ◇ SUPRAX	Tab, Coated	Cefixime 400 mg	Suprax by PDRX	55289-0954	Antibiotic
LL400 ◇ SUPRAX	Tab, Rounded Corners, Coated, Scored	Cefixime 400 mg	Suprax by Quality Care	60346-0846	Antibiotic
LL400 ◇ SUPRAX	Tab, Coated	Cefixime 400 mg	Suprax by Lederle	00005-3897	Antibiotic
LL400 ◇ SUPRAX	Tab, Coated, Scored	Cefixime 400 mg	Suprax by Physicians Total Care	54868-1383	Antibiotic
LL400 ◇ SUPRAX	Tab, Coated	Cefixime 400 mg	Suprax by Allscripts	54569-2861	Antibiotic
LL400 ◇ SUPRAX	Tab, Coated	Cefixime 400 mg	Suprax by Dept Health Central Pharm	53808-0062	Antibiotic
LL50	Tab, White, Round	Levothyroxine Sodium 50 mcg	Levo-T by Lederle		Antithyroid
LL50 ◇ A15	Tab	Amoxapine 50 mg	Asendin by Lederle	00005-5390	Antidepressant
LL50A15	Tab, Orange, Heptagonal, LL50/A15	Amoxapine 50 mg	by Wyeth-Ayerst	Canadian	Antidepressant
LL50X4	Tab, White, Round, LL/50/x/4	Loxapine 50 mg	by Wyeth-Ayerst	Canadian	Antipsychotic
LL5C33	Tab, Yellow, Round, LL5/C33	Leucovorin 5 mg	Leucovorin by Immunex		Antineoplastic
LL5X1	Tab, Yellow, Round, LL/5/x/1	Loxapine 5 mg	by Wyeth-Ayerst	Canadian	Antipsychotic
LL75	Tab, Lavender, Round	Levothyroxine Sodium 75 mcg	Levo-T by Lederle		Antithyroid
LLA1	Tab, Yellow, Oblong	Triamcinolone 1 mg	Aristocort by Lederle		Steroid
LLA10	Tab, White, Round	Aminocaproic Acid 500 mg	Amicar by Lederle		Hemostatic
LLA11	Tab, White, Round, LA/A11	Trihexyphenidyl HCl 2 mg	Artane by Lederle		Antiparkinson
LLA11 ◇ ARTANE2	Tab	Trihexyphenidyl HCl 2 mg	Artane by Lederle	00005-4434	Antiparkinson
LLA11 ◇ ARTANE2	Tab, LL over A11 ◇ Artane over 2	Trihexyphenidyl HCl 2 mg	by UDL	51079-0115	Antiparkinson
LLA11 ◇ ARTANE2	Tab, LL over A11 ◇ Artane over 2	Trihexyphenidyl HCl 2 mg	Artane by Amerisource	62584-0434	Antiparkinson
LLA11ARTANE2	Tab, White, Round, LL/A11/Artane 2	Trihexyphenidyl 2 mg	by Wyeth-Ayerst	Canadian	Antiparkinson
LLA12	Tab, White, Round, LL/A12	Trihexyphenidyl HCl 5 mg	Artane by Lederle		Antiparkinson
LLA12 ◇ ARTANE5	Tab, White, LL over A12 ◇ Artane over 5	Trihexyphenidyl HCl 5 mg	Artane by Lederle	00005-4436	Antiparkinson
LLA12 ◇ ARTANE5	Tab, LL over A12 ◇ Artane over 5	Trihexyphenidyl HCl 5 mg	by UDL	51079-0124	Antiparkinson
LLA12ARTANE5	Tab, Pink, Round, LL/A12/Artane 5	Trihexyphenidyl 5 mg	by Wyeth-Ayerst	Canadian	Antiparkinson
LLA14	Tab, Yellow, Round, LL-A14	Amiloride HCl 5 mg, Hydrochlorothiazide 50 mg	Moduretic 5/50 by Lederle		Diuretic
LLA16	Tab, White, Oblong	Triamcinolone 16 mg	Aristocort by Lederle		Steroid
LLA2	Tab, White, Oblong, LL/A2	Triamcinolone 2 mg	Aristocort by Glades	Canadian	Steroid
LLA2	Tab, Pink, Oblong	Triamcinolone 2 mg	Aristocort by Lederle		Steroid
LLA23	Tab, White, Round	Acetaminophen 300 mg, Codeine 30 mg	Tylenol #3 by Lederle		Analgesic; C III
LLA24	Tab, Pink, Round	Amitriptyline HCl 10 mg	Elavil by Lederle		Antidepressant

ID FRONT <> BACK	DESCRIPTION FRONT <> BACK	INGREDIENT & STRENGTH	BRAND (OR EQUIV.) & FIRM	NDC#	CLASS; SCH.
LLA25	Tab, Green, Round	Amitriptyline HCl 25 mg	Elavil by Lederle		Antidepressant
LLA26	Tab, Brown, Round	Amitriptyline HCl 50 mg	Elavil by Lederle		Antidepressant
LLA27	Tab, Purple, Round	Amitriptyline HCl 75 mg	Elavil by Lederle		Antidepressant
LLA28	Tab, Orange, Round	Amitriptyline HCl 100 mg	Elavil by Lederle		Antidepressant
LLA353	Tab, White, Round, LL A 35-3	Aspirin 325 mg, Codeine 30 mg	Empirin #3 by Lederle		Analgesic; C III
LLA36	Tab, White, Round, LL-A36	Ascorbic Acid 250 mg	Vitamin C by Lederle		Vitamin
LLA37	Tab, White, Round, LL-A37	Ascorbic Acid 500 mg	Vitamin C by Lederle		Vitamin
LLA38	Tab, White, Round, LL-A38	Ascorbic Acid 1000 mg	Vitamin C by Lederle		Vitamin
LLA4	Tab, Red, Oblong, LL/A4	Triamcinolone 4 mg	Aristocort by Glades	Canadian	Steroid
LLA4	Tab, White, Oblong	Triamcinolone 4 mg	Aristocort by Lederle		Steroid
LLA43	Tab, White, Round	Allopurinol 100 mg	Zyloprim by Lederle		Antigout
LLA44	Tab, White, Round	Allopurinol 300 mg	Zyloprim by Lederle		Antigout
LLA45	Tab, White, Round, LL-A45	Albuterol Sulfate 2 mg	Proventil by Lederle		Antiasthmatic
LLA46	Tab, White, Round, LL-A46	Albuterol Sulfate 4 mg	Proventil by Lederle		Antiasthmatic
LLA49	Tab	Atenolol 50 mg	by Med Pro	53978-1199	Antihypertensive
LLA52	Tab	Alprazolam 0.5 mg	by Zenith Goldline	00182-0028	Antianxiety; C IV
LLA53	Tab	Alprazolam 1 mg	by Zenith Goldline	00182-0029	Antianxiety; C IV
LLA54	Tab, Green, Rectangular	Alprazolam 2 mg	Xanax by Lederle		Antianxiety; C IV
LLA7	Tab	Atenolol 25 mg	by PDRX	55289-0227	Antihypertensive
LLA7	Tab, White, Round	Atenolol 50 mg	by Southwood Pharms	58016-0333	Antihypertensive
LLA8	Tab, Yellow, Oblong	Triamcinolone 8 mg	Aristocort by Lederle		Steroid
LLALL <> ARTANE2	Tab	Trihexyphenidyl HCl 2 mg	Artane by Thrift Drug	59198-0006	Antiparkinson
LLB1	Tab, Pink, Heart Shaped	Bisoprolol Fumarate 5 mg	Zebeta by Lederle		Antihypertensive
LLB10	Tab, White, Oval	Benztropine Mesylate 1 mg	Cogentin by Lederle		Antiparkinson
LLB11	Tab, White, Round	Benztropine Mesylate 2 mg	Cogentin by Lederle		Antiparkinson
LLB14	Tab, White, Round	Bisoprolol 10 mg, Hydrochlorothiazide 6.25 mg	Ziac by Lederle		Antihypertensive; Diuretic
LLB3	Tab, White, Heart Shaped	Bisoprolol Fumarate 10 mg	Zebeta by Lederle		Antihypertensive
LLC13	Tab, White, Round	Chlorothiazide 250 mg	Diuril by Lederle		Diuretic
LLC14	Tab, White, Round	Chlorothiazide 500 mg	Diuril by Lederle		Diuretic
LLC15	Tab, Blue, Round	Chlorthalidone 50 mg	Hygroton by Lederle		Diuretic
LLC16	Tab, Yellow, Round	Chlorpheniramine Maleate 4 mg	Chlor-trimeton by Lederle		Antihistamine
LLC19	Tab, Yellow, Round	Chlorzoxazone 250 mg, Acetaminophen 300 mg	Parafon Forte by Lederle		Muscle Relaxant
LLC22	Tab, Tan, Round	Chlorpromazine 25 mg	Thorazine by Lederle		Antipsychotic
LLC23	Tab, Tan, Round	Chlorpromazine 50 mg	Thorazine by Lederle		Antipsychotic
LLC24	Tab, Tan, Round	Chlorpromazine 100 mg	Thorazine by Lederle		Antipsychotic
LLC25	Tab, Tan, Round	Chlorpromazine 200 mg	Thorazine by Lederle		Antipsychotic
LLC37	Tab, Green, Round	Chlorpropamide 100 mg	Diabinese by Lederle		Antidiabetic
LLC38	Tab, Green, Round	Chlorpropamide 250 mg	Diabinese by Lederle		Antidiabetic
LLC42	Tab, White, Round	Clonidine HCl 0.1 mg	Catapres by Lederle		Antihypertensive
LLC43	Tab, Debossed	Clonidine HCl 0.2 mg	by Quality Care	60346-0787	Antihypertensive
LLC44	Tab, Green, Round	Clonidine HCl 0.3 mg	Catapres by Lederle		Antihypertensive
LLC66	Tab, White, Round	Carbamazepine 200 mg	Tegretol by Lederle		Anticonvulsant
LLC67	Tab, Green, Round	Chlordiazepoxide HCl 5 mg, Amitriptyline 12.5 mg	Limbitrol by Lederle		Antianxiety; C IV
LLC68	Tab, White, Round	Chlordiazepoxide HCl 10 mg, Amitriptyline 25 mg	Limbitrol DS by Lederle		Antianxiety; C IV
LLC69	Tab, Blue, Round	Clorazepate Dipotassium 30.75 mg	Tranxene by Lederle		Antianxiety; C IV
LLC7	Tab, Orange, Round	Chlorthalidone 25 mg	Hygroton by Lederle		Diuretic
LLC70	Tab, Peach, Round	Clorazepate Dipotassium 7.5 mg	Tranxene by Lederle		Antianxiety; C IV
LLC71	Tab, Lavender, Round	Clorazepate Dipotassium 15 mg	Tranxene by Lederle		Antianxiety; C IV
LLD11	Tab, Red, Round	Demeclocycline HCl 150 mg	Declomycin by Wyeth-Ayerst	Canadian	Antibiotic
LLD11	Tab, Red, Round	Demeclocycline HCl 150 mg	Declomycin by Lederle		Antibiotic
LLD12	Tab, Red, Round	Demeclocycline HCl 300 mg	Declomycin by Wyeth-Ayerst	Canadian	Antibiotic

ID FRONT <> BACK	DESCRIPTION FRONT <> BACK	INGREDIENT & STRENGTH	BRAND (OR EQUIV.) & FIRM	NDC#	CLASS; SCH.
LLD12	Tab, Red, Round	Demeclocycline HCl 300 mg	Declomycin by Lederle		Antibiotic
LLD2 <> DIAMOX250	Tab, LL in Upper Right Quadrant, D2 in Lower Left Quadrant <> Diamox 250	Acetazolamide 250 mg	Diamox by Thrift Drug	59198-0186	Diuretic
LLD2 <> DIAMOX250	Tab	Acetazolamide 250 mg	Diamox by Storz Ophtha	57706-0755	Diuretic
LLD24	Tab, Blue, Round	Decyclomine HCl 20 mg	Bentyl by Lederle		Gastrointestinal
LLD27	Tab, White, Round	Ergoloid Mesylates Sublingual 0.5 mg	Hydergine by Lederle		Ergot
LLD2DIAMOX250	Tab, White, Round, LLD2/Diamox 250	Acetazolamide 250 mg	by Storz	Canadian	Diuretic
LLD31	Tab, White, Round	Diphenoxylate HCl 2.5 mg, Atropine Sulfate 0.025 mg	Lomotil by Lederle		Antidiarrheal; C V
LLD32	Cap, Red	DSS 100 mg	Colace by Lederle		Sleep Aid
LLD34	Cap, Maroon	DSS 100 mg, Casanthranol 30 mg	Peri-Colace by Lederle		Sleep Aid
LLD41	Tab, Green, Round	Doxycycline Hyclate 100 mg	Vibra-Tab by Lederle		Antibiotic
LLD45	Tab, Lavender, Round	Dipyridamole 50 mg	Persantine by Lederle		Antiplatelet
LLD71	Tab, Film Coated	Diltiazem HCl 30 mg	by Zenith Goldline	00182-1937	Antihypertensive
LLD71	Tab, Light Blue, Film Coated	Diltiazem HCl 30 mg	by PDRX	55289-0335	Antihypertensive
LLD71	Tab, Coated	Diltiazem HCl 30 mg	by Med Pro	53978-2064	Antihypertensive
LLD72	Tab, Film Coated	Diltiazem HCl 60 mg	by Zenith Goldline	00182-1938	Antihypertensive
LLD72	Tab, Film Coated	Diltiazem HCl 60 mg	by Nat Pharmpak Serv	55154-5523	Antihypertensive
LLD72	Tab, Film Coated	Diltiazem HCl 60 mg	by Med Pro	53978-1235	Antihypertensive
LLD75	Tab, Coated	Diltiazem HCl 90 mg	by Zenith Goldline	00182-1939	Antihypertensive
LLD77	Tab, Coated	Diltiazem HCl 120 mg	by Zenith Goldline	00182-1940	Antihypertensive
LLE10	Tab, Beige, Oblong	Erythromycin Ethylsuccinate 400 mg	EES 400 by Lederle		Antibiotic
LLE2	Tab, Pink, Round	Erythromycin Stearate 250 mg	Erythrocin by Lederle		Antibiotic
LLE27	Tab, White, Round	Ergoloid Mesylates SL 0.5 mg	Hydergine by Lederle		Ergot
LLE28	Tab, White, Oval	Ergoloid Mesylates SL 1 mg	Hydergine by Lederle		Ergot
LLE3	Tab, White, Round	Ergoloid Mesylates Oral 1 mg	Hydergine by Lederle		Ergot
LLE5	Tab, Yellow, Oval	Erythromycin Stearate 500 mg	Erythrocin by Lederle		Antibiotic
LLF1	Tab, Orange, Round	Folic Acid 1 mg	Folvite by Lederle		Vitamin
LLF13	Tab	Furosemide 80 mg	by Med Pro	53978-0927	Diuretic
LLF2	Tab, Green, Oblong, LL-F2	Vitamin, Mineral	Ferro Sequels by Lederle		Vitamin
LLF20	Tab, Green, Round, LL/F20	Ferrous Sulfate 300 mg	Feosol by Lederle		Mineral
LLF21	Tab, White, Round, LL/F21	Ferrous Gluconate 300 mg	Fergon by Lederle		Mineral
LLF4	Tab, Pink, Oblong, LL-F4	Prenatal Vitamin, Mineral	Filibon by Lederle		Vitamin
LLF5	Tab, Pink, Oblong	Prenatal Vitamin Combination	Filibon FA by Lederle		Vitamin
LLF6	Tab, Pink, Oblong	Prenatal Vitamin Combination	Filibon FORTE by Lederle		Vitamin
LLF7	Tab, Pink, Oblong, LL-F7	Prenatal Vitamin, Mineral	Filibon OT by Lederle		Vitamin
LLH1	Tab, White, Round	Quinethazone 50 mg	Hydromox by Lederle		Diuretic
LLH17	Tab, Lavender, Round	Hydroxyzine HCl 10 mg	Atarax by Lederle		Antihistamine
LLH18	Tab, Fuchsia, Round	Hydroxyzine HCl 25 mg	Atarax by Lederle		Antihistamine
LLH2	Tab, Yellow, Round	Quinethazone 50 mg, Reserpine 0.125 mg	Hydromox R by Lederle		Diuretic; Antihypertensive
LLH21	Tab, Purple, Round	Hydroxyzine HCl 50 mg	Atarax by Lederle		Antihistamine
LLH22	Tab, Brown, Round	Reserpine 0.1 mg, Hydralazine HCl 25 mg, Hydrochlorothiazide 15 mg	Ser- by Lederle		Antihypertensive
LLH25	Tab, Orange, Round	Haloperidol 0.5 mg	Haldol by Lederle		Antipsychotic
LLH26	Tab, Orange, Round	Haloperidol 1 mg	Haldol by Lederle		Antipsychotic
LLH27	Tab, Orange, Round	Haloperidol 2 mg	Haldol by Lederle		Antipsychotic
LLH28	Tab, Orange, Round	Haloperidol 5 mg	Haldol by Lederle		Antipsychotic
LLH29	Tab, Green, Round	Haloperidol 10 mg	Haldol by Lederle		Antipsychotic
LLH5	Tab, White, Round	Diethylcarbamazine Citrate 50 mg	Hetrazan by Lederle		Antiparasitic
LLI11	Tab, Yellow, Round	Imipramine HCl 10 mg	Tofranil by Lederle		Antidepressant
LLI12	Tab, Salmon, Round	Imipramine HCl 25 mg	Tofranil by Lederle		Antidepressant
LLI13	Tab, Green, Round	Imipramine HCl 50 mg	Tofranil by Lederle		Antidepressant
LLI15	Tab, Pink, Round	Isosorbide Dinitrate 5 mg	Isordil by Lederle		Antianginal

ID FRONT <> BACK	DESCRIPTION FRONT <> BACK	INGREDIENT & STRENGTH	BRAND (OR EQUIV.) & FIRM	NDC#	CLASS; SCH.
LLI16	Tab, White, Round	Isosorbide Dinitrate 10 mg	Isordil by Lederle		Antianginal
LLI21	Tab, White, Round	Isoxsuprine HCl 10 mg	Vasodilin by Lederle		Vasodilator
LLI22	Tab, White, Round	Isoxsuprine HCl 20 mg	Vasodilan by Lederle		Vasodilator
LLI23	Tab, Green, Round	Isosorbide Dinitrate SA 40 mg	Isordil by Lederle		Antianginal
LLI24	Tab, Green, Round	Isosorbide Dinitrate 20 mg	Isordil by Lederle		Antianginal
LLI27	Tab, Orange, Round	Ibuprofen 200 mg	Advil by Lederle		NSAID
LLI28	Tab, White, Round	Ibuprofen 400 mg	Motrin by Lederle		NSAID
LLI29	Tab, White, Oval	Ibuprofen 600 mg	Motrin by Lederle		NSAID
LLI30	Tab, White, Oblong	Ibuprofen 800 mg	Motrin by Lederle		NSAID
LLJ1	Tab, White, Square	Methazolamide 25 mg	Neptazane by Lederle		Diuretic
LLJ2	Tab, White, Round	Methazolamide 50 mg	Neptazane by Lederle		Diuretic
LLL10	Tab, White, Round	Penicillin V Potassium 250 mg	Ledercillin by Lederle		Antibiotic
LLL10	Tab, Brown, Round, LL/L10	Potassium Phenoxymethyl Penicillin 400, 000 Units	Ledercillin VK by Wyeth-Ayerst	Canadian	Antibiotic
LLL17	Tab, Blue, Round	Levothyroxine Sodium 0.15 mg	Synthroid by Lederle		Antithyroid
LLL30	Tab, White, Round	Lorazepam 0.5 mg	Ativan by Lederle		Sedative/Hypnotic; C IV
LLL31	Tab, White, Round	Lorazepam 1 mg	Ativan by Lederle		Sedative/Hypnotic; C IV
LLL32	Tab, White, Round	Lorazepam 2 mg	Ativan by Lederle		Sedative/Hypnotic; C IV
LLL6	Cap, White, LL/L6	Vitamin	Lederplex by Lederle		Vitamin
LLL9	Tab, White, Round	Penicillin V Potassium 500 mg	Ledercillin by Lederle		Antibiotic
LLM	Tab	Ethambutol HCl 400 mg	Myambutol by Leiner	59606-0737	Antituberculosis
LLM <> 7	Tab, White, Round, Scored, Film Coated	Ethambutol HCl 400 mg	Myambutol by Dura	51479-0047	Antituberculosis
LLM1	Tab, White, Round	Methotrexate 2.5 mg	Rheumatrex by Lederle		Antineoplastic
LLM12	Tab, Yellow, Oval	Meclizine HCl 12.5 mg	Antivert by Lederle		Antiemetic
LLM13	Tab, White & Yellow, Oval	Meclizine HCl 25 mg	Antivert by Lederle		Antiemetic
LLM21	Tab, Peach, Round	Methyldopa 125 mg	Aldomet by Lederle		Antihypertensive
LLM25	Tab, Blue, Round	Methyclothiazide 5 mg	Enduron by Lederle		Diuretic
LLM26	Tab, White, Round	Metronidazole 250 mg	Flagyl by Lederle		Antibiotic
LLM27	Tab, White, Oval	Metronidazole 500 mg	Flagyl by Lederle		Antibiotic
LLM28	Tab, White, Round	Metoclopramide 10 mg	Reglan by Lederle		Gastrointestinal
LLM3	Tab, Orange, Round	Minocycline HCl 50 mg	Minocin by Lederle		Antibiotic
LLM35	Tab, White, Round	Medroxyprogesterone Acetate 10 mg	Provera by Lederle		Progestin
LLM36	Tab, Chartreuse, Round	Methyldopa 250 mg, Hydrochlorothiazide 15 mg	Aldoril by Lederle		Antihypertensive
LLM37	Tab, Pink, Round	Methyldopa 250 mg, Hydrochlorothiazide 25 mg	Aldoril by Lederle		Antihypertensive
LLM5	Tab, Orange, Round	Minocycline HCl 100 mg	Minocin by Lederle		Antibiotic
LLM7	Tab, White, Round	Ethambutol HCl 400 mg	by Dept Health Central Pharm	53808-0006	Antituberculosis
LLM7	Tab, White, Round, LL/M7	Ethambutol HCl 400 mg	by Wyeth-Ayerst	Canadian	Antituberculosis
LLM8 <> MAXZIDE	Tab, LL/M8	Hydrochlorothiazide 50 mg, Triamterene 75 mg	Maxzide by Nat Pharmpak Serv	55154-1705	Diuretic
LLM9 <> MAXZIDE	Tab, Bowtie Shaped	Hydrochlorothiazide 25 mg, Triamterene 37.5 mg	Maxzide 25 by Allscripts	54569-2320	Diuretic
LLN1	Tab, White, Round, LL/N/1	Methazolamide 50 mg	Neptazane by Storz	Canadian	Diuretic
LLN1	Tab, White, Round	Methazolamide 50 mg	Neptazane by Lederle		Diuretic
LLN10	Tab, White, Round	Neomycin Sulfate 500 mg	Neomycin by Lederle		Antibiotic
LLN2	Tab, White, Square, LL/N2	Methazolamide 25 mg	Neptazane by Storz	Canadian	Diuretic
LLN23	Tab, White, Round	Nylidrin HCl 6 mg	Arlidin by Lederle		Vasodilator
LLN24	Tab, White, Round	Nylidrin HCl 12 mg	Arlidin by Lederle		Vasodilator
LLN5	Tab, Pink, Round	Nystatin Oral 500,000 Units	Nilstat by Lederle		Antifungal
LLO4LEDERLE	Tab, Red & White, Oval	Vitamin, Mineral	Ocuvite by Lederle		Vitamin
LLP	Tab, White, Round	Scopolamine Hydrobromide 0.0065 mg, Hyoscyamine Sulfate 0.1037 mg, Atropine Sulfate 0.0194 mg	Colytrol by Llorens Pharm	54859-0704	Gastrointestinal
LLP	Tab, White, Round	Scopolamine Hydrobromide 0.0065 mg, Hyoscyamine Sulfate 0.1037 mg, Atropine Sulfate 0.0194 mg	Colytrol by Lex Pharm	49523-0169	Gastrointestinal
LLP13	Tab, White, Round	Papaverine HCl 100 mg	by Lederle		Vasodilator
LLP24	Tab, White, Round	Prednisone 5 mg	Deltasone by Lederle		Steroid

ID FRONT <> BACK	DESCRIPTION FRONT <> BACK	INGREDIENT & STRENGTH	BRAND (OR EQUIV.) & FIRM	NDC#	CLASS; SCH.
LLP25	Tab, Orange, Oblong	Probenecid 500 mg	Benemid by Lederle		Antigout
LLP26	Tab, White, Oblong	Probenecid 500 mg, Colchicine 0.5 mg	ColBenemid by Lederle		Antigout
LLP33	Tab, White, Round	Propylthiouracil 50 mg	by Lederle		Antithyroid
LLP34	Tab, White, Round	Pseudoephedrine HCl 60 mg	Sudafed by Lederle		Decongestant
LLP35	Tab, Red, Round	Pseudoephedrine HCl 30 mg	Sudafed by Lederle		Decongestant
LLP37	Tab, White, Round, LL-P37	Pyridoxine HCl 25 mg	Betalin by Lederle		Vitamin
LLP38	Tab, White, Round, LL-P38	Pyridoxine HCl 50 mg	Hexa Betalin by Lederle		Vitamin
LLP39	Tab, White, Oblong	Propoxyphene Napsylate 100 mg, Acetaminophen 650 mg	Darvocet N 100 by Lederle		Analgesic; C IV
LLP4	Tab, Pink, Round	Tridihexethyl Chloride 25 mg	Pathilon by Lederle		Antispasmodic
LLP44	Tab, Gray, Round	Propranolol HCl 10 mg	Inderal by Lederle		Antihypertensive
LLP45	Tab, Lavender, Round	Propranolol HCl 20 mg	Inderal by Lederle		Antihypertensive
LLP46	Tab, Brown, Round	Propranolol HCl 40 mg	Inderal by Lederle		Antihypertensive
LLP47	Tab, Blue, Round	Propranolol HCl 80 mg	Inderal by Lederle		Antihypertensive
LLP48	Tab, Blue, Oval	Procainamide HCl SR 250 mg	Procan SR by Lederle		Antiarrhythmic
LLP49	Tab, Pink, Oval	Procainamide HCl SR 500 mg	Procan SR by Lederle		Antiarrhythmic
LLP50	Tab, Tan, Oval	Procainamide HCl SR 750 mg	Procan SR by Lederle		Antiarrhythmic
LLP65	Tab, White, Round	Propranolol HCl 60 mg	Inderal by Lederle		Antihypertensive
LLP67	Tab, White, Round	Propranolol HCl 40 mg, Hydrochlorthiazide 25 mg	Inderide by Lederle		Antihypertensive
LLP68	Tab, White, Round	Propranolol HCl 80 mg, Hydrochlorthiazide 25 mg	Inderide by Lederle		Antihypertensive
LLP7	Cap, Red	Vitamin Combination, Stool Softener	Perihemin by Lederle		Vitamin
LLP72	Tab, Blue, Round	Perphenazine 2 mg, Amitriptyline HCl 10 mg	Triavil by Lederle		Antipsychotic; Antidepressant
LLP73	Tab, Orange, Round	Perphenazine 2 mg, Amitriptyline HCl 25 mg	Triavil by Lederle		Antipsychotic; Antidepressant
LLP74	Tab, Salmon, Round	Perphenazine 4 mg, Amitriptyline HCl 10 mg	Triavil by Lederle		Antipsychotic; Antidepressant
LLP75	Tab, Yellow, Round	Perphenazine 4 mg, Amitriptyline HCl 25 mg	Triavil by Lederle		Antipsychotic; Antidepressant
LLP76	Tab, Orange, Round	Perphenazine 4 mg, Amitriptyline HCl 50 mg	Triavil by Lederle		Antipsychotic; Antidepressant
LLP8	Tab, Maroon, Oblong	Vitamin, Mineral	Peritinic by Lederle		Vitamin
LLP9	Cap, White	Vitamin Combination	Pronemia by Lederle		Vitamin
LLQ11	Tab, White, Round	Quinidine Sulfate 200 mg	by Lederle		Antiarrhythmic
LLQ13	Tab, White, Round	Quinidine Gluconate SR 324 mg	Quinaglute by Lederle		Antiarrhythmic
LLS1	Tab, Orange, Oblong	Vitamin	Stresstab 600 by Lederle		Vitamin
LLS11	Tab, White, Round	Selegiline HCl 5 mg	by ESI Lederle		Antiparkinson
LLS12	Tab, White, Round	Spironolactone 25 mg, Hydrochlorothiazide 25 mg	Aldactazide by Lederle		Diuretic
LLS13	Tab, White, Round	Spironolactone 25 mg	Aldactone by Lederle		Diuretic
LLS14	Tab, Brown, Round	Sulfasalazine 500 mg	Azulfidine by Lederle		Gastrointestinal
LLS2	Tab, Red, Oblong	Vitamin, Mineral	Stresstab 600 FE by Lederle		Vitamin
LLS3	Tab, Peach, Oblong	Vitamin, Mineral	Stresstab 600 Zn by Lederle		Vitamin
LLT1	Tab, Red, Oblong	Vitamin Combination	Trihemic 600 by Lederle		Vitamin
LLT10	Tab, Orange, Round	Thioridazine HCl 10 mg	Mellaril by Lederle		Antipsychotic
LLT11	Tab, White, Round	Thiamine HCl 50 mg	Betalin by Lederle		Vitamin
LLT12	Tab, White, Round	Thiamine HCl 100 mg	Betalin by Lederle		Vitamin
LLT13	Tab, White, Round	Sulfamethoxazole 400 mg, Trimethoprim 80 mg	Bactrim by Lederle		Antibiotic
LLT14	Tab, Tan, Round	Thyroid 65 mg	by Lederle		Thyroid
LLT16	Tab, White, Oval	Sulfamethoxazole 800 mg, Trimethoprim 160 mg	Bactrim DS by Lederle		Antibiotic
LLT17	Tab, White, Round	Tolbutamide 500 mg	Orinase by Lederle		Antidiabetic
LLT19	Tab, White, Round	Tolazamide 100 mg	Tolinase by Lederle		Antidiabetic
LLT20	Tab, White, Round	Tolazamide 250 mg	Tolinase by Lederle		Antidiabetic
LLT22	Tab, White, Round	Tolazamide 500 mg	Tolinase by Lederle		Antidiabetic

ID FRONT <> BACK	DESCRIPTION FRONT <> BACK	INGREDIENT & STRENGTH	BRAND (OR EQUIV.) & FIRM	NDC#	CLASS; SCH.
LLT23	Tab, White, Round	Triprolidine HCl 2.5 mg, Pseudoephedrine HCl 60 mg	Actifed by Lederle		Cold Remedy
LLT25	Tab, Orange, Round	Thioridazine HCl 25 mg	Mellaril by Lederle		Antipsychotic
LLT29	Tab, White, Round	Trazodone HCl 50 mg	Desyrel by Lederle		Antidepressant
LLT30	Tab, White, Round	Trazodone HCl 100 mg	Desyrel by Lederle		Antidepressant
LLT3150100	Tab, White, Rectangular, LL T31-50/100	Trazodone HCl 150 mg	Desyrel by Lederle		Antidepressant
LLT34	Tab, White, Round	Theophylline CR 100 mg	Theo-Dur by Lederle		Antiasthmatic
LLT35	Tab, White, Oval	Theophylline CR 200 mg	Theo-Dur by Lederle		Antiasthmatic
LLT36	Tab, White, Oblong	Theophylline CR 300 mg	Theo-Dur by Lederle		Antiasthmatic
LLU1	Tab, Yellow, Round	Folic Acid 5 mg	Folvite by Wyeth-Ayerst	Canadian	Vitamin
LLU13	Tab, White, Round, LL/U13	Calcium Carbimide 50 mg	Temposil by Wyeth-Ayerst	Canadian	Vitamin/Mineral
LLU4	Tab, White, Round	Aminophylline 100 mg	by Lederle		Antiasthmatic
LLU5	Tab, White, Round	Aminophylline 200 mg	by Lederle		Antiasthmatic
LLUSV	Tab, White, Round, LL/USV	Levothyroxine Sodium 50 mcg	Levothroid by Forest	00456-0321	Antithyroid
LLV4	Tab, White, Round	Verapamil HCl 80 mg	Isoptin by Lederle		Antihypertensive
LLV5	Tab, White, Round	Verapamil HCl 120 mg	Isoptin by Lederle		Antihypertensive
LM	Tab, Lavender, Round, Abbott Logo	Warfarin Sodium 2 mg	Panwarfin by Abbott		Anticoagulant
LMUSV	Tab, Yellow, Round, LM/USV	Levothyroxine Sodium 100 mcg	Levothroid by Forest	00456-0323	Antithyroid
LN	Tab, Orange, Round, Abb. Logo	Warfarin Sodium 2.5 mg	Panwarfin by Abbott		Anticoagulant
LN259724	Cap	Amoxicillin 250 mg	by United Res	00677-0660	Antibiotic
LN382	Cap, Yellow	Clofibrate 500 mg	Atromid S by Novopharm	43806-0382	Antihyperlipidemic
LN42025	Cap, Green, L/N 420-25	Indomethacin 25 mg	Indocin by MP		NSAID
LN43950	Cap, Green, L/N 439-50	Indomethacin 50 mg	Indocin by MP		NSAID
LN716500	Cap	Amoxicillin 500 mg	by United Res	00677-0661	Antibiotic
LN72Y <> 250	Cap	Amoxicillin 250 mg	by Geneva	00781-2020	Antibiotic
LNK25	Cap, Clear & Pink	Diphenhydramine HCl 25 mg	by Allscripts	54569-0239	Antihistamine
LNK25	Cap	Diphenhydramine HCl 25 mg	by Zenith Goldline	00182-0492	Antihistamine
LNK50	Cap	Diphenhydramine HCl 50 mg	by Zenith Goldline	00182-0135	Antihistamine
LNK50	Cap	Diphenhydramine HCl 50 mg	by LNK	50844-0108	Antihistamine
LNUSV	Tab, Light Blue, Round, LN/USV	Levothyroxine Sodium 150 mcg	Levothroid by Forest	00456-0325	Antithyroid
LO	Tab, Peach, Round, Abbott Logo	Warfarin Sodium 5 mg	Panwarfin by Abbott		Anticoagulant
LOBAC0176 <> SEATRACE	Cap, Egg Shell, Lobac-0176 <> Seatrace	Acetaminophen 300 mg, Phenyltoloxamine Citrate 20 mg, Salicylamide 200 mg	Lobac by Seatrace	00551-0176	Analgesic
LODINE200	Cap, Gray	Etodolac 200 mg	Lodine by Wyeth Pharms	52903-0738	NSAID
LODINE300	Cap, Gray, Lodine 300 with One Wide Red Band <> Two Narrow Red Bands	Etodolac 300 mg	Lodine by Heartland	61392-0909	NSAID
LODINE300	Cap, Wide Red Band <> 2 Narrow Red Bands	Etodolac 300 mg	Lodine by Quality Care	60346-0076	NSAID
LODINE300	Cap, Gray	Etodolac 300 mg	Lodine by Wyeth Pharms	52903-0739	NSAID
LODINE300	Cap, Gray, Red Bands	Etodolac 300 mg	Lodine by Allscripts	54569-3264	NSAID
LODINE400	Tab, Yellowish Orange, Film Coated	Etodolac 400 mg	Lodine by Allscripts	54569-3764	NSAID
LODINE400	Tab, Yellow-Orange, Film Coated	Etodolac 400 mg	Lodine by Quality Care	60346-0878	NSAID
LODINE400	Tab, Yellowish Orange, Film Coated	Etodolac 400 mg	Lodine by PDRX	55289-0644	NSAID
LODINE400	Tab, Orange, Oval	Etodolac 400 mg	Lodine by Wyeth Pharms	52903-0761	NSAID
LODINE500	Tab, Blue, Oval, Film Coated	Etodolac 500 mg	by HJ Harkins	52959-0445	NSAID
LODINE500	Tab, Coated	Etodolac 500 mg	Lodine by Ayerst	00046-0787	NSAID
LODINE500	Tab, Film Coated	Etodolac 500 mg	Lodine by PDRX	55289-0197	NSAID
LODINE500	Tab, Coated, Ayerst Logo	Etodolac 500 mg	Lodine by Allscripts	54569-4416	NSAID
LODINE500	Tab, Film Coated	Etodolac 500 mg	Lodine by Wyeth	52903-0787	NSAID
LODINE500	Tab, Coated	Etodolac 500 mg	Lodine by Physicians Total Care	54868-3856	NSAID
LODINEXL400	Tab, Orangish Red, Film Coated	Etodolac 400 mg	Lodine XL by Caremark	00339-5710	NSAID
LODINEXL400	Tab, Orangish Red, Film Coated	Etodolac 400 mg	Lodine XL by PDRX	55289-0237	NSAID
LODINEXL400	Tab, Film Coated	Etodolac 400 mg	Lodine XL by Physicians Total Care	54868-3901	NSAID
LODINEXL400	Tab, Red, Oval, Convex, Film Coated	Etodolac 400 mg	Lodine XL by Heartland	61392-0843	NSAID

ID FRONT ⬦ BACK	DESCRIPTION FRONT ⬦ BACK	INGREDIENT & STRENGTH	BRAND (OR EQUIV.) & FIRM	NDC#	CLASS; SCH.
LODINEXL400	Tab, Orange, Oval, Convex, Film	Etodolac 400 mg	Lodine XL by Heartland	61392-0834	NSAID
LODINEXL400	Tab, Film Coated	Etodolac 400 mg	Lodine XL by Murfreesboro	51129-1145	NSAID
LODINEXL400	Tab, Film Coated	Etodolac 400 mg	Lodine XL by Ayerst	00046-0829	NSAID
LODINEXL500	Tab, Green, Oval, Film Coated	Etodolac 500 mg	Lodine XL by Heartland	61392-0836	NSAID
LODINEXL500	Tab, Grayish Green	Etodolac 500 mg	Lodine XL by Ayerst	00046-0839	NSAID
LODINEXL500	Tab, Grayish Green	Etodolac 500 mg	Lodine XL by Wyeth	52903-0839	NSAID
LODINEXL600	Tab, Gray, Oval	Etodolac 600 mg	Lodine XL by Wyeth Pharms	52903-0831	NSAID
LODINEXL600	Tab, Film Coated	Etodolac 600 mg	Lodine XL by Ayerst	00046-0831	NSAID
LODOSYN ⬦ 511	Tab, Orange, Round, Scored	Carbidopa 25 mg	Lodosyn by DuPont Pharma	00056-0511	Antiparkinson
LOGO ⬦ 3875500	Tab, 387 5 Over 500	Acetaminophen 500 mg, Hydrocodone Bitartrate 5 mg	by Quality Care	60346-0442	Analgesic; C III
LOGO001 ⬦ 3	Tab, Logo 001	Acetaminophen 300 mg, Codeine Phosphate 30 mg	by Quality Care	60346-0059	Analgesic; C III
LOGO063	Tab, White, Round, Scored, Logo 063	Lorazepam 2 mg	by Nat Pharmpak Serv	55154-1350	Sedative/Hypnotic; C IV
LOGO277	Tab, Logo 277	Isoniazid 300 mg	Isoniazid by Quality Care	60346-0483	Antimycobacterial
LOGOZENITH20MG ⬦ 4288	Cap, Opaque & White, Logo Zenith 20 MG	Nicardipine HCl 20 mg	by Par	49884-0590	Antihypertensive
LOP2MG	Cap, Light Green, LOP/2/mg	Loperamide HCl 2 mg	by Novopharm	Canadian	Antidiarrheal
LOPID ⬦ PD737	Tab, Elliptical, Film Coated, P-D 737	Gemfibrozil 600 mg	Lopid by Parke Davis	00071-0737	Antihyperlipidemic
LOPID600MG ⬦ PARKEDAVIS	Tab, White, Ellipsoid, Film Coated	Gemfibrozil 600 mg	by Parke-Davis	Canadian DIN# 00659606	Antihyperlipidemic
LORABID200MG ⬦ LILLY3170	Cap, Blue-Gray, Bullet Shaped	Loracarbef	Lorabid by Allscripts	54569-3659	Antibiotic
LORABID200MG ⬦ LILLY3170	Cap, Blue & Gray, Lorabid 200 mg ⬦ Lilly 3170	Loracarbef 200 mg	Lorabid by Eli Lilly	00002-3170	Antibiotic
LORABID400MG ⬦ LILLY3171	Cap, Lorabid 400 mg ⬦ Lilly 3171	Loracarbef 400 mg	Lorabid by Eli Lilly	00002-3171	Antibiotic
LORABID400MG ⬦ LILLY3171	Cap, Coated, Lorabid 400 mg ⬦ Lilly 3171	Loracarbef 400 mg	Lorabid by Allscripts	54569-4219	Antibiotic
LORELCO250	Tab, White, Round	Probucol 250 mg	Lorelco by Marion Merrell Dow	Canadian	Antihyperlipidemic
LOSEC10	Tab, Pink, Round	Omeprazole Magnesium 10 mg	Losec by Astra	Canadian	Gastrointestinal
LOSEC20	Tab, Brown & Red, Round	Omeprazole Magnesium 20 mg	Losec by Astra	Canadian	Gastrointestinal
LOTENSIN ⬦ 10	Tab, Dark Yellow, Coated	Benazepril HCl 10 mg	Lotensin by DRX	55045-2374	Antihypertensive
LOTENSIN ⬦ 10	Tab, Coated	Benazepril HCl 10 mg	Lotensin by Quality Care	60346-0833	Antihypertensive
LOTENSIN ⬦ 10	Tab, Dark Yellow, Coated	Benazepril HCl 10 mg	Lotensin by PDRX	55289-0109	Antihypertensive
LOTENSIN ⬦ 10	Tab, Dark Yellow, Coated	Benazepril HCl 10 mg	Lotensin by Pharm Utilization	60491-0383	Antihypertensive
LOTENSIN ⬦ 10	Tab, Coated	Benazepril HCl 10 mg	Lotensin by Amerisource	62584-0063	Antihypertensive
LOTENSIN ⬦ 10	Tab, Dark Yellow	Benazepril HCl 10 mg	Lotensin by Novartis	00083-0063	Antihypertensive
LOTENSIN ⬦ 10	Tab, Coated	Benazepril HCl 10 mg	Lotensin by Allscripts	54569-3423	Antihypertensive
LOTENSIN ⬦ 10MG	Tab, Dark Yellow	Benazepril HCl 10 mg	Lotensin by Southwood Pharms	58016-0420	Antihypertensive
LOTENSIN ⬦ 20	Tab, Coated	Benazepril HCl 20 mg	Lotensin by Quality Care	60346-0892	Antihypertensive
LOTENSIN ⬦ 20	Tab, Coated	Benazepril HCl 20 mg	Lotensin by PDRX	55289-0086	Antihypertensive
LOTENSIN ⬦ 20	Tab, Coated	Benazepril HCl 20 mg	Lotensin by Amerisource	62584-0079	Antihypertensive
LOTENSIN ⬦ 20	Tab, Beige Pink	Benazepril HCl 20 mg	Lotensin by Novartis	00083-0079	Antihypertensive
LOTENSIN ⬦ 20	Tab, Coated	Benazepril HCl 20 mg	Lotensin by Allscripts	54569-3359	Antihypertensive
LOTENSIN ⬦ 40	Tab, Red, Round	Benazepril HCl 40 mg	Lotensin by Phy Total Care	54868-2352	Antihypertensive
LOTENSIN ⬦ 40	Tab, Dark Rose	Benazepril HCl 40 mg	Lotensin by Novartis	00083-0094	Antihypertensive
LOTENSIN ⬦ 5	Tab, Light Yellow	Benazepril HCl 5 mg	Lotensin by Novartis	00083-0059	Antihypertensive
LOTENSIN ⬦ 5MG	Tab, Yellow	Benazepril HCl 5 mg	Lotensin by Southwood Pharms	58016-0264	Antihypertensive
LOTENSINHCT ⬦ 57	Tab, White, Oblong, Scored	Benazepril HCl 5 mg, Hydrochlorothiazide 6.25 mg	Lotensin HCT by Novartis	00083-0057	Antihypertensive; Diuretic
LOTENSINHCT ⬦ 57	Tab, White, Oblong, Coated	Benazepril HCl 5 mg, Hydrochlorothiazide 6.25 mg	Lotensin HCT by Novartis	17088-0057	Antihypertensive; Diuretic

ID FRONT <> BACK	DESCRIPTION FRONT <> BACK	INGREDIENT & STRENGTH	BRAND (OR EQUIV.) & FIRM	NDC#	CLASS; SCH.
LOTENSINHCT <> 72	Tab, Light Pink, Oblong, Scored	Benazepril HCl 10 mg, Hydrochlorothiazide 12.5 mg	Lotensin HCT by Novartis	00083-0072	Antihypertensive; Diuretic
LOTENSINHCT <> 72	Tab, Light Pink, Oblong, Coated	Benazepril HCl 10 mg, Hydrochlorothiazide 12.5 mg	Lotensin HCT by Novartis	17088-0072	Antihypertensive; Diuretic
LOTENSINHCT <> 74	Tab, Grayish Violet, Oblong, Scored	Benazepril HCl 20 mg, Hydrochlorothiazide 12.5 mg	Lotensin HCT by Novartis	00083-0074	Antihypertensive; Diuretic
LOTENSINHCT <> 74	Tab, Grayish Violet, Oblong, Coated	Benazepril HCl 20 mg, Hydrochlorothiazide 12.5 mg	Lotensin HCT by Novartis	17088-0074	Antihypertensive; Diuretic
LOTENSINHCT <> 75	Tab, Red, Oblong, Scored	Benazepril HCl 20 mg, Hydrochlorothiazide 25 mg	Lotensin HCT by Novartis	00083-0075	Antihypertensive; Diuretic
LOTENSINHCT <> 75	Tab, Red, Oblong	Benazepril HCl 20 mg, Hydrochlorothiazide 25 mg	Lotensin HCT by Novartis	17088-0075	Antihypertensive; Diuretic
LOTREL	Cap, 2 Gold Bands	Amlodipine Besylate 2.5 mg, Benazepril HCl 10 mg	Lotrel 2.5/10 by Pharm Utilization	60491-0807	Antihypertensive
LOTREL <> 2260	Cap, Brown, 2 White Bands	Amlodipine Besylate 5 mg, Benazepril HCl 10 mg	Lotrel 5/10 by Barr	00555-0512	Antihypertensive
LOTREL2255	Cap, White with 2 Gold Bands	Amlodipine Besylate 2.5 mg, Benazepril HCl 10 mg	Lotrel by Novartis	00083-2255	Antihypertensive
LOTREL2260	Cap, Light Brown with 2 White Bands	Amlodipine Besylate 5 mg, Benazepril HCl 10 mg	Lotrel by Novartis	00083-2260	Antihypertensive
LOTREL2260	Cap, Lotrel 2260 <> 2 White Bands	Amlodipine Besylate 5 mg, Benazepril HCl 10 mg	Lotrel by Caremark	00339-6100	Antihypertensive
LOTREL2265	Cap, Pink with 2 White Bands	Amlodipine Besylate 5 mg, Benazepril HCl 20 mg	Lotrel by Novartis	00083-2265	Antihypertensive
LOX10 <> NU	Tab, Green, Round, Film Coated, Scored, Lox over 10 <> NU	Loxapine Succinate 10 mg	by Nu Pharm	Canadian DIN# 02237535	Antipsychotic
LOX25 <> NU	Tab, Pink, Round, Film Coated, Scored, Lox over 25 <> NU	Loxapine Succinate 25 mg	by Nu Pharm	Canadian DIN# 02237535	Antipsychotic
LOX5 <> NU	Tab, Yellow, Round, Film Coated, Scored, Lox over 5 <> NU	Loxapine Succinate 5 mg	by Nu Pharm	Canadian DIN# 02237534	Antipsychotic
LOX50 <> NU	Tab, White, Round, Film Coated, Scored, Lox over 50 <> NU	Loxapine Succinate 50 mg	by Nu Pharm	Canadian DIN# 02237536	Antipsychotic
LOXAPINE10PMS	Tab, Light Green, Round, Loxapine 10/pms	Loxapine 10 mg	by Pharmascience	Canadian	Antipsychotic
LOXAPINE25PMS	Tab, Pink, Round, Loxapine 2/pms	Loxapine 25 mg	by Pharmascience	Canadian	Antipsychotic
LOXAPINE50PMS	Tab, Yellow, Round, Loxapine 50/pms	Loxapine 50 mg	by Pharmascience	Canadian	Antipsychotic
LOXAPINE5PMS	Tab, Yellow, Round, Loxapine 5/pms	Loxapine 5 mg	by Pharmascience	Canadian	Antipsychotic
LOXITANE10MG <> WATSON	Cap, Yellow & Dark Green, Opaque, Loxitane over 10 mg <> Logo over Watson	Loxapine Succinate 10 mg	Loxitane by Watson	52544-0495	Antipsychotic
LOXITANE25MG <> WATSON	Cap, Dark Green & Light Green, Opaque, Loxitane over 25 mg <> Logo over Watson	Loxapine Succinate 25 mg	Loxitane by Watson	52544-0496	Antipsychotic
LOXITANE50MG <> WATSON	Cap, Blue & Dark Green, Opaque, Loxitane over 50 mg <> Logo over Watson	Loxapine Succinate 50 mg	Loxitane by Watson	52544-0497	Antipsychotic
LOXITANE5MG <> WATSON	Cap, Dark Green, Opaque, Loxitane over 5 mg <> Logo over Watson	Loxapine Succinate 5 mg	Loxitane by Watson	52544-0494	Antipsychotic
LP <> GEIGY	Tab, White, Round, Film Coated	Clomipramine HCl 50 mg	Anafranil by Novartis	Canadian DIN# 00402591	OCD
LR	Tab, Yellow, Round, Abbott Logo	Warfarin Sodium 7.5 mg	Panwarfin by Abbott		Anticoagulant
LRUSV	Tab, Pink, Round, LR/USV	Levothyroxine Sodium 200 mcg	Levothroid by Forest	00456-0327	Antithyroid
LS	Tab, Yellow, Square, Scored, Grooved, LS over Abbott Logo	Methyclothiazide 5 mg, Deserpidine 0.25 mg	Enduronyl by Abbott	00074-6838	Diuretic; Antihypertensive
LSUSV	Tab, Lime Green, Round, LS/USV	Levothyroxine Sodium 300 mcg	Levothroid by Forest	00456-0328	Antithyroid
LT	Tab, Gray, Square, Scored, LT over Abbott Logo	Methyclothiazide 5 mg, Deserpidine 0.5 mg	Enduronyl Forte by Abbott	00074-6854	Diuretic; Antihypertensive

ID FRONT <> BACK	DESCRIPTION FRONT <> BACK	INGREDIENT & STRENGTH	BRAND (OR EQUIV.) & FIRM	NDC#	CLASS; SCH.
LTUSV	Tab, Gray, Round, LT/USV	Levothyroxine Sodium 75 mcg	Levothroid by Forest	00456-0322	Antithyroid
LU	Tab, Yellow, Oblong, Abbott Logo	Estropipate 0.625 mg	Ogen by Abbott		Hormone
LUCHEM110	Tab, White, Oblong, with Pink Specks, Luchem Logo 110	Yohimbine HCl 5.4 mg	Yocon by LuChem		Impotence Agent
LUCHEM5	Tab	Acetaminophen 500 mg, Hydrocodone Bitartrate 5 mg	by Pharmedix	53002-0119	Analgesic; C III
LUCHEM5	Tab	Acetaminophen 500 mg, Hydrocodone Bitartrate 5 mg	by Quality Care	60346-0442	Analgesic; C III
LUCHEM5	Tab, White, Oblong	Hydrocodone Bitatrate 5 mg, Acetaminophen 500 mg	Zydone by LuChem		Analgesic; C III
LUCHEM649	Tab, Green, Round	Pseudoephedrine, Dexbrompheniramine TR	Drixoral by Norton		Cold Remedy
LUCHEM663	Cap	Acetaminophen 500 mg, Hydrocodone Bitartrate 5 mg	by Zenith Goldline	00182-0156	Analgesic; C III
LUCHEM663	Cap, Black & Red	Hydrocodone Bitartrate 5 mg, Acetaminophen 500 mg	Zydone by LuChem		Analgesic; C III
LUCHEM741	Tab, Blue, Oval	Phenylpropanolamine HCl 75 mg, Guaifenesin LA 400 mg	Entex LA by LuChem		Cold Remedy
LUCHEM743	Tab	Chlorpheniramine Tannate 8 mg, Phenylephrine Tannate 25 mg, Pyrilamine Tannate 25 mg	by Zenith Goldline	00182-1912	Cold Remedy
LUCHEM746	Cap	Guaifenesin 200 mg, Phenylephrine HCl 5 mg, Phenylpropanolamine HCl 45 mg	by Pharmedix	53002-0518	Cold Remedy
LUCHEM746	Cap, Luchem over 746	Guaifenesin 200 mg, Phenylephrine HCl 5 mg, Phenylpropanolamine HCl 45 mg	Enomine by Quality Care	60346-0725	Cold Remedy
LUCHEM992	Cap, Clear & Green	Chlorpheniramine Maleate 12 mg	Teldrin by LuChem		Antihistamine
LUNSCO <> 0127	Tab, Film Coated	Acetaminophen 500 mg, Chlorpheniramine Maleate 8 mg, Phenylephrine HCl 40 mg	Protid by Lunsco	10892-0127	Cold Remedy
LUNSCO <> 0127	Tab, Film Coated	Acetaminophen 500 mg, Chlorpheniramine Maleate 8 mg, Phenylephrine HCl 40 mg	by Mikart	46672-0161	Cold Remedy
LUNSCO <> 151	Cap	Acetaminophen 300 mg, Phenyltoloxamine Citrate 20 mg, Salicylamide 200 mg	Anabar by Seatrace	00551-0151	Analgesic
LUNSCO <> 151	Cap	Acetaminophen 300 mg, Phenyltoloxamine Citrate 20 mg, Salicylamide 200 mg	Anabar by Lunsco	10892-0151	Analgesic
LUNSCO <> LUNSCO	Cap, Green Print	Acetaminophen 325 mg, Butalbital 50 mg, Caffeine 40 mg	Pacaps by Lunsco	10892-0116	Analgesic
LV	Tab, Peach, Oblong, Abbott Logo	Estropipate 1.25 mg	Ogen by Abbott		Hormone
LV <> CG	Tab, Light Yellow, Cap Shaped, Film Coated	Benazepril HCl 5 mg	Lotensin by Geigy	Canadian DIN# 00885835	Antihypertensive
LX	Tab, Blue, Oblong, Abbott Logo	Estropipate 2.5 mg	Ogen by Abbott		Hormone
LY	Tab, Green, Oblong, Abbott Logo	Estropipate 5 mg	Ogen by Abbott		Hormone
M	Tab, Green, Round	Bismuth Subgalate 324 mg	by Bryant	63629-1381	Gastrointestinal
M	Tab, Pink, Round, M underlined Logo	Benzocaine 10 mg, Cetylpyridinium Chloride 0.4 mg	Max Lozenger by Century	00436-0663	Anesthetic; Antiseptic
M	Tab, Yellow, Round	Meloxicam 7.5 mg	Mobic by Boehringer Pharms	00597-0029	NSAID
M	Tab, Yellow, Round	Meloxicam 7.5 mg	Mobic by Boehringer Ingelheim	12714-0126	NSAID
M	Tab, White	Theophylline 118 mg, Ephedrine 24 mg, Phenobarbital 8 mg	Tedral by Parke-Davis	Canadian	Antiasthmatic
M <> 057	Tab, White, Oblong, Scored	Sucralfate 1 gm	by Sidmark		Gastrointestinal
M <> 057	Tab, White, Oblong, Scored	Sucralfate 1 gm	by SKB	00029-4153	Gastrointestinal
M <> 10	Tab, White, Round, Scored	Methylphenidate HCl 10 mg	Methylin ER by D M Graham	00756-0284	Stimulant; C II
M <> 10	Tab, White, Round, Scored	Methylphenidate HCl 10 mg	Methylin ER by Mallinckrodt Hobart	00406-1122	Stimulant; C II
M <> 1202MJ	Tab, Lower Case M	Fosinopril Sodium 40 mg	Monopril by Quality Care	62682-6027	Antihypertensive
M <> 1202MJ	Tab	Fosinopril Sodium 40 mg	Monopril by Bristol Myers	15548-0202	Antihypertensive
M <> 132	Tab	Nadolol 80 mg	Nadolol by Qualitest	00603-4742	Antihypertensive
M <> 1423	Tab, White, Round	Methylphenidate HCl 20 mg	Methylin ER by D M Graham	00756-0285	Stimulant; C II
M <> 1423	Tab, White, Round	Methylphenidate HCl 10 mg	by Mallinckrodt Hobart	00406-1423	Stimulant; C II
M <> 1451	Tab, White, Round	Methylphenidate HCl 20 mg	by Mallinckrodt Hobart	00406-1451	Stimulant; C II
M <> 158MJ	Tab, Off-White to White, Scored	Fosinopril Sodium 10 mg	Monopril by Nat Pharmpak Serv	55154-2015	Antihypertensive
M <> 171	Tab	Nadolol 40 mg	Nadolol by Qualitest	00603-4741	Antihypertensive
M <> 2	Tab, White, Round	Hydromorphone HCl 2 mg	by Mallinckrodt Hobart	00406-3243	Analgesic; C II
M <> 2	Tab, White, Round	Hydromorphone HCl 2 mg	by Murfreesboro	51129-1465	Analgesic; C II
M <> 2	Tab, White, Round	Hydromorphone HCl 4 mg	by Murfreesboro	51129-1466	Analgesic; C II
M <> 20	Tab, White, Round, Scored	Methylphenidate HCl 20 mg	Methylin ER by Mallinckrodt Hobart	00406-1124	Stimulant; C II
M <> 204	Tab, White, Round	Diclofenac Sodium 50 mg	by Martec Pharms	65413-0001	NSAID
M <> 205	Tab, White, Round	Diclofenac Sodium 75 mg	by Martec Pharms	65413-0002	NSAID
M <> 231	Tab, 231 Above the Score	Atenolol 50 mg	by Heartland	61392-0543	Antihypertensive
M <> 231	Tab	Atenolol 50 mg	by Quality Care	60346-0719	Antihypertensive
M <> 231	Tab, White, Scored	Atenolol 50 mg	by Mylan	00378-0231	Antihypertensive

ID FRONT <> BACK	DESCRIPTION FRONT <> BACK	INGREDIENT & STRENGTH	BRAND (OR EQUIV.) & FIRM	NDC#	CLASS; SCH.
M <> 231	Tab	Atenolol 50 mg	by Allscripts	54569-3432	Antihypertensive
M <> 231	Tab, Scored	Atenolol 50 mg	by UDL	51079-0684	Antihypertensive
M <> 231	Tab, White, Round, Scored	Atenolol 50mg	Tenormin by UDL	51079-0684	Antihypertensive
M <> 28	Tab	Nadolol 20 mg	Nadolol by Qualitest	00603-4740	Antihypertensive
M <> 317	Tab, Film Coated	Cimetidine 300 mg	by Quality Care	60346-0944	Gastrointestinal
M <> 317	Tab, Green, Film Coated	Cimetidine 300 mg	by Nat Pharmpak Serv	55154-5560	Gastrointestinal
M <> 317	Tab, Green, Film Coated	Cimetidine 300 mg	by Mylan	00378-0317	Gastrointestinal
M <> 317	Tab, Green, Pentagonal, Film Coated	Cimetidine 300 mg	Tagamet by UDL	51079-0807	Gastrointestinal
M <> 317	Tab, Pentagonal, Film Coated	Cimetidine 300 mg	by HJ Harkins Co	52959-0345	Gastrointestinal
M <> 317	Tab, Film Coated	Cimetidine 300 mg	by Murfreesboro	51129-1181	Gastrointestinal
M <> 321	Tab, Beveled Edge	Lorazepam 0.5 mg	by Mylan	00378-0321	Sedative/Hypnotic; C IV
M <> 321	Tab	Lorazepam 0.5 mg	by Murfreesboro	51129-1344	Sedative/Hypnotic; C IV
M <> 321	Tab	Lorazepam 0.5 mg	by Vangard	00615-0450	Sedative/Hypnotic; C IV
M <> 321	Tab, White, Round	Lorazepam 0.5 mg	Ativan by UDL	51079-0417	Sedative/Hypnotic; C IV
M <> 3354	Tab, White & Yellow, Round	Orphenadrine Citrate 25 mg, Aspirin 385 mg, Caffeine 30 mg	Norgesic Forte by Perrigo	00113-0427	Muscle Relaxant
M <> 3354	Tab, White & Yellow	Orphenadrine Citrate 25 mg, Aspirin 385 mg, Caffeine 30 mg	by Mylan	00378-3354	Muscle Relaxant
M <> 3356	Tab, White & Yellow	Orphenadrine Citrate 25 mg, Aspirin 770 mg, Caffeine 60 mg	by Mylan	00378-3356	Muscle Relaxant
M <> 3356	Tab, White & Yellow, Oblong, Scored	Orphenadrine Citrate 50 mg, Aspirin 770 mg, Caffeine 60 mg	Norgesic Forte by Perrigo	00113-0454	Muscle Relaxant
M <> 3358	Tab, White, Round	Orphenadrine Citrate 100 mg	by Phy Total Care	54868-4102	Muscle Relaxant
M <> 3358	Tab, White	Orphenadrine Citrate 100 mg	by Mylan		Muscle Relaxant
M <> 3358	Tab, White, Round	Orphenadrine Citrate ER 100 mg	Norgesic by 3M	00089-1221	Muscle Relaxant
M <> 341	Tab, Orange & Red, Round, Film	Ranitidine HCl 150 mg	Ranitidine USP by RX PAK	65084-0170	Gastrointestinal
M <> 361	Tab, Blue, Oblong, Scored	Hydrocodone Bitartrate 10 mg, Acetaminophen 650 mg	by Southwood Pharms	58016-0232	Analgesic; C III
M <> 372	Tab, Film Coated, Scored	Cimetidine 400 mg	by Nat Pharmpak Serv	55154-5555	Gastrointestinal
M <> 372	Tab, Film Coated	Cimetidine 400 mg	by Quality Care	60346-0945	Gastrointestinal
M <> 372	Tab, Green, Pentagonal, Coated, Scored	Cimetidine 400 mg	by Allscripts	54569-3838	Gastrointestinal
M <> 372	Tab, Green, Film Coated, Scored	Cimetidine 400 mg	by Mylan	00378-0372	Gastrointestinal
M <> 372	Tab, Pentagonal, Film Coated, Scored	Cimetidine 400 mg	by HJ Harkins Co	52959-0375	Gastrointestinal
M <> 372	Tab, Green, Pentagonal, Film Coated	Cimetidine 400 mg	Tagamet by UDL	51079-0808	Gastrointestinal
M <> 372	Tab, Film Coated, Scored	Cimetidine 400 mg	by Murfreesboro	51129-1179	Gastrointestinal
M <> 373	Tab, Film Coated	Hydroxychloroquine 155 mg	by Mylan	00378-0373	Antimalarial
M <> 373	Tab, White	Hydroxychloroquine Sulfate 200 mg	by Mylan		Antimalarial
M <> 4	Tab, White, Triangular, Film Coated	Fluphenazine HCl 1 mg	Prolixin by UDL	51079-0485	Antipsychotic
M <> 4	Tab, White, Triangular	Fluphenazine HCl 1 mg	Prolixin by Mylan		Antipsychotic
M <> 4	Tab, White, Coated	Fluphenazine HCl 1 mg	by Mylan	00378-6004	Antipsychotic
M <> 4	Tab, White, Round	Hydromorphone HCl 4 mg	by Mallinckrodt Hobart	00406-3244	Analgesic; C II
M <> 423	Tab, Orange & Red, Round, Film	Ranitidine HCl 300 mg	Ranitidine USP by RX PAK	65084-0172	Gastrointestinal
M <> 433	Tab, Peach, Round, Film Coated	Bupropion 75 mg	Wellbutrin by UDL	51079-0943	Antidepressant
M <> 435	Tab, Light Blue, Round, Film Coated	Bupropion 100 mg	Wellbutrin by UDL	51079-0944	Antidepressant
M <> 454	Tab, Round	Pindolol 5 mg	by Merckle	58107-0004	Antihypertensive
M <> 455	Tab, Round	Pindolol 10 mg	by Merckle	58107-0005	Antihypertensive
M <> 5	Tab, White, Round	Methylphenidate HCl 5 mg	Ritalin by Mallinckrodt Hobart	00406-1121	Stimulant; C II
M <> 501	Tab, Orange, Round, Film Coated	Bisoprolol Fumarate 2.5 mg, Hydrochlorothiazide 6.25 mg	Ziac by UDL	51079-0954	Antihypertensive; Diuretic
M <> 503	Tab, Blue, Round, Film Coated	Bisoprolol Fumarate 5 mg;Hydrochlorothiazide 6.25 mg	Ziac by UDL	51079-0955	Antihypertensive; Diuretic
M <> 505	Tab, White, Round, Film Coated	Bisoprolol Fumarate 10 mg; Hydrochlorothiazide	Ziac by UDL	51079-0956	Antihypertensive; Diuretic
M <> 53	Tab, Pentagonal, Film Coated	Cimetidine 200 mg	by HJ Harkins Co	52959-0374	Gastrointestinal
M <> 53	Tab, House Shaped, Film Coated	Cimetidine 200 mg	by Heartland	61392-0194	Gastrointestinal
M <> 53	Tab, Film Coated	Cimetidine 200 mg	by Murfreesboro	51129-1177	Gastrointestinal
M <> 53	Tab, Green, Film Coated	Cimetidine 200 mg	by Mylan	00378-0053	Gastrointestinal

ID FRONT <> BACK	DESCRIPTION FRONT <> BACK	INGREDIENT & STRENGTH	BRAND (OR EQUIV.) & FIRM	NDC#	CLASS; SCH.
M <> 537	Tab, Light Blue, Beveled Edge, Film Coated	Naproxen Sodium 275 mg	by Mylan	00378-0537	NSAID
M <> 537	Tab, Light Blue, Film Coated	Naproxen Sodium 275 mg	by HJ Harkins Co	52959-0357	NSAID
M <> 537	Tab, Film Coated	Naproxen Sodium 275 mg	by Allscripts	54569-3761	NSAID
M <> 57	Tab, Round	Sucralfate 1000 mg	by Merckle	58107-0001	Gastrointestinal
M <> 57	Tab, White, Oblong, Scored	Sucralfate 1000 mg	by Warrick Pharms	59930-1532	Gastrointestinal
M <> 60	Tab, White, Beveled Edge, Coated, 6 on Left, 0 on Right of Score	Maprotiline HCl 25 mg	by Mylan	00378-0060	Antidepressant
M <> 609MJ	Tab, Lower Case M	Fosinopril Sodium 20 mg	Monopril by Quality Care	62682-6026	Antihypertensive
M <> 69	Tab, Pink, Film Coated	Indapamide 1.25 mg	by Mylan	00378-0069	Diuretic
M <> 7113	Tab, White, Round, Scored	Meperidine HCl 50 mg	by D M Graham	00756-0286	Analgesic; C II
M <> 7113	Tab, Yellow, Cap Shaped, Scored	Meperidine HCl 50 mg	Demerol by Mallinckrodt Hobart	00406-7113	Analgesic; C II
M <> 7115	Tab, Yellow, Cap Shaped, Scored	Meperidine HCl 100 mg	Demerol by Mallinckrodt Hobart	00406-7115	Analgesic; C II
M <> 733	Tab, Light Blue, Beveled Edge, Film Coated	Naproxen Sodium 550 mg	by Mylan	00378-0733	NSAID
M <> 74	Tab, Green, Triangular, Film Coated	Fluphenazine HCl 5 mg	Prolixin by UDL	51079-0487	Antipsychotic
M <> 74	Tab, Light Green, Coated	Fluphenazine HCl 5 mg	by Mylan	00378-6074	Antipsychotic
M <> 751	Tab, Film Coated	Cyclobenzaprine HCl 10 mg	by Kaiser	00179-1140	Muscle Relaxant
M <> 751	Tab, Butterscotch Yellow, Film Coated	Cyclobenzaprine HCl 10 mg	by Mylan	00378-0751	Muscle Relaxant
M <> 751	Tab, Film Coated	Cyclobenzaprine HCl 10 mg	by Physicians Total Care	54868-1110	Muscle Relaxant
M <> 751	Tab, Film Coated	Cyclobenzaprine HCl 10 mg	by Allscripts	54569-3193	Muscle Relaxant
M <> 751	Tab, Film Coated	Cyclobenzaprine HCl 10 mg	by Allscripts	54569-2573	Muscle Relaxant
M <> 751	Tab, Butterscotch Yellow, Round, Film Coated	Cyclobenzaprine HCl 10 mg	Flexeril by UDL	51079-0644	Muscle Relaxant
M <> 751	Tab, Film Coated	Cyclobenzaprine HCl 10 mg	by Kaiser	62224-7559	Muscle Relaxant
M <> 751	Tab, Butterscotch Yellow, Film Coated	Cyclobenzaprine HCl 10 mg	by Quality Care	60346-0581	Muscle Relaxant
M <> 751	Tab, Film Coated	Cyclobenzaprine HCl 10 mg	by PDRX	55289-0567	Muscle Relaxant
M <> 751	Tab, Yellow, Round, Film Coated	Cyclobenzaprine HCl 10 mg	by DJ Pharma	64455-0028	Muscle Relaxant
M <> 751	Tab, Yellow, Round	Cyclobenzaprine HCl 10 mg	by Va Cmop	65243-0022	Muscle Relaxant
M <> 751	Tab, Yellow, Round, Film Coated	Cyclobenzaprine HCl 10 mg	by DJ Pharma	64455-0034	Muscle Relaxant
M <> 757	Tab	Atenolol 100 mg	by Quality Care	60346-0914	Antihypertensive
M <> 757	Tab	Atenolol 100 mg	by Diversified Hlthcare Serv	55887-0998	Antihypertensive
M <> 757	Tab, White	Atenolol 100 mg	by Mylan	00378-0757	Antihypertensive
M <> 757	Tab	Atenolol 100 mg	by Allscripts	54569-3654	Antihypertensive
M <> 757	Tab, White, Round	Atenolol 100 mg	Tenormin by UDL	51079-0685	Antihypertensive
M <> 80	Tab, White, Beveled Edge, Coated	Indapamide 2.5 mg	by Mylan	00378-0080	Diuretic
M <> 80	Tab, White, Round, Film-Coated, M <> 80	Indapamide 2.5 mg	Lozol by UDL	51079-0868	Diuretic
M <> 80	Tab, Coated	Indapamide 2.5 mg	by DRX	55045-2385	Diuretic
M <> 87	Tab, Blue, Round, Film Coated, Scored	Maprotiline HCl 50 mg	by Murfreesboro Ph	51129-1679	Antidepressant
M <> 87	Tab, Blue, Beveled Edge, Coated, 8 to Left, 7 to Right of Score	Maprotiline HCl 50 mg	by Mylan	00378-0087	Antidepressant
M <> 9	Tab, Yellow, Triangular, Film Coated	Fluphenazine HCl 2.5 mg	Prolixin by UDL	51079-0486	Antipsychotic
M <> 9	Tab, Yellow, Triangular	Fluphenazine HCl 2.5 mg	Prolixin by Mylan		Antipsychotic
M <> 9	Tab, Yellow	Fluphenazine HCl 2.5 mg	by Mylan	00378-6009	Antipsychotic
M <> 92	Tab, White, Beveled Edge, Coated, 9 to Left, 2 to Right of Score	Maprotiline HCl 75 mg	by Mylan	00378-0092	Antidepressant
M <> 93	Tab, Coated	Flurbiprofen 100 mg	by Quality Care	60346-0968	NSAID
M <> 97	Tab, Orange, Triangular, Film Coated	Fluphenazine HCl 10 mg	Prolixin by UDL	51079-0488	Antipsychotic
M <> 97	Tab, Orange, Coated	Fluphenazine HCl 10 mg	by Mylan	00378-6097	Antipsychotic
M <> 97	Tab, Orange, Triangular, Film Coated	Fluphenazine HCl 10 mg	by Invamed	52189-0312	Antipsychotic
M <> 970	Tab, White, Round	Acetaminophen 325 mg; Caffeine 40 mg; Butalbital 50 mg	by Mallinckrodt Hobart	00406-0970	Analgesic
M <> A2	Tab, White	Atenolol 25 mg	by Mylan		Antihypertensive
M <> A2	Tab, White, Round	Atenolol 25 mg	Tenormin by UDL	51079-0759	Antihypertensive
M <> C11	Tab, Green, Round, Scored	Clozapine 100 mg	by UDL	51079-0922	Antipsychotic
M <> C11	Tab, Green	Clozapine 100 mg	by Mylan		Antipsychotic
M <> C13	Tab, Yellow	Clonazepam 0.5 mg	by Mylan		Anticonvulsant; C IV
M <> C13	Tab, Yellow, Round, Scored, M <> C over 13	Clonazepam 0.5 mg	by UDL		Anticonvulsant; C IV
M <> C13	Tab, Yellow, Round, Scored	Clonazepam 0.5 mg	Clonazepam by D M Graham	00756-0266	Anticonvulsant; C IV

ID FRONT <> BACK	DESCRIPTION FRONT <> BACK	INGREDIENT & STRENGTH	BRAND (OR EQUIV.) & FIRM	NDC#	CLASS; SCH.
M <> C13	Tab, Yellow, Round, Scored, M <> C over 13	Clonazepam 0.5 mg	Klonopin by UDL	51079-0881	Anticonvulsant; C IV
M <> C14	Tab, Green, Round, Scored	Clonazepam 1 mg	Clonazepam by D M Graham	00756-0267	Anticonvulsant; C IV
M <> C14	Tab, Light Green	Clonazepam 1 mg	by Mylan		Anticonvulsant; C IV
M <> C14	Tab, Light Green, Round, Scored, M <> C over 14	Clonazepam 1 mg	Klonopin by UDL	51079-0882	Anticonvulsant; C IV
M <> C15	Tab, White	Clonazepam 2 mg	by Mylan		Anticonvulsant; C IV
M <> C15	Tab, White, Round, Scored	Clonazepam 2 mg	Clonazepam by D M Graham	00756-0268	Anticonvulsant; C IV
M <> C15	Tab, White, Round, Scored, M <> C over 15	Clonazepam 2 mg	Klonopin by UDL	51079-0883	Anticonvulsant; C IV
M <> C7	Tab, Peach, Round, Scored, M <> C/7	Clozapine 25 mg	by UDL	51079-0921	Antipsychotic
M <> C7	Tab, Peach	Clozapine 25 mg	by Mylan		Antipsychotic
M <> D5	Tab, White	Diclofenac Potassium 50 mg	by Mylan		NSAID
M <> DP	Tab, Mottled Pink, D-P	Aspirin 500 mg, Hydrocodone Bitartrate 5 mg	Damason P by Quality Care	60346-0748	Analgesic; C III
M <> DP	Tab	Aspirin 500 mg, Hydrocodone Bitartrate 5 mg	Damason P by Mason Pharmaceuticals	12758-0057	Analgesic; C III
M <> E3	Tab, Off-White	Estradiol 0.5 mg	by Mylan	00378-1452	Hormone
M <> E4	Tab, Pink	Estradiol 1 mg	by Mylan	00378-1454	Hormone
M <> E5	Tab, Pale Blue	Estradiol 2 mg	by Mylan		Hormone
M <> E5	Tab, Blue, Round	Estradiol 2 mg	by Mylan Pharms	00378-1458	Hormone
M <> G4	Tab, White	Guanfacine 1 mg	by Mylan		Antihypertensive
M <> G4	Tab	Guanfacine HCl	by Mylan	00378-1160	Antihypertensive
M <> G5	Tab	Guanfacine HCl	by Mylan	00378-1190	Antihypertensive
M <> G5	Tab, Blue	Guanfacine 2 mg	by Mylan		Antihypertensive
M <> MJ609	Tab, Coated	Fosinopril Sodium 20 mg	Monopril by Allscripts	54569-3809	Antihypertensive
M <> MSD917	Tab, Peach, Diamond Shaped	Amiloride HCl 5 mg, Hydrochlorothiazide 50 mg	Moduretic by Merck	00006-0917	Diuretic
M <> MYSOLINE250	Tab	Primidone 250 mg	Mysoline by Wal Mart	49035-0169	Anticonvulsant
M <> MYSOLINE250	Tab	Primidone 250 mg	Mysoline by Murfreesboro	51129-1168	Anticonvulsant
M <> MYSOLINE250	Tab	Primidone 250 mg	Mysoline by Thrift Drug	59198-0181	Anticonvulsant
M <> MYSOLINE50	Tab	Primidone 50 mg	Mysoline by Wal Mart	49035-0168	Anticonvulsant
M <> P1	Tab, Maroon, Round, Film Coated	Prochlorperazine Maleate 5 mg	Compazine by UDL	51079-0541	Antiemetic
M <> P2	Tab, Maroon, Round, Film Coated	Prochlorperazine Maleate 10 mg	Compazine by UDL	51079-0542	Antiemetic
M <> P2	Tab, Maroon, Film Coated	Prochlorperazine Maleate 10 mg	by Mylan	00378-5110	Antiemetic
M <> PI	Tab, Maroon, Film Coated	Prochlorperazine Maleate 5 mg	by Mylan	00378-5105	Antiemetic
M <> T3	Tab, White, Round, Film Coated	Trifluoperazine HCl 1 mg	Stelazine by UDL	51079-0572	Antipsychotic
M <> T3	Tab, White, Beveled Edge, Film Coated	Trifluoperazine HCl	by Mylan	00378-2401	Antipsychotic
M <> T4	Tab, White, Round, Film Coated	Trifluoperazine HCl 2 mg	Stelazine by UDL	51079-0573	Antipsychotic
M <> T4	Tab, White, Round, Film Coated	Trifluoperazine HCl 2 mg	by Dixon Shane	17236-0293	Antipsychotic
M <> T4	Tab, White, Beveled Edge, Film Coated	Trifluoperazine HCl	by Mylan	00378-2402	Antipsychotic
M <> T5	Tab, Lavender, Round, Film Coated	Trifluoperazine HCl 5 mg	Stelazine by UDL	51079-0574	Antipsychotic
M <> T5	Tab, Purple, Round, Film Coated	Trifluoperazine HCl 5 mg	by Dixon Shane	17236-0296	Antipsychotic
M <> T5	Tab, Lavender, Beveled Edge, Film Coated	Trifluoperazine HCl	by Mylan	00378-2405	Antipsychotic
M <> T6	Tab, Purple, Round, Film Coated	Trifluoperazine HCl 10 mg	by Dixon Shane	17236-0334	Antipsychotic
M <> T6	Tab, Lavender, Round, Film Coated	Trifluoperazine HCl 5 mg	Stelazine by UDL	51079-0575	Antipsychotic
M <> T6	Tab, Lavender, Film Coated	Trifluoperazine HCl	by Mylan	00378-2410	Antipsychotic
M 15	Tab	Atropine Sulfate 0.025 mg, Diphenoxylate HCl 2.5 mg	by Physicians Total Care	54868-0032	Antidiarrheal; C V
M 2	Tab, White, Round	Furosemide 20 mg	Lasix by Mylan	00378-0208	Diuretic
M006	Tab, White, Round	Atenolol 50 mg	Tenormin by Mylan		Antihypertensive
M007	Tab, White, Round	Atenolol 100 mg	Tenormin by Mylan		Antihypertensive
M01 <> MOVA	Tab, White, Oval, Scored	Captopril 12.5 mg	Capoten by Mova	55370-0164	Antihypertensive
M018	Cap, Clear & Green	Codeine Phosphate 20 mg, Pseudoephedrine HCl 60 mg	Nucofed by King	61570-0018	Cold Remedy; C III
M019	Tab, Ivory	Theophylline 300 mg	Quibron-T/SR by Monarch	54092-0070	Antiasthmatic
M020	Tab, Ivory	Theophylline 300 mg	Quibron-T by Monarch	54092-0069	Antiasthmatic
M022	Cap, Opaque & Yellow	Theophylline 150 mg, Guaifenesin 90 mg	Quibron by Monarch	54092-0067	Antiasthmatic
M022	Cap, Yellow	Theophylline 150 mg, Guaifenesin 90 mg	Quibron by Talbert Med	44514-0469	Antiasthmatic
M024	Tab, White, Oval, M over 024	Chlorthalidone 15 mg	Thalitone by Compumed	00403-0044	Diuretic

ID FRONT <> BACK	DESCRIPTION FRONT <> BACK	INGREDIENT & STRENGTH	BRAND (OR EQUIV.) & FIRM	NDC#	CLASS; SCH.
M0315 <> Z	Tab, White, Oval, Scored	Glyburide 1.5 mg	Glycron by Mova Pharms	55370-0592	Antidiabetic
M0361	Tab, M on One Side of the Score and 0361 on the Opposite Side	Acetaminophen 650 mg, Hydrocodone Bitartrate 10 mg	by King	60793-0849	Analgesic; C III
M0361	Tab, Blue, Cap Shaped, Scored	Acetaminophen 650 mg, Hydrocodone Bitartrate 10 mg	Lorcet by Geneva	00781-1524	Analgesic; C III
M0362	Tab, White, Oblong, M/0362	Hydrocodone Bitartrate 10 mg, Acetaminophen 660 mg	Vicodin HP by Mallinckrodt		Analgesic; C III
M0421	Tab, Blue & Clear, M/0421	Chlorpheniramine Maleate 12 mg, Phenylpropanolam Hydro. 75 mg	Ornade by Mallinckrodt		Cold Remedy
M0421	Cap, Blue & Clear	Chlorpheniramine Maleate 12 mg, Phenylpropanolamine HCl 75 mg	Ornade by Mallinckrodt Hobart	00406-0421	Cold Remedy
M0430 <> Z	Tab, Blue, Oval, Scored	Glyburide 3 mg	Glycron by Mova Pharms	55370-0594	Antidiabetic
M057	Tab, White, Oblong, Scored	Sucralfate 1 gm	Carafate by Merckle/Martec	52555-0057	Gastrointestinal
M0645 <> Z	Tab, Green, Oval, Scored	Glyburide 4.5 mg	Glycron by Mova Pharms	55370-0595	Antidiabetic
M0760 <> Z	Tab, Yellow, Oval, Scored	Glyburide 6 mg	Glycron by Mova Pharms	55370-0596	Antidiabetic
M1	Tab, Scored, M over 1	Chlorthalidone 15 mg, Clonidine HCl 0.1 mg	by Mylan	00378-0001	Diuretic; Antihypertensive
M1	Tab	Chlorthalidone 15 mg, Clonidine HCl 0.1 mg	by Med Pro	53978-0851	Diuretic; Antihypertensive
M1	Tab, Yellow, Round	Clonidine HCl 0.1 mg, Chlorthalidone 15 mg	Combipres by Mylan		Antihypertensive; Diuretic
M1	Tab, Yellow, Round, Scored	Clonidine HCl 0.1 mg, Chlorthalidone 15 mg	Clorpres by DHHS Prog	11819-0120	Antihypertensive; Diuretic
M1	Tab, Purple, Oval, Film Coated	Methenamine Mandelate 1 gm	Mandelamine by Able	53265-0160	Antibiotic; Urinary Tract
M1	Tab, Purple, Oval, Film Coated	Methenamine Mandelate 1 mg	by Nat Pharmpak Serv	55154-9002	Antibiotic; Urinary Tract
M10	Tab	Buspirone HCl 10 mg	Buspar by Med Pro	53978-2036	Antianxiety
M10	Tab, White, Round, Scored	Methimazole 10 mg	Methimazole by Jones Pharma	00689-1085	Antithyroid
M10	Tab, Orange, Round	Propranolol 10 mg	Inderal by Martec		Antihypertensive
M100	Cap, White, Film Coated, Scored	Ibuprofen 100 mg	Junior Strength Motrin by McNeil	Canadian DIN# 02240527	NSAID
M100	Tab, Film Coated	Ibuprofen 100 mg	Motrin by McNeil	50580-0445	NSAID
M100	Tab	Levothyroxine Sodium 100 mcg	Euthyrox by Em Pharma	63254-0439	Antithyroid
M100	Tab, Yellow, Scored	Levothyroxine Sodium 100 mcg	by Altimed	Canadian DIN# 02237216	Antithyroid
M10061	Tab, Film Coated, M 100 61	Thioridazine HCl 100 mg	by Med Pro	53978-2007	Antipsychotic
M100G	Cap, Orange, M 100/G	Minocycline HCl 100 mg	by Genpharm	Canadian	Antibiotic
M100LEVOT	Tab, Yellow, Round	Levothyroxine Sodium 0.1 mg	Synthroid by Mova		Antithyroid
M11	Tab	Penicillin V Potassium 250 mg	by Mylan	00378-0111	Antibiotic
M11	Tab	Penicillin V Potassium 250 mg	by Prescription Dispensing	61807-0003	Antibiotic
M112	Tab, Rose, Scored	Levothyroxine Sodium 112 mcg	by Altimed	Canadian DIN# 02237217	Antithyroid
M113	Tab, White	Glyburide 1.5 mg	by Mylan	00378-1113	Antidiabetic
M118	Tab, Light Yellow, Cap Shaped, Scored	Pentazocine HCl 50 mg, Naloxone 0.5 mg	by Mallinckrodt Hobart	00406-3118	Analgesic; C IV
M118	Tab, Yellow, Oblong	Pentazocine HCl 50 mg, Naloxone HCl 0.5 mg	by Ohm	51660-0506	Analgesic; C IV
M12	Tab, Film Coated	Penicillin V Potassium	by Med Pro	53978-5055	Antibiotic
M12	Tab, M to Left, 12 to Right of Score	Penicillin V Potassium 500 mg	by Mylan	00378-0112	Antibiotic
M12	Tab, Film Coated, M 12	Verapamil HCl 80 mg	by Med Pro	53978-7001	Antihypertensive
M125	Tab, Light Yellow	Glyburide 3 mg	by Mylan	00378-1125	Antidiabetic
M125	Tab, Tan, Round	Levothyroxine Sodium 0.125 mg	Synthroid by Duramed		Antithyroid
M125	Tab, Brown, Scored	Levothyroxine Sodium 125 mcg	by Altimed	Canadian DIN# 02237218	Antithyroid
M125LEVOT	Tab, Brown, Round	Levothyroxine Sodium 0.125 mg	Synthroid by Mova		Antithyroid
M127	Tab, White, Round, Scored	Pindolol 10 mg	by Mylan	55160-0133	Antihypertensive

ID FRONT <> BACK	DESCRIPTION FRONT <> BACK	INGREDIENT & STRENGTH	BRAND (OR EQUIV.) & FIRM	NDC#	CLASS; SCH.
M127	Tab, White, M Above Score, 127 Below	Pindolol 10 mg	by Mylan	00378-0127	Antihypertensive
M13	Tab, White to Off White, Round, Scored, M/13	Tolbutamide 500 mg	Orinase	51079-0560	Antidiabetic
M13	Tab, Compressed, M-13	Tolbutamide 500 mg	by Kaiser	00179-0198	Antidiabetic
M13	Tab, Off-White to White, M to Left, 13 to Right of Score	Tolbutamide 500 mg	by Mylan	00378-0215	Antidiabetic
M13	Tab	Tolbutamide 500 mg	by Pharmedix	53002-0519	Antidiabetic
M132	Tab, Yellow, Beveled Edge, M Over 132	Nadolol 80 mg	Nadolol by Mylan	00378-1132	Antihypertensive
M132	Tab	Nadolol 80 mg	Nadolol by Physicians Total Care	54868-3721	Antihypertensive
M132	Tab, Yellow, Round, Scored, M Over 132	Nadolol 80 mg	Corgard by UDL	51079-0814	Antihypertensive
M132	Tab	Nadolol 80 mg	Nadolol by Med Pro	53978-2019	Antihypertensive
M134	Tab, White, Beveled Edge, Film Coated, M Over 134	Ketorolac Tromethamine 10 mg	by Mylan	00378-1134	NSAID
M135	Tab, Film Coated	Diltiazem HCl 90 mg	by Heartland	61392-0146	Antihypertensive
M135	Tab, Film Coated	Diltiazem HCl 90 mg	by Heartland	61392-0055	Antihypertensive
M135	Tab, White, Film Coated	Diltiazem HCl 90 mg	by Mylan	00378-0135	Antihypertensive
M135	Tab, White, Cap Shaped, Scored, Film Coated	Diltiazem HCl 90 mg	Cardizem by UDL	51079-0747	Antihypertensive
M135	Tab, White, Oblong, Scored, Film Coated	Diltiazem HCl 90 mg	by Egis	48581-6123	Antihypertensive
M139	Tab, White, Round, M-139	Sulfamethoxazole 400 mg, Trimethoprim 80 mg	Bactrim by Mylan		Antibiotic
M14	Tab, M Over 14	Methotrexate Sodium	by Allscripts	54569-1818	Antineoplastic
M14	Tab, Orange, M Over 14	Methotrexate Sodium 2.5 mg	by Mylan	00378-0014	Antineoplastic
M14	Tab, Orange, Round, Scored, M Over 14	Methotrexate Sodium 2.5 mg	Methotrexate by UDL	51079-0670	Antineoplastic
M140	Tab, White, Round, M-140	Sulfamethoxazole 800 mg, Trimethoprim 160 mg	Bactrim DS by Mylan		Antibiotic
M15	Tab	Atropine Sulfate 0.025 mg, Diphenoxylate HCl 2.5 mg	by Nat Pharmpak Serv	55154-5563	Antidiarrheal; C V
M15	Tab	Atropine Sulfate 0.025 mg, Diphenoxylate HCl 2.5 mg	Lonox by Quality Care	60346-0437	Antidiarrheal; C V
M15	Tab, M/15	Atropine Sulfate 0.025 mg, Diphenoxylate HCl 2.5 mg	by Kaiser	00179-0276	Antidiarrheal; C V
M15	Tab, White, M over 15	Atropine Sulfate 0.025 mg, Diphenoxylate HCl 2.5 mg	by Mylan	00378-0415	Antidiarrheal; C V
M15	Tab	Atropine Sulfate 0.025 mg, Diphenoxylate HCl 2.5 mg	by Vangard	00615-0429	Antidiarrheal; C V
M15	Tab	Atropine Sulfate 0.025 mg, Diphenoxylate HCl 2.5 mg	by Allscripts	54569-0222	Antidiarrheal; C V
M15	Tab	Atropine Sulfate 0.025 mg, Diphenoxylate HCl 2.5 mg	by Murfreesboro	51129-1343	Antidiarrheal; C V
M15	Tab	Atropine Sulfate 0.025 mg, Diphenoxylate HCl 2.5 mg	by Urgent Care Ctr	50716-0477	Antidiarrheal; C V
M15	Tab, White, Round, M over 15	Atropine Sulfate 0.025 mg, Diphenoxylate HCl 2.5 mg	by Patient	57575-0074	Antidiarrheal; C V
M15	Tab, White, Round	Diphenoxylate 2.5 mg, Atropine 0.025 mg	Benadryl by UDL	51079-0067	Antidiarrheal; C V
M150	Tab, Blue, Round	Levothyroxine Sodium 0.15 mg	by Geneva	00781-2054	Antidiarrheal; C V
M150	Tab, Blue, Scored	Levothyroxine Sodium 150 mcg	Synthroid by Duramed		Antithyroid
M150LEVOT	Tab, Blue, Round	Levothyroxine Sodium 0.15 mg	by Altimed	Canadian DIN# 02237219	Antithyroid
M158	Tab, White, Diamond	Fosinopril Sodium 10 mg	Synthroid by Mova		Antithyroid
M171	Tab, Yellow, Beveled Edge, M Over 171	Nadolol 40 mg	Monopril by MJ		Antihypertensive
M171	Tab	Nadolol 40 mg	Nadolol by Mylan	00378-1171	Antihypertensive
M171	Tab	Nadolol 40 mg	Nadolol by Allscripts	54569-3790	Antihypertensive
M171	Tab, Yellow, Round, Scored, M Over 171	Nadolol 40 mg	Nadolol by Med Pro	53978-2018	Antihypertensive
M175	Tab, Lilac, Scored	Levothyroxine Sodium 175 mcg	Corgard by UDL	51079-0813	Antihypertensive
M18	Tab, White, Round, M18/+	Guaifenesin 200 mg, Ephedrine 25 mg	by Altimed	Canadian DIN# 02237220	Antithyroid
M187 <> TIGAN	Cap, Blue, Opaque	Trimethobbenzamide HCl 250 mg	by PDK Labs		Cold Remedy
M187 <> TIGAN	Cap, Blue, Opaque	Trimethobbenzamide HCl 250 mg	Tigan by King	54092-0186	Antiemetic
M19 <> LL	Tab	Methocarbamol 500 mg	Tigan by King	61570-0187	Antiemetic
M19 <> LL	Tab, Lederle Logo	Methocarbamol 500 mg	by Lederle	00005-3562	Muscle Relaxant
M19 <> LL	Tab	Methocarbamol 500 mg	by Quality Care	60346-0080	Muscle Relaxant
M19 <> LL	Tab, White, Round, Scored	Methocarbamol 500 mg	by Nat Pharmpak Serv	55154-5541	Muscle Relaxant
M19 <> LL	Tab, M Over 19	Methocarbamol 500 mg	by Neuman Distr	64579-0010	Muscle Relaxant
		Methocarbamol 500 mg	by UDL	51079-0091	Muscle Relaxant

ID FRONT <> BACK	DESCRIPTION FRONT <> BACK	INGREDIENT & STRENGTH	BRAND (OR EQUIV.) & FIRM	NDC#	CLASS; SCH.
M1LL	Tab, Yellow, Round, M1/LL	Methotrexate Sodium 2.5 mg	Rheumatrex by Wyeth-Ayerst	Canadian	Antineoplastic
M2	Tab	Furosemide 20 mg	by Heartland	61392-0256	Diuretic
M2	Tab	Furosemide 20 mg	by Quality Care	60346-0761	Diuretic
M2	Tab	Furosemide 20 mg	by Kaiser	62224-1220	Diuretic
M2	Tab	Furosemide 20 mg	by PDRX	55289-0593	Diuretic
M2	Tab, White, Round, M-2	Furosemide 20 mg	Lasix by Martec		Diuretic
M2	Tab, M-2	Furosemide 20 mg	by Allscripts	54569-0572	Diuretic
M2	Tab, White, Round	Furosemide 20 mg	Lasix by UDL	51079-0072	Diuretic
M2	Tab, White, Round	Furosemide 20 mg	by JB	51111-0480	Diuretic
M2	Tab	Furosemide 40 mg	by PDRX	55289-0118	Diuretic
M2	Tab, White, Round, M/2	Hydromorphone HCl 2 mg	Dilaudid by Mallinckrodt		Analgesic; C II
M2 <> M2	Tab	Furosemide 20 mg	by Diversified Hlthcare Serv	55887-0997	Diuretic
M20	Tab	Methocarbamol 750 mg	by Lederle	00005-3563	Muscle Relaxant
M20	Tab	Methocarbamol 750 mg	by Physicians Total Care	54868-1103	Muscle Relaxant
M20	Tab, Blue, Round	Propranolol 20 mg	Inderal by Martec		Antihypertensive
M20 <> LL	Tab, White, Oblong, Scored	Methocarbamol 750 mg	by Neuman Distr	64579-0008	Muscle Relaxant
M20 <> LL	Tab, M/20	Methocarbamol 750 mg	by UDL	51079-0092	Muscle Relaxant
M200	Tab	Levothyroxine Sodium 200 mcg	Euthyrox by Em Pharma	63254-0444	Antithyroid
M200	Tab, Pink, Scored	Levothyroxine Sodium 200 mcg	by Altimed	Canadian DIN# 02237221	Antithyroid
M200LEVOT	Tab, Pink, Round	Levothyroxine Sodium 0.2 mg	Synthroid by Mova		Antithyroid
M204	Tab, White, Round, M/204	Diclofenac Sodium 50 mg	Voltaren by Martec	52555-0204	NSAID
M205	Tab, White, Round, M/205	Diclofenac Sodium 75 mg	Voltaren by Martec	52555-0205	NSAID
M21	Tab, White, Round	Penicillin G Potassium 250,000 Units	Pentids by Mylan		Antibiotic
M21ICN	Tab, White, Round, M21/ICN	Metformin HCl 500 mg	by ICN	Canadian	Antidiabetic
M22 <> LL	Tab, Coated	Methyldopa 250 mg	by UDL	51079-0200	Antihypertensive
M22 <> LL	Tab, Coated	Methyldopa 250 mg	by Lederle	00005-3850	Antihypertensive
M221	Tab, Green, Round, Scored, M 221	Timolol Maleate 10 mg	by Teva	00480-0088	Antihypertensive
M221	Tab, Green, Beveled Edge, M Above Score, 221 Below	Timolol Maleate 10 mg	by Mylan	00378-0221	Antihypertensive
M221	Tab, M 221	Timolol Maleate 10 mg	by Med Pro	53978-2021	Antihypertensive
M23	Tab, Film Coated	Diltiazem HCl 30 mg	by Heartland	61392-0053	Antihypertensive
M23	Tab, White, Round, Film	Diltiazem HCl 30 mg	by Elan Hold	60274-0880	Antihypertensive
M23	Tab, Coated, M Over 23	Diltiazem HCl 30 mg	by Quality Care	60346-0960	Antihypertensive
M23	Tab, White, Film Coated, M over 23	Diltiazem HCl 30 mg	by Mylan	00378-0023	Antihypertensive
M23	Tab, White, Round, Film Coated, M over 23	Diltiazem HCl 30 mg	Cardizem by UDL	51079-0745	Antihypertensive
M23	Tab, Film Coated, M over 23	Diltiazem HCl 30 mg	by Allscripts	54569-3665	Antihypertensive
M23	Tab, Film Coated	Diltiazem HCl 30 mg	by PDRX	55289-0335	Antihypertensive
M23	Tab, White, Round, Film Coated	Diltiazem HCl 30 mg	by Vangard Labs	00615-3548	Antihypertensive
M23	Tab, White, Round	Ephedrine 25 mg, Guiafenisin 100 mg	Two Way Tab by PDK		Cold Remedy
M23 <> LL	Tab, Coated	Methyldopa 500 mg	by UDL	51079-0201	Antihypertensive
M23 <> LL	Tab, Coated	Methyldopa 500 mg	by Lederle	00005-3851	Antihypertensive
M23 <> LL	Tab, Coated	Methyldopa 500 mg	by Caremark	00339-5231	Antihypertensive
M25	Tab, Peach, Round	Levothyroxine Sodium 0.025 mg	Synthroid by Duramed		Antithyroid
M25	Tab, Orange, Scored	Levothyroxine Sodium 25 mcg	by Altimed	Canadian DIN# 02237213	Antithyroid
M25	Tab, Yellow, Round, M 2.5	Methotrexate 2.5 mg	Methotrexate Tab by Faulding	Canadian	Antineoplastic
M25	Tab	Methyclothiazide 5 mg	by Med Pro	53978-2016	Diuretic
M253	Tab, White	Acyclovir 400 mg	by Mylan	00378-0253	Antiviral
M255	Tab, White, M/255	Albuterol Sulfate 2 mg	by Mylan	00378-0255	Antiasthmatic
M255	Tab, White, Round, Scored, M over 255	Albuterol Sulfate 2 mg	by UDL	51079-0657	Antiasthmatic

ID FRONT <> BACK	DESCRIPTION FRONT <> BACK	INGREDIENT & STRENGTH	BRAND (OR EQUIV.) & FIRM	NDC#	CLASS; SCH.
M255	Tab	Albuterol Sulfate 2 mg	by Allscripts	54569-3409	Antiasthmatic
M2558	Tab, Film Coated	Thioridazine HCl 25 mg	by Med Pro	53978-2005	Antipsychotic
M259 <> MONODOX100	Cap, Brown & White Print	Doxycycline Monohydrate	Monodox by Oclassen	55515-0259	Antibiotic
M259 <> MONODOX100	Cap, Brown & White	Doxycycline Monohydrate	Monodox by Eckerd Drug	19458-0838	Antibiotic
M259 <> MONODOX100	Cap, Brown & Yellow	Doxycycline Monohydrate 100 mg	Monodox by Thrift Services	59198-0363	Antibiotic
M259 <> MONODOX100	Cap, Brown & Yellow	Doxycycline Monohydrate 100 mg	by West Pharm	52967-0302	Antibiotic
M259 <> MONODOX100	Cap	Doxycycline Monohydrate	by Vintage	00254-4316	Antibiotic
M260 <> MONODOX50	Cap, Brown Print	Doxycycline Monohydrate	Monodox by Oclassen	55515-0260	Antibiotic
M260 <> MONODOX50	Cap	Doxycycline Monohydrate	Monodox by Vintage	00254-4315	Antibiotic
M260 <> MONODOX50	Cap, White & Yellow	Doxycycline Monohydrate 50 mg	by West Pharm	52967-0301	Antibiotic
M27	Tab, Scored, M over 27	Chlorthalidone 15 mg, Clonidine HCl 0.2 mg	by Mylan	00378-0027	Diuretic; Antihypertensive
M27	Tab, M 27	Chlorthalidone 15 mg, Clonidine HCl 0.2 mg	by Med Pro	53978-2030	Diuretic; Antihypertensive
M27	Tab, Yellow, Round, Scored	Clonidine HCl 0.2 mg, Chlorthalidone 15 mg	Clorpres by DHHS Prog	11819-0121	Antihypertensive; Diuretic
M28	Tab, Yellow, Beveled Edge, M Over 28	Nadolol 20 mg	Nadolol by Mylan	00378-0028	Antihypertensive
M28	Tab	Nadolol 20 mg	Nadolol by Med Pro	53978-2017	Antihypertensive
M28	Tab, Yellow, Round, Scored, M Over 28	Nadolol 20 mg	Corgard by UDL	51079-0812	Antihypertensive
M29	Tab, Blue, Beveled Edge, M Above Score, 29 Below	Methyclothiazide 5 mg	by Mylan	00378-0160	Diuretic
M29	Tab	Methyclothiazide 5 mg	by Pharmedix	53002-1044	Diuretic
M2A357344	Tab, White, Round, M2A3 over 57344	Acetaminophen 325 mg	by Marlex Co	10135-0123	Antipyretic
M2MIN50MG	Cap, Orange, M2/MIN 50 mg	Minocycline 50 mg	by Altimed	Canadian	Antibiotic
M30	Tab, Blue, Round, Scored, M over 30	Clorazepam Dipotassium 3.75 mg	Tranxene by UDL	51079-0633	Sedative
M30	Tab, Blue, Scored, M over 30	Clorazepate Dipotassium 3.75 mg	by Mylan	00378-0030	Antianxiety; C IV
M30	Tab	Clorazepate Dipotassium 3.75 mg	by Allscripts	54569-0952	Antianxiety; C IV
M300	Tab, Green, Round	Levothyroxine Sodium 0.3 mg	Synthroid by Duramed		Antithyroid
M300	Tab, Green, Scored	Levothyroxine Sodium 300 mcg	by Altimed	Canadian DIN# 02237222	Antithyroid
M300LEVOT	Tab, Green, Round	Levothyroxine Sodium 0.3 mg	Synthroid by Mova		Antithyroid
M31	Tab	Allopurinol 100 mg	by Kaiser	62224-7111	Antigout
M31	Tab	Allopurinol 100 mg	by Heartland	61392-0103	Antigout
M31	Tab	Allopurinol 100 mg	by Nat Pharmpak Serv	55154-5534	Antigout
M31	Tab, White, Round, Scored, M/31	Allopurinol 100 mg	by UDL	51079-0205	Antigout
M31	Tab, White	Allopurinol 100 mg	by Mylan	00378-0137	Antigout
M31	Tab, Coated, M 31 on One Side Only	Mephobarbital 32 mg	Mebaral by Bayer	00280-1231	Sedative/Hypnotic; C IV
M312	Tab, Blue, Oval, Scored, Film-Coated, M/312	Verapamil HCl 180 mg	Isoptin SR by UDL	51079-0899	Antihypertensive
M312	Tab, Blue, Round	Verapamil HCl 180 mg	by Mylan	00378-1180	Antihypertensive
M312	Tab, Blue, Oblong, Film	Verapamil HCl 180 mg	by Thrift Drug	59198-0319	Antihypertensive
M313	Tab, Beige, Oval, Film	Tolmetin 600 mg	by Teva	00480-0102	NSAID
M313	Tab, Beige, Oval, Film, M 313	Tolmetin Sodium 600 mg	by Teva	00480-0106	NSAID
M313	Tab, Blue, Film Coated	Tolmetin Sodium 735 mg	by Mylan	00378-0313	NSAID
M317	Tab, House Shaped, Film Coated, M/317	Cimetidine 300 mg	by Heartland	61392-0197	Gastrointestinal
M317	Tab, Coated, M/317	Cimetidine 300 mg	by Qualitest	00603-2891	Gastrointestinal
M317	Tab, Film Coated	Cimetidine 300 mg	by Allscripts	54569-3837	Gastrointestinal
M32	Tab, Coated, M 32	Mephobarbital 50 mg	Mebaral by Bayer	00280-1232	Sedative/Hypnotic; C IV
M32	Tab, Pink, Beveled Edge, Film Coated, M Over 32	Metoprolol Tartrate 50 mg	by Mylan	00378-0032	Antihypertensive
M32	Tab, Film Coated, M Over 32	Metoprolol Tartrate 50 mg	by Caremark	00339-5861	Antihypertensive
M32	Tab, Film Coated, M Over 32	Metoprolol Tartrate 50 mg	by Allscripts	54569-3787	Antihypertensive
M32	Tab, Film Coated	Metoprolol Tartrate 50 mg	by Med Pro	53978-2058	Antihypertensive
M32	Tab, Pink, Round, Scored, Film Coated, M Over 32	Metoprolol Tartrate 50 mg	Lopressor by UDL	51079-0801	Antihypertensive

ID FRONT <> BACK	DESCRIPTION FRONT <> BACK	INGREDIENT & STRENGTH	BRAND (OR EQUIV.) & FIRM	NDC#	CLASS; SCH.
M32	Tab, Film Coated	Metoprolol Tartrate 50 mg	by Heartland	61392-0286	Antihypertensive
M32	Tab, Film Coated, M Over 32	Metoprolol Tartrate 50 mg	by Nat Pharmpak Serv	55154-5512	Antihypertensive
M32	Tab, Film Coated, M over 32	Metoprolol Tartrate 50 mg	by Kaiser	62224-4446	Antihypertensive
M321	Tab, M 321	Lorazepam 0.5 mg	by Caremark	00339-4018	Sedative/Hypnotic; C IV
M321	Tab	Lorazepam 0.5 mg	by Nat Pharmpak Serv	55154-5550	Sedative/Hypnotic; C IV
M321	Tab, Coated	Lorazepam 0.5 mg	by Quality Care	60346-0363	Sedative/Hypnotic; C IV
M33	Tab, Scored	Chlorothiazide 250 mg, Reserpine 0.125 mg	by Mylan	00378-0175	Diuretic; Antihypertensive
M33	Tab, Coated, M 33	Mephobarbital 100 mg	Mebaral by Bayer	00280-1233	Sedative/Hypnotic; C IV
M35	Tab, Light Yellow	Chlorthalidone 25 mg	by Mylan	00378-0222	Diuretic
M35	Tab	Chlorthalidone 25 mg	by Allscripts	54569-0552	Diuretic
M35	Tab, Yellow, Round	Chlorthalidone 25 mg	Hygroton by UDL	51079-0058	Diuretic
M35	Tab	Chlorthalidone 25 mg	by Med Pro	53978-0032	Diuretic
M357	Tab, White, Cap Shaped, Scored	Acetaminophen 500 mg, Hydrocodone Bitartrate 5 mg	by Allscripts	54569-0303	Analgesic; C III
M357	Tab, White, Cap Shaped, Scored	Acetaminophen 500 mg, Hydrocodone Bitartrate 5 mg	Vicodin by Geneva	00781-1606	Analgesic; C III
M357	Tab, White, Cap Shaped, Scored	Acetaminophen 500 mg; Hydrocodone Bitartrate 5 mg	Lortab, Vicodin by Mallinckrodt Hobart	00406-0357	Analgesic; C III
M357	Tab, Beige, Beveled Edge, Film Coated	Hydrocodone 5 mg, Acetaminophen 500 mg	by Mallinckrodt		Analgesic; C III
M357	Tab, White, Oblong, Scored, M 357	Hydrocodone Bitartrate 5 mg, Acetaminophen 500 mg	by Murfreesboro	51129-1445	Analgesic; C III
M357	Tab, White, Oblong, Scored, M 357	Hydrocodone Bitartrate 5 mg, Acetaminophen 500 mg	by Murfreesboro	51129-1453	Analgesic; C III
M357	White, Oblong, Scored	Hydrocodone Bitartrate 5 mg, Acetaminophen 500 mg	by D M Graham	00756-0276	Analgesic; C III
M358	Tab, Coated, M 358	Acetaminophen 500 mg, Hydrocodone Bitartrate 7.5 mg	by King	60793-0889	Analgesic; C III
M358	Tab, White, Cap Shaped, Scored	Acetaminophen 500 mg, Hydrocodone Bitartrate 7.5 mg	by Allscripts	54569-3911	Analgesic; C III
M358	Tab, White, Cap Shaped, Scored	Acetaminophen 500 mg, Hydrocodone Bitartrate 7.5 mg	by Mallinckrodt Hobart	00406-0358	Analgesic; C III
M358	Tab, White, Oblong, Scored	Hydrocodone Bitartrate 7.5 mg, Acetaminophen 500 mg	by Murfreesboro	51129-1455	Analgesic; C III
M358	Tab, White, Oblong, Scored	Hydrocodone Bitartrate 7.5 mg, Acetaminophen 500 mg	by D M Graham	00756-0282	Analgesic; C III
M358	Tab, White, Oblong, Bisected	Hydrocodone Bitartrate 7.5 mg, Acetaminophen 500 mg	by Geneva Pharms	00781-1513	Analgesic; C III
M359	Tab, White, Cap Shaped, Scored	Acetaminophen 650 mg, Hydrocodone Bitartrate 7.5 mg	Lorcet Plus by Mallinckrodt Hobart	00406-0359	Analgesic; C III
M359	Tab, White, Oblong, Scored	Hydrocodone Bitartrate 7.5 mg, Acetaminophen 650 mg	by D M Graham	00756-0281	Analgesic; C III
M36	Tab, Film Coated, M Over 36	Amitriptyline HCl 50 mg	by Quality Care	60346-0673	Antidepressant
M36	Tab, Brown, Round, Film Coated, M over 36	Amitriptyline HCl 50 mg	Elavil by UDL	51079-0133	Antidepressant
M36	Tab, Brown, Coated, M over 36	Amitriptyline HCl 50 mg	by Mylan	00378-2650	Antidepressant
M360	Tab, White, Cap Shaped, Scored	Acetaminophen 750 mg, Hydrocodone Bitartrate 7.5 mg; Acetaminophen 750 mg, Hydrocodone Bitartrate 7.5 mg	Vicodin ES by Mallinckrodt Hobart	00406-0360	Analgesic; C III
M360	Tab, White, Oblong, Scored	Hydrocodone Bitartrate 7.5 mg, Acetaminophen 750 mg	by D M Graham	00756-0280	Analgesic; C III
M361	Tab, Blue, Cap Shaped, Scored	Acetaminophen 650 mg, Hydrocodone Bitartrate 10 mg	by Mallinckrodt Hobart	00406-0361	Analgesic; C III
M361	Tab, Blue, Oblong, Scored	Hydrocodone Bitartrate 10 mg, Acetaminophen 650 mg	by D M Graham	00756-0279	Analgesic; C III
M362	Tab, White, Cap Shaped, Scored	Acetaminophen 660 mg, Hydrocodone Bitartrate 10 mg	Vicodin HP by Mallinckrodt Hobart	00406-0362	Analgesic; C III
M362	White, Oblong, Scored	Hydrocodone Bitartrate 10 mg, Acetaminophen 660 mg	by D M Graham	00756-0278	Analgesic; C III
M363	Tab, White, Cap Shaped, Scored	Acetaminophen 500 mg, Hydrocodone Bitartrate 10 mg	by Mallinckrodt Hobart	00406-0363	Analgesic; C III
M363	Tab, White, Oblong, M/363	Hydrocodone Bitartrate 10 mg, Acetaminophen 500 mg	Lortab by Mallinckrodt		Analgesic; C III
M363	Tab, White, Oblong, Scored	Hydrocodone Bitartrate 10 mg, Acetaminophen 500 mg	by King Pharms	60793-0890	Analgesic; C III
M363	White, Oblong, Scored	Hydrocodone Bitartrate 10 mg, Acetaminophen 500 mg	by D M Graham	00756-0277	Analgesic; C III
M367	Tab, White, Cap Shaped, Scored	Acetaminophen 325 mg, Hydrocodone Bitartrate 10 mg	Lortab by Mallinckrodt Hobart	00406-0367	Analgesic; C III
M37	Tab, Blue, Round, Film Coated, M over 37	Amitriptyline 75 mg	Elavil by UDL	51079-0147	Antidepressant
M37	Tab, Coated	Amitriptyline 75 mg	by Caremark	00339-5016	Antidepressant
M37	Tab, Blue, Coated, M over 37	Amitriptyline HCl 75 mg	by Mylan	00378-2675	Antidepressant
M372	Tab, Film Coated, M/372	Cimetidine 400 mg	by Heartland	61392-0200	Gastrointestinal
M372	Tab, Coated, M/372	Cimetidine 400 mg	by Qualitest	00603-2892	Gastrointestinal
M38	Tab, Orange, Round, Film Coated, M over 38	Amitriptyline HCl 100 mg	Elavil by UDL	51079-0563	Antidepressant
M38	Tab, Orange, Coated, M over 38	Amitriptyline HCl 100 mg	by Mylan	00378-2685	Antidepressant
M38	Tab, Coated	Amitriptyline HCl 100 mg	by Caremark	00339-5018	Antidepressant
M39	Tab, Flesh, Cap Shaped, Film Coated	Amitriptyline HCl 150 mg	Elavil by UDL	51079-0564	Antidepressant

ID FRONT <> BACK	DESCRIPTION FRONT <> BACK	INGREDIENT & STRENGTH	BRAND (OR EQUIV.) & FIRM	NDC#	CLASS; SCH.
M39	Tab, Flesh, Coated	Amitriptyline HCl 150 mg	by Mylan	00378-2695	Antidepressant
M4	Tab, Coated	Fluphenazine HCl 1 mg	by Heartland	61392-0057	Antipsychotic
M4	Tab, White, Round, M/4	Hydromorphone HCl 4 mg	Dilaudid by Mallinckrodt		Analgesic; C II
M40	Tab, Peach, Round, Scored, M over 40	Clorazepam Dipotassium 7.5 mg	Tranxene by UDL	51079-0634	Sedative
M40	Tab, Peach, Round, Scored	Clorazepate Dipotassium 7.5 mg	by Murfreesboro Ph	51129-1355	Antianxiety; C IV
M40	Tab, White, Oblong	Clorazepate Dipotassium 7.5 mg	by Mylan	00378-0040	Antianxiety; C IV
M40	Tab	Clorazepate Dipotassium 7.5 mg	by Allscripts	54569-0951	Antianxiety; C IV
M400	Tab, Film Coated	Erythromycin 500 mg	by Quality Care	60346-0646	Antibiotic
M400	Tab, Film Coated	Erythromycin Ethylsuccinate	by Allscripts	54569-3531	Antibiotic
M400	Tab, Film Coated	Erythromycin Ethylsuccinate	by Med Pro	53978-0022	Antibiotic
M400	Tab, Film Coated	Erythromycin Ethylsuccinate	by Physicians Total Care	54868-0018	Antibiotic
M400	Tab, Film Coated	Erythromycin Ethylsuccinate	by Allscripts	54569-2507	Antibiotic
M400	Tab, Beige, Oblong, Film Coated	Erythromycin Ethylsuccinate 400 mg	by Direct Dispensing	57866-0351	Antibiotic
M400	Tab, Peach, Film Coated	Erythromycin Ethylsuccinate 400 mg	by Mylan	00378-6400	Antibiotic
M400 <> BAYER	Tab, Red, Oblong, Film Coated	Moxifloxacin HCl 400 mg	by Bayer (GM)	12527-8581	Antibiotic
M400 <> BAYER	Tab, Red, Oblong, Film Coated	Moxifloxacin HCl 400 mg	Avelox by Bayer	00026-8581	Antibiotic
M41	Tab, Ivory, Round, M Over 41	Hydrochlorothiazide 25 mg, Spironolactone 25 mg	Aldactazide by UDL	51079-0104	Diuretic; Antihypertensive
M41	Tab	Hydrochlorothiazide 25 mg, Spironolactone 25 mg	by Allscripts	54569-0502	Diuretic; Antihypertensive
M411	Tab, Blue, Oblong, Scored, Film Coated	Verapamil HCl 240 mg	by Teva	00480-1005	Antihypertensive
M411	Tab, Blue, Oblong, Film Coated	Verapamil HCl 240 mg	by Ther Rx	64011-0019	Antihypertensive
M411	Tab, Blue, Film Coated, M 411	Verapamil HCl 240 mg	by Mylan	00378-0411	Antihypertensive
M411	Tab, Blue, Modified Cap Shaped, Film Coated, M/411	Verapamil HCl 240 mg	Isoptin SR by UDL	51079-0869	Antihypertensive
M411	Tab, Film Coated	Verapamil HCl 240 mg	by Direct Dispensing	57866-6914	Antihypertensive
M411	Tab, Blue, Oblong, Film Coated, Scored	Verapamil HCl 240 mg	by Compumed	00403-5198	Antihypertensive
M43	Tab, Scored	Chlorothiazide 500 mg, Reserpine 0.125 mg	by Mylan	00378-0176	Diuretic; Antihypertensive
M4357	Cap, White Print	Acetaminophen 500 mg, Hydrocodone Bitartrate 5 mg	by D M Graham	00756-0253	Analgesic; C III
M4357	Cap, Maroon, Gelatin	Acetaminophen 500 mg, Hydrocodone Bitartrate 5 mg	by Mallinckrodt Hobart	00406-4357	Analgesic; C III
M4358	Cap, White, Hard Gel, M Inside a Square and 4358 Imprinted in Red	Hydrocodone Bitartrate 5 mg, Acetaminophen 500 mg	by Murfreesboro	51129-1444	Analgesic; C III
M44	Tab, White, Round	Cyproheptadine HCl 4 mg	Periactin by Mylan		Antihistamine
M45	Tab, White, Film Coated, M over 45	Diltiazem HCl 60 mg	by Mylan	00378-0045	Antihypertensive
M45	Tab, Film Coated	Diltiazem HCl 60 mg	by Nat Pharmpak Serv	55154-5523	Antihypertensive
M45	Tab, Film Coated	Diltiazem HCl 60 mg	by Kaiser	62224-9337	Antihypertensive
M45	Tab, Beveled Edge, Film Coated, M Over 45	Diltiazem HCl 60 mg	by Amerisource	62584-0367	Antihypertensive
M45	Tab, White, Round, Scored, Film	Diltiazem HCl 60 mg	by Elan Hold	60274-0882	Antihypertensive
M45	Tab, Film Coated	Diltiazem HCl 60 mg	by Heartland	61392-0054	Antihypertensive
M45	Tab, Film Coated	Diltiazem HCl 60 mg	by Allscripts	54569-3667	Antihypertensive
M45	Tab, White, Round, Scored, Film Coated, M over 45	Diltiazem HCl 60 mg	Cardizem by UDL	51079-0746	Antihypertensive
M45	Tab, Film Coated	Diltiazem HCl 60 mg	by Med Pro	53978-1235	Antihypertensive
M45	Tab, White, Round, Film Coated, Scored	Diltiazem HCl 60 mg	by Vangard Labs	00615-3549	Antihypertensive
M450	Tab, White, Round, Scored	Atenolol 50 mg, Chlorthalidone 25 mg	Tenoretic by Merckle/Martec	52555-0450	Antihypertensive; Diuretic
M450	Tab, White, Round, Film Coated	Atenolol 50 mg; Chlorthalidone 25 mg	by Merckle	58107-0002	Antihypertensive; Diuretic
M451	Tab, White, Round	Atenolol 100 mg, Chlorthalidone 25 mg	Tenoretic by Merckle/Martec	52555-0451	Antihypertensive; Diuretic
M451	Tab, White, Round, Film Coated	Atenolol 100 mg; Chlorthalidone 25 mg	by Merckle	58107-0003	Antihypertensive; Diuretic
M454	Tab, White, Round, Scored	Pindolol 5 mg	Visken by Merckle/Martec	52555-0454	Antihypertensive

ID FRONT <> BACK	DESCRIPTION FRONT <> BACK	INGREDIENT & STRENGTH	BRAND (OR EQUIV.) & FIRM	NDC#	CLASS; SCH.
M455	Tab, White, Round, Scored	Pindolol 10 mg	Visken by Merckle/Martec	52555-0455	Antihypertensive
M47	Tab, Film Coated, M over 47	Metoprolol Tartrate 50 mg	by Kaiser	62224-4442	Antihypertensive
M47	Tab, Light Blue, Beveled Edge, Film Coated, M Over 47	Metoprolol Tartrate 100 mg	by Mylan	00378-0047	Antihypertensive
M47	Tab, Film Coated, M Over 47	Metoprolol Tartrate 100 mg	by Allscripts	54569-3788	Antihypertensive
M47	Tab, Light Blue, Round, Scored, Film Coated, M Over 47	Metoprolol Tartrate 100 mg	Lopressor by UDL	51079-0802	Antihypertensive
M47	Tab, Light Blue, Film Coated	Metoprolol Tartrate 100 mg	by Heartland	61392-0280	Antihypertensive
M471	Tab, Film Coated	Fenoprofen Calcium	by St Marys Med	60760-0471	NSAID
M471	Tab, Orange, Oblong, Film Coated, Scored	Fenoprofen Calcium	by HJ Harkins	52959-0067	NSAID
M471	Tab, Film Coated	Fenoprofen Calcium	by UDL	51079-0477	NSAID
M471	Tab, Light Orange, Film Coated	Fenoprofen Calcium 600 mg	by Mylan	00378-0471	NSAID
M471	Tab, Film Coated	Fenoprofen Calcium 691.8 mg	by Allscripts	54569-2105	NSAID
M5	Tab, White, Round, Scored	Methimazole 5 mg	Methimazole by Jone's Pharma	00689-1084	Antithyroid
M5	Tab, Brown, Oval, Film Coated	Methenamine Mandelate 0.5 gm	by Able	53265-0159	Antibiotic; Urinary Tract
M50	Tab, White	Chlorothiazide 250 mg	by Mylan	00378-0150	Diuretic
M50	Tab, White, Round, Scored, M/50	Chlorothiazide 250 mg	Diuril by by UDL	51079-0060	Diuretic
M50	Tab, White, Scored	Levothyroxine Sodium 50 mcg	by Altimed	Canadian DIN# 02237214	Antithyroid
M5059	Tab, Film Coated	Thioridazine HCl 50 mg	by Med Pro	53978-2006	Antipsychotic
M50G	Cap, Orange, M/50/G	Minocycline HCl 50 mg	by Genpharm	Canadian	Antibiotic
M50LEVOT	Tab, White, Round	Levothyroxine Sodium 0.05 mg	Synthroid by Mova		Antithyroid
M51	Tab, Film Coated	Amitriptyline HCl 25 mg	by Prescription Dispensing	61807-0129	Antidepressant
M51	Tab, Film Coated	Amitriptyline HCl 25 mg	by Diversified Hlthcare Serv	55887-0986	Antidepressant
M51	Tab, Light Green, Film Coated, M over 51	Amitriptyline HCl 25 mg	by Mylan	00378-2625	Antidepressant
M51	Tab, Light Green, Round, Film Coated, M over 51	Amitriptyline HCl 25 mg	Elival by UDL	51079-0107	Antidepressant
M51 <> M51	Tab, Film Coated	Amitriptyline HCl 25 mg	by Caremark	00339-5015	Antidepressant
M52	Tab, White, Round, Scored	Pindolol 5 mg	by Mylan	55160-0132	Antihypertensive
M52	Tab, White, M Above Score, 52 Below	Pindolol 5 mg	by Mylan	00378-0052	Antihypertensive
M525	Tab, Film Coated	Diltiazem HCl 120 mg	by Heartland	61392-0056	Antihypertensive
M525	Tab, Film Coated	Diltiazem HCl 120 mg	by Heartland	61392-0145	Antihypertensive
M525	Tab, White, Film Coated	Diltiazem HCl 120 mg	by Mylan	00378-0525	Antihypertensive
M53	Tab, Coated, M/53	Cimetidine 200 mg	by Qualitest	00603-2890	Gastrointestinal
M532	Cap, Beige & Red	Acetaminophen 500 mg, Oxycodone HCl 5 mg	Tylox by Mallinckrodt Hobart	00406-0532	Analgesic; C II
M532	Tab, Beige & Red, Hard Gel, M Inside a Square and 532	Oxycodone 5 mg, Acetaminophen 500 mg	by Pharmafab	62542-0255	Analgesic; C II
M54 <> 10	Tab, Orange, Round, Film Coated	Thioridazine HCl 10 mg	by Dixon Shane	17236-0318	Antipsychotic
M54 <> 10	Tab, Orange, Round, Film Coated, M over 54 <> 10	Thioridazine HCl 10 mg	Mellaril by UDL	51079-0565	Antipsychotic
M54 <> 10	Tab, Film Coated, M Over 54	Thioridazine HCl 10 mg	by Mylan	00378-0612	Antipsychotic
M54 <> 10	Tab, Film Coated	Thioridazine HCl 10 mg	by Qualitest	00603-5992	Antipsychotic
M54 <> 10	Tab, Coated	Thioridazine HCl 10 mg	by Vangard	00615-2504	Antipsychotic
M541	Tab, Film Coated, M 541 Across the Partial Score	Cimetidine 800 mg	by Quality Care	60346-0209	Gastrointestinal
M541	Tab, Film Coated, M /541	Cimetidine 800 mg	by Heartland	61392-0203	Gastrointestinal
M541	Tab, Coated	Cimetidine 800 mg	by Qualitest	00603-2893	Gastrointestinal
M541	Tab, Green, Film Coated, Scored	Cimetidine 800 mg	by Mylan	00378-0541	Gastrointestinal
M541	Tab, Green, Oval, Scored, Film Coated, M/541	Cimetidine 800 mg	Tagamet by UDL	51079-0809	Gastrointestinal
M541	Tab, Film Coated, Scored, M/541	Cimetidine 800 mg	by Murfreesboro	51129-1178	Gastrointestinal
M5410	Tab, Film Coated	Thioridazine HCl 10 mg	by Med Pro	53978-2004	Antipsychotic
M55	Tab, Green, Beveled Edge, M Over 55	Timolol Maleate 5 mg	by Mylan	00378-0055	Antihypertensive
M55	Tab, Green, Round, M 55	Timolol Maleate 5 mg	by Teva	00480-0076	Antihypertensive
M572	Tab, White, M/572	Albuterol Sulfate 4 mg	by Mylan	00378-0572	Antiasthmatic
M572	Tab, White, Round, Scored, M over 255	Albuterol Sulfate 4 mg	by UDL	51079-0658	Antiasthmatic
M572	Tab	Albuterol Sulfate 4.8 mg	by Allscripts	54569-2874	Antiasthmatic
M577	Tab	Amiloride HCl 5 mg, Hydrochlorothiazide 50 mg	by Kaiser	62224-7115	Diuretic

ID FRONT <> BACK	DESCRIPTION FRONT <> BACK	INGREDIENT & STRENGTH	BRAND (OR EQUIV.) & FIRM	NDC#	CLASS; SCH.
M577	Tab, Light Orange, Round, Scored, M over 577	Amiloride HCl 5 mg, Hydrochlorothiazide 50 mg	by UDL	51079-0421	Diuretic
M577	Tab, Light Orange, M/577	Amiloride HCl 5 mg, Hydrochlorothiazide 50 mg	by Mylan	00378-0577	Diuretic
M58 <> 25	Tab, Orange, Film Coated, M Over 58	Thioridazine HCl 25 mg	by Mylan	00378-0614	Antipsychotic
M58 <> 25	Tab, Film Coated	Thioridazine HCl 25 mg	by Quality Care	60346-0839	Antipsychotic
M58 <> 25	Tab, Orange, Round, Film Coated	Thioridazine HCl 25 mg	by Dixon Shane	17236-0301	Antipsychotic
M58 <> 25	Tab, Coated	Thioridazine HCl 25 mg	by Vangard	00615-2506	Antipsychotic
M58 <> 25	Tab, Orange, Round, Film Coated, M over 58 <> 25	Thioridazine HCl 25 mg	Mellaril by UDL	51079-0566	Antipsychotic
M59 <> 50	Tab, Orange, Round, Film Coated, M over 59 <> 50	Thioridazine HCl 50 mg	Mellaril by UDL	51079-0567	Antipsychotic
M59 <> 50	Tab, Orange, Film Coated, M Over 59	Thioridazine HCl 50 mg	by Mylan	00378-0616	Antipsychotic
M59 <> 50	Tab, Film Coated, M Over 59	Thioridazine HCl 50 mg	by Quality Care	60346-0840	Antipsychotic
M59 <> 50	Tab, Film Coated	Thioridazine HCl 50 mg	by Vangard	00615-2507	Antipsychotic
M59 <> 50	Tab, Orange, Round, Film Coated	Thioridazine HCl 50 mg	by Dixon Shane	17236-0302	Antipsychotic
M59 <> 50	Tab, Film Coated	Thioridazine HCl 50 mg	by Qualitest	00603-5994	Antipsychotic
M6	Tab, Pink, Round	Erythromycin Stearate 250 mg	Erythrocin by Mylan		Antibiotic
M6	Tab, Yellow, Round	Erythromycin Stearate 250 mg	Erythrocin by Mylan		Antibiotic
M6 <> LL	Tab, White, Round, Convex, Film Coated	Ethambutol HCl 100 mg	Myambutol by Heartland	61392-0718	Antituberculosis
M6 <> LL	Tab, White, Round	Ethambutol HCl 100 mg	Myambutol by Lederle Pharm	00005-5015	Antituberculosis
M6 <>LL	Tab, White, Round, Scored, Film Coated	Ethambutol HCl 100 mg	Myambutol by Dura	51479-0046	Antituberculosis
M61 <> 100	Tab, Orange, Round, Film Coated, M over 61 <> 100	Thioridazine HCl 100 mg	Mellaril by UDL	51079-0580	Antipsychotic
M61 <> 100	Tab, Orange, Film Coated, M Over 61	Thioridazine HCl 100 mg	by Mylan	00378-0618	Antipsychotic
M61 <> 100	Tab, Orange, Round, Film Coated	Thioridazine HCl 100 mg	by Dixon Shane	17236-0305	Antipsychotic
M61 <> 100	Tab, Film Coated	Thioridazine HCl 100 mg	by Qualitest	00603-5995	Antipsychotic
M61 <> 100	Tab, Film Coated	Thioridazine HCl 100 mg	by Vangard	00615-2508	Antipsychotic
M6110	Tab, Orange, Round, M 61/10	Thioridazine HCl 100 mg	Mellaril by Roxane		Antipsychotic
M62	Tab, White, Round	Chlorothiazide 500 mg	Diuril by Mylan		Diuretic
M63	Tab, M over 63	Atenolol 50 mg, Chlorthalidone 25 mg	by Caremark	00339-5839	Antihypertensive; Diuretic
M63	Tab, White, Scored, M over 63	Atenolol 50 mg, Chlorthalidone 25 mg	by Mylan	00378-2063	Antihypertensive; Diuretic
M64	Tab, White, M over 64	Atenolol 100 mg, Chlorthalidone 25 mg	by Mylan	00378-2064	Antihypertensive; Diuretic
M65	Tab, Orange, Oblong	Propoxyphene HCl 65 mg, Acetaminophen. 650 mg	Wygesic by Mylan		Analgesic; C IV
M7	Tab, M/7 <> Lederle Logo	Ethambutol HCl 400 mg	Myambutol by Lederle	00005-5084	Antituberculosis
M7	Tab, M over 7 <> Logo	Ethambutol HCl 400 mg	Myambutol by Nat Pharmpak Serv	55154-1709	Antituberculosis
M7	Tab, Pink, Oval	Erythromycin Stearate 500 mg	Erythrocin by Mylan		Antibiotic
M7	Tab, Yellow, Oval	Erythromycin Stearate 500 mg	Erythrocin by Mylan		Antibiotic
M7 <> LL	Tab	Ethambutol HCl 400 mg	Myambutol by Allscripts	54569-3070	Antituberculosis
M7 <> LL	Tab, White, Round, Convex, Scored, Film Coated	Ethambutol HCl 400 mg	Myambutol by Heartland	61392-0728	Antituberculosis
M7 <> LL	Tab, White, Round, Film Coated, Scored	Ethambutol HCl 400 mg	Myambutol by DRX Pharm Consults	55045-2763	Antituberculosis
M70	Tab, White, Round, Scored	Clorazepate Dipotassium 15 mg	by Murfreesboro Ph	51129-1354	Antianxiety; C IV
M70	Tab, White, Round, Scored	Clorazepate Dipotassium 15 mg	by Allscripts	54569-4586	Antianxiety; C IV
M70	Tab, White, Scored, M over 70	Clorazepate Dipotassium 15 mg	by Mylan	00378-0070	Antianxiety; C IV
M70	Tab, White, Round, Scored, M over 70	Clorazepate Dipotassium 15 mg	Tranxene by UDL	51079-0635	Antianxiety; C IV
M70	Tab, White, Round, Scored	Clorazepate Dipotassium 15 mg	by DHHS Prog	11819-0150	Antianxiety; C IV
M71	Tab	Allopurinol 300 mg	by Kaiser	62224-7113	Antigout
M71	Tab	Allopurinol 300 mg	by Heartland	61392-0104	Antigout
M71	Tab, White, Round, Scored, M/71	Allopurinol 300 mg	by UDL	51079-0206	Antigout
M71	Tab, White, Scored	Allopurinol 300 mg	by Mylan	00378-0181	Antigout
M715	Tab, Green, Beveled Edge, M to Left, 715 to Right of Score	Timolol Maleate 20 mg	by Mylan	00378-0715	Antihypertensive
M715	Tab, M 715	Timolol Maleate 20 mg	by Med Pro	53978-2022	Antihypertensive
M72	Tab, Scored, M over 72	Chlorthalidone 15 mg, Clonidine HCl 0.3 mg	by Mylan	00378-0072	Diuretic; Antihypertensive

ID FRONT <> BACK	DESCRIPTION FRONT <> BACK	INGREDIENT & STRENGTH	BRAND (OR EQUIV.) & FIRM	NDC#	CLASS; SCH.
M72	Tab, Yellow, Round, Scored	Clonidine HCl 0.3 mg, Chlorthalidone 15 mg	Clorpres USP by DHHS Prog	11819-0130	Antihypertensive; Diuretic
M74	Tab, Coated	Fluphenazine HCl 5 mg	by Heartland	61392-0059	Antipsychotic
M74	Tab, Coated	Fluphenazine HCl 5 mg	by Heartland	61392-0151	Antipsychotic
M75	Tab	Chlorthalidone 50 mg	by Med Pro	53978-0033	Diuretic
M75	Tab	Chlorthalidone 50 mg	by Allscripts	54569-0554	Diuretic
M75	Tab, Green, Round, Scored	Chlorthalidone 50 mg	by Compumed	00403-0046	Diuretic
M75	Tab, Light Green, Scored	Chlorthalidone 50 mg	by Mylan	00378-0213	Diuretic
M75	Tab, Green, Round, Scored, M/75	Chlorthalidone 50 mg	Hygroton by UDL	51079-0059	Diuretic
M75	Tab, Pink, Oblong, Film Coated	Estrogens, Esterified 2.5 mg	Menest by Monarch Pharms	61570-0075	Hormone
M75	Tab, Pink, Oblong, Film Coated	Estrogens, Esterified 2.5 mg	Menest by King	61570-0075	Hormone
M75	Tab, Violet, Scored	Levothyroxine Sodium 75 mcg	by Altimed	Canadian DIN# 02237215	Antithyroid
M751	Tab, Film Coated	Cyclobenzaprine HCl 10 mg	by Pharmedix	53002-0308	Muscle Relaxant
M751	Tab, Coated	Cyclobenzaprine HCl 10 mg	by Med Pro	53978-1035	Muscle Relaxant
M76	Tab, Beige, Round	Flurbiprofen 100 mg	by PDRX Pharms	55289-0561	NSAID
M76	Tab, Beige, Film Coated, M over 76	Flurbiprofen 50 mg	by Mylan	00378-0076	NSAID
M76	Tab, Film Coated, M over 76	Flurbiprofen 50 mg	by Allscripts	54569-3857	NSAID
M77	Tab, White, Round, Film Coated	Amitriptyline HCl 10 mg	Elavil by UDL	51079-0131	Antidepressant
M77	Tab, White, Coated	Amitriptyline HCl 10 mg	by Mylan	00378-2610	Antidepressant
M81	Tab, White	Captopril 25 mg, Hydrochlorothiazide 15 mg	by Mylan	00378-0081	Antihypertensive; Diuretic
M83	Tab, Peach	Captopril 25 mg, Hydrochlorothiazide 25 mg	by Mylan	00378-0083	Antihypertensive; Diuretic
M84	Tab, White, Scored	Captopril 50 mg, Hydrochlorothiazide 15 mg	by Mylan	00378-0084	Antihypertensive; Diuretic
M86	Tab, Peach, Scored	Captopril 50 mg, Hydrochlorothiazide 25 mg	by Mylan	00378-0086	Antihypertensive; Diuretic
M87 <> W	Tab, M/87 <>	Ambenonium Chloride 10 mg	Mytelase Chloride by Sanofi	00024-1287	Myasthenia Gravis
M87 <> W	Tab, Coated, M/87 <> W	Ambenonium Chloride 10 mg	Mytelase by Bayer	00280-1287	Myasthenia Gravis
M93	Tab, Beige, Film Coated, Scored, M over 93	Flurbiprofen 100 mg	by Mylan	00378-0093	NSAID
M93	Tab, Film Coated, M over 93	Flurbiprofen 100 mg	by Physicians Total Care	54868-3362	NSAID
M93	Tab, Beige, Round, Film Coated, M over 93	Flurbiprofen 100 mg	Ansaid by UDL	51079-0815	NSAID
M93	Tab, Film Coated	Flurbiprofen 100 mg	by Allscripts	54569-3858	NSAID
M95	Tab, M to Left, 95 to Right of Score	Penicillin V Potassium	by Mylan	00378-0195	Antibiotic
M97	Tab, Coated	Fluphenazine HCl 10 mg	by Heartland	61392-0150	Antipsychotic
M97	Tab, Coated	Fluphenazine HCl 10 mg	by Heartland	61392-0060	Antipsychotic
M970	Tab, White, Round, M/970	Butalbital 50 mg, Acetaminophen 325 mg, Caffeine 40 mg	Fioricet by Mallinckrodt		Analgesic
M98	Tab	Penicillin V Potassium	by Mylan	00378-0198	Antibiotic
M98	Tab	Penicillin V Potassium	by Prescription Dispensing	61807-0004	Antibiotic
M9B <> MAXZIDE	Tab, M9B <> Maxzide	Hydrochlorothiazide 25 mg, Triamterene 37.5 mg	Maxzide by Eckerd Drug	19458-0845	Diuretic
MAALOXAG150	Tab, Pink, Round	Simethicone 150 mg	Maalox by Ciba	Canadian	Antiflatulent
MAALOXAG80	Tab, Pink, Round	Simethicone 80 mg	Maalox by Ciba	Canadian	Antiflatulent
MAALOXHRF	Tab, Green, Round	Alginate Compound 250 mg	Maalox by Ciba	Canadian	Gastrointestinal
MAALOXTC	Tab, White, Round, Mallox TC/Novartis Logo	Aluminum Hydroxide 300 mg	by Novartis	Canadian	Gastrointestinal
MACRO100MG <> 01490009	Cap, Macro100MG <> 0149 0009	Nitrofurantoin 100 mg	Macrodantin by Quality Care	60346-0651	Antibiotic
MACROBID <> NORWICHEAT	Cap	Nitrofurantoin 100 mg	Macrobid by Quality Care	60346-0289	Antibiotic
MACROBID <> NORWICHEATON	Cap, Black & Yellow	Nitrofurantoin 100 mg	Macrobid by Promex Medcl	62301-0039	Antibiotic

ID FRONT <> BACK	DESCRIPTION FRONT <> BACK	INGREDIENT & STRENGTH	BRAND (OR EQUIV.) & FIRM	NDC#	CLASS; SCH.
MACROBID <> NORWICHEATON	Cap, Black & Yellow	Nitrofurantoin 100 mg	Macrobid by Southwood Pharms	58016-0260	Antibiotic
MACROBID <> NORWICHEATON	Cap, Black & Yellow w/ Grey lines & Grey ink, Opaque	Nitrofurantoin Monohydrate 100 mg	Macrobid by Procter & Gamble	00149-0710	Antibiotic
MACROBID <> NORWICHEATON	Cap, Norwich Eaton	Nitrofurantoin 100 mg	Macrobid by Allscripts	54569-3544	Antibiotic
MACROBID <> NORWICHEATON	Cap	Nitrofurantoin 100 mg	Macrobid by DRX	55045-2341	Antibiotic
MACRODANTIN <> 100MGSAMPLE	Cap, White w/ Yellow Powder, Opaque	Nitrofurantoin 100 mg	Macrodantin by Procter & Gamble	00149-0009	Antibiotic
MACRODANTIN <> 25MGSAMPLE	Cap, White w/ Yellow Powder, Opaque	Nitrofurantoin 25 mg	Macrodantin by Procter & Gamble	00149-0007	Antibiotic
MACRODANTIN <> 50MGSAMPLE	Cap, White w/ Yellow Powder, Opaque	Nitrofurantoin 50 mg	Macrodantin by Procter & Gamble	00149-0008	Antibiotic
MACRODANTIN100	Cap, Yellow	Nitrofurantoin Macrocrystalline 100 mg	by Rightpak	65240-0688	Antibiotic
MACRODANTIN100 <> 01490009	Cap	Nitrofurantoin 100 mg	Macrodantin by Pharmedix	53002-0273	Antibiotic
MACRODANTIN100 <> 01490009	Cap, 3 Black Lines Encircling the Capsule	Nitrofurantoin 100 mg	Macrodantin by Pharm Utilization	60491-0389	Antibiotic
MACRODANTIN100 <> 01490009	Cap, Macrodantin 100 mg, 3 Black Lines Encircling the Capsule <> 0149-0009	Nitrofurantoin 100 mg	Macrodantin by Quality Care	60346-0651	Antibiotic
MACRODANTIN100M <> 01490009	Cap, Macrodantin 100 mg 0149-0009 <> 3 Black Lines Encircling Capsule	Nitrofurantoin 100 mg	Macrodantin by Thrift Drug	59198-0057	Antibiotic
MACRODANTIN100M <> 01490009	Cap, Macrodantin over 100 mg <> 0149 Over 0009 with 3 Black Lines Encircling	Nitrofurantoin 100 mg	Macrodantin by Amerisource	62584-0009	Antibiotic
MACRODANTIN50MG	Cap, White & Yellow	Nitrofurantoin Macrocrystalline 50 mg	by Rightpak	65240-0687	Antibiotic
MACRODANTIN50MG <> 01490008	Cap, Opaque & White & Yellow, Macrodantin 50 mg <> 0149-0008	Nitrofurantoin 50 mg	Macrodantin by PDRX	55289-0239	Antibiotic
MACRODANTIN50MG <> 01490008	Cap, Macrodantin 50 mg <> 0149-0008 with 2 Black Lines	Nitrofurantoin 50 mg	Macrodantin by Thrift Drug	59198-0056	Antibiotic
MACRODANTIN50MG <> 01490008	Cap, Opaque Yellow, 2 Black Lines Encircling the Capsule, Macrodantin 50 mg <> 0149-0008	Nitrofurantoin 50 mg	Macrodantin by Quality Care	60346-0318	Antibiotic
MACRODANTIN50MG <> 01490008	Cap, Macrodantin over 50 mg <> 0149 Over 0008 with 2 Black Lines Encircling	Nitrofurantoin 50 mg	Macrodantin by Amerisource	62584-0008	Antibiotic
MACRODANTIN50MG <> 1490008	Cap, White & Yellow	Nitrofurantoin Macrocrystalline 50 mg	Macrodantin by Med-Pro	53978-3397	Antibiotic
MACRODANTIN50MG <> LINES01490008	Cap, Macrodantin 50 mg <> Lines/01490008	Nitrofurantoin 50 mg	Macrodantin by Nat Pharmpak Serv	55154-2301	Antibiotic
MAJOR <> 0058	Cap, Ex Release	Chlorpheniramine Maleate 8 mg, Pseudoephedrine HCl 120 mg	Pseudo Chlor by Sovereign	58716-0014	Cold Remedy
MARAX <> ROERIG254	Tab	Ephedrine Sulfate 25 mg, Hydroxyzine HCl 10 mg, Theophylline 130 mg	Marax by Roerig	00049-2540	Antiasthmatic
MARCPM	Tab, Off-White, MAR-CPM	Chlorpheniramine Maleate 8 mg, Methscopolamine Nitrate 2.5 mg, Phenylephrine HCl 20 mg	Prehist by Anabolic	00722-6280	Cold Remedy
MAREZINE	Tab, Round	Cyclizine HCl 50 mg	Marezine by Himmel		Antiemetic
MARGESIC <> MARNEL	Cap, Green Print	Acetaminophen 325 mg, Butalbital 50 mg, Caffeine 40 mg	Margesic by Marnel	00682-0804	Analgesic
MARGESICH	Cap, White Print	Acetaminophen 500 mg, Hydrocodone Bitartrate 5 mg	Margesic H by Marnel	00682-0808	Analgesic; C III
MARION <> 1771	Tab, Green, Coated	Diltiazem HCl 30 mg	Cardizem by Hoechst Roussel	00088-1771	Antihypertensive
MARION <> 1772	Tab, Yellow	Diltiazem HCl 60 mg	Cardizem by Hoechst Marion Roussel	00088-1772	Antihypertensive
MARION <> 1772	Tab, Coated	Diltiazem HCl 60 mg	Cardizem by Drug Distr	52985-0191	Antihypertensive
MARION120MG	Tab, Yellow, Oblong	Diltiazem HCl 120 mg	Cardizem by Marion	00088-1792	Antihypertensive
MARION1375	Tab, Blue, Round	Oxybutynin 5 mg	Ditropan by Marion		Urinary
MARION1555	Cap, Brown & Clear	Papaverine HCl 150 mg	Pavabid by Hoechst Marion Roussel		Vasodilator
MARION1712	Tab, Pink, Oblong, Marion/1712	Sucralfate 1 gm	Carafate by Marion		Gastrointestinal

ID FRONT <> BACK	DESCRIPTION FRONT <> BACK	INGREDIENT & STRENGTH	BRAND (OR EQUIV.) & FIRM	NDC#	CLASS; SCH.
MARION90MG	Tab, Green, Oblong	Diltiazem HCl 90 mg	Cardizem by Marion	00088-1791	Antihypertensive
MARNATALF	Tab, Film Coated, Marnatal-F	Ascorbic Acid 100 mg, Calcium 250 mg, Copper 2 mg, Cyanocobalamin 12 mcg, Folic Acid 1 mg, Iodine 0.2 mg, Iron 60 mg, Magnesium 25 mg, Niacinamide 20 mg, Pyridoxine HCl 5 mg, Riboflavin 3.4 mg, Thiamine HCl 3 mg, Vitamin A 4000 Units, Vitamin D 400 Units, Vitamin E 30 Units, Zinc 25 mg	Marnatal F by Lini	58215-0309	Vitamin
MARNEL <> MARGESIC	Cap, Green Print	Acetaminophen 325 mg, Butalbital 50 mg, Caffeine 40 mg	Margesic by Marnel	00682-0804	Analgesic
MARNEL <> MARNEL	Cap, White Beads, Black Print	Chlorpheniramine Maleate 8 mg, Phenylephrine HCl 20 mg	Prehist by		Cold Remedy
MARSAM0530	Cap, Purple	Cefaclor 250 mg	Ceclor by Marsam		Antibiotic
MARSAM0531	Cap, Purple & Yellow	Cefaclor 500 mg	Ceclor by Marsam		Antibiotic
MARSAM530	Cap, Purple	Cefaclor 250 mg	Ceclor by Schein		Antibiotic
MARTEC972	Cap, Ivory & Red, Martec/972	Piroxicam 10 mg	Feldene by Martec	52555-0972	NSAID
MARTEC973	Cap	Piroxicam 20 mg	by Med Pro	53978-1255	NSAID
MARTEC973	Cap, Red, Martec/973	Piroxicam 20 mg	Feldene by Martec	52555-0973	NSAID
MATERNA U24	Tab, Pink, Oval	Multi Vitamin	Materna by Wyeth-Ayerst	Canadian	Vitamin
MATULANEROCHE	Cap, Matulane/Roche	Procarbazine HCl 50	Matulane by Hoffmann La Roche	00004-0053	Antineoplastic
MATULANESIGMATU	Cap, Ivory	Procarbazine HCl 50 mg	Matulane by Ranbaxy	54907-0608	Antineoplastic
MAXALT <> MRK267	Tab, Pale Pink, Cap-Shaped, MRK 267	Rizatriptan Benzoate 14.53 mg	Maxalt by Merck	00006-0267	Antimigraine
MAXALT <> MRK267	Tab, MRK 267	Rizatriptan Benzoate 14.53 mg	by Merck & Sharp & Dohme	60312-0267	Antimigraine
MAXAQUIN400	Tab, White, Oval, Scored	Lomefloxacin HCl 400 mg	Maxaquin by West Pharm	52967-0283	Antibiotic
MAXAQUIN400	Tab, White, Oval, Film Coated	Lomefloxacin HCl mg	Maxaquin by Unimed	00051-1651	Antibiotic
MAXIDONE634	Tab, Yellow, Cap Shaped, Scored	Acetaminophen 750 mg, Hydrocodone Bitartrate 10 mg	Maxidone by Watson	52544-0634	Analgesic; C III
MAXIFEDDM <> MCR526	Tab, Scored	Guaifenesin 500 mg; Pseudoephedrine HCl 60 mg; Dextromethorphan Hydrobromide 30 mg	Maxifed DM by AM Pharms	58605-0526	Cold Remedy
MAXIFEDDM <> MCR526	Tab, Scored	Guaifenesin 500 mg; Pseudoephedrine HCl 60 mg; Dextromethorphan Hydrobromide 30 mg	by Pfab	62542-0772	Cold Remedy
MAXZIDE <> BM8	Tab, B On the Left and M8 On the Right of Score	Hydrochlorothiazide 50 mg, Triamterene 75 mg	Maxzide by Mylan	00378-7550	Diuretic
MAXZIDE <> BM8	Tab, Beveled Edge <> B On Left, M8 On Right of Score	Hydrochlorothiazide 50 mg, Triamterene 75 mg	Maxzide by Bertek	62794-0460	Diuretic
MAXZIDE <> BM9	Tab, B/M9	Hydrochlorothiazide 25 mg, Triamterene 37.5 mg	Maxzide by Caremark	00339-6094	Diuretic
MAXZIDE <> BM9	Tab, Beveled, B/M9	Hydrochlorothiazide 25 mg, Triamterene 37.5 mg	Maxide 25 by Direct Dispensing	57866-6801	Diuretic
MAXZIDE <> BM9	Tab, Beveled Edge, B/M9	Hydrochlorothiazide 25 mg, Triamterene 37.5 mg	Maxzide 25 by Bertek	62794-0464	Diuretic
MAXZIDE <> BM9	Tab, Bowtie Shaped, <> B/M9	Hydrochlorothiazide 25 mg, Triamterene 37.5 mg	Maxzide by Eckerd Drug	19458-0845	Diuretic
MAXZIDE <> LLM8	Tab, LL/M8	Hydrochlorothiazide 50 mg, Triamterene 75 mg	Maxzide by Nat Pharmpak Serv	55154-1705	Diuretic
MAXZIDE <> LLM9	Tab, Bowtie Shaped	Hydrochlorothiazide 25 mg, Triamterene 37.5 mg	Maxzide 25 by Allscripts	54569-2320	Diuretic
MAXZIDEBM9	Tab, Light Green, Bowtie-Shaped, Scored	Hydrochlorothiazide 25 mg, Triamterene 37.5 mg	by Allscripts	54569-2320	Diuretic
MC	Tab, White, Round, Abbott Logo	Methamphetamine HCl LR 5 mg	Desoxyn by Abbott	00074-6941	Stimulant; C II
MC <> 10	Tab, White, Round, Scored, M/C	Isoxsuprine HCl 10 mg	by Murfreesboro	51129-1584	Vasodilator
MC <> 20	Tab, White, Round, Scored	Isoxsuprine HCl 20 mg	by Murfreesboro	51129-1585	Vasodilator
MC <> 20	Tab, M/C	Isoxsuprine HCl 20 mg	by Shire Richwood	58521-0576	Vasodilator
MC1	Tab, White, Oblong, Scored	Captopril 12.5 mg	Capoten by Mylan	00378-3007	Antihypertensive
MC1	Tab, White, Oval, M/C1	Captopril 12.5 mg	Capoten by UDL	51079-0863	Antihypertensive
MC2	Tab, M Over C2	Captopril 25 mg	by Quality Care	60346-0778	Antihypertensive
MC2	Tab, M over C2	Captopril 25 mg	by Direct Dispensing	57866-6106	Antihypertensive
MC2	Tab, M Over C2	Captopril 25 mg	by Heartland	61392-0605	Antihypertensive
MC2	Tab, White, Round	Captopril 25 mg	Capoten by Mylan		Antihypertensive
MC2	Tab, White, Round, Scored, M over C2	Captopril 25 mg	Capoten by UDL	51079-0864	Antihypertensive
MC3	White, Round, Scored, M over C3	Captopril 50 mg	Capoten by Mylan	00378-3017	Antihypertensive
MC3	Tab, White, Round, Scored	Captopril 50 mg	by Heartland Healthcare	61392-0147	Antihypertensive
MC3	Tab, White, Round, Scored	Captopril 50 mg	by Southwood Pharms	58016-0165	Antihypertensive
MC4	Tab, White, Round, Scored, M over C4	Captopril 100 mg	Capoten by Mylan	00378-3022	Antihypertensive
MCG 219	Cap	Phenylpropanolamine 75 mg, Chlorpheniramine 8 mg, Methscop. 2.5 mg	Rhinolar by McGregor		Cold Remedy

ID FRONT <> BACK	DESCRIPTION FRONT <> BACK	INGREDIENT & STRENGTH	BRAND (OR EQUIV.) & FIRM	NDC#	CLASS; SCH.
MCNEIL	Tab, Light Green, Round, Scored	Acetaminophen 300 mg, Chloroxazone 250 mg	Parafon Forte by Johnson & Johnson	Canadian DIN# 02229946	Muscle Relaxant
McNEIL	Tab	Acetaminophen 300 mg, Codeine Phosphate 30 mg	Tylenol Codeine No 3 by Nat Pharmpak Serv	55154-1908	Analgesic; C III
McNEIL	Tab, Green, Round	Chlorzoxazone 250 mg	Parafon Forte by McNeil	Canadian	Muscle Relaxant
McNEIL	Tab, Peach, Round	Pimozide 10 mg	Orap by McNeil	Canadian	Antipsychotic
McNEIL	Tab, White, Round	Pimozide 2 mg	Orap by McNeil	Canadian	Antipsychotic
McNEIL	Tab, Green, Round	Pimozide 4 mg	Orap by McNeil	Canadian	Antipsychotic
MCNEIL <> 659	Tab, White, Cap-Shaped, Film Coated	Tramadol HCl 50 mg	Ultram by McNeil	00045-0659	Analgesic
MCNEIL <> 659	Tab, Film Coated	Tramadol HCl 50 mg	Ultram by Ortho	00062-0659	Analgesic
MCNEIL <> 659	Tab, White, Oblong, Film	Tramadol HCl 50 mg	by Teva	00480-0148	Analgesic
MCNEIL <> 659	Tab, Film Coated	Tramadol HCl 50 mg	Ultram by Caremark	00339-6099	Analgesic
MCNEIL <> 659	Tab, Film Coated	Tramadol HCl 50 mg	Ultram by DRX	55045-2219	Analgesic
MCNEIL <> 659	Tab, Film Coated	Tramadol HCl 50 mg	Ultram by Northeast	58163-0659	Analgesic
MCNEIL <> 659	Tab, Film Coated	Tramadol HCl 50 mg	Ultram by HJ Harkins Co	52959-0414	Analgesic
MCNEIL <> 659	Tab, Film Coated	Tramadol HCl 50 mg	Ultram by McNeil	52021-0659	Analgesic
MCNEIL <> 659	Tab, Film Coated	Tramadol HCl 50 mg	Ultram by Allscripts	54569-4089	Analgesic
MCNEIL <> 659	Tab, Film Coated	Tramadol HCl 50 mg	Ultram by Heartland	61392-0625	Analgesic
MCNEIL <> 659	Tab, Film Coated	Tramadol HCl 50 mg	Ultram by Prescription Dispensing	61807-0128	Analgesic
MCNEIL <> 659	Tab, Film Coated	Tramadol HCl 50 mg	Ultram by PDRX	55289-0650	Analgesic
MCNEIL <> 659	Tab, Film Coated	Trazodone HCl 50 mg	by Nat Pharmpak Serv	55154-1910	Antidepressant
MCNEIL <> NO1	Cap, White, Film Coated, McNeil <> No. 1	Acetaminophen 300 mg, Caffeine 15 mg, Codeine Phosphate 8 mg	Tylenol No. 1 by McNeil	Canadian DIN# 02181061	Analgesic
MCNEIL <> NO1FORTE	Cap, White, Film Coated, McNeil <> No. 1 Forte	Acetaminophen 500 mg, Caffeine 15 mg, Codeine Phosphate 8 mg	Tylenol No. 1 Forte by McNeil	Canadian DIN# 02181088	Analgesic
MCNEIL <> PANCREASE	Cap, Delayed Release	Amylase 20000 Units, Lipase 4500 Units, Protease 25000 Units	Pancrease by Leiner	59606-0714	Gastrointestinal
MCNEIL <> PANCREASE	Cap	Amylase 20000 Units, Lipase 4500 Units, Protease 25000 Units	Pancrease by Prestige Packaging	58056-0350	Gastrointestinal
MCNEIL <> PANCREASE	Cap, White, Red Print	Amylase 20000 Units, Lipase 4500 Units, Protease 25000 Units	Pancrease by McNeil	00045-0095	Gastrointestinal
MCNEIL <> PANCREASE	Cap	Amylase 20000 Units, Lipase 4500 Units, Protease 25000 Units	Pancrease by McNeil	52021-0095	Gastrointestinal
MCNEIL <> PANCREASE	Cap, Clear & White	Lipase 4,500 Units, Amylase 20,000 Units, Protease 25,000 Units	Pancrease by Murfreesboro	51129-9416	Gastrointestinal
MCNEIL <> PANCREASEMT10	Cap, Clear & Pink	Amylase 30000 Units, Lipase 10000 Units, Protease 30000 Units	Pancrease Mt 10 by McNeil	00045-0342	Gastrointestinal
MCNEIL <> PANCREASEMT10	Cap	Amylase 30000 Units, Lipase 10000 Units, Protease 30000 Units	Pancrease Mt 10 by McNeil	52021-0342	Gastrointestinal
MCNEIL <> PANCREASEMT16	Cap, Clear & Salmon	Amylase 48000 Units, Lipase 16000 Units, Protease 48000 Units	Pancrease Mt 16 by McNeil	00045-0343	Gastrointestinal
MCNEIL <> PANCREASEMT16	Cap	Amylase 48000 Units, Lipase 16000 Units, Protease 48000 Units	Pancrease Mt 16 by McNeil	52021-0343	Gastrointestinal
MCNEIL <> PANCREASEMT16	Cap, Clear & Peach	Lipase 16000 Unt, Amylase 48000 Unt, Protease 48000 Unt	Pancrease MT by Murfreesboro Ph	51129-1171	Gastrointestinal
MCNEIL <> PANCREASEMT20	Cap, White, Yellow Band, Yellow Beads	Amylase 56000 Units, Lipase 20000 Units, Protease 44000 Units	Pancrease Mt 20 by McNeil	00045-0346	Gastrointestinal
MCNEIL <> PANCREASEMT20	Cap, Yellow Band	Amylase 56000 Units, Lipase 20000 Units, Protease 44000 Units	Pancrease Mt 20 by McNeil	52021-0346	Gastrointestinal

ID FRONT <> BACK	DESCRIPTION FRONT <> BACK	INGREDIENT & STRENGTH	BRAND (OR EQUIV.) & FIRM	NDC#	CLASS; SCH.
MCNEIL <> PANCREASEMT4	Cap, Clear & Yellow	Amylase 12000 Units, Lipase 4000 Units, Protease 12000 Units	Pancrease Mt 4 by McNeil	00045-0341	Gastrointestinal
MCNEIL <> PANCREASEMT4	Cap	Amylase 12000 Units, Lipase 4000 Units, Protease 12000 Units	Pancrease Mt 4 by McNeil	52021-0341	Gastrointestinal
MCNEIL <> PARAFONFORTEDSC	Tab, Light Green, Coated, Parafon Forte DSC	Chlorzoxazone 500 mg	Parafon Forte DSC by Thrift Drug	59198-0089	Muscle Relaxant
MCNEIL <> PARAFONFORTEDSC	Tab, Lime Green, Coated, McNeil <> Parafon over Forte DSC	Chlorzoxazone 500 mg	Parafon Forte DSC by McNeil	00045-0325	Muscle Relaxant
MCNEIL <> PARAFONFORTEDSC	Tab, Coated	Chlorzoxazone 500 mg	Parafon Forte DSC by Allscripts	54569-1506	Muscle Relaxant
MCNEIL <> PARAFONFORTEDSC	Tab, Coated	Chlorzoxazone 500 mg	Parafon Forte DSC by Nat Pharmpak Serv	55154-1907	Muscle Relaxant
MCNEIL <> TOLECTIN200	Tab, White	Tolmetin Sodium 246 mg	Tolectin 200 by McNeil	00045-0412	NSAID
MCNEIL <> TOLECTIN600	Tab, Film Coated	Tolmetin Sodium 738 mg	by Pharmedix	53002-0597	NSAID
MCNEIL <> TOLECTINDS	Cap	Sodium 36 mg, Tolmetin Sodium 490 mg	Tolectin Ds by Thrift Drug	59198-0127	NSAID
MCNEIL <> TOLECTINDS	Cap, Orange, Gray Band	Tolmetin Sodium 400 mg	Tolectin Ds by McNeil	00045-0414	NSAID
MCNEIL <> TOLECTINDS	Cap	Tolmetin Sodium 492 mg	by Pharmedix	53002-0318	NSAID
MCNEIL <> TOLECTINDS	Cap, Contrasting Parallel Band	Tolmetin Sodium 492 mg	Tolectin Ds by Amerisource	62584-0414	NSAID
MCNEIL <> TYLCODEINE3	Tab, Tyl over Codeine 3	Acetaminophen 300 mg, Codeine Phosphate 30 mg	Tylenol Codeine No 3 by Quality Care	60346-0853	Analgesic; C III
MCNEIL <> TYLENOL3CODEINE	Tab, White	Acetaminophen 300 mg, Codeine Phosphate 30 mg	Tylenol Codeine No 3 by McNeil	00045-0513	Analgesic; C III
MCNEIL <> TYLENOL4CODEINE	Tab, White	Acetaminophen 300 mg, Codeine Phosphate 60 mg	Tylenol Codeine No 4 by McNeil	00045-0515	Analgesic; C III
MCNEIL <> TYLENOLCODEINE2	Tab, White	Acetaminophen 300 mg, Codeine Phosphate 15 mg	Tylenol Codeine No 2 by McNeil	00045-0511	Analgesic; C III
MCNEIL <> TYLENOLCODEINE2	Tab	Acetaminophen 300 mg, Codeine Phosphate 15 mg	Tylenol Codeine No 2 by Murfreesboro	51129-1393	Analgesic; C III
MCNEIL <> TYLENOLCODEINE3	Tab	Acetaminophen 300 mg, Codeine Phosphate 30 mg	Tylenol Codeine No 3 by Allscripts	54569-0024	Analgesic; C III
MCNEIL <> TYLENOLCODEINE3	Tab	Acetaminophen 300 mg, Codeine Phosphate 30 mg	Tylenol Codeine No 3 by Med Pro	53978-3087	Analgesic; C III
MCNEIL <> TYLENOLCODEINE4	Tab	Acetaminophen 300 mg, Codeine Phosphate 60 mg	Tylenol Codeine No 4 by Med Pro	53978-3094	Analgesic; C III
MCNEIL <> TYLENOLCODEINE4	Tab, White, Round	Codeine Phosphate 60 mg; Acetaminophen 300 mg	by Natl Pharmpak	55154-1916	Analgesic; C III
MCNEIL1520 <> 250	Tab, Coated	Levofloxacin 250 mg	Levaquin by McNeil	00045-1520	Antibiotic
MCNEIL1520 <> 250	Tab, Pink, Modified Rectangular, Film Coated	Levofloxacin 250 mg	Levaquin by Ortho	00062-1520	Antibiotic
MCNEIL1520 <> 250	Tab, Film Coated	Levofloxacin 250 mg	Levaquin by Johnson & Johnson	59604-0520	Antibiotic
MCNEIL1525 <> 500	Tab, Film Coated	Levofloxacin 500 mg	Levaquin by McNeil	00045-1525	Antibiotic
MCNEIL1525 <> 500	Tab, Peach, Modified Rectangular, Film Coated	Levofloxacin 500 mg	Levaquin by Ortho	00062-1525	Antibiotic
MCNEIL1525 <> 500	Tab, Film Coated	Levofloxacin 500 mg	Levaquin by Allscripts	54569-4489	Antibiotic
MCNEIL1525 <> 500	Tab, Peach, Rectangle, Film Coated	Levofloxacin 500 mg	Levaquin by Murfreesboro	51129-1629	Antibiotic
MCNEIL1525 <> 500	Tab, Film Coated	Levofloxacin 500 mg	Levaquin by Johnson & Johnson	59604-0525	Antibiotic
MCNEIL2	Tab, White, Round, McNeil/2	Acetaminophen 300 mg, Caffeine 15 mg, Codeine 15 mg	by McNeil	Canadian	Analgesic
MCNEIL3	Tab, White, Round, McNeil/3	Acetaminophen 300 mg, Caffeine 15 mg, Codeine 30 mg	by McNeil	Canadian	Analgesic

ID FRONT <> BACK	DESCRIPTION FRONT <> BACK	INGREDIENT & STRENGTH	BRAND (OR EQUIV.) & FIRM	NDC#	CLASS; SCH.
MCNEIL4	Tab, White, Round, McNeil/4	Acetaminophen 300 mg, Codeine 60 mg	by McNeil	Canadian	Analgesic
MCNEIL425200	Tab, White, Round, McNeil 425/200	Anhydrous Theophylline 100 mg	Duraphyl by Forest	00456-0632	Antiasthmatic
MCNEIL426200	Tab, White, Cap Shaped, McNeil 426/200	Anhydrous Theophylline 200 mg	Duraphyl by Forest	00456-0633	Antiasthmatic
MCNEIL427200	Tab, White, Cap Shaped, McNeil 427/200	Anhydrous Theophylline 300 mg	Duraphyl by Forest	00456-0634	Antiasthmatic
MCNEILHALDOL05MG	Tab, H Symbol, McNeil Haldol 0.5 mg	Haloperidol 0.5 mg	Haldol by McNeil	52021-0240	Antipsychotic
MCNEILHALDOL1	Tab, H Symbol	Haloperidol 1 mg	Haldol by HJ Harkins Co	52959-0356	Antipsychotic
MCNEILHALDOL10	Tab, H Symbol	Haloperidol 10 mg	Haldol by McNeil	52021-0246	Antipsychotic
MCNEILHALDOL1MG	Tab, H Symbol	Haloperidol 1 mg	Haldol by McNeil	52021-0241	Antipsychotic
MCNEILHALDOL20	Tab, H Symbol	Haloperidol 20 mg	Haldol by McNeil	52021-0248	Antipsychotic
MCNEILHALDOL2MG	Tab, H Symbol	Haloperidol 2 mg	Haldol by McNeil	52021-0242	Antipsychotic
MCNEILHALDOL5MG	Tab, H Symbol	Haloperidol 5 mg	Haldol by McNeil	52021-0245	Antipsychotic
McNEILPANCREASE	Cap, Clear & Natural, McNeil-Pancrease	Pancrelipase 4000 Units	Pancrease by McNeil	Canadian	Gastrointestinal
MCR <> TIMEHIST	Cap	Chlorpheniramine Maleate 8 mg, Pseudoephedrine HCl 120 mg	Time Hist by Sovereign	58716-0016	Cold Remedy
MCR513 <> ALLFEN	Tab, White, Oblong, Scored	Guaifenesin 1000 mg	by Pfab	62542-0907	Expectorant
MCR513 <> ALLFEN	Tab, White, Oblong	Guaifenesin 1000 mg	Allfen by AM Pharms	58605-0513	Expectorant
MCR514 <> MAXIFEDG	Tab, White, Oblong, Scored	Guaifenesin 550 mg; Pseudoephedrine HCl 60 mg	by Pfab	62542-0750	Cold Remedy
MCR514 <> MAXIFEDG	Tab, White, Oblong	Pseudoephedrine HCl 60 mg, Guaifenesin 550 mg	Maxifed G by RX PAK	65084-0109	Cold Remedy
MCR520 <> MAXIFED	Tab, Green, Oblong, Scored	Guaifenesin 700 mg, Pseudoephedrine HCl 80 mg	GFN 700 PSEH 80 by Med Pro	53978-3359	Cold Remedy
MCR520 <> MAXIFED	Tab, Green, Oblong, Scored	Pseudoephedrine HCl 80 mg, Guaifenesin 700 mg	Maxifed by RX PAK	65084-0110	Cold Remedy
MCR521 <> ALLFENDM	Tab, White, Oblong, Scored, MCR over 521 <> Allfen DM	Dextromethorphan Hydrobromide 50 mg, Guaifenesin 1000 mg	Allfen DM by DRX	55045-2650	Cold Remedy
MCR521 <> ALLFENDM	Tab, White, Oblong, Scored, MCR over 521 <> Allfen DM	Guaifenesin 1000 mg, Dextromethorphan Hydriodide 50 mg	GFN 1000 DTMH 50 by Mallinckrodt Hobart	00406-1122	Cold Remedy
MCR526 <> MAXIFEDDM	Tab, Scored	Guaifenesin 500 mg; Pseudoephedrine HCl 60 mg; Dextromethorphan Hydrobromide 30 mg	Maxifed DM by AM Pharms	58605-0526	Cold Remedy
MCR526 <> MAXIFEDDM	Tab, Scored	Guaifenesin 500 mg; Pseudoephedrine HCl 60 mg; Dextromethorphan Hydrobromide 30 mg	by Pfab	62542-0772	Cold Remedy
MD <> 450	Tab	Diethylpropion HCl 75 mg	by Jones	52604-9160	Antianorexiant; C IV
MD <> 502	Tab, Dark Green	Dextromethorphan Hydrobromide 30 mg, Guaifenesin 600 mg	Humigen DM by MD	43567-0502	Cold Remedy
MD <> 530	Tab, Light Blue, Round, Scored	Hethylphenidate HCl 10 mg	by Altimed	Canadian DIN# 02230321	CNS Stimulant
MD <> 530	Tab, Blue, Round, Scored	Methylphenidate HCl 10 mg	by Apothecon	59772-8841	Stimulant; C II
MD <> 530	Tab, Pale Blue & Green	Methylphenidate HCl 10 mg	by Medeva	53014-0530	Stimulant; C II
MD <> 530	Tab	Methylphenidate HCl 10 mg	by Qualitest	00603-4570	Stimulant; C II
MD <> 531	Tab, Yellow	Methylphenidate HCl 5 mg	by Medeva	53014-0531	Stimulant; C II
MD <> 531	Tab	Methylphenidate HCl 5 mg	by Qualitest	00603-4569	Stimulant; C II
MD <> 532	Tab, Orange, Round, Scored	Methylphenidate HCl 20 mg	by Apothecon	59772-8842	Stimulant; C II
MD <> 532	Tab, Orange	Methylphenidate HCl 20 mg	by Medeva	53014-0532	Stimulant; C II
MD <> 532	Tab, Orange, Round, Scored	Methylphenidate HCl 20 mg	by Altimed	Canadian DIN# 02230322	Stimulant
MD <> 535	Tab	Atropine Sulfate 0.025 mg, Diphenoxylate HCl 2.5 mg	Lonox by Quality Care	60346-0437	Antidiarrheal; C V
MD <> 562	Tab, White, Extended Release	Methylphenidate HCl 20 mg	by Medeva	53014-0562	Stimulant; C II
MD10	Tab, Pink, Round, Scored, M over D10	Doxazosin Mesylate 2mg	Cardura by UDL	51079-0958	Antihypertensive
MD11	Tab, Blue, Round, Scored, M over D11	Doxazosin Mesylate 4mg	Cardura by UDL	51079-0959	Antihypertensive
MD20	Tab, Purple, Oval	Hyoscyamine Sulfate 0.12 mg, Methenamine 81.6 mg, Methylene Blue 10.8 mg, Phenyl Salicylate 36.2 mg, Sodium Phosphate, Monobasic 40.8 mg	MD 20 by	00131-2093	Gastrointestinal
MD20	Tab, Coated, Imprinted MD-20	Hyoscyamine Sulfate 0.12 mg, Methenamine 81.6 mg, Methylene Blue 10.8 mg, Phenyl Salicylate 36.2 mg, Sodium Phosphate, Monobasic 40.8 mg	Urogesic Blue by Edwards	00485-0051	Gastrointestinal
MD20	Tab, Purple, Oval	Hyoscyamine Sulfate 0.12 mg, Methenamine 81.6 mg, Methylene Blue 10.8 mg, Phenyl Salicylate 36.2 mg, Sodium Phosphate, Monobasic 40.8 mg	Urogesic by Murfreesboro	51129-1504	Gastrointestinal

ID FRONT <> BACK	DESCRIPTION FRONT <> BACK	INGREDIENT & STRENGTH	BRAND (OR EQUIV.) & FIRM	NDC#	CLASS; SCH.
MD20	Tab, MD-20	Hyoscyamine Sulfate 0.12 mg, Methenamine 81.6 mg, Methylene Blue 10.8 mg, Phenyl Salicylate 36.2 mg, Sodium Phosphate, Monobasic 40.8 mg	Urimar T by Shire Richwood	58521-0945	Gastrointestinal
MD20	Tab, Sugar Coated, Imprinted MD-20	Hyoscyamine Sulfate 0.12 mg, Methenamine 81.6 mg, Methylene Blue 10.8 mg, Phenyl Salicylate 36.2 mg, Sodium Phosphate, Monobasic 40.8 mg	Urimar T by Marnel	00682-0333	Gastrointestinal
MD20	Tab, Coated, Imprinted MD-20	Hyoscyamine Sulfate 0.12 mg, Methenamine 81.6 mg, Methylene Blue 10.8 mg, Phenyl Salicylate 36.2 mg, Sodium Phosphate, Monobasic 40.8 mg	Uro Blue by RA McNeil	12830-0301	Gastrointestinal
MD451	Tab, Blue, Oblong, MD/451	Guaifenesin 600 mg, Pseudoephedrine HCl 120 mg	Entex PSE by MD		Cold Remedy
MD518	Tab, MD Over 518	Diethylpropion HCl 25 mg	by Quality Care	60346-0060	Antianorexiant; C IV
MD530	Tab, White, Round, MD/530	Methylphenidate 10 mg	by Technilab	Canadian	Stimulant
MD531	Tab	Methylphenidate HCl 5 mg	by Schein	00364-0561	Stimulant; C II
MD532	Tab	Methylphenidate HCl 20 mg	by Schein	00364-0562	Stimulant; C II
MD532	Tab, Debossed 532 and MD	Methylphenidate HCl 20 mg	by Zenith Goldline	00182-1174	Stimulant; C II
MD538	Tab, Pink, Round	Amitriptyline HCl 10 mg	Elavil by MD		Antidepressant
MD539	Tab, Green, Round	Amitriptyline HCl 25 mg	Elavil by MD		Antidepressant
MD540	Tab, Brown, Round	Amitriptyline HCl 50 mg	Elavil by MD		Antidepressant
MD541	Tab, Purple, Round	Amitriptyline HCl 75 mg	Elavil by MD		Antidepressant
MD542	Tab, Orange, Round	Amitriptyline HCl 100 mg	Elavil by MD		Antidepressant
MD543	Tab, Flesh, Round	Amitriptyline HCl 150 mg	Elavil by MD		Antidepressant
MD562	Tab, White, Round, MD/562	Methylphenidate HCl ER 20 mg	Ritalin SR by MD		Stimulant; C II
MD6	Tab, Blue, Round, M over D6	Dicyclomine HCl 20 mg	by UDL	51079-0119	Gastrointestinal
MD711	Tab, White, Round	Triprolidine 2.5 mg, Pseudoephedrine 60 mg	Actifed by MD		Cold Remedy
MD9	Tab, White to Off-White, Round, Scored, M over D9	Doxazosin Mesylate 1 mg	Cardura by UDL	51079-0957	Antihypertensive
MDC	Tab, Blue, Round, M D-C	Hydrocodone Bitartrate 5 mg, Acetaminophen 500 mg	Doucet by Mason		Analgesic; C III
MDP	Tab, Pink, Round, M D-P	Hydrocodone Bitartrate 5 mg, Aspirin 224 mg, Caffeine 32 mg	Damason-P by Mason		Analgesic; C III
ME	Tab, Orange, Round, Abbott Logo	Methamphetamine HCl LR 10 mg	Desoxyn by Abbott	00074-6948	Stimulant; C II
ME15	Tab, White, Round, Scored, M over E15	Enalapril Maleate 2.5 mg	Vasotec by UDL	51079-0950	Antihypertensive
ME16	Tab, White, Round, Scored, M over E 16	Enalapril Maleate 5 mg	Vasotec by UDL	51079-0951	Antihypertensive
ME17	Tab, Light Blue, Round, M over E 17	Enalapril Maleate 10 mg	Vasotec by UDL	51079-0952	Antihypertensive
ME18	Tab, Medium Blue, Round, M over E 18	Enalapril Maleate 20 mg	Vasotec by UDL	51079-0953	Antihypertensive
ME7	Tab, Yellow, Round, Scored	Estropipate 0.75 mg	by Mylan	55160-0134	Hormone
ME7	Tab, Yellow, Round, Scored	Estropipate 0.75 mg	by Mylan Pharms	00378-4551	Hormone
ME8	Tab, Peach, Round, Scored	Estropipate 1.5 mg	by Mylan	55160-0135	Hormone
ME8	Tab, Peach, Round, Scored	Estropipate 1.5 mg	by Mylan Pharms	00378-4553	Hormone
ME9	Tab, Blue, Round, Scored	Estropipate 3 mg	by Mylan	55160-0136	Hormone
ME9	Tab, Blue, Round, Scored	Estropipate 3 mg	by Mylan Pharms	00378-4555	Hormone
MEDEVA <> 012	Tab, Green, Oblong, Scored,	Guaifenesin 600 mg	Humibid LA by Lilly	00110-0894	Expectorant
MEDEVA <> 012	Tab, Light Green, Scored	Guaifenesin 600 mg	Humibid LA by Medeva	53014-0012	Expectorant
MEDEVA <> 012	Tab, Light Green, Scored	Guaifenesin 600 mg	Humibid LA by Adams	53014-0012	Expectorant
MEDEVA <> 012	Tab, Light Green, Scored	Guaifenesin 600 mg (PM Tablet)	Syn-Rx by Medeva	53014-0308	Expectorant
MEDEVA <> 012	Tab	Guaifenesin 600 mg, Pseudoephedrine HCl 60 mg	Syn Rx by Adams	53014-0308	Cold Remedy
MEDEVA <> 015	Tab, Light Blue, Scored,	Guaifenesin 400 mg, Pseudoephedrine HCl 120 mg	Deconsal LA by Medeva	53014-0015	Cold Remedy
MEDEVA <> 015	Tab, Scored	Guaifenesin 400 mg, Pseudoephedrine HCl 120 mg	Deconsal LA by Adams	53014-0015	Cold Remedy
MEDEVA <> 017	Tab, Scored	Guaifenesin 600 mg, Pseudoephedrine HCl 60 mg	Deconsal II by Mallinckrodt Hobart	00406-0552	Cold Remedy
MEDEVA <> 017	Tab, Scored	Guaifenesin 600 mg, Pseudoephedrine HCl 60 mg	Deconsal II by Adams	53014-0017	Cold Remedy
MEDEVA <> 017	Tab, Dark Blue, Scored	Guaifenesin 600 mg, Pseudoephedrine HCl 60 mg	Deconsal II by Medeva	53014-0017	Cold Remedy
MEDEVA <> 017	Tab	Guaifenesin 600 mg, Pseudoephedrine HCl 60 mg	Syn Rx by Adams	53014-0308	Cold Remedy
MEDEVA <> 017	Tab, Dark Blue, Scored	Psuedoephedrine HCl 60 mg, Guaifenesin 600 mg (AM tablet)	Syn-Rx by Medeva	53014-0308	Cold Remedy
MEDEVA <> 030	Tab, Green, Oblong, Scored	Dextromethorphan Hydrobromide 30 mg, Guaifenesin 600 mg	Humibid DM by DRX	55045-2634	Cold Remedy
MEDEVA <> 030	Tab, Dark Green, Scored	Dextromethorphan Hydrobromide 30 mg, Guaifenesin 600 mg	Humibid DM by Medeva	53014-0030	Cold Remedy
MEDEVA <> 030	Tab, Dark Green, Scored	Dextromethorphan Hydrobromide 30 mg, Guaifenesin 600 mg	Humibid DM by Adams	53014-0030	Cold Remedy
MEDEVA <> 12	Tab, Green, Oblong, Scored	Guaifenesin 600 mg	Humibid LA by Phy Total Care	54868-1777	Expectorant
MEDEVA <> 12	Tab, Green, Oblong, Scored	Guaifenesin 600 mg	Humabid LA by Adams Labs	63824-0012	Expectorant

ID FRONT ◇ BACK	DESCRIPTION FRONT ◇ BACK	INGREDIENT & STRENGTH	BRAND (OR EQUIV.) & FIRM	NDC#	CLASS; SCH.
MEDEVA ◇ 12	Tab, Green, Oblong, Scored	Guaifenesin 600 mg	Humibid LA by Compumed	00403-1009	Expectorant
MEDEVA ◇ 12	Tab, Green, Oblong, Scored	Guaifenesin 600 mg; Pseudoephedrine HCl 60 mg	Syn Rx by Adams Labs	63824-0308	Cold Remedy
MEDEVA ◇ 15	Tab, Blue, Scored	Guaifenesin 400 mg; Pseudoephedrine HCl 120 mg	Deconsal LA by Adams Labs	63824-0015	Cold Remedy
MEDEVA ◇ 17	Tab, Blue, Oblong, Scored	Guaifenesin 600 mg; Pseudoephedrine HCl 60 mg	Syn Rx by Adams Labs	63824-0308	Cold Remedy
MEDEVA ◇ 17	Tab, Blue, Scored	Guaifenesin 600 mg; Pseudoephedrine HCl 60 mg	Deconsal LA by Adams Labs	63824-0017	Cold Remedy
MEDEVA ◇ 30	Tab, Green, Oblong, Scored	Guaifenesin 600 mg; Dextromethorphan Hydrobromide 30 mg	Humibid DM by Adams Labs	63824-0030	Cold Remedy
MEDEVA ◇ 309	Tab	Dextromethorphan Hydrobromide 30 mg, Guaifenesin 600 mg, Pseudoephedrine HCl 60 mg	Syn Rx DM by Adams	53014-0311	Cold Remedy
MEDEVA ◇ 309	Tab, Yellow, Scored	Dextromethorphan Hydrobromide 30 mg, Guaifenesin 600 mg, Pseudoephedrine HCl 60 mg	Syn Rx DM by Medeva	53014-0311	Cold Remedy
MEDEVA ◇ 309	Tab, Yellow, Oblong, Scored	Guaifenesin 600 mg; Pseudoephedrine HCl 60 mg; Dextromethorphan Hydrobromide 30 mg	Syn Rx by Adams Labs	63824-0311	Cold Remedy
MEDEVA ◇ 310	Tab	Dextromethorphan Hydrobromide 30 mg, Guaifenesin 600 mg, Pseudoephedrine HCl 60 mg	Syn Rx DM by Adams	53014-0311	Cold Remedy
MEDEVA ◇ 310	Tab, Light Blue, Scored,	Dextromethorphan Hydrobromide 30 mg, Guaifenesin 600 mg, Pseudoephedrine HCl 60 mg	Syn Rx DM by Medeva	53014-0311	Cold Remedy
MEDEVA ◇ 310	Tab, Blue, Oblong, Scored	Guaifenesin 600 mg; Pseudoephedrine HCl 60 mg; Dextromethorphan Hydrobromide 30 mg	Syn Rx by Adams Labs	63824-0311	Cold Remedy
MEDEVA ◇ 400	Cap, White & Yellow	Chlorpheniramine Maleate 4 mg, Pseudoephedrine HCl 60 mg	Atrohist Ped by Medeva	53014-0400	Cold Remedy
MEDEVA ◇ 400	Cap	Chlorpheniramine Maleate 4 mg, Pseudoephedrine HCl 60 mg	Atrohist Ped by Adams	53014-0400	Cold Remedy
MEDEVA ◇ 400	Cap, White & Yellow	Pseudoephedrine HCl 60 mg, Chlorpheniramine Maleate 4 mg	Atrohist by Adams Labs	63824-0400	Cold Remedy
MEDEVA ◇ 402	Cap, Clear & Green	Guaifenesin 300 mg	Humibid by Adams Labs	63824-0402	Expectorant
MEDEVA ◇ 402	Cap	Guaifenesin 300 mg	Humibid Ped by Adams	53014-0402	Expectorant
MEDEVA ◇ 402	Cap, Clear & Green, White Beads	Guaifenesin 300 mg	Humibid Ped by Medeva	53014-0402	Expectorant
MEDEVA ◇ SEMPREXD	Cap, Printed in White Ink ◇ Semprex-D	Acrivastine 8 mg, Pseudoephedrine HCl 60 mg	Semprex D by Catalytica	63552-0404	Cold Remedy
MEDEVA ◇ SEMPREXD	Cap, Dark Green & White, Yellow Band	Acrivastine 8 mg, Pseudoephedrine HCl 60 mg	Semprex D by Medeva	53014-0404	Cold Remedy
MEDEVA012	Tab	Guaifenesin 600 mg, Pseudoephedrine HCl 60 mg	Syn Rx by Medeva	53014-0308	Cold Remedy
MEDEVA017	Tab, Blue, Medeva/017	Pseudophedrine HCl 60 mg, Guaifenesin 600 mg	Deconsal II by Medeva		Cold Remedy
MEDEVA024	Tab, Yellow, Medeva/0 24	Pheny. HCl 25 mg, Phenypr. HCl 50 mg, Chlorphen. Mal 8 mg, Hyso 0.19 mg, Atro 0.04 mg, Scopolamine HBr 0.01 mg	Atrohist Plus by Medeva	53014-0024	Cold Remedy
MEDEVA401	Cap, Blue & Clear, with White Beads	Phenylephrine HCl 10 mg, Guaifenesin 300 mg	Deconsal Ped by Medeva	53014-0401	Cold Remedy
MEDICIS ◇ 049750MG	Cap, 0497 50MG	Minocycline HCl	Dynacin by Thrift Drug	59198-0276	Antibiotic
MEDICIS ◇ 0498100MG	Cap, 0498 100 MG	Minocycline HCl	Dynacin by Medicis	99207-0498	Antibiotic
MEDICIS ◇ 0498100MG	Cap, 0498 100MG	Minocycline HCl	Dynacin by Thrift Drug	59198-0277	Antibiotic
MEDROL16	Tab, White, Elliptical, Scored	Methylprednisolone 16 mg	by Upjohn	Canadian DIN# 00036129	Steroid
MEDROL8	Tab	Methylprednisolone 8 mg	Medrol by Allscripts	54569-4516	Steroid
MEDTEK	Tab, Med/Tek	Acetaminophen 500 mg, Chlorpheniramine Maleate 2 mg, Pseudoephedrine HCl 30 mg	Lorsin by Pharmafab	62542-0800	Cold Remedy
MEDTEK	Tab, Med/Tek	Acetaminophen 500 mg, Chlorpheniramine Maleate 2 mg, Pseudoephedrine HCl 30 mg	Sinumed by Anabolic	00722-6315	Cold Remedy
MEDTEK	Tab, MED/TEK	Hyoscyamine Sulfate 0.125 mg	Medispaz by Anabolic	00722-6352	Gastrointestinal
MEDTEK	Tab, MED/TEK	Meclizine HCl 30 mg	Medivert by Anabolic	00722-6312	Antiemetic
MEGACE ◇ 40	Tab, Light Blue, Flat-faced, Bevel-edged	Megestrol Acetate 40 mg	Megace by Mead Johnson	00015-0596	Progestin
MEGESTROL40 ◇ PCH	Tab, White, Scored	Megestrol Acetate 40 mg	by Pharmachemie NI	57527-0513	Progestin

ID FRONT <> BACK	DESCRIPTION FRONT <> BACK	INGREDIENT & STRENGTH	BRAND (OR EQUIV.) & FIRM	NDC#	CLASS; SCH.
MEGESTROL40 <> PCH	Tab, White, Scored, Megestrol over 40 <> PCH	Megestrol Acetate 40 mg	by Teva Pharms	00093-5138	Progestin
MELLARIL100 <> S	Tab, Coated, Mellaril 100 <> S in triangle	Thioridazine HCl 100 mg	Mellaril by Novartis	00078-0005	Antipsychotic
MELLARIL25 <> S	Tab, Coated, Mellaril 25 <> S in triangle	Thioridazine HCl 25 mg	Mellaril by Novartis	00078-0003	Antipsychotic
MELLARIL50 <> S	Tab, Coated, Mellaril 50 <> S in triangle	Thioridazine HCl 50 mg	Mellaril by Novartis	00078-0004	Antipsychotic
MEPHYTON <> MSD43	Tab	Phytonadione 5 mg	Mephyton by Quality Care	60346-0696	Vitamin
MEPROSPAN200	Cap, Yellow	Meprobamate 200 mg	Meprospan by Wallace	00037-1401	Sedative/Hypnotic; C IV
MEPROSPAN400	Cap, Blue	Meprobamate 400 mg	Meprospan by Wallace	00037-1301	Sedative/Hypnotic; C IV
MERICON	Tab, Tan, Merigon Logo	Ginkgo Biloba 60 mg	Ginkgo by Mericon		Supplement
MERICONLOGO	Tab, Brown	Zinc 10 mg	Orazinc by Mericon		Mineral Supplement
MERIDIA <> 10	Cap, Blue & White	Sibutramine HCl 10 mg	Meridia by Knoll	00048-0610	Anorexiant; C IV
MERIDIA <> 10	Cap	Sibutramine HCl 10 mg	Meridia by DRX	55045-2555	Anorexiant; C IV
MERIDIA <> 10	Cap	Sibutramine HCl 10 mg	Meridia by Quality Care	62682-7049	Anorexiant; C IV
MERIDIA <> 10	Cap, -10-	Sibutramine HCl 10 mg	Meridia by BASF	10117-0610	Anorexiant; C IV
MERIDIA <> 10	Cap, Blue & White	Sibutramine HCl 10 mg	Meridia by Compumed	00403-5373	Anorexiant; C IV
MERIDIA <> 10	Cap, Blue & White	Sibutramine HCl 10 mg	Meridia by PDRX Pharms	55289-0375	Anorexiant; C IV
MERIDIA <> 10	Cap, Blue & White	Sibutramine HCl 10 mg	Meridia by Apotheca	12634-0534	Anorexiant; C IV
MERIDIA <> 15	Cap, White & Yellow	Sibutraline HCl 15 mg	Meridia by PDRX Pharms	55289-0380	Anorexiant; C IV
MERIDIA <> 15	Cap, White & Yellow	Sibutramine HCl 15 mg	Meridia by Apotheca	12634-0545	Anorexiant; C IV
MERIDIA <> 15	Cap, Yellow & White	Sibutramine HCl 15 mg	Meridia by Knoll	00048-0615	Anorexiant; C IV
MERIDIA <> 15	Cap, White & Yellow	Sibutramine HCl 15 mg	Meridia		Anorexiant; C IV
MERIDIA <> 15	Cap	Sibutramine HCl 15 mg	Meridia by Quality Care	62682-7050	Anorexiant; C IV
MERIDIA <> 15	Cap, -15-	Sibutramine HCl 15 mg	Meridia by BASF	10117-0615	Anorexiant; C IV
MERIDIA <> 15	Cap, White & Yellow	Sibutramine HCl 15 mg	Meridia by Compumed	00403-5375	Anorexiant; C IV
MERIDIA <> 5	Cap, Blue & Yellow	Sibutramine HCl 5 mg	Meridia by Knoll	00048-0605	Anorexiant; C IV
MERIDIA <> 5	Cap, Blue & Yellow	Sibutramine HCl 5 mg	Meridia		Anorexiant; C IV
MERIDIA <> 5	Cap	Sibutramine HCl 5 mg	Meridia by Quality Care	62682-7048	Anorexiant; C IV
MERIDIA <> 5	Cap, Blue & Yellow	Sibutramine HCl 5 mg	Meridia by Compumed	00403-5371	Anorexiant; C IV
MERIDIA <> 5	Cap, -5-	Sibutramine HCl 5 mg	Meridia by BASF	10117-0605	Anorexiant; C IV
MERIDIA <> 5	Cap, Blue & Yellow	Sibutramine HCl 5 mg	Meridia by PDRX Pharms	55289-0377	Anorexiant; C IV
MERRELL277	Tab, Yellow, Oblong	Methenamine Hippurate 1 GM	Hiprex by Hoechst Marion Roussel	00068-0277	Antibiotic; Urinary Tract
MERRELL37	Tab, Yellow, Round	Metenzolate Bromide 25 mg	Cantil by Hoechst Marion Roussel	00068-0037	Antispasmodic
MERRELL62	Tab, Pink, Round	Trichlormethiazide 2 mg	Metahydrin by Hoechst Marion Roussel		Diuretic
MERRELL63	Tab, Blue, Round	Trichlormethiazide 4 mg	Metahydrin by Hoechst Marion Roussel		Diuretic
MERRELL64	Tab, Yellow, Round	Trichlormethiazide 2 mg, Reserpine 0.1 mg	Metatensin #2 by Hoechst Marion Roussel		Diuretic; Antihypertensive
MERRELL65	Tab, Lavender, Round	Trichlormethiazide 4 mg, Reserpine 0.1 mg	Metatensin #4 by Hoechst Marion Roussel		Diuretic; Antihypertensive
MERRELL69	Cap, Clear & Green	Chlorotrianisene 12 mg	by RP Scherer	11014-0152	Hormone
MERRELL690	Cap, Clear & Forest Green, Gelatin	Chlorotrianisene 12 mg	Tace Twelve by RP Scherer	11014-1224	Hormone
MERRELL691	Cap, Green	Chlorotrianisene 25 mg	Tace by Merrell		Hormone
MERRELL692	Cap, Green & Yellow	Chlorotrianisene 72 mg	Tace by Merrell		Hormone
MERRELL697	Tab, White, Round	Diethylpropion HCl 25 mg	Tenuate by Hoechst Marion Roussel	00068-0697	Antianorexiant; C IV
MERRELL698	Tab, White, Oblong	Diethylpropion HCl 75 mg	Tenuate Dospan by Hoechst Marion Roussel	00068-0698	Antianorexiant; C IV
MERRELL725	Tab, White, Round	Terbutaline Sulfate 2.5 mg	Bricanyl by Merrell		Antiasthmatic
MESLON10	Cap, White, M-Eslon 10	Morphine Sulfate 10 mg	M-Eslon by Rhone-Poulenc Rorer	Canadian	Analgesic
MESLON100	Cap, White, M-Eslon 100	Morphine Sulfate 100 mg	M-Eslon by Rhone-Poulenc Rorer	Canadian	Analgesic
MESLON30	Cap, White, M-Eslon 30	Morphine Sulfate 30 mg	M-Eslon by Rhone-Poulenc Rorer	Canadian	Analgesic
MESLON60	Cap, White, M-Eslon 60	Morphine Sulfate 60 mg	M-Eslon by Rhone-Poulenc Rorer	Canadian	Analgesic
MESTINON60ICN	Tab, White, Mestinon 60-ICN	Pyridostigmine 60 mg	by ICN	Canadian	Muscle Stimulant
MET10832	Tab, White, Round, MET-10/832	Metoclopramide HCl 10 mg	Reglan by Rosemont		Gastrointestinal

425

ID FRONT <> BACK	DESCRIPTION FRONT <> BACK	INGREDIENT & STRENGTH	BRAND (OR EQUIV.) & FIRM	NDC#	CLASS; SCH.
METHADOSE10	Tab, White, Round	Methadone HCl 10 mg	Dolophine by Mallinckrodt		Analgesic; C II
METHADOSE10	Tab, White, Round, Scored	Methadone HCl 10 mg	Dolophine by Mallinckrodt Hobart	00406-3454	Analgesic; C II
METHADOSE40	Tab, White, Round	Methadone HCl 40 mg	Disket by Mallinckrodt		Analgesic; C II
METHADOSE40	Tab, White, Round, Quadrisected	Methadone HCl 40 mg	Dolophine by Mallinckrodt Hobart	00406-0540	Analgesic; C II
METHADOSE5	Tab, White, Round	Methadone HCl 5 mg	Dolophine by Mallinckrodt		Analgesic; C II
METHADOSE5	Tab, White, Round, Scored	Methadone HCl 5 mg	Dolophine by Mallinckrodt Hobart	00406-6974	Analgesic; C II
METOPBPPMS100S	Tab, White, Circular, Metop-B/pPMS 100s	Metoprolol Tartrate 100 mg	by Pharmascience	Canadian	Antihypertensive
METOPBSPMS50S	Tab, White, Circular, Metop-B/pPMS 50s	Metoprolol Tartrate 50 mg	by Pharmascience	Canadian	Antihypertensive
MEVACOR <> MSD730	Tab, Peach, Octagonal	Lovastatin 10 mg	Mevacor by Merck	00006-0730	Antihyperlipidemic
MEVACOR <> MSD730	Tab, MSD/730	Lovastatin 10 mg	by Kaiser	00179-1209	Antihyperlipidemic
MEVACOR <> MSD731	Tab, Blue, Octagonal, MSD 731 <> Mevacor	Lovastatin 20 mg	by Allscripts	54569-0613	Antihyperlipidemic
MEVACOR <> MSD731	Tab, Blue, Octagon	Lovastatin 20 mg	Mevacor by Va Cmop	65243-0045	Antihyperlipidemic
MEVACOR <> MSD731	Tab	Lovastatin 20 mg	by Nat Pharmpak Serv	55154-5004	Antihyperlipidemic
MEVACOR <> MSD731	Tab	Lovastatin 20 mg	Mevacor by Allscripts	54569-0613	Antihyperlipidemic
MEVACOR <> MSD731	Tab	Lovastatin 20 mg	by Pharmedix	53002-0570	Antihyperlipidemic
MEVACOR <> MSD731	Tab, MSD 731	Lovastatin 20 mg	by Amerisource	62584-0426	Antihyperlipidemic
MEVACOR <> MSD731	Tab, Green, Octagon	Lovastatin 40 mg	Mevacor by PDRX Pharms	55289-0548	Antihyperlipidemic
MEVACOR <> MSD732	Tab, Green, Octagonal	Lovastatin 40 mg	Mevacor by Merck	00006-0732	Antihyperlipidemic
MEVACOR <> MSD732	Tab	Lovastatin 40 mg	by Allscripts	54569-3256	Antihyperlipidemic
MF	Tab, Yellow, Round, Abbott Logo	Methamphetamine HCl LR 15 mg	Desoxyn by Abbott	00074-6959	Stimulant; C II
MF1	Tab, White, MF/1	Metformin HCl 500 mg	by Genpharm	Canadian	Antidiabetic
MFG	Tab, White, MF/G	Metformin HCl 500 mg	by BDH	Canadian	Antidiabetic
MGH	Cap, Lavender, White Print	Acetaminophen 500 mg, Hydrocodone Bitartrate 5 mg	Dolorex Forte by A G Marin	12539-0984	Analgesic; C III
MGI <> 705	Tab, Film Coated	Pilocarpine HCl 5 mg	Salagen by MGI	58063-0705	Cholinergic Agonist
MGI705	Tab, Film Coated	Pilocarpine HCl 5 mg	Salagen by Physicians Total Care	54868-3447	Cholinergic Agonist
MIA <> 093	Tab	Chlorpheniramine Tannate 8 mg, Phenylephrine Tannate 25 mg, Pyrilamine Tannate 25 mg	by Zenith Goldline	00182-1912	Cold Remedy
MIA <> 093	Tab	Chlorpheniramine Tannate 8 mg, Phenylephrine Tannate 25 mg, Pyrilamine Tannate 25 mg	Rhinatate by Major	00904-1669	Cold Remedy
MIA <> 093	Tab	Chlorpheniramine Tannate 8 mg, Phenylephrine Tannate 25 mg, Pyrilamine Tannate 25 mg	Histatan by Zenith Goldline	00172-4376	Cold Remedy
MIA <> 108	Tab	Acetaminophen 500 mg, Hydrocodone Bitartrate 5 mg	by Zenith Goldline	00172-5643	Analgesic; C III
MIA <> 110	Tab	Acetaminophen 325 mg, Butalbital 50 mg, Caffeine 40 mg	by Quality Care	60346-0703	Analgesic
MIA <> 253	Cap, White Print	Acetaminophen 325 mg, Dichloralantipyrine 100 mg, Isometheptene Mucate 65 mg	Midrin by Carnrick	00086-0120	Analgesic
MIA <> 253	Cap, White Print	Acetaminophen 325 mg, Dichloralantipyrine 100 mg, Isometheptene Mucate 65 mg	Migratine by Major	00904-7622	Cold Remedy
MIA093	Tab, Beige, Cap-Shaped, MIA/093	Phenylephrine Tannate 25 mg, Chlorpheniramine Tannate 8 mg, Pyrilamine Tannate 25 mg	Tanamine by Mikart	46672-0093	Cold Remedy
MIA106	Tab	Acetaminophen 325 mg, Butalbital 50 mg	Marten Tab by Marnel	00682-1400	Analgesic
MIA106	Tab, MIA/106	Acetaminophen 325 mg, Butalbital 50 mg	by Mikart	46672-0099	Analgesic
MIA108	Tab, White, Cap Shaped, Scored, MIA/108	Acetaminophen 500 mg, Hydrocodone 5 mg	by Inwood	00258-3666	Analgesic; C III
MIA108	Tab, White, Cap Shaped	Acetaminophen 500 mg, Hydrocodone Bitartrate 5 mg	by Inwood	00258-3666	Analgesic; C III
MIA108	Tab	Acetaminophen 500 mg, Hydrocodone Bitartrate 5 mg	by Mikart	46672-0052	Analgesic; C III
MIA108	Tab, MIA 108	Acetaminophen 500 mg, Hydrocodone Bitartrate 5 mg	by Quality Care	60346-0442	Analgesic; C III
MIA110	Tab	Acetaminophen 325 mg, Butalbital 50 mg, Caffeine 40 mg	Bac by Diversified Healthcare Serv	55887-0988	Analgesic
MIA110	Tab	Acetaminophen 325 mg, Butalbital 50 mg, Caffeine 40 mg	by Zenith Goldline	00182-1274	Analgesic
MIA110	Tab, MIA/110	Acetaminophen 325 mg, Butalbital 50 mg, Caffeine 40 mg	by Qualitest	00603-2547	Analgesic
MIA110	Tab	Acetaminophen 325 mg, Butalbital 50 mg, Caffeine 40 mg	by Geneva	00781-1901	Analgesic
MIA110	Tab, White, Cap Shaped, Scored, MIA/110	Acetaminophen 325 mg, Butalbital 50 mg, Caffeine 40 mg	by Inwood	00258-3665	Analgesic
MIA110	Tab, MIA/110	Acetaminophen 325 mg, Butalbital 50 mg, Caffeine 40 mg	by Rugby	00536-5567	Analgesic
MIA110	Tab, White, Cap Shaped, MIA/110	Acetaminophen 325 mg, Butalbital 50 mg, Caffeine 40 mg	Fioricet by Martec	52555-0647	Analgesic
MIA110	Tab, White, Cap Shaped	Acetaminophen 325 mg, Butalbital 50 mg, Caffeine 40 mg	by Mikart	46672-0053	Analgesic
MIA110	Tab	Aspirin 325 mg, Butalbital 50 mg, Caffeine 40 mg	by Physicians Total Care	54868-1075	Analgesic; C III

ID FRONT <> BACK	DESCRIPTION FRONT <> BACK	INGREDIENT & STRENGTH	BRAND (OR EQUIV.) & FIRM	NDC#	CLASS; SCH.
MIA111	Tab, White, Round	Yohimbine HCl 5.4 mg	Yocon by Mikart		Impotence Agent
MIA112	Tab, Debossed	Acetaminophen 650 mg, Butalbital 50 mg	Dolgic by CTEX	62022-0073	Analgesic
MIA112	Tab, MIA/112	Acetaminophen 650 mg, Butalbital 50 mg	by Mikart	46672-0098	Analgesic
MIA112	Tab, Blue, Oblong	Butalbital 50 mg; Acetaminophen 650 mg	Promacet by AM Pharms	58605-0524	Analgesic
MIA253	Cap	Acetaminophen 325 mg, Dichloralantipyrine 100 mg, Isometheptene Mucate 65 mg	Migquin by Qualitest	00603-4664	Cold Remedy
MICRIZIDE125	Cap, Green	Hydrochlorothiazide 12.5 mg	Microzide by Allscripts	54569-4912	Diuretic
MICROK <> AHR5720	Cap, ER, Micro K <> AHR 5720	Potassium Chloride 600 mg	Micro K by A H Robins	00031-5720	Electrolytes
MICROK <> AHR5720	Cap, ER, Micro-K	Potassium Chloride 600 mg	by Med Pro	53978-0155	Electrolytes
MICROK <> AHR5720	Cap, ER, Micro K <> AHR 5720	Potassium Chloride 600 mg	Micro K by Thrift Drug	59198-0310	Electrolytes
MICROK <> AHR5720	Cap, Orange	Potassium Chloride 600 mg	Micro K Extencaps by Promeco SA	64674-0019	Electrolytes
MICROK <> AHR5720	Cap, ER, AHR/5720	Potassium Chloride 600 mg	Micro K by Nat Pharmpak Serv	55154-3010	Electrolytes
MICROK <> AHR5730	Cap, Micro-K <> AHR/5730	Potassium Chloride 750 mg	Micro K 10 by Allscripts	54569-0660	Electrolytes
MICROK <> AHR5730	Cap, ER	Potassium Chloride 600 mg	Micro K by Leiner	59606-0691	Electrolytes
MICROK <> THERRX010	Cap, Orange, Gelatin, Micro-K <> Ther-Rx 010	Potassium Chloride 600 mg	by KV Pharmaceutical	64011-0010	Electrolytes
MICROK10	Cap, Pale Orange, Ex Release, Micro-K 10	Potassium Chloride 750 mg	Micro K by Nat Pharmpak Serv	55154-3009	Electrolytes
MICROK10 <> AHR5	Cap, ER, Micro-K 10 <> AHR 5	Potassium Chloride 750 mg	by Med Pro	53978-5044	Electrolytes
MICROK10 <> AHR5730	Cap, ER, Micro-K 10 <> AHR 5730	Potassium Chloride 750 mg	Micro K 10 by A H Robins	00031-5730	Electrolytes
MICROK10 <> AHR5730	Cap, ER, AHR/5730	Potassium Chloride 750 mg	Micro K 10 by Wal Mart	49035-0153	Electrolytes
MICROK10 <> AHR5730	Cap, ER	Potassium Chloride 750 mg	Micro K by PDRX	55289-0899	Electrolytes
MICROK10 <> AHR5730	Cap, ER, Micro-K 10 <> AHR 5730	Potassium Chloride 750 mg	Micro K by Nat Pharmpak Serv	55154-3012	Electrolytes
MICROK10 <> AHR5730	Cap, ER, Micro-K 10 <> AHR 5730	Potassium Chloride 750 mg	Micro K 10 by Amerisource	62584-0730	Electrolytes
MICROK10 <> AHR5730	Cap, Micro-K 10 <> AHR/5730	Potassium Chloride 750 mg	Micro K 10 by Leiner	59606-0772	Electrolytes
MICROK10 <> AHR5730	Cap, ER, Micro-K 10 <> AHR 5730	Potassium Chloride 750 mg	Micro K 10 by Thrift Drug	59198-0229	Electrolytes
MICROK10 <> THERRX009	Cap, Orange & White, Opaque, Gelatin, Micro-K 10 <> Ther-Rx 009	Potassium Chloride 750 mg	Micro K by Ther Rx	64011-0009	Electrolytes
MICROK10 <> THERRX009	Cap, Light Orange & White, Micro-K 10 <> Ther-Rx 009	Potassium Chloride 750 mg	by Allscripts	54569-0660	Electrolytes
MICROK10AHR5730	Cap, Orange & White	Potassium Chloride 750 mg	Micro K by Rx Pac	65084-0193	Electrolytes
MICROKAHR5720	Cap, Pale Orange, Ex Release	Potassium Chloride 600 mg	Micro K by Caremark	00339-5239	Electrolytes
MICROKAHR5720	Cap, Pale Orange, Ex Release, Micro-K AHR Over 5720	Potassium Chloride 600 mg	Micro K by Amerisource	62584-0720	Electrolytes
MICRONASE	Tab	Glyburide 2.5 mg	by Med Pro	53978-0693	Antidiabetic
MICRONASE25	Tab, Mlicronase/2.5	Glyburide 2.5 mg	Micronase by Nat Pharmpak Serv	55154-3916	Antidiabetic
MICRONASE25	Tab, Micronase/2.5	Glyburide 2.5 mg	Micronase by Pharmacia & Upjohn	00009-0141	Antidiabetic
MICRONASE5	Tab	Glyburide 5 mg	Micronase by Nat Pharmpak Serv	55154-3905	Antidiabetic
MICRONASE5	Tab, Blue, Round, Scored	Glyburide 5 mg	Micronase by Kiel	59063-0113	Antidiabetic
MICRONASE5	Tab	Glyburide 5 mg	Micronase by Quality Care	60346-0662	Antidiabetic
MICRONASE5	Tab, Blue, Round, Scored	Glyburide 5 mg	Micronase by Rightpak	65240-0690	Antidiabetic
MICRONASE5	Tab	Glyburide 5 mg	Micronase by Amerisource	62584-0171	Antidiabetic
MICRONASE5	Tab, Blue, Round, Scored	Glyburide 5 mg	Micronase by Thrift Services	59198-0335	Antidiabetic
MICRONASE5	Tab, Light Blue	Glyburide 5 mg	Micronase by Pharmacia & Upjohn	00009-0171	Antidiabetic
MICRONASE5	Tab, Blue, Round, Scored	Glyburide 5 mg	Micronase by Kenwood	00482-0440	Antidiabetic
MICRONASE5	Tab, Micronase over 5	Glyburide 5 mg	Micronase by Med Pro	53978-3000	Antidiabetic
MICRONASE5	Tab	Glyburide 5 mg	Micronase by HJ Harkins Co	52959-0177	Antidiabetic
MICRONASE5	Tab	Glyburide 5 mg	by Med Pro	53978-0694	Antidiabetic
MICRONASE5	Tab	Glyburide 5 mg	by Pharmedix	53002-0417	Antidiabetic
MICROZIDE125	Cap, Teal w/ Black Print	Hydrochlorothiazide 12.5 mg	Microzide by Caremark	00339-6188	Diuretic
MICROZIDE125MG	Cap, Microzide 12.5 mg	Hydrochlorothiazide 12.5 mg	Microzide by Watson	52544-0622	Diuretic
MIDOL	Cap, White	Acetaminophen 500 mg, Caffeine 60 mg, Pyrilamine 15 mg	Midol by Bayer	Canadian	Analgesic
MIDOL	Cap, White	Acetaminophen 500 mg, Pamabrom 25 mg, Pyrilamine 15 mg	Midol by Bayer	Canadian	PMS Relief
MIDOL	Cap, White	Aspirin 500 mg, Caffeine Anahydrous 32 mg	by Bayer	Canadian	Analgesic

ID FRONT <> BACK	DESCRIPTION FRONT <> BACK	INGREDIENT & STRENGTH	BRAND (OR EQUIV.) & FIRM	NDC#	CLASS; SCH.
MIDOLMIDOL	Cap, White, Midol/Midol	Aspirin 500 mg, Cinnamedrine 5.5 mg, Caffeine 32.4 mg	Midol by Bayer	Canadian	Analgesic
MIGRALAM	Cap	Acetaminophen 325 mg, Caffeine 100 mg, Isometheptene Mucate (1:1) 65 mg	Migralam by Sovereign	58716-0039	Analgesic
MILES <> 512	Tab, Film Coated	Ciprofloxacin HCl 291.5 mg	Cipro by Quality Care	60346-0433	Antibiotic
MILES <> 513	Tab, Pale Yellow, Film Coated	Ciprofloxacin HCl 583 mg	Cipro by Quality Care	60346-0031	Antibiotic
MILES <> 513	Tab, Film Coated	Ciprofloxacin HCl 583 mg	Ciprobay by Bayer	00026-8513	Antibiotic
MILES <> 513	Tab, Film Coated	Ciprofloxacin HCl 583 mg	Cipro by Nat Pharmpak Serv	55154-4801	Antibiotic
MILES093	Tab, White, Bullet Shaped	Clotrimazole 100 mg	Mycelex G Vaginal by Miles		Antifungal
MILES095	Tab	Clotrimazole 10 mg	by Med Pro	53978-3040	Antifungal
MILES097	Tab, White, Bullet Shaped	Clotrimazole 500 mg	Mycelex G Vaginal by Miles		Antifungal
MILES121	Tab, White, Round	Dehydrocholic Acid 250 mg	Decholin by Miles		Gastrointestinal
MILES132	Tab, White, Round, Gray Specks	Diethylstilbestrol Diphosphate 50 mg	Stilphostrol by Miles		Hormone
MILES20	Tab, Grayish Pink, Round	Nifedipine 20 mg	Adalat PA by Miles		Antihypertensive
MILES30 <> 884	Tab, Pink	Nifedipine 30 mg	Adalat CC by Direct Dispensing	57866-6719	Antihypertensive
MILES30 <> 884	Tab, Film Coated	Nifedipine 30 mg	Adalat CC by Caremark	00339-5976	Antihypertensive
MILES411	Tab, White, Round	Aluminum Sulfate, Calcium Acetate	Domeboro by Miles		Gastrointestinal
MILES514	Tab, White, Oblong	Ciprofloxacin 750 mg	Cipro by Miles		Antibiotic
MILES521	Tab, White, Oblong	Praziquantel 600 mg	Biltricide by Miles		Antihelmintic
MILES60 <> 885	Tab, Film Coated	Nifedipine 60 mg	Adalat CC by Pharm Utilization	60491-0010	Antihypertensive
MILES721	Tab, Yellow, Round	Niclosamide Chewable 500 mg	Niclocide by Miles		Anthelmintic
MILES811 <> ADALAT	Cap	Nifedipine 10 mg	Adalat by Bayer	00026-8811	Antihypertensive
MILES811 <> ADALAT	Cap	Nifedipine 10 mg	Adalat by Nat Pharmpak Serv	55154-4803	Antihypertensive
MILES821 <> ADALAT	Cap	Nifedipine 20 mg	by Med Pro	53978-2050	Antihypertensive
MILES855	Cap, Ivory	Nimodipine 30 mg	Nimotop by Miles		Antihypertensive
MILES855	Cap	Nimodipine 30 mg	Nimodipine by Med Pro	53978-2054	Antihypertensive
MILES90886	Tab, Brown, Round	Nifedipine ER 90 mg	Adalat CC by Miles		Antihypertensive
MILES951	Tab, Green, Round	Lithium Carbonate 300 mg	Lithane by Miles		Antipsychotic
MILESDT	Tab, Grayish Pink, Round	Nifedipine 10 mg	Adalat FT by Miles		Antihypertensive
MINIHR60	Tab, White, Round, Mini/HR60	Pseudoephedrine 60 mg	Mini Pseudo by BDI		Decongestant
MINIPRESS <> PFIZER431	Cap, Pfizer 431	Prazosin HCl 1 mg	Minipress by Pfizer	00663-4310	Antihypertensive
MINIPRESS <> PFIZER437	Cap, Pfizer 437	Prazosin HCl 2 mg	Minipress by Pfizer	00663-4370	Antihypertensive
MINISLIM	Cap, Clear & Red, Red & White Beads	Phenylpropanolamine 75 mg	Mini Slims by BDI		Decongestant; Appetite Suppressant
MINITHIN	Cap, Red Brown	Ephedrine group alkaloids 25 mg, Kola Nut Extract 100 mg	Mini Thin 25/50 by BDI		Dietary Supplement
MINOCYCLINE100 <> DAN5694	Cap, Dark Gray	Minocycline HCl	by Danbury	00591-5695	Antibiotic
MINOCYCLINE100 <> DAN5695	Cap	Minocycline HCl	by Danbury	61955-2498	Antibiotic
MINOCYCLINE50 <> DAN5694	Cap	Minocycline HCl	by Danbury	00591-5694	Antibiotic
MINOCYCLINE50 <> DAN5694	Cap	Minocycline HCl	by Danbury	61955-2497	Antibiotic
MINOXIDIL10 <> PAR257	Tab	Minoxidil 10 mg	by Physicians Total Care	54868-3467	Antihypertensive
MINOXIDIL10 <> PAR257	Tab	Minoxidil 10 mg	by Par	49884-0257	Antihypertensive
MINOXIDIL10 <> PAR257	Tab	Minoxidil 10 mg	by Qualitest	00603-4688	Antihypertensive
MINOXIDIL10 <> PAR257	Tab, Debossed	Minoxidil 10 mg	by HL Moore	00839-7342	Antihypertensive

ID FRONT <> BACK	DESCRIPTION FRONT <> BACK	INGREDIENT & STRENGTH	BRAND (OR EQUIV.) & FIRM	NDC#	CLASS; SCH.
MINOXIDIL10 <> PAR257	Tab	Minoxidil 10 mg	by United Res	00677-1162	Antihypertensive
MINOXIDIL212 <> PAR256	Tab, Minoxidil 2 1/2 <> Par 256	Minoxidil 2.5 mg	by Par	49884-0256	Antihypertensive
MINOXIDIL212 <> PAR256	Tab, Minoxidil 2 1/2 <> Par 256	Minoxidil 2.5 mg	by Qualitest	00603-4687	Antihypertensive
MINTEZOL <> MSD907	Tab, White, Round, Chew	Thiabendazole 500 mg	Mintezol by Merck	00006-0907	Antihelmintic
MISSION <> 610	Tab	Potassium Citrate 1080 mg	Urocit K by Mission	00178-0610	Electrolytes
MJ	Tab, White, Rectangle, Scored, Logo	Buspirone HCl 10 mg	Buspar by Thrift Services	59198-0370	Antianxiety
MJ	Tab, White, Square, Scored	Buspirone HCl 10 mg	Buspar by Va Cmop	65243-0016	Antianxiety
MJ	Tab, White, Rectangle, Scored	Buspirone HCl 10 mg	Buspar by Caremark	00339-4106	Antianxiety
MJ	Tab, White, Rectangle, Scored	Buspirone HCl 5 mg	Buspar by Thrift Services	59198-0369	Antianxiety
MJ <> 468	Tab, Chewable	Ascorbic Acid 60 mg, Cholecalciferol 400, Cyanocobalamin 4.5 mcg, Folic Acid 0.3 mg, Niacin 13.5 mg, Niacinamide, Pyridoxine HCl, Riboflavin Phosphate Sodium, Sodium Fluoride, Thiamine Mononitrate, Vitamin A Acetate, Vitamin E 15 Units	Poly Vi Flor by Bristol Myers Squibb	00087-0468	Vitamin
MJ <> 474	Tab, Orange, Pink & Purple, Pillow Shaped, Chewable	Ascorbic Acid 60 mg, Cyanocobalamin 4.5 mcg, Fluoride Ion 1 mg, Folic Acid 0.3 mg, Niacin 13.5 mg, Pyridoxine HCl 1.05 mg, Riboflavin 1.2 mg, Thiamine 1.05 mg, Vitamin A 2500 Units, Vitamin D 400 Units, Vitamin E 15 Units	Poly Vi Flo by Bristol Myers Squibb	00087-0474	Vitamin
MJ <> 476	Tab, Pillow Shaped, Chewable	Ascorbic Acid 60 mg, Copper 1 mg, Cyanocobalamin 4.5 mcg, Fluoride Ion 1 mg, Folic Acid 0.3 mg, Iron 12 mg, Niacin 13.5 mg, Pyridoxine HCl 1.05 mg, Riboflavin 1.2 mg, Thiamine 1.05 mg, Vitamin A 2500 Units, Vitamin D 400 Units, Vitamin E 15 Units, Zinc 10 mg	Poly Vi Flor Iron by Bristol Myers Squibb	00087-0476	Vitamin
MJ <> 477	Tab, Orange, Pink & Purple, Pillow Shaped, Chewable	Ascorbic Acid 60 mg, Cholecalciferol 400 Units, Sodium Fluoride, Vitamin A Acetate 2500 Units	Tri Vi Flor by Bristol Myers Squibb	00087-0477	Vitamin
MJ <> 482	Tab, Pillow Shaped, Chewable	Ascorbic Acid 60 mg, Copper 1 mg, Cyanocobalamin 4.5 mcg, Fluoride Ion 0.5 mg, Folic Acid 0.3 mg, Iron 12 mg, Niacin 13.5 mg, Pyridoxine HCl 1.05 mg, Riboflavin 1.2 mg, Thiamine 1.05 mg, Vitamin A 2500 Units, Vitamin D 400 Units, Vitamin E 15 Units, Zinc 10 mg	Poly Vi Flor Iron by Bristol Myers Squibb	00087-0482	Vitamin
MJ <> 487	Tab, Orange, Pink & Purple, Chewable	Cyanocobalamin 4.5 mcg, Folic Acid 0.3 mg, Niacinamide, Pyridoxine HCl 1.05 mg, Riboflavin 1.2 mg, Sodium Ascorbate, Sodium Fluoride, Thiamine Mononitrate, Vitamin A Acetate, Vitamin D 400 Units, Vitamin E Acetate	Poly Vi Flo by Bristol Myers Squibb	00087-0487	Vitamin
MJ <> 488	Tab, Pillow Shaped, Chewable	Cupric Oxide, Cyanocobalamin 4.5 mcg, Ferrous Fumarate, Folic Acid 0.3 mg, Niacinamide, Pyridoxine HCl 1.05 mg, Riboflavin 1.2 mg, Sodium Ascorbate, Sodium Fluoride, Thiamine Mononitrate, Vitamin A Acetate, Vitamin D 400 Units, Vitamin E Acetate, Zinc Oxide	Poly Vi Flor Iron by Bristol Myers Squibb	00087-0488	Vitamin
MJ <> 583	Tab	Ethinyl Estradiol 0.035 mg, Norethindrone 0.4 mg	Ovcon 35 by Physicians Total Care	54868-0509	Oral Contraceptive
MJ <> 583	Tab, Peach, Round	Ethinyl Estradiol 0.035 mg, Norethindrone 0.4 mg	Ovcon 35 by Heartland	61392-0814	Oral Contraceptive
MJ <> 583	Tab, Peach, Round	Ethinyl Estradiol 0.035 mg, Norethindrone 0.4 mg	Ovcon 35 by Heartland	61392-0818	Oral Contraceptive
MJ <> 583	Tab	Ethinyl Estradiol 0.035 mg, Norethindrone 0.4 mg	Ovcon 35 21 by Bristol Myers Squibb	00087-0583	Oral Contraceptive
MJ <> 583	Tab, MJ Logo	Ethinyl Estradiol 0.035 mg, Norethindrone 0.4 mg	Ovcon 35 28 by Bristol Myers Squibb	00087-0578	Oral Contraceptive
MJ <> 584	Tab	Ethinyl Estradiol 0.035 mg, Norethindrone 0.4 mg	Ovcon 50 28 by Bristol Myers	15548-0579	Oral Contraceptive
MJ <> 584	Tab, MJ Logo	Ethinyl Estradiol 0.035 mg, Norethindrone 0.4 mg	Ovcon 50 28 by Bristol Myers Squibb	00087-0579	Oral Contraceptive
MJ <> 584	Tab	Ethinyl Estradiol 0.035 mg, Norethindrone 0.4 mg	Ovcon 50 by Physicians Total Care	54868-3772	Oral Contraceptive
MJ <> 702	Tab, White, Coated, Speckled	Ascorbic Acid 80 mg, Biotin 0.03 mg, Calcium 200 mg, Copper 3 mg, Cyanocobalamin 2.5 mcg, Folic Acid 1 mg, Iron 54 mg, Magnesium 100 mg, Niacin 17 mg, Pantothenic Acid 7 mg, Pyridoxine HCl 4 mg, Riboflavin 1.6 mg, Thiamine 1.5 mg, Vitamin A 4000 Units, Vitamin D 400 Units, Vitamin E 15 Units, Zinc 25 mg	Natalins Tablets Rx by Bristol Myers Squibb	00087-0702	Vitamin
MJ <> 755	Tab	Estradiol 1 mg	by Quality Care	60346-0375	Hormone
MJ <> 756	Tab, Blue, Round, Scored	Estradiol 2 mg	Estrace by Rx Pac	65084-0187	Hormone
MJ <> 822	Tab, White, Scored	Buspirone HCl 15 mg	Buspar by Direct Dispensing	57866-0904	Antianxiety
MJ <> 850	Tab, Green, Round	Ethinyl Estradiol 0.035 mg, Norethindrone 0.4 mg	Ovcon 35 by Heartland	61392-0809	Oral Contraceptive

ID FRONT <> BACK	DESCRIPTION FRONT <> BACK	INGREDIENT & STRENGTH	BRAND (OR EQUIV.) & FIRM	NDC#	CLASS; SCH.
MJ <> 850	Tab, Green, Round	Ethinyl Estradiol 0.035 mg, Norethindrone 0.4 mg	Ovcon 35 by Heartland	61392-0817	Oral Contraceptive
MJ <> 850	Tab, MJ Logo	Ethinyl Estradiol 0.035 mg, Norethindrone 0.4 mg	Ovcon 35 28 by Bristol Myers Squibb	00087-0578	Oral Contraceptive
MJ <> 850	Tab	Ethinyl Estradiol 0.035 mg, Norethindrone 0.4 mg	Ovcon 35 by Physicians Total Care	54868-0509	Oral Contraceptive
MJ <> 850	Tab, MJ Logo	Ethinyl Estradiol 0.05 mg, Norethindrone 1 mg	Ovcon 50 28 by Bristol Myers Squibb	00087-0579	Oral Contraceptive
MJ <> 850	Tab	Ethinyl Estradiol 0.05 mg, Norethindrone 1 mg	Ovcon 50 by Physicians Total Care	54868-3772	Oral Contraceptive
MJ <> 850	Tab	Inert	Ovcon 50 28 by Bristol Myers	15548-0579	Placebo
MJ <> BUSPAR5MG	Tab, White, Rectangle, Scored, MJ Logo <> Buspar 5 mg	Buspirone HCl 5 mg	Buspar by Caremark	00339-4110	Antianxiety
MJ021	Tab, White	Estradiol 0.5 mg	Estrace by Bristol Myers Squibb	00087-0021	Hormone
MJ10 <> BUSPAR	Tab, MJ Logo 10	Buspirone HCl 10 mg	Buspar by Quality Care	60346-0162	Antianxiety
MJ10 <> BUSPAR	Tab, MJ Logo, Strength	Buspirone HCl 10 mg	Buspar by Heartland	61392-0602	Antianxiety
MJ10 <> BUSPAR	Tab, White, Ovoid-Rectangular, Scored	Buspirone HCl 10 mg	Buspar by Bristol Myers Squibb	00087-0819	Antianxiety
MJ10 <> BUSPAR	Tab, White, Rectangle, Scored	Buspirone HCl 10 mg	Buspar by Caremark	00339-4109	Antianxiety
MJ10 <> BUSPAR	Tab	Buspirone HCl 10 mg	Buspar by Pharmedix	53002-1017	Antianxiety
MJ10 <> BUSPAR	Tab	Buspirone HCl 10 mg	Buspar by CVS Revco	00894-5215	Antianxiety
MJ10BUSPAR	Tab, MJ Logo	Buspirone HCl 10 mg	Buspar by Allscripts	54569-1606	Antianxiety
MJ10BUSPAR	Tab, MJ Logo	Buspirone HCl 10 mg	Buspar by Bristol Myers	15548-0819	Antianxiety
MJ10MGBUSPAR	Tab, White, Oval	Buspirone HCl 10 mg	Buspar by Rightpak	65240-0618	Antianxiety
MJ1202M	Tab, White, Hexagonal	Fosinopril Sodium 40 mg	Monopril by BMS		Antihypertensive
MJ158	Tab, White, Diamond	Fosinopril Sodium 10 mg	Monopril by MJ		Antihypertensive
MJ158M	Tab, Off-White, MJ 158/M	Fosinopril Sodium 10 mg	Monopril by Allscripts	54569-3808	Antihypertensive
MJ5	Tab, White, Rectangular	Buspirone HCl 5 mg	Buspar by BMS		Antianxiety
MJ5 <> BUSPAR	Tab, Rectangular, <> MJ Logo Then 5	Buspirone HCl 5 mg	Buspar by Heartland	61392-0601	Antianxiety
MJ5 <> BUSPAR	Tab, White, Ovoid-Rectangular, Scored	Buspirone HCl 5 mg	Buspar by Bristol Myers Squibb	00087-0818	Antianxiety
MJ503 <> 50	Tab	Cyclophosphamide 50 mg	Cytoxan by Mead Johnson	00015-0503	Antineoplastic
MJ504 <> 25	Tab	Cyclophosphamide 25 mg	Cytoxan by Mead Johnson	00015-0504	Antineoplastic
MJ543 <> 10	Tab	Isoxsuprine HCl 10 mg	Vasodilan by Bristol Myers Squibb	00087-0543	Vasodilator
MJ544 <> 20	Tab	Isoxsuprine HCl 20 mg	Vasodilan by Bristol Myers Squibb	00087-0544	Vasodilator
MJ595	Tab	Megestrol Acetate 20 mg	Megace by Mead Johnson	00015-0595	Progestin
MJ596	Tab, Blue, Round	Megestrol Acetate 40 mg	Megace by BM		Progestin
MJ5BUSPAR	Tab, MJ Logo	Buspirone HCl 5 mg	Buspar by Nat Pharmpak Serv	55154-2008	Antianxiety
MJ5BUSPAR	Tab, MJ Logo	Buspirone HCl 5 mg	Buspar by Bristol Myers	15548-0818	Antianxiety
MJ5MGBUSPAR	Tab, White, Oval	Buspirone HCl 5 mg	Buspar by Rightpak	65240-0617	Antianxiety
MJ5MGBUSPAR	Tab, White, Oval	Buspirone HCl 5 mg	Buspar by Direct Dispensing	57866-0902	Antianxiety
MJ609 <> M	Tab, Coated	Fosinopril Sodium 20 mg	Monopril by Allscripts	54569-3809	Antihypertensive
MJ755	Tab, Lavender, MJ/755	Estradiol 1 mg	Estrace by Bristol Myers Squibb	00087-0755	Hormone
MJ755	Tab, Lavender, MJ/755	Estradiol 1 mg	by Nat Pharmpak Serv	55154-2013	Hormone
MJ756	Tab, Turquoise Blue, MJ 756	Estradiol 2 mg	by Quality Care	60346-0029	Hormone
MJ756	Tab, Turquoise, MJ 756	Estradiol 2 mg	Estrace by Bristol Myers Squibb	00087-0756	Hormone
MJ756	Tab, Turquoise, MJ/756	Estradiol 2 mg	by Nat Pharmpak Serv	55154-2012	Hormone
MJ756	Tab	Estradiol 2 mg	by Bristol Myers	15548-0756	Hormone
MJ775 <> DESYREL	Tab, Film Coated	Trazodone HCl 50 mg	Desyrel by Leiner	59606-0629	Antidepressant
MJ775 <> DESYREL	Tab, Film Coated	Trazodone HCl 50 mg	Desyrel by Amerisource	62584-0775	Antidepressant
MJ776 <> DESYREL	Tab, Film Coated	Trazodone HCl 100 mg	Desyrel by Amerisource	62584-0776	Antidepressant
MJ778 <> 505050	Tab, Orange, Scored	Trazodone HCl 150 mg	Desyrel by Rx Pac	65084-0221	Antidepressant
MJ778 <> 505050	Tab, Orange	Trazodone HCl 150 mg	Desyrel by Rightpak	65240-0631	Antidepressant
MJ778 <> 505050	Tab, Orange, Rectangle, Scored	Trazodone HCl 150 mg	Desyrel by Thrift Services	59198-0374	Antidepressant
MJ778 <> 505050	Tab, MJ 778 <> 50/50/50	Trazodone HCl 150 mg	Desyrel Dividose by Bristol Myers Squibb	00087-0778	Antidepressant
MJ778 <> 505050	Tab	Trazodone HCl 150 mg	Desyrel by Physicians Total Care	54868-2549	Antidepressant
MJ778 <> 505050	Tab, MJ/778 <> 50/50/50	Trazodone HCl 150 mg	Desyrel by Nat Pharmpak Serv	55154-2011	Antidepressant
MJ778 <> 505050	Tab	Trazodone HCl 150 mg	Desyrel Dividose by Amerisource	62584-0778	Antidepressant
MJ778 <> 505050	Tab, Dividose	Trazodone HCl 150 mg	Desyrel by Pharm Utilization	60491-0912	Antidepressant

ID FRONT <> BACK	DESCRIPTION FRONT <> BACK	INGREDIENT & STRENGTH	BRAND (OR EQUIV.) & FIRM	NDC#	CLASS; SCH.
MJ778 <> 505050	Tab	Trazodone HCl 150 mg	Desyrel by Leiner	59606-0631	Antidepressant
MJ784	Cap, Red & White	Cefadroxil 500 mg	Duricef by BMS		Antibiotic
MJ785	Tab, White, Oval	Cefadroxil 1 GM	Duricef by BMS		Antibiotic
MJ796 <> 100100100	Tab	Trazodone HCl 300 mg	Desyrel by Bristol Myers Squibb	00087-0796	Antidepressant
MJ822 <> 5	Tab, White, Rectangular, Scored	Buspirone HCl 15 mg	Buspar by Murfreesboro Ph	51129-1375	Antianxiety
MJ822 <> 5	Tab, White, Rectangle, Scored	Buspirone HCl 15 mg	Buspar by Caremark	00339-4105	Antianxiety
MJ822 <> 555	Tab, White, Rectangle, Scored	Buspirone HCl 15 mg	Buspar by WalMart	49035-0188	Antianxiety
MJ822555	Tab, White, Rectangular, MJ 822 5-5-5	Buspirone HCl 15 mg	Buspar by BMS	15548-0822	Antianxiety
MJBUSPAR	Tab	Buspirone HCl 5 mg	Buspar by Med Pro	53978-2044	Antianxiety
MJBUSPAR10	Tab, White, Rectangular, Scored	Buspirone HCl 15 mg	Buspar by PDRX Pharms	55289-0556	Antianxiety
MLA05250	Cap, Blue & White, Opaque, ML-A05 250	Cefaclor 250 mg	Ceclor by Caremark	00339-6150	Antibiotic
MLA06500	Cap, Blue & Gray, Opaque, ML-A06 500	Cefaclor 500 mg	Ceclor by Caremark	00339-6151	Antibiotic
MLA07	Cap, Green & White	Cephalexin Monohydrate 250 mg	by Southwood Pharms	58016-0138	Antibiotic
MLA08	Cap, Green	Cephalexin Monohydrate 500 mg	by Southwood Pharms	58016-0139	Antibiotic
MM35	Cap, Light Green	Acetaminophen 300 mg, Phenyltoloxamine Citrate 20 mg, Salicylamide 200 mg	Cetazone T by Marnel	00682-1444	Analgesic
MM35	Cap	Acetaminophen 300 mg, Phenyltoloxamine Citrate 20 mg, Salicylamide 200 mg	Cetazone T by Seatrace	00551-1444	Analgesic
MMDC	Tab, White, Round	Metformin 500 mg	Glucophage by Marion Merrel Dow	Canadian	Antidiabetic
MMDC	Tab, White, Round, Scored	Metoclopramide 10 mg	by Hoechst Marion Roussel	Canadian	Gastrointestinal
MMDC30	Tab, Green, MMDC/30	Diltiazem 30 mg	by Hoechst Marion Roussel	Canadian	Antihypertensive
MMDC60	Tab, Yellow, MMDC/60	Diltiazem 60 mg	by Hoechst Marion Roussel	Canadian	Antihypertensive
MMDC850	Tab, White, Oval, MMDC/850	Metformin 850 mg	Glucophage by Marion Merrel Dow	Canadian	Antidiabetic
MMS830	Cap, Clear & Orange	Diazoxide 50 mg	Proglycem by MMS		Diuretic
MMSPBA	Cap, Clear & Orange	Diazoxide 50 mg	Proglycem by MMS		Diuretic
MO315 <> MOVA	Tab, White, Oval, MO3 1.5 <> Mova	Glyburide 1.5 mg	Glynase by Watson	52544-0558	Antidiabetic
MO315 <> MOVA	Tab, White, Oval, Scored, MO31.5 <> Mova	Glyburide 1.5 mg	Glynase PresTab by MOVA	55370-0146	Antidiabetic
MO430 <> MOVA	Tab, Blue, Oval, Scored, MO43.0 <> Mova	Glyburide 3 mg	Glynase PresTab by MOVA	55370-0147	Antidiabetic
MO430 <> MOVA	Tab, Blue, Oval, MO4 3.0 <> Mova	Glyburide 3 mg	Glynase by Watson	52544-0559	Antidiabetic
MO430 <> MOVA	Tab, MO4 3.0	Glyburide 3.15 mg	by Caremark	00339-5910	Antidiabetic
MO52 <> MO52	Tab, Pink, Round, Scored	Trimethoprim 80 mg, Sulfamethoxazole 400 mg	Septra by King Pharms	60793-0899	Antibiotic
MO53 <> MO53	Tab, Pink, Oval, Scored	Trimethoprim 160 mg, Sulfamethoxazole 800 mg	Septra DS by King Pharms	60793-0900	Antibiotic
MO645 <> MOVA	Tab, MO6 4.5	Glyburide 4.725 mg	by MOVA	55370-0149	Antidiabetic
MO760 <> MOVA	Tab, Light Yellow, Oval, Scored, MO76.0 <> Mova	Glyburide 6 mg	Glynase PresTab by MOVA	55370-0506	Antidiabetic
MO760 <> MOVA	Tab, Light Yellow, Oval, MO7 6.0 <> Mova	Glyburide 6 mg	Glynase by Watson	52544-0560	Antidiabetic
MOBAN10	Tab	Molindone HCl 10 mg	Moban by Du Pont Pharma	00056-0073	Antipsychotic
MOBAN10	Tab, Lavender, Round	Molindone HCl 10 mg	Moban by Endo	63481-0073	Antipsychotic
MOBAN10 <> GATE	Tab	Molindone HCl 10 mg	Moban by Gate	57844-0915	Antipsychotic
MOBAN100	Tab, Tan, Round, Scored	Molindone HCl 100 mg	Moban by Endo Labs	63481-0077	Antipsychotic
MOBAN100	Tab	Molindone HCl 100 mg	Moban by Du Pont Pharma	00056-0077	Antipsychotic
MOBAN100 <> GATE	Tab	Molindone HCl 100 mg	Moban by Gate	57844-0918	Antipsychotic
MOBAN25	Tab, Green, Round, Scored	Molindone HCl 25 mg	Moban by Endo Labs	63481-0074	Antipsychotic
MOBAN25	Tab, Partial Bisect	Molindone HCl 25 mg	Moban by Du Pont Pharma	00056-0074	Antipsychotic
MOBAN25 <> GATE	Tab	Molindone HCl 25 mg	Moban by Gate	57844-0916	Antipsychotic
MOBAN5	Tab	Molindone HCl 5 mg	Moban by Du Pont Pharma	00056-0072	Antipsychotic
MOBAN5	Tab, Orange, Round	Molindone HCl 5 mg	Moban by Endo	63481-0072	Antipsychotic
MOBAN5 <> GATE	Tab	Molindone HCl 5 mg	Moban by Gate	57844-0914	Antipsychotic
MOBAN50	Tab	Molindone HCl 50 mg	Moban by Du Pont Pharma	00056-0076	Antipsychotic
MOBAN50	Tab, Blue, Round, Scored	Molindone HCl 50 mg	Moban by Endo	63481-0076	Antipsychotic
MOBAN510 <> GATE	Tab	Molindone HCl 50 mg	Moban by Gate	57844-0917	Antipsychotic
MOC150	Tab, Yellow, MOC/150	Moclobemide 150 mg	by Altimed	Canadian DIN# 02218410	Antidepressant

ID FRONT <> BACK	DESCRIPTION FRONT <> BACK	INGREDIENT & STRENGTH	BRAND (OR EQUIV.) & FIRM	NDC#	CLASS; SCH.
MOC300	Tab, White to Yellowish-White, Oval, Film Coated, Scored	Moclobemide 300 mg	by Altimed	Canadian DIN# 02218429	Antidepressant
MOLE	Cap, White	Caffeine 200 mg	by B & M Labs		Stimulant
MOLE	Cap, Black	Caffeine 200 mg	Molie by BDI		Stimulant
MONODOX100 <> M259	Cap, Brown & White Print	Doxycycline Monohydrate	Monodox by Oclassen	55515-0259	Antibiotic
MONODOX100 <> M259	Cap, Brown & White Print	Doxycycline Monohydrate	Monodox by Eckerd Drug	19458-0838	Antibiotic
MONODOX100 <> M259	Cap, Brown & Yellow	Doxycycline Monohydrate 100 mg	Monodox by Thrift Services	59198-0363	Antibiotic
MONODOX100 <> M259	Cap, Brown & Yellow	Doxycycline Monohydrate 100 mg	by West Pharm	52967-0302	Antibiotic
MONODOX100MG <> M259	Cap	Doxycycline Monohydrate	by Vintage	00254-4316	Antibiotic
MONODOX50 <> M260	Cap, Brown Print	Doxycycline Monohydrate	Monodox by Oclassen	55515-0260	Antibiotic
MONODOX50 <> M260	Cap	Doxycycline Monohydrate	Monodox by Vintage	00254-4315	Antibiotic
MONODOX50 <> M260	Cap, White & Yellow	Doxycycline Monohydrate 50 mg	by West Pharm	52967-0301	Antibiotic
MONOPRIL10 <> 158MJ	Tab, Scored	Fosinopril Sodium 10 mg	Monopril by Bristol Myers Squibb	00087-0158	Antihypertensive
MONOPRIL10 <> BMS	Tab, Off White	Fosinopril Sodium 10 mg	Monopril by Direct Dispensing	57866-3800	Antihypertensive
MONOPRIL10 <> BMS	Tab, Off-White, Diamond Shaped	Fosinopril Sodium 10 mg	by Allscripts	54569-3808	Antihypertensive
MONOPRIL10 <> BMS	Tab, White, Diamond	Fosinopril Sodium 10 mg	Monopril by Va Cmop	65243-0092	Antihypertensive
MONOPRIL10 <> BMS	Tab, Off-White, Diamond Shaped	Fosinopril Sodium 10 mg	Monopril by Bristol Myers	00087-0158	Antihypertensive
MONOPRIL10 <> BMS	Tab, Off White, Scored	Fosinopril Sodium 10 mg	Monopril by Caremark	00339-5745	Antihypertensive
MONOPRIL20 <> BMS	Tab	Fosinopril Sodium 20 mg	Monopril by Direct Dispensing	57866-3803	Antihypertensive
MONOPRIL20 <> BMS	Tab, White, Oval	Fosinopril Sodium 20 mg	Monopril by Va Cmop	65243-0093	Antihypertensive
MONOPRIL20 <> BMS	Tab, White to Off-White, Oval	Fosinopril Sodium 20 mg	by Allscripts	54569-3809	Antihypertensive
MONOPRIL20 <> BMS	Tab, Off-White, Oval	Fosinopril Sodium 20 mg	Monopril by Bristol Myers Squibb	00087-0609	Antihypertensive
MONOPRIL20 <> BMS	Tab	Fosinopril Sodium 20 mg	Monopril by Bristol Myers	15548-0609	Antihypertensive
MONOPRIL40 <> BMS	Tab, White, Hexagon	Fosinopril Sodium 40 mg	Monopril by Va Cmop	65243-0094	Antihypertensive
MONOPRIL40 <> BMS	Tab, Off White, Hexagonal	Fosinopril Sodium 40 mg	Monopril by Bristol Myers Squibb	00087-1202	Antihypertensive
MONOPRIL40 <> BMS	Tab	Fosinopril Sodium 40 mg	Monopril by Bristol Myers	15548-0202	Antihypertensive
MOSSR30	Tab, Blue, Round, M.O.S.-SR/30	Morphine HCl 30 mg	by ICN	Canadian	Analgesic
MOSSR60	Tab, Red, Round, M.O.S.-SR/60	Morphine HCl 60 mg	by ICN	Canadian	Analgesic
MOTRIN <> 400MG	Tab, Coated	Ibuprofen 400 mg	Motrin by Allscripts	54569-0284	NSAID
MOTRIN <> 800MG	Tab, Apricot, Coated	Ibuprofen 800 mg	Motrin by Quality Care	60346-0855	NSAID
MOTRIN100	Tab, Chew	Ibuprofen 100 mg	Motrin by McNeil	50580-0431	NSAID
MOTRIN300MG	Tab, White, Round, Film Coated	Ibuprofen 300 mg	Motrin (300 mg) by McNeil	Canadian DIN# 00327794	NSAID
MOTRIN400	Tab	Ibuprofen 400 mg	Motrin by Amerisource	62584-0385	NSAID
MOTRIN400	Tab, White, Round	Ibuprofen 400 mg	Motrin by Compumed	00403-1377	NSAID
MOTRIN400	Tab	Ibuprofen 400 mg	Motrin by Pharmacia & Upjohn	00009-7385	NSAID
MOTRIN400	Tab	Ibuprofen 400 mg	Motrin by Allscripts	54569-4321	NSAID
MOTRIN400	Tab, White, Round	Ibuprofen 400 mg	Motrin by Murfreesboro	51129-1511	NSAID
MOTRIN400	Tab, Coated, Motrin 400 <> Pharmacia/Up John	Ibuprofen 400 mg	Motrin by Thrift Drug	59198-0071	NSAID
MOTRIN400	Tab	Ibuprofen 400 mg	Motrin by Nat Pharmpak Serv	55154-3906	NSAID
MOTRIN400	Tab	Ibuprofen 400 mg	Motrin by DRX	55045-2422	NSAID
MOTRIN400MG	Tab, Orange, Round, Film Coated	Ibuprofen 400 mg	Motrin (400 mg) by McNeil	Canadian DIN# 00364142	NSAID
MOTRIN400MG	Tab, Orange	Ibuprofen 400 mg	by Pharmacia	Canadian	NSAID
MOTRIN400MG	Tab, Coated	Ibuprofen 400 mg	Motrin by Pharmacia & Upjohn	00009-0750	NSAID
MOTRIN50	Tab, Chew	Ibuprofen 50 mg	Motrin by McNeil	50580-0361	NSAID
MOTRIN600	Tab, White	Ibuprofen 600 mg	Motrin by Rightpak	65240-0695	NSAID

ID FRONT <> BACK	DESCRIPTION FRONT <> BACK	INGREDIENT & STRENGTH	BRAND (OR EQUIV.) & FIRM	NDC#	CLASS; SCH.
MOTRIN600	Tab	Ibuprofen 600 mg	by Kaiser	00179-1277	NSAID
MOTRIN600	Tab, White, Oval	Ibuprofen 600 mg	Motrin by Murfreesboro	51129-1510	NSAID
MOTRIN600	Tab	Ibuprofen 600 mg	Motrin by Thrift Drug	59198-0072	NSAID
MOTRIN600	Tab	Ibuprofen 600 mg	Motrin by Amerisource	62584-0386	NSAID
MOTRIN600MG	Tab, Peach, Oval, Film Coated	Ibuprofen 600 mg	Motrin (600 mg)	Canadian DIN# 00484911	NSAID
MOTRIN600MG	Tab, Peach	Ibuprofen 600 mg	by Pharmacia	Canadian	NSAID
MOTRIN600MG	Tab, Coated	Ibuprofen 600 mg	Motrin by Pharmacia & Upjohn	00009-0742	NSAID
MOTRIN600MG	Tab, Coated	Ibuprofen 600 mg	by Kaiser	00179-1100	NSAID
MOTRIN600MG	Tab	Ibuprofen 600 mg	Motrin by Pharmacia & Upjohn	00009-7386	NSAID
MOTRIN600MG	Tab, Film Coated	Ibuprofen 600 mg	by Med Pro	53978-5006	NSAID
MOTRIN600MG	Tab, Coated	Ibuprofen 600 mg	Motrin by Nat Pharmpak Serv	55154-3907	NSAID
MOTRIN800	Tab, Coated	Ibuprofen 800 mg	by Med Pro	53978-0118	NSAID
MOTRIN800	Tab, White, Oval	Ibuprofen 800 mg	Motrin by Murfreesboro	51129-1509	NSAID
MOTRIN800	Tab	Ibuprofen 800 mg	Motrin by Smiths Food & Drug	58341-0060	NSAID
MOTRIN800	Tab	Ibuprofen 800 mg	Motrin by Amerisource	62584-0387	NSAID
MOTRIN800	Tab, Elliptical Shaped, Coated	Ibuprofen 800 mg	Motrin by Thrift Drug	59198-0073	NSAID
MOTRIN800	Tab, Coated	Ibuprofen 800 mg	Motrin by Nat Pharmpak Serv	55154-3908	NSAID
MOTRIN800	Tab, White	Ibuprofen 800 mg	Motrin by Rightpak	65240-0696	NSAID
MOTRIN800	Tab	Ibuprofen 800 mg	Motrin by Pharmacia & Upjohn	00009-7387	NSAID
MOTRIN800MG	Tab	Ibuprofen 800 mg	by Kaiser	00179-1142	NSAID
MOTRIN800MG	Tab, Apricot, Elliptical Shaped, Coated	Ibuprofen 800 mg	Motrin by Pharmacia & Upjohn	00009-0725	NSAID
MOTRINIB	Cap, Orange & White, Gelatin	Ibuprofen 200 mg	Motrin IB by McNeil	Canadian DIN# 01983873	NSAID
MOTRINIB	Tab, White, Round, Film Coated	Ibuprofen 200 mg	Motrin IB by McNeil	Canadian DIN# 02186934	NSAID
MOTRINIB	Cap, White, Film Coated	Ibuprofen 200 mg	Motrin by McNeil	Canadian DIN# 02187124	NSAID
MOTRINIB	Cap, Orange & White	Ibuprofen 200 mg	Motrin IB by McNeil	Canadian	NSAID
MOVA <> 100M10	Tab, White, Cap Shaped	Captopril 100 mg	Capoten by Mova	55370-0145	Antihypertensive
MOVA <> 250M25	Tab	Naproxen 250 mg	by Caremark	00339-5870	NSAID
MOVA <> 250M25	Tab	Naproxen 250 mg	by Martec	52555-0712	NSAID
MOVA <> 250M25	Tab, Rose, Round	Naproxen 250 mg	Naprosyn by Mova	55370-0139	NSAID
MOVA <> 300M30	Tab, White, Round	Cimetidine 300 mg	Tagamet by Mova	55370-0135	Gastrointestinal
MOVA <> 375M37	Tab	Naproxen 375 mg	by Caremark	00339-5872	NSAID
MOVA <> 375M37	Tab	Naproxen 375 mg	by Martec	52555-0713	NSAID
MOVA <> 375M37	Tab, White, Cap Shaped	Naproxen 375 mg	Naprosyn by Mova	55370-0140	NSAID
MOVA <> 400M40	Tab, Coated, Mova <> 400/M40	Cimetidine 400 mg	by Rosemont	00832-0103	Gastrointestinal
MOVA <> 400M4O	Tab, White, Cap Shaped, Scored	Cimetidine 400 mg	Tagamet by Mova	55370-0136	Gastrointestinal
MOVA <> 500M50	Tab, Rose, Cap Shaped	Naproxen 500 mg	Naprosyn by Mova	55370-0141	NSAID
MOVA <> 500M50	Tab	Naproxen 500 mg	by Martec	52555-0714	NSAID
MOVA <> 500M50	Tab	Naproxen 500 mg	by Caremark	00339-5874	NSAID
MOVA <> 500M50	Tab, Rose	Naproxen 500 mg	by Quality Care	60346-0815	NSAID
MOVA <> 500M50	Tab, Pink, Oblong	Naproxen 500 mg	by Compumed	00403-1442	NSAID
MOVA <> 50MO	Tab, Debossed	Captopril 50 mg	by Quality Care	60346-0868	Antihypertensive
MOVA <> 50MO5	Tab, White, Cap Shaped	Captopril 50 mg	Capoten by Mova	55370-0144	Antihypertensive
MOVA <> 800M80	Tab, White, Cap Shaped, Scored	Cimetidine 800 mg	Tagamet by Mova	55370-0137	Gastrointestinal
MOVA <> M01	Tab, White, Oval, Scored	Captopril 12.5 mg	Capoten by Mova	55370-0164	Antihypertensive

ID FRONT <> BACK	DESCRIPTION FRONT <> BACK	INGREDIENT & STRENGTH	BRAND (OR EQUIV.) & FIRM	NDC#	CLASS; SCH.
MOVA <> MO1	Tab, Mova <> MO1	Captopril 12.5 mg	by Caremark	00339-6121	Antihypertensive
MOVA <> MO315	Tab, White, Oval, Scored, Mova <> MO31.5	Glyburide 1.5 mg	Glynase PresTab by Mova	55370-0146	Antidiabetic
MOVA <> MO430	Tab, Blue, Oval, Scored, Mova <> MO43.0	Glyburide 3 mg	Glynase PresTab by Mova	55370-0147	Antidiabetic
MOVA <> MO430	Tab, MO4 3.0	Glyburide 3.15 mg	by Caremark	00339-5910	Antidiabetic
MOVA <> MO645	Tab, MO6 4.5	Glyburide 4.725 mg	by Mova	55370-0149	Antidiabetic
MOVA <> MO760	Tab, Light Yellow, Oval, Scored, Mova <> MO76.0	Glyburide 6 mg	Glynase PresTab by Mova	55370-0506	Antidiabetic
MOVA25	Tab, Quadrisect Bar	Captopril 25 mg	by Quality Care	60346-0778	Antihypertensive
MOVA25	Tab	Captopril 25 mg	by Caremark	00339-6122	Antihypertensive
MOVA25	Tab, White, Round	Captopril 25 mg	Capoten by Mova	55370-0142	Antihypertensive
MOVA50M05	Tab	Captopril 50 mg	by Caremark	00339-6123	Antihypertensive
MOXY <> 5	Tab, White, Round, M-OXY	Oxycodone HCl 5 mg	by Pharmafab	62542-0258	Analgesic; C II
MOXY <> 5	Tab, White, Round, Scored, M-OXY <> 5	Oxycodone HCl 5 mg	Roxicodone/Percolone by Mallinckrodt Hobart	00406-0552	Analgesic; C II
MP	Tab	Albuterol Sulfate 2.4 mg	by Patient	57575-0018	Antiasthmatic
MP	Tab, Film Coated	Doxycycline Hyclate	by Pharmedix	53002-0271	Antibiotic
MP	Tab, Orange, Oblong, M/P	Guaifenesin 400 mg, Pseudophedrine 60 mg, Dextromethorphan 20 mg	Anatuss DM by Merz		Cold Remedy
MP	Tab, Sugar Coated	Hydroxyzine HCl 25 mg	by Patient	57575-0064	Antihistamine
MP <> 0331	Tab, Red, Film Coated	Calcium Carbonate 312 mg, Cyanocobalamin 3 mcg, Ferric Polysaccharide Complex, Folic Acid 1 mg, Niacinamide 10 mg, Pyridoxine HCl 2 mg, Riboflavin 3 mg, Sodium Ascorbate, Thiamine Mononitrate 3 mg, Vitamin A 4000 Units, Vitamin D 400 Units	Nu Iron V by	00131-2306	Vitamin/Mineral
MP <> 0331	Tab, Coated	Calcium Carbonate 312 mg, Cyanocobalamin 3 mcg, Ferric Polysaccharide Complex, Folic Acid 1 mg, Niacinamide 10 mg, Pyridoxine HCl 2 mg, Riboflavin 3 mg, Sodium Ascorbate, Thiamine Mononitrate 3 mg, Vitamin A 4000 Units, Vitamin D 400 Units	Nu Iron V by Merz	00259-0331	Vitamin/Mineral
MP <> 112	Tab, Yellow, Round	Sulindac 150 mg	by St. Marys Med	60760-0415	NSAID
MP <> 114	Tab, White, Round, Coated, Scored	Trazodone HCl 100 mg	by Allscripts	54569-1999	Antidepressant
MP <> 52	Tab, White, Round, Scored	Prednisone 10 mg	by Allscripts	54569-3302	Steroid
MP <> 52	Tab, White, Round, Scored	Prednisone 10 mg	by Allscripts	54569-0331	Steroid
MP <> 53	Tab, Peach, Round, Scored	Prednisone 20 mg	by Allscripts	54569-0332	Steroid
MP <> 66	Tab, Off White, Ex Release	Quinidine Gluconate 324 mg	by Quality Care	60346-0555	Antiarrhythmic
MP <> ALTACE5MG	Cap, Red, Gelatin	Ramipril 5 mg	by Allscripts	54569-3714	Antihypertensive
MP <> ELDERCAPS	Cap	Ascorbic Acid 200 mg, Calcium Pantothenate 10 mg, Cholecalciferol 400 Units, Folic Acid 1 mg, Magnesium Sulfate, Manganese Sulfate, Niacinamide 25 mg, Pyridoxine HCl 2 mg, Riboflavin 5 mg, Thiamine Mononitrate 10 mg, Vitamin A 4000 Units, Vitamin E 25 Units, Zinc Sulfate	Eldercaps by Merz	00259-0393	Vitamin
MP <> ELDERCAPS	Cap	Ascorbic Acid 200 mg, Calcium Pantothenate 10 mg, Cholecalciferol 400 Units, Folic Acid 1 mg, Magnesium Sulfate, Manganese Sulfate, Niacinamide 25 mg, Pyridoxine HCl 2 mg, Riboflavin 5 mg, Thiamine Mononitrate 10 mg, Vitamin A 4000 Units, Vitamin E 25 Units, Zinc Sulfate	Eldercaps by Anabolic	00722-6386	Vitamin
MP 25	Tab, Film Coated	Amitriptyline HCl 25 mg	by Kaiser	62224-7117	Antidepressant
MP 26	Tab, Film Coated	Amitriptyline HCl 50 mg	by Kaiser	62224-7220	Antidepressant
MP0384	Cap, Brown, Oval	Vitamin E 100 IU, Vitamin C 120, Beta-Carotene 25 mg	Antiox by Scherer		Vitamin
MP10	Tab, Coated, MP Over 10	Amitriptyline HCl 10 mg	by Quality Care	60346-0354	Antidepressant
MP10	Tab, Film Coated	Amitriptyline HCl 10 mg	by United Res	00677-0475	Antidepressant
MP10	Tab, Pink, Round, Film Coated	Amitriptyline HCl 10 mg	by Mutual	53489-0104	Antidepressant
MP108	Tab, White, Round, Scored	Quinidine Sulfate 200 mg	by Mutual	53489-0461	Antiarrhythmic
MP108	Tab	Quinidine Sulfate 200 mg	by United Res	00677-0122	Antiarrhythmic
MP11	Tab, Film Coated, MP Over 11	Dipyridamole 25 mg	by Quality Care	60346-0789	Antiplatelet
MP11	Tab, Film Coated	Dipyridamole 25 mg	by Mutual	53489-0115	Antiplatelet
MP111 <> 2	Tab	Acetaminophen 300 mg, Codeine 15 mg	by United Res	00677-0611	Analgesic; C III
MP111 <> 2	Tab	Acetaminophen 300 mg, Codeine Phosphate 15 mg	by Pharmedix	53002-0122	Analgesic; C III
MP1112	Tab, MP111 over 2	Acetaminophen 300 mg, Codeine Phosphate 15 mg	by Mutual	53489-0159	Analgesic; C III
MP1112	Tab, White, Round, MP 111 Over 2	Acetaminophen 300 mg, Codeine 15 mg	Acetaminophen W COD by Amerisource	62584-0058	Analgesic; C III

ID FRONT <> BACK	DESCRIPTION FRONT <> BACK	INGREDIENT & STRENGTH	BRAND (OR EQUIV.) & FIRM	NDC#	CLASS; SCH.
MP112	Tab, Yellow, Round	Sulindac 150 mg	by Southwood Pharms	58016-0743	NSAID
MP112	Tab, MP/112	Sulindac 150 mg	by Rugby	00536-4621	NSAID
MP112	Tab, Yellow, Round	Sulindac 150 mg	by Mutual	53489-0478	NSAID
MP112	Tab	Sulindac 150 mg	by Prescription Dispensing	61807-0036	NSAID
MP112	Tab	Sulindac 150 mg	by Quality Care	60346-0044	NSAID
MP112	Tab, MP Over 112	Sulindac 150 mg	by Direct Dispensing	57866-4621	NSAID
MP112	Tab	Sulindac 150 mg	by United Res	00677-1173	NSAID
MP112	Tab	Sulindac 150 mg	by Qualitest	00603-5872	NSAID
MP114	Tab, White, Round, Scored	Trazodone HCl 100 mg	Desyrel by Martec	52555-0728	Antidepressant
MP114	Tab, White, Round, Scored, Film Coated	Trazodone HCl 100 mg	by Teva	00480-0318	Antidepressant
MP114	Tab, White, Round, Scored, Film Coated	Trazodone HCl 100 mg	by Mutual	53489-0511	Antidepressant
MP114	Tab, Film Coated	Trazodone HCl 100 mg	by PDRX	55289-0223	Antidepressant
MP114	Tab, Film Coated	Trazodone HCl 100 mg	by Med Pro	53978-0563	Antidepressant
MP114	Tab, Film Coated	Trazodone HCl 100 mg	by Quality Care	60346-0014	Antidepressant
MP114	Tab, Film Coated	Trazodone HCl 100 mg	by United Res	00677-1134	Antidepressant
MP116	Tab, Yellow, Round, Scored	Sulindac 200 mg	by Allscripts	54569-4032	NSAID
MP116	Tab, Yellow, Round, Scored	Sulindac 200 mg	by Direct Dispensing	57866-4622	NSAID
MP116	Tab, Yellow, Round, Scored	Sulindac 200 mg	by Southwood Pharms	58016-0294	NSAID
MP116	Tab	Sulindac 200 mg	by Zenith Goldline	00182-1706	NSAID
MP116	Tab	Sulindac 200 mg	by Rugby	00536-4622	NSAID
MP116	Tab, Yellow, Round, Scored	Sulindac 200 mg	by Mutual	53489-0479	NSAID
MP116	Tab	Sulindac 200 mg	by Quality Care	60346-0686	NSAID
MP116	Tab	Sulindac 200 mg	by United Res	00677-1174	NSAID
MP116	Tab	Sulindac 200 mg	by Qualitest	00603-5873	NSAID
MP118	Tab, White, Round, Film Coated, Scored	Trazodone HCl 50 mg	by Allscripts	54569-1470	Antidepressant
MP118	Tab, White, Round, Scored	Trazodone HCl 50 mg	Desyrel by Martec	52555-0727	Antidepressant
MP118	Tab, White, Round, Scored, Film Coated	Trazodone HCl 50 mg	by Teva	00480-0294	Antidepressant
MP118	Tab, White, Round, Scored, Film Coated	Trazodone HCl 50 mg	by Mutual	53489-0510	Antidepressant
MP118	Tab, Film Coated	Trazodone HCl 50 mg	by United Res	00677-1133	Antidepressant
MP12	Tab, Yellow, Film Coated	Thioridazine HCl 10 mg	by Taro	52549-4030	Antipsychotic
MP12	Tab, Yellow, Round, Film Coated	Thioridazine HCl 10 mg	by Mutual	53489-0148	Antipsychotic
MP12	Tab, Film Coated	Thioridazine HCl 10 mg	by Qualitest	00603-5992	Antipsychotic
MP12	Tab, Coated	Thioridazine HCl 10 mg	by United Res	00677-0823	Antipsychotic
MP12	Tab, Film Coated, Debossed	Thioridazine HCl 10 mg	by Major	00904-5240	Antipsychotic
MP122 <> 3	Tab	Acetaminophen 300 mg, Codeine 30 mg	by United Res	00677-0612	Analgesic; C III
MP122 <> 3	Tab, MP Over 122	Acetaminophen 300 mg, Codeine Phosphate 30 mg	by Quality Care	60346-0059	Analgesic; C III
MP1223	Tab, MP 122 over 3	Acetaminophen 300 mg, Codeine Phosphate 30 mg	by Mutual	53489-0160	Analgesic; C III
MP124	Tab, White, Round, Scored	Quinidine Sulfate 300 mg	by Mutual	53489-0460	Antiarrhythmic
MP124	Tab	Quinidine Sulfate 300 mg	by United Res	00677-1209	Antiarrhythmic
MP124	Tab	Quinidine Sulfate 300 mg	by Qualitest	00603-5595	Antiarrhythmic
MP127 <> 4	Tab	Acetaminophen 300 mg, Codeine 60 mg	by United Res	00677-0632	Analgesic; C III
MP1274	Tab, MP 127 over 4	Acetaminophen 300 mg, Codeine Phosphate 60 mg	by Mutual	53489-0161	Analgesic; C III
MP1274	Tab, White, Round, MP 127 Over 4	Acetaminophen 300 mg, Codeine 60 mg	by Amerisource	62584-0065	Analgesic; C lll
MP13	Tab, Purple, Round, Scored, Film Coated	Hydroxyzine HCl 50 mg	by Mutual	53489-0128	Antihistamine
MP13	Tab, Purple, Round, Film Coated	Hydroxyzine HCl 50 mg	by Murfreesboro	51129-1474	Antihistamine
MP13	Tab, Coated	Hydroxyzine HCl 50 mg	by Quality Care	60346-0796	Antihistamine
MP13	Tab, Sugar Coated	Hydroxyzine HCl 50 mg	by United Res	00677-0606	Antihistamine
MP135	Tab, White, Round	Acetaminophen 325 mg	Tylenol by Mutual		Antipyretic
MP14	Tab, Yellow, Round, Film Coated	Thioridazine HCl 25 mg	by Mutual	53489-0149	Antipsychotic
MP14	Tab, Yellow, Film Coated	Thioridazine HCl 25 mg	by Taro	52549-4031	Antipsychotic
MP14	Tab, Film Coated	Thioridazine HCl 25 mg	by Quality Care	60346-0839	Antipsychotic
MP14	Tab, Film Coated	Thioridazine HCl 25 mg	by United Res	00677-0824	Antipsychotic

ID FRONT <> BACK	DESCRIPTION FRONT <> BACK	INGREDIENT & STRENGTH	BRAND (OR EQUIV.) & FIRM	NDC#	CLASS; SCH.
MP14	Tab, Film Coated, Debossed	Thioridazine HCl 25 mg	by Major	00904-5241	Antipsychotic
MP141	Tab, MP Over 141	Acetazolamide 250 mg	by Quality Care	60346-0734	Diuretic
MP141	Tab	Acetazolamide 250 mg	by Mutual	53489-0167	Diuretic
MP142	Tab	Benztropine Mesylate 2 mg	by Mutual	53489-0184	Antiparkinson
MP142	Tab	Benztropine Mesylate 2 mg	by United Res	00677-0995	Antiparkinson
MP146	Tab, MP 146	Atenolol 50 mg	by Quality Care	60346-0719	Antihypertensive
MP146	Tab, Debossed	Atenolol 50 mg	by Darby Group	66467-3330	Antihypertensive
MP146	Tab	Atenolol 50 mg	by Qualitest	00603-2371	Antihypertensive
MP146	Tab	Atenolol 50 mg	by United Res	00677-1478	Antihypertensive
MP146	Tab, White, Round, Scored	Atenolol 50 mg	by Mutual	53489-0529	Antihypertensive
MP146	Tab, White, Round, Scored	Atenolol 50 mg	Ternormin by Martec	52555-0673	Antihypertensive
MP147	Tab, MP 147	Atenolol 100 mg	by Quality Care	60346-0914	Antihypertensive
MP147	Tab	Atenolol 100 mg	by Qualitest	00603-2372	Antihypertensive
MP147	Tab	Atenolol 100 mg	by United Res	00677-1479	Antihypertensive
MP147	Tab, White, Round, Scored	Atenolol 100 mg	Tenormin by Martec	52555-0674	Antihypertensive
MP147	Tab, White, Round	Atenolol 100 mg	by Mutual	53489-0530	Antihypertensive
MP147	Tab	Atenolol 100 mg	by Talbert Med	44514-0885	Antihypertensive
MP148	Tab, White, Round, Debossed	Metoclopramide HCl 5 mg	by Mutual	53489-0384	Gastrointestinal
MP148	Tab, Debossed	Metoclopramide HCl	by Rugby	00536-4038	Gastrointestinal
MP148	Tab, Debossed	Metoclopramide HCl	by Major	00904-1069	Gastrointestinal
MP15	Tab, Film Coated	Dipyridamole 50 mg	by Mutual	53489-0116	Antiplatelet
MP151	Tab, Beveled Bisect	Prednisone 5 mg	by Apotheca	12634-0184	Steroid
MP152	Tab	Atenolol 100 mg, Chlorthalidone 25 mg	by PDRX	55289-0988	Antihypertensive; Diuretic
MP152	Tab	Atenolol 100 mg, Chlorthalidone 25 mg	by Zenith Goldline	00182-1943	Antihypertensive; Diuretic
MP152	Tab	Atenolol 100 mg, Chlorthalidone 25 mg	by United Res	00677-1481	Antihypertensive; Diuretic
MP152	Tab, White	Atenolol 100 mg, Chlorthalidone 25 mg	by Mutual	53489-0532	Antihypertensive; Diuretic
MP153	Tab	Atenolol 50 mg, Chlorthalidone 25 mg	by PDRX	55289-0993	Antihypertensive; Diuretic
MP153	Tab	Atenolol 50 mg, Chlorthalidone 25 mg	by Zenith Goldline	00182-1942	Antihypertensive; Diuretic
MP153	Tab	Atenolol 50 mg, Chlorthalidone 25 mg	by Geneva	00781-1315	Antihypertensive; Diuretic
MP153	Tab	Atenolol 50 mg, Chlorthalidone 25 mg	by United Res	00677-1480	Antihypertensive; Diuretic
MP153	Tab, White, Scored	Atenolol 50 mg, Chlorthalidone 25 mg	by Mutual	53489-0531	Antihypertensive; Diuretic
MP153	Tab	Atenolol 50 mg, Chlorthalidone 25 mg	by Murfreesboro	51129-1328	Antihypertensive; Diuretic
MP155	Tab	Quinine Sulfate 260 mg	by Mutual	53489-0462	Antimalarial
MP160	Tab, Yellow, Round, Film Coated	Thioridazine HCl 100 mg	by Mutual	53489-0500	Antipsychotic
MP160	Tab, Film Coated	Thioridazine HCl 100 mg	by Qualitest	00603-5995	Antipsychotic
MP160	Tab, Film Coated, Debossed	Thioridazine HCl 100 mg	by Major	00904-5243	Antipsychotic
MP160	Tab, Film Coated	Thioridazine HCl 100 mg	by United Res	00677-0832	Antipsychotic
MP167	Tab, Film Coated	Fenoprofen Calcium 691.8 mg	by Mutual	53489-0287	NSAID
MP168	Tab, White, Round, Scored	Trazodone HCl 150 mg	Desyrel by Martec	52555-0729	Antidepressant
MP168	Tab, White, Round, Divided Dose	Trazodone HCl 150 mg	by Mutual	53489-0517	Antidepressant
MP168	Tab, MP 168 <> Circle Divided Into 4 25/25/50/50	Trazodone HCl 150 mg	by Major	00904-5221	Antidepressant
MP168 <> 25255050	Tab, 25 in 2 Quadrants and 50 in Two Quadrants	Trazodone HCl 150 mg	by Rugby	00536-4691	Antidepressant

ID FRONT <> BACK	DESCRIPTION FRONT <> BACK	INGREDIENT & STRENGTH	BRAND (OR EQUIV.) & FIRM	NDC#	CLASS; SCH.
MP168 <> 25255050	Tab, 25 25 / 50 50	Trazodone HCl 150 mg	by Allscripts	54569-3732	Antidepressant
MP17	Tab, Yellow, Round, Film Coated	Thioridazine HCl 50 mg	by Mutual	53489-0150	Antipsychotic
MP17	Tab, Film Coated	Thioridazine HCl 50 mg	by United Res	00677-0825	Antipsychotic
MP17	Tab, Film Coated	Thioridazine HCl 50 mg	by Qualitest	00603-5994	Antipsychotic
MP17	Tab, Film Coated, Debossed	Thioridazine HCl 50 mg	by Major	00904-5242	Antipsychotic
MP174	Tab, Film Coated	Salsalate 500 mg	by Kaiser	00179-1220	NSAID
MP174	Tab, Yellow, Round, Film Coated	Salsalate 500 mg	by Mutual	53489-0465	NSAID
MP177	Tab, Coated	Salsalate 500 mg	by United Res	00677-1024	NSAID
MP177	Tab, Film Coated	Salsalate 750 mg	by Kaiser	00179-1229	NSAID
MP177	Tab, Yellow, Capsule Shape, Film Coated	Salsalate 750 mg	by Mutual	53489-0466	NSAID
MP177	Tab, Film Coated	Salsalate 750 mg	by Med Pro	53978-0399	NSAID
MP177	Tab, Film Coated	Salsalate 750 mg	by Pharmedix	53002-0488	NSAID
MP177	Tab, Film Coated	Salsalate 750 mg	by Kaiser	62224-0559	NSAID
MP177	Tab, Coated	Salsalate 750 mg	by Quality Care	60346-0034	NSAID
MP177	Tab, Film Coated, Debossed	Salsalate 750 mg	by Golden State	60429-0207	NSAID
MP178	Tab, White, Debossed	Pindolol 5 mg	by Mutual	53489-0430	Antihypertensive
MP178	Tab	Pindolol 5 mg	by Qualitest	00603-5220	Antihypertensive
MP178	Tab, Debossed	Pindolol 5 mg	by Major	00904-7893	Antihypertensive
MP178 <> MP178	Tab	Pindolol 5 mg	by United Res	00677-1457	Antihypertensive
MP18	Tab, Film Coated	Dipyridamole 75 mg	by Mutual	53489-0117	Antiplatelet
MP183	Tab, White	Pindolol 10 mg	by Mutual	53489-0431	Antihypertensive
MP183	Tab, Debossed	Pindolol 10 mg	by Major	00904-7894	Antihypertensive
MP183 <> MP183	Tab	Pindolol 10 mg	by United Res	00677-1458	Antihypertensive
MP184	Tab, Orange, Cap-Shape, Scored, Film Coated	Metoprolol Tartrate 50 mg	by Mutual	53489-0366	Antihypertensive
MP184	Tab, Film Coated, Debossed	Metoprolol Tartrate 50 mg	by Quality Care	60346-0523	Antihypertensive
MP184	Tab, Film Coated, Debossed	Metoprolol Tartrate 50 mg	by Major	00904-7772	Antihypertensive
MP185	Tab, Film Coated	Metoprolol Tartrate 100 mg	by Murfreesboro	51129-1109	Antihypertensive
MP185	Tab, Film Coated	Metoprolol Tartrate 100 mg	by Rugby	00536-5605	Antihypertensive
MP185	Tab, Yellow, Cap-Shape, Scored, Film Coated	Metoprolol Tartrate 100 mg	by Mutual	53489-0367	Antihypertensive
MP185	Tab, Film Coated, Debossed	Metoprolol Tartrate 100 mg	by PDRX	55289-0093	Antihypertensive
MP185	Tab, Film Coated	Metoprolol Tartrate 100 mg	by United Res	00677-1483	Antihypertensive
MP185	Tab, Film Coated, Debossed	Metoprolol Tartrate 100 mg	by Major	00904-7773	Antihypertensive
MP20	Tab, White, Round	Dihydro-Alpha-Ergocryptine Mesylate 0.222 mg, Dihydro-Beta-Ergocryptine Mesylate 0.111 mg, Dihydroergocornine Mesylate 0.333 mg, Dihydroergocristine Mesylate 0.333 mg	Ergoloid Mesylates by Mutual	53489-0281	Ergot
MP20	Tab	Dihydro-Alpha-Ergocryptine Mesylate 0.222 mg, Dihydro-Beta-Ergocryptine Mesylate 0.111 mg, Dihydroergocornine Mesylate 0.333 mg, Dihydroergocristine Mesylate 0.333 mg	Ergoloid Mesylates by Zenith Goldline	00182-1518	Ergot
MP20	Tab	Dihydro-Alpha-Ergocryptine Mesylate 0.222 mg, Dihydro-Beta-Ergocryptine Mesylate 0.111 mg, Dihydroergocornine Mesylate 0.333 mg, Dihydroergocristine Mesylate 0.333 mg	Ergoloid Mesylates by Qualitest	00603-3527	Ergot
MP20	Tab	Dihydro-Alpha-Ergocryptine Mesylate 0.222 mg, Dihydro-Beta-Ergocryptine Mesylate 0.111 mg, Dihydroergocornine Mesylate 0.333 mg, Dihydroergocristine Mesylate 0.333 mg	Ergoloid Mesylates by United Res	00677-0782	Ergot
MP20	Tab, MP Over 20	Dihydro-Alpha-Ergocryptine Mesylate 0.222 mg, Dihydro-Beta-Ergocryptine Mesylate 0.111 mg, Dihydroergocornine Mesylate 0.333 mg, Dihydroergocristine Mesylate 0.333 mg	Ergoloid Mesylates by UDL	51079-0110	Ergot
MP20	Tab, White, Round	Ergoloid Mesylate 1 mg	Ergoloid by Direct Dispensing	57866-0303	Ergot
MP20	Tab	Ergoloid Mesylates 1 mg	Gerimal by Rugby	00536-3856	Ergot
MP22	Tab, Film Coated	Hydralazine HCl 10 mg	by Mutual	53489-0123	Antihypertensive
MP25	Tab, Coated, MP Over 25	Amitriptyline HCl 25 mg	by Quality Care	60346-0027	Antidepressant
MP25	Tab, Film Coated	Amitriptyline HCl 25 mg	by Kaiser	00179-0042	Antidepressant

ID FRONT <> BACK	DESCRIPTION FRONT <> BACK	INGREDIENT & STRENGTH	BRAND (OR EQUIV.) & FIRM	NDC#	CLASS; SCH.
MP25	Tab, Film Coated	Amitriptyline HCl 25 mg	by United Res	00677-0476	Antidepressant
MP25	Tab, Green, Round, Film Coated	Amitriptyline HCl 25 mg	by Mutual	53489-0105	Antidepressant
MP26	Tab, Film Coated, MP Over 26	Amitriptyline HCl 50 mg	by Quality Care	60346-0673	Antidepressant
MP26	Tab, Film Coated	Amitriptyline HCl 50 mg	by United Res	00677-0477	Antidepressant
MP26	Tab, Brown, Round, Film Coated	Amitriptyline HCl 50 mg	by Mutual	53489-0106	Antidepressant
MP27	Tab, Film Coated	Amitriptyline HCl 75 mg	by United Res	00677-0478	Antidepressant
MP27	Tab, Purple, Round, Film Coated	Amitriptyline HCl 75 mg	by Mutual	53489-0107	Antidepressant
MP271	Tab, White, Scored, Film Coated	Labetalol 200 mg	by Mutual	53489-0355	Antihypertensive
MP271	Tab, White, Round, Scored	Labetalol HCl 200 mg	by United Res Labs	00677-1702	Antihypertensive
MP271	Tab, White, Round, Scored, Film Coated	Labetalol HCl 200 mg	Labetalol HCl by Murfreesboro	51129-1609	Antihypertensive
MP272	Tab, Blue, Film Coated	Labetalol 300 mg	by Mutual	53489-0356	Antihypertensive
MP272	Tab, Blue, Round	Labetalol 300 mg	by United Res Tabs	00677-1703	Antihypertensive
MP272	Tab, Blue, Round, Film Coated	Labetalol HCl 300 mg	Labetalol HCl by Murfreesboro	51129-1611	Antihypertensive
MP277	Tab, Beige, Scored, Film Coated	Labetalol 100 mg	Normodyne by Mutual	53489-0354	Antihypertensive
MP277	Tab, Beige, Round, Scored, Film Coated	Labetalol HCl 100 mg	Labetalol HCl by Murfreesboro	51129-1608	Antihypertensive
MP28	Tab	Amitriptyline HCl 100 mg	by United Res	00677-0568	Antidepressant
MP28	Tab, Orange, Round, Film Coated	Amitriptyline HCl 100 mg	by Mutual	53489-0108	Antidepressant
MP29	Tab, Film Coated	Amitriptyline HCl 150 mg	by United Res	00677-0645	Antidepressant
MP29	Tab, Peach, Cap Shaped, Film Coated	Amitriptyline HCl 150 mg	by Mutual	53489-0109	Antidepressant
MP3	Tab, Purple or White, Round	Hydroxyzine 10 mg	by Allscripts	54569-0406	Antihistamine
MP3	Tab, Purple, Round	Hydroxyzine HCl 10 mg	Atarax by Mutual		Antihistamine
MP3	Tab, Film Coated	Hydroxyzine HCl 10 mg	by Pharmedix	53002-0390	Antihistamine
MP3	Tab, Sugar Coated	Hydroxyzine HCl 10 mg	by United Res	00677-0604	Antihistamine
MP30	Tab	Chlorthalidone 25 mg	by Mutual	53489-0111	Diuretic
MP303	Tab, White, Oval, Scored, Film Coated	Spironolactone 100 mg	by Sidmark		Diuretic
MP303	Tab, White, Oval, Film Coated, Scored	Spironolactone 100 mg	by United Res	00677-1708	Diuretic
MP303	Tab, White, Oval, Scored, Film Coated	Spironolactone 100 mg	Spironolactone by Sidmark		Diuretic
MP303	Tab, White, Oval, Scored, Film Coated	Spironolactone 50 mg	by Mutual	53489-0329	Diuretic
MP35	Tab, White, Round	Spironolactone 25 mg	by Allscripts	54569-0505	Diuretic
MP35	Tab, White, Round, Debossed	Spironolactone 25 mg	by Mutual	53489-0143	Diuretic
MP35	Tab	Spironolactone 25 mg	by Pharmedix	53002-0472	Diuretic
MP35	Tab	Spironolactone 25 mg	by Quality Care	60346-0810	Diuretic
MP35	Tab	Spironolactone 25 mg	by Qualitest	00603-5766	Diuretic
MP36	Tab	Metoclopramide 10 mg	by Mutual	53489-0385	Gastrointestinal
MP37	Cap, Light Orange, MP 37	Doxycycline Hyclate	by Quality Care	60346-0449	Antibiotic
MP37	Tab, Film Coated, MP 37	Doxycycline Hyclate	by Golden State	60429-0069	Antibiotic
MP37	Tab, Film Coated	Doxycycline Hyclate	by Darby Group	66467-0340	Antibiotic
MP37	Tab, Light Orange, Film Coated	Doxycycline 100 mg	by Allscripts	54569-0118	Antibiotic
MP37	Tab, Film Coated	Doxycycline Hyclate	by United Res	00677-0799	Antibiotic
MP37	Tab, Film Coated	Doxycycline Hyclate	by Qualitest	00603-3482	Antibiotic
MP37	Tab, Film Coated	Doxycycline Hyclate	by HJ Harkins Co	52959-0474	Antibiotic
MP37	Cap	Doxycycline Hyclate	by Major	00904-0430	Antibiotic
MP37	Tab, Light Orange, Round	Doxycycline Hyclate 100 mg	Vibra-Tabs by Mutual	53489-0120	Antibiotic
MP37 <> MP37	Tab, Film Coated	Doxycycline Hyclate	by Dept Health Central Pharm	53808-0041	Antibiotic
MP39	Tab, White, Round, Scored	Lorazepam 1 mg	by Mutual	53489-0358	Sedative/Hypnotic; C IV
MP39	Tab	Lorazepam 1 mg	by United Res	00677-1057	Sedative/Hypnotic; C IV
MP392	Tab	Acetaminophen 650 mg, Butalbital 50 mg	Sedapap by Merz	00259-0392	Analgesic
MP392	Tab	Acetaminophen 650 mg, Butalbital 50 mg	by Mikart	46672-0164	Analgesic
MP4	Tab, Yellow, Round	Imipramine HCl 10 mg	by United Res Labs	00677-0421	Antidepressant
MP4	Tab, Yellow, Round	Imipramine HCl 10 mg	Tofranil by Mutual		Antidepressant
MP4	Tab, Yellow, Film Coated	Imipramine HCl 10 mg	by Mutual	53489-0330	Antidepressant
MP4	Tab, Film Coated	Imipramine HCl 10 mg	by Qualitest	00603-4043	Antidepressant

ID FRONT <> BACK	DESCRIPTION FRONT <> BACK	INGREDIENT & STRENGTH	BRAND (OR EQUIV.) & FIRM	NDC#	CLASS; SCH.
MP40	Tab, Buff, Round	Hydrochlorothiazide 25 mg, Spironolactone 25 mg	by Allscripts	54569-0502	Diuretic; Antihypertensive
MP40	Tab	Hydrochlorothiazide 25 mg, Spironolactone 25 mg	by Zenith Goldline	00182-1158	Diuretic; Antihypertensive
MP40	Tab, Buff, Round	Hydrochlorothiazide 25 mg, Spironolactone 25 mg	by Mutual	53489-0144	Diuretic; Antihypertensive
MP40	Tab, Buff	Hydrochlorothiazide 25 mg, Spironolactone 25 mg	by Quality Care	60346-0811	Diuretic; Antihypertensive
MP40	Tab	Hydrochlorothiazide 25 mg, Spironolactone 25 mg	by Geneva	00781-1149	Diuretic; Antihypertensive
MP40	Tab	Hydrochlorothiazide 25 mg, Spironolactone 25 mg	by United Res	00677-0624	Diuretic; Antihypertensive
MP423	Tab, Cap Shaped, Scored	Guaifenesin 600 mg	by Mutual	53489-0423	Expectorant
MP424	Tab, Film Coated	Guaifenesin 600 mg, Pseudoephedrine HCl 120 mg	by United Res	00677-1476	Cold Remedy
MP424	Tab, White, Oval, Scored	Guaifenesin 600 mg, Pseudoephedrine HCl 120 mg	by Mutual	53489-0424	Cold Remedy
MP425	Tab	Guaifenesin 600 mg, Pseudoephedrine HCl 60 mg	by United Res	00677-1487	Cold Remedy
MP425	Tab, Blue, Cap Shaped	Guaifenesin 600 mg, Pseudoephedrine HCl 60 mg	by Mutual	53489-0425	Cold Remedy
MP43	Tab	Chlorthalidone 50 mg	by Mutual	53489-0112	Diuretic
MP44	Tab	Benztropine Mesylate 1 mg	by Quality Care	60346-0776	Antiparkinson
MP44	Tab	Benztropine Mesylate 1 mg	by Mutual	53489-0183	Antiparkinson
MP44	Tab	Benztropine Mesylate 1 mg	by United Res	00677-0993	Antiparkinson
MP45	Tab, White, Round	Metronidazole 250 mg	by Neuman Distr	64579-0108	Antibiotic
MP45	Tab	Metronidazole 250 mg	by Pharmedix	53002-0221	Antibiotic
MP45	Tab, White	Metronidazole 250 mg	by Mutual	53489-0135	Antibiotic
MP45	Tab, White, Round	Metronidazole 250 mg	Flagyl by Martec	52555-0725	Antibiotic
MP45	Tab	Metronidazole 250 mg	by Quality Care	60346-0592	Antibiotic
MP46	Tab, White, Cap Shaped	Metronidazole 500 mg	Flagyl by Martec	52555-0726	Antibiotic
MP46	Tab, White, Oblong	Metronidazole 500 mg	by Neuman Distr	64579-0110	Antibiotic
MP46	Tab	Metronidazole 500 mg	by Pharmedix	53002-0247	Antibiotic
MP46	Tab, White, Cap-Shaped	Metronidazole 500 mg	by Mutual	53489-0136	Antibiotic
MP46	Tab, Coated	Metronidazole 500 mg	by Quality Care	60346-0507	Antibiotic
MP47	Tab	Albuterol Sulfate	by PDRX	55289-0363	Antiasthmatic
MP47	Tab, White, Round, Scored	Albuterol Sulfate 2 mg	by Mutual	53489-0176	Antiasthmatic
MP47	Tab	Albuterol Sulfate 2.4 mg	by United Res	00677-1359	Antiasthmatic
MP47	Tab, MP/47	Albuterol Sulfate 2.4 mg	by Major	00904-2876	Antiasthmatic
MP48	Tab, White, Round, Scored	Albuterol Sulfate 4 mg	by Mutual	53489-0177	Antiasthmatic
MP50	Tab, Off-White, Round, Scored	Tolmetin Sodium 200 mg	by Mutual	53489-0506	NSAID
MP50	Tab	Tolmetin Sodium 246 mg	by United Res	00677-1425	NSAID
MP500	Tab, White to Off-White, Round, Scored	Ketoconazole 200 mg	Nizoral by Mutual	53489-0554	Antifungal
MP500	Tab, White, Round, Scored	Ketoconazole 200 mg	by Murfreesboro	51129-1594	Antifungal
MP500	Tab, White, Round, Scored	Ketoconazole 200 mg	Ketoconazole by Murfreesboro	51129-1592	Antifungal
MP51	Tab, MP/51	Prednisone 5 mg	by Darby Group	66467-4324	Steroid
MP51	Tab, White, Round, Scored, MP/51	Prednisone 5 mg	by Allscripts	54569-0330	Steroid
MP51	Tab, MP/51	Prednisone 5 mg	by Qualitest	00603-5332	Steroid
MP51	Tab, White, Round, Scored, Debossed MP/51	Prednisone 5 mg	by Qualitest	00603-3459	Steroid
MP51	Tab	Prednisone 5 mg	by Pharmedix	53002-0352	Steroid
MP51	Tab, White, Round, Scored, MP over 51	Prednisone 5 mg	Deltasone by UDL	51079-0032	Steroid
MP51	Tab, Beveled Bisect <> MP/51	Prednisone 5 mg	by HJ Harkins Co	52959-0220	Steroid
MP51	Tab, White, Round, Scored	Prednisone 5 mg	by Mutual	53489-0138	Steroid
MP51	Tab, MP Over 51	Prednisone 5 mg	by PDRX	55289-0438	Steroid
MP51	Tab	Prednisone 5 mg	by Prescription Dispensing	61807-0044	Steroid
MP51	Tab, MP/51	Prednisone 5 mg	by Quality Care	60346-0515	Steroid

ID FRONT <> BACK	DESCRIPTION FRONT <> BACK	INGREDIENT & STRENGTH	BRAND (OR EQUIV.) & FIRM	NDC#	CLASS; SCH.
MP51	Tab	Prednisone 5 mg	by United Res	00677-0117	Steroid
MP51	Tab, White, Round, Flat, Scored, MP/51	Prednisone 5 mg	by Qualitest	00603-5025	Steroid
MP51	Tab, White, Round, Scored, MP/51	Prednisone 5 mg	by Qualitest	00603-4235	Steroid
MP51	Tab, Beveled Bisect, Compressed	Prednisone 5 mg	by Major	00904-2157	Steroid
MP52	Tab	Prednisone 10 mg	by Darby Group	66467-4325	Steroid
MP52	Tab, Coated, MP/52	Prednisone 10 mg	by Qualitest	00603-5333	Steroid
MP52	Tab, Beveled, MP/52	Prednisone 10 mg	by HJ Harkins Co	52959-0126	Steroid
MP52	Tab	Prednisone 10 mg	by Pharmedix	53002-0309	Steroid
MP52	Tab, White, Round, Scored	Prednisone 10 mg	by Mutual	53489-0139	Steroid
MP52	Tab, White, Round, Scored, MP over 52	Prednisone 10 mg	Deltasone by UDL	51079-0033	Steroid
MP52	Tab, MP/52	Prednisone 10 mg	by Quality Care	60346-0058	Steroid
MP52	Tab, MP/52	Prednisone 10 mg	by Major	00904-2141	Steroid
MP52	Tab	Prednisone 10 mg	by United Res	00677-0698	Steroid
MP53	Tab, Flat Faced, Beveled Bisect, MP/53	Prednisone 20 mg	by Quality Care	60346-0094	Steroid
MP53	Tab, Beveled Bisect	Prednisone 20 mg	by Major	00904-2140	Steroid
MP53	Tab	Prednisone 20 mg	by United Res	00677-0427	Steroid
MP53	Tab, Peach, Round, Scored	Prednisone 20 mg	by Qualitest	00603-3763	Steroid
MP53	Tab, Peach, Round, Scored, MP over 53	Prednisone 20 mg	Deltasone by UDL	51079-0022	Steroid
MP53	Tab	Prednisone 20 mg	by PDRX	55289-0352	Steroid
MP53	Tab, Peach, Round, Scored	Prednisone 20 mg	by Mutual	53489-0140	Steroid
MP53	Tab	Prednisone 20 mg	by Prescription Dispensing	61807-0067	Steroid
MP53	Tab	Prednisone 20 mg	by St Marys Med	60760-0002	Steroid
MP53	Tab, Peach, Round, Scored	Prednisone 20 mg	by Allscripts	54569-3043	Steroid
MP53	Tab, Peach, Scored	Prednisone 20 mg	by Direct Dispensing	57866-4326	Steroid
MP53 <> 1332	Tab, Peach, Scored	Prednisone 20 mg	by Southwood Pharms	58016-0217	Steroid
MP542	Tab, White, Round, Scored, Film Coated	Spironolactone 50 mg	by Mutual	53489-0328	Diuretic
MP542	Tab, White, Round, Scored, Film Coated	Spironolactone 50 mg	by Sidmark		Diuretic
MP542	Tab, White, Round, Scored, Film Coated	Spironolactone 50 mg	Spironolactone by Sidmark	50111-0615	Diuretic
MP55	Tab	Hydralazine HCl 50 mg	by Kaiser	00179-0345	Antihypertensive
MP55	Tab	Hydralazine HCl 50 mg	by Mutual	53489-0125	Antihypertensive
MP58	Tab, White, Round	Carisoprodol 350 mg	by Allscripts	54569-3403	Muscle Relaxant
MP58	Tab, White, Round	Carisoprodol 350 mg	by Allscripts	54569-1709	Muscle Relaxant
MP58	Tab	Carisoprodol 350 mg	by Kaiser	00179-0171	Muscle Relaxant
MP58	Tab	Carisoprodol 350 mg	by Zenith Goldline	00182-1079	Muscle Relaxant
MP58	Tab	Carisoprodol 350 mg	by Qualitest	00603-2582	Muscle Relaxant
MP58	Tab	Carisoprodol 350 mg	by United Res	00677-0589	Muscle Relaxant
MP58	Tab	Carisoprodol 350 mg	by Urgent Care Ctr	50716-0202	Muscle Relaxant
MP58	Tab, White, Round, MP over 58	Carisoprodol 350 mg	Soma by UDL	51079-0055	Muscle Relaxant
MP58	Tab	Carisoprodol 350 mg	by HJ Harkins Co	52959-0026	Muscle Relaxant
MP58	Tab	Carisoprodol 350 mg	by Pharmedix	53002-0356	Muscle Relaxant
MP58	Tab, White, Round	Carisoprodol 350 mg	by Mutual	53489-0110	Muscle Relaxant
MP58	Tab	Carisoprodol 350 mg	by PDRX	55289-0049	Muscle Relaxant
MP58	Tab	Carisoprodol 350 mg	by Kaiser	62224-7333	Muscle Relaxant
MP58	Tab	Carisoprodol 350 mg	by Quality Care	60346-0635	Muscle Relaxant
MP58	Tab	Carisoprodol 350 mg	by Direct Dispensing	57866-3435	Muscle Relaxant
MP58	Tab	Carisoprodol 350 mg	by Prescription Dispensing	61807-0047	Muscle Relaxant
MP58	Tab	Carisoprodol 350 mg	by Nat Pharmpak Serv	55154-5515	Muscle Relaxant
MP58	Tab, MP 58	Carisoprodol 350 mg	by Darby Group	66467-3435	Muscle Relaxant
MP6	Tab, White, Round	Lorazepam 0.5 mg	by Mutual	53489-0357	Sedative/Hypnotic; C IV
MP6	Tab	Lorazepam 0.51 mg	by United Res	00677-1056	Sedative/Hypnotic; C IV
MP64	Tab	Hydralazine HCl 25 mg	by Kaiser	00179-0344	Antihypertensive
MP64	Tab	Hydralazine HCl 25 mg	by United Res	00677-0447	Antihypertensive

ID FRONT <> BACK	DESCRIPTION FRONT <> BACK	INGREDIENT & STRENGTH	BRAND (OR EQUIV.) & FIRM	NDC#	CLASS; SCH.
MP64	Tab	Hydralazine HCl 25 mg	by Pharmedix	53002-0429	Antihypertensive
MP64	Tab	Hydralazine HCl 25 mg	by Mutual	53489-0124	Antihypertensive
MP65	Tab, MP/65	Acetazolamide 125 mg	by Quality Care	60346-0773	Diuretic
MP65	Tab	Acetazolamide 125 mg	by United Res	00677-1248	Diuretic
MP65	Tab, White, Scored	Acetazolamide 125 mg	by Mutual	53489-0166	Diuretic
MP66	Tab, Cream, Round, MP/66	Quinidine Gluconate 324 mg	by RX PAK	65084-0130	Antiarrhythmic
MP66	Tab, White, Round, MP/66	Quinidine Gluconate 324 mg	by RX PAK	65084-0131	Antiarrhythmic
MP66	Tab, Ex Release	Quinidine Gluconate 324 mg	by Zenith Goldline	00182-1382	Antiarrhythmic
MP66	Tab, ER	Quinidine Gluconate 324 mg	by Rugby	00536-4434	Antiarrhythmic
MP66	Tab, White to Off-White, Round	Quinidine Gluconate 324 mg	by Mutual	53489-0141	Antiarrhythmic
MP66	Tab, White-Off White, Round, MP Over 66	Quinidine Gluconate 324 mg	Quinaglute by UDL	51079-0027	Antiarrhythmic
MP66	Tab, Ex Release	Quinidine Gluconate 324 mg	by Qualitest	00603-5598	Antiarrhythmic
MP66	Tab, ER	Quinidine Gluconate 324 mg	by United Res	00677-0675	Antiarrhythmic
MP68	Tab	Tolazamide 100 mg	by Mutual	53489-0151	Antidiabetic
MP69	Tab, Film Coated	Verapamil HCl 80 mg	by Mutual	53489-0154	Antihypertensive
MP7	Tab, Sugar Coated	Hydroxyzine HCl 25 mg	by United Res	00677-0605	Antihistamine
MP7	Tab, Purple, Round, Scored, Film Coated	Hydroxyzine HCl 25 mg	Atarax by Mutual	53489-0127	Antihistamine
MP7	Tab, Film Coated	Hydroxyzine HCl 25 mg	by Pharmedix	53002-0320	Antihistamine
MP70	Tab	Tolazamide 250 mg	by Mutual	53489-0152	Antidiabetic
MP71	Tab	Allopurinol 100 mg	by Qualitest	00603-2117	Antigout
MP71	Tab	Allopurinol 100 mg	by United Res	00677-0870	Antigout
MP71	Tab, White, Round, Scored	Allopurinol 100 mg	by Mutual	53489-0156	Antigout
MP71	Tab, Debossed	Allopurinol 100 mg	by Major	00904-2613	Antigout
MP72	Tab	Tolazamide 500 mg	by Mutual	53489-0153	Antidiabetic
MP74	Tab	Chlorzoxazone 500 mg	by Mutual	53489-0193	Muscle Relaxant
MP74	Tab	Chlorzoxazone 500 mg	by United Res	00677-1221	Muscle Relaxant
MP76	Tab, Film Coated	Verapamil HCl 120 mg	by Mutual	53489-0155	Antihypertensive
MP77	Tab, White, Round	Ibuprofen 200 mg	Advil by Mutual		NSAID
MP79	Tab, Green, Round, Film Coated	Imipramine HCl 50 mg	by Allscripts	54569-0196	Antidepressant
MP79	Tab, Green, Round	Imipramine HCl 50 mg	by United Res Labs	00677-0423	Antidepressant
MP79	Tab, Green, Film Coated	Imipramine HCl 50 mg	by Mutual	53489-0332	Antidepressant
MP79	Tab, Film Coated	Imipramine HCl 50 mg	by Qualitest	00603-4045	Antidepressant
MP8	Tab, Brown, Round, Film-Coated	Imipramine HCl 25 mg	by Allscripts	54569-0194	Antidepressant
MP8	Tab, Brown, Round, Film Coated	Imipramine HCl 25 mg	Tofranil by Mutual	53489-0331	Antidepressant
MP8	Tab, Sugar Coated	Imipramine HCl 25 mg	by United Res	00677-0422	Antidepressant
MP80	Tab	Allopurinol 300 mg	by Golden State	60429-0014	Antigout
MP80	Tab, Apricot, MP/80	Allopurinol 300 mg	by Kaiser	00179-1212	Antigout
MP80	Tab	Allopurinol 300 mg	by Qualitest	00603-2118	Antigout
MP80	Tab	Allopurinol 300 mg	by United Res	00677-0871	Antigout
MP80	Tab, Orange, Round, Scored	Allopurinol 300 mg	by Mutual	53489-0157	Antigout
MP80	Tab	Allopurinol 300 mg	by Pharmedix	53002-0482	Antigout
MP80	Tab	Allopurinol 300 mg	by Major	00904-2614	Antigout
MP81	Tab	Sulfamethoxazole 400 mg, Trimethoprim 80 mg	by Darby Group	66467-4692	Antibiotic
MP81	Tab	Sulfamethoxazole 400 mg, Trimethoprim 80 mg	by Rugby	00536-4692	Antibiotic
MP81	Tab	Sulfamethoxazole 800 mg, Trimethoprim 160 mg	SMZ TMP DS by Quality Care	60346-0087	Antibiotic
MP81	Tab, Compressed, MP/81	Sulfamethoxazole 400 mg, Trimethoprim 80 mg	by Kaiser	00179-0371	Antibiotic
MP81	Tab	Sulfamethoxazole 400 mg, Trimethoprim 80 mg	by Zenith Goldline	00182-1478	Antibiotic
MP81	Tab, Debossed	Sulfamethoxazole 400 mg, Trimethoprim 80 mg	by ESI Lederle	59911-5859	Antibiotic
MP81	Tab, Debossed	Sulfamethoxazole 400 mg, Trimethoprim 80 mg	by Major	00904-2726	Antibiotic
MP81	Tab	Sulfamethoxazole 400 mg, Trimethoprim 80 mg	by United Res	00677-0783	Antibiotic
MP81	Tab, White, Round, Scored	Sulfamethoxazole 400 mg, Trimethoprim 800 mg	Bactrim by Mutual	53489-0145	Antibiotic
MP81	Tab, White, Round, Scored	Sulfamethoxazole 400 mg; Trimethoprim 80 mg	by Murfreesboro Ph	51129-1438	Antibiotic

ID FRONT <> BACK	DESCRIPTION FRONT <> BACK	INGREDIENT & STRENGTH	BRAND (OR EQUIV.) & FIRM	NDC#	CLASS; SCH.
MP81	Tab, White, Round, Scored	Trimethoprim 80 mg, Sulfamethoxazole 400 mg	SMZ TMP by Southwood Pharms	58016-0171	Antibiotic
MP83	Tab, Brown, Round, Film Coated	Nystatin 500 MU	by Mutual	53489-0400	Antifungal
MP83	Tab, Film Coated	Nystatin 500000 Units	by United Res	00677-0613	Antifungal
MP83	Tab, Film Coated, Debossed	Nystatin 500000 Units	by Major	00904-0672	Antifungal
MP83	Tab, Brown, Round, Film Coated	Nystatin 500000 Unt	by Murfreesboro Ph	51129-1360	Antifungal
MP84	Tab, White, Round	Minoxidil 2.5 mg	Loniten by Mutual		Antihypertensive
MP84	Tab, White	Minoxidil 2.5 mg	by Mutual	53489-0386	Antihypertensive
MP85	Tab	Sulfamethoxazole 800 mg, Trimethoprim 160 mg	by West Ward	00143-1625	Antibiotic
MP85	Tab	Sulfamethoxazole 800 mg, Trimethoprim 160 mg	by Rugby	00536-4693	Antibiotic
MP85	Tab, White, Oval, Scored	Sulfaamethoxazole 800 mg, Trimethoprim 160 mg	Bactrim DS by Mutual	53489-0146	Antibiotic
MP85	Tab, White, Oval, Scored, MP/85	Sulfamethoxazole 800 mg, Trimethoprim 160 mg	Bactrim by UDL	51079-0128	Antibiotic
MP85	Tab	Sulfamethoxazole 800 mg, Trimethoprim 160 mg	Trimeth Sulfa DS by Pharmedix	53002-0210	Antibiotic
MP85	Tab, White, Oval, Scored	Sulfamethoxazole 800 mg, Trimethoprim 160 mg	by St. Marys Med	60760-0076	Antibiotic
MP85	Tab	Sulfamethoxazole 800 mg, Trimethoprim 160 mg	by ESI Lederle	59911-5860	Antibiotic
MP85	Tab	Sulfamethoxazole 800 mg, Trimethoprim 160 mg	by Golden State	60429-0170	Antibiotic
MP85	Tab	Sulfamethoxazole 800 mg, Trimethoprim 160 mg	by Apotheca	12634-0177	Antibiotic
MP85	Tab	Sulfamethoxazole 800 mg, Trimethoprim 160 mg	by Qualitest	00603-5779	Antibiotic
MP85	Tab	Sulfamethoxazole 800 mg, Trimethoprim 160 mg	by United Res	00677-0784	Antibiotic
MP88	Tab, Coated, MP 88	Albuterol Sulfate 4.8 mg	by Quality Care	60346-0285	Antiasthmatic
MP88	Tab	Albuterol Sulfate 4.8 mg	by United Res	00677-1360	Antiasthmatic
MP88	Tab, Debossed	Albuterol Sulfate 4.8 mg	by Major	00904-2877	Antiasthmatic
MP89	Tab, White, Round	Minoxidil 10 mg	Loniten by Mutual		Antihypertensive
MP89	Tab, White, Scored	Minoxidil 10 mg	by Mutual	53489-0387	Antihypertensive
MP9	Tab	Atenolol 25 mg	by United Res	00677-1633	Antihypertensive
MP9	Tab, White, Round, Scored	Atenolol 25 mg	Tenormin by Martec	52555-0689	Antihypertensive
MP9	Tab, White, Round,	Atenolol 25 mg	by Mutual	53489-0536	Antihypertensive
MP91	Tab	Sulfasalazine 500 mg	by Zenith Goldline	00182-1016	Gastrointestinal
MP91	Tab, Yellow, Round, Scored	Sulfasalazine 500 mg	by Mutual	53489-0147	Gastrointestinal
MP91	Tab, Golden Yellow	Sulfasalazine 500 mg	by Quality Care	60346-0812	Gastrointestinal
MP91	Tab	Sulfasalazine 500 mg	by Qualitest	00603-5802	Gastrointestinal
MP91	Tab	Sulfasalazine 500 mg	by United Res	00677-0483	Gastrointestinal
MP91	Tab	Sulfasalazine 500 mg	by Darby Group	66467-4617	Gastrointestinal
MP91	Tab, Yellow, Round, Scored	Sulfasalazine 500 mg	by Murfreesboro Ph	51129-1408	Gastrointestinal
MP93	Tab	Quinidine Sulfate 100 mg	by Mutual	53489-0459	Antiarrhythmic
MP94	Tab, White, Round	Ibuprofen 300 mg	Motrin by Mutual		NSAID
MP95	Tab, Film Coated	Ibuprofen 400 mg	by United Res	00677-1031	NSAID
MP95	Tab, Film Coated	Ibuprofen 400 mg	by West Ward	00143-1300	NSAID
MP96	Tab, White, Round, Scored	Lorazepam 2 mg	by United Res Labs	00677-1058	Sedative/Hypnotic; C IV
MP96	Tab, White, Round, Scored	Lorazepam 2 mg	by Mutual	53489-0359	Sedative/Hypnotic; C IV
MP98	Tab, Film Coated	Ibuprofen 600 mg	by West Ward	00143-1302	NSAID
MP98	Tab, Film Coated	Ibuprofen 600 mg	by United Res	00677-1032	NSAID
MP99	Tab, Film Coated	Ibuprofen 800 mg	by West Ward	00143-1304	NSAID
MP99	Tab, Film Coated	Ibuprofen 800 mg	by St Marys Med	60760-0119	NSAID
MP99 <> 800	Tab, Film Coated	Ibuprofen 800 mg	by United Res	00677-1119	NSAID
MPC <> 500	Tab	Acetohydroxamic Acid 250 mg	Lithostat by Mission	00178-0500	Analgesic
MPC <> 600	Tab, ER	Potassium Citrate 540 mg	Urocit K by Mission	00178-0600	Electrolytes
MPC100	Tab	Chlorpheniramine 4 mg, Hydrocodone Bitartrate 5 mg, Pseudoephedrine HCl 60 mg	Tussend by King	60793-0856	Cold Remedy; C III
MPC100	Tab, Yellow, Cap Shaped	Chlorpheniramine 4 mg, Hydrocodone Bitartrate 5 mg, Pseudoephedrine HCl 60 mg	Tussend by Monarch	61570-0011	Cold Remedy; C III
MPC100	Tab, Yellow, Scored, MPC/100	Chlorpheniramine 4 mg, Hydrocodone Bitartrate 5 mg, Pseudoephedrine HCl 60 mg	Tussend by King	61570-0004	Cold Remedy; C III
MPC188 <> ANEXSIA	Tab	Acetaminophen 650 mg, Hydrocodone Bitartrate 7.5 mg	Anexsia by Nat Pharmpak Serv	55154-7101	Analgesic; C III
MPC188 <> ANEXSIA	Tab	Acetaminophen 650 mg, Hydrocodone Bitartrate 7.5 mg	Anexsia by King	60793-0843	Analgesic; C III
MPC188 <> ANEXSIA	Tab	Acetaminophen 650 mg, Hydrocodone Bitartrate 7.5 mg	Anexsia by Mallinckrodt Hobart	00406-5362	Analgesic; C III

ID FRONT <> BACK	DESCRIPTION FRONT <> BACK	INGREDIENT & STRENGTH	BRAND (OR EQUIV.) & FIRM	NDC#	CLASS; SCH.
MPC188 <> ANEXSIA	Tab	Acetaminophen 650 mg, Hydrocodone Bitartrate 7.5 mg	Anexsia by Med Pro	53978-3309	Analgesic; C III
MPC207 <> ANEXSIA	Tab	Acetaminophen 500 mg, Hydrocodone Bitartrate 5 mg	Anexsia 5/500 by King	60793-0842	Analgesic; C III
MPC207 <> ANEXSIA	Tab	Acetaminophen 500 mg, Hydrocodone Bitartrate 5 mg	Anexsia by Mallinckrodt Hobart	00406-5361	Analgesic; C III
MPC7	Tab, Coated	Calcium Ascorbate, Calcium Carbonate, Precipitated, Cupric Oxide, Cyanocobalamin 8 mcg, Ferrous Fumarate, Folic Acid 1 mg, Niacinamide, Potassium Iodide, Pyridoxine HCl, Riboflavin 2 mg, Thiamine Mononitrate, Vitamin A Acetate, Vitamin D 400 Units, Zinc Sulfate	Mission Prenatal Rx by Mission	00178-0007	Vitamin/Mineral
MPELDERCAPS	Tab, Red, Oblong	Multivitamin With Folic Acid 1 mg	Eldercaps by Merz		Vitamin
MPIII <> 2	Tab, MP III	Acetaminophen 300 mg, Codeine Phosphate 15 mg	by Quality Care	60346-0015	Analgesic; C III
MR	Tab	Acetaminophen 325 mg, Dextromethorphan Hydrobromide 15 mg, Guaifenesin 100 mg, Phenylpropanolamine HCl 25 mg	Anatuss by Merz	00259-2244	Cold Remedy
MR	Tab, White, Oblong, M/R	Guaifenesin 200 mg	Glytuss by Merz		Expectorant
MR <> 0379	Tab, Off-White, Film Coated	Guaifenesin 400 mg, Pseudoephedrine HCl 120 mg	Anatuss LA by Merz	00259-0379	Cold Remedy
MR <> GEIGY	Tab, White w/ Red Specks, Round, Scored	Carbamazepine 100 mg	Tegretol Chewtabs by Novartis	Canadian DIN# 00369810	Anticonvulsant
MR0382	Tab, Orange, M/R 0382	Guaifenesin 400 mg, Dextromethorphan 20 mg, Pseudoephedrine 60 mg	Anatuss DM by Vintage		Cold Remedy
MR1278	Tab, White, Oblong	Butalbital 50 mg, Acetaminohen 650 mg	Sedapap by Merz		Analgesic
MRK <> 266	Tab, Pale Pink, Cap Shaped	Rizatriptan Benzoate 7.265 mg	Maxalt by Merck	00006-0266	Antimigraine
MRK <> 266	Tab	Rizatriptan Benzoate 7.265 mg	by Merck Sharp & Dohme	60312-0266	Antimigraine
MRK <> 951	Tab, Light Green, Teardrop Shaped, Film Coated	Losartan Potassium 25 mg	Cozaar by Merck	00006-0951	Antihypertensive
MRK <> 951	Tab, Green, Oval, Scored, Film	Losartan Potassium 25 mg	by Nat Pharmpak Serv	55154-2713	Antihypertensive
MRK <> 951	Tab, Light Green, Teardrop Shaped, Film Coated	Losartan Potassium 25 mg	Cozaar by Nat Pharmpak Serv	55154-5009	Antihypertensive
MRK <> 952	Tab, Green, Teardrop Shaped, Film Coated	Losartan Potassium 50 mg	Cozaar by Merck	00006-0952	Antihypertensive
MRK110	Tab, Yellow, Round	Rofecoxib 25 mg	Vioxx by Allscripts	54569-4759	NSAID
MRK110 <> VIOXX	Tab, Yellow, Round	Rofecoxib 25 mg	Vioxx by RX PAK	65084-0201	NSAID
MRK110 <> VIOXX	Tab, Yellow, Round	Rofecoxib 25 mg	Vioxx by Merck	00006-0110	NSAID
MRK117 <> SINGULAIR	Tab, Beige, Square, Film Coated	Montelukast Sodium 10 mg	Singulair by Murfreesboro Ph	51129-1398	Antiasthmatic
MRK117 <> SINGULAIR	Tab, Beige, Round, Square Shaped	Montelukast Sodium 10 mg	Singulair by Merck	00006-0117	Antiasthmatic
MRK212 <> FOSOMAX	Tab, White, Triangular, Bone Print	Alendronate Sodium 40 mg	Fosamax by Merck	00006-0212	Antiosteoporosis
MRK212FOSAMAX	Tab, White, Triangle, MRK 212/Fosamax	Alendronate 40 mg	by MSD	Canadian	Antiosteoporosis
MRK267 <> MAXALT	Tab, Pale Pink, Cap Shaped	Rizatriptan Benzoate 14.53 mg	Maxalt by Merck	00006-0267	Antimigraine
MRK267 <> MAXALT	Tab, MRK 267	Rizatriptan Benzoate 14.53 mg	by Merck Sharp & Dohme	60312-0267	Antimigraine
MRK275 <> SINGULAIR	Tab, Pink, Round, Biconvex Shaped	Montelukast Sodium 5 mg	Singulair by Merck	00006-0275	Antiasthmatic
MRK275 <> SINGULAIR	Tab, Pink, Round	Montelukast Sodium 5 mg	Singulair Chewable by Neuman Distr	64579-0348	Antiasthmatic
MRK71 <> PROPECIA	Tab, Tan, Octagonal	Finasteride 1 mg	Propecia by Southwood Pharms	58016-0329	Antiandrogen
MRK71 <> PROPECIA1	Tab, Tan, Octagonal	Finasteride 1 mg	Propecia by Phy Total Care	54868-4120	Antiandrogen
MRK71 <> PROPECIA1	Tab, Tan, Octagonal, Film Coated	Finasteride 1 mg	Propecia by Merck	00006-0071	Antiandrogen
MRK711	Tab, Pink, Oval	Montelukast Sodium 4 mg	Singulair by Merck	00006-0711	Antiasthmatic
MRK717 <> HYZAAR	Tab, Yellow, Teardrop Shape, Film Coated	Hydrochlorothiazide 12.5 mg, Losartan Potassium 50 mg	Hyzaar by Merck	00006-0717	Diuretic; Antihypertensive
MRK717 <> HYZAAR	Tab, Yellow, Oval, Film	Losartan Potassium 50 mg, Hydrochlorothiazide 12.5 mg	Hyzaar by Nat Pharmpak Serv	55154-3011	Antihypertensive
MRK717 <> HYZAAR	Tab, Yellow, Oval, Film Coated	Losartan Potassium 50 mg; Hydrochlorothiazide 12.5 mg	Hyzaar by Allscripts	54569-4722	Antihypertensive
MRK717HYZAAR	Tab, Yellow, Teardrop, MRK717/Hyzaar	Losartan Potassium 50 mg, Hydrochlorothiazide 12.5 mg	by MSD	Canadian	Antihypertensive
MRK74 <> VIOXX	Tab, Beige, Round	Rofecoxib 12.5 mg	Vioxx by DRX Pharm Consults	55045-2720	NSAID
MRK74 <> VIOXX	Tab, Cream, Round	Rofecoxib 12.5 mg	Vioxx by Allscripts	54569-4758	NSAID
MRK74 <> VIOXX	Tab, Cream, Round	Rofecoxib 12.5 mg	Vioxx by Phy Total Care	54868-4148	NSAID
MRK74 <> VIOXX	Tab, White, Round, MRK 74	Rofecoxib 12.5 mg	Vioxx by RX PAK	65084-0199	NSAID
MRK74 <> VIOXX	Tab, Cream, Round	Rofecoxib 12.5 mg	Vioxx by Merck	00006-0074	NSAID
MRK925	Tab, White, Round	Alendronate Sodium 5 mg	Fosamax by Murfreesboro Ph	51129-1356	Antiosteoporosis
MRK925	Tab, White, Round, MRK 925 <> Bone Print	Alendronate Sodium 5 mg	Fosamax by Merck	00006-0925	Antiosteoporosis
MRK936 <> FOSAMAX	Tab, MRK 936 Bone Image <> Fosamax Bone Image	Alendronate Sodium 13.05 mg	Fosamax by Physicians Total Care	54868-3857	Antiosteoporosis

ID FRONT <> BACK	DESCRIPTION FRONT <> BACK	INGREDIENT & STRENGTH	BRAND (OR EQUIV.) & FIRM	NDC#	CLASS; SCH.
MRK936 <> FOSAMAX	Tab, White, Round	Alendronate Sodium 10 mg	Fosamax by Heartland Hlthcare	61392-0854	Antiosteoporosis
MRK936 <> FOSAMAX	Tab, White, Round, Bone Image	Alendronate Sodium 10 mg	Fosamax by Merck	00006-0936	Antiosteoporosis
MRK936FOSAMAX	Tab, White, Round, MRK 936/Fosamax	Alendronate 10 mg	by MSD	Canadian	Antiosteoporosis
MRK952 <> COZAAR	Tab, Green, Oval, Film Coated	Losartan Potassium 50 mg	Cozaar by Phy Total Care	54868-3726	Antihypertensive
MRK952 <> COZAAR	Tab, Teardrop, Film Coated	Losartan Potassium 50 mg	Cozaar by Nat Pharmpak Serv	55154-5016	Antihypertensive
MRK952 <> COZAAR	Tab, Green, Oval, Film, MRK 952	Losartan Potassium 50 mg	Cozaar by Nat Pharmpak Serv	55154-2714	Antihypertensive
MRK952COZAAR	Tab, Green, Teardrop, MRK952/Cozaar	Losartan Potassium 50 mg	by MSD	Canadian	Antihypertensive
MS958	Tab, White, Round	Aspirin 325 mg	by MS		Analgesic
MSAP	Tab, White, Oblong	Aspirin 500 mg	APF by Medtech		Analgesic
MSD	Tab, White	Ethacrynic 50 mg	by MSD	Canadian	Diuretic
MSD	Cap, Blue & White	Indomethacin 25 mg	Indocid by MSD	Canadian	NSAID
MSD	Cap, Opaque Blue & White	Indomethacin 50 mg	Indocid by MSD	Canadian	NSAID
MSD	Tab	Phytonadione 5 mg	Mephyton by HJ Harkins Co	52959-0424	Vitamin
MSD <> 15	Tab, White, Round	Lisinopril 2.5 mg	by Allscripts	54569-4721	Antihypertensive
MSD <> 173	Tab, Green, Squared Cap Shape	Enalapril Maleate 5 mg, Hydrochlorothiazide 12.5 mg	Vaseretic 5 12.5 by Merck	00006-0173	Antihypertensive; Diuretic
MSD <> 32	Tab, White, Round	Ivermectin 3 mg	Stromectil by Merck	00006-0032	Antiparasitic
MSD <> 32	Tab, White, Round, Flat	Ivermectin 3 mg	Stromectol by Murfreesboro	51129-1590	Antiparasitic
MSD 102	Tab, Beige, Discoid	Amitriptyline 75 mg	Elavil by MSD	Canadian	Antidepressant
MSD 23	Tab, Blue, Discoid	Amitriptyline 10 mg	Elavil by MSD	Canadian	Antidepressant
MSD 405 <> DIUPRES	Tab	Chlorothiazide 500 mg, Reserpine 0.125 mg	Diupres-500 by Merck	00006-0405	Diuretic; Antihypertensive
MSD 430	Tab, Orange, Discoid	Amitriptyline HCl 75 mg	by MSD	Canadian	Antidepressant
MSD 432 <> DIURIL	Tab, White, Round	Chlorothiazide 500 mg	Diuril by Merck	00006-0432	Diuretic
MSD 45	Tab, Yellow, Discoid	Amitriptyline 25 mg	Elavil by MSD	Canadian	Antidepressant
MSD 60	Tab, White, Discoid	Benztropine Mesylate 2 mg	by MSD	Canadian	Antiparkinson
MSD 92	Tab, Yellow, Diamond	Amiloride 5 mg	by MSD	Canadian	Diuretic
MSD 921	Tab, Orange, Triangular	Amitriptyline HCl 25 mg, Perphenazine 2 mg	Elavil Plus by MSD	Canadian	Antipsychotic
MSD105	Tab, Peach	Hydrochlorothiazide 50 mg	HydroDiuril by MSD	Canadian	Diuretic
MSD105 <> HYDRODIURL	Tab, Peach, Round, MSD on Left, 105 on Right	Hydrochlorothiazide 50 mg	Hydrodiuril by Merck	00006-0105	Diuretic
MSD106	Tab, Yellow	Lisinopril 10 mg	Prinivil by Amerisource Health	62584-0925	Antihypertensive
MSD106 <> PRINIVIL	Tab, Yellow, Triangle	Lisinopril 10 mg	Prinivil by Phcy Care	65070-0012	Antihypertensive
MSD106 <> PRINIVIL	Tab, Light Yellow, Shield-Shaped	Lisinopril 10 mg	Prinivil by Merck	00006-0106	Antihypertensive
MSD106 <> PRINIVIL	Tab, Pale Yellow, Four Sides	Lisinopril 10 mg	Prinivil by Merck	00006-0106	Antihypertensive
MSD106 <> PRINIVIL	Tab, Shield Shape	Lisinopril 10 mg	Prinivil by DRX	55045-2292	Antihypertensive
MSD106 <> PRINIVIL	Tab	Lisinopril 10 mg	Prinivil by Nat Pharmpak Serv	55154-5015	Antihypertensive
MSD106 <> PRINIVIL	Tab	Lisinopril 10 mg	Lisinopril by Med Pro	53978-3015	Antihypertensive
MSD106 <> PRINIVIL	Tab, Shield Shaped	Lisinopril 10 mg	Prinivil by PDRX	55289-0929	Antihypertensive
MSD106 <> PRINIVIL	Tab	Lisinopril 10 mg	Prinivil by Quality Care	60346-0972	Antihypertensive
MSD126	Tab, White, Discoid	Cortisone Acetate 5 mg	Cortisone Tablets by MSD	Canadian	Steroid
MSD135 <> ALDOMET	Tab, Yellow, Round	Methyldopa 125 mg	Aldomet by Merck	00006-0135	Antihypertensive
MSD136 <> BLOCADREN	Tab, Light Blue, Cap Shaped	Timolol Maleate 10 mg	Blocadren by Merck	00006-0136	Antihypertensive
MSD139	Tab, White, Round	Ivermectin 6 mg	Stromectol by Merck	00006-0139	Anithelmintic
MSD139	Tab	Ivermectin 6 mg	Mectizan by Merck Sharp and Dohme	52888-8107	Anithelmintic
MSD139	Tab	Ivermectin 6 mg	Stromectol by Merck Sharp and Dohme	52888-0139	Anithelmintic
MSD14 <> VASOTEC	Tab, Yellow, Oblong, Scored	Enalapril Maleate 2.5 mg	Vasotec by Southwood Pharms	58016-0882	Antihypertensive
MSD14 <> VASOTEC	Tab	Enalapril Maleate 2.5 mg	Vasotec by Amerisource	62584-0482	Antihypertensive
MSD14 <> VASOTEC	Tab, Yellow, Barrel Shaped	Enalapril Maleate 2.5 mg	Vasotec by Merck	00006-0014	Antihypertensive
MSD14 <> VASOTEC	Tab	Enalapril Maleate 2.5 mg	Vasotec by Caremark	00339-5413	Antihypertensive
MSD14 <> VASOTEC	Tab	Enalapril Maleate 2.5 mg	Vasotec by Allscripts	54569-3258	Antihypertensive

ID FRONT ◇ BACK	DESCRIPTION FRONT ◇ BACK	INGREDIENT & STRENGTH	BRAND (OR EQUIV.) & FIRM	NDC#	CLASS; SCH.
MSD14 ◇ VASOTEC	Tab, Yellow, Round	Enalapril Maleate 2.5 mg	Vasotec by H J Harkins Co	52959-0507	Antihypertensive
MSD14 ◇ VASOTEC	Tab	Enalapril Maleate 2.5 mg	Vasotec by Nat Pharmpak Serv	55154-5008	Antihypertensive
MSD140 ◇ PRINZIDE	Tab, Yellow, Round	Lisinopril 20 mg, Hydrochlorothiazide 12.5 mg	Prinzide by Merck	00006-0140	Antihypertensive
MSD140PRINZIDE	Tab, Yellow, Round, MSD 140/Prinzide	Lisinopril 20 mg, Hydrochlorothiazide 12.5 mg	Prinzide by MSD	Canadian	Antihypertensive
MSD142 ◇ PRINZIDE	Tab, Peach, Round	Lisinopril 20 mg, Hydrochlorothiazide 25 mg	Prinzide by Merck	00006-0142	Antihypertensive
MSD142PRINZIDE	Tab, Orange, Round, MSD 142/Prinzide	Lisinopril 20 mg, Hydrochlorothiazide 25 mg	Prinzide by MSD	Canadian	Antihypertensive
MSD145 ◇ PRINZIDE	Tab, Blue, Hexagon Shaped	Lisinopril 10 mg, Hydrochlorothiazide 12.5 mg	Prinzide by Merck	00006-0145	Antihypertensive
MSD145 ◇ PRINZIDE	Tab, Blue, Hexagon	Lisinopril 10 mg; Hydrochlorothiazide 12.5 mg	Prinzide by Murfreesboro Ph	51129-1397	Antihypertensive
MSD145PRINZIDE	Tab, Blue, Hexagonal, MSD 145/Prinzide	Lisinopril 10 mg, Hydrochlorothiazide 12.5 mg	Prinzide by MSD	Canadian	Antihypertensive
MSD14VASOTEC	Tab	Enalapril Maleate 2.5 mg	by Med Pro	53978-1122	Antihypertensive
MSD19 ◇ PRINIVIL	Tab, White, Triangle, Scored	Lisinopril 5 mg	Prinivil by Phcy Care	65070-0014	Antihypertensive
MSD19 ◇ PRINIVIL	Tab, White, Shield-Shaped	Lisinopril 5 mg	Prinivil by Merck	00006-0019	Antihypertensive
MSD19 ◇ PRINIVIL	Tab	Lisinopril 5 mg	Prinivil by Nat Pharmpak Serv	55154-5006	Antihypertensive
MSD207 ◇ PRINIVIL	Tab, Peach, Triangle	Lisinopril 20 mg	Prinivil by Phcy Care	65070-0013	Antihypertensive
MSD207 ◇ PRINIVIL	Tab, Peach, Shield-Shaped	Lisinopril 20 mg	Prinivil by Merck	00006-0207	Antihypertensive
MSD207 ◇ PRINIVIL	Tab	Lisinopril 20 mg	Lisinopril by Med Pro	53978-3017	Antihypertensive
MSD207 ◇ PRINIVIL	Tab	Lisinopril 20 mg	Prinivil by Nat Pharmpak Serv	55154-5011	Antihypertensive
MSD21 ◇ COGENTIN	Tab, White, Round	Benztropine Mesylate 0.5 mg	Cogentin by Merck	00006-0021	Antiparkinson
MSD214 ◇ DIURIL	Tab, White, Round	Chlorothiazide 250 mg	Diuril by Merck	00006-0214	Diuretic
MSD219	Tab, White, Discoid	Cortisone Acetate 25 mg	Cortisone Tablets by MSD	Canadian	Steroid
MSD219 ◇ CORTONE	Tab	Cortisone Acetate 25 mg	by Merck	00006-0219	Steroid
MSD25 ◇ INDOCIN	Cap, Light Blue & White	Indomethacin 25 mg	Indocin by Merck	00006-0025	NSAID
MSD26 ◇ VIVACTIL	Tab, Orange, Oval, Film Coated	Protriptyline HCl 5 mg	Vivactil by Merck	00006-0026	Antidepressant
MSD401 ◇ ALDOMET	Tab, Yellow, Round, Film	Methyldopa 250 mg	Aldomet by Neuman Distr	64579-0017	Antihypertensive
MSD401 ◇ ALDOMET	Tab, Yellow, Round, Film Coated	Methyldopa 250 mg	Aldomet by Merck	00006-0401	Antihypertensive
MSD403 ◇ URECHOLINE	Tab, White	Bethanechol Chloride 5 mg	Urecholine by Merck	00006-0403	Urinary Tract
MSD41	Tab, White, Pentagonal	Dexamethasone 0.5 mg	Decadron by MSD	Canadian	Steroid
MSD41 ◇ DECADRON	Tab, Yellow, Pentagonal	Dexamethasone 0.5 mg	Decadron by Merck	00006-0041	Steroid
MSD410	Tab, Peach	Hydrochlorothiazide 100 mg	HydroDiuril by MSD	Canadian	Diuretic
MSD42	Tab, Peach	Hydrochlorothiazide 25 mg	HydroDiuril by MSD	Canadian	Diruetic
MSD42 ◇ HYDRODIURIL	Tab, Peach, Round	Hydrochlorothiazide 25 mg	Hydrodiuril by Merck	00006-0042	Diuretic
MSD423	Tab, Salmon, Biconvex	Methyldopa 250 mg, Hydrochlorothiazide 15 mg	Aldoril 15 by MSD	Canadian	Antihypertensive
MSD423 ◇ ALDORIL	Tab, Salmon, Round, Film Coated	Hydrochlorothiazide 15 mg, Methyldopa 250 mg	Aldoril 15 by Merck	00006-0423	Diuretic; Antihypertensive
MSD43	Tab, Compressed	Phytonadione 5 mg	Mephyton by PDRX	55289-0793	Vitamin
MSD43 ◇ MEPHYTON	Tab, Yellow, Round	Phytonadione 5 mg	Mephyton by Merck	00006-0043	Vitamin
MSD43 ◇ MEPHYTON	Tab	Phytonadione 5 mg	Mephyton by Quality Care	60346-0696	Vitamin
MSD437 ◇ BLOCADREN	Tab, Light Blue, Cap Shaped	Timolol Maleate 20 mg	Blocadren by Merck	00006-0437	Antihypertensive
MSD456	Tab, White, Biconvex	Methyldopa 250 mg, Hydrochlorothiazide 25 mg	Aldoril 25 by MSD	Canadian	Antihypertensive
MSD456 ◇ ALDORIL	Tab, White, Round	Methyldopa 250 mg, Hydrochlorothiazide 15 mg	Aldoril by Merck	00006-0456	Antihypertensive
MSD47	Tab, White, Round	Protriptyline HCl 10 mg	by MSD	Canadian	Antidepressant
MSD47 ◇ VIVACTIL	Tab, Yellow, Oval, Film Coated	Protriptyline HCl 10 mg	Vivactil by Merck	00006-0047	Antidepressant
MSD49 ◇ DARANIDE	Tab, Yellow, Round	Dichlorphenamide 50 mg	Daranide by Merck	00006-0050	Carbonic Anhydrase Inhibitor
MSD50 ◇ INDOCIN	Cap, Blue & White	Indomethacin 50 mg	Indocin by Merck	00006-0050	NSAID
MSD501	Tab, White, Round	Probenecid 500 mg	Benemid by MSD	Canadian	Antigout
MSD516 ◇ ALDOMET	Tab, Yellow, Round, Film Coated	Methyldopa 500 mg	Aldomet by Merck	00006-0516	Antihypertensive
MSD543 ◇ 80	Tab, Brick Red, Cap Shaped, Film Coated	Simvastatin 80 mg	Zocor by Merck	00006-0543	Antihyperlipidemic
MSD543 ◇ 80	Tab, Film Coated	Simvastatin 80 mg	Simvastatin by Merck Sharp Dohme	60312-0543	Antihyperlipidemic

ID FRONT ⟷ BACK	DESCRIPTION FRONT ⟷ BACK	INGREDIENT & STRENGTH	BRAND (OR EQUIV.) & FIRM	NDC#	CLASS; SCH.
MSD59 ⟷ BLOCADREN	Tab, Light Blue, Round	Timolol Maleate 5 mg	Blocadren by Merck	00006-0059	Antihypertensive
MSD60 ⟷ COGENTIN	Tab, White, Round	Benztropine Mesylate 2 mg	Cogentin by Merck	00006-0060	Antiparkinson
MSD602	Cap, Ivory	Penicillamine 250 mg	by MSD	Canadian	Chelating Agent
MSD602 ⟷ CUPRIMINE	Cap, Ivory	Penicillamine 250 mg	Cuprimine by Merck	00006-0602	Chelating Agent
MSD612	Tab, Coated	Chlorothiazide 150 mg, Methyldopa 250 mg	Aldoclor 150 by Merck	00006-0612	Diuretic; Antihypertensive
MSD619	Tab, White, Oval	Hydrocortisone 10 mg	Hydrocortone by Merck	00006-0619	Steroid
MSD62	Tab, White, Round, Scored	Cyproheptadine HCl 4 mg	Periactin by Johnson & Johnson	Canadian DIN# 00016454	Antihistamine
MSD62 ⟷ PERIACTIN	Tab, White, Round	Cyproheptadine HCl 4 mg	Periactin by Merck	00006-0062	Antihistamine
MSD63 ⟷ DECADRON	Tab, Bluish-Green	Dexamethasone 0.75 mg	Decadron by Merck	00006-0063	Steroid
MSD634	Tab, Green, Oval, Film Coated	Chlorothiazide 250 mg, Methyldopa 250 mg	Aldoclor by Merck	00006-0634	Diuretic; Antihypertensive
MSD635 ⟷ COGENTIN	Tab, White, Oval	Benztropine Mesylate 1 mg	Cogentin by Merck	00006-0635	Antiparkinson
MSD65 ⟷ EDECRIN	Tab, White, Cap Shaped	Ethacrynic Acid 25 mg	Edecrin by Merck	00006-0065	Diuretic
MSD661 ⟷ SYPRINE	Cap, Light Brown	Trientine HCl 250 mg	Syprine by Merck	00006-0661	Chelating Agent
MSD67 ⟷ TIMOLIDE	Tab, Light Blue, Hexagonal-Shaped	Timolol Maleate 10 mg, Hydrochlorothiazide 25 mg	Timolide by Merck	00006-0067	Antihypertensive
MSD672	Cap, Gray & Yellow	Penicillamine 125 mg	by MSD	Canadian	Chelating Agent
MSD672	Cap	Penicillamine 125 mg	Cuprimine by DRX	55045-2486	Chelating Agent
MSD672 ⟷ CUPRIMINE	Cap, Gray & Ivory	Penicillamine 125 mg	Cuprimine by Merck	00006-0672	Chelating Agent
MSD675 ⟷ DOLOBID	Tab, Peach, Cap Shaped, Film Coated	Diflunisal 250 mg	Dolobid by Merck	00006-0675	NSAID
MSD690 ⟷ DEMSER	Cap, Two-Tone	Methyrosine 250 mg	Demser by Merck	00006-0690	Antipheochromocytoma
MSD693	Cap, Clear & Opaque	Indomethacin 75 mg	Indocin SR by MSD	Canadian	NSAID
MSD693 ⟷ INDOCINSR	Cap, Blue & Clear	Indomethacin 75 mg	Indocin SR by Merck	00006-0693	NSAID
MSD694 ⟷ ALDORIL	Tab, Salmon, Round	Methyldopa 500 mg, Hydrochlorothiazide 30 mg	Aldoril by Merck	00006-0694	Antihypertensive
MSD697 ⟷ DOLOBID	Tab, Film Coated	Diflunisal 500 mg	Dolobid by Quality Care	60346-0940	NSAID
MSD697 ⟷ DOLOBID	Tab, Orange, Cap Shaped	Diflunisal 500 mg	Dolobid by Merck	00006-0697	NSAID
MSD697 ⟷ DOLOBID	Tab, Film Coated	Diflunisal 500 mg	Dolobid by Allscripts	54569-0296	NSAID
MSD705	Tab, White, Oval	Norfloxacin 400 mg	by MSD	Canadian	Antibiotic
MSD705 ⟷ NOROXIN	Tab, Dark Pink, Oval	Norfloxacin 400 mg	Noroxin by Merck	00006-0705	Antibiotic
MSD705 ⟷ NOROXIN	Tab, Film Coated	Norfloxacin 400 mg	Noroxin by Allscripts	54569-0191	Antibiotic
MSD705 ⟷ NOROXIN	Tab, Film Coated	Norfloxacin 400 mg	Noroxin by Roberts	54092-0097	Antibiotic
MSD705 ⟷ NOROXIN	Tab, Film Coated	Norfloxacin 400 mg	Noroxin by Quality Care	60346-0563	Antibiotic
MSD705 ⟷ NOROXIN	Tab, Dark Pink, Film Coated	Norfloxacin 400 mg	Noroxin by DRX	55045-2419	Antibiotic
MSD712	Tab	Enalapril Maleate 5 mg	Vasotec by Pharmedix	53002-1021	Antihypertensive
MSD712 ⟷ VASOTEC	Tab, Barrel Shaped	Enalapril Maleate 5 mg	Vasotec by Quality Care	60346-0612	Antihypertensive
MSD712 ⟷ VASOTEC	Tab, Barrel Shaped	Enalapril Maleate 5 mg	Vasotec by PDRX	55289-0622	Antihypertensive
MSD712 ⟷ VASOTEC	White, Oblong, Scored	Enalapril Maleate 5 mg	Vasotec by Southwood Pharms	58016-0572	Antihypertensive
MSD712 ⟷ VASOTEC	Tab	Enalapril Maleate 5 mg	Vasotec by Amerisource	62584-0483	Antihypertensive
MSD712 ⟷ VASOTEC	Tab, White, Barrel Shaped	Enalapril Maleate 5 mg	Vasotec by Merck	00006-0712	Antihypertensive
MSD712 ⟷ VASOTEC	Tab, Barrel Shaped	Enalapril Maleate 5 mg	Vasotec by DRX	55045-2319	Antihypertensive
MSD712 ⟷ VASOTEC	Tab, White, Round	Enalapril Maleate 5 mg	Vasotec by H J Harkins Co	52959-0531	Antihypertensive
MSD712 ⟷ VASOTEC	Tab	Enalapril Maleate 5 mg	Vasotec by Nat Pharmpak Serv	55154-5001	Antihypertensive
MSD712 ⟷ VASOTEC	Tab, Barrel Shaped	Enalapril Maleate 5 mg	Vasotec by Allscripts	54569-0606	Antihypertensive
MSD713 ⟷ VASOTEC	Tab, Salmon, Barrel Shaped	Enalapril Maleate 10 mg	Vasotec by Quality Care	60346-0901	Antihypertensive
MSD713 ⟷ VASOTEC	Pink, Oblong	Enalapril Maleate 10 mg	Vasotec by Southwood Pharms	58016-0569	Antihypertensive
MSD713 ⟷ VASOTEC	Tab, Salmon	Enalapril Maleate 10 mg	Vasotec by Amerisource	62584-0484	Antihypertensive
MSD713 ⟷ VASOTEC	Tab, Salmon, Barrel Shaped	Enalapril Maleate 10 mg	Vasotec by Merck	00006-0713	Antihypertensive
MSD713 ⟷ VASOTEC	Tab, Pink, Round	Enalapril Maleate 10 mg	Vasotec by H J Harkins Co	52959-0505	Antihypertensive
MSD713 ⟷ VASOTEC	Tab, Salmon	Enalapril Maleate 10 mg	Vasotec by Nat Pharmpak Serv	55154-5003	Antihypertensive
MSD713 ⟷ VASOTEC	Tab	Enalapril Maleate 10 mg	by Med Pro	53978-3013	Antihypertensive

ID FRONT <> BACK	DESCRIPTION FRONT <> BACK	INGREDIENT & STRENGTH	BRAND (OR EQUIV.) & FIRM	NDC#	CLASS; SCH.
MSD713 <> VASOTEC	Tab, Salmon, Barrel Shaped	Enalapril Maleate 10 mg	Vasotec by Allscripts	54569-0607	Antihypertensive
MSD714 <> VASOTEC	Tab	Enalapril Maleate 20 mg	Vasotec by Quality Care	60346-0534	Antihypertensive
MSD714 <> VASOTEC	Tab, Peach, Oblong	Enalapril Maleate 20 mg	Vasotec by Southwood Pharms	58016-0571	Antihypertensive
MSD714 <> VASOTEC	Tab, Peach, Barrel Shaped	Enalapril Maleate 20 mg	Vasotec by Merck	00006-0714	Antihypertensive
MSD714 <> VASOTEC	Tab	Enalapril Maleate 20 mg	Vasotec by Caremark	00339-5415	Antihypertensive
MSD714 <> VASOTEC	Tab	Enalapril Maleate 20 mg	Vasotec by DRX	55045-2364	Antihypertensive
MSD714 <> VASOTEC	Tab	Enalapril Maleate 20 mg	Vasotec by Nat Pharmpak Serv	55154-5013	Antihypertensive
MSD714 <> VASOTEC	Tab	Enalapril Maleate 20 mg	by Med Pro	53978-3016	Antihypertensive
MSD714 <> VASOTEC	Tab, Barrel Shaped	Enalapril Maleate 20 mg	Vasotec by Allscripts	54569-0612	Antihypertensive
MSD72 <> PROSCAR	Tab, Blue, Round, Film	Finasteride 5 mg	by Integrity	64731-0754	Antiandrogen
MSD72 <> PROSCAR	Tab, Blue, Round, Film Coated	Finasteride 5 mg	Proscar by Phy Total Care	54868-2719	Antiandrogen
MSD72 <> PROSCAR	Tab, Blue, Apple Shaped	Finasteride 5 mg	Proscar by Merck	00006-0072	Antiandrogen
MSD720 <> VASERETIC	Tab, Rust, Squared Cap Shape	Enalapril Maleate 10 mg, Hydrochlorothiazide 25 mg	Vaseretic by Merck	00006-0720	Antihypertensive; Diuretic
MSD726 <> ZOCOR	Tab, Buff, Shield-Shaped, Film Coated	Simvastatin 5 mg	Zocor by Merck	00006-0726	Antihyperlipidemic
MSD72PROSCAR	Tab, Blue, Apple, MSD 72/Proscar	Finasteride 5 mg	by MSD	Canadian	Antiandrogen
MSD730 <> MEVACOR	Tab, Peach, Octagonal	Lovastatin 10 mg	Mevacor by Merck	00006-0730	Antihyperlipidemic
MSD730 <> MEVACOR	Tab, MSD/730	Lovastatin 10 mg	by Kaiser	00179-1209	Antihyperlipidemic
MSD730 <> MEVACOR	Tab, Peach, Octagon	Lovastatin 10 mg	by Nat Pharmpak Serv	55154-3618	Antihyperlipidemic
MSD731	Tab, Blue, Octagon	Lovastatin 20 mg	by Nat Pharmpak Serv	55154-3605	Antihyperlipidemic
MSD731	Tab, Blue, Octagon	Lovastatin 20 mg	Mevacor by Nat Pharmpak Serv	55154-3421	Antihyperlipidemic
MSD731 <> MEVACOR	Tab, Blue, Octagon	Lovastatin 20 mg	Mevacor by Va Cmop	65243-0045	Antihyperlipidemic
MSD731 <> MEVACOR	Tab, Blue, Octagonal	Lovastatin 20 mg	by Allscripts	54569-0613	Antihyperlipidemic
MSD731 <> MEVACOR	Tab, Light Blue, Octagonal	Lovastatin 20 mg	Mevacor by Merck	00006-0731	Antihyperlipidemic
MSD731 <> MEVACOR	Tab	Lovastatin 20 mg	by Nat Pharmpak Serv	55154-5004	Antihyperlipidemic
MSD731 <> MEVACOR	Tab	Lovastatin 20 mg	Mevacor by Allscripts	54569-0613	Antihyperlipidemic
MSD731 <> MEVACOR	Tab	Lovastatin 20 mg	by Pharmedix	53002-0570	Antihyperlipidemic
MSD731 <> MEVACOR	Tab	Lovastatin 20 mg	by Amerisource	62584-0426	Antihyperlipidemic
MSD732 <> MEVACOR	Tab, Green, Octagon	Lovastatin 40 mg	Mevacor by PDRX Pharms	55289-0548	Antihyperlipidemic
MSD732 <> MEVACOR	Tab, Green, Octagonal	Lovastatin 40 mg	Mevacor by Merck	00006-0732	Antihyperlipidemic
MSD732 <> MEVACOR	Tab	Lovastatin 40 mg	by Allscripts	54569-3256	Antihyperlipidemic
MSD735	Tab, Peach, Trapezoid, Film Coated	Simvastatin 10 mg	by		Antihyperlipidemic
MSD735 <> ZOCOR	Tab, Peach	Simvastatin 10 mg	Zocor by Southwood Pharms	58016-0364	Antihyperlipidemic
MSD735 <> ZOCOR	Tab, Peach	Simvastatin 10 mg	Zocor by Va Cmop	65243-0064	Antihyperlipidemic
MSD735 <> ZOCOR	Tab, Peach, Shield Shaped, Film Coated	Simvastatin 10 mg	Zocor by Merck	00006-0735	Antihyperlipidemic
MSD735 <> ZOCOR	Tab, Film Coated	Simvastatin 10 mg	Zocor by Caremark	00339-5795	Antihyperlipidemic
MSD735 <> ZOCOR	Tab, Film Coated	Simvastatin 10 mg	Simvastatin by Med Pro	53978-3069	Antihyperlipidemic
MSD735 <> ZOCOR	Tab, Film Coated	Simvastatin 10 mg	Zocor by Nat Pharmpak Serv	55154-5012	Antihyperlipidemic
MSD735 <> ZOCOR	Tab, Shield Shaped, Film Coated	Simvastatin 10 mg	Zocor by Allscripts	54569-4180	Antihyperlipidemic
MSD735 <> ZOCOR	Tab, Shield Shaped, Film Coated	Simvastatin 10 mg	Zocor by DRX	55045-2316	Antihyperlipidemic
MSD740 <> ZOCOR	Tab, Tan	Simvastatin 20 mg	Zocor by Southwood Pharms	58016-0385	Antihyperlipidemic
MSD740 <> ZOCOR	Tab, Tan	Simvastatin 20 mg	Zocor by Va Cmop	65243-0065	Antihyperlipidemic
MSD740 <> ZOCOR	Tab, Tan	Simvastatin 20 mg	Simvastatin by Med-Pro	53978-3370	Antihyperlipidemic
MSD740 <> ZOCOR	Tab, Tan, Shield Shaped, Film Coated	Simvastatin 20 mg	Zocor by Merck	00006-0740	Antihyperlipidemic
MSD740 <> ZOCOR	Tab, Tan, Trapezoid, Film Coated	Simvastatin 20 mg	by		Antihyperlipidemic
MSD740 <> ZOCOR	Tab, Shield Shaped, Film Coated	Simvastatin 20 mg	Zocor by Physicians Total Care	54868-3104	Antihyperlipidemic
MSD742	Cap, Amethyst, Delayed Release	Omeprazole 20 mg	Prilosec by Astra Merck	00186-0742	Gastrointestinal
MSD742	Cap, Amethyst	Omeprazole 20 mg	Prilosec by Nat Pharmpak Serv	55154-5002	Gastrointestinal
MSD747 <> HYZAAR	Tab, Light Yellow, Teardrop-Shaped	Losartan Potassium 100 mg, Hydrochlorothiazide 25 mg	Hyzaar by Merck	00006-0747	Antihypertensive
MSD749 <> ZOCOR	Tab, Red	Simvastatin 40 mg	Zocor by Va Cmop	65243-0082	Antihyperlipidemic
MSD749 <> ZOCOR	Tab, Brick Red, Shield Shaped	Simvastatin 40 mg	Zocor by Merck	00006-0749	Antihyperlipidemic
MSD749 <> ZOCOR	Tab, Film Coated	Simvastatin 40 mg	Zocor by Caremark	00339-5798	Antihyperlipidemic

ID FRONT <> BACK	DESCRIPTION FRONT <> BACK	INGREDIENT & STRENGTH	BRAND (OR EQUIV.) & FIRM	NDC#	CLASS; SCH.
MSD749 <> ZOCOR	Tab, Red, Film Coated	Simvastatin 40 mg	Zocor by Kaiser Fdn	00179-1331	Antihyperlipidemic
MSD90 <> EDECRIN	Tab, Green, Cap Shaped	Ethacrynic Acid 50 mg	Edecrin by Merck	00006-0090	Diuretic
MSD907 <> MINTEZOL	Tab, Chew	Thiabendazole 500 mg	Mintezol by Merck	00006-0907	Antihelmintic
MSD917 <> M	Tab, Peach, Diamond Shaped	Amiloride HCl 5 mg, Hydrochlorothiazide 50 mg	Moduretic by Merck	00006-0917	Diuretic
MSD92 <> MIDAMOR	Tab, Yellow, Diamond Shaped	Amiloride HCl 5 mg	Midamor by Merck	00006-0092	Diuretic
MSD931	Tab, Yellow, D-Shaped, Film	Cyclobenzaprine HCl 10 mg	Flexeril by DJ Pharma	64455-0014	Muscle Relaxant
MSD931 <> FLEXERIL	Tab, Butterscotch Yellow, D-Shaped, Film Coated	Cyclobenzaprine HCl 10 mg	Flexeril by Merck	00006-0931	Muscle Relaxant
MSD931 <> FLEXERIL	Tab, D-Shaped, Film Coated	Cyclobenzaprine HCl 10 mg	Flexeril by Allscripts	54569-0835	Muscle Relaxant
MSD931 <> FLEXERIL	Tab, Film Coated	Cyclobenzaprine HCl 10 mg	Flexeril by Nat Pharmpak Serv	55154-5007	Muscle Relaxant
MSD931 <> FLEXERIL	Tab, D-Shaped, Film Coated	Cyclobenzaprine HCl 10 mg	Flexeril by Allscripts	54569-4008	Muscle Relaxant
MSD931 <> FLEXERIL	Tab, Butterscotch Yellow, D-Shaped, Film Coated	Cyclobenzaprine HCl 10 mg	Flexeril by Quality Care	60346-0471	Muscle Relaxant
MSD935 <> ALDORIL	Tab, White, Oval	Methyldopa 500 mg, Hydrochlorothiazide 50 mg	Aldoril by Merck	00006-0935	Antihypertensive
MSD941 <> CLINORIL	Tab, Bright Yellow, Hexagon-Shaped	Sulindac 200 mg	Clinoril by Merck	00006-0941	NSAID
MSD942 <> CLINORIL	Tab, Bright Yellow, Hexagon-Shaped	Sulindac 200 mg	Clinoril by Merck	00006-0942	NSAID
MSD942 <> CLINORIL	Tab	Sulindac 200 mg	Clinoril by Allscripts	54569-0268	NSAID
MSD942 <> CLINORIL	Tab	Sulindac 200 mg	Clinoril by Merck Sharp and Dohme	62904-0941	NSAID
MSD942 <> CLINORIL	Tab	Sulindac 200 mg	Clinoril by Merck Sharp and Dohme	62904-0942	NSAID
MSD960 <> COZAAR	Tab, Dark Green, Teardrop-Shaped	Losartan Potassium 100 mg	Cozaar by Merck	00006-0960	Antihypertensive
MSD963 <> PEPCID	Tab, U-Shaped, Film Coated	Famotidine 20 mg	Pepcid by Amerisource	62584-0440	Gastrointestinal
MSD963 <> PEPCID	Tab, Beige, U-Shaped	Famotidine 20 mg	Pepcid by Merck	00006-0963	Gastrointestinal
MSD963 <> PEPCID	Tab, Film Coated	Famotidine 20 mg	Pepcid by Nat Pharmpak Serv	55154-5005	Gastrointestinal
MSD963 <> PEPCID	Tab, U-Shaped, Film Coated, MSD/963	Famotidine 20 mg	Pepcid by Allscripts	54569-2352	Gastrointestinal
MSD963 <> PEPCID	Tab, U-Shaped, Film Coated	Famotidine 20 mg	Pepcid by PDRX	55289-0162	Gastrointestinal
MSD963 <> PEPCID	Tab, U Shaped, Film Coated	Famotidine 20 mg	Pepcid by HJ Harkins Co	52959-0465	Gastrointestinal
MSD963 <> PEPCID	Tab, Film Coated	Famotidine 20 mg	by Med Pro	53978-0518	Gastrointestinal
MSD964 <> PEPCID	Tab, Light Brownish-Orange, U-Shaped	Famotidine 40 mg	Pepcid by Merck	00006-0964	Gastrointestinal
MSD964 <> PEPCID	Tab, U-Shaped, Coated	Famotidine 40 mg	Pepcid by Allscripts	54569-0431	Gastrointestinal
MSD964 <> PEPCID	Tab, Brownish Orange, U-Shaped, Coated	Famotidine 40 mg	Pepcid by PDRX	55289-0146	Gastrointestinal
MSD97	Tab, White, Pentagonal	Dexamethasone 4 mg	Decadron by MSD	Canadian	Steroid
MSD97 <> DECADRON	Tab, Blue-Green, Pentagonal	Dexamethasone 4 mg	Decadron by Merck	00006-0097	Steroid
MSM	Tab, White, Football	Magnesium Salicylate 467 mg	Momentum by Whitehall Robins		Analgesic
MSM	Tab, White, Oval	Magnesium Salicylate 580 mg	MD Mentom by Medtech		Analgesic
MSTSM <> 500	Cap, Green, Film Coated	Acetaminophen 500 mg, Pseudoephedrine HCl 30 mg	Extra Strength Tylenol Sinus	Canadian DIN# 00663980	Cold Remedy
MT20 <> ULTRASE	Cap, Gray & Yellow	Pancrelipase (Amylase 65000 U, Lipase 20000 U, Protease 65000 U)	Ultrase MT 20 by Eurand	57298-0052	Gastrointestinal
MT20ULTRACE	Cap, Gray & Yellow, Oblong	Lipase 20,000 Units	Ultrace MT 20 by Scandipharm	58914-0004	Gastrointestinal
MUCOFEN800	Tab, White, Elliptical, Scored	Guaifenesin 800 mg	Muco-Fen 800 by Wakefield	59310-0109	Expectorant
MUCOFEN800	Tab, White, Oval, Scored, Mucofen over 800	Guaifenesin 800 mg	GFN 800 by Lilly	00002-4006	Expectorant
MUCOFEN800DM	Tab, White, Elliptical	Guaifenesin 800 mg, Dextromethorphan HBr 60 mg	Muco-Fen by Wakefield	59310-0114	Cold Remedy
MUCOFEN800DM	Tab, White, Oval, Scored, Mucofen over 800 DM	Guaifenesin 800 mg, Dextromethorphan Hydrobromide 60 mg	GFN 800 DM 60 by Med Pro	53978-3360	Cold Remedy
MUCOFENDM	Tab, Ex Release	Dextromethorphan Hydrobromide 30 mg, Guaifenesin 600 mg	Muco Fen DM by Wakefield	59310-0108	Cold Remedy
MUCOFENDM	Tab	Dextromethorphan Hydrobromide 30 mg, Guaifenesin 600 mg	Mucofen DM by Anabolic	00722-6355	Cold Remedy
MUCOFENDM	Tab, White, Scored	Guaifenesin 600 mg; Dextromethorphan Hydrobromide 30 mg	by Pfab	62542-0726	Cold Remedy
MUCOFENLA	Tab, Ex Release	Guaifenesin 600 mg	Muco-Fen-LA by Wakefield	59310-0102	Expectorant
MUCOFENLA	Tab, White, Oblong	Guaifenesin 600 mg	by Pfab	62542-0706	Expectorant
MUCOFENLA	Tab	Guaifenesin 600 mg	Muco Fen LA by Anabolic	00722-6249	Expectorant
MURO120250 <> GUAIFED	Cap, Ex Release, Muro 120-250	Guaifenesin 250 mg, Pseudoephedrine HCl 120 mg	Guaifed by Thrift Drug	59198-0192	Cold Remedy
MURO120250 <> GUAIFED	Cap, Muro 120-250 <> Guaifed	Guaifenesin 250 mg, Pseudoephedrine HCl 120 mg	Guaifed by Muro	00451-4002	Cold Remedy

ID FRONT <> BACK	DESCRIPTION FRONT <> BACK	INGREDIENT & STRENGTH	BRAND (OR EQUIV.) & FIRM	NDC#	CLASS; SCH.
MURO120250 <> GUAIFED	Cap, Muro 120-250 <> Guaifed	Guaifenesin 250 mg, Pseudoephedrine HCl 120 mg	Guaifed by Nat Pharmpak Serv	55154-4302	Cold Remedy
MURO12120 <> BROMFED	Cap, Light Green, Ex Release, MURO 12-120 <>	Brompheniramine Maleate 12 mg, Pseudoephedrine HCl 120 mg	Bromfed by Thrift Drug	59198-0190	Cold Remedy
MURO12120 <> BROMFED	Cap, Muro 12-120 <> Bromfed	Brompheniramine Maleate 12 mg, Pseudoephedrine HCl 120 mg	Bromfed by Muro	00451-4000	Cold Remedy
MURO40060	Tab, Purple, Muro 400/60	Pseudoephedrine HCl 60 mg, Guaifenesin 400 mg	Guaitab by Central		Cold Remedy
MURO4060	Tab	Brompheniramine Maleate 4 mg, Pseudoephedrine HCl 60 mg	Bromfed by PDRX	55289-0807	Cold Remedy
MURO4060	Tab	Brompheniramine Maleate 4 mg, Pseudoephedrine HCl 60 mg	Bromfed by		Cold Remedy
MURO60300 <> GUAIFEDPD	Cap, Ex Release, Muro 60-300 <> Guaifed PD	Guaifenesin 300 mg, Pseudoephedrine HCl 60 mg	Guaifed PD by Thrift Drug	59198-0191	Cold Remedy
MURO60300 <> GUAIFEDPD	Cap, Muro 60-300 <> Guaifed PD	Guaifenesin 300 mg, Pseudoephedrine HCl 60 mg	Guaifed PD by Muro	00451-4003	Cold Remedy
MURO60300 <> GUAIFEDPD	Cap, Muro 60-300 <> Guaifed PD	Guaifenesin 300 mg, Pseudoephedrine HCl 60 mg	Guaifed PD by Nat Pharmpak Serv	55154-4303	Cold Remedy
MURO60300 <> GUAIFEDPD	Cap	Guaifenesin 300 mg, Pseudoephedrine HCl 60 mg	by Pharmedix	53002-0623	Cold Remedy
MURO660 <> BROMFEDPD	Cap, Muro 6-60 <> Bromfed-PD	Brompheniramine Maleate 6 mg, Pseudoephedrine HCl 60 mg	Bromfed PD by Nat Pharmpak Serv	55154-4301	Cold Remedy
MURO660 <> BROMFEDPD	Cap, Dark Green, Ex Release, Muro 6-60 <> Bromfed-PD	Brompheniramine Maleate 6 mg, Pseudoephedrine HCl 60 mg	Bromfed PD by Thrift Drug	59198-0189	Cold Remedy
MURO660 <> BROMFEDPD	Cap, Muro 6-60 <> Bromfed-PD	Brompheniramine Maleate 6 mg, Pseudoephedrine HCl 60 mg	Bromfed-PD by Muro	00451-4001	Cold Remedy
MUTUAL <> 101	Cap	Indomethacin 25 mg	by Quality Care	60346-0684	NSAID
MUTUAL <> 105	Cap, Light Blue	Doxycycline Hyclate	by Quality Care	60346-0109	Antibiotic
MUTUAL <> 106	Cap	Indomethacin 50 mg	by Quality Care	60346-0733	NSAID
MUTUAL100	Cap, Blue & White	Doxycycline Hyclate 50 mg	by DRX Pharm Consults	55045-2731	Antibiotic
MUTUAL100	Cap, Light Blue & White, Opaque	Doxycycline Hyclate 50 mg	Vibramycin by Mutual	53489-0118	Antibiotic
MUTUAL100	Cap, Blue & White	Doxycycline 50 mg	by Allscripts	54569-0147	Antibiotic
MUTUAL100	Cap, Light Blue	Doxycycline Hyclate	by Qualitest	00603-3480	Antibiotic
MUTUAL100	Cap	Doxycycline Hyclate	by United Res	00677-0598	Antibiotic
MUTUAL101	Cap	Indomethacin 25 mg	by Pharmedix	53002-0305	NSAID
MUTUAL101	Cap	Indomethacin 25 mg	by Mutual	53489-0133	NSAID
MUTUAL101	Cap	Indomethacin 25 mg	by United Res	00677-0872	NSAID
MUTUAL102	Cap, Clear	Quinine Sulfate 324 mg	by RX PAK	65084-0136	Antimalarial
MUTUAL102	Cap, Clear	Quinine Sulfate 324 mg	by Mutual	53489-0221	Antimalarial
MUTUAL102	Cap	Quinine Sulfate 324 mg	by United Res	00677-1647	Antimalarial
MUTUAL102	Cap, Clear	Quinine Sulfate 325 mg	by Allscripts	54569-2096	Antimalarial
MUTUAL102	Cap, Clear	Quinine Sulfate 324 mg	by RX PAK	65084-0138	Antimalarial
MUTUAL103	Cap, Mutual Over 103	Diphenhydramine HCl 25 mg	by Quality Care	60346-0589	Antihistamine
MUTUAL103	Cap, Pink	Diphenhydramine HCl 25 mg	by Direct Dispensing	57866-3594	Antihistamine
MUTUAL103	Cap	Diphenhydramine HCl 25 mg	by United Res	00677-0063	Antihistamine
MUTUAL103	Cap	Diphenhydramine HCl 25 mg	by Pharmedix	53002-0314	Antihistamine
MUTUAL103	Cap	Diphenhydramine HCl 25 mg	by Allscripts	54569-0239	Antihistamine
MUTUAL103	Cap, Clear & Pink	Diphenhydramine HCl 25 mg	by Mutual	53489-0113	Antihistamine
MUTUAL105	Cap	Doxycycline Hyclate	by St Marys Med	60760-0562	Antibiotic
MUTUAL105	Cap, Light Blue, Opaque	Doxycycline Hyclate	by Allscripts	54569-1840	Antibiotic
MUTUAL105	Cap, Opaque Light Blue	Doxycycline Hyclate	by Darby Group	66467-0230	Antibiotic
MUTUAL105	Cap	Doxycycline Hyclate	by Qualitest	00603-3481	Antibiotic
MUTUAL105	Cap	Doxycycline Hyclate	by United Res	00677-0562	Antibiotic
MUTUAL105	Cap	Doxycycline Hyclate	by HJ Harkins Co	52959-0055	Antibiotic
MUTUAL105	Cap, Blue	Doxycycline Hyclate 100 mg	by Direct Dispensing	57866-0341	Antibiotic

ID FRONT <> BACK	DESCRIPTION FRONT <> BACK	INGREDIENT & STRENGTH	BRAND (OR EQUIV.) & FIRM	NDC#	CLASS; SCH.
MUTUAL105	Cap, Light Blue, Opaque	Doxycycline Hyclate 100 mg	by Mutual	53489-0119	Antibiotic
MUTUAL106	Cap	Indomethacin 50 mg	by Mutual	53489-0134	NSAID
MUTUAL106	Cap	Indomethacin 50 mg	by Pharmedix	53002-0350	NSAID
MUTUAL106	Cap	Indomethacin 50 mg	by Talbert Med	44514-0453	NSAID
MUTUAL106	Cap	Indomethacin 50 mg	by United Res	00677-0873	NSAID
MUTUAL107	Cap, Mutual over 107	Diphenhydramine HCl 50 mg	by Quality Care	60346-0045	Antihistamine
MUTUAL107	Cap	Diphenhydramine HCl 50 mg	by United Res	00677-0064	Antihistamine
MUTUAL107	Cap	Diphenhydramine HCl 50 mg	by Pharmedix	53002-0331	Antihistamine
MUTUAL107	Cap, Pink	Diphenhydramine HCl 50 mg	by Mutual	53489-0114	Antihistamine
MUTUAL107	Cap	Diphenhydramine HCl 50 mg	by Allscripts	54569-0241	Antihistamine
MUTUAL165	Cap	Piroxicam 10 mg	by United Res	00677-1430	NSAID
MUTUAL166	Cap, Lavender, Mutual over 166	Piroxicam 20 mg	by Quality Care	60346-0676	NSAID
MUTUAL166	Cap	Piroxicam 20 mg	by United Res	00677-1431	NSAID
MUTUAL179	Cap	Tolmetin Sodium 400 mg	by Allscripts	54569-3730	NSAID
MUTUAL179	Cap	Tolmetin Sodium 492 mg	by Mutual	53489-0507	NSAID
MUTUAL179	Cap, Mutual over 179	Tolmetin Sodium 492 mg	by Quality Care	60346-0615	NSAID
MUTUAL179	Cap	Tolmetin Sodium 492 mg	by United Res	00677-1424	NSAID
MUTUAL400	Cap, Blue, Mutual over 400	Trimethobenzamide HCl 250 mg	by Mutual	53489-0293	Antiemetic
MUTUAL400	Cap	Trimethobenzamide HCl 250 mg	by United Res	00677-1383	Antiemetic
MUTUAL400	Cap, Mutual over 400	Trimethobenzamide HCl 250 mg	by Qualitest	00603-6256	Antiemetic
MUTUAL688	Cap, White	Lipase 4500 Unt; Amylase 20000 Unt; Protease 25000 Unt	Pancrelipase by United Res	00677-1653	Gastrointestinal
MUTUAL688	Cap, White	Pancrelipase 4500I Units	by Mutual	53489-0320	Gastrointestinal
MUTUAL689	Cap, Brown, Scored	Lipase 10000 Unt, Protease 37500 Unt, Amylase 33200 Unt	Pancrelipase by United Res	00677-1654	Gastrointestinal
MUTUAL689	Cap, Light Brown	Pancrelipase 10000I Units	by Mutual	53489-0321	Gastrointestinal
MUTUAL690	Cap, Light Orange	Pancrelipase 16000I Units	by Mutual	53489-0322	Gastrointestinal
MUTUAL691	Cap, Orange, Enteric Coated	Lipase 20000 Unt, Protease 75000 Unt, Amylase 66400 Unt	Microspheres by Mutual Pharm	53489-0323	Gastrointestinal
MUTUAL691	Cap, Orange, Enteric Coated	Lipase 20000 Unt, Protease 75000 Unt, Amylase 66400 Unt	Microspheres by United Res	00677-1656	Gastrointestinal
MX <> 511	Tab, Yellow, Round, Scored	Methotrexate Sodium 2.5 mg	by Lederle Pharm	00005-5874	Antineoplastic
MX <> 511	Tab, Yellow, Round, Scored	Methotrexate Sodium 2.5 mg	by ESI Lederle	59911-5874	Antineoplastic
MX225	Tab, White, Oblong, MX/225	Guaifenesin 500 mg, Pseudoephedrine 120 mg	Nasatab LA by ECR		Cold Remedy
MX225	Tab, Ex Release, MX/225	Guaifenesin 500 mg, Pseudoephedrine HCl 120 mg	Nasatab LA by Sovereign	58716-0669	Cold Remedy
MX225	Tab, White, Capsule-shaped, Scored	Pseudoephedrine 120 mg, Guaifenesin 500 mg	Nasatab LA by ECR	00095-0225	Cold Remedy
MYCELEX10	Tab	Clotrimazole 10 mg	by Med Pro	53978-3040	Antifungal
MYCELEX10	Tab	Clotrimazole 10 mg	Mycelex Troche by Eckerd Drug	19458-0858	Antifungal
MYCELEX10	Tab, White	Clotrimazole 10 mg	Mycelex Troche by DHHS Prog	11819-0163	Antifungal
MYCELEX10	Tab, White, Round	Clotrimazole 10 mg	Mycelex Troche by DHHS Prog	11819-0164	Antifungal
MYCOBUTIN	Cap, Red-Brown, Mycobutin/Pharmacia	Rifabutin 150 mg	Mycobutin by Pharmacia & Upjohn	00013-5301	Antibiotic
MYKROX <> 12	Tab, White, Mykrox <> 1/2	Metolazone 0.5 mg	Mykrox by Medeva	53014-0847	Diuretic
MYLAN <> 1101	Cap	Prazosin HCl 1 mg	by Quality Care	60346-0572	Antihypertensive
MYLAN <> 115	Cap, Scarlet	Ampicillin Trihydrate	by Quality Care	60346-0082	Antibiotic
MYLAN <> 1155	Tab, White	Propoxyphene Napsylate 100 mg, Acetaminophen 650 mg	by Mylan		Analgesic; C IV
MYLAN <> 1155	Tab, White, Capsule Shaped, Film Coated	Propoxyphene Napsylate 100 mg, Acetaminophen 650 mg	Darvocet-N by UDL	51079-0934	Analgesic; C IV
MYLAN <> 129	Cap	Aspirin 389 mg, Caffeine 32.4 mg, Propoxyphene HCl 65 mg	by Qualitest	00603-5460	Analgesic; C IV
MYLAN <> 130	Tab	Acetaminophen 650 mg, Propoxyphene HCl 65 mg	by Quality Care	60346-0909	Analgesic; C IV
MYLAN <> 130	Tab	Acetaminophen 650 mg, Propoxyphene HCl 65 mg	by Qualitest	00603-5463	Analgesic; C IV
MYLAN <> 130	Tab, Orange, Coated	Acetaminophen 650 mg, Propoxyphene HCl 65 mg	by Mylan	00378-0130	Analgesic; C IV
MYLAN <> 130	Tab, Orange, Cap Shaped, Film Coated	Acetaminophen 650 mg, Propoxyphene HCl 65 mg	Wygesic by UDL	51079-0741	Analgesic; C IV
MYLAN <> 155	Tab, Coated	Acetaminophen 650 mg, Propoxyphene Napsylate 100 mg	by Qualitest	00603-5466	Analgesic; C IV
MYLAN <> 155	Tab	Acetaminophen 650 mg, Propoxyphene Napsylate 100 mg	by Vangard	00615-0455	Analgesic; C IV
MYLAN <> 155	Tab, Pink, Coated	Acetaminophen 650 mg, Propoxyphene Napsylate 100 mg	by Mylan	00378-0155	Analgesic; C IV
MYLAN <> 155	Tab, Coated	Acetaminophen 650 mg, Propoxyphene Napsylate 100 mg	Propoxacet N by Quality Care	60346-0628	Analgesic; C IV
MYLAN <> 155	Tab, Coated	Acetaminophen 650 mg, Propoxyphene Napsylate 100 mg	by UDL	51079-0322	Analgesic; C IV

ID FRONT ⬦ BACK	DESCRIPTION FRONT ⬦ BACK	INGREDIENT & STRENGTH	BRAND (OR EQUIV.) & FIRM	NDC#	CLASS; SCH.
MYLAN ⬦ 155	Tab, Pink, Oblong, Film	Acetaminophen 650 mg, Propoxyphene Napsylate 100 mg	by Abbott	00074-3975	Analgesic; C IV
MYLAN ⬦ 155	Tab, Coated	Acetaminophen 650 mg, Propoxyphene Napsylate 100 mg	by Allscripts	54569-0015	Analgesic; C IV
MYLAN ⬦ 2020	Cap, Green	Piroxicam 20 mg	by Va Cmop	65243-0057	NSAID
MYLAN ⬦ 2020	Cap	Piroxicam 20 mg	by Quality Care	60346-0676	NSAID
MYLAN ⬦ 211	Tab, Green, Coated	Amitriptyline HCl 12.5 mg, Chlordiazepoxide 5 mg	by Mylan	00378-0211	Antianxiety; C IV
MYLAN ⬦ 2200	Cap, Lavender, Opaque	Acyclovir 200 mg	by Allscripts	54569-4482	Antiviral
MYLAN ⬦ 237	Tab, White, Film Coated	Etodolac 400 mg	by Mylan	00378-0237	NSAID
MYLAN ⬦ 237	Tab, White, Oval, Convex, Film	Etodolac 400 mg	by Hoechst Marion Roussel	64734-0002	NSAID
MYLAN ⬦ 242	Tab, Pink, Oval, Convex, Film	Etodolac 500 mg	Etodolac by Heartland	61392-0912	NSAID
MYLAN ⬦ 242	Tab, Pink	Etodolac 500 mg	by Mylan		NSAID
MYLAN ⬦ 244	Tab, Film Coated	Verapamil HCl 120 mg	by Murfreesboro	51129-1298	Antihypertensive
MYLAN ⬦ 244	Tab, Blue, Oval, Film Coated	Verapamil HCl 120 mg	Isoptin SR by UDL	51079-0894	Antihypertensive
MYLAN ⬦ 244	Tab, Blue, Beveled Edge, Film Coated	Verapamil HCl 120 mg	by Mylan	00378-1120	Antihypertensive
MYLAN ⬦ 245	Tab, Light Green	Bumetanide 0.5 mg	by Hoffmann La Roche	00004-0290	Diuretic
MYLAN ⬦ 245	Tab, Light Green, Scored	Bumetanide 0.5 mg	by Mylan	00378-0245	Diuretic
MYLAN ⬦ 277	Tab, White, Coated	Amitriptyline HCl 25 mg, Chlordiazepoxide 10 mg	by Mylan	00378-0277	Antianxiety; C IV
MYLAN ⬦ 3000	Cap, Coral	Meclofenamate Sodium	by Quality Care	60346-0350	NSAID
MYLAN ⬦ 302	Tab, White	Acyclovir 800 mg	by Mylan	00378-0302	Antiviral
MYLAN ⬦ 330	Tab, White, Coated	Amitriptyline HCl 10 mg, Perphenazine 2 mg	by Mylan	00378-0330	Antipsychotic
MYLAN ⬦ 357	Tab, Lavender, Film Coated	Pentoxifylline 400 mg	by Mylan	00378-0357	Anticoagulent
MYLAN ⬦ 357	Tab, Labender, Capsule Shaped, Film Coated	Pentoxifylline 400 mg	Trental by UDL	51079-0889	Anticoagulent
MYLAN ⬦ 370	Tab, Yellow, Round	Bumetanide 1 mg	by UDL	51079-0892	Diuretic
MYLAN ⬦ 370	Tab, Yellow, Scored	Bumetanide 1 mg	by Mylan	00378-0370	Diuretic
MYLAN ⬦ 3725	Tab, Beveled Edge, 37 to Left, 25 to Right of Score	Hydrochlorothiazide 25 mg, Triamterene 37.5 mg	Maxzide 25 by Mylan	00378-3725	Diuretic
MYLAN ⬦ 377	Tab, White	Naproxen 250 mg	by Mylan	00378-0377	NSAID
MYLAN ⬦ 377	Tab	Naproxen 250 mg	by Kaiser	00179-1186	NSAID
MYLAN ⬦ 377	Tab, White, Round	Naproxen 250 mg	Naprosyn by UDL	51079-0793	NSAID
MYLAN ⬦ 377	Tab	Naproxen 250 mg	by HJ Harkins Co	52959-0190	NSAID
MYLAN ⬦ 377	Tab	Naproxen 250 mg	by Allscripts	54569-3758	NSAID
MYLAN ⬦ 377	Tab	Naproxen 250 mg	by Quality Care	60346-0816	NSAID
MYLAN ⬦ 377	Tab, White, Round	Naproxen 250 mg	by Novartis	17088-0014	NSAID
MYLAN ⬦ 377	Tab, White, Round	Naproxen 250 mg	by Dixon Shane	17236-0076	NSAID
MYLAN ⬦ 401	Tab, Beveled Edge, Coated	Ibuprofen 400 mg	by Mylan	00378-0401	NSAID
MYLAN ⬦ 4010	Cap, Peach	Temazepam 15 mg	by Natl Pharmpak	55154-5591	Sedative/Hypnotic; C IV
MYLAN ⬦ 417	Tab, Peach, Oval, Scored	Bumetanide 2 mg	by Caraco	57664-0367	Diuretic
MYLAN ⬦ 417	Tab, Peach, Scored	Bumetanide 2 mg	Bumex by Capellon	64543-0112	Diuretic
MYLAN ⬦ 417	Tab, Peach, Scored	Bumetanide 2 mg	by Mylan	00378-0417	Diuretic
MYLAN ⬦ 421	Tab, Beige, Capsule-Shaped, Film-Coated	Methyldopa 500 mg	Aldomet by UDL	51079-0201	Antihypertensive
MYLAN ⬦ 421	Tab, Beige, Beveled Edge, Coated	Methyldopa 500 mg	by Mylan	00378-0421	Antihypertensive
MYLAN ⬦ 427	Tab, Yellowish Orange	Sulindac 150 mg	by Mylan	00378-0427	NSAID
MYLAN ⬦ 427	Tab, Yellow-Orange, Round	Sulindac 150 mg	Clinoril by UDL	51079-0666	NSAID
MYLAN ⬦ 427	Tab	Sulindac 150 mg	by Quality Care	60346-0044	NSAID
MYLAN ⬦ 442	Tab, Purple, Coated	Amitriptyline HCl 25 mg, Perphenazine 2 mg	by Mylan	00378-0442	Antipsychotic
MYLAN ⬦ 442	Tab, Purple, Round, Film	Perphenazine 2 mg, Amitriptyline HCl 25 mg	by Pharmafab	62542-0914	Antipsychotic; Antidepressant
MYLAN ⬦ 451	Tab	Naproxen 500 mg	by Kaiser	00179-1188	NSAID
MYLAN ⬦ 451	Tab, White, Capsule-Shaped	Naproxen 500 mg	Naprosyn by UDL	51079-0795	NSAID
MYLAN ⬦ 451	Tab	Naproxen 500 mg	by Murfreesboro	51129-1314	NSAID
MYLAN ⬦ 451	Tab	Naproxen 500 mg	by Allscripts	54569-3760	NSAID
MYLAN ⬦ 451	Tab, White, Oblong	Naproxen 500 mg	by OHM	51660-0701	NSAID
MYLAN ⬦ 451	Tab	Naproxen 500 mg	by Allscripts	54569-4255	NSAID
MYLAN ⬦ 451	Tab, White	Naproxen 500 mg	by Mylan	00378-0451	NSAID

ID FRONT <> BACK	DESCRIPTION FRONT <> BACK	INGREDIENT & STRENGTH	BRAND (OR EQUIV.) & FIRM	NDC#	CLASS; SCH.
MYLAN <> 451	Tab	Naproxen 500 mg	by St Marys Med	60760-0451	NSAID
MYLAN <> 451	Tab	Naproxen 500 mg	by Quality Care	60346-0815	NSAID
MYLAN <> 451	Tab	Naproxen 500 mg	by Kaiser	62224-2119	NSAID
MYLAN <> 451	Tab, White, Oblong	Naproxen 500 mg	by Dixon Shane	17236-0078	NSAID
MYLAN <> 451	Tab	Naproxen 500 mg	by Talbert Med	44514-0651	NSAID
MYLAN <> 457	Tab	Lorazepam 1 mg	by Vangard	00615-0451	Sedative/Hypnotic; C IV
MYLAN <> 507	Tab, Green, Beveled Edge, Coated	Hydrochlorothiazide 15 mg, Methyldopa 250 mg	by Mylan	00378-0507	Diuretic; Antihypertensive
MYLAN <> 517	Tab, White, Film Coated, Scored	Gemfibrozil 600 mg	by Mylan	00378-0517	Antihyperlipidemic
MYLAN <> 521	Tab, Coated	Acetaminophen 650 mg, Propoxyphene Napsylate 100 mg	by Mylan	00378-0521	Analgesic; C IV
MYLAN <> 5375	Cap	Doxepin HCl	by PDRX	55289-0258	Antidepressant
MYLAN <> 555	Tab, White, Oblong	Naproxen 375 mg	by Novartis	61615-0016	NSAID
MYLAN <> 555	Tab	Naproxen 375 mg	by Kaiser	62224-4552	NSAID
MYLAN <> 555	Tab, MYLAN	Naproxen 375 mg	by Quality Care	60346-0817	NSAID
MYLAN <> 555	Tab, White, Oblong	Naproxen 375 mg	by Dixon Shane	17236-0077	NSAID
MYLAN <> 555	Tab	Naproxen 375 mg	by Mylan	00378-0555	NSAID
MYLAN <> 555	Tab	Naproxen 375 mg	by Kaiser	00179-1187	NSAID
MYLAN <> 555	Tab	Naproxen 375 mg	by Allscripts	54569-3759	NSAID
MYLAN <> 555	Tab, White, Capsule-Shaped	Naproxen 375 mg	Naprosyn by UDL	51079-0794	NSAID
MYLAN <> 555	Tab	Naproxen 375 mg	by HJ Harkins Co	52959-0191	NSAID
MYLAN <> 574	Tab, Orange, Film Coated	Amitriptyline HCl 25 mg, Perphenazine 4 mg	by Mylan	00378-0574	Antipsychotic
MYLAN <> 601	Tab, Beveled Edge, Coated	Ibuprofen 600 mg	by Mylan	00378-0601	NSAID
MYLAN <> 611	Tab, Beige, Round, Film Coated	Methyldopa 250 mg	by Allscripts	54569-0508	Antihypertensive
MYLAN <> 611	Tab, Beige, Round, Film Coated	Methyldopa 250 mg	Aldomet by UDL	51079-0200	Antihypertensive
MYLAN <> 611	Tab, Beige, Beveled Edge, Film Coated	Methyldopa 250 mg	by Mylan	00378-0611	Antihypertensive
MYLAN <> 611	Tab, Film Coated	Methyldopa 250 mg	by Murfreesboro	51129-1293	Antihypertensive
MYLAN <> 711	Tab, Green, Beveled Edge, Coated	Hydrochlorothiazide 25 mg, Methyldopa 250 mg	by Mylan	00378-0711	Diuretic; Antihypertensive
MYLAN <> 711	Tab, Coated	Hydrochlorothiazide 25 mg, Methyldopa 250 mg	by Allscripts	54569-0513	Diuretic; Antihypertensive
MYLAN <> 727	Tab, Film Coated	Amitriptyline HCl 10 mg, Perphenazine 4 mg	by Mylan	00378-0042	Antipsychotic
MYLAN <> 73	Tab, Coated	Amitriptyline HCl 50 mg, Perphenazine 4 mg	by Mylan	00378-0073	Antipsychotic
MYLAN <> 733	Tab, Film Coated	Naproxen Sodium 550 mg	by Allscripts	54569-3762	NSAID
MYLAN <> 733	Tab, Film Coated	Naproxen Sodium 550 mg	by Quality Care	60346-0826	NSAID
MYLAN <> 777	Tab	Lorazepam 2 mg	by Vangard	00615-0452	Sedative/Hypnotic; C IV
MYLAN <> 801	Tab, Beveled Edge, Coated	Ibuprofen 800 mg	by Mylan	00378-0801	NSAID
MYLAN <> 94	Tab, Purple, Oval, Scored, Mylan <> 9/4	Carbidopa 50 mg; Levodopa 200 mg, ER	by UDL	51079-0923	Antiparkinson
MYLAN <> CYSTA50	Cap, Cysta over 50	Cysteamine Bitartrate	Cystagon by Mylan	00378-9040	Nephropathic Cystimosis
MYLAN <> CYSTAGON150	Cap, White	Cystagon 150 mg	by Mylan		Urinary Tract
MYLAN <> CYSTAGON150	Cap, Cystagon over 150	Cysteamine Bitartrate	Cystagon by Mylan	00378-9045	Nephropathic Cystimosis
MYLAN <> CYSTAGON50	Cap, White	Cystagon 50 mg	by Mylan		Urinary Tract
MYLAN <> TH1	Tab, Green, Round, Beveled Edge, TH/1	Hydrochlorothiazide 25 mg, Triamterene 37.5 mg	Maxzide-25 by Mylan	00378-1352	Diuretic
MYLAN <> TH1	Tab, Green, Round, TH Over 1	Hydrochlorothiazide 25 mg, Triamterene 37.5 mg	Maxzide-25 by Mylan	55160-0126	Diuretic
MYLAN <> TH2	Tab, Yellow, Round, Scored, Mylan <> TH over 2	Hydrochlorothiazide 50 mg, Triamterene 75 mg	Maxzide by UDL	51079-0433	Diuretic
MYLAN <> TH2	Tab, Yellow, Beveled Edge TH/2	Hydrochlorothiazide 50 mg, Triamterene 75 mg	by Mylan	00378-1355	Diuretic
MYLAN <> TH2	Tab, Yellow, TH Over 2	Hydrochlorothiazide 50 mg, Triamterene 75 mg	by Mylan	55160-0127	Diuretic
MYLAN 148	Tab, Blue, Oblong	Doxycycline Hyclate 100 mg	by Family Hlth Phcy	65149-0554	Antibiotic
MYLAN 186	Tab	Clonidine HCl 0.2 mg	by Kaiser	62224-7555	Antihypertensive

ID FRONT <> BACK	DESCRIPTION FRONT <> BACK	INGREDIENT & STRENGTH	BRAND (OR EQUIV.) & FIRM	NDC#	CLASS; SCH.
MYLAN 216 <> 40	Tab	Furosemide 40 mg	by Kaiser	62224-1222	Diuretic
MYLAN 2200	Cap, Lavender, Mylan over 2200	Acyclovir 200 mg	by Mylan	00378-2200	Antiviral
MYLAN1001	Cap, Caramel & Powder Blue, Mylan over 1001	Thiothixene 1 mg	Navane by UDL	51079-0586	Antipsychotic
MYLAN1001	Cap, Caramel & Powder Blue, Mylan over 1001 in Black Ink	Thiothixene 1 mg	by Mylan	00378-1001	Antipsychotic
MYLAN1001	Cap, Caramel	Thiothixene 1 mg	by Med Pro	53978-2003	Antipsychotic
MYLAN1001	Cap, Caramel	Thiothixene 1 mg	by Dixon Shane	17236-0465	Antipsychotic
MYLAN101	Cap, Medium Orange & Yellow, Mylan over 1001 in Black Ink	Tetracycline HCl 250 mg	by Mylan	00378-0101	Antibiotic
MYLAN101	Cap	Tetracycline HCl 500 mg	by Urgent Care Ctr	50716-0782	Antibiotic
MYLAN1010	Cap, Dark Green & Olive, Mylan over 1010	Piroxicam 10 mg	Feldine by UDL	51079-0742	NSAID
MYLAN1010	Cap, Dark Green & Olive, Mylan over 1010	Piroxicam 10 mg	by Mylan	55160-0128	NSAID
MYLAN1010	Cap, Dark Green & Olive, Mylan over 1010	Piroxicam 10 mg	by Mylan	00378-1010	NSAID
MYLAN1010	Cap, Olive	Piroxicam 10 mg	by Allscripts	54569-3974	NSAID
MYLAN1010	Cap, Dark Green & Olive, Mylan over 1010	Piroxicam 10 mg	by HJ Harkins Co	52959-0398	NSAID
MYLAN1010	Cap, Olive, Mylan over 1010	Piroxicam 10 mg	by Mylan	55160-0128	NSAID
MYLAN1010	Cap, Mylan over 1010	Piroxicam 10 mg	by Quality Care	60346-0737	NSAID
MYLAN102	Cap, Black & Yellow, Mylan over 102 in White Ink	Tetracycline HCl 500 mg	by Mylan	00378-0102	Antibiotic
MYLAN1020	Cap, Medium Blue Green & Ivory	Nicardipine HCl 20 mg	Cardene by Mylan		Antihypertensive
MYLAN1020	Cap, Green & Ivory	Nicardipine HCl 20 mg	by Murfreesboro Ph	51129-1372	Antihypertensive
MYLAN1020	Cap, Mylan over 1020 in Black Ink	Nicardipine HCl 20 mg	by Mylan	00378-1020	Antihypertensive
MYLAN1049	Cap	Doxepin HCl	by Pharmedix	53002-0489	Antidepressant
MYLAN1049	Cap	Doxepin HCl	by Major	00904-1260	Antidepressant
MYLAN1049	Cap, Buff, Mylan over 1049	Doxepin HCl 10 mg	Sinequan by UDL	51079-0436	Antidepressant
MYLAN1049	Cap, Buff, Black Print	Doxepin HCl 10 mg	by Mylan	00378-1049	Antidepressant
MYLAN106 <> 250	Tab, Film Coated, Mylan over 106 <> 250	Erythromycin Stearate	by Diversified Hlthcare Serv	55887-0994	Antibiotic
MYLAN106 <> 250	Tab, Film Coated	Erythromycin Stearate	by Quality Care	60346-0580	Antibiotic
MYLAN106 <> 250	Tab, Film Coated, Mylan over 106 <> 250	Erythromycin Stearate	by Prescription Dispensing	61807-0013	Antibiotic
MYLAN106 <> 250	Tab, Yellow, Film Coated, Mylan over 106 <> 250	Erythromycin Stearate 250 mg	by Mylan	00378-0106	Antibiotic
MYLAN107 <> 500	Tab, Coated	Erythromycin Stearate	by PDRX	55289-0705	Antibiotic
MYLAN107 <> 500	Tab, Film Coated, Mylan over 107 <> 500	Erythromycin Stearate	by Prescription Dispensing	61807-0015	Antibiotic
MYLAN107 <> 500	Tab, Coated	Erythromycin Stearate	by Quality Care	60346-0645	Antibiotic
MYLAN107 <> 500	Tab, Film Coated, Mylan over 107 <> 500	Erythromycin Stearate	by St Marys Med	60760-0107	Antibiotic
MYLAN107 <> 500	Tab, Coated	Erythromycin Stearate	by Direct Dispensing	57866-0265	Antibiotic
MYLAN107 <> 500	Tab, Film Coated, Mylan over 107 <> 500	Erythromycin Stearate	by DRX	55045-1113	Antibiotic
MYLAN107 <> 500	Tab, Film Coated	Erythromycin Stearate	by Med Pro	53978-0026	Antibiotic
MYLAN107 <> 500	Tab, Yellow, Film Coated, Mylan over 107 <> 500	Erythromycin Stearate 500 mg	by Mylan	00378-0107	Antibiotic
MYLAN1101	Cap	Prazosin HCl	by Med Pro	53978-5045	Antihypertensive
MYLAN1101	Cap	Prazosin HCl	by Pharmedix	53002-0499	Antihypertensive
MYLAN1101	Cap	Prazosin HCl	by Kaiser	62224-0119	Antihypertensive
MYLAN1101	Cap, Light Brown & Dark Green, Mylan over 1101 in White Ink	Prazosin HCl 1 mg	by Mylan	00378-1101	Antihypertensive
MYLAN1101	Cap, Dark Green & Light Brown, Mylan over 1101	Prazosin HCl 1 mg	Minipress by UDL	51079-0630	Antihypertensive
MYLAN1101	Cap	Prazosin HCl	by Allscripts	54569-2582	Antihypertensive
MYLAN111250	Tab, White, Oval, Mylan 111/250	Penicillin V Potassium 250 mg	V-Cillin K by Mylan		Antibiotic
MYLAN112500	Tab, White, Round, Mylan 112/500	Penicillin V Potassium 500 mg	V-Cillin K by Mylan		Antibiotic
MYLAN115	Cap	Ampicillin Trihydrate 250 mg	by Med Pro	53978-5018	Antibiotic
MYLAN115	Cap, Scarlet, Mylan over 115	Ampicillin Trihydrate 250 mg	by Mylan	00378-0115	Antibiotic
MYLAN1155	Tab, White, Oblong	Propoxyphene Napsylate 100 mg, Acetaminophen 650 mg	Darvocet N 100 by Mylan		Analgesic; C IV
MYLAN116	Cap	Ampicillin Trihydrate 500 mg	by Apotheca	12634-0168	Antibiotic
MYLAN116	Cap, Scarlet, Mylan over 116	Ampicillin Trihydrate 500 mg	by Mylan	00378-0116	Antibiotic
MYLAN1200	Cap, Orange, Black Print	Acebutolol HCl 200 mg	by Mylan	00378-1200	Antihypertensive
MYLAN121	Tab, White, Round	Penicillin G Potassium 250,000 Units	Pentids by Mylan		Antibiotic
MYLAN122	Tab, White, Round	Penicillin G Potassium 400,000 Units	Pentids by Mylan		Antibiotic
MYLAN129	Cap, Pink, Coated, Mylan over 129 in Black Ink	Propoxyphene HCl 65 mg	by Mylan	00378-0129	Analgesic; C IV

ID FRONT <> BACK	DESCRIPTION FRONT <> BACK	INGREDIENT & STRENGTH	BRAND (OR EQUIV.) & FIRM	NDC#	CLASS; SCH.
MYLAN129	Cap, Pink	Propoxyphene HCl 65 mg	by Ranbaxy	63304-0701	Analgesic; C IV
MYLAN130	Tab, Coated	Acetaminophen 650 mg, Propoxyphene HCl 6.5 mg	by Allscripts	54569-2588	Analgesic; C IV
MYLAN130	Tab, Coated	Acetaminophen 650 mg, Propoxyphene HCl 65 mg	by Heartland	61392-0148	Analgesic; C IV
MYLAN130	Tab, Coated,	Acetaminophen 650 mg, Propoxyphene HCl 65 mg	by Med Pro	53978-2020	Analgesic; C IV
MYLAN131	Cap	Aspirin 389 mg, Caffeine 32.4 mg, Propoxyphene HCl 65 mg	Propoxyphene Compd 65 by Quality Care	60346-0682	Analgesic; C IV
MYLAN131	Cap, Gray & Red, Mylan over 131	Aspirin 389 mg, Caffeine 32.4 mg, Propoxyphene HCl 65 mg	by Mylan	00378-0131	Analgesic; C IV
MYLAN1400	Cap, Orange	Acebutolol HCl 400 mg	Sectral by Mylan		Antihypertensive
MYLAN1400	Cap, Orange, Black Print	Acebutolol HCl 400 mg	by Mylan	00378-1400	Antihypertensive
MYLAN1400	Cap, Mylan over 1400 <> Mylan over 1400	Acebutolol HCl	by Caremark	00339-6092	Antihypertensive
MYLAN1400	Cap, Opaque & Orange, Mylan over 1400	Acebutolol HCl 400 mg	by ABG	60999-0900	Antihypertensive
MYLAN1401	Tab, White, Beveled Edge, Coated, Mylan over 1401 in Black Ink	Ibuprofen 400 mg	by Mylan	00378-1401	NSAID
MYLAN141	Tab, Ivory, Round	Spironolactone 25 mg, Hydrochlorothiazide 25 mg	Aldactazide by Mylan		Diuretic
MYLAN1410	Cap, Swedish Orange, in White Ink	Nortriptyline HCl 10 mg	by Mylan	00378-1410	Antidepressant
MYLAN1410	Cap, Orange, Opaque, Mylan over 1410	Nortriptyline HCl 10 mg	Pamelar by UDL	51079-0803	Antidepressant
MYLAN1410	Cap, Orange	Nortriptyline HCl 10 mg	by Dixon Shane	17236-0003	Antidepressant
MYLAN143	Cap, Light Green, Mylan Over 143	Indomethacin 25 mg	Indocin by UDL	51079-0190	NSAID
MYLAN143	Cap, Light Green, Mylan over 143 in Black Ink	Indomethacin 25 mg	by Mylan	00378-0143	NSAID
MYLAN1430	Cap, Bluish Green & Yellow	Nicardipine HCl 30 mg	Cardene by Mylan		Antihypertensive
MYLAN1430	Cap, Mylan over 1430 in Black Ink	Nicardipine HCl 30 mg	by Mylan	00378-1430	Antihypertensive
MYLAN145	Cap, Aqua Blue & White, Mylan over 145	Doxycycline Hyclate 50 mg	by Mylan	00378-0145	Antibiotic
MYLAN146 <> 25	Tab, White, Mylan over 146	Spironolactone 25 mg	by Mylan	00378-2146	Diuretic
MYLAN146 <> 25	Tab	Spironolactone 25 mg	by Vangard	00615-1535	Diuretic
MYLAN146 <> 25	Tab, White, Round, Scored, Mylan over 146 <> 25	Spironolactone 25 mg	Aldactone by UDL	51079-0103	Diuretic
MYLAN146 <> 25	Tab	Spironolactone 25 mg	by Nat Pharmpak Serv	55154-5517	Diuretic
MYLAN146 <> 25	Tab	Spironolactone 25 mg	by Heartland	61392-0083	Diuretic
MYLAN146 <> 25	Tab, White, Round, Scored	Spironolactone 25 mg	by Sidmark		Diuretic
MYLAN146 <> 25	Tab	Spironolactone 25 mg	by Qualitest	00603-5766	Diuretic
MYLAN14625	Tab, Mylan 146/25	Spironolactone 25 mg	by Allscripts	54569-0505	Diuretic
MYLAN14625	Tab	Spironolactone 25 mg	by Pharmedix	53002-0472	Diuretic
MYLAN147	Cap, Light Green, Mylan Over 147	Indomethacin 50 mg	Indocin by UDL	51079-0191	NSAID
MYLAN147	Cap, Light Green	Indomethacin 50 mg	by Mylan	00378-0147	NSAID
MYLAN147	Cap	Indomethacin 50 mg	by St Marys Med	60760-0147	NSAID
MYLAN148	Cap, Aqua Blue	Doxycycline Hyclate 100 mg	by Mylan	00378-0148	Antibiotic
MYLAN148	Cap, Aqua Blue, Mylan over 148	Doxycycline Hyclate 100 mg	Vibramycin by UDL	51079-0522	Antibiotic
MYLAN148	Cap, Aqua Blue	Doxycycline Hyclate	by Diversified Hlthcare Serv	55887-0979	Antibiotic
MYLAN150250	Tab, White, Round, Mylan 150/250	Chlorothiazide 250 mg	Diuril by Mylan		Diuretic
MYLAN152	Tab	Clonidine HCl 0.1 mg	by Kaiser	62224-7551	Antihypertensive
MYLAN152	Tab	Clonidine HCl 0.1 mg	by Nat Pharmpak Serv	55154-5561	Antihypertensive
MYLAN152	Tab	Clonidine HCl 0.1 mg	by Prepackage Spec	58864-0110	Antihypertensive
MYLAN152	Tab	Clonidine HCl 0.1 mg	by Quality Care	60346-0786	Antihypertensive
MYLAN152	Tab	Clonidine HCl 0.1 mg	by PDRX	55289-0073	Antihypertensive
MYLAN152	Tab, White, Round, Scored	Clonidine HCl 0.1 mg	by Allscripts	54569-0478	Antihypertensive
MYLAN152	Tab, White, Round, Scored	Clonidine HCl 0.1 mg	by Southwood Pharms	58016-0517	Antihypertensive
MYLAN152	Tab, White, Round, Scored, Mylan over 152	Clonidine HCl 0.1 mg	Catapres by UDL	51079-0299	Antihypertensive
MYLAN152	Tab, White, Mylan over 152	Clonidine HCl 0.1 mg	by Mylan	00378-0152	Antihypertensive
MYLAN152	Tab	Clonidine HCl 0.1 mg	by Nat Pharmpak Serv	55154-5228	Antihypertensive
MYLAN152	Tab	Clonidine HCl 0.1 mg	by Med Pro	53978-0936	Antihypertensive
MYLAN152	Tab	Clonidine HCl 0.1 mg	by Pharmedix	53002-0414	Antihypertensive
MYLAN152	Tab, White, Round	Clonidine HCl 0.1 mg	Clonidine HCl USP by DHHS Prog	11819-0100	Antihypertensive
MYLAN152	Tab, White, Round, Scored	Clonidine HCl 0.2 mg	by Southwood Pharms	58016-0518	Antihypertensive
MYLAN155	Tab, Coated	Acetaminophen 650 mg, Propoxyphene Napsylate 100 mg	by Med Pro	53978-5013	Analgesic; C IV

ID FRONT <> BACK	DESCRIPTION FRONT <> BACK	INGREDIENT & STRENGTH	BRAND (OR EQUIV.) & FIRM	NDC#	CLASS; SCH.
MYLAN156 <> 500	Tab, Yellow, Film Coated	Probenecid 500 mg	by Mylan	00378-0156	Antigout
MYLAN156 <> 500	Tab, Film Coated	Probenecid 500 mg	by Med Pro	53978-0014	Antigout
MYLAN156 <> 500	Tab, Film Coated	Probenecid 500 mg	by Quality Care	60346-0768	Antigout
MYLAN1570	Cap, Light Lavender, Mylan over 1570	Terazosin HCl 10 mg	Hytrin by UDL	51079-0939	Antihypertensive
MYLAN159	Cap, Maroon & White	Disopyramide Phosphate 100 mg	Norpace by Mylan		Antiarrhythmic
MYLAN1601	Tab, White, Beveled Edge, Coated, Mylan over 1601 in Black Ink	Ibuprofen 600 mg	by Mylan	00378-1601	NSAID
MYLAN161	Cap, Maroon	Disopyramide Phosphate 150 mg	Norpace by Mylan		Antiarrhythmic
MYLAN1610	Cap, Blue, Mylan over 1610	Dicyclomine HCl 10 mg	by UDL	51079-0118	Gastrointestinal
MYLAN162	Tab, White, Scored	Chlorothiazide 500 mg	by Mylan	00378-0162	Diuretic
MYLAN162	Tab	Chlorothiazide 500 mg	by Med Pro	53978-0020	Diuretic
MYLAN162	Tab, White, Round, Scored, Mylan over 162	Chlorothiazide 500 mg	Diuril by UDL	51079-0061	Diuretic
MYLAN162	Tab	Chlorothiazide 500 mg	by Allscripts	54569-0537	Diuretic
MYLAN1650	Cap, Light Brown, Opaque	Nitrofurantoin 50 mg	by Allscripts	54569-0181	Antibiotic
MYLAN1650	Cap, Light Brown, Opaque, Mylan over 1650	Nitrofurantoin 50 mg	Macrodantin by UDL	51079-0584	Antibiotic
MYLAN1650	Cap, Light Brown, Mylan over 1650 in Black Ink	Nitrofurantoin 50 mg	by Mylan	00378-1650	Antibiotic
MYLAN167 <> 100	Tab, Beige, Film Coated, Mylan over 167 <> 100	Doxycycline Hyclate 100 mg	by Mylan	00378-0167	Antibiotic
MYLAN167 <> 100	Tab, Beige, Round, Film Coated, Mylan over 167 <> 100	Doxycycline Hyclate 100 mg	Vibra-Tabs by UDL	51079-0554	Antibiotic
MYLAN1700	Cap, Gray, Opaque, Mylan over 1700	Nitrofurantoin 100 mg	Macrodantin by UDL	51079-0585	Antibiotic
MYLAN1700	Cap, Gray, Mylan over 1700 in Black Ink	Nitrofurantoin 100 mg	by Mylan	00378-1700	Antibiotic
MYLAN175	Tab, Orange, Round	Chlorothiazide 250 mg, Reserpine 0.125 mg	Diupres by Mylan		Diuretic; Antihypertensive
MYLAN176	Tab, Orange, Round	Chlorothiazide 500 mg, Reserpine 0.125 mg	Diupres by Mylan		Diuretic; Antihypertensive
MYLAN1801	Tab, White, Beveled Edge, Coated, Mylan over 1801 in Black Ink	Ibuprofen 800 mg	by Mylan	00378-1801	NSAID
MYLAN182 <> 10	Tab, Orange, Round, Scored, Mylan over 182 <> 10	Propranolol HCl 10 mg	Inderal by UDL	51079-0277	Antihypertensive
MYLAN182 <> 10	Tab, Orange, Beveled Edge, Mylan over 182	Propranolol HCl 10 mg	by Mylan	00378-0182	Antihypertensive
MYLAN182 <> 10	Tab, Mylan 182	Propranolol HCl 10 mg	by Quality Care	60346-0570	Antihypertensive
MYLAN183 <> 20	Tab, Blue, Round, Scored, Mylan over 183 <> 20	Propranolol HCl 20 mg	Inderal by UDL	51079-0278	Antihypertensive
MYLAN183 <> 20	Tab, Blue, Beveled Edge, Mylan over 184	Propranolol HCl 20 mg	by Mylan	00378-0183	Antihypertensive
MYLAN184 <> 40	Tab, Green, Beveled Edge, Mylan over 184	Propranolol HCl 40 mg	by Mylan	00378-0184	Antihypertensive
MYLAN184 <> 40	Tab, Green, Round, Scored, Mylan over 184 <> 40	Propranolol HCl 40 mg	Inderal by UDL	51079-0279	Antihypertensive
MYLAN185 <> 80	Tab, Yellow, Round, Scored, Mylan over 185 <> 80	Propranolol HCl 80 mg	Inderal by UDL	51079-0280	Antihypertensive
MYLAN185 <> 80	Tab, Yellow, Beveled Edge, Mylan over 185	Propranolol HCl 80 mg	by Mylan	00378-0185	Antihypertensive
MYLAN186	Tab, Scored, Mylan over 186	Clonidine HCl 0.2 mg	by Amerisource	62584-0339	Antihypertensive
MYLAN186	Tab, White	Clonidine HCl 0.2 mg	by Quality Care	60346-0787	Antihypertensive
MYLAN186	Tab	Clonidine HCl 0.2 mg	by Prepackage Spec	58864-0111	Antihypertensive
MYLAN186	Tab	Clonidine HCl 0.2 mg	by Nat Pharmpak Serv	55154-5562	Antihypertensive
MYLAN186	Tab, White, Round, Scored, Mylan over 186	Clonidine HCl 0.2 mg	Catapres by UDL	51079-0300	Antihypertensive
MYLAN186	Tab, White, Scored, Mylan over 186	Clonidine HCl 0.2 mg	by Mylan	00378-0186	Antihypertensive
MYLAN186	Tab	Clonidine HCl 0.2 mg	by Med Pro	53978-0816	Antihypertensive
MYLAN186	Tab	Clonidine HCl 0.2 mg	by Nat Pharmpak Serv	55154-5229	Antihypertensive
MYLAN186	Tab, White, Round, Scored	Clonidine HCl 0.2 mg	by Vangard Labs	00615-2573	Antihypertensive
MYLAN186	Tab, White, Round, Scored	Clonidine HCl 0.2 mg	by DHHS Prog	11819-0112	Antihypertensive
MYLAN189	Tab	Clonidine HCl 0.3 mg	by Med Pro	53978-1099	Antihypertensive
MYLAN195250	Tab, White, Round, Mylan 195/250	Penicillin V Potassium 250 mg	V-Cillin K by Mylan		Antibiotic
MYLAN197 <> 100	Tab, Green, Round, Scored, Mylan over 197 <> 100	Chlorpropamide 100 mg	Diabinese by UDL	51079-0202	Antidiabetic
MYLAN197 <> 100	Tab, Green, Scored, Mylan over 197 <> 100	Chlorpropamide 100 mg	by Mylan	00378-0197	Antidiabetic
MYLAN197100	Tab	Chlorpropamide 100 mg	by Allscripts	54569-2017	Antidiabetic
MYLAN198500	Tab, White, Oval, Mylan 198/500	Penicillin V Potassium 500 mg	V-Cillin K by Mylan		Antibiotic
MYLAN199	Tab, White, Round, Scored	Clonidine HCl 0.3 mg	by Natl Pharmpak	55154-5570	Antihypertensive
MYLAN199	Tab, White, Round, Scored, Mylan over 199	Clonidine HCl 0.3 mg	Catapres by UDL	51079-0301	Antihypertensive
MYLAN199	Tab, White	Clonidine HCl 0.3 mg	by Mylan	00378-0199	Antihypertensive

ID FRONT <> BACK	DESCRIPTION FRONT <> BACK	INGREDIENT & STRENGTH	BRAND (OR EQUIV.) & FIRM	NDC#	CLASS; SCH.
MYLAN2002	Cap, Caramel & Yellow, Mylan over 2002	Thiothixene 2 mg	Navane by UDL	51079-0587	Antipsychotic
MYLAN2002	Cap, Caramel & Yellow, Mylan over 2002 in Black Ink	Thiothixene 2 mg	by Mylan	00378-2002	Antipsychotic
MYLAN2002	Cap, Caramel	Thiothixene 2 mg	by Med Pro	53978-2000	Antipsychotic
MYLAN2002	Cap, Mylan over 2002	Thiothixene 2 mg	by Quality Care	60346-0841	Antipsychotic
MYLAN2002	Cap, Caramel	Thiothixene 2 mg	by Dixon Shane	17236-0466	Antipsychotic
MYLAN2020	Cap, Medium Green, Imprint in Black Ink	Piroxicam 20 mg	by Mylan	00378-2020	NSAID
MYLAN2020	Cap	Piroxicam 20 mg	by Allscripts	54569-3693	NSAID
MYLAN2020	Cap, Green, Opaque, Mylan over 2020	Piroxicam 20 mg	Feldine by UDL	51079-0743	NSAID
MYLAN2020	Cap, Green	Piroxicam 20 mg	by Compumed	00403-0880	NSAID
MYLAN204	Cap	Amoxicillin Trihydrate	by Pharmedix	53002-0208	Antibiotic
MYLAN204	Cap, Buff & Caramel, Mylan over 204	Amoxicillin Trihydrate	by Mylan	00378-0204	Antibiotic
MYLAN205	Cap	Amoxicillin Trihydrate	by Pharmedix	53002-0216	Antibiotic
MYLAN205	Cap, Buff, Mylan over 205	Amoxicillin Trihydrate	by Mylan	00378-0205	Antibiotic
MYLAN20820	Tab, White, Round, Mylan 208/20	Furosemide 20 mg	Lasix by Mylan		Diuretic
MYLAN210 <> 250	Tab, Green, Round, Scored, Mylan over 210 <> 250	Chlorpropamide 250 mg	Diabinese by UDL	51079-0203	Antidiabetic
MYLAN210 <> 250	Tab, Green, Scored, Mylan over 210 <> 250	Chlorpropamide 250 mg	by Mylan	00378-0210	Antidiabetic
MYLAN210 <> 250	Tab	Chlorpropamide 250 mg	by Physicians Total Care	54868-0036	Antidiabetic
MYLAN2100	Cap, Brown	Loperamide HCl 2 mg	by Mylan	55160-0137	Antidiarrheal
MYLAN2100	Cap, Light Brown, Mylan over 2100 in Black Ink	Loperamide HCl 2 mg	by Mylan	00378-2100	Antidiarrheal
MYLAN2100	Cap, Light Brown, Mylan Over 2100	Loperamide HCl 2 mg	Imodium by UDL	51079-0690	Antidiarrheal
MYLAN2100	Cap	Loperamide 2 mg	by Vangard	00615-0362	Antidiarrheal
MYLAN2100	Cap, Brown	Loperamide HCl 2 mg	by Mylan	00378-3272	Antidiarrheal
MYLAN2100	Cap	Loperamide HCl 2 mg	by Med Pro	53978-3009	Antidiarrheal
MYLAN2100	Cap	Loperamide HCl 2 mg	by Quality Care	60346-0046	Antidiarrheal
MYLAN2100	Cap, Brown	Loperamide HCl 2 mg	by Compumed	00403-1046	Antidiarrheal
MYLAN211	Tab, Coated, Mylan over 211	Amitriptyline HCl 12.5 mg, Chlordiazepoxide 5 mg	by Quality Care	60346-0923	Antianxiety; C IV
MYLAN211	Tab, Coated	Amitriptyline HCl 12.5 mg, Chlordiazepoxide 5 mg	by Physicians Total Care	54868-2206	Antianxiety; C IV
MYLAN211	Tab, Green, Round	Chlordiazepoxide 5 mg, Amitriptyline HCl 12.5 mg	Limbitrol by Mylan		Antianxiety; C IV
MYLAN21350	Tab, Green, Round, Mylan 213/50	Chlorthalidone 50 mg	Hygroton by Mylan		Diuretic
MYLAN214	Tab	Haloperidol 2 mg	by Heartland	61392-0269	Antipsychotic
MYLAN214	Tab, Orange, Mylan over 214	Haloperidol 2 mg	by Mylan	00378-0214	Antipsychotic
MYLAN215	Tab, White, Round	Tolbutamide 500 mg	Orinase by Mylan		Antidiabetic
MYLAN2150	Cap, Coral	Meclofenamate Sodium	by Med Pro	53978-2015	NSAID
MYLAN2150	Cap, Cora	Meclofenamate Sodium	by Qualitest	00603-4344	NSAID
MYLAN2150	Cap, Coral, Mylan over 2150 in Black Ink	Meclofenamate Sodium 50 mg	by Mylan	00378-2150	NSAID
MYLAN216 <> 40	Tab	Furosemide 40 mg	by Quality Care	60346-0487	Diuretic
MYLAN216 <> 40	Tab, White, Round, Scored	Furosemide 40 mg	by Murfreesboro Ph	51129-1389	Diuretic
MYLAN216 <> 40	Tab, White, Scored, Mylan over 216 <> 40	Furosemide 40 mg	by Mylan	00378-0216	Diuretic
MYLAN216 <> 40	Tab, White, Round, Scored, Mylan over 216 <> 40	Furosemide 40 mg	Lasix by UDL	51079-0073	Diuretic
MYLAN216 <> 40	Tab	Furosemide 40 mg	by Allscripts	54569-0574	Diuretic
MYLAN21640	Tab, Mylan 216/40	Furosemide 40 mg	by Heartland	61392-0253	Diuretic
MYLAN217 <> 250	Tab, White, Mylan over 217	Tolazamide 250 mg	by Mylan	00378-0217	Antidiabetic
MYLAN2200	Cap, Lavender, Mylan over 2200	Acyclovir 200 mg	by Quality Care	62682-1021	Antiviral
MYLAN2200	Cap, Opaque & Purple, Mylan over 2200 in Black Ink	Acyclovir 200 mg	by Amerisource	62584-0694	Antiviral
MYLAN2200	Cap, Lavender	Acyclovir 200 mg	by Direct Dispensing	57866-6950	Antiviral
MYLAN2200	Cap, Purple, Gelatin	Acyclovir 200 mg	by Phy Total Care	54868-3996	Antiviral
MYLAN22225	Tab, Yellow, Round, Mylan 222/25	Chlorthalidone 25 mg	Hygroton by Mylan		Diuretic
MYLAN2260	Cap, Light Lavender & Yellow, Opaque, Mylan over 2260	Terazosin HCl 1 mg	Hytrin by UDL	51079-0936	Antihypertensive
MYLAN2264	Cap, Black & Light Lavender, Opaque, Mylan over 2264	Terazosin HCl 2 mg	Hytrin by UDL	51079-0937	Antihypertensive
MYLAN2268	Cap, Gray & Light Lavender, Opaque, Mylan over 2268	Terazosin HCl 5 mg	Hytrin by UDL	51079-0938	Antihypertensive
MYLAN2302	Cap	Prazosin HCl	by Caremark	00339-6020	Antihypertensive
MYLAN2302	Cap, Light Brown, Mylan over 2302 in White Ink	Prazosin HCl	by Mylan	00378-2302	Antihypertensive

456

ID FRONT <> BACK	DESCRIPTION FRONT <> BACK	INGREDIENT & STRENGTH	BRAND (OR EQUIV.) & FIRM	NDC#	CLASS; SCH.
MYLAN2302	Cap	Prazosin HCl	by Med Pro	53978-1077	Antihypertensive
MYLAN2302	Cap	Prazosin HCl	by Pharmedix	53002-0453	Antihypertensive
MYLAN2302	Cap	Prazosin HCl	by Kaiser	62224-0115	Antihypertensive
MYLAN2302	Cap, Brown & Light Brown, Mylan over 2302	Prazosin HCl 2 mg	Minipress by UDL	51079-0631	Antihypertensive
MYLAN2302	Cap, Light Brown, Mylan over 2302	Prazosin HCl	by Mylan	00378-2302	Antihypertensive
MYLAN2302	Cap	Prazosin HCl	by Allscripts	54569-2583	Antihypertensive
MYLAN2302	Cap, Brown	Prazosin HCl 2 mg	by Purepac		Antihypertensive
MYLAN232 <> 80	Tab, White, Round, Scored, Mylan over 232 <> 80	Furosemide 80 mg	Lasix by UDL	51079-0527	Diuretic
MYLAN232 <> 80	Tab, White, Mylan over 232 <> 80	Furosemide 80 mg	by Mylan	00378-0232	Diuretic
MYLAN2325	Cap, Orange & Swedish Orange, Imprint in White Ink	Nortriptyline HCl 25 mg	by Mylan	00378-2325	Antidepressant
MYLAN2325	Cap, Orange, Opaque, Mylan over 2325	Nortriptyline HCl 25 mg	Pamelar by UDL	51079-0804	Antidepressant
MYLAN2325	Cap, Orange	Nortriptyline HCl 25 mg	by Dixon Shane	17236-0005	Antidepressant
MYLAN2325	Cap	Nortriptyline HCl	by Quality Care	60346-0757	Antidepressant
MYLAN2325	Cap	Nortriptyline HCl	by Medirex	57480-0824	Antidepressant
MYLAN23280	Tab, MYLAN 232/80	Furosemide 80 mg	by Heartland	61392-0254	Diuretic
MYLAN245	Tab, Green, Oval, Scored	Bumetanide 0.5 mg	by Caraco	57664-0317	Diuretic
MYLAN245	Tab, Mylan/245	Bumetanide 0.5 mg	by Heartland	61392-0048	Diuretic
MYLAN251	Tab, Beveled Edge, Coated, Mylan over 251	Trazodone HCl 50 mg	by Mylan	00378-0251	Antidepressant
MYLAN252	Tab, Beveled Edge, Coated, Mylan over 252	Trazodone HCl 100 mg	by Mylan	00378-0252	Antidepressant
MYLAN2537	Cap, Olive & Rich Yellow, Marked in Black Ink with Mylan over 2537	Hydrochlorothiazide 25 mg, Triamterene 37.5 mg	by Mylan	55160-0125	Diuretic
MYLAN2537	Cap, Olive & Yellow, Opaque, Mylan over 2537	Triamterene 37.5 mg, Hydrochlorothiazide 25 mg	Dyazide by UDL	51079-0935	Diuretic
MYLAN2537	Cap, Green & Opaque & Yellow	Triamterene 37.5 mg, Hydrochlorothiazide 25 mg	by Teva	00480-0734	Diuretic
MYLAN257	Tab	Haloperidol 1 mg	by Heartland	61392-0266	Antipsychotic
MYLAN257	Tab, Orange, Mylan over 257	Haloperidol 1 mg	by Mylan	00378-0257	Antipsychotic
MYLAN271	Tab, White, Round, Scored	Diazepam 2 mg	by Allscripts	54569-0947	Antianxiety; C IV
MYLAN271	Tab, White, Round, Scored, Mylan over 271	Diazepam 2 mg	Valium by UDL	51079-0284	Antianxiety; C IV
MYLAN271	Tab, White, Mylan over 271	Diazepam 2 mg	by Mylan	00378-0271	Antianxiety; C IV
MYLAN277	Tab, Coated, Mylan Over 277	Amitriptyline HCl 25 mg, Chlordiazepoxide 10 mg	by Quality Care	60346-0921	Antianxiety; C IV
MYLAN3000	Cap	Meclofenamate Sodium	by Med Pro	53978-0660	NSAID
MYLAN3000	Cap	Meclofenamate Sodium	by Pharmedix	53002-0400	NSAID
MYLAN3000	Cap, Coral	Meclofenamate Sodium	by Qualitest	00603-4345	NSAID
MYLAN3000	Cap, Coral & White, Mylan over 3000 in Black Ink <> Mylan over 3000 in Black Ink	Meclofenamate Sodium 100 mg	by Mylan	00378-3000	NSAID
MYLAN3000	Cap, Coral, Mylan over 3000	Meclofenamate Sodium 100 mg	by Allscripts	54569-2526	NSAID
MYLAN3000	Cap, Coral, Mylan over 3000	Meclofenamate Sodium	by Mylan	00378-3000	NSAID
MYLAN3005	Cap, Caramel & White, Mylan over 3005 in Black Ink	Thiothixene 5 mg	by Mylan	00378-3005	Antipsychotic
MYLAN3005	Cap, Caramel	Thiothixene 5 mg	by Med Pro	53978-2001	Antipsychotic
MYLAN3005	Cap	Thiothixene 5 mg	by Quality Care	60346-0842	Antipsychotic
MYLAN3005	Cap, Caramel & White, Mylan over 3005	Thiothixene 5 mg	Navane by UDL	51079-0588	Antipsychotic
MYLAN3005	Cap, Caramel	Thiothixene 5 mg	by Dixon Shane	17236-0467	Antipsychotic
MYLAN3025	Cap, Flesh & Medium Orange	Clomipramine HCl 25 mg	by Mylan	00378-3025	OCD
MYLAN3050	Cap, Flesh & Yellow, Mylan over 3050	Clomipramine HCl 50 mg	by Mylan	00378-3050	OCD
MYLAN3075	Cap, Flesh & Swedish Orange, Mylan over 3075	Clomipramine HCl 75 mg	by Mylan	00378-3075	OCD
MYLAN3125	Cap, Mylan Over 3125	Doxepin HCl	by Quality Care	60346-0553	Antidepressant
MYLAN3125	Cap	Doxepin HCl	by Pharmedix	53002-0490	Antidepressant
MYLAN3125	Cap	Doxepin HCl	by Major	00904-1261	Antidepressant
MYLAN3125	Cap, Ivory & White, Mylan over 3125	Doxepin HCl 25 mg	Sinequan by UDL	51079-0437	Antidepressant
MYLAN3125	Cap, Ivory & White, Mylan over 3125	Doxepin HCl 25 mg	by Mylan	00378-3125	Antidepressant
MYLAN3125	Cap	Doxepin HCl 25 mg	by Allscripts	54569-2179	Antidepressant
MYLAN3125	Cap, Ivory & Yellow	Doxepin HCl 25 mg	by H J Harkins Co	52959-0280	Antidepressant
MYLAN3205	Cap, Light Blue & Light Brown, Mylan over 3205 in White Ink	Prazosin HCl 5 mg	by Mylan	00378-3205	Antihypertensive

ID FRONT <> BACK	DESCRIPTION FRONT <> BACK	INGREDIENT & STRENGTH	BRAND (OR EQUIV.) & FIRM	NDC#	CLASS; SCH.
MYLAN3205	Cap, Brown	Prazosin HCl 5 mg	by Allscripts	54569-2584	Antihypertensive
MYLAN3205	Cap, Light Blue & Light Brown, Mylan over 3205	Prazosin HCl 5 mg	Minipress by UDL	51079-0632	Antihypertensive
MYLAN3205	Cap, Blue & Brown	Prazosin HCl	by Caremark	00339-6069	Antihypertensive
MYLAN3205	Cap	Prazosin HCl	by Med Pro	53978-2047	Antihypertensive
MYLAN3205	Cap	Prazosin HCl	by Kaiser	62224-0111	Antihypertensive
MYLAN3250	Cap, Swedish Orange & Yellow, Imprint in White Ink	Nortriptyline HCl 50 mg	by Mylan	00378-3250	Antidepressant
MYLAN3250	Cap, Orange & Yellow, Opaque, Mylan over 3250	Nortriptyline HCl 50 mg	Pamelar by UDL	51079-0805	Antidepressant
MYLAN3250	Cap, Orange & Yellow	Nortriptyline HCl 50 mg	by Dixon Shane	17236-0006	Antidepressant
MYLAN327	Tab	Haloperidol 5 mg	by Heartland	61392-0272	Antipsychotic
MYLAN327	Tab, Orange, Mylan over 327	Haloperidol 5 mg	by Mylan	00378-0327	Antipsychotic
MYLAN327	Tab	Haloperidol 5 mg	by Vangard	00615-2597	Antipsychotic
MYLAN327	Tab	Haloperidol 5 mg	by Murfreesboro	51129-1244	Antipsychotic
MYLAN330	Tab, White, Round	Perphenazine 2 mg; Amitriptyline HCl 10 mg	by Direct Dispensing	57866-3077	Antipsychotic; Antidepressant
MYLAN345	Tab, Orange, Round, Scored	Diazepam 5 mg	by DRX	55045-2666	Antianxiety; C IV
MYLAN345	Tab, Orange, Round, Scored	Diazepam 5 mg	by Allscripts	54569-0949	Antianxiety; C IV
MYLAN345	Tab, Orange, Round, Scored	Diazepam 5 mg	by HJ Harkins	52959-0047	Antianxiety; C IV
MYLAN345	Tab, Orange, Round, Scored, Mylan over 345	Diazepam 5 mg	Valium by UDL	51079-0285	Antianxiety; C IV
MYLAN345	Tab, Orange, Mylan over 345	Diazepam 5 mg	by Mylan	00378-0345	Antianxiety; C IV
MYLAN347	Tab, White, Mylan over 347	Hydrochlorothiazide 25 mg, Propranolol HCl 80 mg	by Mylan	00378-0347	Diuretic; Antihypertensive
MYLAN351	Tab	Haloperidol 0.5 mg	by Heartland	61392-0263	Antipsychotic
MYLAN351	Tab, Orange, Mylan over 351	Haloperidol 0.5 mg	by Mylan	00378-0351	Antipsychotic
MYLAN370	Tab, Mylan/370	Bumetanide 1 mg	by Heartland	61392-0049	Diuretic
MYLAN370	Tab	Bumetanide 1 mg	by Hoffmann La Roche	00004-0291	Diuretic
MYLAN370	Tab	Bumetanide 1 mg	by Caremark	00339-6030	Diuretic
MYLAN377	Tab, Green, Round, Scored	Diazepam 10 mg	by Allscripts	54569-0936	Antianxiety; C IV
MYLAN4010	Cap, Peach, Mylan over 4010 in Black Ink	Temazepam 15 mg	Tem by Mylan	00378-4010	Sedative/Hypnotic; C IV
MYLAN4010	Cap, Peach, Mylan over 4010	Temazepam 15 mg	Restoril by UDL	51079-0418	Sedative/Hypnotic; C IV
MYLAN4010	Cap, Peach	Temazepam 15 mg	by St. Marys Med	60760-0607	Sedative/Hypnotic; C IV
MYLAN4010	Cap	Temazepam 15 mg	Tem by Vangard	00615-0470	Sedative/Hypnotic; C IV
MYLAN4010	Cap, Peach	Temazepam 15 mg	by Direct Dispensing	57866-4628	Sedative/Hypnotic; C IV
MYLAN4070	Cap, Light Celery	Ketoprofen 50 mg	Ketoprofen by Mylan	00378-4070	NSAID
MYLAN41	Tab, Mylan over 41	Hydrochlorothiazide 25 mg, Spironolactone 25 mg	by Mylan	00378-0141	Diuretic; Antihypertensive
MYLAN415	Tab, White, Round	Diphenoxylate HCl 2.5 mg, Atropine Sulfate 0.025 mg	Lomotil by Mylan		Antidiarrheal; C V
MYLAN417	Tab, Mylan/417	Bumetanide 2 mg	by Heartland	61392-0050	Diuretic
MYLAN417	Cap	Bumetanide 2 mg	by Caremark	00339-6031	Diuretic
MYLAN4175	Cap	Nortriptyline HCl	by Medirex	57480-0826	Antidepressant
MYLAN4175	Cap, Brown & Swedish Orange	Nortriptyline HCl 75 mg	by Mylan	00378-4175	Antidepressant
MYLAN4175	Cap, Brown & Orange	Nortriptyline HCl 75 mg	by Dixon Shane	17236-0007	Antidepressant
MYLAN4250	Cap	Doxepin HCl	by Quality Care	60346-0269	Antidepressant
MYLAN4250	Cap, Ivory, Mylan over 4250	Doxepin HCl 50 mg	Sinequan by UDL	51079-0438	Antidepressant
MYLAN4250	Cap, Ivory, Black Print	Doxepin HCl 50 mg	by Mylan	00378-4250	Antidepressant
MYLAN4415	Cap, Powder Blue & White, Mylan over 4415	Flurazepam HCl 15 mg	by Mylan	00378-4415	Hypnotic; C IV
MYLAN4415	Cap, Powder Blue, Mylan over 4415	Flurazepam HCl 15 mg	by Quality Care	60346-0239	Hypnotic; C IV
MYLAN4415	Cap, Powder Blue & White, Opaque, Mylan over 4415	Flurazepam HCl 15 mg	Dalmane by UDL	51079-0302	Hypnotic; C IV
MYLAN4415	Tab, Blue & White, Oblong	Flurazepam HCl 15 mg	by Southwood Pharms	58016-0811	Hypnotic; C IV
MYLAN4430	Cap, Powder Blue	Flurazepam HCl 30 mg	by Quality Care	60346-0762	Hypnotic; C IV
MYLAN4430	Cap, Powder Blue, Opaque, Mylan over 4430	Flurazepam HCl 30 mg	Dalmane by UDL	51079-0303	Hypnotic; C IV
MYLAN4430	Cap, Powder Blue, Mylan over 4430	Flurazepam HCl 30 mg	by Mylan	00378-4430	Hypnotic; C IV
MYLAN4430	Cap	Flurazepam HCl 30 mg	by Allscripts	54569-0898	Hypnotic; C IV

ID FRONT <> BACK	DESCRIPTION FRONT <> BACK	INGREDIENT & STRENGTH	BRAND (OR EQUIV.) & FIRM	NDC#	CLASS; SCH.
MYLAN4430	Tab, Blue, Oblong	Flurazepam HCl 30 mg	by Southwood Pharms	58016-0812	Hypnotic; C IV
MYLAN451	Tab	Naproxen 500 mg	by Med Pro	53978-2083	NSAID
MYLAN457	Tab, White, Round, Scored	Lorazepam 1 mg	by Nat Pharmpak Serv	55154-2418	Sedative/Hypnotic; C IV
MYLAN457	Tab	Lorazepam 1 mg	by Allscripts	54569-1585	Sedative/Hypnotic; C IV
MYLAN457	Tab, White, Round, Scored	Lorazepam 1 mg	by Nat Pharmpak Serv	55154-1609	Sedative/Hypnotic; C IV
MYLAN457	Tab	Lorazepam 1 mg	by PDRX	55289-0487	Sedative/Hypnotic; C IV
MYLAN457	Tab, White	Lorazepam 1 mg	by Nat Pharmpak Serv	55154-0250	Sedative/Hypnotic; C IV
MYLAN457	Tab	Lorazepam 1 mg	by Quality Care	60346-0047	Sedative/Hypnotic; C IV
MYLAN457	Tab, White, Round, Scored	Lorazepam 1 mg	by Murfreesboro Ph	51129-1401	Sedative/Hypnotic; C IV
MYLAN457	Tab, White, Round, Scored, Mylan over 457	Lorazepam 1 mg	Ativan by UDL	51079-0386	Sedative/Hypnotic; C IV
MYLAN457	Tab, White, Beveled Edge, Mylan over 457	Lorazepam 1 mg	by Mylan	00378-0457	Sedative/Hypnotic; C IV
MYLAN457	Tab	Lorazepam 1 mg	by Caremark	00339-4020	Sedative/Hypnotic; C IV
MYLAN4700	Tab, Mylan over 4700	Gemfibrozil 300 mg	by Mylan	00378-4700	Antihyperlipidemic
MYLAN477	Tab, Mylan over 477	Diazepam 10 mg	by Pharm Serv Ctr	00855-3243	Antianxiety; C IV
MYLAN477	Tab, Green, Round, Scored, Mylan over 477	Diazepam 10 mg	Valium by UDL	51079-0286	Antianxiety; C IV
MYLAN477	Tab, Green, Mylan over 477	Diazepam 10 mg	by Mylan	00378-0477	Antianxiety; C IV
MYLAN5010	Cap, Caramel	Thiothixene 10 mg	by Med Pro	53978-2002	Antipsychotic
MYLAN5010	Cap, Light Orange, Mylan over 5010	Thiothixene 10 mg	by Quality Care	60346-0843	Antipsychotic
MYLAN5010	Cap, Caramel	Thiothixene 10 mg	by Dixon Shane	17236-0468	Antipsychotic
MYLAN5010	Cap, Caramel & Peach, Mylan over 5010	Thiothixene 10 mg	Navane by UDL	51079-0589	Antipsychotic
MYLAN5010	Cap, Caramel, Mylan over 5010	Thiothixene 10 mg	by Mylan	00378-5010	Antipsychotic
MYLAN5050	Cap, Yellow	Temazepam 30 mg	by HJ Harkins	52959-0459	Sedative/Hypnotic; C IV
MYLAN5050	Cap, Yellow, Mylan over 5050	Temazepam 30 mg	Restoril by UDL	51079-0419	Sedative/Hypnotic; C IV
MYLAN5050	Cap, Yellow, Mylan over 5050 Black Ink	Temazepam 30 mg	Tem by Mylan	00378-5050	Sedative/Hypnotic; C IV
MYLAN5050	Cap, Yellow	Temazepam 30 mg	by St. Marys Med	60760-0618	Sedative/Hypnotic; C IV
MYLAN5050	Cap	Temazepam 30 mg	Tem by Quality Care	60346-0005	Sedative/Hypnotic; C IV
MYLAN5050	Cap, Yellow	Temazepam 30 mg	by Direct Dispensing	57866-4629	Sedative/Hypnotic; C IV
MYLAN5050	Cap	Temazepam 30 mg	Tem by Vangard	00615-0471	Sedative/Hypnotic; C IV
MYLAN512	Tab, White, Round, Scored, Film-Coated, Mylan over 512	Verapamil HCl 80 mg	Calan/Isoptin by UDL	51079-0682	Antihypertensive
MYLAN512	Tab, White, Beveled Edge, Coated, Mylan over 512	Verapamil HCl 80 mg	by Mylan	00378-0512	Antihypertensive
MYLAN512	Tab, Coated, Debossed	Verapamil HCl 80 mg	by Allscripts	54569-0639	Antihypertensive
MYLAN512	Tab, White, Round, Scored, Film	Verapamil HCl 80 mg	by Thrift Drug	59198-0317	Antihypertensive
MYLAN517	Tab, White, Oval	Gemfibrozil 600 mg	Lopid by Mylan		Antihyperlipidemic
MYLAN5200	Cap, Light Blue, Mylan over 5200 in Black Ink	Tolmetin Sodium 492 mg	by Mylan	00378-5200	NSAID
MYLAN5200	Cap, Mylan over 5200	Tolmetin Sodium 492 mg	by Quality Care	60346-0615	NSAID
MYLAN5220	Cap, Flesh & Pink, Opaque, Mylan over 5220	Diltiazem HCl 120 mg	Dilacor XR by UDL	51079-0947	Antihypertensive
MYLAN5220	Cap, Flesh & Light Pink, Mylan over 5220	Diltiazem HCl 120 mg	by Mylan	00378-5220	Antihypertensive
MYLAN5280	Cap, Flesh & Lavender, Opaque, Mylan over 5280	Diltiazem HCl 180 mg	Dilacor XR by UDL	51079-0948	Antihypertensive
MYLAN5280	Cap, Beige & Purple	Diltiazem HCl 180 mg	by Phy Total Care	54868-4186	Antihypertensive
MYLAN5280	Cap, Beige & Purple	Diltiazem HCl 180 mg	by Murfreesboro Ph	51129-1681	Antihypertensive
MYLAN5280	Cap, Flesh & Lavender, Mylan over 5280	Diltiazem HCl 180 mg	by Mylan	00378-5280	Antihypertensive
MYLAN531	Tab, Yellow-Orange, Round, Scored, Mylan over 531	Sulindac 200 mg	Clinoril by UDL	51079-0667	NSAID
MYLAN531	Tab, Yellowish Orange, Mylan over 531	Sulindac 200 mg	by Mylan	00378-0531	NSAID
MYLAN5340	Cap, Blue	Diltiazem HCl 240 mg	by Phy Total Care	54868-4184	Antihypertensive
MYLAN5340	Cap, Flesh & Light Blue, Opaque, Mylan over 5340	Diltiazem HCl 240 mg	Dilacor XR by UDL	51079-0949	Antihypertensive
MYLAN5340	Cap, Flesh & Light Blue, Mylan over 5340	Diltiazem HCl 240 mg	by Mylan	00378-5340	Antihypertensive
MYLAN5340	Tab, Blue & Tan, Oblong	Diltiazem HCl 240 mg	by Egis	48581-6122	Antihypertensive
MYLAN5375	Cap, Bright Green & Bright Light Green, Black Print	Doxepin HCl 75 mg	by Mylan	00378-5375	Antidepressant
MYLAN5375	Cap, Light Green, Mylan over 5375	Doxepin HCl 75 mg	Sinequan by UDL	51079-0645	Antidepressant
MYLAN5375	Cap	Doxepin HCl 75 mg	by Major	00904-1263	Antidepressant
MYLAN551	Tab, White, Mylan over 551	Tolazamide 500 mg	by Mylan	00378-0551	Antidiabetic
MYLAN574	Tab, Film Coated	Amitriptyline HCl 25 mg, Perphenazine 4 mg	by PDRX	55289-0185	Antipsychotic

ID FRONT <> BACK	DESCRIPTION FRONT <> BACK	INGREDIENT & STRENGTH	BRAND (OR EQUIV.) & FIRM	NDC#	CLASS; SCH.
MYLAN5750	Cap, Light Aqua	Ketoprofen 75 mg	Ketoprofen by Mylan	00378-5750	NSAID
MYLAN5750	Cap, Aqua	Ketoprofen 75 mg	by Murfreesboro Ph	51129-1382	NSAID
MYLAN5750	Cap, Blue	Ketoprofen 75 mg	by Direct Dispensing	57866-4639	NSAID
MYLAN6025	Cap, Dark Blue & White, Coated, Mylan over 6025	Cephalexin Monohydrate 250 mg	by Mylan	00378-6025	Antibiotic
MYLAN6050	Cap, Dark Blue & Light Blue, Coated, Mylan over 6050	Cephalexin Monohydrate 500 mg	by Mylan	00378-6050	Antibiotic
MYLAN6060	Cap, Coral & Ivory, Mylan over 6060	Diltiazem HCl 60 mg	by Mylan	00378-6060	Antihypertensive
MYLAN6060	Cap, Coral & White, Opaque, Mylan over 6060	Diltiazem HCl 60 mg	by UDL	51079-0924	Antihypertensive
MYLAN6060	Cap, Pink & White, Opaque, Mylan over 6060	Diltiazem HCl 60 mg	by Egis	48581-6121	Antihypertensive
MYLAN6090	Cap, Coral & Ivory, Opaque, Mylan over 6090	Diltiazem HCl 90 mg	by UDL	51079-0925	Antihypertensive
MYLAN6090	Cap, Pink & White	Diltiazem HCl 90 mg	by Murfreesboro Ph	51129-1365	Antihypertensive
MYLAN6090	Cap, Coral & Ivory, Mylan over 6090	Diltiazem HCl 90 mg	by Mylan	00378-6090	Antihypertensive
MYLAN611	Tab, Film Coated	Methyldopa 250 mg	by Heartland	61392-0184	Antihypertensive
MYLAN6120	Cap, Coral, Mylan over 6120	Diltiazem HCl 120 mg	by Mylan	00378-6120	Antihypertensive
MYLAN6120	Cap, Coral, Opaque, Mylan over 6120	Diltiazem HCl 120 mg	by UDL	51079-0926	Antihypertensive
MYLAN6120	Cap, Orange, Mylan over 6120	Diltiazem HCl 120 mg	by Eisai	62856-0243	Antihypertensive
MYLAN6120	Cap, Coral, Mylan over 6120	Diltiazem HCl 120 mg	by Mylan	00378-6120	Antihypertensive
MYLAN62	Tab	Glipizide 10 mg	by Med Pro	53978-2014	Antidiabetic
MYLAN6320	Cap, Bluish Green & White	Verapamil HCl 120 mg	by Mylan		Antihypertensive
MYLAN6320	Cap, Bluish Green & White, Opaque, Mylan over 6320	Verapamil HCl ER 120 mg	Verelan by UDL	51079-0917	Antihypertensive
MYLAN6380	Cap, Bluish Green & Light Green	Verapamil HCl 180 mg	by Mylan		Antihypertensive
MYLAN6380	Cap, Bluish Green & Light Green, Opaque, Mylan over 6380	Verapamil HCl ER 180 mg	Verelan by UDL	51079-0918	Antihypertensive
MYLAN6410	Cap	Doxepin HCl	by Major	00904-1264	Antidepressant
MYLAN6410	Cap, Bright Light Green & White, Black Print	Doxepin HCl 100 mg	by Mylan	00378-6410	Antidepressant
MYLAN6410	Cap, Light Green & White, Mylan over 6410	Doxepin HCl 100 mg	Sinequan by UDL	51079-0651	Antidepressant
MYLAN6440	Cap, Bluish Green	Verapamil HCl 240 mg	by Mylan		Antihypertensive
MYLAN6440	Cap, Bluish Green, Opaque	Verapamil HCl ER 240 mg	Verelan by UDL	51079-0919	Antihypertensive
MYLAN7200	Cap, Brown, Mylan over 7200	Etodolac 200 mg	by Mylan	00378-7200	NSAID
MYLAN7200	Cap	Etodolac 200 mg	by Murfreesboro	51129-1274	NSAID
MYLAN7233	Cap, Brown	Etodolac 300 mg	by DRX Pharm Consults	55045-2592	NSAID
MYLAN7233	Cap, Light Brown, Mylan over 7233	Etodolac 300 mg	by Mylan	00378-7233	NSAID
MYLAN7233	Cap, Brown	Etodolac 300 mg	by HJ Harkins	52959-0483	NSAID
MYLAN7233	Cap, MYLAN over 7233	Etodolac 300 mg	by Allscripts	54569-4545	NSAID
MYLAN7250	Cap, Mylan 7250	Cefaclor Monohydrate	by Qualitest	00603-2586	Antibiotic
MYLAN7250	Cap, Pink & White	Cefaclor Monohydrate 250 mg	by Mylan	00378-7250	Antibiotic
MYLAN7250	Cap	Cefaclor Monohydrate 250 mg	by Quality Care	60346-0202	Antibiotic
MYLAN73	Tab, Coated	Amitriptyline HCl 50 mg, Perphenazine 4 mg	by Med Pro	53978-2010	Antipsychotic
MYLAN731	Tab, White, Mylan over 731	Hydrochlorothiazide 25 mg, Propranolol HCl 40 mg	by Mylan	00378-0731	Diuretic; Antihypertensive
MYLAN7500	Cap, Mylan 7500	Cefaclor Monohydrate	by Qualitest	00603-2587	Antibiotic
MYLAN7500	Cap, Gray & Pink	Cefaclor Monohydrate 500 mg	by Mylan	00378-7500	Antibiotic
MYLAN7500	Cap	Cefaclor Monohydrate	by Quality Care	62682-1023	Antibiotic
MYLAN7500	Cap, Gray & Pink	Cefaclor Monohydrate 500 mg	Cefaclor by Compumed	00403-0038	Antibiotic
MYLAN772	Tab, White, Round, Film Coated, Mylan over 772	Verapamil HCl 120 mg	Calan/Isotin by UDL	51079-0683	Antihypertensive
MYLAN772	Tab, Film Coated	Verapamil HCl 120 mg	by Allscripts	54569-0646	Antihypertensive
MYLAN772	Tab, White, Beveled Edge, Film Coated, Mylan over 772	Verapamil HCl 120 mg	by Mylan	00378-0772	Antihypertensive
MYLAN777	Tab, White, Round, Scored, Mylan over 777	Lorazepam 2 mg	Ativan by UDL	51079-0387	Sedative/Hypnotic; C IV
MYLAN777	Tab	Lorazepam 2 mg	by Caremark	00339-4022	Sedative/Hypnotic; C IV
MYLAN777	Tab, White, Beveled Edge, Mylan over 777	Lorazepam 2 mg	by Mylan	00378-0777	Sedative/Hypnotic; C IV
MYLAN777	Tab	Lorazepam 2 mg	by Allscripts	54569-2173	Sedative/Hypnotic; C IV
MYLAN777	Tab, White, Round, Flat, Scored, Mylan over 777	Lorazepam 2 mg	by Nat Pharmpak Serv	55154-0913	Sedative/Hypnotic; C IV
MYLAN777	Tab	Lorazepam 2 mg	by Quality Care	60346-0800	Sedative/Hypnotic; C IV
MYLAN777	Tab, White, Round, Scored	Lorazepam 2 mg	by Compumed	00403-0012	Sedative/Hypnotic; C IV

ID FRONT <> BACK	DESCRIPTION FRONT <> BACK	INGREDIENT & STRENGTH	BRAND (OR EQUIV.) & FIRM	NDC#	CLASS; SCH.
MYLANA	Tab, Coated, Mylan over A	Alprazolam 0.25 mg	by Quality Care	60346-0876	Antianxiety; C IV
MYLANA	Tab, White, Round, Scored, Mylan over A	Alprazolam 0.25 mg	Zanax by UDL	51079-0788	Antianxiety; C IV
MYLANA	Tab, White, Round	Alprazolam 0.25 mg	Xanax by Mylan		Antianxiety; C IV
MYLANA	Tab, Mylan over A	Alprazolam 0.25 mg	by Kaiser	00179-1183	Antianxiety; C IV
MYLANA	Tab, Mylan over A	Alprazolam 0.25 mg	by Mylan	00378-4001	Antianxiety; C IV
MYLANA	Tab, Mylan over A	Alprazolam 0.25 mg	by Allscripts	54569-3755	Antianxiety; C IV
MYLANA	Tab, White, Round, Scored	Alprazolam 0.25 mg	by Apotheca	12634-0533	Antianxiety; C IV
MYLANA1	Tab, Blue, Oval	Alprazolam 1 mg	by Compumed	00403-4578	Antianxiety; C IV
MYLANA1	Tab, Mylan over A1	Alprazolam 1 mg	by PDRX	55289-0920	Antianxiety; C IV
MYLANA1	Tab, Blue, Round, Scored, Mylan over A1	Alprazolam 1 mg	Zanax by UDL	51079-0790	Antianxiety; C IV
MYLANA1	Tab, Blue	Alprazolam 1 mg	by Mylan		Antianxiety; C IV
MYLANA1	Tab, Light Blue, Mylan over A1	Alprazolam 1 mg	by Kaiser	00179-1185	Antianxiety; C IV
MYLANA1	Tab, Mylan over A1	Alprazolam 1 mg	by Mylan	00378-4005	Antianxiety; C IV
MYLANA3	Tab, Mylan over A3	Alprazolam 0.5 mg	by PDRX	55289-0945	Antianxiety; C IV
MYLANA3	Tab, Peach	Alprazolam 0.5 mg	by Mylan		Antianxiety; C IV
MYLANA3	Tab, Mylan over A3	Alprazolam 0.5 mg	by Kaiser	00179-1184	Antianxiety; C IV
MYLANA3	Tab, Mylan over A3	Alprazolam 0.5 mg	by Mylan	00378-4003	Antianxiety; C IV
MYLANA3	Tab, Mylan over A3	Alprazolam 0.5 mg	by Allscripts	54569-3756	Antianxiety; C IV
MYLANA3	Tab	Alprazolam 0.5 mg	by Murfreesboro	51129-1200	Antianxiety; C IV
MYLANA3	Tab, Peach, Round, Scored	Alprazolam 0.5 mg	by Apotheca	12634-0525	Antianxiety; C IV
MYLANA3	Tab, Peach, Round, Scored, Mylan over A3	Alprazolam 0.5 mg	Zanax by UDL	51079-0789	Antianxiety; C IV
MYLANA4	Tab, White	Alprazolam 2 mg	by Mylan		Antianxiety; C IV
MYLANA4	Tab, Mylan over A4	Alprazolam 2 mg	by Mylan	00378-4007	Antianxiety; C IV
MYLAND <> 237	Tab, White, Oval, Film Coated	Etodolac 400 mg	by Allscripts	54569-4468	NSAID
MYLAND327	Tab, Orange, Round, Scored	Haloperidol 5 mg	by Allscripts	54569-2883	Antipsychotic
MYLANG1	Tab, Mylan/61	Glipizide 5 mg	by Kaiser	00179-1207	Antidiabetic
MYLANG1	Tab, Mylan over G1	Glipizide 5 mg	by Mylan	00378-1105	Antidiabetic
MYLANG1	Tab	Glipizide 5 mg	by Med Pro	53978-2013	Antidiabetic
MYLANG1	Tab	Glipizide 5 mg	by Allscripts	54569-3841	Antidiabetic
MYLANG1	Tab, White, Round, Scored, Mylan over G1	Glipizide 5 mg	Glucotrol by UDL	51079-0810	Antidiabetic
MYLANG1	Tab, Mylan over G1	Glipizide 5 mg	by Nat Pharmpak Serv	55154-5224	Antidiabetic
MYLANG1	Tab, White, Round, Scored	Glipizide 5 mg	by Compumed	00403-0920	Antidiabetic
MYLANG1	Tab, White, Round, Scored	Glipizide 5 mg	by Dixon Shane	17236-0441	Antidiabetic
MYLANG1	Tab, White, Round	Glipizide 5 mg	by Mylan	55160-0122	Antidiabetic
MYLANG1	Tab, Mylan over G1	Glipizide 5 mg	by Heartland	61392-0063	Antidiabetic
MYLANG2	Tab, Mylan over G2	Glipizide 10 mg	by Heartland	61392-0064	Antidiabetic
MYLANG2	Tab, Mylan over G2	Glipizide 10 mg	by Quality Care	62682-5004	Antidiabetic
MYLANG2	Tab, Mylan/62	Glipizide 10 mg	by Kaiser	00179-1208	Antidiabetic
MYLANG2	Tab, White, Round	Glipizide 10 mg	Glucotrol by Mylan	00378-1110	Antidiabetic
MYLANG2	Tab	Glipizide 10 mg	by Allscripts	54569-3842	Antidiabetic
MYLANG2	Tab, White, Round, Scored, Mylan over G2	Glipizide 10 mg	Glucotrol by UDL	51079-0811	Antidiabetic
MYLANG2	Tab, White, Round, Scored	Glipizide 10 mg	by Dixon Shane	17236-0442	Antidiabetic
MYLANTM1	Tab, Green, Round	Triamterene 37.5 mg, Hydrochlorothiazide 25 mg	Maxzide 25 by Mylan		Diuretic
MYLANTM2	Tab, Yellow, Round	Triamterene 75 mg, Hydrochlorothiazide 50 mg	Maxzide by Mylan		Diuretic
MYLERAN <> K2A	Tab	Busulfan 2 mg	Myleran by Catalytica	63552-0713	Antineoplastic
MYLERAN K2A	Tab, White, Biconvex	Busulfan 2 mg	by Glaxo	Canadian	Antineoplastic
MYOGESIC	Tab, Green	Magnesium Salicylate 600 mg; Phenyltoloxamine Citrate 25 mg	Myogesic by A J Bart	49326-0182	NSAID; Antihistamine
MYSOLINE250	Tab, Yellow, Square, Scored	Primidone 250 mg	Mysoline by Rightpak	65240-0697	Anticonvulsant
MYSOLINE250	Tab	Primidone 250 mg	Mysoline by Leiner	59606-0697	Anticonvulsant
MYSOLINE250 <> M	Tab	Primidone 250 mg	Mysoline by Wal Mart	49035-0169	Anticonvulsant
MYSOLINE250 <> M	Tab	Primidone 250 mg	Mysoline by Murfreesboro	51129-1168	Anticonvulsant

ID FRONT <> BACK	DESCRIPTION FRONT <> BACK	INGREDIENT & STRENGTH	BRAND (OR EQUIV.) & FIRM	NDC#	CLASS; SCH.
MYSOLINE250 <> M	Tab	Primidone 250 mg	Mysoline by Thrift Drug	59198-0181	Anticonvulsant
MYSOLINE50 <> M	Tab	Primidone 50 mg	Mysoline by Wal Mart	49035-0168	Anticonvulsant
N	Tab, White, Round	Aspirin 325 mg	by PG		Analgesic
N	Tab, White, Oval, Scored	Cimetidine 800 mg	by Novopharm (Ca)	43806-0305	Gastrointestinal
N	Tab, Blue	Diphenhydramine 50 mg	by Block Drug	Canadian	Antihistamine
N	Tab, White	Diphenhydramine 25 mg	by Block Drug	Canadian	Antihistamine
N	Tab, Cream, Round	Spironolactone 100 mg	Novo Spiroton by Novopharm	Canadian	Diuretic
N <> 125	Cap, Pink	Amoxicillin Trihydrate 250 mg	by Southwood Pharms	58016-0103	Antibiotic
N <> 15	Tab, White, Round	Codeine Phosphate 15 mg	by Altimed	Canadian DIN# 00779458	Analgesic
N <> 2	Cap	Loperamide HCl 2 mg	by Rugby	00536-3974	Antidiarrheal
N <> 2	Cap	Loperamide HCl 2 mg	by Mova	55370-0169	Antidiarrheal
N <> 2	Cap, White	Loperamide HCl 2 mg	by Novopharm	55953-0020	Antidiarrheal
N <> 2	Cap	Loperamide HCl 2 mg	by HL Moore	00839-7623	Antidiarrheal
N <> 20	Cap	Piroxicam 20 mg	by Prescription Dispensing	61807-0039	NSAID
N <> 200	Cap, Blue, Convex	Acyclovir 200 mg	by Amerisource	62584-0707	Antiviral
N <> 500	Cap, Brown	Amoxicillin 500 mg	by Natl Pharmpak	55154-1750	Antibiotic
N <> 500	Cap	Cephalexin Monohydrate 541 mg	by Prescription Dispensing	61807-0006	Antibiotic
N 25	Tab, Orange, Round	Dipyridamole 25 mg	Novo Dipiradol by Novopharm	Canadian	Antiplatelet
N 342 <> 125	Tab, N 342 <> 1.25	Glyburide 1.25 mg	by Warrick	59930-1592	Antidiabetic
N 50	Tab, Brown, Round	Dipyridamole 50 mg	Novo Dipiradol by Novopharm	Canadian	Antiplatelet
N 75	Tab, Orange, Round	Dipyridamole 75 mg	Novo Dipiradol by Novopharm	Canadian	Antiplatelet
N0172MG	Tab, Green, Oblong, N 017/2 mg	Loperamide 2 mg	Imodium by Novopharm		Antidiarrheal
N020 <> 2	Cap, Opaque White, N Over 020 <> 2	Loperamide HCl 2 mg	by Mylan	00378-3260	Antidiarrheal
N020 <> 2	Cap, N Over 020 <> 2	Loperamide HCl 2 mg	by Allscripts	54569-3707	Antidiarrheal
N020 <> 2	Cap, N Over 020 <> 2	Loperamide HCl 2 mg	by Martec	52555-0519	Antidiarrheal
N020 <> 2	Cap, Opaque White, 2 <> N Over 020	Loperamide HCl 2 mg	by Quality Care	60346-0046	Antidiarrheal
N020 <> 2	Cap, N Over 020	Loperamide HCl 2 mg	by Medirex	57480-0830	Antidiarrheal
N020 <> 2	Cap	Loperamide HCl 2 mg	by Heartland	61392-0336	Antidiarrheal
N020 <> 2	Cap, N Over 020 <> 2	Loperamide HCl 2 mg	by Amerisource	62584-0768	Antidiarrheal
N020 <> 2	Cap, N Over 020 <> 2	Loperamide HCl 2 mg	by Major	00904-7617	Antidiarrheal
N020 <> 2	Cap	Loperamide HCl 2 mg	by DHHS Prog	11819-0036	Antidiarrheal
N02705	Tab, Orange, Oval, Scored, N 027/0.5	Clonazepam 0.5 mg	by Novopharm	55953-0027	Anticonvulsant; C IV
N02705	Tab, Orange, Oval, N 027/0.5	Clonazepam 0.5 mg	by Novopharm	43806-0027	Anticonvulsant; C IV
N02810	Tab, Blue, Oval, Scored, N 028/1.0	Clonazepam 1.0 mg	by Novopharm	55953-0028	Anticonvulsant; C IV
N02810	Tab, Blue, Oval, N 028/1.0	Clonazepam 1.0 mg	by Novopharm	43806-0028	Anticonvulsant; C IV
N02920	Tab, White, Oval, Scored, N 029/2.0	Clonazepam 2 mg	by Novopharm	55953-0029	Anticonvulsant; C IV
N02920	Tab, White, Oval, N 029/2.0	Clonazepam 2 mg	by Novopharm	43806-0029	Anticonvulsant; C IV
N031 <> 25	Cap, Bright Yellow & Deep Orange, N over 031 <> 25	Clomipramine HCl 25 mg	by Novopharm	55953-0031	OCD
N031 <> 25	Cap, Bright Yellow & Deep Orange, N over 031 <> 25	Clomipramine HCl 25 mg	by Novopharm	43806-0031	OCD
N032 <> 50	Cap, Bright Yellow & Turquoise, N over 032 <> 50	Clomipramine HCl 50 mg	by Novopharm	55953-0032	OCD
N032 <> 50	Cap, Bright Yellow & Turquoise, N over 032 <> 50	Clomipramine HCl 50 mg	by Novopharm	43806-0032	OCD
N033 <> 75	Cap, Bright Yellow, N over 033 <> 75	Clomipramine HCl 75 mg	by Novopharm	55953-0033	OCD
N033 <> 75	Cap, Bright Yellow, N over 033 <> 75	Clomipramine HCl 75 mg	by Novopharm	43806-0033	OCD
N039 <> 50	Tab, N Over 039 and 50 On Opposing Sides	Atenolol 50 mg	by Quality Care	60346-0719	Antihypertensive
N039 <> 50	Tab, N over 039 <> 50	Atenolol 50 mg	by Medirex	57480-0446	Antihypertensive
N039 <> 50	Tab, White, Round, N over 039 <> 50	Atenolol 50 mg	by Novopharm	55953-0039	Antihypertensive
N039 <> 50	Tab, White, Round, Scored	Atenolol 50 mg	by Novopharm (US)	62528-0039	Antihypertensive
N039 <> 50	Tab, N over 039 <> 50	Atenolol 50 mg	by DRX	55045-1860	Antihypertensive
N039 <> 50	Tab, N over 039 <> 50	Atenolol 50 mg	by Apotheca	12634-0436	Antihypertensive
N03950	Tab	Atenolol 50 mg	by Qualitest	00603-2371	Antihypertensive

ID FRONT ⟷ BACK	DESCRIPTION FRONT ⟷ BACK	INGREDIENT & STRENGTH	BRAND (OR EQUIV.) & FIRM	NDC#	CLASS; SCH.
N03950	Tab	Atenolol 50 mg	by Med Pro	53978-1199	Antihypertensive
N084 ⟷ 250	Cap, N Over 084	Cephalexin Monohydrate	by St Marys Med	60760-0008	Antibiotic
N084 ⟷ 250	Cap, N over 084 ⟷ 250	Cephalexin Monohydrate	by HJ Harkins Co	52959-0030	Antibiotic
N084 ⟷ 250	Cap, N over 084 ⟷ 250	Cephalexin Monohydrate	by Apotheca	12634-0433	Antibiotic
N084 ⟷ 250	Cap, Gray & Swedish Orange, N over 084 ⟷ 250	Cephalexin Monohydrate	by Novopharm	43806-0084	Antibiotic
N084 ⟷ 250	Cap, Gray & Swedish Orange	Cephalexin Monohydrate 250 mg	by Novopharm	43806-0084	Antibiotic
N084250	Cap	Cephalexin Monohydrate	by United Res	00677-1158	Antibiotic
N084250 ⟷ 250	Cap, N Over 084 ⟷ Imprinted 250 on Body	Cephalexin Monohydrate	by Prescription Dispensing	61807-0005	Antibiotic
N084250 ⟷ N084250	Cap, Swedish Orange, N Over 084 and 250 ⟷ N Over 084 250	Cephalexin Monohydrate	by Quality Care	60346-0441	Antibiotic
N0885	Tab	Pindolol 5 mg	by Med Pro	53978-2046	Antihypertensive
N0885	Tab, White, Round, N088/5	Pindolol 5 mg	Visken by Novopharm	43806-0088	Antihypertensive
N093 ⟷ 10	Tab,	Pindolol 10 mg	by Med Pro	53978-2025	Antihypertensive
N09310	Tab, White, Round, N093/10	Pindolol 10 mg	Visken by Novopharm	43806-0093	Antihypertensive
N1	Tab, White, N/1	Acetaminophen 300 mg, Caffeine 15 mg, Codeine Phosphate 8 mg	Novo Gesic C8 by Novopharm	Canadian	Analgesic
N1	Tab	Ammonium Iodide 0.15 gr, Ammonium Tri-Iodide 0.35 gr	Iodide by Nadin	14836-1001	Cold Remedy
N1	Tab	Ammonium Iodide 0.15 gr, Ammonium Tri-Iodide 0.35 gr	Nadin by Vitaminerals	11359-0013	Cold Remedy
N1	Tab, White, Oblong	Lorazepam 1 mg	Novo Lorazem by Novopharm	Canadian	Sedative/Hypnotic
N10	Tab, Yellow, Round, N/10	Hydralazine HCl 10 mg	Novo Hylazin by Novopharm	Canadian	Antihypertensive
N10	Tab, Cream, Round, N/10	Maprotiline 10 mg	by Novopharm	Canadian	Antidepressant
N10	Cap, Brown, Soft Gel	Nifedipine 10 mg	by HJ Harkins	52959-0273	Antihypertensive
N10	Cap	Nifedipine 10 mg	by Med Pro	53978-1189	Antihypertensive
N10	Tab, White, Round, N/10	Tamoxifen Citrate 10 mg	Novo Tamoxifen by Novopharm	Canadian	Antiestrogen
N10 ⟷ N171	Cap, N/171	Nifedipine 10 mg	by Allscripts	54569-3121	Antihypertensive
N100	Tab, Blue, Oval, N/100	Flurbiprofen 100 mg	by Novopharm	Canadian	NSAID
N100	Tab, Light Blue, Oblong, N/100	Metoprolol Tartrate 100 mg	by Novopharm	Canadian	Antihypertensive
N100	Tab, White, Round, N/100	Metoprolol Tartrate 100 mg	by Novopharm	Canadian	Antihypertensive
N100	Cap, Yellow, N/100	Nitrofurantoin 100 mg	by Novopharm	Canadian	Antibiotic
N100	Tab, White, Round, N/100	Sulfinpyrazone 100 mg	Novo Pyrazone by Novopharm	Canadian	Uricosuric
N11 ⟷ LL	Tab, N Over 11	Naproxen 250 mg	by UDL	51079-0793	NSAID
N110	Tab, White, Barrel, N/110	Buspirone 10 mg	by Novopharm	Canadian	Antianxiety
N114 ⟷ 500	Cap, Orange	Cephalexin 500 mg	by Caremark	00339-6168	Antibiotic
N114 ⟷ 500	Cap	Cephalexin Monohydrate	by Quality Care	60346-0055	Antibiotic
N114 ⟷ 500	Cap, N over 114 ⟷ 500	Cephalexin Monohydrate	by Apotheca	12634-0434	Antibiotic
N114 ⟷ 500	Cap, Swedish Orange, N over 114 ⟷ 500	Cephalexin Monohydrate 541 mg	by Novopharm	55953-0114	Antibiotic
N114 ⟷ 500	Cap, N over 114 ⟷ 500	Cephalexin Monohydrate 541 mg	by HJ Harkins Co	52959-0031	Antibiotic
N114500	Tab, Coated	Cephalexin Monohydrate	by Med Pro	53978-5021	Antibiotic
N125 ⟷ 2	Tab, White, N over 125 ⟷ 2	Alprazolam 2 mg	by Novopharm	55953-8125	Antianxiety; C IV
N126 ⟷ 025	Tab, Coated, N Over 126 ⟷ 0.25	Alprazolam 0.25 mg	by Quality Care	60346-0876	Antianxiety; C IV
N126 ⟷ 025	Tab, N over 126 ⟷ 0.25	Alprazolam 0.25 mg	by PDRX	55289-0962	Antianxiety; C IV
N126 ⟷ 025	Tab, N over 126 ⟷ 0.25	Alprazolam 0.25 mg	by Medirex	57480-0520	Antianxiety; C IV
N126 ⟷ 025	Tab, White, Round, Scored, N over 126 ⟷ 0.25	Alprazolam 0.25 mg	by Novopharm	55953-8131	Antianxiety; C IV
N127 ⟷ 05	Tab, N over 127 ⟷ 0.5	Alprazolam 0.5 mg	by Medirex	57480-0521	Antianxiety; C IV
N127 ⟷ 05	Tab, N over 127 ⟷ 0.5	Alprazolam 0.5 mg	by HL Moore	00839-7852	Antianxiety; C IV
N127 ⟷ 05	Tab, Orange, Round, Scored, N over 127 ⟷ 0.5	Alprazolam 0.5 mg	by Novopharm	55953-8127	Antianxiety; C IV
N131 ⟷ 10	Tab, N over 131 ⟷ 1.0	Alprazolam 1 mg	by Medirex	57480-0522	Antianxiety; C IV
N131 ⟷ 10	Tab, Blue, Round, Scored, N over 131 ⟷ 1.0	Alprazolam 1 mg	by Novopharm	55953-0131	Antianxiety; C IV
N132 ⟷ 125	Tab, Scored, N over 132 ⟷ 12.5	Captopril 12.5 mg	by Medirex	57480-0838	Antihypertensive
N132 ⟷ 125	Tab, White, Oval, Scored, N over 132 ⟷ 12.5	Captopril 12.5 mg	by Novopharm	55953-0132	Antihypertensive
N132 ⟷ 125	Tab, Scored, N over 132 ⟷ 12.5	Captopril 12.5 mg	by Major	00904-5045	Antihypertensive
N132 ⟷ 125	Tab, White, Oval, Scored, N over 132 ⟷ 12.5	Captopril 12.5 mg	by Novopharm	43806-0132	Antihypertensive
N132125	Tab, White, Oval, N 132/12.5	Captopril 12.5 mg	Capoten by Novopharm	43806-0132	Antihypertensive
N133	Tab, Quadrisected, N over 133	Captopril 25 mg	by Medirex	57480-0839	Antihypertensive

ID FRONT ⟺ BACK	DESCRIPTION FRONT ⟺ BACK	INGREDIENT & STRENGTH	BRAND (OR EQUIV.) & FIRM	NDC#	CLASS; SCH.
N133	Tab	Captopril 25 mg	by Quality Care	60346-0778	Antihypertensive
N133	Tab, N over 133	Captopril 25 mg	by HL Moore	00839-7995	Antihypertensive
N133	Tab, N over 133	Captopril 25 mg	by Major	00904-5046	Antihypertensive
N134 ⟺ 50	Tab, White, Oblong, Scored	Captopril 50 mg	by Caremark	00339-5916	Antihypertensive
N134 ⟺ 50	Tab, Scored, N over 134	Captopril 50 mg	by HL Moore	00839-7996	Antihypertensive
N134 ⟺ 50	Tab, White, Oval, N over 134 ⟺ 50	Captopril 50 mg	by Novopharm	43806-0134	Antihypertensive
N134 ⟺ 50	Tab, N over 134 ⟺ 50	Captopril 50 mg	by Major	00904-5047	Antihypertensive
N134 ⟺ 50	Tab, Scored, N over 134 ⟺ 50	Captopril 50 mg	by Medirex	57480-0840	Antihypertensive
N134 ⟺ 50	Tab, White, Oval, N over 134 ⟺ 50	Captopril 50 mg	by Novopharm	55953-0134	Antihypertensive
N135 ⟺ 100	Tab, Scored, N over 135 ⟺ 100	Captopril 100 mg	by Medirex	57480-0841	Antihypertensive
N135 ⟺ 100	Tab, White, Oval, N over 135 ⟺ 100	Captopril 100 mg	by Novopharm	43806-0135	Antihypertensive
N135 ⟺ 100	Tab, N over 135 ⟺ 100	Captopril 100 mg	by Major	00904-5048	Antihypertensive
N144500 ⟺ L	Cap	Cephalexin Monohydrate 541 mg	by United Res	00677-1159	Antibiotic
N15	Tab, White	Codeine Phosphate 15 mg	by Rougier	Canadian	Analgesic
N150	Tab, Yellow, Hexagonal, N/150	Sulindac 150 mg	Novo Sundac by Novopharm	Canadian	NSAID
N15034	Tab, White, Oval, N/1.5-034	Glyburide 1.5 mg	by Novopharm	43806-0034	Antidiabetic
N15034	Tab, White, Oval, Scored, N/1.5-034	Glyburide Micronized 1.5 mg	by Novopharm	55953-0034	Antidiabetic
N160	Tab, White, Oval, N/160	Trimethoprim 160 mg, Sulfamethoxazole 800 mg	by Novopharm	Canadian	Antibiotic
N17 ⟺ LL	Tab	Naproxen 375 mg	by Physicians Total Care	54868-2965	NSAID
N17 ⟺ LL	Tab, Lavender	Naproxen 375 mg	by UDL	51079-0794	NSAID
N171 ⟺ 10	Cap	Nifedipine 10 mg	by HL Moore	00839-7564	Antihypertensive
N171 ⟺ 10	Cap, Soft Gelatin, N Over 171 ⟺ 10	Nifedipine 10 mg	by Quality Care	60346-0803	Antihypertensive
N171 ⟺ 10	Cap	Nifedipine 10 mg	by Warrick	59930-1618	Antihypertensive
N171 ⟺ 10	Cap, Brown, N Over 171 ⟺ 10	Nifedipine 10 mg	by Novopharm	55953-0171	Antihypertensive
N171 ⟺ N10	Cap, N/171	Nifedipine 10 mg	by Allscripts	54569-3121	Antihypertensive
N17110	Cap, N Over 171 10	Nifedipine 10 mg	by PDRX	55289-0907	Antihypertensive
N179 ⟺ 5	Tab, N Over 179	Selegiline HCl 5 mg	by Warrick	59930-1537	Antiparkinson
N179 ⟺ 5	Tab, White, Round, Beveled Edge, N Over 179 ⟺	Selegiline HCl 5 mg	by Novopharm	55953-0179	Antiparkinson
N179 ⟺ 5	Tab, White, Round, N Over 179	Selegiline HCl 5 mg	by Novopharm	43806-0179	Antiparkinson
N179 ⟺ 5	Tab	Selegiline HCl 5 mg	by Major	00904-5206	Antiparkinson
N181 ⟺ 200	Tab, Green, Oval, Film Coated	Cimetidine 200 mg	by Novopharm	55953-0181	Gastrointestinal
N181 ⟺ 200	Tab, Coated	Cimetidine 200 mg	by Brightstone	62939-2111	Gastrointestinal
N181 ⟺ 200	Tab, Film Coated, Engraved	Cimetidine 200 mg	by Darby Group	66467-3480	Gastrointestinal
N181 ⟺ 200	Tab, Coated	Cimetidine 200 mg	by United Res	00677-1527	Gastrointestinal
N181200	Tab, Film Coated	Cimetidine 200 mg	by Geneva	00781-1447	Gastrointestinal
N192 ⟺ 300	Tab, Film Coated	Cimetidine 300 mg	by Warrick	59930-1801	Gastrointestinal
N192 ⟺ 300	Tab, Light Green, Film Coated	Cimetidine 300 mg	by Quality Care	60346-0944	Gastrointestinal
N192 ⟺ 300	Tab, Film Coated	Cimetidine 300 mg	by Medirex	57480-0813	Gastrointestinal
N192 ⟺ 300	Tab, Dark Green, Oval, Film Coated	Cimetidine 300 mg	by Novopharm	55953-0192	Gastrointestinal
N192 ⟺ 300	Tab, Green, Oval, Film Coated	Cimetidine 300 mg	by Nat Pharmpak Serv	55154-9303	Gastrointestinal
N192 ⟺ 300	Tab, Coated, N/192	Cimetidine 300 mg	by Brightstone	62939-2121	Gastrointestinal
N192 ⟺ 300	Tab, Coated	Cimetidine 300 mg	by United Res	00677-1528	Gastrointestinal
N192 ⟺ 300	Tab, Film Coated	Cimetidine 300 mg	by DRX	55045-2272	Gastrointestinal
N192 ⟺ 300	Tab, Green, Oval, Film Coated	Cimetidine 300 mg	by Dixon Shane	17236-0171	Gastrointestinal
N192300	Tab, Film Coated	Cimetidine 300 mg	by Geneva	00781-1448	Gastrointestinal
N2	Tab, White, N/2	Acetaminophen 300 mg, Caffeine 15 mg, Codeine Phosphate 15 mg	Novo Gesic C15 by Novopharm	Canadian	Analgesic
N2	Tab	Ammonium Iodide 0.05 gr, Ammonium Tri-Iodide 0.117 gr	Nadin by Vitaminerals	11359-0014	Cold Remedy
N2	Tab	Ammonium Iodide 0.05 gr, Ammonium Tri-Iodide 0.117 gr	Iodide by Nadin	14836-1002	Cold Remedy
N2	Tab	Ammonium Iodide 0.15 gr, Ammonium Tri-Iodide 0.35 gr	Nadin by Nadin	14836-7001	Cold Remedy
N2	Tab, White, Oval	Lorazepam 2 mg	Novo Lorazem by Novopharm	Canadian	Sedative/Hypnotic
N2	Tab, Pink, Round	Salbutamol Sulfate 2 mg	Novo Salmol by Novopharm	Canadian	Antiasthmatic
N20	Tab, White, Round, N/20	Tamoxifen Citrate 20 mg	Novo Tamoxifen by Novopharm	Canadian	Antiestrogen

ID FRONT <> BACK	DESCRIPTION FRONT <> BACK	INGREDIENT & STRENGTH	BRAND (OR EQUIV.) & FIRM	NDC#	CLASS; SCH.
N20	Tab, Yellow, Oval, N/20	Tenoxicam 20 mg	Mobiflex by Roche	Canadian	NSAID
N200	Tab, Yellow, Hexagonal, N/200	Sulindac 200 mg	Novo Sundac by Novopharm	Canadian	NSAID
N200 <> 940	Cap, Blue, Opaque, N 200 over 940	Acyclovir 200 mg	by Novopharm	55953-0940	Antiviral
N200 <> N200	Cap, Blue, Opaque	Acyclovir 200 mg	by Novopharm	55953-8940	Antiviral
N200940	Cap, Blue, Opaque, N 200 over 940	Acyclovir 200 mg	by Novopharm	55953-0940	Antiviral
N204 <> 400	Tab, Film Coated, Scored	Cimetidine 400 mg	by Prescription Dispensing	61807-0066	Gastrointestinal
N204 <> 400	Tab, Film Coated, Scored	Cimetidine 400 mg	by Warrick	59930-1802	Gastrointestinal
N204 <> 400	Tab, Film Coated, Scored	Cimetidine 400 mg	by Medirex	57480-0814	Gastrointestinal
N204 <> 400	Tab, Green, Oval, Film Coated, Scored	Cimetidine 400 mg	by Novopharm	55953-0204	Gastrointestinal
N204 <> 400	Tab, Coated, N/204	Cimetidine 400 mg	by Brightstone	62939-2131	Gastrointestinal
N204 <> 400	Tab, Green, Oval, Film Coated	Cimetidine 400 mg	by Compumed	00403-1005	Gastrointestinal
N204 <> 400	Tab, Coated	Cimetidine 400 mg	by United Res	00677-1529	Gastrointestinal
N204400	Tab, Film Coated	Cimetidine 400 mg	by Geneva	00781-1449	Gastrointestinal
N21	Tab, White, Round	Nitrazepam 5 mg	by ICN	Canadian	Sedative/Hypnotic
N21 <> W	Tab, Light Buff, N/21	Nalidixic Acid 250 mg	Neggram by Sanofi	00024-1321	Antibiotic
N214 <> 200	Tab, Pink, Oval, Scored	Amiodarone HCl 200 mg	by Novopharm	55953-0214	Antiarrhythmic
N214200	Tab, Pink, Oval, N 214/200	Amiodarone 200 mg	by Novopharm	43806-0214	Antiarrhythmic
N22	Tab, White, Round	Nitrazepam 10 mg	by ICN	Canadian	Sedative/Hypnotic
N22 <> W	Tab, Light Buff, N/22	Nalidixic Acid 500 mg	Neggram by Sanofi	00024-1322	Antibiotic
N22W	Cap, Yellow, N/22/W	Nalidixic Acid 500 mg	by Sanofi	Canadian	Antibiotic
N23 <> W	Tab, Light Buff, N/23	Nalidixic Acid 1 gm	Neggram by Sanofi	00024-1323	Antibiotic
N235 <> 800	Tab, Film Coated, Scored	Cimetidine 800 mg	by Warrick	59930-1803	Gastrointestinal
N235 <> 800	Tab, Coated, N/235	Cimetidine 800 mg	by Brightstone	62939-2141	Gastrointestinal
N235 <> 800	Tab, Coated	Cimetidine 800 mg	by United Res	00677-1530	Gastrointestinal
N235800	Tab, Coated	Cimetidine 800 mg	Tagamet by Zenith Goldline	00182-1986	Gastrointestinal
N25	Tab, Blue, Round, N/25	Hydralazine HCl 25 mg	Novo Hylazin by Novopharm	Canadian	Antihypertensive
N25	Tab, Orange, Round, N/25	Maprotiline 25 mg	by Novopharm	Canadian	Antidepressant
N25	Tab, Pink, Round, N/250	Trimipramine Maleate 25 mg	Novo Tripramine by Novopharm	Canadian	Antidepressant
N250	Cap, Gray	Cephalexin Monohydrate 500 mg	by Southwood Pharms	58016-0139	Antibiotic
N250	Tab, White, N/250	Metronidazole 250 mg	Novo Nidazol by Novopharm	Canadian	Antibiotic
N250 <> N250	Cap, Gray	Cephalexin Monohydrate 250 mg	by Southwood Pharms	58016-0138	Antibiotic
N251 <> 500	Cap	Cefaclor Monohydrate	by Warrick	59930-1536	Antibiotic
N251 <> 500	Cap, N over 251 <> 500	Cefaclor Monohydrate	by Qualitest	00603-2587	Antibiotic
N251 <> 500	Cap	Cefaclor Monohydrate	by Rugby	00536-1375	Antibiotic
N251 <> 500	Cap, Gray & Light Orange, N over 251 <> 500	Cefaclor Monohydrate	by Novopharm	43806-0251	Antibiotic
N251 <> 500	Cap, N over 251 <> 500	Cefaclor Monohydrate	by Major	00904-5205	Antibiotic
N251 <> 500	Cap, Bright Orange & Gray, Opaque, N over 251 <> 500	Cefaclor Monohydrate 500 mg	Ceclor by UDL	51079-0618	Antibiotic
N251500 <> N251500	Cap, N over 251 500	Cefaclor Monohydrate	by Novopharm	55953-0251	Antibiotic
N253 <> 250	Cap	Cefaclor Monohydrate	by Novopharm	55953-0253	Antibiotic
N253 <> 250	Cap, N over 253 <> 250	Cefaclor Monohydrate	by Qualitest	00603-2586	Antibiotic
N253 <> 250	Cap	Cefaclor Monohydrate	by Rugby	00536-1365	Antibiotic
N253 <> 250	Cap, N over 253 <> 250	Cefaclor Monohydrate	by HJ Harkins Co	52959-0367	Antibiotic
N253 <> 250	Cap, Light Orange & White	Cefaclor Monohydrate	by Novopharm	43806-0253	Antibiotic
N253 <> 250	Cap, N over 253 <> 250	Cefaclor Monohydrate	by Major	00904-5204	Antibiotic
N253 <> 250	Cap, Bright Orange & White, Opaque, N over 253 <> 250	Cefaclor Monohydrate 250 mg	Ceclor by UDL	51079-0617	Antibiotic
N3	Tab, White, Round, N/3	Acetaminophen 300 mg, Caffeine 15 mg, Codeine Phosphate 30 mg	Novo Gesic C30 by Novopharm	Canadian	Analgesic
N30	Tab, White	Codeine Phosphate 30 mg	by Rougier	Canadian	Analgesic
N3035	Tab, Pale Blue, Oval, N/3-035	Glyburide 3 mg	by Novopharm	43806-0035	Antidiabetic
N3035	Tab, Pale Blue, Oval, Scored, N/3-035	Glyburide Micronized 3.0 mg	by Novopharm	55953-0035	Antidiabetic
N305800	Tab, White, Oval, Scored, N305/800	Cimetidine 800 mg	by Novopharm	55953-0305	Gastrointestinal
N325	Tab, White, Round	Aspirin 325 mg	by P&G		Analgesic
N3325	Tab, White, Round, N 133/25	Captopril 25 mg	Capoten by Novopharm	43806-0133	Antihypertensive

ID FRONT <> BACK	DESCRIPTION FRONT <> BACK	INGREDIENT & STRENGTH	BRAND (OR EQUIV.) & FIRM	NDC#	CLASS; SCH.
N342 <> 125	Tab, White, Round, N over 342 <> 1.25	Glyburide 1.25 mg	by Novopharm	55953-0342	Antidiabetic
N342 <> 125	Tab, N/342	Glyburide 1.25 mg	by Brightstone	62939-3211	Antidiabetic
N342 <> 125	Tab, N 342 <> 1.25	Glyburide 1.25 mg	by HL Moore	00839-8039	Antidiabetic
N342 <> 125	Tab, N over 342 <> 1.25	Glyburide 1.25 mg	by Qualitest	00603-3762	Antidiabetic
N342 <> 125	Tab, N over 342 <> 1.25	Glyburide 1.25 mg	by Zenith Goldline	00182-2645	Antidiabetic
N342 <> 125	Tab, White, Round, Scored, N over 342 <> 1.25	Glyburide 1.25 mg	by KV	10609-1437	Antidiabetic
N342 <> 125	Tab, N 342 <> 1.25	Glyburide 1.25 mg	by Major	00904-5075	Antidiabetic
N342 <> 125	Tab, White, Round, N/342 <> 1.25	Glyburide 1.25 mg	by Novopharm	43806-0342	Antidiabetic
N342125	Tab, White, Round, N 342/1.25	Glyburide 1.25 mg	Micronase by Novopharm	43806-0342	Antidiabetic
N343 <> 25	Tab, Peach, Round, Convex, Scored, N 3443 <> 2.5	Glyburide 2.5 mg	by Kaiser	62224-4559	Antidiabetic
N343 <> 25	Tab, Scored, N over 343 <> 2.5	Glyburide 2.5 mg	by Medirex	57480-0408	Antidiabetic
N343 <> 25	Tab, Peach, Round, N over 343 <> 2.5	Glyburide 2.5 mg	by Novopharm	55953-0343	Antidiabetic
N343 <> 25	Tab, N 343 <> 2.5	Glyburide 2.5 mg	by Warrick	59930-1622	Antidiabetic
N343 <> 25	Tab, N 343 <> 2.5	Glyburide 2.5 mg	by Kaiser	62224-1331	Antidiabetic
N343 <> 25	Tab, Pale Peach, Round, Scored, N 343 <> 2.5	Glyburide 2.5 mg	by Allscripts	54569-3830	Antidiabetic
N343 <> 25	Tab, Peach, Round, Scored	Glyburide 2.5 mg	by Murfreesboro Ph	51129-1405	Antidiabetic
N343 <> 25	Tab, N Over 343 <> 2.5	Glyburide 2.5 mg	by Quality Care	62682-5006	Antidiabetic
N343 <> 25	Tab, Peach, Round	Glyburide 2.5 mg	by Heartland Healthcare	61392-0709	Antidiabetic
N343 <> 25	Tab, N/343 <> 2.5	Glyburide 2.5 mg	by Brightstone	62939-3221	Antidiabetic
N343 <> 25	Tab, N over 343 <> 2.5	Glyburide 2.5 mg	by Zenith Goldline	00182-2646	Antidiabetic
N343 <> 25	Tab, N 343 <> 2.5	Glyburide 2.5 mg	by HL Moore	00839-8040	Antidiabetic
N343 <> 25	Tab, Peach, Round, Scored, N over 343 <> 2.5	Glyburide 2.5 mg	Micronase by UDL	51079-0872	Antidiabetic
N343 <> 25	Tab, N 343 <> 2.5	Glyburide 2.5 mg	by Major	00904-5076	Antidiabetic
N343 <> 25	Tab, Peach, Round, N 343 <> 2.5	Glyburide 2.5 mg	by Novopharm	43806-0343	Antidiabetic
N34325	Tab, Peach, Round, N 343/2.5	Glyburide 2.5 mg	Micronase by Novopharm	43806-0343	Antidiabetic
N344 <> 5	Tab, Light Green, Round, Scored	Glyburide 5 mg	by Novopharm	43806-0344	Antidiabetic
N344 <> 5	Tab	Glyburide 5 mg	by Talbert Med	44514-0385	Antidiabetic
N344 <> 5	Tab, Light Green, Round, Scored, N over 344 <> 5	Glyburide 5.1 mg	by Novopharm	55953-0344	Antidiabetic
N344 <> 5	Tab, Light Green, Round, N Horizontal Bisect 344	Glyburide 5.1 mg	by Novopharm	62528-0344	Antidiabetic
N344 <> 5	Tab, Scored, N over 344 <> 5	Glyburide 5 mg	by Medirex	57480-0409	Antidiabetic
N344 <> 5	Tab, N over 344 <> 5	Glyburide 5 mg	by PDRX	55289-0892	Antidiabetic
N344 <> 5	Tab	Glyburide 5 mg	by Warrick	59930-1639	Antidiabetic
N344 <> 5	Tab, Green, Round, Scored	Glyburide 5 mg	by Murfreesboro Ph	51129-1288	Antidiabetic
N344 <> 5	Tab, N/344	Glyburide 5 mg	by Brightstone	62939-3231	Antidiabetic
N344 <> 5	Tab, Light Green, Round, Scored	Glyburide 5 mg	by Allscripts	54569-3831	Antidiabetic
N344 <> 5	Tab, N/344	Glyburide 5 mg	by Kaiser	00179-1205	Antidiabetic
N344 <> 5	Tab, Green, Round, Scored, N over 344 <> 5	Glyburide 5 mg	by Lederle	00005-5886	Antidiabetic
N344 <> 5	Tab	Glyburide 5 mg	by HL Moore	00839-8041	Antidiabetic
N344 <> 5	Tab	Glyburide 5 mg	by Qualitest	00603-3764	Antidiabetic
N344 <> 5	Tab, N over 344 <> 5	Glyburide 5 mg	by Zenith Goldline	00182-2647	Antidiabetic
N344 <> 5	Tab, Light Green, Round, Scored, N over 344 <> 5	Glyburide 5 mg	Micronase by UDL	51079-0873	Antidiabetic
N344 <> 5	Tab	Glyburide 5 mg	by Major	00904-5077	Antidiabetic
N344 <> 5	Tab, Green, Round	Glyburide 5 mg	by KV	10609-1429	Antidiabetic
N382	Cap	Clofibrate 500 mg	by Qualitest	00603-2932	Antihyperlipidemic
N392 <> 500	Tab, White, Round	Etodolac 500 mg	by Novopharm	55953-0392	NSAID
N392 <> 500	Tab, White, Oval	Etodolac 500 mg	by Novopharm	43806-0392	NSAID
N393400	Tab, Orange, Round, N 393/400	Etodolac 400 mg	by Novopharm	43806-0393	NSAID
N393400	Tab, Orange, Round, N 393/400	Etodolac 400 mg	by Novopharm	55953-0393	NSAID
N397300	Cap, Opaque & Red, Hard Gel, N397 Over 300 in Gray Ink	Etodolac 300 mg	Etodolac by Heartland	61392-0885	NSAID
N399200	Cap, Opaque & Red, Hard Gel, N 399 Over 200 in Gray Ink	Etodolac 200 mg	Etodolac by Heartland	61392-0903	NSAID
N399200	Cap, Opaque & Red, Hard Gel, N 399 Over 200 in Gray Ink, 2 Dark Red Bands	Etodolac 200 mg	Etodolac by Heartland	61392-0904	NSAID

ID FRONT <> BACK	DESCRIPTION FRONT <> BACK	INGREDIENT & STRENGTH	BRAND (OR EQUIV.) & FIRM	NDC#	CLASS; SCH.
N4	Tab, Pink, Round	Salbutamol Sulfate 4 mg	Novo Salmol by Novopharm	Canadian	Antiasthmatic
N401 <> 100	Tab, N over 401 <> 100	Atenolol 100 mg	by Medirex	57480-0447	Antihypertensive
N401 <> 100	Tab, N Over 401	Atenolol 100 mg	by Quality Care	60346-0914	Antihypertensive
N401 <> 100	Tab, White, Round, N over 401 <> 100	Atenolol 100 mg	by Novopharm	55953-0401	Antihypertensive
N401 <> 100	Tab, White, Round	Atenolol 100 mg	by Novopharm (US)	62528-0401	Antihypertensive
N401 <> 100	Tab, White, Round	Atenolol 100 mg	by Allscripts	54569-3654	Antihypertensive
N401100	Tab, N over 401 100	Atenolol 100 mg	by Qualitest	00603-2372	Antihypertensive
N420 <> 25	Cap, Light Green	Indomethacin 25 mg	by Allscripts	54569-0277	NSAID
N420 <> 25	Cap, Green, N Over 420	Indomethacin 25 mg	by Murfreesboro	51129-1549	NSAID
N420 <> 25	Cap, Light Green	Indomethacin 25 mg	by Quality Care	60346-0684	NSAID
N420 <> 25	Cap	Indomethacin 25 mg	by Apotheca	12634-0455	NSAID
N42025	Cap, Light Green, N 420/25	Indomethacin 25 mg	by Novopharm	43806-0420	NSAID
N439 <> 50	Cap, Green	Indomethacin 50 mg	by Allscripts	54569-0275	NSAID
N43950	Cap, Green, N 439-50	Indomethacin 50 mg	Indocin by Novopharm	43806-0439	NSAID
N463	Tab, White, Round, N/463	Methyldopa 125 mg	Aldomet by Novopharm		Antihypertensive
N471	Tab, White, Round, N/471	Methyldopa 250 mg	Aldomet by Novopharm		Antihypertensive
N480	Tab	Albuterol Sulfate 2.4 mg	by Apotheca	12634-0090	Antiasthmatic
N480 <> 2	Tab, White, Round, Scored	Albuterol Sulfate 2 mg	by Amerisource	62584-0821	Antiasthmatic
N480 <> 2	Tab, White, Round, Scored	Albuterol Sulfate 2 mg	by Anabolic	00722-6436	Antiasthmatic
N480 <> 2	Tab, White, Round, N over 480 <> 2	Albuterol Sulfate 2.4 mg	by Novopharm	55953-0480	Antiasthmatic
N480 <> 2	Tab	Albuterol Sulfate 2.4 mg	by Heartland	61392-0567	Antiasthmatic
N4802	Tab, N 480/2	Albuterol Sulfate 2.4 mg	by Qualitest	00603-2093	Antiasthmatic
N498	Tab, White, Round, N/498	Methyldopa 500 mg	Aldomet by Novopharm		Antihypertensive
N499 <> 4	Tab, White, Round, Scored	Albuterol 4 mg	by Allscripts	54569-2874	Antiasthmatic
N499 <> 4	Tab, White, Round, Scored	Albuterol Sulfate 4 mg	by Anabolic	00722-6437	Antiasthmatic
N499 <> 4	Tab	Albuterol Sulfate 4.8 mg	by Heartland	61392-0570	Antiasthmatic
N499 <> 4	Tab, White, Round, N over 499 <> 4	Albuterol Sulfate 4.8 mg	by Novopharm	55953-0499	Antiasthmatic
N499 <> 4	Tab	Albuterol Sulfate 4.8 mg	by Medirex	57480-0423	Antiasthmatic
N499 <> 4	Tab, Coated, N 499	Albuterol Sulfate 4.8 mg	by Quality Care	60346-0285	Antiasthmatic
N499 <> 4	Tab, N over 499 <> 4	Albuterol Sulfate 4.8 mg	by DRX	55045-2283	Antiasthmatic
N4994	Tab, N 499/4	Albuterol Sulfate 4.8 mg	by Qualitest	00603-2094	Antiasthmatic
N5	Cap, Gray & Red, N/5	Flunarizine HCl 5 mg	by Novopharm	Canadian	Entry Blocker
N5	Tab, White, Round, N/.5	Lorazepam 0.5 mg	Novo Lorazem by Novopharm	Canadian	Sedative/Hypnotic; C IV
N5	Cap, Tan	Nifedipine 5 mg	Novo Nifedin by Novopharm	Canadian	Antihypertensive
N50	Tab, White, Oval, N/50	Flurbiprofen 50 mg	by Novopharm	Canadian	NSAID
N50	Tab, Pink, Round, N/50	Hydralazine HCl 50 mg	Novo Hylazin by Novopharm	Canadian	Antihypertensive
N50	Tab, Orange, Round, N/50	Maprotiline 50 mg	by Novopharm	Canadian	Antidepressant
N50	Tab, White, Round, N/50	Metoprolol Tartrate 50 mg	by Novopharm	Canadian	Antihypertensive
N50	Cap, Pink, N/50	Metoprolol Tartrate 50 mg	by Novopharm	Canadian	Antihypertensive
N50	Cap, White & Yellow	Nitrofurantoin 50 mg	by Novopharm	Canadian	Antibiotic
N500	Cap, Orange	Cephalexin Monohydrate 541 mg	by DRX Pharm Consults	55045-2787	Antibiotic
N517 <> 250	Tab, Yellow, Oval	Naproxen 250 mg	by OHM	51660-0714	NSAID
N517 <> 250	Tab, Light Yellow	Naproxen 250 mg	by Quality Care	60346-0816	NSAID
N517 <> 250	Tab, Peach & Yellow, N Over 517	Naproxen 250 mg	by Novopharm	55953-0517	NSAID
N517 <> 520	Tab, Film Coated	Naproxen Sodium 550 mg	by United Res	00677-1514	NSAID
N518 <> 375	Tab, N Over 518	Naproxen 375 mg	by Medirex	57480-0834	NSAID
N518 <> 375	Tab, Pink, N Over 518	Naproxen 375 mg	by Novopharm	55953-0518	NSAID
N520 <> 500	Tab, Yellow, Oval	Naproxen 500 mg	by Opti Med	63369-0071	NSAID
N520 <> 500	Tab, N Over 520	Naproxen 500 mg	by Medirex	57480-0835	NSAID
N520 <> 500	Tab, Peach & Yellow, N Over 520	Naproxen 500 mg	by Novopharm	55953-0520	NSAID
N520 <> 500	Tab, Light Yellow, N Over 520	Naproxen 500 mg	by Quality Care	60346-0815	NSAID
N524 <> 5	Tab, White, Oval, Scored	Glipizide 5 mg	by Novopharm (CA)	43806-0524	Antidiabetic

ID FRONT <> BACK	DESCRIPTION FRONT <> BACK	INGREDIENT & STRENGTH	BRAND (OR EQUIV.) & FIRM	NDC#	CLASS; SCH.
N525 <> 10	Tab, White, Oval, Scored	Glipizide 10 mg	by Novopharm (CA)	43806-0525	Antidiabetic
N531 <> 275	Tab, White, Round, Film Coated, N Over 531	Naproxen Sodium 275 mg	by Novopharm	55953-0531	NSAID
N531 <> 275	Tab, Film Coated	Naproxen Sodium 275 mg	by Major	00904-5040	NSAID
N531 <> 275	Tab, Film Coated	Naproxen Sodium 275 mg	by HL Moore	00839-7889	NSAID
N533 <> 550	Tab, Film Coated	Naproxen Sodium 550 mg	by Major	00904-5041	NSAID
N533 <> 550	Tab, White, Round, Film Coated, N Over 533	Naproxen Sodium 550 mg	by Novopharm	55953-0533	NSAID
N533 <> 550	Tab, Film Coated, N Over 533	Naproxen Sodium 550 mg	by Quality Care	60346-0826	NSAID
N533 <> 550	Tab, Light Blue, Film Coated	Naproxen Sodium 550 mg	by HL Moore	00839-7890	NSAID
N544 <> 150	Tab, White, Round, Film Coated, N over 544 <> 150	Ranitidine HCl 150 mg	Zantac by UDL	51079-0879	Gastrointestinal
N544 <> 150	Tab, White, Round, Film Coated	Ranitidine HCl	by Natl Pharmpak	55154-5581	Gastrointestinal
N544 <> 150	Tab, Film Coated, N Over 544 <> 150	Ranitidine HCl	by Med Pro	53978-2075	Gastrointestinal
N544 <> 150	Tab, Film Coated, N Over 544	Ranitidine HCl	by Allscripts	54569-4507	Gastrointestinal
N544 <> 150	Tab, Round, Film Coated, N Over 544	Ranitidine HCl	by Novopharm	55953-0544	Gastrointestinal
N544 <> 150	Tab, White, Round, Film Coated, N Over 544	Ranitidine HCl	by Novopharm	43806-0544	Gastrointestinal
N544 <> 150	Tab, White, Round, Convex, Film, N Over 544	Ranitidine HCl 150 mg	Ranitidine by RX PAK	65084-0177	Gastrointestinal
N544 <> 150	Tab, White, Round, Convex, Film, N Over 544	Ranitidine HCl 150 mg	by RX PAK	65084-0165	Gastrointestinal
N544 <> 150	Tab, White, Round, Convex, Film, N Over 544	Ranitidine HCl 150 mg	by RX PAK	65084-0180	Gastrointestinal
N544 <> 150	Tab, White, Round, Film Coated	Ranitidine HCl 150 mg	by Murfreesboro Ph	51129-1197	Gastrointestinal
N544 <> 150	Tab, White, Round	Ranitidine HCl 150 mg	by Phcy Care	65070-0053	Gastrointestinal
N547 <> 300	Tab, White, Oblong, Film Coated, N Over 547	Ranitidine HCl 300 mg	by RX PAK	65084-0166	Gastrointestinal
N547 <> 300	Tab, White, Oblong, Film Coated, Debossed N Over 547 <> 300	Ranitidine HCl 300 mg	by RX PAK	65084-0163	Gastrointestinal
N547 <> 300	Tab, Film Coated, N Over 547	Ranitidine HCl 336 mg	by UDL	51079-0880	Gastrointestinal
N547 <> 300	Tab, Film Coated, N Over 547	Ranitidine HCl 336 mg	by Allscripts	54569-4508	Gastrointestinal
N547 <> 300	Tab, White, Cap Shaped, Film Coated, N Over 547	Ranitidine HCl 336 mg	by Novopharm	55953-0547	Gastrointestinal
N547 <> 300	Tab, White, Cap Shaped, Film Coated, N Over 547	Ranitidine HCl 336 mg	by Novopharm	43806-0547	Gastrointestinal
N557 <> 100	Tab, Blue, Round, Film Coated	Flurbiprofen 100 mg	by Invamed	52189-0392	NSAID
N573 <> 50	Tab, Film Coated	Flurbiprofen 50 mg	by Warrick	59930-1771	NSAID
N573 <> 50	Tab, Film Coated	Flurbiprofen 50 mg	by HL Moore	00839-8003	NSAID
N57350	Tab, White, Round, N 573/50	Flurbiprofen 50 mg	by Novopharm	43806-0573	NSAID
N577 <> 100	Tab, Film Coated	Flurbiprofen 100 mg	by Warrick	59930-1772	NSAID
N577 <> 100	Tab, Dark Blue, Round, Film Coated	Flurbiprofen 100 mg	by Allscripts	54569-3858	NSAID
N577 <> 100	Tab, Coated	Flurbiprofen 100 mg	by Quality Care	60346-0968	NSAID
N577 <> 100	Tab, Film Coated	Flurbiprofen 100 mg	by Qualitest	00603-3700	NSAID
N577 <> 100	Tab, Film Coated	Flurbiprofen 100 mg	by HL Moore	00839-8004	NSAID
N577100	Tab, Deep Blue, Round, N 577/100	Flurbiprofen 100 mg	by Novopharm	43806-0577	NSAID
N6036	Tab, Dark Blue, Oval, N/6-036	Glyburide 6 mg	by Novopharm	43806-0036	Antidiabetic
N6036	Tab, Dark Blue, Oval, Scored, N/6-036	Glyburide Micronized 6 mg	by Novopharm	55953-0036	Antidiabetic
N617 <> 10	Cap	Piroxicam 10 mg	by Heartland	61392-0398	NSAID
N617 <> 10	Cap	Piroxicam 10 mg	by HL Moore	00839-7773	NSAID
N61710	Cap, Gray & Dark Green, N617/10	Piroxicam 10 mg	by Novopharm	55953-0617	NSAID
N61710	Cap, Light Gray & Dark Green, Oblong, N 617/10	Piroxicam 10 mg	by Novopharm	43806-0617	NSAID
N634	Tab, Green, Round, N/634	Methyldopa 250 mg, Hydrochlorothiazide 15 mg	Aldoril by Novopharm		Antihypertensive
N635	Tab, Green, Round, N/635	Methyldopa 500 mg, Hydrochlorothiazide 30 mg	Aldoril by Novopharm		Antihypertensive
N640 <> 20	Cap, Dark Green	Piroxicam 20 mg	by Heartland	61392-0401	NSAID
N640 <> 20	Cap	Piroxicam 20 mg	by HL Moore	00839-7774	NSAID
N64020	Cap	Piroxicam 20 mg	by Med Pro	53978-1255	NSAID
N64020	Cap, Dark Green, N640/20	Piroxicam 20 mg	by Novopharm	55953-0640	NSAID
N64020	Cap, Dark Green, N Over 640 on Opposing Cap and Body Portions	Piroxicam 20 mg	by Quality Care	60346-0676	NSAID
N64020	Cap, Dark Green, Oblong, N 640/20	Piroxicam 20 mg	by Novopharm	43806-0640	NSAID
N642	Tab, White, Round, N/642	Methyldopa 250 mg, Hydrochlorothiazide 25 mg	Aldoril by Novopharm		Antihypertensive
N643	Tab, White, Round, N/643	Methyldopa 500 mg, Hydrochlorothiazide 50 mg	Aldoril by Novopharm		Antihypertensive

ID FRONT <> BACK	DESCRIPTION FRONT <> BACK	INGREDIENT & STRENGTH	BRAND (OR EQUIV.) & FIRM	NDC#	CLASS; SCH.
N716 <> 500	Cap, Buff, Opaque, N over 716 <> 500	Amoxicillin 500 mg	by Novopharm	43806-0716	Antibiotic
N716 <> 500	Cap	Amoxicillin Trihydrate	by Qualitest	00603-2267	Antibiotic
N716 <> 500	Cap, Buff & Opaque	Amoxicillin 500 mg	by Quality Care	60346-0634	Antibiotic
N716 <> 500	Cap, N Over 716	Amoxicillin 500 mg	by St Marys Med	60760-0716	Antibiotic
N716 <> 500	Cap	Amoxicillin 500 mg	by Casa De Amigos	62138-0601	Antibiotic
N716500	Cap	Amoxicillin 500 mg	by Dept Health Central Pharm	53808-0040	Antibiotic
N716500	Cap	Amoxicillin Trihydrate	by Med Pro	53978-5003	Antibiotic
N716500 <> N716500	Cap, Buff	Amoxicillin 500 mg	by Prescription Dispensing	61807-0002	Antibiotic
N724 <> 250	Cap, Buff & Caramel	Amoxicillin 250 mg	by Quality Care	60346-0655	Antibiotic
N724 <> 250	Cap, N over 724 <> 250	Amoxicillin Trihydrate	by Qualitest	00603-2266	Antibiotic
N724 <> 250	Cap, Buff & Caramel, N over 724 <> 250	Amoxicillin 250 mg	by Novopharm	43806-0724	Antibiotic
N724 <> 250	Cap, N over 724 <> 250	Amoxicillin 250 mg	by Apotheca	12634-0185	Antibiotic
N724250	Cap, Novapharm Logo N724/250	Amoxicillin 250 mg	by Rugby	00536-0070	Antibiotic
N724250	Cap	Amoxicillin 250 mg	by Dept Health Central Pharm	53808-0039	Antibiotic
N727 <> 50	Tab, White, Oblong, Scored, Film, N 727	Metoprolol Tartrate 50 mg	by Neuman Distr	64579-0095	Antihypertensive
N727 <> 50	Tab, White, Oblong, Scored	Metoprolol Tartrate 50 mg	by Va Cmop	65243-0048	Antihypertensive
N727 <> 50	Tab, Film Coated, N 727	Metoprolol Tartrate 50 mg	by Brightstone	62939-2211	Antihypertensive
N727 <> 50	Tab, White, Cap Shaped, Film Coated, Engraved N 727	Metoprolol Tartrate 50 mg	by Novopharm	55953-0727	Antihypertensive
N727 <> 50	Tab, Film Coated	Metoprolol Tartrate 50 mg	by Medirex	57480-0802	Antihypertensive
N727 <> 50	Tab, Film Coated, Engraved N 727	Metoprolol Tartrate 50 mg	by Major	00904-7946	Antihypertensive
N734	Tab, White, Oblong, Scored	Metoprolol Tartrate 100 mg	by Va Cmop	65243-0091	Antihypertensive
N734 <> 100	Tab, White, Oblong, Scored, Film Coated, N 734	Metoprolol Tartrate 100 mg	Metoprolol Tartrate by Neuman Distr	64579-0079	Antihypertensive
N734 <> 100	Tab, Film Coated, N 734	Metoprolol Tartrate 100 mg	by Brightstone	62939-2221	Antihypertensive
N734 <> 100	Tab, Film Coated	Metoprolol Tartrate 100 mg	by Medirex	57480-0803	Antihypertensive
N734 <> 100	Tab, White, Cap Shaped, Film Coated, Engraved	Metoprolol Tartrate 100 mg	by Novopharm	55953-0734	Antihypertensive
N734 <> 100	Tab, Film Coated	Metoprolol Tartrate 100 mg	by Direct Dispensing	57866-6579	Antihypertensive
N735 <> 50	Tab, Dark Orange, Round, Film Coated	Diclofenac Sodium 50 mg	by Allscripts	54569-4165	NSAID
N73550	Tab, Orange, Round, N 735/50	Diclofenac Sodium 50 mg	by Novopharm	55953-0735	NSAID
N73550	Tab, Orange, Round, N 735/50	Diclofenac Sodium 50 mg	by Novopharm	43806-0735	NSAID
N737 <> 75	Tab, N over 737 <> 75	Diclofenac Sodium 75 mg	by HJ Harkins Co	52959-0423	NSAID
N737 <> 75	Tab, N over 737 <> 75	Diclofenac Sodium 75 mg	by DRX	55045-2247	NSAID
N737 <> 75	Tab, White, Round	Diclofenac Sodium 75 mg	by Novopharm	43806-0737	NSAID
N737 <> 75	Tab, White, Round	Diclofenac Sodium 75 mg	by Novopharm	55953-0737	NSAID
N737 <> 75	Tab, Delayed Release, N Over 737	Diclofenac Sodium 75 mg	by Warrick	59930-1642	NSAID
N737 <> 75	Tab, Delayed Release	Diclofenac Sodium 75 mg	by Prescription Dispensing	61807-0088	NSAID
N737 <> 75	Tab, White, Round, Film Coated	Diclofenac Sodium 75 mg	by Allscripts	54569-4166	NSAID
N739 <> 150	Cap, Tan & Orange, Gelatin	Acetaminophen 400 mg, Hydrocodone Bitartrate 10 mg	by Allscripts	54569-4732	Analgesic; C III
N739 <> 150	Cap, N Over 739	Mexiletine HCl 150 mg	by Physicians Total Care	54868-3776	Antiarrhythmic
N739 <> 150	Cap, Black Ink	Mexiletine HCl 150 mg	by Warrick	59930-1685	Antiarrhythmic
N739 <> 150	Tab, Orange & Tan, Oblong, N Over 739	Mexiletine HCl 150 mg	by Neuman Distr	64579-0186	Antiarrhythmic
N739 <> 150	Cap	Mexiletine HCl 150 mg	by Brightstone	62939-2312	Antiarrhythmic
N739 <> 150	Cap, Light Orange & Tan, White Granular Powder, in Black Ink	Mexiletine HCl 150 mg	by Novopharm	55953-0739	Antiarrhythmic
N739 <> 150	Cap, N Over 739 in Black Ink	Mexiletine HCl 150 mg	by Medirex	57480-0836	Antiarrhythmic
N740 <> 200	Cap, Light Orange, with White Beads	Mexiletine HCl 200 mg	by Novopharm	55953-0740	Antiarrhythmic
N740 <> 200	Cap, Black Ink	Mexiletine HCl 200 mg	by Warrick	59930-1686	Antiarrhythmic
N740 <> 200	Cap	Mexiletine HCl 200 mg	by Brightstone	62939-2322	Antiarrhythmic
N740 <> 200	Cap, N Over 740 in Black Ink	Mexiletine HCl 200 mg	by Medirex	57480-0837	Antiarrhythmic
N741 <> 250	Cap, Dark Green & Light Orange	Mexiletine HCl 250 mg	by Novopharm	55953-0741	Antiarrhythmic
N741 <> 250	Cap	Mexiletine HCl 250 mg	by Brightstone	62939-2332	Antiarrhythmic
N741 <> 250	Cap, Black Ink	Mexiletine HCl 250 mg	by Warrick	59930-1687	Antiarrhythmic
N747 <> 125	Tab, Pink, Round, N over 747 <> 125	Amoxicillin Trihydrate 125 mg	by Novopharm	43806-0747	Antibiotic
N747 <> 125	Tab, Cherry & Rose, Chewable, N over 747 <> 25	Amoxicillin Trihydrate 155 mg	by Novopharm	55953-0747	Antibiotic

ID FRONT <> BACK	DESCRIPTION FRONT <> BACK	INGREDIENT & STRENGTH	BRAND (OR EQUIV.) & FIRM	NDC#	CLASS; SCH.
N747 <> 125	Tab, Chewable	Amoxicillin Trihydrate 155 mg	by Warrick	59930-1573	Antibiotic
N75	Tab, Red, Round, N/75	Maprotiline 75 mg	by Novopharm	Canadian	Antidepressant
N751 <> 250	Tab, Cherry & Rose, Chewable, N over 751 <> 250	Amoxicillin Trihydrate 250 mg	by Novopharm	55953-0751	Antibiotic
N751 <> 250	Tab, Pink, Rond, Scored, N over 751 <> 250	Amoxicillin Trihydrate 250 mg	by Novopharm	43806-0751	Antibiotic
N751 <> 250	Tab, Chew, N/751	Amoxicillin Trihydrate 310 mg	by Warrick	59930-1611	Antibiotic
N77 <> LL	Tab	Naproxen 500 mg	by UDL	51079-0795	NSAID
N77 <> LL	Tab	Naproxen 500 mg	by St Marys Med	60760-0452	NSAID
N80	Tab, White, Round, N/80	Trimethoprim 80 mg, Sulfamethoxazole 400 mg	by Novopharm	Canadian	Antibiotic
N815 <> 400	Cap, Red	Tolmetin Sodium 400 mg	by Allscripts	54569-3730	NSAID
N815 <> 400	Cap, N Over 815 and 400	Tolmetin Sodium 492 mg	by Quality Care	60346-0615	NSAID
N815 <> 400	Cap, N Over 815	Tolmetin Sodium 492 mg	by United Res	00677-1424	NSAID
N815 <> 400	Cap, Red, N Over 815	Tolmetin Sodium 492 mg	by Novopharm	43806-0815	NSAID
N815400	Cap, N 815 400	Tolmetin Sodium 492 mg	by Qualitest	00603-6130	NSAID
N827 <> 200	Tab, Yellow, Round, Scored, Debossed, N Over 827	Ketoconazole 200 mg	by Murfreesboro	51129-1591	Antifungal
N827200	Tab, Light Peach, Round, N827/200	Ketoconazole 200 mg	by Novopharm	55953-0827	Antifungal
N827200	Tab, Light Peach, Round, N 827/200	Ketoconazole 200 mg	by Novopharm	43806-0827	Antifungal
N837 <> 25	Tab, Film Coated, N837 <> 2.5	Indapamide 2.5 mg	by Novopharm	55953-0837	Diuretic
N837 <> 25	Tab, Film Coated, N837 <> 2.5	Indapamide 2.5 mg	by Novopharm	43806-0837	Diuretic
N853 <> 125	Tab, Light Yellow, Film Coated, N853 <> 1.25	Indapamide 1.25 mg	by Novopharm	55953-0853	Diuretic
N853 <> 125	Tab, Light Yellow, Film Coated, N853 <> 1.25	Indapamide 1.25 mg	by Novopharm	43806-0853	Diuretic
N940 <> 200	Cap	Acyclovir 200 mg	by Warrick	59930-1538	Antiviral
N940 <> 200	Cap, Blue, Gelatin	Acyclovir 200 mg	by Phy Total Care	54868-3996	Antiviral
N940 <> 200	Cap, Blue, Gelatin	Acyclovir 200 mg	by Murfreesboro Ph	51129-1359	Antiviral
N940 <> 200	Cap, Blue, Opaque, N over 940 <> 200	Acyclovir 200 mg	by UDL	51079-0876	Antiviral
N940 <> 200	Cap	Acyclovir 200 mg	by Allscripts	54569-4482	Antiviral
N940 <> 200	Cap	Acyclovir 200 mg	by Major	00904-5231	Antiviral
N940 <> 200	Cap, Blue, N over 940 <> 200	Acyclovir 200 mg	by Novopharm	43806-0940	Antiviral
N943 <> 400	Tab, Deep Blue, Cap Shaped, N over 943 <> 400	Acyclovir 400 mg	by Novopharm	55953-0943	Antiviral
N943 <> 400	Tab, Blue, Oblong, Convex	Acyclovir 400 mg	by Amerisource	62584-0437	Antiviral
N943 <> 400	Tab	Acyclovir 400 mg	by Warrick	59930-1576	Antiviral
N943 <> 400	Tab, Blue, Oblong	Acyclovir 400 mg	by Allscripts	54569-4765	Antiviral
N943 <> 400	Tab, Blue, Cap Shaped, N over 943 <> 400	Acyclovir 400 mg	by UDL	51079-0877	Antiviral
N943 <> 400	Tab	Acyclovir 400 mg	by Major	00904-5232	Antiviral
N943 <> 400	Tab, Deep Blue, Cap Shaped, N over 943 <> 400	Acyclovir 400 mg	by Novopharm	43806-0943	Antiviral
N947 <> 800	Tab, White, Oblong, N Over 947	Acyclovir 800 mg	by Amerisource	62584-0789	Antiviral
N947 <> 800	Tab, Off-White to White, Cap Shaped, N over 947 <> 800	Acyclovir 800 mg	by UDL	51079-0878	Antiviral
N947 <> 800	Tab, White, Cap Shaped, N over 947 <> 800	Acyclovir 800 mg	by Novopharm	43806-0947	Antiviral
N947 <> 800	Tab, White to Off-White, Cap Shaped	Acyclovir 800 mg	by Novopharm	55953-0947	Antiviral
N947 <> 800	Tab	Acyclovir 800 mg	by Warrick	59930-1584	Antiviral
N947 <> 800	Tab, White, Oblong, Convex	Acyclovir 800 mg	by Amerisource	62584-0429	Antiviral
N947 <> 800	Tab, White, Oblong, Convex	Acyclovir 800 mg	by Amerisource	62584-0605	Antiviral
N947 <> 800	Tab, White, Cap Shaped	Acyclovir 800 mg	by Allscripts	54569-4724	Antiviral
N9615	Tab, White, Round, N 961-5	Timolol Maleate 5 mg	Blocadren by Novopharm		Antihypertensive
N97210	Tab, White, Round, N 972-10	Timolol Maleate 10 mg	Blocadren by Novopharm		Antihypertensive
N98420	Tab, White, Round, N 984-20	Timolol Maleate 20 mg	Blocadren by Novopharm		Antihypertensive
NA	Tab, Pink, Round, Abbott Logo	Pargyline HCl 10 mg	Eutonyl by Abbott		Antihypertensive
NALDECON <> BLN1	Tab, White, Red Specks, Naldecon around Perimeter <> BL over N1	Chlorpheniramine Maleate 5 mg, Phenylephrine HCl 10 mg, Phenylpropanolamine HCl 40 mg, Phenyltoloxamine Citrate 15 mg	Naldecon by Mead Johnson	00015-5600	Cold Remedy
NALEXJR <> BLANSETT33	Cap, Green & White Print	Guaifenesin 300 mg, Pseudoephedrine HCl 60 mg	Nalex Jr by Sovereign	58716-0006	Cold Remedy
NALFON <> DISTAH77	Cap	Fenoprofen Calcium 324 mg	Nalfon by Dista Prod	00777-0877	NSAID
NALFON <> DISTAH77	Cap	Fenoprofen Calcium 324 mg	Nalfon by Physicians Total Care	54868-0856	NSAID

ID FRONT <> BACK	DESCRIPTION FRONT <> BACK	INGREDIENT & STRENGTH	BRAND (OR EQUIV.) & FIRM	NDC#	CLASS; SCH.
NAPROSYN <> 250	Tab	Naproxen 250 mg	Naprosyn by HJ Harkins Co	52959-0110	NSAID
NAPROSYN <> 375	Tab	Naproxen 375 mg	Naprosyn by Amerisource	62584-0273	NSAID
NAPROSYN <> 375	Tab	Naproxen 375 mg	Naprosyn by Nat Pharmpak Serv	55154-3803	NSAID
NAPROSYN <> 375	Tab	Naproxen 375 mg	Naprosyn by Quality Care	60346-0636	NSAID
NAPROSYN <> 375	Tab, Debossed	Naproxen 375 mg	Naprosyn by Syntex	18393-0273	NSAID
NAPROSYN <> 375	Tab, Peach, Oblong	Naproxen 375 mg	Naprosyn by Rightpak	65240-0700	NSAID
NAPROSYN <> 375	Tab	Naproxen 375 mg	Naprosyn by Allscripts	54569-0293	NSAID
NAPROSYN <> 375	Tab, Peach, Oblong	Naproxen 375 mg	Naprosyn by Par	49884-0566	NSAID
NAPROSYN <> 375	Tab	Naproxen 375 mg	Naprosyn by HJ Harkins Co	52959-0192	NSAID
NAPROSYN <> 375	Tab, Debossed	Naproxen 375 mg	Naprosyn by Thrift Drug	59198-0238	NSAID
NAPROSYN <> 500	Tab, Yellow, Oblong	Naproxen 500 mg	Naprosyn by Par	49884-0565	NSAID
NAPROSYN <> 500	Tab	Naproxen 500 mg	Naprosyn by HJ Harkins Co	52959-0111	NSAID
NAPROSYN <> 500	Tab, Yellow, Round, Scored	Naproxen 500 mg	by HJ Harkins	52959-0516	NSAID
NAPROSYN <> 500	Tab, Yellow, Oblong	Naproxen 500 mg	Naprosyn by Rightpak	65240-0701	NSAID
NAPROSYN <> 500	Tab	Naproxen 500 mg	Naprosyn by Allscripts	54569-0294	NSAID
NAPROSYN <> 500	Tab	Naproxen 500 mg	Naprosyn by Quality Care	60346-0637	NSAID
NAPROSYN <> 500	Tab	Naproxen 500 mg	Naprosyn by Nat Pharmpak Serv	55154-3804	NSAID
NAPROSYN <> 500	Tab, Debossed	Naproxen 500 mg	Naprosyn by Thrift Drug	59198-0239	NSAID
NAPROSYN <> 500	Tab, Yellow, Oblong	Naproxen 500 mg	Naprosyn by Novopharm	43806-0139	NSAID
NAPROSYN <> 500	Tab, Bone	Naproxen 500 mg	Naprosyn by Syntex	18393-0277	NSAID
NAPROSYN250 <> ROCHE	Tab	Naproxen 250 mg	Naprosyn by Allscripts	54569-0292	NSAID
NAPROSYN250 <> ROCHE	Tab	Naproxen 250 mg	Naprosyn by Amerisource	62584-0272	NSAID
NAPROSYN250 <> ROCHE	Tab	Naproxen 250 mg	Naprosyn by Thrift Drug	59198-0237	NSAID
NAPROSYN250 <> ROCHE	Tab, Debossed	Naproxen 250 mg	Naprosyn by Syntex	18393-0272	NSAID
NAPROSYN250 <> SYNTEX	Tab	Naproxen 250 mg	Naprosyn by Quality Care	60346-0092	NSAID
NAPROSYN500	Tab	Naproxen 500 mg	by Pharmedix	53002-0311	NSAID
NAPROXEN <> 375	Tab	Naproxen 375 mg	by Quality Care	60346-0817	NSAID
NAPROXEN250 <> SYNTEX	Tab	Naproxen 250 mg	by Pharmedix	53002-0324	NSAID
NAPROXEN375	Tab	Naproxen 375 mg	by Pharmedix	53002-0310	NSAID
NASABID <> SR	Tab, Nasabid <> S/R	Guaifenesin 600 mg, Pseudoephedrine HCl 90 mg	Nasabid Sr by Anabolic	00722-6356	Cold Remedy
NASABID <> SR	Tab, Yellow, Oval, Scored	Guaifenesin 600 mg, Pseudoephedrine HCl 90 mg	Nasabid Sr by Jones	52604-0600	Cold Remedy
NATAFORT	Tab, Film Coated	Ascorbic Acid 120 mg, Cholecalciferol 400 Units, Cyanocobalamin 12 mcg, Folic Acid 1 mg, Iron 60 mg, Niacinamide 20 mg, Pyridoxine HCl 10 mg, Riboflavin 3 mg, Thiamine Mononitrate 2 mg, Vitamin A 1000 Units, Vitamin E 11 Units	Natafort by Amide	52152-0176	Vitamin
NATURALMINI	Tab, White, Film Coated, Natural/Mini	Ephedra Alkaloids 12.5 mg, Kola Nut Extract 80 mg 50%	Mini Natural by BDI		Supplement
NATURETIN10 <> PPP618	Tab, Naturetin 10 <> PPP 618	Bendroflumethiazide 10 mg	Naturetin by ER Squibb	00003-0618	Diuretic
NATURETIN5 <> PPP606	Tab, Naturetin 5 <> PPP over 606	Bendroflumethiazide 5 mg	Naturetin by ER Squibb	00003-0606	Diuretic
NAVANE <> ROERIG572	Cap, Blue & Yellow	Thiothixene HCl 2 mg	Navane by Roerig	00049-5720	Antipsychotic
NAVANE <> ROERIG573	Cap, Orange & White	Thiothixene HCl 5 mg	Navane by Roerig	00049-5730	Antipsychotic
NAXEN	Tab, Yellow, Oblong	Naproxen 500 mg	Navalbine by B.W. Inc	Canadian	NSAID

ID FRONT <> BACK	DESCRIPTION FRONT <> BACK	INGREDIENT & STRENGTH	BRAND (OR EQUIV.) & FIRM	NDC#	CLASS; SCH.
NAXEN250	Tab, Yellow, Round, Naxen/250	Naxen 250 mg	by Altimed	Canadian DIN# 00615315	NSAID
NAXEN375	Tab, Pink, Oval, Naxen/375	Naxen 375 mg	by Altimed	Canadian DIN# 00615323	NSAID
NAXEN500	Tab, Yellow, Oblong, Naxen/500	Naxen 500 mg	by Altimed	Canadian DIN# 00615331	NSAID
NB	Tab, Apricot, Round, Abbott Logo	Pargyline HCl 25 mg	Eutonyl by Abbott		Antihypertensive
ND	Tab, Orange, Round, Abbott Logo	Imipramine 10 mg	Janimine by Abbott		Antidepressant
NDESEF	Cap, Yellow, ND ES/EF	D-Pseudoephedrine 30 mg, Acetaminophen 500 mg	by Whitehall-Robins	Canadian	Analgesic
NE	Tab, Yellow, Round, Abbott Logo	Imipramine 25 mg	Janimine by Abbott		Antidepressant
NE	Tab, Blue	Phenypropanolamine HCl 75 mg, Guaifenesin 600 mg	Entocort by Astra	Canadian	Cold Remedy
NE <> 406	Tab, N E	Etidronate Disodium 400 mg	Didronel by Pharm Utilization	60491-0802	Calcium Metabolism
NE <> 406	Tab, White, Cap Shaped, Scored	Etidronate Disodium 400 mg	Didronel by Procter & Gamble	00149-0406	Calcium Metabolism
NE1	Tab, White, Cap Shaped, Scored, Obtained in a kit containing NE2	Etidronate Disodium 400 mg	Didrocal by Proctor & Gambel	Canadian DIN# 02176017	Calcium Metabolism
NE10G	Cap, Mustard, Opaque, NE 10/G	Nifedipine 10 mg	by Genpharm	Canadian	Antihypertensive
NE10G	Cap, Mustard, Opaque, NE/10/G	Nifedipine 10 mg	Gen Nifedipine by Genpharm	Canadian	Antihypertensive
NE2	Tab, Blue, Cap Shaped, Film Coated, NE2 <> NE2, Obtained in a kit containing NE1	Calcium Carbonate 500 mg	Didrocal by Proctor & Gamble	Canadian DIN# 02176017	Vitamin/Mineral
NE406	Tab, White, Pillow	Etidronate Disodium 400 mg	Didronel by Norwich		Calcium Metabolism
NE560	Tab, Green, Oblong	Esterified Estrogen 1.25 mg, Methyltestosterone 2.5 mg	Estratest by Econolab		Hormone
NE570	Tab, Green, Oblong	Esterified Estrogen 0.625 mg, Methyltestosterone 1.25 mg	Estratest by Econolab		Hormone
NEORAL <> 25MG	Cap	Cyclosporine 25 mg	Sandimmun Neoral B63 by RP Scherer	11014-1197	Immunosuppressant
NEORAL100MG	Cap, Neoral over 100 mg	Cyclosporine 100 mg	Neoral by Nat Pharmpak Serv	55154-3419	Immunosuppressant
NEORAL100MG	Cap, Bluish Gray, Oblong, Red Print, Neoral over 100 mg	Cyclosporine 100 mg	Neoral by Novartis	00078-0248	Immunosuppressant
NEORAL25	Tab, Blue, Oval, Neoral over 25	Cyclosporine 25 mg	by Drug Distr	52985-0230	Immunosuppressant
NEORAL25MG	Cap, Gelatin Coated, Neoral over 25 mg	Cyclosporine 25 mg	Neoral by Nat Pharmpak Serv	55154-3418	Immunosuppressant
NEORAL25MG	Cap, Bluish Gray, Oval, Red Print, Neoral over 25 mg	Cyclosporine 25 mg	Neoral by Novartis	00078-0246	Immunosuppressant
NEURONTIN100MG	Cap, Scored, Neurontin over 100 mg	Gabapentin 100 mg	Neurontin by Nat Pharmpak Serv	55154-2414	Anticonvulsant
NEURONTIN100MG <> PD	Cap, White, Hard Gel	Gabapentin 100 mg	Neurontin by Johnson & Johnson	59604-0301	Anticonvulsant
NEURONTIN100MG <> PD	Cap, White, Opaque, Neurontin/100 mg <> PD	Gabapentin 100 mg	Neurontin by Parke-Davis	Canadian DIN# 02084260	Anticonvulsant
NEURONTIN100MG <> PD	Cap, White, Gelatin	Gabapentin 100 mg	Neurontin by HJ Harkins	52959-0506	Anticonvulsant
NEURONTIN100MG <> PD	Cap, White	Gabapentin 100 mg	Neurontin by Amerisource Health	62584-0083	Anticonvulsant
NEURONTIN100MG <> PD	Cap, White, Nuerontin/100 mg <> Parke Davis Logo	Gabapentin 100 mg	Neurontin by Parke Davis	00071-0803	Anticonvulsant
NEURONTIN300MG <> PD	Cap, Yellow	Gabapentin 300 mg	Neurontin by Heartland Healthcare	61392-0716	Anticonvulsant
NEURONTIN300MG <> PD	Cap, Yellow	Gabapentin 300 mg	Neurontin by Amerisource Health	62584-0085	Anticonvulsant
NEURONTIN300MG <> PD	Cap, Yellow, Gelatin	Gabapentin 300 mg	Neurontin by HJ Harkins	52959-0434	Anticonvulsant

ID FRONT <> BACK	DESCRIPTION FRONT <> BACK	INGREDIENT & STRENGTH	BRAND (OR EQUIV.) & FIRM	NDC#	CLASS; SCH.
NEURONTIN300MG <> PD	Cap, Yellow, Opaque, Neurontin/300 mg <> PD	Gabapentin 300 mg	Neurontin by Parke-Davis	Canadian DIN# 02084279	Anticonvulsant
NEURONTIN300MG <> PD	Cap, Yellow, Nuerontin/300 mg <> Parke Davis Logo	Gabapentin 300 mg	Neurontin by Parke Davis	00071-0805	Anticonvulsant
NEURONTIN300MG <> PD	Cap, Neurontin 300 mg <> PD	Gabapentin 300 mg	Neurontin by Nat Pharmpak Serv	55154-2415	Anticonvulsant
NEURONTIN300MG <> PD	Cap, Neurontin/300 mg	Gabapentin 300 mg	by Med Pro	53978-3020	Anticonvulsant
NEURONTIN300MG <> PD	Cap, Neurontin/300 mg <> PD	Gabapentin 300 mg	by Pharm Packaging Ctr	54383-0080	Anticonvulsant
NEURONTIN300MG <> PD	Cap	Gabapentin 300 mg	Neurontin by Physicians Total Care	54868-3768	Anticonvulsant
NEURONTIN400MG <> PD	Cap	Gabapentin 400 mg	Neurontin by DRX	55045-2545	Anticonvulsant
NEURONTIN400MG <> PD	Cap, Orange, Hard Gel	Gabapentin 400 mg	Neurontin by Amerisource Health	62584-0086	Anticonvulsant
NEURONTIN400MG <> PD	Cap, Orange, Gelatin	Gabapentin 400 mg	Neurontin by Natl Pharmpak	55154-2417	Anticonvulsant
NEURONTIN400MG <> PD	Cap, Orange, Opaque, Neurontin/400 mg <> PD	Gabapentin 400 mg	Neurontin by Parke-Davis	Canadian DIN# 02084287	Anticonvulsant
NEURONTIN600	Tab, White, Elliptical, Film Coated	Gabapentin 600 mg	Neurontin by Parke-Davis	Canadian DIN# 02239717	Anticonvulsant
NEURONTIN600MG	Tab, White, Elliptical, Black Print	Gabapentin 600 mg	Neurontin by Parke Davis	00071-0416	Anticonvulsant
NEURONTIN800	Tab, White, Elliptical, Film Coated	Gabapentin 800 mg	Neurontin by Parke-Davis	Canadian DIN# 02239718	Anticonvulsant
NEURONTIN800MG	Tab, White, Elliptical, Black Print	Gabapentin 800 mg	Neurontin by Parke Davis	00071-0426	Anticonvulsant
NEURONTINR300MG <> PD	Cap, Neurontin R/300 mg <> PD	Gabapentin 300 mg	Neurontin by Caremark	00339-6101	Anticonvulsant
NEUROTIN400MG <> PD	Cap, Orange, Neurotin/400 mg <> PD	Gabapentin 400 mg	Neurontin by Kaiser	00179-1280	Anticonvulsant
NEUROTIN400MG <> PD	Cap, Orange, Neurontin/400 mg <> Parke Davis Logo	Gabapentin 400 mg	Neurontin by Parke Davis	00071-0806	Anticonvulsant
NF	Tab, Green, Abbott Logo	Hexocyclium Methylsulfate 25 mg	Tral by Abbott		Antispasmodic
NHA <> HNA	Cap, HN-A	Terazosin HCl 10 mg	Terazosin by RP Scherer	11014-1034	Antihypertensive
NICHE	Cap, Yellow	Magnesium L-lactate Dihydrate 84 mg	Mag-Tab SR by Niche	59016-0420	Mineral
NIFED2030	Cap, Nifed./20-30	Nifedipine 20 mg	by RP Scherer	11014-0873	Antihypertensive
NIFEDIPINE <> 100364	Cap, 10-0364	Nifedipine 10 mg	by Schein	00364-2376	Antihypertensive
NIFEDIPINE10 <> 0364	Cap	Nifedipine 10 mg	by Nat Pharmpak Serv	55154-5206	Antihypertensive
NIFEDIPINE10 <> 0364	Cap	Nifedipine 10 mg	by Quality Care	60346-0803	Antihypertensive
NIFEDIPINE10 <> 0364	Cap	Nifedipine 10 mg	by Amerisource	62584-0802	Antihypertensive
NIFEDIPINE20 <> 0364	Cap	Nifedipine 20 mg	by Schein	00364-2377	Antihypertensive
NIFEDIPINE20 <> 0364	Cap	Nifedipine 20 mg	by Allscripts	54569-3122	Antihypertensive
NIFEDIPINE20 <> 0364	Cap	Nifedipine 20 mg	by Amerisource	62584-0803	Antihypertensive
NIMOTOP	Cap, Ivory	Nimodipine 30 mg	Nimotop by Bayer	Canadian	Antihypertensive
NIMOTOP	Cap, Ivory	Nimodipine 30 mg	Nimotop by Par	49884-0632	Antihypertensive
NIMOTOP	Cap, Ivory, Soft Gel	Nimodipine 30 mg	Nimotop by Par	49884-0643	Antihypertensive
NIMOTOP	Cap, Off White	Nimodipine 30 mg	Nimotop by RP Scherer	11014-0781	Antihypertensive

ID FRONT <> BACK	DESCRIPTION FRONT <> BACK	INGREDIENT & STRENGTH	BRAND (OR EQUIV.) & FIRM	NDC#	CLASS; SCH.
NITROFURANTOIN MACRO	Cap, Yellow	Nitrofurantoin Macrocrystal Ca 100 mg	by Schein	00364-2557	Antibiotic
NITROFURANTOIN MACRO	Cap, White	Nitrofurantoin Macrocrystal Ca 25 mg	by Schein	00364-2555	Antibiotic
NITROFURANTOIN MACRO	Cap, White & Yellow	Nitrofurantoin Macrocrystal Ca 50 mg	by Schein	00364-2556	Antibiotic
NITROGLYN25MG	Cap, ER	Nitroglycerin 2.5 mg	Nitroglyn by Kenwood	00482-1025	Vasodilator
NITROGLYN65MG	Cap, ER	Nitroglycerin 6.5 mg	Nitroglyn by Kenwood	00482-1065	Vasodilator
NITROGLYN9MG	Cap, ER, White Beads	Nitroglycerin 9 mg	Nitroglyn by Kenwood	00482-1090	Vasodilator
NIZORAL <> JANSSEN	Tab, White, Scored	Ketoconazole 200 mg	Nizoral by HJ Harkins	52959-0197	Antifungal
NIZORAL <> JANSSEN	Tab	Ketoconazole 200 mg	Nizoral by Janssen	50458-0220	Antifungal
NIZORAL <> JANSSEN	Tab	Ketoconazole 200 mg	Nizoral by Johnson & Johnson	59604-0220	Antifungal
NIZORAL <> JANSSEN	Tab, Debossed	Ketoconazole 200 mg	Nizoral by Direct Dispensing	57866-6570	Antifungal
NIZORAL <> JANSSEN	Tab	Ketoconazole 200 mg	Nizoral by Pharm Utilization	60491-0454	Antifungal
NIZORAL <> JANSSEN	Tab	Ketoconazole 200 mg	Nizoral by Quality Care	60346-0247	Antifungal
NJ	Tab, Green, Oval, Abbott Logo	Vitamin Combination	Cefol by Abbott	00074-6089	Vitamin
NJ	Tab, Green, Film Coated	Vitamin Combination	Cefol by Abbott	00074-6089	Vitamin
NK	Tab, Purple, Oval, Abb. Logo	Pargyline HCl 25 mg, Methyclothiazide 5 mg	Eutron by Abbott		Antihypertensive
NL	Tab, Peach, Oval, Abb. Logo	Imipramine 50 mg	Janimine by Abbott		Antidepressant
NL <> 175	Tab, White, Oval	Guaifenesin 600 mg; Phenylpropanolamine HCl 37.5 mg	by Neil Labs	60242-0700	Cold Remedy
NM	Tab, Yellow, Ovaloid, Film Coated, NM <> Abbott Logo	Potassium Chloride 750 mg	K-Tab ER by Abbott	00074-7804	Electrolytes
NMI	Tab, Coated	Ascorbic Acid 50 mg, Calcium Carbonate, Cholecalciferol, Cupric Sulfate, Ferrous Fumarate, Folic Acid 1 mg, Magnesium Oxide, Pyridoxine HCl 2 mg, Tocopheryl Acetate, Zinc Sulfate	Precare Prenatal by Northampton Med	58436-0071	Vitamin
NMI	Tab, Peach, Coated, Brown Specks	Ascorbic Acid 50 mg, Calcium Carbonate, Cholecalciferol, Cupric Sulfate, Ferrous Fumarate, Folic Acid 1 mg, Magnesium Oxide, Pyridoxine HCl 2 mg, Tocopheryl Acetate, Zinc Sulfate	Precare by		Vitamin
NMI	Tab, Coated	Ascorbic Acid 50 mg, Calcium Carbonate, Cholecalciferol, Cupric Sulfate, Ferrous Fumarate, Folic Acid 1 mg, Magnesium Oxide, Pyridoxine HCl 2 mg, Tocopheryl Acetate, Zinc Sulfate	Precare by Physicians Total Care	54868-3787	Vitamin
NMI	Cap, Peach, Scored, Film	Vitamin D 6 mcg, Vitamin E 3.5 mg, Ascorbic Acid 50 mg, Folic Acid 1 mg, Pyridoxine HCl 2 mg, Calcium 50 mg, Magnesium 50 mg, Iron 40 mg, Zinc 15 mg, Copper 2 mg	Precare by Thrift Drug	59198-0340	Vitamin
NN160	Tab, Light Blue, Round, N/N/160	Sotalol HCl 160 mg	by Novopharm	Canadian	Antiarrhythmic
NN2	Tab, White, Square	Methazolamide 25 mg	Neptazane by Lederle		Diuretic
NN5	Tab, Blue, Round, N/N/5	Oxybutynin Chloride 5 mg	by Novopharm	Canadian	Urinary
NO1 <> MCNEIL	Cap, White, Film Coated, No. 1 <> McNeil	Acetaminophen 300 mg, Caffeine 15 mg, Codeine Phosphate 8 mg	Tylenol No. 1 by McNeil	Canadian DIN# 02181061	Analgesic
NO1FORTE <> MCNEIL	Cap, White, Film Coated, No. 1 Forte <> McNeil	Acetaminophen 500 mg, Caffeine 15 mg, Codeine Phosphate 8 mg	Tylenol No. 1 Forte by McNeil	Canadian DIN# 02181088	Analgesic
NOLVADEX 10	Tab, White, Round	Tamoxifen Citrate 15.2 mg	by Zeneca	Canadian	Antiestrogen
NOLVADEX600	Tab	Tamoxifen 10 mg	by Pharmedix	53002-1032	Antiestrogen
NOLVADEX600	Tab	Tamoxifen 10 mg	Nolvadex by Amerisource	62584-0600	Antiestrogen
NOLVADEX600	Tab, White, Round	Tamoxifen Citrate 10 mg	Nolvadex by St. Marys Med	60760-0460	Antiestrogen
NOLVADEX600	Tab, White, Round	Tamoxifen Citrate 15.2 mg	Nolvadex by AstraZeneca	00310-0600	Antiestrogen
NOLVADEX604	Tab, White, Round	Tamoxifen Citrate 20 mg	Nolvadex by AstraZeneca	00310-0604	Antiestrogen
NORCO539	Tab, Yellow, Cap Shaped, Scored	Acetaminophen 325 mg, Hydrocodone Bitartrate 10 mg	Norco by Watson	52544-0539	Analgesic; C III
NORCO539	Tab, Yellow	Hydrocodone Bitartrate 10 mg, Acetaminophen 325 mg	Norco by Natl Pharmpak	55154-1150	Analgesic; C III
NORCO539	Tab, Yellow, Oblong, Bisected	Hydrocodone Bitartrate 10 mg, Acetaminophen 325 mg	Norco by Allscripts	54569-4685	Analgesic; C III
NORCO539	Tab, Yellow, Oblong, Scored	Hydrocodone Bitartrate 10 mg, Acetaminophen 325 mg	Norco by Eckerd	19458-0916	Analgesic; C III

ID FRONT <> BACK	DESCRIPTION FRONT <> BACK	INGREDIENT & STRENGTH	BRAND (OR EQUIV.) & FIRM	NDC#	CLASS; SCH.
NORCO539	Tab, Yellow, Oblong, Scored	Hydrocodene Bitartrate 10 mg, Acetaminophin 325 mg	Norco by Murfreesboro	51129-1425	Analgesic; C lll
NORCO729	Tab, Light Orange, Cap Shaped, Scored	Acetaminophen 325 mg, Hydrocodone Bitartrate 7.5 mg	Norco by Watson	52544-0729	Analgesic; C lll
NORGESIC <> 3M	Tab, White & Yellow, Round	Aspirin 385 mg, Caffeine 30 mg, Orphenadrine Citrate 25 mg	Norgesic by 3M	00089-0231	Analgesic; Muscle Relaxant
NORGESICFORTE	Tab, White, Oblong, Scored	Orphenadrine Citrate 50 mg, Caffeine 60 mg, Aspirin 770 mg	Norgesic Forte by Rightpak	65240-0704	Muscle Relaxant
NORGESICFORTE <> 3M	Tab, Light Green & White & Yellow, Layered, Norgesic over Forte <> 3M	Aspirin 770 mg, Caffeine 60 mg, Orphenadrine Citrate 50 mg	Norgesic Forte by Quality Care	60346-0185	Analgesic
NORGESICFORTE <> 3M	Tab, Light Green, Layered, Norgesic over Forte <> 3M	Aspirin 770 mg, Caffeine 60 mg, Orphenadrine Citrate 50 mg	Norgesic Forte by Amerisource	62584-0233	Analgesic
NORGESICFORTE <> 3M	Tab, Green & White, Cap Shaped, Scored	Aspirin 770 mg, Caffeine 60 mg, Orphenadrine Citrate 50 mg	Norgesic Forte by 3M	00089-0233	Analgesic
NORGESICFORTE <> 3M	Tab, Light Green, White & Yellow	Aspirin 770 mg, Caffeine 60 mg, Orphenadrine Citrate 50 mg	Norgesic Forte by Allscripts	54569-0840	Analgesic
NORGESICFORTE <> 3M	Tab, Light Green & White & Yellow, Layered	Aspirin 770 mg, Caffeine 60 mg, Orphenadrine Citrate 50 mg	Norgesic Forte by Thrift Drug	59198-0158	Analgesic
NORGESICFORTE <> 3M	Tab, Green & White	Aspirin 770 mg, Caffeine 60 mg, Orphenadrine Citrate 50 mg	Norgesic Forte by Nat Pharmpak Serv	55154-2905	Analgesic
NORGESICFORTE <> 3M	Tab, Green & White	Aspirin 770 mg, Caffeine 60 mg, Orphenadrine Citrate 50 mg	Norgesic Forte by CVS	51316-0050	Analgesic
NORGESICFORTE <> 3M	Tab	Aspirin 770 mg, Caffeine 60 mg, Orphenadrine Citrate 50 mg	Norgesic Forte by CVS Revco	00894-6767	Analgesic
NORGESICFORTE <> 3M	Tab, White & Yellow, Oblong	Orphenadrine Citrate 50 mg, Caffeine 60 mg, Aspirin 770 mg	Norgesic Forte by Med-Pro	53978-3384	Muscle Relaxant
NORGESICFORTE <> RIKER	Tab, Green	Aspirin 770 mg, Caffeine 60 mg, Orphenadrine Citrate 50 mg	Orphengesic Forte by Pharmedix	53002-0376	Analgesic
NORINYLSYNTEX	Tab, White, Circular, Norinyl/Syntex	Norethindrone 1 mg, Mestranol 0.05 mg	by Novartis	Canadian	Oral Contraceptive
NORMODYNE <> SCHERING244	Tab, Film Coated	Labetalol HCl 100 mg	Normodyne by Med Pro	53978-0696	Antihypertensive
NORMODYNE <> SCHERING438	Tab, Blue, Round	Labetalol HCl 300 mg	Normodyne by Rx Pac	65084-0230	Antihypertensive
NORMODYNE <> SCHERING7	Tab, Film Coated	Labetalol HCl 200 mg	Normodyne by Pharmedix	53002-1046	Antihypertensive
NORMODYNE <> SCHERING752	Tab, Film Coated	Labetalol HCl 200 mg	Normodyne by Med Pro	53978-0697	Antihypertensive
NORMODYNE100 <> SCHERING244	Tab, Light Brown, Round, Film Coated, Normodyne/100 <> Schering/244	Labetalol HCl 100 mg	Normodyne by Schering	00085-0244	Antihypertensive
NORMODYNE100 <> SCHERING244	Tab, Film Coated	Labetalol HCl 100 mg	Normodyne by Caremark	00339-5265	Antihypertensive
NORMODYNE100 <> SCHERING244	Tab, Film Coated	Labetalol HCl 100 mg	Normodyne by Rite Aid	11822-5260	Antihypertensive
NORMODYNE200 <> SCHERING752	Tab, White, Round, Film Coated	Labetalol HCl 200 mg	Normodyne by Schering	00085-0752	Antihypertensive
NORMODYNE200 <> SCHERING752	Tab, Film Coated	Labetalol HCl 200 mg	Normodyne by Nat Pharmpak Serv	55154-3506	Antihypertensive
NORMODYNE200 <> SCHERING752	Tab, Film Coated	Labetalol HCl 200 mg	Normodyne by Rite Aid	11822-5234	Antihypertensive
NORMODYNE300 <> SCHERING438	Tab, Blue, Round, Film Coated	Labetalol HCl 300 mg	Normodyne by Schering	00085-0438	Antihypertensive
NORMODYNE300 <> SCHERING438	Tab, Film Coated	Labetalol HCl 300 mg	Normodyne by Leiner	59606-0670	Antihypertensive
NOROXIN <> MSD705	Tab, Film Coated	Norfloxacin 400 mg	Noroxin by Roberts	54092-0097	Antibiotic
NOROXIN <> MSD705	Tab, Film Coated	Norfloxacin 400 mg	Noroxin by Allscripts	54569-0191	Antibiotic

ID FRONT <> BACK	DESCRIPTION FRONT <> BACK	INGREDIENT & STRENGTH	BRAND (OR EQUIV.) & FIRM	NDC#	CLASS; SCH.
NOROXIN <> MSD705	Tab, Film Coated	Norfloxacin 400 mg	Noroxin by Quality Care	60346-0563	Antibiotic
NOROXIN <> MSD705	Tab, Dark Pink, Film Coated	Norfloxacin 400 mg	Noroxin by DRX	55045-2419	Antibiotic
NORPACE100MG <> SEARLE2732	Cap, Light Green, Ex Release	Disopyramide Phosphate	Norpace CR by Amerisource	62584-0732	Antiarrhythmic
NORPACE100MG <> SEARLE2752	Cap	Disopyramide Phosphate	Norpace by Amerisource	62584-0753	Antiarrhythmic
NORPACE100MG <> SEARLE2752	Cap, Orange & White, Norpace 100 mg <> Searle 2752	Disopyramide Phosphate	Norpace by GD Searle	00025-2752	Antiarrhythmic
NORPACE100MG <> SEARLE2752	Cap	Disopyramide Phosphate	Norpace by Leiner	59606-0707	Antiarrhythmic
NORPACE100MG <> SEARLE2752	Cap	Disopyramide Phosphate	Norpace by Thrift Drug	59198-0083	Antiarrhythmic
NORPACE100MG <> SEARLE2752	Cap	Disopyramide Phosphate	Norpace by Nat Pharmpak Serv	55154-3607	Antiarrhythmic
NORPACE150MG <> SEARLE2742	Cap, Brown & Light Green	Disopyramide Phosphate	Norpace CR by GD Searle	00014-2742	Antiarrhythmic
NORPACE150MG <> SEARLE2762	Cap	Disopyramide Phosphate	Norpace by Leiner	59606-0708	Antiarrhythmic
NORPACE150MG <> SEARLE2762	Cap	Disopyramide Phosphate	Norpace by Amerisource	62584-0762	Antiarrhythmic
NORPACE150MG <> SEARLE2762	Cap, Brown & Orange, Norpace 150 mg <> Searle 2762	Disopyramide Phosphate	Norpace by GD Searle	00025-2762	Antiarrhythmic
NORPACE150MG <> SEARLE2762	Cap	Disopyramide Phosphate	Norpace by Thrift Drug	59198-0084	Antiarrhythmic
NORPACECR100MG <> SEARLE2732	Cap, Ex Release	Disopyramide Phosphate	Norpace CR by Leiner	59606-0709	Antiarrhythmic
NORPACECR100MG <> SEARLE2732	Cap, Light Green & White, Norpace CR 100 mg <> Searle 2732	Disopyramide Phosphate	Norpace CR by GD Searle	00025-2732	Antiarrhythmic
NORPACECR100MG <> SEARLE2732	Cap, Light Green, Ex Release	Disopyramide Phosphate	Norpace CR by Thrift Drug	59198-0164	Antiarrhythmic
NORPACECR100MG <> SEARLE2732	Cap	Disopyramide Phosphate	Norpace CR by Nat Pharmpak Serv	55154-3609	Antiarrhythmic
NORPACECR150MG <> SEARLE2742	Cap, Ex Release	Disopyramide Phosphate	Norpace CR by Leiner	59606-0710	Antiarrhythmic
NORPACECR150MG <> SEARLE2742	Cap, Light Green, Ex Release	Disopyramide Phosphate	Norpace CR by Amerisource	62584-0742	Antiarrhythmic
NORPACECR150MG <> SEARLE2742	Cap, Brown & Light Green, Norpace CR 150 mg <> Searle 2742	Disopyramide Phosphate	Norpace CR by GD Searle	00025-2742	Antiarrhythmic
NORPACECR150MG <> SEARLE2742	Cap, Light Green, Ex Release	Disopyramide Phosphate	Norpace CR by Thrift Drug	59198-0085	Antiarrhythmic
NORPACECR150MG <> SEARLE2742	Cap	Disopyramide Phosphate	Norpace CR by Nat Pharmpak Serv	55154-3610	Antiarrhythmic
NORPACECR150MG <> SEARLE2762	Cap	Disopyramide Phosphate	Norpace by Nat Pharmpak Serv	55154-3608	Antiarrhythmic
NORPRAMIN 25	Tab, Yellow, Round	Desipramine HCl 25 mg	Norpramin by Marion Merrell Dow	Canadian	Antidepressant
NORPRAMIN 75	Tab, Orange, Round	Desipramine HCl 75 mg	Norpramin by Marion Merrell Dow	Canadian	Antidepressant
NORPRAMIN100	Tab, Peach, Round	Desipramine HCl 100 mg	Norpramin by Marion Merrell Dow	Canadian	Antidepressant
NORPRAMIN100	Tab, Peach	Desipramine HCl 100 mg	Norpramin by Hoechst Marion Roussel	00068-0020	Antidepressant
NORPRAMIN150	Tab, White	Desipramine HCl 150 mg	Norpramin by Hoechst Marion Roussel	00068-0021	Antidepressant
NORPRAMIN25	Tab, Yellow	Desipramine HCl 25 mg	Norpramin by Hoechst Marion Roussel	00068-0011	Antidepressant
NORPRAMIN50	Tab, Green, Round	Desipramine HCl 50 mg	Norpramin by Marion Merrell Dow	Canadian	Antidepressant
NORPRAMIN50	Tab, Green	Desipramine HCl 50 mg	Norpramin by Hoechst Marion Roussel	00068-0015	Antidepressant

ID FRONT <> BACK	DESCRIPTION FRONT <> BACK	INGREDIENT & STRENGTH	BRAND (OR EQUIV.) & FIRM	NDC#	CLASS; SCH.
NORPRAMIN75	Tab, Orange	Desipramine HCl 75 mg	Norpramin by Hoechst Marion Roussel	00068-0019	Antidepressant
NORTRIPTYLI <> DAN25MG	Cap, Opaque Deep Green & Opaque White	Nortriptyline HCl	by Quality Care	60346-0757	Antidepressant
NORTRIPTYLINE <> DAN10MG	Cap, Green & White	Nortriptyline HCl 10 mg	by Allscripts	54569-4146	Antidepressant
NORTRIPTYLINE <> DAN10MG	Cap, Green & Opaque & White	Nortriptyline HCl 10 mg	by PDRX	55289-0405	Antidepressant
NORTRIPTYLINE <> DAN10MG	Cap, Deep Green	Nortriptyline HCl	by Danbury	00591-5786	Antidepressant
NORTRIPTYLINE <> DAN10MG	Cap	Nortriptyline HCl	by Heartland	61392-0361	Antidepressant
NORTRIPTYLINE <> DAN10MG	Cap, Deep Green	Nortriptyline HCl	by Danbury	61955-2508	Antidepressant
NORTRIPTYLINE <> DAN25	Cap	Nortriptyline HCl	by Nat Pharmpak Serv	55154-5220	Antidepressant
NORTRIPTYLINE <> DAN25MG	Cap	Nortriptyline HCl	by Danbury	61955-2509	Antidepressant
NORTRIPTYLINE <> DAN25MG	Cap	Nortriptyline HCl	by Heartland	61392-0364	Antidepressant
NORTRIPTYLINE <> DAN25MG	Cap, Deep Green	Nortriptyline HCl	by Danbury	00591-5787	Antidepressant
NORTRIPTYLINE <> DAN50MG	Cap	Nortriptyline HCl	by Danbury	61955-2510	Antidepressant
NORTRIPTYLINE <> DAN50MG	Cap, White	Nortriptyline HCl 50 mg	by PDRX	55289-0386	Antidepressant
NORTRIPTYLINE <> DAN50MG	Cap	Nortriptyline HCl	by Danbury	00591-5788	Antidepressant
NORTRIPTYLINE <> DAN50MG	Cap	Nortriptyline HCl	by Heartland	61392-0367	Antidepressant
NORTRIPTYLINE <> DAN50MG	Cap	Nortriptyline HCl	by Danbury	61955-2511	Antidepressant
NORTRIPTYLINE <> DAN75MG	Cap	Nortriptyline HCl	by Danbury	00591-5789	Antidepressant
NORTRIPTYLINE <> DAN75MG	Cap	Nortriptyline HCl	by Heartland	61392-0370	Antidepressant
NORTRIPTYLINE <> DAN75MG	Cap, Green	Nortriptyline HCl 75 mg	by Apothecon	62269-0331	Antidepressant
NORTRIPTYLINE <> INV75	Cap, Green	Nortriptyline HCl 75 mg	by Invamed	52189-0331	Antidepressant
NORTRIPTYLINE <> INV75	Cap, Green & White	Nortriptyline HCl 10 mg	by HJ Harkins	52959-0358	Antidepressant
NORTRIPTYLINE10 <> 250	Cap	Nortriptyline 10 mg	by Creighton Prod	50752-0250	Antidepressant
NORTRIPTYLINE10 <> CP250	Cap, Green & White	Nortriptyline HCl 25 mg	by HJ Harkins	52959-0359	Antidepressant
NORTRIPTYLINE25 <> 251	Cap, Black & White Print	Nortriptyline HCl 25 mg	by Prescription Dispensing	61807-0142	Antidepressant
NORTRIPTYLINE25 <> 251CP	Cap, Opaque Green & White, Black & White Print	Nortriptyline HCl	by Quality Care	60346-0757	Antidepressant
NORTRIPTYLINE25 <> CP251	Cap, Deep Green, Opaque	Nortriptyline HCl 10 mg	by Schein	00364-2508	Antidepressant
NORTRIPTYLINEDAN1	Cap, Deep Green, Opaque	Nortriptyline HCl 25 mg	by Schein	00364-2509	Antidepressant
NORTRIPTYLINEDAN2	Cap, White, Opaque	Nortriptyline HCl 50 mg	by Schein	00364-2510	Antidepressant
NORTRIPTYLINEDAN5					

ID FRONT <> BACK	DESCRIPTION FRONT <> BACK	INGREDIENT & STRENGTH	BRAND (OR EQUIV.) & FIRM	NDC#	CLASS; SCH.
NORTRIPTYLINEDAN7	Cap, Deep Green, Opaque	Nortriptyline HCl 75 mg	by Schein	00364-2511	Antidepressant
NORTRIPTYLINEIN	Cap, Green & White	Nortriptyline HCl 10 mg	by Apothecon	62269-0328	Antidepressant
NORTRIPTYLINEIN	Cap, Green & White	Nortriptyline HCl 10 mg	by Invamed	52189-0328	Antidepressant
NORTRIPTYLINEIN	Cap, Green & White	Nortriptyline HCl 25 mg	by Apothecon	62269-0329	Antidepressant
NORTRIPTYLINEIN	Cap, Green & White	Nortriptyline HCl 25 mg	by Invamed	52189-0329	Antidepressant
NORTRIPTYLINEIN	Cap, White	Nortriptyline HCl 50 mg	by Invamed	52189-0330	Antidepressant
NORTRIPTYLINEIN	Cap, White	Nortriptyline HCl 50 mg	by Apothecon	62269-0330	Antidepressant
NORVASC	Tab, Flat Faced, Beveled Edged	Amlodipine Besylate	Norvasc by Amerisource	62584-0540	Antihypertensive
NORVASC <> 25	Tab, Norvasc <> 2.5	Amlodipine Besylate 2.5 mg	Norvasc by DRX	55045-2377	Antihypertensive
NORVASC <> 25	Tab, White, Diamond Shaped, Norvasc <> 2.5	Amlodipine Besylate 2.5 mg	Norvasc by Pfizer	00069-1520	Antihypertensive
NORVASC <> 25	Tab, White, Diamond Shaped, Norvasc <> 2.5	Amlodipine Besylate 2.5 mg	by Barr	00555-0582	Antihypertensive
NORVASC <> 25	Tab, Norvasc <> 2.5	Amlodipine Besylate 2.5 mg	Norvasc by Murfreesboro	51129-1260	Antihypertensive
NORVASC <> 25	Tab, Norvasc <> 2.5	Amlodipine Besylate 2.5 mg	Norvasc by Physicians Total Care	54868-3853	Antihypertensive
NORVASC <> 5	Tab	Amlodipine Besylate 5 mg	Norvasc by Nat Pharmpak Serv	55154-2708	Antihypertensive
NORVASC10	Tab, White, Round	Amlodipine Besylate 10 mg	Norvaxs by Va Cmop	65243-0009	Antihypertensive
NORVASC10	Tab, White, Round	Amlodipine Besylate 10 mg	Norvasc by PDRX Pharms	55289-0549	Antihypertensive
NORVASC10	Tab, White, Round	Amlodipine Besylate 10 mg	Norvasc by Direct Dispensing	57866-6626	Antihypertensive
NORVASC10	Tab, White, Round, Norvasc/10	Amlodipine Besylate 10 mg	Norvasc by Pfizer	00069-1540	Antihypertensive
NORVASC10	Tab	Amlodipine Besylate 10 mg	Norvasc by Nat Pharmpak Serv	55154-2710	Antihypertensive
NORVASC10	Tab	Amlodipine Besylate 10 mg	by Med Pro	53978-3073	Antihypertensive
NORVASC10	Tab	Amlodipine Besylate 10 mg	Norvasc by Allscripts	54569-4472	Antihypertensive
NORVASC10	Tab	Amlodipine Besylate 10 mg	Norvasc by DRX	55045-2305	Antihypertensive
NORVASC10	Tab	Amlodipine Besylate 10 mg	Norvasc by Physicians Total Care	54868-3464	Antihypertensive
NORVASC5	Tab, Beveled Edged	Amlodipine Besylate 5 mg	Norvasc by Amerisource	62584-0530	Antihypertensive
NORVASC5	Tab, White, Octagon	Amlodipine Besylate 5 mg	Norvasc by Heartland Hlthcare	61392-0711	Antihypertensive
NORVASC5	Tab, White, Octagonal	Amlodipine Besylate 5 mg	Norvasc by Direct Dispensing	57866-6625	Antihypertensive
NORVASC5	Tab, White, Octagon	Amlodipine Besylate 5 mg	Norvasc by Va Cmop	65243-0008	Antihypertensive
NORVASC5	Tab, White, Octagon	Amlodipine Besylate 5 mg	Norvasc by Rightpac	65240-0794	Antihypertensive
NORVASC5	Tab, White, Octagon	Amlodipine Besylate 5 mg	Norvasc by Pfizer	00069-1530	Antihypertensive
NORVASC5	Tab, White, Octagon, Flat, Norvasc 5	Amlodipine Besylate 5 mg	Norvasc by B F Ascher	00225-0570	Antihypertensive
NORVASC5	Tab, Elongated Octagon	Amlodipine Besylate 5 mg	Norvasc by Wal Mart	49035-0185	Antihypertensive
NORVASC5	Tab	Amlodipine Besylate 5 mg	Norvasc by Med Pro	53978-2045	Antihypertensive
NORVASC5	Tab	Amlodipine Besylate 5 mg	Norvasc by Repack Co of Amer	55306-1530	Antihypertensive
NORVASC5	Tab	Amlodipine Besylate 5 mg	Norvasc by Allscripts	54569-3866	Antihypertensive
NORVASC5	Tab	Amlodipine Besylate 5 mg	Norvasc by Drug Distr	52985-0229	Antihypertensive
NORVASC5	Tab	Amlodipine Besylate 5 mg	by Med Pro	53978-3053	Antihypertensive
NORVASC5	Tab, White, Rectangle	Amlodipine Besylate 5 mg	Norvasc by Compumed	00403-0933	Antihypertensive
NORVASC5	Tab	Amlodipine Besylate 5 mg	Norvasc by CVS Revco	00894-6780	Antihypertensive
NORVASC5	Tab, White, Octagonal	Amlodipine Besylate 5 mg	Norvasc by Astra Zeneca	17228-1587	Antihypertensive
NORVASC5	Tab, White, Octagonal	Amlodipine Besylate 5 mg	Norvasc by Astra Zeneca	17228-1549	Antihypertensive
NORVASC5	Tab, White, Octagonal	Amlodipine Besylate 5 mg	Norvasc by Astra Zeneca	17228-1502	Antihypertensive
NORVASC5 <> PLAIN	Tab, Octagonal	Amlodipine Besylate 5 mg	Norvasc by PDRX	55289-0103	Antihypertensive
NORWICH EATON <> MACROBID	Cap	Nitrofurantoin 100 mg	Macrobid by DRX	55045-2341	Antibiotic
NORWICHEAT <> MACROBID	Cap	Nitrofurantoin 100 mg	Macrobid by Quality Care	60346-0289	Antibiotic
NORWICHEATON <> MACROBID	Cap, Black & Yellow	Nitrofurantoin 100 mg	Macrobid by Promex Medcl	62301-0039	Antibiotic
NORWICHEATON <> MACROBID	Cap, Black & Yellow	Nitrofurantoin 100 mg	Macrobid by Southwood Pharms	58016-0260	Antibiotic
NORWICHEATON <> MACROBID	Cap	Nitrofurantoin 100 mg	Macrobid by Allscripts	54569-3544	Antibiotic

ID FRONT <> BACK	DESCRIPTION FRONT <> BACK	INGREDIENT & STRENGTH	BRAND (OR EQUIV.) & FIRM	NDC#	CLASS; SCH.
NOVAFEDA	Cap, Orange & Red	Pseudoephedrine 120 mg, Chlorpheniramine Maleate 8 mg	Novafed A by Hoechst Marion Roussel	00068-0106	Cold Remedy
NOVALDEXD	Tab, White, Octagonal	Tamoxifen Citrate 30.4 mg	by Zeneca	Canadian	Antiestrogen
NOVO	Tab, Rose, Oval	Amoxicillin 125 mg	by Novopharm	Canadian	Antibiotic
NOVO	Tab, White, Round	Carbamazepine 200 mg	by Novopharm	Canadian	Anticonvulsant
NOVO	Tab, White, Round, Scored	Metformin HCl 500 mg	by Novopharm	Canadian	Antidiabetic
NOVO	Tab, White, Oblong	Sucralfate 1g	Novo Sucralate by Novopharm	Canadian	Gastrointestinal
NOVO 180	Cap, Blue	Doxycycline Hyclate 100 mg	Novo Doxylin by Novopharm	Canadian	Antibiotic
NOVO 250	Cap, Black & Red	Ampicillin 250 mg	Novo Ampicillin by Novopharm	Canadian	Antibiotic
NOVO 250	Cap, Clear & Orange	Erythromycin 250 mg	Novo Rythro Enca by Novopharm	Canadian	Antibiotic
NOVO 500	Cap, Black & Red	Ampicillin 500 mg	Novo Ampicillin by Novopharm	Canadian	Antibiotic
NOVO01	Tab, White, Round, No/Vo/0.1	Clonidine 0.1 mg	by Novopharm	Canadian	Antihypertensive
NOVO0125	Tab, Violet, Oval, Novo/0.125	Triazolam 0.125 mg	by Novopharm	Canadian	Sedative/Hypnotic
NOVO02	Tab, Orange, Round, No/Vo/0.2	Clonidine 0.2 mg	by Novopharm	Canadian	Antihypertensive
NOVO025	Tab, White, Oval, no/vo/0.25	Alprazolam 0.25 mg	by Novopharm	Canadian	Antianxiety
NOVO025	Tab, Powder Blue, Oval, Novo/0.25	Triazolam 0.25 mg	by Novopharm	Canadian	Sedative/Hypnotic
NOVO05	Tab, Peach, Oval, no/vo/0.5	Alprazolam 0.5 mg	by Novopharm	Canadian	Antianxiety
NOVO1	Tab, Peach, Oblong, Novo/1	Prazosin HCl 1 mg	Novo Prazin by Novopharm	Canadian	Antihypertensive
NOVO10	Tab, White, Oval, novo/10	Baclofen 10 mg	by Novopharm	Canadian	Muscle Relaxant
NOVO10	Tab, Light Yellow, Triangle, Novo/10	Clomipramine 10 mg	by Novopharm	Canadian	OCD
NOVO10	Tab, Blue, Round, Novo/10	Desipramine 10 mg	by Novopharm	Canadian	Antidepressant
NOVO10	Cap, Gray & Green, novo/10	Fluoxetine HCl 10 mg	by Novopharm	Canadian	Antidepressant
NOVO10	Tab, Cream, Round, Novo/10	Maprotiline HCl 10 mg	Novo Maprotiline by Novopharm	Canadian	Antidepressant
NOVO10	Tab, White, Round, Novo/10	Medroxyprogesterone Acetate 10 mg	by Novopharm	Canadian	Progestin
NOVO10	Cap, Tan	Nifedipine 10 mg	Novo Nifedin by Novopharm	Canadian	Antihypertensive
NOVO10	Tab, White, Round	Pindolol 10 mg	Novo Pindol by Novopharm	Canadian	Antihypertensive
NOVO10	Cap, Blue & Maroon	Piroxicam 10 mg	Novo Pirocam by Novopharm	Canadian	NSAID
NOVO10	Tab, Light Blue, Round, Novo/10	Timolol Maleate 10 mg	Novo Timol by Novopharm	Canadian	Antihypertensive
NOVO100	Tab, White, novo/100	Atenolol 100 mg	Novo Atenol by Novopharm	Canadian	Antihypertensive
NOVO100	Tab, White, Oval, novo/100	Captopril 100 mg	by Novopharm	Canadian	Antihypertensive
NOVO100	Cap, Blue & Pink, Novo/100	Doxepin HCl 100 mg	Novo Doxepin by Novopharm	Canadian	Antidepressant
NOVO100	Cap, Blue	Doxycycline Hyclate 100 mg	by Novopharm	Canadian	Antibiotic
NOVO100	Tab, Blue, Oval, novo/100	Flurbiprofen 100 mg	Novo Flurprofen by Novopharm	Canadian	NSAID
NOVO100	Tab, Yellow, Round, Novo/100	Ketoprofen 100 mg	Novo Keto EC by Novopharm	Canadian	NSAID
NOVO100	Tab, Blue, Oblong	Metoprolol Tartrate 100 mg	Novo Metoprol by Novopharm	Canadian	Antihypertensive
NOVO100	Cap, Orange & Scarlet, Novo/100	Mexiletine HCl 100 mg	by Novopharm	Canadian	Antiarrhythmic
NOVO100	Cap, Orange & Purple, Novo/100	Minocycline HCl 100 mg	by Novopharm	Canadian	Antibiotic
NOVO100	Tab, White, Round, Novo/100	Theophylline Anhydrous 100 mg	by Novopharm	Canadian	Antiasthmatic
NOVO100	Tab, Pink, Round, Novo/100	Trimipramine Maleate 100 mg	Novo Trimipramine100 by Novopharm	Canadian	Antidepressant
NOVO100	Cap, Blue & White, Novo/100	Zidovudine 100 mg	by Novopharm	Canadian	Antiviral
NOVO120	Tab, White, Round	Verapamil HCl 120 mg	Novo Veramil by Novopharm	Canadian	Antihypertensive
NOVO125	Tab, White, Oblong, novo/12.5	Captopril 12.5 mg	by Novopharm	Canadian	Antihypertensive
NOVO125	Tab, Yellow, Round, Novo/125	Methyldopa 125 mg	by Novopharm	Canadian	Antihypertensive
NOVO125	Tab, Green, Oval	Naproxen 125 mg	Novo Naprox by Novopharm	Canadian	NSAID
NOVO15	Tab, White, Round	Pindolol 15 mg	Novo Pindol by Novopharm	Canadian	Antihypertensive
NOVO15	Cap, Flesh & Maroon, Novo/15	Temazepam 15 mg	by Novopharm	Canadian	Sedative/Hypnotic
NOVO150	Cap, Pink, Novo/150	Doxepin HCl 150 mg	Novo Doxepin by Novopharm	Canadian	Antidepressant
NOVO2	Tab, White, Round, Novo/2	Prazosin HCl 2 mg	Novo Prazin by Novopharm	Canadian	Antihypertensive
NOVO20	Tab, White, Oblong, novo/20	Baclofen 20 mg	by Novartis	Canadian	Muscle Relaxant
NOVO20	Tab, Beige, D-Shaped, Novo/20	Famotidine 20 mg	Novo Famotidine by Novopharm	Canadian	Gastrointestinal
NOVO20	Cap, Green & Ivory, novo/20	Fluoxetine HCl 20 mg	by Novopharm	Canadian	Antidepressant
NOVO20	Tab, Light Blue, Oblong, Novo/20	Timolol Maleate 20 mg	Novo Timol by Novopharm	Canadian	Antihypertensive
NOVO200	Cap, Scarlet, Novo/200	Mexiletine HCl 200 mg	by Novopharm	Canadian	Antiarrhythmic

ID FRONT <> BACK	DESCRIPTION FRONT <> BACK	INGREDIENT & STRENGTH	BRAND (OR EQUIV.) & FIRM	NDC#	CLASS; SCH.
NOVO200	Tab, White, Round	Sulfinpyrazone 200 mg	Novo Pyrazone by Novopharm	Canadian	Uricosuric
NOVO200	Tab, White, Oval, Novo/200	Theophylline Anhydrous 200 mg	by Novopharm	Canadian	Antiasthmatic
NOVO200	Tab, White, Novo/200	Tiaprofenic Acid 200 mg	by Novopharm	Canadian	NSAID
NOVO25	Tab, Yellow, Round, Novo/25	Desipramine 25 mg	by Novopharm	Canadian	Antidepressant
NOVO25	Tab, White, Round, Novo/2.5	Glyburide 2.5 mg	Novo Glyburide by Novopharm	Canadian	Antidiabetic
NOVO25	Cap, Opaque	Indomethacin 25 mg	Novo Methacin by Novopharm	Canadian	NSAID
NOVO25	Tab, Orange, Round, Novo/25	Maprotiline HCl 25 mg	Novo Maprotiline by Novopharm	Canadian	Antidepressant
NOVO25	Tab, Peach, Round, Novo/2.5	Medroxyprogesterone Acetate 2.5 mg	by Novopharm	Canadian	Progestin
NOVO25	Tab, Cream, Round, Novo/25	Spironolactone 25 mg	Novo Spiroton by Novopharm	Canadian	Diuretic
NOVO250	Tab, Orange, Oblong, novo/250	Cephalexin 250 mg	Novo Lexin by Novopharm	Canadian	Antibiotic
NOVO250	Tab, Peach, Oblong, Novo/250	Diflunisal 250 mg	Novo Diflunisal by Novopharm	Canadian	NSAID
NOVO250	Tab, Light Yellow, Round, novo/250	Flutamide 250 mg	by Novopharm	Canadian	Antiandrogen
NOVO250	Tab, Yellow, Round, Novo/250	Methyldopa 250 mg	by Novopharm	Canadian	Antihypertensive
NOVO250	Tab, Yellow, Oval	Naproxen 250 mg	Novo Naprox by Novopharm	Canadian	NSAID
NOVO250	Cap, Orange & Yellow	Tetracycline HCl 250 mg	Novo Tetra by Novopharm	Canadian	Antibiotic
NOVO25MG	Cap, Blue & Pink	Doxepin HCl 25 mg	Novo Doxepin by Novopharm	Canadian	Antidepressant
NOVO275	Tab, Blue, Oblong	Naproxen Sodium 275 mg	Novo Naprox Sod by Novopharm	Canadian	NSAID
NOVO288 <> APISBULL	Tab, White, Round, Film Coated	Estradiol 1 mg; Norethindrone Acetate 0.5 mg	Activella by Novo Nordisk	00420-5174	Hormone
NOVO288 <> APISBULL	Tab, White, Round, Film Coated	Estradiol 1 mg; Norethindrone Acetate 0.5 mg	Activella by Pharmacia & Upjohn	00009-5174	Hormone
NOVO2MG	Tab, Light Green, Oblong, Novo/2 mg	Loperamide HCl 2 mg	Novo Loperamide by Novopharm	Canadian	Antidiarrheal
NOVO3	Tab, Pink, Round, novo/3	Bromazepam 3 mg	by Novopharm	Canadian	Sedative
NOVO30	Tab, Green, Round, Novo/30	Diltiazem HCl 30 mg	Novo Diltiazem by Novopharm	Canadian	Antihypertensive
NOVO30	Cap, Blue & Maroon, Novo/30	Temazepam 30 mg	by Novopharm	Canadian	Sedative/Hypnotic
NOVO300	Tab, White, Oblong, Novo/300	Theophylline Anhydrous 300 mg	by Novopharm	Canadian	Antiasthmatic
NOVO300	Tab, White, Novo/300	Tiaprofenic Acid 300 mg	by Novopharm	Canadian	NSAID
NOVO375	Tab, Peach, Oblong	Naproxen 375 mg	Novo Naprox by Novopharm	Canadian	NSAID
NOVO40	Tab, Brown & Orange, D-Shaped, novo/40	Famotidine 40 mg	Novo Famotidine by Novopharm	Canadian	Gastrointestinal
NOVO40	Tab, White, Round, Novo/40	Nadolol 40 mg	Novo Nadolol by Novopharm	Canadian	Antihypertensive
NOVO400	Cap, Opaque & Orange, Novo/400	Tolmetin Sodium 400 mg	Novo Tripramine by Novopharm	Canadian	NSAID
NOVO5	Tab, White, Oblong, Novo/5	Glyburide 5 mg	Novo Glyburide by Novopharm	Canadian	Antidiabetic
NOVO5	Tab, Blue, Round, Novo/5	Medroxyprogesterone Acetate 5 mg	by Novopharm	Canadian	Progestin
NOVO5	Tab, White, Round	Pindolol 5 mg	Novo Pindol by Novopharm	Canadian	Antihypertensive
NOVO5	Tab, White, Diamond, Novo/5	Prazosin HCl 5 mg	Novo Prazin by Novopharm	Canadian	Antihypertensive
NOVO5	Tab, White, Round, Novo/5	Timolol Maleate 5 mg	Novo Timol by Novopharm	Canadian	Antihypertensive
NOVO50	Tab, White, novo/50	Atenolol 50 mg	Novo Atenol by Novopharm	Canadian	Antihypertensive
NOVO50	Tab, White, Oval, novo/50	Captopril 50 mg	by Novopharm	Canadian	Antihypertensive
NOVO50	Tab, Green, Round, Novo/50	Desipramine 50 mg	by Novopharm	Canadian	Antidepressant
NOVO50	Tab, White, Oval, novo/50	Flurbiprofen 50 mg	Novo Flurprofen by Novopharm	Canadian	NSAID
NOVO50	Cap, Blue & White	Indomethacin 50 mg	Novo Methacin by Novopharm	Canadian	NSAID
NOVO50	Tab, Yellow, Round, Novo/50	Ketoprofen 50 mg	Novo Keto by Novopharm	Canadian	NSAID
NOVO50	Tab, Orange, Round, Novo/50	Maprotiline HCl 50 mg	Novo Maprotiline by Novopharm	Canadian	Antidepressant
NOVO50	Tab, Pink, Oblong	Metoprolol Tartrate 50 mg	Novo Metoprol by Novopharm	Canadian	Antihypertensive
NOVO50	Cap, Orange, Novo/50	Minocycline HCl 50 mg	by Novopharm	Canadian	Antibiotic
NOVO50	Tab, Pink, Round, Novo/50	Trimipramine Maleate 50 mg	Novo Tripramine by Novopharm	Canadian	Antidepressant
NOVO50	Tab, Light Orange, Round, Novo/50	Trazodone HCl 50 mg	Novo Trazadone by Novopharm	Canadian	Antidepressant
NOVO500	Tab, Orange, Oblong, novo/500	Cephalexin 500 mg	Novo Lexin by Novopharm	Canadian	Antibiotic
NOVO500	Tab, Orange, Oblong, Novo/500	Diflunisal 500 mg	Novo Diflunisal by Novopharm	Canadian	NSAID
NOVO500	Tab, Yellow, Round, Novo/500	Methyldopa 500 mg	by Novopharm	Canadian	Antihypertensive
NOVO500	Tab, Yellow, Oval	Naproxen 500 mg	Novo Naprox by Novopharm	Canadian	NSAID
NOVO50MG	Cap, Pink	Doxepin HCl 50 mg	Novo Doxepin by Novopharm	Canadian	Antidepressant
NOVO6	Tab, Green, Round, novo/6	Bromazepam 6 mg	by Novopharm	Canadian	Sedative
NOVO60	Tab, Yellow, Round, Novo/60	Diltiazem HCl 60 mg	Novo Diltiazem by Novopharm	Canadian	Antihypertensive

ID FRONT <> BACK	DESCRIPTION FRONT <> BACK	INGREDIENT & STRENGTH	BRAND (OR EQUIV.) & FIRM	NDC#	CLASS; SCH.
NOVO600	Tab, White, Oval, Novo/600	Gemfibrozil 600 mg	by Novopharm	Canadian	Antihyperlipidemic
NOVO75	Tab, Orange, Round, Novo/75	Desipramine 75 mg	by Novopharm	Canadian	Antidepressant
NOVO75	Tab, Orange & Red, Round, Novo/75	Maprotiline HCl 75 mg	Novo Maprotiline by Novopharm	Canadian	Antidepressant
NOVO75MG	Cap, Pink	Doxepin HCl 75 mg	Novo Doxepin by Novopharm	Canadian	Antidepressant
NOVO80	Tab, White, Round, Novo/80	Nadolol 80 mg	Novo Nadolol by Novopharm	Canadian	Antihypertensive
NOVO80	Tab, Light Blue, Oblong, Novo/80	Sotalol HCl 80 mg	by Novopharm	Canadian	Antiarrhythmic
NOVO80	Tab, Yellow, Round	Verapamil HCl 80 mg	Novo Veramil by Novopharm	Canadian	Antihypertensive
NOVOl	Tab, White, Round, Novo/l	Ketotifen Fumarate 1.38 mg	by Novopharm	Canadian	Antiasthmatic
NP	Tab	Ascorbic Acid 60 mg, Biotin 300 mcg, Calcium Pantothenate, Cyanocobalamin 6 mcg, Folic Acid 1 mg, Niacinamide 20 mg, Pyridoxine HCl 10 mg, Riboflavin 1.7 mg, Thiamine Mononitrate 1.5 mg	Nephplex Rx by Nephro Tech	59528-0317	Vitamin
NP	Tab, N-P	Ascorbic Acid 60 mg, Biotin 300 mcg, Calcium Pantothenate, Cyanocobalamin 6 mcg, Folic Acid 1 mg, Niacinamide 20 mg, Pyridoxine HCl 10 mg, Riboflavin 1.7 mg, Thiamine Mononitrate 1.5 mg	Nephplex Rx by Anabolic	00722-6396	Vitamin
NPL430	Tab, White, Round	Chlorpheniramine Maleate 4 mg, Pseudoephedrine HCl 60 mg	Deconamine by Nutripharm Labs, Inc.		Cold Remedy
NPL510	Tab, White	Carbinoxamine Maleate 4 mg, Pseudoephedrine 60 mg	Carbiset by Nutripharm Labs, Inc.		Cold Remedy
NPL51081424	Cap, White, NPL 51081/424	Isometheptene 65 mg, Dichloralphenzaone 100 mg, Acetaminophen 325 mg	Isocom by Nutripharm Labs, Inc.		Analgesic
NPL512	Tab, White	Carbinoxamine Maleate 8 mg, Pseudoephedrine 120 mg	Carbiset-TR by Nutripharm Labs, Inc.		Cold Remedy
NPREC250	Tab, Round	Naproxen 250 mg	Naprosyn E by Roche	Canadian	NSAID
NPREC375	Tab, Oval	Naproxen 375 mg	Naprosyn E by Roche	Canadian	NSAID
NPREC500	Tab, Oblong	Naproxen 500 mg	Naprosyn E by Roche	Canadian	NSAID
NPRLE250	Tab, Yellow, Oval	Naproxen 250 mg	Naprosyn by Roche	Canadian	NSAID
NPRLE375	Tab, Pink, Oval	Naproxen 375 mg	Naprosyn by Roche	Canadian	NSAID
NPRLE500	Tab, Yellow, Oblong	Naproxen 500 mg	Naprosyn by Roche	Canadian	NSAID
NPRSR750	Tab, Peach, Oval	Naproxen 750 mg	by Roche	Canadian	NSAID
NPS275	Tab, Blue, Oval, NPS-275	Naprosyn Sodium 275 mg	Anaprox by Roche	Canadian	NSAID
NPS550	Tab, Dark Blue, Oblong, NPS-550	Naprosyn Sodium 550 mg	Anaprox DS by Roche	Canadian	NSAID
NR	Tab, Delayed Release, Abbott Logo	Divalproex Sodium	Depakote by Amerisource	62584-0356	Anticonvulsant
NR	Tab, Delayed Release, Logo NR	Divalproex Sodium	Depakote by Quality Care	62682-7028	Anticonvulsant
NR	Tab, Peach, Oval, NR over Abbott Logo	Divalproex Sodium 250 mg	Depakote by Abbott	00074-6214	Anticonvulsant
NRV 5PFIZER	Tab, White, Octagonal	Amlodipine Besylate 5 mg	by Pfizer	Canadian	Antihypertensive
NRV10 <> PFIZER	Tab, White, Octagonal	Amiodipine 10 mg	Norvasc by Pfizer	Canadian DIN# 00878936	Antihypertensive
NRV10PFIZER	Tab, White, Octagonal, NRV 10/Pfizer	Amlodipine Besylate 10 mg	by Pfizer	Canadian	Antihypertensive
NRV5 <> PFIZER	Tab, White, Octagonal, Scored	Amiodipine 5 mg	Norvasc by Pfizer	Canadian DIN# 00878928	Antihypertensive
NS	Tab, Lavender, Oval, NS over Abbott Logo	Divalproex Sodium 500 mg	Depakote by Abbott	00074-6215	Anticonvulsant
NT	Tab, N/T	Ascorbic Acid 40 mg, Biotin 300 mcg, Cyanocobalamin 6 mcg, Docusate Sodium 75 mg, Ferrous Fumarate 200 mg, Folic Acid 1 mg, Niacinamide 20 mg, Pantothenic Acid 10 mg, Pyridoxine HCl 10 mg, Riboflavin 1.7 mg, Thiamine Mononitrate 1.5 mg	Nephron Fa by Anabolic	00722-6392	Vitamin
NT	Tab, Salmon Pink, Oval, NT over Abbott Logo	Divalproex Sodium 125 mg	Depakote by Abbott	00074-6212	Anticonvulsant
NT	Tab	Divalproex Sodium 125 mg	Depakote by Allscripts	54569-4134	Anticonvulsant
NT <> V	Tab, N/T	Ascorbic Acid 40 mg, Biotin 300 mcg, Cyanocobalamin 6 mcg, Docusate Sodium 75 mg, Ferrous Fumarate 200 mg, Folic Acid 1 mg, Niacinamide 20 mg, Pantothenic Acid 10 mg, Pyridoxine HCl 10 mg, Riboflavin 1.7 mg, Thiamine Mononitrate 1.5 mg	Nephron Fa by Nephro Tech	59528-4456	Vitamin
NT112 <> JMI	Tab, NT Over 1 1/2	Thyroid 97.2 mg	Nature Thyroid by JMI Canton	00252-3304	Thyroid
NT112 <> JMI	Tab, NT Over 1 1/2	Thyroid 97.2 mg	Nature Thyroid by Jones	52604-3304	Thyroid
NT12 <> JMI	Tab, NT Over 1/2	Thyroid 32.4 mg	Nature Thyroid by JMI Canton	00252-3299	Thyroid

ID FRONT <> BACK	DESCRIPTION FRONT <> BACK	INGREDIENT & STRENGTH	BRAND (OR EQUIV.) & FIRM	NDC#	CLASS; SCH.
NT12 <> JMI	Tab, NT Over 1/2	Thyroid 32.4 mg	Nature Thyroid by Jones	52604-3299	Thyroid
NT3 <> JMI	Tab	Thyroid 3 gr	Nature Thyroid by Jones	52604-3312	Thyroid
NTRDUPONT	Tab, Orange, Round, NTR/DuPont	Naltrexone HCl 50 mg	Revia by DuPont Pharma	Canadian	Opiod Antagonist
NU <> 05	Tab, White, Round, NU <> 0.5	Lorazepam 0.5 mg	by Nu-Pharm	Canadian DIN# 00865672	Sedative/Hypnotic
NU <> 10	Tab, White, Round, Film Coated	Domperidone Maleate 10 mg	by Nu Pharm	Canadian DIN# 02231477	Gastrointestinal
NU <> 10	Tab, Grayish-Pink, Round, Film Coated	Nifedipine 10 mg	by Nu Pharm	Canadian DIN# 02212102	Antihypertensive
NU <> 100	Tab, White, Oval, Film Coated	Fluvoxamine Maleate 100 mg	by Nu Pharm	Canadian DIN# 02231193	OCD
NU <> 10010	Tab, Blue, Oval, Scored, NU <> 100 over 10	Carbidopa 10 mg, Levodopa 100 mg	by Nu Pharm	Canadian DIN# 02182831	Antiparkinson
NU <> 125	Tab, White, Cap Shaped, Scored, NU <> 12.5	Captopril 12.5 mg	Nu Capto by Nu-Pharm	Canadian DIN# 01913824	Antihypertensive
NU <> 20	Tab, Grayish-Pink, Round, Film Coated	Nifedipine 20 mg	by Nu Pharm	Canadian DIN# 02200937	Antihypertensive
NU <> 250	Tab, White, Oval	Ticlopidine HCl 250 mg	by Nu Pharm	Canadian DIN# 02237560	Anticoagulant
NU <> 25025	Tab, Blue, Oval, Scored, NU <> 250 over 50	Carbidopa 25 mg, Levodopa 250 mg	by Nu Pharm	Canadian DIN# 02182831	Antiparkinson
NU <> 400	Tab, Pink, Cap Shaped	Pentoxifylline 400 mg	by Nu Pharm	Canadian DIN# 02230401	Anticoagulent
NU <> 50	Tab, White, Round, Film Coated	Fluvoxamine Maleate 50 mg	by Nu Pharm	Canadian DIN# 02231192	OCD
NU <> 850	Tab, White, Cap Shaped	Meftormin HCl 850 mg	by Nu Pharm	Canadian DIN# 02229517	Antidiabetic
NU <> BU10	Tab, White, Rectangular, Scored	Buspirone 10 mg	by Nu Pharm	Canadian DIN# 02207672	Antianxiety
NU <> D500	Tab, Orange, Cap Shaped, Film Coated	Diflusinal 500 mg	by Nu Pharm	Canadian DIN# 02058413	NSAID
NU <> LOX10	Tab, Green, Round, Film Coated, Scored, NU <> Lox over 10	Loxapine Succinate 10 mg	by Nu Pharm	Canadian DIN# 02237535	Antipsychotic
NU <> LOX25	Tab, Pink, Round, Film Coated, Scored, NU <> Lox over 25	Loxapine Succinate 25 mg	by Nu Pharm	Canadian DIN# 02237535	Antipsychotic

ID FRONT <> BACK	DESCRIPTION FRONT <> BACK	INGREDIENT & STRENGTH	BRAND (OR EQUIV.) & FIRM	NDC#	CLASS; SCH.
NU <> LOX5	Tab, Yellow, Round, Film Coated, Scored, NU <> Lox over 5	Loxapine Succinate 5 mg	by Nu Pharm	Canadian DIN# 02237534	Antipsychotic
NU <> LOX50	Tab, White, Round, Film Coated, Scored, NU <> Lox over 50	Loxapine Succinate 50 mg	by Nu Pharm	Canadian DIN# 02237536	Antipsychotic
NU <> T1	Tab, White, Round	Terazosin HCl 1 mg	by Nu Pharm	Canadian DIN# 02233047	Antihypertensive
NU <> T10	Tab, Blue, Round	Terazosin HCl 10 mg	by Nu Pharm	Canadian DIN# 02233050	Antihypertensive
NU <> T2	Tab, Orange, Round	Terazosin HCl 2 mg	by Nu Pharm	Canadian DIN# 02233048	Antihypertensive
NU <> T5	Tab, Tan, Round	Terazosin HCl 5 mg	by Nu Pharm	Canadian DIN# 02233049	Antihypertensive
NU 500	Tab, Orange, Oblong	Diflunisal 500 mg	by Nu-Pharm	Canadian	NSAID
NU01	Tab, White, Round, Scored, NU over 0.1	Clonidine 0.1 mg	by Nu Pharm	Canadian DIN# 01913786	Antihypertensive
NU01	Tab, White, Round, NU/0.1	Clonidine HCl 0.1 mg	Nu Clonidine by Nu-Pharm	Canadian	Antihypertensive
NU02	Tab, Orange, Round, Scored, NU over 0.2	Clonidine 0.2 mg	by Nu Pharm	Canadian DIN# 01913220	Antihypertensive
NU02	Tab, Orange, Round, N NU/0.2	Clonidine HCl 0.2 mg	Nu Clonidine by Nu-Pharm	Canadian	Antihypertensive
NU05	Tab, Peach, Oval, Scored, NU over 0.5	Alprazolam 0.5 mg	Nu Alpraz by Nu-Pharm	Canadian DIN# 01913247	Antianxiety
NU1	Tab, White, Cap Shaped, Scored, NU over 1	Lorazepam 1 mg	by Nu-Pharm	Canadian DIN# 00865680	Sedative/Hypnotic
NU1	Tab, Peach, Cap Shaped, Scored	Prazosin HCl 1 mg	Nu Prazo by Nu-Pharm	Canadian DIN# 01913794	Antihypertensive
NU10	Tab, White to Off-White, Oval, Scored	Baclofen 10 mg	by Nu-Pharm	Canadian DIN# 02136090	Muscle Relaxant
NU10	Tab, Yellow, D-Shaped, Film Coated, NU over 10	Cyclobenzaprine HCl 10 mg	by Nu Pharm	Canadian DIN# 002171848	Muscle Relaxant
NU10	Cap, Gray & Light Green, Opaque, Gelatin	Fluoxetine HCl 10 mg	by Nu Pharm	Canadian DIN# 02192756	Antidepressant
NU10	Tab, Yellow, Round, Scored, NU over 10	Hydralazine HCl 10 mg	by Nu Pharm	Canadian DIN# 01913204	Antihypertensive
NU10	Tab, White, Round, Film Coated, NU over 10	Ketorolac Tromethamine 10 mg	by Nu Pharm	Canadian DIN# 02237910	NSAID

ID FRONT <> BACK	DESCRIPTION FRONT <> BACK	INGREDIENT & STRENGTH	BRAND (OR EQUIV.) & FIRM	NDC#	CLASS; SCH.
NU10	Cap, Dark Yellow, Gelatin	Nifedipine 10 mg	Nu Nifed by Nu-Pharm	Canadian DIN# 00865591	Antihypertensive
NU10	Cap, White & Yellow, Opaque, Gelatin	Nortriptyline HCl 10 mg	by Nu Pharm	Canadian DIN# 02223139	Antidepressant
NU10	Tab, White, Round, Scored, NU over 10	Pindolol 10 mg	Nu Pindol by Nu-Pharm	Canadian DIN# 00886009	Antihypertensive
NU10	Tab, Peachish Orange, Round, Film Coated, NU over 10	Prochlorperazine 10 mg	Nu Prochlor by Nu-Pharm	Canadian DIN# 01964402	Antiemetic
NU10	Cap, Blue & Maroon, Gelatin	Piroxicam 10 mg	Nu Pirox by Nu-Pharm	Canadian DIN# 00865761	NSAID
NU10	Tab, Orange, Round, NU/10	Propranolol HCl 10 mg	Nu Propanolol by Nu-Pharm	Canadian	Antihypertensive
NU10	Tab, Light Blue, Round, Scored, NU over 10	Timolol Maleate 10 mg	Nu Timolol by Nu-Pharm	Canadian DIN# 02044617	Antihypertensive
NU100	Tab, White, Round, Film Coated, Scored, NU over 100	Acebutolol HCl 100 mg	by Nu Pharm	Canadian DIN# 02165546	Antihypertensive
NU100	Tab, White, Round, Scored, NU over 100	Atenolol 100 mg	Nu Atenol by Nu-Pharm	Canadian DIN# 00886122	Antihypertensive
NU100	Tab, White, Oval, Scored	Captopril 100 mg	Nu Capto by Nu-Pharm	Canadian DIN# 01913859	Antihypertensive
NU100	Cap, Blue, Opaque, Gelatin	Doxycycline Hyclate 100 mg	by Nu-Pharm	Canadian DIN# 02044668	Antibiotic
NU100	Tab, Light Orange, Round, Film Coated, NU over 100	Doxycycline Hyclate 100 mg	by Nu-Pharm	Canadian DIN# 02044676	Antibiotic
NU100	Tab, Blue, Oval	Flurbiprofen 100 mg	by Nu-Pharm	Canadian	NSAID
NU100	Cap, White, Opaque, Gelatin	Fenofibrate 100 mg	by Nu Pharm	Canadian DIN# 02223600	Antihyperlipidemic
NU100	Tab, Blue, Oval, Film Coated, NU over 100	Flurbiprofen 100 mg	by Nu-Pharm	Canadian DIN# 02020688	NSAID
NU100	Tab, Orange, Oval, Film Coated, Scored, NU over 100	Moclobemide 100 mg	by Nu Pharm	Canadian DIN# 02237111	Antidepressant
NU100	Tab, White, Round, Scored, NU over 100	Sulfinpyrazone 100 mg	Nu Sulfinpyrazone by Nu-Pharm	Canadian DIN# 02045680	Uricosuric
NU100	Tab, Pink, Round, NU/100	Trimipramine Maleate 100 mg	by Nu-Pharm	Canadian	Antidepressant
NU120	Cap, Light Turquoise, Opaque, Gelatin	Diltiazem HCl 120 mg	by Nu Pharm	Canadian DIN# 02231052	Antihypertensive
NU120	Tab, Rose, Round, NU/120	Propranolol HCl 120 mg	Nu Propanolol by Nu-Pharm	Canadian	Antihypertensive

ID FRONT <> BACK	DESCRIPTION FRONT <> BACK	INGREDIENT & STRENGTH	BRAND (OR EQUIV.) & FIRM	NDC#	CLASS; SCH.
NU120	Tab, White, Round, Film Coated, NU over 120	Verapamil HCl 120 mg	by Nu-Pharm	Canadian DIN# 00886041	Antihypertensive
NU125	Tab, Yellow, Round, NU/125	Methyldopa 125 mg	by Nu-Pharm	Canadian	Antihypertensive
NU125	Tab, Green, Oval, NU-125	Naproxen 125 mg	Nu Naprox by Nu-Pharm	Canadian	NSAID
NU15	Tab, White, Round, Scored, NU over 15	Pindolol 15 mg	Nu Pindol by Nu-Pharm	Canadian DIN# 00886130	Antihypertensive
NU15	Cap, Maroon & Pink, Opaque, Gelatin	Temazepam 15 mg	by Nu Pharm	Canadian DIN# 02223570	Sedative/Hypnotic
NU150	Tab, Pale Yellow, Oval, Film Coated, Scored, NU over 150	Moclobemide 150 mg	by Nu Pharm	Canadian DIN# 02237112	Antidepressant
NU150	Tab, White, Round, Film Coated, NU over 150	Ranitidine HCl 150 mg	Nu Ranit by Nu-Pharm	Canadian DIN# 00865737	Gastrointestinal
NU150	Tab, Dark Yellow, Hexagonal, Scored, NU over 150	Sulindac 150 mg	by Nu-Pharm	Canadian DIN# 02042576	NSAID
NU150 <> 50252550	Tab, Pale Orange, Rectangular, Scored, NU-150 <> 50 over 25 over 25 over 50	Trazodone HCl 150 mg	by Nu Pharm	Canadian DIN# 02165406	Antidepressant
NU160	Tab, White, Oval, Scored	Megesterol Acetate 160 mg	by Nu Pharm	Canadian DIN# 02185423	Progestin
NU160	Tab, Blue, Cap Shaped, NU-160	Sotalol 160 mg	by Nu Pharm	Canadian DIN# 02163772	Antiarrhythmic
NU180	Cap, Light Blue & Turquoise, Opaque, Gelatin	Diltiazem HCl 180 mg	by Nu Pharm	Canadian DIN# 02231053	Antihypertensive
NU1G	Tab, White, Cap Shaped, Scored, NU-1g	Sucralfate 1 g	by Nu Pharm	Canadian DIN# 02134829	Gastrointestinal
NU2	Tab, White, Oval, Scored	Lorazepam 2 mg	by Nu-Pharm	Canadian DIN# 00865699	Sedative/Hypnotic
NU2	Tab, White, Round, Scored, NU over 2	Prazosin HCl 2 mg	Nu Prazo by Nu-Pharm	Canadian DIN# 01913808	Antihypertensive
NU20	Tab, White to Off-White, Oval, Scored	Baclofen 20 mg	by Nu-Pharm	Canadian DIN# 02136104	Muscle Relaxant
NU20	Tab, Beige, D-Shaped, Film Coated, NU over 20	Famotidine 20 mg	by Nu-Pharm	Canadian DIN# 02024195	Gastrointestinal
NU20	Cap, Green & Ivory, Opaque, Gelatin	Fluoxetine HCl 20 mg	by Nu Pharm	Canadian DIN# 02192764	Antidepressant

ID FRONT <> BACK	DESCRIPTION FRONT <> BACK	INGREDIENT & STRENGTH	BRAND (OR EQUIV.) & FIRM	NDC#	CLASS; SCH.
NU20	Cap, Maroon, Gelatin	Piroxicam 20 mg	Nu Pirox by Nu-Pharm	Canadian DIN# 00865788	NSAID
NU20	Tab, Blue, Hexagonal, Scored, NU over 20	Propranolol HCl 20 mg	Nu Propanolol by Nu-Pharm	Canadian DIN# 02044692	Antihypertensive
NU20	Tab, Light Blue, Oblong, NU/20	Timolol Maleate 20 mg	Nu Timolol by Nu-Pharm	Canadian	Antihypertensive
NU200	Tab, White, Oval, Film Coated, Scored	Acebutolol HCl 200 mg	by Nu Pharm	Canadian DIN# 02165554	Antihypertensive
NU200	Tab, Blue, Round, NU over 200	Acyclovir 200 mg	by Nu Pharm	Canadian DIN# 02197405	Antiviral
NU200	Tab, White, Round, Scored	Carbamazepine 200 mg	by Taro	Canadian DIN# 02042568	Anticonvulsant
NU200	Tab, Pale Green, Round, Film Coated, NU over 200	Cimetidine 200 mg	Nu Cimet by Nu-Pharm	Canadian DIN# 00865796	Gastrointestinal
NU200	Tab, White, Round, Scored, NU over 200	Sulfinpyrazone 200 mg	Nu Sulfinpyrazone by Nu-Pharm	Canadian DIN# 02045699	Uricosuric
NU200	Tab, Dark Yellow, Hexagonal, Scored, NU over 200	Sulindac 200 mg	by Nu-Pharm	Canadian DIN# 02042584	NSAID
NU240	Cap, Light Blue, Opaque, Gelatin	Diltiazem HCl 240 mg	by Nu Pharm	Canadian DIN# 02231054	Antihypertensive
NU25	Tab, White, Oval, Scored, NU over .25	Alprazolam 0.25 mg	Nu Alpraz by Nu-Pharm	Canadian DIN# 01913239	Antianxiety
NU25	Tab, White, Square, Quadrisected, NU over 25	Captopril 25 mg	Nu Capto by Nu-Pharm	Canadian DIN# 01913832	Antihypertensive
NU25	Tab, Yellow, Barrel Shaped, Scored, NU over 2.5	Enalapril Maleate 2.5 mg	by Nu Pharm	Canadian DIN# 02239498	Antihypertensive
NU25	Tab, White, Round, Scored, NU over 2.5	Glyburide 2.5 mg	by Nu-Pharm	Canadian DIN# 02020734	Antidiabetic
NU25	Cap, Blue & White, Opaque, Gelatin	Indomethacin 25 mg	by Nu-Pharm	Canadian DIN# 00865850	NSAID
NU25	Cap, White & Yellow, Opaque, Gelatin	Nortriptyline HCl 25 mg	by Nu Pharm	Canadian DIN# 02223147	Antidepressant
NU250	Cap, Gold & Red, Opaque, Gelatin	Amoxicillin Trihydrate 250 mg	Nu Amoxi by Nu-Pharm	Canadian DIN# 00865567	Antibiotic
NU250	Cap, Purple & White, Opaque, Gelatin	Cefaclor 250 mg	by Nu Pharm	Canadian DIN# 02231432	Antibiotic

ID FRONT <> BACK	DESCRIPTION FRONT <> BACK	INGREDIENT & STRENGTH	BRAND (OR EQUIV.) & FIRM	NDC#	CLASS; SCH.
NU250	Cap, Black & Red, Opaque, Gelatin	Ampicillin Trihydrate 250 mg	Nu Ampi by Nu-Pharm	Canadian DIN# 00717657	Antibiotic
NU250	Tab, Orange, Cap Shaped, Film Coated, NU-250	Cephalexin 250 mg	Nu Cephalex by Nu-Pharm	Canadian DIN# 00865877	Antibiotic
NU250	Cap, Black & Orange, Gelatin	Cloxacillin Sodium 250 mg	Nu Cloxi by Nu-Pharm	Canadian DIN# 00717584	Antibiotic
NU250	Tab, Orange, Oblong, NU-250	Diflunisal 250 mg	by Nu-Pharm	Canadian	NSAID
NU250	Tab, Bright Pink, Round, Film Coated, NU over 250	Erythromycin 250 mg	by Nu-Pharm	Canadian DIN# 02051850	Antibiotic
NU250	Cap, Blue & Yellow, Opaque, Gelatin	Mefenamic Acid 250 mg	by Nu Pharm	Canadian DIN# 02229569	NSAID
NU250	Tab, Yellow, Round, Film Coated	Methyldopa 250 mg	by Nu-Pharm	Canadian DIN# 00717509	Antihypertensive
NU250	Tab, Yellow, Oval, NU-250	Naproxen 250 mg	Nu Naprox by Nu-Pharm	Canadian DIN# 08865648	NSAID
NU250	Cap, Orange & Yellow, Opaque, Gelatin	Tetracycline HCl 250 mg	Nu Tetra by Nu-Pharm	Canadian DIN# 00717606	Antibiotic
NU30	Tab, Light Green, Round, Film Coated, NU over 30	Diltiazem HCl 30 mg	by Nu-Pharm	Canadian DIN# 00886068	Antihypertensive
NU30	Cap, Light Blue & Maroon, Opaque, Gelatin	Temazepam 30 mg	by Nu Pharm	Canadian DIN# 02223589	Sedative/Hypnotic
NU300	Tab, Pale Green, Round, Film Coated, NU over 300	Cimetidine 300 mg	Nu Cimet by Nu-Pharm	Canadian DIN# 00865818	Gastrointestinal
NU300	Cap, Maroon & White, Opaque, Gelatin	Gemfibrozil 300 mg	by Nu-Pharm	Canadian DIN# 02058456	Antihyperlipidemic
NU300	Tab, White, Round, Film Coated, NU over 300	Ibuprofen 300 mg	by Nu-Pharm	Canadian DIN# 02020696	NSAID
NU300	Tab, Orange, Round, Film Coated, NU over 300	Penicillan V Potassium 300 mg	by Nu-Pharm	Canadian DIN# 00717568	Antibiotic
NU300	Tab, White, Cap Shaped, Film Coated	Ranitidine 300 mg	Nu Ranit by Nu-Pharm	Canadian DIN# 00865745	Gastrointestinal
NU300	Tab, White, Round, Film Coated, Scored, NU over 300	Tiaprofenic Acid 300 mg	by Nu Pharm	Canadian DIN# 02146886	NSAID
NU375	Tab, Peach, Cap Shaped, Scored	Naproxen 375 mg	Nu Naprox by Nu-Pharm	Canadian DIN# 00865656	NSAID

ID FRONT <> BACK	DESCRIPTION FRONT <> BACK	INGREDIENT & STRENGTH	BRAND (OR EQUIV.) & FIRM	NDC#	CLASS; SCH.
NU40	Tab, Light Brown, D-Shaped, Film Coated, NU over 40	Famotidine 40 mg	by Nu-Pharm	Canadian DIN# 02024209	Gastrointestinal
NU40	Tab, Light Blue, Round, Scored, NU over 40	Megesterol Acetate 40 mg	by Nu Pharm	Canadian DIN# 02185415	Progestin
NU40	Tab, Green, Round, NU/40	Propranolol HCl 40 mg	Nu Propanolol by Nu-Pharm	Canadian	Antihypertensive
NU400	Tab, White, Cap Shaped, Film Coated, Scored	Acebutolol HCl 200 mg	by Nu Pharm	Canadian DIN# 02165562	Antihypertensive
NU400	Tab, Pink, Round, NU over 400	Acyclovir 400 mg	by Nu Pharm	Canadian DIN# 02197413	Antiviral
NU400	Tab, Pale Green, Oblong, Film Coated, NU-400	Cimetidine 400 mg	Nu Cimet by Nu-Pharm	Canadian DIN# 00865826	Gastrointestinal
NU400	Tab, Orange, Round, Film Coated, NU over 400	Ibuprofen 400 mg	by Nu-Pharm	Canadian DIN# 02020718	NSAID
NU40080	Tab, White, Round, Scored, NU over 400-80	Sulfamethoxazole 400 mg, Trimethoprim 80 mg	Nu Cotrimix by Nu-Pharm	Canadian DIN# 00865753	Antibiotic
NU5	Tab, White, Cap Shaped, Scored	Glyburide 5 mg	by Nu-Pharm	Canadian DIN# 02020742	Antidiabetic
NU5	Tab, White, Round, Scored, NU over 5	Pindolol 5 mg	Nu-Pindol by Nu-Pharm	Canadian DIN# 00886149	Antihypertensive
NU5	Tab, Blue, Round, Scored, NU over 5	Oxybutynin Chloride 5 mg	by Nu Pharm	Canadian DIN# 02158590	Urinary
NU5	Tab, Peachish Orange, Round, Film Coated, NU over 5	Prochlorperazine Maleate 5 mg	Nu Prochlor by Nu-Pharm	Canadian DIN# 01964399	Antiemetic
NU5	Tab, White, Diamond Shaped, Scored, NU over 5	Prazosin HCl 5 mg	Nu Prazo by Nu-Pharm	Canadian DIN# 01913816	Antihypertensive
NU50	Tab, White, Round, Scored, NU over 50	Atenolol 50 mg	Nu Atenol by Nu-Pharm	Canadian DIN# 00886114	Antihypertensive
NU50	Tab, White, Oval, Scored, NU-50	Captopril 50 mg	Nu Capto by Nu-Pharm	Canadian DIN# 01913840	Antihypertensive
NU50	Tab, White, Oval, Film Coated, NU over 50	Flurbiprofen 50 mg	by Nu-Pharm	Canadian DIN# 02020661	NSAID
NU50	Cap, Blue & White, Opaque, Gelatin	Indomethacin 50 mg	by Nu-Pharm	Canadian DIN# 00865869	NSAID
NU50	Cap, Green & Ivory, NU-50	Ketoprofen 50 mg	by Nu-Pharm	Canadian	NSAID
NU50	Tab, Pink, Round, NU/50	Trimipramine Maleate 50 mg	by Nu-Pharm	Canadian	Antidepressant

ID FRONT <> BACK	DESCRIPTION FRONT <> BACK	INGREDIENT & STRENGTH	BRAND (OR EQUIV.) & FIRM	NDC#	CLASS; SCH.
NU500	Cap, Gold & Red, Opaque, Gelatin	Amoxicillin Trihydrate 500 mg	Nu Amoxi by Nu-Pharm	Canadian DIN# 00865575	Antibiotic
NU500	Cap, Black & Red, Opaque, Gelatin	Ampicillin Trihydrate 500 mg	Nu Ampi by Nu-Pharm	Canadian DIN# 00717673	Antibiotic
NU500	Cap, Gray & Purple, Opaque, Gelatin	Cefaclor 500 mg	by Nu Pharm	Canadian DIN# 02231433	Antibiotic
NU500	Tab, Orange, Cap Shaped, Film Coated, Scored, NU-500	Cephalexin 500 mg	Nu Cephalex by Nu-Pharm	Canadian DIN# 00865885	Antibiotic
NU500	Cap, Black & Orange, Gelatin	Cloxacillin Sodium 500 mg	Nu Cloxi by Nu-Pharm	Canadian DIN# 00717592	Antibiotic
NU500	Tab, Yellow, Round, Film Coated	Methyldopa 500 mg	by Nu-Pharm	Canadian DIN# 00717576	Antihypertensive
NU500	Tab, Yellow, Cap Shaped, Scored	Naproxen 500 mg	Nu Naprox by Nu-Pharm	Canadian DIN# 00865664	NSAID
NU550	Tab, Peach, Diamond Shaped, Scored, NU above score, 5/50 below score	Amiloride HCl 5 mg, Hydrochlorothiazide 50 mg	Nu Amilzide by Nu-Pharm	Canadian DIN# 00886106	Diuretic
NU60	Tab, Yellow, Round, Film Coated, Scored, NU over 60	Diltiazem HCl 60 mg	by Nu-Pharm	Canadian DIN# 00886076	Antihypertensive
NU600	Tab, Pale Green, Oblong, Film Coated, NU-600	Cimetidine 600 mg	Nu Cimet by Nu-Pharm	Canadian DIN# 00865834	Gastrointestinal
NU600	Tab, White, Oval, Film Coated, NU-600	Gemfibrozil 600 mg	by Nu-Pharm	Canadian DIN# 02058464	Antihyperlipidemic
NU600	Tab, Light Orange, Oval, Film Coated, NU-600	Ibuprofen 600 mg	by Nu-Pharm	Canadian DIN# 02020726	NSAID
NU75	Tab, Light Pink, Triangular, Film Coated, NU over 75	Diclofenac Sodium 75 mg	by Nu Pharm	Canadian DIN# 02228203	NSAID
NU75	Tab, Blue, Oval, Film Coated, Scored, NU 7.5	Zopiclone 7.5 mg	by Nu Pharm	Canadian DIN# 02228270	Hypnotic
NU80	Tab, Yellow, Round, NU/80	Propranolol HCl 80 mg	Nu Propanolol by Nu-Pharm	Canadian	Antihypertensive
NU80	Tab, Blue, Cap Shaped, NU-80	Sotalol 80 mg	by Nu Pharm	Canadian DIN# 02200996	Antiarrhythmic
NU80	Tab, Yellow, Round, Film Coated, NU over 80	Verapamil HCl 80 mg	by Nu-Pharm	Canadian DIN# 00886033	Antihypertensive
NU800	Tab, Blue, Oval, Scored	Acyclovir 800 mg	by Nu Pharm	Canadian DIN# 02197421	Antiviral

ID FRONT <> BACK	DESCRIPTION FRONT <> BACK	INGREDIENT & STRENGTH	BRAND (OR EQUIV.) & FIRM	NDC#	CLASS; SCH.
NUB15	Tab, White, Round, Scored, NU over B-1.5	Bromazepam 1.5 mg	by Nu Pharm	Canadian DIN# 02171856	Sedative
NUB3	Tab, Pink, Round, Scored, NU over B-3	Bromazepam 3 mg	by Nu Pharm	Canadian DIN# 02171864	Sedative
NUB6	Tab, Green, Round, Scored, NU over B-6	Bromazepam 6 mg	by Nu Pharm	Canadian DIN# 02171872	Sedative
NUC05	Tab, Orange, Round, Scored, NU over C-0.5	Clonazepam 0.5 mg	by Nu Pharm	Canadian DIN# 02173344	Anticonvulsant
NUC2	Tab, White, Round, Scored, NU over C-2	Clonazepam 2 mg	by Nu Pharm	Canadian DIN# 02173352	Anticonvulsant
NUDS	Tab, White, Cap Shaped, Scored, NU-DS	Sulfamethoxazole 800 mg, Trimethoprim 160 mg	Nu Cotrimix by Nu-Pharm	Canadian DIN# 00865729	Antibiotic
NUE10	Tab, White, Barrel Shaped, Scored, NU over E10	Enalapril Maleate 10 mg	by Nu Pharm	Canadian DIN# 02239500	Antihypertensive
NUE25	Tab, Dark Pink, Barrel Shaped, Scored, NU over E25	Enalapril Maleate 20 mg	by Nu Pharm	Canadian DIN# 02239501	Antihypertensive
NUE5	Tab, White, Barrel Shaped, Scored, NU over E5	Enalapril Maleate 5 mg	by Nu Pharm	Canadian DIN# 02239599	Antihypertensive
NUIRON1500291	Tab, Red & White, Oblong	Elemental Iron 150 mg	Nu Iron 150 by Merz		Mineral
NUM10	Tab, White, Round, NU over M10	Metoclopramide HCl 10 mg	by Nu-Pharm	Canadian DIN# 02143283	Gastrointestinal
NUM5	Tab, White, Square, NU over M5	Metoclopramide HCl 5 mg	by Nu-Pharm	Canadian DIN# 02143275	Gastrointestinal
NUM500	Tab, White, Round, Scored, NU over M500	Meftormin HCl 500 mg	by Nu Pharm	Canadian DIN# 02162822	Antidiabetic
NUMARK <> 1039	Tab, Soluble	Chlorpheniramine Maleate 4 mg, Phenylephrine HCl 10 mg, Phenylpropanolamine HCl 50 mg, Pyrilamine Maleate 25 mg	Histalet Forte by Numark	55499-1039	Cold Remedy; C III
NUMARK <> 1039	Tab, Soluble, Numark <> 10/39	Chlorpheniramine Maleate 4 mg, Phenylephrine HCl 10 mg, Phenylpropanolamine HCl 50 mg, Pyrilamine Maleate 25 mg	by Mikart	46672-0021	Cold Remedy; C III
NUMARK <> 1091	Tab	Hydrocodone Bitartrate 5 mg, Pseudoephedrine HCl 60 mg	P V Tussin by Numark	55499-1091	Analgesic; C III
NUMARK <> 1091	Tab, 10/91	Hydrocodone Bitartrate 5 mg, Pseudoephedrine HCl 60 mg	by Mikart	46672-0133	Analgesic; C III
NUMARK1050	Tab	Guaifenesin 400 mg, Pseudoephedrine HCl 120 mg	Histalet X by Numark	55499-1050	Cold Remedy
NUMARK1050	Tab	Guaifenesin 400 mg, Pseudoephedrine HCl 120 mg	by Mikart	46672-0162	Cold Remedy
NUMARK1082	Cap, Orange, Coated	Phendimetrazine Tartrate 105 mg	Melfiat 105 by Eon	00185-2053	Anorexiant; C III
NUMARK1082	Cap, Coated	Phendimetrazine Tartrate 105 mg	Melifiat 105 by Numark	55499-1082	Anorexiant; C III
NUT	Tab, Light Orange, Round, Scored, NU over T	Triamterene 50 mg, Hydrochlorothiazide 25 mg	by Nu-Pharm	Canadian DIN# 00865532	Diuretic

ID FRONT <> BACK	DESCRIPTION FRONT <> BACK	INGREDIENT & STRENGTH	BRAND (OR EQUIV.) & FIRM	NDC#	CLASS; SCH.
NUT100	Tab, White to Off-White, Round, Scored, NU over T100	Trazodone HCl 100 mg	by Nu Pharm	Canadian DIN# 02165392	Antidepressant
NUT5	Tab, White, Round, Scored, NU over T5	Timolol Maleate 5 mg	Nu Timolol by Nu-Pharm	Canadian DIN# 02044609	Antihypertensive
NUT50	Tab, Pale Orange, Round, Scored, NU over T50	Trazodone HCl 50 mg	by Nu Pharm	Canadian DIN# 02165384	Antidepressant
NYTOL	Cap, Blue	Diphenhydramine 50 mg	by Block Drug	Canadian	Antihistamine
O1A	Cap, Ivory & Red, Gelatin	Dipyridamole 200 mg; Aspirin 25 mg	Aggrenox by Boehringer Pharms	00597-0001	Antiplatelet
O1O1 <> BIOCRAFT	Cap	Amoxicillin Trihydrate	by Urgent Care Ctr	50716-0606	Antibiotic
O2C <> SEPTRADS	Tab	Sulfamethoxazole 800 mg, Trimethoprim 160 mg	Septra DS by Leiner	59606-0733	Antibiotic
OC <> 10	Tab, White, Round	Oxycodone HCl 10 mg	Oxycontin by PF Labs	48692-0710	Analgesic; C II
OC <> 10	Tab, White, Round	Oxycodone HCl 10 mg	Oxycontin by PF Labs	48692-0670	Analgesic; C II
OC <> 10	Tab, White, Round, Convex, Film	Oxycodone HCl 10 mg	Oxy-Contin by Pharmacia & Upjohn	00009-5088	Analgesic; C II
OC <> 10	Tab, Film Coated	Oxycodone HCl 10 mg	Oxycontin by Physicians Total Care	54868-3813	Analgesic; C II
OC <> 10	Tab, White, Round, Convex	Oxycodone HCl 10 mg	OxyContin CR by Pharmafab	62542-0108	Analgesic; C II
OC <> 20	Tab, Pink, Round	Oxycodone HCl 20 mg	Oxycontin by PF Labs	48692-0711	Analgesic; C II
OC <> 20	Tab, Pink, Round	Oxycodone HCl 20 mg	Oxycontin by PF Labs	48692-0601	Analgesic; C II
OC <> 20	Tab, Film Coated	Oxycodone HCl 20 mg	Oxycontin by Physicians Total Care	54868-3814	Analgesic; C II
OC <> 20	Tab, Pink, Round, Convex, Film	Oxycodone HCl 20 mg	OxyContin CR by Pharmacia & Upjohn	59632-5000	Analgesic; C II
OC <> 20	Tab, Pink, Round, Convex	Oxycodone HCl 20 mg	OxyContin CR by Pharmafab	62542-0157	Analgesic; C II
OC <> 40	Tab, Yellow, Round	Oxycodone HCl 40 mg	Oxycontin by PF Labs	48692-0712	Analgesic; C II
OC <> 40	Tab, Yellow, Round	Oxycodone HCl 40 mg	Oxycontin by PF Labs	48692-0672	Analgesic; C II
OC <> 40	Tab, Film Coated	Oxycodone HCl 40 mg	Oxycontin by Physicians Total Care	54868-3815	Analgesic; C II
OC <> 40	Tab, Yellow, Round, Convex, Film	Oxycodone HCl 40 mg	OxyContin CR by Pharmafab	62542-0158	Analgesic; C II
OC <> 80	Tab, Green, Round	Oxycodone HCl 80 mg	Oxycontin by Phy Total Care	54868-3986	Analgesic; C II
OC <> 80	Tab	Oxycodone HCl 80 mg	Oxycontin by PF	48692-0005	Analgesic; C II
OC <> 80	Tab	Oxycodone HCl 80 mg	Oxycontin by Purdue Pharma	59011-0107	Analgesic; C II
OC40	Tab, Yellow, Round	Oxycodone HCl (CR) 40 mg	OxyContin by PF	48692-0032	Analgesic; C II
OCL55 <> CINOBAC250MG	Cap, OCL 55 <> Cinobac 250 mg	Cinoxacin 250 mg	Cinobac by Eli Lilly	00002-3055	Antibiotic
OCL55 <> CINOBAC250MG	Cap, OCL 55 <> Cinobac 250 mg	Cinoxacin 250 mg	Cinobac by Eli Lilly	00002-0055	Antibiotic
OCL55 <> CINOBAC25OMG	Cap	Cinoxacin 250 mg	Cinobac by Oclassen	55515-0055	Antibiotic
OCL56 <> CINOBAC500MG	Cap	Cinoxacin 500 mg	Cinobac by Oclassen	55515-0056	Antibiotic
OCL56 <> CINOBAC500MG	Cap, OCL 56 <> Cinobac 500 mg	Cinoxacin 500 mg	Cinobac by Eli Lilly	00002-0056	Antibiotic
OCL56 <> CINOBAC500MG	Cap, Green & Orange	Cinoxacin 500 mg	Cinobac by Compumed	00403-2041	Antibiotic
OCTK0	Tab, White, Round, Scored, Coated	Acetaminophen 325 mg	Tylenol by Geneva		Antipyretic
OCTK10	Tab, White, Round, Coated	Acetaminophen 500 mg	Tylenol by Geneva		Antipyretic
OCTK48	Tab, White, Film Coated	Aspirin Buffered 325 mg	by Geneva		Analgesic
OHM010	Tab, White, Round, Scored, OHM over 010	Acetaminophen 325 mg	by UDL	51079-0002	Antipyretic
OHM010	Tab	Acetaminophen 325 mg	by Allscripts	54569-1533	Antipyretic
OHM011	Tab, White, Round	Acetaminophen 500 mg	Tylenol ES by OHM		Antipyretic
OHM021	Tab, White, Round	Aspirin Buffered 325 mg	Bufferin by OHM		Analgesic
OHM045	Tab, White & Yellow, Round	Gendecon	Dristan Adv. Formula by OHM		Cold Remedy
OHM055	Tab, White, Round	Acetaminophen 250 mg, Aspirin 250 mg, Caffeine 65 mg	Headrin by Reese	10956-0739	Analgesic

ID FRONT <> BACK	DESCRIPTION FRONT <> BACK	INGREDIENT & STRENGTH	BRAND (OR EQUIV.) & FIRM	NDC#	CLASS; SCH.
OHM076	Tab, White, Round, OHM/076	Pseudophedrine HCl 60 mg	Sudafed by OHM		Decongestant
OHM078	Tab, Peach, Round	Acetaminophen 325 mg, Phenyltoloxamine 30 mg	Percogesic by OHM		Analgesic
OHM117	Tab, Brown & Green, Round, OHM/117	Senna Concentrate 217 mg	Senokot by OHM		Gastrointestinal
OHM135	Tab, Yellow, Round	Genacol 325 mg	Comtrex by OHM		Cold Remedy
OHM311	Tab, White, Oblong	Acetaminophen 500 mg	Tylenol ES by OHM		Antipyretic
OIR <> PF5MG	Cap, Beige & Orange	Oxycodone HCl 5 mg	Oxynorm by PF Labs	48692-0720	Analgesic; C II
OIR <> PF5MG	Cap, Beige & Orange, O-IR	Oxycodone HCl 5 mg	Oxy IR by PF	48692-0006	Analgesic; C II
OJF547	Cap, Brown & White	Acetaminophen 325 mg, Butalbital 50 mg, Codeine 30 mg	Bancap with Codeine by Forest	00456-0547	Analgesic
OL459743	Cap, OL4/59743	Acetaminophen 325 mg, Butalbital 50 mg, Caffeine 40 mg	by Qualitest	00603-2546	Analgesic
OMNICEF	Cap, Lavender & Turquoise	Cefdinir 300 mg	Omnicef by Parke Davis	00071-0067	Antibiotic
OMNICEF300MG	Cap, Lavender & Turquoise, Omnicef 300 mg <> Abbott Logo	Cefdinir 300 mg	Omnicef by Abbott	00074-3769	Antibiotic
OMNICEFPD	Cap, Lavender & Turquoise, Omnicef/PD	Cefdinir 300 mg	Omnicef by Lilly del Caribe		Antibiotic
OP32	Tab, Blue, Round	Amphetamine, Dextroamphetamine Combination	Adderall by Richwood		Stimulant; C II
OP33	Tab, Orange, Round	Amphetamine, Dextroamphetamine Combination	Adderall by Richwood		Stimulant; C II
OP704	Tab, Yellow, Round	Bethanechol Chloride 25 mg	Urecholine by Odyssey Pharms	65473-0704	Urinary Tract
OPPOSINGCS	Tab, White, Round, Opposing C's	Medroxyyprogesterone Acetate 2.5 mg	Cycrin by ESI Lederle		Progestin
OPPOSINGCS <> CYCRIN	Tab, Opposing C's <> Cycrin	Medroxyprogesterone Acetate 10 mg	by Kaiser	62224-4331	Progestin
OR607	Tab, Light Pink, Round, OR <> 607	Ranitidine HCl 75 mg	by Schein		Gastrointestinal
ORAP1	Tab, White, Oval, Orap 1	Pimozide 1 mg	Orap by Teva	00093-0151	Antipsychotic
ORAP1	Tab, White, Oval, Scored	Pimozide 1 mg	Orap by Gate	57844-0151	Antipsychotic
ORAP2	Tab, White, Oval, Scored	Pimozide 2 mg	Orap by Gate	57844-0187	Antipsychotic
ORAP2 <> LEMMON	Tab, White, Oval, Scored, Orap/2 <> Lemmon	Pimozide 2 mg	Orap by Teva	00093-0187	Antipsychotic
ORAP2 <> LEMMON	Tab	Pimozide 2 mg	Orap by Gate	57844-0187	Antipsychotic
ORETIC	Tab, White, Round, Oretic over Abbott Logo	Hydrochlorothiazide 25 mg	Oretic by Abbott	00074-6978	Diuretic
ORETIC	Tab, Compressed, Abbott Logo	Hydrochlorothiazide 25 mg	by Kaiser	00179-0347	Diuretic
ORETIC	Tab, White, Round, Scored, Oretic over Abbott Logo	Hydrochlorothiazide 50 mg	Oretic by Abbott	00074-6985	Diuretic
ORETIC	Tab, Compressed, Abbott Logo	Hydrochlorothiazide 50 mg	by Kaiser	00179-0352	Diuretic
ORFENAGESIC	Tab	Acetaminophen 500 mg, Orphenadrine Citrate 50 mg	Orfenagesic by Lex	49523-2313	Analgesic; C II
ORG <> ORG	Tab, Green	Ethinyl Estradiol 0.035 mg, Norethindrone 0.5 mg, Norethindrone 1 mg	Jenest-28 by Ortho	00062-1790	Oral Contraceptive
ORG07 <> ORG07	Tab, White	Ethinyl Estradiol 0.035 mg, Norethindrone 0.5 mg, Norethindrone 1 mg	Jenest-28 by Ortho	00062-1790	Oral Contraceptive
ORG14 <> ORG14	Tab, Peach	Ethinyl Estradiol 0.035 mg, Norethindrone 0.5 mg, Norethindrone 1 mg	Jenest-28 by Ortho	00062-1790	Oral Contraceptive
ORG472	Cap, Off-White	Calcifediol, Anhydrous 20 mcg	Sec Calderol by RP Scherer	11014-0763	Vitamin/Mineral
ORG474	Cap	Calcifediol, Anhydrous 50 mcg	Calderol by RP Scherer	11014-0836	Vitamin/Mineral
ORGANON	Cap, Clear, Gelatin w/ Dark Blue Print, Organon Logo	Amylase 30,000 USP, Lipase 8,000 USP, Proteasse 30,000 USP	Cotazym by Organon	Canadian DIN# 00263818	Gastrointestinal
ORGANON <> KH2	Tab, Green, Round	Inate	Marvelon 28 by Organon	Canadian DIN# 02042479	Oral Contraceptive Placebo
ORGANON <> TR5	Tab, White, Round	Desogestrel 0.15 mg, Ethinyl Estradiol 0.03 mg	Marvelon 28 by Organon	Canadian DIN# 02042479	Oral Contraceptive
ORGANON <> 381	Cap	Amylase 30000 Units, Lipase 8000 Units, Protease 30000 Units	Cotazym by Physicians Total Care	54868-3793	Gastrointestinal
ORGANON <> KH2	Tab, Film Coated, Organon <> K H over 2	Desogestrel 0.15 mg, Ethinyl Estradiol 0.02 mg, Ethinyl Estradiol 0.01 mg	Mircette by Organon	00052-0281	Oral Contraceptive
ORGANON <> KH2	Tab, Film Coated, Organon <> K H over 2	Desogestrel 0.15 mg, Ethinyl Estradiol 0.02 mg, Ethinyl Estradiol 0.01 mg	Mircette by NV Organon	12860-0281	Oral Contraceptive
ORGANON <> KH2	Tab, KH Over 2	Desogestrel 0.15 mg, Ethinyl Estradiol 0.03 mg	Desogen by Organon	60889-0261	Oral Contraceptive
ORGANON <> KH2	Tab, Film Coated, KH over 2 <> Organon	Desogestrel 0.15 mg, Ethinyl Estradiol 0.03 mg	Desogen by Organon	00052-0261	Oral Contraceptive
ORGANON <> KS2	Tab, Film Coated, Organon <> K S over 2	Desogestrel 0.15 mg, Ethinyl Estradiol 0.02 mg, Ethinyl Estradiol 0.01 mg	Mircette by Organon	00052-0281	Oral Contraceptive
ORGANON <> KS2	Tab, Film Coated, Organon <> K S over 2	Desogestrel 0.15 mg, Ethinyl Estradiol 0.02 mg, Ethinyl Estradiol 0.01 mg	Mircette by NV Organon	12860-0281	Oral Contraceptive
ORGANON <> TR4	Tab, Film Coated, Organon <> T R over 4	Desogestrel 0.15 mg, Ethinyl Estradiol 0.02 mg, Ethinyl Estradiol 0.01 mg	Mircette by Organon	00052-0281	Oral Contraceptive
ORGANON <> TR4	Tab, Film Coated, Organon <> T R over 4	Desogestrel 0.15 mg, Ethinyl Estradiol 0.02 mg, Ethinyl Estradiol 0.01 mg	Mircette by NV Organon	12860-0281	Oral Contraceptive

ID FRONT <> BACK	DESCRIPTION FRONT <> BACK	INGREDIENT & STRENGTH	BRAND (OR EQUIV.) & FIRM	NDC#	CLASS; SCH.
ORGANON <> TR5	Tab, White, Round	Desogestrel 0.15 mg, Ethinyl 0.03 mg	Marvelon 21 by Organon	Canadian DIN# 02042487	Oral Contraceptive
ORGANON <> TR5	Tab, White, Round, TR Over 5	Desogestrel 0.15 mg, Ethinyl Estradiol 0.03 mg	Desogen by Organon	60889-0261	Oral Contraceptive
ORGANON <> TZ3	Tab, Yellow, Oval	Mirtazapine 15 mg	Remeron by Neuman Distbtrs	64579-0390	Antidepressant
ORGANON <> TZ3	Tab, Yellow, Oval, Film Coated	Mirtazapine 15 mg	Remeron by Organon	00052-0105	Antidepressant
ORGANON <> TZ3	Tab, Film Coated	Mirtazapine 15 mg	Remeron by NV Organon	12860-0105	Antidepressant
ORGANON <> TZ5	Tab, Red-Browned, Film Coated	Mirtazapine 30 mg	Remeron by Organon	00052-0107	Antidepressant
ORGANON <> TZ5	Tab, Red-Browned, Film Coated	Mirtazapine 30 mg	Remeron by NV Organon	12860-0107	Antidepressant
ORGANON <> TZ7	Tab, Film Coated	Mirtazapine 45 mg	Remeron by Organon	00052-0109	Antidepressant
ORGANON <> TZ7	Tab, White, Oval, Film Coated	Mirtazapine 45 mg	Remeron by Nv Organon	12860-0109	Antidepressant
ORGANON381	Cap, Green	Pancrelipase	Cotazyme by Organon		Gastrointestinal
ORGANON388	Cap, Clear	Pancrelipase	Cotazyme-S by Organon		Gastrointestinal
ORGANON393	Cap, Clear & Green	Lipase, Protease, Amylase	Zymase by Organon		Gastrointestinal
ORGANON542	Tab, White, Round	Ergotamine Tartrate 1 mg, Caffeine 100 mg	Wigraine by Organon		Antimigraine
ORGANON790	Tab, Peach, Round	Dexamethasone 1.5 mg	Hexadrol by Organon		Steroid
ORGANON791	Tab, White, Round	Dexamethasone 0.75 mg	Hexadrol by Organon		Steroid
ORGANON792	Tab, Yellow, Round	Dexamethasone 0.5 mg	Hexadrol by Organon		Steroid
ORGANON798	Tab, Green, Round	Dexamethasone 4 mg	Hexadrol by Organon		Steroid
ORGANONKH2	Tab, Green, Round	Inert	Desogen 28 by Organon		Placebo
ORHTO <> ORTHO	Tab	Ethinyl Estradiol 0.035 mg, Norgestimate 0.25 mg	Ortho Cyclen by Physicians Total Care	54868-2606	Oral Contraceptive
ORINASE500	Tab	Tolbutamide 500 mg	by Danbury	00591-5508	Antidiabetic
ORNADESB	Cap, Natural & Red, Ornade/SB	Phenylpropanolamine HCl 12 mg, Chlorphen. Mal. 75 mg	Ornade by SKB	00007-4421	Cold Remedy
ORNEX <> ORNEX	Tab, Blue, Oblong, Cap-Shaped	Pseudoephedrine HCl 30 mg, Acetaminophen 325 mg	Ornex by B F Ascher	00225-0590	Cold Remedy
ORNEXMAX	Tab, White, Oblong, Cap-Shaped	Pseudoephedrine HCl 30 mg, Acetaminophen 500 mg	Ornex-Max by B F Ascher	00225-0600	Cold Remedy
ORTH535	Tab, White	Norethindrone 0.75 mg, Ethinyl Estradiol 0.035 mg	by Kaiser Fdn	00179-1298	Oral Contraceptive
ORTHO	Tab, White, Cap Shaped	Sulfabenzamide 184 mg, Sulfacetamide 143.75 mg, Sulfathiazole 172.5 mg	Sultrin by Ortho	00062-5441	Antibiotic
ORTHO <> 135	Tab	Ethinyl Estradiol 0.035 mg, Norethindrone 1 mg	Ortho Novum 1 Plus 35 by Dept Health Central Pharm	53808-0031	Oral Contraceptive
ORTHO <> 150	Tab	Ethinyl Estradiol 0.035 mg, Norgestimate 0.215 mg, Norgestimate 0.18 mg, Norgestimate 0.25 mg	Ortho Tri Cyclen 28 by Dept Health Central Pharm	53808-0043	Oral Contraceptive
ORTHO <> 150	Tab	Mestranol 0.05 mg, Norethindrone 1 mg	Ortho Novum 1 Plus 50 by Dept Health Central Pharm	53808-0030	Oral Contraceptive
ORTHO <> 35	Tab	Ethinyl Estradiol 0.035 mg, Norethindrone 0.5 mg, Norethindrone 1 mg, Norethindrone 0.75 mg	Ortho Novum 777 by Dept Health Central Pharm	53808-0032	Oral Contraceptive
ORTHO <> 35	Tab	Norethindrone 0.35 mg	Micronor 28 by Dept Health Central Pharm	53808-0029	Oral Contraceptive
ORTHO <> D150	Tab, Orange	Desogestrel 150 mcg, Ethinyl Estradiol 3 mcg	Ortho Cept 28 by Ortho	00062-1796	Oral Contraceptive
ORTHO <> D150	Tab, Peach, Round	Desogestrel 150 mcg, Ethinyl Estradiol 3 mcg	Ortho Cept 21 by Ortho	00062-1795	Oral Contraceptive
ORTHO <> ORTHO	Tab, Green, Round	Ethinyl Estradiol 0.035 mg, Norethindrone 0.5 mg	Modicon 28 by Ortho	00062-1714	Oral Contraceptive
ORTHO <> ORTHO	Tab, Green	Ethinyl Estradiol 0.035 mg, Norethindrone 0.5 mg, Norethindrone 1 mg	Ortho-Novum 10 11 28 by Ortho	00062-1771	Oral Contraceptive
ORTHO <> ORTHO	Tab, Green	Ethinyl Estradiol 0.035 mg, Norethindrone 0.5 mg, Norethindrone 1 mg, Norethindrone 0.75 mg	Ortho-Novum 7 7 7 28 by Ortho	00062-1781	Oral Contraceptive
ORTHO <> ORTHO	Tab, Green, Round	Ethinyl Estradiol 0.035 mg, Norethindrone 1 mg	Ortho Novum 1 35 28 by Ortho	00062-1761	Oral Contraceptive
ORTHO <> ORTHO	Tab, Green, Round	Ethinyl Estradiol 0.035 mg, Norgestimate 0.18 mg, Norgestimate 0.25 mg, Norgestimate 0.215 mg	Ortho Tri Cyclen 28 by Ortho	00062-1903	Oral Contraceptive
ORTHO <> ORTHO	Tab, Green	Ethinyl Estradiol 0.035 mg, Norgestimate 0.25 mg	Ortho-Cyclen-28 by Ortho	00062-1901	Oral Contraceptive
ORTHO <> ORTHO	Tab	Ethinyl Estradiol 0.035 mg, Norgestimate 0.25 mg	Ortho Cyclen by Physicians Total Care	54868-2606	Oral Contraceptive
ORTHO <> ORTHO	Tab	Mestranol 0.05 mg, Norethindrone 1 mg	Ortho-Novum 1/50-28 by Ortho	00062-1332	Oral Contraceptive
ORTHO <> ORTHO	Tab, Green, Round	Placebo	Ortho Novum by McNeil	00062-1770	Placebo
ORTHO <> ORTHO	Tab, Green, Round	Placebo	Ortho Novum by McNeil	00062-1771	Placebo
ORTHO035	Tab, Lime, Round, Ortho 0.35	Norethindrone 0.35 mg	Micronor by Ortho-McNeil		Oral Contraceptive

ID FRONT <> BACK	DESCRIPTION FRONT <> BACK	INGREDIENT & STRENGTH	BRAND (OR EQUIV.) & FIRM	NDC#	CLASS; SCH.
ORTHO035 <> ORTHO035	Tab, Ortho 0.35	Norethindrone 0.35 mg	Micronor by Ortho	00062-1411	Oral Contraceptive
ORTHO1	Tab, White, Round	Norethindrone 1 mg, Mestranol 0.08 mg	Ortho Novum by Ortho-McNeil		Oral Contraceptive
ORTHO135	Tab, Peach	Norethindrone 1 mg, Ethinyl Estradiol 35 mcg	by Janssen	Canadian	Oral Contraceptive
ORTHO135 <> ORTHO135	Tab, Peach	Ethinyl Estradiol 0.035 mg, Norethindrone 0.5 mg, Norethindrone 1 mg	Ortho Novum 10 11 21 by Ortho	00062-1770	Oral Contraceptive
ORTHO135 <> ORTHO135	Tab, Peach	Ethinyl Estradiol 0.035 mg, Norethindrone 0.5 mg, Norethindrone 1 mg	Ortho-Novum 10 11 28 by Ortho	00062-1771	Oral Contraceptive
ORTHO135 <> ORTHO135	Tab, Peach	Ethinyl Estradiol 0.035 mg, Norethindrone 0.5 mg, Norethindrone 1 mg, Norethindrone 0.75 mg	Ortho-Novum 7 7 7 28 by Ortho	00062-1781	Oral Contraceptive
ORTHO135 <> ORTHO135	Tab, Light Peach	Ethinyl Estradiol 0.035 mg, Norethindrone 0.5 mg, Norethindrone 1 mg, Norethindrone 0.75 mg	Ortho-Novum 7 7 7 21 by Ortho	00062-1780	Oral Contraceptive
ORTHO135 <> ORTHO135	Tab, Peach	Ethinyl Estradiol 0.035 mg, Norethindrone 0.5 mg, Norethindrone 1 mg	Ortho Novum 10 11 21 by Ortho	00107-1770	Oral Contraceptive
ORTHO135	Tab	Ethinyl Estradiol 0.035 mg, Norethindrone 0.5 mg, Norethindrone 1 mg, Norethindrone 0.75 mg	Ortho Novum 777 21 by Physicians Total Care	54868-0508	Oral Contraceptive
ORTHO135	Tab, Peach, Round	Ethinyl Estradiol 0.035 mg, Norethindrone 1 mg	Ortho Novum 1 35 28 by Ortho	00062-1761	Oral Contraceptive
ORTHO135	Tab	Ethinyl Estradiol 0.035 mg, Norethindrone 1 mg	Ortho Novum 21 1 35 by Ortho	00062-1760	Oral Contraceptive
ORTHO135	Tab, Peach	Ethinyl Estradiol 0.035 mg, Norethindrone 1 mg, Norethindrone 0.5 mg	Ortho Novum 10 11 28 by Ortho	00107-1771	Oral Contraceptive
ORTHO135	Tab, Peach	Ethinyl Estradiol 35 mcg, Norethindrone 1 mg	Ortho Novum 1 35 21 by Ortho	00062-1760	Oral Contraceptive
ORTHO135	Tab, Peach	Norethindrone 0.5 mg, Ethinyl Estradiol 0.035 mg	Ortho Novum by Kaiser Fdn	00179-1298	Oral Contraceptive
ORTHO135	Tab, Peach	Norethindrone 1 mg, Ethinyl Estradiol 0.035 mg	Ortho Novum by Haines Pharms	59564-0149	Oral Contraceptive
ORTHO135	Tab, Peach	Norethindrone 1 mg, Ethinyl Estradiol 0.035 mg	Ortho Novum by Kaiser Fdn	00179-1297	Oral Contraceptive
ORTHO135	Tab, Light Peach	Ethinyl Estradiol 0.035 mg, Norethindrone 0.5 mg, Norethindrone 1 mg, Norethindrone 0.75 mg	Ortho Novum 777 by Dept Health Central Pharm	53808-0032	Oral Contraceptive
ORTHO150	Tab, Yellow	Norethindrone 1 mg, Mestranol 50 mcg	Ortho-Novum by Ortho	Canadian	Oral Contraceptive
ORTHO150	Tab	Mestranol 0.05 mg, Norethindrone 1 mg	Ortho Novum 21 by Ortho	00062-1331	Oral Contraceptive
ORTHO150	Tab, Pale Yellow, Round	Mestranol 0.05 mg, Norethindrone 1 mg	Ortho-Novum 1/50-28 by Ortho	00062-1332	Oral Contraceptive
ORTHO1570	Tab, White, Oblong	Metronidazole 250 mg	Protostat by Ortho-McNeil	00062-1570	Antibiotic
ORTHO1571	Tab, White, Oblong	Metronidazole 500 mg	Protostat by Ortho-McNeil	00062-1571	Antibiotic
ORTHO1571	Tab, Off White to White	Metronidazole 500 mg	Protostat by Quality Care	60346-0862	Antibiotic
ORTHO180	Tab, White, Round	Ethinyl Estradiol 0.035 mg, Norgestimate 0.18 mg, Norgestimate 0.215 mg, Norgestimate 0.25 mg	Ortho Tri Cyclen 21 by Ortho	00107-1902	Oral Contraceptive
ORTHO180	Tab, White, Round	Ethinyl Estradiol 0.035 mg, Norgestimate 0.18 mg, Norgestimate 0.25 mg, Norgestimate 0.215 mg	Ortho Tri Cyclen 28 by Ortho	00107-1903	Oral Contraceptive
ORTHO180	Tab, White, Round	Ethinyl Estradiol 0.035 mg, Norgestimate 0.18 mg, Norgestimate 0.25 mg, Norgestimate 0.215 mg	Ortho Tri Cyclen 28 by Ortho	00062-1903	Oral Contraceptive
ORTHO180	Tab, White, Round	Ethinyl Estradiol 0.035 mg, Norgestimate 0.18 mg, Norgestimate 0.25 mg, Norgestimate 0.215 mg	Ortho Tri Cyclen 21 by Ortho	00062-1902	Oral Contraceptive
ORTHO180	Tab, White, Round	Ethinyl Estradiol 0.035 mg, Norgestimate 0.215 mg, Norgestimate 0.18 mg, Norgestimate 0.25 mg	Ortho Tri Cyclen 28 by Heartland	61392-0821	Oral Contraceptive
ORTHO1800	Tab, Lavender	Estropipate 1.5 mg	Ortho EST by Ortho	00062-1800	Hormone
ORTHO1801	Tab	Estropipate 0.75 mg	Ortho EST by Ortho	00062-1801	Hormone
ORTHO2	Tab, White, Round	Norethindrone 2 mg, Mestranol 0.1 mg	Ortho Novum by Ortho-McNeil		Oral Contraceptive
ORTHO211	Tab	Griseofulvin, Microsize 250 mg	Grifulvin V by Ortho	00062-0211	Antifungal
ORTHO214	Tab	Griseofulvin, Microsize 500 mg	Grifulvin V by Pharm Utilization	60491-0286	Antifungal
ORTHO214	Tab	Griseofulvin, Microsize 500 mg	Grifulvin V Microsize by PDRX	55289-0857	Antifungal
ORTHO214	Tab	Griseofulvin, Microsize 500 mg	Grifulvin V by Ortho	00062-0214	Antifungal
ORTHO214	Tab	Griseofulvin, Microsize 500 mg	Grifulvin V by Eckerd Drug	19458-0846	Antifungal
ORTHO215	Tab	Ethinyl Estradiol 0.035 mg, Norgestimate 0.215 mg, Norgestimate 0.18 mg, Norgestimate 0.25 mg	Ortho Tri Cyclen 28 by Dept Health Central Pharm	53808-0043	Oral Contraceptive

ID FRONT <> BACK	DESCRIPTION FRONT <> BACK	INGREDIENT & STRENGTH	BRAND (OR EQUIV.) & FIRM	NDC#	CLASS; SCH.
ORTHO215	Tab, Light Blue, Round	Ethinyl Estradiol 0.035 mg, Norgestimate 0.18 mg, Norgestimate 0.215 mg, Norgestimate 0.25 mg	Ortho Tri Cyclen 21 by Ortho	00107-1902	Oral Contraceptive
ORTHO215	Tab, Light Blue, Round	Ethinyl Estradiol 0.035 mg, Norgestimate 0.18 mg, Norgestimate 0.25 mg, Norgestimate 0.215 mg	Ortho Tri Cyclen 28 by Ortho	00107-1903	Oral Contraceptive
ORTHO215	Tab, Blue, Round	Ethinyl Estradiol 0.035 mg, Norgestimate 0.215 mg, Norgestimate 0.18 mg, Norgestimate 0.25 mg	Ortho Tri Cyclen 28 by Heartland	61392-0823	Oral Contraceptive
ORTHO250	Tab	Ethinyl Estradiol 0.035 mg, Norgestimate 0.215 mg, Norgestimate 0.18 mg, Norgestimate 0.25 mg	Ortho Tri Cyclen 28 by Dept Health Central Pharm	53808-0043	Oral Contraceptive
ORTHO250	Tab, Blue	Norgestimate 0.25 mg, Ethinyl Estradiol 35 mcg	by Janssen	Canadian	Oral Contraceptive
ORTHO250	Tab, Blue, Round	Ethinyl Estradiol 0.035 mg, Norgestimate 0.18 mg, Norgestimate 0.215 mg, Norgestimate 0.25 mg	Ortho Tri Cyclen 21 by Ortho	00107-1902	Oral Contraceptive
ORTHO250	Tab, Blue, Round	Ethinyl Estradiol 0.035 mg, Norgestimate 0.18 mg, Norgestimate 0.25 mg, Norgestimate 0.215 mg	Ortho Tri Cyclen 21 by Ortho	00062-1902	Oral Contraceptive
ORTHO250	Tab, Blue, Round	Ethinyl Estradiol 0.035 mg, Norgestimate 0.18 mg, Norgestimate 0.25 mg, Norgestimate 0.215 mg	Ortho Tri Cyclen 28 by Ortho	00107-1903	Oral Contraceptive
ORTHO250	Tab, Blue, Round	Ethinyl Estradiol 0.035 mg, Norgestimate 0.18 mg, Norgestimate 0.25 mg, Norgestimate 0.215 mg	Ortho Tri Cyclen 28 by Ortho	00062-1903	Oral Contraceptive
ORTHO250	Tab, Blue, Round	Ethinyl Estradiol 0.035 mg, Norgestimate 0.215 mg, Norgestimate 0.18 mg, Norgestimate 0.25 mg	Ortho Tri Cyclen 28 by Heartland	61392-0826	Oral Contraceptive
ORTHO250	Tab, Blue	Ethinyl Estradiol 0.035 mg, Norgestimate 0.25 mg	Ortho Cyclen 28 by Ortho	00107-1901	Oral Contraceptive
ORTHO250	Tab	Ethinyl Estradiol 0.035 mg, Norgestimate 0.25 mg	Ortho Cyclen 21 by Ortho	00107-1900	Oral Contraceptive
ORTHO250	Tab	Ethinyl Estradiol 0.035 mg, Norgestimate 0.25 mg	Ortho Cyclen 21 by Ortho	00062-1900	Oral Contraceptive
ORTHO250	Tab, Blue	Ethinyl Estradiol 0.035 mg, Norgestimate 0.25 mg	Ortho-Cyclen-28 by Ortho	00062-1901	Oral Contraceptive
ORTHO250	Tab	Ethinyl Estradiol 0.035 mg, Norgestimate 0.25 mg	Ortho Cyclen by Physicians Total Care	54868-2606	Oral Contraceptive
ORTHO535	Tab, White	Ethinyl Estradiol 0.035 mg, Norethindrone 0.5 mg, Norethindrone 1 mg	Ortho Novum 10 11 21 by Ortho	00062-1770	Oral Contraceptive
ORTHO535	Tab, White	Norethindrone 0.5 mg, Ethinyl Estradiol 35 mcg	by Janssen	Canadian	Oral Contraceptive
ORTHO535	Tab, White, Round	Ethinyl Estradiol 0.035 mg, Norethindrone 0.5 mg	Modicon 28 by Ortho	00062-1714	Oral Contraceptive
ORTHO535	Tab, White, Round	Ethinyl Estradiol 0.035 mg, Norethindrone 0.5 mg	Modicon 21 by Ortho	00107-1712	Oral Contraceptive
ORTHO535	Tab, White, Round	Ethinyl Estradiol 0.035 mg, Norethindrone 0.5 mg	Modicon 21 by Ortho	00062-1712	Oral Contraceptive
ORTHO535	Tab, White, Round	Ethinyl Estradiol 0.035 mg, Norethindrone 0.5 mg	Modicon 28 by Ortho	00107-1714	Oral Contraceptive
ORTHO535	Tab, White	Ethinyl Estradiol 0.035 mg, Norethindrone 0.5 mg, Norethindrone 1 mg	Ortho Novum 10 11 21 by Ortho	00062-1770	Oral Contraceptive
ORTHO535	Tab, White	Ethinyl Estradiol 0.035 mg, Norethindrone 0.5 mg, Norethindrone 1 mg	Ortho-Novum 10 11 28 by Ortho	00062-1771	Oral Contraceptive
ORTHO535	Tab, White	Ethinyl Estradiol 0.035 mg, Norethindrone 0.5 mg, Norethindrone 1 mg, Norethindrone 0.75 mg	Ortho-Novum 7 7 7 21 by Ortho	00062-1780	Oral Contraceptive
ORTHO535	Tab, White	Ethinyl Estradiol 0.035 mg, Norethindrone 0.5 mg, Norethindrone 1 mg, Norethindrone 0.75 mg	Ortho Novum 7 7 7 28 by Ortho	00062-1781	Oral Contraceptive
ORTHO535	Tab	Ethinyl Estradiol 0.035 mg, Norethindrone 0.5 mg, Norethindrone 1 mg, Norethindrone 0.75 mg	Ortho Novum 777 21 by Physicians Total Care	54868-0508	Oral Contraceptive
ORTHO735	Tab, Peach	Norethindrone 0.75 mg, Ethinyl Estradiol 35 mcg	by Janssen	Canadian	Oral Contraceptive
ORTHO75	Tab, Light Peach	Ethinyl Estradiol 0.035 mg, Norethindrone 0.5 mg, Norethindrone 1 mg, Norethindrone 0.75 mg	Ortho Novum 777 by Dept Health Central Pharm	53808-0032	Oral Contraceptive
ORTHO75	Tab, Light Peach	Ethinyl Estradiol 0.035 mg, Norethindrone 0.5 mg, Norethindrone 1 mg, Norethindrone 0.75 mg	Ortho-Novum 7 7 7 28 by Ortho	00062-1781	Oral Contraceptive
ORTHO75	Tab, Peach	Ethinyl Estradiol 0.035 mg, Norethindrone 0.5 mg, Norethindrone 1 mg, Norethindrone 0.75 mg	Ortho-Novum 7 7 7 21 by Ortho	00062-1780	Oral Contraceptive
ORTHO75	Tab, Light Peach	Ethinyl Estradiol 0.035 mg, Norethindrone 0.5 mg, Norethindrone 1 mg, Norethindrone 0.75 mg	Ortho Novum 777 21 by Physicians Total Care	54868-0508	Oral Contraceptive
ORTHO75	Tab, Peach	Norethindrone 1 mg, Ethinyl Estradiol 0.035 mg	Ortho Novum by Kaiser Fdn	00179-1298	Oral Contraceptive
ORTHOP <> ORTHOP	Tab, Green, Round	Desogestrel 150 mcg, Ethinyl Estradiol 3 mcg	Ortho Cept 28 by Ortho	00062-1796	Oral Contraceptive
ORTHOPD150	Tab, Orange, Ortho/p D 150	Desogestrel 0.15 mg, Ethinyl Estradiol 0.03 mg	by Janssen	Canadian	Oral Contraceptive
ORUDIS50	Cap, Green & Ivory	Ketoprofen 50 mg	Orudis by Rhone-Poulenc Rorer	Canadian	NSAID

ID FRONT <> BACK	DESCRIPTION FRONT <> BACK	INGREDIENT & STRENGTH	BRAND (OR EQUIV.) & FIRM	NDC#	CLASS; SCH.
ORUDIS50 <> WYETH4181	Cap, Dark Green & Light Green	Ketoprofen 50 mg	Orudis by Allscripts	54569-2178	NSAID
ORUDIS50 <> WYETH4181	Cap, Dark Green & Light Green	Ketoprofen 50 mg	Orudis by Quality Care	60346-0253	NSAID
ORUDIS75 <> WYETH4187	Cap, Coated	Ketoprofen 75 mg	Orudis by Wyeth Labs	00008-4187	NSAID
ORUDIS75 <> WYETH4187	Cap	Ketoprofen 75 mg	Ketoprofen by Pharmedix	53002-0531	NSAID
ORUDIS75 <> WYETH4187	Cap	Ketoprofen 75 mg	Orudis by Nat Pharmpak Serv	55154-4201	NSAID
ORUDIS75 <> WYETH4187	Cap, Dark Green	Ketoprofen 75 mg	Orudis by Amerisource	62584-0187	NSAID
ORUDIS75 <> WYETH4187	Cap, Dark Green	Ketoprofen 75 mg	Orudis by Thrift Drug	59198-0087	NSAID
ORUDIS75 <> WYETH4187	Cap, Dark Green & White, Coated	Ketoprofen 75 mg	Orudis by Quality Care	60346-0443	NSAID
ORUDISSR200	Tab, White, Round	Ketoprofen 200 mg	Orudis by Rhone-Poulenc Rorer	Canadian	NSAID
ORUVAIL100	Cap, ER, Marked with Two Radial Bands	Ketoprofen 100 mg	Oruvail by Wyeth Labs	00008-0821	NSAID
ORUVAIL100	Cap, ER, Marked with Two Radial Bands	Ketoprofen 100 mg	Oruvail by Wyeth	52903-0821	NSAID
ORUVAIL150	Cap, Pink & White	Ketoprofen 150 mg	Oruvail by May & Baker Pharma	Canadian	NSAID
ORUVAIL150	Cap, ER, Marked with Two Radial Bands	Ketoprofen 150 mg	Oruvail by Wyeth Labs	00008-0822	NSAID
ORUVAIL150	Cap, ER, Marked with Two Radial Bands	Ketoprofen 150 mg	Oruvail by Wyeth	52903-0822	NSAID
ORUVAIL200	Cap, Blue & Pink	Ketoprofen 200 mg	Oruvail by May & Baker Pharma	Canadian	NSAID
ORUVAIL200	Cap, Pink & White	Ketoprofen 200 mg	Oruvail by Wyeth Pharms	52903-0690	NSAID
ORUVAIL200	Cap, Off White, Ex Release	Ketoprofen 200 mg	Oruvail by DRX	55045-2118	NSAID
ORUVAIL200	Cap, Opaque & Pink & White	Ketoprofen 200 mg	Oruvail ER by Murfreesboro	51129-1597	NSAID
ORUVAIL200	Cap, Off White, Ex Release, with 2 Radial Bands, ORUVAIL 200	Ketoprofen 200 mg	Oruvail by Allscripts	54569-3792	NSAID
OSCAL	Tab, Green, Oblong, OS-CAL	Elemental Calcium 500 mg	OS-CAL by Wyeth-Ayerst	Canadian	Mineral
OSCAL	Tab, White, Round, OS-CAL	Elemental Calcium 750 mg	OS-CAL by Wyeth-Ayerst	Canadian	Mineral
OVOL160	Tab, White, Round, Ovol-160	Simethicone 160 mg	Ovol by Horner	Canadian	Antiflatulent
OW	Tab, Pink, Round	Phenolphthalein	Correctol by Barre		Gastrointestinal
P	Tab, White, Round	Docusate Sodium 100 mg	Phillips Liqui Gels by Group Health	58087-0019	Laxative
P	Cap, Orange	Docusate Sodium 200 mg	by Pharmascience	Canadian	Laxative
P	Tab, PRAVACHOL 40	Pravastatin Sodium 40 mg	Pravachol by Bristol Myers	15548-0194	Antihyperlipidemic
P <> 0140	Cap, Gelatin, P in a triangle	Ergocalciferol 1.25 mg	Vitamin D by Banner Pharmacaps	10888-0140	Vitamin
P <> 063	Tab, PUREPAC Logo <> 063 Top Half of Bisect	Lorazepam 2 mg	by Talbert Med	44514-0100	Sedative/Hypnotic; C IV
P <> 11	Tab, Round, Dye Free, Chewable, P <> 1.1	Sodium Fluoride 1.1 mg	Pharmaflur 1.1 by Pharmics	00813-0065	Element
P <> 22	Tab, Round, Dye Free, Chewable, P <> 2.2	Sodium Fluoride 2.21 mg	Pharmaflur by Pharmics	00813-0066	Element
P <> 221	Tab, Partially Bisected	Hydrochlorothiazide 25 mg	Hctz by Quality Care	60346-0184	Diuretic
P <> 3900	Cap, Gelatin, P in a triangle	Guaifenesin 90 mg, Theophylline 150 mg	Bronchial by Banner Pharmacaps	10888-3900	Antiasthmatic
P <> 4600	Cap, Gelatin, P in a triangle	Benzonatate 100 mg	by Banner Pharmacaps	10888-4600	Antitussive
P <> 480	Tab, Film Coated, Purepac Logo	Tolmetin Sodium 735 mg	by Physicians Total Care	54868-2421	NSAID
P <> 500	Cap, Purepac Logo	Prazosin HCl 1 mg	by Quality Care	60346-0572	Antihypertensive
P <> 57	Tab, Coated	Lorazepam 0.5 mg	by Quality Care	60346-0363	Sedative/Hypnotic; C IV
P <> 606	Tab, Purepac Logo	Acyclovir 400 mg	by Golden State	60429-0712	Antiviral
P <> 618	Tab, Yellow, Oblong, Enteric	Naproxen DR 500 mg	by Orion	52483-0014	NSAID
P <> PF	Tab, White, Round	Aminophylline 225 mg	PhylloContin by Purdue Frederick	Canadian	Antiasthmatic
P <> PRAVACHOL10	Tab, Pink to Peach, Oblong	Pravastatin Sodium 10 mg	Pravachol by Bristol Myers	00003-5154	Antihyperlipidemic
P <> PRAVACHOL10	Tab, Pink, Round, Convex	Pravastatin Sodium 10 mg	Pravachol by Purepac		Antihyperlipidemic
P <> PRAVACHOL10	Tab	Pravastatin Sodium 10 mg	Pravachol by Nat Pharmpak Serv	55154-0606	Antihyperlipidemic
P <> PRAVACHOL10	Tab, Peach to Pink, Round, Rectangular-Shaped	Pravastatin Sodium 10 mg	Pravachol by PDRX	55289-0104	Antihyperlipidemic
P <> PRAVACHOL20	Tab, Yellow, Oblong	Pravastatin Sodium 20 mg	Pravachol by Bristol Myers	00003-5178	Antihyperlipidemic

ID FRONT <> BACK	DESCRIPTION FRONT <> BACK	INGREDIENT & STRENGTH	BRAND (OR EQUIV.) & FIRM	NDC#	CLASS; SCH.
P <> PRAVACHOL20	Tab, Rounded Rectangle Shape	Pravastatin Sodium 20 mg	Pravachol by Allscripts	54569-4071	Antihyperlipidemic
P <> PRAVACHOL20	Tab	Pravastatin Sodium 20 mg	Pravachol by Nat Pharmpak Serv	55154-0608	Antihyperlipidemic
P <> PRAVACHOL20	Tab, Yellow, Rectangle	Pravastatin Sodium 20 mg	Pravachol by Squibb Mfg	12783-0178	Antihyperlipidemic
P <> PRAVACHOL40	Tab, Green, Oblong	Pravastatin Sodium 40 mg	Pravachol by Bristol Myers	00003-5194	Antihyperlipidemic
P <> PRAVACHOL40	Tab	Pravastatin Sodium 40 mg	Pravachol by Caremark	00339-5746	Antihyperlipidemic
P <> PRAVACHOL40	Tab, Embossed	Pravastatin Sodium 40 mg	Pravachol by Quality Care	62682-6028	Antihyperlipidemic
P <> R50	Tab, Purepac Logo <> R/50	Lorazepam 1 mg	by Kaiser	00179-1093	Sedative/Hypnotic; C IV
P <> SEARLE	Tab	Ethinyl Estradiol 35 mcg, Ethynodiol Diacetate 1 mg	Demulen 1 35 28 by Pharm Utilization	60491-0181	Oral Contraceptive
P <> SEARLE	Tab, White, Round, Placebo	Ethinyl Estradiol 35 mcg, Ethynodiol Diacetate 1 mg	Demulen 1/35-28 by GD Searle	00025-0161	Oral Contraceptive
P <> SEARLE	Tab	Ethinyl Estradiol 35 mcg, Ethynodiol Diacetate 1 mg	Demulen by Physicians Total Care	54868-0404	Oral Contraceptive
P <> SEARLE	Tab, Blue, Round	Ethinyl Estradiol 35 mcg; Ethynodiol Diacetate 1 mg	Demulen Compack by Rx Pac	65084-0219	Oral Contraceptive
P <> SEARLE	Tab, Placebo	Ethinyl Estradiol 50 mcg, Ethynodiol Diacetate 1 mg	Demulen 1 50 28 by Pharm Utilization	60491-0183	Oral Contraceptive
P <> SEARLE	Tab	Ethinyl Estradiol 50 mcg, Ethynodiol Diacetate 1 mg	Demulen by Physicians Total Care	54868-3790	Oral Contraceptive
P <> SEARLE	Tab, Orange, Round	Inert	Brevicon .5/35 28 day by Pharmacia	Canadian DIN# 02187094	Placebo
P <> SEARLE	Tab, Orange, Round	Inert	Brevicon 1/35 28 day by Pharmacia	Canadian DIN# 02189062	Placebo
P <> SEARLE	Tab, Orange, Round, Film Coated	Inert	Demulen 30 28 day by Pharmacia	Canadian DIN# 0047152	Placebo
P <> SEARLE	Tab, Orange, Round	Inert	Synphasic 28 day by Pharmacia	Canadian DIN# 02187116	Placebo
P <> SEARLE	Tab, Orange, Round	Inert	Select 1/35 28 day by Pharmacia	Canadian DIN# 02199297	Placebo
P <> WATSON	Tab	Ethinyl Estradiol 0.035 mg, Norethindrone 0.5 mg	Necon 0.5 35 28 by Watson	52544-0550	Oral Contraceptive
P <> WATSON	Tab	Ethinyl Estradiol 0.035 mg, Ethynodiol Diacetate 1 mg	Zovia 1 35E 28 by Watson	52544-0383	Oral Contraceptive
P <> WATSON	Tab	Ethinyl Estradiol 0.035 mg, Norethindrone 0.5 mg, Norethindrone 1 mg	Necon 10 11 28 by Watson	52544-0554	Oral Contraceptive
P <> WATSON	Tab	Ethinyl Estradiol 0.035 mg, Norethindrone 1 mg	Necon 1 35 28 by Watson	52544-0552	Oral Contraceptive
P <> WATSON	Tab	Ethinyl Estradiol 0.05 mg, Ethynodiol Diacetate 1 mg	by Watson	52544-0384	Oral Contraceptive
P <> WATSON	Tab	Mestranol 0.05 mg, Norethindrone 1 mg	Necon 1 50 28 by Watson	52544-0556	Oral Contraceptive
P <> WATSON	Tab, White	Norethindrone 1 mg, Mestranol 0.05 mg	Necon by DRX Pharm Consults	55045-2722	Oral Contraceptive
P <> WATSON	Tab, White	Norethidrone 1 mg, Mestranol 50 mcg	Necon by PDRX	55289-0381	Oral Contraceptive
P&G <> 402	Tab, P & G	Etidronate Disodium 200 mg	Didronel by Pharm Utilization	60491-0801	Calcium Metabolism
P0	Tab, Red, Round	Pseudoephedrine HCl 30 mg	Sudafed by PFI		Decongestant
P001 <> 3	Tab, Purepac Logo	Acetaminophen 300 mg, Codeine Phosphate 30 mg	by Talbert Med	44514-0223	Analgesic; C III
P0013	Tab, Purepac Logo 001/3	Acetaminophen 300 mg, Codeine Phosphate 30 mg	by Golden State	60429-0500	Analgesic; C III
P0013	Tab, Purepac Logo P 001/3	Acetaminophen 300 mg, Codeine Phosphate 30 mg	by St Marys Med	60760-0001	Analgesic; C III
P0034	Tab, P003/4 Purepac Logo	Acetaminophen 300 mg, Codeine Phosphate 60 mg	by Quality Care	60346-0632	Analgesic; C III
P012	Tab, White, Round, Triangle over P/012	Acetaminophen 325 mg	by Advance Pharm		Antipyretic
P0140	Cap, Gelatin Coated, P in a triangle	Ergocalciferol 1.25 mg	Vitamin D by Superior	00144-0639	Vitamin
P0140	Cap, Gelatin, Logo P Inside Triangle	Ergocalciferol 1.25 mg	Vitamin D by Rugby	00536-4783	Vitamin
P0140	Cap, Gelatin, P in a triangle	Ergocalciferol 1.25 mg	Vitamin D by Consolidated Midland Corp.	00223-1971	Vitamin
P0140	Cap, Gelatin, P in a triangle	Ergocalciferol 1.25 mg	Vitamin D by United Res	00677-0765	Vitamin
P0140	Cap, Gelatin, P in a triangle 0140	Ergocalciferol 1.25 mg	Vitamin D by Major	00904-0291	Vitamin
P021	Cap, Purepac Logo 21	Flurazepam HCl 15 mg	by Quality Care	60346-0239	Hypnotic; C IV
P022	Cap, Purepad Logo 022	Flurazepam HCl 30 mg	by Quality Care	60346-0762	Hypnotic; C IV
P026	Tab, Light Peach, Cushion, P/026	Phenyltoloxamine 325 mg	by Advance Pharm		Decongestant

ID FRONT <> BACK	DESCRIPTION FRONT <> BACK	INGREDIENT & STRENGTH	BRAND (OR EQUIV.) & FIRM	NDC#	CLASS; SCH.
P026	Tab, Purepac Logo 026	Phenobarbital 15 mg	by Heartland	61392-0382	Sedative/Hypnotic; C IV
P027	Tab, Coated, Embossed, Purepac Logo 027	Alprazolam 0.25 mg	by Quality Care	60346-0876	Antianxiety; C IV
P051	Tab, Purepac Logo 051	Diazepam 2 mg	by Heartland	61392-0726	Antianxiety; C IV
P051	Tab, P, Purepac Logo	Diazepam 2 mg	by Quality Care	60346-0579	Antianxiety; C IV
P052	Tab, Purepac Logo 052	Diazepam 5 mg	by Heartland	61392-0831	Antianxiety; C IV
P052	Tab, Purepac Logo	Diazepam 5 mg	by Physicians Total Care	54868-0059	Antianxiety; C IV
P053	Tab, Purepac Logo 053	Diazepam 10 mg	by Quality Care	60346-0033	Antianxiety; C IV
P063	Tab, Purepac Logo 063	Lorazepam 2 mg	by Quality Care	60346-0800	Sedative/Hypnotic; C IV
P076	Cap, Purepac Logo	Temazepam 15 mg	Tem by Allscripts	54569-0905	Sedative/Hypnotic; C IV
P076	Cap, Purepac Logo	Temazepam 15 mg	Tem by Quality Care	60346-0668	Sedative/Hypnotic; C IV
P085	Tab, Film Coated, Purepac Logo 085	Acetaminophen 650 mg, Propoxyphene Napsylate 100 mg	by Golden State	60429-0518	Analgesic; C IV
P087 <> P087	Cap, White, with Red Bands	Diphenhydramine HCl 25 mg	by Quality Care	60346-0589	Antihistamine
P1	Tab, Brown, Round	Ibuprofen 200 mg	Motrin by PFI		NSAID
P1	Tab, Brown, Round	Prochlorperazine 5 mg	Compazine by Mylan		Antiemetic
P1 <> M	Tab, Maroon, Round, Film Coated	Prochlorperazine Maleate 5 mg	Compazine by UDL	51079-0541	Antiemetic
P1 <> M	Tab, Maroon, Round	Prochlorperazine Maleate 5 mg	Compazine by Mylan		Antiemetic
P10	Tab, Yellow, Round	Meclizine HCl 25 mg	by PFI		Antiemetic
P10 <> G	Tab	Pindolol 10 mg	by Par	49884-0443	Antihypertensive
P10 <> G	Tab	Pindolol 10 mg	by Genpharm	55567-0016	Antihypertensive
P10 <> G	Tab	Pindolol 10 mg	by United Res	00677-1458	Antihypertensive
P10 <> JANSSEN	Tab, P/10 <> Janssen	Cisapride 10 mg	Propulsid by PDRX	55289-0105	Gastrointestinal
P10 <> JANSSEN	Tab, P Over 10	Cisapride 10 mg	Propulsid by Quality Care	60346-0490	Gastrointestinal
P10 <> JANSSEN	Tab, P/10 <> Janssen	Cisapride 10 mg	Propulsid by Nat Pharmpak Serv	55154-1402	Gastrointestinal
P10 <> JANSSEN	Tab, P over 10 <> Janssen	Cisapride 10 mg	by Pharm Packaging Ctr	54383-0077	Gastrointestinal
P10 <> JANSSEN	Tab, P/10	Cisapride 10 mg	Propulsid by Johnson & Johnson	59604-0430	Gastrointestinal
P10 <> JANSSEN	Tab, P/10	Cisapride Monohydrate	Propulsid by Allscripts	54569-4238	Gastrointestinal
P10G	Tab, White, Round, P10/G	Pindolol 10 mg	Gen Pindolol by Genpharm	Canadian	Antihypertensive
P10JANSSEN	Tab, Beige & White, Circular, P/10/Janssen	Cisapride 10 mg	Prepulsid by Janssen	Canadian	Gastrointestinal
P111	Tab, White, Oblong	Acetaminophen 500 mg	Tylenol by PFI		Antipyretic
P112	Tab, White, Oblong	Acetaminophen 325 mg, Pseudoephedrine 30 mg, DM 15 mg	by PFI		Cold Remedy
P114	Tab, Yellow, Round	Caffeine 200 mg	by PFI		Stimulant
P115	Tab, Yellow, Round	Acetaminophen 325 mg, Pseudoephedrine 30 mg, Chlorpheniramine 2 mg, DM 15 mg	by PFI		Cold Remedy
P12	Tab, Blue, Round	Pseudoephedrine 30 mg, Chlorpheniramine 2 mg	by PFI		Cold Remedy
P121	Tab, White, Round	Acetaminophen 500 mg	Tylenol by PFI		Antipyretic
P122	Tab, Green, Oblong	Loperamide 2 mg	Imodium by PFI		Antidiarrheal
P125	Tab, Green, Oblong	Pseudoephedrine 30 mg, Diphenhydramine 12.5 mg, Acetaminophen 500 mg	by PFI		Cold Remedy
P127	Tab, Purepac Logo 127	Clonidine HCl 0.1 mg	by Quality Care	60346-0786	Antihypertensive
P127	Tab, Purepac Logo 127	Clonidine HCl 0.1 mg	by Apotheca	12634-0465	Antihypertensive
P128	Tab, Orange, Round	Clonidine HCl 0.2 mg	Catapres by Purepac		Antihypertensive
P128	Tab, Orange, Round, Scored	Clonidine HCl 0.2 mg	by DHHS Prog	11819-0113	Antihypertensive
P129	Tab, Orange, Round	Clonidine HCl 0.3 mg	Catapres by Purepac		Antihypertensive
P13	Tab, Orange, Round	Aspirin Enteric Coated 500 mg	Ecotrin by PFI		Analgesic
P133	Tab, Reddish Brown, Film Coated, Purepac Logo 133	Amitriptyline HCl 50 mg	by Quality Care	60346-0673	Antidepressant
P14	Tab, Blue, Round	Phenylpropanolamine 25 mg, Brompheniramine 4 mg	by PFI		Cold Remedy
P141	Cap, Yellow	Acetaminophen 500 mg, Pseudoephedrine 30 mg, Chlorpheniramine 2 mg	by PFI		Cold Remedy
P142	Tab, Orange, Ellipse	Acetaminophen 500 mg, Pseudoephedrine 30 mg	by PFI		Cold Remedy
P143	Tab, Coated, Purepac Logo	Carbamazepine 200 mg	by Heartland	61392-0038	Anticonvulsant
P143	Tab, Purepac Logo 143	Carbamazepine 200 mg	by Quality Care	60346-0777	Anticonvulsant
P144	Tab, Purple, Round	Acetaminophen Chewable 160 mg	by PFI		Antipyretic
P147	Tab, Blue, Round	Acetaminophen 500 mg, Pseudoephedrine 30 mg	by PFI		Cold Remedy
P147	Tab, Orange, Oblong	Pseudoephedrine HCl 60 mg, Acetaminophen 500 mg	by PFI		Cold Remedy
P15	Tab, White, Round	Acetaminophen Chewable 80 mg	Tylenol by PFI		Antipyretic

ID FRONT <> BACK	DESCRIPTION FRONT <> BACK	INGREDIENT & STRENGTH	BRAND (OR EQUIV.) & FIRM	NDC#	CLASS; SCH.
P15	Tab, White, Round, P-15	Phenobarbital 15 mg	by Eon		Sedative/Hypnotic; C IV
P151	Tab, Pink, Round	Acetaminophen 325 mg, Pseudoephedrine 30 mg	by PFI		Cold Remedy
P15G	Tab, White, Round, P-15/G	Pindolol 15 mg	Gen Pindolol by Genpharm	Canadian	Antihypertensive
P171	Cap, Yellow	Acetaminophen 650 mg, Pseudoephedrine 60 mg, Dextromethorphan 30 mg	by PFI		Cold Remedy
P172	Cap, Blue	Acetaminophen 650 mg, Pseudoephedrine 60 mg, Diphenhydramine 50 mg	by PFI		Cold Remedy
P174	Tab, White, Oblong	Acetaminophen 325 mg, Pseudoephedrine 30 mg, Chlorpheniramine 2 mg, DM 15 mg	by PFI		Cold Remedy
P177	Tab, White, Oval	Diphenhydramine 25 mg, Pseudoephedrine 60 mg	by PFI		Cold Remedy
P19	Tab, Orange, Round	Aspirin Enteric Coated 325 mg	Ecotrin by PFI		Analgesic
P2	Tab, White, Round	Ibuprofen 200 mg	Advil by PFI		NSAID
P2	Tab, Brown, Round	Prochlorperazine 10 mg	Compazine by Mylan		Antiemetic
P2 <> M	Tab, Maroon, Round, Film Coated	Prochlorperazine Maleate 10 mg	Compazine by UDL	51079-0542	Antiemetic
P2 <> M	Tab, Maroon, Film Coated	Prochlorperazine Maleate 10 mg	by Mylan	00378-5110	Antiemetic
P20	Tab, White, Round	Acetaminophen 325 mg, Phenylpropanolamine 12.5 mg, Chlorpheniramine 2 mg	by PFI		Cold Remedy
P20	Tab, Yellow, Oval, Enteric Coated	Pantoprozole Sodium Sesquihydrate 22.6 mg	Pantoloc by Solvay Pharma 20 mg	Canadian DIN# 02241804	Gastrointestinal
P20	Tab, White, Round, P-20	Pseudoephedrine HCl 60 mg	Sudafed by Circa		Decongestant
P20 <> JANSSEN	Tab, P/20 <> Tab Also Comes in Blue	Cisapride 20 mg	Propulsid by Johnson & Johnson	59604-0440	Gastrointestinal
P20 <> JANSSEN	Tab, P/20 <> Janssen	Cisapride 20 mg	Propulsid by Janssen	50458-0440	Gastrointestinal
P200 <> US0147	Tab, Pink, Round, Scored, P200 <> U-S over 0147	Amidarone HCl 200 mg	Pacerone by Apotheca	12634-0543	Antiarrhythmic
P200 <> US0147	Tab, U-S over 0147	Amiodarone HCl 200 mg	Pacerone by Upsher Smith	00245-0147	Antiarrhythmic
P200 <> USO147	Tab, Pink, Round, Scored	Amiodarone HCl 200 mg	Pacerone by Thrift Services	59198-0362	Antiarrhythmic
P203	Tab, Purepac Logo 20/3	Acetaminophen 300 mg, Codeine Phosphate 30 mg	by McNeil	52021-0020	Analgesic; C III
P207	Tab, White, Oblong	Sucralfate 1000 mg	Carafate by PFI		Gastrointestinal
P21	Tab, Blue, Round	Diphenhydramine HCl 25 mg	by PFI		Antihistamine
P21	Tab, Green, Round, P-21	Imipramine HCl 50 mg	Tofranil by Eon		Antidepressant
P210	Tab, Yellow, Oblong	Phenylpropanolamine HCl 75 mg	by PFI		Decongestant; Appetite Suppressant
P211	Tab, Green, Oblong	Acetaminophen 500 mg, Pseudoephedrine 30 mg	by PFI		Cold Remedy
P2120	Cap, White, Soft Gel, P in an Inverted Triangle 2120	Valproic Acid 250 mg	by Teva	00480-0757	Anticonvulsant
P2120	Cap, Gelatin Coated, P Inside of Upside Down Triangle	Valproic Acid 250 mg	by Banner Pharmacaps	10888-2120	Anticonvulsant
P2120	Cap, Gelatin Coated	Valproic Acid 250 mg	by Qualitest	00603-6334	Anticonvulsant
P2120	Cap, Gelatin Coated, P Inside of Upside Down Triangle	Valproic Acid 250 mg	by HL Moore	00839-7180	Anticonvulsant
P2120	Cap, Gelatin Coated, P Inside of Upside Down Triangle	Valproic Acid 250 mg	by United Res	00677-1079	Anticonvulsant
P214	Tab, P 21/4	Acetaminophen 300 mg, Codeine Phosphate 60 mg	by McNeil	52021-0021	Analgesic; C III
P214	Tab, Orange, Oblong	Acetaminophen 325 mg, Pseudoephedrine 30 mg, Dextromethorphan 10 mg	by PFI		Cold Remedy
P218	Tab, Yellow, Oblong	Triprolidine HCl 2.5 mg, Pseudoephedrine HCl 60 mg	Actifed by PFI		Cold Remedy
P219	Tab, Blue, Oblong	Pseudoephedrine HCl 60 mg, Diphenhydramine HCl 25 mg	by PFI		Cold Remedy
P221	Tab, Orange, Round	Acetaminophen 500 mg, Pseudoephedrine 30 mg	by PFI		Cold Remedy
P221	Tab, Purepac	Hydrochlorothiazide 25 mg	by Apotheca	12634-0445	Diuretic
P221	Tab, Orange, Round	Pseudoephedrine HCl 60 mg, Acetaminophen 500 mg	by PFI		Cold Remedy
P224	Tab, Blue, Oblong	Acetaminophen 500 mg, Phenylpropanolamine 12.5 mg, Brompheniramine 2 mg	by PFI		Cold Remedy
P225	Tab, White, Oblong	Magnesium Salicylate 467 mg	by PFI		Analgesic
P225	Tab, Green, Oblong	Magnesium Salicylate 500 mg	by PFI		Analgesic
P227	Tab, Yellow, Oblong	Phenylpropanolamine 25 mg, Chlorpheniramine 4 mg	by PFI		Cold Remedy
P23	Tab, White, Round	Aspirin 400 mg, Caffeine 32 mg	by PFI		Analgesic
P241	Tab, Yellow, Oblong	Pseudoephedrine HCl 30 mg, Acetaminophen 500 mg	by PFI		Cold Remedy
P243	Tab, White, Oblong	Acetaminophen 500 mg, Pamabrom 25 mg, Pyrilamine 15 mg	by PFI		PMS Relief
P25	Tab, White, Round	Dimenhydrinate 50 mg	Dramamine by PFI		Antiemetic
P25	Tab, Peach, Round, P-25	Hydrochlorothiazide 25 mg	Hydrodiuril by Eon		Diruetic
P250	Cap, Blue & Yellow, p/250	Mefenamic Acid 250 mg	by Pharmascience	Canadian	NSAID
P252	Tab, Yellow, Round	Acetaminophen 325 mg, Pseudoephedrine 30 mg, Chlorpheniramine 2 mg, DM 10 mg	by PFI		Cold Remedy

ID FRONT <> BACK	DESCRIPTION FRONT <> BACK	INGREDIENT & STRENGTH	BRAND (OR EQUIV.) & FIRM	NDC#	CLASS; SCH.
P253	Tab, Yellow, Oblong	Acetaminophen 325 mg, Pseudoephedrine 30 mg, Chlorpheniramine 2 mg, DM 10 mg by PFI			Cold Remedy
P254	Cap, Brown & Ivory	Ibuprofen 200 mg	by Pharmaceutical Formulations		NSAID
P254	Cap, Purple	Ibuprofen 200 mg	Motrin by PFI		NSAID
P255	Tab, White, Ellipse	Pseudoephedrine 30 mg, Acetaminophen 500 mg, Diphenhydramine 12.5 mg	by PFI		Cold Remedy
P262	Tab, Buff, Round	Phenophthalein 90 mg	by PFI		Gastrointestinal
P269	Tab, Biconvex, Purepac Logo	Metoclopramide HCl	by Quality Care	60346-0802	Gastrointestinal
P269	Tab	Metoclopramide HCl 10 mg	by Nat Pharmpak Serv	55154-5510	Gastrointestinal
P27	Tab, Purepac Logo	Propranolol HCl 10 mg	by Golden State	60429-0227	Antihypertensive
P29	Tab, Purepac Logo	Propranolol HCl 20 mg	by Golden State	60429-0164	Antihypertensive
P2M	Tab, Maroon, Round, P2/M	Prochlorperazine Maleate 10 mg	Compazine by Mylan		Antiemetic
P3	Tab, White, Oblong	Acetaminophen 160 mg	Revinol Jr. by PFI		Antipyretic
P30	Tab, Tan, Oblong, Brown Specks	Calcium Polycarbophil 625 mg	Fiberlax by PFI		Vitamin/Mineral
P30	Cap, Maroon	Docusate Sodium 100 mg, Casanthranol 30 mg	Peri-Colace by Paddock		Laxative
P30	Tab, White, Round, P-30	Phenobarbital 30 mg	by Eon		Sedative/Hypnotic; C IV
P300	Cap, Green & Ivory	Acetaminophen 325 mg, Pseudoephedrine 30 mg, Chlorpheniramine 2 mg	by PFI		Cold Remedy
P301	Cap, Green & White	Acetaminophen 500 mg, Pseudoephedrine 30 mg	by PFI		Cold Remedy
P31	Tab, Coated, Purepac Logo	Amitriptyline HCl 10 mg	by Quality Care	60346-0354	Antidepressant
P316	Cap, Red & White	Acetaminophen 500 mg	Tylenol by PFI		Antipyretic
P32	Tab, Coated, Purepac Logo 32	Amitriptyline HCl 25 mg	by Quality Care	60346-0027	Antidepressant
P32	Tab, Orange, Round	Aspirin Chewable 81 mg	Tylenol by PFI		Analgesic
P32	Tab, White, Round, P-32	Reserpine 0.1 mg	Serpasil by Eon		Antihypertensive
P325	Tab, Blue, Oblong	Acetaminophen 500 mg, Diphenhydramine 25 mg	by PFI		Cold Remedy
P33	Tab, Purepac Logo 33	Clonazepam 0.5 mg	by Murfreesboro	51129-1140	Anticonvulsant; C IV
P33	Tab, White, Round	Diphenhydramine HCl 25 mg	by PFI		Antihistamine
P33 <> LL	Tab	Propylthiouracil 50 mg	by Physicians Total Care	54868-1752	Antithyroid
P334	Tab, Blue, Round	Acetaminophen 500 mg, Diphenhydramine 25 mg	by PFI		Cold Remedy
P337	Tab, White, Oblong	Acetaminophen 500 mg, Pseudoephedrine 30 mg, Dextromethorphan 15 mg	by PFI		Cold Remedy
P34	Tab, Pink, Round	Acetaminophen 325 mg, Pseudoephedrine 30 mg, Chlorpheniramine 2 mg	by PFI		Cold Remedy
P34	Tab, Yellow, Round, Scored	Clonazepam 1 mg	by Danbury	61955-2667	Anticonvulsant; C IV
P345	Tab, Aqua & Ivory, Oblong	Calcium Carbonate 311 mg, Magnesium Carbonate 232 mg	by PFI		Vitamin/Mineral
P346	Cap, Orange & Red	Acetaminophen 325 mg, Pseudoephedrine 30 mg, Dextromethorphan 15 mg	by PFI		Cold Remedy
P349	Cap, Blue	Acetaminophen 500 mg, Diphenhydramine 25 mg	by PFI		Cold Remedy
P35	Tab, White, Round, Scored	Clonazepam 2 mg	by Phcy Svc Ctr	00855-0762	Anticonvulsant; C IV
P35	Tab, Red, Round	Pseudoephedrine HCl 30 mg	Sudafed by Circa		Decongestant
P350 <> PF	Tab, White, Square	Aminophylline 350 mg	PhylloContin-350 by Purdue Frederick	Canadian	Antiasthmatic
P36 <> LL	Tab	Pyrazinamide 500 mg	by Lederle	00005-5093	Antibiotic
P36 <> LL	Tab	Pyrazinamide 500 mg	by PDRX	55289-0283	Antibiotic
P36 <> LL	Tab	Pyrazinamide 500 mg	by Allscripts	54569-3950	Antibiotic
P36 <> LL	Tab, White, Round, Scored, P over 36 <> LL	Pyrazinamide 500 mg	Lederle by UDL	51079-0691	Antibiotic
P36 <> LL	Tab	Pyrazinamide 500 mg	by Amerisource	62584-0848	Antibiotic
P384	Tab, Purple, Round	Acetaminophen 80 mg, Pseudoephedrine 7.5 mg, Chlorpheniramine 0.5 mg	by PFI		Cold Remedy
P4	Tab, White, Round	Pseudoephedrine 30 mg, Chlorpheniramine 4 mg	by PFI		Cold Remedy
P40	Tab, Yellow, Oval, Enteric Coated	Pantroprazole Sodium Sesquihydrate 45.1 mg	Pantoloc by Solvay Pharma	Canadian DIN# 02229453	Gastrointestinal
P406	Cap, Hard Gelatin, Logo <> Purepac	Tetracycline HCl 500 mg	by Quality Care	60346-0435	Antibiotic
P41	Tab, White, Round	Acetaminophen 325 mg	Tylenol by PFI		Antipyretic
P411	Tab, Pink, Oval	Diphenhydramine HCl 25 mg	by PFI		Antihistamine
P412	Tab, White, Round	Aspirin 250 mg, Acetaminophen 250 mg, Caffeine 65 mg	by PFI		Analgesic
P416	Tab, Blue, Round	Phenophthalein 135 mg	by PFI		Gastrointestinal
P419	Cap, Clear & Red	Acetaminophen 650 mg, Pseudoephedrine 30 mg, Dextromethorphan 15 mg	by PFI		Cold Remedy
P42	Tab, White, Oblong	Ibuprofen 200 mg	Advil by PFI		NSAID

ID FRONT <> BACK	DESCRIPTION FRONT <> BACK	INGREDIENT & STRENGTH	BRAND (OR EQUIV.) & FIRM	NDC#	CLASS; SCH.
P420	Cap, Beige	Acetaminophen 500 mg, Pseudoephedrine 30 mg, Diphenhydramine 25 mg	by PFI		Cold Remedy
P422	Tab, White, Round	Acetaminophen 500 mg, Pseudoephedrine 30 mg, Dextromethorphan 15 mg	by PFI		Cold Remedy
P43	Tab, Brown, Oblong	Ibuprofen 200 mg	Advil by PFI		NSAID
P431	Tab, Blue, Oblong	Acetaminophen 500 mg, Pseudoephedrine 30 mg, Diphenhydramine 25 mg	by PFI		Cold Remedy
P434	Tab, Blue, Round	Naproxen Sodium 200 mg	by PFI		NSAID
P439	Tab, Coated, Purepac Logo 439	Trazodone HCl 50 mg	by Quality Care	60346-0620	Antidepressant
P44	Tab, Blue, Round	Diphenhydramine HCl 50 mg	by PFI		Antihistamine
P440	Tab, White, Oblong	Acetaminophen 500 mg, Pamabrom 25 mg, Pyrilamine 15 mg	by PFI		PMS Relief
P441	Tab, Orange, Oblong	Pseudoephedrine HCl 30 mg, Acetaminophen 500 mg	by PFI		Cold Remedy
P445	Tab, Blue, Oblong	Naproxen Sodium 200 mg	by PFI		NSAID
P452	Tab, Red, Round	Acetaminophen 80 mg, Pseudoephedrine 7.5 mg, Dextromethorphan 2.5 mg	by PFI		Cold Remedy
P454	Tab, Blue, Oblong	Acetaminophen 500 mg, Phenylpropanolamine 12.5 mg, Chlorpheniramine 2 mg, DM 15 mg	by PFI		Cold Remedy
P457	Tab, Maroon, Round	Acetaminophen 500 mg, Diphenhydramine 50 mg	by PFI		Cold Remedy
P458	Tab, Blue, Round	Acetaminophen 500 mg, Diphenhydramine Citrate 38 mg	by PFI		Cold Remedy
P459	Tab, Purple, Round	Diphenhydramine HCl 12.5 mg	Benadryl by PFI		Antihistamine
P460	Tab, Yellow, Oblong	Acetaminophen 500 mg, Diphenhydramine 12.5 mg	by PFI		Cold Remedy
P4600	Cap, Football Shaped, Gelatin Coated	Benzonatate 100 mg	by Quality Care	60346-0101	Antitussive
P4600	Cap, Gelatin, P in a triangle 4600	Benzonatate 100 mg	by Murfreesboro	51129-1148	Antitussive
P4600	Cap, Gelatin, P in a triangle 4600	Benzonatate 100 mg	by Kaiser	00179-1256	Antitussive
P4600	Cap, Gelatin, P in a triangle	Benzonatate 100 mg	by Warner Chilcott	00047-0048	Antitussive
P4600	Cap, P in a triangle	Benzonatate 100 mg	by United Res	00677-1472	Antitussive
P4600	Cap, Gelatin, P Inside of Triangle	Benzonatate 100 mg	by Qualitest	00603-2426	Antitussive
P4600	Cap, Gelatin Coated, P in a triangle	Benzonatate 100 mg	by Martec	52555-0484	Antitussive
P4600	Cap, Gelatin Coated, P in a triangle 4600	Benzonatate 100 mg	by PDRX	55289-0175	Antitussive
P467	Tab, White, Round	Acetaminophen 500 mg, Pseudoephedrine 30 mg, Dextromethorphan 15 mg	by PFI		Cold Remedy
P47	Tab, Purple, Round	Acetaminophen Chewable 80 mg	Tylenol by PFI		Antipyretic
P475	Tab, Coated	Verapamil HCl 120 mg	by Prepackage Spec	58864-0530	Antihypertensive
P480	Tab, Film Coated	Tolmetin Sodium 735 mg	by Zenith Goldline	00182-1932	NSAID
P484	Tab, White, Round	Acetaminophen 250 mg, Aspirin 250 mg, Caffeine 65 mg	by PFI		Analgesic
P485	Tab, Yellow, Round	Bisacodyl 5 mg	Dulcolax by PFI		Gastrointestinal
P497	Cap, Yellow, Soft Gel, Purepac Logo 497	Nifedipine 10 mg	by Par	49884-0619	Antihypertensive
P497	Cap, Purepac Logo 497	Nifedipine 10 mg	by Quality Care	60346-0803	Antihypertensive
P497	Cap, Purepac Logo	Nifedipine 10 mg	by Golden State	60429-0138	Antihypertensive
P5 <> G	Tab	Pindolol 5 mg	by Par	49884-0442	Antihypertensive
P5 <> G	Tab	Pindolol 5 mg	by Genpharm	55567-0015	Antihypertensive
P5 <> G	Tab	Pindolol 5 mg	by United Res	00677-1457	Antihypertensive
P50	Tab, Pink, Round	Diphenhydramine HCl 25 mg	by PFI		Antihistamine
P500	Cap, Purepac Logo	Prazosin HCl	by Golden State	60429-0159	Antihypertensive
P501	Cap, Purepac Logo	Prazosin HCl	by Golden State	60429-0160	Antihypertensive
P502	Cap, Purepac Logo	Prazosin HCl	by Golden State	60429-0161	Antihypertensive
P51	Cap, Red	Docusate Sodium 100 mg	Colace by Paddock		Laxative
P511	Tab, White & Yellow, Round	Acetaminophen 325 mg, Phenylephrine 5 mg, Chlorpheniramine 2 mg	by PFI		Cold Remedy
P513	Tab, Pink, Round	Calcium Carbonate 400 mg	by PFI		Vitamin/Mineral
P514	Tab, Orange, Round	Pseudoephedrine HCl (Chewable) 15 mg	by PFI		Decongestant
P515	Tab, Yellow, Oblong	Guaifensin 200 mg, Pseudoephedrine 30 mg, Acetaminophen 325 mg, Dextromethorphan 15 mg	by PFI		Cold Remedy
P516	Tab, Orange, Round	Calcium Carbonate 400 mg	by PFI		Vitamin/Mineral
P52	Tab, White, Oblong	Acetaminophen 500 mg, Calcium Carbonate 250 mg	by PFI		Analgesic
P530	Cap, Brown, P 530	Nifedipine 20 mg	by Par	49884-0620	Antihypertensive
P530	Cap, Brown, Soft Gel	Nifedipine 20 mg	by Par	49884-0624	Antihypertensive
P530	Cap, Purepac Logo	Nifedipine 20 mg	by Golden State	60429-0139	Antihypertensive

ID FRONT <> BACK	DESCRIPTION FRONT <> BACK	INGREDIENT & STRENGTH	BRAND (OR EQUIV.) & FIRM	NDC#	CLASS; SCH.
P530	Cap, Reddish Brown, Purepac Logo looks like R 530 <>	Nifedipine 20 mg	by Heartland	61392-0353	Antihypertensive
P530	Cap, Reddish Brown, Purepac Logo 530	Nifedipine 20 mg	by Quality Care	60346-0845	Antihypertensive
P537	Tab, Ivory & Orange, Oblong	Acetaminophen 500 mg	Tylenol by PFI		Antipyretic
P547	Tab, Film Coated	Naproxen Sodium 275 mg	by Quality Care	60346-0875	NSAID
P550	Tab, Black Ink, Purepac Logo, Delayed Release	Diclofenac Sodium 50 mg	by Quality Care	60346-0238	NSAID
P550	Tab, Purepac Logo	Diclofenac Sodium 50 mg	by PDRX	55289-0166	NSAID
P551	Tab, Purepac Logo	Diclofenac Sodium 75 mg	by PDRX	55289-0150	NSAID
P551	Tab, Black Ink, Purepac Logo, Delayed Release	Diclofenac Sodium 75 mg	by Quality Care	60346-0463	NSAID
P553	Cap, White, Delayed Release, Enteric Coated Pellets	Erythromycin 250 mg	by Quality Care	60346-0017	Antibiotic
P553	Cap	Erythromycin 250 mg	by Zenith Goldline	00182-1398	Antibiotic
P553	Cap	Erythromycin 250 mg	by Pharmedix	53002-0252	Antibiotic
P555	Tab, Embossed, Film Coated	Metoprolol Tartrate 100 mg	by Talbert Med	44514-0515	Antihypertensive
P59	Tab, Purepac Logo 59	Lorazepam 1 mg	by Golden State	60429-0512	Sedative/Hypnotic; C IV
P59	Tab, Purepac Logo P	Lorazepam 1 mg	by Quality Care	60346-0047	Sedative/Hypnotic; C IV
P6	Tab, White, Round	Cimetidine 100 mg	Tagamet HB by PFI		Gastrointestinal
P605	Cap, Purepac Logo P 605	Acyclovir 200 mg	by Golden State	60429-0711	Antiviral
P607	Tab, Pastel Green, Purepac Logo P 607	Acyclovir 800 mg	by Golden State	60429-0713	Antiviral
P611	Tab, Film Coated	Pentoxifylline 400 mg	by Phcy Care	65070-0030	Anticoagulent
P611	Tab, Film Coated, P is Purepac Logo, looks like R	Pentoxifylline 400 mg	by Murfreesboro	51129-1100	Anticoagulent
P611	Tab, Yellow, Oblong, Film Coated, Purepac Logo and 611	Pentoxifylline 400 mg	by Pharmafab	62542-0753	Anticoagulent
P611	Tab, Film Coated, Purepac Logo then 611	Pentoxifylline 400 mg	by Heartland	61392-0833	Anticoagulent
P62	Cap, Red	Docusate Sodium 250 mg	by Paddock		Laxative
P64	Tab, Pink, Round	Acetaminophen Chewable 80 mg	by PFI		Antipyretic
P67	Tab, White, Oval	Cimetidine 200 mg	Tagamet by PFI		Gastrointestinal
P69 <> LEDERLE	Cap, Flesh	Prazosin HCl 1 mg	by Quality Care	60346-0572	Antihypertensive
P7	Tab, Yellow, Round	Chlorpheniramine Maleate 4 mg	Chlor-Trimeton by PFI		Antihistamine
P70 <> LEDERLE	Cap	Prazosin HCl	by Quality Care	60346-0805	Antihypertensive
P73	Tab, Yellow, Round	Aspirin EC 81 mg	by PFI		Analgesic
P75	Tab, Green, Oval	Magnesium Salicylate 325 mg	by PFI		Analgesic
P77	Tab, White, Round	Aspirin 325 mg	by PFI		Analgesic
P77 <> 511	Tab, White, Oblong	Pentoxifylline 400 mg	by ESI Lederle	59911-3290	Anticoagulent
P771	Tab, White, Round	Diphenoxylate HCl 2.5 mg; Atropine Sulfate 0.25 mg	by Par Pharm	49884-0771	Antidiarrheal; C V
P8	Tab, White, Round	Triprolidine HCl 2.5 mg, Pseudoephedrine HCl 60 mg	Actifed by PFI		Cold Remedy
P9	Tab, Brown, Round, P-9	Imipramine HCl 25 mg	Tofranil by Eon		Antidepressant
P912	Tab, Pink, Round	Docusate Sodium 100 mg, Phenophthalein 65 mg	Correctol by PFI		Laxative
P9523	Tab, White, Round	Phenobarbital 16 mg	Solfoton by Poythress		Sedative/Hypnotic; C IV
P97	Tab, Coated, Logo	Primaquine Phosphate 26.3 mg	by Quality Care	60346-0744	Antimalarial
P97 <> W	Tab, in Black Ink, Coated	Primaquine Phosphate 26.3 mg	by Sanofi	00024-1596	Antimalarial
P97 <> W	Tab, in Black Ink, Coated	Primaquine Phosphate 26.3 mg	by Bayer	00280-1596	Antimalarial
PAL <> 0016	Cap, White Print	Acetaminophen 356.4 mg, Caffeine 30 mg, Dihydrocodeine Bitartrate 16 mg	Panlor DC by Pan Am	00525-0016	Analgesic; C III
PAL <> 0016	Cap	Acetaminophen 356.4 mg, Caffeine 30 mg, Dihydrocodeine Bitartrate 16 mg	by Mikart	46672-0267	Analgesic; C III
PAL <> 0305	Cap, White	Dyphylline 200 mg, Guaifenesin 100 mg	Panfil G by Pan Am	00525-0305	Antiasthmatic
PAL <> 0775	Tab, Pal <> 07/75	Guaifenesin 600 mg, Pseudoephedrine HCl 90 mg	Panmist LA by Sovereign	58716-0658	Cold Remedy
PAL <> 0775	Tab, Pal <> 07/75	Guaifenesin 600 mg, Pseudoephedrine HCl 90 mg	Panmist LA by Pan Am	00525-0775	Cold Remedy
PAL <> 0780	Tab, Green Speckled	Chlorpheniramine Maleate 8 mg, Methscopolamine Nitrate 2.5 mg, Phenylpropanolamine HCl 75 mg	Pannaz by Pan Am	00525-0780	Cold Remedy
PAL <> 0780	Tab, White, Green Specks	Chlorpheniramine Maleate 8 mg, Methscopolamine Nitrate 2.5 mg, Phenylpropanolamine HCl 75 mg	Pannaz by Anabolic	00722-6337	Cold Remedy
PAL <> 32	Tab, Purple, Oval, Scored	Acetaminophen 712.8 mg; Caffeine 60 mg; Dihydrocodeine Bitartrate 32 mg	by Mikart	46672-0141	Analgesic; C III
PAL <> 32	Tab, Purple, Oval, Scored	Acetaminophen 712.8 mg; Caffeine 60 mg; Dihydrocodeine Bitartrate 32 mg	Panlor SS by Pan Am Labs	00525-0032	Analgesic; C III
PAL <> 6121	Tab, White, Oblong, Scored	Carbinoxamine Maleate 8 mg; Pseudoephedrine HCl 90 mg	Palgic D by Pan Am Labs	00525-6121	Cold Remedy
PAL <> 762	Tab, White, Oblong	Pseudoephedrine HCl 45 mg, Guaifenesin 600 mg	Panmist Jr by Sovereign Pharms	58716-0680	Cold Remedy

ID FRONT <> BACK	DESCRIPTION FRONT <> BACK	INGREDIENT & STRENGTH	BRAND (OR EQUIV.) & FIRM	NDC#	CLASS; SCH.
PAL <> 762	Tab, White, Oblong	Pseudoephedrine HCl 45 mg, Guaifenesin 600 mg	Panmist JR by Pan Am Labs	00525-0762	Cold Remedy
PAL <> 780	Tab, Green, Oblong, Scored	Methscopolamine Nitrate 2.5 mg; Chlorpheniramine Maleate 8 mg; Phenylpropanolamine HCl 75 mg	Pannaz by Murfreesboro Ph	51129-1429	Cold Remedy
PAL <> JUL42	Tab, White, Scored	Pseudoephedrine HCl 80 mg; Guaifenesin 800 mg	Panmist LA by Sovereign Pharms	58716-0692	Cold Remedy
PAL0016	Cap, Red	Acetaminophrn 356.4 mg, Caffeine 30 mg, Dyhydro Bitrate 16 mg	by Pan American		Analgesic
PAL0305	Cap, Green	Dyphylline 200 mg, Guafenesin 100 mg	by Pan American		Antiasthmatic
PAL0305	Cap, White Print	Dyphylline 200 mg, Guafenesin 100 mg	by Mikart	46672-0202	Antiasthmatic
PAL0754	Tab, Green, Oblong, Scored	Pseudoephedrine HCl 45 mg, Guaifenesin 600 mg, Dextromethorphan Hydrobromide 30 mg	Panmist DM by Sovereign Pharms	58716-0687	Cold Remedy
PAL0754	Tab, Green, Oblong, Scored	Pseudoephedrine HCl 45 mg, Guaifenesin 600 mg, Dextromethorphan Hydrobromide 30 mg	Panmist DM by Pan Am Labs	00525-0754	Cold Remedy
PAL0775	Tab, White, Oblong, PAL 07/75	Pseudoephedrine HCl 90 mg, Guaifenesin 600 mg	by Pan American		Cold Remedy
PAL0780	Tab, White/Green	Phenylpropanolamine HCl 75 mg, Chlorphen Mal 8 mg, Meth Nit 2.5 mg	by Pan American		Cold Remedy
PAMELOR25MG <> SANDOZ	Cap, Pamelor 25 MG	Nortriptyline HCl 25 mg	Pamelor by Novartis	00078-0087	Antidepressant
PAMINE	Tab	Methscopolamine Bromide 2.5 mg	Pamine by Kenwood	00482-0061	Gastrointestinal
PAMPRIN	Cap, White	Acetaminophen 500 mg, Pamabrom 25 mg, Pyrilamine Maleate 15 mg	Pamprin ES by Chattem	Canadian DIN# 00718130	PMS Relief
PAMPRIN	Cap, Yellow/Red	Pamabrom 25 mg, Pyrilamine Maleate 15 mg, Acetaminophen 500 mg	Pamprin ES by Chattem	Canadian	PMS Relief
PAMPRINPMS	Cap, White	Acetaminophen 500 mg, Pamabrom 25 mg, Pyrilamine Maleate 15 mg	Pamprin PMS by Chattem	Canadian DIN# 02240359	PMS Relief
PAN2000	Cap, White, PAN/2000	Pancrelipase EC	Pancrease by Jones		Gastrointestinal
PAN2001	Cap, Delayed Release, PAN/2001	Pancreatin 195.73 mg	Pancrelipase by JMI Canton	00252-2001	Gastrointestinal
PAN2001	Cap, Delayed Release, PAN/2001	Pancreatin 195.73 mg	Pancrelipase by Jones	52604-2001	Gastrointestinal
PANCREASE <> MCNEIL	Cap	Amylase 20000 Units, Lipase 4500 Units, Protease 25000 Units	Pancrease by Prestige Packaging	58056-0350	Gastrointestinal
PANCREASE <> MCNEIL	Cap, Delayed Release	Amylase 20000 Units, Lipase 4500 Units, Protease 25000 Units	Pancrease by Leiner	59606-0714	Gastrointestinal
PANCREASE <> MCNEIL	Cap, White, Red Print	Amylase 20000 Units, Lipase 4500 Units, Protease 25000 Units	Pancrease by McNeil	00045-0095	Gastrointestinal
PANCREASE <> MCNEIL	Cap	Amylase 20000 Units, Lipase 4500 Units, Protease 25000 Units	Pancrease by McNeil	52021-0095	Gastrointestinal
PANCREASEMT10 <> MCNEIL	Cap	Amylase 30000 Units, Lipase 10000 Units, Protease 30000 Units	Pancrease Mt 10 by McNeil	00045-0342	Gastrointestinal
PANCREASEMT10 <> MCNEIL	Cap	Amylase 30000 Units, Lipase 10000 Units, Protease 30000 Units	Pancrease Mt 10 by McNeil	52021-0342	Gastrointestinal
PANCREASEMT16 <> MCNEIL	Cap, Salmon	Amylase 48000 Units, Lipase 16000 Units, Protease 48000 Units	Pancrease Mt 16 by McNeil	00045-0343	Gastrointestinal
PANCREASEMT16 <> MCNEIL	Cap	Amylase 48000 Units, Lipase 16000 Units, Protease 48000 Units	Pancrease Mt 16 by McNeil	52021-0343	Gastrointestinal
PANCREASEMT16 <> MCNEIL	Cap, Clear & Peach	Lipase 16000 Unt, Amylase 48000 Unt, Protease 48000 Unt	Pancrease MT by Murfreesboro Ph	51129-1171	Gastrointestinal
PANCREASEMT20 <> MCNEIL	Cap, Yellow Band	Amylase 56000 Units, Lipase 20000 Units, Protease 44000 Units	Pancrease Mt 20 by McNeil	00045-0346	Gastrointestinal
PANCREASEMT20 <> MCNEIL	Cap, Yellow Band	Amylase 56000 Units, Lipase 20000 Units, Protease 44000 Units	Pancrease Mt 20 by McNeil	52021-0346	Gastrointestinal
PANCREASEMT20 <> MCNEIL	Cap, White, Opaque	Lipase 20,000 Units, Protease 44,000 Units, Amylase 56,000 Units	Pancrease MT 20 by Murfreesboro	51129-2530	Gastrointestinal
PANCREASEMT4 <> MCNEIL	Cap	Amylase 12000 Units, Lipase 4000 Units, Protease 12000 Units	Pancrease Mt 4 by McNeil	00045-0341	Gastrointestinal

ID FRONT <> BACK	DESCRIPTION FRONT <> BACK	INGREDIENT & STRENGTH	BRAND (OR EQUIV.) & FIRM	NDC#	CLASS; SCH.
PANCREASEMT4 <> MCNEIL	Cap	Amylase 12000 Units, Lipase 4000 Units, Protease 12000 Units	Pancrease Mt 4 by McNeil	52021-0341	Gastrointestinal
PANCRECARBMS4 <> DCI	Cap, Blue Ink, Delayed Release	Amylase 25000 Units, Lipase 4000 Units, Protease 25000 Units	Pancrecarb Ms-4 by Digestive Care	59767-0002	Gastrointestinal
PANCRECARBMS8 <> DCI	Cap, Delayed Release	Amylase 40000 Units, Lipase 8000 Units, Protease 45000 Units	Pancrecarb Ms-8 by Digestive Care	59767-0001	Gastrointestinal
PANDG <> 402	Tab	Etidronate Disodium 200 mg	Didronel by DRX	55045-2326	Calcium Metabolism
PAR <> 012	Tab, Coated	Hydroxyzine HCl 10 mg	by Par	49884-0012	Antihistamine
PAR <> 013	Tab, Coated	Hydroxyzine HCl 25 mg	by Par	49884-0013	Antihistamine
PAR <> 014	Tab, Coated	Hydroxyzine HCl 50 mg	by Par	49884-0014	Antihistamine
PAR <> 015	Tab, Layered	Meclizine HCl 50 mg	by Par	49884-0015	Antiemetic
PAR <> 016	Tab	Chlorzoxazone 250 mg	by Par	49884-0016	Muscle Relaxant
PAR <> 034	Tab, Blue & White, Oval	Meclizine HCl 12.5 mg	Antivert by UDL	51079-0089	Antiemetic
PAR <> 034	Tab, Layered	Meclizine HCl 12.5 mg	by Schein	00364-0411	Antiemetic
PAR <> 034	Tab, Blue/White, Multilayer	Meclizine HCl 12.5 mg	by Par	49884-0034	Antiemetic
PAR <> 034	Tab	Meclizine HCl 12.5 mg	by Vangard	00615-1553	Antiemetic
PAR <> 035	Tab, Yellow & White, Pumpkin Seed Shaped	Meclizine HCl 25 mg	Antivert by UDL	51079-0090	Antiemetic
PAR <> 035	Tab, Layered	Meclizine HCl 25 mg	by Schein	00364-0412	Antiemetic
PAR <> 035	Tab, Layered	Meclizine HCl 25 mg	by Par	49884-0035	Antiemetic
PAR <> 035	Tab	Meclizine HCl 25 mg	by Vangard	00615-1554	Antiemetic
PAR <> 061	Tab, Film Coated	Fluphenazine HCl 1 mg	by Schein	00364-2265	Antipsychotic
PAR <> 061	Tab, Film Coated	Fluphenazine HCl 1 mg	by Qualitest	00603-3666	Antipsychotic
PAR <> 062	Tab, Coated	Fluphenazine HCl 2.5 mg	by Qualitest	00603-3667	Antipsychotic
PAR <> 062	Tab, Coated	Fluphenazine HCl 2.5 mg	by Schein	00364-2266	Antipsychotic
PAR <> 064	Tab, Film Coated	Fluphenazine HCl 10 mg	by Qualitest	00603-3669	Antipsychotic
PAR <> 064	Tab, Film Coated	Fluphenazine HCl 10 mg	by Schein	00364-2268	Antipsychotic
PAR <> 076	Tab, Film Coated	Fluphenazine HCl 5 mg	by Qualitest	00603-3668	Antipsychotic
PAR <> 076	Tab, Film Coated	Fluphenazine HCl 5 mg	by Schein	00364-2267	Antipsychotic
PAR <> 104	Tab	Allopurinol 100 mg	by Quality Care	60346-0774	Antigout
PAR <> 114	Tab, Coated, Debossed	Metronidazole 500 mg	by Quality Care	60346-0507	Antibiotic
PAR <> 187	Tab, Film Coated	Hydrochlorothiazide 25 mg, Methyldopa 250 mg	by Par	49884-0187	Diuretic; Antihypertensive
PAR <> 188	Tab, Coated	Hydrochlorothiazide 30 mg, Methyldopa 500 mg	by Par	49884-0188	Diuretic; Antihypertensive
PAR <> 193	Cap	Flurazepam HCl 15 mg	by Qualitest	00603-3691	Hypnotic; C IV
PAR <> 194	Cap	Flurazepam HCl 30 mg	by Qualitest	00603-3692	Hypnotic; C IV
PAR <> 217	Cap, Buff	Doxepin HCl	by Qualitest	00603-3455	Antidepressant
PAR <> 218	Cap	Doxepin HCl	by Qualitest	00603-3456	Antidepressant
PAR <> 219	Cap	Doxepin HCl	by Qualitest	00603-3457	Antidepressant
PAR <> 220	Cap, Green	Doxepin HCl	by Qualitest	00603-3458	Antidepressant
PAR <> 222	Cap	Doxepin HCl	by Schein	00364-2525	Antidepressant
PAR <> 222	Cap	Doxepin HCl	by Qualitest	00603-3460	Antidepressant
PAR <> 225	Tab	Haloperidol 2 mg	by Zenith Goldline	00182-1264	Antipsychotic
PAR <> 246	Tab, Lavender	Aspirin 325 mg, Carisoprodol 200 mg	by Schein	00364-2524	Analgesic; Muscle Relaxant
PAR <> 265	Tab, Coated	Amitriptyline HCl 14.145 mg, Chlordiazepoxide 5 mg	by Par	49884-0265	Antianxiety; C IV
PAR <> 266	Tab, Coated	Amitriptyline HCl 25 mg, Chlordiazepoxide 10 mg	by Par	49884-0266	Antianxiety; C IV
PAR <> 289	Tab	Megestrol Acetate 20 mg	by Schein	00364-2235	Progestin
PAR <> 290	Tab	Megestrol Acetate 40 mg	by Schein	00364-2234	Progestin
PAR <> 467	Tab, Film Coated	Ibuprofen 400 mg	by Quality Care	60346-0430	NSAID
PAR <> 468	Tab, Elongated Shape, Film Coated	Ibuprofen 600 mg	by Quality Care	60346-0556	NSAID
PAR <> 469	Tab, Film Coated	Ibuprofen 400 mg	by Quality Care	60346-0030	NSAID

ID FRONT <> BACK	DESCRIPTION FRONT <> BACK	INGREDIENT & STRENGTH	BRAND (OR EQUIV.) & FIRM	NDC#	CLASS; SCH.
PAR <> 473	Tab, Green & White, Oblong, Scored	Orphenadrine Citrate 50 mg; Aspirin 770 mg; Caffeine 60 mg	Orphengesic Forte by Par Pharm	49884-0473	Muscle Relaxant
PAR <> 54	Tab, Yellow, Triangular, Sugar Coated	Imipramine 10 mg	by Allscripts	54569-2726	Antidepressant
PAR <> 54	Tab, Sugar Coated	Imipramine HCl 10 mg	by Par	49884-0054	Antidepressant
PAR <> 54	Tab, Sugar Coated	Imipramine HCl 10 mg	by Quality Care	60346-0718	Antidepressant
PAR <> 54	Tab, Yellow, Triangle	Impramine HCl 10 mg	by Murfreesboro	51129-1534	Antidepressant
PAR <> 55	Tab, Sugar Coated	Imipramine HCl 25 mg	by Par	49884-0055	Antidepressant
PAR <> 56	Tab, Sugar Coated	Imipramine HCl 50 mg	by Par	49884-0056	Antidepressant
PAR <> 56	Tab, Sugar Coated, 56 Printed in Black Ink	Imipramine HCl 50 mg	by Amerisource	62584-0751	Antidepressant
PAR <> 56	Tab, Sugar Coated, 56 Printed in Black Ink	Imipramine HCl 50 mg	by Quality Care	60346-0709	Antidepressant
PAR009	Tab, Blue, Round, Scored	Isosorbide Dinitrate 30 mg	by Murfreesboro	51129-1565	Antianginal
PAR009	Tab, PAR 009	Isosorbide Dinitrate 30 mg	by United Res	00677-0786	Antianginal
PAR009	Tab	Isosorbide Dinitrate 30 mg	by Qualitest	00603-4119	Antianginal
PAR009	Tab	Isosorbide Dinitrate 30 mg	by Major	00904-2682	Antianginal
PAR009	Tab	Isosorbide Dinitrate 30 mg	by Par	49884-0009	Antianginal
PAR018	Cap, Blue & White, Par/018	Doxycycline Hyclate 50 mg	Vibramycin by Par		Antibiotic
PAR019	Cap, Blue, Par/019	Doxycycline Hyclate 100 mg	Vibramycin by Par		Antibiotic
PAR020	Tab	Isosorbide Dinitrate 5 mg	by Zenith Goldline	00182-0550	Antianginal
PAR020	Tab	Isosorbide Dinitrate 5 mg	by Par	49884-0020	Antianginal
PAR020	Tab, Debossed	Isosorbide Dinitrate 5 mg	by Amerisource	62584-0761	Antianginal
PAR020	Tab	Isosorbide Dinitrate 5 mg	by Baker Cummins	63171-0550	Antianginal
PAR020	Tab, Par over 020	Isosorbide Dinitrate 5 mg	by UDL	51079-0084	Antianginal
PAR021	Tab	Isosorbide Dinitrate 10 mg	by Zenith Goldline	00182-0514	Antianginal
PAR021	Tab, Par over 021	Isosorbide Dinitrate 10 mg	by UDL	51079-0029	Antianginal
PAR021	Tab	Isosorbide Dinitrate 10 mg	by Par	49884-0021	Antianginal
PAR021	Tab, Debossed	Isosorbide Dinitrate 10 mg	by Amerisource	62584-0763	Antianginal
PAR021	Tab	Isosorbide Dinitrate 10 mg	by Quality Care	60346-0577	Antianginal
PAR021	Tab	Isosorbide Dinitrate 10 mg	by Nat Pharmpak Serv	55154-5532	Antianginal
PAR021	Tab	Isosorbide Dinitrate 10 mg	by Heartland	61392-0305	Antianginal
PAR022	Tab, Par over 022	Isosorbide Dinitrate 20 mg	by UDL	51079-0085	Antianginal
PAR022	Tab	Isosorbide Dinitrate 20 mg	by Zenith Goldline	00182-0868	Antianginal
PAR022	Tab	Isosorbide Dinitrate 20 mg	by PDRX	55289-0174	Antianginal
PAR022	Tab	Isosorbide Dinitrate 20 mg	by Par	49884-0022	Antianginal
PAR022	Tab, Debossed	Isosorbide Dinitrate 20 mg	by Baker Cummins	63171-0868	Antianginal
PAR022	Tab	Isosorbide Dinitrate 20 mg	by Heartland	61392-0321	Antianginal
PAR022	Tab	Isosorbide Dinitrate 20 mg	by Quality Care	60346-0798	Antianginal
PAR022	Tab, Debossed	Isosorbide Dinitrate 20 mg	by Amerisource	62584-0764	Antianginal
PAR025	Tab, Green, Round, Par/025	Isosorbide Dinitrate Sustained Action 40 mg	Isordil by Par		Antianginal
PAR027	Tab	Hydralazine HCl 25 mg	by Quality Care	60346-0824	Antihypertensive
PAR027	Tab	Hydralazine HCl 25 mg	by Qualitest	00603-3831	Antihypertensive
PAR027	Tab	Hydralazine HCl 25 mg	by Allscripts	54569-0515	Antihypertensive
PAR027	Tab	Hydralazine HCl 25 mg	by Physicians Total Care	54868-1949	Antihypertensive
PAR027	Tab	Hydralazine HCl 25 mg	by Par	49884-0027	Antihypertensive
PAR028	Tab	Hydralazine HCl 50 mg	by Qualitest	00603-3832	Antihypertensive
PAR028	Tab	Hydralazine HCl 50 mg	by Par	49884-0028	Antihypertensive
PAR029	Tab, Light Pink, Round, Par/029	Hydralazine HCl 10 mg	Apresoline by Par		Antihypertensive
PAR0299	Tab	Hydralazine HCl 10 mg	by Qualitest	00603-3830	Antihypertensive
PAR030	Tab, White/Blue-Green Speckles, Par/030	Phenylprop. 40 mg, Phenyleph. 10 mg, Phenyltolox. 15 mg, Chlorphenir. 5 mg	Naldecon by Par		Cold Remedy
PAR034	Tab	Meclizine HCl 12.5 mg	by Zenith Goldline	00182-0871	Antiemetic
PAR034	Tab, Par over 034	Meclizine HCl 12.5 mg	by Quality Care	60346-0056	Antiemetic
PAR034	Tab, Blue & White	Meclizine HCl 12.5 mg	by PDRX	55289-0982	Antiemetic
PAR034	Tab, Debossed, Multiple Layered	Meclizine HCl 12.5 mg	by Amerisource	62584-0772	Antiemetic
PAR034	Tab, Layered	Meclizine HCl 12.5 mg	by United Res	00677-0418	Antiemetic

ID FRONT <> BACK	DESCRIPTION FRONT <> BACK	INGREDIENT & STRENGTH	BRAND (OR EQUIV.) & FIRM	NDC#	CLASS; SCH.
PAR034	Tab, Debossed, Layered	Meclizine HCl 12.5 mg	by Major	00904-2384	Antiemetic
PAR034	Tab	Meclizine HCl 12.5 mg	by Qualitest	00603-4319	Antiemetic
PAR035	Tab	Meclizine HCl 25 mg	by Zenith Goldline	00182-0872	Antiemetic
PAR035	Tab, Layered	Meclizine HCl 25 mg	by Pharmedix	53002-0351	Antiemetic
PAR035	Tab, Multiple Layered <> Debossed	Meclizine HCl 25 mg	by Amerisource	62584-0774	Antiemetic
PAR035	Tab, Par over 035	Meclizine HCl 25 mg	by Quality Care	60346-0694	Antiemetic
PAR035	Tab	Meclizine HCl 25 mg	by Qualitest	00603-4320	Antiemetic
PAR035	Tab	Meclizine HCl 25 mg	by United Res	00677-0419	Antiemetic
PAR035	Tab, Layered	Meclizine HCl 25 mg	by Apotheca	12634-0424	Antiemetic
PAR036	Tab	Methocarbamol 500 mg	by Par	49884-0036	Muscle Relaxant
PAR037	Tab	Methocarbamol 750 mg	by Par	49884-0037	Muscle Relaxant
PAR038	Tab	Trichlormethiazide 2 mg	by Par	49884-0038	Diuretic
PAR039	Tab	Trichlormethiazide 4 mg	by Par	49884-0039	Diuretic
PAR043	Tab	Cyproheptadine HCl 4 mg	by Amerisource	62584-0355	Antihistamine
PAR043	Tab	Cyproheptadine HCl 4 mg	by Par	49884-0043	Antihistamine
PAR053	Tab, Orange, Oblong	B Complex, Folic Acid	Berocca by Par		Vitamin
PAR06	Tab, White, Oval	Dexchlorpheniramine Maleate TD 6 mg	Polaramine by Par		Antihistamine
PAR061	Tab, Film Coated	Fluphenazine HCl 1 mg	by Par	49884-0061	Antipsychotic
PAR061	Tab, White, Round, Film Coated	Fluphenazine HCl 1 mg	by Dixon Shane	17236-0489	Antipsychotic
PAR061	Tab, Film Coated, Debossed	Fluphenazine HCl 1 mg	by Major	00904-3673	Antipsychotic
PAR061	Tab, Film Coated	Fluphenazine HCl 1 mg	by Baker Cummins	63171-1365	Antipsychotic
PAR061	Tab, Film Coated	Fluphenazine HCl 1 mg	by Zenith Goldline	00182-1365	Antipsychotic
PAR062	Tab, Coated	Fluphenazine HCl 2.5 mg	by Amerisource	62584-0699	Antipsychotic
PAR062	Tab, Coated	Fluphenazine HCl 2.5 mg	by Baker Cummins	63171-1366	Antipsychotic
PAR062	Tab, Coated	Fluphenazine HCl 2.5 mg	by Zenith Goldline	00182-1366	Antipsychotic
PAR062	Tab, Coated	Fluphenazine HCl 2.5 mg	by United Res	00677-1218	Antipsychotic
PAR062	Tab, Coated	Fluphenazine HCl 2.5 mg	by Par	49884-0062	Antipsychotic
PAR062	Tab, Blue, Round, Film Coated	Fluphenazine HCl 2.5 mg	by Dixon Shane	17236-0490	Antipsychotic
PAR064	Tab, Film Coated	Fluphenazine HCl 10 mg	by Amerisource	62584-0704	Antipsychotic
PAR064	Tab, Film Coated	Fluphenazine HCl 10 mg	by Zenith Goldline	00182-1368	Antipsychotic
PAR064	Tab, Film Coated	Fluphenazine HCl 10 mg	by Vangard	00615-3574	Antipsychotic
PAR064	Tab, Film Coated	Fluphenazine HCl 10 mg	by Par	49884-0064	Antipsychotic
PAR064	Tab, Orange, Round, Film Coated	Fluphenazine HCl 10 mg	by Dixon Shane	17236-0492	Antipsychotic
PAR066	Tab, Round	Doxylamine Succinate 25 mg	Unisom by Par		Sleep Aid
PAR067	Cap	Indomethacin 25 mg	by Par	49884-0067	NSAID
PAR068	Cap	Indomethacin 50 mg	by Par	49884-0068	NSAID
PAR069	Cap, Green, Par/069	Hydroxyzine Pamoate 25 mg	Vistaril by Par		Antihistamine
PAR070	Cap, White & Green, Par/070	Hydroxyzine Pamoate 50 mg	Vistaril by Par		Antihistamine
PAR071	Cap, Gray & Green, Par/071	Hydroxyzine Pamoate 100 mg	Vistaril by Par		Antihistamine
PAR076	Tab, Film Coated, Par over 076	Fluphenazine HCl 5 mg	by Quality Care	60346-0980	Antipsychotic
PAR076	Tab, Dark Pink, Film Coated	Fluphenazine HCl 5 mg	by Amerisource	62584-0703	Antipsychotic
PAR076	Tab, Film Coated	Fluphenazine HCl 5 mg	by Zenith Goldline	00182-1367	Antipsychotic
PAR076	Tab, Coated	Fluphenazine HCl 5 mg	by Vangard	00615-1501	Antipsychotic
PAR076	Tab, Film Coated	Fluphenazine HCl 5 mg	by Par	49884-0076	Antipsychotic
PAR076	Tab, Pink, Round, Film Coated	Fluphenazine HCl 5 mg	by Invamed	52189-0314	Antipsychotic
PAR076	Tab, Pink, Round, Film Coated	Fluphenazine HCl 5 mg	by Dixon Shane	17236-0491	Antipsychotic
PAR077	Tab	Chlorpropamide 100 mg	by Par	49884-0077	Antidiabetic
PAR078	Tab	Chlorpropamide 250 mg	by Par	49884-0078	Antidiabetic
PAR083	Tab	Dexamethasone 0.25 mg	by Par	49884-0083	Steroid
PAR084	Tab	Dexamethasone 0.5 mg	by Zenith Goldline	00182-1612	Steroid
PAR084	Tab, Par/084	Dexamethasone 0.5 mg	by Qualitest	00603-3190	Steroid
PAR084	Tab	Dexamethasone 0.5 mg	by Par	49884-0084	Steroid

ID FRONT <> BACK	DESCRIPTION FRONT <> BACK	INGREDIENT & STRENGTH	BRAND (OR EQUIV.) & FIRM	NDC#	CLASS; SCH.
PAR084	Tab	Dexamethasone 0.5 mg	by Major	00904-0243	Steroid
PAR085	Tab	Dexamethasone 0.75 mg	by Quality Care	60346-0550	Steroid
PAR085	Tab, Blue, Scored	Dexamethasone 0.75 mg	by DRX	55045-2597	Steroid
PAR085	Tab	Dexamethasone 0.75 mg	by Zenith Goldline	00182-0488	Steroid
PAR085	Tab, Coated, Par/085	Dexamethasone 0.75 mg	by Qualitest	00603-3191	Steroid
PAR085	Tab	Dexamethasone 0.75 mg	by Par	49884-0085	Steroid
PAR085	Tab	Dexamethasone 0.75 mg	by Physicians Total Care	54868-0916	Steroid
PAR086	Tab, Pink, Pentagon, Scored	Dexamethasone 1.5 mg	DexPak Taperpak by ECR	00095-0086	Steroid
PAR086	Tab	Dexamethasone 1.5 mg	by Zenith Goldline	00182-1613	Steroid
PAR086	Tab, Par/086	Dexamethasone 1.5 mg	by Qualitest	00603-3192	Steroid
PAR086	Tab	Dexamethasone 1.5 mg	by Par	49884-0086	Steroid
PAR086	Tab	Dexamethasone 1.5 mg	by Physicians Total Care	54868-1744	Steroid
PAR087	Tab	Dexamethasone 4 mg	by Quality Care	60346-0479	Steroid
PAR087	Tab, White, Pentagonal, Scored	Dexamethasone 4 mg	by DRX	55045-2596	Steroid
PAR087	Tab	Dexamethasone 4 mg	by Zenith Goldline	00182-1614	Steroid
PAR087	Tab, Par/087	Dexamethasone 4 mg	by Qualitest	00603-3194	Steroid
PAR087	Tab	Dexamethasone 4 mg	by Rugby	00536-3580	Steroid
PAR087	Tab	Dexamethasone 4 mg	by United Res	00677-0849	Steroid
PAR087	Tab	Dexamethasone 4 mg	by Pharmedix	53002-0508	Steroid
PAR087	Tab	Dexamethasone 4 mg	by Par	49884-0087	Steroid
PAR087	Tab, White, Scored	Dexamethasone 4 mg	by Compumed	00403-0752	Steroid
PAR095	Tab, White, Round	Metronidazole 250 mg	Metronidazole by Neuman Distr	64579-0106	Antibiotic
PAR095	Tab	Metronidazole 250 mg	by Par	49884-0095	Antibiotic
PAR095	Tab	Metronidazole 250 mg	by Quality Care	60346-0592	Antibiotic
PAR101	Tab, Orange, Round, Par/101	Thioridazine HCl 100 mg	Mellaril by Par		Antipsychotic
PAR102	Tab, Orange, Round	Thioridazine HCl 150 mg	Mellaril by Par		Antipsychotic
PAR103	Tab, Orange, Round	Thioridazine HCl 200 mg	Mellaril by Par		Antipsychotic
PAR104	Tab	Allopurinol 100 mg	by Nat Pharmpak Serv	55154-5534	Antigout
PAR104	Tab, White, Round, Flat, Scored	Allopurinol 100 mg	by Allscripts	54569-0233	Antigout
PAR104	Tab, Debossed, Flat Bevel	Allopurinol 100 mg	by Amerisource	62584-0607	Antigout
PAR104	Tab, Par/104	Allopurinol 100 mg	by UDL	51079-0205	Antigout
PAR104	Tab	Allopurinol 100 mg	by Zenith Goldline	00182-1481	Antigout
PAR104	Tab, Par/104	Allopurinol 100 mg	by Qualitest	00603-2117	Antigout
PAR104	Tab	Allopurinol 100 mg	by Med Pro	53978-5000	Antigout
PAR104	Tab, Par over 104	Allopurinol 100 mg	by Par	49884-0104	Antigout
PAR104	Tab, White, Round	Allopurinol 100 mg	by Caremark	00339-6179	Antigout
PAR105	Tab	Allopurinol 300 mg	by Quality Care	60346-0638	Antigout
PAR105	Tab, Debossed	Allopurinol 300 mg	by Amerisource	62584-0608	Antigout
PAR105	Tab	Allopurinol 300 mg	by Baker Cummins	63171-1482	Antigout
PAR105	Tab, Orange, Round, Scored	Allopurinol 300 mg	by Allscripts	54569-0235	Antigout
PAR105	Tab, Orange, Round, Scored	Allopurinol 300 mg	by Va Cmop	65243-0004	Antigout
PAR105	Tab, Par over 105	Allopurinol 300 mg	by UDL	51079-0206	Antigout
PAR105	Tab	Allopurinol 300 mg	by Zenith Goldline	00182-1482	Antigout
PAR105	Tab, Par/105	Allopurinol 300 mg	by Qualitest	00603-2118	Antigout
PAR105	Tab	Allopurinol 300 mg	by Par	49884-0105	Antigout
PAR105	Tab	Allopurinol 300 mg	by Med Pro	53978-5001	Antigout
PAR105	Tab, Orange, Round, Scored	Allopurinol 300 mg	by Caremark	00339-6180	Antigout
PAR106	Tab	Propranolol HCl 10 mg	by Par	49884-0106	Antihypertensive
PAR107	Tab	Propranolol HCl 20 mg	by Par	49884-0107	Antihypertensive
PAR108	Tab	Propranolol HCl 40 mg	by Par	49884-0108	Antihypertensive
PAR109	Tab	Propranolol HCl 80 mg	by Par	49884-0109	Antihypertensive
PAR110	Tab	Clonidine HCl 0.1 mg	by Quality Care	60346-0786	Antihypertensive

ID FRONT <> BACK	DESCRIPTION FRONT <> BACK	INGREDIENT & STRENGTH	BRAND (OR EQUIV.) & FIRM	NDC#	CLASS; SCH.
PAR111	Tab, Yellow, Round, Par/111	Clonidine HCl 0.2 mg	Catapres by Par		Antihypertensive
PAR112	Tab, Blue, Round, Par/112	Clonidine HCl 0.3 mg	Catapres by Par		Antihypertensive
PAR112	Tab	Clonidine HCl 0.3 mg	by Zenith Goldline	00182-1252	Antihypertensive
PAR113	Tab	Chlorthalidone 15 mg, Clonidine HCl 0.1 mg	by Par	49884-0113	Diuretic; Antihypertensive
PAR114	Tab	Metronidazole 500 mg	by Par	49884-0114	Antibiotic
PAR114	Tab	Metronidazole 500 mg	by Dept Health Central Pharm	53808-0053	Antibiotic
PAR115	Tab	Chlorthalidone 15 mg, Clonidine HCl 0.2 mg	by Par	49884-0115	Diuretic; Antihypertensive
PAR116	Tab	Chlorthalidone 15 mg, Clonidine HCl 0.3 mg	by Zenith Goldline	00182-1277	Diuretic; Antihypertensive
PAR116	Tab	Chlorthalidone 15 mg, Clonidine HCl 0.3 mg	by Par	49884-0116	Diuretic; Antihypertensive
PAR117	Tab	Amiloride HCl 5 mg	by Zenith Goldline	00182-1828	Diuretic
PAR117	Tab	Amiloride HCl 5 mg	by Qualitest	00603-2187	Diuretic
PAR117	Tab	Amiloride HCl 5 mg	by Par	49884-0117	Diuretic
PAR118	Tab, Peach, Round, Par/118	Propantheline Bromide 15 mg	Pro-Banthine by Par		Gastrointestinal
PAR119	Tab, Film Coated	Nystatin 500,000 Units	by Allscripts	54569-0270	Antifungal
PAR119	Tab, Film Coated	Nystatin 500000 Units	by Zenith Goldline	00182-1369	Antifungal
PAR119	Tab, Film Coated	Nystatin 500000 Units	by Par	49884-0119	Antifungal
PAR119	Tab, Film Coated	Nystatin 500000 Units	by Qualitest	00603-4830	Antifungal
PAR121	Tab	Hydralazine HCl 100 mg	by Qualitest	00603-3833	Antihypertensive
PAR121	Tab, Par over 121	Hydralazine HCl 100 mg	by Par	49884-0121	Antihypertensive
PAR121	Tab, Coated, Par over 121	Hydralazine HCl 50 mg	by UDL	51079-0076	Antihypertensive
PAR122	Tab	Tolazamide 100 mg	by Par	49884-0122	Antidiabetic
PAR123	Tab	Tolazamide 250 mg	by Par	49884-0123	Antidiabetic
PAR124	Tab	Tolazamide 500 mg	by Par	49884-0124	Antidiabetic
PAR125	Cap	Valproic Acid 250 mg	by Par	49884-0125	Anticonvulsant
PAR127	Tab, Pink, Round, Par/127	Propranolol HCl 60 mg	Inderal by Par		Antihypertensive
PAR128	Tab	Amiloride HCl 5 mg, Hydrochlorothiazide 50 mg	Hydro Ride by Par	49884-0128	Diuretic
PAR129	Tab	Dexamethasone 6 mg	by Par	49884-0129	Steroid
PAR130	Tab, Coated	Metronidazole 250 mg	by Par	49884-0229	Antibiotic
PAR131	Tab, Coated	Metronidazole 500 mg	by Par	49884-0230	Antibiotic
PAR132	Tab, White, Round, Par/132	Metoclopramide HCl 10 mg	Reglan by Par		Gastrointestinal
PAR133	Tab, Pink, Round, Par/133	Amitriptyline HCl 10 mg	Elavil by Par		Antidepressant
PAR134	Tab, Green, Round, Par/134	Amitriptyline HCl 25 mg	Elavil by Par		Antidepressant
PAR135	Tab, Brown, Round, Par/135	Amitriptyline HCl 50 mg	Elavil by Par		Antidepressant
PAR136	Tab, Purple, Round, Par/136	Amitriptyline HCl 75 mg	Elavil by Par		Antidepressant
PAR137	Tab, Orange, Round, Par/137	Amitriptyline HCl 100 mg	Elavil by Par		Antidepressant
PAR138	Tab, Peach, Round	Amitriptyline HCl 150 mg	Elavil by Par		Antidepressant
PAR139	Tab	Sulfamethoxazole 400 mg, Trimethoprim 80 mg	by Par	49884-0139	Antibiotic
PAR140	Tab	Sulfamethoxazole 800 mg, Trimethoprim 160 mg	by Par	49884-0140	Antibiotic
PAR143	Cap	Hydralazine HCl 25 mg, Hydrochlorothiazide 25 mg	by Zenith Goldline	00182-1509	Antihypertensive
PAR143	Cap	Hydralazine HCl 25 mg, Hydrochlorothiazide 25 mg	by United Res	00677-0773	Antihypertensive
PAR143	Cap	Hydralazine HCl 25 mg, Hydrochlorothiazide 25 mg	by Qualitest	00603-3834	Antihypertensive
PAR143	Cap	Hydralazine HCl 25 mg, Hydrochlorothiazide 25 mg	Hydra Zide by Par	49884-0143	Antihypertensive
PAR144	Cap	Hydralazine HCl 50 mg, Hydrochlorothiazide 50 mg	by Zenith Goldline	00182-1510	Antihypertensive
PAR144	Cap	Hydralazine HCl 50 mg, Hydrochlorothiazide 50 mg	by Qualitest	00603-3835	Antihypertensive
PAR144	Cap	Hydralazine HCl 50 mg, Hydrochlorothiazide 50 mg	Hydra Zide by Par	49884-0144	Antihypertensive
PAR145	Cap, Light Blue	Hydralazine HCl 100 mg, Hydrochlorothiazide 50 mg	by Qualitest	00603-3836	Antihypertensive
PAR145	Cap	Hydralazine HCl 100 mg, Hydrochlorothiazide 50 mg	Hydra Zide by Par	49884-0145	Antihypertensive
PAR147	Tab	Hydroflumethiazide 50 mg	by Par	49884-0147	Diuretic

ID FRONT <> BACK	DESCRIPTION FRONT <> BACK	INGREDIENT & STRENGTH	BRAND (OR EQUIV.) & FIRM	NDC#	CLASS; SCH.
PAR148	Tab	Hydroflumethiazide 50 mg, Reserpine 0.125 mg	by Par	49884-0148	Diuretic; Antihypertensive
PAR150	Tab, Coated	Methyldopa 125 mg	by Par	49884-0150	Antihypertensive
PAR151	Tab, Coated	Methyldopa 250 mg	by Par	49884-0151	Antihypertensive
PAR152	Tab, Coated	Methyldopa 500 mg	by Par	49884-0152	Antihypertensive
PAR153	Tab	Disulfiram 250 mg	by Par	49884-0153	Antialcoholism
PAR154	Tab	Disulfiram 500 mg	by Par	49884-0154	Antialcoholism
PAR158	Tab	Methylprednisolone 16 mg	by Par	49884-0158	Steroid
PAR159	Tab	Methylprednisolone 24 mg	by Par	49884-0159	Steroid
PAR160	Tab	Methylprednisolone 32 mg	by Par	49884-0160	Steroid
PAR161	Tab, Film Coated	Fluphenazine HCl 1 mg	by Amerisource	62584-0698	Antipsychotic
PAR161300	Tab, White, Round, Par/161 300	Ibuprofen 300 mg	Motrin by Par		NSAID
PAR162 <> 400	Tab, Coated	Ibuprofen 400 mg	by Prescription Dispensing	61807-0027	NSAID
PAR162 <> 400	Tab, White, Round, Film Coated, Par over 162 <> 400	Ibuprofen 400 mg	Rufen/Motrin by UDL	51079-0281	NSAID
PAR162 <> 400	Tab, Film Coated	Ibuprofen 400 mg	by Zenith Goldline	00172-4018	NSAID
PAR162 <> 400	Tab, White, Round	Ibuprofen 400 mg	Ibuprofen by Murfreesboro	51129-1524	NSAID
PAR162 <> 400	Tab, Film Coated, Par over 162 <> 400	Ibuprofen 400 mg	by Par	49884-0162	NSAID
PAR162 <> 400	Tab, Film Coated, Debossed	Ibuprofen 400 mg	by Amerisource	62584-0746	NSAID
PAR162 <> 400	Tab, Film Coated	Ibuprofen 400 mg	by PDRX	55289-0590	NSAID
PAR162 <> 400	Tab, Film Coated	Ibuprofen 400 mg	by Quality Care	60346-0430	NSAID
PAR162 <> 400	Tab, White, Round, Film Coated	Ibuprofen 400 mg	by Goldline Labs	00182-1809	NSAID
PAR163 <> 600	Tab, White, Oval, Film Coated, Par over 163 <> 600	Ibuprofen 600 mg	Rufen/Motrin by Udl	51079-0282	NSAID
PAR163 <> 600	Tab, Film Coated	Ibuprofen 600 mg	by Zenith Goldline	00172-3646	NSAID
PAR163 <> 600	Tab, Film Coated	Ibuprofen 600 mg	by Pharmedix	53002-0301	NSAID
PAR163 <> 600	Tab, Film Coated	Ibuprofen 600 mg	by Par	49884-0163	NSAID
PAR163 <> 600	Tab, Film Coated	Ibuprofen 600 mg	by Quality Care	60346-0556	NSAID
PAR163600	Tab, Film Coated	Ibuprofen 600 mg	by Med Pro	53978-5006	NSAID
PAR164	Tab	Benztropine Mesylate 0.5 mg	by Baker Cummins	63171-1299	Antiparkinson
PAR164	Tab, Debossed	Benztropine Mesylate 0.5 mg	by Amerisource	62584-0625	Antiparkinson
PAR164	Tab, White, Round, Scored	Benztropine Mesylate 0.5 mg	by Bryant	63629-0350	Antiparkinson
PAR164	Tab, White, Round, Scored	Benztropine Mesylate 0.5 mg	by Bryant	63629-0349	Antiparkinson
PAR164	Tab, Par over 164	Benztropine Mesylate 0.5 mg	by UDL	51079-0220	Antiparkinson
PAR164	Tab	Benztropine Mesylate 0.5 mg	by Zenith Goldline	00182-1299	Antiparkinson
PAR164	Tab	Benztropine Mesylate 0.5 mg	by Rugby	00536-3370	Antiparkinson
PAR164	Tab, Par/164	Benztropine Mesylate 0.5 mg	by Qualitest	00603-2430	Antiparkinson
PAR164	Tab	Benztropine Mesylate 0.5 mg	by Par	49884-0164	Antiparkinson
PAR164	Tab, White, Round, Scored	Benztropine Mesylate 0.5 mg	by Vangard Labs	00615-2547	Antiparkinson
PAR164	Tab	Benztropine Mesylate 0.5 mg	by Major	00904-1055	Antiparkinson
PAR165	Tab	Benztropine Mesylate 1 mg	by Quality Care	60346-0776	Antiparkinson
PAR165	Tab, White, Pumpkin Seed Shaped, Scored	Benztropine Mesylate 1 mg	by Bryant	63629 -0630	Antiparkinson
PAR165	Tab, Compressed	Benztropine Mesylate 1 mg	by Baker Cummins	63171-1700	Antiparkinson
PAR165	Tab, Debossed	Benztropine Mesylate 1 mg	by Amerisource	62584-0626	Antiparkinson
PAR165	Tab, Par/165	Benztropine Mesylate 1 mg	by UDL	51079-0221	Antiparkinson
PAR165	Tab	Benztropine Mesylate 1 mg	by Zenith Goldline	00182-1700	Antiparkinson
PAR165	Tab, Par/165	Benztropine Mesylate 1 mg	by Qualitest	00603-2431	Antiparkinson
PAR165	Tab	Benztropine Mesylate 1 mg	by Vangard	00615-2548	Antiparkinson
PAR165	Tab, Pumpkin Seed Shaped	Benztropine Mesylate 1 mg	by Rugby	00536-3371	Antiparkinson
PAR165	Tab	Benztropine Mesylate 1 mg	by Med Pro	53978-3045	Antiparkinson
PAR165	Tab	Benztropine Mesylate 1 mg	by Par	49884-0165	Antiparkinson
PAR165	Tab	Benztropine Mesylate 1 mg	by Major	00904-1056	Antiparkinson
PAR166	Tab	Benztropine Mesylate 2 mg	by Quality Care	60346-0699	Antiparkinson
PAR166	Tab, Debossed	Benztropine Mesylate 2 mg	by Amerisource	62584-0627	Antiparkinson

ID FRONT ◇ BACK	DESCRIPTION FRONT ◇ BACK	INGREDIENT & STRENGTH	BRAND (OR EQUIV.) & FIRM	NDC#	CLASS; SCH.
PAR166	Tab	Benztropine Mesylate 2 mg	by Baker Cummins	63171-1701	Antiparkinson
PAR166	Tab, Par over 166	Benztropine Mesylate 2 mg	by UDL	51079-0222	Antiparkinson
PAR166	Tab	Benztropine Mesylate 2 mg	by Zenith Goldline	00182-1701	Antiparkinson
PAR166	Tab	Benztropine Mesylate 2 mg	by Vangard	00615-2549	Antiparkinson
PAR166	Tab, Par/166	Benztropine Mesylate 2 mg	by Qualitest	00603-2432	Antiparkinson
PAR166	Tab	Benztropine Mesylate 2 mg	by Par	49884-0166	Antiparkinson
PAR166	Tab	Benztropine Mesylate 2 mg	by Allscripts	54569-2862	Antiparkinson
PAR166	Tab	Benztropine Mesylate 2 mg	by Med Pro	53978-2093	Antiparkinson
PAR166	Tab	Benztropine Mesylate 2 mg	by Major	00904-1057	Antiparkinson
PAR170	Tab	Sulfinpyrazone 100 mg	by Par	49884-0170	Uricosuric
PAR171	Cap	Sulfinpyrazone 200 mg	by Par	49884-0171	Uricosuric
PAR176	Tab, Green/Orange, Round, Par/176	Meprobamate 200 mg, Aspirin 325 mg	Equagesic by Par		Sedative/Hypnotic; C IV
PAR177	Tab	Methyclothiazide 2.5 mg	by Par	49884-0177	Diuretic
PAR178	Tab	Methyclothiazide 5 mg	by Par	49884-0178	Diuretic
PAR181	Tab, Blue, Round, Par/181	Perphenazine 2 mg, Amitriptyline 10 mg	Triavil by Par		Antipsychotic; Antidepressant
PAR182	Tab, Orange, Round, Par/182	Perphenazine 2 mg, Amitriptyline 25 mg	Triavil by Par		Antipsychotic; Antidepressant
PAR183	Tab, Salmon, Round, Par/183	Perphenazine 4 mg, Amitriptyline 10 mg	Triavil by Par		Antipsychotic; Antidepressant
PAR184	Tab, Yellow, Round, Par/184	Perphenazine 4 mg, Amitriptyline 25 mg	Triavil by Par		Antipsychotic; Antidepressant
PAR185	Tab, Orange, Round, Par/185	Perphenazine 4 mg, Amitriptyline 50 mg	Triavil by Par		Antipsychotic; Antidepressant
PAR186	Tab, Film Coated	Hydrochlorothiazide 15 mg, Methyldopa 250 mg	by Zenith Goldline	00182-1830	Diuretic; Antihypertensive
PAR186	Tab, Film Coated	Hydrochlorothiazide 15 mg, Methyldopa 250 mg	by Par	49884-0186	Diuretic; Antihypertensive
PAR189	Tab, Coated	Hydrochlorothiazide 50 mg, Methyldopa 500 mg	by Par	49884-0189	Diuretic; Antihypertensive
PAR190 ◇ DIAZEPAM2	Tab	Diazepam 2 mg	by Par	49884-0190	Antianxiety; C IV
PAR191 ◇ DIAZEPAM5	Tab	Diazepam 5 mg	by Par	49884-0191	Antianxiety; C IV
PAR192 ◇ DIAZEPAM10	Tab	Diazepam 10 mg	by Par	49884-0192	Antianxiety; C IV
PAR193	Cap	Flurazepam HCl 15 mg	by Par	49884-0193	Hypnotic; C IV
PAR193	Cap, Powder Blue, Par over 193	Flurazepam HCl 15 mg	by Quality Care	60346-0239	Hypnotic; C IV
PAR193 ◇ PAR193	Cap, Powder Blue	Flurazepam HCl 15 mg	by Amerisource	62584-0705	Hypnotic; C IV
PAR194	Cap, Powder Blue, Par Over 194	Flurazepam HCl 30 mg	by Quality Care	60346-0762	Hypnotic; C IV
PAR194	Cap	Flurazepam HCl 30 mg	by Par	49884-0194	Hypnotic; C IV
PAR202	Tab, Beige, Round, Par/202	Methyldopa 250 mg, Chlorothiazide 150 mg	Aldoclor 150 by Par		Antihypertensive
PAR203	Tab, Green, Round, Par/203	Methyldopa 250 mg, Chlorothiazide 250 mg	Aldoclor 250 by Par		Antihypertensive
PAR206	Tab, White, Round, Par/206	Lorazepam 0.5 mg	Ativan by Par		Sedative/Hypnotic; C IV
PAR207	Tab, White, Round, Par/207	Lorazepam 1 mg	Ativan by Par		Sedative/Hypnotic; C IV
PAR208	Tab, White, Round, Par/208	Lorazepam 2 mg	Ativan by Par		Sedative/Hypnotic; C IV
PAR213	Tab, White & Green, Round, Par/213	Orphenadrine 25 mg, Aspirin 325 mg, Caffeine 30 mg	Orphengesic by Par		Muscle Relaxant
PAR214	Tab, White & Green, Oblong, Par/214	Orphenadrine 50 mg, Aspirin 770 mg, Caffeine 60 mg	Orphengesic Forte by Par		Muscle Relaxant
PAR216	Tab, Film Coated	Ibuprofen 800 mg	by Med Pro	53978-5007	NSAID
PAR216 ◇ 800	Tab, Coated, Debossed, Par over 216 ◇ 800	Ibuprofen 800 mg	by Zenith Goldline	00182-1297	NSAID
PAR216 ◇ 800	Tab, Film Coated	Ibuprofen 800 mg	by Zenith Goldline	00172-3648	NSAID
PAR216 ◇ 800	Tab, Film Coated, Par over 216 ◇ 800	Ibuprofen 800 mg	by PDRX	55289-0140	NSAID
PAR216 ◇ 800	Tab, Coated	Ibuprofen 800 mg	by Par	49884-0216	NSAID
PAR216 ◇ 800	Tab, Coated, Par over 216 ◇ 800	Ibuprofen 800 mg	by Nat Pharmpak Serv	55154-5565	NSAID
PAR216 ◇ 800	Tab, Film Coated	Ibuprofen 800 mg	by Quality Care	60346-0030	NSAID

ID FRONT <> BACK	DESCRIPTION FRONT <> BACK	INGREDIENT & STRENGTH	BRAND (OR EQUIV.) & FIRM	NDC#	CLASS; SCH.
PAR216 <> 800	Tab, White, Capsule Shaped, Film-Coated, Par over 216 <> 800	Ibuprofen 800 mg	Rufen/Motrin by UDL	51079-0596	NSAID
PAR216 <> 800	Tab, Coated, Par over 216 <> 800	Ibuprofen 800 mg	by Baker Cummins	63171-1297	NSAID
PAR217	Cap	Doxepin HCl 10 mg	by Zenith Goldline	00182-1325	Antidepressant
PAR217	Cap	Doxepin HCl 10 mg	by Par	49884-0217	Antidepressant
PAR217	Cap, Buff, Par/217	Doxepin HCl 10 mg	Sinequan by Martec	52555-0447	Antidepressant
PAR217 <> PAR217	Cap, Buff, Par 217	Doxepin HCl 10 mg	by Quality Care	60346-0793	Antidepressant
PAR217 <> PAR217	Cap, Buff, Opaque	Doxepin HCl 10 mg	by Amerisource	62584-0686	Antidepressant
PAR217 <> PAR217	Cap, Beige, Opaque	Doxepin HCl 10 mg	Doxepin HCl USP by H J Harkins Co	52959-0077	Antidepressant
PAR217 <> PAR217	Cap, Beige, Opaque	Doxepin HCl 10 mg	by H J Harkins Co	52959-0133	Antidepressant
PAR217 <> PAR217	Tab, Tan, Oval, Opaque	Doxepin HCl 10 mg	by H J Harkins Co	52959-0211	Antidepressant
PAR217 <> PAR217	Cap	Doxepin HCl 10 mg	by H J Harkins Co	52959-0343	Antidepressant
PAR217 <> PAR217	Cap, Tan, Opaque	Doxepin HCl 10 mg	by H J Harkins Co	52959-0347	Antidepressant
PAR217 <> PAR217	Cap	Doxepin HCl 10 mg	by Major	00904-1260	Antidepressant
PAR218	Cap, Par over 218	Doxepin HCl 25 mg	by Quality Care	60346-0553	Antidepressant
PAR218	Cap	Doxepin HCl 25 mg	by Zenith Goldline	00182-1326	Antidepressant
PAR218	Cap	Doxepin HCl 25 mg	by United Res	00677-1102	Antidepressant
PAR218	Cap, Ivory & White, Par/218	Doxepin HCl 25 mg	Sinequan by Martec	52555-0448	Antidepressant
PAR218 <> PAR218	Cap, Par over 218 <> Par over 218	Doxepin HCl 25 mg	by Quality Care	60346-0553	Antidepressant
PAR218 <> PAR218	Cap, Opaque	Doxepin HCl 25 mg	by Amerisource	62584-0687	Antidepressant
PAR218 <> PAR218	Cap	Doxepin HCl 25 mg	by Par	49884-0218	Antidepressant
PAR218 <> PAR218	Cap, Ivory & White, Opaque	Doxepin HCl 25 mg	Doxepin HCl USP by H J Harkins Co	52959-0042	Antidepressant
PAR218 <> PAR218	Cap, White & Ivory, Opaque	Doxepin HCl 25 mg	by H J Harkins Co	52959-0161	Antidepressant
PAR218 <> PAR218	Cap	Doxepin HCl 25 mg	by Major	00904-1261	Antidepressant
PAR219	Cap, Ivory	Doxepin HCl 50mg	by Direct Dispensing	57866-4565	Antidepressant
PAR219	Cap	Doxepin HCl 50 mg	by Quality Care	60346-0269	Antidepressant
PAR219	Cap	Doxepin HCl 50 mg	by Zenith Goldline	00182-1327	Antidepressant
PAR219	Cap	Doxepin HCl 50 mg	by United Res	00677-1103	Antidepressant
PAR219	Cap, Ivory, Par/219	Doxepin HCl 50 mg	Sinequan by Martec	52555-0449	Antidepressant
PAR219 <> PAR219	Cap, Opaque	Doxepin HCl 50 mg	by Amerisource	62584-0688	Antidepressant
PAR219 <> PAR219	Cap, Ivory, Opaque	Doxepin HCl 50 mg	Doxepin HCl USP by H J Harkins Co	52959-0050	Antidepressant
PAR219 <> PAR219	Cap	Doxepin HCl 50 mg	by Physicians Total Care	54868-1964	Antidepressant
PAR219 <> PAR219	Cap	Doxepin HCl 50 mg	by Par	49884-0219	Antidepressant
PAR219 <> PAR219	Cap, Ivory, Opaque	Doxepin HCl 50 mg	by H J Harkins Co	52959-0193	Antidepressant
PAR220	Cap, Opaque	Doxepin HCl 75 mg	by Amerisource	62584-0689	Antidepressant
PAR220	Cap, Light Green, Par/220	Doxepin HCl 75 mg	Sinequan by Martec	52555-0331	Antidepressant
PAR220	Cap	Doxepin HCl 75 mg	by Zenith Goldline	00182-1328	Antidepressant
PAR220	Cap	Doxepin HCl 75 mg	by Par	49884-0220	Antidepressant
PAR220 <> PAR220	Cap, White & Green, Opaque	Doxepin HCl 100 mg	Doxepin HCl by H J Harkins Co	52959-0069	Antidepressant
PAR220 <> PAR220	Cap, Green, Opaque	Doxepin HCl 75 mg	Doxepin HCl by H J Harkins Co	52959-0066	Antidepressant
PAR221	Cap	Doxepin HCl 100 mg	by Zenith Goldline	00182-1329	Antidepressant
PAR221	Cap	Doxepin HCl 100 mg	by Par	49884-0221	Antidepressant
PAR221 <> PAR221	Cap, Opaque	Doxepin HCl 100 mg	by Amerisource	62584-0690	Antidepressant
PAR221 <> PAR221	Cap, Green & White, Opaque	Doxepin HCl 100 mg	by H J Harkins Co	52959-0022	Antidepressant
PAR221 <> PAR221	Cap, White & Green, Opaque	Doxepin HCl 100 mg	by H J Harkins Co	52959-0216	Antidepressant
PAR221 <> PAR221	Cap, Green & White	Doxepin HCl 100 mg	by H J Harkins Co	52959-0208	Antidepressant
PAR221 <> PAR221	Cap	Doxepin HCl 100 mg	by Major	00904-1264	Antidepressant
PAR222	Cap, Blue & White, Par/222	Doxepin HCl 150 mg	Sinequan by Martec	52555-0322	Antidepressant
PAR222	Cap	Doxepin HCl 150 mg	by Zenith Goldline	00182-1878	Antidepressant
PAR222	Cap	Doxepin HCl 150 mg	by Par	49884-0222	Antidepressant
PAR222 <> PAR222	Cap, White & Blue, Opaque	Doxepin HCl 150 mg	Doxepin HCl by H J Harkins Co	52959-0087	Antidepressant
PAR223	Tab, Debossed	Haloperidol 0.5 mg	by Amerisource	62584-0724	Antipsychotic
PAR223	Tab	Haloperidol 0.5 mg	by Zenith Goldline	00182-1262	Antipsychotic

ID FRONT ⬦ BACK	DESCRIPTION FRONT ⬦ BACK	INGREDIENT & STRENGTH	BRAND (OR EQUIV.) & FIRM	NDC#	CLASS; SCH.
PAR223	Tab	Haloperidol 0.5 mg	by Vangard	00615-2594	Antipsychotic
PAR223	Tab	Haloperidol 0.5 mg	by Qualitest	00603-3782	Antipsychotic
PAR223	Tab, White, Round, Scored	Haloperidol 0.5 mg	by Merck Sharp & Dohme	52888-0032	Antipsychotic
PAR223	Tab	Haloperidol 0.5 mg	by Par	49884-0223	Antipsychotic
PAR223	Tab	Haloperidol 0.5 mg	by Major	00904-1830	Antipsychotic
PAR224	Tab	Haloperidol 1 mg	by Quality Care	60346-0819	Antipsychotic
PAR224	Tab	Haloperidol 1 mg	by Zenith Goldline	00182-1263	Antipsychotic
PAR224	Tab	Haloperidol 1 mg	by Qualitest	00603-3783	Antipsychotic
PAR224	Tab	Haloperidol 1 mg	by Par	49884-0224	Antipsychotic
PAR224	Tab, Yellow, Round, Scored	Haloperidol 1 mg	by Mikart	46672-0172	Antipsychotic
PAR224	Tab, Yellow, Round, Scored	Haloperidol 1 mg	by Vangard Labs	00615-2595	Antipsychotic
PAR224	Tab	Haloperidol 1 mg	Haloperido by Major	00904-1831	Antipsychotic
PAR224	Tab, Yellow, Round, Scored	Haloperidol 1 mg	by Mikart	46672-0171	Antipsychotic
PAR225	Tab	Haloperidol 2 mg	by Quality Care	60346-0820	Antipsychotic
PAR225	Tab, Debossed	Haloperidol 2 mg	by Amerisource	62584-0726	Antipsychotic
PAR225	Tab, Lavender	Haloperidol 2 mg	by Qualitest	00603-3784	Antipsychotic
PAR225	Tab	Haloperidol 2 mg	by Vangard	00615-2596	Antipsychotic
PAR225	Tab	Haloperidol 2 mg	by Par	49884-0225	Antipsychotic
PAR226	Tab	Haloperidol 5 mg	by Quality Care	60346-0821	Antipsychotic
PAR226	Tab, Debossed	Haloperidol 5 mg	by Amerisource	62584-0727	Antipsychotic
PAR226	Tab	Haloperidol 5 mg	by Zenith Goldline	00182-1265	Antipsychotic
PAR226	Tab	Haloperidol 5 mg	by Qualitest	00603-3785	Antipsychotic
PAR226	Tab	Haloperidol 5 mg	by Par	49884-0226	Antipsychotic
PAR227	Tab	Haloperidol 10 mg	by Quality Care	60346-0822	Antipsychotic
PAR227	Tab, Debossed	Haloperidol 10 mg	by Amerisource	62584-0728	Antipsychotic
PAR227	Tab	Haloperidol 10 mg	by Zenith Goldline	00182-1854	Antipsychotic
PAR227	Tab	Haloperidol 10 mg	by Qualitest	00603-3786	Antipsychotic
PAR227	Tab	Haloperidol 10 mg	by Par	49884-0227	Antipsychotic
PAR227	Tab	Haloperidol 10 mg	by HL Moore	00839-7398	Antipsychotic
PAR228	Tab, Salmon, Round, Par/228	Haloperidol 20 mg	Haldol by Par		Antipsychotic
PAR237	Tab	Leucovorin Calcium	by Par	49884-0237	Antineoplastic
PAR238	Tab	Leucovorin Calcium	by Par	49884-0238	Antineoplastic
PAR239	Tab	Propranolol HCl 90 mg	by Par	49884-0239	Antihypertensive
PAR240	Cap	Temazepam 15 mg	Tem by Par	49884-0240	Sedative/Hypnotic; C IV
PAR240	Cap	Temazepam 15 mg	Tem by Qualitest	00603-5895	Sedative/Hypnotic; C IV
PAR240 ⬦ PAR240	Cap, White/Dark Green, Opaque	Temazepam 15 mg	Tem by Quality Care	60346-0668	Sedative/Hypnotic; C IV
PAR240 ⬦ PAR240	Cap, Opaque	Temazepam 15 mg	by Amerisource	62584-0860	Sedative/Hypnotic; C IV
PAR241	Cap	Temazepam 30 mg	Tem by Par	49884-0241	Sedative/Hypnotic; C IV
PAR241	Cap, Par over 241	Temazepam 30 mg	Tem by Quality Care	60346-0005	Sedative/Hypnotic; C IV
PAR241	Cap	Temazepam 30 mg	Tem by Qualitest	00603-5896	Sedative/Hypnotic; C IV
PAR241 ⬦ PAR241	Cap, White	Temazepam 30 mg	by Southwood Pharms	58016-0831	Sedative/Hypnotic; C IV
PAR241 ⬦ PAR241	Cap	Temazepam 30 mg	Tem by Quality Care	60346-0005	Sedative/Hypnotic; C IV
PAR241 ⬦ PAR241	Cap	Temazepam 30 mg	by Amerisource	62584-0862	Sedative/Hypnotic; C IV
PAR241 ⬦ PAR241	Cap	Temazepam 30 mg	Tem by Major	00904-2811	Sedative/Hypnotic; C IV
PAR246	Tab	Aspirin 325 mg, Carisoprodol 200 mg	by Zenith Goldline	00182-1821	Analgesic; Muscle Relaxant
PAR246	Tab, Lavender, Par/246	Aspirin 325 mg, Carisoprodol 200 mg	by Qualitest	00603-2583	Analgesic; Muscle Relaxant
PAR246	Tab, Light Lavender & White	Aspirin 325 mg, Carisoprodol 200 mg	by HJ Harkins Co	52959-0454	Analgesic; Muscle Relaxant
PAR246	Tab	Aspirin 325 mg, Carisoprodol 200 mg	by Par	49884-0246	Analgesic; Muscle Relaxant

ID FRONT <> BACK	DESCRIPTION FRONT <> BACK	INGREDIENT & STRENGTH	BRAND (OR EQUIV.) & FIRM	NDC#	CLASS; SCH.
PAR247	Tab, Coated	Salsalate 500 mg	by Par	49884-0247	NSAID
PAR248	Tab, Coated	Salsalate 750 mg	by Par	49884-0248	NSAID
PAR249	Tab	Aspirin 325 mg, Methocarbamol 400 mg	by DRX	55045-2551	Analgesic; Muscle Relaxant
PAR249	Tab	Aspirin 325 mg, Methocarbamol 400 mg	by Quality Care	60346-0956	Analgesic; Muscle Relaxant
PAR249	Tab	Aspirin 325 mg, Methocarbamol 400 mg	by Qualitest	00603-4489	Analgesic; Muscle Relaxant
PAR249	Tab	Aspirin 325 mg, Methocarbamol 400 mg	by Allscripts	54569-2893	Analgesic; Muscle Relaxant
PAR249	Tab	Aspirin 325 mg, Methocarbamol 400 mg	by Par	49884-0249	Analgesic; Muscle Relaxant
PAR249	Tab	Aspirin 325 mg, Methocarbamol 400 mg	by Major	00904-0227	Analgesic; Muscle Relaxant
PAR25	Tab, White, Round, Par/25	Dipyridamole 25 mg	Persantine by Par		Antiplatelet
PAR250	Cap, Gray & Orange, Par/250	Cephalexin 250 mg	Keflex by Par		Antibiotic
PAR256	Tab	Minoxidil 2.5 mg	by Zenith Goldline	00182-1602	Antihypertensive
PAR256 <> MINOXIDIL212	Tab, Par 256 <> Minoxidil 2 1/2	Minoxidil 2.5 mg	by Par	49884-0256	Antihypertensive
PAR256 <> MINOXIDIL212	Tab, Par 256 <> Minoxidil 2 1/2	Minoxidil 2.5 mg	by Qualitest	00603-4687	Antihypertensive
PAR257 <> MINOXIDIL10	Tab	Minoxidil 10 mg	by Par	49884-0257	Antihypertensive
PAR257 <> MINOXIDIL10	Tab	Minoxidil 10 mg	by Physicians Total Care	54868-3467	Antihypertensive
PAR257 <> MINOXIDIL10	Tab	Minoxidil 10 mg	by United Res	00677-1162	Antihypertensive
PAR257 <> MINOXIDIL10	Tab, Debossed	Minoxidil 10 mg	by HL Moore	00839-7342	Antihypertensive
PAR257 <> MINOXIDIL10	Tab	Minoxidil 10 mg	by Qualitest	00603-4688	Antihypertensive
PAR258	Tab	Metaproterenol Sulfate 10 mg	by Par	49884-0258	Antiasthmatic
PAR258	Tab	Metaproterenol Sulfate 10 mg	by Pharm Packaging Ctr	54383-0090	Antiasthmatic
PAR259	Tab	Metaproterenol Sulfate 20 mg	by Par	49884-0259	Antiasthmatic
PAR263	Cap, Maroon & Pink, Par/263	Meclofenamate Sodium 50 mg	Meclomen by Par		NSAID
PAR264	Cap, Maroon & White, Par/264	Meclofenamate Sodium 100 mg	Meclomen by Par		NSAID
PAR279	Tab	Hydrochlorothiazide 50 mg, Triamterene 75 mg	by Quality Care	60346-0704	Diuretic
PAR286	Tab, Coated	Fenoprofen Calcium	by Par	49884-0286	NSAID
PAR287	Cap	Fenoprofen Calcium	by Par	49884-0287	NSAID
PAR288	Cap	Fenoprofen Calcium	by Par	49884-0288	NSAID
PAR289	Tab, White, Round, Scored	Megestrol Acetate 20 mg	by Murfreesboro Ph	51129-1305	Progestin
PAR289	Tab, Par over 289	Megestrol Acetate 20 mg	by UDL	51079-0434	Progestin
PAR289	Tab	Megestrol Acetate 20 mg	by Zenith Goldline	00182-1863	Progestin
PAR289	Tab, Flat-faced, Beveled Edge	Megestrol Acetate 20 mg	by Par	49884-0289	Progestin
PAR289	Tab, Debossed, Beveled Edged	Megestrol Acetate 20 mg	by Amerisource	62584-0777	Progestin
PAR289	Tab, White, Round, Flat, Scored	Megestrol Acetate 20 mg	Megestrol Acetate by Nat Pharmpak Serv	55154-5583	Progestin
PAR289	Tab	Megestrol Acetate 20 mg	by Qualitest	00603-4391	Progestin
PAR290	Tab, Par over 290	Megestrol Acetate 40 mg	by UDL	51079-0435	Progestin
PAR290	Tab	Megestrol Acetate 40 mg	by Zenith Goldline	00182-1864	Progestin
PAR290	Tab	Megestrol Acetate 40 mg	by Rugby	00536-4822	Progestin
PAR290	Tab, Debossed, Beveled Edged	Megestrol Acetate 40 mg	by Med Pro	53978-3010	Progestin

ID FRONT <> BACK	DESCRIPTION FRONT <> BACK	INGREDIENT & STRENGTH	BRAND (OR EQUIV.) & FIRM	NDC#	CLASS; SCH.
PAR290	Tab, Flat-faced, Beveled Edge	Megestrol Acetate 40 mg	by Par	49884-0290	Progestin
PAR290	Tab, Beveled Edged	Megestrol Acetate 40 mg	by Amerisource	62584-0779	Progestin
PAR290	Tab, White, Round, Flat, Scored	Megestrol Acetate 40 mg	Megestrol Acetate by Nat Pharmpak Serv	55154-5584	Progestin
PAR290	Tab, White, Round, Flat, Scored	Megestrol Acetate 40 mg	by Nat Pharmpak Serv	55154-5582	Progestin
PAR290	Tab	Megestrol Acetate 40 mg	by Nat Pharmpak Serv	55154-5516	Progestin
PAR290	Tab, White, Round, Scored	Megestrol Acetate 40 mg	by Vangard Labs	00615-3570	Progestin
PAR290	Tab	Megestrol Acetate 40 mg	by United Res	00677-1206	Progestin
PAR304	Tab, Peach, Round	Divalproex sodium 250 mg	Depakote by Par		Anticonvulsant
PAR305	Tab, Lavender, Round	Divalproex sodium 500 mg	Depakote by Par		Anticonvulsant
PAR4	Tab, Yellow, Oval, Par/4	Dexchlorpheniramine Maleate 4 mg	Polaramine Repetabs by Par		Antihistamine
PAR412	Tab, Film Coated	Metoprolol Tartrate 50 mg	by Par	49884-0412	Antihypertensive
PAR413	Tab, Blue, Round, Scored, Film	Metoprolol Tartrate 100 mg	by Neuman Distr	64579-0059	Antihypertensive
PAR413	Tab, Coated	Metoprolol Tartrate 100 mg	by Par	49884-0413	Antihypertensive
PAR444	Tab, Scored	Captopril 12.5 mg	by Par	49884-0444	Antihypertensive
PAR445	Tab	Captopril 25 mg	by Par	49884-0445	Antihypertensive
PAR446	Tab	Captopril 50 mg	by Par	49884-0446	Antihypertensive
PAR447	Tab	Captopril 100 mg	by Par	49884-0447	Antihypertensive
PAR467	Tab, Film Coated	Ibuprofen 400 mg	IBU Ibuprofen by Par	49884-0467	NSAID
PAR467	Tab, White, Oblong, Film Coated	Ibuprofen 400 mg	by Dixon Shane	17236-0568	NSAID
PAR468	Tab, Film Coated	Ibuprofen 600 mg	by Quality Care	60346-0556	NSAID
PAR468	Tab, Film Coated	Ibuprofen 600 mg	by Prepackage Spec	58864-0286	NSAID
PAR468	Tab, Printed in Black, Film Coated	Ibuprofen 600 mg	by Amerisource	62584-0747	NSAID
PAR468	Tab, White, Oblong, Film Coated	Ibuprofen 600 mg	by Dixon Shane	17236-0569	NSAID
PAR469	Tab, Film Coated	Ibuprofen 800 mg	IBU Ibuprofen by Par	49884-0469	NSAID
PAR469	Tab, Printed in Black, Film Coated	Ibuprofen 800 mg	by Amerisource	62584-0748	NSAID
PAR469	Tab, White, Oblong, Film Coated	Ibuprofen 800 mg	by Dixon Shane	17236-0570	NSAID
PAR472	Tab, Green & White, Round	Orphenadrine Citrate 25 mg; Aspirin 385 mg; Caffeine 30 mg	Orphengesic by Par Pharm	49884-0472	Muscle Relaxant
PAR50	Tab, White, Round, Par/50	Dipyridamole 50 mg	Persantine by Par		Antiplatelet
PAR500	Cap, Orange, Par/500	Cephalexin 500 mg	Keflex by Par		Antibiotic
PAR54	Tab, Sugar Coated	Imipramine HCl 10 mg	by Zenith Goldline	00182-0826	Antidepressant
PAR544	Tab, Peach, Round	Ranitidine HCl 150 mg	Ranitidine HCl by RX PAK	65084-0175	Gastrointestinal
PAR545	Tab, Peach, Oval	Ranitidine HCl 300 mg	Ranitidine HCl by RX PAK	65084-0176	Gastrointestinal
PAR55	Tab, Sugar Coated	Imipramine HCl 25 mg	by Zenith Goldline	00182-0827	Antidepressant
PAR55	Tab, Printed in Black Ink, Sugar Coated	Imipramine HCl 25 mg	by Amerisource	62584-0750	Antidepressant
PAR55	Tab, Sugar Coated	Imipramine HCl 25 mg	by United Res	00677-0422	Antidepressant
PAR56	Tab, Round, Sugar Coated	Imipramine HCl 50 mg	by United Res Labs	00677-0423	Antidepressant
PAR56	Tab, Sugar Coated	Imipramine HCl 50 mg	by Zenith Goldline	00182-0828	Antidepressant
PAR6	Tab, White, Oval, Par/6	Dexchlorpheniramine Maleate 6 mg	Polaramine Repetabs by Par		Antihistamine
PAR75	Tab, White, Round, Par/75	Dipyridamole 75 mg	Persantine by Par		Antiplatelet
PAR96	Tab, Orange, Round, Par/96	Thioridazine HCl 10 mg	Mellaril by Par		Antipsychotic
PAR97	Tab, Orange, Round, Par/97	Thioridazine HCl 15 mg	Mellaril by Par		Antipsychotic
PAR98	Tab, Orange, Round, Par/98	Thioridazine HCl 25 mg	Mellaril by Par		Antipsychotic
PAR99	Tab, Orange, Round, Par/99	Thioridazine HCl 50 mg	Mellaril by Par		Antipsychotic
PARAFLEX	Tab, Peach, Cap Shaped	Chlorzoxazone 250 mg	Paraflex by McNeil	00045-0317	Muscle Relaxant
PARAFONFORTEC8M	Tab, Pink/White, Round	Acetaminophen 300 mg, Chlorzoxazone 250 mg, Codeine 8 mg	Parafon Forte C8 by Johnson & Johnson	Canadian	Muscle Relaxant
PARAFONFORTEDSC	Tab, Green, Oblong, Scored	Chlorzoxazone 500 mg	Parafon Forte DSC by Rightpac	65240-0715	Muscle Relaxant
PARAFONFORTEDSC <> MCNEIL	Tab, Light Green, Coated	Chlorzoxazone 500 mg	Parafon Forte DSC by Thrift Drug	59198-0089	Muscle Relaxant
PARAFONFORTEDSC <> MCNEIL	Tab, Lime Green, Coated, Parafon over Forte DSC <> McNeil	Chlorzoxazone 500 mg	Parafon Forte DSC by McNeil	00045-0325	Muscle Relaxant

ID FRONT <> BACK	DESCRIPTION FRONT <> BACK	INGREDIENT & STRENGTH	BRAND (OR EQUIV.) & FIRM	NDC#	CLASS; SCH.
PARAFONFORTEDSC <> MCNEIL	Cap, Green, Scored	Chlorzoxazone 500 mg	Parafon Forte DSC by Compumed	00403-0261	Muscle Relaxant
PARAFONFORTEDSC <> MCNEIL	Tab, Coated	Chlorzoxazone 500 mg	Parafon Forte DSC by Allscripts	54569-1506	Muscle Relaxant
PARAFONFORTEDSC <> MCNEIL	Tab, Coated	Chlorzoxazone 500 mg	Parafon Forte DSC by Nat Pharmpak Serv	55154-1907	Muscle Relaxant
PARAONFORTEC8M	Tab, Pink/White, Round, Paraon Forte C8/M	Chlorzoxazone 250 mg, Acetaminophen 300 mg, Codeine Phosphate 8 mg	Parafon Forte C8 by McNeil	Canadian	Muscle Relaxant
PARKEDAVIS	Cap, Green & Pink, <ParkeDavis>	Caffeine 100 mg, Diphenhydamine 25 mg, Ergotamine 1 mg	Ergodryl by Pfizer	Canadian DIN# 00156086	Antimigraine
PARKEDAVIS	Cap, Clear & Yellow, Opaque	Erythromycin 333 mg	Eryc by Parke-Davis	Canadian DIN# 00873454	Antibiotic
PARKEDAVIS	Cap, Aqua Blue & Ivory, Opaque	Mefenamic Acid 250 mg	Ponston by Pfizer	Canadian DIN# 00155225	NSAID
PARKEDAVIS	Cap, Orange & Yellow	Methsuximide 300 mg	Celontin by Pfizer	Canadian DIN# 00022802	Anticonvulsant
PARKEDAVIS <> LOPID600MG	Tab, White, Ellipsoid, Film Coated	Gemfibrozil 600 mg	Lopid by Parke-Davis	Canadian DIN# 00659606	Antihyperlipidemic
PARKEDAVISPD100	Cap, Orange & White, Parke-Davis P-D 100	Phenytoin Sodium 100 mg	Dilantin by Parke-Davis	Canadian DIN# 00022780	Anticonvulsant
PARKEDAVISPD30	Cap, Pink & White Parke-Davis P-D 30	Phenytoin Sodium 30 mg	Dilantin by Parke-Davis	Canadian DIN# 00022772	Anticonvulsant
PARLODEL	Tab, White, Oval, Scored	Bromocriptine Mesylate 5 mg	Parlodel by Sandoz	Canadian DIN# 00371033	Antiparkinson
PARLODEL212	Tab, Parlodel 2 1/2	Bromocriptine Mesylate	Parlodel by Pharm Utilization	60491-0497	Antiparkinson
PARLODEL5MG	Cap, Caramel & White	Bromocriptine Mesylate 5 mg	Parlodel by Sandoz	Canadian DIN# 00568643	Antiparkinson
PARLODEL5MG <> S	Cap, Caramel, S in a triangle	Bromocriptine Mesylate 5.74 mg	Parlodel by Pharm Utilization	60491-0499	Antiparkinson
PARLODEL5MG <> S	Cap, Light Brown, Parlodel 5 mg <> S in a Triangle	Bromocriptine Mesylate 5.74 mg	Parlodel by Novartis	00078-0102	Antiparkinson
PARNATESB	Tab, Pink, Round, Parnate/SB	Tranylcypromine Sulfate 10 mg	Parnate by SKB	00007-4471	Antidepressant
PARNATESR	Tab, Red, Round, Film Coated	Tranylcypromine Sulfate 10 mg	Partnate by Teva	00480-0149	Antidepressant
PAXIL	Tab, Film Coated	Paroxetine HCl 10 mg	by Med Pro	53978-2059	Antidepressant
PAXIL <> 10	Tab, Yellow, Oval	Paroxetine HCl 10 mg	Paxil by Phcy Care	65070-0144	Antidepressant
PAXIL <> 10	Tab, Yellow, Oval, Film Coated	Paroxetine HCl 10 mg	Paxil by SKB	00029-3210	Antidepressant
PAXIL <> 10	Tab, Film Coated	Paroxetine HCl 10 mg	Paxil by SB	59742-3210	Antidepressant
PAXIL <> 10	Tab, Yellow, Oval	Paroxetine HCl 10 mg	Paxil by Pharmafab	62542-0405	Antidepressant
PAXIL <> 20	Tab, Pink, Oval, Film Coated	Paroxetine HCl 20 mg	Paxil by SKB	00029-3211	Antidepressant
PAXIL <> 20	Tab, Film Coated	Paroxetine HCl 20 mg	Paxil by Kaiser	00179-1182	Antidepressant
PAXIL <> 20	Tab, Film Coated	Paroxetine HCl 20 mg	Paxil by Nat Pharmpak Serv	55154-4504	Antidepressant
PAXIL <> 20	Tab, Film Coated	Paroxetine HCl 20 mg	Paxil by Allscripts	54569-3810	Antidepressant
PAXIL <> 20	Tab, Film Coated	Paroxetine HCl 20 mg	Paxil by HJ Harkins Co	52959-0360	Antidepressant
PAXIL <> 20	Tab, Pink, Oblong	Paroxetine HCl 20 mg	Paxil by Pharmafab	62542-0352	Antidepressant
PAXIL <> 20	Tab, Film Coated	Paroxetine HCl 20 mg	by Kaiser	62224-2340	Antidepressant
PAXIL <> 20	Tab, Film Coated	Paroxetine HCl 20 mg	Paxil by Amerisource	62584-0211	Antidepressant

ID FRONT <> BACK	DESCRIPTION FRONT <> BACK	INGREDIENT & STRENGTH	BRAND (OR EQUIV.) & FIRM	NDC#	CLASS; SCH.
PAXIL <> 20	Tab, Pink, Oval, Scored, Film Coated	Paroxetine HCl 20 mg	Paxil by Pharmafab	62542-0404	Antidepressant
PAXIL <> 20	Tab, Film Coated	Paroxetine HCl 20 mg	Paxil by SB	59742-3211	Antidepressant
PAXIL <> 30	Tab, Blue, Oval, Coated	Paroxetine HCl 30 mg	Paxil by SKB	00029-3212	Antidepressant
PAXIL <> 30	Tab, Coated	Paroxetine HCl 30 mg	Paxil by Physicians Total Care	54868-3526	Antidepressant
PAXIL <> 30	Tab, Coated	Paroxetine HCl 30 mg	Paxil by SB	59742-3212	Antidepressant
PAXIL <> 40	Tab, Green, Oval, Film Coated	Paroxetine HCl 40 mg	Paxil by SKB	00029-3213	Antidepressant
PAXIL <> 40	Tab, Film Coated	Paroxetine HCl 40 mg	Paxil by SB	59742-3213	Antidepressant
PAXIL20MG	Tab, Pink, Oval, Paxil/20 mg	Paroxetine HCl 20 mg	Paxil by SmithKline SKB	Canadian	Antidepressant
PAXIL30MG	Tab, Blue, Oval, Paxil 30 mg	Paroxetine HCl 30 mg	Paxil by SmithKline SKB	Canadian	Antidepressant
PCE	Tab, White w/ Pink Speckles, Oval, PCE over Abbott Logo	Erythromycin 333 mg	PCE by Abbott	00074-6290	Antibiotic
PCE	Tab, Pink, White Specks, Abbott Logo	Erythromycin 333 mg	Pce Dispertab by Allscripts	54569-0157	Antibiotic
PCE <> A	Tab, Pink Specks, Abbott Logo	Erythromycin 333 mg	PCE by Pharmedix	53002-0253	Antibiotic
PCH <> MEGESTROL40	Tab, White, Scored	Megestrol Acetate 40 mg	by Pharmachemie NI	57527-0513	Progestin
PCH <> MEGESTROL40	Tab, White, Scored, PCH <> Megestrol over 40	Megestrol Acetate 40 mg	by Teva Pharms	00093-5138	Progestin
PCHRES25	Tab, Yellow & White, Round, PCH/RES/25	Leucovorin 25 mg	by Astra		Antineoplastic
PCHRES5	Tab, Yellow & White, Round, PCH/RES/5	Leucovorin Calcium 5 mg	by Astra		Antineoplastic
PD	Tab, Tan	Dessicated Thyroid 30 mg	Thyroid by Parke-Davis	Canadian	Thyroid
PD	Tab, Mottled Salmon	Nitroglycerom 5 mg	Norutate by Nitrostat	Canadian DIN# 00023760	PD
PD	Tab, Salmon	Northindrone Acetate 5 mg	by Parke-Davis	Canadian	Hormone
PD	Tab, Tan	Thyroid Hormone 125 mg	Thyroid by Pfizer	Canadian DIN# 00023965	Thyroid
PD	Tab, Tan	Thyroid Hormone 30 mg	Thyroid by Pfizer	Canadian DIN# 00023949	Thyroid
PD	Tab, Tan	Thyroid Hormone 60 mg	Thyroid by Pfizer	Canadian DIN# 00023957	Thyroid
PD <> 144	Tab, White, D-Shaped	Ethinyl Estradiol 5 mcg, Norethindrone Acetate 1 mg	FemHRT by Pfizer	Canadian DIN# 02242531	Oral Contraceptive
PD <> NEURONTIN100MG	Cap, White, Opaque, PD <> Neurontin/100 mg	Gabapentin 100 mg	Neurontin by Parke-Davis	Canadian DIN# 02084260	Anticonvulsant
PD <> NEURONTIN100MG	Cap, White, Gelatin	Gabapentin 100 mg	Neurontin by HJ Harkins	52959-0506	Anticonvulsant
PD <> NEURONTIN100MG	Cap, White	Gabapentin 100 mg	Neurontin by Amerisource Health	62584-0083	Anticonvulsant
PD <> NEURONTIN100MG	Cap, White, Parke Davis Logo <> Nuerontin/100 mg	Gabapentin 100 mg	Neurontin by Parke Davis	00071-0803	Anticonvulsant
PD <> NEURONTIN300MG	Cap, Yellow, Hard Gel, Neurontin/300 mg	Gabapentin 300 mg	Neurontin by Johnson & Johnson	59604-0302	Anticonvulsant
PD <> NEURONTIN300MG	Cap, Yellow, Opaque, PD <> Neurontin/300 mg	Gabapentin 300 mg	Neurontin by Parke-Davis	Canadian DIN# 02084279	Anticonvulsant
PD <> NEURONTIN300MG	Cap, Yellow	Gabapentin 300 mg	Neurontin by Heartland Healthcare	61392-0716	Anticonvulsant
PD <> NEURONTIN300MG	Cap, Yellow	Gabapentin 300 mg	Neurontin by Amerisource Health	62584-0085	Anticonvulsant

ID FRONT <> BACK	DESCRIPTION FRONT <> BACK	INGREDIENT & STRENGTH	BRAND (OR EQUIV.) & FIRM	NDC#	CLASS; SCH.
PD <> NEURONTIN300MG	Cap, Yellow, Gelatin	Gabapentin 300 mg	Neurontin by HJ Harkins	52959-0434	Anticonvulsant
PD <> NEURONTIN300MG	Cap, Yellow	Gabapentin 300 mg	Neurontin by JB	51111-0498	Anticonvulsant
PD <> NEURONTIN300MG	Cap, Yellow, Parke Davis Logo <> Neurontin/300 mg	Gabapentin 300 mg	Neurontin by Parke Davis	00071-0805	Anticonvulsant
PD <> NEURONTIN300MG	Cap, Neurontin/300 mg	Gabapentin 300 mg	by Med Pro	53978-3020	Anticonvulsant
PD <> NEURONTIN300MG	Cap, PD <> Neurontin 300 mg	Gabapentin 300 mg	Neurontin by Nat Pharmpak Serv	55154-2415	Anticonvulsant
PD <> NEURONTIN300MG	Cap, PD <> Neurontin/300 mg	Gabapentin 300 mg	by Pharm Packaging Ctr	54383-0080	Anticonvulsant
PD <> NEURONTIN300MG	Cap	Gabapentin 300 mg	Neurontin by Physicians Total Care	54868-3768	Anticonvulsant
PD <> NEURONTIN400MG	Cap	Gabapentin 400 mg	Neurontin by DRX	55045-2545	Anticonvulsant
PD <> NEURONTIN400MG	Cap, Orange, Gelatin	Gabapentin 400 mg	Neurontin by Natl Pharmpak	55154-2417	Anticonvulsant
PD <> NEURONTIN400MG	Cap, Orange, Opaque, PD <> Neurontin/400 mg	Gabapentin 400 mg	Neurontin by Parke-Davis	Canadian DIN# 02084287	Anticonvulsant
PD <> NEURONTIN400MG	Cap, Orange, Hard Gel	Gabapentin 400 mg	Neurontin by Amerisource Health	62584-0086	Anticonvulsant
PD <> NEURONTINR300MG	Cap, PD <> Neurontin R/300 mg	Gabapentin 300 mg	Neurontin by Caremark	00339-6101	Anticonvulsant
PD <> NEUROTIN400MG	Cap, Orange, Parke Davis Logo <> Neurontin/400 mg	Gabapentin 400 mg	Neurontin by Parke Davis	00071-0806	Anticonvulsant
PD001	Tab, Green, Round, P-D 001	Pentaerythritol Tetranitrate 20 mg	Peritrate by PD		Antianginal
PD004	Tab, Green, Round, P-D 004	Pentaerythritol Tetranitrate SA 80 mg	Peritrate SA by PD		Antianginal
PD007	Tab, Chew, P-D 007	Phenytoin 50 mg	Dilantin Infatabs by Parke Davis	00071-0007	Anticonvulsant
PD007	Tab, Chew, P-D 007	Phenytoin 50 mg	Dilantin Infatabs by Nat Pharmpak Serv	55154-2416	Anticonvulsant
PD008	Tab, Coral, Round, P-D 008	Pentaerythritol Tetranitrate 40 mg	Peritrate by PD		Antianginal
PD013	Tab, Green, Round, P-D 013	Pentaerythritol Tetranitrate 10 mg	Peritrate by PD		Antianginal
PD070	Tab, White, Round, P-D 070	Propranolol 10 mg	Inderal by PD		Antihypertensive
PD071	Tab, White, Round, P-D 071	Propranolol 20 mg	Inderal by PD		Antihypertensive
PD072	Tab, White, Round, P-D 072	Propranolol 40 mg	Inderal by PD		Antihypertensive
PD073	Tab, White, Round, P-D 073	Propranolol 60 mg	Inderal by PD		Antihypertensive
PD074	Tab, White, Round, P-D 074	Propranolol 80 mg	Inderal by PD		Antihypertensive
PD111	Tab, Orange, Round, P-D 111	Ergotamine Tartrate SL 2 mg	Ergostat SL by PD		Antimigraine
PD121	Tab, Blue, Round, P-D 121	Chlorthalidone 50 mg	Hygroton by PD		Diuretic
PD123	Tab, Orange, Round, P-D 123	Chlorthalidone 25 mg	Hygroton by PD		Diuretic
PD1412	Tab, White, Oval, P-D 141/2	Diazepam 2 mg	Valium by PD		Antianxiety; C IV
PD1425	Tab, White, Triangular, P-D 142/5	Diazepam 5 mg	Valium by PD		Antianxiety; C IV
PD14310	Tab, White, Round, P-D 143/10	Diazepam 10 mg	Valium by PD		Antianxiety; C IV
PD15	Tab, Pink	Phenobarbital 15 mg	by Parke-Davis	Canadian	Sedative/Hypnotic
PD155 <> 10	Tab, White, Elliptical, Film Coated	Atorvastatin 10 mg	Lipitor by Parke-Davis	Canadian DIN# 02230711	Antihyperlipidemic
PD155 <> 10	Tab, Film Coated, PD 155	Atorvastatin Calcium 10 mg	Lipitor by Pharm Utilization	60491-0803	Antihyperlipidemic
PD155 <> 10	Tab, White, Elliptical, Film Coated	Atorvastatin Calcium 10 mg	Lipitor by Parke Davis	00071-0155	Antihyperlipidemic
PD155 <> 10	Tab, Film Coated	Atorvastatin Calcium 10 mg	Lipitor by Goedecke	53869-0155	Antihyperlipidemic
PD155 <> 10	Tab, Film Coated	Atorvastatin Calcium 10 mg	Lipitor by Allscripts	54569-4466	Antihyperlipidemic

ID FRONT <> BACK	DESCRIPTION FRONT <> BACK	INGREDIENT & STRENGTH	BRAND (OR EQUIV.) & FIRM	NDC#	CLASS; SCH.
PD156 <> 20	Tab, White, Elliptical, Film-Coated	Atorvastatin 20 mg	Lipitor by Parke-Davis	Canadian DIN# 02230713	Antihyperlipidemic
PD156 <> 20	Tab, Film Coated, PD 156	Atorvastatin Calcium 20 mg	Lipitor by Pharm Utilization	60491-0804	Antihyperlipidemic
PD156 <> 20	Tab, White	Atorvastatin Calcium 20 mg	Lipitor by Phy Total Care	54868-3946	Antihyperlipidemic
PD156 <> 20	Tab, White, Elliptical, Film Coated	Atorvastatin Calcium 20 mg	Lipitor by Parke Davis	00071-0156	Antihyperlipidemic
PD156 <> 20	Tab, Film Coated	Atorvastatin Calcium 20 mg	Lipitor by Goedecke	53869-0156	Antihyperlipidemic
PD156 <> 20	Tab, Film Coated	Atorvastatin Calcium 20 mg	Lipitor by Allscripts	54569-4467	Antihyperlipidemic
PD157 <> 40	Tab, White, Elliptical, Film Coated	Atorvastatin 40 mg	Lipitor by Parke-Davis	Canadian DIN# 02230714	Antihyperlipidemic
PD157 <> 40	Tab, White, Oval, Film Coated	Atorvastatin Calcium 40 mg	Lipitor by Murfreesboro Ph	51129-1424	Antihyperlipidemic
PD157 <> 40	Tab, White	Atorvastatin Calcium 40 mg	Lipitor by Phy Total Care	54868-4229	Antihyperlipidemic
PD157 <> 40	Tab, White, Elliptical, Film Coated	Atorvastatin Calcium 40 mg	Lipitor by Parke Davis	00071-0157	Antihyperlipidemic
PD157 <> 40	Tab, Film Coated	Atorvastatin Calcium 40 mg	Lipitor by Goedecke	53869-0157	Antihyperlipidemic
PD166	Tab, Brown, Oval, P-D 166	Methenamine Mandelate 500 mg	Mandelamine by PD		Antibiotic; Urinary Tract
PD167	Tab, Purple, Oval, P-D 167	Methenamine Mandelate 1000 mg	Mandelamine by PD		Antibiotic; Urinary Tract
PD177	Tab, Pink, Oval, P-D 177	Phenylpropanolamine 100 mg, Phenyltoloxamine 66 mg, Acetaminophen 600 mg	Sinubid by PD		Cold Remedy
PD180	Tab, Reddish Brown, Coated	Phenazopyridine HCl 100 mg	Pyridium by Parke-Davis	Canadian DIN# 00476714	Urinary Analgesic
PD180	Tab, Maroon, Round, P-D 180	Phenazopyridine HCl 100 mg	Pyridium by PD		Urinary Analgesic
PD181	Tab, Reddish Brown, Coated	Phenazopyridine HCl 200 mg	Pyridium by Parke-Davis	Canadian DIN# 00476722	Urinary Analgesic
PD181	Tab, P-D 181, Coated	Phenazopyridine HCl 200 mg	Pyridium by Allscripts	54569-0089	Urinary Analgesic
PD181	Tab, Coated	Phenazopyridine HCl 200 mg	Pyridium by Urgent Care Ctr	50716-0181	Urinary Analgesic
PD182	Tab, Maroon, Square, P-D 182	Phenazopyridine HCl 150 mg, Hyoscyamine HBr 0.3 mg, Butabarbital 15 mg	Pyridium Plus by PD		Urinary
PD200	Tab, Salmon, Round, P-D 200	Oxtriphylline 200 mg, Guaifenesin 100 mg	Brondecon by PD		Antiasthmatic
PD202	Tab, Green, Oval, P-D 202	Procainamide HCl SR 250 mg	Procan SR by PD		Antiarrhythmic
PD204	Tab, Yellow, Oval, P-D 204	Procainamide HCl SR 500 mg	Procan SR by PD		Antiarrhythmic
PD205	Tab, Orange, Oval, P-D 205	Procainamide HCl SR 750 mg	Procan SR by PD		Antiarrhythmic
PD207	Tab, Red, Oblong, P-D 207	Procainamide HCl SR 1000 mg	Procan SR by PD		Antiarrhythmic
PD210	Tab, Red, Round, P-D 210	Oxtriphylline 100 mg	Choledyl by PD		Antiasthmatic
PD211	Tab, Yellow, Round, P-D 211	Oxtriphylline 200 mg	Choledyl by PD		Antiasthmatic
PD214	Tab, Elliptical-Shaped, Film Coated, P-D 214	Oxtriphylline 400 mg	Choledyl SA by Parke Davis	00071-0214	Antiasthmatic
PD220	Tab, Pink, Triangular, Scored, Film Coated	Hydrochlorothiazide 12.5 mg, Quinapril 20 mg	Accuretic by Park-Davis	Canadian DIN# 02237368	Diuretic; Antihypertensive
PD221	Tab, Elliptical-Shaped, Film Coated, P-D 221	Oxtriphylline 600 mg	Choledyl SA by Parke Davis	00071-0221	Antiasthmatic
PD222	Tab, Pink, Elliptical, Scored, Film Coated	Hydrochlorothiazide 12.5 mg, Quinapril 10 mg	Accuretic by Park-Davis	Canadian DIN# 02237367	Diuretic; Antihypertensive
PD223	Tab, Pink, Round, Scored, Film Coated	Hydrochlorothiazide 25 mg, Quinapril 20 mg	Accuretic by Parke-Davis	Canadian	Diuretic; Antihypertensive
PD230	Tab, White, Round	Phenobarbital 8 mg, Theophylline 130 mg, Ephedrine 24 mg	Tedral by PD		Antiasthmatic; C IV
PD231	Tab, Coral & White, Round, P-D 231	Theophylline 180 mg, Ephedrine 48 mg, Phenobarbital SA 25 mg	Tedral SA by PD		Antiasthmatic
PD237	Cap, P-D 237	Ethosuximide 250 mg	Zarontin by Parke Davis	00071-0237	Anticonvulsant
PD237	Cap, P-D/237	Ethosuximide 250 mg	Zarontin by RP Scherer	11014-0121	Anticonvulsant
PD237	Cap, Clear, Gelatin, P-D/237	Ethosuximide 250 mg	Zarontin S.G. No. 237 by RP Scherer	11014-0771	Anticonvulsant
PD251	Tab, Gray, Round, P-D 251	Thyroglobulin 32 mg	Proloid by PD		Thyroid
PD252	Tab, Gray, Round, P-D 252	Thyroglobulin 65 mg	Proloid by PD		Thyroid

ID FRONT <> BACK	DESCRIPTION FRONT <> BACK	INGREDIENT & STRENGTH	BRAND (OR EQUIV.) & FIRM	NDC#	CLASS; SCH.
PD253	Tab, Gray, Round, P-D 253	Thyroglobulin 100 mg	Proloid by PD		Thyroid
PD254	Tab, Gray, Round, P-D 254	Thyroglobulin 200 mg	Proloid by PD		Thyroid
PD257	Tab, Gray, Round, P-D 257	Thyroglobulin 130 mg	Proloid by PD		Thyroid
PD260	Tab, Peach, Square, P-D 260	Liotrix	Euthroid 1/2 by PD		Antithyroid
PD261	Tab, Tan, Square, P-D 261	Liotrix	Euthroid 1 by PD		Antithyroid
PD262	Tab, Lavender, Square, P-D 262	Liotrix	Euthroid 2 by PD		Antithyroid
PD263	Tab, Gray, Square, P-D 263	Liotrix	Euthroid 3 by PD		Antithyroid
PD270	Tab, Sugar Coated, P-D 270	Phenelzine Sulfate 1000	Nardil by Parke Davis	00071-0270	Antidepressant
PD271	Tab, Dark Yellow, Round, P-D 271	Amitriptyline 100 mg	Elavil by PD		Antidepressant
PD272	Tab, Tan, Round, P-D 272	Amitriptyline 10 mg	Elavil by PD		Antidepressant
PD273	Tab, Coral, Round, P-D 273	Amitriptyline 25 mg	Elavil by PD		Antidepressant
PD274	Tab, Blue & Purple, Round, P-D 274	Amitriptyline 50 mg	Elavil by PD		Antidepressant
PD275	Tab, Green, Round, P-D 275	Amitriptyline 75 mg	Elavil by PD		Antidepressant
PD276	Tab, Blue, Round, P-D 276	Prazepam 10 mg	Centrax by PD		Sedative/Hypnotic; C IV
PD278	Tab, Orange, Oval, P-D 278	Amitriptyline 150 mg	Elavil by PD		Antidepressant
PD282	Tab, Yellow, Oblong, P-D 282	Prenatal Vitamin Combination	Natafort Filmseals by PD		Vitamin
PD30	Tab, Yellow	Phenobarbital 30 mg	by Parke-Davis	Canadian	Sedative/Hypnotic
PD320	Tab, White, Round, P-D 320	Ethopropazine 10 mg	Parsidol by PD		Antiparkinson
PD321	Tab, White, Round, P-D 321	Ethopropazine 50 mg	Parsidol by PD		Antiparkinson
PD337	Cap, Blue, P-D 337	Vitamin Combination	Eldec by PD		Vitamin
PD352 <> 200	Tab, Yellow, Oval, Film Coated	Troglitazone 200 mg	Rezulin by Murfreesboro Ph	51129-1286	Antidiabetic
PD352 <> 200	Tab, Yellow, Oval, Film Coated, PD 352	Troglitazone 200 mg	Rezulin by Parke Davis	00071-0352	Antidiabetic
PD352200MG	Tab, Yellow, Oval	Troglitazone 200 mg	Rezulin by PD		Antidiabetic
PD353 <> 400	Tab, Tan, Oval, Coated, PD 353	Troglitazone 400 mg	Rezulin by Parke Davis	00071-0353	Antidiabetic
PD353 <> 400	Tab, Tan, Oval, Film Coated, PD 353	Troglitazone 400 mg	Rezulin by Teva	00480-0756	Antidiabetic
PD353400MG	Tab, Tan, Oval	Troglitazone 400 mg	Rezulin by PD		Antidiabetic
PD357 <> 300	Tab, White, Oval, Film Coated	Troglitazone 300 mg	Rezulin by Murfreesboro Ph	51129-1423	Antidiabetic
PD357 <> 300	Tab, White, Oval, Debossed, Film Coated	Troglitazone 300 mg	Rezulin by Parke Davis	00071-0357	Antidiabetic
PD357300MG	Tab, White, Oval	Troglitazone 300 mg	Rezulin by PD		Antidiabetic
PD362	Cap, Orange Band, Ex Release	Phenytoin Sodium 100 mg	Dilantin by Pharmedix	53002-0415	Anticonvulsant
PD362	Cap, Orange Band, Ex Release	Phenytoin Sodium 100 mg	by Med Pro	53978-0298	Anticonvulsant
PD362	Cap, White with Orange Band, Ex Release	Phenytoin Sodium 100 mg	Dilantin by Allscripts	54569-0161	Anticonvulsant
PD362 <> PD362	Cap, Clear with Orange Band, Ex Release, PD 362	Phenytoin Sodium 100 mg	Dilantin by Parke Davis	00071-0362	Anticonvulsant
PD362 <> PD362	Cap, Orange Band, Black Imprint, Ex Release	Phenytoin Sodium 100 mg	Dilantin by Kaiser	00179-0222	Anticonvulsant
PD362 <> PD362	Cap, ER, PD 362	Phenytoin Sodium 100 mg	Dilantin by Nat Pharmpak Serv	55154-2404	Anticonvulsant
PD362 <> PD362	Cap, Transparent with Orange Band, PD 362 <> Printed in middle of band, Ex Release	Phenytoin Sodium 100 mg	Dilantin by Quality Care	60346-0428	Anticonvulsant
PD365	Cap, White, Pink Band, P-D 365	Extended Phenytoin Sodium 30 mg	Dilantin by PD		Anticonvulsant
PD365	Cap, White with Pink Band, P-D 365	Phenytoin Sodium 30 mg	Dilantin by Parke Davis	00071-0365	Anticonvulsant
PD373	Cap, Pink with White Band, P-D 373	Diphenhydramine HCl 50 mg	Benadryl by Parke Davis	00071-0373	Antihistamine
PD375	Cap, White/Red Band, P-D 375	Phenytoin Sodium 100 mg, Phenobarbital 16 mg	Dilantin with PB by PD		Anticonvulsant; C IV
PD379	Cap, White with Gray Band, P-D 379	Chloramphenicol 250 mg	Chloromycetin by Parke Davis	00071-0379	Antibiotic
PD389	Cap, P-D 389	Bromodiphenhydramine 25 mg	Ambodryl by PD		Antihistamine
PD390	Cap, Pink & Blue	Vitamin, Mineral Combination	Natabec by PD		Vitamin
PD393	Cap, Orange, P-D 393	Phensuximide 500 mg	Milontin by PD		Anticonvulsant
PD402	Cap, Blue & Gray, P-D 402	Ampicillin 250 mg	Amcill by PD		Antibiotic
PD404	Cap, Blue & Gray, P-D 404	Ampicillin 500 mg	Amcill by PD		Antibiotic
PD407	Cap, Red & White, P-D 407	Tetracycline HCl 250 mg	Achromycin V by PD		Antibiotic
PD425	Tab, White, Square	Norethindrone 1 mg, Ethinyl Estradiol 30 mcg	Estrostep by PD		Oral Contraceptive
PD427	Tab, White, Triangular	Norethindrone 1 mg, Ethinyl Estradiol 20 mcg	Estrostep by PD		Oral Contraceptive
PD437	Tab, Blue, Round, P-D 437	Quinestrol 100 mcg	Estrovis by PD		Hormone
PD440	Tab, White, Oval, P-D 440	Furosemide 20 mg	Lasix by Watson		Diuretic

ID FRONT <> BACK	DESCRIPTION FRONT <> BACK	INGREDIENT & STRENGTH	BRAND (OR EQUIV.) & FIRM	NDC#	CLASS; SCH.
PD441	Tab, White, Round, P-D 441	Furosemide 40 mg	Lasix by PD		Diuretic
PD442	Tab, White, Round, P-D 442	Furosemide 80 mg	Lasix by PD		Diuretic
PD443	Tab, Pink, Round, P-D 443	Clonidine HCl 0.1 mg	Catapres by PD		Antihypertensive
PD444	Tab, White, Round, P-D 444	Clonidine HCl 0.2 mg	Catapres by PD		Antihypertensive
PD445	Tab, White, Round, P-D 445	Clonidine HCl 0.3 mg	Catapres by PD		Antihypertensive
PD471	Cap, P-D 471	Diphenhydramine HCl 25 mg	Benadryl by Parke Davis	00071-0471	Antihistamine
PD490	Tab, Rose, Elliptical	Aspirin Delayed Release 975 mg	Easprin by PD		Analgesic
PD525	Cap, Transparent Yellow with Orange Band, P-D 525	Methsuximide 300 mg	Celontin by Parke Davis	00071-0525	Anticonvulsant
PD527 <> 5	Tab, Brown	Quinapril HCl 5 mg	Accupril by PDRX Pharms	55289-0552	Antihypertensive
PD527 <> 5	Tab, Brown, Elliptical-Shaped, Coated	Quinapril HCl 5 mg	Accupril by Parke Davis	00071-0527	Antihypertensive
PD527 <> 5	Tab, Coated	Quinapril HCl 5 mg	Accupril by Pharm Utilization	60491-0001	Antihypertensive
PD527 <> 5	Tab, Brown, Elliptical, Scored, Film Coated, PD/527 <> 5	Quinapril 5 mg	Accupril by Parke-Davis	Canadian DIN# 01947664	Antihypertensive
PD529	Cap, Black & Yellow, Opaque	Paromomycin 250 mg	Humantin by Pfizer	Canadian DIN# 02078759	Antibiotic
PD529	Cap, P-D 529	Paromomycin Sulfate 250	Humatin by Parke Davis	00071-0529	Antibiotic
PD529	Cap, Yellow & Brown	Paromomycin Sulfate 250 mg	Humatin by Monarch	61570-0529	Antibiotic
PD530 <> 10	Tab, Brown, Triangular, Coated	Quinapril HCl 10 mg	Accupril by Parke Davis	00071-0530	Antihypertensive
PD530 <> 10	Tab, PD 530, Coated	Quinapril HCl 10 mg	Accupril by Allscripts	54569-3984	Antihypertensive
PD530 <> 10	Tab, Brown, Triangular, Film Coated, PD/530 <> 10	Quinapril 10 mg	Accupril by Parke-Davis	Canadian DIN# 01947672	Antihypertensive
PD530 <> 10	Tab, Brown, Triangle	Quinapril HCl 10 mg	Accupril by PDRX Pharms	55289-0553	Antihypertensive
PD530 <> 10	Tab, Brown, Triangle, Film Coated	Quinapril HCl 10 mg	Accupril by RX PAK	65084-0124	Antihypertensive
PD530 <> 10	Tab, Brown, Triangle	Quinapril HCl 10 mg	Accupril by Direct Dispensing	57866-4420	Antihypertensive
PD531	Cap, White/Black Band, P-D 531	Phenytoin Sodium 100 mg, Phenobarbital 32 mg	Dilantin with PB by PD		Anticonvulsant; C IV
PD532	Tab, Brown, Round, Film Coated	Quinapril HCl 20 mg	Accupril by RX PAK	65084-0120	Antihypertensive
PD532 <> 20	Tab, Brown, Round, Film Coated, PD 532	Quinapril HCl 20 mg	Accupril by RX PAK	65084-0117	Antihypertensive
PD532 <> 20	Tab, Brown, Round	Quinapril HCl 20 mg	Accupril by PDRX Pharms	55289-0554	Antihypertensive
PD532 <> 20	Tab, Brown, Round, Coated	Quinapril HCl 20 mg	Accupril by Parke Davis	00071-0532	Antihypertensive
PD532 <> 20	Tab, Coated	Quinapril HCl 20 mg	Accupril by Allscripts	54569-3985	Antihypertensive
PD532 <> 20	Tab, Brown, Round, Film Coated, PD/532 <> 20	Quinapril 20 mg	Accupril by Parke-Davis	Canadian DIN# 01947680	Antihypertensive
PD534	Cap, Pink & Purple, P-D 534	Prenatal Vitamin Combination, Fluoride	Natabec Fluoride by PD		Vitamin
PD534	Cap, Pink & Red	Vitamin, Mineral Combination	Natabec Fluoride by PD		Vitamin
PD535 <> 40	Tab, Brown	Quinapril HCl 40 mg	Accupril by PDRX Pharms	55289-0555	Antihypertensive
PD535 <> 40	Tab, Brown, Elliptical-Shaped, Coated	Quinapril HCl 40 mg	Accupril by Parke Davis	00071-0535	Antihypertensive
PD535 <> 40	Tab, Brown, Elliptical, Film Coated, PD/535 <> 40	Quinapril 40 mg	Accupril by Parke-Davis	Canadian DIN# 01947699	Antihypertensive
PD537	Cap, Cream/Gray Band, P-D 537	Methsuximide 150 mg	Celontin by PD		Anticonvulsant
PD540	Cap, Cream/Blue, P-D 540	Mefenamic Acid 250 mg	Ponstel by PD		NSAID
PD540 <> PONSTEL	Cap, Yellow with Blue Band, P-D 540	Mefenamic Acid 250 mg	Ponstel by Parke Davis	00071-0540	NSAID
PD540PONSTEL	Cap, Yellow & Blue, P-D 540/Ponstel	Mefenamic Acid 250 mg	Ponstel Kapseals by Parke-Davis		NSAID
PD541	Cap, Pink & White	Vitamin, Mineral Combination	Natabec FA by PD		Vitamin
PD544	Cap, Blue & Yellow	Vitamin, Mineral Combination	Geriplex-FS by PD		Vitamin
PD547	Cap, Blue & White Band, P-D 547	Prenatal Vitamin Combination	Natabec RX by PD		Vitamin
PD552	Cap, Celery	Prazepam 5 mg	Centrax by PD		Sedative/Hypnotic; C IV
PD553	Cap, Aqua	Prazepam 10 mg	Centrax by PD		Sedative/Hypnotic; C IV

ID FRONT <> BACK	DESCRIPTION FRONT <> BACK	INGREDIENT & STRENGTH	BRAND (OR EQUIV.) & FIRM	NDC#	CLASS; SCH.
PD554	Cap, Ivory	Prazepam 20 mg	Centrax by PD		Sedative/Hypnotic; C IV
PD555	Tab, White, Round	Norethindrone 1 mg, Ethinyl Estradiol 35 mcg	Estrostep by PD		Oral Contraceptive
PD557	Tab, White, Round, P-D 557	Verapamil 80 mg	Isoptin by PD		Antihypertensive
PD573	Tab, White, Round, P-D 573	Verapamil 120 mg	Isoptin by PD		Antihypertensive
PD60	Tab, Light Green	Phenobarbital 60 mg	by Parke-Davis	Canadian	Sedative/Hypnotic
PD607	Tab, White, Round, P-D 607	Phenobarbital 60 mg	by PD		Sedative/Hypnotic; C IV
PD618	Tab, White, Round, P-D 618	Placebo	by PD		Placebo
PD622	Tab, Brown, Round, P-D 622	Ferrous Fumarate 75 mg	by PD		Mineral
PD634	Tab, White, Round, P-D 634	Acetaminophen 300 mg, Codeine 15 mg	Tylenol #2 by PD		Analgesic; C III
PD635	Tab, White, Round, P-D 635	Acetaminophen 300 mg, Codeine 30 mg	Tylenol #3 by PD		Analgesic; C III
PD637	Tab, White, Round, P-D 637	Acetaminophen 300 mg, Codeine 60 mg	Tylenol #4 by PD		Analgesic; C III
PD638	Tab, Brown, Oval, P-D 638	Vitamin Combination	Tabron by PD		Vitamin
PD648	Tab, White, Oval, P-D 648	Penicillin V Potassium 250 mg	V-Cillin K by PD		Antibiotic
PD663	Cap, Orange, Clear	Erythromycin Delayed Release 125 mg	Eryc by PD		Antibiotic
PD672	Tab, Yellow, Round, P-D 672	Erythromycin Stearate 250 mg	Erythrocin by PD		Antibiotic
PD673	Tab, White, Oval, P-D 673	Penicillin V Potassium 500 mg	V-Cillin K by PD		Antibiotic
PD692	Cap, P-D 692	Propoxyphene HCl 65 mg	Darvon by PD		Analgesic; C IV
PD696 <> ERYC	Cap, Clear & Orange	Erythromycin 250 mg	Eryc by Murfreesboro Ph	51129-1422	Antibiotic
PD696 <> ERYC	Cap, Clear & Orange, Opaque	Erythromycin 250 mg	Eryc by Parke-Davis	Canadian DIN# 00607142	Antibiotic
PD696 <> ERYC	Cap, P-D 696	Erythromycin 250 mg	Eryc by Parke Davis	00071-0696	Antibiotic
PD696 <> ERYC	Cap, P-D 696	Erythromycin 250 mg	Eryc by Allscripts	54569-0131	Antibiotic
PD697	Cap, Orange & White, P-D 697	Tetracycline HCl 500 mg	Achromycin V by PD		Antibiotic
PD698	Tab, White, Round, P-D 698	Phenobarbital 100 mg	by PD		Sedative/Hypnotic; C IV
PD699	Tab, White, Round, P-D 699	Phenobarbital 15 mg	by PD		Sedative/Hypnotic; C IV
PD700	Tab, White, Round, P-D 700	Phenobarbital 30 mg	by PD		Sedative/Hypnotic; C IV
PD702	Tab, White, Round, P-D 702	Hydrochlorothiazide 25 mg	Hydrodiuril by PD		Diuretic
PD710	Tab, White, Round, P-D 710	Hydrochlorothiazide 50 mg	Hydrodiuril by PD		Diuretic
PD712	Tab, White, Round, P-D 712	Spironolactone 25 mg, Hydrochlorothiazide 25 mg	Aldactazide by PD		Diuretic
PD713	Tab, White, Round, P-D 713	Spironolactone 25 mg	Aldactone by PD		Diuretic
PD725	Tab, White, Round, P-D 725	Aspirin 325 mg, Codeine Phosphate 15 mg	Empirin #2 by PD		Analgesic; C III
PD726	Tab, White, Round, P-D 726	Aspirin 325 mg, Codeine Phosphate 30 mg	Empirin #3 by PD		Analgesic; C III
PD727	Tab, White, Round, P-D 727	Aspirin 325 mg, Codeine Phosphate 60 mg	Empirin #4 by PD		Analgesic; C III
PD730	Cap, Pink & Red, P-D 730	Amoxicillin 250 mg	Amoxil by PD		Antibiotic
PD731	Cap, Pink & Red, P-D 731	Amoxicillin 500 mg	Amoxil by PD		Antibiotic
PD737 <> LOPID	Tab, Elliptical, Film Coated, P-D 737	Gemfibrozil 600 mg	Lopid by Parke Davis	00071-0737	Antihyperlipidemic
PD737LOPID	Tab, White, P-D 737/Lopid	Gemfibrozil 600 mg	Lopid by Parke-Davis		Antihyperlipidemic
PD813	Tab, Orange, Round, P-D 813	Doxycycline Hyclate 100 mg	Vibra-Tab by PD		Antibiotic
PD829	Cap, Aqua & Cream, P-D 829	Doxycycline Hyclate 50 mg	Vibramycin by PD		Antibiotic
PD830	Cap, Aqua, P-D 830	Doxycycline Hyclate 100 mg	Vibramycin by PD		Antibiotic
PD849	Tab, White, Round, P-D 849	Quinidine Sulfate 200 mg	Quinidine by PD		Antiarrhythmic
PD850	Tab, White, Round, P-D 850	Quinidine Gluconate 330 mg	Duraquin by PD		Antiarrhythmic
PD865	Tab, Blue, Round, P-D 865	Methyldopa 250 mg	Aldomet by PD		Antihypertensive
PD866	Tab, Blue, Round, P-D 866	Methyldopa 500 mg	Aldomet by PD		Antihypertensive
PD882	Tab, White, Round, P-D 882	Norethindrone 5 mg	Norlutin by PD		Oral Contraceptive
PD887	Cap, Blue & Aqua, P-D 887	Indomethacin 25 mg	Indocin by PD		NSAID
PD888	Cap, Blue & Aqua, P-D 888	Indomethacin 50 mg	Indocin by PD		NSAID
PD901	Tab, Pink, Round, P-D 901	Norethindrone Acetate 2.5 mg, Ethinyl Estradiol 50 mcg	Norlestrin 2.5/50 by PD		Oral Contraceptive
PD904	Tab, Yellow, Round, P-D 904	Norethindrone Acetate 1 mg, Ethinyl Estradiol 50 mcg	Norlestrin 1/50 by PD		Oral Contraceptive
PD915	Tab, White, P-D 915	Ethinyl Estradiol 20 mcg, Norethindrone Acetate 1 mg	Loestrin 21 1/20 by Parke Davis	00071-0915	Oral Contraceptive
PD916	Tab, Green, Round, P-D 916	Norethindrone Acetate 1.5 mg, Ethinyl Estradiol 30 mcg	Loestrin 1.5/30 by PD		Oral Contraceptive

ID FRONT <> BACK	DESCRIPTION FRONT <> BACK	INGREDIENT & STRENGTH	BRAND (OR EQUIV.) & FIRM	NDC#	CLASS; SCH.
PD917	Tab, Green, P-D 917	Ethinyl Estradiol 30 mcg, Norethindrone Acetate 1.5 mg	Loestrin Fe 1.5/30 by Parke Davis	00071-0917	Oral Contraceptive
PD918	Tab, Pink, Round, P-D 918	Norethindrone Acetate 5 mg	Norlutate by PD		Oral Contraceptive
PD919	Tab, Yellow, Oval, P-D 919	Erythromycin Stearate 500 mg	Erythrocin by PD		Antibiotic
PEC <> 103	Tab, Coated	Ascorbic Acid 120 mg, Calcium 250 mg, Cholecalciferol 400 Units, Copper 2 mg, Cyanocobalamin 12 mcg, Docusate Sodium 50 mg, Folic Acid 1 mg, Iodine 150 mcg, Iron 90 mg, Niacinamide 20 mg, Pyridoxine HCl 20 mg, Riboflavin 3.4 mg, Thiamine HCl 3 mg, Vitamin A 4000 Units, Vitamin E 30 Units, Zinc 25 mg	Maternity 90 Prenatal by Qualitest	00603-5355	Vitamin
PEC <> 111	Cap, Gray, Pink & White Beads	Chlorpheniramine Maleate 12 mg, Phenylpropanolamine HCl 75 mg	Ordrine by Mutual	53489-0302	Cold Remedy
PEC <> 122	Cap, Orange Opaque <> Orange Clear, Delayed Release	Amylase 48000 Units, Lipase 16000 Units, Protease 48000 Units	Pancrelipase 16,000 by Pecos	59879-0122	Gastrointestinal
PEC <> 122	Cap, Clear & Orange, Opaque	Amylase 48000 Units, Lipase 16000 Units, Protease 48000 Units	Pancrelipase 16000 by Lini	58215-0300	Gastrointestinal
PEC <> 122	Cap, Orange Clear & Orange Opaque	Amylase 48000 Units, Lipase 16000 Units, Protease 48000 Units	Pancrelipase 16000 by Mutual	53489-0247	Gastrointestinal
PEC <> 122	Cap, Clear & Orange, Opaque	Amylase 48000 Units, Lipase 16000 Units, Protease 48000 Units	Pancrelipase 16000 by United Res	00677-1543	Gastrointestinal
PEC <> 128	Tab, Film Coated	Ascorbic Acid 120 mg, Biotin 30 mcg, Calcium 200 mg, Chromium 25 mcg, Copper 2 mg, Cyanocobalamin 12 mcg, Folic Acid 1 mg, Iodine 150 mcg, Iron 27 mg, Magnesium 25 mg, Manganese 5 mg, Molybdenum 25 mcg, Niacinamide 20 mg, Pantothenic Acid 10 mg, Pyridoxine HCl 10 mg, Riboflavin 3.4 mg, Selenium 20 mcg, Thiamine HCl 3 mg, Vitamin A 5000 Units, Vitamin D 400 Units, Vitamin E 30 Units, Zinc 25 mg	Prenatal M New Form by Pecos	59879-0128	Vitamin
PEC <> 505	Cap	Amylase 33200 Units, Lipase 10000 Units, Protease 37500 Units	Pancrelipase 10000 by Mutual	53489-0246	Gastrointestinal
PEC <> 505	Cap	Amylase 33200 Units, Lipase 10000 Units, Protease 37500 Units	Pancreatin 10 by HL Moore	00839-8016	Gastrointestinal
PEC101	Tab, Coated, PEC/101	Ascorbic Acid 100 mg, Biotin 0.03 mg, Calcium Carbonate, Precipitated, Calcium Pantothenate, Cholecalciferol, Chromium 0.025 mg, Cupric Oxide, Cyanocobalamin 0.012 mg, Ferrous Fumarate, Folic Acid 1 mg, Magnesium Oxide, Manganese Sulfate Monohydrate, Niacinamide 20 mg, Potassium Iodide, Pyridoxine HCl 10 mg, Riboflavin 3.4 mg, Sodium Molybdate, Thiamine Mononitrate, Vitamin A Acetate 5000 Units, Zinc Oxide	Pecos Prenatal No 101 by Anabolic	00722-6266	Vitamin
PEC101	Tab, Scored	Ascorbic Acid 100 mg, Biotin, D- 30 mcg, Calcium 250 mg, Calcium Pantothenate 10 mg, Cholecalciferol 400 Units, Chromium 25 mcg, Copper 2 mg, Cyanocobalamin 12 mcg, Folic Acid 1 mg, Iodine 150 mcg, Iron 60 mg, Magnesium 25 mg, Manganese 5 mg, Molybdenum 25 mcg, Niacin 20 mg, Pyridoxine HCl 10 mg, Riboflavin 3.4 mg, Thiamine HCl 3 mg, Vitamin A 5000 Units, Vitamin E 30 Units, Zinc 25 mg	Prenatal M by Mutual	53489-0300	Vitamin
PEC101 <> PEC101	Tab, PEC/101 <> PEC/101	Ascorbic Acid 100 mg, Biotin, D- 30 mcg, Calcium 250 mg, Calcium Pantothenate 10 mg, Cholecalciferol 400 Units, Chromium 25 mcg, Copper 2 mg, Cyanocobalamin 12 mcg, Folic Acid 1 mg, Iodine 150 mcg, Iron 60 mg, Magnesium 25 mg, Manganese 5 mg, Molybdenum 25 mcg, Niacin 20 mg, Pyridoxine HCl 10 mg, Riboflavin 3.4 mg, Thiamine HCl 3 mg, Vitamin A 5000 Units, Vitamin E 30 Units, Zinc 25 mg	Materna Type by Contract	10267-1371	Vitamin
PEC102	Tab, Scored	Ascorbic Acid 120 mg, Calcium 250 mg, Copper 2 mg, Cyanocobalamin 12 mcg, Docusate Sodium 50 mg, Folic Acid 1 mg, Iodine 0.15 mg, Iron 90 mg, Niacinamide 20 mg, Pyridoxine HCl 20 mg, Riboflavin 3.4 mg, Thiamine HCl 3 mg, Vitamin A 4000 Units, Vitamin D 400 Units, Vitamin E 30 Units, Zinc 25 mg	Maternal Plus 90 by Zenith Goldline	00182-4387	Vitamin
PEC102	Tab, Film Coated, Scored	Ascorbic Acid 120 mg, Calcium 250 mg, Copper 2 mg, Cyanocobalamin 12 mcg, Docusate Sodium 50 mg, Folic Acid 1 mg, Iodine 0.15 mg, Iron 90 mg, Niacinamide 20 mg, Pyridoxine HCl 20 mg, Riboflavin 3.4 mg, Thiamine HCl 3 mg, Vitamin A 4000 Units, Vitamin D 400 Units, Vitamin E 30 Units, Zinc 25 mg	Prenatal 90 by Mutual	53489-0301	Vitamin
PEC102	Tab, Film Coated, Scored	Ascorbic Acid 120 mg, Calcium 250 mg, Copper 2 mg, Cyanocobalamin 12 mcg, Docusate Sodium 50 mg, Folic Acid 1 mg, Iodine 0.15 mg, Iron 90 mg, Niacinamide 20 mg, Pyridoxine HCl 20 mg, Riboflavin 3.4 mg, Thiamine HCl 3 mg, Vitamin A 4000 Units, Vitamin D 400 Units, Vitamin E 30 Units, Zinc 25 mg	Prenate 90 by Lini	58215-0307	Vitamin
PEC104	Tab	Ascorbic Acid 70 mg, Calcium 200 mg, Cyanocobalamin 2.2 mcg, Folic Acid 1 mg, Iodine 175 mcg, Iron 65 mg, Magnesium 100 mg, Niacin 17 mg, Pyridoxine HCl 2.2 mg, Riboflavin 1.6 mg, Selenium 65 mcg, Thiamine Mononitrate 1.5 mg, Vitamin A 4000 Units, Vitamin D 400 Units, Vitamin E 10 Units, Zinc 15 mg	Z+ Prenatal by Qualitest	00603-6476	Vitamin

ID FRONT <> BACK	DESCRIPTION FRONT <> BACK	INGREDIENT & STRENGTH	BRAND (OR EQUIV.) & FIRM	NDC#	CLASS; SCH.
PEC105	Cap, Orange & Brown	Polysaccharide Iron Complex	Niferex-150 by Pecos Pharmaceuticals		Vitamin
PEC106	Cap, ER	Pheniramine Maleate 8 mg, Phenylpropanolamine HCl 25 mg, Phenyltoloxamine Citrate 8 mg, Pyrilamine Maleate 8 mg	Multihist D Ped by Mutual	53489-0267	Cold Remedy
PEC106	Cap, ER	Pheniramine Maleate 8 mg, Phenylpropanolamine HCl 25 mg, Phenyltoloxamine Citrate 8 mg, Pyrilamine Maleate 8 mg	Multihistamine D Ped by Lini	58215-0323	Cold Remedy
PEC108	Tab, White, Oblong	Guiavent	by Lini		Cold Remedy
PEC108	Tab	Guaifenesin 600 mg, Phenylpropanolamine HCl 75 mg	Guaivent by Pecos	59879-0108	Cold Remedy
PEC108	Tab	Guaifenesin 600 mg, Phenylpropanolamine HCl 75 mg	by Zenith Goldline	00182-2626	Cold Remedy
PEC108	Tab	Guaifenesin 600 mg, Phenylpropanolamine HCl 75 mg	Guaivent by HL Moore	00839-8018	Cold Remedy
PEC108	Tab	Guaifenesin 600 mg, Phenylpropanolamine HCl 75 mg	Guaivent by Lini	58215-0321	Cold Remedy
PEC109	Cap, ER	Hyoscyamine Sulfate 0.375 mg	by Qualitest	00603-4004	Gastrointestinal
PEC110	Tab, Sugar Coated	Atropine Sulfate 0.0582 mg, Hyoscyamine Sulfate 0.3111 mg, Phenobarbital 48.6 mg, Scopolamine Hydrobromide 0.0195 mg	Phenobel by Pecos	59879-0110	Gastrointestinal; C IV
PEC110	Tab, Sugar Coated	Atropine Sulfate 0.0582 mg, Hyoscyamine Sulfate 0.3111 mg, Phenobarbital 48.6 mg, Scopolamine Hydrobromide 0.0195 mg	Antispasmodic by HL Moore	00839-7974	Gastrointestinal; C IV
PEC110	Tab	Atropine Sulfate 0.0582 mg, Hyoscyamine Sulfate 0.311 mg, Phenobarbital 48.6 mg, Scopolamine Hydrobromide 0.0195 mg	Phenobel by Physicians Total Care	54868-3622	Gastrointestinal; C IV
PEC110	Tab, Sugar Coated	Atropine Sulfate 0.0582 mg, Hyoscyamine Sulfate 0.3111 mg, Phenobarbital 48.6 mg, Scopolamine Hydrobromide 0.0195 mg	Donnatal by Lini	58215-0303	Gastrointestinal; C IV
PEC110	Tab, Green, Round	Belladonna Alkaloids, Phenobarbital ER	Donnatal Extentab by Pecos Pharmaceuticals		Gastrointestinal; C IV
PEC111	Cap	Chlorpheniramine Maleate 12 mg, Phenylpropanolamine HCl 75 mg	Ornade Type by Lini	58215-0329	Cold Remedy
PEC111	Cap	Chlorpheniramine Maleate 12 mg, Phenylpropanolamine HCl 75 mg	Ordrine by Pecos	59879-0111	Cold Remedy
PEC111	Cap, Maroon, Opaque	Chlorpheniramine Maleate 12 mg, Phenylpropanolamine HCl 75 mg	Ordrine Extended Release by Circa	71114-4209	Cold Remedy
PEC111	Cap	Chlorpheniramine Maleate 12 mg, Phenylpropanolamine HCl 75 mg	Or Phen Ade by Qualitest	00603-4862	Cold Remedy
PEC111	Cap, Red	Phenylpropanolamine HCl 75 mg, Chlorpheniramine Maleate 12 mg	Ornade by Breckenridge	51991-0150	Cold Remedy
PEC112	Tab, Film Coated	Guaifenesin 600 mg, Pseudoephedrine HCl 120 mg	Entex PSE by Lini	58215-0310	Cold Remedy
PEC112	Tab	Guaifenesin 600 mg, Pseudoephedrine HCl 120 mg	Enomine PSE by Quality Care	60346-0933	Cold Remedy
PEC112	Tab, Film Coated	Guaifenesin 600 mg, Pseudoephedrine HCl 120 mg	Guaifed PSE by Pecos	59879-0112	Cold Remedy
PEC112	Tab, Film Coated	Guaifenesin 600 mg, Pseudoephedrine HCl 120 mg	by United Res	00677-1476	Cold Remedy
PEC114	Tab, Ex Release, PEC 114	Hyoscyamine Sulfate 0.375 mg	by Mutual	53489-0241	Gastrointestinal
PEC114	Tab, Ex Release, PEC 114	Hyoscyamine Sulfate 0.375 mg	by United Res	00677-1611	Gastrointestinal
PEC114	Tab, Ex Release, PEC 114	Hyoscyamine Sulfate 0.375 mg	by Lini	58215-0331	Gastrointestinal
PEC114	Tab, Ex Release, PEC/114	Hyoscyamine Sulfate 0.375 mg	by Sovereign	58716-0679	Gastrointestinal
PEC114	Tab, Ex Release, PEC 114	Hyoscyamine Sulfate 0.375 mg	by Pecos	59879-0114	Gastrointestinal
PEC115	Cap	Trimethobenzamide HCl 250 mg	by Rugby	00536-4727	Antiemetic
PEC115	Cap	Trimethobenzamide HCl 250 mg	by Lini	58215-0320	Antiemetic
PEC115	Cap	Trimethobenzamide HCl 250 mg	by Pecos	59879-0115	Antiemetic
PEC115	Cap	Trimethobenzamide HCl 250 mg	by Qualitest	00603-6256	Antiemetic
PEC115	Cap	Trimethobenzamide HCl 250 mg	by United Res	00677-1383	Antiemetic
PEC116	Tab, Dark Blue	Guaifenesin 600 mg, Pseudoephedrine HCl 60 mg	Decongestant II by Pecos	59879-0116	Cold Remedy
PEC116	Tab, Dark Blue	Guaifenesin 600 mg, Pseudoephedrine HCl 60 mg	by United Res	00677-1487	Cold Remedy
PEC116	Tab, Dark Blue	Guaifenesin 600 mg, Pseudoephedrine HCl 60 mg	Decongestant II by Lini	58215-0318	Cold Remedy
PEC117	Cap, ER, PEC 117	Pheniramine Maleate 16 mg, Phenylpropanolamine HCl 50 mg, Phenyltoloxamine Citrate 16 mg, Pyrilamine Maleate 16 mg	Multihist D by Mutual	53489-0266	Cold Remedy
PEC117	Cap, ER, PEC 117	Pheniramine Maleate 16 mg, Phenylpropanolamine HCl 50 mg, Phenyltoloxamine Citrate 16 mg, Pyrilamine Maleate 16 mg	Poly D by Qualitest	00603-5230	Cold Remedy
PEC117	Cap, ER	Pheniramine Maleate 16 mg, Phenylpropanolamine HCl 50 mg, Phenyltoloxamine Citrate 16 mg, Pyrilamine Maleate 16 mg	Multihistamine D by Lini	58215-0317	Cold Remedy
PEC118	Cap, Burgundy	Vitamin, Iron	Chromagen by Pecos Pharmaceuticals		Vitamin
PEC121	Tab	Belladonna Alkaloids 0.2 mg, Ergotamine Tartrate 0.6 mg, Phenobarbital 40 mg	Bellaphen S by Pecos	59879-0121	Gastrointestinal; C IV
PEC121	Tab	Belladonna Alkaloids 0.2 mg, Ergotamine Tartrate 0.6 mg, Phenobarbital 40 mg	by Mutual	53489-0232	Gastrointestinal; C IV

ID FRONT ◇ BACK	DESCRIPTION FRONT ◇ BACK	INGREDIENT & STRENGTH	BRAND (OR EQUIV.) & FIRM	NDC#	CLASS; SCH.
PEC121	Tab	Belladonna Alkaloids 0.2 mg, Ergotamine Tartrate 0.6 mg, Phenobarbital 40 mg	Phenerbel S by Rugby	00536-4234	Gastrointestinal; C IV
PEC121	Tab, Bluish Green	Belladonna Alkaloids 0.2 mg, Ergotamine Tartrate 0.6 mg, Phenobarbital 40 mg	Phenarbal S by Lini	58215-0304	Gastrointestinal; C IV
PEC122	Cap, Orange & Clear	Pancrelipase 16000 U	Pancrease MT 16 by Pecos Pharmaceuticals		Gastrointestinal
PEC123	Tab, White, Oval	Prenatal Vitamin	Prenate Ultra by Pecos Pharmaceuticals		Vitamin
PEC126	Cap	Amylase 66400 Units, Lipase 20000 Units, Protease 75000 Units	Pancrelipase 20000 by Lini	58215-0332	Gastrointestinal
PEC126	Cap, Delayed Release	Amylase 66400 Units, Lipase 20000 Units, Protease 75000 Units	Pancron 20 by Pecos	59879-0126	Gastrointestinal
PEC126	Cap,	Amylase 66400 Units, Lipase 20000 Units, Protease 75000 Units	Pancrelipase 20000 by United Res	00677-1631	Gastrointestinal
PEC126	Cap	Amylase 66400 Units, Lipase 20000 Units, Protease 75000 Units	Pancrelipase 20000 by Mutual	53489-0303	Gastrointestinal
PEC126	Cap, White & Opaque	Pancron 20	Creon 20 by Pecos Pharmaceuticals		Gastrointestinal
PEC301	Tab, PEC 301	Hyoscyamine Sulfate 0.125 mg	by Mutual	53489-0239	Gastrointestinal
PEC301	Tab, PEC/301	Hyoscyamine Sulfate 0.125 mg	by Sovereign	58716-0651	Gastrointestinal
PEC505	Cap	Amylase 33200 Units, Lipase 10000 Units, Protease 37500 Units	Pancron 10 Pancreatin by Pecos	59879-0505	Gastrointestinal
PEC505	Cap	Amylase 33200 Units, Lipase 10000 Units, Protease 37500 Units	Pancrelipase 10000 by United Res	00677-1576	Gastrointestinal
PEC505	Cap	Amylase 33200 Units, Lipase 10000 Units, Protease 37500 Units	Pancrelipase 10000 by Lini	58215-0322	Gastrointestinal
PEC505	Cap, Brown & Clear	Encron-10	Creon 10 by Pecos Pharmaceuticals		Enzyme
PEC506	Cap, ER	Pheniramine Maleate 8 mg, Phenylpropanolamine HCl 25 mg, Phenyltoloxamine Citrate 8 mg, Pyrilamine Maleate 8 mg	Uni Multihist D Ped by United Res	00677-1575	Cold Remedy
PEC512	Tab	Codeine Phosphate 10 mg, Guaifenesin 300 mg	by Pecos	59879-0512	Cold Remedy; C III
PEC512	Tab, Film Coated	Codeine Phosphate 10 mg, Guaifenesin 300 mg	by Anabolic	00722-6373	Cold Remedy; C III
PENGLOBE	Tab, White/Yellow, Oval, Pen/Globe	Bacampicillin 400 mg	Penglobe by Astra	Canadian	Antibiotic
PENGLOBE	Tab, White/Yellow, Oval, Pen/Globe	Bacampicillin 800 mg	Penglobe by Astra	Canadian	Antibiotic
PENGLOBE	Tab, White/Yellow, Pen/Globe	Bacampicillin HCl 371 mg	Penglobe by Astra	Canadian	Antibiotic
PENGLOBE	Tab, White/Yellow, Pen/Globe	Bacampicillin HCl 742 mg	Penglobe by Astra	Canadian	Antibiotic
PENTASA250	Tab, Gray & Light Brown, Pentasa/250	5-Aminosalicylic Acid 250 mg	Pentasa by Marion Merrell Dow	Canadian	Gastrointestinal
PENTASA250	Tab, Gray/Light Brown, Pentasa/250	5-Aminosalicylic Acid 250 mg	by Hoechst Marion Roussel	Canadian	Gastrointestinal
PENTASA250MG	Cap, Green & Blue	5-Aminosalicylic Acid 250 mg	by Hoechst Marion Roussel	Canadian	Gastrointestinal
PENTASA250MG ◇ 2010	Cap, Blue & Green	Mesalamine 250 mg	Pentasa by Natl Pharmpak	55154-2216	Gastrointestinal
PENTASA500	Tab, Gray/Light Brown, Pentasa/500	5-Aminosalicylic Acid 250 mg	by Hoechst Marion Roussel	Canadian	Gastrointestinal
PENTASA500	Tab, Gray/Light Brown, Pentasa/500	5-Aminosalicylic Acid 250 mg	Pentasa by Marion Merrell Dow	Canadian	Gastrointestinal
PENTOX ◇ 672	Tab, White, Oblong, Film Coated	Pentoxifylline 400 mg	by Blue Ridge	59273-0018	Anticoagulent
PENTOX ◇ 672	Tab, Film Coated	Pentoxifylline 400 mg	by Merrell	00068-0672	Anticoagulent
PENTOX ◇ 672	Tab, White, Oblong, Film Coated	Pentoxifylline 400 mg	by Pharmafab	62542-0781	Anticoagulent
PENTOX ◇ 672	Tab, White, Oblong, Film Coated	Pentoxifylline 400 mg	by Pharmafab	62542-0761	Anticoagulent
PENTOX ◇ 672	Tab, Film Coated	Pentoxifylline 400 mg	by Copley	38245-0672	Anticoagulent
PENTOX672	Tab, White, Oval	Pentoxifylline 400 mg	Pentox by Merrell		Anticoagulent
PENVEE300	Tab, Orange, Round, PEN VEE/300	Penicillin V 300 mg	Pen-Vee by Wyeth-Ayerst	Canadian	Antibiotic
PEPCID ◇ MSD963	Tab, U-Shaped, Film Coated	Famotidine 20 mg	Pepcid by Amerisource	62584-0440	Gastrointestinal
PEPCID ◇ MSD963	Tab, Beige, U-Shaped	Famotidine 20 mg	Pepcid by Merck	00006-0963	Gastrointestinal
PEPCID ◇ MSD963	Tab, Film Coated	Famotidine 20 mg	by Med Pro	53978-0518	Gastrointestinal
PEPCID ◇ MSD963	Tab, Film Coated	Famotidine 20 mg	Pepcid by Nat Pharmpak Serv	55154-5005	Gastrointestinal
PEPCID ◇ MSD963	Tab, U-Shaped, Film Coated, MSD/963	Famotidine 20 mg	Pepcid by Allscripts	54569-2352	Gastrointestinal
PEPCID ◇ MSD963	Tab, U Shaped, Film Coated	Famotidine 20 mg	Pepcid by HJ Harkins Co	52959-0465	Gastrointestinal
PEPCID ◇ MSD963	Tab, U-Shaped, Film Coated	Famotidine 20 mg	Pepcid by PDRX	55289-0162	Gastrointestinal
PEPCID ◇ MSD964	Tab, U-Shaped, Coated	Famotidine 40 mg	Pepcid by Allscripts	54569-0431	Gastrointestinal
PEPCID ◇ MSD964	Tab, Brownish Orange, U-Shaped, Coated	Famotidine 40 mg	Pepcid by PDRX	55289-0146	Gastrointestinal
PEPCIDAC	Tab, Pink, Square, Film Coated	Famotidine 10 mg	Pepcid AC by Johnson & Johnson	Canadian DIN# 02185938	Gastrointestinal

ID FRONT <> BACK	DESCRIPTION FRONT <> BACK	INGREDIENT & STRENGTH	BRAND (OR EQUIV.) & FIRM	NDC#	CLASS; SCH.
PEPCIDAC	Tab, Pink, Round, Chewable	Famotidine 10 mg	by Johnson & Johnson	Canadian DIN# 02185911	Gastrointestinal
PERCOCET <> 10	Tab, Yellow, Oval	Acetaminophen 650 mg; Oxycodone HCl 10 mg	Percocet by Dupont Pharma	00056-0622	Analgesic; C II
PERCOCET <> 10	Tab, Yellow, Oval	Acetaminophen 650 mg; Oxycodone HCl 10 mg	Percocet by West Pharm	52967-0280	Analgesic; C II
PERCOCET <> 10	Tab, Yellow, Oval	Oxycodone HCl 10 mg, Acetaminophen 650 mg	Percocet by Endo	63481-0622	Analgesic; C II
PERCOCET <> 25	Tab, Pink, Oval	Acetaminophen 325 mg, Oxycodone HCl 2.5 mg	Percocet by Allscripts	54569-4695	Analgesic; C II
PERCOCET <> 25	Tab, White, Round, Scored	Clorazepate Dipotassium 15 mg	Percocet by Allscripts	54569-4586	Antianxiety; C IV
PERCOCET <> 25	Tab, Pink, Oval, Percocet <> 2.5	Oxycodone HCl 5 mg, Acetaminophen 325 mg	Percocet by West Pharm	52967-0278	Analgesic; C II
PERCOCET <> 25	Tab, Pink, Oval, Percocet <> 2.5	Oxycodone HCl 2.5 mg, Acetaminophen 325 mg	Percocet by Endo	63481-0627	Analgesic; C II
PERCOCET <> 75	Tab, Peach, Cap Shaped, Percocet <> 7.5	Oxycodone HCl 7.5 mg, Acetaminophen 500 mg	Percocet by Endo	63481-0621	Analgesic; C II
PERCOCET <> 75	Tab, Peach, Oblong	Oxycodone HCl 7.5 mg, Acetaminophen 500 mg	Percocet by West Pharm	52967-0279	Analgesic; C II
PERCOCET <> DUPONT	Tab	Acetaminophen 325 mg, Oxycodone HCl 5 mg	Percocet by Dupont	00590-0127	Analgesic; C II
PERCOCET5	Tab	Alprazolam 1 mg	Percocet by Allscripts	54569-4619	Antianxiety; C IV
PERCOCET5	Tab, White, Round, Percocet/5	Oxycodone 5 mg, Acetaminophen 325 mg	Percocet by Endo		Analgesic; C II
PERCOCET5	Tab, Blue, Round, Scored	Oxycodone HCl 5 mg, Acetaminophen 325 mg	Percocet by Endo	63481-0623	Analgesic; C II
PERCOCET5	Tab, Blue, Round, Scored	Oxycodone HCl 5 mg; Acetaminophen 325 mg	Percocet by Phy Total Care	54868-0510	Analgesic; C II
PERCOCET5	Tab, Blue, Oval, Scored	Sildenafil Citrate 25 mg	Percocet by Allscripts	54569-4568	Impotence Agent
PERCOCETDEMI	Tab, Blue, Percocet-Demi	Oxycodone HCl 2.5 mg, Acetaminophen 325 mg	Percocet by Dupont	Canadian	Analgesic; C II
PERCOCETDUPONT	Tab, White, Percocet/Dupont	Oxycodone HCl 5 mg, Acetaminophen 325 mg	Percocet by Dupont	Canadian	Analgesic; C II
PERCODAN	Tab, Yellow, Round, Scored	Aspirin 325 mg, Oxycodone HCl 4.5 mg, Oxycodone Terephthalate 0.38 mg	Percodan by Endo	63481-0135	Analgesic; C II
PERCODAN	Tab	Aspirin 325 mg, Oxycodone HCl 4.5 mg, Oxycodone Terephthalate 0.38 mg	Percodan by Dupont	00590-0135	Analgesic; C II
PERCODAN	Tab, Yellow, Round	Oxycodone 4.5 mg, Aspirin 325 mg	Percodan by Endo		Analgesic; C II
PERCODANDEMI	Tab, White, Round, Scored	Aspirin 325 mg, Oxycodone HCl 2.25 mg, Oxycodone Terephthalate 0.19 mg	Percodan Demi by Endo Labs	63481-0166	Analgesic; C II
PERCODANDEMI	Tab, White, Round, Percodan/Demi	Oxycodine 2.25 mg, Aspirin 325 mg	Percodan by Endo		Analgesic; C II
PERCODANDEMI	Tab, Pink, Percodan-Demi	Oxycodone 2.5 mg, Aspirin 325 mg	Percodan by DuPont Pharma	Canadian	Analgesic; C II
PERCODANDEMI <> DUPONT	Tab, Percodan-Demi <> Dupont	Aspirin 325 mg, Oxycodone HCl 2.25 mg, Oxycodone Terephthalate 0.19 mg	Percodan Demi by Dupont	00590-0166	Analgesic; C II
PERCODANDUPONT	Tab, Yellow, Percodan/Dupont	Oxycodone 5 mg, Aspirin 325 mg	Percodan by DuPont Pharma	Canadian	Analgesic; C II
PERCODENDUPONT	Tab, Yellow, Percodan/Dupont	Oxycodone HCl 5 mg, Acetaminophen 325 mg	Percodan by Dupont	Canadian	Analgesic; C II
PERGOSEC	Tab, Orange, Round	Acetaminophen 325 mg, Phenyltoloxamine 30 mg	Perogesic by Medtech		Analgesic
PERIACTIN <> MSD62	Tab	Cyproheptadine HCl 4 mg	Periactin by Merck	00006-0062	Antihistamine
PF	Tab, Blue	Phenylpropanolamine 75 mg, Guaifenesin 600 mg	Entex by Purdue Frederick	Canadian	Cold Remedy
PF <> 10	Tab, White, Round	Morphine Sulfate Pentahydrate 10 mg	MS IR by Purdue Frederick	Canadian	Analgesic
PF <> 100MG	Tab, Gray, Round	Morphine Sulfate 100 mg	MS Contin by Purdue Frederick	Canadian	Analgesic
PF <> 15MG	Tab, Green, Round	Morphine Sulfate 15 mg	MS Contin by Purdue Frederick	Canadian	Analgesic
PF <> 20	Tab, White, Oblong	Morphine Sulfate Pentahydrate 20 mg	MS IR by Purdue Frederick	Canadian	Analgesic
PF <> 200	Tab, Red, Oblong	Morphine Sulfate 200 mg	MS Contin by Purdue Frederick	Canadian	Analgesic
PF <> 200	Tab, Green, Oblong, Film Coated	Morphine Sulfate 200 mg	MS Contin by Novartis	00067-0149	Analgesic; C II
PF <> 200	Tab, ER	Morphine Sulfate 200 mg	Ms Contin by Purdue Frederick	00034-0513	Analgesic; C II
PF <> 30	Tab, White, Oblong	Morphine Sulfate Pentahydrate 30 mg	MS IR by Purdue Frederick	Canadian	Analgesic
PF <> 30MG	Tab, Violet, Round	Morphine Sulfate 30 mg	MS Contin by Purdue Frederick	Canadian	Analgesic
PF <> 5	Tab, White, Round	Morphine Sulfate Pentahydrate 5 mg	MS IR by Purdue Frederick	Canadian	Analgesic
PF <> 60MG	Tab, Orange, Round	Morphine Sulfate 60 mg	MS Contin by Purdue Frederick	Canadian	Analgesic
PF <> C275	Tab, Bone	Quinidine Polygalacturonate 275 mg	Cardioquin by Purdue Frederick	00034-5470	Antiarrhythmic
PF <> CC 100	Tab, Yellow, Round	Codeine Monohydrate 53 mg, Codeine Sulfate 62.7 mg	Codeine Contin by Purdue Frederick	Canadian	Analgesic
PF <> CC 150	Tab, Red, Round	Codeine Monohydrate 79.5 mg, Codeine Sulfate 94.1 mg	Codeine Contin by Purdue Frederick	Canadian	Analgesic
PF <> CC 200	Tab, Orange, Oblong	Codeine Monohydrate 106 mg, Codeine Sulfate 125.4 mg	Codeine Contin by Purdue Frederick	Canadian	Analgesic
PF <> CC 50	Tab, Blue, Round	Codeine Monohydrate 26.5 mg, Codeine Sulfate 31.35 mg	Codeine Contin by Purdue Frederick	Canadian	Analgesic
PF <> M 60	Tab, Orange, Round	Morphine Sulfate 60 mg	MS Contin by PF	48692-0010	Analgesic; C II
PF <> M100	Tab, Orange, Round	Morphine Sulfate 100 mg	MS Contin by PF	48692-0011	Analgesic; C II

ID FRONT <> BACK	DESCRIPTION FRONT <> BACK	INGREDIENT & STRENGTH	BRAND (OR EQUIV.) & FIRM	NDC#	CLASS; SCH.
PF <> M15	Tab, Blue, Round	Morphine Sulfate 15 mg	MS Contin by PF	48692-0008	Analgesic; C II
PF <> M30	Tab, Lavender, Round	Morphine Sulfate CR 30 mg	MS Contin by PF	48692-0009	Analgesic; C II
PF <> T 500	Tab, Peach, Oblong	Choline Magnesium Trisalicylate 500 mg	Trilisate by PF	48692-0020	NSAID
PF <> T1000	Tab, Red, Oblong	Choline Magnesium Trisalicylate 1000 mg	Trilisate by PF	48692-0022	NSAID
PF <> T750	Tab, White, Oblong	Choline Magnesium Trisalicylate 750 mg	Trilisate by PF	48692-0021	NSAID
PF <> T750	Tab, Film Coated	Choline Magnesium Trisalicylate 750 mg	Trilisate by Purdue Frederick	00034-0505	NSAID
PF <> T750	Tab, Film Coated	Choline Magnesium Trisalicylate 750 mg	Trilisate 750 by Allscripts	54569-2493	NSAID
PF <> U400	Tab, Ex Release, U 400	Theophylline Anhydrous 400 mg	Uniphyl by Purdue Frederick	00034-7004	Antiasthmatic
PF <> U600	Tab	Theophylline Anhydrous 600 mg	Uniphyl by PF	48692-0004	Antiasthmatic
PF <> U600	Tab, P, Vertical Score, F	Theophylline Anhydrous 600 mg	Uniphyl by Purdue Frederick	00034-7006	Antiasthmatic
PF1	Tab, Ex Release, PF/1	Atropine Sulfate 0.04 mg, Chlorpheniramine Maleate 8 mg, Hyoscyamine Sulfate 0.19 mg, Phenylephrine HCl 25 mg, Phenylpropanolamine HCl 50 mg, Scopolamine Hydrobromide 0.01 mg	by Pharmafab	62542-0001	Cold Remedy
PF1	Tab, PF/1	Atropine Sulfate 0.04 mg, Chlorpheniramine Maleate 8 mg, Hyoscyamine Sulfate 0.19 mg, Phenylephrine HCl 25 mg, Phenylpropanolamine HCl 50 mg, Scopolamine Hydrobromide 0.01 mg	Phenchlor Sha by Rugby	00536-4410	Cold Remedy
PF100	Tab, Gray, Round, PF/100	Morphine Sulfate CR 100 mg	MSCONTIN by Purdue Pharma		Analgesic; C II
PF12MG <> HYDROMORPHCONTIN	Cap, Orange	Hydromorphone 12 mg	Hydromorph Contin by Purdue Frederick	Canadian	Analgesic
PF24MG <> HYDROMORPHCONTIN	Cap, Gray	Hydromorphone 24 mg	Hydromorph Contin by Purdue Frederick	Canadian	Analgesic
PF30MG <> HYDROMORPHCONTIN	Cap, Red	Hydromorphone HCl 30 mg	Hydromorph Contin by Purdue Frederick	Canadian	Analgesic
PF3MG <> HYDROMORPHCONTIN	Cap, Green	Hydromorphone 3 mg	Hydromorph Contin by Purdue Frederick	Canadian	Analgesic
PF5MG <> OIR	Cap, Beige & Orange	Oxycodone HCl 5 mg	Oxynorm by PF Labs	48692-0720	Analgesic; C II
PF5MG <> OIR	Cap, O-IR	Oxycodone HCl 5 mg	Oxy IR by PF	48692-0006	Analgesic; C II
PF6MG <> HYDROMORPHCONTIN	Cap, Pink	Hydromorphone 6 mg	Hydromorph Contin by Purdue Frederick	Canadian	Analgesic
PFE	Tab, Red, Round, Coated, P-Fe	Iron 106 mg	Ferretts by Pharmics	00813-0012	Mineral
PFI440 <> PFI440	Cap, ER, PFI 440	Pheniramine Maleate 16 mg, Phenylpropanolamine HCl 50 mg, Phenyltoloxamine Citrate 16 mg, Pyrilamine Maleate 16 mg	Poly D Sr by Pharmafab	62542-0440	Cold Remedy
PFIZER	Tab, Yellow, Oval	Chlorpropamide 100 mg	Diabinese by Pfizer	Canadian	Antidiabetic
PFIZER	Tab, White, Oval	Chlorpropamide 250 mg	Diabinese by Pfizer	Canadian	Antidiabetic
PFIZER	Tab, Orange, Scored	Prazosin 1 mg	Minipress by Pfizer	Canadian DIN# 00560952	Antihypertensive
PFIZER	Tab, White, Round, Scored	Prazosin 2 mg	Minipress by Pfizer	Canadian DIN# 00560960	Antihypertensive
PFIZER	Tab, White, Diamond, Scored	Prazosin 5 mg	Minipress by Pfizer	Canadian DIN# 00560979	Antihypertensive
PFIZER	Cap, Flesh, Pfizer Logo	Doxepin 10 mg	Sinequan by Pfiser	Canadian DIN# 00024325	Antidepressant
PFIZER	Cap, Blue & Flesh, Pfizer Logo	Doxepin 100 mg	Sinequan by Pfiser	Canadian DIN# 00326925	Antidepressant
PFIZER	Cap, Blue & Pink, Pfizer Logo	Doxepin 25 mg	Sinequan by Pfiser	Canadian DIN# 00024333	Antidepressant

ID FRONT ⬥ BACK	DESCRIPTION FRONT ⬥ BACK	INGREDIENT & STRENGTH	BRAND (OR EQUIV.) & FIRM	NDC#	CLASS; SCH.
PFIZER	Cap, Flesh & Pink, Pfizer Logo	Doxepin 50 mg	Sinequan by Pfiser	Canadian DIN# 00024341	Antidepressant
PFIZER	Cap, Pink & Scarlet, Pfizer Logo	Doxepin 75 mg	Sinequan by Pfixer	Canadian DIN# 00400750	Antidepressant
PFIZER	Cap, Orange, Gelatin, Pfizer Logo	Thiothixene 10 mg	by Navane	Canadian DIN# 00024457	Antipsychotic
PFIZER	Cap, White, Gelatin, Pfizer Logo	Thiothixene 2 mg	by Navane	Canadian DIN# 00024430	Antipsychotic
PFIZER	Cap, Orange & White, Gelatin, Pfizer Logo	Thiothixene 5 mg	by Navane	Canadian DIN# 00024449	Antipsychotic
PFIZER ⬥ 305	Cap	Azithromycin Dihydrate	Zithromax by Quality Care	60346-0670	Antibiotic
PFIZER ⬥ 306	Tab, Red, Film Coated	Azithromycin Dihydrate	Zithromax by Pfizer	00069-3060	Antibiotic
PFIZER ⬥ 306	Tab, Film Coated	Azithromycin Dihydrate	Zithromax by Allscripts	54569-4522	Antibiotic
PFIZER ⬥ 306	Tab, Pink, Cap Shaped, Film Coated, Scored	Azithromycin Dihydrate 250 mg	Zithromax by Pfizer	Canadian DIN# 02212021	Antibiotic
PFIZER ⬥ 306	Tab, Red, Oblong	Azithromycin Dihydrate 250 mg	ZPAK by Phy Total Care	54868-4183	Antibiotic
PFIZER ⬥ 308	Tab, White, Cap Shaped, Film Coated	Azithromycin Dihydrate 600 mg	Zithromax by Pfizer	Canadian DIN# 02231143	Antibiotic
PFIZER ⬥ 378	Tab, Blue, Round	Trovafloxacin 100 mg	Trovan by Pfizer	Canadian DIN# 02239191	Antibiotic
PFIZER ⬥ 378	Tab, Blue, Round, Delayed Release	Trovafloxacin Mesylate	Trovan by Roerig	00049-3780	Antibiotic
PFIZER ⬥ 379	Tab, Blue, Oval	Trovafloxacin 200 mg	Trovan by Pfizer	Canadian DIN# 02239192	Antibiotic
PFIZER ⬥ 379	Tab, Blue, Delayed Release, Modified IV	Trovafloxacin Mesylate	Trovan by Roerig	00049-3790	Antibiotic
PFIZER ⬥ 411	Tab	Glipizide 5 mg	Glucotrol by Allscripts	54569-0206	Antidiabetic
PFIZER ⬥ 412	Tab	Glipizide 5 mg	Glucotrol by Med Pro	53978-0226	Antidiabetic
PFIZER ⬥ 550	Tab, White, Rectangular	Cetirizine HCl 5 mg	Zyrtec by Pfizer	00069-5500	Antihistamine
PFIZER ⬥ 551	Tab, Rounded Rectangle, Film Coated	Cetirizine HCl 10 mg	Zyrtec by PDRX	55289-0108	Antihistamine
PFIZER ⬥ 551	Tab, Rounded Off Rectangular-Shape, Film Coated	Cetirizine HCl 10 mg	Zyrtec by Quality Care	60346-0036	Antihistamine
PFIZER ⬥ 551	Tab, White, Rectangular, Film Coated	Cetirizine HCl 10 mg	Zyrtec by Pfizer	00069-5510	Antihistamine
PFIZER ⬥ 551	Tab, Rectangular, Film Coated	Cetirizine HCl 10 mg	Zyrtec by Caremark	00339-6097	Antihistamine
PFIZER ⬥ 551	Tab, Rounded Rectangular, Film Coated	Cetirizine HCl 10 mg	Zyrtec by Physicians Total Care	54868-3876	Antihistamine
PFIZER ⬥ 551	Tab, Film Coated	Cetirizine HCl 10 mg	Zyrtec by Allscripts	54569-4290	Antihistamine
PFIZER ⬥ DIFLUCAN100	Tab, Pink, Trapezold	Fluconazole 100 mg	Diflucan by Pfizer	Canadian DIN# 00891819	Antifungal
PFIZER ⬥ NRV10	Tab, White, Octagonal	Amiodipine 10 mg	Norvasc by Pfizer	Canadian DIN# 00878936	Antihypertensive
PFIZER ⬥ NRV5	Tab, White, Octagonal, Scored	Amiodipine 5 mg	Norvasc by Pfizer	Canadian DIN# 00878928	Antihypertensive

ID FRONT <> BACK	DESCRIPTION FRONT <> BACK	INGREDIENT & STRENGTH	BRAND (OR EQUIV.) & FIRM	NDC#	CLASS; SCH.
PFIZER <> TVN100	Tab, Blue, Round	Trovafloxacin 100 mg	Trovan by Pfizer	Canadian DIN# 02239191	Antibiotic
PFIZER <> TVN200	Tab, Blue, Oval	Trovafloxacin 200 mg	Trovan by Pfizer	Canadian DIN# 02239192	Antibiotic
PFIZER <> VGR100	Tab, Blue, Diamond Shaped	Sildenafil 100 mg	Viagra by Pfizer	Canadian DIN# 02239768	Impotence Agent
PFIZER <> VGR100	Tab, Blue, Diamond	Sildenafil Citrate 100 mg	Viagra by Southwood Pharms	58016-0371	Impotence Agent
PFIZER <> VGR100	Tab, Blue, Rounded Diamond-Shape, Film Coated	Sildenafil Citrate 100 mg	Viagra by Pfizer	00069-4220	Impotence Agent
PFIZER <> VGR100	Tab, Rounded Diamond-Shape, Film Coated	Sildenafil Citrate 100 mg	Viagra by Allscripts	54569-4570	Impotence Agent
PFIZER <> VGR100	Tab, Blue, Diamond, Film Coated	Sildenafil Citrate 100 mg	Viagra by Compumed	00403-1989	Impotence Agent
PFIZER <> VGR25	Tab, Blue, Diamond Shaped	Sildenafil 25 mg	Viagra by Pfizer	Canadian DIN# 02239766	Impotence Agent
PFIZER <> VGR25	Tab, Blue, Rounded Diamond-Shape, Delayed Release	Sildenafil Citrate	Viagra by Pfizer	00069-4200	Impotence Agent
PFIZER <> VGR25	Tab, Blue, Rounded-Diamond-Shaped, Film Coated	Sildenafil Citrate 25 mg	by Allscripts	54569-4568	Impotence Agent
PFIZER <> VGR50	Tab, Blue, Diamond Shaped	Sildenafil 50 mg	Viagra by Pfizer	Canadian DIN# 02239767	Impotence Agent
PFIZER <> VGR50	Tab, Blue, Rounded Diamond-Shape, Film Coated	Sildenafil Citrate	Viagra by Pfizer	00069-4210	Impotence Agent
PFIZER <> VGR50	Tab, Rounded Diamond-Shape, Film Coated	Sildenafil Citrate	Viagra by Allscripts	54569-4569	Impotence Agent
PFIZER <> VGR50	Tab, Blue, Diamond	Sildenafil Citrate 50 mg	Viagra by Southwood Pharms	58016-0355	Impotence Agent
PFIZER <> VGR50	Tab, Blue, Diamond, Film Coated	Sildenafil Citrate 50 mg	Viagra by Compumed	00403-1947	Impotence Agent
PFIZER 375	Tab, White, Round	Polythiazide 1 mg	Renese by Pfizer	00069-3750	Diuretic
PFIZER 376	Tab, Yellow, Round	Polythiazide 2 mg	Renese by Pfizer	00069-3760	Diuretic
PFIZER 377	Tab, White, Round	Polythiazide 4 mg	Renese by Pfizer	00069-3770	Diuretic
PFIZER 436	Cap, Blue-Green & Blue	Prazosin 5 mg, Polythiazide 0.5 mg	Minizide 5 by Pfizer	00069-4360	Antihypertensive
PFIZER <> DIFLUCAN50	Tab, Pink, Trapezold	Fluconazole 50 mg	Diflucan by Pfizer	Canadian DIN# 00891800	Antifungal
PFIZER092	Cap, Yellow & Green	Oxytetracycline 250 mg, Sulfamethizole 250 mg, Phenazopyridine 50 mg	Urobiotic by Roerig	00049-0920	Antibiotic
PFIZER094	Cap, Blue & White	Doxycycline Hyclate 50 mg	Vibramycin by Pfizer	00069-0940	Antibiotic
PFIZER095 <> VIBRA	Cap, Light Blue	Doxycycline Hyclate	Vibramycin by Pfizer	00069-0950	Antibiotic
PFIZER099 <> VIBRATA3 Tab, Salmon, Round, Film Coated, Pfizer 099 <> Vibra TA3		Doxycycline Hyclate	Vibra by Pfizer	00069-0990	Antibiotic
PFIZER099 <> VIBRATAB Tab, Orange, Film Coated		Doxycycline Hyclate 100 mg	Vibra-Tabs by Pfizer	Canadian DIN# 00578452	Antibiotic
PFIZER128	Tab, Blue, Round	Glipizide Extended Release 2.5 mg	Glucotrol XL by Roerig	00049-1620	Antidiabetic
PFIZER305	Cap	Azithromycin Dihydrate	Zithromax by PDRX	55289-0004	Antibiotic
PFIZER305	Cap	Azithromycin Dihydrate	Zithromax by Pfizer	00069-3050	Antibiotic
PFIZER306	Tab, Film Coated	Azithromycin Dihydrate	Zithromax by DRX	55045-2492	Antibiotic
PFIZER306	Tab, Film Coated	Azithromycin Dihydrate	Zithromax by Quality Care	62682-1022	Antibiotic
PFIZER308	Tab, White	Azithromycin 600 mg	Zithromax by Pfizer	00069-3080	Antibiotic
PFIZER322	Cap, Maroon & Blue	Piroxicam 10 mg	Feldene by Pfizer	00069-3220	NSAID
PFIZER323 <> FELDENE Cap, Maroon		Piroxicam 20 mg	Feldene by Pfizer	00069-3230	NSAID
PFIZER323 <> FELDENE Cap		Piroxicam 20 mg	Feldene by Allscripts	54569-0272	NSAID
PFIZER323 <> FELDENE Cap		Piroxicam 20 mg	by Pharmedix	53002-0389	NSAID
PFIZER323 <> FELDENE Cap		Piroxicam 20 mg	Feldene by Nat Pharmpak Serv	55154-2702	NSAID
PFIZER323 <> FELDENE Cap		Piroxicam 20 mg	Feldene by Quality Care	60346-0241	NSAID
PFIZER323 <> FELDENE Cap		Piroxicam 20 mg	Feldene by Amerisource	62584-0230	NSAID

ID FRONT <> BACK	DESCRIPTION FRONT <> BACK	INGREDIENT & STRENGTH	BRAND (OR EQUIV.) & FIRM	NDC#	CLASS; SCH.
PFIZER393	Tab, Blue, D-Shaped	Chlorpropamide 100 mg	Diabinese by Pfizer	00069-3930	Antidiabetic
PFIZER394	Tap, Blue, D-Shaped	Chlorpropamide 250 mg	Diabinese by Pfizer	00069-3940	Antidiabetic
PFIZER394	Tab	Chlorpropamide 250 mg	Diabinese by Pfizer	00663-3940	Antidiabetic
PFIZER411	Tab, White, Diamond, Scored	Glipizide 5 mg	Glucotrol by Rightpak	65240-0651	Antidiabetic
PFIZER411	Tab, White, Diamond Shaped	Glipizide 5 mg	Glucotrol by Roerig	00049-4110	Antidiabetic
PFIZER411	White, Diamond, Scored, Pfizer over 411	Glipizide 5 mg	Glucotrol by Kaiser	00179-1296	Antidiabetic
PFIZER411	Tab	Glipizide 5 mg	by Pharmedix	53002-0446	Antidiabetic
PFIZER411	Tab	Glipizide 5 mg	Glucotrol by Amerisource	62584-0110	Antidiabetic
PFIZER411	Tab, Pfizer/411	Glipizide 5 mg	Glucotrol by Nat Pharmpak Serv	55154-3213	Antidiabetic
PFIZER412	Tab	Glipizide 10 mg	Glucotrol by Quality Care	60346-0613	Antidiabetic
PFIZER412	Tab, Pfizer/412	Glipizide 10 mg	Glucotrol by Nat Pharmpak Serv	55154-3212	Antidiabetic
PFIZER412	Tab	Glipizide 10 mg	Glucotrol by Amerisource	62584-0120	Antidiabetic
PFIZER412	Tab, White, Diamond, Scored	Glipizide 10 mg	Glucotrol by Rightpak	65240-0652	Antidiabetic
PFIZER412	White, Diamond, Scored	Glipizide 10 mg	Glucotrol by Kaiser	00179-1299	Antidiabetic
PFIZER412	Tab, White, Diamond Shaped	Glipizide 10 mg	Glucotrol by Roerig	00049-4120	Antidiabetic
PFIZER412	Tab, Red Print	Glipizide 10 mg	Glucotrol by Med Pro	53978-0183	Antidiabetic
PFIZER430	Cap, Blue-Green	Prazosin 1 mg, Ploythiazide 0.5 mg	Minizide 1 by Pfizer	00069-4300	Antihypertensive
PFIZER431	Cap, White	Prazosin HCl 1 mg	Minipress by Pfizer	00069-4310	Antihypertensive
PFIZER431 <> MINIPRESS	Cap	Prazosin HCl 1 mg	Minipress by Pfizer	00663-4310	Antihypertensive
PFIZER432	Cap, Blue-Green & Pink	Prazosin 2 mg, Polythiazide 0.5 mg	Minizide 2 by Pfizer	00069-4320	Antihypertensive
PFIZER437	Cap, White & Pink	Prazosin HCl 2 mg	Minipress by Pfizer	00069-4370	Antihypertensive
PFIZER437 <> MINIPRESS	Cap	Prazosin HCl 2 mg	Minipress by Pfizer	00663-4370	Antihypertensive
PFIZER438	Cap, White & Pink	Prazosin HCl 5 mg	Minipress by Pfizer	00069-4380	Antihypertensive
PFIZER441	Tab, Yellow, Oval	Rescinnamine 0.25 mg	Moderil by Pfizer		Antihypertensive
PFIZER442	Tab, Salmon, Oval	Rescinnamine 0.5 mg	Moderil by Pfizer		Antihypertensive
PFIZER446	Tab, Blue, Round	Polythiazide 2 mg, Reserpine 0.25 mg	Renese R by Pfizer		Duiretic; Antihypertensive
PFIZER541 <> VISTARIL	Cap, Dark Green & Light Green	Hydroxyzine Pamoate	Vistaril by Pfizer	00069-5410	Antihistamine
PFIZER542 <> VISTARIL	Cap, Dark Green	Hydroxyzine Pamoate	Vistaril by Pfizer	00069-5420	Antihistamine
PFIZER543	Cap, Dark Green & Pink	Hydroxyzine Pamoate 100 mg	Vistaril by Pfizer	00069-5430	Antihistamine
PFIZER641	Cap, Green & Yellow	Oxamniquine 250 mg	Vansil by Pfizer		Antihelmintic
PFIZERDIFLUCAN150	Cap, White, Gelatin	Fluconazole 150 MG	Diflucan by Pfizer	Canadian DIN# 02141442	Antifungal
PFIZERLITHANE150MG	Cap, Ivory, Gelatin	Lithium Carbonate 150 mg	LITHANE By Pfizer	Canadian DIN# 02013231	Antipsychotic
PFIZERLITHANE300MG	Cap, Green & Ivory, Gelatin	Lithium Carbonate 300 mg	LITHANE By Pfizer	Canadian DIN# 00406775	Antipsychotic
PFIZERZOLOFT100MG	Cap, Orange	Sertraline 100 mg	Zoloft by Pfizer	Canadian DIN# 01962779	Antidepressant
PFIZERZOLOFT25MG	Cap, Yellow	Sertraline 25 mg	Zoloft by Pfizer	Canadian DIN# 02132702	Antidepressant
PFIZERZOLOFT50MG	Cap, White & Yellow	Sertraline 50 mg	Zoloft by Pfizer	Canadian DIN# 01962816	Antidepressant
PFM15	Tab, White, Round	Morphine Sulfate 15 mg	MSIR by PF		Analgesic; C II

ID FRONT <> BACK	DESCRIPTION FRONT <> BACK	INGREDIENT & STRENGTH	BRAND (OR EQUIV.) & FIRM	NDC#	CLASS; SCH.
PFM30	Tab, White, Oblong	Morphine Sulfate 30 mg	MSIR by PF		Analgesic; C II
PFMI15	Tab, White, Round, PF/MI 15	Morphine Sulfate 15 mg	MSIR by Purdue Pharma		Analgesic; C II
PFMI30	Tab, White, Oblong, PF/MI 30	Morphine Sulfate 30 mg	MSIR by Purdue Pharma		Analgesic; C II
PFMSIR15	Cap, White-Blue	Morphine Sulfate 15 mg	MSIR by Purdue Pharma		Analgesic; C II
PFMSIR30	Cap, Gray-Lavender	Morphine Sulfate 30 mg	MSIR by Purdue Pharma		Analgesic; C II
PFMSIR30 <> THISENDUP	Cap	Morphine Sulfate 30 mg	Msir by PF	48692-0001	Analgesic; C II
PFMSIR30 <> THISENDUP	Cap, Lavender	Morphine Sulfate 30 mg	Msir by Purdue Frederick	00034-1026	Analgesic; C II
PFNZ	Tab, Yellow, Round	Thiethylperazine Maleate 10 mg	Norzine by PF		Antiemetic
PFT750	Tab, Film Coated	Choline Magnesium Trisalicylate 750 mg	by Med Pro	53978-1306	NSAID
PFU200	Tab, White, Round	Theophylline 200 mg	T-Phyl by PF		Antiasthmatic
PG <> 402	Tab, White, Rectangular	Etidronate Disodium 200 mg	Didronel by Procter & Gamble	Canadian	Calcium Metabolism
PG <> 402	Tab, White, Pillow shaped, P & G <> 402	Etidronate Disodium 200 mg	Didronel by Procter & Gamble	00149-0405	Calcium Metabolism
PG <> 402	Tab, White, Rectangular	Etidronate Disodium 200 mg	Didronel by Procter & Gamble	Canadian DIN# 01997629	Calcium Metabolism
PG10	Tab, Pink, Round, Chewable	Bismuth Subsalicylate 262 mg	Helidac Therapy Kit by Procter & Gamble	00149-0495	Gastrointestinal
PG11	Tab, White, Round, Chew	Metronidazole 250 mg	Helidac Therapy Kit by Procter & Gamble	00149-0495	Antibiotic
PG12	Cap, Pink	Tetracycline 500 mg	Sumycin by Procter & Gamble		Antibiotic
PG12	Cap, Pale Orange & White	Tetracycline HCl 500 mg	Helidac Therapy Kit by Procter & Gamble	00149-0495	Antibiotic
PG402	Tab, White, Rectangular, P & G 402	Etidronate Disodium 200 mg	Didronel by Norwich		Calcium Metabolism
PHARMACIA <> EMCYT140MG	Cap	Estramustine Phosphate Sodium	Emcyt by Pharmacia & Upjohn	00013-0132	Antineoplastic
PHARMACIA MYCOBUTIN	Cap, Brownish Red, Opaque, Gelatin, Pharmacia/ Mycobutin w/ White Ink	Rifabutin 150 mg	by Pharmacia	Canadian DIN# 02063786	Antibiotic
PHARMICS	Tab, Yellow, Oblong, Coated	Ascorbic Acid 300 mg, Lemon Bioflavonoid Complex 200 mg, Riboflavin 10 mg, Thiamine HCl 25 mg, Calcium Pantothenate 10 mg, Niacinamide 50 mg	B-Scorbic by Pharmics	00813-0070	Vitamin
PHARMICS	Tab, Yellow, Oblong	Ascorbic Acid 300 mg, Lemon Bioflavonoid Complex 200 mg, Riboflavin 10 mg, Thiamine HCl 25 mg, Calcium Pantothenate 10 mg, Niacinamide 50 mg	B-Scorbic by Pharmics	00831-0070	Vitamin
PHARMICS	Tab, Pink, Oblong, Coated	Ascorbic Acid 120 mg, Calcium Carbonate, Precipitated, Calcium Pantothenate, Cupric Oxide, Cyanocobalamin 12 mcg, Ergocalciferol 400 Units, Ferrous Fumarate, Folic Acid 1 mg, Magnesium 100 mg, Niacinamide 20 mg, Potassium Iodide, Pyridoxine HCl 12 mg, Riboflavin 3.4 mg, Thiamine Mononitrate, Vitamin A Acetate, Vitamin E 30 Units, Zinc Oxide	Par F by Pharmics	00813-0076	Vitamin
PHARMICS	Tab, Off-White, Oblong, Chewable	Ascorbic Acid 60 mg, Cyanocobalamin 4.5 mcg, Folic Acid 0.3 mg, Niacinamide 13.5 mg, Pyridoxine HCl 1.05 mg, Riboflavin 1.2 mg, Sodium Fluoride 2.21 mg, Thiamine Mononitrate 1.05 mg, Vitamin A Acetate 2500 Units, Vitamin D 400 Units, Vitamin E Acetate 15 Units	Soluvite C T by Pharmics	00813-0078	Vitamin
PHARMICS	Tab, Clear, Oblong	Ascorbic Acid 90 mg, Calcium Carbonate 200 mg, Copper 2 mg, Cyanocobalamin 12 mcg, Ergocalciferol 400 Units, Ferrous Fumarate 200 mg, Folic Acid 1 mg, Iodine 150 mcg, Magnesium Oxide 100 mg, Niacinamide 20 mg, Pyridoxine HCl 4 mg, Riboflavin 3 mg, Sodium Fluoride 1.1 mg, Thiamine HCl 3 mg, Vitamin A Acetate 5000 Units, Vitamin E Acetate 400 Units, Zinc 15 mg	O Cal F A by Pharmics	00813-0038	Vitamin
PHARMICS <> 0025	Tab, 00 Over 25	Acetaminophen 500 mg, Hydrocodone Bitartrate 5 mg	by Quality Care	60346-0442	Analgesic; C III
PHI	Tab, Yellow, Round, Scored	Acetaminophen 375 mg, Caffeine 15 mg, Codeine Phosphate 15 mg	by Frosst	Canadian	Analgesic
PHI292	Tab, Peach, Round, Scored, PHI over 292	Acetaminophen 375 mg, Caffeine 15 mg, Codeine Phosphate 30 mg	by Frosst	Canadian	Analgesic
PHILLIPSPHILLIPS	Tab, White, Round, Phillips/Phillips	Magnesium Hydroxide 311 mg	Phillips by Bayer	Canadian	Mineral

ID FRONT <> BACK	DESCRIPTION FRONT <> BACK	INGREDIENT & STRENGTH	BRAND (OR EQUIV.) & FIRM	NDC#	CLASS; SCH.
PHOSCHOL	Cap, Amber	Soybean Lecithin	Phoschol by American Lecithin		Supplement
PHPH	Tab, Green, Round	pHos-pHaid 250 mg	pHos-pHaid by Guardian		Urinary
PHPH	Tab, Blue, Round	pHos-pHaid 500 mg	pHos-pHaid by Guardian		Urinary
PHPH	Tab, Orange, Round	pHos-pHaid 500 mg	pHos-pHaid by Guardian		Urinary
PI	Tab, Red, Round, Scored	Ferrous Fumarate 150 mg; Ascorbic Acid 500 mg; Cyanocobalamin 60 mcg; Intrinsic Factor, Concentrate 75 mg; Folic Acid 1 mg; Vitamin E 30 unt; Docusate Sodium 50 mg	Genhemat by Pharmakon	55422-0220	Mineral
PI <> M	Tab, Film Coated	Prochlorperazine Maleate	by Mylan	00378-5105	Antiemetic
PLACIDYL	Cap, Red	Ethchlorvynol 500 mg	Placidyl by Abbott	00074-6685	Hypnotic; C IV
PLACIDYLI	Cap, Green	Ethchlorvynol 750 mg	Placidyl by Abbott	00074-6630	Hypnotic; C IV
PLAIN <> GG 60	Tab, Scored	Allopurinol 300 mg	by Golden State	60429-0014	Antigout
PLAIN <> GG242	Tab	Methyclothiazide 5 mg	by Geneva	00781-1810	Diuretic
PLAIN <> GG244	Tab	Methyclothiazide 2.5 mg	by Geneva	00781-1803	Diuretic
PLAIN <> GG250	Tab, ER	Quinidine Gluconate 324 mg	by Golden State	60429-0167	Antiarrhythmic
PLAIN <> GG288	Tab, Coated	Cyclobenzaprine HCl 10 mg	by Golden State	60429-0052	Muscle Relaxant
PLAIN <> NORVASC5	Tab, Octagonal	Amlodipine Besylate	Norvasc by PDRX	55289-0103	Antihypertensive
PLAQUENIL	Tab, White, Peanut Shaped	Hydroxychloroquine Sulfate 200 mg	Plaquenil by Sanofi	Canadian	Antimalarial
PLAQUENIL	Tab, Dog Bone-Shaped	Hydroxychloroquine Sulfate 200 mg	Plaquenil Sulfate by Pharmedix	53002-0485	Antimalarial
PLENDIL <> 450	Tab, Sugar Coated	Felodipine 2.5 mg	Plendil by Merck	00006-0450	Antihypertensive
PLENDIL <> 450	Tab, Sugar Coated	Felodipine 2.5 mg	Plendil by Murfreesboro	51129-1248	Antihypertensive
PLENDIL <> 451	Tab, Red-Brown, Ex Release	Felodipine 5 mg	Plendil by Promex Med	62301-0029	Antihypertensive
PLENDIL <> 451	Tab, Red, Round	Felodipine 5 mg	by Va Cmop	65243-0028	Antihypertensive
PLENDIL <> 452	Tab, Red, Round, Film Coated	Felodipine 10 mg	Plendil by ICN	00187-4051	Antihypertensive
PLENDIL <> 452	Tab	Felodipine 10 mg	Plendil by Allscripts	54569-3719	Antihypertensive
PLENDIL <> 452	Tab	Felodipine 10 mg	Plendil ER by Physicians Total Care	54868-2168	Antihypertensive
PLENDIL451	Tab	Felodipine 5 mg	Plendil by Allscripts	54569-3718	Antihypertensive
PLETAL 100	Tab, White, Round	Cilostazol 100 mg	PLETAL by Otsuka	59148-0002	Antiplatelet
PLETAL 50	Tab, White, Triangular	Cilostazol 50 mg	PLETAL by Otsuka	59148-0003	Antiplatelet
PLETAL100	Tab, White, Round	Cilostazol 100 mg	Pletal by Compumed	00403-0803	Antiplatelet
PLETAL50	Tab, White, Triangular	Cilostazol 50 mg	Pletal by Compumed	00403-0994	Antiplatelet
PM200 <> PM200	Cap, Ex Release	Chlorpheniramine Maleate 8 mg, Pseudoephedrine HCl 120 mg	by Pharma	62441-0200	Cold Remedy
PM200 <> PM200	Cap, Black Print	Chlorpheniramine Maleate 8 mg, Pseudoephedrine HCl 120 mg	by Kaiser	00179-0376	Cold Remedy
PM200 <> PM200	Cap, Clear	Chlorpheniramine Maleate 8 mg, Pseudoephedrine HCl 120 mg	CPM PSEH 07 by Compumed	00403-0010	Cold Remedy
PM200 <> PM200	Cap, Clear	Chlorpheniramine Maleate 8 mg; Pseudoephedrine HCl 120 mg	Pseudofed CPM by Kaiser Fdn Hlth	62224-0448	Cold Remedy
PMS	Tab, White, Round	Acetaminophen 325 mg	by Pharmascience	Canadian	Antipyretic
PMS	Tab, White, Round	Acetaminophen 500 mg	by Pharmascience	Canadian	Antipyretic
PMS	Tab, Pink	Amitriptylline HCl 2 mg, Perphenazine 25 mg	by Pharmascience	Canadian	Antipsychotic
PMS	Tab, Red	Amitriptylline HCl 4 mg, Perphenazine 25 mg	by Pharmascience	Canadian	Antipsychotic
PMS	Tab, Dark Pink	Fluphenazine HCl 2 mg	by Pharmascience	Canadian	Antipsychotic
PMS	Tab, White	Fluphenazine HCl 5 mg	by Pharmascience	Canadian	Antipsychotic
PMS	Tab, Pink	Fluphenazine HCl 1 mg	by Pharmascience	Canadian	Antipsychotic
PMS	Tab, Yellow, Round	Flutamide 250 mg	by Pharmascience	Canadian	Antiandrogen
PMS	Tab, White, Round	Isoniazid 100 mg	by Pharmascience	Canadian	Antimycobacterial
PMS	Tab, White, Round	Isoniazid 300 mg	by Pharmascience	Canadian	Antimycobacterial
PMS	Tab, White, Round	Isoniazid 50 mg	by Pharmascience	Canadian	Antimycobacterial
PMS	Tab, White	Magnesium Gluconate 500 mg	by Pharmascience	Canadian	Mineral
PMS	Tab, White, Round	Metoclopramide 10 mg	by Pharmascience	Canadian	Gastrointestinal
PMS	Tab, White, Round	Metoclopramide 5 mg	by Pharmascience	Canadian	Gastrointestinal
PMS	Tab, Orange, Round, Scored	Procyclidine HCl 2.5 mg	by Pharmascience	Canadian	Antiemetic
PMS	Tab, Round, Scored	Propranolol HCl 10 mg	by Pharmascience	Canadian	Antihypertensive
PMS	Tab, White, Round	Pyrazinamide 500 mg	by Pharmascience	Canadian	Antibiotic
PMS	Tab, Yellow, Round, Scored	Salicylazosulfapyridine 500 mg	by Pharmascience	Canadian	Gastrointestinal

ID FRONT <> BACK	DESCRIPTION FRONT <> BACK	INGREDIENT & STRENGTH	BRAND (OR EQUIV.) & FIRM	NDC#	CLASS; SCH.
PMS	Tab, White, Round, Scored	Tiaprofenic Acid 200 mg	by Pharmascience	Canadian	NSAID
PMS	Tab, White, Round	Zinc Sulfate 220 mg	by Pharmascience	Canadian	Mineral Supplement
PMS10	Tab, Peach, Round, PMS/10	Bethanechol Chloride 10 mg	by Pharmascience	Canadian	Urinary Tract
PMS10	Tab, Blue, Round, PMS-10	Desipramine HCl 10 mg	by Pharmascience	Canadian	Antidepressant
PMS10	Tab, Peach, Round, PMS/10	Prochlorperazine 10 mg	by Pharmascience	Canadian	Antiemetic
PMS100	Cap, Orange	Docusate Sodium 100 mg	by Pharmascience	Canadian	Laxative
PMS100	Tab, Yellow, Round, Logo pms/100	Ketoprofen 100 mg	by Pharmascience	Canadian	NSAID
PMS10110	Tab, Blue/Green, Round, pms/10 110	Methylphenidate HCl 10 mg	by Pharmascience	Canadian	Stimulant
PMS10BACLOFEN	Tab, White, Oval, pms/10/Baclofen	Baclofen 10 mg	by Pharmascience	Canadian	Muscle Relaxant
PMS150LITH	Cap, Orange, pms/150/Lith	Lithium Carbonate 150 mg	by Pharmascience	Canadian	Antipsychotic
PMS20BACLOFEN	Tab, White, Oblong, pms/20/Baclofen	Baclofen 20 mg	by Pharmascience	Canadian	Muscle Relaxant
PMS240	Cap, Red	Docusate Calcium 240 mg	by Pharmascience	Canadian	Laxative
PMS25	Tab, White, Round, PMS/25	Bethanechol Chloride 25 mg	by Pharmascience	Canadian	Urinary Tract
PMS25	Tab, Yellow, Round, pms-25	Desipramine HCl 25 mg	by Pharmascience	Canadian	Antidepressant
PMS300LITH	Cap, Flesh, pms/300/Lith	Lithium Carbonate 300 mg	by Pharmascience	Canadian	Antipsychotic
PMS403	Tab, Pink, PMS/403	Sennosides 12 mg	by Pharmascience	Canadian	Gastrointestinal
PMS411	Tab, Gray, PMS/411	Sennosides 8.6 mg	by Pharmascience	Canadian	Gastrointestinal
PMS488	Tab, Yellow, Oval, PMS/488	Salicylazosulfapyridine 500 mg	by Pharmascience	Canadian	Gastrointestinal
PMS5	Tab, Peach, Round, PMS/5	Prochlorperazine 5 mg	by Pharmascience	Canadian	Antiemetic
PMS50	Tab, Beige, Round, PMS/50	Bethanechol Chloride 50 mg	by Pharmascience	Canadian	Urinary Tract
PMS50	Tab, Green, Round, pms-50	Desipramine HCl 50 mg	by Pharmascience	Canadian	Antidepressant
PMS50	Tab, Logo pms/50	Ketoprofen 50 mg	by Pharmascience	Canadian	NSAID
PMS600LITH	Cap, Blue, pms/600/Lith	Lithium Carbonate 600 mg	by Pharmascience	Canadian	Antipsychotic
PMS75	Tab, Orange, Round, pms-75	Desipramine HCl 75 mg	by Pharmascience	Canadian	Antidepressant
PMSB5	Tab, White, Round, pms/B/5	Buspirone 5 mg	by Pharmascience	Canadian	Antianxiety
PMSF250	Cap, Orange	Valproic Acid 250 mg	by Pharmascience	Canadian	Anticonvulsant
PMSTRAZODONE125	Tab, Pink, Round, pms/Trazodone/12.5	Trazodone HCl 12.5 mg	by Pharmascience	Canadian	Antidepressant
PMSTRAZODONE25	Tab, Blue, Round, pms/Trazodone/25	Trazodone HCl 25 mg	by Pharmascience	Canadian	Antidepressant
PMSYOHIMBINE	Tab, Pink, Round, PMS/Yohimbine	Yohimbine HCl 6 mg	by Pharmascience	Canadian	Impotence Agent
PN <> CIBA	Tab, Pale Yellow, Round, Scored	Methylphenidate HCl 20 mg	Ritalin by Novartis	Canadian DIN# 00005614	Stimulant
PN <> SANOFI	Tab, Coated	Ascorbic Acid 120 mg, Calcium Citrate 200 mg, Cholecalciferol 400 Units, Cupric Oxide 2 mg, Cyanocobalamin 12 mcg, Docusate Sodium 50 mg, Folic Acid 1 mg, Iron Pentacarbonyl 90 mg, Niacinamide 20 mg, Potassium Iodide 150 mcg, Pyridoxine HCl 20 mg, Riboflavin 3.4 mg, Thiamine HCl 3 mg, Vitamin A 2700 Units, Vitamin E 30 Units, Zinc Oxide 25 mg	Prenate Ultra by Sanofi	00024-1730	Vitamin
PN90 <> BOCK	Tab, PN/90	Ascorbic Acid 120 mg, Calcium 250 mg, Cholecalciferol 10 mcg, Copper 2 mg, Cyanocobalamin 12 mcg, Docusate Sodium 50 mg, Folic Acid 1 mg, Iodine 150 mcg, Iron 90 mg, Niacinamide 20 mg, Pyridoxine HCl 20 mg, Riboflavin 3.4 mg, Thiamine Mononitrate 3 mg, Vitamin A Acetate 1.2 mg, Vitamin E Acetate 30 mg, Zinc 25 mg	Prenate 90 by Physicians Total Care	54868-2703	Vitamin
PNAXEN250S	Tab, Yellow, Round	Naproxen 250 mg	by AltiMed	Canadian	NSAID
PNAXEN375S	Tab, Pink, Oval	Naproxen 375 mg	by AltiMed	Canadian	NSAID
PNAXEN500S	Tab, Yellow, Oblong	Naproxen 500 mg	by AltiMed	Canadian	NSAID
POLY0101	Tab, Poly over 0101, Ex Release	Chlorpheniramine Maleate 4 mg, Phenylephrine HCl 10 mg, Phenylpropanolamine HCl 50 mg, Pyrilamine Maleate 25 mg	Poly Hist Forte by Pharmafab	62542-0903	Cold Remedy; C III
POLY500 <> FLEXTRADS	Tab, Orange & Red, Oblong, Scored, Poly/500<>Flextra-DS	Acetaminophen	Flextra DS by ABG	60999-0901	Antipyretic
POLYVENT <> 675	Tab, 6 Over 75, Ex Release	Guaifenesin 600 mg, Phenylpropanolamine HCl 75 mg	Poly Vent by Pharmafab	62542-0780	Cold Remedy
POLYVENT <> 675	Tab, Poly-Vent <> 6 over 75	Guaifenesin 600 mg, Phenylpropanolamine HCl 75 mg	Poly Vent by Poly	50991-0408	Cold Remedy
PONSTEL <> PD540	Cap, Yellow with Blue Band, <> P-D 540, Cap	Mefenamic Acid 250 mg	Ponstel by Parke Davis	00071-0540	NSAID

ID FRONT <> BACK	DESCRIPTION FRONT <> BACK	INGREDIENT & STRENGTH	BRAND (OR EQUIV.) & FIRM	NDC#	CLASS; SCH.
PP	Tab, White, P/P	Proguanil 100 mg	Paludrine by Wyeth-Ayerst	Canadian	Antimalarial
PP040	Tab, White, Round, PP-040	Furosemide 40 mg	Lasix by Eon		Diuretic
PP052	Tab	Diazepam 5 mg	by Pharmedix	53002-0334	Antianxiety; C IV
PP071	Tab, Blue, Round, PP-071	Chlorthalidone 50 mg	Hygroton by Eon		Diuretic
PP073	Tab, White, Round, PP/073	Chlorthalidone 100 mg	Hygroton by Eon		Diuretic
PP081	Tab, Yellow, Round, PP-081	Folic Acid 1 mg	Folvite by Eon		Vitamin
PP111	Tab, White, Round, PP-111	Sulfamethoxazole 400 mg, Trimethoprim 80 mg	Bactrim by Eon		Antibiotic
PP112	Tab, Eon Logo	Sulfamethoxazole 800 mg, Trimethoprim 160 mg	Trimeth Sulfa DS by Pharmedix	53002-0210	Antibiotic
PP12	Tab, Red, Round, PP-12	Ferrous Sulfate 325 mg	Feosol by Eon		Mineral
PP1217	Cap, Green & Yellow, PP-1217	Nitroglycerin 9 mg	Nitrobid by Eon		Vasodilator
PP1235	Cap, ER, Eon Logo	Nitroglycerin 6.5 mg	by United Res	00677-0486	Vasodilator
PP125	Tab, White, Oval, PP-125	Methylprednisolone 4 mg	Medrol by Eon		Steroid
PP13	Tab, Green, Round, PP-13	Ferrous Sulfate 325 mg	Feosol by Eon		Mineral
PP1303	Cap, Clear	Quinine Sulfate 325 mg	by Eon		Antimalarial
PP1304	Cap	Chlorpheniramine Maleate 8 mg, Pseudoephedrine HCl 120 mg	Pseudo Chlor by Geneva	00781-2915	Cold Remedy
PP134	Tab, White, Round, PP-134	Reserpine 0.25 mg	Serpasil by Eon		Antihypertensive
PP14	Tab, Yellow, Round	Chlorpheniramine 4 mg	Chlor-Trimeton by Eon		Antihistamine
PP16	Tab, White, Round, PP-16	Triprolidine 2.5 mg, Pseudoephedrine 60 mg	Actifed by Eon		Cold Remedy
PP17	Tab, White, Round, PP-17	Baclofen 10 mg	Lioresal by Eon		Muscle Relaxant
PP18	Tab, White, Round, PP-18	Baclofen 20 mg	Lioresal by Eon		Muscle Relaxant
PP2007	Cap, Brown & Clear	Papaverine HCl 150 mg	Pavabid by Pioneer		Vasodilator
PP212	Tab, Blue, Round, PP-212	Butabarbital Sodium 30 mg	Butisol by Eon		Sedative; C III
PP220	Tab, Blue, Round, PP-220	Urinary Antiseptic #2	Atrosept by Eon		Urinary Tract
PP226	Tab, Green, Round, PP-226	Chlorzoxazone 250 mg, Acetaminophen 300 mg	Parafon Forte by Eon		Muscle Relaxant
PP250	Cap, Blue & Yellow, PP-250	Mefenamic Acid 250 mg	Ponstel by Eon		NSAID
PP256	Cap, Blue & Clear, PP-256	Chlorpheniramine Maleate 12 mg, Phenylpropanolamine HCl 75 mg	Ordrine by Eon		Cold Remedy
PP257	Tab, Yellow, Oblong, PP-257	Prenatal Vitamin	by Eon		Vitamin
PP259	Tab, Yellow, Oblong	Prenatal Vitamin	Stuartnatal 1+1 by Eon		Vitamin
PP29	Tab, White, Round, PP-29	Desipramine HCl 10 mg	Norpramine by Eon		Antidepressant
PP29	Tab, Purepac Logo	Propranolol HCl 20 mg	by Pharmedix	53002-0360	Antihypertensive
PP3	Tab, White, Round, PP-3	Dipyridamole 25 mg	Persantine by Eon		Antiplatelet
PP3001	Tab, White with Red Specks, Round	Phenylprop. 40 mg, phenyleph. 10 mg, phenyltolox. 15 mg, chlorphenir. 5 mg	Naldecon by Pioneer		Cold Remedy
PP3008	Tab, Blue, Round	Brompheniramine 12 mg, Phenylephrine 15 mg, Phenylpropanolamine 15 mg	Dimetapp by Pioneer		Cold Remedy
PP333	Tab, White/Green, Round, PP-333	Meprobamate 200 mg, Aspirin 325 mg	Equagesic by Eon		Sedative/Hypnotic; C IV
PP345	Cap, Clear & White	Phenylpropanolamine HCl 75 mg, Caramiphen Edisylate 40 mg	Tuss-Omade by Eon		Cold Remedy
PP3602	Tab, White, Round, PP-360 & 2	Acetaminophen 300 mg, Codeine 15 mg	Tylenol #2 by Eon		Analgesic; C III
PP3653	Tab, White, Round, PP-365 & 3	Acetaminophen 300 mg, Codeine 30 mg	Tylenol #3 by Eon		Analgesic; C III
PP3704	Tab, White, Round, PP-370 & 4	Acetaminophen 300 mg, Codeine 60 mg	Tylenol #4 by Eon		Analgesic; C III
PP4001	Cap, Blue	Cyclandelate 200 mg	Cyclospasmol by Pioneer		Vasodilator
PP4002	Cap, Blue & Red	Cyclandelate 400 mg	Cyclospasmol by Pioneer		Vasodilator
PP4005	Cap, Green	Indomethacin 25 mg	Indocin by Pioneer		NSAID
PP4006	Cap, Green	Indomethacin 50 mg	Indocin by Pioneer		NSAID
PP4008	Cap, Pink	Diphenhydramine 50 mg	Benadryl by Pioneer		Antihistamine
PP4009	Cap, Green	Chlordiazepoxide 5 mg, Clidinium Bromide 2.5 mg	Librax by Pioneer		Gastrointestinal; C IV
PP4010	Cap, Green & Yellow	Chlordiazepoxide HCl 5 mg	Librium by Pioneer		Antianxiety; C IV
PP4011	Cap, Black & Green	Chlordiazepoxide HCl 10 mg	Librium by Pioneer		Antianxiety; C IV
PP4012	Cap, Green & White	Chlordiazepoxide HCl 25 mg	Librium by Pioneer		Antianxiety; C IV
PP4013	Cap, Clear & Pink	Diphenhydramine 25 mg	Benadryl by Pioneer		Antihistamine
PP4017	Cap, Blue	Decyclomine HCl 10 mg	Bentyl by Pioneer		Gastrointestinal
PP497	Tab, White, Round, PP-497	Diphenoxylate HCl 2.5 mg, Atropine Sulfate 0.025 mg	Lomotil by Eon		Antidiarrheal; C V
PP50	Tab, PP/50	Hydrochlorothiazide 50 mg	Aquazide H by JMI Canton	00252-9783	Diuretic
PP50	Tab, PP/50	Hydrochlorothiazide 50 mg	Aquazide by Jones	52604-9783	Diuretic

ID FRONT <> BACK	DESCRIPTION FRONT <> BACK	INGREDIENT & STRENGTH	BRAND (OR EQUIV.) & FIRM	NDC#	CLASS; SCH.
PP5000	Cap	Phentermine HCl 30 mg	by Geneva	00781-2415	Anorexiant; C IV
PP5023	Tab, Yellow, Oblong	Vitamin Combination	Strovite by Pioneer		Vitamin
PP511	Tab, White, Round, PP-511	Quinidine Sulfate 200 mg	by Eon		Antiarrhythmic
PP512	Tab, White, Round, PP-512	Quinidine Sulfate 300 mg	Quinidine Sulfate by Eon		Antiarrhythmic
PP5156	Cap, Brown & Clear, PP-5156	Papaverine HCl 150 mg	Pavabid by Eon		Vasodilator
PP5174	Cap, ER, Eon Logo	Nitroglycerin 2.5 mg	by United Res	00677-0485	Vasodilator
PP5254	Cap, Brown & Clear, PP-5254	Phendimetrazine Tartrate TR 105 mg	by Eon		Anorexiant; C III
PP53	Tab, Pink, Oblong, PP-53	Prenatal Vitamin, Folic Acid	by Eon		Vitamin
PP53010	Tab, White, Round, PP-530 & 10	Isoxsuprine HCl 10 mg	Vasodilan by Eon		Vasodilator
PP53120	Tab, White, Round, PP-31 & 20	Isoxsuprine HCl 20 mg	Vasodilan by Eon		Vasodilator
PP535	Tab, White, Round, PP-535	Tolbutamide 500 mg	Orinase by Eon		Antidiabetic
PP5380	Cap, Red & Maroon	Multivitamin, Mineral	Trinsicon by Eon		Vitamin
PP54	Tab, Yellow, Round, PP-54	Triamterene 75 mg, Hydrochlorothiazide 50 mg	Maxzide by Eon		Diuretic
PP551	Tab, White, Round, PP-551	Metronidazole 250 mg	Flagyl by Eon		Antibiotic
PP5511	Cap, Clear & Green, PP-5511	Chlorpheniramine Maleate SR 8 mg	Teldrin by Eon		Antihistamine
PP5512	Cap, Clear & Green, PP-5512	Chlorpheniramine Maleate SR 12 mg	Teldrin by Eon		Antihistamine
PP555	Tab, Eon Logo	Metronidazole 500 mg	by Pharmedix	53002-0247	Antibiotic
PP5730	Cap, Blue & Clear, PP-5730	Phendimetrazine Tartrate 35 mg	by Eon		Anorexiant; C III
PP5740	Cap, Orange/Clear, PP-5740	Phendimetrazine Tartrate 35 mg	by Eon		Anorexiant; C III
PP58	Tab, Yellow, Round, PP-58	Hydroxyzine HCl 50 mg	Atarax by Eon		Antihistamine
PP585	Tab, White, Round	Methocarbamol 500 mg	Robaxin by Eon		Muscle Relaxant
PP587	Tab, White, Oblong	Methocarbamol 750 mg	Robaxin by Eon		Muscle Relaxant
PP59	Tab, Green, Round, PP-59	Hydroxyzine HCl 25 mg	Atarax by Eon		Antihistamine
PP60	Tab, Orange, Round, PP-60	Hydroxyzine HCl 10 mg	Atarax by Eon		Antihistamine
PP6001	Tab, Blue, Round	Ephedrine 25 mg, Hydroxyzine 10 mg, Theophylline 130 mg	Marax by Pioneer		Antiasthmatic
PP6004	Tab, Yellow, Round	Folic Acid 1 mg	Folvite by Pioneer		Vitamin
PP6007	Tab, White, Round	Diazepam 2 mg	Valium by Pioneer		Antianxiety; C IV
PP6008	Tab, White, Round	Diazepam 5 mg	Valium by Pioneer		Antianxiety; C IV
PP6009	Tab, Blue, Round	Diazepam 10 mg	Valium by Pioneer		Antianxiety; C IV
PP6012	Tab, Peach, Round	Chlorzoxazone 250 mg	Parafon by Pioneer		Muscle Relaxant
PP6013	Tab, Blue, Round	Decyclomine HCl 20 mg	Bentyl by Pioneer		Gastrointestinal
PP6015	Tab, White, Round	Cyproheptadine HCl 4 mg	Periactin by Pioneer		Antihistamine
PP6017	Tab, Green, Round	Chlorzoxazone 250 mg, Acetaminophen 300 mg	Parafon Forte by Pioneer		Muscle Relaxant
PP6018	Tab, White, Round	Carisoprodol 350 mg	Soma by Pioneer		Muscle Relaxant
PP6026	Tab, Yellow, Round	Chlorpheniramine Maleate 4 mg	Chlor-trimeton by Pioneer		Antihistamine
PP6031	Tab, Orange, Round	Brompheniramine Maleate 4 mg	Dimetane by Pioneer		Antihistamine
PP6036	Tab, White, Round	Methocarbamol 500 mg	Robaxin by Pioneer		Muscle Relaxant
PP6038	Tab, White, Oblong	Methocarbamol 750 mg	Robaxin by Pioneer		Muscle Relaxant
PP6048	Tab, Green, Oblong	Chlorzoxazone 500 mg	Parafon DSC by Pioneer		Muscle Relaxant
PP605	Cap, Green & Yellow, PP-605	Chlordiazepoxide HCl 5 mg	Librium by Eon		Antianxiety; C IV
PP6062	Tab, Peach, Round	Chlorthalidone 25 mg	Hygroton by Pioneer		Diuretic
PP6063	Tab, Blue, Round	Chlorthalidone 50 mg	Hygroton by Pioneer		Diuretic
PP610	Cap, Black & Green, PP-610	Chlordiazepoxide HCl 10 mg	Librium by Eon		Antianxiety; C IV
PP613	Cap, Green & Green, PP-613	Hydroxyzine Pamoate 25 mg	Vistaril by Eon		Antihistamine
PP615	Cap, Green & White, PP-615	Hydroxyzine Pamoate 50 mg	Vistaril by Eon		Antihistamine
PP617	Cap, White, PP-617	Chlordiazepoxide HCl 5 mg, Clidinium Bromide 2.5 mg	Librax by Eon		Gastrointestinal; C IV
PP625	Cap, Green & White, PP-625	Chlordiazepoxide 25 mg	Librium by Eon		Antianxiety; C IV
PP6265	Cap, Black & Orange, PP-6265	Phendimetrazine Tartrate 35 mg	by Eon		Anorexiant; C III
PP630	Cap, Pink, PP-630	Propoxyphene HCl 65 mg	Darvon by Eon		Analgesic; C IV
PP635	Cap, Red/Black, PP-635	Phentermine HCl 30 mg	by Eon		Anorexiant; C IV
PP640	Cap, Black, PP-640	Phentermine HCl 30 mg	Phentermine HCl by Eon		Anorexiant; C IV
PP647	Cap, Yellow/Yellow, PP-647	Phentermine HCl 30 mg	Ionamin by Eon		Anorexiant; C IV

ID FRONT <> BACK	DESCRIPTION FRONT <> BACK	INGREDIENT & STRENGTH	BRAND (OR EQUIV.) & FIRM	NDC#	CLASS; SCH.
PP648	Cap, Clear & Pink	Diphenhydramine HCl 25 mg	Benadryl by Eon		Antihistamine
PP649	Cap, Pink	Diphenhydramine HCl 50 mg	Benadryl by Eon		Antihistamine
PP670	Cap, Yellow/Orange, PP-670	Tetracycline 250 mg	Achromycin V by Eon		Antibiotic
PP671	Cap, Black & Yellow, PP-671	Tetracycline 500 mg	Achromycin V by Eon		Antibiotic
PP686	Cap, Red/Gray, PP-686	Propoxyphene HCl 65 mg, Aspirin 389 mg, Caffeine 32.4 mg	Darvon Compound 65 by Eon		Analgesic; C IV
PP698	Cap, Blue & White, PP-698	Doxycycline Hyclate 50 mg	Vibramycin by Eon		Antibiotic
PP699	Cap, Blue, PP-699	Doxycycline Hyclate 100 mg	Vibramycin by Eon		Antibiotic
PP711	Tab, Green, Round	Salsalate 500 mg	Disalcid by Eon		NSAID
PP712	Tab, Green, Oblong	Salsalate 750 mg	Disalcid by Eon		NSAID
PP713	Tab, Green/White, Round, PP-713	Orphenadrine 25 mg, Aspirin 385 mg, Caffeine 60 mg	Norgesic by Eon		Muscle Relaxant
PP714	Tab, Green/White, Round, PP-714	Orphenadrine 50 mg, Aspirin 770 mg, Caffeine 60 mg	Norgesic Forte by Eon		Muscle Relaxant
PP716	Tab, White, Round, PP-716	Meprobamate 200 mg	Equanil by Eon		Sedative/Hypnotic; C IV
PP717	Tab, White, Round, PP-717	Meprobamate 400 mg	Equanil by Eon		Sedative/Hypnotic; C IV
PP717	Tab, Film Coated	Salsalate 750 mg	by Pharmedix	53002-0488	NSAID
PP718	Cap, Green & Opaque, PP-718	Indomethacin 25 mg	Indocin by Eon		NSAID
PP719	Cap, Green & Opaque, PP-719	Indomethacin 50 mg	Indocin by Eon		NSAID
PP720	Cap, Green & Clear, PP-720	Indomethacin SR 75 mg	Indocin SR by Eon		NSAID
PP721	Tab, Blue, Round	Desipramine HCl 50 mg	Norpramin by Eon		Antidepressant
PP722	Tab, Blue, Round, PP-722	Desipramine HCl 75 mg	Norpramin by Eon		Antidepressant
PP723	Tab, White, Round, PP-723	Carisoprodol 350 mg	Soma by Eon		Muscle Relaxant
PP725	Cap, Rust, PP-725	Meclofenamate Sodium 50 mg	Meclomen by Eon		NSAID
PP726	Cap, Rust/White, PP-726	Meclofenamate Sodium 100 mg	Meclomen by Eon		NSAID
PP736	Tab, Blue, Round, PP-736	Desipramine HCl 100 mg	Norpramin by Eon		Antidepressant
PP737	Cap, Green & Pink, PP-737	Cephradine 250 mg	Anspor by Eon		Antibiotic
PP738	Cap, Green, PP-738	Cephradine 500 mg	Anspor by Eon		Antibiotic
PP739	Cap, Yellow & White	Trimipramine Maleate 25 mg	Surmontil by Eon		Antidepressant
PP740	Cap, Orange & White	Trimipramine Maleate 50 mg	Surmontil by Eon		Antidepressant
PP741	Cap, White, PP-741	Trimipramine Maleate 100 mg	Surmontil by Eon		Antidepressant
PP743	Cap, Green & Clear	Niacin SR 250 mg	Nicobid by Eon		Vitamin
PP745	Tab	Guaifenesin 400 mg, Phenylpropanolamine HCl 75 mg	by Pharmedix	53002-0323	Cold Remedy
PP75	Tab, Pink/White/Blue, Oblong, PP-75	Phendimetrazine Tartrate 35 mg	by Eon		Anorexiant; C III
PP750	Tab, Brown, Round, PP/750	Nystatin Oral 500,000 Units	Mycostatin by Eon		Antifungal
PP7512	Tab, White, Round, PP-753 4	Aspirin 325 mg, Codeine 15 mg	by Eon		Analgesic; C III
PP7523	Tab, White, Round, PP-753 3	Aspirin 325 mg, Codeine 30 mg	by Eon		Analgesic; C III
PP7534	Tab, White, Round, PP-753 4	Aspirin 325 mg, Codeine 60 mg	by Eon		Analgesic; C III
PP754	Cap, Flesh	Clindamycin HCl 75 mg	Cleocin by Eon		Antibiotic
PP755	Cap, Flesh & Lavender	Clindamycin HCl 150 mg	Cleocin by Eon		Antibiotic
PP756	Cap, Red, PP-756	Triamterene 50 mg, Hydrochlorothiazide 25 mg	Dyazide by Eon		Diuretic
PP760	Tab, White, Round, PP-760	Desipramine HCl 150 mg	Norpramin by Eon		Antidepressant
PP761	Tab, Yellow, Round	Salsalate 500 mg	Disalcid by Eon		NSAID
PP762	Tab, Yellow, Oblong	Salsalate 750 mg	Disalcid by Eon		NSAID
PP777	Tab, Yellow, Diamond-Shaped, PP-777	Nystatin Vaginal 100,000 Units	Mycostatin by Eon		Antifungal
PP8	Tab, Yellow, Round	Imipramine HCl 10 mg	Tofranil by Eon		Antidepressant
PP84	Tab, Orange, Round	Iodinated Glycerol 30 mg	Organidin by Eon		Expectorant
PP856	Tab, Blue, Round	Salsalate 500 mg	Disalcid by Eon		NSAID
PP857	Tab, Blue, Oblong	Salsalate 750 mg	Disalcid by Eon		NSAID
PP882	Cap, PP 882	Phentermine HCl 15 mg	by Quality Care	60346-0133	Anorexiant; C IV
PP968	Cap, Green	Chlordiazepoxide HCl 5 mg, Clidinium Bromide 2.5 mg	Librax by Eon		Gastrointestinal; C IV
PP970	Cap, Red & Gray, PP-970	Cephalexin 250 mg	Keflex by Eon		Antibiotic
PP971	Cap, Red, PP-971	Cephalexin 500 mg	Keflex by Eon		Antibiotic
PP988	Tab, White, Round	Quinine Sulfate 260 mg	Quinamm by Eon		Antimalarial
PP995	Tab, Yellow, Oblong	Choline Magnesium Trisalicylate 500 mg	Trilisate by Eon		NSAID

ID FRONT <> BACK	DESCRIPTION FRONT <> BACK	INGREDIENT & STRENGTH	BRAND (OR EQUIV.) & FIRM	NDC#	CLASS; SCH.
PP996	Tab, Blue, Oblong	Choline Magnesium Trisalicylate 750 mg	Trilisate by Eon		NSAID
PP997	Tab, Pink, Oblong	Choline Magnesium Trisalicylate 1000 mg	Trilisate by Eon		NSAID
PPIROXICAM10	Cap, Blue & Maroon, P/Piroxicam/10	Piroxicam 10 mg	by Pharmascience	Canadian	NSAID
PPIROXICAM20	Cap, Blue & Maroon, P/Piroxicam/20	Piroxicam 20 mg	by Pharmascience	Canadian	NSAID
PPL54	Tab, Yellow, Round	Triamterene 75 mg, Hydrochlorothiazide 10 mg	Maxzide by Eon		Diuretic
PPP207 <> CORGARD40	Tab	Nadolol 40 mg	Nadolol by Pharmedix	53002-1018	Antihypertensive
PPP208	Tab, Blue, Oblong	Nadolol 120 mg	Corgard by BMS		Antihypertensive
PPP232	Tab, Blue, Round	Nadolol 20 mg	Corgard by BMS		Antihypertensive
PPP241	Tab, Blue, Round	Nadolol 80 mg	Corgard by BMS		Antihypertensive
PPP246	Tab, Blue, Oblong	Nadolol 160 mg	Corgard by BMS		Antihypertensive
PPP283	Tab, Blue Specks	Bendroflumethiazide 5 mg, Nadolol 40 mg	Corzide 40 5 by Pharmedix	53002-1038	Diuretic; Antihypertensive
PPP284	Tab, White/Blue Specks, Round	Nadolol 80 mg, Bendroflumethiazide 5 mg	Corzide by BMS		Antihypertensive
PPP431	Tab, Coated, PPP Over 431 in Black Ink	Procainamide HCl 250 mg	Pronestyl by ER Squibb	00003-0431	Antiarrhythmic
PPP434	Tab, Light Orange, Coated, PPP Over 434 in Black Ink	Procainamide HCl 375 mg	Pronestyl by ER Squibb	00003-0434	Antiarrhythmic
PPP438	Tab, PPP Over 438 in Black Ink	Procainamide HCl 500 mg	Pronestyl by ER Squibb	00003-0438	Antiarrhythmic
PPP606 <> NATURETIN5	Tab, PPP over 606 <> Naturetin 5	Bendroflumethiazide 5 mg	Naturetin by ER Squibb	00003-0606	Diuretic
PPP618 <> NATURETIN10	Tab, PPP 618 <> Naturetin 10	Bendroflumethiazide 10 mg	Naturetin by ER Squibb	00003-0618	Diuretic
PPP769	Tab, White Print, PPP over 769	Bendroflumethiazide 4 mg, Rauwolfia Serpentina 50 mg	Rauzide by ER Squibb	00003-0769	Diuretic
PPP775	Tab, Greenish Yellow, Ex Release, PPP Over 775 in Black Ink	Procainamide HCl 500 mg	Pronestyl SR by ER Squibb	00003-0775	Antiarrhythmic
PPP784 <> DURICEF500	Cap, PPP over 784 <> Duricef over 500	Cefadroxil 500 mg	Duricef by Nat Pharmpak Serv	55154-2009	Antibiotic
PPP784 <> DURICEF500MG	Cap	Cefadroxil 500 mg	Duricef by Prestige Packaging	58056-0348	Antibiotic
PPP784 <> DURICEF500MG	Cap	Cefadroxil 500 mg	Duricef by Bristol Myers Barcelaneta	55961-0784	Antibiotic
PPP784 <> DURICEF500MG	Cap, PPP 784 <> Duricef 500 mg	Cefadroxil 500 mg	Duricef by Bristol Myers Squibb	00087-0784	Antibiotic
PPP784 <> DURICEF500MG	Cap	Cefadroxil 500 mg	Duricef by Allscripts	54569-0108	Antibiotic
PPP784 <> DURICEF500MG	Cap, Duricef over 500 MG	Cefadroxil Monohydrate	Duricef by Quality Care	60346-0641	Antibiotic
PPP785	Tab, Film Coated, PPP/785	Cefadroxil 1 gm	Duricef by Bristol Myers Barcelaneta	55961-0785	Antibiotic
PPP785	Tab, Film Coated, Scored	Cefadroxil 1 gm	Duricef by Quality Care	60346-0700	Antibiotic
PPP785	Tab, Coated	Cefadroxil 1 gm	Duricef by Bristol Myers Squibb	00087-0785	Antibiotic
PPP785	Tab, Film Coated	Cefadroxil 1 gm	Duricef by Allscripts	54569-0110	Antibiotic
PPP863	Tab, Film Coated	Fluphenazine HCl 1 mg	Prolixin by ER Squibb	00003-0863	Antipsychotic
PPP864	Tab, Coated	Fluphenazine HCl 2.5 mg	Prolixin by ER Squibb	00003-0864	Antipsychotic
PPP877	Tab, Sugar Coated, Dark Green Print	Fluphenazine HCl 5 mg	Prolixin by ER Squibb	00003-0877	Antipsychotic
PPP956	Tab, Coral, Film Coated, Dark Green Print, PPP over 956	Fluphenazine HCl 10 mg	Prolixin by ER Squibb	00003-0956	Antipsychotic
PPRAVACHOL10	Tab, Peach & Pink, Round, P/Pravachol 10	Pravastatin Sodium 10 mg	by Squibb	Canadian	Antihyperlipidemic
PPRAVACHOL20	Tab, Yellow, Rectangular, P/Pravachol 20	Pravastatin Sodium 20 mg	by Squibb	Canadian	Antihyperlipidemic
PPRAVACHOL40	Tab, Green, Rectangular, P/Pravachol 40	Pravastatin Sodium 40 mg	by Squibb	Canadian	Antihyperlipidemic
PRATT155	Tab, White, Round	Glipizide Extended Release 5 mg	Glucotrol XL by Roerig	00049-1550	Antidiabetic
PRATT156	Tab, White, Round	Glipizide Extended Release 10 mg	Glucotrol XL by Roerig	00049-1560	Antidiabetic
PRAVACHOL10 <> P	Tab, Pink to Peach, Oblong	Pravastatin Sodium 10 mg	Pravachol by Bristol Myers	00003-5154	Antihyperlipidemic
PRAVACHOL10 <> P	Tab, Pink/Peach, Rounded, Rectangular-Shaped	Pravastatin Sodium 10 mg	Pravachol by PDRX	55289-0104	Antihyperlipidemic
PRAVACHOL10 <> P	Tab	Pravastatin Sodium 10 mg	Pravachol by Nat Pharmpak Serv	55154-0606	Antihyperlipidemic
PRAVACHOL20 <> P	Tab, Yellow, Oblong	Pravastatin Sodium 20 mg	Pravachol by Bristol Myers	00003-5178	Antihyperlipidemic

ID FRONT <> BACK	DESCRIPTION FRONT <> BACK	INGREDIENT & STRENGTH	BRAND (OR EQUIV.) & FIRM	NDC#	CLASS; SCH.
PRAVACHOL20 <> P	Tab, Pravachol 20 <> Rounded Rectangle Shape	Pravastatin Sodium 20 mg	Pravachol by Allscripts	54569-4071	Antihyperlipidemic
PRAVACHOL20 <> P	Tab	Pravastatin Sodium 20 mg	Pravachol by Nat Pharmpak Serv	55154-0608	Antihyperlipidemic
PRAVACHOL20 <> P	Tab, Yellow, Rectangle	Pravastatin Sodium 20 mg	Pravachol by Squibb Mfg	12783-0178	Antihyperlipidemic
PRAVACHOL40 <> P	Tab, Green, Oblong	Pravastatin Sodium 40 mg	Pravachol by Bristol Myers	00003-5194	Antihyperlipidemic
PRAVACHOL40 <> P	Tab, Pravachol 40	Pravastatin Sodium 40 mg	Pravachol by Caremark	00339-5746	Antihyperlipidemic
PRAVACHOL40 <> P	Tab, Embossed	Pravastatin Sodium 40 mg	Pravachol by Quality Care	62682-6028	Antihyperlipidemic
PRECOSE <> 25	Tab	Acarbose 25 mg	Precose by Bayer	00026-2863	Antidiabetic
PRECOSE <> 50	Tab, Whitish Yellow	Acarbose 50 mg	Precose by Physicians Total Care	54868-3823	Antidiabetic
PRECOSE100	Tab, Whitish Yellow Tinged	Acarbose 100 mg	Precose by Bayer	00026-2862	Antidiabetic
PRECOSE50	Tab, Whitish Yellow Tinged	Acarbose 50 mg	Precose by Bayer	00026-2861	Antidiabetic
PRECOSE50	Tab, Whitish Yellow	Acarbose 50 mg	Precose by Caremark	00339-6105	Antidiabetic
PRECOSE50	Tab, Whitish Yellow	Acarbose 50 mg	Precose by Allscripts	54569-4501	Antidiabetic
PREGNANTLADY	Cap, White, Scored	Thalidomide 50 mg	Thalomid by Celgene		Immunomodulator
PREMARIN	Tab, Green, Oval	Conjugated Estrogens 0.3 mg	Premarin by Wyeth-Ayerst	Canadian	Estrogen
PREMARIN	Tab, Maroon, Oval	Conjugated Estrogens 0.625 mg	Premarin by Wyeth-Ayerst	Canadian	Estrogen
PREMARIN	Tab, Pink, Oval	Conjugated Estrogens 0.9 mg	Premarin by Wyeth-Ayerst	Canadian	Estrogen
PREMARIN	Tab, Yellow, Oval	Conjugated Estrogens 1.25 mg	Premarin by Wyeth-Ayerst	Canadian	Estrogen
PREMARIN	Tab, Purple, Oval	Conjugated Estrogens 2.5 mg	Premarin by Wyeth-Ayerst	Canadian	Estrogen
PREMARIN <> 0625	Tab, Coated, 0.625	Estrogens, Conjugated 0.625 mg	Premarin by Quality Care	60346-0599	Hormone
PREMARIN <> 0625	Tab, Coated	Estrogens, Conjugated 0.625 mg	Premarin by Med Pro	53978-0189	Hormone
PREMARIN <> 25	Tab, Coated, 2.5	Estrogens, Conjugated 2.5 mg	Premarin by Quality Care	60346-0859	Hormone
PREMARIN03	Tab, Green, Oval, Premarin over 0.3	Conjugated Estrogens 0.3 mg	Premarin by Respa	60575-0078	Estrogen
PREMARIN03	Tab, Coated, Premarin/0.3	Estrogens, Conjugated 0.3 mg	Premarin by Kaiser	00179-1173	Hormone
PREMARIN03	Tab, Dark Green, Coated, Premarin 0.3	Estrogens, Conjugated 0.3 mg	Premarin by Ayerst	00046-0868	Hormone
PREMARIN03	Tab, Coated, Premarin 0.3	Estrogens, Conjugated 0.3 mg	Premarin by Allscripts	54569-0811	Hormone
PREMARIN0625	Tab, Maroon, Oval, Premarin 0.625	Conjugated Estrogens 0.625 mg	Premarin by DJ Pharma	64455-0006	Estrogen
PREMARIN0625	Tab, Maroon, Oval, Premarin over 0.625	Estrogens, Conjugated 0.625 mg	Premarin by Heartland	61392-0418	Hormone
PREMARIN0625	Tab, Coated, Premarin 0.625	Estrogens, Conjugated 0.625 mg	Premarin by Thrift Drug	59198-0092	Hormone
PREMARIN0625	Tab, Coated, Premarin 0.625	Estrogens, Conjugated 0.625 mg	Premarin by Prepackage Spec	58864-0422	Hormone
PREMARIN0625	Tab, Coated, Premarin over 0.625	Estrogens, Conjugated 0.625 mg	Premarin by Nat Pharmpak Serv	55154-0213	Hormone
PREMARIN0625	Tab, Maroon, Oval	Estrogens, Conjugated 0.625 mg	Premarin by HJ Harkins	52959-0223	Hormone
PREMARIN0625	Tab, Coated, Premarin/0.625	Estrogens, Conjugated 0.625 mg	Premarin by Ayerst	00046-0867	Hormone
PREMARIN0625	Tab, Coated, Premarin/0.625	Estrogens, Conjugated 0.625 mg	Premarin by Kaiser	00179-1172	Hormone
PREMARIN0625	Tab, Coated, Premarin 0.625	Estrogens, Conjugated 0.625 mg	Premarin by Allscripts	54569-0812	Hormone
PREMARIN0625	Tab, Coated	Estrogens, Conjugated 0.625 mg	by Talbert Med	44514-0493	Hormone
PREMARIN0625	Tab, Coated, Premarin 0.625	Estrogens, Conjugated 0.625 mg	Premarin by Apotheca	12634-0409	Hormone
PREMARIN0625MG	Tab, Coated, Premarin 0.625 mg	Estrogens, Conjugated 0.625 mg	Premarin by Rite Aid	11822-5207	Hormone
PREMARIN09	Tab, Coated, Premarin 0.9	Estrogens, Conjugated 0.9 mg	Premarin by Allscripts	54569-0849	Hormone
PREMARIN125	Tab, Sugar Coated, Premarin over 1.25	Estrogens, Conjugated 1.25 mg	Premarin by Quality Care	60346-0847	Hormone
PREMARIN125	Tab, Sugar Coated, Premarin 1.25	Estrogens, Conjugated 1.25 mg	Premarin by Nat Pharmpak Serv	55154-0211	Hormone
PREMARIN125	Tab, Sugar Coated, Premarin 1.25	Estrogens, Conjugated 1.25 mg	Premarin by Thrift Drug	59198-0093	Hormone
PREMARIN125	Tab, Sugar Coated, Premarin 1.25	Estrogens, Conjugated 1.25 mg	Premarin by Ayerst	00046-0866	Hormone
PREMARIN125	Tab, Sugar Coated, Premarin 1.25	Estrogens, Conjugated 1.25 mg	Premarin by Kaiser	00179-1239	Hormone
PREMARIN125	Tab, Sugar Coated, Premarin 1.25	Estrogens, Conjugated 1.25 mg	Premarin by Allscripts	54569-0813	Hormone
PREMARIN125	Tab, Sugar Coated, Premarin/1.25	Estrogens, Conjugated 1.25 mg	Premarin by Med Pro	53978-0190	Hormone
PREMARIN125	Tab, Film Coated, Premarin 1.25	Estrogens, Conjugated 1.25 mg	Premarin 1-25 by Rite Aid	11822-5200	Hormone
PREMARIN25	Tab, Coated, Premarin 2.5	Estrogens, Conjugated 2.5 mg	Premarin by Thrift Drug	59198-0094	Hormone
PREMARIN25	Tab, Coated, Premarin over 2.5	Estrogens, Conjugated 2.5 mg	Premarin by Prestige Packaging	58056-0353	Hormone
PREMARIN25	Tab, Coated, Premarin 2.5	Estrogens, Conjugated 2.5 mg	Premarin by Nat Pharmpak Serv	55154-0212	Hormone
PREMARIN25	Tab, Coated, Premarin 2.5	Estrogens, Conjugated 2.5 mg	Premarin by Amerisource	62584-0865	Hormone
PREMARIN25	Tab, Coated, Premarin 2.5	Estrogens, Conjugated 2.5 mg	Premarin by Ayerst	00046-0865	Hormone
PREMARIN25	Tab, Coated, Premarin 2.5	Estrogens, Conjugated 2.5 mg	Premarin by Kaiser	00179-1240	Hormone

ID FRONT <> BACK	DESCRIPTION FRONT <> BACK	INGREDIENT & STRENGTH	BRAND (OR EQUIV.) & FIRM	NDC#	CLASS; SCH.
PREMARIN25	Tab, Coated, Premarin over 2.5	Estrogens, Conjugated 2.5 mg	Premarin by Repack Co of Amer	55306-0865	Hormone
PREMPRO	Tab	Estrogens, Conjugated 0.625 mg, Medroxyprogesterone Acetate 2.5 mg	Prempro by DRX	55045-2561	Hormone
PRENATE	Tab, White, Oval	Iron Pentacarbonyl 90 mg, Calcium Carbonate 200 mg, Cupric Oxide 2 mg; Zinc Oxide 25 mg; Folic Acid 1 mg; Beta-Carotene 2700 Unt; Cholecalciferol 400 Unt; Tocopherol Acetate 30 Unt; Ascorbic Acid 120 mg; Thiamine Mononitrate 3 mg, Riboflavin 3.4 mg	Prenatal Vitamin by Patheon Niagara	52814-1727	Vitamin/Mineral
PREVACID15	Cap, Delayed Release, Prevacid 15 <> Logo	Lansoprazole 15 mg	Prevacid by Murfreesboro	51129-1147	Antiulcer
PREVACID15	Cap, Green & Pink	Lansoprazole 15 mg	Prevacid by DRX Pharm Consults	55045-2740	Gastrointestinal
PREVACID15	Cap, Green & Pink, Opaque, Gelatin, Tap Logo	Lansoprazole 15 mg	Prevacid by Tap Pharmaceutical	00300-1541	Gastrointestinal
PREVACID15 <> TAP	Cap, Green & Pink	Lansoprazole 15 mg	Prevacid by Abbott	00074-1541	Gastrointestinal
PREVACID30	Cap, Black & Pink, Opaque, Gelatin, Tap Logo	Lansoprazole 30 mg	Prevacid by Tap Pharmaceutical	00300-3046	Gastrointestinal
PREVACID30	Cap, Pink & Black, Opaque, Enteric, Tap Logo	Lansoprazole 30 mg	Prevacid Starter Kit by Murfreesboro	51129-1626	Gastrointestinal
PREVACID30 <> TAP	Cap, Black & Pink	Lansoprazole 30 mg	Prevacid by Va Cmop	65243-0044	Gastrointestinal
PREVACID30 <> TAP	Cap, Black & Pink	Lansoprazole 30 mg	Prevacid by Compumed	00403-2121	Gastrointestinal
PREVACID30 <> TAP	Cap, Black & Pink, Hard Gel	Lansoprazole 30 mg	Prevacid by Abbott	00074-3046	Gastrointestinal
PRIFTIN <> 150	Tab, Dark Pink	Rifapentine 150 mg	Priftin by Gruppo Lepetit	12522-8598	Antibiotic
PRILOSEC10 <> 606	Cap, Delayed Release	Omeprazole 10 mg	Prilosec by Merck	00006-0606	Gastrointestinal
PRILOSEC10 <> 606	Cap, Delayed Release, Prilosec 10	Omeprazole 10 mg	Prilosec by Astra Merck	00186-0606	Gastrointestinal
PRILOSEC10 <> 606	Cap, Delayed Release	Omeprazole 10 mg	Omeprazole by Kaiser	62224-2226	Gastrointestinal
PRILOSEC20 <> 742	Cap, Purple	Omeprazole 20 mg	Prilosec by Amerisource Hlth	62584-0451	Gastrointestinal
PRILOSEC20 <> 742	Cap, Purple	Omeprazole 20 mg	Prilosec by Southwood Pharms	58016-0327	Gastrointestinal
PRILOSEC20 <> 742	Cap, Delayed Release, Prilosec 20	Omeprazole 20 mg	Omeprazole by Kaiser	00179-1245	Gastrointestinal
PRILOSEC20 <> 742	Cap, Delayed Release, Prilosec 20	Omeprazole 20 mg	Prilosec by Caremark	00339-5695	Gastrointestinal
PRILOSEC20 <> 742	Cap, Delayed Release, On Body <> On Cap	Omeprazole 20 mg	Prilosec by Allscripts	54569-3267	Gastrointestinal
PRILOSEC20 <> 742	Cap, Delayed Release, On Body <> On Cap	Omeprazole 20 mg	Omeprazole by Med Pro	53978-1129	Gastrointestinal
PRILOSEC20 <> 742	Cap, Delayed Release, Prilosec 20	Omeprazole 20 mg	Prilosec by Quality Care	62682-4001	Gastrointestinal
PRILOSEC20 <> 742	Cap, Delayed Release, Code on Body <> Code on Cap	Omeprazole 20 mg	Prilosec by Kaiser	62224-8111	Gastrointestinal
PRILOSEC40 <> 743	Cap, Delayed Release, Prilosec 40	Omeprazole 40 mg	Prilosec by Merck	00006-0743	Gastrointestinal
PRILOSEC40 <> 743	Cap, Delayed Release, Prilosec 40	Omeprazole 40 mg	Prilosec by Astra Merck	00186-0743	Gastrointestinal
PRINIVIL <> MSD106	Tab, Yellow, Triangle	Lisinopril 10 mg	Prinivil by Phcy Care	65070-0012	Antihypertensive
PRINIVIL <> MSD106	Tab, Light Yellow, Shield-Shaped	Lisinopril 10 mg	Prinivil by Merck	00006-0106	Antihypertensive
PRINIVIL <> MSD106	Tab	Lisinopril 10 mg	Prinivil by Nat Pharmpak Serv	55154-5015	Antihypertensive
PRINIVIL <> MSD106	Tab, Shield-Shaped	Lisinopril 10 mg	Prinivil by DRX	55045-2292	Antihypertensive
PRINIVIL <> MSD106	Tab	Lisinopril 10 mg	Lisinopril by Med Pro	53978-3015	Antihypertensive
PRINIVIL <> MSD106	Tab, Shield-Shaped	Lisinopril 10 mg	Prinivil by PDRX	55289-0929	Antihypertensive
PRINIVIL <> MSD106	Tab	Lisinopril 10 mg	Prinivil by Quality Care	60346-0972	Antihypertensive
PRINIVIL <> MSD19	Tab, White, Triangle, Scored	Lisinopril 5 mg	Prinivil by Phcy Care	65070-0014	Antihypertensive
PRINIVIL <> MSD19	Tab, White, Shield-Shaped	Lisinopril 5 mg	Prinivil by Merck	00006-0019	Antihypertensive
PRINIVIL <> MSD19	Tab	Lisinopril 5 mg	Prinivil by Nat Pharmpak Serv	55154-5006	Antihypertensive
PRINIVIL <> MSD207	Tab, Peach, Triangle	Lisinopril 20 mg	Prinivil by Phcy Care	65070-0013	Antihypertensive
PRINIVIL <> MSD207	Tab, Rose Red, Shield-Shaped	Lisinopril 20 mg	Prinivil by Merck	00006-0207	Antihypertensive
PRINIVIL <> MSD207	Tab	Lisinopril 20 mg	Lisinopril by Med Pro	53978-3017	Antihypertensive
PRINIVIL <> MSD207	Tab	Lisinopril 20 mg	Prinivil by Nat Pharmpak Serv	55154-5011	Antihypertensive
PRINIVIL106	Tab, Yellow, Shield-Shaped	Lisonopril 10 mg	by MSD	Canadian	Antihypertensive
PRINIVIL207	Tab, Peach, Shield-Shaped	Lisonopril 20 mg	by MSD	Canadian	Antihypertensive
PRINZIDE <> MSD145	Tab, Blue, Hexagon	Lisinopril 10 mg; Hydrochlorothiazide 12.5 mg	Prinzide by Murfreesboro Ph	51129-1397	Antihypertensive
PROCANBID <> 1000	Tab, Gray, Oval, Film Coated	Procainamide HCl 1000 mg	Procanbid by Monarch Pharms	61570-0071	Antiarrhythmic
PROCANBID <> 1000	Tab, Elliptical-Shaped, Film Coated	Procainamide HCl 1000 mg	Procanbid by Parke Davis	00071-0564	Antiarrhythmic
PROCANBID <> 1000	Tab, Gray, Film Coated	Procainamide HCl 1000 mg	Procanbid by Ranbaxy	54907-0604	Antiarrhythmic
PROCANBID <> 500	Tab, White, Elliptical	Procanamide HCl 500 mg	Procanbid by Monarch	61570-0069	Antiarrhythmic
PROCANBID <> 500	Tab, Elliptical-Shaped, Film Coated	Procainamide HCl 500 mg	Procanbid by Parke Davis	00071-0562	Antiarrhythmic
PROCANBID1000	Tab, Gray, Elliptical, Procanbid/1000	Procanamide HCl 1000 mg	Procanbid by Monarch	00071-0564	Antiarrhythmic

ID FRONT <> BACK	DESCRIPTION FRONT <> BACK	INGREDIENT & STRENGTH	BRAND (OR EQUIV.) & FIRM	NDC#	CLASS; SCH.
PROCANBID1000	Tab, Gray	Procainamide HCl 1000 mg	Procanbid by Parke-Davis		Antiarrhythmic
PROCANBID500	Blue	Procainamide HCl 500 mg	Procanbid by Parke-Davis		Antiarrhythmic
PROCANSR250MG	Tab, Green, Ellipitical, Film Coated	Procainamide HCl 250 mg	Procan SR by Parke-Davis	Canadian DIN# 00638692	Antiarrhythmic
PROCANSR500MG	Tab, Green, Elliptical, Film Coated	Procainamide HCl 500 mg	Procan by Parke-Davis	Canadian DIN# 00638676	Antiarrhythmic
PROCANSR750MG	Tab, Orange, Elliptical, Film Coated	Procainamide HCl 750 mg	Procan SR by Parke-Davis	Canadian DIN# 00638684	Antiarrhythmic
PROCARDIA20PFIZ	Cap, Dark Orange, Procardia 20 Pfizer 261	Nifedipine 20 mg	Procardia by Pfizer	00069-2610	Antihypertensive
PROCARDIAPFIZER	Cap, Orange & Light Brown, Procardia Pfizer 260	Nifedipine 10 mg	Procardia by Pfizer	00069-2600	Antihypertensive
PROCARDIAPFIZER	Cap, Procardia Pfizer 260	Nifedipine 10 mg	Procardia by Allscripts	54569-0643	Antihypertensive
PROCARDIAXL <> 30	Tab, Pink, Round, Ex Release, Procardia XL	Nifedipine 30 mg	Procardia XL by Pfizer	00069-2650	Antihypertensive
PROCARDIAXL <> 30	Tab, Ex Release, Procardia XL	Nifedipine 30 mg	Procardia XL by Nat Pharmpak Serv	55154-2706	Antihypertensive
PROCARDIAXL <> 30	Tab, Ex Release, Procardia XL	Nifedipine 30 mg	Procardia XL by Amerisource	62584-0650	Antihypertensive
PROCARDIAXL <> 60	Tab, Pink, Round, Ex Release, Procardia XL	Nifedipine 60 mg	Procardia XL by Pfizer	00069-2660	Antihypertensive
PROCARDIAXL <> 60	Tab, Ex Release, Procardia XL	Nifedipine 60 mg	Procardia XL by Nat Pharmpak Serv	55154-2707	Antihypertensive
PROCARDIAXL <> 60	Tab, Ex Release, Procardia XL	Nifedipine 60 mg	Procardia XL by Amerisource	62584-0660	Antihypertensive
PROCARDIAXL30	Tab, ER	Nifedipine 30 mg	Procardia XL by Giant Food	11146-0270	Antihypertensive
PROCARDIAXL30	Tab, Ex Release, Procardia XL 30	Nifedipine 30 mg	Procardia XL by Allscripts	54569-2780	Antihypertensive
PROCARDIAXL30	Tab, ER	Nifedipine 30 mg	Procardia XL by Pharmedix	53002-1054	Antihypertensive
PROCARDIAXL30	Tab, Ex Release, Procardia XL 30	Nifedipine 30 mg	Procardia XL by Med Pro	53978-3035	Antihypertensive
PROCARDIAXL30 <> 30	Tab, ER	Nifedipine 30 mg	by Med Pro	53978-1107	Antihypertensive
PROCARDIAXL60	Tab, Ex Release, Procardia XL 60	Nifedipine 60 mg	Procardia XL by Allscripts	54569-2781	Antihypertensive
PROCARDIAXL60	Tab, Ex Release, Mfr is Pfizer	Nifedipine 60 mg	Procardia XL by Med Pro	53978-3036	Antihypertensive
PROCARDIAXL60	Tab, Pink, Round, Convex, Film Coated, Procardia XL Over 60	Nifedipine 60 mg	Procardia XL by Par	49884-0623	Antihypertensive
PROCARDIAXL90	Tab, Film Coated	Nifedipine 90 mg	Procardia XL by Allscripts	54569-3055	Antihypertensive
PROCARDIAXL90	Tab, Rose Pink, Film Coated	Nifedipine 90 mg	Procardia XL by Quality Care	60346-0186	Antihypertensive
PRODM	Tab, Ex Release, Pro DM	Dextromethorphan Hydrobromide 30 mg, Guaifenesin 600 mg, Pseudoephedrine HCl 60 mg	Protuss DM by Horizon	59630-0160	Cold Remedy
PRODM	Tab	Dextromethorphan Hydrobromide 30 mg, Guaifenesin 600 mg, Pseudoephedrine HCl 60 mg	Protuss DM by Anabolic	00722-6370	Cold Remedy
PROFENFORTE	Tab, White, Scored	Guaifenesin 800 mg, Pseudoephedrine HCl 90 mg	by Wakefield	59310-0315	Cold Remedy
PROFENFORTEDM	Tab, White, Cap Shaped, Scored	Dextromethorphan HBr 60 mg, Guaifenesin 800 mg, Pseudoephedrine HCl 90 mg	by Wakefield	59310-0316	Cold Remedy
PROFENII	Tab	Guaifenesin 600 mg, Phenylpropanolamine HCl 37.5 mg	Profen II by Anabolic	00722-6351	Cold Remedy
PROFENII	Tab, White, Scored	Guaifenesin 800 mg, Pseudoephedrine HCl 45 mg	by Wakefield	59310-0307	Cold Remedy
PROFENII	Tab, White, Elliptical	Phenylpropanolamine HCl 37.5 mg, Guaifenesin 600 mg	Profen II by Wakefield	59310-0107	Cold Remedy
PROFENIIDM	Tab, White, Cap Shaped, Scored	Dextromethorphan HBr 30 mg, Guaifenesin 800 mg, Pseudoephedrine HCl 45 mg	by Wakefield	59310-0310	Cold Remedy
PROFENIIDM	Tab, White, Oblong, Scored	Guaifenesin 600 mg, Phenylpropanolamine HCl 37.5 mg, Dextromethorphan Hydrobromide 30 mg	GFN PPAH DM by Med Pro	53978-3329	Cold Remedy
PROFENLA	Tab, Ex Release	Guaifenesin 600 mg, Phenylpropanolamine HCl 75 mg	Profen LA by Sage	59243-0906	Cold Remedy
PROFENLA	Tab, White, Elliptical, Ex Release, Profen-LA	Guaifenesin 600 mg, Phenylpropanolamine HCl 75 mg	Profen LA by Wakefield	59310-0104	Cold Remedy
PROFENLA	Tab, Profen-LA	Guaifenesin 600 mg, Phenylpropanolamine HCl 75 mg	Profen LA by Anabolic	00722-6397	Cold Remedy
PROFENLA	Tab, White, Oval, Scored	Guaifenesin 600 mg, Phenylpropanolamine HCl 75 mg	GFN PPAH by Med Pro	53978-3316	Cold Remedy
PROFENIIDM	Tab, White, Elliptical	Dextromethorphan 30 mg	Profen II DM by Wakefield	59310-0110	Antitussive
PROLEXD	Tab, White, Oval, Scored	Phenylephrine HCl 20 mg, Guaifenesin 600 mg	Prolex D by Sovereign Pharms	58716-0686	Cold Remedy
PROLEXD	Tab, White, Oval, Scored	Phenylephrine HCl 20 mg, Guaifenesin 600 mg	Prolex D by Blansett Pharma	51674-0124	Cold Remedy
PROLOPRIM09A	Tab, White, Biconvex	Trimethoprim 100 mg	Proloprim by B.W. Inc	Canadian	Antibiotic
PROLOPRIM09A	Tab	Trimethoprim 100 mg	Proloprim by Catalytica	63552-0820	Antibiotic
PROLOPRIM09A	Tab, White, Round, Scored	Trimethoprim 100 mg	Proloprim by Monarch Pharms	61570-0057	Antibiotic

ID FRONT <> BACK	DESCRIPTION FRONT <> BACK	INGREDIENT & STRENGTH	BRAND (OR EQUIV.) & FIRM	NDC#	CLASS; SCH.
PROLOPRIM200	Tab	Trimethoprim 200 mg	Proloprim by Catalytica	63552-0825	Antibiotic
PROLOPRIM200	Tab, White, Round	Trimethoprim 200 mg	Proloprim by Monarch	61570-0058	Antibiotic
PROLOPRIMO9A	Tab, White, Round	Trimethoprim 100 mg	Proloprim by Monarch	00173-0820	Antibiotic
PROLOPRIMR2C	Tab, Yellow, Round	Trimethoprim 200 mg	Proloprim by B.W. Inc	Canadian	Antibiotic
PROPACET	Tab, White, Oblong, Film Coated	Acetaminophen 650 mg, Propoxyphene Napsylate 100 mg	Propacet by Teva	00093-0590	Analgesic; C IV
PROPACET	Tab, Coated	Acetaminophen 650 mg, Propoxyphene Napsylate 100 mg	Propoxy N APAP by Quality Care	60346-0610	Analgesic; C IV
PROPACET	Tab, Coated	Acetaminophen 650 mg, Propoxyphene Napsylate 100 mg	by Patient	57575-0019	Analgesic; C IV
PROPECIA <> MRK71	Tab, Tan, Octagonal	Finasteride 1 mg	Propecia by Southwood Pharms	58016-0329	Antiandrogen
PROPECIA1 <> MRK71	Tab, Tan, Octagonal	Finasteride 1 mg	Propecia by Phy Total Care	54868-4120	Antiandrogen
PROPECIA1 <> MRK71	Tab, Tan, Octagonal, Film Coated	Finasteride 1 mg	Propecia by Merck	00006-0071	Antiandrogen
PROSCAR <> MSD72	Tab, Blue, Round, Film Coated	Finasteride 5 mg	Proscar by Phy Total Care	54868-2719	Antiandrogen
PROSEDDS	Tab, Deep Blue, Round, Coated, Prosed/DS	Methenamine 81.6 mg, Phenyl Salicylate 36.2 mg, Methylene Blue 10.8 mg	Prosed DS by Star	00076-0108	Antibiotic; Urinary Tract
PROTONIX	Tab, Yellow, Oval	Pantoprazole Sodium 40 mg	Protonix by BYK Gulden	47234-0001	Gastrointestinal
PROVENTIL <> 4	Tab, Film Coated	Albuterol 4 mg	Proventil by Nat Pharmpak Serv	55154-3507	Antiasthmatic
PROVENTIL2 <> 252252	Tab, Off-White, Round, Proventil 2 <> 252 over 252	Albuterol Sulfate 2.41 mg	Proventil by Schering	00085-0252	Antiasthmatic
PROVENTIL4 <> 573	Tab, Film Coated	Albuterol 4 mg	Proventil by PDRX	55289-0634	Antiasthmatic
PROVENTIL4 <> 573	Tab, Film Coated	Albuterol 4 mg	Proventil by Amerisource	62584-0463	Antiasthmatic
PROVENTIL4 <> 573	Tab, White, Round, Scored	Albuterol Sulfate 4 mg	Proventil Repetabs by Amide	52152-0188	Antiasthmatic
PROVENTIL4 <> 573573	Tab, Off-White, Round, Proventil 4 <> 573/573	Albuterol Sulfate 4.8 mg	Proventil by Schering	00085-0573	Antiasthmatic
PROVERA <> 25	Tab, UPJOHN <> 2.5, Tab	Medroxyprogesterone Acetate 2.5 mg	Provera by Quality Care	60346-0848	Progestin
PROVERA <> 5	Tab	Medroxyprogesterone Acetate 5 mg	Provera by Quality Care	60346-0603	Progestin
PROVERA10	Tab, Provera 10	Medroxyprogesterone Acetate 10 mg	Provera by Thrift Drug	59198-0197	Progestin
PROVERA10	Tab, Provera 10	Medroxyprogesterone Acetate 10 mg	Provera by Nat Pharmpak Serv	55154-3913	Progestin
PROVERA10	Tab, Provera 10	Medroxyprogesterone Acetate 10 mg	Provera by Pharmacia & Upjohn	00009-0050	Progestin
PROVERA10	Tab	Medroxyprogesterone Acetate 10 mg	Provera by Allscripts	54569-0816	Progestin
PROVERA10MG	Tab, Provera 10	Medroxyprogesterone Acetate 10 mg	Provera by Murfreesboro	51129-9005	Progestin
PROVERA25	Tab	Medroxyprogesterone Acetate 10 mg	Provera by Rite Aid	11822-5269	Progestin
PROVERA25	Tab, Provera 2.5	Medroxyprogesterone Acetate 2.5 mg	Provera by Murfreesboro	51129-0064	Progestin
PROVERA25	Tab, Provera 2.5	Medroxyprogesterone Acetate 2.5 mg	Provera by Pharmacia & Upjohn	00009-0064	Progestin
PROVERA25	Tab, Provera 2.5	Medroxyprogesterone Acetate 2.5 mg	Provera by Thrift Drug	59198-0198	Progestin
PROVERA25	Tab, Provera 2.5	Medroxyprogesterone Acetate 2.5 mg	Provera by Nat Pharmpak Serv	55154-3911	Progestin
PROVERA5	Tab	Medroxyprogesterone Acetate 2.5 mg	Provera by Rite Aid	11822-5267	Progestin
PROVERA5	Tab, Provera 5	Medroxyprogesterone Acetate 5 mg	Provera by Pharmacia & Upjohn	00009-0286	Progestin
PROVERA5	Tab	Medroxyprogesterone Acetate 5 mg	Provera by Allscripts	54569-1779	Progestin
PROVERA5	Tab, Provera 5	Medroxyprogesterone Acetate 5 mg	Provera by Thrift Drug	59198-0199	Progestin
PROVERA5	Tab, Provera 5	Medroxyprogesterone Acetate 5 mg	Provera by Nat Pharmpak Serv	55154-3912	Progestin
PROVERA5	Tab	Medroxyprogesterone Acetate 5 mg	Provera by Rite Aid	11822-5268	Progestin
PROVIGIL <> 100MG	Tab, White, Cap-Shaped	Modafinil 100 mg	Provigil by Cephalon	63459-0100	Stimulant; C IV
PROVIGIL <> 100MG	Tab, White, Oblong, Uncoated	Modafinil 100 mg	by Neuman Distr	64579-0319	Stimulant; C IV
PROVIGIL <> 200MG	Tab, White, Cap-Shaped	Modafinil 200 mg	Provigil by Cephalon	63459-0200	Stimulant; C IV
PROVIGIL <> 200MG	Tab, White, Oblong, Uncoated	Modafinil 200 mg	by Neuman Distr	64579-0324	Stimulant; C IV
PROZAC10	Tab, Green, Elliptical, Scored	Fluoxetine 10 mg	Prozac by Lilly	00002-4006	Antidepressant
PROZAC10	Tab, Green, Oval, Scored	Fluoxetine HCl 10 mg	Prozac by International Processing	59885-3513	Antidepressant
PROZAC10 <> DISTA3104	Cap, Prozac 10 <> Dista over 3104	Fluoxetine HCl	Prozac by Quality Care	60346-0971	Antidepressant
PROZAC10 <> DISTA3104	Cap	Fluoxetine HCl	Prozac by Kaiser	00179-1252	Antidepressant
PROZAC10MG <> DISTA3104	Cap	Fluoxetine HCl	by Kaiser	62224-1115	Antidepressant
PROZAC10MG <> DISTA3104	Cap, Green	Fluoxetine HCl	Prozac by Eli Lilly	00002-3104	Antidepressant

ID FRONT <> BACK	DESCRIPTION FRONT <> BACK	INGREDIENT & STRENGTH	BRAND (OR EQUIV.) & FIRM	NDC#	CLASS; SCH.
PROZAC10MG <> DISTA3104	Cap	Fluoxetine HCl	Prozac by Dista Prod	00777-3104	Antidepressant
PROZAC10MG <> DISTA3104	Cap	Fluoxetine HCl	Prozac by Allscripts	54569-4129	Antidepressant
PROZAC20 <> DISTA3105	Cap, Beige & Green	Fluoxetine 20 mg	Prozac by Southwood Pharms	58016-0828	Antidepressant
PROZAC20MG <> DISTA3105	Cap, Off-White, Gelatin Coated	Fluoxetine 20 mg	Prozac by Quality Care	60346-0004	Antidepressant
PROZAC20MG <> DISTA3105	Cap, Gelatin Coated	Fluoxetine 20 mg	Prozac by Promex Med	62301-0008	Antidepressant
PROZAC20MG <> DISTA3105	Cap, Gelatin Coated	Fluoxetine 20 mg	Prozac by Heartland	61392-0235	Antidepressant
PROZAC20MG <> DISTA3105	Cap, Green & White	Fluoxetine 20 mg	Prozac by Va Cmop	65243-0031	Antidepressant
PROZAC20MG <> DISTA3105	Cap, Green & White	Fluoxetine 20 mg	Prozac by Eli Lilly	00002-3105	Antidepressant
PROZAC20MG <> DISTA3105	Cap, Green & Yellow, Gelatin	Fluoxetine 20 mg	Prozac by Dista Prod	00777-3105	Antidepressant
PROZAC20MG <> DISTA3105	Cap, Gelatin	Fluoxetine 20 mg	Prozac by Pharmedix	53002-1016	Antidepressant
PROZAC20MG <> DISTA3105	Cap, Gelatin	Fluoxetine 20 mg	by Med Pro	53978-1033	Antidepressant
PROZAC20MG <> DISTA3105	Cap, Gelatin Coated	Fluoxetine 20 mg	Prozac by Allscripts	54569-1732	Antidepressant
PROZAC20MG <> DISTA3106	Cap, Gelatin Coated, Prozac/20 mg <> Dista/3105	Fluoxetine 20 mg	Prozac by Kaiser	00179-1159	Antidepressant
PROZAC40MG <> DISTA3107	Cap, Green & Orange, Opaque	Fluoxetine HCl 40 mg	Prozac by Invamed	52189-0311	Antidepressant
PROZAC40MG DISTA3107	Cap, Green & Orange, Opaque	Fluoxetine 40 mg	Prozac by Dista Prod	00777-3107	Antidepressant
PSA	Tab, White, Oblong, Film Coated	Acetaminophen 300 mg, Phenyltoloxamine Citrate 20 mg, Salicylamide 200 mg	Cetazone T by ABG	60999-0904	Analgesic
PSEARLE930S	Tab, White, Circular	Ethynodiol Diacetate 2 mg	by Searle	Canadian	Oral Contraceptive
PT <> 150	Cap	Chlorpheniramine Maleate 12 mg, Phenylpropanolamine HCl 75 mg	by Kaiser	00179-1136	Cold Remedy
PT <> 150	Cap, Clear, P/T <> 150	Chlorpheniramine Maleate 12 mg, Phenylpropanolamine HCl 75 mg	Drize by Jones	52604-0405	Cold Remedy
PT <> GLYNASE3	Tab, Coated, Glynase 3	Glyburide 3 mg	Glynase Prestab by Thrift Drug	59198-0171	Antidiabetic
PT <> GLYNASE3PT	Tab, Coated, PT <> Glynase 3/PT	Glyburide 3 mg	Glynase by Allscripts	54569-3690	Antidiabetic
PT <> GLYNASE6PT	Tab, Yellow, Scored	Glyburide 6 mg	Glynase by Rightpac	65240-0723	Antidiabetic
PT150	Cap, Ex Release, P/T-150	Chlorpheniramine Maleate 12 mg, Phenylpropanolamine HCl 75 mg	Propade by Kaiser	62224-2444	Cold Remedy
PTGLYNASE3	Tab, Coated, PT <> Glynase 3	Glyburide 3 mg	Glynase Prestab by Quality Care	60346-0513	Antidiabetic
PTP710	Tab, PTP Over 710	Acetaminophen 500 mg, Hydrocodone Bitartrate 10 mg	by Peachtree	62793-0710	Analgesic; C III
PTP710	Tab, PTP/710	Acetaminophen 500 mg, Hydrocodone Bitartrate 10 mg	by D M Graham	00756-0257	Analgesic; C III
PTP775	Tab, PTP Over 775	Acetaminophen 650 mg, Hydrocodone Bitartrate 7.5 mg	by Peachtree	62793-0775	Analgesic; C III
PTPT <> GLYNASE3	Tab, Coated, PT Score PT	Glyburide 3 mg	Glynase Prestab by Amerisource	62584-0352	Antidiabetic
PTPT <> GLYNASE3	Tab, Coated, PT/PT <> Glynase/3	Glyburide 3 mg	Glynase Prestab by Nat Pharmpak Serv	55154-3909	Antidiabetic
PTPT <> GLYNASE3	Tab, Coated	Glyburide 3 mg	Glynase Prestab by Pharmacia & Upjohn	00009-0352	Antidiabetic
PTPT <> GLYNASE3	Tab, Coated, Scored	Glyburide 3 mg	Glynase by Physicians Total Care	54868-3017	Antidiabetic
PTPT <> GLYNASE6	Tab, Coated	Glyburide 6 mg	Glynase Prestabs by Nat Pharmpak Serv	55154-3917	Antidiabetic
PTPT <> GLYNASE6	Tab, Coated, PT/PT <> Glynase 6	Glyburide 6 mg	Glynase Prestabs by Thrift Drug	59198-0003	Antidiabetic
PTPT <> GLYNASE6	Tab, Yellow, Oblong, Scored	Glyburide 6 mg	by Allscripts	54569-4695	Antidiabetic

ID FRONT <> BACK	DESCRIPTION FRONT <> BACK	INGREDIENT & STRENGTH	BRAND (OR EQUIV.) & FIRM	NDC#	CLASS; SCH.
PTPT <> GLYNASE6	Tab, Coated	Glyburide 6 mg	Glynase Prestab by Pharmacia & Upjohn	00009-3449	Antidiabetic
PTPT <> GLYNASE6	Tab, Coated, PT PT <> Glynase over 6	Glyburide 6 mg	Glynase Prestab by Physicians Total Care	54868-3711	Antidiabetic
PU <> 700	Tab	Cabergoline 0.5 mg	Dostinex by Pharmacia & Upjohn	00013-7001	Antiparkinson
PU <> 700	Tab	Cabergoline 0.5 mg	Dostinex by Pharmacia & Upjohn	10829-7001	Antiparkinson
PU <> 700	Tab, White, Cap Shaped, Scored	Cabergoline 0.5 mg	by Pharmacia	Canadian DIN# 02242471	Antiparkinson
PU <> GEIGY	Tab, White w/ Red Specks, Oval, Scored	Carbamazepine 200 mg	Tegretol Chewtabs by Novartis	Canadian DIN# 00665088	Anticonvulsant
PURDUE	Cap, Bluish Green	Dihydrocodeine Bitartrate 16 mg, Acetaminophen 356.4 mg, Caffeine 30 mg	DHCplus by Purdue Pharma		Analgesic
PURINETHOL <> 04A	Tab	Mercaptopurine 50 mg	Purinethol by Catalytica	63552-0807	Antineoplastic
PURINETHOL <> 04A	Tab	Mercaptopurine 50 mg	Purinethol by Glaxo	00173-0807	Antineoplastic
PURINETHOLO4A	Tab, Yellow, Purinethol/O4A	Mercaptopurine 50 mg	by Wyeth-Ayerst	Canadian	Antineoplastic
PURINETHOLO4A	Tab, Yellow, Round	Mercaptopurine 50 mg	Purinethol by Glaxo Wellcome		Antineoplastic
PVK250	Tab, Off-White, Round, Scored, Film Coated	Penicillin 250 mg	Pen Vee K by Geneva	00781-1205	Antibiotic
PVK500	Tab, Off-White, Round, Scored, Film Coated	Penicillin 500 mg	Pen Vee K by Geneva	00781-1655	Antibiotic
Q	Tab, White, Oblong	Anhydrous Cholestyramine Resin 800 mg	Questran by Apothecon		Antihyperlipidemic
Q11 <> LL	Tab, Q Over 11	Quinidine Sulfate 200 mg	by UDL	51079-0031	Antiarrhythmic
Q2542 <> Q2542	Cap, White, Opaque, in Black	Acetaminophen 650 mg, Butalbital 50 mg	by American Pharm	58605-0520	Analgesic
Q2542Q2542	Cap, White, Opaque, Q2542/Q2542	Acetaminophen 650 mg, Butalbital 50 mg	by Alza	17314-9400	Analgesic
QPL114	Tab, Brown, Round, QPL-114	Nystatin Oral 500,000 Units	Mycostatin by Quantum		Antifungal
QPL115Q	Tab, White, Round	Benztropine Mesylate 2 mg	Cogentin by Quantum		Antiparkinson
QPL116Q	Tab, White, Round, QPL-116 Q	Benztropine Mesylate 0.5 mg	Cogentin by Quantum		Antiparkinson
QPL117Q	Tab, White, Oval, QPL-117 Q	Benztropine Mesylate 1 mg	Cogentin by Quantum		Antiparkinson
QPL154	Tab, Maroon, Round	Phenazopyridine HCl 100 mg	Pyridium by Quantum		Urinary Analgesic
QPL155	Tab, Maroon, Round	Phenazopyridine HCl 200 mg	Pyridium by Quantum		Urinary Analgesic
QPL156Q	Tab, White, Round, QPL/156 Q	Lorazepam 0.5 mg	Ativan by Quantum		Sedative/Hypnotic; C IV
QPL157Q	Tab, White, Round, QPL/157 Q	Lorazepam 1 mg	Ativan by Quantum		Sedative/Hypnotic; C IV
QPL158Q	Tab, White, Round, QPL/158 Q	Lorazepam 2 mg	Ativan by Quantum		Sedative/Hypnotic; C IV
QPL171	Tab, Green/Yellow, Round	Meprobamate 200 mg, Aspirin 325 mg	Equagesic by Quantum		Sedative/Hypnotic; C IV
QPL179	Cap, Blue & Clear, QPL-179	Phentermine Resin Complex	Ionamin by Quantum		Anorexiant; C IV
QPL194Q	Tab, White, Round, QPL-194/Q	Haloperidol 0.5 mg	Haldol by Quantum		Antipsychotic
QPL195Q	Tab, Yellow, Round, QPL-195/Q	Haloperidol 1 mg	Haldol by Quantum		Antipsychotic
QPL196Q	Tab, Lavender, Round, QPL-196/Q	Haloperidol 2 mg	Haldol by Quantum		Antipsychotic
QPL197Q	Tab, Green, Round, QPL-197/Q	Haloperidol 5 mg	Haldol by Quantum		Antipsychotic
QPL207	Cap, Green & Yellow, QPL-207	Oxazepam 30 mg	Serax by Quantum		Sedative/Hypnotic; C IV
QPL208	Cap, Green & White, QPL-208	Oxazepam 15 mg	Serax by Quantum		Sedative/Hypnotic; C IV
QPL209	Cap, Green/Black, QPL-209	Oxazepam 10 mg	Serax by Quantum		Sedative/Hypnotic; C IV
QPL212	Tab, Green/Yellow, Round	Meprobamate 200 mg, Aspirin 325 mg	Equagesic by Quantum		Sedative/Hypnotic; C IV
QPL213Q	Tab, White, Round, QPL/213 Q	Trazodone HCl 50 mg	Desyrel by Quantum		Antidepressant
QPL214Q	Tab, White, Round, QPL/214 Q	Trazodone HCl 100 mg	Desyrel by Quantum		Antidepressant
QPL217Q	Tab, White, Round, QPL217/Q	Metoclopramide 10 mg	Reglan by Quantum		Gastrointestinal
QPL2181Q	Tab, White, Round, QPL/2/181 Q	Diazepam 2 mg	Valium by Quantum		Antianxiety; C IV
QPL220Q	Tab, Yellow, Round, QPL-220/Q	Triamterene 75 mg, Hydrochlorothiazide 50 mg	Maxzide by Quantum		Diuretic
QPL225Q	Tab, Blue, Round, QPL-225 Q	Clorazepate Dipotassium 30.75 mg	Tranxene by Quantum		Antianxiety; C IV
QPL226Q	Tab, Peach, Round, QPL-226 Q	Clorazepate Dipotassium 7.5 mg	Tranxene by Quantum		Antianxiety; C IV
QPL227Q	Tab, Lavender, Round, QPL-227 Q	Clorazepate Dipotassium 15 mg	Tranxene by Quantum		Antianxiety; C IV
QPL236Q	Cap, Flesh & Lavender, QPL-236/Q	Fenoprofen Calcium 200 mg	Nalfon by Quantum		NSAID
QPL237Q	Cap, Flesh & Orange, QPL-237/Q	Fenoprofen Calcium 300 mg	Nalfon by Quantum		NSAID

ID FRONT <> BACK	DESCRIPTION FRONT <> BACK	INGREDIENT & STRENGTH	BRAND (OR EQUIV.) & FIRM	NDC#	CLASS; SCH.
QPL238Q	Tab, Peach, QPL-238/Q	Fenoprofen Calcium 600 mg	Nalfon by Quantum		NSAID
QPL242Q	Tab, Green/Yellow, Round, QPL242/Q	Meprobamate 400 mg, Aspirin 325 mg	Equagesic by Quantum		Sedative/Hypnotic; C IV
QPL24325	Tab, White, Round, QPL-243/2.5	Minoxidil 2.5 mg	Loniten by Quantum		Antihypertensive
QPL245Q	Tab, White, Round, QPL/245-Q	Oxybutynin Chloride 5 mg	Ditropan by Quantum		Urinary
QPL270Q	Tab, Pink, Round, QPL-270/Q	Metoclopramide HCl 5 mg	Reglan by Quantum		Gastrointestinal
QPL273Q	Tab, Green, Round, QPL-273/Q	Timolol Maleate 5 mg	Blocadren by Quantum		Antihypertensive
QPL274Q	Tab, Green, Round, QPL-274/Q	Timolol Maleate 10 mg	Blocadren by Quantum		Antihypertensive
QPL275Q	Tab, Green, Round, QPL-275/Q	Timolol Maleate 20 mg	Blocadren by Quantum		Antihypertensive
QUANTUM10183	Tab, Blue, Round, Quantum/10/183	Diazepam 10 mg	Valium by Quantum		Antianxiety; C IV
QUANTUM5182	Tab, Yellow, Round, Quantum/5/182	Diazepam 5 mg	Valium by Quantum		Antianxiety; C IV
QUINIDEX <> AHR	Tab, White, Round	Quinidine Sulfate 300 mg	Quinidex Extentabs by RX PAK	65084-0133	Antiarrhythmic
QUINIDEXAHR	Tab, White, Round	Quinidine Sulfate 300 mg	Quinidex Extend by Wyeth-Ayerst	Canadian	Antiarrhythmic
QUINIDEXAHR	Tab, White, Round	Quinidine Sulfate 300 mg	Quinidex by Rightpac	65240-0728	Antiarrhythmic
QUINIDEXAHR	Tab	Quinidine Sulfate 300 mg	Quindex by A H Robins	00031-6649	Antiarrhythmic
QUINIDEXAHR	Tab, Ex Release	Quinidine Sulfate 300 mg	Quindex by Leiner	59606-0728	Antiarrhythmic
QUINIDEXAHR	Tab, Ex Release, Quinidex over AHR	Quinidine Sulfate 300 mg	Quindex by Amerisource	62584-0649	Antiarrhythmic
QUINIDEXAHR	Tab, Sugar-Coated	Quinidine Sulfate 300 mg	Quindex by Thrift Drug	59198-0098	Antiarrhythmic
QUINIDEXAHR	Tab	Quinidine Sulfate 300 mg	Quindex by Nat Pharmpak Serv	55154-3003	Antiarrhythmic
R	Tab, Compressed, Debossed	Atropine Sulfate 0.0194 mg, Hyoscyamine Sulfate 0.1037 mg, Phenobarbital 16.2 mg, Scopolamine Hydrobromide 0.0065 mg	Donnatal by Leiner	59606-0778	Gastrointestinal; C IV
R	Tab, Coated	Chlorophyllin Copper Complex 100 mg	by Pharm Packaging Ctr	54383-0076	Gastrointestinal
R	Tab, White, Round	Phenobarbital, Hyoscyamine, Atropine, Scopolamine	Donnatal by A.H.Robins		Gastrointestinal; C IV
R <> 023	Tab, White, Round	Aspirin 325 mg, Butalbital 50 mg, Caffeine 40 mg	by Purepac	00228-2023	Analgesic; C III
R <> 026	Tab, White, Round	Phenobarbital 15 mg	by Purepac	00228-2026	Sedative/Hypnotic; C IV
R <> 026	Tab, White, Round, Scored	Phenobarbital 15 mg	by UDL	51079-0094	Sedative/Hypnotic; C IV
R <> 026	Tab	Phenobarbital 17.01 mg	by Vangard	00615-0420	Sedative/Hypnotic; C IV
R <> 027	Tab, White, Round, Scored	Alprazolam 0.25 mg	by Purepac	00228-2027	Antianxiety; C IV
R <> 028	Tab, White, Round, Scored	Phenobarbital 30 mg		51079-0095	Sedative/Hypnotic; C IV
R <> 028	Tab, White, Round, Scored	Phenobarbital 30 mg	by Purepac	00228-2028	Sedative/Hypnotic; C IV
R <> 028	Tab	Phenobarbital 30 mg	by Vangard	00615-0421	Sedative/Hypnotic; C IV
R <> 029	Tab, Peach, Round, Scored	Alprazolam 0.5 mg	by Purepac	00228-2029	Antianxiety; C IV
R <> 031	Tab, Blue, Round, Scored	Alprazolam 1 mg	by Purepac	00228-2031	Antianxiety; C IV
R <> 051	Tab, White, Round, Scored	Diazepam 2 mg	by Purepac	00228-2051	Antianxiety; C IV
R <> 052	Tab, Yellow, Round, Scored	Diazepam 5 mg	by Purepac	00228-2052	Antianxiety; C IV
R <> 052	Tab	Diazepam 5 mg	by Urgent Care Ctr	50716-0132	Antianxiety; C IV
R <> 053	Tab, Blue, Round, Scored	Diazepam 10 mg	by Purepac	00228-2053	Antianxiety; C IV
R <> 063	Tab, White, Round	Lorazepam 2 mg	by Purepac	00228-2063	Sedative/Hypnotic; C IV
R <> 085	Tab, Pink, Cap Shaped, Film Coated	Acetaminophen 650 mg, Propoxyphene Napsylate 100 mg	by Purepac	00228-2085	Analgesic; C IV
R <> 127	Tab, Orange, Round	Clonidine HCl 0.1 mg	by Purepac	00228-2127	Antihypertensive
R <> 143	Tab	Carbamazepine 200 mg	by Vangard	00615-3505	Anticonvulsant
R <> 143	Tab, White, Round	Carbamazepine 200 mg	by Purepac	00228-2143	Anticonvulsant
R <> 183	Tab, Coated	Dipyridamole 50 mg	by Vangard	00615-1573	Antiplatelet
R <> 221	Tab, Peach, Round, Scored	Hydrochlorothiazide 25 mg	by Purepac	00228-2221	Diuretic
R <> 222	Tab, Peach, Round, Scored	Hydrochlorothiazide 50 mg	by Purepac	00228-2222	Diuretic
R <> 269	Tab, White, Round, Scored	Metoclopramide HCl 10 mg	Reglan by UDL	51079-0283	Gastrointestinal
R <> 269	Tab, White, Round, Scored	Metoclopramide HCl 10 mg	by Purepac	00228-2269	Gastrointestinal
R <> 27	Tab, Orange, Round	Propranolol HCl 10 mg	by Purepac	00228-2327	Antihypertensive
R <> 321	Tab, Pink, Round	Propranolol HCl 60 mg	by Purepac	00228-2321	Antihypertensive
R <> 333	Tab, Yellow, Round	Propranolol HCl 80 mg	by Purepac	00228-2333	Antihypertensive
R <> 337	Tab, Peach, Round	Prednisone 20 mg	by Purepac	00228-2337	Steroid
R <> 338	Tab, White, Round	Prednisone 10 mg	by Purepac	00228-2338	Steroid
R <> 34625	Tab, Film Coated, Royce Logo, <> 346 25	Hydroxyzine HCl 25 mg	by Quality Care	60346-0086	Antihistamine

ID FRONT <> BACK	DESCRIPTION FRONT <> BACK	INGREDIENT & STRENGTH	BRAND (OR EQUIV) & FIRM	NDC#	CLASS, SCH.
R <> 348	Tab, White, Round, Scored	Propylthiouracil 50 mg	by Purepac	00228-2348	Antithyroid
R <> 4382	Cap, R in a Diamond	Propoxyphene HCl 65 mg	by Teva	00093-0741	Analgesic; C IV
R <> 439	Tab	Trazodone HCl 50 mg	by UDL	51079-0427	Antidepressant
R <> 439	Tab, White, Round, Film Coated	Trazodone HCl 50 mg	by Vangard	00615-2578	Antidepressant
R <> 439	Tab, Coated	Trazodone HCl 50 mg	by Purepac	00228-2439	Antidepressant
R <> 441	Tab, White, Round, Film Coated	Trazodone HCl 100 mg	by Purepac	00228-2441	Antidepressant
R <> 441	Tab	Trazodone HCl 100 mg	by UDL	51079-0428	Antidepressant
R <> 441	Tab, Coated	Trazodone HCl 100 mg	by Vangard	00615-2579	Antidepressant
R <> 473	Tab, White, Round, Bisected, Film Coated	Verapamil HCl 80 mg	by Purepac	00228-2473	Antihypertensive
R <> 475	Tab, White, Round, Bisected, Film Coated	Verapamil HCl 120 mg	by Purepac	00228-2475	Antihypertensive
R <> 480	Tab, White, Oval, Film Coated	Tolmetin Sodium 600 mg	by Purepac	00228-2480	NSAID
R <> 538	Tab, Mottled Dark Blue, Round, Scored	Carbidopa 10 mg, Levodopa 100 mg	by Purepac	00228-2538	Antiparkinson
R <> 538	Tab	Carbidopa 10 mg, Levodopa 100 mg	by Murfreesboro	51129-1301	Antiparkinson
R <> 539	Tab, Mottled Yellow, Round, Scored	Carbidopa 25 mg, Levodopa 100 mg	by Purepac	00228-2539	Antiparkinson
R <> 540	Tab, Mottled Light Blue, Round, Scored	Carbidopa 25 mg, Levodopa 250 mg	by Purepac	00228-2540	Antiparkinson
R <> 540	Tab	Carbidopa 25 mg, Levodopa 250 mg	by Murfreesboro	51129-1292	Antiparkinson
R <> 545	Tab, R <> Purepac Logo 545	Diflunisal 250 mg	by Purepac	00228-2545	NSAID
R <> 550	Tab, White, Round, Enteric Coated	Diclofenac Sodium 50 mg	DR by Purepac	00228-2550	NSAID
R <> 551	Tab, White, Round, Enteric Coated	Diclofenac Sodium 75 mg	DR by Purepac	00228-2551	NSAID
R <> 554	Tab, Film Coated	Metoprolol Tartrate 50 mg	by Vangard	00615-3552	Antihypertensive
R <> 57	Tab, White, Round, Coated	Lorazepam 0.5 mg	by Purepac	00228-2057	Sedative/Hypnotic; C IV
R <> 57	Tab, Engraved, Coated	Lorazepam 0.5 mg	by Kaiser	00179-1174	Sedative/Hypnotic; C IV
R <> 571	Tab, White, Round, Coated	Indapamide 2.5 mg	by Purepac	00228-2571	Diuretic
R <> 59	Tab, White, Round, Scored	Lorazepam 0.5 mg	by Allscripts	54569-2687	Sedative/Hypnotic; C IV
R <> 59	Tab, White, Round	Lorazepam 1 mg	by Purepac	00228-2059	Sedative/Hypnotic; C IV
R <> 597	Tab, Orange, Round, Coated	Indapamide 1.25 mg	by Purepac	00228-2597	Diuretic
R <> 606	Tab, White, Round, Purepac Logo, Scrolled P with Arm Extension	Acyclovir 400 mg	by Purepac	00228-2606	Antiviral
R <> 611	Tab, Purepac Logo, Film Coated	Pentoxifylline 400 mg	by Murfreesboro	51129-1121	Anticoagulant
R <> 611	Tab, Yellow, Oblong, Film Coated	Pentoxifylline 400 mg	ER by Purepac	00228-2611	Anticoagulant
R <> 613	Tab, White, Oval, Film Coated	Ticlopidine HCl 250 mg	by Purepac	00228-2613	Anticoagulant
R <> 617	Tab, Yellow, Cap Shaped, Black Print	Naproxen 375 mg	DR by Purepac	00228-2617	NSAID
R <> 618	Tab, Yellow, Cap Shaped, Black Print	Naproxen 500 mg	DR by Purepac	00228-2618	NSAID
R <> 63	Tab, White, Round, Scored	Lorazepam 2 mg	by Compumed	00403-0012	Sedative/Hypnotic; C IV
R <> 650	Tab, Yellow, Cap Shaped, Film Coated	Bisoprolol Fumarate 2.5 mg, Hydrochlorothiazide 6.25 mg	by Purepac	00228-2650	Antihypertensive; Diuretic
R <> 651	Tab, Pink, Cap Shaped, Film Coated	Bisoprolol Fumarate 5 mg, Hydrochlorothiazide 6.25 mg	by Purepac	00228-2651	Antihypertensive; Diuretic
R <> 652	Tab, White, Cap Shaped, Film Coated	Bisoprolol Fumarate 10 mg, Hydrochlorothiazide 6.25 mg	by Purepac	00228-2652	Antihypertensive; Diuretic
R <> 7	Tab, Orange, Octagon-Shaped, Film	Indapamide 1.25 mg	Lozol by Murfreesboro	51129-1538	Diuretic
R <> 7	Tab, Film Coated	Indapamide 1.25 mg	Lozol by Thrift Drug	59198-0263	Diuretic
R <> 7	Tab, Film Coated	Indapamide 1.25 mg	Lozol by Amerisource	62584-0700	Diuretic
R <> 7	Tab, Orange, Octagon-Shaped, Film Coated	Indapamide 1.25 mg	Lozol by RPR	00801-0700	Diuretic
R <> 7	Tab, Film Coated	Indapamide 1.25 mg	Lozol by RPR	00075-0700	Diuretic
R <> 704	Tab, Green, Cap Shaped, Film Coated	Fluvoxamine Maleate 25 mg	by Purepac	00228-2704	OCD
R <> 8	Tab, Film Coated	Indapamide 2.5 mg	Lozol by RPR	00075-0082	Diuretic
R <> 8	Tab, Film Coated	Indapamide 2.5 mg	Lozol by Nat Pharmpak Serv	55154-4011	Diuretic
R <> 8	Tab, Film Coated	Indapamide 2.5 mg	Lozol by Drug Distr	52985-0062	Diuretic
R <> 8	Tab, Film Coated	Indapamide 2.5 mg	Lozol by Allscripts	54569-0579	Diuretic
R <> 8	Tab, Film Coated	Indapamide 2.5 mg	Lozol by Thrift Drug	59198-0174	Diuretic
R <> 8	Tab, Film Coated	Indapamide 2.5 mg	Lozol by Pharm Utilization	60491-0382	Diuretic
R <> 8	Tab, White, Octagon-Shaped, Film Coated	Indapamide 2.5 mg	Lozol by RPR	00801-0082	Diuretic

ID FRONT <> BACK	DESCRIPTION FRONT <> BACK	INGREDIENT & STRENGTH	BRAND (OR EQUIV.) & FIRM	NDC#	CLASS; SCH.
R 3487	Cap, Chelsea Logo	Chlordiazepoxide HCl 25 mg	by Quality Care	60346-0260	Antianxiety; C IV
R001 <> 3	Tab	Acetaminophen 300 mg, Codeine Phosphate 30 mg	by Purepac	00228-2001	Analgesic; C III
R001 <> 3	Tab	Acetaminophen 300 mg, Codeine Phosphate 30 mg	by Vangard	00615-0430	Analgesic; C III
R001 <> 3	Tab, Purepac Logo	Acetaminophen 300 mg, Codeine Phosphate 30 mg	by Pharmedix	53002-0101	Analgesic; C III
R0013	Tab	Acetaminophen 300 mg, Codeine 30 mg	by Zenith Goldline	00182-0948	Analgesic; C III
R0013	Tab	Acetaminophen 300 mg, Codeine Phosphate 30 mg	by Allscripts	54569-0025	Analgesic; C III
R003 <> 4	Tab	Acetaminophen 300 mg, Codeine Phosphate 60 mg	by Purepac	00228-2003	Analgesic; C III
R0034	Tab	Acetaminophen 300 mg, Codeine 60 mg	by Zenith Goldline	00182-1338	Analgesic; C III
R0034	Tab, White, Round	Acetaminophen 300 mg, Codeine Phosphate 60 mg	by Allscripts	54569-0302	Analgesic; C III
R012	Cap, Green	Chloral Hydrate 500 mg	Noctec by Rondex		Sedative/Hypnotic; C IV
R012	Tab, White, Round	Meprobamate 200 mg	Miltown by Rondex		Sedative/Hypnotic; C IV
R016	Tab, White, Round	Meprobamate 200 mg	Miltown by Purepac		Sedative/Hypnotic; C IV
R018	Tab, White, Round	Meprobamate 400 mg	Miltown by Purepac		Sedative/Hypnotic; C IV
R021	Cap, Blue & White	Flurazepam HCl 15 mg	by Purepac	00228-2021	Hypnotic; C IV
R022	Cap, Blue	Flurazepam HCl 30 mg	by Purepac	00228-2022	Hypnotic; C IV
R027	Tab	Alprazolam 0.25 mg	by Zenith Goldline	00182-0027	Antianxiety; C IV
R028	Tab, R 028	Phenobarbital 30 mg	by Heartland	61392-0391	Sedative/Hypnotic; C IV
R029	Tab	Alprazolam 0.5 mg	by Zenith Goldline	00182-0028	Antianxiety; C IV
R031	Tab	Alprazolam 1 mg	by Zenith Goldline	00182-0029	Antianxiety; C IV
R039	Tab	Alprazolam 2 mg	by Zenith Goldline	00182-0030	Antianxiety; C IV
R039	Tab, Yellow, Rectangular, Scored	Alprazolam 2 mg	by Purepac	00228-2039	Antianxiety; C IV
R051	Tab, White, Round	Diazepam 2 mg	by Purepac	00228-2051	Antianxiety; C IV
R052	Tab, Yellow, Round	Diazepam 5 mg	by Purepac	00228-2052	Antianxiety; C IV
R052	Tab	Diazepam 5 mg	by Allscripts	54569-0949	Antianxiety; C IV
R053	Tab, Purepac Logo	Diazepam 10 mg	by HJ Harkins Co	52959-0306	Antianxiety; C IV
R053	Tab, Blue	Diazepam 10 mg	by Purepac	00228-2053	Antianxiety; C IV
R067	Cap, Pink, Opaque	Oxazepam 10 mg	by PF	48692-0031	Sedative/Hypnotic; C IV
R067	Cap, Pink, Opaque	Oxazepam 10 mg	by Purepac	00228-2067	Sedative/Hypnotic; C IV
R067	Cap, R 067	Oxazepam 10 mg	by Direct Dispensing	57866-6970	Sedative/Hypnotic; C IV
R069	Cap, Red, Opaque	Oxazepam 15 mg	by Purepac	00228-2069	Sedative/Hypnotic; C IV
R073	Cap, Maroon, Opaque	Oxazepam 30 mg	by Purepac	00228-2073	Sedative/Hypnotic; C IV
R076	Cap	Temazepam 15 mg	Tem by Zenith Goldline	00182-1822	Sedative/Hypnotic; C IV
R076	Cap, Green & White, Opaque	Temazepam 15 mg	Tem by Purepac	00228-2076	Sedative/Hypnotic; C IV
R076	Cap, Green & White, R-076	Temazepam 15 mg	by Allscripts	54569-0905	Sedative/Hypnotic; C IV
R076 <> R076	Cap	Temazepam 15 mg	by UDL	51079-0418	Sedative/Hypnotic; C IV
R077	Cap, White	Temazepam 30 mg	by Direct Dispensing	57866-4629	Sedative/Hypnotic; C IV
R077	Cap, White, Opaque	Temazepam 30 mg	Tem by Purepac	00228-2077	Sedative/Hypnotic; C IV
R077	Cap	Temazepam 30 mg	Tem by Zenith Goldline	00182-1823	Sedative/Hypnotic; C IV
R077 <> R077	Cap	Temazepam 30 mg	Tem by UDL	51079-0419	Sedative/Hypnotic; C IV
R078	Tab, Blue, Round	Clorazepate Dipotassium 30.75 mg	Tranxene by Purepac		Antianxiety; C IV
R081	Tab, Peach, Round	Clorazepate Dipotassium 7.5 mg	Tranxene by Purepac		Antianxiety; C IV
R082	Cap, Pink	Propoxyphene HCl 65 mg	Darvon 65 by Purepac		Analgesic; C IV
R083	Tab, Pink, Round	Clorazepate Dipotassium 15 mg	Tranxene by Purepac		Antianxiety; C IV
R085	Tab, Coated, Purepac Logo	Acetaminophen 650 mg, Propoxyphene Napsylate 100 mg	by Rugby	00536-4361	Analgesic; C IV
R085	Tab, Pink, Cap Shaped, Film Coated	Acetaminophen 650 mg, Propoxyphene Napsylate 100 mg	by Purepac	00228-2085	Analgesic; C IV
R085	Tab, Coated, Purepac Logo	Acetaminophen 650 mg, Propoxyphene Napsylate 100 mg	Propoxacet N by Quality Care	60346-0628	Analgesic; C IV
R085	Tab, Coated, Purepac Logo 085	Acetaminophen 650 mg, Propoxyphene Napsylate 100 mg	by Urgent Care Ctr	50716-0364	Analgesic; C IV
R085	Tab, Pink, Cap-Shaped, Film Coated	Propoxyphene Hapslate 100 mg, Acetaminophen 650 mg	by Purepac		Analgesic; C IV
R1	Tab, R/1	Chlorpheniramine Tannate 8 mg, Phenylephrine Tannate 25 mg	Ricobid by Teral	51234-0154	Cold Remedy
R1 <> JANSSEN	Tab, White	Risperidone 1 mg	Risperdal by Va Cmop	65243-0061	Antipsychotic
R1 <> JANSSEN	Tab, White, Coated, Oblong, R/1	Risperidone 1 mg	Risperdal by Janssen	50458-0300	Antipsychotic
R1 <> JANSSEN	Tab, Coated	Risperidone 1 mg	Risperdal by Johnson & Johnson	59604-0300	Antipsychotic

ID FRONT <> BACK	DESCRIPTION FRONT <> BACK	INGREDIENT & STRENGTH	BRAND (OR EQUIV.) & FIRM	NDC#	CLASS; SCH.
R10	Tab, Black, Round	Charcoal	by Requa	10961-0010	Gastrointestinal
R102	Tab, White, Round	Allopurinol 100 mg	Zyloprim by Purepac		Antigout
R103	Tab, Peach, Round	Allopurinol 300 mg	Zyloprim by Purepac		Antigout
R11	Tab, Blue, Round	Verapamil 40 mg	Isoptin by Rugby		Antihypertensive
R1103	Tab, White, Round	Acetaminophen 325 mg	Tylenol by Purepac		Antipyretic
R111	Tab, White, Oval	Ibuprofen 800 mg	Motrin by Purepac		NSAID
R118	Tab, White, Round	Belladonna Alkaloids, Phenobarbital	by Purepac		Gastrointestinal; C IV
R124	Tab, White, Round	Ibuprofen 400 mg	Motrin by Purepac		NSAID
R125	Tab, White, Oval	Ibuprofen 600 mg	Motrin by Purepac		NSAID
R127	Tab, R=Purepac Logo	Clonidine HCl 0.1 mg	by Golden State	60429-0050	Antihypertensive
R127	Tab	Clonidine HCl 0.1 mg	by Heartland	61392-0513	Antihypertensive
R127	Tab, Purepac Logo	Clonidine HCl 0.1 mg	by PDRX	55289-0073	Antihypertensive
R127	Tab, Orange, Round, Scored	Clonidine HCl 0.1 mg	by Purepac	00228-2127	Antihypertensive
R127	Tab	Clonidine HCl 0.1 mg	by Vangard	00615-2572	Antihypertensive
R127	Tab	Clonidine HCl 0.1 mg	by Qualitest	00603-2954	Antihypertensive
R127	Tab, R/127	Clonidine HCl 0.1 mg	by Allscripts	54569-0478	Antihypertensive
R128	Tab, Purepac Logo 128	Clonidine HCl 0.2 mg	by Quality Care	60346-0787	Antihypertensive
R128	Tab, R=Purepac Logo	Clonidine HCl 0.2 mg	by Golden State	60429-0051	Antihypertensive
R128	Tab	Clonidine HCl 0.2 mg	by Heartland	61392-0516	Antihypertensive
R128	Tab, Orange, Round, Scored	Clonidine HCl 0.2 mg	by Purepac	00228-2128	Antihypertensive
R128	Tab	Clonidine HCl 0.2 mg	by Qualitest	00603-2955	Antihypertensive
R128	Tab, Purepac Logo	Clonidine HCl 0.2 mg	by Allscripts	54569-1853	Antihypertensive
R128	Tab	Clonidine HCl 0.3 mg	by Heartland	61392-0519	Antihypertensive
R129	Tab, Orange, Round	Clonidine HCl 0.3 mg	by Allscripts	54569-2801	Antihypertensive
R129	Tab	Clonidine HCl 0.3 mg	by Qualitest	00603-2956	Antihypertensive
R129	Tab, Orange, Round, Scored	Clonidine HCl 0.3 mg	by Purepac	00228-2129	Antihypertensive
R133	Tab, Coated	Amitriptyline HCl 50 mg	by Purepac	00228-2133	Antidepressant
R134	Tab, Coated	Amitriptyline HCl 75 mg	by Purepac	00228-2134	Antidepressant
R135	Tab, Coated	Amitriptyline HCl 100 mg	by Purepac	00228-2135	Antidepressant
R143	Tab, Coated, Purepac Logo	Carbamazepine 200 mg	by PDRX	55289-0210	Anticonvulsant
R147	Tab, Blue, Oblong	Prenatal Vitamins	Pramet FA by Ross		Vitamin
R1507	Tab, White, Round	Quinine Sulfate 200 mg	by Purepac		Antimalarial
R1511	Tab, White, Round	Quinine Sulfate 325 mg	by Purepac		Antimalarial
R161	Tab, Yellow, Round	Chlorthalidone 25 mg	Hygroton by Purepac		Diuretic
R163	Tab, Green, Round	Chlorthalidone 50 mg	Hygroton by Purepac		Diuretic
R176	Tab, Pink, Round	Digitoxin 0.1 mg	Crystodigin by Purepac		Cardiac Agent
R178	Tab, White, Round	Digitoxin 0.2 mg	Crystodigin by Purepac		Cardiac Agent
R185	Tab, White, Round	Dipyridamole 75 mg	Persantine by Purepac		Antiplatelet
R191	Cap, Clear & Pink, R/191	Diphenhydramine HCl 25 mg	by Pharmascience	Canadian	Antihistamine
R191	Cap, Clear & Pink	Diphenhydramine HCl 25 mg	Benadryl by Purepac		Antihistamine
R192	Cap, Pink, R/192	Diphenhydramine HCl 50 mg	by Pharmascience	Canadian	Antihistamine
R192	Cap, Pink	Diphenhydramine HCl 50 mg	Benadryl by Purepac		Antihistamine
R193	Tab, White, Round	Dipyridamole 25 mg	Persantine by Purepac		Antiplatelet
R194	Cap, Aqua & White	Doxycycline Hyclate 50 mg	Vibramycin by Purepac		Antibiotic
R195	Cap, Blue	Doxycycline Hyclate 100 mg	Vibramycin by Purepac		Antibiotic
R2	Tab, Ex Release, R/2	Guaifenesin 600 mg, Phenylephrine HCl 15 mg	Numonyl Sr by Sovereign	58716-0629	Cold Remedy
R2	Tab, Yellow, Round	Isosorbide Dinitrate SL 2.5 mg	Isordil by Rugby		Antianginal
R2 <> JANSSEN	Tab, Coated	Risperidone 2 mg	Risperdal by Janssen	50458-0320	Antipsychotic
R2 <> JANSSEN	Tab, Coated	Risperidone 2 mg	Risperdal by Johnson & Johnson	59604-0320	Antipsychotic
R20 <> 3	Tab, White, Round	Acetaminophen 300 mg, Codeine Phosphate 30 mg	by Purepac		Analgesic; C III
R20 <> 3	Tab, White, Round	Acetaminophen 300 mg, Codeine Phosphate 30 mg	by Purepac	00228-3020	Analgesic; C III
R203	Tab, White, Round	Acetaminophen 300 mg; Codeine Phosphate 30 mg	by Heartland Hlthcare	61392-0714	Analgesic; C III

ID FRONT ⟷ BACK	DESCRIPTION FRONT ⟷ BACK	INGREDIENT & STRENGTH	BRAND (OR EQUIV.) & FIRM	NDC#	CLASS; SCH.
R204	Tab, Pink, Round	Erythromycin Stearate 250 mg	Erythrocin by Purepac		Antibiotic
R21 ⟷ 4	Tab, White, Round	Acetaminophen 300 mg, Codeine Phosphate 60 mg	by Purepac	00228-3021	Analgesic; C III
R210	Tab, Yellow, Round	Folic Acid 1 mg	Folvite by Purepac		Vitamin
R212	Tab, White, Round, R/212	Hydrocortisone 10 mg	Hydrocortone by Rondex		Steroid
R212	Tab, White, Round	Hydrocortisone 10 mg	Hydrocortone by Purepac		Steroid
R214	Tab, White, Round, R 21/4	Acetaminophen 300 mg, Codeine Phosphate 60 mg	by Purepac		Analgesic; C III
R214	Tab, White, Round	Hydrocortisone 20 mg	Hydrocortone by Purepac		Steroid
R219	Tab, Green, Round	Hydralazine HCl 25 mg	Apresoline by Purepac		Antihypertensive
R220	Tab, Green, Round	Hydralazine HCl 50 mg	Apresoline by Purepac		Antihypertensive
R221	Tab, Peach, Round, Scored	Hydrochlorothiazide 25 mg	by HJ Harkins	52959-0132	Diuretic
R222	Tab, R/222	Hydrochlorothiazide 50 mg	by Allscripts	54569-0549	Diuretic
R227	Tab, Salmon, Round	Hydrochlorothiazide 15 mg, Reserpine 0.1 mg, Hydralazine 25 mg	Ser- by Rondex		Diuretic; Antihypertensive
R247	Tab, White, Round	Methocarbamol 500 mg	Robaxin by Purepac		Muscle Relaxant
R249	Tab, White, Oblong	Methocarbamol 750 mg	Robaxin by Purepac		Muscle Relaxant
R253	Tab, Beige, Round	Methyldopa 250 mg	Aldomet by Rondex		Antihypertensive
R253	Tab, White, Round	Methyldopa 250 mg	Aldomet by Purepac		Antihypertensive
R255	Tab, White, Round	Methyldopa 500 mg	Aldomet by Purepac		Antihypertensive
R255	Tab, Beige, Oblong	Methyldopa 500 mg	Aldomet by Rondex		Antihypertensive
R25710	Tab, Coated	Cyclobenzaprine HCl 10 mg	by Zenith Goldline	00182-1919	Muscle Relaxant
R2577	Cap, Blue & Green	Diltiazem HCl 180 mg	by Heartland Healthcare	61392-0962	Antihypertensive
R2577	Cap, Aqua Blue & Dark Green	Diltiazem HCl 180 mg	by Purepac	00228-2577	Antihypertensive
R2578	Cap, Green	Diltiazem HCl 240 mg	by Heartland Hlthcare	61392-0963	Antihypertensive
R2578	Cap, Dark Green	Diltiazem HCl 240 mg	by Purepac	00228-2578	Antihypertensive
R2579	Cap, Green	Diltiazem HCl 300 mg	by Heartland Healthcare	61392-0964	Antihypertensive
R2579	Cap, Dark Green & Light Gray	Diltiazem HCl 300 mg	by Purepac	00228-2579	Antihypertensive
R2588	Cap, Gray	Diltiazem HCl 120 mg	by Heartland Healthcare	61392-0961	Antihypertensive
R2588	Cap, Light Gray	Diltiazem HCl 120 mg	by Purepac	00228-2588	Antihypertensive
R2598	Cap, Clear & Yellow	Doxycycline Hyclate Delayed Release 100 mg	Doryx by Faulding		Antibiotic
R2598	Cap, White	Doxycycline Hyclate 100 mg	by Faulding Pharms (AS)	50546-0470	Antibiotic
R261	Tab, Tan, Round	Methyldopa 250 mg, Hydrochlorothiazide 15 mg	Aldoril 15 by Purepac		Antihypertensive
R263	Tab, White, Round	Methyldopa 250 mg, Hydrochlorothiazide 25 mg	Aldoril 25 by Purepac		Antihypertensive
R265	Tab, Tan, Oval	Methyldopa 500 mg, Hydrochlorothiazide 30 mg	Aldoril by Purepac		Antihypertensive
R267	Tab, White, Oval	Methyldopa 500 mg, Hydrochlorothiazide 50 mg	Aldoril by Purepac		Antihypertensive
R269	Tab	Metoclopramide HCl 10 mg	by Med Pro	53978-5011	Gastrointestinal
R269	Tab	Metoclopramide HCl 10 mg	by Heartland	61392-0558	Gastrointestinal
R27	Tab	Propranolol HCl 10 mg	by Med Pro	53978-0034	Antihypertensive
R27	Tab	Propranolol HCl 10 mg	by Heartland	61392-0420	Antihypertensive
R276	Tab, White, Round	Reserpine 0.25 mg	Serpasil by Rondex		Antihypertensive
R278	Cap, Yellow	Oxytetracycline 250 mg	Terramycin by Rondex		Antibiotic
R280	Tab, Yellow, Round	Haloperidol 1 mg	Haldol by Purepac		Antipsychotic
R281	Tab, Pink, Round	Haloperidol 2 mg	Haldol by Purepac		Antipsychotic
R282	Tab, Green, Round	Haloperidol 5 mg	Haldol by Purepac		Antipsychotic
R286	Tab, Aqua, Round	Haloperidol 10 mg	Haldol by Purepac		Antipsychotic
R287	Tab, Salmon, Round	Haloperidol 20 mg	Haldol by Purepac		Antipsychotic
R289	Tab, White, Round	Haloperidol 0.5 mg	Haldol by Purepac		Antipsychotic
R29	Tab	Propranolol HCl 20 mg	by Purepac	00228-2329	Antihypertensive
R29	Tab	Propranolol HCl 20 mg	by Med Pro	53978-5014	Antihypertensive
R29	Tab, R/29	Propranolol HCl 20 mg	by Allscripts	54569-0559	Antihypertensive
R29	Tab	Propranolol HCl 20 mg	by Heartland	61392-0423	Antihypertensive
R292	Cap, Brown & Clear	Papaverine HCl SR 150 mg	Pavabid by Purepac		Vasodilator
R296	Tab, White, Round	Penicillin G Potassium 200,000 Units	Pentids by Rondex		Antibiotic

ID FRONT <> BACK	DESCRIPTION FRONT <> BACK	INGREDIENT & STRENGTH	BRAND (OR EQUIV.) & FIRM	NDC#	CLASS; SCH.
R3 <> JANSSEN	Tab, Coated	Risperidone 3 mg	Risperdal by Janssen	50458-0330	Antipsychotic
R3 <> JANSSEN	Tab, Coated	Risperidone 3 mg	Risperdal by Johnson & Johnson	59604-0330	Antipsychotic
R303 <> 325	Cap	Quinine Sulfate 325 mg	by Zenith Goldline	00172-4172	Antimalarial
R31	Tab, Coated	Amitriptyline HCl 10 mg	by Heartland	61392-0143	Antidepressant
R31	Tab, Coated	Amitriptyline HCl 10 mg	by Purepac	00228-2131	Antidepressant
R316	Tab, White, Oblong, Scored	Phentermine HCl 37.5 mg	by Allscripts	54569-4860	Anorexiant; C IV
R316	Tab, White, Cap-Shaped, Scored	Phentermine HCl 37.5 mg	by Purepac	00228-3016	Anorexiant; C IV
R317	Tab, Yellow, Cap Shaped, Scored, Coated	Fenoprofen Calcium 600 mg	by Purepac	00228-2317	NSAID
R317	Tab, Film Coated	Fenoprofen Calcium 691.8 mg	by Quality Care	60346-0233	NSAID
R317	Tab	Fenoprofen Calcium 691.8 mg	by Pharmedix	53002-0367	NSAID
R32	Tab, Film Coated	Amitriptyline HCl 25 mg	by Heartland	61392-0140	Antidepressant
R32	Tab, Film Coated	Amitriptyline HCl 25 mg	by Purepac	00228-2132	Antidepressant
R33	Tab, Red-Brown, Coated	Amitriptyline HCl 50 mg	by Heartland	61392-0141	Antidepressant
R33	Tab, R=Purepac Logo	Clonazepam 0.5 mg	by Golden State	60429-0524	Anticonvulsant; C IV
R33	Tab, Pink, Round, Scored	Clonazepam 0.5 mg	by Purepac	00228-3003	Anticonvulsant; C IV
R330	Tab, White, Round	Penicillin V Potassium 500 mg	V-Cillin K by Rondex		Antibiotic
R331	Tab, Green, Round	Propranolol HCl 40 mg	by Purepac	00228-2331	Antihypertensive
R331	Tab	Propranolol HCl 40 mg	by Allscripts	54569-0561	Antihypertensive
R331	Tab	Propranolol HCl 40 mg	by Prepackage Spec	58864-0431	Antihypertensive
R331	Tab	Propranolol HCl 40 mg	by Heartland	61392-0430	Antihypertensive
R336	Tab, White, Round	Prednisone 5 mg	Deltasone by Purepac		Steroid
R34	Tab, Yellow, Round, Scored	Clonazepam 1 mg	by Purepac	00228-3004	Anticonvulsant; C IV
R34	Tab, R=Purepac Logo	Clonazepam 1 mg	by Golden State	60429-0525	Anticonvulsant; C IV
R34	Tab, Yellow, Round, Scored	Clonazepam 1 mg	by Southwood Pharms	58016-0186	Anticonvulsant; C IV
R346	Cap, Orange	Procainamide HCl 500 mg	Pronestyl by Rondex		Antiarrhythmic
R3487	Cap, Rugby 3487	Chlordiazepoxide HCl 5 mg	by Rugby	00536-3487	Antianxiety; C IV
R3487	Cap, R in a Diamond-Shape	Chlordiazepoxide HCl 5 mg	by Chelsea	46193-0944	Antianxiety; C IV
R3488	Cap, R inside of a Diamond-Shape	Chlordiazepoxide HCl 10 mg	by Quality Care	60346-0052	Antianxiety; C IV
R3488	Cap, Rugby 3488	Chlordiazepoxide HCl 10 mg	by Rugby	00536-3488	Antianxiety; C IV
R3488	Cap	Chlordiazepoxide HCl 10 mg	by Chelsea	46193-0945	Antianxiety; C IV
R3489	Cap, R in a Diamond Shape	Chlordiazepoxide HCl 25 mg	by Rugby	00536-3489	Antianxiety; C IV
R3489	Cap	Chlordiazepoxide HCl 25 mg	by Chelsea	46193-0946	Antianxiety; C IV
R35	Tab, R=Purepac Symbol	Clonazepam 2 mg	by Golden State	60429-0526	Anticonvulsant; C IV
R35	Tab, White, Round, Scored	Clonazepam 2 mg	by Purepac	00228-3005	Anticonvulsant; C IV
R356	Tab, White, Round	Quinidine Sulfate 200 mg	by Purepac		Antiarrhythmic
R358	Tab, White, Round, Scored	Hydrochlorothiazide 25 mg, Propranolol HCl 40 mg	by Purepac	00228-2358	Diuretic; Antihypertensive
R360	Tab, White, Round, Scored	Hydrochlorothiazide 25 mg, Propranolol HCl 80 mg	by Purepac	00228-2360	Diuretic; Antihypertensive
R368	Tab, Red, Round	Rauwolfia Serpentina 50 mg	Raudixin by Purepac		Antihypertensive
R370	Tab, Red, Round	Rauwolfia Serpentina 100 mg	Raudixin by Purepac		Antihypertensive
R374	Tab, White, Round	Reserpine 0.1 mg	Serpasil by Purepac		Antihypertensive
R376	Tab, White, Round	Reserpine 0.25 mg	Serpasil by Purepac		Antihypertensive
R386	Tab, White, Round	Sulfisoxazole 500 mg	Gantrisin by Purepac		Antibiotic
R388	Tab, White, Round	Spironolactone 25 mg	Aldactone by Purepac		Diuretic
R390	Cap, White, Round	Spironolactone 25 mg, Hydrochlorothiazide 25 mg	Aldactazide by Purepac		Diuretic
R3924	Cap	Butalbital 50 mg, Aspirin 40 mg, Caffeine 325 mg	Fiorinal by Rugby		Analgesic
R397	Cap, Green	Doxepin HCl 75 mg	Sinequan by Purepac		Antidepressant
R398	Cap, Green & White	Doxepin HCl 100 mg	Sinequan by Purepac		Antidepressant
R4	Tab, Ex Release, R-4	Guaifenesin 675 mg	Numobid by Sovereign	58716-0607	Expectorant
R4 <> JANSSEN	Tab, Coated	Risperidone 4 mg	Risperdal by Janssen	50458-0350	Antipsychotic
R4 <> JANSSEN	Tab, Coated	Risperidone 4 mg	Risperdal by Johnson & Johnson	59604-0350	Antipsychotic

ID FRONT <> BACK	DESCRIPTION FRONT <> BACK	INGREDIENT & STRENGTH	BRAND (OR EQUIV.) & FIRM	NDC#	CLASS; SCH.
R400	Cap, White	Doxepin HCl 150 mg	Sinequan by Purepac		Antidepressant
R404	Cap, Orange & Yellow	Tetracycline HCl 250 mg	Tetracyn by Purepac		Antibiotic
R406	Cap, Black & Yellow	Tetracycline HCl 500 mg	Tetracyn by Purepac		Antibiotic
R409	Cap, Gray & Orange	Cephalexin 250 mg	Keflex by Rondex		Antibiotic
R418	Cap, Orange	Cephalexin 500 mg	Keflex by Rondex		Antibiotic
R4250	Tab, White, Round	Phenobarbital, Hyoscyamine, Atropine, Scopolamine	Donnatal by A.H.Robins		Gastrointestinal; C IV
R4264	Tab, Round	Phenobarbital, Hyoscyamine, Atropine, Scopolamine	Donnatal #2 by A.H.Robins		Gastrointestinal; C IV
R4306	Tab, White, Round	Promethazine 25 mg	Phenergan by Richlyn		Antiemetic; Antihistamine
R4322	Tab, White, Round	Propylthiouracil 50 mg	Propylthiouracil by Richlyn		Antithyroid
R4374	Cap	Aspirin 389 mg, Caffeine 32.4 mg, Propoxyphene HCl 65 mg	by Allscripts	54569-0301	Analgesic; C IV
R4388	Tab, Burgundy, Round	Phenazopyridine HCl 100 mg	Pyridium by Rugby		Urinary Analgesic
R439	Tab, Film Coated	Trazodone HCl 50 mg	by Heartland	61392-0487	Antidepressant
R4392	Tab, Burgundy, Round	Phenazopyridine HCl 200 mg	Pyridium by Rugby		Urinary Analgesic
R440	Tab, White, Round	Tolbutamide 500 mg	Orinase by Purepac		Antidiabetic
R441	Tab	Trazodone HCl 100 mg	by Heartland	61392-0490	Antidepressant
R4429	Tab, R inside of a Diamond-Shape 4429	Quinidine Sulfate 300 mg	by Rugby	00536-4429	Antiarrhythmic
R473	Tab, Film Coated, R/473	Verapamil HCl 80 mg	by Heartland	61392-0493	Antihypertensive
R475	Tab, Film Coated, R/475	Verapamil HCl 120 mg	by Heartland	61392-0496	Antihypertensive
R480	Tab, Film Coated	Tolmetin Sodium 735 mg	by Qualitest	00603-6131	NSAID
R497	Cap, Light Yellow	Nifedipine 10 mg	by RP Scherer	11014-0870	Antihypertensive
R497	Cap, R 497	Nifedipine 10 mg	by Baker Cummins	63171-1547	Antihypertensive
R497	Cap, R 497	Nifedipine 10 mg	by Murfreesboro	51129-1133	Antihypertensive
R497	Cap, Yellow, Softgel	Nifedipine 10 mg	by Purepac	00228-2497	Antihypertensive
R497	Cap	Nifedipine 10 mg	by Vangard	00615-0360	Antihypertensive
R497	Cap	Nifedipine 10 mg	by Zenith Goldline	00182-1547	Antihypertensive
R497	Cap, Purepac Logo	Nifedipine 10 mg	by Med Pro	53978-1189	Antihypertensive
R497	Cap, R 497	Nifedipine 10 mg	by UDL	51079-0664	Antihypertensive
R497	Cap, Purepac Logo 497	Nifedipine 10 mg	by PDRX	55289-0907	Antihypertensive
R497	Cap	Nifedipine 10 mg	by Heartland	61392-0356	Antihypertensive
R5	Tab, Ex Release, R/5	Dextromethorphan Hydrobromide 30 mg, Guaifenesin 675 mg	Numobid Dx by Sovereign	58716-0637	Cold Remedy
R5	Tab, White, Round	Isosorbide Dinitrate SL 5 mg	Isordil by Rugby		Antianginal
R50 <> P	Tab, R/50 <> Purepac Logo	Lorazepam 1 mg	by Kaiser	00179-1093	Sedative/Hypnotic; C IV
R500	Cap, White	Prazosin HCl	by Purepac	00228-2500	Antihypertensive
R500	Cap	Prazosin HCl 1 mg	by Qualitest	00603-5286	Antihypertensive
R500 <> R500	Cap	Prazosin HCl	by Heartland	61392-0115	Antihypertensive
R501	Cap, Pink	Prazosin HCl	by Purepac	00228-2501	Antihypertensive
R501 <> R501	Cap	Prazosin HCl	by Heartland	61392-0118	Antihypertensive
R502	Cap	Prazosin HCl 5 mg	by Qualitest	00603-5288	Antihypertensive
R502	Cap, Blue	Prazosin HCl	by Purepac	00228-2502	Antihypertensive
R520	Cap, Orange & White	Tolmetin Sodium 400 mg	by Purepac	00228-2520	NSAID
R521	Tab, White, Round	Naproxen 250 mg	Naprosyn by Purepac		NSAID
R522	Tab, White, Oblong	Naproxen 375 mg	Naprosyn by Purepac		NSAID
R523	Tab, White, Oblong	Naproxen 500 mg	Naprosyn by Purepac		NSAID
R530	Cap, Reddish Brown, R 530 <>	Nifedipine 20 mg	by Baker Cummins	63171-1548	Antihypertensive
R530	Cap, Reddish Brown, Softgel	Nifedipine 20 mg	by Purepac	00228-2530	Antihypertensive
R530	Cap	Nifedipine 20 mg	by Vangard	00615-0359	Antihypertensive
R530	Cap	Nifedipine 20 mg	by Zenith Goldline	00182-1548	Antihypertensive
R530	Cap, Reddish Brown, R 530	Nifedipine 20 mg	by UDL	51079-0665	Antihypertensive
R530	Cap	Nifedipine 20 mg	by Med Pro	53978-2038	Antihypertensive
R530	Cap, Reddish Brown, R 530	Nifedipine 20 mg	by Quality Care	60346-0845	Antihypertensive
R534	Tab, White, Round	Pindolol 5 mg	Visken by Purepac		Antihypertensive

ID FRONT ⟷ BACK	DESCRIPTION FRONT ⟷ BACK	INGREDIENT & STRENGTH	BRAND (OR EQUIV.) & FIRM	NDC#	CLASS; SCH.
R535	Tab, White, Round	Pindolol 10 mg	Visken by Purepac		Antihypertensive
R538	Tab	Carbidopa 10 mg, Levodopa 100 mg	by Zenith Goldline	00182-1948	Antiparkinson
R538	Tab	Carbidopa 10 mg, Levodopa 100 mg	by Qualitest	00603-2568	Antiparkinson
R538	Tab	Carbidopa 10 mg, Levodopa 100 mg	by Heartland	61392-0177	Antiparkinson
R539	Tab	Carbidopa 25 mg, Levodopa 100 mg	by Heartland	61392-0180	Antiparkinson
R539	Tab	Carbidopa 25 mg, Levodopa 100 mg	by Zenith Goldline	00182-1949	Antiparkinson
R539	Tab	Carbidopa 25 mg, Levodopa 100 mg	by Qualitest	00603-2569	Antiparkinson
R539	Tab	Carbidopa 25 mg, Levodopa 100 mg	by Med Pro	53978-2078	Antiparkinson
R540	Tab, Light Blue	Carbidopa 25 mg, Levodopa 250 mg	by Heartland	61392-0183	Antiparkinson
R540	Tab	Carbidopa 25 mg, Levodopa 250 mg	by Zenith Goldline	00182-1950	Antiparkinson
R540	Tab	Carbidopa 25 mg, Levodopa 250 mg	by Qualitest	00603-2570	Antiparkinson
R546	Tab, Orange, Round	Diflunisal 500 mg	Dolobid by Purepac		NSAID
R547	Tab, White, Oval	Naproxen Sodium 275 mg	Anaprox by Purepac		NSAID
R548	Tab, White, Oval	Naproxen Sodium 550 mg	Anaprox by Purepac		NSAID
R550	Tab, Black Print	Diclofenac Sodium 50 mg	by Zenith Goldline	00182-2618	NSAID
R550	Tab	Diclofenac Sodium 50 mg	by CVS Revco	00894-5841	NSAID
R551	Tab, Black Print	Diclofenac Sodium 75 mg	by Rugby	00536-5738	NSAID
R551	Tab, Black Print	Diclofenac Sodium 75 mg	by Zenith Goldline	00182-2619	NSAID
R551	Tab, Black Print	Diclofenac Sodium 75 mg	by DRX	55045-2247	NSAID
R551	Tab	Diclofenac Sodium 75 mg	by CVS Revco	00894-5846	NSAID
R552	Tab, Film Coated	Gemfibrozil 600 mg	by Zenith Goldline	00182-1956	Antihyperlipidemic
R553	Cap, Clear with White Beads	Erythromycin 250 mg	by Purepac	00228-2553	Antibiotic
R553	Cap	Erythromycin 250 mg	by Qualitest	00603-3548	Antibiotic
R553 ⟷ R553	Cap, Clear	Erythromycin 250 mg	by Faulding Pharms (AS)	50546-0350	Antibiotic
R554	Tab, Film Coated	Metoprolol Tartrate 50 mg	by Zenith Goldline	00182-1987	Antihypertensive
R554	Tab, Film Coated	Metoprolol Tartrate 50 mg	by Talbert Med	44514-0514	Antihypertensive
R555	Tab, Film Coated	Metoprolol Tartrate 100 mg	by Zenith Goldline	00182-1988	Antihypertensive
R5726	Tab, Tan, Oblong	Carbinoxamine Maleate 4 mg, Pseudoephedrine 60 mg	Rondec by Ross		Cold Remedy
R599	Tab, Football-Shaped, Film Coated, Purepac Logo	Etodolac 400 mg	by Allscripts	54569-4468	NSAID
R599	Tab, Gray, Oblong, Film	Etodolac 400 mg	by Heartland	61392-0908	NSAID
R599	Tab, Light Gray, Football Shaped, Film Coated, Purepac Logo	Etodolac 400 mg	by DRX	55045-2490	NSAID
R599	Tab, Light Gray, Football Shaped, Film Coated, Purepac Logo	Etodolac 400 mg	by Purepac	00228-2599	NSAID
R60	Tab, Yellow, Round	Phendimetrazine 35 mg	Plegine by Rugby		Anorexiant; C III
R60	Tab, R 60	Phendimetrazine Tartrate 35 mg	by Quality Care	60346-0562	Anorexiant; C III
R605 ⟷ R605	Cap, Green, Black Print	Acyclovir 200 mg	by Purepac	00228-2605	Antiviral
R607	Tab, Pastel Green, Oval	Acyclovir 800 mg	by Purepac	00228-2607	Antiviral
R617	Tab, Yellow, Oblong, R/617	Naproxen 375 mg	by Purepac		NSAID
R618	Tab, Yellow, Oblong, R/618	Naproxen 500 mg	by Purepac		NSAID
R620	Tab, Blue, Round	Isosorbide Mononitrate 20 mg	by Purepac		Antianginal
R620	Tab, Blue, Round, Scored	Isosorbide Mononitrate 20 mg	by Purepac	00228-2620	Antianginal
R6240	Tab, Ex Release	Carbinoxamine Maleate 8 mg, Pseudoephedrine HCl 120 mg	Rondec TR by Abbott	60692-6240	Cold Remedy
R63	Tab	Clonazepam 0.5 mg	by Pharm Serv Ctr	00855-9215	Anticonvulsant; C IV
R631	Tab, Blue, Round, Scored	Isosorbide Mononitrate 10 mg	by Purepac	00228-2631	Antianginal
R632	Tab, White, Oval, Film, R 632	Etodolac 500 mg	by Heartland	61392-0905	NSAID
R632	Tab, White, Football Shaped, Film Coated	Etodolac 500 mg	by Purepac	00228-2632	NSAID
R642	Tab, White, Round, Scored	Doxazosin Mesylate 1 mg	by Purepac	00228-2642	Antihypertensive
R643	Tab, White, Cap Shaped, Scored	Doxazosin Mesylate 2 mg	by Purepac	00228-2643	Antihypertensive
R644	Tab, White, Cap Shaped, Scored	Doxazosin Mesylate 4 mg	by Purepac	00228-2644	Antihypertensive
R645	Tab, White, Round, Scored	Doxazosin Mesylate 8 mg	by Purepac	00228-2645	Antihypertensive
R655	Tab, Blue, Cap Shaped, Film Coated, Scored	Fluvoxamine Maleate 50 mg	by Purepac	00228-2655	OCD
R656	Tab, White, Cap Shaped, Film Coated, Scored	Fluvoxamine Maleate 100 mg	by Purepac	00228-2656	OCD
R671	Tab, Peach, Oval, Film Coated	Etodolac 400 mg	ER by Purepac	00228-2671	NSAID

ID FRONT <> BACK	DESCRIPTION FRONT <> BACK	INGREDIENT & STRENGTH	BRAND (OR EQUIV.) & FIRM	NDC#	CLASS; SCH.
R672	Tab, White, Oval, Scored, Film Coated	Spironolactone 50 mg	by Purepac	00228-2672	Diuretic
R673	Tab, White, Round, Scored, Film Coated	Spironolactone 100 mg	by Purepac	00228-2673	Diuretic
R7	Tab, Orange, Octagonal	Indapamide 1.25 mg	Lozol by RPR		Diuretic
R70	Tab, White, Round	Dipyridamole 25 mg	Persantine by Rugby		Antiplatelet
R711	Tab, Beige, Oval, Film Coated, Scored	Isosorbide Mononitrate 60 mg	ER by Purepac	00228-2711	Antianginal
R713	Tab, White, Oval, Film Coated, Scored	Isosorbide Mononitrate 30 mg	ER by Purepac	00228-2713	Antianginal
R7621	Tab, Maroon, Oval	Multivitamin, Fluoride, Iron	ViDaylin F with Iron by Ross		Vitamin
R7626	Tab, Yellow, Oval	Multivitamin, Fluoride	ViDaylin F by Ross		Vitamin
R8	Tab, White, Octagon	Indapamide 2.5 mg	Lozol by Rightpak	65240-0685	Diuretic
R8	Tab, White, Octagonal, Film Coated, R Over 8	Indapamide 2.5 mg	Lozol by Amerisource	62584-0082	Diuretic
RAFTON	Tab, White, Round	Alginates	Rafton by Ferring	Canadian	Gastrointestinal
RAFTONRAFTON	Tab, Round, Rafton/Rafton	Alginic Acid 200 mg, Aluminum Hydroxide 80 mg	Rafton by Ferring	Canadian	Gastrointestinal
RAM017 <> RAM017	Tab	Yohimbine HCl 5.4 mg	Yovital by Kenwood	00482-0017	Impotence Agent
RAM020	Tab, Sugar Coated	Bile Salts 150 mg, Pancreatin 300 mg, Pepsin 250 mg	Digepepsin by Lini	58215-0302	Gastrointestinal
RAPIDE50 <> VOLTAREN	Tab, Reddish-Brown, Round, Sugar Coated	Diclofenac Potassium 50 mg	Voltaren Rapide by Novartis	Canadian DIN# 00881635	NSAID
RC	Tab, Purple, Round, RC/+	Diphenhydramine HCl 25 mg, Pseudoephed HCl 60 mg, Acetamino 500 mg	Cold Control by Reese	10956-0589	Cold Remedy
RC22	Tab, Coated	Penbutolol Sulfate 20 mg	Levatol		Antihypertensive
RCA	Tab, White, RC/A	Acetaminophen 650 mg	Pain-Eze+ by Reese		Antipyretic
RCAPP	Cap, Orange, RC/APP	Phenylpropanolamine HCl 25 mg, Acetaminophen 500 mg	Tetra Caps by Reese	10956-0706	Cold Remedy
RCCGUF	Cap, Pink, RCC/GUF	Guaifenesin 200 mg	Refenesen by Reese	10956-0700	Expectorant
RCD	Tab, Yellow, Round, RC/D	Diphenhydramine HCl 50 mg	Sleep-Ettes D by Reese	10956-0601	Antihistamine
RCE	Cap, Orange, RC/E	Guaifenesin 200 mg, Phenylpropanolamine HCl 37.5 mg	Rephenyl by Reese	10956-0685	Cold Remedy
RCGGP	Cap, White, RC/GGP	Guaifenesin 400 mg, Pseudoephedrine HCl 60 mg	Refenesen Plus by Reese	10956-0724	Cold Remedy
RCNS	Tab, Green, Round, RC/NS	Acetaminophen 500 mg, Pseudoeph HCl 60 mg, Dexbromphen Mal 2 mg	Sinadrin Plus by Reese	10956-0636	Cold Remedy
RCP	Cap, Yellow, RC/P	Guaifenesin 200 mg, Dextromethorphan HBr 15 mg	Recofen by Reese	10956-0659	Cold Remedy
RCP	Cap, Yellow, RC/P	Pyrantel Pamoate 180 mg	Reese's Pinworm by Reese	10956-0658	Antihelmintic
RCSS	Tab, Yellow, Round	Acetaminophen 500 mg, Phenylprop HCl 25 mg, Chlorphen Maleate 4 mg	Spr Stren Sinadrin by Reese	10956-0697	Cold Remedy
RCTC	Cap, Yellow, RC/TC	Acetamin 500 mg, Phenylpro HCl 37.5 mg, Pyrilam Mal 50 mg, Dextrom HBr 30 mg	Theracaps by Reese	10956-0637	Cold Remedy
RD12	Tab, Film Coated	Ascorbic Acid 60 mg, Biotin, D- 300 mcg, Calcium Pantothenate 10 mg, Cyanocobalamin 6 mcg, Folic Acid 1 mg, Niacinamide 20 mg, Pyridoxine HCl 10 mg, Riboflavin 1.7 mg, Thiamine Mononitrate 1.5 mg	Nephro Vite Rx by Anabolic	00722-6191	Vitamin
RD12	Tab, Film Coated	Ascorbic Acid 60 mg, Biotin, D- 300 mcg, Calcium Pantothenate 10 mg, Cyanocobalamin 6 mcg, Folic Acid 1 mg, Niacinamide 20 mg, Pyridoxine HCl 10 mg, Riboflavin 1.7 mg, Thiamine Mononitrate 1.5 mg	Nephro Vite Rx by R & D	54391-1002	Vitamin
RD23	Tab, Film Coated	Ascorbic Acid 60 mg, Biotin 0.3 mg, Calcium Pantothenate, Cyanocobalamin 0.006 mg, Ferrous Fumarate, Folic Acid 1 mg, Niacinamide 20 mg, Pyridoxine HCl, Riboflavin 1.7 mg, Thiamine Mononitrate	Nephro Vite Rx Iron by Anabolic	00722-6244	Vitamin
RD23	Tab, Film Coated	Ascorbic Acid 60 mg, Biotin 0.3 mg, Calcium Pantothenate, Cyanocobalamin 0.006 mg, Ferrous Fumarate, Folic Acid 1 mg, Niacinamide 20 mg, Pyridoxine HCl, Riboflavin 1.7 mg, Thiamine Mononitrate	Nephro Vite Fe by R & D	54391-2213	Vitamin
RD33	Tab, Film Coated	Ferrous Fumarate 324 mg, Folic Acid 1 mg	Nephro Fer Rx by Anabolic	00722-6262	Mineral
RD33	Tab, Film Coated	Ferrous Fumarate 324 mg, Folic Acid 1 mg	Nephro Fer Rx by R & D	54391-1313	Mineral
REBETOL200	Cap, Rebetol 200 <> Schering Logo	Ribavirin 200 mg	Rebetol by Schering	53922-1194	Antiviral
REGLAN <> AHR10	Tab, AHR to Left, 10 to the Right	Metoclopramide HCl 10 mg	Reglan by A H Robins	00031-6701	Gastrointestinal
REGLAN <> AHR10	Tab	Metoclopramide HCl 10 mg	Reglan by Wal Mart	49035-0157	Gastrointestinal
REGLAN <> AHR10	Tab, AHR 10	Metoclopramide HCl 10 mg	Reglan by Thrift Drug	59198-0099	Gastrointestinal
REGLAN <> AHR10	Tab, AHR 10	Metoclopramide HCl 10 mg	Reglan by Nat Pharmpak Serv	55154-3004	Gastrointestinal
RELAFEN <> 500	Tab, Oval, Film Coated	Nabumetone 500 mg	Relafen by SKB	00029-4851	NSAID
RELAFEN <> 500	Tab, Film Coated	Nabumetone 500 mg	Relafen by HJ Harkins Co	52959-0227	NSAID
RELAFEN <> 500	Tab, Film Coated	Nabumetone 500 mg	Relafen by Nat Pharmpak Serv	55154-4505	NSAID

ID FRONT <> BACK	DESCRIPTION FRONT <> BACK	INGREDIENT & STRENGTH	BRAND (OR EQUIV.) & FIRM	NDC#	CLASS; SCH.
RELAFEN <> 500	Tab, Film Coated	Nabumetone 500 mg	Relafen by Quality Care	60346-0316	NSAID
RELAFEN <> 500	Tab, Film Coated	Nabumetone 500 mg	Relafen by SB	59742-4851	NSAID
RELAFEN <> 500	Tab, Film Coated	Nabumetone 500 mg	Relafen by Amerisource	62584-0851	NSAID
RELAFEN <> 750	Tab, Oval, Film Coated	Nabumetone 750 mg	Relafen by SKB	00029-4852	NSAID
RELAFEN <> 750	Tab, Film Coated	Nabumetone 750 mg	Relafen by HJ Harkins Co	52959-0373	NSAID
RELAFEN <> 750	Tab, Film Coated	Nabumetone 750 mg	Relafen by Quality Care	60346-0925	NSAID
RELAFEN <> 750	Tab, Film Coated	Nabumetone 750 mg	Relafen by SB	59742-4852	NSAID
RELAFEN <> 750	Tab, Film Coated	Nabumetone 750 mg	Relafen by DRX	55045-2440	NSAID
RELAFEN500	Tab, White, Pillow, Relafen/500	Nabilone 500 mg	by Lilly	Canadian	Antiemetic
RELAFEN500	Tab, White, Pillow, Relafen/500	Nabumetone 500 mg	Relafen by SmithKline SKB	Canadian	NSAID
RELAFEN500	Tab, White, Oval, Relafen/500	Nabumetone 500 mg	Relafen by SKB		NSAID
RELAFEN500	Tab, Film Coated	Nabumetone 500 mg	Relafen by PDRX	55289-0015	NSAID
RELAFEN500	Tab, Film Coated	Nabumetone 500 mg	Relafen by Allscripts	54569-3535	NSAID
RELAFEN500	Tab, Film Coated, SmithKline	Nabumetone 500 mg	Relafen by Prescription Dispensing	61807-0051	NSAID
RELAFEN750	Tab, Beige, Oval, Relafen/750	Nabumetone 750 mg	Relafen by SKB		NSAID
RELAFEN750	Tab, Film Coated, SmithKline	Nabumetone 750 mg	Relafen by Prescription Dispensing	61807-0059	NSAID
RELAFEN750	Tab, Film Coated	Nabumetone 750 mg	Relafen by Allscripts	54569-3845	NSAID
RENAGEL400	Tab, Off-White with Black Print, Oval, Film Coated	Sevelamer HCl 400 mg	Renagel by Genzyme/GelTex	58468-0020	Phosphate Binder
RENAGEL800	Tab, Off-White with Black Print, Oval, Film Coated	Sevelamer HCl 800 mg	Renagel by Genzyme/GelTex	58468-0021	Phosphate Binder
REQUA	Cap, Pink	Charcocaps	by Requa	10961-0030	Gastrointestinal
RESCON	Tab, Ex Release, Res/Con	Chlorpheniramine Maleate 8 mg, Methscopolamine Nitrate 2.5 mg, Pseudoephedrine HCl 120 mg	Rescon MX by Sovereign	58716-0674	Cold Remedy
RESCON	Tab	Chlorpheniramine Maleate 8 mg, Methscopolamine Nitrate 2.5 mg, Pseudoephedrine HCl 120 mg	Rescon MX by ION	11808-0088	Cold Remedy
RESCON	Tab, White, Oblong, Scored, Res/Con	Chlorpheniramine Maleate 8 mg, Methscopolamine Nitrate 2.5 mg, Pseudoephedrine HCl 120 mg	Rescon MX SR by Compumed	00403-0002	Cold Remedy
RESCON	Cap, Printed in White, Ex Release	Chlorpheniramine Maleate 12 mg, Pseudoephedrine HCl 120 mg	Rescon Sr by Sovereign	58716-0023	Cold Remedy
RESCONED	Cap, Ex Release, Rescon ED	Chlorpheniramine Maleate 8 mg, Pseudoephedrine HCl 120 mg	Rescon ED by Sovereign	58716-0021	Cold Remedy
RESCONED	Cap, Green & Clear, Black Ink	Pseudoephedrine HCl 120 mg, Chlorpheniramine Malate 8 mg	Rescon ED by RX PAK	65084-0112	Cold Remedy
RESCONJR	Cap, Ex Release, Rescon-JR	Chlorpheniramine Maleate 4 mg, Pseudoephedrine HCl 60 mg	Rescon Jr by Sovereign	58716-0022	Cold Remedy
RESPA <> 789	Cap, Ex Release	Brompheniramine Maleate 6 mg, Pseudoephedrine HCl 60 mg	Respahist by Pharmafab	62542-0102	Cold Remedy
RESPA733	Tab, White, Oblong, Scored	Dextromethorphan Hydrobromide 30 mg, Guaifenesin 600 mg, Pseudoephedrine HCl 37.5 mg	Trikof D by DRX	55045-2649	Cold Remedy
RESPA733	Tab, White, Oblong, Scored, Respa over 733	Guaifenesin 600 mg, Phenylpropanolamine HCl 37.5 mg, Pseudoephedrine HCl 37.5 mg	GFN PPAH DTMH 00 by Med Pro	53978-3328	Cold Remedy
RESPA78	Tab, White, Oblong, Scored	Dextromethorphan Hydrobromide 28 mg, Guaifenesin 600 mg	Respa DM by DRX	55045-2617	Cold Remedy
RESPA78	Tab, White, Oblong, Scored	Guaifenesin 600 mg, Dextromethorphan Hydriodide 28 mg	GFN DTMH 05 by Med Pro	53978-0903	Cold Remedy
RESPA786	Tab, Embossed, Ex Release, Respa over 786	Guaifenesin 600 mg	Respa GF by Pharmafab	62542-0702	Expectorant
RESPA786	Tab, Respa/786	Guaifenesin 600 mg	Respa GF by Anabolic	00722-6334	Expectorant
RESPA787	Tab, Ex Release	Guaifenesin 600 mg, Pseudoephedrine HCl 60 mg	Respa 1st by Respa	60575-0108	Cold Remedy
RESPA787	Tab, Ex Release, Respa over 787	Guaifenesin 600 mg, Pseudoephedrine HCl 60 mg	Respa 1st by Pharmafab	62542-0742	Cold Remedy
RESPA787	Tab	Guaifenesin 600 mg, Pseudoephedrine HCl 60 mg	Respa 1st by Anabolic	00722-6350	Cold Remedy
RESPA788	Tab, Ex Release, Respa/788	Dextromethorphan Hydrobromide 30 mg, Guaifenesin 600 mg	Respa-DM by Respa	60575-0123	Cold Remedy
RESPA788	Tab, Ex Release, Respa/788	Dextromethorphan Hydrobromide 30 mg, Guaifenesin 600 mg	Respa DM by Pharmafab	62542-0721	Cold Remedy
RESPA788	Tab, Respa/788	Dextromethorphan Hydrobromide 30 mg, Guaifenesin 600 mg	Respa DM by Anabolic	00722-6349	Cold Remedy
RESPA790	Tab, Ex Release	Belladonna Alkaloids 0.24 mg, Chlorpheniramine Maleate 8 mg, Phenylephrine HCl 25 mg, Phenylpropanolamine HCl 50 mg	Respa ARM by Respa	60575-0790	Cold Remedy
RESPA790	Tab	Belladonna Alkaloids 0.24 mg, Chlorpheniramine Maleate 8 mg, Phenylephrine HCl 25 mg, Phenylpropanolamine HCl 50 mg	Respa ARM by Anabolic	00722-6371	Cold Remedy
RESPA87	Tab, White, Oblong, Scored	Guaifenesin 600 mg, Pseudoephedrine HCl 58 mg	Respa 1ST by Med Pro	53978-3357	Cold Remedy
RESPA87	Tab, White, Oblong, Scored	Guaifenesin 600 mg, Pseudoephedrine HCl 58 mg	GFN 600 PSEH 58 04 by Med Pro	53978-3347	Cold Remedy

ID FRONT <> BACK	DESCRIPTION FRONT <> BACK	INGREDIENT & STRENGTH	BRAND (OR EQUIV.) & FIRM	NDC#	CLASS; SCH.
RESTORIL15MG <> FORSLEEP	Cap, Restoril 15 MG Above Restoril 15 MG <> For Sleep Above For Sleep	Temazepam 15 mg	Restoril by Novartis	00078-0098	Sedative/Hypnotic; C IV
RESTORIL15MG <> FORSLEEP	Cap, For Sleep is Imprinted Twice on Capsule	Temazepam 15 mg	Restoril by Med Pro	53978-3080	Sedative/Hypnotic; C IV
RESTORIL30MG <> FORSLEEP	Cap, Restoril 30 MG Above Restoril 30 MG <> For Sleep Above For Sleep	Temazepam 30 mg	Restoril by Novartis	00078-0099	Sedative/Hypnotic; C IV
RESTORIL30MG <> FORSLEEP	Cap, For Sleep is Imprinted Twice on Capsule	Temazepam 30 mg	Restoril by Med Pro	53978-3081	Sedative/Hypnotic; C IV
RETE	Tap, Blue, Round	Caffeine 65 mg, Potassium Salicylate 75 mg, Salicylamide 3.0 mg	Trim-Elim by Reese	10956-0647	Diuretic
RGP <> BM	Cap	Acetaminophen 300 mg, Phenyltoloxamine Citrate 20 mg, Salicylamide 200 mg	by Pharmakon	55422-0411	Analgesic
RGP <> BM	Cap	Acetaminophen 300 mg, Phenyltoloxamine Citrate 20 mg, Salicylamide 200 mg	by Seatrace	00551-0411	Analgesic
RH	Tab, Pink, Round	Trimipramine 12.5 mg	Rhotrimine by Rhodiapharm	Canadian	Antidepressant
RH100RHOTRAL	Tab, White, Shield, RH/100-Rhotral	Acebutolol HCl 100 mg	Rhotral by Rhodiapharm	Canadian	Antihypertensive
RH200RHOTRAL	Tab, Blue, Shield, RH/200-Rhotral	Acebutolol HCl 200 mg	Rhotral by Rhodiapharm	Canadian	Antihypertensive
RH400RHOTRAL	Tab, White, Shield, RH/400-Rhotral	Acebutolol HCl 400 mg	Rhotral by Rhodiapharm	Canadian	Antihypertensive
RHO05	Tab, Orange, Round, RHO/0.5	Clorazepam 0.5 mg	Rho-Clonazepam by Rhoxal Pharma	Canadian	Sedative
RHO1	Tab, Green, Round, RHO/1	Clorazepam 1 mg	Rho-Clonazepam by Rhoxal Pharma	Canadian	Sedative
RHO10	Tab, White, Round, RHO/10	Nitrazepam 10 mg	Rho-Nitrazepam by Rhoxal Pharma	Canadian	Sedative/Hypnotic
RHO160	Tab, Light Blue, Oblong, RHO-160	Sotalol HCl 160 mg	Rho-Sotalol by Rhoxal Pharma	Canadian	Antiarrhythmic
RHO2	Tab, White, Round, RHO/2	Clorazepam 2 mg	Rho-Clonazepam by Rhoxal Pharma	Canadian	Sedative
RHO2	Tab, Green, Oblong, RHO-2	Loperamide HCl 2 mg	Rho-Loperamide by Rhoxal Pharma	Canadian	Antidiarrheal
RHO5	Tab, White, Round, RHO/5	Nitrazepam 5 mg	Rho-Nitrazepam by Rhoxal Pharma	Canadian	Sedative/Hypnotic
RHO500	Tab, White, Round, RHO/500	Metformin HCl 500 mg	Rho-Metformin by Rhoxal Pharma	Canadian	Antidiabetic
RHO80	Tab, Light Blue, Oblong, RHO-80	Sotalol HCl 80 mg	Rho-Sotalol by Rhoxal Pharma	Canadian	Antiarrhythmic
RHODOX 50	Cap, Pink/Salmon, RHO/DOX 50	Doxepin HCl 50 mg	Rho Doxepin by Rhodiapharm	Canadian	Antidepressant
RHODOX10	Cap, Pink & Red, RHO/DOX 10	Doxepin HCl 10 mg	Rho Doxepin by Rhodiapharm	Canadian	Antidepressant
RHODOX25	Cap, Blue & Pink, RHO/DOX 25	Doxepin HCl 25 mg	Rho Doxepin by Rhodiapharm	Canadian	Antidepressant
RHODXY100	Tab, Orange, RHO/DXY 200	Doxycycline Hyclate 100 mg	Rho Doxycin Tabs by Rhodiapharm	Canadian	Antibiotic
RHODXY100	Cap, Blue & Opaque, RHO/DXY 100	Doxycycline Hyclate 100 mg	Rho Doxycin by Rhodiapharm	Canadian	Antibiotic
RHOPIR10	Cap, Maroon/Blue, RHO/PIR 10	Piroxicam 10 mg	Rho Piroxicam by Rhodiapharm	Canadian	NSAID
RHOPIR20	Cap, Maroon/Opaque, RHO/PIR 20	Piroxicam 20 mg	Rho Piroxicam by Rhodiapharm	Canadian	NSAID
RHOPRA1	Cap, Orange, RHO/PRA 1	Prazosin HCl 1 mg	Rho Prazosin by Rhodiapharm	Canadian	Antihypertensive
RHOPRA2	Tab, White, Round, RHO/PRA 2	Prazosin HCl 2 mg	Rho Prazosin by Rhodiapharm	Canadian	Antihypertensive
RHOPRA5	Tab, White, Diamond, RHO/PRA 5	Prazosin HCl 5 mg	Rho Prazosin by Rhodiapharm	Canadian	Antihypertensive
RHOVAIL150MG	Cap, Pink & White, Rhovail/150 mg	Ketoprofen 150 mg	Rhovail by Rho-Pharm	Canadian	NSAID
RHOVAIL200MG	Cap, Pink & Blue, Rhovail/200 mg	Ketoprofen 200 mg	Rhovail by Rho-Pharm	Canadian	NSAID
RHRHODISSR200	Tab, White, Round, RH-Rhodis SR 200	Ketoprofen 200 mg	Rhodis-SR by Rhodiapharm	Canadian	NSAID
RHRHRHOVANE	Tab, Blue, Oval, RH/RH-Rhovane	Zopiclone 7.5 mg	Rhovane by Rhodiapharm	Canadian	Hypnotic
RIDAURA	Cap, Tan/Brown	Auranofin 3 mg	by SmithKline SKB	Canadian	Antiarthritic
RIDAURA	Cap	Auranofin 3 mg	Ridaura by Connetics	63032-0011	Antiarthritic
RIFADIN	Cap, Scarlet	Rifampin 150 mg	by Dept Health Central Pharm	53808-0011	Antibiotic
RIFADIN	Cap, Scarlet	Rifampin 300 mg	by Dept Health Central Pharm	53808-0012	Antibiotic
RIFADIN150	Cap, Scarlet	Rifampin 150 mg	Rifadin by Allscripts	54569-4113	Antibiotic
RIFADIN150	Cap	Rifampin 150 mg	Rifadin by Merrell	00068-0510	Antibiotic
RIFADIN150	Cap, Maroon & Scarlet	Rifampin 150 mg	Rifadin by HJ Harkins Co	52959-0461	Antibiotic
RIFADIN300	Cap, Maroon & Red	Rifampin 150 mg	Rifadin by Quality Care	60346-0970	Antibiotic
RIFADIN300	Cap, Scarlet	Rifampin 300 mg	Rifadin by Merrell	00068-0508	Antibiotic
RIFADIN300	Cap, Scarlet	Rifampin 300 mg	Rifadin by Allscripts	54569-0295	Antibiotic
RIFAMATE	Cap, Red	Rifampin 300 mg, Isoniazid 150 mg	Rifamate by Hoechst Marion Roussel	00068-0509	Antibiotic
RIFATER	Tab, Light Beige, Round, In Black Ink, Sugar Coated	Isoniazid 50 mg, Pyrazinamide 300 mg, Rifampin 120 mg	Rifater by Hoechst Roussel	00088-0576	Antimycobacterial
RIFATER	Tab, In Black Ink, Sugar Coated	Isoniazid 50 mg, Pyrazinamide 300 mg, Rifampin 120 mg	Rifater by Gruppo Lepetit	12522-8576	Antimycobacterial

ID FRONT <> BACK	DESCRIPTION FRONT <> BACK	INGREDIENT & STRENGTH	BRAND (OR EQUIV.) & FIRM	NDC#	CLASS; SCH.
RIKER <> NORGESICFORTE	Tab, Green	Aspirin 770 mg, Caffeine 60 mg, Orphenadrine Citrate 50 mg	Orphengesic Forte by Pharmedix	53002-0376	Analgesic
RIKER125PLUS	Tab, White, Round, Riker/125 Plus	Theophylline 125 mg, Guaifenesin 100 mg	Theolair-Plus by Riker		Antiasthmatic
RIKER161	Tab, Green, Round, Riker/161	Orphenadrine HCl 50 mg	Disipal by 3M		Muscle Relaxant
RIKER250PLUS	Cap, White, Riker/250 Plus	Theophylline 250 mg, Guaifenesin 200 mg	Theolair-Plus by Riker		Antiasthmatic
RIKER265	Tab, Brown, Round, Riker/265	Rauwolfia Serpentina 2 mg	Rauwiloid by 3M		Antihypertensive
RILUTEK <> RPR202	Tab, Film Coated	Riluzole 50 mg	Rilutek by RPR	62047-7700	Amyotrophic Lateral Sclerosis Agent
RIOPANPLUS	Tab, White, Round	Magaldrate 480 mg	Riopan by Whitehall-Robbins	Canadian	Gastrointestinal
RIS <> JANSSEN	Tab, Yellow	Risperidone 0.25 mg	Risperdal by Janssen Cilag	62579-0301	Antipsychotic
RIS1JANSSEN	Tab, White, Oblong, Ris 1/Janssen	Risperidone 1 mg	Risperidal by Janssen	Canadian	Antipsychotic
RIS2JANSSEN	Tab, Orange, Oblong, Ris 2/Janssen	Risperidone 2 mg	Risperidal by Janssen	Canadian	Antipsychotic
RIS3JANSSEN	Tab, Yellow, Oblong, Ris 3/Janssen	Risperidone 3 mg	Risperidal by Janssen	Canadian	Antipsychotic
RIS4JANSSEN	Tab, Green, Oblong, Ris 4/Janssen	Risperidone 4 mg	Risperidal by Janssen	Canadian	Antipsychotic
RIVA	Tab, Green	Calcium Carbonate 1250 mg	by Riva	Canadian	Vitamin/Mineral
RIVA	Tab, Yellow	Calcium Carbonate 1250 mg	by Riva	Canadian	Vitamin/Mineral
RIVOTRIL05ROCHE	Tab, Orange, Cylindrical, Rivotril/0.5/Roche	Clonazepam 0.5 mg	Rivotril by Roche	Canadian	Anticonvulsant
RL	Cap	Delta-9-Tetrahydrocannabinol 10 mg	Dronabinol by Banner Pharmacaps	10888-1039	Antiemetic
RL	Cap	Delta-9-Tetrahydrocannabinol 2.5 mg	Dronabinol by Banner Pharmacaps	10888-1037	Antiemetic
RL	Cap	Delta-9-Tetrahydrocannabinol 5 mg	Dronabinol by Banner Pharmacaps	10888-1038	Antiemetic
RL	Cap, Orange	Dronabinol 10 mg	by Sanofi	Canadian	Antiemetic
RL	Cap, Orange, Gelatin, Round	Dronabinol 10 mg	by Roxane	00054-2603	Antiemetic; C III
RL	Cap, White	Dronabinol 2.5 mg	by Sanofi	Canadian	Antiemetic
RL	Cap, White, Gelatin, Round	Dronabinol 2.5 mg	by Roxane	00054-2601	Antiemetic; C III
RL	Cap, Brown	Dronabinol 5 mg	by Sanofi	Canadian	Antiemetic
RL	Cap, Dark Brown, Gelatin, Round	Dronabinol 5 mg	by Roxane	00054-2602	Antiemetic; C III
RO26	Tab, White, Round	Phenobarbital 15 mg	by Rondex		Sedative/Hypnotic; C IV
RO28	Tab, White, Round	Phenobarbital 30 mg	by Rondex		Sedative/Hypnotic; C IV
ROA10	Cap, Purple, ROA/10	Isotretinoin 10 mg	Accutane by Roche	Canadian	Dermatologic
ROA40	Cap, Yellow, ROA/40	Isotretinoin 40 mg	Accutane by Roche	Canadian	Dermatologic
ROBAXIN750 <> AHR	Tab, Film Coated, Robaxin 750	Methocarbamol 750 mg	Robaxin by A H Robins	00031-7449	Muscle Relaxant
ROBAXIN750 <> AHR	Tab, Film Coated, Robaxin-750	Methocarbamol 750 mg	Robaxin by Thrift Drug	59198-0182	Muscle Relaxant
ROBAXIN750 <> AHR	Tab, Film Coated, Robaxin Over 750	Methocarbamol 750 mg	Robaxin by Amerisource	62584-0450	Muscle Relaxant
ROBAXIN750 <> AHR	Tab, Film Coated	Methocarbamol 750 mg	Robaxin 750 by Leiner	59606-0730	Muscle Relaxant
ROBAXINAHR	Tab, Coated, Robaxin AHR	Methocarbamol 500 mg	Robaxin by A H Robins	00031-7429	Muscle Relaxant
ROBAXINAHR	Tab, Orange, Round	Methocarbamol 750 mg	Robaxin by Rightpac	65240-0730	Muscle Relaxant
ROBAXINAHR	Tab, Orange, Round, Scored, Film Coated	Methcarbamol 500 mg	Robaxin by Nat Pharmpak Serv	55154-9001	Muscle Relaxant
ROBAXISALAHR	Tab	Aspirin 325 mg, Methocarbamol 400 mg	Robaxisal by A H Robins	00031-7469	Analgesic; Muscle Relaxant
ROBERTS <> COMHISTLA	Cap	Chlorpheniramine Maleate 4 mg, Phenylephrine HCl 20 mg, Phenyltoloxamine Citrate 50 mg	Comhist LA by Roberts	54092-0065	Cold Remedy; C III
ROBERTS <> ETHMOZINE200	Tab, Film Coated	Moricizine HCl 200 mg	by Roberts	54092-0046	Antiarrhythmic
ROBERTS <> ETHMOZINE250	Tab, Film Coated	Moricizine HCl 250 mg	by Roberts	54092-0047	Antiarrhythmic
ROBERTS <> ETHMOZINE300	Tab, Film Coated	Moricizine HCl 300 mg	by Roberts	54092-0048	Antiarrhythmic
ROBERTS063	Cap, White & Opaque	Anagrelide 0.5 mg	by Roberts	Canadian	Antiplatelet Agent
ROBERTS063	Cap	Anagrelide HCl	Agrylin by D M Graham	00756-0251	Antiplatelet Agent
ROBERTS063	Cap, Black Print	Anagrelide HCl	Agrylin by Roberts	54092-0063	Antiplatelet Agent
ROBERTS064	Cap	Anagrelide HCl	Agrylin by D M Graham	00756-0252	Antiplatelet Agent
ROBERTS064	Cap, Black Print	Anagrelide HCl	Agrylin by Roberts	54092-0064	Antiplatelet Agent

ID FRONT <> BACK	DESCRIPTION FRONT <> BACK	INGREDIENT & STRENGTH	BRAND (OR EQUIV.) & FIRM	NDC#	CLASS; SCH.
ROBERTS067	Cap	Guaifenesin 91.44 mg, Theophylline 152.4 mg	Quibron by Bristol Myers Squibb	00087-0516	Antiasthmatic
ROBERTS067	Cap	Guaifenesin 91.44 mg, Theophylline 152.4 mg	Quibron by RP Scherer	11014-0543	Antiasthmatic
ROBERTS067	Cap, Yellow	Theophylline Anhydrous 150 mg, Guaifenesin 90 mg	Quibron by Monarch		Antiasthmatic
ROBERTS068	Cap	Guaifenesin 183 mg, Theophylline 305 mg	Quibron by Bristol Myers Squibb	00087-0515	Antiasthmatic
ROBERTS068	Cap, Light Beige	Guaifenesin 183 mg, Theophylline 305 mg	Quibron 300 by RP Scherer	11014-0730	Antiasthmatic
ROBERTS068	Cap, White & Yellow	Theophylline Anhydrous 300 mg, Guaifenesin 180 mg	Quibron by Monarch		Antiasthmatic
ROBERTS103 <> 50	Tab	Bethanechol Chloride 50 mg	Duvoid by Pharm Utilization	60491-0221	Urinary Tract
ROBERTS130	Tab	Furazolidone 100 mg	Furoxone by Roberts	54092-0130	Antibiotic
ROBERTS135 <> CHLORAFEDHS	Cap, White, Beads, Black Print	Chlorpheniramine Maleate 4 mg, Pseudoephedrine HCl 60 mg	Chlorafed		Cold Remedy
ROBERTS136 <> CHLORAFED	Cap, Black Print, White Beads	Chlorpheniramine Maleate 8 mg, Pseudoephedrine HCl 120 mg	Chlorafed	00131-4513	Cold Remedy
ROBERTS138 <> DOLACET	Cap	Acetaminophen 500 mg, Hydrocodone Bitartrate 5 mg	Dolacet by Roberts	54092-0138	Analgesic; C III
ROBERTS138 <> DOLACET	Cap	Acetaminophen 500 mg, Hydrocodone Bitartrate 5 mg	by Mikart	46672-0247	Analgesic; C III
ROBERTS151	Cap, White Beads, Black Print	Guaifenesin 300 mg, Pseudoephedrine HCl 60 mg	Sinufed by		Cold Remedy
ROBERTS186 <> TIGAN	Cap	Trimethobenzamide HCl 100 mg	Tigan by Roberts	54092-0186	Antiemetic
ROBERTS187 <> TIGAN	Cap, Roberts 187	Trimethobenzamide HCl 250 mg	Tigan by King	60793-0885	Antiemetic
ROBITAB8217	Tab, White, Round	Penicillin VK 250 mg	Robicillin by A.H.Robins		Antibiotic
ROBITAB8227	Tab, White, Round	Penicillin VK 500 mg	Robicillin by A.H.Robins		Antibiotic
ROCALTROL05ROC	Cap, Rocaltrol 0.5 Roche	Calcitriol 0.5 mcg	Rocaltrol by Pharm Utilization	60491-0562	Vitamin/Mineral
ROCHE	Cap, White	Clodronate Disodium 400 mg	Ostac by Roche	Canadian	Bone Metab. Regul
ROCHE	Cap, Blue & Caramel	Levodopa 100 mg, Benseazide 25 mg	Prolopa by Roche	Canadian	Antiparkinson
ROCHE	Tab, White, Cylindrical	Mefloquine 250 mg	Lariam by Roche	Canadian	Antiprotozoal
ROCHE	Tab, White	Sulfadoxine 500 mg	by Roche	Canadian	Antimalarial
ROCHE	Tab, White	Sulfadoxine 500 mg, Pyrimethamine 25 mg	Fansidar by Roche	Canadian	Antimalarial
ROCHE	Tab, White, Round	Sulfamethoxazole 400 mg, Trimethoprim 80 mg	Bactrim by Roche	Canadian	Antibiotic
ROCHE	Tab, Yellowish-Buff, Round	Tetrabenazine 25 mg	Nitoman by Roche	Canadian	Agent for Dyskinesia
ROCHE	Tab, Yellow, Oblong	Tenoxicam 20 mg	Mobiflex by Roche	Canadian	NSAID
ROCHE <> 0245	Cap	Saquinavir Mesylate 200 mg	Invirase by Hoffmann La Roche	00004-0245	Antiviral
ROCHE <> 0245	Cap, ROCHE	Saquinavir Mesylate 200 mg	Invirase by Physicians Total Care	54868-3699	Antiviral
ROCHE <> 1KLONOPIN	Tab, Blue, Round	Clonazepam 1 mg	by Allscripts	54569-2727	Anticonvulsant; C IV
ROCHE <> 274	Tab, Light Blue, Oval, Film Coated	Naproxen Sodium 275 mg	Anaprox by Allscripts	54569-0264	NSAID
ROCHE <> 274	Tab, Light Blue, Film Coated	Naproxen Sodium 275 mg	Anaprox by Syntex	18393-0274	NSAID
ROCHE <> 5VALIUM	Tab, V Design	Diazepam 5 mg	Valium by PDRX	55289-0117	Antianxiety; C IV
ROCHE <> 75MG	Cap, Gray & Yellow, Hard Gel	Oseltamivir Phosphate 75 mg	Tamiflu by Perrigo	00113-0527	Antiviral
ROCHE <> 75MG	Cap, Gray & Yellow, Hard Gel, Roche in Blue Ink<> 75 MG in Blue Ink	Oseltamivir Phosphate 75 mg	Tamiflu by Perrigo	00113-0477	Antiviral
ROCHE <> ANAPROX	Tab, Film Coated	Naproxen Sodium 275 mg	Anaprox by HJ Harkins Co	52959-0015	NSAID
ROCHE <> ANAPROXDS	Tab, Film Coated	Naproxen Sodium 550 mg	Anaprox DS by Allscripts	54569-1763	NSAID
ROCHE <> ANAPROXDS	Tab, Dark Blue, Film Coated, Anaprox DS	Naproxen Sodium 550 mg	Anaprox DS by Syntex	18393-0276	NSAID
ROCHE <> ANAPROXDS	Tab, Dark Blue, Debossed <> Anaprox DS, Film Coated	Naproxen Sodium 550 mg	Anaprox DS by Thrift Drug	59198-0244	NSAID
ROCHE <> ANAPROXDS	Tab, Film Coated	Naproxen Sodium 550 mg	Anaprox DS by Quality Care	60346-0035	NSAID
ROCHE <> ANAPROXDS	Tab, Film Coated, Anaprox DS	Naproxen Sodium 550 mg	Anaprox DS by Nat Pharmpak Serv	55154-3805	NSAID
ROCHE <> ANAPROXDS	Tab, Blue, Oblong	Naproxen Sodium 550 mg	Anaprox DS by Rightpak	65240-0603	NSAID

ID FRONT <> BACK	DESCRIPTION FRONT <> BACK	INGREDIENT & STRENGTH	BRAND (OR EQUIV.) & FIRM	NDC#	CLASS; SCH.
ROCHE <> ANAPROXDS	Tab, Blue, Oblong	Naproxen Sodium 550 mg	Anaprox DS by Med-Pro	53978-3369	NSAID
ROCHE <> ANAPROXDS	Tab, Blue, Oblong, Film Coated, Anaprox DS	Naproxen Sodium 550 mg	Anaprox DS by Par	49884-0497	NSAID
ROCHE <> ANAPROXDS	Tab, Blue, Oblong, Film Coated, Anaprox Over DS	Naproxen Sodium 550 mg	Anaprox DS by Par	49884-0496	NSAID
ROCHE <> ANAPROXDS	Tab, Dark Blue, Film Coated, Anaprox DS	Naproxen Sodium 550 mg	Anaprox DS by HJ Harkins Co	52959-0016	NSAID
ROCHE <> BACTRIMDS	Tab, Bactrim DS	Sulfamethoxazole 800 mg, Trimethoprim 160 mg	Bactrim DS by Hoffmann La Roche	00004-0117	Antibiotic
ROCHE <> BACTRIMDS	Tab	Sulfamethoxazole 800 mg, Trimethoprim 160 mg	Bactrim DS by DRX	55045-2291	Antibiotic
ROCHE <> BACTRIMDS	Tab	Sulfamethoxazole 800 mg, Trimethoprim 160 mg	Bactrim DS by Amerisource	62584-0117	Antibiotic
ROCHE <> BACTRIMDS	Tab, Bactrim-DS	Sulfamethoxazole 800 mg, Trimethoprim 160 mg	Bactrim DS by Thrift Drug	59198-0258	Antibiotic
ROCHE <> BACTRIMDS	Tab, Bactrim-DS	Sulfamethoxazole 800 mg, Trimethoprim 160 mg	Bactrim DS by Nat Pharmpak Serv	55154-3101	Antibiotic
ROCHE <> BUMEX	Tab	Bumetanide 2 mg	Bumex by Med Pro	53978-2035	Diuretic
ROCHE <> BUMEX05	Tab, Light Green, Bumex 0.5	Bumetanide 0.5 mg	Bumex by Thrift Drug	59198-0257	Diuretic
ROCHE <> BUMEX05	Tab, Roche <> Bumex 0.5	Bumetanide 0.5 mg	Bumex by Nat Pharmpak Serv	55154-3103	Diuretic
ROCHE <> BUMEX05	Tab, Roche <> Bumex 0.5	Bumetanide 0.5 mg	Bumex by Hoffmann La Roche	00004-0125	Diuretic
ROCHE <> BUMEX1	Tab, Bumex 1	Bumetanide 1 mg	Bumex by Thrift Drug	59198-0256	Diuretic
ROCHE <> BUMEX1	Tab	Bumetanide 1 mg	Bumex by Nat Pharmpak Serv	55154-3104	Diuretic
ROCHE <> BUMEX1	Tab	Bumetanide 1 mg	Bumex by Hoffmann La Roche	00004-0121	Diuretic
ROCHE <> BUMEX1	Tab, Roche <> Bumex/1	Bumetanide 1 mg	Bumex by Med Pro	53978-0241	Diuretic
ROCHE <> BUMEX2	Tab, Bumex 2	Bumetanide 2 mg	Bumex by Thrift Drug	59198-0101	Diuretic
ROCHE <> BUMEX2	Tab	Bumetanide 2 mg	Bumex by Nat Pharmpak Serv	55154-3105	Diuretic
ROCHE <> BUMEX2	Tab	Bumetanide 2 mg	Bumex by Quality Care	60346-0310	Diuretic
ROCHE <> BUMEX2	Tab, Peach, Bumex 2	Bumetanide 2 mg	Bumex by Capellon	64543-0121	Diuretic
ROCHE <> BUMEX2	Tab, Bumex 2	Bumetanide 2 mg	Bumex by Amerisource	62584-0162	Diuretic
ROCHE <> BUMEX2	Tab	Bumetanide 2 mg	Bumex by Hoffmann La Roche	00004-0162	Diuretic
ROCHE <> CARDENE	Cap, Blue	Nicardipine HCl 30 mg	Cardene by ICN Dutch Holdings	64158-0437	Antihypertensive
ROCHE <> CARDENE20	Cap, Blue Band	Nicardipine HCl 20 mg	Cardene by Repack Co of Amer	55306-2437	Antihypertensive
ROCHE <> CARDENE20MG	Cap, Blue Band, Cardene 20mg	Nicardipine HCl 20 mg	Cardene by Murfreesboro	51129-1125	Antihypertensive
ROCHE <> CARDENE20MG	Cap, Brilliant Blue Band, Blue Band <> Cardene 20mg	Nicardipine HCl 20 mg	Cardene by Hoffmann La Roche	00004-0183	Antihypertensive
ROCHE <> CARDENE20MG	Cap	Nicardipine HCl 20 mg	Cardene by Syntex	18393-0437	Antihypertensive
ROCHE <> CARDENE30MG	Cap, Brilliant Blue Band, Blue Band <> Cardene 30mg, Gelatin Coated	Nicardipine HCl 30 mg	Cardene by Hoffmann La Roche	00004-0184	Antihypertensive
ROCHE <> CARDENE30MG	Cap, Blue Band	Nicardipine HCl 30 mg	Cardene by Repack Co of Amer	55306-2438	Antihypertensive
ROCHE <> CARDENE30MG	Cap, Brilliant Blue Band, Blue Band <> Cardene 30mg, Gelatin Coated	Nicardipine HCl 30 mg	Cardene by Murfreesboro	51129-1206	Antihypertensive
ROCHE <> CARDENE30MG	Cap, Gelatin Coated	Nicardipine HCl 30 mg	Cardene by Syntex	18393-0438	Antihypertensive
ROCHE <> CARDENESR30MG	Cap, ER	Nicardipine HCl 30 mg	Cardene SR by Hoffmann La Roche	00004-0180	Antihypertensive
ROCHE <> CARDENESR45MG	Cap, ER	Nicardipine HCl 45 mg	Cardene SR by Hoffmann La Roche	00004-0181	Antihypertensive
ROCHE <> CARDENESR60MG	Cap, ER	Nicardipine HCl 60 mg	Cardene SR by Hoffmann La Roche	00004-0182	Antihypertensive
ROCHE <> CELLCEPT250	Cap, Printed in Black	Mycophenolate Mofetil 250 mg	Cellcept by Syntex	18393-0259	Immunosuppressant

ID FRONT <> BACK	DESCRIPTION FRONT <> BACK	INGREDIENT & STRENGTH	BRAND (OR EQUIV.) & FIRM	NDC#	CLASS; SCH.
ROCHE <> CELLCEPT250	Cap, Blue & Brown, Hard Gel	Mycophenolate Mofetil 250 mg	Cellcept by Murfreesboro Ph	51129-1358	Immunosuppressant
ROCHE <> CELLCEPT250	Cap	Mycophenolate Mofetil 250 mg	Cellcept by Hoffmann La Roche	00004-0259	Immunosuppressant
ROCHE <> CELLCEPT500	Tab, Lavender, Coated	Mycophenolate Mofetil 500 mg	Cellcept by Hoffmann La Roche	00004-0260	Immunosuppressant
ROCHE <> CELLCEPT500	Tab, Coated	Mycophenolate Mofetil 500 mg	Cellcept by Syntex	18393-0923	Immunosuppressant
ROCHE <> CYTOVENE250	Cap, Gelatin Coated	Ganciclovir 250 mg	Cytovene by Hoffmann La Roche	00004-0269	Antiviral
ROCHE <> CYTOVENE250	Cap	Ganciclovir 250 mg	Cytovene by Syntex	18393-0269	Antiviral
ROCHE <> CYTOVENE50	Cap, Dark Blue Print, 2 Blue Bands	Ganciclovir 500 mg	Cytovene by Syntex	18393-0914	Antiviral
ROCHE <> CYTOVENE500	Cap	Ganciclovir 500 mg	Cytovene by Hoffmann La Roche	00004-0278	Antiviral
ROCHE <> HIVID0375	Tab, Film Coated, Roche <> Hivid 0.375	Zalcitabine 0.375 mg	Hivid by Hoffmann La Roche	00004-0220	Antiviral
ROCHE <> HIVID0375	Tab, Film Coated, Roche <> Hivid 0.375	Zalcitabine 0.375 mg	Hivid by Pharm Utilization	60491-0296	Antiviral
ROCHE <> HIVID0750	Tab, Coated, Roche <> Hivid 0.750	Zalcitabine 0.75 mg	Hivid by Allscripts	54569-3877	Antiviral
ROCHE <> HIVID0750	Tab, Coated, Roche <> Hivid 0.750	Zalcitabine 0.75 mg	Hivid by Pharm Utilization	60491-0297	Antiviral
ROCHE <> NAPROSYN250	Tab	Naproxen 250 mg	Naprosyn by Allscripts	54569-0292	NSAID
ROCHE <> NAPROSYN250	Tab	Naproxen 250 mg	Naprosyn by Thrift Drug	59198-0237	NSAID
ROCHE <> NAPROSYN250	Tab	Naproxen 250 mg	Naprosyn by Amerisource	62584-0272	NSAID
ROCHE <> NAPROSYN250	Tab, Debossed	Naproxen 250 mg	Naprosyn by Syntex	18393-0272	NSAID
ROCHE <> TASMAR100	Tab, Film Coated	Tolcapone 100 mg	Tasmar by Hoffmann La Roche	00004-5920	Antiparkinson
ROCHE <> TASMAR200	Tab, Reddish-Brown, <> Tasmar 200, Film Coated	Tolcapone 200 mg	Tasmar by Hoffmann La Roche	00004-5921	Antiparkinson
ROCHE <> TORADOL	Tab, Roche Inside T Logo <> Toradol Inside T Logo, Film Coated	Ketorolac Tromethamine 10 mg	Toradol by Murfreesboro	51129-1151	NSAID
ROCHE <> TORADOL	Tab, Film Coated	Ketorolac Tromethamine 10 mg	Toradol by Quality Care	60346-0446	NSAID
ROCHE <> XENICAL120	Cap, Blue, Hard Gel, Opaque	Orlistat 120 mg	Xenical by Pegasus	55246-0020	Lipase Inhibitor
ROCHE <> XENICAL120	Cap, Blue	Orlistat 120 mg	Xenical by PDRX	55289-0512	Lipase Inhibitor
ROCHE 5	Tab, Red & Brown, Oval	Cilazapril 5 mg	Inhibace by Roche	Canadian	Antihypertensive
ROCHE0245	Cap, Green/Tan	Saquinavir 200 mg	Invirase by Roche		Antiviral
ROCHE0245	Cap, Light Brown & Green	Saquinavir Mesylate 200 mg	Invirase by Pharm Utilization	60491-0336	Antiviral
ROCHE0245	Cap, Roche over 0245	Saquinavir Mesylate 200 mg	Invirase by Quality Care	62682-1018	Antiviral
ROCHE0246	Cap, Beige	Saquinavir 200 mg	Fortovase by Roche	Canadian	Antiviral
ROCHE0246	Cap	Saquinavir 200 mg	Fortovase by Hoffmann La Roche	00004-0246	Antiviral
ROCHE1	Tab, Yellow, Oval	Cilazapril 1 mg	Inhibace by Roche	Canadian	Antihypertensive
ROCHE10	Tab, Light Blue, Cylindrical, Roche/10	Diazepam 10 mg	Valium Roche by Roche	Canadian	Antianxiety
ROCHE100	Tab, Orange, Roche/100	Moclobemide 100 mg	Manerix by Roche	Canadian	Antidepressant
ROCHE100	Tab, Light Yellow, Hexagonal	Tolcapone 100 mg	Tasmar by Roche	Canadian	Antiparkinson
ROCHE15	Tab, White, Cylindrical, Roche 1.5	Bromazepam 1.5 mg	Lectopam by Roche	Canadian	Sedative
ROCHE150	Tab, Yellow, Biconvex, Roche/150	Moclobemide 150 mg	Manerix by Roche	Canadian	Antidepressant
ROCHE2	Tab, White, Cylindrical, Roche/2	Clonazepam 2 mg	Rivotril by Roche	Canadian	Anticonvulsant
ROCHE200	Tab, Brown/Orange, Hexagonal	Tolcapone 200 mg	Tasmar by Roche	Canadian	Antiparkinson
ROCHE25	Tab, Pink, Oval, Tabish Brown, Roche 2.5	Cilazapril 2.5 mg	Inhibace by Roche	Canadian	Antihypertensive
ROCHE3	Tab, Pink, Cylindrical, Roche/3	Bromazepam 3 mg	Lectopam by Roche	Canadian	Sedative

ID FRONT <> BACK	DESCRIPTION FRONT <> BACK	INGREDIENT & STRENGTH	BRAND (OR EQUIV.) & FIRM	NDC#	CLASS; SCH.
ROCHE300	Tab, White, Biconvex, Roche/300	Moclobemide 300 mg	Manerix by Roche	Canadian	Antidepressant
ROCHE5	Tab, Yellow, Cylindrical	Diazepam 5 mg	Valium Roche by Roche	Canadian	Antianxiety
ROCHE6	Tab, Green, Cylindrical, Roche/6	Bromazepam 6 mg	Lectopam by Roche	Canadian	Sedative
ROCHE800160	Tab, White, Oval, Roche 800 + 160	Sulfamethoxazole 800 mg, Trimethoprim 160 mg	Bactrim DS by Roche	Canadian	Antibiotic
ROCHEBUMEX05	Tab, Roche Bumex 0.5	Bumetanide 0.5 mg	Bumex by Amerisource	62584-0125	Diuretic
ROCHEBUMEX05	Tab, Green, Round	Bumetanide 0.5 mg	Bumex by Med-Pro	53978-3386	Diuretic
ROCHEBUMEX05	Tab, Green	Bumetanide 0.5 mg	Bumex by Rightpak	65240-0698	Diuretic
ROCHEBUMEX1	Tab	Bumetanide 1 mg	Bumex by Amerisource	62584-0121	Diuretic
ROCHEBUMEX1	Tab	Bumetanide 1 mg	Bumex by Allscripts	54569-0503	Diuretic
ROCHEBUMEX1	Tab	Bumetanide 1 mg	Bumex by Physicians Total Care	54868-1293	Diuretic
ROCHEBUMEX1MG	Tab, Yellow	Bumetanide 1 mg	Bumex by Rightpak	65240-0610	Diuretic
ROCHEBUMEX2	Tab, Peach, Oblong	Bumetanide 2 mg	Bumex by Caraco	57664-0219	Diuretic
ROCHEBUMEX2	Tab	Bumetanide 2 mg	Bumex by Leiner	59606-0716	Diuretic
ROCHEBUMEX2	Tab	Bumetanide 2 mg	Bumex by Drug Distr	52985-0222	Diuretic
ROCHECLIBRAX	Cap, Green, Roche/C/Librax	Chlordiazepoxide 5 mg, Clidinium Bromide 2.5 mg	Librax by Roche	Canadian	Gastrointestinal
ROCHECPROLOPA	Cap, Blue & Flesh, Roche/C/Prolopa	Levodopa 100 mg, Benserazide 25 mg	Prolopa by Roche	Canadian	Antiparkinson
ROCHECPROLOPA	Cap, Light Gray/Blue, Roche/C/Prolopa	Levodopa 50 mg, Benserazide 12.5 mg	Prolopa by Roche	Canadian	Antiparkinson
ROCHECVALIUM5	Tab, Yellow, Cylindrical, Roche/C/Valium/5	Diazepam 5 mg	Valium Roche by Roche	Canadian	Antianxiety
ROCHEHEXAGON	Tab, White, Cylindrical, Roche/Hexagon	Mefloquine 250 mg	Lariam by Roche	Canadian	Antiprotozoal
ROCHEHEXAGON	Tab, White, Roche/Hexagon	Sulfadoxine 500 mg, Pyramethamine 25 mg	Fansidar by Roche	Canadian	Antimalarial
ROCHEROCHE	Cap, Brown & White, Roche/Roche	Acitretin 10 mg	Soriatane by Roche	Canadian	Dermatologic
ROCHEROCHE	Cap, Brown & Yellow, Roche/Roche	Acitretin 25 mg	Soriatane by Roche	Canadian	Dermatologic
ROCHEROCHE <> 5VALIUM	Tab, Round with Cut Out V Design	Diazepam 5 mg	Valium by Quality Care	60346-0439	Antianxiety; C IV
ROCHEROCHE <> 5VALIUM	Tab, V Design	Diazepam 5 mg	Valium by Caremark	00339-4073	Antianxiety; C IV
ROCHEROCHE <> 5VALIUM	Tab, Scored, Roche over Roche <> V over Valium	Diazepam 5 mg	Valium by Allscripts	54569-0948	Antianxiety; C IV
ROCHEVROCHE <> 10VVALIUM	Tab, Roche V Roche <> 10 over V over Valium	Diazepam 10 mg	Valium by Roche	00140-0006	Antianxiety; C IV
ROCHEVROCHE <> 2VVALIUM	Tab, Roche V Roche <> 2 over V Logo Valium	Diazepam 2 mg	Valium by Roche	00140-0004	Antianxiety; C IV
ROCHEVROCHE <> 5VVALIUM	Tab, Roche V Roche <> 2 over V Logo Valium	Diazepam 5 mg	Valium by Roche	00140-0005	Antianxiety; C IV
ROCHEXENICAL120	Cap, Turquoise, Roche Xenical 120	Orlistat 120 mg	Xenical by Roche	Canadian	Lipase Inhibitor
ROCHEXENICAL120	Cap, Dark Blue, Gelatin	Orlistat 120 mg	by Allscripts	54569-4742	Lipase Inhibitor
ROCHEXENICAI120	Cap, Blue	Orlistat 120 mg	Xenical by Southwood Pharms	58016-0361	Lipase Inhibitor
ROERIG <> DIFLUCAN100	Tab, Coated, Diflucan/100	Fluconazole 100 mg	Diflucan by Amerisource	62584-0362	Antifungal
ROERIG <> DIFLUCAN100	Tab, Coated, Roerig <> Diflucan/100	Fluconazole 100 mg	Diflucan by Nat Pharmpak Serv	55154-3214	Antifungal
ROERIG <> DIFLUCAN100	Tab, Pink, Trapezoidal, Coated, Roerig <> Diflucan/100	Fluconazole 100 mg	Diflucan by Roerig	00049-3420	Antifungal
ROERIG <> DIFLUCAN100	Tab, Coated	Fluconazole 100 mg	by Med Pro	53978-3012	Antifungal
ROERIG <> DIFLUCAN100	Tab, Coated	Fluconazole 100 mg	Diflucan by Allscripts	54569-3926	Antifungal
ROERIG <> DIFLUCAN200	Tab, Coated	Fluconazole 200 mg	Diflucan by Nat Pharmpak Serv	55154-3215	Antifungal
ROERIG <> DIFLUCAN200	Tab, Coated, Diflucan/200	Fluconazole 200 mg	Diflucan by Amerisource	62584-0363	Antifungal

ID FRONT <> BACK	DESCRIPTION FRONT <> BACK	INGREDIENT & STRENGTH	BRAND (OR EQUIV.) & FIRM	NDC#	CLASS; SCH.
ROERIG <> DIFLUCAN200	Tab, Pink, Trapezoidal, Coated, Roerig <> Diflucan/200	Fluconazole 200 mg	Diflucan by Roerig	00049-3430	Antifungal
ROERIG <> DIFLUCAN200	Tab, Coated	Fluconazole 200 mg	by Med Pro	53978-3105	Antifungal
ROERIG <> DIFLUCAN200	Tab	Fluconazole 200 mg	Diflucan by Allscripts	54569-3269	Antifungal
ROERIG <> DIFLUGAN50	Tab, Coated	Fluconazole 50 mg	Diflucan by Pharm Utilization	60491-0194	Antifungal
ROERIG143	Tab, Yellow, Oblong	Carbenicillin Indanyl 382 mg	Geocillin by Pfizer		Antibiotic
ROERIG143	Tab, Yellow, Cap Shaped	Carbenicillin Indanyl Sodium Equivalent to 382 mg Carbenicillin	Geocillin by Roerig	00049-1430	Antibiotic
ROERIG159	Cap, White	Troleandomycin 250 mg	Tao by Roerig	00049-1590	Antibiotic
ROERIG210	Tab, Blue & White, Oblong	Meclizine HCl 12.5 mg	Antivert by Roerig	00049-2100	Antiemetic
ROERIG211	Tab, Blue & Yellow, Oblong	Meclizine HCl 25 mg	Antivert by Roerig	00049-2110	Antiemetic
ROERIG214	Tab, Blue & Yellow, Oblong	Meclizine HCl 50 mg	Antivert by Roerig	00049-2140	Antiemetic
ROERIG254 <> MARAX	Tab	Ephedrine Sulfate 25 mg, Hydroxyzine HCl 10 mg, Theophylline 130 mg	Marax by Roerig	00049-2540	Antiasthmatic
ROERIG341	Tab, Pink, Trapezoidal	Fluconazole 50 mg	Diflucan by Roerig	00049-3410	Antifungal
ROERIG350	Tab, Pink, Oval	Fluconazole 150 mg	Diflucan by Roerig	00049-3500	Antifungal
ROERIG491	Tab, Yellow, Cap-Shaped	Sertraline HCl 100 mg	Zoloft by Roerig	00049-4910	Antidepression
ROERIG534	Cap, Pink & Red	Doxepin HCl 10 mg	Sinequan by Roerig	00049-5340	Antidepressant
ROERIG534 <>	Cap	Doxepin HCl	Sinequan by Roerig Pfizer	00662-5340	Antidepressant
ROERIG535 SINEQUAN	Cap, Blue & Pink	Doxepin HCl 25 mg	Sinequan by Roerig	00049-5350	Antidepressant
ROERIG535 <> SINEQUAN	Cap	Doxepin HCl	Sinequan by Nat Pharmpak Serv	55154-3209	Antidepressant
ROERIG535 <> SINEQUAN	Cap, Roerig over 535 <> Sinequan	Doxepin HCl	Sinequan by Roerig Pfizer	00662-5350	Antidepressant
ROERIG535 <> SINEQUAN	Cap, Blue & Pink	Doxepin HCl 25 mg	Sinequan by Rightpac	65240-0734	Antidepressant
ROERIG536	Cap, Pink & White	Doxepin HCl 50 mg	Sinequan by Roerig	00049-5360	Antidepressant
ROERIG536 <> SINEQUAN	Cap	Doxepin HCl	Sinequan by Nat Pharmpak Serv	55154-3210	Antidepressant
ROERIG536 <> SINEQUAN	Cap, Bright Pink & Pale Pink, Roerig over 536 <> Sinequan	Doxepin HCl	Sinequan by Roerig Pfizer	00662-5360	Antidepressant
ROERIG536 <> SINEQUAN	Cap, Pink	Doxepin HCl 50 mg	Sinequan by Rightpac	65240-0735	Antidepressant
ROERIG537	Cap, Blue	Doxepin HCl 150 mg	Sinequan by Roerig	00049-5370	Antidepressant
ROERIG538	Cap, Blue & White	Doxepin HCl 100 mg	Sinequan by Roerig	00049-5380	Antidepressant
ROERIG539	Cap, White	Doxepin HCl 75 mg	Sinequan by Roerig	00049-5390	Antidepressant
ROERIG539 <> SINEQUAN	Cap	Doxepin HCl	Sinequan by Roerig Pfizer	00662-5390	Antidepressant
ROERIG562	Tab, Yellow, Triangle-Shaped	Hydroxyzine HCl 50 mg	Atarax by Roerig	00049-5620	Antihistamine
ROERIG563	Tab, Red, Triangle-Shaped	Hydroxyzine HCl 100 mg	Atarax by Roerig	00049-5630	Antihistamine
ROERIG571	Cap, Orange & Yellow	Thiothixene 1 mg	Navane by Roerig	00049-5710	Antipsychotic
ROERIG572 <> NAVANE	Cap, Blue & Yellow, Roerig 572	Thiothixene HCl 2 mg	Navane by Roerig	00049-5720	Antipsychotic
ROERIG573 <> NAVANE	Cap, Orange & White, Roerig573	Thiothixene HCl 5 mg	Navane by Roerig	00049-5730	Antipsychotic
ROERIG574	Cap, Blue & White	Thiothixene 10 mg	Navane by Roerig	00049-5740	Antipsychotic
ROERIG577	Cap, Blue & Green	Thiothixene 20 mg	Navane by Roerig	00049-5770	Antipsychotic
RONDEX278	Cap, Yellow	Oxytetracycine 250 mg	Terramycin by Rondex		Antibiotic
ROSETTE	Tab, White, Round	Pamabrom 25 mg, Pyrilamine Maleate 12.5 mg, Acetaminophen 325 mg	Pamprin by Chattem	Canadian	PMS Relief

ID FRONT <> BACK	DESCRIPTION FRONT <> BACK	INGREDIENT & STRENGTH	BRAND (OR EQUIV.) & FIRM	NDC#	CLASS; SCH.
ROUGIER	Cap, Blue & White, Opaque, Rougier Logo	Acidophilus, Bulgaricus, Lactobacillus, Streptococcus, Thermophilus	by Rougier	Canadian DIN# 00351547	Probiotic
ROUGIER	Cap, Yellow, Opaque, Gelatin, Rougier Logo	Diphenhydramine HCl 50 mg	by Altimed	Canadian DIN# 02153165	Antihistamine
ROUGIER	Tab, Pink, Round, Scored, Rougier Logo	Yohimbine HCl 6 mg	by Altimed	Canadian DIN# 00843512	Impotence Agent
ROWELL7720	Tab, White, Round	Chenodiol 250 mg	Chenix by RR		Cholelitholytic
ROYCE <> 377200	Tab, Coated, Royce Logo <> 377,200 and a Partial Score	Hydroxychloroquine Sulfate 200 mg	by Zenith Goldline	00182-2609	Antimalarial
RP <> 51	Tab, Yellow, Round	Dextroamphetamine Sulfate 5 mg	Dextrostat by Shire Richwood	58521-0451	Stimulant; C II
RP <> 52	Tab, Yellow, Round	Dextroamphetamine Sulfate 10 mg	Dextrostat by Shire Richwood	58521-0452	Stimulant; C II
RP069	Tab, Ivory, Round, RP Monarch Logo 069	Anhydrous Theophylline 300 mg	Quibron-T Accud by Monarch		Antiasthmatic
RP069	Tab, RP 069 Debossed, Bevel-edged,	Theophylline 300 mg	Quibron T by Bristol Myers Squibb	00087-0512	Antiasthmatic
RP070	Tab, White, Round, RP Monarch Logo 070	Anhydrous Theophylline 300 mg	Quibron-T/SR Acc by Monarch		Antiasthmatic
RP070	Tab, Ex Release, RP 070 Debossed, Bevel-edged	Theophylline 300 mg	Quibron T Sr by Bristol Myers Squibb	00087-0519	Antiasthmatic
RP5455	Tab, Pink, Round	Methamphetamine HCl 5 mg	by Richwood		Stimulant; C II
RP5456	Tab, Pink, Round	Methamphetamine HCl 10 mg	by Richwood		Stimulant; C II
RP57	Tab, Yellow, Round	Phendimetrazine Tartrate 35 mg	X-Trozine by Richwood		Anorexiant; C III
RP57	Tab, Green, Round	Phendimetrazine Tartrate 35 mg	X-Trozine by Richwood		Anorexiant; C III
RP57	Tab, Blue, Round	Phendimetrazine Tartrate 35 mg	X-Trozine by Richwood		Anorexiant; C III
RP57	Tab, Pink, Round	Phendimetrazine Tartrate 35 mg	X-Trozine by Richwood		Anorexiant; C III
RP600	Tab	Guaifenesin 600 mg	Gua Sr by Seatrace	00551-0189	Expectorant
RPC <> 073	Tab, Sugar Coated	Propantheline Bromide 7.5 mg	Pro Banthine by Roberts	54092-0073	Gastrointestinal
RPC <> 074	Tab, Sugar Coated	Propantheline Bromide 15 mg	Pro Banthine by Roberts	54092-0074	Gastrointestinal
RPC <> 62	Cap, ER	Phendimetrazine Tartrate 105 mg	X Trozine LA by Shire Richwood	58521-0105	Anorexiant; C III
RPC <> 73	Tab, White, Round	Propantheline Bromide 7.5 mg	Pro Banthine by Compumed	00403-5167	Gastrointestinal
RPC 63	Cap, Black	Phendimetrazine Tartrate 35 mg	X-Trozine by Richwood		Anorexiant; C III
RPC 63	Cap, Red & White	Phendimetrazine Tartrate 35 mg	X-Trozine by Richwood		Anorexiant; C III
RPC 63	Cap, Black & Orange	Phendimetrazine Tartrate 35 mg	X-Trozine by Richwood		Anorexiant; C III
RPC055	Tab, RPC Over 055	Hydroflumethiazide 50 mg	Saluron by Mead Johnson	00015-5410	Diuretic; Antihypertensive
RPC055	Tab, RPC Over 055	Hydroflumethiazide 50 mg	Saluron by Roberts	54092-0055	Diuretic
RPC056	Tab, RPC Over 056	Hydroflumethiazide 50 mg, Reserpine 0.125 mg	Salutensin by Mead Johnson	00015-5436	Diuretic; Antihypertensive
RPC056	Tab	Hydroflumethiazide 50 mg, Reserpine 0.125 mg	Salutensin by Roberts	54092-0056	Diuretic; Antihypertensive
RPC057	Tab, Pale Yellow, RPC Over 05	Hydroflumethiazide 25 mg, Reserpine 0.125 mg	Salutensin Demi by Mead Johnson	00015-5455	Diuretic; Antihypertensive
RPC066 <> COMHIST	Tab	Chlorpheniramine Maleate 2 mg, Phenylephrine HCl 10 mg, Phenyltoloxamine Citrate 25 mg	Comhist by Roberts	54092-0066	Cold Remedy
RPC152	Tab, Ex Release, RPC/152	Guaifenesin 600 mg	Sinumist Sr by Sovereign	58716-0602	Expectorant
RPC25 <> 003	Tab, RPC Above Score and 2.5 Below	Midodrine HCl 2.5 mg	Proamatine by Nycomed	57585-0103	Antihypotension
RPC25 <> 003	Tab, RPC Above Score and 2.5 Below <> Biplaner	Midodrine HCl 2.5 mg	Proamatine by Roberts	54092-0003	Antihypotension
RPC25003	Tab, White, Round, RPC 2.5/003	Midodrine HCl 2.5 mg	ProAmatine by Roberts		Antihypotension
RPC5 <> 004	Tab, RPC Above Score and 5 Below	Midodrine HCl 5 mg	Proamatine by Nycomed	57585-0104	Antihypotension
RPC5 <> 004	Tab, RPC Above and 5 Below Score <> Biplanar Tab	Midodrine HCl 5 mg	Proamatine by Roberts	54092-0004	Antihypotension
RPC5 <> 4	Tab, Orange, Round, Scored	Midodrine HCl 5 mg	Proamatine by Murfreesboro Ph	51129-1433	Antihypotension
RPC62	Cap, Brown & Clear	Phendimetrazine Tartrate 105 mg	by Physicians Total Care	54868-1336	Anorexiant; C III
RPC62	Cap, Clear with White Beads, ER, RPC/62 <> Clear with White Beads	Phendimetrazine Tartrate 105 mg	Adipost by Jones	52604-0470	Anorexiant; C III

ID FRONT <> BACK	DESCRIPTION FRONT <> BACK	INGREDIENT & STRENGTH	BRAND (OR EQUIV.) & FIRM	NDC#	CLASS; SCH.
RPC62	Cap, ER	Phendimetrazine Tartrate 105 mg	by DRX	55045-2453	Anorexiant; C III
RPC62	Cap, Brown & Clear	Phendimetrazine Tartrate 105 mg	by Compumed	00403-0016	Anorexiant; C III
RPC69	Cap	Phentermine HCl 30 mg	by Quality Care	62682-7042	Anorexiant; C IV
RPC69	Cap, Yellow	Phentermine HCl 30 mg	Oby Trim by Eon	00185-2061	Anorexiant; C IV
RPC69	Cap	Phentermine HCl 30 mg	by Allscripts	54569-3248	Anorexiant; C IV
RPL1050	Tab, White/Green Specks, Round	Pseudoephedrine HCl 120 mg, Guaifenesin 400 mg	Histalet X by RR		Cold Remedy
RPL1082	Cap, Orange/Clear	Phendimetrazine Tartrate 105 mg	Melfiat-105 by RR		Anorexiant; C III
RPR <> 20R	Tab	Chlorthalidone 50 mg	Hygroton by RPR	00801-0020	Diuretic
RPR <> 20R	Tab, RPR Logo <> 20 in raised H	Chlorthalidone 50 mg	Hygroton by RPR	00075-0020	Diuretic
RPR <> 22R	Tab, RPR Logo <> 22 in raised H	Chlorthalidone 25 mg	Hygroton by RPR	00075-0022	Diuretic
RPR <> 22R	Tab	Chlorthalidone 25 mg	Hygroton by RPR	00801-0022	Diuretic
RPR <> 5100	Tab, Film Coated, RPR Logo <> 5100	Enoxacin Sesquihydrate	Penetrex by RPR	00075-5100	Antibiotic
RPR <> 5100	Tab, Light Blue, Oblong	Enoxacin Sesquihydrate	Penetrex by RPR	00801-5100	Antibiotic
RPR <> 5140	Tab, Film Coated, RPR Logo <> 5140	Enoxacin Sesquihydrate	Penetrex by RPR	00075-5140	Antibiotic
RPR <> 5140	Tab, Dark Blue, Oblong	Enoxacin Sesquihydrate	Penetrex by RPR	00801-5140	Antibiotic
RPR <> DDAVP01	Tab, White, Oblong, RPR <> DDAVP 0.1	Desmopressin Acetate 0.1 mg	DDAVP by RPR	00075-0016	Antidiuretic
RPR <> DDAVP02	Tab, RPR <> DDAVP Over 0.2	Desmopressin Acetate 0.2 mg	DDAVP by Promex Med	62301-0030	Antidiuretic
RPR <> DDAVP02	Tab, White, Oblong, RPR Logo <> DDAVP 0.2	Desmopressin Acetate 0.2 mg	DDAVP by RPR	00075-0026	Antidiuretic
RPR <> DILACORXR120MG	Cap, Gold	Diltiazem HCl 120 mg	Dilacor XR by Thrift Drug	59198-0259	Antihypertensive
RPR <> DILACORXR180MG	Cap, Ex Release	Diltiazem HCl 180 mg	Dilacor XR by Thrift Drug	59198-0260	Antihypertensive
RPR <> SLOBID	Tab, White, Oval, In Red RPR<>SLO-BID	Theophylline 50 mg	Slo Bid by Takeda	64764-0451	Antiasthmatic
RPR <> SLOBID100MG	Cap, ER, RPR Logo <> SLO-BID 100 MG	Theophylline 100 mg	Slo Bid by RPR	00075-0100	Antiasthmatic
RPR <> SLOBID125MG	Cap, White	Theophylline 125 mg	Slo Bid by Murfreesboro Ph	51129-1668	Antiasthmatic
RPR <> SLOBID125MG	Cap, ER, RPR Logo <> SLO-BID 125 MG	Theophylline 125 mg	Slo Bid by RPR	00075-1125	Antiasthmatic
RPR <> SLOBID200MG	Cap, ER, RPR Logo <> SLO-BID 200 MG	Theophylline 200 mg	Slo Bid by RPR	00075-0200	Antiasthmatic
RPR <> SLOBID300MG	Cap, ER, RPR Logo <> SLO-BID 300 MG	Theophylline 300 mg	Slo Bid by RPR	00075-0300	Antiasthmatic
RPR <> SLOBID50MG	Cap, ER	Theophylline 50 mg	Slo Bid by RPR	00075-0057	Antiasthmatic
RPR <> SLOBID75MG	Cap, ER, SLO-BID 75 MG	Theophylline 75 mg	Slo Bid by RPR	00075-1075	Antiasthmatic
RPR 202	Tab, White, Cap-Shaped, Film Coated	Riluzole 50 mg	Rilutek by RPR	00801-7700	Amyotrophic Lateral Sclerosis Agent
RPr 351	Tab, White, Round	Theophylline 100 mg	Slophyllin by RPR		Antiasthmatic
RPr 352	Tab, White, Round	Theophylline 200 mg	Slophyllin by RPR		Antiasthmatic
RPR0251180MG	Cap	Diltiazem HCl 180 mg	Dilacor XR by RPR		Antihypertensive
RPR0252240MG	Cap	Diltiazem HCl 240 mg	Dilacor XR by RPR		Antihypertensive
RPR201	Tab, Film Coated	Sparfloxacin 200 mg	Zagam by RPR	00075-5410	Antibiotic
RPR201	Tab, Film Coated	Sparfloxacin 200 mg	Zagam by RPR	62047-5410	Antibiotic
RPR201	Tab, Film Coated	Sparfloxacin 200 mg	Zagam by RPR	00801-5410	Antibiotic
RPR202	Tab, Film Coated, RPR=Rhone-Poulenc Rorer Logo	Riluzole 50 mg	Rilutek by RPR	00075-7700	Amyotrophic Lateral Sclerosis Agent
RPR202 <> RILUTEK	Tab, Film Coated	Riluzole 50 mg	Rilutek by RPR	62047-7700	Amyotrophic Lateral Sclerosis Agent
RPR21	Tab, White, Round	Chlorthalidone 100 mg	Hygroton by RPR		Diuretic
RPRDILACOR120	Cap, Gold & White, RPR/Dilacor/120	Diltazem 120 mg	Dilacor XR by Watson		Antihypertensive
RPRDILACOR180	Cap, Gold & White, RPR/Dilacor/180	Diltazem 180 mg	Dilacor XR by Watson		Antihypertensive
RPRDILACOR240	Cap, Gold & White, RPR/Dilacor/240	Diltazem 240 mg	Dilacor XR by Watson		Antihypertensive
RPRDILACORXR240	Cap, RPR Dilacor XR 240 mg <> Black Vertical Lines, ER	Diltiazem HCl 240 mg	Dilacor XR by Thrift Drug	59198-0261	Antihypertensive
RPRH20	Tab, Aqua, Square	Chlorthalidone 50 mg	Hygroton by RPR		Diuretic
RPRH22	Tab, Peach, Square	Chlorthalidone 25 mg	Hygroton by RPR		Diuretic
RPRSLOBID200MG	Cap, ER	Theophylline 200 mg	by Talbert Med	44514-0903	Antiasthmatic
RPRSLOBID300MG	Cap, ER	Theophylline 300 mg	by Talbert Med	44514-0904	Antiasthmatic

ID FRONT <> BACK	DESCRIPTION FRONT <> BACK	INGREDIENT & STRENGTH	BRAND (OR EQUIV.) & FIRM	NDC#	CLASS; SCH.
RR	Tab, White, Round	Calcium Sulfate, Belladonna, Potassoum Bromide	Acne Relief Tab by Herbal Harvest		Supplement
RR0840	Cap, Yellow, RR-0840	Acetaminophen 325 mg, Codeine 16 mg, Phenylephrine 10 mg, Chlorphen. 2 mg	Colrex by RR		Analgesic; C III
RR1	Tab, Pink, Round	Prednisone 1 mg	Orasone 1 by RR		Steroid
RR10	Tab, Blue, Round	Prednisone 10 mg	Orasone 10 by RR		Steroid
RR1007	Tab, White, Round	Medroxyprogestrone Acetate 10 mg	Curretab by RR		Progestin
RR1014	Tab, Blue, Round	Esterified Estrogens 0.3 mg	Estratab by RR		Hormone
RR1022	Tab, Yellow, Round	Esterified Estrogens 0.625 mg	Estratab by RR		Hormone
RR1023	Tab, Green, Oblong	Esterified Estrogens 0.625 mg, Methyltestosterone 2.5 mg	Estratest by RR		Hormone
RR1024	Tab, Red, Round	Esterified Estrogens 1.25 mg	Estratab by RR		Hormone
RR1025	Tab, Pink, Round	Esterified Estrogens 2.5 mg	Estratab by RR		Hormone
RR1026	Tab, Green, Oblong	Esterified Estrogens 1.25 mg, Methyltestosterone 2.5 mg	Estratest by RR		Hormone
RR1039	Tab, White/Blue Specks, Oblong	Phenylpropanolamine 50 mg, Pyrilamine 25 mg, Chlorophen 4 mg, Phenylep 10 mg	Histalet Forte by RR		Cold Remedy
RR1088	Tab, Brown, Rectangular	Hydrocodone Bitartrate 5 mg, Phenindamine 25 mg, Guaifenesin 200 mg	P-V-Tussin by RR		Analgesic; C III
RR1132	Tab, Yellow, Round	Hydralazine 25 mg, Reserpine 0.1 mg, Hydrochlorothiazide 15 mg	Unipres by RR		Antihypertensive
RR1146	Tab, Blue, Oblong	Prenatal Vitamin	Zenate by RR		Vitamin
RR1216	Cap, Brown	Vitamin Combination	Vio-Bec by RR		Vitamin
RR1218	Tab, Brown, Oblong	Vitamin Combination	Vio-Bec Forte by RR		Vitamin
RR1611	Tab, Peach, Oval	Vitamin, Mineral Comb.	Norlac RX by RR		Vitamin
RR20	Tab, Yellow, Round	Prednisone 20 mg	Orasone 20 by RR		Steroid
RR3205	Tab, Yellow, Round	Dexamethasone 0.5 mg	Decadron by RR		Steroid
RR3210	Tab, Green, Round	Dexamethasone 0.75 mg	Decadron by RR		Steroid
RR3215	Tab, Pink, Round	Dexamethasone 1.5 mg	Decadron by RR		Steroid
RR3220	Tab, White, Round	Dexamethasone 4 mg	Decadron by RR		Steroid
RR40	Cap, Red	Amantidine 100 mg	Symmetrel by Reid-Rowell		Antiviral
RR4020	Cap, Clear	Quinidine Sulfate 300 mg	Cin-Quin by RR		Antiarrhythmic
RR4024	Tab, White, Round	Quinidine Sulfate 100 mg	Cin-Quin by RR		Antiarrhythmic
RR4028	Tab, White, Round	Quinidine Sulfate 200 mg	Cin-Quin by RR		Antiarrhythmic
RR4032	Tab, White, Round	Quinidine Sulfate 300 mg	Cin-Quin by RR		Antiarrhythmic
RR4120	Cap, Orange, Oval	Valproic Acid 250 mg	Depakene by Reid-Rowell		Anticonvulsant
RR4140	Cap, Red, Oval	Amantadine HCl 100 mg	Symadine by Reid-Rowell		Antiviral
RR5	Tab, White, Round	Prednisone 5 mg	Orasone 5 by RR		Steroid
RR50	Tab, White, Round	Prednisone 50 mg	Orasone 50 by RR		Steroid
RR586	Tab, Green, Octagonal	Fluoxymesterone 10 mg	Halotestin by RR		Steroid; C III
RR7025	Tab, Red, Round	Meclizine HCl 20 mg	Ru-Vert M by RR		Antiemetic
RR7512	Cap, Peach	Lithium Carbonate 300 mg	Lithonate by RR		Antipsychotic
RR7516	Tab, White, Round	Lithium Carbonate 300 mg	Lithotab by RR		Antipsychotic
RS <> 301	Tab, White, Round	Diphenoxylate HCl 2.5 mg; Atropine Sulfate 0.025 mg	by R & S Pharma	65162-0301	Antidiarrheal; C V
RS <> 301	Tab, White, Round	Diphenoxylate HCl 2.5 mg; Atropine Sulfate 0.025 mg	by Corepharma	64720-0301	Antidiarrheal; C V
RSN <> 30MG	Tab, White, Oval, Film Coated	Risedronate Sodium 30 mg	Actonel by Procter & Gamble	Canadian DIN# 02239146	Bisphosphonate
RSN <> 30MG	Tab, Yellow, Oval, Film Coated	Risedronate Sodium 30 mg	Actonel by Procter & Gamble	00149-0470	Bisphosphonate
RSN <> 5MG	Tab, Yellow, Oval, Film-Coated	Risedronate Sodium 5 mg	Actonel by Procter & Gamble	Canadian DIN# 02242531	Bisphosphonate
RSN <> 5MG	Tab, Yellow, Oval, Film Coated	Risedronate Sodium 5 mg	Actonel by Procter & Gamble	Canadian DIN# 02242518	Bisphosphonate
RSN <> 5MG	Tab, Yellow, Oval, Film Coated	Risedronate Sodium 5 mg	Actonel by Procter Gamble Pharm	00149-0471	Bisphosphonate
RSTSM <> 325	Cap, Green, Film Coated	Acetaminophen 325 mg, Pseudoephedrine HCl 30 mg	Regular Tylenol Sinus	Canadian DIN# 00778400	Cold Remedy

ID FRONT <> BACK	DESCRIPTION FRONT <> BACK	INGREDIENT & STRENGTH	BRAND (OR EQUIV.) & FIRM	NDC#	CLASS; SCH.
RUFEN400	Tab, Magenta, Round	Ibuprofen 400 mg	Rufen by Boots		NSAID
RUFEN6	Tab, White, Elongated	Ibuprofen 600 mg	Rufen by Boots		NSAID
RUFEN8	Tab, White, Elongated	Ibuprofen 800 mg	Rufen by Boots		NSAID
RUGBY	Tab	Captopril 100 mg	by Rugby	00536-3474	Antihypertensive
RUGBY <> 3109	Tab	Clomiphene Citrate 50 mg	by Rugby	00536-3109	Infertility
RUGBY <> 3367	Cap	Decyclomine HCl 10 mg	by Chelsea	46193-0105	Gastrointestinal
RUGBY <> 3377	Tab	Decyclomine HCl 20 mg	by Heartland	61392-0041	Gastrointestinal
RUGBY <> 3377	Tab	Decyclomine HCl 20 mg	by Quality Care	60346-0912	Gastrointestinal
RUGBY <> 3377	Tab	Decyclomine HCl 20 mg	by DRX	55045-1467	Gastrointestinal
RUGBY <> 3377	Tab	Dicyclomine HCl 20 mg	by Allscripts	54569-0419	Gastrointestinal
RUGBY <> 3840	Tab	Furosemide 20 mg	by Rugby	00536-3840	Diuretic
RUGBY <> 3841	Tab	Furosemide 40 mg	by Rugby	00536-3841	Diuretic
RUGBY <> 3914	Tab	Acetaminophen 500 mg, Hydrocodone Bitartrate 7.5 mg	by Rugby	00536-5507	Analgesic; C III
RUGBY <> 3918	Tab, 39/18	Hyoscyamine Sulfate 0.125 mg	by Anabolic	00722-6286	Gastrointestinal
RUGBY <> 3920	Tab	Atropine Sulfate 0.0194 mg, Hyoscyamine Sulfate 0.1037 mg, Phenobarbital 16.2 mg, Scopolamine Hydrobromide 0.0065 mg	Belladonna PB by Quality Care	60346-0042	Gastrointestinal; C IV
RUGBY <> 3922	Tab	Hydrochlorothiazide 25 mg	by Heartland	61392-0011	Diuretic
RUGBY <> 4012	Tab, Film Coated	Etodolac 400 mg	by Rugby	00536-4012	NSAID
RUGBY <> 4012	Tab, Film Coated	Etodolac 400 mg	by Chelsea	46193-0584	NSAID
RUGBY <> 4025	Tab	Methyclothiazide 5 mg	by Chelsea	46193-0525	Diuretic
RUGBY <> 4328	Tab, White, Scored	Prednisone 50 mg	by Allscripts	54569-0333	Steroid
RUGBY <> 4432	Tab	Quinidine Sulfate 200 mg	by Quality Care	60346-0627	Antiarrhythmic
RUGBY <> 4617	Tab, Partial Score	Sulfasalazine 500 mg	by Murfreesboro	51129-1338	Gastrointestinal
RUGBY <> 4840	Tab, Film Coated	Cyclobenzaprine HCl 10 mg	by Quality Care	60346-0581	Muscle Relaxant
RUGBY <> 4843	Tab	Naproxen 375 mg	by Quality Care	60346-0817	NSAID
RUGBY <> 5574	Cap	Nicardipine HCl 30 mg	by Chelsea	46193-0560	Antihypertensive
RUGBY <> 5663	Tab, Film Coated	Cimetidine 400 mg	by Quality Care	60346-0945	Gastrointestinal
RUGBY <> 5721	Tab, White, Round	Ketorolac Tromethamine 10 mg	by Murfreesboro	51129-1605	NSAID
RUGBY <> 5721	Tab, Film Coated	Ketorolac Tromethamine 10 mg	by Rugby	00536-5721	NSAID
RUGBY <> 5721	Tab, Film Coated	Ketorolac Tromethamine 10 mg	by Chelsea	46193-0564	NSAID
RUGBY <> 5725	Cap	Acyclovir 200 mg	by Rugby	00536-5725	Antiviral
RUGBY <> 5725	Cap	Acyclovir 200 mg	by Chelsea	46193-0569	Antiviral
RUGBY <> 5925	Tab, White, Round	Diethylpropion HCl 25 mg	by Blue Ridge	59273-0007	Antianorexiant; C IV
RUGBY <> 5925	Tab, White, Round	Diethylpropion HCl 25 mg	by Dupont Pharma	00056-0675	Antianorexiant; C IV
RUGBY <> 5925	Tab, White, Round	Diethylpropion HCl 25 mg	by Dupont Pharma	00056-0669	Antianorexiant; C IV
RUGBY0070	Cap	Amoxicillin 250 mg	Amoxil by Rugby		Antibiotic
RUGBY0080	Cap, Cream	Amoxicillin 500 mg	Amoxil by Rugby		Antibiotic
RUGBY0120	Cap, Gray & Red	Cephalexin 250 mg	Keflex by Rugby		Antibiotic
RUGBY0130	Cap, Red	Cephalexin 500 mg	Keflex by Rugby		Antibiotic
RUGBY0230	Cap, Blue	Doxycycline Hyclate 100 mg	Vibramycin by Rugby		Antibiotic
RUGBY0250	Tab, Pink, Round	Erythromycin Stearate 250 mg	Erythrocin by Rugby		Antibiotic
RUGBY0265	Tab, Pink, Oval	Erythromycin Stearate 500 mg	Erythrocin by Rugby		Antibiotic
RUGBY0280	Cap, Aqua & White	Doxycycline Hyclate 50 mg	Vibramycin by Rugby		Antibiotic
RUGBY0340	Tab, Buff	Doxycycline Hyclate 100 mg	Vibra-Tab by Rugby		Antibiotic
RUGBY0390	Tab, Buff	Doxycycline Hyclate 50 mg	Vibra-Tab by Rugby		Antibiotic
RUGBY10	Tab, White, Round	Isoxsuprine HCl 10 mg	Vasodilan by Rugby		Vasodilator
RUGBY1003027	Tab, White, Round, Rugby 100/3027	Allopurinol 100 mg	Zyloprim by Rugby		Antigout
RUGBY1820	Cap, Orange & Yellow	Tetracycline HCl 250 mg	Achromycin V by Rugby		Antibiotic
RUGBY1830	Cap, Black & Yellow	Tetracycline HCl 250 mg	Achromycin V by Rugby		Antibiotic
RUGBY1870	Cap, Black & Yellow	Tetracycline HCl 500 mg	Achromycin V by Rugby		Antibiotic
RUGBY20	Tab, White, Round	Isoxsuprine HCl 20 mg	Vasodilan by Rugby		Vasodilator
RUGBY212	Tab, White, Round	Terfenadine 60 mg	Seldane by Rugby		Antihistamine

ID FRONT <> BACK	DESCRIPTION FRONT <> BACK	INGREDIENT & STRENGTH	BRAND (OR EQUIV.) & FIRM	NDC#	CLASS; SCH.
RUGBY23228	Tab, White, Round, Rugby 2/3228	Acetaminophen 300 mg, Codeine 15 mg	Tylenol #2 by Rugby		Analgesic; C III
RUGBY3003028	Tab, Peach, Round, Rugby 300/3028	Allopurinol 300 mg	Zyloprim by Rugby		Antigout
RUGBY3007	Tab, White, Round, Rugby Logo 3007	Acetazolamide 250 mg	Diamox by Rugby		Diuretic
RUGBY3018	Tab, White, Round	Triprolidine HCl 2.5 mg, Pseudoephedrine HCl 60 mg	Actifed by Rugby		Cold Remedy
RUGBY3021	Tab, White, Round	Triprolidine HCl 2.5 mg, Pseudoephedrine HCl 60 mg	Actifed by Rugby		Cold Remedy
RUGBY3044	Tab, Yellow, Round	Amiloride 5 mg, Hydrochlorothiazide 50 mg	Moduretic by Rugby		Diuretic
RUGBY3046	Tab, White, Round	Aminophylline 100 mg	Aminophyllin by Rugby		Antiasthmatic
RUGBY3060	Tab, White, Round	Aminophylline 200 mg	Aminophyllin by Rugby		Antiasthmatic
RUGBY3071	Tab, Pink, Round	Amitriptyline 10 mg	Elavil by Rugby		Antidepressant
RUGBY3072	Tab, Green, Round	Amitriptyline 25 mg	Elavil by Rugby		Antidepressant
RUGBY3073	Tab, Brown, Round	Amitriptyline 50 mg	Elavil by Rugby		Antidepressant
RUGBY3074	Tab, Lavender, Round	Amitriptyline 75 mg	Elavil by Rugby		Antidepressant
RUGBY3075	Tab, Orange, Round	Amitriptyline 100 mg	Elavil by Rugby		Antidepressant
RUGBY3076	Tab, Peach, Round	Amitriptyline 150 mg	Elavil by Rugby		Antidepressant
RUGBY3077	Tab, Blue, Round	Amitriptyline HCl 10 mg, Perphenazine 2 mg	Triavil by Rugby		Antipsychotic
RUGBY3078	Tab, Salmon, Round	Amitriptyline HCl 10 mg, Perphenazine 4 mg	Triavil by Rugby		Antipsychotic
RUGBY3082	Tab, Orange, Round	Amitriptyline HCl 25 mg, Perphenazine 2 mg	Triavil by Rugby		Antipsychotic
RUGBY3083	Tab, Yellow, Round	Amitriptyline HCl 25 mg, Perphenazine 4 mg	Triavil by Rugby		Antipsychotic
RUGBY3084	Tab, Orange, Round	Amitriptyline HCl 50 mg, Perphenazine 4 mg	Triavil by Rugby		Antipsychotic
RUGBY3218	Tab, White, Oblong	Acetaminophen 500 mg	Tylenol by Rugby		Antipyretic
RUGBY3222	Tab, White, Rugby Logo 3222	Acetaminophen 325 mg	Tylenol by Rugby		Antipyretic
RUGBY3231	Tab, Rugby Logo 3231	Acetaminophen 500 mg	Tylenol by Rugby		Antipyretic
RUGBY3235	Tab, White, Round	Alprazolam 0.25 mg	Xanax by Rugby		Antianxiety; C IV
RUGBY3236	Tab, Orange, Round	Alprazolam 0.5 mg	Xanax by Rugby		Antianxiety; C IV
RUGBY3237	Tab, Blue, Round	Alprazolam 1 mg	Xanax by Rugby		Antianxiety; C IV
RUGBY3279	Tab	Hydralazine 25 mg, Hydrochlorothiazide 15 mg	Apresoline-Esidrix by Rugby		Antihypertensive
RUGBY33227	Tab, White, Round, Rugby 3/3227	Acetaminophen 300 mg, Codeine 30 mg	Tylenol #3 by Rugby		Analgesic; C III
RUGBY3325	Tab, White, Round	Atenolol 25 mg	Tenormin by Rugby		Antihypertensive
RUGBY3329	Tab, White, Round	Aspirin 325 mg, Codeine 60 mg	by Rugby		Analgesic; C III
RUGBY3360	Tab	Belladonna, Phenobarbital	by Rugby		Gastrointestinal; C IV
RUGBY3364	Tab	Bethanechol Chloride 5 mg	Urecholine by Rugby		Urinary Tract
RUGBY3365	Tab, White, Round	Bethanechol Chloride 10 mg	Urecholine by Rugby		Urinary Tract
RUGBY3367	Cap	Decyclomine HCl 10 mg	by Rugby	00536-3367	Gastrointestinal
RUGBY3367	Cap	Decyclomine HCl 10 mg	by Pharmedix	53002-0329	Gastrointestinal
RUGBY3369	Tab, Yellow, Round	Bethanechol Chloride 25 mg	Urecholine by Rugby		Urinary Tract
RUGBY3370	Tab, White, Round	Benztropine Mesylates 0.5 mg	Cogentin by Rugby		Antiparkinson
RUGBY3371	Tab, White, Round	Benztropine Mesylates 1 mg	Cogentin by Rugby		Antiparkinson
RUGBY3372	Tab	Benztropine Mesylate 2 mg	by Rugby	00536-3372	Antiparkinson
RUGBY3377	Tab	Decyclomine HCl 20 mg	by Rugby	00536-3377	Gastrointestinal
RUGBY3377	Tab	Decyclomine HCl 20 mg	by Pharmedix	53002-0345	Gastrointestinal
RUGBY3377	Tab	Decyclomine HCl 20 mg	by Chelsea	46193-0115	Gastrointestinal
RUGBY3406	Cap	Clorazepate Dipotassium 30.75 mg	Tranxene by Rugby		Antianxiety; C IV
RUGBY3407	Cap	Clorazepate Dipotassium 7.5 mg	Tranxene by Rugby		Antianxiety; C IV
RUGBY3408	Cap	Clorazepate Dipotassium 15 mg	Tranxene by Rugby		Antianxiety; C IV
RUGBY3414	Tab, White, Round	Calcium Carbonate 650 mg	by Rugby		Vitamin/Mineral
RUGBY3415	Tab, White	Carbamazepine 200 mg	Tegretol by Rosemont		Anticonvulsant
RUGBY3420	Cap, Blue & Clear	Pseudoephedrine HCl 120 mg, Chlorpheniramine 8 mg	Novafed A by Rugby		Cold Remedy
RUGBY3435	Tab	Carisoprodol 350 mg	by Rugby	00536-3435	Muscle Relaxant
RUGBY3435	Tab	Carisoprodol 350 mg	by Chelsea	46193-0500	Muscle Relaxant
RUGBY3444	Tab	Chlorzoxazone 500 mg	by Rugby	00536-3444	Muscle Relaxant
RUGBY3444	Tab	Chlorzoxazone 500 mg	by Chelsea	46193-0809	Muscle Relaxant
RUGBY3450	Tab	Chlorzoxazone 250 mg, Acetaminophen 300 mg	Parafon Forte by Rugby		Muscle Relaxant

ID FRONT <> BACK	DESCRIPTION FRONT <> BACK	INGREDIENT & STRENGTH	BRAND (OR EQUIV.) & FIRM	NDC#	CLASS; SCH.
RUGBY3455	Tab, Butterscotch Yellow, Round	Chlorpromazine 25 mg	Thorazine by Rugby		Antipsychotic
RUGBY3456	Tab, Butterscotch Yellow, Round	Chlorpromazine 50 mg	Thorazine by Rugby		Antipsychotic
RUGBY3457	Tab, Butterscotch Yellow, Round	Chlorpromazine 100 mg	Thorazine by Rugby		Antipsychotic
RUGBY3458	Tab, Butterscotch Yellow, Round	Chlorpromazine 200 mg	Thorazine by Rugby		Antipsychotic
RUGBY3460	Tab, White, Round	Chlorothiazide 250 mg	Diuril by Rugby		Diuretic
RUGBY3461	Tab, White, Round	Chlorothiazide 500 mg	Diuril by Rugby		Diuretic
RUGBY3462	Tab, Blue, Round	Chlorpropamide 100 mg	Diabinese by Rugby		Antidiabetic
RUGBY3465	Tab, Blue, Round	Chlorpropamide 250 mg	Diabinese by Rugby		Antidiabetic
RUGBY3466	Cap, Yellow	Clofibrate 500 mg	Atromid-S by Rugby		Antihyperlipidemic
RUGBY3468	Tab, Blue, Round	Chlorthalidone 50 mg	Hygroton by Rugby		Diuretic
RUGBY3469	Tab, White, Round	Chlorthalidone 100 mg	Hygroton by Rugby		Diuretic
RUGBY3471	Tab	Captopril 12.5 mg	by Rugby	00536-3471	Antihypertensive
RUGBY3471	Tab	Captopril 12.5 mg	by Chelsea	46193-0552	Antihypertensive
RUGBY3472	Tab	Captopril 25 mg	by Rugby	00536-3472	Antihypertensive
RUGBY3472	Tab	Captopril 25 mg	by Chelsea	46193-0553	Antihypertensive
RUGBY3473	Tab	Captopril 50 mg	by Rugby	00536-3473	Antihypertensive
RUGBY3473	Tab	Captopril 50 mg	by Chelsea	46193-0554	Antihypertensive
RUGBY3474	Tab, Yellow, Oval	Captopril 100 mg	Capoten by Rugby		Antihypertensive
RUGBY3474	Tab	Captopril 100 mg	by Rugby	00536-3474	Antihypertensive
RUGBY3474	Tab	Captopril 100 mg	by Chelsea	46193-0555	Antihypertensive
RUGBY3475	Tab, White, Round	Dimenhydrinate 50 mg	Dramamine by Rugby		Antiemetic
RUGBY3477	Cap, Green	Chloral Hydrate 500 mg	Noctec by Rugby		Sedative/Hypnotic; C IV
RUGBY3485	Tab, Yellow	Chlorthalidone 25 mg	Hygroton by Rugby		Diuretic
RUGBY3490	Cap	Chlordiazepoxide HCl 5 mg, Clidinium Bromide 2.5 mg	by Rugby	00536-3490	Gastrointestinal; C IV
RUGBY3494	Tab, White, Round, Rugby Logo 3494	Colchicine 0.6 mg	by West-ward		Antigout
RUGBY3496	Tab, White, Round, Rugby Logo 3496	Conjugated Estrogens 0.3 mg	Premarin by Rugby		Estrogen
RUGBY3497	Tab, White, Round, Rugby Logo 3497	Conjugated Estrogens 0.625 mg	Premarin by Rugby		Estrogen
RUGBY3498	Tab, White, Round, Rugby Logo 3498	Conjugated Estrogens 1.25 mg	Premarin by Rugby		Estrogen
RUGBY3501	Tab, White, Round, Rugby Logo 3501	Conjugated Estrogens 2.5 mg	Premarin by Rugby		Estrogen
RUGBY3515	Tab, White, Round	Cyproheptadine 4 mg	Periactin by Rugby		Antihistamine
RUGBY3516	Tab, White, Round	Conjugated Estrogens 0.625 mg	Premarin by Rugby		Estrogen
RUGBY3517	Tab, White, Round, Rugby Logo 3517	Conjugated Estrogens 0.3 mg	Premarin by Rugby		Estrogen
RUGBY3522	Tab, White, Round	Conjugated Estrogens 1.25 mg	Premarin by Rugby		Estrogen
RUGBY3523	Tab, Orange, Round	Clonidine HCl 0.1 mg	Catapres by Par		Antihypertensive
RUGBY3524	Tab, Orange, Round	Clonidine HCl 0.2 mg	Catapres by Par		Antihypertensive
RUGBY3526	Tab, Orange, Round	Clonidine HCl 0.3 mg	Catapres by Par		Antihypertensive
RUGBY3528	Tab, White, Round	Conjugated Estrogens 2.5 mg	Premarin by Rugby		Estrogen
RUGBY3529	Cap, Red & Blue	Cyclandelate 400 mg	Cyclospasmol by Rugby		Vasodilator
RUGBY3530	Tab	Cortisone Acetate 25 mg	by Rugby	00536-3530	Steroid
RUGBY3531	Cap, Blue	Cyclandelate 200 mg	Cyclospasmol by Rugby		Vasodilator
RUGBY3571	Tab, White, Round	Dipyridamole 50 mg	Persantine by Rugby		Antiplatelet
RUGBY3572	Tab, White, Round	Dipyridamole 75 mg	Persantine by Rugby		Antiplatelet
RUGBY3583	Tab	Dexamethasone 0.75 mg	Decadron by Rugby		Steroid
RUGBY3591	Tab, White, Round	Diazepam 2 mg	Valium by Rugby		Antianxiety; C IV
RUGBY3592	Tab, Yellow, Round	Diazepam 5 mg	Valium by Rugby		Antianxiety; C IV
RUGBY3593	Tab, Blue, Round	Diazepam 10 mg	Valium by Rugby		Antianxiety; C IV
RUGBY3595	Cap, Blue	Disopyramide Phosphate 100 mg	Norpace by Rugby		Antiarrhythmic
RUGBY3596	Cap, Scarlet	Disopyramide Phosphate 150 mg	Norpace by Rugby		Antiarrhythmic
RUGBY3597	Tab, Purple, Oblong	Diphenhydramine HCl 25 mg	Benadryl by Rugby		Antihistamine
RUGBY3728	Cap, Orange	Doxepin HCl 25 mg	Sinequan by Rugby		Antidepressant
RUGBY3729	Cap, Black & White	Doxepin HCl 50 mg	Sinequan by Rugby		Antidepressant
RUGBY3730	Cap, Yellow	Doxepin HCl 100 mg	Sinequan by Rugby		Antidepressant

ID FRONT <> BACK	DESCRIPTION FRONT <> BACK	INGREDIENT & STRENGTH	BRAND (OR EQUIV.) & FIRM	NDC#	CLASS; SCH.
RUGBY3736	Cap, Yellow	Doxepin HCl 10 mg	Sinequan by Rugby		Antidepressant
RUGBY3737	Cap, Green	Doxepin HCl 75 mg	Sinequan by Rugby		Antidepressant
RUGBY3738	Cap, Blue & White	Doxepin 150 mg	Sinequan by Rugby		Antidepressant
RUGBY3745	Tab, White, Round	Dimenhydrinate 50 mg	Dramamine by Rugby		Antiemetic
RUGBY3758	Cap, Natural	Diphenhydramine HCl 25 mg	by Rugby	00536-3758	Antihistamine
RUGBY3758	Cap, Pink & White	Diphenoxylate HCl 2.5 mg, Atropine Sulfate 0.025 mg	Lomotil by Rugby		Antidiarrheal; C V
RUGBY3762	Cap	Diphenhydramine HCl 50 mg	by Quality Care	60346-0045	Antihistamine
RUGBY3762	Cap	Diphenhydramine HCl 50 mg	by Rugby	00536-3762	Antihistamine
RUGBY3764	Cap, White	Prompt Phenytoin Sodium 100 mg	by Rugby		Anticonvulsant
RUGBY3767	Tab, White, Round	Disulfiram 250 mg	Antabuse by Rugby		Antialcoholism
RUGBY3768	Tab, White, Round	Disulfiram 500 mg	Antabuse by Rugby		Antialcoholism
RUGBY3770	Tab, Blue/Green	Trichlormethiazide 4 mg	Metahydrin by Par		Diuretic
RUGBY3778	Cap	Ephedrine Sulfate 50 mg	by Rugby		Antiasthmatic
RUGBY3780	Cap	Ephedrine Sulfate 25 mg	by Rugby		Antiasthmatic
RUGBY3795	Cap, Blue & White	Flurazepam HCl 15 mg	Dalmane by Par		Hypnotic; C IV
RUGBY3796	Cap	Flurazepam HCl 30 mg	by Rugby	00536-3796	Hypnotic; C IV
RUGBY3798	Tab, Salmon/Blue Green, Round	Meprobamate 400 mg, Aspirin 325 mg	Equagesic by Quantum		Sedative/Hypnotic; C IV
RUGBY3804	Cap	Vitamin Combination	Trinsicon by Rugby		Vitamin
RUGBY3813	Tab, White, Oval	Fenoprofen 600 mg	Nalfon by Rugby		NSAID
RUGBY3824	Tab, Red, Round	Ferrous Gluconate 5 gr	Fergon by Rugby		Mineral
RUGBY3835	Tab, White	Furosemide 80 mg	Lasix by Rugby		Diuretic
RUGBY3845	Tab	Folic Acid 1 mg	by Rugby	00536-3845	Vitamin
RUGBY3854	Tab, Light Orange, Film Coated, Scored	Gemfibrozil 600 mg	by Rugby	00536-3854	Antihyperlipidemic
RUGBY3854	Tab, Light Orange, Film Coated, Scored	Gemfibrozil 600 mg	by Chelsea	46193-0537	Antihyperlipidemic
RUGBY3856	Tab, White, Round	Ergoloid Mesylates Oral 1 mg	Hydergine by Rugby		Ergot
RUGBY3857	Tab, White, Round	Ergoloid Mesylates SL 1 mg	Hydergine by Rugby		Ergot
RUGBY3859	Tab, White, Round	Ergoloid Mesylates SL 0.5 mg	Hydergine by Rugby		Ergot
RUGBY3862	Tab, Peach, Round	Hydralazine HCl 25 mg	Apresoline by Par		Antihypertensive
RUGBY3863	Tab, Peach, Round	Hydralazine HCl 50 mg	Apresoline by Par		Antihypertensive
RUGBY3871	Tab	Guaifenesin 400 mg, Phenylpropanolamine HCl 75 mg	Guiatex LA by Rugby	00536-3871	Cold Remedy
RUGBY3871	Tab, Peach	Phenylpropanolamine HCl 75 mg, Guaifenesin 400 mg	Entex LA by Rugby		Cold Remedy
RUGBY3874	Tab, Lavender	Hydroxyzine HCl 10 mg	Atarax by Rugby		Antihistamine
RUGBY3875	Tab, Lavender, Round	Hydroxyzine HCl 25 mg	Atarax by Rugby		Antihistamine
RUGBY3876	Tab, Purple, Round	Hydroxyzine HCl 50 mg	Atarax by Rugby		Antihistamine
RUGBY3882	Tab, Peach, Round	Hydroflumethiazide 50 mg	Saluron by Rugby		Diuretic
RUGBY3893	Cap, Dark Green & Light Green	Hydroxyzine Pamoate	by Chelsea	46193-0619	Antihistamine
RUGBY3894	Cap, Dark Green	Hydroxyzine Pamoate	by Rugby	00536-3894	Antihistamine
RUGBY3894	Cap, Dark Green	Hydroxyzine Pamoate	by Chelsea	46193-0623	Antihistamine
RUGBY3894	Cap, Green & White, Opaque, Rugby 3894	Hydroxyzine Pamoate 50 mg	by Murfreesboro	51129-1487	Antihistamine
RUGBY3895	Cap, Green/Gray	Hydroxyzine Pamoate 100 mg	Vistaril by Rugby		Antihistamine
RUGBY3906	Tab, White	Theophylline 130 mg, Ephedrine Sulfate 25 mg, Hydroxyzine HCl 10 mg	Marax by Rugby		Antiasthmatic
RUGBY3915	Tab, Green, Round	Reserpine 0.125 mg, Hydrochlorothiazide 25 mg	Hydropres by Rugby		Antihypertensive
RUGBY3916	Tab, Green, Round	Reserpine 0.125 mg, Hydrochlorothiazide 50 mg	Hydropres by Rugby		Antihypertensive
RUGBY3918	Tab	Hyoscyamine Sulfate 0.125 mg	by Rugby	00536-3918	Gastrointestinal
RUGBY3919	Tab	Hydrochlorothiazide 50 mg	by Rugby	00536-3919	Diuretic
RUGBY3920	Tab	Atropine Sulfate 0.0194 mg, Hyoscyamine Sulfate 0.1037 mg, Phenobarbital 16.2 mg, Scopolamine Hydrobromide 0.0065 mg	Hyosophen by Rugby	00536-3920	Gastrointestinal; C IV
RUGBY3920	Tab, Rugby/3920	Atropine Sulfate 0.0194 mg, Hyoscyamine Sulfate 0.1037 mg, Phenobarbital 16.2 mg, Scopolamine Hydrobromide 0.0065 mg	by JMI Canton	00252-6793	Gastrointestinal; C IV
RUGBY3920	Tab, White, Round	Belladonna Alkaloids, Phenobarbital	Donnatal by Rugby		Gastrointestinal; C IV
RUGBY3921	Tab, Yellow, Round	Hydrochlorothiazide 50 mg	Hydrodiuril by Rugby		Diuretic
RUGBY3922	Tab	Hydrochlorothiazide 25 mg	by Rugby	00536-3922	Diuretic

ID FRONT <> BACK	DESCRIPTION FRONT <> BACK	INGREDIENT & STRENGTH	BRAND (OR EQUIV.) & FIRM	NDC#	CLASS; SCH.
RUGBY3923	Tab, Peach, Round	Hydrochlorothiazide 100 mg	Hydrodiuril by Rugby		Diuretic
RUGBY3927	Tab	Isosorbide Dinitrate 20 mg	by Rugby	00536-3927	Antianginal
RUGBY3929	Tab, Yellow	Imipramine HCl 10 mg	Tofranil by Rugby		Antidepressant
RUGBY3930	Tab, Orange	Imipramine HCl 25 mg	Tofranil by Rugby		Antidepressant
RUGBY3931	Tab, Green	Imipramine HCl 50 mg	Tofranil by Rugby		Antidepressant
RUGBY3933	Cap, White, Round, Rugby Logo R 3933	Butalbital 50 mg, Aspirin 40 mg, Caffeine 325 mg	Fiorinal by Rugby		Analgesic
RUGBY3934	Tab	Ibuprofen 200 mg	Advil by Rugby		NSAID
RUGBY3935	Tab, White, Round	Isoxsuprine 10 mg	Vasodilan by Rugby		Vasodilator
RUGBY3936	Tab, White, Round	Isoxsuprine 20 mg	Vasodilan by Rugby		Vasodilator
RUGBY3937	Tab	Aspirin 325 mg, Butalbital 50 mg, Caffeine 40 mg	by Rugby	00536-3937	Analgesic; C III
RUGBY3938	Tab, Blue	Isosorbide Dinitrate Oral 30 mg	Isordil by Rugby		Antianginal
RUGBY3940	Tab	Isosorbide Dinitrate TR 40 mg	Isordil by Rugby		Antianginal
RUGBY3941	Tab, White, Round	Isoniazide 300 mg	INH by Rugby		Antimycobacterial
RUGBY3943	Tab, White, Round	Isosorbide Dinitrate Oral 10 mg	Isordil by Rugby		Antianginal
RUGBY3946	Tab, Pink, Round	Isosorbide Dinitrate Oral 5 mg	Isordil by Par		Antianginal
RUGBY3947	Tab, Orange, Round	Levothyroxine Sodium 25 mcg	Synthroid by Rugby		Antithyroid
RUGBY3948	Tab, White, Round	Isoniazid 100 mg	INH by Rugby		Antimycobacterial
RUGBY3950	Tab, White, Round	Isosorbide Dinitrate SL 10 mg	Isordil by Rugby		Antianginal
RUGBY3950	Tab, Pink, Round	Levothyroxine Sodium 50 mcg	Synthroid by Rugby		Antithyroid
RUGBY3951	Tab, Round	Levothyroxine Sodium 75 mcg	Synthroid by Rugby		Antithyroid
RUGBY3952	Tab, Yellow, Round	Levothyroxine Sodium 0.1 mg	Synthroid by Rugby		Antithyroid
RUGBY3953	Tab, Blue, Round	Levothyroxine Sodium 0.15 mg	Synthroid by Rugby		Antithyroid
RUGBY3954	Tab, Round	Levothyroxine Sodium 0.2 mg	Synthroid by Rugby		Antithyroid
RUGBY3956	Cap	Lithium Carbonate 300 mg	Eskalith by Rugby		Antipsychotic
RUGBY3957	Cap	Prochlorperazine Maleate 10 mg, Isopropamide Iodide 5 mg	Combid by Rugby		Gastrointestinal
RUGBY3958	Tab, Green, Round	Levothyroxine Sodium 0.3 mg	Synthroid by Rugby		Antithyroid
RUGBY3961	Tab, White, Round	Lorazepam 2 mg	Ativan by Watson		Sedative/Hypnotic; C IV
RUGBY3963	Tab, Beige, Round	Levothyroxine Sodium 125 mcg	Synthroid by Rugby		Antithyroid
RUGBY3976	Tab	Ibuprofen 300 mg	Motrin by Rugby		NSAID
RUGBY3977	Tab, Orange, Round	Ibuprofen 400 mg	Motrin by Rugby		NSAID
RUGBY3978	Tab, Orange, Oval	Ibuprofen 600 mg	Motrin by Rugby		NSAID
RUGBY3979	Tab	Ibuprofen 800 mg	Motrin by Rugby		NSAID
RUGBY3980	Cap, Purple/White	Indomethacin SR 75 mg	Indocin by Rugby		NSAID
RUGBY3981	Cap, Green	Indomethacin 25 mg	Indocin by Rugby		NSAID
RUGBY3982	Cap, Green	Indomethacin 50 mg	Indocin by Rugby		NSAID
RUGBY3985	Tab, White	Meclizine HCl 12.5 mg	Antivert by Rugby		Antiemetic
RUGBY3986	Tab, Blue & White, Multilayer	Meclizine HCl 12.5 mg	by Rugby	00536-3986	Antiemetic
RUGBY3988	Tab, Yellow & White	Meclizine HCl 25 mg	by Rugby	00536-3988	Antiemetic
RUGBY3988	Tab, Yellow & White, Mult-layer	Meclizine HCl 25 mg	by Chelsea	46193-0149	Antiemetic
RUGBY3990	Tab	Meclizine HCl Chewable 25 mg	Antivert by Rugby		Antiemetic
RUGBY3995	Tab, White, Round	Medroxyprogesterone Acetate 10 mg	Provera by Rugby		Progestin
RUGBY3996	Tab	Methyldopa 250 mg, Hydrochlorothiazide 15 mg	Aldoril by Bolar		Antihypertensive
RUGBY3997	Tab	Methyldopa 250 mg, Hydrochlorothiazide 25 mg	Aldoril by Bolar		Antihypertensive
RUGBY4002	Cap, Yellow	Meclofenamate Sodium 50 mg	Meclomen by Rugby		NSAID
RUGBY4003	Cap, Beige/Yellow	Meclofenamate Sodium 100 mg	Meclomen by Rugby		NSAID
RUGBY4005	Tab, White, Round	Meprobamate 200 mg	Equanil by Rugby		Sedative/Hypnotic; C IV
RUGBY4006	Tab, White, Round	Meprobamate 400 mg	Equanil by Rugby		Sedative/Hypnotic; C IV
RUGBY4010	Tab, White, Round	Methyldopa 250 mg	Aldomet by Rugby		Antihypertensive
RUGBY4011	Tab, White, Round	Methyldopa 500 mg	Aldomet by Rugby		Antihypertensive
RUGBY4012	Tab, White, Round	Methyldopa 125 mg	Aldomet by Rugby		Antihypertensive
RUGBY4016	Tab, White, Oval	Methylprednisolone 4 mg	by Rugby	00536-4036	Steroid
RUGBY4016	Tab	Methylprednisolone 4 mg	by Chelsea	46193-0604	Steroid

ID FRONT <> BACK	DESCRIPTION FRONT <> BACK	INGREDIENT & STRENGTH	BRAND (OR EQUIV.) & FIRM	NDC#	CLASS; SCH.
RUGBY4018	Tab, White, Round	Metronidazole 250 mg	Flagyl by Rugby		Antibiotic
RUGBY4019	Tab, White, Oval	Metronidazole 500 mg	Flagyl by Rugby		Antibiotic
RUGBY4020	Tab, Peach, Round	Methyldopa 125 mg	Aldomet by Rugby		Antihypertensive
RUGBY4021	Tab, Peach, Round	Methyldopa 250 mg	Aldomet by Rugby		Antihypertensive
RUGBY4023	Tab, Peach, Round	Methyldopa 500 mg	Aldomet by Rugby		Antihypertensive
RUGBY4025	Tab, Yellow, Round	Methyclothiazide 5 mg	Enduron by Rugby		Diuretic
RUGBY4026	Tab	Methocarbamol 500 mg	by Rugby	00536-4026	Muscle Relaxant
RUGBY4026	Tab	Methocarbamol 500 mg	by Quality Care	60346-0080	Muscle Relaxant
RUGBY4026	Tab	Methocarbamol 500 mg	by Chelsea	46193-0120	Muscle Relaxant
RUGBY4027	Tab	Methocarbamol 750 mg	by Rugby	00536-4027	Muscle Relaxant
RUGBY4027	Tab	Methocarbamol 750 mg	by Chelsea	46193-0121	Muscle Relaxant
RUGBY4028	Tab	Methocarbamol 500 mg, Aspirin 325 mg	Robaxisal by Rugby		Muscle Relaxant
RUGBY4036	Tab	Methylprednisolone 4 mg	Medrol by Rugby		Steroid
RUGBY4040	Tab, Peach, Round	Methyclothiazide 2.5 mg	Enduron by Rugby		Diuretic
RUGBY4041	Tab, Pink, Orange, Round	Methyclothiazide 5 mg	Enduron by Rugby		Diuretic
RUGBY4042	Tab, White, Round	Metoclopramide HCl 10 mg	Reglan by Watson		Gastrointestinal
RUGBY4043	Tab, White, Round	Minoxidil 10 mg	Loniten by Rugby		Antihypertensive
RUGBY4052	Tab	Methyldopa 250 mg, Chlorothiazide 150 mg	Aldochlor by Rugby		Antihypertensive
RUGBY4053	Tab	Methyldopa 250 mg, Chlorothiazide 250 mg	Aldochlor by Rugby		Antihypertensive
RUGBY4081	Tab	Nitrofurantoin 50 mg	Furadantin by Rugby		Antibiotic
RUGBY4082	Tab	Nitrofurantoin 100 mg	Furadantin by Rugby		Antibiotic
RUGBY4083	Cap, Lavender/Clear	Nitroglycerin SR 2.5 mg	Nitrobid by Rugby		Vasodilator
RUGBY4084	Cap, ER	Nitroglycerin 6.5 mg	by Rugby	00536-4084	Vasodilator
RUGBY4090	Cap, ER	Nitroglycerin 9 mg	by Rugby	00536-4090	Vasodilator
RUGBY4091	Tab, Off-White	Nystatin Vaginal 100,000 Units	Mycostatin by Rugby		Antifungal
RUGBY4094	Tab, Brown, Round	Nystatin 500,000 Units	Mycostatin by Lemmon		Antifungal
RUGBY4114	Cap, Pink & Clear	Oxazepam 10 mg	Serax by Rugby		Sedative/Hypnotic; C IV
RUGBY4115	Cap, White	Oxazepam 15 mg	Serax by Rugby		Sedative/Hypnotic; C IV
RUGBY4116	Cap, Clear	Oxazepam 30 mg	Serax by Rugby		Sedative/Hypnotic; C IV
RUGBY4124	Cap, Brown & Clear	Papaverine HCl TD 150 mg	Pavabid by Rugby		Vasodilator
RUGBY4130	Tab	Pentaerythritol Tetranitrate 10 mg	Peritrate by Rugby		Antianginal
RUGBY4131	Tab, Round	Perphenazine 2 mg	Trilafon by Rugby		Antipsychotic
RUGBY4132	Tab, Round	Perphenazine 4 mg	Trilafon by Rugby		Antipsychotic
RUGBY4133	Tab, Round	Perphenazine 8 mg	Trilafon by Rugby		Antipsychotic
RUGBY4134	Tab, Round	Perphenazine 16 mg	Trilafon by Rugby		Antipsychotic
RUGBY4138	Tab	Pentaerythritol Tetranitrate 20 mg	Peritrate by Rugby		Antianginal
RUGBY4147	Tab, White, Round	Perphenazine 8 mg	Trilafon by Rugby		Antipsychotic
RUGBY4148	Tab	Leucovorin 5 mg	Wellcovorin by Rugby		Antineoplastic
RUGBY4149	Tab	Leucovorin 25 mg	Wellcovorin by Rugby		Antineoplastic
RUGBY4160	Tab, Yellow	Phendimetrazine Tartrate 35 mg	Plegine by Rugby		Anorexiant; C III
RUGBY4161	Tab, Gray	Phendimetrazine Tartrate 35 mg	Plegine by Rugby		Anorexiant; C III
RUGBY4162	Tab, Pink	Phendimetrazine Tartrate 35 mg	Plegine by Rugby		Anorexiant; C III
RUGBY4167	Tab, White	Phendimetrazine Tartrate 35 mg	Plegine by Rugby		Anorexiant; C III
RUGBY4224	Tab	Phenobarbital 20 mg	by West-ward		Sedative/Hypnotic; C IV
RUGBY4234	Tab, Blue, Round	Ergotamine 0.6 mg, Phenobarbital 40 mg, Belladonna 0.2	Bellergal S by Rugby		Antispasmodic; C IV
RUGBY4235	Cap, Blue & Clear	Phentermine HCl 30 mg	Fastin by Rugby		Anorexiant; C IV
RUGBY4288	Tab, Green	Phentermine HCl 8 mg	by Rugby		Anorexiant; C IV
RUGBY4290	Tab	Phenylpropanolamine 25 mg	Dexatrim by Rugby		Decongestant; Appetite Suppressant
RUGBY4295	Cap	Phenylbutazone 100 mg	Butazolidin by Rugby		Anti-Inflammatory
RUGBY4298	Tab, Orange, Round	Phenylbutazone 100 mg	Butazolidin by Rugby		Anti-Inflammatory
RUGBY4299	Tab, Red	Phenylbutazone 100 mg	Butazolidin by Rugby		Anti-Inflammatory

ID FRONT <> BACK	DESCRIPTION FRONT <> BACK	INGREDIENT & STRENGTH	BRAND (OR EQUIV.) & FIRM	NDC#	CLASS; SCH.
RUGBY4305	Cap, Orange/Cream	Phenylbutazone 100 mg	Butazolidin by Rugby		Anti-Inflammatory
RUGBY4307	Tab, Chewable	Ascorbic Acid 60 mg, Cyanocobalamin 4.5 mcg, Folic Acid 0.3 mg, Niacinamide, Pyridoxine HCl 1.05 mg, Riboflavin 1.2 mg, Sodium Fluoride, Thiamine Mononitrate, Vitamin A Acetate, Vitamin D 400 Units, Vitamin E Acetate	Poly-Vitamin by Rugby	00536-4307	Vitamin
RUGBY4308	Tab, Chewable	Ascorbic Acid 60 mg, Cupric Oxide, Cyanocobalamin 4.5 mcg, Ferrous Fumarate, Folic Acid 0.3 mg, Niacinamide, Pyridoxine HCl 1.05 mg, Riboflavin 1.2 mg, Sodium Fluoride, Thiamine HCl 1.05 mg, Vitamin A Acetate 2500 Units, Vitamin D 400 Units, Zinc Oxide	Poly-Vitamin by Rugby	00536-4308	Vitamin
RUGBY4309	Tab, Orange, Round	Propranolol HCl 10 mg	Inderal by Rugby		Antihypertensive
RUGBY4312	Tab, Chewable	Ascorbic Acid 60 mg, Cyanocobalamin 4.5 mcg, Fluoride Ion 0.5 mg, Folic Acid 0.3 mg, Niacin 13.5 mg, Pyridoxine HCl 1.05 mg, Riboflavin 1.2 mg, Thiamine Mononitrate 1.05 mg, Vitamin A 2500 Units, Vitamin D 400 Units, Vitamin E 15 Units	Poly-Vitamin by Rugby	00536-4312	Vitamin
RUGBY4313	Tab, Blue, Round	Propranolol HCl 20 mg	Inderal by Rugby		Antihypertensive
RUGBY4314	Tab, Green, Round	Propranolol HCl 40 mg	Inderal by Rugby		Antihypertensive
RUGBY4315	Tab, Pink, Round	Propranolol HCl 60 mg	Inderal by Rugby		Antihypertensive
RUGBY4316	Tab, Yellow, Round	Propranolol HCl 80 mg	Inderal by Rugby		Antihypertensive
RUGBY43215	Tab, White, Round, Rugby 4/3215	Acetaminophen 300 mg, Codeine 60 mg	Tylenol #4 by Rugby		Analgesic; C III
RUGBY4322	Tab, Round	Potassium Chloride 600 mg (8 mEq)	Slow K by Rugby		Electrolytes
RUGBY4324	Tab	Prednisone 5 mg	by Rugby	00536-4324	Steroid
RUGBY4324	Tab	Prednisone 5 mg	by Chelsea	46193-0102	Steroid
RUGBY4325	Tab	Prednisone 10 mg	by Rugby	00536-4325	Steroid
RUGBY4325	Tab	Prednisone 10 mg	by Chelsea	46193-0676	Steroid
RUGBY4326	Tab	Prednisone 20 mg	by Chelsea	46193-0647	Steroid
RUGBY4326	Tab	Prednisone 20 mg	by Rugby	00536-4326	Steroid
RUGBY4328	Tab, White, Round	Prednisone 50 mg	Meticorten by Rugby		Steroid
RUGBY4328	Tab	Prednisone 50 mg	by Rugby	00536-4328	Steroid
RUGBY4335	Tab	Prenatal, Folic Acid, Iron Improved	by Rugby		Vitamin
RUGBY4339	Tab, Yellow	Prenatal, Folic Acid, Iron Plus	Prenatal Plus by Rugby		Vitamin
RUGBY4340	Tab, White	Prednisolone 5 mg	by Rugby		Steroid
RUGBY4346	Tab, Salmon	Prednisolone 5 mg	by Rugby	00536-4346	Steroid
RUGBY4352	Tab, Green	Prednisolone 5 mg	by Rugby		Steroid
RUGBY4360	Tab, Pink, Round	Propoxyphene Napsylate 50 mg, Acetaminophen 325 mg	Darvocet N by Rugby		Analgesic; C IV
RUGBY4361	Tab, Pink, Oblong	Propoxyphene Napsylate 100 mg, Acetaminophen 650 mg	Darvocet N 100 by Rugby		Analgesic; C IV
RUGBY4365	Tab	Probenecid 500 mg, Colchicine 0.5 mg	ColBenemid by Rugby		Antigout
RUGBY4366	Tab	Probenecid 500 mg	Benemid by Rugby		Antigout
RUGBY4367	Cap, Yellow	Procainamide HCl 250 mg	Pronestyl by Rugby		Antiarrhythmic
RUGBY4368	Cap, Orange & Yellow	Procainamide HCl 500 mg	Pronestyl by Rugby		Antiarrhythmic
RUGBY4369	Tab	Promethazine 50 mg	Phenergan by Rugby		Antiemetic; Antihistamine
RUGBY4374	Cap, Red/Gray	Propoxyphene 65 mg, Aspirin 389 mg, Caffeine 32.4 mg	Darvon Compound by Lemmon		Analgesic; C IV
RUGBY4374	Cap	Propoxyphene 65 mg, Aspirin 389 mg, Caffeine 32.4 mg	Darvon Compound 65 by Rugby		Analgesic; C IV
RUGBY4377	Cap, Orange & White	Procainamide HCl 375 mg	Pronestyl by Rugby		Antiarrhythmic
RUGBY4378	Tab	Promethazine 12.5 mg	Phenergan by Rugby		Antiemetic; Antihistamine
RUGBY4379	Tab	Promethazine 25 mg	Phenergan by Rugby		Antiemetic; Antihistamine
RUGBY4380	Tab	Levothyroxine Sodium 0.15 mg	Synthroid by Rugby		Antithyroid
RUGBY4381	Tab, White, Round	Levothyroxine Sodium 0.2 mg	Synthroid by Rugby		Antithyroid
RUGBY4382	Cap, Pink	Propoxyphene HCl 65 mg	Darvon by Lemmon		Analgesic; C IV
RUGBY4384	Tab	Propylthiouracil 50 mg	by Rugby		Antithyroid
RUGBY4387	Tab	Propoxyphene 65 mg, Acetaminophen 650 mg	Wygesic by Rugby		Analgesic; C IV
RUGBY4390	Tab	Pseudoephedrine HCl 60 mg	Sudafed by Rugby		Decongestant

ID FRONT <> BACK	DESCRIPTION FRONT <> BACK	INGREDIENT & STRENGTH	BRAND (OR EQUIV.) & FIRM	NDC#	CLASS; SCH.
RUGBY4391	Tab	Pseudoephedrine HCl 30 mg	Sudafed by Rugby		Decongestant
RUGBY4399	Tab, Round	Pseudoephedrine HCl 60 mg	Sudafed by Rugby		Decongestant
RUGBY4402	Tab, White, Round	Propranolol HCl 40 mg, Hydrochlorothiazide 25 mg	Inderide by Rugby		Antihypertensive
RUGBY4403	Tab, White, Round	Propranolol HCl 80 mg, Hydrochlorothiazide 25 mg	Inderide by Rugby		Antihypertensive
RUGBY4411	Cap	Pyrilamine 25 mg	by Rugby		Antihistamine
RUGBY4426	Tab, White, Round	Quinine Sulfate 260 mg	Quinamm by Rugby		Antimalarial
RUGBY4429	Tab, White, Round	Quinidine Sulfate 300 mg	by Rugby		Antiarrhythmic
RUGBY4432	Tab	Quinidine Sulfate 200 mg	by Rugby	00536-4432	Antiarrhythmic
RUGBY4433	Cap	Quinine Sulfate 325 mg	by Rugby		Antimalarial
RUGBY4434	Tab, White, Round	Quinidine Gluconate SR 324 mg	Quinaglute by Rugby		Antiarrhythmic
RUGBY4447	Tab	Guaifenesin 600 mg	by Rugby	00536-4447	Expectorant
RUGBY4454	Tab	Reserpine 0.1 mg	Serpasil by Rugby		Antihypertensive
RUGBY4455	Tab, Film Coated, Rugby 4455	Ranitidine HCl 168 mg	by Rugby	00536-4455	Gastrointestinal
RUGBY4455	Tab, Film Coated, Rugby 4455	Ranitidine HCl 168 mg	by Chelsea	46193-0575	Gastrointestinal
RUGBY4456	Tab, Film Coated	Ranitidine HCl 336 mg	by Rugby	00536-4456	Gastrointestinal
RUGBY4456	Tab, Film Coated	Ranitidine HCl 336 mg	by Chelsea	46193-0576	Gastrointestinal
RUGBY4458	Tab, White, Round	Reserpine 0.25 mg	Serpasil by Rugby		Antihypertensive
RUGBY4494	Tab, White, Round	Nylidrin 6 mg	Arlidin by Rugby		Vasodilator
RUGBY4495	Tab, White, Round	Nylidrin 12 mg	Arlidin by Rugby		Vasodilator
RUGBY4515	Cap, Yellow	Thiothixene 2 mg	Navane by Rugby		Antipsychotic
RUGBY4516	Cap, Orange	Thiothixene 5 mg	Navane by Rugby		Antipsychotic
RUGBY4517	Cap, Orange & Blue	Thiothixene 10 mg	Navane by Rugby		Antipsychotic
RUGBY4522	Tab	Salicylic Acid 500 mg	Disalcid by Rosemont		NSAID
RUGBY4523	Tab	Salicylic Acid 750 mg	Disalcid by Rosemont		NSAID
RUGBY4547	Tab, Pink, Round	Sodium Fluoride 2.2 mg	Luride by Copley		Element
RUGBY4548	Tab	Sodium Fluoride Chewable 1.1 mg	Luride by Rugby		Element
RUGBY4563	Cap, Buff, Rugby Logo 4563	Doxepin HCl 10 mg	Sinequan by Rugby		Antidepressant
RUGBY4564	Cap, Ivory & White, Rugby Logo 4564	Doxepin HCl 25 mg	Sinequan by Rugby		Antidepressant
RUGBY4565	Cap, Yellow, Rugby Logo 4565	Doxepin HCl 50 mg	Sinequan by Rugby		Antidepressant
RUGBY4566	Cap, Green & White, Rugby Logo 4566	Doxepin HCl 100 mg	Sinequan by Rugby		Antidepressant
RUGBY4575	Tab, White, Round	Spironolactone 25 mg	Aldactone by Rugby		Diuretic
RUGBY4576	Tab, White, Round	Spironolactone 25 mg, Hydrochlorothiazide 25 mg	Aldactazide by Rugby		Diuretic
RUGBY4604	Tab, White, Oval	Ibuprofen 400 mg	Motrin by Rugby		NSAID
RUGBY4605	Tab, White, Oval	Ibuprofen 600 mg	Motrin by Rugby		NSAID
RUGBY4606	Tab, White, Oval	Ibuprofen 800 mg	Motrin by Rugby		NSAID
RUGBY4617	Tab, Mustard	Sulfasalazine 500 mg	by Rugby	00536-4617	Gastrointestinal
RUGBY4617	Tab	Sulfasalazine 500 mg	by Allscripts	54569-0313	Gastrointestinal
RUGBY4617	Tab, Mustard	Sulfasalazine 500 mg	by Chelsea	46193-0166	Gastrointestinal
RUGBY4618	Tab, White, Round	Sulfisoxazole 500 mg	Gantrisin by Rugby		Antibiotic
RUGBY4628	Cap	Temazepam 15 mg	Restoril by Quantum		Sedative/Hypnotic; C IV
RUGBY4629	Cap	Temazepam 30 mg	Restoril by Quantum		Sedative/Hypnotic; C IV
RUGBY4640	Tab, Orange, Round	Thioridazine HCl 15 mg	Mellaril by Rugby		Antipsychotic
RUGBY4641	Tab, Orange, Round	Thioridazine HCl 10 mg	Mellaril by Rugby		Antipsychotic
RUGBY4642	Tab, Orange, Round	Thioridazine HCl 25 mg	Mellaril by Rugby		Antipsychotic
RUGBY4643	Tab, Orange, Round	Thioridazine HCl 50 mg	Mellaril by Rugby		Antipsychotic
RUGBY4644	Tab, Orange, Round	Thioridazine HCl 100 mg	Mellaril by Rugby		Antipsychotic
RUGBY4648	Tab, White, Round	Phenobarbital 8 mg, Theophylline 130 mg, Ephedrine (Azpan) 24 mg	Tedral by Rugby		Antiasthmatic; C IV
RUGBY4649	Cap	Theophylline CR 250 mg	by Rugby		Antiasthmatic
RUGBY4657	Cap	Theophylline CR 300 mg	by Rugby		Antiasthmatic
RUGBY4668	Tab, White, Round	Tolbutamide 500 mg	Orinase by Rugby		Antidiabetic
RUGBY4687	Tab, Peach, Round	Trazodone 50 mg	Desyrel by Rugby		Antidepressant
RUGBY4688	Tab, White, Round	Trazodone 100 mg	Desyrel by Rugby		Antidepressant

ID FRONT <> BACK	DESCRIPTION FRONT <> BACK	INGREDIENT & STRENGTH	BRAND (OR EQUIV.) & FIRM	NDC#	CLASS; SCH.
RUGBY4692	Tab, White, Round	Sulfamethoxazole 400 mg, Trimethoprim 80 mg	Bactrim by Rugby		Antibiotic
RUGBY4693	Tab, White, Oval	Sulfamethoxazole 800 mg, Trimethoprim 160 mg	Bactrim DS by Rugby		Antibiotic
RUGBY4694	Tab	Thyroid 30 mg	by Rugby		Thyroid
RUGBY4698	Tab	Thyroid 30 mg	by Rugby		Thyroid
RUGBY4702	Tab	Thyroid 60 mg	by Rugby		Thyroid
RUGBY4706	Tab	Thyroid 60 mg	by Rugby		Thyroid
RUGBY4710	Tab	Thyroid 125 mg	by Rugby		Thyroid
RUGBY4714	Tab	Thyroid 125 mg	by Rugby		Thyroid
RUGBY4717	Tab	Triamcinolone 4 mg	Aristocort by Rugby		Steroid
RUGBY4720	Tab, Round	Hydrochlorothiazide 15 mg, Hydralazine 25 mg, Reserpine (Hydroserpine Plus) 0.1 mg	Ser- by Rugby		Antihypertensive
RUGBY4721	Tab, White, Round	Hydrochlorothiazide 15 mg, Hydralazine 25 mg, Reserpine 0.1 mg	Ser- by Rugby		Antihypertensive
RUGBY4725	Tab	Phenylprop. 40 mg, phenyleph. 10 mg, phenyltolox. 15 mg, chlorphenir. 5 mg	Naldecon by Rugby		Cold Remedy
RUGBY4729	Tab	Chlorpheniramine Tannate 8 mg, Phenylephrine Tannate 25 mg, Pyrilamine Tannate 25 mg	Tri Tannate by Rugby	00536-4729	Cold Remedy
RUGBY4736	Tab	Tripelennamine 50 mg	PBZ by Rugby		Antihistamine
RUGBY4737	Tab, Chewable	Ascorbic Acid 30 mg, Sodium Ascorbate 33 mg, Sodium Fluoride, Vitamin A Acetate, Vitamin D 400 Units	Tri Vitamins by Rugby	00536-4737	Vitamin
RUGBY4738	Tab	Tolazamide 100 mg	Tolinase by Rugby		Antidiabetic
RUGBY4739	Tab	Tolazamide 250 mg	Tolinase by Rugby		Antidiabetic
RUGBY4744	Tab	Tolazamide 500 mg	Tolinase by Rugby		Antidiabetic
RUGBY4759	Tab	Therapeutic Vitamins	Berocca by Amide		Vitamin
RUGBY4812	Tab, Aqua, Round	Verapamil HCl 80 mg	Calan by Rugby		Antihypertensive
RUGBY4813	Tab, Blue, Round	Verapamil HCl 120 mg	Calan by Rugby		Antihypertensive
RUGBY4840	Tab, White, Round, Rugby Logo 4840	Cyclobenzaprine HCl 10 mg	Flexeril by Rugby		Muscle Relaxant
RUGBY4841	Tab, Film Coated	Naproxen Sodium 275 mg	by Rugby	00536-4841	NSAID
RUGBY4841	Tab, Film Coated	Naproxen Sodium 275 mg	by Chelsea	46193-0530	NSAID
RUGBY4842	Tab	Naproxen 250 mg	by Rugby	00536-4842	NSAID
RUGBY4842	Tab	Naproxen 250 mg	by Chelsea	46193-0527	NSAID
RUGBY4843	Tab	Naproxen 375 mg	by Chelsea	46193-0528	NSAID
RUGBY4843	Tab	Naproxen 375 mg	by Rugby	00536-4843	NSAID
RUGBY4844	Tab	Naproxen 500 mg	by Rugby	00536-4844	NSAID
RUGBY4844	Tab	Naproxen 500 mg	by Chelsea	46193-0529	NSAID
RUGBY4848	Tab, Film Coated	Naproxen Sodium 550 mg	by Rugby	00536-4848	NSAID
RUGBY4848	Tab, Film Coated	Naproxen Sodium 550 mg	by Chelsea	46193-0531	NSAID
RUGBY4861	Tab	Desipramine HCl 25 mg	Norpramin by Rugby		Antidepressant
RUGBY4862	Tab	Desipramine HCl 50 mg	Norpramin by Rugby		Antidepressant
RUGBY4863	Tab	Desipramine HCl 75 mg	Norpramin by Rugby		Antidepressant
RUGBY4864	Tab	Desipramine HCl 100 mg	Norpramin by Rugby		Antidepressant
RUGBY4881	Tab, Yellow, Round	Desipramine HCl 25 mg	Norpramin by Rugby	52544-0808	Antidepressant
RUGBY4881	Tab, Yellow, Rugby over 4881	Desipramine HCl 25 mg	by DRX	55045-2278	Antidepressant
RUGBY4881	Tab, Yellow	Desipramine HCl 25 mg	by Blue Ridge	59273-0009	Antidepressant
RUGBY4882	Tab, Green	Desipramine HCl 50 mg	by Blue Ridge	59273-0010	Antidepressant
RUGBY4882	Tab, Coated	Desipramine HCl 50 mg	by Rugby	00536-4882	Antidepressant
RUGBY4882	Tab, Green, Rugby over 4882	Desipramine HCl 50 mg	by DRX	55045-2352	Antidepressant
RUGBY4883	Tab, Orange, Round	Desipramine HCl 75 mg	Norpramin by Rugby		Antidepressant
RUGBY4884	Tab, Peach, Round, Rugby/4884	Desipramine HCl 50 mg	by DRX	55045-2548	Antidepressant
RUGBY4884	Tab, Peach, Rugby over 4884	Desipramine HCl 100 mg	by DRX	55045-2569	Antidepressant
RUGBY4884	Tab, Peach	Desipramine HCl 100 mg	by Blue Ridge	59273-0012	Antidepressant
RUGBY4884	Tab, Coated	Desipramine HCl 100 mg	by Rugby	00536-4884	Antidepressant
RUGBY4884	Tab, Peach, Round	Desipramine HCl 100 mg	Norpramin by Rugby	51544-0545	Antidepressant
RUGBY4903	Tab, Tan, Round	Chlorpromazine 10 mg	Thorazine by Rosemont		Antipsychotic
RUGBY4903	Tab, Butterscotch Yellow, Round	Chlorpromazine 10 mg	Thorazine by Rugby		Antipsychotic

ID FRONT <> BACK	DESCRIPTION FRONT <> BACK	INGREDIENT & STRENGTH	BRAND (OR EQUIV.) & FIRM	NDC#	CLASS; SCH.
RUGBY4906	Tab, Butterscotch Yellow, Round	Chlorpromazine 25 mg	Thorazine by Rugby		Antipsychotic
RUGBY4906	Tab, Tan, Round	Chlorpromazine 25 mg	Thorazine by Rosemont		Antipsychotic
RUGBY4909	Tab	Reserpine 0.1 mg, Hydralazine HCl 25 mg, Hydrochlorothiazide 15 mg	Serapes by Rugby		Antihypertensive
RUGBY4915	Tab, White, Round	Chlorpromazine 50 mg	Thorazine by Rugby		Antipsychotic
RUGBY4916	Tab, Tan, Round	Chlorpromazine 100 mg	Thorazine by Rosemont		Antipsychotic
RUGBY4916	Tab, Butterscotch Yellow, Round	Chlorpromazine 100 mg	Thorazine by Rugby		Antipsychotic
RUGBY4918	Tab, Butterscotch Yellow, Round	Chlorpromazine 200 mg	Thorazine by Rugby		Antipsychotic
RUGBY4918	Tab, Tan, Round	Chlorpromazine 200 mg	Thorazine by Rosemont		Antipsychotic
RUGBY4926	Cap, Red	Triamterene 50 mg, Hydrochlorothiazide 25 mg	Dyazide by Rugby		Diuretic
RUGBY4930	Cap, White	Triamterene 50 mg, Hydrochlorothiazide 25 mg	Dyazide by Rugby		Diuretic
RUGBY4931	Tab, White, Round	Verapamil HCl 80 mg	Isoptin,Calan by Rugby		Antihypertensive
RUGBY4932	Tab, White, Round	Verapamil HCl 120 mg	Isoptin,Calan by Rugby		Antihypertensive
RUGBY4939	Cap, Clear & Lavender w/ White Beads	Indomethacin 75 mg	by Inwood	00258-3607	NSAID
RUGBY4939	Cap, Purple/White	Indomethacin SR 75 mg	Indocin by Rugby		NSAID
RUGBY4940	Tab, Blue, Round	Clorazepate Dipotassium 30.75 mg	Tranxene by Watson		Antianxiety; C IV
RUGBY4941	Tab, Beige, Round	Clorazepate Dipotassium 7.5 mg	Tranxene by Watson		Antianxiety; C IV
RUGBY4942	Tab, Pink, Round	Clorazepate Dipotassium 15 mg	Tranxene by Watson		Antianxiety; C IV
RUGBY4948	Tab, Round	Desipramine 25 mg	Norpramin by Rugby		Antidepressant
RUGBY4949	Tab, Round	Desipramine 50 mg	Norpramin by Rugby		Antidepressant
RUGBY4950	Tab, White	Theophylline Anhydrous CR 100 mg	Theo-Dur by Rugby		Antiasthmatic
RUGBY4951	Tab, White	Theophylline Anhydrous CR 200 mg	Theo-Dur by Rugby		Antiasthmatic
RUGBY4952	Tab, White	Theophylline Anhydrous CR 300 mg	Theo-Dur by Rugby		Antiasthmatic
RUGBY4956	Tab, Yellow, Round	Triamterene 75 mg, Hydrochlorothiazide 50 mg	Maxzide by Watson		Diuretic
RUGBY4957	Tab, Round	Desipramine 75 mg	Norpramin by Rugby		Antidepressant
RUGBY4958	Tab, Round	Desipramine 100 mg	Norpramin by Rugby		Antidepressant
RUGBY4959	Tab	Baclofen 10 mg	by Chelsea	46193-0869	Muscle Relaxant
RUGBY4960	Tab, Chelsea	Baclofen 20 mg	by Rugby	00536-4960	Muscle Relaxant
RUGBY4960	Tab	Baclofen 20 mg	by Chelsea	46193-0870	Muscle Relaxant
RUGBY4963	Cap	Danazol 200 mg	Danocrine by Rugby		Steroid
RUGBY4989	Tab, White, Round	Yohimbine HCl 5.4 mg	Yocon by Rugby		Impotence Agent
RUGBY4989	Tab	Yohimbine HCl 5.4 mg	by Rugby	00536-4989	Impotence Agent
RUGBY4989 <> EL730	Tab	Yohimbine HCl 5.4 mg	by Pegasus	55246-0947	Impotence Agent
RUGBY4996	Tab, White	Theophylline Anhydrous CR 100 mg	Theo-Dur by Rugby		Antiasthmatic
RUGBY4997	Tab, White	Theophylline Anhydrous CR 200 mg	Theo-Dur by Rugby		Antiasthmatic
RUGBY4998	Tab, White	Theophylline Anhydrous CR 300 mg	Theo-Dur by Rugby		Antiasthmatic
RUGBY5506	Tab, Beige, Round	Levothyroxine Sodium 0.125 mg	Synthroid by Rugby		Antithyroid
RUGBY5535	Tab, Coated	Guaifenesin 600 mg, Pseudoephedrine HCl 120 mg	Guaitex PSE by Rugby	00536-5535	Cold Remedy
RUGBY5573	Cap	Nicardipine HCl 20 mg	by Chelsea	46193-0559	Antihypertensive
RUGBY5575	Tab, Blue/Green	Hyoscyamine Sulfate 0.125 mg	by Rugby	00536-5575	Gastrointestinal
RUGBY5575 <> EL717	Tab	Hyoscyamine Sulfate 0.125 mg	Hyosol SL by Pegasus	55246-0949	Gastrointestinal
RUGBY5595	Tab, White, Round	Clorazepate Dipotassium 15 mg	Tranxene by Rugby		Antianxiety; C IV
RUGBY5661	Tab, White, Round	Cimetidine 200 mg	Tagamet by Rugby		Gastrointestinal
RUGBY5662	Tab, Film Coated	Cimetidine 300 mg	by Rugby	00536-5662	Gastrointestinal
RUGBY5663	Tab, Film Coated	Cimetidine 400 mg	by Rugby	00536-5663	Gastrointestinal
RUGBY5664	Tab, Film Coated	Cimetidine 800 mg	by Rugby	00536-5664	Gastrointestinal
RUGBY5670	Tab, White, Round	Oxycodone HCl 5 mg, Acetaminophen 325 mg	Percocet by Rugby		Analgesic; C II
RUGBY5673	Tab, White, Oblong	Diethylpropion HCl 75 mg	by Blue Ridge	59273-0008	Antianorexiant; C IV
RUGBY5673	Tab, White, Oblong	Diethylpropion HCl 75 mg	by Dupont Pharma	00056-0668	Antianorexiant; C IV
RUGBY5673	Tab	Diethylpropion HCl 75 mg	by Rugby	00536-5673	Antianorexiant; C IV
RUGBY5673	Tab, White, Oblong	Diethylpropion HCl 75 mg	by Dupont Pharma	00590-0623	Antianorexiant; C IV
RUGBY5673	Tab, White, Cap Shaped	Diethylpropion HCl 75 mg	by Allscripts	54569-0396	Antianorexiant; C IV
RUGBY5683	Tab, Yellow	Prenatal, Beta Carotene	Prenatal Plus by Rugby		Vitamin

ID FRONT <> BACK	DESCRIPTION FRONT <> BACK	INGREDIENT & STRENGTH	BRAND (OR EQUIV.) & FIRM	NDC#	CLASS; SCH.
RUGBY5925	Tab, White, Round	Diethylpropion 25 mg	by Allscripts	54569-2059	Antianorexiant; C IV
RUGBY5925	Tab, Rugby over 5925	Diethylpropion HCl 25 mg	by Merrell	00068-5925	Antianorexiant; C IV
RUGBY5925	Tab, Rugby over 5925	Diethylpropion HCl 25 mg	by Rugby	00536-5925	Antianorexiant; C IV
RUGBYR3702	Tab, Rugby Logo R 3702	Diethylpropion HCl 25 mg	Tenuate by Rugby		Antianorexiant; C IV
RUGBYR3763	Tab, Rugby Logo R 3763	Diphenoxylate HCl 2.5 mg, Atropine Sulfate 0.025 mg	Lomotil by Rugby		Antidiarrheal; C V
RUGBYR3870	Tab, Rugby Logo R 3870	Glutethimide 500 mg	Doriden by Rugby		Hypnotic
RUSS316	Cap, Orange/Black	Vitamin, Mineral Comb.	Vicon Forte by Eon		Vitamin
RUSS500	Tab, Pink, Oblong	Hydrocodone Bitartrate 5 mg, Aspirin 500 mg	Lortab ASA by Russ		Analgesic; C III
RUSS901	Tab, White/Pink Specks, Oblong	Hydrocodone Bitartrate 2.5 mg, Acetaminophen 500 mg	Lortab by Russ		Analgesic; C III
RUSS902	Tab, White/Blue Specks, Oblong	Hydrocodone Bitartrate 5 mg, Acetaminophen 500 mg	Lortab-5 by Russ		Analgesic; C III
RUSS903	Tab, White/Green Specks, Oblong	Hydrocodone Bitartrate 7.5 mg, Acetaminophen 500 mg	Lortab 7.5 by Russ		Analgesic; C III
RUSS906	Tab, White/Green Specks, Oblong	Hydrocodone Bitartrate 7.5 mg, Acetaminophen 500 mg	Lortab-7 by Russ		Analgesic; C III
RW 2	Tab, Orange, Round	Hydromorphone HCl 2 mg	Dilaudid by Richwood		Analgesic; C II
RW 4	Tab, Yellow, Round	Hydromorphone HCl 4 mg	Dilaudid by Richwood		Analgesic; C II
RW81	Tab, White, Round	Aspirin 81 mg	Acuprin by Richwood		Analgesic
RX 743	Tab, White, Round, Scored	Phenobarbital 60 mg	by Ranbaxy		Sedative/Hypnotic; C IV
RX504	Tab, White, Oval	Acyclovir 400 mg	by Ranbaxy Pharms	63304-0504	Antiviral
RX504	Tab, White, Oval	Acyclovir 400 mg	by Eli Lilly	00002-0504	Antiviral
RX505	Tab, White, Oval	Acyclovir 800 mg	by Eli Lilly	00002-0505	Antiviral
RX505	Tab, White, Oval	Acyclovir 800 mg	by Ranbaxy Pharms	63304-0505	Antiviral
RX512	Tab, White, Oblong, Scored, Film Coated	Cefadroxil 1 gm	Cefadroxil by Caremark	00339-6156	Antibiotic
RX512	Tab, White, Oblong, Scored, Film Coated	Cefadroxil 1 gm	Cefadroxil by Caremark	00339-6152	Antibiotic
RX512	Tab, White, Oblong, Scored, Film Coated	Cefadroxil 1 gm	Cefadroxil by Caremark	00339-6157	Antibiotic
RX514	Tab, Mottled Pink, Oval, Chewable	Amoxicillin 125 mg	by Purepac	00228-2639	Antibiotic
RX514	Tab, Pink, Oval, Scored	Amoxicillin Trihydrate	by Ranbaxy Pharms	63304-0514	Antibiotic
RX514	Tab, Pink, Oval, Scored	Amoxicillin Trihydrate 125 mg	by Ranbaxy Labs	54907-5140	Antibiotic
RX515	Tab, Pink, Round	Amoxicillin Trihydrate	by Ranbaxy Pharms	63304-0515	Antibiotic
RX515	Tab, Pink, Round	Amoxicillin Trihydrate 250 mg	by Ranbaxy Labs	54907-5150	Antibiotic
RX515	Tab, Mottled Pink, Oval, Chewable	Amoxicillin 250 mg	by Purepac	00228-2640	Antibiotic
RX522	Tab, Yellow, Round, Scored	Enalapril Maleate 2.5 mg	by Ranbaxy Pharms	63304-0522	Antihypertensive
RX522	Tab, Yellow, Round, Scored	Enalapril Maleate 2.5 mg	by OHM	51660-0522	Antihypertensive
RX522	Tab, Yellow, Round, Biconvex, Scored	Enalapril Maleate 2.5 mg	by Purepac	00228-2658	Antihypertensive
RX523	Tab, White, Round, Scored	Enalapril Maleate 5 mg	by OHM	51660-0523	Antihypertensive
RX523	Tab, White, Round, Scored	Enalapril Maleate 5 mg	by Ranbaxy Pharms	63304-0523	Antihypertensive
RX523	Tab, White, Round, Biconvex, Scored	Enalapril Maleate 5 mg	by Purepac	00228-2659	Antihypertensive
RX524	Tab, Brown, Round	Enalapril Maleate 10 mg	by Ranbaxy Pharms	63304-0524	Antihypertensive
RX524	Tab, Brown, Round, Scored	Enalapril Maleate 10 mg	by OHM	51660-0524	Antihypertensive
RX524	Tab, Reddish Brown, Round	Enalapril Maleate 10 mg	by Purepac	00228-2660	Antihypertensive
RX525	Tab, Orange, Round	Enalapril Maleate 20 mg	by OHM	51660-0525	Antihypertensive
RX525	Tab, Orange, Round	Enalapril Maleate 20 mg	by Ranbaxy Pharms	63304-0525	Antihypertensive
RX525	Tab, Orange, Round	Enalapril Maleate 20 mg	by Purepac	00228-2661	Antihypertensive
RX652 <> RX652	Cap, White	Acyclovir 200 mg	by Ranbaxy Pharms	63304-0652	Antiviral
RX652 <> RX652	Cap, White	Acyclovir 200 mg	by Eli Lilly	00002-0652	Antiviral
RX654	Cap, Yellow, Opaque	Amoxicillin 250 mg	by Allscripts	54569-1746	Antibiotic
RX654	Cap, Yellow, Opaque	Amoxicillin 250 mg	by Purepac	00228-2688	Antibiotic
RX654 <> RX654	Cap, Yellow, Opaque	Amoxicillin 250 mg	Amoxicillin USP by Bayer	00026-5012	Antibiotic
RX654 <> RX654	Cap, Yellow, Opaque	Amoxicillin 250 mg	by Barr	00555-0899	Antibiotic
RX654 <> RX654	Cap, Yellow, Opaque	Amoxicillin 250 mg	Amoxicillin USP by Barr	00555-0926	Antibiotic
RX655	Cap, Maroon & Yellow, Opaque	Amoxicillin 500 mg	by Allscripts	54569-1861	Antibiotic
RX655	Cap, Maroon & Yellow, Opaque	Amoxicillin 500 mg	by Purepac	00228-2689	Antibiotic
RX655 <> RX655	Cap, Maroon & Yellow, Opaque	Amoxicillin 500 mg	Amoxicillin USP by Bayer	00026-5013	Antibiotic
RX655 <> RX655	Cap, Maroon & Yellow, Opaque	Amoxicillin 500 mg	Amoxicillin USP by Bayer	00026-2885	Antibiotic

ID FRONT <> BACK	DESCRIPTION FRONT <> BACK	INGREDIENT & STRENGTH	BRAND (OR EQUIV.) & FIRM	NDC#	CLASS; SCH.
RX655 <> RX655	Cap, Maroon & Yellow, Opaque	Amoxicillin 500 mg	by Barr	00555-0925	Antibiotic
RX656 <> RX656	Cap, Green & White	Cephalexin Monohydrate 250 mg	by Ranbaxy Pharms	54907-6560	Antibiotic
RX656 <> RX656	Cap, Green & White	Cephalexin Monohydrate 250 mg	by Ranbaxy Pharms	63304-0656	Antibiotic
RX657 <> RX657	Cap, Green	Cephalexin Monohydrate 500 mg	by Ranbaxy Pharms	54907-6570	Antibiotic
RX657 <> RX657	Cap, Green	Cephalexin Monohydrate 500 mg	by Ranbaxy Pharms	63304-0657	Antibiotic
RX658	Cap	Cefaclor 250 mg	by Ranbaxy	54907-6580	Antibiotic
RX658	Cap, Blue & Green	Cefaclor Monohydrate 250 mg	by Allscripts	54569-3901	Antibiotic
RX658 <> RX658	Cap	Cefaclor 250 mg	by Ranbaxy	63304-0658	Antibiotic
RX659	Cap	Cefaclor 500 mg	by Ranbaxy	63304-0659	Antibiotic
RX659	Cap	Cefaclor 500 mg	by Ranbaxy	54907-6590	Antibiotic
RX659	Cap, Blue & Green	Cefaclor Monohydrate 500 mg	by Allscripts	54569-3902	Antibiotic
RX675 <> RX675	Cap, Imprint in Edible Black Ink	Cephalexin Monohydrate 250 mg	by Ranbaxy	63304-0675	Antibiotic
RX675 <> RX675	Cap, Green & White	Cephalexin Monohydrate 250 mg	by Eli Lilly	00002-0675	Antibiotic
RX676 <> RX676	Cap, Dark Green & Light Green	Cephalexin Monohydrate 500 mg	by Ranbaxy	63304-0676	Antibiotic
RX676 <> RX676	Cap, Dark Green & Light Green	Cephalexin Monohydrate 500 mg	by Eli Lilly	00002-0676	Antibiotic
RX677 <> RX677	Cap, Using Edible Black Ink	Propoxyphene HCl 65 mg	by Ranbaxy	63304-0677	Analgesic; C IV
RX677 <> RX677	Cap, Pink, Black Ink	Propoxyphene HCl 65 mg	by Eli Lilly	00002-0677	Analgesic; C IV
RX678 <> RX678	Cap, Using Edible Black Ink	Aspirin 389 mg, Caffeine 32.4 mg, Propoxyphene HCl 65 mg	by Ranbaxy	63304-0678	Analgesic; C IV
RX678 <> RX678	Cap, Gray & Red, Black Print	Aspirin 389 mg, Caffeine 32.4 mg, Propoxyphene HCl 65 mg	by Eli Lilly	00002-0678	Analgesic; C IV
RX679 <> RX679	Cap, Orange	Secobarbital Sodium 100 mg	by Ranbaxy Pharms	63304-0679	Sedative/Hypnotic; C II
RX679 <> RX679	Cap, Orange	Secobarbital Sodium 100 mg	Seconal by Eli Lilly	00002-0679	Sedative/Hypnotic; C II
RX680	Cap, Blue & Orange	Amobarbital Sodium 50 mg; Secobarbital 50 mg	Tuinal by Ranbaxy Pharms	63304-0680	Sedative/Hypnotic; C II
RX680 <> RX680	Cap, Blue & Orange	Amobarbital Sodium 50 mg; Secobarbital 50 mg	Tuinal by Eli Lilly	00002-0680	Sedative/Hypnotic; C II
RX701	Tab, Yellow, Oval, Film Coated	Etodolac 400 mg	by Heartland	61392-0913	NSAID
RX701	Tab, Yellow, Oval, Film Coated	Etodolac 400 mg	Etodolac by Heartland	61392-0920	NSAID
RX714	Tab, Blue, Oval, Film Coated	Etodolac 500 mg	by Heartland	61392-0914	NSAID
RX714	Tab, Blue, Oval, Film Coated	Etodolac 500 mg	Etodolac by Hoechst Marion Roussel	64734-0001	NSAID
RX742	Tab, White, Round	Phenobarbital 30 mg	by Eli Lilly	00002-0742	Sedative/Hypnotic; C IV
RX756	Tab, Yellow, Round, Film Coated	Ranitidine 150 mg	by Ranbaxy Labs	54907-0756	Gastrointestinal
RX757	Tab, Yellow, Oblong	Ranitidine 300 mg	by Ranbaxy Labs	54907-0757	Gastrointestinal
RX770	Tab, White, Round, Film Coated	Ranitidine 150 mg	by Ranbaxy Labs	54907-0770	Gastrointestinal
RX771	Tab, White, Oblong	Ranitidine 300 mg	by Ranbaxy Labs	54907-0771	Gastrointestinal
RYNATAN711	Tab, Coral, Sugar Coated, Black Print	Azatadine Maleate 1 mg, Pseudoephedrine Sulfate 120 mg	Rynatan by Wallace	00037-0711	Cold Remedy
RYR	Tab, White, Circular, RY R/Roussel Logo	Disopyramide Phosphate 250 mg	by Hoechst Marion Roussel	Canadian	Antiarrhythmic
S	Tab, White, Round	Acetaminophen 325 mg, Codeine Phosph 8 mg, Doxylamine Succ 5 mg	Mersyndol by Marion Merrell Dow	Canadian	Analgesic
S	Tab, Dark Green, Light Yellow & Orange, Speckled, Scored, S in a Triangle	Belladonna 0.2 mg, Ergotamine 0.6 mg, Phenobarbital 40 mg	by Novartis	Canadian DIN# 00176141	Gastrointestinal
S	Tab, White, Round	Clomiphene Citrate 50 mg	Serophene by Serono	Canadian	Infertility
S	Tab, Light-Brown	Standardized Sennosides 8.6 mg	Senokot by Purdue Frederick	Canadian	Gastrointestinal
S	Tab, White, Round, Scored	Clomiphene Citrate 50 mg	by Serono	Canadian DIN# 00893722	Hormone
S <> 0770	Tab	Isosorbide Dinitrate 5 mg	Sorbitrate by Zeneca	00310-0770	Antianginal
S <> 256	Tab, White to Off-White, Round	Betahistine Dihydrochloride 8 mg	by Solvay	Canadian DIN# 02240601	Antivertigo
S <> 291291	Tab, White, Round, Scored, Film Coated	Fluvoxamine Maleate 50 mg	Luvox by Solvay Pharma	Canadian DIN# 01919342	OCD

ID FRONT <> BACK	DESCRIPTION FRONT <> BACK	INGREDIENT & STRENGTH	BRAND (OR EQUIV.) & FIRM	NDC#	CLASS; SCH.
S <> 313313	Tab, White, Oval, Scored, Film Coated	Fluvoxamine Maleate 100 mg	Luvox by Solvay Pharma	Canadian DIN# 01919369	OCD
S <> 5	Tab, White, Shield-Shaped	Selegiline HCl 5 mg	Eldepryl by Watson	52544-0136	Antiparkinson
S <> 50	Tab, Orange, Round, Film Coated, S over Triangle <> 50	Pinaverium Bromide 50 mg	Dicetel by Solvay Pharma	Canadian DIN# 01950592	Gastrointestinal
S <> 773	Tab	Isosorbide Dinitrate 30 mg	Sorbitrate by Zeneca	00310-0773	Antianginal
S <> 774	Tab, Light Blue	Isosorbide Dinitrate 40 mg	Sorbitrate by Zeneca	00310-0774	Antianginal
S <> 780	Tab	Isosorbide Dinitrate 10 mg	Sorbitrate by Zeneca	00310-0780	Antianginal
S <> 782	Tab, Light Green, Coated, S in Triangle <> 78-2	Thioridazine HCl 10 mg	Mellaril by Novartis	00078-0002	Antipsychotic
S <> 810	Tab, Chewable	Isosorbide Dinitrate 5 mg	Sorbitrate by Zeneca	00310-0810	Antianginal
S <> 815	Tab, Chewable	Isosorbide Dinitrate 10 mg	Sorbitrate by Zeneca	00310-0815	Antianginal
S <> 820	Tab	Isosorbide Dinitrate 20 mg	Sorbitrate by Zeneca	00310-0820	Antianginal
S <> 820	Tab	Isosorbide Dinitrate 20 mg	Sorbitrate by Nat Pharmpak Serv	55154-4402	Antianginal
S <> 853	Tab	Isosorbide Dinitrate 2.5 mg	Sorbitrate by Zeneca	00310-0853	Antianginal
S <> FIORINAL	Tab, White, Round, Fiorinal <> S in a triangle	Butalbital 50 mg, Caffeine 40 mg, Aspirin 330 mg	by Novartis	Canadian DIN# 00275328	Analgesic
S <> G	Tab, White, Oblong, Scored	Sotalol HCl 80 mg	by Par Pharm	49884-0582	Antiarrhythmic
S <> HYDERGINE	Tab, White, Round	Ergoloid Mesylates 1 mg	Hydergine by Novartis Pharms (Ca)	61615-0102	Ergot
S <> LESCOLLESCOL	Cap, Brown, S in a triangle <> S in a triangle Lescol Lescol	Fluvastatin Sodium 40 mg	Lescol by Inwood	00258-3657	Antihyperlipidemic
S <> MELLARIL100	Tab, Coated, S in Triangle <> Mellaril 100	Thioridazine HCl 100 mg	Mellaril by Novartis	00078-0005	Antipsychotic
S <> MELLARIL25	Tab, Coated, S in Triangle <> Mellaril 25	Thioridazine HCl 25 mg	Mellaril by Novartis	00078-0003	Antipsychotic
S <> MELLARIL50	Tab, Coated, S in Triangle <> Mellaril 50	Thioridazine HCl 50 mg	Mellaril by Novartis	00078-0004	Antipsychotic
S <> PARLODEL5MG	Cap, Caramel, S in Triangle <> Parlodel 5 mg	Bromocriptine Mesylate 5.74 mg	Parlodel by Pharm Utilization	60491-0499	Antiparkinson
S <> PARLODEL5MG	Cap, Light Brown, S in Triangle <> Parlodel 5 mg	Bromocriptine Mesylate 5.74 mg	Parlodel by Novartis	00078-0102	Antiparkinson
S <> S	Cap, Off-White	Ergoloid Mesylates 1 mg	Hydergine by RP Scherer	11014-0775	Ergot
S <> S80	Tab, White, Oblong	Sotalol HCl 80 mg	by Genpharm	55567-0057	Antiarrhythmic
S0260	Cap, Gelatin	Ascorbic Acid 250 mg, Cyanocobalamin 10 mcg, Ferrous Fumarate 200 mg, Zinc Sulfate 25 mg	Chromagen by RP Scherer	11014-1173	Vitamin
S0262	Cap, Gelatin	Ascorbic Acid 60 mg, Cyanocobalamin 10 mcg, Ferrous Fumarate 460 mg, Folic Acid 1 mg	Chromagen by RP Scherer	11014-1176	Vitamin
S1 <> GPI	Tab, White with Green Specks	Acetaminophen 325 mg, Phenylephrine HCl 5 mg, Chlorpheniramine Maleate 2 mg	Super Cold Tabs by Reese	10956-0771	Cold Remedy
S100MG	Cap, Blueish-Gray, S in a triangle	Cyclosporin 100 mg	Neoral by Novartis	Canadian DIN# 02150670	Immunosuppressant
S103	Tab, Brown, Round, S-103	Chlorpheniramine 8 mg, Phenylephrine 20 mg, Methscopolamine 2.5 mg	Dura- by Dura		Cold Remedy
S10MG	Cap, Yellowish-White, Oval, S in a triangle	Cyclosporin 10 mg	Neoral by Novartis	Canadian DIN# 02237671	Immunosuppressant
S11 <> LL	Tab, White, Round, Scored	Selegiline HCl 5 mg	by Lederle Pharm	00005-3254	Antiparkinson
S11 <> LL	Tab, White, Round	Selegiline HCl 5 mg	by ESI Lederle	59911-3254	Antiparkinson
S1124	Tab, Pink, Dark Pink Specks, S over 1124	Dyphylline 200 mg, Guaifenesin 200 mg	Dilor-G by Savage	00281-1124	Antiasthmatic
S120 <> G	Tab, White, Oblong	Sotalol HCl 120 mg	by Genpharm	55567-0076	Antiarrhythmic
S120 <> G	Tab, White, Oblong	Sotalol HCl 120 mg	by Par Pharm	49884-0583	Antiarrhythmic
S15WYETH317	Tab, Yellow, Pentagonal, S15/Wyeth 317	Oxazepam 15 mg	Serax by Wyeth		Sedative/Hypnotic; C IV
S16 <> LL	Tab	Sulindac 150 mg	by Lederle	00005-3550	NSAID
S16 <> LL	Tab	Sulindac 150 mg	by Caremark	00339-5696	NSAID
S16 <> LL	Tab, S Over 16	Sulindac 150 mg	by UDL	51079-0666	NSAID
S16 <> LL	Tab	Sulindac 150 mg	by Quality Care	60346-0044	NSAID
S160 <> G	Tab, White, Oblong	Sotalol HCl 160 mg	by Par Pharm	49884-0584	Antiarrhythmic

ID FRONT <> BACK	DESCRIPTION FRONT <> BACK	INGREDIENT & STRENGTH	BRAND (OR EQUIV.) & FIRM	NDC#	CLASS; SCH.
S160 <> G	Tab, White, Oblong	Sotalol HCl 160 mg	by Genpharm	55567-0058	Antiarrhythmic
S17 <> LL	Tab	Sulindac 200 mg	by Quality Care	60346-0686	NSAID
S20 <> LESCOL	Cap, S inside Triangle & 20 imprinted Twice <> Lescol & Lescol Logo Printed Twice	Fluvastatin Sodium 20 mg	Lescol by Pharm Utilization	60491-0355	Antihyperlipidemic
S2020 <> LESCOLLESCOL	Cap, Light Brown & Brown, Gelatin, S in triangle 20 20 <> Lescol Logo	Fluvastatin Sodium 20 mg	Lescol by Novartis	Canadian DIN# 02061562	Antihyperlipidemic
S240 <> G	Tab, White, Oblong	Sotalol HCl 240 mg	by Par Pharm	49884-0585	Antiarrhythmic
S240 <> G	Tab, White, Oblong	Sotalol HCl 240 mg	by Genpharm	55567-0059	Antiarrhythmic
S25MG	Cap, Blueish-Gray, Oval, S in a triangle	Cyclosporin 25 mg	Neoral by Novartis	Canadian DIN# 02150689	Immunosuppressant
S3A <> KEMADRIN	Tab	Procyclidine HCl 5 mg	Kemadrin by Catalytica	63552-0604	Antiparkinson
S3A <> KEMADRIN	Tab, White	Procyclidine HCl 5 mg	Kemadrin by Monarch	61570-0059	Antiparkinson
S40 <> LESCOL	Cap, Gold, Sandoz Logo 40 Sandoz Logo 40 <> Lescol Logo	Fluvastatin Sodium 40 mg	Lescol by DRX	55045-2369	Antihyperlipidemic
S40 <> LESCOL	Cap, S inside Triangle & 40 imprinted Twice <> Lescol Over Lescol Logo Twice	Fluvastatin Sodium 40 mg	Lescol by Pharm Utilization	60491-0356	Antihyperlipidemic
S40 <> S	Cap, Brown & Yellow, Lescol Logo 40	Fluvastatin Sodium 40 mg	Lescol by Inwood	00258-3711	Antihyperlipidemic
S4040 <> LESCOLLESCOL	Cap, Gold & Brown, Gelatin, S in triangle 40 40 <> Lescol Logo	Fluvastatin Sodium 40 mg	Lescol by Novartis	Canadian DIN# 02061570	Antihyperlipidemic
S4140	Cap	Amantadine HCl 100 mg	by United Res	00677-1452	Antiviral
S4140	Cap	Amantadine HCl 100 mg	by Pharmedix	53002-0375	Antiviral
S4140	Cap, Dark Red	Amantadine HCl 100 mg	by RP Scherer	11014-0813	Antiviral
S4140 <> S4140	Cap, Gelatin	Amantadine HCl 100 mg	by Qualitest	00603-2163	Antiviral
S5	Tab, White, Round	Selegiline HCl 5 mg	Selegilineby Apotex	Canadian DIN# 02230717	Antiparkinson
S50MG	Cap, Yellowish-White, Oval, S in a triangle	Cyclosporin 50 mg	Neoral by Novartis	Canadian DIN# 02150662	Immunosuppressant
S547	Tab, Aqua, Clover-Shaped	Trichlormethiazide 4 mg	Naqua by Schering	00085-0547	Diuretic
S5E <> G	Tab, White, Round	Selegiline HCl 5 mg	by Par Pharm	49884-0610	Antiparkinson
S760	Tab, Pink, Round	Isosorbide Dinitrate SL 5 mg	Sorbitrate by Zeneca		Antianginal
S761	Tab, Yellow, Round	Isosorbide Dinitrate SL 10 mg	Sorbitrate by Zeneca		Antianginal
S770	Tab, Green, Oval	Isosorbide Dinitrate Oral 5 mg	Sorbitrate by Zeneca		Antianginal
S7720	Tab, White, Round	Chenodiol 250 mg	Chenix by Solvay		Cholelitholytic
S7830	Tab, White, Round, S 78-30	Belladonna Alkaloids 0.25 mg	Bellafoline by Sandoz		Gastrointestinal
S7836	Tab, Green, Round, S 78-36	Ergotamine 1 mg, Caffeine 100 mg, Bellafoline 0.125 mg, Pentobarbital 30 mg	Cafergot Pb by Sandoz		Antimigraine; C IV
S788	Tab, Rose, Round. S 78-8	Thioridazine HCl 15 mg	Mellaril by Sandoz		Antipsychotic
S80 <> S	Tab, White, Oblong	Sotalol HCl 80 mg	by Genpharm	55567-0057	Antiarrhythmic
S822	Tab, Pink, Clover-Shaped	Trichlormethiazide 2 mg	Naqua by Schering		Diuretic
S880	Tab, Yellow, Round	Isosorbide Dinitrate SR Oral 40 mg	Sorbitrate SA by Zeneca		Antianginal
SABRIL	Tab, White, Oval	Vigabatrin 500 mg	Sabril by Marion Merrell Dow	Canadian	Antiepileptic
SAHG	Tab, Pink, Clover-Shaped	Trichlormethiazide 2 mg	Naqua by Schering		Diuretic
SAHH	Tab, Aqua, Clover-Shaped	Trichlormethiazide 4 mg	Naqua by Schering	00085-0547	Diuretic
SAL <> 5	Tab, White, Round, Film Coated	Pilocarpine HCl 5 mg	by Pharmacia	Canadian DIN# 02216345	Cholinergic Agonist
SAL5	Tab, White, Round, SAL/5	Pilocarpine HCl 5 mg	by Pharmacia	Canadian	Cholinergic Agonist
SAMPLE <> 4	Tab, Film Coated	Ondansetron HCl	Zofran by Glaxo Wellcome	00173-0446	Antiemetic
SAMPLE <> 8	Tab	Ondansetron HCl 8 mg	Zofran by Glaxo Wellcome	00173-0447	Antiemetic

ID FRONT <> BACK	DESCRIPTION FRONT <> BACK	INGREDIENT & STRENGTH	BRAND (OR EQUIV.) & FIRM	NDC#	CLASS; SCH.
SAMPLE <> ZOFRAN	Tab	Ondansetron HCl 8 mg	Zofran by Glaxo Wellcome	00173-0447	Antiemetic
SAMPLE <> ZOFRAN	Tab, Film Coated	Ondansetron HCl	Zofran by Glaxo Wellcome	00173-0446	Antiemetic
SANDOZ	Tab, Green/Yellow, Circular, SAN/DOZ	Methysergide Maleate 2 mg	Sansert by Sandoz	Canadian	Antimigraine
SANDOZ	Tab, Coated	Methylergonovine Maleate 0.2 mg	Methergine by Apotheca	12634-0179	Ergot
SANDOZ	Tab, Red	Mesoridazine Besylate 10 mg	Serentil by Sandoz	Canadian	Antipsychotic
SANDOZ	Tab, White, Round, Scored	Pizotifen 1 mg	Sandomigran DS by Sandoz	Canadian DIN# 00511552	Antimigraine
SANDOZ <> 25	Tab, Red, Round, Sugar Coated	Mesoridazine Besylate 25 mg	Serentil by Novartis	Canadian DIN# 00027456	Antipsychotic
SANDOZ <> 50MG	Cap	Cyclosporine 50 mg	Sandimmun Neoral B17 by RP Scherer	11014-1196	Immunosuppressant
SANDOZ <> 7854	Tab, Orchid, Coated, 78-54 in Black Ink	Methylergonovine Maleate 0.2 mg	Methergine by Kaiser	00179-0432	Ergot
SANDOZ <> 7854	Tab, Coated	Methylergonovine Maleate 0.2 mg	Methergine by Allscripts	54569-3920	Ergot
SANDOZ <> 7854	Tab, Coated	Methylergonovine Maleate 0.2 mg	Methergine by Allscripts	54569-0973	Ergot
SANDOZ <> 7854	Tab, Coated, 78-54	Methylergonovine Maleate 0.2 mg	Methergine by Quality Care	60346-0028	Ergot
SANDOZ <> 7854	Tab, Coated	Methylergonovine Maleate 0.2 mg	Methergine by PDRX	55289-0708	Ergot
SANDOZ <> 7858	Tab, Sandoz <> 78-58	Methysergide Maleate 2 mg	Sansert by Novartis	00078-0058	Antimigraine
SANDOZ <> BC	Tab, Ivory, Round, Sugar Coated	Pizotifen 0.5 mg	Sandomigran by Novartis	Canadian DIN# 00329320	Antimigraine
SANDOZ <> PAMELOR25MG	Cap, Pamelor 25 MG	Nortriptyline HCl 25 mg	Pamelor by Novartis	00078-0087	Antidepressant
SANDOZ <> VJ	Tab, White, Round	Ergoloid Mesylates 1 mg	Hydergine by Novartis	Canadian DIN# 00176176	Ergot
SANDOZ10	Tab, Red, Round, Sandoz/10	Mesoridazine Besylate 10 mg	Serentil by Novartis	Canadian	Antipsychotic
SANDOZ10MG	Cap, Yellow-Orange & White, Pamelor Logo <> Sandoz 10 mg	Nortriptyline HCl 10 mg	Pamelor by Allscripts	54569-0225	Antidepressant
SANDOZ50	Tab, Red, Round, Sandoz/50	Mesoridazine Besylate 50 mg	Serentil by Novartis	Canadian	Antipsychotic
SANDOZ78107 <> FC	Cap, Sandoz 78-107 <> Sandoz Logo F-C	Aspirin 325 mg, Butalbital 50 mg, Caffeine 40 mg, Codeine Phosphate 30 mg	Fiorinal w Codeine #3 by Allscripts	54569-0341	Analgesic; C III
SANDOZ78107 <> SFC	Cap, Sandoz 78-107 <> S in Triangle F-C	Aspirin 325 mg, Butalbital 50 mg, Caffeine 40 mg, Codeine Phosphate 30 mg	Fiorinal w Codeine No 3 by Physicians Total Care	54868-0530	Analgesic; C III
SANDOZ7858	Tab, Yellow, Round, Sandoz 78-58	Methysergide 2 mg	Sansert by Sandoz		Antimigraine
SANDOZ7866	Tab, White, Round, Sandoz 78-66	Mazindol 2 mg	Sanorex by Sandoz		Anorexiant
SANDOZME100	Tab, Blue/Green, Circular, SAN/DOZ/MEL100	Thioridazine HCl 100 mg	Mellaril by Sandoz	Canadian	Antipsychotic
SANDOZMEL10	Tab, Light Green, Circular, SAN/DOZ/MEL/10	Thioridazine HCl 10 mg	Mellaril by Sandoz	Canadian	Antipsychotic
SANDOZMEL25	Tab, Light Brown, Circular, SAN/DOZ/MEL/25	Thioridazine HCl 25 mg	Mellaril by Sandoz	Canadian	Antipsychotic
SANDOZMEL50	Tab, White, Circular, SAN/DOZ/MEL/50	Thioridazine HCl 50 mg	Mellaril by Sandoz	Canadian	Antipsychotic
SANDOZRESTORIL15	Cap, Flesh & Maroon, Gelatin	Temazepam 15 mg	Restoril by Sandoz	Canadian DIN# 00604453	Sedative/Hypnotic
SANDOZRESTORIL30	Cap, Blue & Maroon, Gelatin	Temazepam 30 mg	Restoril by Sandoz	Canadian DIN# 00604461	Sedative/Hypnotic
SANDZO <> 7854	Tab, Purple, Round	Methylergonovine Maleate 0.2 mg	Methergine by Novartis Pharms (Ca)	61615-0107	Ergot
SANOFI <> PN	Tab, Coated	Ascorbic Acid 120 mg, Calcium Citrate 200 mg, Cholecalciferol 400 Units, Cupric Oxide 2 mg, Cyanocobalamin 12 mcg, Docusate Sodium 50 mg, Folic Acid 1 mg, Iron Pentacarbonyl 90 mg, Niacinamide 20 mg, Potassium Iodide 150 mcg, Pyridoxine HCl 20 mg, Riboflavin 3.4 mg, Thiamine HCl 3 mg, Vitamin A 2700 Units, Vitamin E 30 Units, Zinc Oxide 25 mg	Prenate Ultra by Sanofi	00024-1730	Vitamin
SANOREX	Tab	Mazindol 1 mg	Sanorex by Allscripts	54569-4517	Anorexiant
SANOREX <> 7871	Tab, White, Eliptical, Sanorex <> 78-71	Mazindol 1 mg	by Allscripts	54569-4517	Anorexiant

ID FRONT <> BACK	DESCRIPTION FRONT <> BACK	INGREDIENT & STRENGTH	BRAND (OR EQUIV.) & FIRM	NDC#	CLASS; SCH.
SANOREX <> JC	Tab, Peach, Round, Scored	Mazindol 2 mg	Sanorex by Novartis	Canadian DIN# 00285544	Anorexiant
SB <> 2	Tab, Pink, Pentagon, Film	Rosiglitazone Maleate 2 mg	Avandia by RX PAK	65084-0207	Antidiabetic
SB <> 2	Tab, Pink, Pentagon, Film	Rosiglitazone Maleate 2 mg	Avandia by RX PAK	65084-0209	Antidiabetic
SB <> 39	Tab, Film Coated	Carvedilol 3.125 mg	Coreg by Murfreesboro	51129-1126	Antihypertensive
SB <> 4	Tab, Orange, Pentagon, Film Coated	Rosiglitazone Maleate 4 mg	Avandia by RX PAK	65084-0210	Antidiabetic
SB <> 8	Tab, Brown, Pentagon, Film Coated	Rosiglitazone Maleate 8 mg	Avandia by RX PAK	65084-0208	Antidiabetic
SB <> 8	Tab, Red, Pentagon	Rosiglitazone Maleate 8 mg	Avandia by RX PAK	65084-0215	Antidiabetic
SB <> AUGMENTIN875	Tab, White, Cap Shaped, Coated	Amoxicillin Trihydrate, Clavulanate Potassium	Augmentin by SKB	00029-6086	Antibiotic
SB <> AUGMENTIN875	Tab, Coated	Amoxicillin Trihydrate, Clavulanate Potassium	Augmentin by HJ Harkins Co	52959-0478	Antibiotic
SB <> DYAZIDE	Cap	Hydrochlorothiazide 25 mg, Triamterene 37.5 mg	Dyazide by Allscripts	54569-3824	Diuretic
SB <> DYAZIDE	Cap, Opaque	Hydrochlorothiazide 25 mg, Triamterene 37.5 mg	Dyazide by Amerisource	62584-0365	Diuretic
SB 2	Tab, Pink, Pentagon	Rosiglitazone Maleate 2 mg	Avandia by SKB	00029-3158	Antidiabetic
SB 4	Tab, Orange, Pentagon	Rosiglitazone Maleate 4 mg	Avandia by SKB	00029-3159	Antidiabetic
SB 4142	Tab, White, Oval	Carvedilol 25 mg	Coreg by SKB	00007-4142	Antihypertensive
SB 8	Tab, Red-Brown, Pentagon	Rosiglitazone Maleate 8 mg	Avandia by SKB	00029-3160	Antidiabetic
SB10MG <> 334410MG	Cap, Ivory & Natural, Ex Release, Yellow & White Pellets	Prochlorperazine Maleate 16.2 mg	Compazine by SKB	00007-3344	Antiemetic
SB10MG <> 351310MG	Cap, Ivory & Natural, 3513/10 mg	Dextroamphetamine Sulfate 10 mg	Dexedrine by SKB	00007-3513	Stimulant; C II
SB10MG334610MG	Cap, Black/Natural, SB 10mg/3346 10mg	Prochlorperazine 15 mg	Compazine Spansule by SKB		Antiemetic
SB15MG351415MG	Cap, Brown & Natural	Dextroamphetamine Sulfate 15 mg	Dexedrine Spansule by SKB	00007-3514	Stimulant; C II
SB4141	Tab, White, Oval	Carvedilol 12.5 mg	Coreg by SKB	00007-4141	Antihypertensive
SB4890	Tab, White, Pentagonal	Ropinirole HCl 0.25 mg	Requip by SKB	00007-4890	Antiparkinson
SB4890	Tab, Coated, SB 4890	Ropinirole HCl 0.25 mg	Requip by SKB	00007-4890	Antiparkinson
SB4890	Tab, Coated	Ropinirole HCl 0.25 mg	Requip by SKB	60351-4890	Antiparkinson
SB4890	Tab, Coated	Ropinirole HCl 0.5 mg	Requip by SKB	00007-4891	Antiparkinson
SB4891	Tab, Yellow, Pentagonal	Ropinirole HCl 0.5 mg	Requip by SKB	00007-4891	Antiparkinson
SB4891	Tab, Coated	Ropinirole HCl 0.5 mg	Requip by SKB	60351-4891	Antiparkinson
SB4892	Tab, Pale Green, Coated	Ropinirole HCl 1 mg	Requip by SKB	00007-4892	Antiparkinson
SB4892	Tab, Coated	Ropinirole HCl 1 mg	Requip by SKB	60351-4892	Antiparkinson
SB4892	Tab, Green, Pentagonal	Ropinirole HCl 1.0 mg	Requip by SKB	00007-4892	Antiparkinson
SB4893	Tab, Yellowish Pink, Coated	Ropinirole HCl 2 mg	Requip by SKB	00007-4893	Antiparkinson
SB4893	Tab, Pale Yellowish Pink, Coated	Ropinirole HCl 2 mg	Requip by SKB	60351-4893	Antiparkinson
SB4893	Tab, Yellow & Pink, Pentagonal	Ropinirole HCl 2.0 mg	Requip by SKB	00007-4893	Antiparkinson
SB4894	Tab, Pale Blue, Coated	Ropinirole HCl 5 mg	Requip by SKB	00007-4894	Antiparkinson
SB4894	Tab, Pale Blue, Coated	Ropinirole HCl 5 mg	Requip by SKB	60351-4894	Antiparkinson
SB4894	Tab, Blue, Pentagonal	Ropinirole HCl 5.0 mg	Requip by SKB	00007-4894	Antiparkinson
SB4896	Tab, Brown, Pentagon, Beveled, Film, SB Over 4896	Ropinirole HCl 4 mg	Requip by RX PAK	65084-0205	Antiparkinson
SB4896	Tab, Brown, Pentagon, Beveled, Film, SB Over 4896	Ropinirole HCl 4 mg	Requip by RX PAK	65084-0204	Antiparkinson
SB5043	Tab, White, Oval, Film Coated, SB5043 <> SB5043	Eprosartan Mesylate 300 mg	Teveten by Solvay Pharma	Canadian DIN# 02240431	Antihypertensive
SB5044	Tab, Pink, Oval, Film Coated, SB5044 <> SB5044	Eprosartan Mesylate 400 mg	Teveten by Solvay Pharma	Canadian DIN# 02240432	Antihypertensive
SB5500	Tab, White, Round, SB/5500	Albendazole 200 mg	Albenza by SKB	00007-5500	Antihelmintic
SB5MG <> 35125MG	Cap, Brown & Natural, 5 mg/SB <> 5 mg/3512	Dextroamphetamine Sulfate 5 mg	Dexedrine Spansule by SKB	00007-3512	Stimulant; C II
SCF	Cap, Blue	Orlistat 120 mg	Contac Severe Cold by Allscripts	54569-4742	Lipase Inhibitor
SCHEIN <> 0765400	Tab, Film Coated, 0765/400	Ibuprofen 400 mg	by Schein	00364-0765	NSAID
SCHEIN0765400	Tab, Film Coated, Schein Over 0765/400	Ibuprofen 400 mg	by Nat Pharmpak Serv	55154-5214	NSAID
SCHEIN0765400	Tab, Mnfrs - Knoll and Upjohn For Schein	Ibuprofen 400 mg	by Med Pro	53978-5005	NSAID
SCHEIN0765400	Tab, White, Film, Schein 0765/400 Black Ink	Ibuprofen 400 mg	by Murfreesboro	51129-1512	NSAID

ID FRONT <> BACK	DESCRIPTION FRONT <> BACK	INGREDIENT & STRENGTH	BRAND (OR EQUIV.) & FIRM	NDC#	CLASS; SCH.
SCHEIN0766 <> 600	Tab, Film Coated	Ibuprofen 600 mg	by Quality Care	60346-0556	NSAID
SCHEIN0766600	Tab, White, Film, Schein Over 0766/600 in Black Ink	Ibuprofen 600 mg	by Murfreesboro	51129-1514	NSAID
SCHEIN0766600	Tab, Schein Over 0766/600, Printed in Black on one Face, Film Coated	Ibuprofen 600 mg	by Nat Pharmpak Serv	55154-5207	NSAID
SCHEIN0766600	Tab, White, Round, Film Coated, Schein Over 0766/600	Ibuprofen 600 mg	by Murfreesboro	51129-1530	NSAID
SCHEIN0766600	Tab	Ibuprofen 600 mg	by Talbert Med	44514-0636	NSAID
SCHEIN20	Cap, Schein Over 20	Nifedipine 10 mg	by RP Scherer	11014-0955	Antihypertensive
SCHEIN2137 <> 800	Tab, Film Coated	Ibuprofen 400 mg	by Quality Care	60346-0030	NSAID
SCHEIN2137800	Tab, Schein/2137/800, Film Coated	Ibuprofen 800 mg	by Schein	00364-2137	NSAID
SCHEIN2137800	Tab, Film Coated, Knoll For Schein	Ibuprofen 800 mg	by Med Pro	53978-5007	NSAID
SCHEIN2137800	Tab, White, Oblong, Film Coated, Schein Over 2137/800	Ibuprofen 800 mg	by Murfreesboro	51129-1531	NSAID
SCHEIN2137800	Tab, White, Oblong, Film Coated, Schein Over 2137/800	Ibuprofen 800 mg	by Murfreesboro	51129-1516	NSAID
SCHEIN2137800	Tab, Schein Over 2137/800, Film Coated	Ibuprofen 800 mg	by Nat Pharmpak Serv	55154-5233	NSAID
SCHEIN2137800	Tab, White, Film Coated, Schein Over 2137/800 in Black Ink	Ibuprofen 800 mg	by Murfreesboro	51129-1515	NSAID
SCHEIN2137800	Tab	Ibuprofen 800 mg	by Talbert Med	44514-0637	NSAID
SCHEIN2137800	Tab, White, Oblong, Film Coated	Ibuprofen 800 mg	By Heartland Healthcare	61392-0528	NSAID
SCHEIN600 <> 0766	Tab, Film Coated	Ibuprofen 600 mg	by Schein	00364-0766	NSAID
SCHERING	Tab, Blue, Round	Betamethasone 1 mg	Celestone by Schering	Canadian	Steroid
SCHERING <> 100NORMODYNE	Tab, Light Brown, Film Coated	Labetalol HCl 100 mg	Normodyne by Pharm Utilization	60491-0458	Antihypertensive
SCHERING <> 496	Tab, White, Mortar and Pestle to Right of Schering	Griseofulvin, Microsize 500 mg	Fulvicin-U/F by Schering	00085-0496	Antifungal
SCHERING <> 948	Tab, White, Mortar and Pestle to Right of Schering	Griseofulvin, Microsize 250 mg	Fulvicin UF by Schering	00085-0948	Antifungal
SCHERING244	Tab, Light Brown, Round	Labetalol 100 mg	Normodyne by Schering		Antihypertensive
SCHERING244 <> 100	Tab, Brown, Round, Scored	Labetalol HCl 100 mg	Normodyne by Rightpak	65240-0705	Antihypertensive
SCHERING244 <> 100NORMODYNE	Tab, Film Coated	Labetalol HCl 100 mg	Normodyne by Nat Pharmpak Serv	55154-3511	Antihypertensive
SCHERING244 <> 100NORMODYNE	Tab, Film Coated	Labetalol HCl 100 mg	Normodyne by Amerisource	62584-0244	Antihypertensive
SCHERING244 <> 100NORMODYNE	Tab, Light Brown, Film Coated, Schering 244 <> 100 Normodyne	Labetalol HCl 100 mg	Normodyne by Thrift Drug	59198-0080	Antihypertensive
SCHERING244 <> 100NORMODYNE	Tab, Brown, Round, Scored, Film Coated, 100 Normodyne	Labetolol HCl 100 mg	Normodyne by Murfreesboro	51129-1618	Antihypertensive
SCHERING244 <> NORMODYNE	Tab, Film Coated	Labetalol HCl 100 mg	Normodyne by Med Pro	53978-0696	Antihypertensive
SCHERING244 <> NORMODYNE100	Tab, Light Brown, Round, Film Coated, Schering/244 <> Normodyne/100	Labetalol HCl 100 mg	Normodyne by Schering	00085-0244	Antihypertensive
SCHERING244 <> NORMODYNE100	Tab, Film Coated	Labetalol HCl 100 mg	Normodyne by Caremark	00339-5265	Antihypertensive
SCHERING244 <> NORMODYNE100	Tab, Film Coated	Labetalol HCl 100 mg	Normodyne by Rite Aid	11822-5260	Antihypertensive
SCHERING396	Tab, White, Bullet Shaped	Clotrimazole 500 mg	Gyne Lotrimin by Schering		Antifungal
SCHERING438	Tab, Blue, Round	Labetalol 300 mg	Normodyne by Schering		Antihypertensive
SCHERING438 <> 300	Tab, Blue, Round	Labetalol HCl 300 mg	Normdyne by Rightpak	65240-0670	Antihypertensive
SCHERING438 <> 300NORMODYNE	Tab, Blue, Round, Film, Schering 438 <> 300 Normodyne	Labetalol 300 mg	Normodyne by Murfreesboro	51129-1607	Antihypertensive
SCHERING438 <> 300NORMODYNE	Tab, Blue, Round, Film Coated	Labetalol 300 mg	Normodyne by Murfreesboro	51129-1606	Antihypertensive
SCHERING438 <> 300NORMODYNE	Tab, Coated, Schering 438 <> 300 Normodyne	Labetalol HCl 300 mg	Normodyne by Thrift Drug	59198-0082	Antihypertensive
SCHERING438 <> NORMODYNE	Tab, Blue, Round	Labetalol HCl 300 mg	Normodyne by Rx Pac	65084-0230	Antihypertensive

ID FRONT <> BACK	DESCRIPTION FRONT <> BACK	INGREDIENT & STRENGTH	BRAND (OR EQUIV.) & FIRM	NDC#	CLASS; SCH.
SCHERING438 <> NORMODYNE300	Tab, Blue, Round, Film Coated	Labetalol HCl 300 mg	Normodyne by Schering	00085-0438	Antihypertensive
SCHERING438 <> NORMODYNE300	Tab, Film Coated	Labetalol HCl 300 mg	Normodyne by Leiner	59606-0670	Antihypertensive
SCHERING525	Cap, Brown, Opaque	Flutamide 125 mg	Eulexin by Schering	00085-0525	Antiandrogen
SCHERING525	Cap, Brown, Opaque, Schering Logo 525	Flutamide 125 mg	Eulexin by Inwood	00258-3613	Antiandrogen
SCHERING525	Cap, Creamed	Flutamide 125 mg	by Med Pro	53978-2031	Antiandrogen
SCHERING525 <> SCHERING525	Cap, Red & White, Schering/525 <> Schering/525	Flutamide 125 mg	Eulexin by Eckerd	19458-0919	Antiandrogen
SCHERING7 <> NORMODYNE	Tab, Film Coated	Labetalol HCl 200 mg	Normodyne by Pharmedix	53002-1046	Antihypertensive
SCHERING703	Tab, Sugar Coated	Azatadine Maleate 1 mg, Pseudoephedrine Sulfate 120 mg	Trinalin by Pharmedix	53002-0413	Cold Remedy
SCHERING752	Tab, White, Round	Labetalol 200 mg	Normodyne by Schering		Antihypertensive
SCHERING752 <> 200	Tab, White, Round, Scored	Labetalol HCl 200 mg	Normodyne by Rightpak	65240-0706	Antihypertensive
SCHERING752 <> 200NORMODYNE	Tab, Film Coated, Schering 752 <> 200 Normodyne	Labetalol HCl 200 mg	Normodyne by Thrift Drug	59198-0081	Antihypertensive
SCHERING752 <> 200NORMODYNE	Tab, White, Round, Scored, Film Coated, Schering 752 <> 200 Normodyne	Labetolol HCl 200 mg	Normodyne by Murfreesboro	51129-1617	Antihypertensive
SCHERING752 <> NORMODYNE	Tab, Film Coated, Schering 752	Labetalol HCl 200 mg	Normodyne by Med Pro	53978-0697	Antihypertensive
SCHERING752 <> NORMODYNE 200	Tab, Film Coated, Schering 438 <> Normodyne 300	Labetalol HCl 200 mg	Normodyne by Schering	53922-0752	Antihypertensive
SCHERING752 <> NORMODYNE 200	Tab, Film Coated	Labetalol HCl 200 mg	Normodyne by Amerisource	62584-0752	Antihypertensive
SCHERING752 <> NORMODYNE200	Tab, White, Round, Film Coated	Labetalol HCl 200 mg	Normodyne by Schering	00085-0752	Antihypertensive
SCHERING752 <> NORMODYNE200	Tab, Film Coated, Schering 752 <> Normodyne 200	Labetalol HCl 200 mg	Normodyne by Nat Pharmpak Serv	55154-3506	Antihypertensive
SCHERING752 <> NORMODYNE200	Tab, Film Coated	Labetalol HCl 200 mg	Normodyne by Rite Aid	11822-5234	Antihypertensive
SCHERINGGROOVE	Tab, Blue, Round, Schering/Groove	Betamethasone 0.5 mg	Celestone by Schering	Canadian	Steroid
SCHERINGLOGO	Tab, Orange, Round, Schering Logo	Chlorpheniramine Maleate 12 mg	Chlor-Tripolon by Schering	Canadian	Antihistamine
SCHWARTZ <> 0920	Tab, Pink & Clear, Opaque, Oblong	Isosorbide Dinitrate 40 mg	Dilatrate SR by Murfreesboro	51129-1564	Antianginal
SCHWARTZ <> 532	Cap, Pale Blue-Green	Hyoscyamine Sulfate 0.125 mg	Levsin SI by Thrift Drug	59198-0173	Gastrointestinal
SCHWARZ <> 525	Cap, White	Pancrelipase (Amylase 30000 unt, Lipase 8000 unt, Protease 8000 unt)	Kuzyme HP by Schwarz Pharma Mfg	00131-3525	Gastrointestinal
SCHWARZ <> 531	Tab, White, Scored	Hyoscyamine Sulfate 0.125 mg	Levsin by Schwarz Pharma	00091-3531	Gastrointestinal
SCHWARZ <> 531	Tab	Hyoscyamine Sulfate 0.125 mg	Levsin by Prestige Packaging	58056-0351	Gastrointestinal
SCHWARZ <> 531	Tab	Hyoscyamine Sulfate 0.125 mg	Levsin by Thrift Drug	59198-0287	Gastrointestinal
SCHWARZ <> 532	Tab, Green, Octagon, Scored	Hyoscyamine Sulfate 0.125 mg	Levsin SL by Natl Pharmpak	55154-0952	Gastrointestinal
SCHWARZ <> 532	Tab, Blue, Octagon, Scored	Hyoscyamine Sulfate 0.125 mg	Levsin SL by Med-Pro	53978-3372	Gastrointestinal
SCHWARZ <> 532	Tab, White, Octagonal, Scored	Hyoscyamine Sulfate 0.125 mg	Levsin SL by Schwarz Pharma	00091-3532	Gastrointestinal
SCHWARZ <> 532	Tab, Pale Blue-Green	Hyoscyamine Sulfate 0.125 mg	Levsin SI by Physicians Total Care	54868-1767	Gastrointestinal
SCHWARZ <> 532	Tab, Blue, Octagon, Scored	Hyoscyamine Sulfate 0.125 mg	Levsin SL sublingual by Murfreesboro	51129-1489	Gastrointestinal
SCHWARZ <> 532	Tab, Pale Blue-Green	Hyoscyamine Sulfate 0.125 mg	Levsin SI by Quality Care	60346-0998	Gastrointestinal
SCHWARZ <> 532	Tab	Hyoscyamine Sulfate 0.125 mg	Levsin SI by Amerisource	62584-0007	Gastrointestinal
SCHWARZ <> 532	Tab, Blue-Green, Embossed	Hyoscyamine Sulfate 0.125 mg	Levsin SI by Prestige Packaging	58056-0352	Gastrointestinal
SCHWARZ <> 534	Tap, Pink	Hyoscyamine Sulfate 0.125 mg, Phenobarbital 15 mg	Levsin Phenobarb by Schwarz Pharma	00091-3534	Gastrointestinal; C IV
SCHWARZ <> 537	Cap, Brown & Clear, Ex Release	Hyoscyamine Sulfate 0.375 mg	Levsinex by Thrift Drug	59198-0288	Gastrointestinal
SCHWARZ 522	Cap, Yellow & White, Opaque	Amylase 30 mg, Cellulase 2 mg, Lipase 1200 Units, Protease 6 mg	Ku-Zyme by Schwarz Pharma	00091-3522	Gastrointestinal
SCHWARZ053	Cap, White & Yellow	Pseudoephedrine HCl 65 mg, Chlorpheniramine 10 mg	Fedahist Gyrocaps by Schwarz Pharma		Cold Remedy
SCHWARZ055	Cap, Clear	Pseudoephedrine HCl 120 mg, Chlorpheniramine 8 mg	Fedahist Timecaps by Schwarz Pharma		Cold Remedy
SCHWARZ0920	Cap, Clear & Pink, Opaque w/ White Beads	Isosorbide Dinitrate 40 mg	Dilatrate SR by Eon	00091-0920	Antianginal

ID FRONT <> BACK	DESCRIPTION FRONT <> BACK	INGREDIENT & STRENGTH	BRAND (OR EQUIV.) & FIRM	NDC#	CLASS; SCH.
SCHWARZ2489 <> VERELAN180MG	Cap, Gray & Yellow, Schwarz over 2489 <> Verelan over 180 mg	Verapamil HCl 180 mg	Verelan by Schwarz Pharma	00091-2489	Antihypertensive
SCHWARZ2490 <> VERELAN120MG	Cap, Yellow, Schwarz over 2490 <> Verelan over 120 mg	Verapamil HCl 120 mg	Verelan by Schwarz Pharma	00091-2490	Antihypertensive
SCHWARZ2491 <> VERELAN240MG	Cap, Blue & Yellow, Schwarz over 2491 <> Verelan over 240 mg	Verapamil HCl 240 mg	Verelan by Schwarz Pharma	00091-2491	Antihypertensive
SCHWARZ2495 <> VERELAN360MG	Cap, Lavender & Yellow, Schwarz over 2495 <> Verelan over 360 mg	Verapamil HCl 360 mg	Verelan by Schwarz Pharma	00091-2495	Antihypertensive
SCHWARZ4085 <> 100MG	Cap, Purple & White, Opaque, Hard Gel	Verapamil HCl 100 mg	Verelan Sustained Release by Teva	00480-0832	Antihypertensive
SCHWARZ4085 <> 100MG	Cap, Amethyst & White, Opaque	Verapamil HCl 100 mg	Verelan PM by Schwarz Pharma	00091-4085	Antihypertensive
SCHWARZ4086 <> 200MG	Cap, Purple, Opaque, Hard Gel	Verapamil HCl 200 mg	Verelan Sustained Release by Teva	00480-0833	Antihypertensive
SCHWARZ4086 <> 200MG	Cap, Amethyst, Opaque	Verapamil HCl 200 mg	Verelan PM by Schwarz Pharma	00091-4086	Antihypertensive
SCHWARZ4087 <> 300MG	Cap, Purple, Opaque, Hard Gel	Verapamil HCl 300 mg	Verelan Sustained Release by Teva	00480-0834	Antihypertensive
SCHWARZ4087 <> 300MG	Cap, Amethyst & Lavender, Opaque	Verapamil HCl 300 mg	Verelan PM by Schwarz Pharma	00091-4087	Antihypertensive
SCHWARZ4122	Cap, White	Amylase 15000 unt; Lipase 1200 unt; Protease 15000 unt	Ku Zyme by Schwarz Pharma Mfg	00131-4122	Gastrointestinal
SCHWARZ4122	Cap, Green & White	Amylase 3000 unt; Lipase 2400 unt; Protease 3000 unt	Kutrase by Schwarz Pharma Mfg	00131-4175	Gastrointestinal
SCHWARZ4122	Cap, White & Yellow, Opaque	Pancreatin: Lipase 1200 units, Amylase 15000 units, Protease 15000 units	Ku-Zyme by Schwarz Pharma	00091-4122	Gastrointestinal
SCHWARZ4175	Cap, Green & White	Amylase 30,000 USP, Lipase 2,400 USP, Protease 30,000 USP	Kutrase by Schwarz Pharma	00091-4175	Gastrointestinal
SCHWARZ475	Cap, Green & White, Opaque	Amylase 30 mg, Cellulase 2 mg, Hyoscyamine Sulfate 0.0625 mg, Lipase 1200 Units, Phenyltoloxamine Citrate 15 mg, Protease 6 mg	Kutrase by Schwarz Pharma	00091-3475	Gastrointestinal
SCHWARZ505	Cap, Orange & White	Lactase Enzyme 250 mg	Lactrase by Schwarz Pharma		Gastrointestinal
SCHWARZ505	Cap, Orange & White, Opaque	Lactase Enzyme 250 mg	Lactrase by Schwarz Pharma	00091-3505	Gastrointestinal
SCHWARZ525	Cap, White, Opaque	Pancreatin Lipase 8000 units, Protease 30000 units, Amylase 30000 units	Ku-Zyme HP by Schwarz	00091-3525	Gastrointestinal
SCHWARZ537	Cap, Brown & White, Schwarz 537	Hyoscyamine Sulfate 0.375 mg	Levsinex ER by Schwarz Pharma	00091-3537	Gastrointestinal
SCHWARZ537	Cap, ER, Schwarz 537	Hyoscyamine Sulfate 0.375 mg	Levsinex by CVS	51316-0251	Gastrointestinal
SCHWARZ537	Cap, Brown & White	Hyoscyamine Sulfate 0.375 mg	Levsinex Timecaps by Schwarz Pharma		Gastrointestinal
SCHWARZ537	Cap, ER, Schwarz 537	Hyoscyamine Sulfate 0.375 mg	Levsinex by Amerisource	62584-0010	Gastrointestinal
SCHWARZ537	Cap, Brown and Clear, Ex Release	Hyoscyamine Sulfate 0.375 mg	Levsinex by Eckerd Drug	19458-0836	Gastrointestinal
SCHWARZ537	Cap, Brown & Clear	Hyoscyamine Sulfate 0.375 mg	Levsinex by Natl Pharmpak	55154-0950	Gastrointestinal
SCHWARZ537	Cap, Brown & Clear	Hyoscyamine Sulfate 0.375 mg	Levsinex by Med-Pro	53978-3399	Gastrointestinal
SCHWARZ610 <> 10	Tab, White, Scored	Isosorbide Mononitrate 10 mg	Monoket by Schwarz Pharma	00091-3610	Antianginal
SCHWARZ620 <> 20	Tab, White, Round, Scored	Isosorbide Mononitrate 20 mg	Monoket by Heartland Healthcare	61392-0630	Antianginal
SCHWARZ620 <> 20	Tab, White, Round, Scored	Isosorbide Mononitrate 20 mg	Monoket by Schwarz Pharma Mfg	00131-3620	Antianginal
SCHWARZ620 <> 20	Tab, White, Scored	Isosorbide Mononitrate 20 mg	Monoket by Schwarz Pharma	00091-3620	Antianginal
SCORED <> C	Tab	Estrogens, Conjugated 0.625 mg, Medroxyprogesterone Acetate 2.5 mg	Prempro by Pharm Utilization	60491-0904	Hormone
SCS <> 1530	Tab	Ethinyl Estradiol 0.03 mg, Levonorgestrel 0.15 mg	Levora by Patheon	63285-0100	Oral Contraceptive
SCS <> 550	Tab, White, Round, SCS <> 5/50	Ogestral (Norgestrel 0.5 mg Ethinyl Estradiol .05 mg)	Ovral by Watson	52544-0848	Hormone
SCS <> 5752	Cap, Orange, <> Searle Canada Inc	Piroxicam 10 mg	by Quality Care	60346-0737	NSAID
SCS <> 5752	Cap	Piroxicam 10 mg	by SCS	00905-5752	NSAID
SCS <> 5762	Cap	Piroxicam 20 mg	by SCS	00905-5762	NSAID
SCS12530	Tab, Pink, Round, SCS 125/30	Levonorgestrel 0.125 mg, Ethinyl Estradiol 0.03 mg	Trivora by Watson		Oral Contraceptive
SCS1530	Tab, Round, SCS/15/30	Levonorgestrel 0.15 mg, Ethinyl Estradiol 30 mcg	Levora by Watson		Oral Contraceptive
SCS221	Tab, Round	Norethindrone 1 mg, Ethinyl Estradiol 35 mcg	Norethin 1/35E by Searle		Oral Contraceptive
SCS431	Tab, Round	Norethindrone 1 mg, Mestranol 50 mcg	Norethin 1/50M by Searle		Oral Contraceptive
SCS5030	Tab, Round, SCS 50/30	Levonorgestrel 0.05 mg, Ethinyl Estradiol 0.03 mg	Trivora by Watson		Oral Contraceptive
SCS7540	Tab, Round, SCS 75/40	Levonorgestrel 0.075 mg, Ethinyl Estradiol 0.04 mg	Trivora by Watson		Oral Contraceptive

ID FRONT <> BACK	DESCRIPTION FRONT <> BACK	INGREDIENT & STRENGTH	BRAND (OR EQUIV.) & FIRM	NDC#	CLASS; SCH.
SCSP	Tab, Peach, Round, SCS>P	Placebo	by Watson	n/a	Placebo
SCSP	Tab, Round, SCS/P	Placebo	Levora by Watson		Placebo
SE5G	Tab, White, SE/5/G	Selegiline HCl 5 mg	by Draxis	Canadian	Antiparkinson
SEARLE	Tab, Blue, Round	Placebo	by Searle		Placebo
SEARLE <> 1	Tab	Mestranol 0.05 mg, Norethindrone 1 mg	Norinyl 1 50 21 Day by GD Searle	00025-0263	Oral Contraceptive
SEARLE <> 1451	Tab	Misoprostol 100 mcg	Cytotec by GD Searle	00025-1451	Gastrointestinal
SEARLE <> 1451	Tab	Misoprostol 100 mcg	Cytotec by HJ Harkins Co	52959-0353	Gastrointestinal
SEARLE <> 1451	Tab	Misoprostol 200 mcg	Cytotec by GD Searle	00025-1461	Gastrointestinal
SEARLE <> 1451	Tab	Misoprostol 200 mcg	Cytotec by Nat Pharmpak Serv	55154-3613	Gastrointestinal
SEARLE <> 151	Tab	Ethinyl Estradiol 35 mcg, Ethynodiol Diacetate 1 mg	Demulen 1 35 28 by Nat Pharmpak Serv	55154-3612	Oral Contraceptive
SEARLE <> 151	Tab, Placebo	Ethinyl Estradiol 35 mcg, Ethynodiol Diacetate 1 mg	Demulen 1 35 28 by Pharm Utilization	60491-0181	Oral Contraceptive
SEARLE <> 151	Tab, White, Round, Searle Logo <> 151	Ethinyl Estradiol 35 mcg, Ethynodiol Diacetate 1 mg	Demulen 1/35-21 by GD Searle	00025-0151	Oral Contraceptive
SEARLE <> 151	Tab, White, Round, Searle Logo <> 151	Ethinyl Estradiol 35 mcg, Ethynodiol Diacetate 1 mg	Demulen 1/35-28 by GD Searle	00025-0161	Oral Contraceptive
SEARLE <> 151	Tab	Ethinyl Estradiol 35 mcg, Ethynodiol Diacetate 1 mg	Demulen by Physicians Total Care	54868-0404	Oral Contraceptive
SEARLE <> 151	Tab, White, Round	Ethinyl Estradiol 35 mcg; Ethynodiol Diacetate 1 mg	Demulen Compack by Rx Pac	65084-0219	Oral Contraceptive
SEARLE <> 6	Tab	Ethinyl Estradiol 0.035 mg, Norethindrone 0.5 mg	Tri Norinyl 21 Day by GD Searle	00025-0272	Oral Contraceptive
SEARLE <> 6	Tab, Searle <> Underlined 6	Ethinyl Estradiol 0.035 mg, Norethindrone 0.5 mg	Brevicon 21 Day by GD Searle	00025-0252	Oral Contraceptive
SEARLE <> 61	Tab	Atropine Sulfate 0.025 mg, Diphenoxylate HCl 2.5 mg	Lomotil by Nat Pharmpak Serv	55154-3614	Antidiarrheal; C V
SEARLE <> 61	Tab	Atropine Sulfate 0.025 mg, Diphenoxylate HCl 2.5 mg	Lomotil by St Marys Med	60760-0061	Antidiarrheal; C V
SEARLE <> 61	Tab	Atropine Sulfate 0.025 mg, Diphenoxylate HCl 2.5 mg	Lomotil by Amerisource	62584-0027	Antidiarrheal; C V
SEARLE <> 61	Tab	Atropine Sulfate 0.025 mg, Diphenoxylate HCl 2.5 mg	Lomotil by GD Searle	00014-0061	Antidiarrheal; C V
SEARLE <> 61	Tab	Atropine Sulfate 0.025 mg, Diphenoxylate HCl 2.5 mg	Lomotil by GD Searle	00025-0061	Antidiarrheal; C V
SEARLE <> 61	Tab	Atropine Sulfate 0.025 mg, Diphenoxylate HCl 2.5 mg	Lomotil by Med Pro	53978-3088	Antidiarrheal; C V
SEARLE <> 61	Tab, White, Round	Diphenoxylate HCl 2.5 mg	Lomotil by Searle	Canadian DIN# 00036323	Antidiarrheal
SEARLE <> 7	Tab, Yellowish Green	Ethinyl Estradiol 0.035 mg, Norethindrone 0.5 mg, Norethindrone 1 mg	Tri Norinyl 21 Day by GD Searle	00025-0272	Oral Contraceptive
SEARLE <> 7	Tab, Yellowish Green	Ethinyl Estradiol 0.035 mg, Norethindrone 1 mg	Norinyl 1 35 21 Day by GD Searle	00025-0257	Oral Contraceptive
SEARLE <> 71	Tab	Ethinyl Estradiol 50 mcg, Ethynodiol Diacetate 1 mg	Demulen 1 50 28 by Pharm Utilization	60491-0183	Oral Contraceptive
SEARLE <> 71	Tab, White, Round	Ethinyl Estradiol 50 mcg, Ethynodiol Diacetate 1 mg	Demulen 1/50-21 by GD Searle	00025-0071	Oral Contraceptive
SEARLE <> 71	Tab	Ethinyl Estradiol 50 mcg, Ethynodiol Diacetate 1 mg	Demulen by Physicians Total Care	54868-3790	Oral Contraceptive
SEARLE <> ALDACTONE	Tab, Film Coated	Spironolactone 25 mg	Aldactone by Nat Pharmpak Serv	55154-3602	Diuretic
SEARLE <> BX	Tab, White, Round	Norethindrone, Ethinyl Estradiol	Synphasic 21 day by Pharmacia	Canadian DIN# 02187108	Oral Contraceptive
SEARLE <> BX	Tab, Blue, Round	Norethindrone, Ethinyl Estradiol	Synphasic 28 day by Pharmacia	Canadian DIN# 02187116	Oral Contraceptive
SEARLE <> BX	Tab, Blue, Round	Norethindrone, Ethinyl Estradiol	Synphasic 21 day by Pharmacia	Canadian DIN# 02187108	Oral Contraceptive
SEARLE <> BX	Tab, White, Round	Norethindrone, Ethinyl Estradiol	Synphasic 28 day by Pharmacia	Canadian DIN# 02187116	Oral Contraceptive
SEARLE <> BX	Tab, Blue, Round	Norethindrone, Ethinyl Estradiol 0.5, 35	Brevicon .5/35 21 day by Pharmacia	Canadian DIN# 02187068	Oral Contraceptive
SEARLE <> BX	Tab, Blue, Round	Norethindrone, Ethinyl Estradiol 0.5/35	Brevicon .5/35 28 day by Pharmacia	Canadian DIN# 02187094	Oral Contraceptive

ID FRONT <> BACK	DESCRIPTION FRONT <> BACK	INGREDIENT & STRENGTH	BRAND (OR EQUIV.) & FIRM	NDC#	CLASS; SCH.
SEARLE <> BX	Tab, White, Round	Norethindrone, Ethinyl Estradiol 1/35	Select 1/35 21 day by Pharmacia	Canadian DIN# 02197502	Oral Contraceptive
SEARLE <> BX	Tab, White, Round	Norethindrone, Ethinyl Estradiol 1/35	Brevicon 1/35 28 day by Pharmacia	Canadian DIN# 02189062	Oral Contraceptive
SEARLE <> BX	Tab, White, Round	Norethindrone, Ethinyl Estradiol 1/35	Brevicon 1/35 21 day by Pharmacia	Canadian DIN# 02189054	Oral Contraceptive
SEARLE <> BX	Tab, White, Round	Norethindrone, Ethinyl Estradiol 1/35	Select 1/35 28 day by Pharmacia	Canadian DIN# 02199297	Oral Contraceptive
SEARLE <> CYTOTEC	Tab, White to Off-White, Round	Misoprostol 100 mcg	by Pharmacia	Canadian DIN# 00813966	Gastrointestinal
SEARLE <> P	Tab	Ethinyl Estradiol 35 mcg, Ethynodiol Diacetate 1 mg	Demulen 1 35 28 by Pharm Utilization	60491-0181	Oral Contraceptive
SEARLE <> P	Tab, White, Round, Placebo	Ethinyl Estradiol 35 mcg, Ethynodiol Diacetate 1 mg	Demulen 1/35-28 by GD Searle	00025-0161	Oral Contraceptive
SEARLE <> P	Tab	Ethinyl Estradiol 35 mcg, Ethynodiol Diacetate 1 mg	Demulen by Physicians Total Care	54868-0404	Oral Contraceptive
SEARLE <> P	Tab, Blue, Round	Ethinyl Estradiol 35 mcg; Ethynodiol Diacetate 1 mg	Demulen Compack by Rx Pac	65084-0219	Oral Contraceptive
SEARLE <> P	Tab, Placebo	Ethinyl Estradiol 50 mcg, Ethynodiol Diacetate 1 mg	Demulen 1 50 28 by Pharm Utilization	60491-0183	Oral Contraceptive
SEARLE <> P	Tab	Ethinyl Estradiol 50 mcg, Ethynodiol Diacetate 1 mg	Demulen by Physicians Total Care	54868-3790	Oral Contraceptive
SEARLE <> P	Tab, Orange, Round	Inert	Brevicon 1/35 28 day by Pharmacia	Canadian DIN# 02189062	Placebo
SEARLE <> P	Tab, Orange, Round, Film Coated	Inert	Demulen 30 28 day by Pharmacia	Canadian DIN# 0047152	Placebo
SEARLE <> P	Tab, Orange, Round	Inert	Brevicon .5/35 28 day by Pharmacia	Canadian DIN# 02187094	Placebo
SEARLE <> P	Tab, Orange, Round	Inert	Synphasic 28 day by Pharmacia	Canadian DIN# 02187116	Placebo
SEARLE <> P	Tab, Orange, Round	Inert	Select 1/35 28 day by Pharmacia	Canadian DIN# 02199297	Placebo
SEARLE1001 <> ALDACTONE25	Tab, Yellow, Round, Film Coated	Spironolactone 25 mg	Aldactone by DRX Pharm Consults	55045-2716	Diuretic
SEARLE1001 <> ALDACTONE25	Tab, Yellow, Round	Spironolactone 25 mg	Aldactone by Rightpak	65240-0601	Diuretic
SEARLE1001 <> ALDACTONE25	Tab, Light Yellow, Round, Film Coated, Searle 1001 <> Aldactone 25	Spironolactone 25 mg	Aldactone by GD Searle	00025-1001	Diuretic
SEARLE1001 <> ALDACTONE25	Tab, Light Yellow, Film Coated	Spironolactone 25 mg	Aldactone by Caremark	00339-5531	Diuretic
SEARLE1001 <> ALDACTONE25	Tab, Film Coated, Debossed	Spironolactone 25 mg	Aldactone by Thrift Drug	59198-0001	Diuretic
SEARLE1001 <> ALDACTONE25	Tab, Film Coated, Debossed	Spironolactone 25 mg	Aldactone by Amerisource	62584-0001	Diuretic
SEARLE1001 <> ALDACTONE25	Tab, Yellow, Round, Film Coated	Spironolactone 25 mg	Aldactone by Rx Pac	65084-0106	Diuretic
SEARLE101	Tab, Brown, Round	Norethynodrel 10 mg, Mestranol 75 mcg	Enovid 10mg by Searle		Oral Contraceptive

ID FRONT <> BACK	DESCRIPTION FRONT <> BACK	INGREDIENT & STRENGTH	BRAND (OR EQUIV.) & FIRM	NDC#	CLASS; SCH.
SEARLE1011 <> ALDACTAZIDE25	Tab, Tan, Round, Film Coated, Searle 1011 <> Aldactazide 25	Hydrochlorothiazide 25 mg, Spironolactone 25 mg	Aldactazide by GD Searle	00025-1011	Diuretic; Antihypertensive
SEARLE1011 <> ALDACTAZIDE25	Tab, Searle 1011 <> Aldactazide 25, Film Coated	Hydrochlorothiazide 25 mg, Spironolactone 25 mg	Aldactazide by Nat Pharmpak Serv	55154-3601	Diuretic; Antihypertensive
SEARLE1011 <> ALDACTAZIDE25	Tab, Tan, Round, Film Coated, Searle 1011 <> Aldactazide 25	Hydrochlorothiazide 25 mg, Spironolactone 25 mg	Aldactazide by Murfreesboro	51129-1377	Diuretic; Antihypertensive
SEARLE1011 <> ALDACTAZIDE25	Tab, Searle 1011 Debossed <> Aldactazide 25, Film Coated	Hydrochlorothiazide 25 mg, Spironolactone 25 mg	Aldactazide by Thrift Drug	59198-0170	Diuretic; Antihypertensive
SEARLE1011 <> ALDACTAZIDE25	Tab, Film Coated	Hydrochlorothiazide 25 mg, Spironolactone 25 mg	Aldactazide by Amerisource	62584-0011	Diuretic; Antihypertensive
SEARLE1011 <> ALDACTAZIDE25	Tab, Tan, Round	Spironolactone 25 mg; Hydrochlorothiazide 25 mg	Aldactazide by Med-Pro	53978-3382	Antihypertensive; Diuretic
SEARLE1021 <> ALDACTAZIDE50	Tab, Tan, Oblong, Coated, Searle 1021 <> Aldactazide 50	Hydrochlorothiazide 50 mg, Spironolactone 50 mg	Aldactazide by GD Searle	00025-1021	Diuretic; Antihypertensive
SEARLE1021 <> ALDACTAZIDE50	Tab, Tan, Oblong, Scored	Spironolactone 25 mg; Hydrochlorothiazide 25 mg	Aldactazide by Rightpak	65240-0600	Diuretic
SEARLE1031 <> ALDACTONE100	Tab, Peach, Round, Coated, Searle 1031 <> Aldactone 100	Spironolactone 100 mg	Aldactone by GD Searle	00025-1031	Diuretic
SEARLE1031 <> ALDACTONE100	Tab, Peach, Round, Scored, Film Coated, Debossed, Searle and 1031 <> Aldactone 100	Spironolactone 100 mg	Aldactone by Sidmark		Diuretic
SEARLE1041 <> ALDACTONE50	Tab, Light Orange, Oval, Coated, Searle 1041 <> Aldactone 50	Spironolactone 50 mg	Aldactone by GD Searle	00025-1041	Diuretic
SEARLE1231	Tab, White, Round	Aminophylline 100 mg	Aminophyllin by Searle		Antiasthmatic
SEARLE1251	Tab, White, Oval	Aminophylline 200 mg	Aminophyllin by Searle		Antiasthmatic
SEARLE131	Tab, Peach, Round	Norethynodrel 2.5 mg, Mestranol 0.1 mg	Enovid-E by Searle		Oral Contraceptive
SEARLE1401	Tab, White, Oval	Oxandrolone 2.5 mg	Anavar by Searle		Steroid
SEARLE1411 <> A	Tab, White to Off-White, Round, Searle over 1411 <> A around the circumference	Diclofenac Sodiummisoprostol 50 mg	by Pharmacia	Canadian DIN# 01917056	NSAID
SEARLE1411 <> AAAA50	Tab, Off-White, Round, Film Coated, Searle 1411 <> A's around 50	Diclofenac Sodium 50 mg, Misoprostol 200 mcg	Arthrotec 50 by GD Searle	00025-1411	NSAID
SEARLE1411 <> AAAA50	Tab, Film Coated, Searle 1411 <> A's around 50	Diclofenac Sodium 50 mg, Misoprostol 200 mcg	Arthrotec 50 by GD Searle	00014-1411	NSAID
SEARLE1411 <> AAAA50	Tab, Film Coated, Searle 1411 <> A's around 50	Diclofenac Sodium 50 mg, Misoprostol 200 mcg	Arthrotec 50 by Searle	51227-6169	NSAID
SEARLE1411AAAA	Tab, White, Round, Searle/1411/AAAA	Diclofenac 50 mg, Misoprostol 200 mcg	by Searle	Canadian	NSAID
SEARLE1421 <> 75A	Tab, White to Off-White, Round, Searle over 1421 <> A around the circumference, 75 in the middle	Diclofenac Sodiummisoprostol 75 mg	by Pharmacia	Canadian DIN# 02229837	NSAID
SEARLE1421 <> AAAA75	Tab, Off-White, Round, Film Coated, Searle 1421 <> A's around 75	Diclofenac Sodium 75 mg, Misoprostol 200 mcg	Arthrotec 75 by GD Searle	00025-1421	NSAID
SEARLE1421 <> AAAA75	Tab, Film Coated, Searle 1421 <> A's around 75	Diclofenac Sodium 75 mg, Misoprostol 200 mcg	Arthrotec 75 by GD Searle	00014-1421	NSAID
SEARLE1421 <> AAAA75	Tab, Film Coated, Searle 1421 <> A's around 75	Diclofenac Sodium 75 mg, Misoprostol 200 mcg	Arthrotec 75 by Searle	51227-6179	NSAID
SEARLE14214A75	Tab, White, Round, Searle/1421/4A/75	Diclofenac Sodium 75 mg	by Searle	Canadian	NSAID
SEARLE1461	Tab, Design	Misoprostol 200 mcg	Cytotec by GD Searle	00025-1461	Gastrointestinal
SEARLE1461	Tab, Searle Above and 1461 Below the Line <> A Double Stomach Debossed	Misoprostol 200 mcg	Cytotec by HJ Harkins Co	52959-0354	Gastrointestinal
SEARLE1461	Tab, Debossed with Double Stomach	Misoprostol 200 mcg	Cytotec by Nat Pharmpak Serv	55154-3613	Gastrointestinal

ID FRONT <> BACK	DESCRIPTION FRONT <> BACK	INGREDIENT & STRENGTH	BRAND (OR EQUIV.) & FIRM	NDC#	CLASS; SCH.
SEARLE1461	Tab, White to Off-White, Hexagonal	Misoprostol 200 mcg	by Pharmacia	Canadian DIN# 00632600	Gastrointestinal
SEARLE1461	Tab	Misoprostol 200 mcg	Misoprostol by Apotheca	12634-0502	Gastrointestinal
SEARLE1461	Tab, White, Hexagon, Searle Over 1461<> Double Stomach, Searle/1461	Misoprostol 200 mg	Cytotec by Neuman Distr	64579-0314	Gastrointestinal
SEARLE1501	Tab, Peach, Round	Methantheline Bromide 50 mg	Banthine by Searle		Gastrointestinal
SEARLE1701	Tab, White, Round	Dimenhydrinate 50 mg	Dramamine by Searle		Antiemetic
SEARLE1831 <> FLAGYL250	Tab, Blue, Round, Film, Searle and 1831 <> Flagyl and 250	Metronidazole 250 mg	Flagyl by Neuman Distr	64579-0102	Antibiotic
SEARLE1831 <> FLAGYL250	Tab, Searle Over 1831 <> Flagyl Over 250, Film Coated	Metronidazole 250 mg	Flagyl by GD Searle	00025-1831	Antibiotic
SEARLE1831 <> FLAGYL250	Tab, Searle 1831 <> Flagyl 250, Film Coated	Metronidazole 250 mg	Flagyl by Thrift Drug	59198-0311	Antibiotic
SEARLE1831 <> FLAGYL250	Tab, Film Coated, Debossed	Metronidazole 250 mg	Flagyl by Amerisource	62584-0831	Antibiotic
SEARLE1961 <> FLAGYLER	Tab, Blue, Oval, Film Coated	Metronidazole 750 mg	Flagyl by Mova Pharms	55370-0562	Antibiotic
SEARLE1961 <> FLAGYLER	Tab, Searle 1961 <> Flagyler, Film Coated	Metronidazole 750 mg	Flagyl ER by GD Searle	00025-1961	Antibiotic
SEARLE201	Tab, White, Round	Spironolactone 25 mg, Hydrochlorothiazide 25 mg	Aldactazide by Searle		Diuretic
SEARLE2011	Tab, Blue, Round, Film Coated	Verapamil HCl 180 mg	by Pharmacia	Canadian DIN# 02231676	Antihypertensive
SEARLE2021	Tab, White, Round, Film Coated	Verapamil HCl 240 mg	by Pharmacia	Canadian DIN# 02231677	Antihypertensive
SEARLE205	Tab, White to Off-White, Round	Spironolactone 25 mg	Aldactone by Searle	Canadian DIN# 00028606	Diuretic
SEARLE210	Tab, White to Off-White, Round	Spironolactone 100 mg	Aldactone by Searle	Canadian DIN# 00285455	Diuretic
SEARLE221	Tab, White, Round	Norethindrone 1 mg, Ethinyl Estradiol 35 mcg	Norethin 1/35 by Searle		Oral Contraceptive
SEARLE235	Tab, Yellow, Round, Searle/235	Norethindrone 0.35 mg	Nor-QD by Watson		Oral Contraceptive
SEARLE244	Tab, White, Round	Spironolactone 50 mg, Hydrochlorothiazide 50 mg	Aldactazide by Searle		Diuretic
SEARLE2732 <> NORPACE100MG	Cap, Light Green, Ex Release	Disopyramide Phosphate	Norpace CR by Amerisource	62584-0732	Antiarrhythmic
SEARLE2732 <> NORPACECR100MG	Cap, White & Light Green, Searle 2732 <> Norpace CR 100 mg	Disopyramide Phosphate	Norpace CR by GD Searle	00025-2732	Antiarrhythmic
SEARLE2732 <> NORPACECR100MG	Cap, Light Green, Ex Release	Disopyramide Phosphate	Norpace CR by Thrift Drug	59198-0164	Antiarrhythmic
SEARLE2732 <> NORPACECR100MG	Cap, Ex Release	Disopyramide Phosphate	Norpace CR by Leiner	59606-0709	Antiarrhythmic
SEARLE2732 <> NORPACECR100MG	Cap	Disopyramide Phosphate	Norpace CR by Nat Pharmpak Serv	55154-3609	Antiarrhythmic
SEARLE2732 <> NORPACECR100MG	Cap, White & Green, Searle over 2732 <> Norpace CR over 100 mg	Disopyramide Phosphate 100 mg	Norpace CR by Glaxo Wellcome	00173-0672	Antiarrhythmic
SEARLE2732 <> NORPACECR100MG	Tab, White & Green, Oblong	Disopyramide Phosphate 100 mg	Norpace CR by Glaxo Wellcome	51947-8310	Antiarrhythmic
SEARLE2732NORPE	Cap, Green & White	Disopyramide Phosphate 100 mg	Norpace CR by Rightpak	65240-0709	Antiarrhythmic

ID FRONT <> BACK	DESCRIPTION FRONT <> BACK	INGREDIENT & STRENGTH	BRAND (OR EQUIV.) & FIRM	NDC#	CLASS; SCH.
SEARLE2742 <> NORPACE150MG	Cap, Brown & Light Green	Disopyramide Phosphate	Norpace CR by GD Searle	00014-2742	Antiarrhythmic
SEARLE2742 <> NORPACECR150MG	Cap, Ex Release	Disopyramide Phosphate	Norpace CR by Leiner	59606-0710	Antiarrhythmic
SEARLE2742 <> NORPACECR150MG	Cap, Light Green, Ex Release	Disopyramide Phosphate	Norpace CR by Amerisource	62584-0742	Antiarrhythmic
SEARLE2742 <> NORPACECR150MG	Cap, Brown & Light Green, Searle 2742 <> Norpace CR 150 mg	Disopyramide Phosphate	Norpace CR by GD Searle	00025-2742	Antiarrhythmic
SEARLE2742 <> NORPACECR150MG	Cap, Light Green, Ex Release	Disopyramide Phosphate	Norpace CR by Thrift Drug	59198-0085	Antiarrhythmic
SEARLE2742 <> NORPACECR150MG	Cap	Disopyramide Phosphate	Norpace CR by Nat Pharmpak Serv	55154-3610	Antiarrhythmic
SEARLE2742 <> NORPACECR150MG	Tab, Brown & Green, Oblong, Searle 2742<> Norpace CR 150 MG	Disopyramide Phosphate 150 mg	Norpace CR by Golden State	60429-0703	Antiarrhythmic
SEARLE2752 <> NORPACE100MG	Cap	Disopyramide Phosphate	Norpace by Leiner	59606-0707	Antiarrhythmic
SEARLE2752 <> NORPACE100MG	Cap	Disopyramide Phosphate	Norpace by Amerisource	62584-0753	Antiarrhythmic
SEARLE2752 <> NORPACE100MG	Cap, White & Orange, Searle 2752 <> Norpace 100 mg	Disopyramide Phosphate	Norpace by GD Searle	00025-2752	Antiarrhythmic
SEARLE2752 <> NORPACE100MG	Cap	Disopyramide Phosphate	Norpace by Thrift Drug	59198-0083	Antiarrhythmic
SEARLE2752 <> NORPACE100MG	Cap	Disopyramide Phosphate	Norpace by Nat Pharmpak Serv	55154-3607	Antiarrhythmic
SEARLE2752 <> NORPACE100MG	Cap, Orange & White, Searle over 2752 <> Norpace over 100 mg	Disopyramide Phosphate 100 mg	Norpace by Glaxo Wellcome	00173-0679	Antiarrhythmic
SEARLE2752NORP	Cap, White	Disopyramide Phosphate 100 mg	Norpace by Rightpak	65240-0707	Antiarrhythmic
SEARLE2762 <> NORPACE150MG	Cap	Disopyramide Phosphate	Norpace by Amerisource	62584-0762	Antiarrhythmic
SEARLE2762 <> NORPACE150MG	Cap, Brown & Orange, Searle 2762 <> Norpace 150 mg	Disopyramide Phosphate	Norpace by GD Searle	00025-2762	Antiarrhythmic
SEARLE2762 <> NORPACE150MG	Cap	Disopyramide Phosphate	Norpace by Leiner	59606-0708	Antiarrhythmic
SEARLE2762 <> NORPACE150MG	Cap	Disopyramide Phosphate	Norpace by Thrift Drug	59198-0084	Antiarrhythmic
SEARLE2762 <> NORPACECR150MG	Cap	Disopyramide Phosphate	Norpace by Nat Pharmpak Serv	55154-3608	Antiarrhythmic
SEARLE2762NORP	Cap, Brown & Orange	Disopyramide Phosphate 150 mg	Norpace CR by Rightpak	65240-0710	Antiarrhythmic
SEARLE2762NORP	Cap, Brown	Disopyramide Phosphate 150 mg	Norpace by Rightpak	65240-0708	Antiarrhythmic
SEARLE401	Tab, White, Pentagonal	Ethynodiol Diacetate 1 mg, Mestranol 0.1 mg	Ovulen by Searle		Oral Contraceptive
SEARLE431	Tab, White, Round	Norethindrone 1 mg, Mestranol 50 mcg	Norethin 1/50 by Searle		Oral Contraceptive
SEARLE501	Tab, Rose, Round	Metolazone 2.5 mg	Diulo by Searle		Diuretic
SEARLE51	Tab, Tan, Round	Norethynodrel 5 mg, Mestranol 75 mcg	Enovid 5mg by Searle		Oral Contraceptive
SEARLE511	Tab, Blue, Round	Metolazone 5 mg	Diulo by Searle		Diuretic
SEARLE521	Tab, Yellow, Round	Metolazone 10 mg	Diulo by Searle		Diuretic
SEARLE531	Tab, Yellow, Round	Chlorthalidone 25 mg	Hygroton by Searle		Diuretic
SEARLE541	Tab, Green, Round	Chlorthalidone 50 mg	Hygroton by Searle		Diuretic
SEARLE571	Tab, White, Round	Furosemide 20 mg	Lasix by Searle		Diuretic
SEARLE581	Tab, White, Round	Furosemide 40 mg	Lasix by Searle		Diuretic
SEARLE601	Tab, Peach, Round	Propantheline Bromide 15 mg	Pro-Banthine by Searle		Gastrointestinal
SEARLE611	Tab, White, Round	Propantheline Bromide 7.5 mg	Pro-Banthine by Searle		Gastrointestinal
SEARLE71	Tab, White, Round, Searle/71	Ethynodiol Diacetate 1 mg	by Searle	Canadian	Oral Contraceptive

ID FRONT <> BACK	DESCRIPTION FRONT <> BACK	INGREDIENT & STRENGTH	BRAND (OR EQUIV.) & FIRM	NDC#	CLASS; SCH.
SEARLE831	Tab, White, Round	Haloperidol 0.5 mg	Haldol by Searle		Antipsychotic
SEARLE841	Tab, White, Round	Haloperidol 1 mg	Haldol by Searle		Antipsychotic
SEARLE851	Tab, White, Round	Haloperidol 2 mg	Haldol by Searle		Antipsychotic
SEARLE861	Tab, White, Round	Haloperidol 5 mg	Haldol by Searle		Antipsychotic
SEARLE871	Tab, White, Round	Haloperidol 10 mg	Haldol by Searle		Antipsychotic
SEARLE881	Tab, White, Round	Haloperidol 20 mg	Haldol by Searle		Antipsychotic
SEARLE930	Tab, White, Round, Film Coated	Norethindrone, Ethinyl Estradiol 30	Demulen 30 28 dayby Pharmacia	Canadian DIN# 0047152	Oral Contraceptive
SEARLE930	Tab, White, Round, Film Coated	Norethindrone, Ethinyl Estradiol 30	Demulen 30 21 dayby Pharmacia	Canadian DIN# 00469327	Oral Contraceptive
SEARLECYOTEC	Tab, White, Round, Searle/Cyotec	Misoprostol 100 mcg	Cyotec by Searle	Canadian	Gastrointestinal
SEATRACE <> LOBAC0176	Cap, Egg Shell, Seatrace<> Lobac-0176	Acetaminophen 300 mg, Phenyltoloxamine Citrate 20 mg, Salicylamide 200 mg	Lobac by Seatrace	00551-0176	Analgesic
SEATRACE <> SEATRACE	Cap, Blue Print	Acetaminophen 500 mg, Hydrocodone Bitartrate 5 mg	Ceta-Plus by Seatrace	00551-0180	Analgesic; C III
SEATRACE <> TENAKE	Cap, Green Print	Acetaminophen 325 mg, Butalbital 50 mg, Caffeine 40 mg	Tenake by Seatrace	00551-0181	Analgesic
SECTRAL 100	Tab, White, Shield	Acebutolol 100 mg	Sectral by Rhone-Poulenc Rorer	Canadian	Antihypertensive
SECTRAL 200	Tab, Blue, Shield	Acebutolol 200 mg	Sectral by Rhone-Poulenc Rorer	Canadian	Antihypertensive
SECTRAL200 <> WYETH4177	Cap, Orange & Purple	Acebutolol HCl 200 mg	Sectral by Wyeth Pharms	52903-4177	Antihypertensive
SECTRAL400	Tab, White, Shield	Acebutolol 400 mg	Sectral by Rhone-Poulenc Rorer	Canadian	Antihypertensive
SECTRAL400	Tab, White, Shield, Rorer Logo	Acebutolol HCl 400 mg	by Rhone-Poulenc Rorer	Canadian	Antihypertensive
SECTRAL400 <> WYETH4179	Cap, Brown & Orange	Acebutolol HCl 400 mg	Sectral by Wyeth Pharms	52903-4179	Antihypertensive
SELDANE	Tab	Terfenadine 60 mg	by Pharmedix	53002-0409	Antihistamine
SELDANE	Tab	Terfenadine 60 mg	Seldane by Quality Care	60346-0569	Antihistamine
SELDANED	Tab, Seldane Over D, Ex Release	Pseudoephedrine HCl 120 mg, Terfenadine 60 mg	Seldane D by Quality Care	60346-0664	Cold Remedy
SEMPREXD <> MEDEVA	Cap, SEMPREX-D in White Ink	Acrivastine 8 mg, Pseudoephedrine HCl 60 mg	Semprex D by Catalytica	63552-0404	Cold Remedy
SEMPREXD <> MEDEVA	Cap, White Print	Acrivastine 8 mg, Pseudoephedrine HCl 60 mg	Semprex D by Medeva	53014-0404	Cold Remedy
SEPTRADS	Tab, Pink, Oval	Trimethoprim 160 mg, Sulfamethoxazole 800 mg	Septra DS by Monarch	61570-0053	Antibiotic
SEPTRADS <> 02C	Tab, Glaxo	Sulfamethoxazole 800 mg, Trimethoprim 160 mg	Septra DS by Nat Pharmpak Serv	55154-0703	Antibiotic
SEPTRADS <> O2C	Tab	Sulfamethoxazole 800 mg, Trimethoprim 160 mg	Septra DS by Leiner	59606-0733	Antibiotic
SEPTRADS02C	Tab	Sulfamethoxazole 800 mg, Trimethoprim 160 mg	Septra DS by Catalytica	63552-0853	Antibiotic
SEPTRADS02C	Tab, Septra DS Over 02C	Sulfamethoxazole 800 mg, Trimethoprim 160 mg	Septra DS by Amerisource	62584-0853	Antibiotic
SEPTRADS02C	Tab, Septra DS 02C	Sulfamethoxazole 800 mg, Trimethoprim 160 mg	Septra DS by Thrift Drug	59198-0212	Antibiotic
SEPTRADS02C	Tab	Sulfamethoxazole 800 mg, Trimethoprim 160 mg	Septra DS by Monarch	61570-0053	Antibiotic
SEPTRADSO2C	Tab, Septra DS 02C	Sulfamethoxazole 800 mg, Trimethoprim 160 mg	Septra DS by Pharm Utilization	60491-0581	Antibiotic
SEPTRADSO2C	Tab, Oval	Trimethoprim 160 mg, Sulfamethoxazole 800 mg	by Glaxo	Canadian	Antibiotic
SEPTRADSO2C	Tab, Pink, Oval, Scored	Trimethoprim 160 mg, Sulfamethoxazole 800 mg	Septra DS by Thrift Services	59198-0322	Antibiotic
SEPTRAY2B	Tab, Septra Y2B	Sulfamethoxazole 400 mg, Trimethoprim 80 mg	Septra by Catalytica	63552-0852	Antibiotic
SEPTRAY2B	Tab, Septra Y2B	Sulfamethoxazole 400 mg, Trimethoprim 80 mg	Septra by Monarch	61570-0052	Antibiotic
SEPTRAY2B	Tab, Round	Trimethoprim 80 mg, Sulfamethoxazole 400 mg	by Glaxo	Canadian	Antibiotic
SEPTRAY2B	Tab, Pink, Round	Trimethoprim 80 mg, Sulfamethoxazole 400 mg	Septra by Monarch	61570-0052	Antibiotic
SERAX	Tab, Light Yellow	Oxazepam 10 mg	Serax by Wyeth-Ayerst	Canadian	Sedative/Hypnotic; C IV
SERAX10 <> SERAX51	Cap, Pink & White	Oxazepam 10 mg	Serax by Wyeth Pharms	52903-0051	Sedative/Hypnotic; C IV
SERAX10 <> WYETH51	Cap, Serax 10 Printed 5 Times <> Wyeth-51 Printed 3 Times with Ten Connected Triangles, Coated	Oxazepam 10 mg	Serax by Wyeth Labs	00008-0051	Sedative/Hypnotic; C IV
SERAX15	Tab, Yellow, Serax/15	Oxazepam 15 mg	by Wyeth-Ayerst	Canadian	Sedative/Hypnotic; C IV

ID FRONT <> BACK	DESCRIPTION FRONT <> BACK	INGREDIENT & STRENGTH	BRAND (OR EQUIV.) & FIRM	NDC#	CLASS; SCH.
SERAX15 <> WYETH6	Cap, Serax 15 Printed 5 Times <> Wyeth-6 Printed 3 Times and Ten Connected Triangles, Coated	Oxazepam 15 mg	Serax by Wyeth Labs	00008-0006	Sedative/Hypnotic; C IV
SERAX30	Tab, Peach, Serax/30	Oxazepam 30 mg	by Wyeth-Ayerst	Canadian	Sedative/Hypnotic; C IV
SERAX51 <> SERAX10	Cap, Pink & White	Oxazepam 10 mg	Serax by Wyeth Pharms	52903-0051	Sedative/Hypnotic; C IV
SEROQUEL100	Tab, Yellow, Round, Seroquel 100, Film Coated	Quetiapine Fumarate 100 mg	Seroquel by AstraZeneca	00310-0271	Antipsychotic
SEROQUEL200	Tab, White, Round, Seroquel 200, Film Coated	Quetiapine Fumarate 200 mg	Seroquel by AstraZeneca	00310-0272	Antipsychotic
SEROQUEL25	Tab, Peach, Round, Film Coated	Quetiapine Fumarate 25 mg	Seroquel by Murfreesboro Ph	51129-1559	Antipsychotic
SEROQUEL25	Tab, Peach, Round, Film Coated, Seroquel 25	Quetiapine Fumarate 25 mg	Seroquel by AstraZeneca	00310-0275	Antipsychotic
SEROQUEL25	Tab, Peach, Round, Convex, Film, Seroquel 25	Quetiapine Fumarate 25 mg	Seroquel by RX PAK	65084-0115	Antipsychotic
SEROQUEL25	Tab, Peach, Round, Convex, Film, Seroquel 25 One Side	Quetiapine Fumarate 25 mg	Seroquel by RX PAK	65084-0113	Antipsychotic
SEROQUELAND100	Tab, Yellow, Round	Quetiapine Fumarate 100 mg	Seroquel by Direct Dispensing	57866-1032	Antipsychotic
SFC <> SANDOZ78107	Cap, S in triangle F-C <> Sandoz 78-107	Aspirin 325 mg, Butalbital 50 mg, Caffeine 40 mg, Codeine Phosphate 30 mg	Fiorinal w Codeine No 3 by Physicians Total Care	54868-0530	Analgesic; C III
SFC3512	Cap, Maroon, SFC-3512	Docusate Calcium 60 mg, Phenolphthalein 65 mg	Doxidan by Chase		Laxative
SGP0535	Tab, White, Round, SGP 0.5/35	Genora 0.5 mg	Modicon by Searle		Oral Contraceptive
SGP135	Tab, Blue, Round, SGP 1/35	Genora	Ortho Novum by Searle		Oral Contraceptive
SGP150	Tap, White, Round, SGP 1/50	Genora	Ortho Novum by Searle		Oral Contraceptive
Shire Logo	Cap, Teal & Black	Carbamazepine 300 mg	Carbatrol by Shire Richwood	58521-0173	Anticonvulsant
SHIRE LOGO	Cap, Teal & Gray	Carbamazepine 200 mg	Carbatrol by Shire Richwood	58521-0172	Anticonvulsant
SHIRE LOGO	Cap, Black, Printed with the Athena Logo in White Ink	Carbamazepine 300 mg	Carbatrol by Shire Richwood	59075-0672	Anticonvulsant
SHIRE LOGO	Cap, Light Gray, Print with the Athena Logo in White Ink	Carbamazepine 200 mg	Carbatrol by Shire Richwood	59075-0671	Anticonvulsant
SHN <>	Cap, ER, Ketoprofen ER 200 MG	Ketoprofen 200 mg	Ketoprofen by Schein	00364-2667	NSAID
SHN <> KETOPROFENER200	Cap, ER, Ketoprofen ER 200 MG	Ketoprofen 200 mg	Ketoprofen by Danbury	00591-8847	NSAID
SHN <> KETOPROFENER200	Cap, ER, Ketoprofen ER 200	Ketoprofen 200 mg	Ketoprofen by Elan	56125-0102	NSAID
SIDMAK <> 375	Tab	Nystatin 100000 Units	by Qualitest	00603-4831	Antifungal
SIDMAK <> 375	Tab, Off-White, Oval	Nystatin Vaginal 100000 Units	Mycostatin by Sidmak	50111-0375	Antifungal
SINEMET <> 647	Tab, Dark Dapple Blue, Oval	Carbidopa 10 mg, Levodopa 100 mg	Sinemet by Dupont Pharma	00056-0647	Antiparkinson
SINEMET <> 650	Tab, Yellow, Oval	Carbidopa 25 mg, Levodopa 100 mg	Sinemet by Dupont Pharma	00056-0650	Antiparkinson
SINEMET <> 654	Tab, Light Dapple Blue, Oval	Carbidopa 25 mg, Levodopa 250 mg	Sinemet by Dupont Pharma	00056-0654	Antiparkinson
SINEMET10010	Tab, Blue, Oval, Sinemet/100/10	Levodopa 100 mg, Carbidopa 10 mg	Sinemet by Dupont Pharma	Canadian	Antiparkinson
SINEMET650	Tab, Yellow, Oval	Levodopa 100 mg, Carbidopa 25 mg	Sinemet by Dupont Pharma	Canadian	Antiparkinson
SINEMET654	Tab, Blue, Oval	Levodopa 250 mg, Carbidopa 25 mg	Sinemet by Dupont Pharma	Canadian	Antiparkinson
SINEMETCR <> 521	Cap, Sinemet over CR <> 521	Carbidopa 50 mg, Levodopa 200 mg	Sinemet CR by Nat Pharmpak Serv	55154-7705	Antiparkinson
SINEMETCR <> 521	Tab, Peach, Oval	Carbidopa 50 mg, Levodopa 200 mg	Sinemet CR by Dupont Pharma	00056-0521	Antiparkinson
SINEMETCR <> 521	Tab, Peach, Oval, Convex, Scored	Carbidopa 50 mg, Levodopa 200 mg	Sinemet CR SR by Caremark	00339-6140	Antiparkinson
SINEMETCR <> 521	Tab, Peach, Oval, Scored	Carbidopa 50 mg; Levodopa 200 mg	Sinemet by WalMart	49035-0189	Antiparkinson
SINEMETCR <> 601	Tab, Pink, Oval	Carbidopa 25 mg, Levodopa 100 mg	Sinemet CR by DuPont Pharma	00056-0601	Antiparkinson
SINEMETCR521521	Tab, Peach, Oval, Sinemet CR/521/521	Levodopa 200 mg, Carbidopa 50 mg	Sinemet CR by Dupont Pharma	Canadian	Antiparkinson
SINEMETCR601	Tab, Pink, Oval, Sinemet CR/601	Levodopa 100 mg, Carbidopa 25 mg	Sinemet CR by Dupont Pharma	Canadian	Antiparkinson
SINEQUAN <> ROERIG534	Cap	Doxepin HCl	Sinequan by Roerig Pfizer	00662-5340	Antidepressant
SINEQUAN <> ROERIG535	Cap	Doxepin HCl	Sinequan by Nat Pharmpak Serv	55154-3209	Antidepressant
SINEQUAN <> ROERIG535	Cap, Sinequan <> Roerig over 535	Doxepin HCl	Sinequan by Roerig Pfizer	00662-5350	Antidepressant
SINEQUAN <> ROERIG535	Cap, Blue & Pink	Doxepin HCl 25 mg	Sinequan by Rightpac	65240-0734	Antidepressant
SINEQUAN <> ROERIG536	Cap	Doxepin HCl	Sinequan by Nat Pharmpak Serv	55154-3210	Antidepressant

ID FRONT <> BACK	DESCRIPTION FRONT <> BACK	INGREDIENT & STRENGTH	BRAND (OR EQUIV.) & FIRM	NDC#	CLASS; SCH.
SINEQUAN <> ROERIG536	Cap, Bright Pink & Pale Pink, Sinequan <> Roerig over 536	Doxepin HCl	Sinequan by Roerig Pfizer	00662-5360	Antidepressant
SINEQUAN <> ROERIG536	Cap, Pink	Doxepin HCl 50 mg	Sinequan by Rightpac	65240-0735	Antidepressant
SINEQUAN <> ROERIG539	Cap	Doxepin HCl	Sinequan by Roerig Pfizer	00662-5390	Antidepressant
SINGULAIR <> MRK117	Tab, Beige, Square, Film Coated	Montelukast Sodium 10 mg	Singulair by Murfreesboro Ph	51129-1398	Antiasthmatic
SINUPAN <> SINUPAN	Cap, Ex Release	Guaifenesin 200 mg, Phenylephrine HCl 40 mg	by Sovereign	58716-0013	Cold Remedy
SINUTAB	Cap, Orange	Acetaminophen Compound 325 mg	Sinutab by Warner Wellcome	Canadian	Antipyretic
SINUTAB	Cap, Yellow	Acetaminophen Compound 500 mg	Sinutab by Warner Wellcome	Canadian	Antipyretic
SINUTAB	Cap, Orange	Acetaminophen Compound 500 mg	Sinutab by Warner Wellcome	Canadian	Antipyretic
SJ <> 630	Cap, Blue Print, S-J <> 630	Acetaminophen 500 mg, Hydrocodone Bitartrate 5 mg	Ugesic by Stewart Jackson	45985-0630	Analgesic; C III
SJ631	Tab, Pink Specks	Guaifenesin 600 mg	Bidex Sr by Anabolic	00722-6348	Expectorant
SJ631	Tab	Guaifenesin 800 mg	Bidex by Stewart Jackson	45985-0637	Expectorant
SJ631	Tab	Guaifenesin 800 mg	by Mikart	46672-0167	Expectorant
SJ638	Tab, White, Oblong, Scored	Guaifenesin 800 mg; Dextromethorphan Hydriodide 30 mg	Bidex DM by Stewart-Jackson	45985-0638	Cold Remedy
SJ638	Tab, White, Oblong	Guaifenesin 800 mg; Dextromethorphan Hydrobromide 300 mg	by Pfab	62542-0916	Cold Remedy
SJ641	Tab, White, Oval, Scored	Guaifenesin 800 mg; Pseudoephedrine HCl 60 mg; Dextromethorphan Hydrobromide 30 mg	by Pfab	62542-0775	Cold Remedy
SJ641	Tab, White, Oblong	Guaifenesin 800 mg; Pseudoephedrine HCl 60 mg; Dextromethorphan Hydrobromide 30 mg	Medent DM by Stewart-Jackson	45985-0641	Cold Remedy
SJ642	Tab, White, Oval, Scored	Guaifenesin 800 mg; Pseudoephedrine HCl 60 mg	by Pfab	62542-0754	Cold Remedy
SJ642	Tab, White, Oblong	Guaifenesin 800 mg; Pseudoephedrine HCl 60 mg	Medent LD by Stewart-Jackson	45985-0642	Cold Remedy
SJGEIGY	Tab, Peach, Round, SJ/Geigy	Desipramine HCl 50 mg	Pertofrane by Geigy	Canadian	Antidepressant
SKF	Tab, Coated	Prochlorperazine Maleate 8.1 mg	Compazine by Patient	57575-0099	Antiemetic
SKF	Tab, Peach, Round	Triamterene 50 mg, Hydrochlorothiazide 25 mg	by SmithKline SKB	Canadian	Diuretic
SKF <> C66	Tab, Yellow-Green, Coated	Prochlorperazine Maleate 8.1 mg	Compazine by Allscripts	54569-0352	Antiemetic
SKF <> C66	Tab, Coated	Prochlorperazine Maleate 8.1 mg	Compazine by Quality Care	60346-0271	Antiemetic
SKF <> C67	Tab, Yellow-Green, Coated	Prochlorperazine Maleate 16.2 mg	Compazine by Quality Care	60346-0860	Antiemetic
SKF <> E12	Cap	Dextroamphetamine Sulfate 5 mg	Dexedrine by Physicians Total Care	54868-3402	Stimulant; C II
SKF <> E19	Tab	Dextroamphetamine Sulfate 5 mg	Dexedrine by SKF	00074-3241	Stimulant; C II
SKF <> E33	Cap, Red	Phenoxybenzamine HCl 10 mg	Dibenzyline by Wellspring Pharm	65197-0001	Antihypertensive
SKF E13	Cap, Brown	Dextroamphetamine Sulfate 10 mg	by SmithKline SKB	Canadian	Stimulant
SKF1	Tab, Yellow, Round	Isopropamide Iodide 5 mg, Trifluoperazine HCl 1 mg	Stelabid by SKB		Antipsychotic
SKF1	Tab, Blue, Round	Trifluoperazine HCl 1 mg	Stelazine by SKB	00108-4903	Antipsychotic
SKF1	Tab, Blue, Round, SKF/1	Trifluoperazine 1 mg	Stelazine by SmithKline SKB	Canadian	Antipsychotic
SKF10	Tab, Blue, Round, SKF/10	Trifluoperazine 10 mg	Stelazine by SmithKline SKB	Canadian	Antipsychotic
SKF2	Tab, Blue, Round	Trifluoperazine HCl 2 mg	Stelazine by SKB	00108-4904	Antipsychotic
SKF2	Tab, Blue, Round, SKF/2	Trifluoperazine 2 mg	Stelazine by SmithKline SKB	Canadian	Antipsychotic
SKF200	Tab, Green, Round	Cimetidine 200 mg	Tagamet by SKB		Gastrointestinal
SKF25	Tab, Yellow, Round	Diphenidol 25 mg	Vontrol by SKB		Antiemetic
SKF300	Tab, Green, Round, SK & F/300	Cimetidine 300 mg	Tagamet by Frosst	Canadian	Gastrointestinal
SKF300TAGAMENT	Tab, Green, Round, SK & F/300/Tagament	Cimetidine 300 mg	by SmithKline SKB	Canadian	Gastrointestinal
SKF400	Tab, Green, Ovoid, SK & F/400	Cimetidine 400 mg	Tagamet by Frosst	Canadian	Gastrointestinal
SKF400TAGAMENT	Tab, Green, Ovoid, SK & F/400/Tagament	Cimetidine 400 mg	by SmithKline SKB	Canadian	Gastrointestinal
SKF5	Tab, Blue, Round	Trifluoperazine HCl 5 mg	Stelazine by SKB		Antipsychotic
SKF5	Tab, Blue, Round, SKF/5	Trifluoperazine 5 mg	Stelazine by SmithKline SKB	Canadian	Antipsychotic
SKF600	Tab, Green, Ovoid SK & F/600	Cimetidine 600 mg	Tagamet by Frosst	Canadian	Gastrointestinal
SKF600TAGAMENT	Tab, Green, Ovoid, SK & F/600/Tagament	Cimetidine 600 mg	by SmithKline SKB	Canadian	Gastrointestinal
SKFC44	Cap, Black/Natural	Prochlorperazine 10 mg	Compazine Spansule by SKB		Antiemetic
SKFC44	Cap, Clear Black with Beads, Ex Release, SKF Over C44 <>	Prochlorperazine Maleate 16.2 mg	Compazine by Quality Care	60346-0434	Antiemetic
SKFC46	Cap, Black/Natural	Prochlorperazine 15 mg	Compazine Spansule by SKB		Antiemetic

ID FRONT <> BACK	DESCRIPTION FRONT <> BACK	INGREDIENT & STRENGTH	BRAND (OR EQUIV.) & FIRM	NDC#	CLASS; SCH.
SKFC47	Cap, Black/Natural	Prochlorperazine 30 mg	Compazine Spansule by SKB		Antiemetic
SKFC66	Tab, Yellow-Green, Coated, in Black Print SKF/C66 <>	Prochlorperazine Maleate 8.1 mg	Compazine by SKB	00007-3366	Antiemetic
SKFC66	Tab, Yellow-Green, Coated	Prochlorperazine Maleate 8.1 mg	Compazine by PDRX	55289-0113	Antiemetic
SKFC67	Tab, Green, Round, SKF Over C67	Prochlorperazine 10 mg	Compazine by Ranbaxy	54907-5120	Antiemetic
SKFC67	Tab, Yellow-Green, Round, Coated, SKF/C67 in Black Print	Prochlorperazine Maleate 16.2 mg	Compazine by SKB	00007-3367	Antiemetic
SKFC67	Tab, Film Coated, SKF/C67	Prochlorperazine Maleate 16.2 mg	Compazine by Nat Pharmpak Serv	55154-4502	Antiemetic
SKFC67 <> SKFC67	Tab, Coated	Prochlorperazine Maleate 16.2 mg	Compazine by Allscripts	54569-0351	Antiemetic
SKFC69	Tab, Yellow, Round	Prochlorperazine 25 mg	Compazine by SKB		Antiemetic
SKFD11	Tab, Yellow, Round	Triamterene 50 mg	Dyrenium by SmithKline SKB	Canadian	Diuretic
SKFD14	Tab, White, Round	Liothyronine 5 mcg	Cytomel by SmithKline SKB	Canadian	Antithyroid
SKFD14	Tab, Off-White, SKF D14,	Liothyronine Sodium	Cytomel by Allscripts	54569-2968	Antithyroid
SKFD16	Tab, White, Round	Liothyronine 25 mcg	by SmithKline SKB	Canadian	Antithyroid
SKFD16	Tab, SKF D16	Liothyronine Sodium	Cytomel by Allscripts	54569-2053	Antithyroid
SKFD17	Tab, SKF D17	Liothyronine Sodium	Cytomel by Allscripts	54569-2980	Antithyroid
SKFD62	Tab, Pink, Round	Isopropamide Iodide 5 mg	Darbid by SKB		Antipsychotic
SKFE12	Cap, Brown & Natural	Dextroamphetamine Sulfate 5 mg	Dexedrine Spansule by SKB		Stimulant; C II
SKFE13	Cap, Brown & Natural	Dextroamphetamine Sulfate 10 mg	Dexedrine Spansule by SKB		Stimulant; C II
SKFE14	Cap, Brown	Dextroamphetamine Sulfate 15 mg	by SmithKline SKB	Canadian	Stimulant
SKFE14	Cap, Brown & Natural	Dextroamphetamine Sulfate 15 mg	Dexedrine Spansule by SKB		Stimulant; C II
SKFE19	Tab, Orange, Heart	Dextroamphetamine Sulfate 5 mg	by SmithKline SKB	Canadian	Stimulant
SKFE33	Cap, Red	Phenoxybenzamine HCl 10 mg	Dibenzyline by SKB		Antihypertensive
SKFE93	Tab, Peach, Round, SKF/E93	Triamterene 50 mg, Hydrochlorothiazide 25 mg	Maxzide 25 by SKB		Diuretic
SKFH10	Tab, Yellow, Round	Triamterene 100 mg	by SmithKline SKB	Canadian	Diuretic
SKFH10	Cap, Red, SKF/H10	Triamterene 100 mg	Dyrenium by SKB		Diuretic
SKFH10	Tab, Yellow, Round, SKF/H10	Triamterene 100 mg	Dyrenium by SKB		Diuretic
SKFH11	Tab, Yellow, Round	Triamterene 50 mg	by SmithKline SKB	Canadian	Diuretic
SKFH11	Cap, Red, SKF/H11	Triamterene 50 mg	Dyrenium by SKB		Diuretic
SKFH11	Tab, Yellow, Round, SKF/H11	Triamterene 50 mg	Dyrenium by SKB		Diuretic
SKFJ09	Tab, Gray, Round	Lithium Carbonate 300 mg	Eskalith by SKB		Antipsychotic
SKFJ10	Tab, Buff, Round	Lithium Carbonate 450 mg	Eskalith CR by SKB	00007-4010	Antipsychotic
SKFN30	Cap, Blue & Clear, SKF/N30	Phenylpropanolamine 75 mg, Chlorpheniramine Maleate 8 mg	Ornade by SKB		Cold Remedy
SKFN31	Cap, Orange & Clear, SKF/N31	Phenylpropanolamine 75 mg, Chlorpheniramine Maleate 12 mg	Ornade by SKB		Cold Remedy
SKFN71	Tab, Red, Round	Tranylcypromine 10 mg	Parnate by SmithKline SKB	Canadian	Antidepressant
SKFN71	Tab, Rose, Round	Tranylcypromine Sulfate 10 mg	Parnate by SKB	00007-4471	Antidepressant
SKFP90	Tab, Maize, Round	Isopropamide 5 mg, Trifluoperazine 1 mg	Stelabid by SmithKline SKB	Canadian	Antipsychotic
SKFP90	Tab, Yellow, Round	Isopropamide Iodide 5 mg	Stelabid No 1 by SKB		Antipsychotic
SKFP90	Tab, Yellow, Round	Isopropamide Iodide 5 mg, Trifluoperazine HCl 1 mg	Stelabid No 1 by SKB		Antipsychotic
SKFP91	Tab, Maize, Round	Isopropamide 5 mg, Trifluoperazine 2 mg	Stelabid by SmithKline SKB	Canadian	Antipsychotic
SKFP91	Tab, Yellow, Round	Isopropamide Iodide 5 mg, Trifluoperazine HCl 2 mg	Stelabid No 2 by SKB		Antipsychotic
SKFP92	Tab, Maize, Round	Isopropamide 7.5 mg, Trifluoperazine 2 mg	Stelabid by SmithKline SKB	Canadian	Antipsychotic
SKFP92	Tab, Yellow, Round	Isopropamide Iodide 7.5 mg, Trifluoperazine HCl 2 mg	Stelabid Forte by SKB		Antipsychotic
SKFP93	Tab, Yellow, Round	Isopropamide Iodide 10 mg, Trifluoperazine HCl 2 mg	Stelabid Ultra by SKB		Antipsychotic
SKFS03	Tab, Blue, Round	Trifluoperazine HCl 1 mg	Stelazine by SKB	00108-4903	Antipsychotic
SKFS04	Tab, Blue, Round	Trifluoperazine HCl 2 mg	Stelazine by SKB	00108-4904	Antipsychotic
SKFS06	Tab, Blue, Round	Trifluoperazine HCl 5 mg	Stelazine by SKB	00108-4906	Antipsychotic
SKFS07	Tab, Blue, Round	Trifluoperazine HCl 10 mg	Stelazine by SKB	00108-4907	Antipsychotic
SKFT12	Tab, Green, Round	Cimetidine 200 mg	Tagamet by SKB		Gastrointestinal
SKFT13	Tab, Green, Round	Cimetidine 300 mg	Tagamet by SKB		Gastrointestinal
SKFT25	Tab, Orange, Round	Diphenidol HCl 25 mg	Vontrol by SKB		Antiemetic
SKFT63	Cap, Natural & Orange	Chlorpromazine HCl 30 mg	Thorazine Spansule by SKB	00007-5063	Antipsychotic
SKFT64	Cap, Natural & Orange	Chlorpromazine HCl 75 mg	Thorazine Spansule by SKB	00007-5064	Antipsychotic
SKFT66	Cap, Natural & Orange	Chlorpromazine HCl 150 mg	Thorazine Spansule by SKB	00007-5066	Antipsychotic

ID FRONT <> BACK	DESCRIPTION FRONT <> BACK	INGREDIENT & STRENGTH	BRAND (OR EQUIV.) & FIRM	NDC#	CLASS; SCH.
SKFT67	Cap, Natural & Orange	Chlorpromazine HCl 200 mg	Thorazine Spansule by SKB		Antipsychotic
SKFT69	Cap, Natural & Orange	Chlorpromazine HCl 300 mg	Thorazine Spansule by SKB		Antipsychotic
SKFT73	Tab, Orange, Round	Chlorpromazine HCl 10 mg	Thorazine by SKB	00007-5073	Antipsychotic
SKFT74	Tab, Orange, Round	Chlorpromazine HCl 25 mg	Thorazine by SKB	00007-5074	Antipsychotic
SKFT76	Tab, Orange, Round	Chlorpromazine HCl 50 mg	Thorazine by SKB	00007-5076	Antipsychotic
SKFT77	Tab, Orange, Round	Chlorpromazine HCl 100 mg	Thorazine by SKB	00007-5077	Antipsychotic
SKFT79	Tab, Orange, Round	Chlorpromazine HCl 200 mg	Thorazine by SKB	00007-5079	Antipsychotic
SKFV36	Cap, White	Phenylpropanolamine 50 mg, Caraminphen 20 mg, Chlorpheniramine 8 mg	Tuss-Ornade by SKB		Cold Remedy
SKFX42	Tab, Yellow, Round	Diphenidol 25 mg	Vontrol by SKB		Antiemetic
SL	Cap, Light Blue, Film Coated	Diphenhydramine HCl 25 mg	Simply Sleep by McNeil	Canadian DIN# 02239548	Antihistamine
SL	Tab, Film Coated	Guaifenesin 400 mg, Phenylpropanolamine HCl 75 mg	Contuss-XT by Patient	57575-0090	Cold Remedy
SL <> 07	Tab, Sugar Coated, Imprint in Black Ink	Hydroxyzine HCl 10 mg	by Kaiser	00179-0294	Antihistamine
SL <> 07	Tab, White, Round	Hydroxyzine HCl 10 mg	by Murfreesboro	51129-1475	Antihistamine
SL <> 07	Tab, White, Round, Sugar Coated	Hydroxyzine HCl 10 mg	Atarax by Sidmak	50111-0307	Antihistamine
SL <> 07	Tab, White, Round	Hydroxyzine HCl 10 mg	by Murfreesboro	51129-1478	Antihistamine
SL <> 07	Tab, Sugar Coated	Hydroxyzine HCl 10 mg	by Qualitest	00603-3970	Antihistamine
SL <> 07	Tab, Sugar Coated	Hydroxyzine HCl 10 mg	by Talbert Med	44514-0418	Antihistamine
SL <> 08	Tab, White, Round	Hydroxyzine HCl 25 mg	by Murfreesboro	51129-1476	Antihistamine
SL <> 08	Tab, White, Round, Sugar Coated	Hydroxyzine HCl 25 mg	Atarax by Sidmak	50111-0308	Antihistamine
SL <> 08	Tab, Sugar Coated, Imprint in Black Ink	Hydroxyzine HCl 25 mg	by Kaiser	00179-0295	Antihistamine
SL <> 08	Tab, White, Round	Hydroxyzine HCl 25 mg	by Murfreesboro	51129-1481	Antihistamine
SL <> 08	Tab, Sugar Coated	Hydroxyzine HCl 25 mg	by Talbert Med	44514-0419	Antihistamine
SL <> 08	Tab, Light Blue, Sugar Coated	Hydroxyzine HCl 25 mg	by Qualitest	00603-3971	Antihistamine
SL <> 11	Tab, Sugar Coated	Dipyridamole 25 mg	by Sidmak	50111-0311	Antiplatelet
SL <> 309	Tab, White, Round, Sugar Coated	Hydroxyzine HCl 50 mg	by Allscripts	54569-0409	Antihistamine
SL <> 309	Tab, White, Round, Sugar Coated	Hydroxyzine HCl 50 mg	Atarax by Sidmak	50111-0309	Antihistamine
SL <> 309	Tab, White, Round, Sugar Coated	Hydroxyzine HCl 50 mg	by Murfreesboro	51129-1473	Antihistamine
SL <> 309	Tab, Sugar Coated	Hydroxyzine HCl 50 mg	by Qualitest	00603-3972	Antihistamine
SL <> 312	Tab, Sugar Coated	Dipyridamole 50 mg	by Sidmak	50111-0312	Antiplatelet
SL <> 313	Tab, Sugar Coated	Dipyridamole 75 mg	by Sidmak	50111-0313	Antiplatelet
SL <> 333	Tab, Film Coated	Metronidazole 250 mg	by Diversified Hlthcare Serv	55887-0978	Antibiotic
SL <> 342	Tab	Sulfamethoxazole 800 mg, Trimethoprim 160 mg	SMZ TMP DS by Quality Care	60346-0087	Antibiotic
SL <> 36	Tab, Light Yellow, Sugar Coated	Desipramine HCl 25 mg	by Schein	00364-2209	Antidepressant
SL <> 36	Tab, Light Yellow, Round, Sugar Coated	Desipramine HCl 25 mg	Norpramin by Sidmak	50111-0436	Antidepressant
SL <> 368	Tab, Brown, Round, Film Coated	Amitriptyline HCl 50 mg	Elavil by Sidmak	50111-0368	Antidepressant
SL <> 387	Tab, Film Coated, Debossed	Ibuprofen 400 mg	by Sidmak	50111-0387	NSAID
SL <> 388	Tab, Film Coated	Ibuprofen 600 mg	by Sidmak	50111-0388	NSAID
SL <> 406	Cap	Indomethacin 25 mg	by Quality Care	60346-0684	NSAID
SL <> 437	Tab, Light Green, Sugar Coated	Desipramine HCl 50 mg	by Schein	00364-2210	Antidepressant
SL <> 437	Tab, Light Green, Round, Sugar Coated	Desipramine HCl 50 mg	Norpramin by Sidmak	50111-0437	Antidepressant
SL <> 438	Tab, Light Orange, Sugar Coated	Desipramine HCl 75 mg	by Schein	00364-2243	Antidepressant
SL <> 438	Tab, Light Orange, Round, Sugar Coated	Desipramine HCl 75 mg	Norpramin by Sidmak	50111-0438	Antidepressant
SL <> 451	Tab, Film Coated, Debossed	Ibuprofen 800 mg	by Sidmak	50111-0451	NSAID
SL <> 467	Tab	Propranolol HCl 10 mg	by Zenith Goldline	00182-1812	Antihypertensive
SL <> 468	Tab	Propranolol HCl 20 mg	by Zenith Goldline	00182-1813	Antihypertensive
SL <> 469	Tab	Propranolol HCl 40 mg	by Zenith Goldline	00182-1814	Antihypertensive
SL <> 471	Tab	Propranolol HCl 80 mg	by Zenith Goldline	00182-1815	Antihypertensive
SL <> 546	Tab, Peach, Round, Film Coated	Diclofenac Sodium 50 mg	Voltaren by Sidmak Labs	50111-0546	NSAID
SL <> 547	Tab, Beige, Round, Film Coated	Diclofenac Sodium 75 mg	Voltaren by Sidmak Labs	50111-0547	NSAID
SL <> 557	Tab, Debossed	Naproxen 500 mg	by Sidmak	50111-0557	NSAID

ID FRONT <> BACK	DESCRIPTION FRONT <> BACK	INGREDIENT & STRENGTH	BRAND (OR EQUIV.) & FIRM	NDC#	CLASS; SCH.
SL <> 563	Tab, Yellow, Round, Film Coated	Cyclobenzaprine HCl 10 mg	Flexeril by Sidmak	50111-0563	Muscle Relaxant
SL <> 604	Tab, Green, Oval, Film Coated, Scored	Guaifenesin 600 mg, Pseudoephedrine HCl 120 mg	Entex PSE by Sidmak	50111-0604	Cold Remedy
SL <> 608	Tab, White, Round, Film Coated	Ketorolac Tromethamine 10 mg	Toradol by Sidmak Labs	50111-0608	NSAID
SL <> 66	Tab, Film Coated	Amitriptyline HCl 10 mg	by Vangard	00615-0828	Antidepressant
SL <> 66	Tab, Pink, Round, Film Coated	Amitriptyline HCl 10 mg	Elavil by Sidmak	50111-0366	Antidepressant
SL <> 67	Tab, Film Coated	Amitriptyline HCl 25 mg	by Nat Pharmpak Serv	55154-5814	Antidepressant
SL <> 67	Tab, Film Coated	Amitriptyline HCl 25 mg	by Kaiser	00179-1275	Antidepressant
SL <> 67	Tab, Film Coated	Amitriptyline HCl 25 mg	by Zenith Goldline	00182-1019	Antidepressant
SL <> 67	Tab, Film Coated	Amitriptyline HCl 25 mg	by Vangard	00615-0829	Antidepressant
SL <> 67	Tab, Green, Round, Film Coated	Amitriptyline HCl 25 mg	Elavil by Sidmak	50111-0367	Antidepressant
SL07	Tab, Purple or White, Round	Hydroxyzine 10 mg	by Allscripts	54569-0406	Antihistamine
SL07	Tab, Sugar Coated	Hydroxyzine HCl 10 mg	by Darby Group	66467-4567	Antihistamine
SL07	Tab, White, Round	Hydroxyzine HCl 10 mg	by Direct Dispensing	57866-3875	Antihistamine
SL07	Tab, Sugar Coated, SL Over 07	Hydroxyzine HCl 10 mg	by Baker Cummins	63171-1492	Antihistamine
SL07	Tab, Sugar Coated	Hydroxyzine HCl 10 mg	by Zenith Goldline	00182-1492	Antihistamine
SL07	Tab, Film Coated, Sidmak	Hydroxyzine HCl 10 mg	by Pharmedix	53002-0390	Antihistamine
SL07	Tab, White, Round, SL/07	Hydroxyzine HCl 10 mg	by Murfreesboro	51129-1479	Antihistamine
SL07	Tab, Sugar Coated, SL/07	Hydroxyzine HCl 10 mg	by HJ Harkins Co	52959-0481	Antihistamine
SL07	Tab, Sugar Coated, SL/07	Hydroxyzine HCl 10 mg	by Richmond	54738-0317	Antihistamine
SL07	Tab, Sugar Coated, SL/07	Hydroxyzine HCl 10 mg	by St Marys Med	60760-0307	Antihistamine
SL07	Tab, Film Coated, Sugar-Coated, SL/07	Hydroxyzine HCl 10 mg	by Quality Care	60346-0795	Antihistamine
SL07	Tab, Sugar Coated	Hydroxyzine HCl 10 mg	by Geneva	00781-1332	Antihistamine
SL07	Tab, Sugar Coated	Hydroxyzine HCl 10 mg	by HL Moore	00839-7437	Antihistamine
SL07	Tab, Sugar Coated	Hydroxyzine HCl 10 mg	by Major	00904-0357	Antihistamine
SL07	Tab, Sugar Coated, SL/07	Hydroxyzine HCl 10 mg	by United Res	00677-0604	Antihistamine
SL08	Tab, Sugar Coated, SL/08	Hydroxyzine HCl 25 mg	by Apotheca	12634-0474	Antihistamine
SL08	Tab, Film Coated, Sidmak	Hydroxyzine HCl 25 mg	by Pharmedix	53002-0320	Antihistamine
SL08	Tab, Sugar Coated, SL/08	Hydroxyzine HCl 25 mg	by HJ Harkins Co	52959-0074	Antihistamine
SL08	Tab, Sugar Coated, SL/08	Hydroxyzine HCl 25 mg	by Med Pro	53978-3066	Antihistamine
SL08	Tab, Sugar Coated, SL/08	Hydroxyzine HCl 25 mg	by Amerisource	62584-0743	Antihistamine
SL08	Tab, Sugar Coated	Hydroxyzine HCl 25 mg	by Darby Group	66467-4568	Antihistamine
SL08	Tab, Sugar Coated	Hydroxyzine HCl 25 mg	by Baker Cummins	63171-1493	Antihistamine
SL08	Tab, White, Round, Sugar Coated	Hydroxyzine 25 mg	by Allscripts	54569-0413	Antihistamine
SL08	Tab, Sugar Coated, SL/08	Hydroxyzine HCl 25 mg	by Zenith Goldline	00182-1493	Antihistamine
SL08	Tab, Coated, SL/08	Hydroxyzine HCl 25 mg	by Physicians Total Care	54868-0063	Antihistamine
SL08	Tab, Sugar Coated, SL/08	Hydroxyzine HCl 25 mg	by Richmond	54738-0308	Antihistamine
SL08	Tab, Film Coated, Sugar-Coated, SL/08	Hydroxyzine HCl 25 mg	by Quality Care	60346-0086	Antihistamine
SL08	Tab, Film Coated, Sidmak	Hydroxyzine HCl 25 mg	by Prescription Dispensing	61807-0032	Antihistamine
SL08	Tab, Sugar Coated	Hydroxyzine HCl 25 mg	by HL Moore	00839-7438	Antihistamine
SL08	Tab, Sugar Coated	Hydroxyzine HCl 25 mg	by Geneva	00781-1334	Antihistamine
SL08	Tab, Sugar Coated	Hydroxyzine HCl 25 mg	by Major	00904-0358	Antihistamine
SL08 <> SL08	Tab, Sugar Coated	Hydroxyzine HCl 25 mg	by Caremark	00339-6009	Antihistamine
SL11	Tab, Film Coated, SL Over 11	Dipyridamole 25 mg	by Quality Care	60346-0789	Antiplatelet
SL125	Tab, Green, Round, Scored	Hyoscyamine Sulfate 0.125 mg	Symax SL by Murfreesboro	51129-1491	Gastrointestinal
SL125	Tab, SL 125	Hyoscyamine Sulfate 0.125 mg	Symax SL by Sovereign	58716-0670	Gastrointestinal
SL236	Tab, Red, Round	Pseudoephedrine HCl 30 mg	by Sidmak		Decongestant
SL253	Tab, Orange, Oblong, Film Coated	Protriptyline HCl 5 mg	Vivactil by Sidmak	50111-0523	Antidepressant
SL301	Cap, Lavender/Clear	Nitroglycerin TD 2.5 mg	Nitro-Bid by Sidmak		Vasodilator
SL302	Cap, Blue & Clear	Nitroglycerin TD 6.5 mg	Nitro-Bid by Sidmak		Antianginal
SL303	Cap, Green & Yellow	Nitroglycerin TD 9 mg	Nitro-Bid by Sidmak		Antianginal
SL309	Tab, Sugar Coated	Hydroxyzine HCl 50 mg	by Darby Group	66467-4569	Antihistamine
SL309	Tab, White, Round	Hydroxyzine HCl 50 mg	by Direct Dispensing	57866-3876	Antihistamine

ID FRONT <> BACK	DESCRIPTION FRONT <> BACK	INGREDIENT & STRENGTH	BRAND (OR EQUIV.) & FIRM	NDC#	CLASS; SCH.
SL309	Tab, Sugar Coated, SL Over 309	Hydroxyzine HCl 50 mg	by Baker Cummins	63171-1494	Antihistamine
SL309	Tab, Sugar Coated, SL/309	Hydroxyzine HCl 50 mg	by Zenith Goldline	00182-1494	Antihistamine
SL309	Tab, Sugar Coated, SL/309	Hydroxyzine HCl 50 mg	by Richmond	54738-0309	Antihistamine
SL309	Tab, Coated, SL 309	Hydroxyzine HCl 50 mg	by Quality Care	60346-0796	Antihistamine
SL309	Tab, Sugar Coated	Hydroxyzine HCl 50 mg	by Geneva	00781-1336	Antihistamine
SL309	Tab, Sugar Coated	Hydroxyzine HCl 50 mg	by HL Moore	00839-7439	Antihistamine
SL309	Tab, Sugar Coated	Hydroxyzine HCl 50 mg	by Major	00904-0359	Antihistamine
SL314	Tab	Cyproheptadine 4 mg	by Direct Dispensing	57866-3515	Antihistamine
SL314	Tab, Sidmak Logo	Cyproheptadine 4 mg	by Major	00904-1145	Antihistamine
SL314	Tab, SL 314	Cyproheptadine HCl 4 mg	by Quality Care	60346-0788	Antihistamine
SL314	Tab, SL/314	Cyproheptadine HCl 4 mg	by Heartland	61392-0209	Antihistamine
SL314	Tab, SL/314	Cyproheptadine HCl 4 mg	by Amerisource	62584-0355	Antihistamine
SL314	Tab, Sidmak, SL-314	Cyproheptadine HCl 4 mg	by Zenith Goldline	00182-1132	Antihistamine
SL314	Tab	Cyproheptadine HCl 4 mg	by HL Moore	00839-7866	Antihistamine
SL314	Tab	Cyproheptadine HCl 4 mg	by Qualitest	00603-3098	Antihistamine
SL314	Tab, White, Round, Scored	Cyproheptadine HCl 4 mg	Periactin by Sidmak	50111-0314	Antihistamine
SL318	Cap, White Beads, Ex Release	Papaverine HCl 150 mg	by Sidmak	50111-0318	Vasodilator
SL318	Cap, ER	Papaverine HCl 150 mg	by United Res	00677-0171	Vasodilator
SL32	Tab	Bethanechol Chloride 5 mg	by Qualitest	00603-2455	Urinary Tract
SL320	Tab, White, Round, Orange Specks	Florvite Chewable	Poly-Vi-Flor by Sidmak		Mineral
SL32110	Tab, White, Round	Isoxsuprine HCl 10 mg	Vasodilan by Sidmak		Vasodilator
SL32220	Tab, White, Round	Isoxsuprine HCl 20 mg	Vasodilan by Sidmak		Vasodilator
SL323	Tab, SL over 323	Bethanechol Chloride 5 mg	by UDL	51079-0053	Urinary Tract
SL323	Tab	Bethanechol Chloride 5 mg	by Sidmak	50111-0323	Urinary Tract
SL324	Tab	Bethanechol Chloride 10 mg	by United Res	00677-0506	Urinary Tract
SL324	Tab	Bethanechol Chloride 10 mg	by Qualitest	00603-2456	Urinary Tract
SL324	Tab, SL over 324	Bethanechol Chloride 10 mg	by UDL	51079-0054	Urinary Tract
SL324	Tab	Bethanechol Chloride 10 mg	by Med Pro	53978-3072	Urinary Tract
SL324	Tab	Bethanechol Chloride 10 mg	by Sidmak	50111-0324	Urinary Tract
SL324	Tab	Bethanechol Chloride 10 mg	by Major	00904-0591	Urinary Tract
SL325	Tab	Bethanechol Chloride 25 mg	by Major	00904-0592	Urinary Tract
SL325	Tab	Bethanechol Chloride 50 mg	by United Res	00677-0940	Urinary Tract
SL325	Tab, Yellow, Round, Scored, SL/325	Bethanechol Chloride 25 mg	by Bryant	63629-0387	Urinary Tract
SL325	Tab	Bethanechol Chloride 25 mg	by United Res	00677-0507	Urinary Tract
SL325	Tab	Bethanechol Chloride 25 mg	by Qualitest	00603-2457	Urinary Tract
SL325	Tab, SL over 325	Bethanechol Chloride 25 mg	by UDL	51079-0123	Urinary Tract
SL325	Tab	Bethanechol Chloride 25 mg	by Sidmak	50111-0325	Urinary Tract
SL326	Tab	Bethanechol Chloride 50 mg	by Qualitest	00603-2458	Urinary Tract
SL326	Tab, SL over 326	Bethanechol Chloride 50 mg	by UDL	51079-0056	Urinary Tract
SL326	Tab, SL over 326	Bethanechol Chloride 50 mg	by Sidmak	50111-0326	Urinary Tract
SL327	Tab, SL 327	Hydralazine HCl 25 mg	by Heartland	61392-0043	Antihypertensive
SL327	Tab	Hydralazine HCl 25 mg	by Nat Pharmpak Serv	55154-5821	Antihypertensive
SL327	Tab, SL 327	Hydralazine HCl 25 mg	by Quality Care	60346-0824	Antihypertensive
SL327	Tab, Orange, Round	Hydralazine HCl 25 mg	by Allscripts	54569-0515	Antihypertensive
SL327	Tab, SL 327	Hydralazine HCl 25 mg	by Baker Cummins	63171-0554	Antihypertensive
SL327	Tab	Hydralazine HCl 25 mg	by Zenith Goldline	00182-0554	Antihypertensive
SL327	Tab	Hydralazine HCl 25 mg	by Qualitest	00603-3831	Antihypertensive
SL327	Tab, Film Coated	Hydralazine HCl 25 mg	by Med Pro	53978-3051	Antihypertensive
SL327	Tab	Hydralazine HCl 25 mg	by Richmond	54738-0327	Antihypertensive
SL327	Tab, Orange, Round	Hydralazine HCl 25 mg	Apresoline by Sidmak	50111-0327	Antihypertensive
SL327	Tab, Orange, Round	Hydralazine HCl 25 mg	by Kaiser Fdn	00179-1290	Antihypertensive
SL327	Tab	Hydralazine HCl 25 mg	by Major	00904-5170	Antihypertensive

ID FRONT <> BACK	DESCRIPTION FRONT <> BACK	INGREDIENT & STRENGTH	BRAND (OR EQUIV.) & FIRM	NDC#	CLASS; SCH.
SL328	Tab, SL/328	Hydralazine HCl 50 mg	by Nat Pharmpak Serv	55154-5818	Antihypertensive
SL328	Tab, Orange, Round	Hydralazine HCl 50 mg	Hydralazine HCl by Monarch	61570-0022	Antihypertensive
SL328	Tab	Hydralazine HCl 50 mg	by Quality Care	60346-0825	Antihypertensive
SL328	Tab	Hydralazine HCl 50 mg	by Kaiser	00179-1274	Antihypertensive
SL328	Tab	Hydralazine HCl 50 mg	by Zenith Goldline	00182-0555	Antihypertensive
SL328	Tab	Hydralazine HCl 50 mg	by Qualitest	00603-3832	Antihypertensive
SL328	Tab	Hydralazine HCl 50 mg	by HL Moore	00839-1363	Antihypertensive
SL328	Tab	Hydralazine HCl 50 mg	by Med Pro	53978-3001	Antihypertensive
SL328	Tab	Hydralazine HCl 50 mg	by Allscripts	54569-0517	Antihypertensive
SL328	Tab, Orange, Round	Hydralazine HCl 50 mg	Apresoline by Sidmak	50111-0328	Antihypertensive
SL328	Tab	Hydralazine HCl 50 mg	by Richmond	54738-0328	Antihypertensive
SL329	Cap, Orange	Cyclandelate 200 mg	Cyclospasmol by Sidmak		Vasodilator
SL330	Cap, Green & White	Cyclandelate 400 mg	Cyclospasmol by Sidmak		Vasodilator
SL331	Tab	Disulfiram 250 mg	by DRX	55045-2423	Antialcoholism
SL331	Tab	Disulfiram 250 mg	by Qualitest	00603-3431	Antialcoholism
SL331	Tab	Disulfiram 250 mg	by Geneva	00781-1060	Antialcoholism
SL331	Tab, White, Round	Disulfiram 250 mg	Antabuse by Sidmak	50111-0331	Antialcoholism
SL331	Tab	Disulfiram 250 mg	by Major	00904-1180	Antialcoholism
SL332	Tab	Disulfiram 500 mg	by Zenith Goldline	00182-0533	Antialcoholism
SL332	Tab, White, Round, Scored	Disulfiram 500 mg	Antabuse by Sidmak	50111-0332	Antialcoholism
SL333	Tab	Metronidazole 250 mg	by Baker Cummins	63171-1330	Antibiotic
SL333	Tab	Metronidazole 250 mg	by Darby Group	66467-4032	Antibiotic
SL333	Tab	Metronidazole 250 mg	by Rugby	00536-4032	Antibiotic
SL333	Tab	Metronidazole 250 mg	by Zenith Goldline	00182-1330	Antibiotic
SL333	Tab	Metronidazole 250 mg	by Med Pro	53978-0215	Antibiotic
SL333	Tab, White, Round	Metronidazole 250 mg	Flagyl by Sidmak	50111-0333	Antibiotic
SL333	Tab, SL/333	Metronidazole 250 mg	by Physicians Total Care	54868-0108	Antibiotic
SL333	Tab	Metronidazole 250 mg	by Prescription Dispensing	61807-0023	Antibiotic
SL333	Tab	Metronidazole 250 mg	by St Marys Med	60760-0333	Antibiotic
SL333	Tab, Sidmak Labs	Metronidazole 250 mg	by Quality Care	60346-0592	Antibiotic
SL333	Tab, Sidmak	Metronidazole 250 mg	by Apotheca	12634-0165	Antibiotic
SL333	Tab	Metronidazole 250 mg	by Major	00904-1453	Antibiotic
SL333	Tab	Metronidazole 250 mg	by Qualitest	00603-4640	Antibiotic
SL333	Tab	Metronidazole 250 mg	by United Res	00677-0690	Antibiotic
SL333	Tab	Metronidazole 250 mg	by HL Moore	00839-6415	Antibiotic
SL333	Tab, White, Round	Metronidazole 250 mg	by Southwood Pharms	58016-0129	Antibiotic
SL334	Tab	Metronidazole 500 mg	by Baker Cummins	63171-1517	Antibiotic
SL334	Tab	Metronidazole 500 mg	by Zenith Goldline	00182-1517	Antibiotic
SL334	Tab	Metronidazole 500 mg	by HJ Harkins Co	52959-0102	Antibiotic
SL334	Tab	Metronidazole 500 mg	by Dept Health Central Pharm	53808-0053	Antibiotic
SL334	Tab	Metronidazole 500 mg	by Martec	52555-0114	Antibiotic
SL334	Tab	Metronidazole 500 mg	by Med Pro	53978-3056	Antibiotic
SL334	Tab, White, Oblong	Metronidazole 500 mg	Flygyl by Sidmak	50111-0334	Antibiotic
SL334	Tab	Metronidazole 500 mg	by Prescription Dispensing	61807-0024	Antibiotic
SL334	Tab	Metronidazole 500 mg	by St Marys Med	60760-0641	Antibiotic
SL334	Tab, Debossed, Coated	Metronidazole 500 mg	by Quality Care	60346-0507	Antibiotic
SL334	Tab, White, Oblong	Metronidazole 500 mg.	by Dixon Shane	17236-0304	Antibiotic
SL334	Tab, Sidmak	Metronidazole 500 mg	by Apotheca	12634-0172	Antibiotic
SL334	Tab	Metronidazole 500 mg	by HL Moore	00839-6620	Antibiotic
SL334	Tab	Metronidazole 500 mg	by United Res	00677-0816	Antibiotic
SL334	Tab	Metronidazole 500 mg	by Qualitest	00603-4641	Antibiotic
SL335	Cap, Blue & Clear	Ethaverine HCl TD 100 mg	by Sidmak		Vasodilator

ID FRONT <> BACK	DESCRIPTION FRONT <> BACK	INGREDIENT & STRENGTH	BRAND (OR EQUIV.) & FIRM	NDC#	CLASS; SCH.
SL337	Tab, White, Round	Nylidrin HCl 6 mg	Arlidin by Sidmak		Vasodilator
SL338	Tab, White, Round	Nylidrin HCl 12 mg	Arlidin by Sidmak		Vasodilator
SL339	Tab, Film Coated	Procainamide HCl 250 mg	by Sidmak	50111-0339	Antiarrhythmic
SL340	Tab	Metoclopramide HCl 10 mg	by United Res	00677-1039	Gastrointestinal
SL340	Tab, ER	Procainamide HCl 500 mg	by Sidmak	50111-0340	Antiarrhythmic
SL341	Tab	Sulfamethoxazole 400 mg, Trimethoprim 80 mg	by Rugby	00536-4692	Antibiotic
SL341	Tab, SL/341	Sulfamethoxazole 400 mg, Trimethoprim 80 mg	by Sidmak	50111-0341	Antibiotic
SL341	Tab	Sulfamethoxazole 400 mg, Trimethoprim 80 mg	SMZ TMP by Casa De Amigos	62138-7383	Antibiotic
SL341	Tab, SL Over 341	Sulfamethoxazole 400 mg, Trimethoprim 80 mg	by Amerisource	62584-0856	Antibiotic
SL341	Tab	Sulfamethoxazole 400 mg, Trimethoprim 80 mg	by Major	00904-2726	Antibiotic
SL341	Tab	Sulfamethoxazole 400 mg, Trimethoprim 80 mg	by Geneva	00781-1062	Antibiotic
SL341	Tab	Sulfamethoxazole 400 mg, Trimethoprim 80 mg	by Qualitest	00603-5778	Antibiotic
SL341	Tab	Sulfamethoxazole 400 mg, Trimethoprim 80 mg	by HL Moore	00839-6487	Antibiotic
SL342	Tab	Sulfamethoxazole 800 mg, Trimethoprim 160 mg	by Urgent Care Ctr	50716-0163	Antibiotic
SL342	Tab, Sidmak	Sulfamethoxazole 800 mg, Trimethoprim 160 mg	Trimeth Sulfa DS by Pharmedix	53002-0210	Antibiotic
SL342	Tab	Sulfamethoxazole 800 mg, Trimethoprim 160 mg	by Sidmak	50111-0342	Antibiotic
SL342	Tab, SL/342	Sulfamethoxazole 800 mg, Trimethoprim 160 mg	by UDL	51079-0128	Antibiotic
SL342	Tab, SL 342	Sulfamethoxazole 800 mg, Trimethoprim 160 mg	SMZ TMP DS by Quality Care	60346-0087	Antibiotic
SL342	Tab, SL/342	Sulfamethoxazole 800 mg, Trimethoprim 160 mg	by Amerisource	62584-0857	Antibiotic
SL342	Tab	Sulfamethoxazole 800 mg, Trimethoprim 160 mg	by Talbert Med	44514-0826	Antibiotic
SL342	Tab, Sidmak	Sulfamethoxazole 800 mg, Trimethoprim 160 mg	by Apotheca	12634-0177	Antibiotic
SL342	Tab	Sulfamethoxazole 800 mg, Trimethoprim 160 mg	by Qualitest	00603-5779	Antibiotic
SL342	Tab, SL/342	Sulfamethoxazole 800 mg, Trimethoprim 160 mg	by Major	00904-2725	Antibiotic
SL343	Tab, Peach, Oval	Papaverine HCl HP 300 mg	Pavabid HP by Sidmak		Vasodilator
SL346	Tab, White, Round	Isosorbide Dinitrate SL 10 mg	Isordil by Sidmak		Antianginal
SL347	Tab, Pink, Round	Isosorbide Dinitrate 5 mg	Isordil by Sidmak		Antianginal
SL348	Tab, Sugar Coated	Desipramine HCl 75 mg	by Zenith Goldline	00182-1335	Antidepressant
SL348	Tab, White, Round	Isosorbide Dinitrate 10 mg	Isordil by Sidmak		Antianginal
SL349	Tab, Green, Round	Isosorbide Dinitrate 20 mg	Isordil by Sidmak		Antianginal
SL350	Tab, Blue, Round	Isosorbide Dinitrate 30 mg	Isordil by Sidmak		Antianginal
SL351	Tab, Yellow, Round	Isosorbide Dinitrate SR 40 mg	Isordil by Sidmak		Antianginal
SL353	Tab, Sidmak	Meclizine HCl 12.5 mg	by Zenith Goldline	00182-0871	Antiemetic
SL353	Tab, Blue & White, Oval	Meclizine HCl 12.5 mg	Antivert by Sidmak	50111-0353	Antiemetic
SL353	Tab, SL 353 <> Double Layered	Meclizine HCl 12.5 mg	by Heartland	61392-0338	Antiemetic
SL353	Tab, SL Over 353	Meclizine HCl 12.5 mg	by Baker Cummins	63171-0871	Antiemetic
SL353	Tab, SL Over 353, 2 Layer	Meclizine HCl 12.5 mg	by Quality Care	60346-0056	Antiemetic
SL353	Tab, SL/353 <> Mfr is Sidmak, Layered	Meclizine HCl 12.5 mg	by United Res	00677-0418	Antiemetic
SL353	Tab, Sidmak	Meclizine HCl 12.5 mg	by Qualitest	00603-4319	Antiemetic
SL354	Tab, Sidmak	Meclizine HCl 25 mg	by Zenith Goldline	00182-0872	Antiemetic
SL354	Tab, Layered, Sidmak	Meclizine HCl 25 mg	by Pharmedix	53002-0351	Antiemetic
SL354	Tab, Double Layered	Meclizine HCl 25 mg	by HJ Harkins Co	52959-0033	Antiemetic
SL354	Tab, Yellow & White, Oval	Meclizine HCl 25 mg	Antivert by Sidmak	50111-0354	Antiemetic
SL354	Tab	Meclizine HCl 25 mg	by Heartland	61392-0339	Antiemetic
SL354	Tab, Double Layered <> Sidmak	Meclizine HCl 25 mg	by Quality Care	60346-0694	Antiemetic
SL354	Tab	Meclizine HCl 25 mg	by Qualitest	00603-4320	Antiemetic
SL354	Tab, Yellow White, <> Mfr is Sidmak	Meclizine HCl 25 mg	by United Res	00677-0419	Antiemetic
SL354	Tab, White & Yellow, Oval, Scored	Meclizine HCl 25 mg	by Major Pharms	00904-5363	Antiemetic
SL354	Tab, Yellow & White, Oval, Scored	Meclizine HCl 25 mg	by Nat Pharmpak Serv	55154-5559	Antiemetic
SL355	Tab, Chewable	Meclizine HCl 25 mg	by Sidmak	50111-0355	Antiemetic
SL359	Tab, Pink, Oval	Dexchlorpheniramine Maleate 2 mg	Polaramine by Sidmak		Antihistamine
SL36	Tab, Sugar Coated	Desipramine HCl 25 mg	by Warner Chilcott	00047-0594	Antidepressant
SL36	Tab, Sugar Coated	Desipramine HCl 25 mg	by Qualitest	00603-3166	Antidepressant

ID FRONT <> BACK	DESCRIPTION FRONT <> BACK	INGREDIENT & STRENGTH	BRAND (OR EQUIV.) & FIRM	NDC#	CLASS; SCH.
SL36	Tab, Sugar Coated	Desipramine HCl 25 mg	by United Res	00677-1198	Antidepressant
SL36	Tab, Sugar Coated	Desipramine HCl 25 mg	by Richmond	54738-0436	Antidepressant
SL36	Tab, Light Yellow, Sugar Coated, SL Over 36	Desipramine HCl 25 mg	by Quality Care	60346-0731	Antidepressant
SL36	Tab, Sugar Coated	Desipramine HCl 25 mg	by Amerisource	62584-0661	Antidepressant
SL36	Tab, Yellow, Oval	Ethaverine HCl 100 mg	Ethatab by Sidmak		Vasodilator
SL362	Tab, Light Orange, Round	Chlorthalidone 25 mg	by Allscripts	54569-0552	Diuretic
SL362	Tab	Chlorthalidone 25 mg	by Zenith Goldline	00182-1434	Diuretic
SL362	Tab	Chlorthalidone 25 mg	by Qualitest	00603-2860	Diuretic
SL362	Tab, Light Orange, Round	Chlorthalidone 25 mg	Hygroton by Sidmak	50111-0362	Diuretic
SL362	Tab	Chlorthalidone 25 mg	by Major	00904-1349	Diuretic
SL363	Tab, Blue, Round, Scored	Chlorthalidone 50 mg	Hygroton by Martec	52555-0373	Diuretic
SL363	Tab, Light Blue, Round, Scored	Chlorthalidone 50 mg	Hygroton by Sidmak	50111-0363	Diuretic
SL363	Tab	Chlorthalidone 50 mg	by Major	00904-1350	Diuretic
SL363	Tab, Light Blue, Round, Scored	Chlorthalidone 50 mg	by Allscripts	54569-0554	Diuretic
SL363	Tab	Chlorthalidone 50 mg	by Zenith Goldline	00182-1435	Diuretic
SL363	Tab	Chlorthalidone 50 mg	by Qualitest	00603-2861	Diuretic
SL364	Tab	Chlorthalidone 100 mg	by Qualitest	00603-2862	Diuretic
SL364	Tab, White, Round, Scored	Chlorthalidone 100 mg	Hygroton by Sidmak	50111-0364	Diuretic
SL364	Tab	Chlorthalidone 100 mg	by Major	00904-1351	Diuretic
SL368	Tab, Film Coated, SL/368	Amitriptyline HCl 50 mg	by Quality Care	60346-0673	Antidepressant
SL368	Tab, Film Coated, SL over 368	Amitriptyline HCl 50 mg	by Nat Pharmpak Serv	55154-5809	Antidepressant
SL368	Tab, Brown, Round, Film Coated	Amitriptyline HCl 50 mg	by Apothecon	59772-8554	Antidepressant
SL368	Tab, Brown, Round, Film Coated	Amitriptyline HCl 50 mg	by Natl Pharmpak	55154-9307	Antidepressant
SL368	Tab, Film Coated, SL Over 368	Amitriptyline HCl 50 mg	by Baker Cummins	63171-1020	Antidepressant
SL368	Tab, Film Coated, SL/368	Amitriptyline HCl 50 mg	by Amerisource	62584-0308	Antidepressant
SL368	Tab, Film Coated	Amitriptyline HCl 50 mg	by Zenith Goldline	00182-1020	Antidepressant
SL368	Tab, Film Coated, SL/368	Amitriptyline HCl 50 mg	by Qualitest	00603-2214	Antidepressant
SL368	Tab, Brown, Round, Film Coated	Amitriptyline HCl 50 mg	by Astra Zeneca	00186-0450	Antidepressant
SL368	Tab, Rust, Film Coated	Amitriptyline HCl 50 mg	by Allscripts	54569-1519	Antidepressant
SL368	Tab, Film Coated	Amitriptyline HCl 50 mg	by HJ Harkins Co	52959-0514	Antidepressant
SL368	Tab, Film Coated, SL/368	Amitriptyline HCl 75 mg	by Qualitest	00603-2215	Antidepressant
SL369	Tab, Film Coated	Amitriptyline HCl 50 mg	by Major	00904-0202	Antidepressant
SL369	Tab, Film Coated	Amitriptyline HCl 75 mg	by Quality Care	60346-0785	Antidepressant
SL369	Tab, Lavender, Film Coated, SL Over 369	Amitriptyline HCl 75 mg	by Baker Cummins	63171-1021	Antidepressant
SL369	Tab, Film Coated	Amitriptyline HCl 75 mg	by Zenith Goldline	00182-1021	Antidepressant
SL369	Tab, Film Coated	Amitriptyline HCl 75 mg	by Parmed	00349-1043	Antidepressant
SL369	Tab, Lavender, Round, Film Coated	Amitriptyline HCl 75 mg	Elavil by Sidmak	50111-0369	Antidepressant
SL369	Tab, Film Coated, SL/369	Amitriptyline HCl 75 mg	by HJ Harkins Co	52959-0284	Antidepressant
SL369	Tab, Film Coated	Amitriptyline HCl 75 mg	by Allscripts	54569-1864	Antidepressant
SL369	Tab, Purple, Round, Film Coated	Amitriptyline HCl 75 mg	by Compumed	00403-0792	Antidepressant
SL370	Tab, Film Coated	Amitriptyline HCl 100 mg	by Zenith Goldline	00182-1063	Antidepressant
SL370	Tab, Film Coated, SL/370	Amitriptyline HCl 100 mg	by Qualitest	00603-2216	Antidepressant
SL370	Tab, Orange, Round, Film Coated	Amitriptyline HCl 100 mg	Elavil by Sidmak	50111-0370	Antidepressant
SL370	Tab, Film Coated, SL/370	Amitriptyline HCl 100 mg	by Major	00904-0204	Antidepressant
SL371	Tab, Film Coated	Amitriptyline HCl 150 mg	by Zenith Goldline	00182-1486	Antidepressant
SL371	Tab, Film Coated	Amitriptyline HCl 150 mg	by HL Moore	00839-6401	Antidepressant
SL371	Tab, Film Coated, SL/371	Amitriptyline HCl 150 mg	by Qualitest	00603-2217	Antidepressant
SL371	Tab, Light Peach, Oval, Film Coated	Amitriptyline HCl 150 mg	Elavil by Sidmak	50111-0371	Antidepressant
SL371	Tab, Film Coated	Amitriptyline HCl 150 mg	by Major	00904-0205	Antidepressant
SL372	Tab, Blue, Scored, SL/372	Chlorpropamide 100 mg	by Compumed		Antidiabetic
SL372	Tab	Chlorpropamide 100 mg	by Zenith Goldline	00182-1851	Antidiabetic
SL372	Tab	Chlorpropamide 100 mg	by Qualitest	00603-2835	Antidiabetic

ID FRONT <> BACK	DESCRIPTION FRONT <> BACK	INGREDIENT & STRENGTH	BRAND (OR EQUIV.) & FIRM	NDC#	CLASS; SCH.
SL372	Tab, Blue, Round, Scored	Chlorpropamide 100 mg	Diabinese by Sidmak	50111-0372	Antidiabetic
SL372	Tab	Chlorpropamide 100 mg	by Major	00904-0225	Antidiabetic
SL372	Tab	Chlorpropamide 100 mg	by HL Moore	00839-7011	Antidiabetic
SL372	Tab, Blue, Round, Scored	Chlorpropramide 100 mg	by Allscripts	54569-2017	Antidiabetic
SL373	Tab	Chlorpropamide 250 mg	by Zenith Goldline	00182-1852	Antidiabetic
SL373	Tab	Chlorpropamide 250 mg	by Qualitest	00603-2836	Antidiabetic
SL373	Tab	Chlorpropamide 250 mg	by Pharmedix	53002-0347	Antidiabetic
SL373	Tab	Chlorpropamide 250 mg	by Allscripts	54569-0203	Antidiabetic
SL373	Tab, SL/373	Chlorpropamide 250 mg	by Quality Care	60346-0633	Antidiabetic
SL373	Tab, Blue, Round, Scored	Chlorpropamide 250 mg	by Compumed		Antidiabetic
SL373	Tab, Blue, Round, Scored	Chlorpropamide 250 mg	Diabinese by Sidmak	50111-0373	Antidiabetic
SL373	Tab, SL/373	Chlorpropamide 250 mg	by HL Moore	00839-7012	Antidiabetic
SL375	Tab, Green, Oblong, Scored, SL/375	Hyoscyamine Sulfate 0.375 mg	Symax SR by Murfreesboro	51129-1492	Gastrointestinal
SL375	Tab	Nystatin 100000 Units	by Zenith Goldline	00182-0981	Antifungal
SL375	Tab	Nystatin 100000 Units	by United Res	00677-1165	Antifungal
SL377	Cap, Lemon Yellow & Teal Blue, Coated	Doxycycline Hyclate 125 mg	by Sidmak	50111-0377	Antibiotic
SL381	Tab, Blue with Blue Specks, Round	Phenylprop. 40 mg, Phenyleph. 10 mg, Phenyltolox. 15 mg, Chlorphenir. 5 mg	Naldecon by Sidmak		Cold Remedy
SL383	Tab, White, Round	Pseudoephedrine, Dexbrompheniramine TR	Drixoral by Sidmak		Cold Remedy
SL384	Tab, Pink, Round	Isosorbide Dinitrate SR 20 mg	Isordil by Sidmak		Antianginal
SL385	Tab	Guaifenesin 400 mg, Phenylpropanolamine HCl 75 mg	Enomine LA by Quality Care	60346-0339	Cold Remedy
SL385	Tab	Guaifenesin 400 mg, Phenylpropanolamine HCl 75 mg	Phenylfenesin LA by Zenith Goldline	00172-4370	Cold Remedy
SL385	Tab	Guaifenesin 400 mg, Phenylpropanolamine HCl 75 mg	by United Res	00677-1026	Cold Remedy
SL385	Tab	Guaifenesin 400 mg, Phenylpropanolamine HCl 75 mg	Ulr LA by Geneva	00781-1503	Cold Remedy
SL385	Tab, Blue, Oval, Scored	Guaifenesin 400 mg, Phenylpropanolamine HCl 75 mg	Entex LA by Sidmak	50111-0385	Cold Remedy
SL385	Tab	Guaifenesin 400 mg, Phenylpropanolamine HCl 75 mg	by Talbert Med	44514-0348	Cold Remedy
SL387	Tab, Coated, Sidmak	Ibuprofen 400 mg	by Pharmedix	53002-0337	NSAID
SL388	Tab, Film Coated, Sidmak	Ibuprofen 600 mg	by Pharmedix	53002-0301	NSAID
SL390	Tab, Film Coated	Salsalate 500 mg	by Zenith Goldline	00182-1802	NSAID
SL390	Tab, Film Coated	Salsalate 500 mg	Salflex by Carnrick	00086-0071	NSAID
SL390	Tab, Yellow, Round, Film Coated	Salsalate 500 mg	Disalcid by Sidmak	50111-0390	NSAID
SL390	Tab, Film Coated	Salsalate 500 mg	by Richmond	54738-0306	NSAID
SL390	Tab, Film Coated	Salsalate 500 mg	by PDRX	55289-0275	NSAID
SL391	Tab, Sidmak	Levothyroxine Sodium 0.1 mg	by Apotheca	12634-0431	Antithyroid
SL391	Tab, Yellow, Oblong, Film Coated	Salsalate 750 mg	by RX PAK	65084-0218	NSAID
SL391	Tab, Film Coated	Salsalate 750 mg	by Zenith Goldline	00182-1803	NSAID
SL391	Tab, Film Coated	Salsalate 750 mg	by Allscripts	54569-1712	NSAID
SL391	Tab, Coated	Salsalate 750 mg	by DRX	55045-1935	NSAID
SL391	Tab, Yellow, Cap Shaped, Film Coated	Salsalate 750 mg	Disalcid by Sidmak	50111-0391	NSAID
SL391	Tab, Film Coated	Salsalate 750 mg	by Med Pro	53978-0399	NSAID
SL391	Tab, Coated	Salsalate 750 mg	by Quality Care	60346-0034	NSAID
SL391	Tab	Salsalate 750 mg	by HL Moore	00839-7168	NSAID
SL391	Tab, Yellow, Oblong, Film Coated	Salsalate 750 mg	by Compumed	00403-0088	NSAID
SL391	Tab, Sidmak, Film Coated	Salsalate 750 mg	by Apotheca	12634-0463	NSAID
SL391	Tab, Yellow, Oblong, Film Coated	Salsalate 750 mg	by RX PAK	65084-0217	NSAID
SL393	Tab, SL/393	Benztropine Mesylate 0.5 mg	by Qualitest	00603-2430	Antiparkinson
SL393	Tab, White, Round, Scored	Benztropine Mesylate 0.5 mg	Cogentin by Sidmak	50111-0393	Antiparkinson
SL394	Tab, SL/394	Benztropine Mesylate 1 mg	by Qualitest	00603-2431	Antiparkinson
SL394	Tab, White, Oval, Scored	Benztropine Mesylate 1 mg	Cogentin by Sidmak	50111-0394	Antiparkinson
SL395	Tab, White, Round, Scored	Benztropine Mesylate 2 mg	by Allscripts	54569-2862	Antiparkinson
SL395	Tab, SL/395	Benztropine Mesylate 2 mg	by Qualitest	00603-2432	Antiparkinson
SL395	Tab, White, Round, Scored	Benztropine Mesylate 2 mg	Congentin by Sidmak	50111-0395	Antiparkinson
SL396	Tab, Peach, Oval	Procainamide HCl SR 750 mg	Procan SR by Sidmak		Antiarrhythmic

ID FRONT <> BACK	DESCRIPTION FRONT <> BACK	INGREDIENT & STRENGTH	BRAND (OR EQUIV.) & FIRM	NDC#	CLASS; SCH.
SL397	Tab	Hydralazine HCl 100 mg	by Zenith Goldline	00182-1553	Antihypertensive
SL397	Tab	Hydralazine HCl 100 mg	by Qualitest	00603-3833	Antihypertensive
SL397	Tab, Orange, Round	Hydralazine HCl 100 mg	Apresoline by Sidmak	50111-0397	Antihypertensive
SL398	Tab, Orange, Round	Hydralazine HCl 10 mg	by Monarch	61570-0024	Antihypertensive
SL398	Tab	Hydralazine HCl 10 mg	by Quality Care	60346-0823	Antihypertensive
SL398	Tab	Hydralazine HCl 10 mg	by Baker Cummins	63171-0905	Antihypertensive
SL398	Tab, Orange, Round	Hydralazine HCl 10 mg	by Natl Pharmpak	55154-5827	Antihypertensive
SL398	Tab	Hydralazine HCl 10 mg	by Zenith Goldline	00182-0905	Antihypertensive
SL398	Tab	Hydralazine HCl 10 mg	by Qualitest	00603-3830	Antihypertensive
SL398	Tab	Hydralazine HCl 10 mg	by Richmond	54738-0398	Antihypertensive
SL398	Tab, Orange, Round	Hydralazine HCl 10 mg	Apresoline by Sidmak	50111-0398	Antihypertensive
SL404	Cap, White	Extended Phenytoin Sodium 100 mg	Dilantin by Sidmak		Anticonvulsant
SL406	Cap	Indomethacin 25 mg	by Richmond	54738-0406	NSAID
SL406	Cap, Green, Gelatin	Indomethacin 25 mg	Indocin by Sidmak	50111-0406	NSAID
SL406	Cap	Indomethacin 25 mg	by HJ Harkins Co	52959-0080	NSAID
SL406	Cap, Green, Hard Gel	Indomethacin 25 mg	by Murfreesboro	51129-1552	NSAID
SL406	Cap	Indomethacin 25 mg	by United Res	00677-0872	NSAID
SL406	Cap	Indomethacin 25 mg	by Qualitest	00603-4067	NSAID
SL407	Cap	Indomethacin 50 mg	by Richmond	54738-0407	NSAID
SL407	Cap, Green, Gelatin	Indomethacin 50 mg	Indocin by Sidmak	50111-0407	NSAID
SL407	Cap, SL 407 <> Sidmark	Indomethacin 50 mg	by United Res	00677-0873	NSAID
SL407	Cap, SL 407 <> Sidmak	Indomethacin 50 mg	by Qualitest	00603-4068	NSAID
SL410	Tab	Carbamazepine 200 mg	by Sidmak	50111-0410	Anticonvulsant
SL415	Tab	Griseofulvin, Ultramicrosize 165 mg	by Sidmak	50111-0415	Antifungal
SL416	Tab	Griseofulvin, Ultramicrosize 330 mg	by Sidmak	50111-0416	Antifungal
SL425	Tab, Pink, Oblong, SL/425	Aspirin Enteric Coated 975 mg	Easprin by Sidmak		Analgesic
SL427	Cap, Orange/Beige, Oblong	Phenylpropanolamine 45 mg, PE 5 mg, Guaifenesin 200 mg	Entex by Sidmak		Cold Remedy
SL430	Tab, White, Round, Scored	Metoclopramide HCl	by Allscripts	54569-0434	Gastrointestinal
SL430	Tab	Metoclopramide HCl	by Zenith Goldline	00182-1789	Gastrointestinal
SL430	Tab	Metoclopramide HCl	by Richmond	54738-0430	Gastrointestinal
SL430	Tab, Sidmak	Metoclopramide HCl	by Quality Care	60346-0802	Gastrointestinal
SL430	Tab, SL/430	Metoclopramide HCl	by Major	00904-1070	Gastrointestinal
SL430	Tab	Metoclopramide HCl	by Qualitest	00603-4617	Gastrointestinal
SL430	Tab, White, Round, Scored	Metoclopramide HCl 10 mg	by Neuman Distr	64579-0048	Gastrointestinal
SL430	Tab, White, Round, Scored	Metoclopramide HCl 10 mg	Reglan by Sidmak	50111-0430	Gastrointestinal
SL430	Tab, White, Round	Metoclopramide HCl 10 mg	Reglan by Martec	52555-0658	Gastrointestinal
SL433	Tab	Trazodone HCl 50 mg	by Major	00904-3990	Antidepressant
SL433	Tab, White, Round, Scored	Trazodone HCl 50 mg	by Direct Dispensing	57866-4715	Antidepressant
SL433	Tab	Trazodone HCl 50 mg	by Warner Chilcott	00047-0577	Antidepressant
SL433	Tab	Trazodone HCl 50 mg	by Rugby	00536-4715	Antidepressant
SL433	Tab, SL/433, Compressed	Trazodone HCl 50 mg	by Kaiser	00179-1118	Antidepressant
SL433	Tab	Trazodone HCl 50 mg	by Zenith Goldline	00182-1259	Antidepressant
SL433	Tab	Trazodone HCl 50 mg	by Martec	52555-0260	Antidepressant
SL433	Tab, White, Round, Scored	Trazodone HCl 50 mg	Desyrel by Sidmak	50111-0433	Antidepressant
SL433	Tab	Trazodone HCl 50 mg	by HJ Harkins Co	52959-0378	Antidepressant
SL433	Tab	Trazodone HCl 50 mg	by DRX	55045-1715	Antidepressant
SL433	Tab, Coated	Trazodone HCl 50 mg	by Quality Care	60346-0620	Antidepressant
SL433	Tab, Debossed	Trazodone HCl 50 mg	by Baker Cummins	63171-1259	Antidepressant
SL433	Tab	Trazodone HCl 50 mg	by Prescription Dispensing	61807-0143	Antidepressant
SL433	Tab, Debossed <> Underscored	Trazodone HCl 50 mg	by Kaiser	62224-0555	Antidepressant
SL433	Tab	Trazodone HCl 50 mg	by HL Moore	00839-7251	Antidepressant
SL433	Tab	Trazodone HCl 50 mg	by Qualitest	00603-6144	Antidepressant

ID FRONT <> BACK	DESCRIPTION FRONT <> BACK	INGREDIENT & STRENGTH	BRAND (OR EQUIV.) & FIRM	NDC#	CLASS; SCH.
SL434	Tab	Trazodone HCl 100 mg	by Warner Chilcott	00047-0578	Antidepressant
SL434	Tab	Trazodone HCl 100 mg	by Zenith Goldline	00182-1260	Antidepressant
SL434	Tab, White, Round, Scored	Trazodone HCl 100 mg	by Teva	00480-0293	Antidepressant
SL434	Tab, White, Round, Scored	Trazodone 100 mg	by Teva	00480-0280	Antidepressant
SL434	Tab, White, Round, Scored	Trazodone HCl 100 mg	Desyrel by Sidmak	50111-0434	Antidepressant
SL434	Tab	Trazodone HCl 100 mg	by Martec	52555-0261	Antidepressant
SL434	Tab, Debossed	Trazodone HCl 100 mg	by Amerisource	62584-0883	Antidepressant
SL434	Tab	Trazodone HCl 100 mg	by Baker Cummins	63171-1260	Antidepressant
SL434	Tab, Film Coated, SL Over 434	Trazodone HCl 100 mg	by Quality Care	60346-0014	Antidepressant
SL434	Tab	Trazodone HCl 100 mg	by Qualitest	00603-6145	Antidepressant
SL436	Tab, Sugar Coated	Desipramine HCl 25 mg	by Zenith Goldline	00182-1332	Antidepressant
SL437	Tab, Light Green, Coated, SL Over 437	Desipramine HCl 50 mg	by Quality Care	60346-0732	Antidepressant
SL437	Tab, Light Green, Sugar Coated	Desipramine HCl 50 mg	by Warner Chilcott	00047-0595	Antidepressant
SL437	Tab, Sugar Coated	Desipramine HCl 50 mg	by Zenith Goldline	00182-1333	Antidepressant
SL437	Tab, Sugar Coated, SL/437	Desipramine HCl 50 mg	by Qualitest	00603-3167	Antidepressant
SL437	Tab, Sugar Coated	Desipramine HCl 50 mg	by United Res	00677-1199	Antidepressant
SL437	Tab, Sugar Coated	Desipramine HCl 50 mg	by Richmond	54738-0437	Antidepressant
SL437	Tab, Sugar Coated	Desipramine HCl 50 mg	by Med Pro	53978-2077	Antidepressant
SL437	Tab, Green, Round	Desipramine HCl 50 mg	by DRX	55045-1909	Antidepressant
SL437	Tab, Light Green, Sugar Coated	Desipramine HCl 50 mg	by Martec	52555-0287	Antidepressant
SL437	Tab, Sugar Coated	Desipramine HCl 50 mg	by HL Moore	00839-7552	Antidepressant
SL438	Tab, Sugar Coated	Desipramine HCl 75 mg	by Warner Chilcott	00047-0596	Antidepressant
SL438	Tab, Sugar Coated	Desipramine HCl 75 mg	by Qualitest	00603-3168	Antidepressant
SL438	Tab, Sugar Coated	Desipramine HCl 75 mg	by Martec	52555-0288	Antidepressant
SL438	Tab, Sugar Coated	Desipramine HCl 75 mg	by HL Moore	00839-7553	Antidepressant
SL439	Tab, Peach, Round, Sugar Coated	Desipramine HCl 100 mg	Norpramin by Sidmak	50111-0439	Antidepressant
SL440	Tab, White, Round, Sugar Coated	Desipramine HCl 150 mg	Norpramin by Sidmak	50111-0440	Antidepressant
SL441 <> 50100	Tab, White, Trapezoid, Scored, SL 441<>50/100	Trazodone 150 mg	by Teva	00480-0154	Antidepressant
SL441 <> 50100	Tab	Trazodone HCl 150 mg	by Physicians Total Care	54868-1959	Antidepressant
SL441 <> 50100	Tab, SL/441 Debossed <> 50/100 Debossed	Trazodone HCl 150 mg	by Heartland	61392-0179	Antidepressant
SL441 <> 50100	Tab, White, Trapezoid, Scored, SL 441 <> 50 100	Trazodone HCl 150 mg	Desyrel by Sidmak	50111-0441	Antidepressant
SL441 <> 505050	Tab, 50/50/50	Trazodone HCl 100 mg	by Major	00904-3991	Antidepressant
SL441 <> 505050	Tab, 50/50/50	Trazodone HCl 100 mg	by Qualitest	00603-6145	Antidepressant
SL441 <> 505050	Tab, 50/50/50	Trazodone HCl 150 mg	by Warner Chilcott	00047-0716	Antidepressant
SL441 <> 505050	Tab, 50/50/50	Trazodone HCl 150 mg	by Zenith Goldline	00182-1298	Antidepressant
SL441 <> 505050	Tab, 50/50/50	Trazodone HCl 150 mg	by Schein	00364-2300	Antidepressant
SL441 <> 505050	Tab, 50/50/50	Trazodone HCl 150 mg	by Parmed	00349-8824	Antidepressant
SL441 <> 505050	Tab, 50/50/50	Trazodone HCl 150 mg	by Martec	52555-0132	Antidepressant
SL441 <> 505050	Tab, 50/50/50	Trazodone HCl 150 mg	by Geneva	00781-1826	Antidepressant
SL441 <> 505050	Tab, 50/50/50	Trazodone HCl 150 mg	by Major	00904-3992	Antidepressant
SL441 <> 505050	Tab, 50/50/50	Trazodone HCl 150 mg	by Qualitest	00603-6146	Antidepressant
SL441 <> 505050	Tab, White, Trapezoid, Scored, Debossed <> 50 50 50	Trazodone HCl 150 mg	Desyrel by Sidmak	50111-0441	Antidepressant
SL441 <> 505050	Tab, 50/50/50	Trazodone HCl 150 mg	by HL Moore	00839-7507	Antidepressant
SL441 <> 505050	Tab, 50/50/50	Trazodone HCl 150 mg	by United Res	00677-1302	Antidepressant
SL44150100TRPZ	Tab, White, Trapezoidal, Scored, Compressed, SL 441 50/100 TRPZ	Trazodone HCl 150 mg	Desyrel by Geneva	00781-1826	Antidepressant
SL443 <> 505050	Tab, 50/50/50	Trazodone HCl 100 mg	by Rugby	00536-4688	Antidepressant
SL451	Tab, White, Oblong	Ibuprofen 800 mg	Motrin by Sidmak		NSAID
SL454	Cap, Red	Ethchlorvynol 500 mg	Placidyl by Rosemont		Hypnotic; C IV
SL455	Cap, Green	Ethchlorvynol 750 mg	Placidyl by Rosemont		Hypnotic; C IV
SL456	Tab, Blue, Round, Scored	Oxybutynin Chloride 5 mg	by Pharmacia & Upjohn	00009-5013	Urinary
SL456	Tab	Oxybutynin Chloride 5 mg	by Zenith Goldline	00182-1289	Urinary

ID FRONT <> BACK	DESCRIPTION FRONT <> BACK	INGREDIENT & STRENGTH	BRAND (OR EQUIV.) & FIRM	NDC#	CLASS; SCH.
SL456	Tab, Pale Blue	Oxybutynin Chloride 5 mg	by Richmond	54738-0456	Urinary
SL456	Tab, Pale Blue, SL Over 456	Oxybutynin Chloride 5 mg	by UDL	51079-0628	Urinary
SL456	Tab, SL Over 456	Oxybutynin Chloride 5 mg	by Nat Pharmpak Serv	55154-5537	Urinary
SL456	Tab	Oxybutynin Chloride 5 mg	by Baker Cummins	63171-1289	Urinary
SL456	Tab	Oxybutynin Chloride 5 mg	by Heartland	61392-0138	Urinary
SL456	Tab, Pale Blue	Oxybutynin Chloride 5 mg	by Quality Care	60346-0832	Urinary
SL456	Tab	Oxybutynin Chloride 5 mg	by Amerisource	62584-0815	Urinary
SL456	Tab	Oxybutynin Chloride 5 mg	by Vangard	00615-3512	Urinary
SL456	Tab, Light Blue	Oxybutynin Chloride 5 mg	by Qualitest	00603-4975	Urinary
SL456	Tab, Pale Blue, Round, Scored	Oxybutynin Chloride 5 mg	Ditropan by Sidmak	50111-0456	Urinary
SL456	Tab	Oxybutynin Chloride 5 mg	by Major	00904-2821	Urinary
SL456	Tab	Oxybutynin Chloride 5 mg	by United Res	00677-1255	Urinary
SL458	Tab, White, Oblong	Theophylline TD 300 mg	Theodur by Sidmak		Antiasthmatic
SL459	Tab	Theophylline Anhydrous 300 mg	by Heartland	61392-0017	Antiasthmatic
SL459	Tab, ER	Theophylline Anhydrous 300 mg	by Geneva	00781-1005	Antiasthmatic
SL459	Tab, Ex Release	Theophylline Anhydrous 300 mg	by DEY LP	49502-0433	Antiasthmatic
SL459	Tab, ER	Theophylline Anhydrous 300 mg	by Warner Chilcott	00047-0592	Antiasthmatic
SL459	Tab, SL/459	Theophylline Anhydrous 300 mg	by Allscripts	54569-2483	Antiasthmatic
SL459	Tab, Scored	Theophylline Anhydrous 300 mg	by Martec	52555-0704	Antiasthmatic
SL459	Tab	Theophylline Anhydrous 300 mg	by Med Pro	53978-0320	Antiasthmatic
SL459	Tab, Ex Release, Sidmak	Theophylline 300 mg	by Pharmedix	53002-0335	Antiasthmatic
SL459	Tab	Theophylline 300 mg	by Quality Care	60346-0596	Antiasthmatic
SL459	Tab, Ex Release, Sidmak Labs is MFG	Theophylline 300 mg	by United Res	00677-0817	Antiasthmatic
SL459	Tab, ER	Theophylline 300 mg	by Qualitest	00603-5946	Antiasthmatic
SL459	Tab, White, Cap Shaped, Scored	Theophylline Anhydrous 300 mg	Theo-Dur by Sidmak	50111-0459	Antiasthmatic
SL460	Tab, Green, Round	Clonidine HCl 0.1 mg	Catapres by Sidmak		Antihypertensive
SL461	Tab, Yellow, Round	Clonidine HCl 0.2 mg	Catapres by Sidmak		Antihypertensive
SL462	Tab, Blue, Round	Clonidine HCl 0.3 mg	Catapres by Sidmak		Antihypertensive
SL463	Tab, Pink, Round	Clonidine HCl 0.1 mg, Chlorthalidone 15 mg	Combipres by Sidmak		Antihypertensive; Diuretic
SL464	Tab, Blue, Round	Clonidine HCl 0.2 mg, Chlorthalidone 15 mg	Combipres by Sidmak		Antihypertensive; Diuretic
SL465	Tab, White, Round	Clonidine HCl 0.3 mg, Chlorthalidone 15 mg	Combipres by Sidmak		Antihypertensive; Diuretic
SL467	Tab, SL Over 467	Propranolol HCl 10 mg	by Baker Cummins	63171-1812	Antihypertensive
SL467	Tab	Propranolol HCl 10 mg	by Warner Chilcott	00047-0070	Antihypertensive
SL467	Tab, SL/467 Debossed, Compressed	Propranolol HCl 10 mg	by Kaiser	00179-1088	Antihypertensive
SL467	Tab	Propranolol HCl 10 mg	by Zenith Goldline	00182-1758	Antihypertensive
SL467	Tab	Propranolol HCl 10 mg	by Richmond	54738-0467	Antihypertensive
SL467	Tab	Propranolol HCl 10 mg	by Allscripts	54569-0557	Antihypertensive
SL467	Tab, SL/467	Propranolol HCl 10 mg	by Med Pro	53978-0034	Antihypertensive
SL467	Tab	Propranolol HCl 10 mg	by Quality Care	60346-0570	Antihypertensive
SL467	Tab, SL/467	Propranolol HCl 10 mg	by Kaiser	62224-0224	Antihypertensive
SL467	Tab	Propranolol HCl 10 mg	by Major	00904-0411	Antihypertensive
SL467	Tab, Orange, Round, Scored	Propranolol HCl 10 mg	Inderal by Sidmak	50111-0467	Antihypertensive
SL467	Tab	Propranolol HCl 10 mg	by Qualitest	00603-5489	Antihypertensive
SL467	Tab	Propranolol HCl 10 mg	by Vangard	00615-2561	Antihypertensive
SL467	Tab	Propranolol HCl 10 mg	by Geneva	00781-1344	Antihypertensive
SL468	Tab, SL/468	Propranolol HCl 20 mg	by Warner Chilcott	00047-0071	Antihypertensive
SL468	Tab, Blue, Round, Scored	Propranolol HCl 20 mg	by Allscripts	54569-0559	Antihypertensive
SL468	Tab, SL/468	Propranolol HCl 20 mg	by Baker Cummins	63171-1813	Antihypertensive
SL468	Tab, SL/468 Debossed, Compressed	Propranolol HCl 40 mg	by Kaiser	00179-1090	Antihypertensive

ID FRONT <> BACK	DESCRIPTION FRONT <> BACK	INGREDIENT & STRENGTH	BRAND (OR EQUIV.) & FIRM	NDC#	CLASS; SCH.
SL468	Tab, SL/468 Debossed, Compressed	Propranolol HCl 20 mg	by Kaiser	00179-1089	Antihypertensive
SL468	Tab	Propranolol HCl 20 mg	by Zenith Goldline	00182-1759	Antihypertensive
SL468	Tab, Sidmak	Propranolol HCl 20 mg	by PDRX	55289-0233	Antihypertensive
SL468	Tab	Propranolol HCl 20 mg	by Med Pro	53978-5014	Antihypertensive
SL468	Tab	Propranolol HCl 20 mg	by Richmond	54738-0468	Antihypertensive
SL468	Tab, SL/468	Propranolol HCl 20 mg	by HJ Harkins Co	52959-0212	Antihypertensive
SL468	Tab	Propranolol HCl 20 mg	by Quality Care	60346-0598	Antihypertensive
SL468	Tab, SL/468	Propranolol HCl 20 mg	by Kaiser	62224-0222	Antihypertensive
SL468	Tab	Propranolol HCl 20 mg	by Qualitest	00603-5490	Antihypertensive
SL468	Tab	Propranolol HCl 20 mg	by Major	00904-0412	Antihypertensive
SL468	Tab, Blue, Round, Scored	Propranolol HCl 20 mg	Inderal by Sidmak	50111-0468	Antihypertensive
SL468	Tab	Propranolol HCl 20 mg	by Geneva	00781-1354	Antihypertensive
SL469	Tab, SL/469	Propranolol HCl 40 mg	by Warner Chilcott	00047-0072	Antihypertensive
SL469	Tab	Propranolol HCl 40 mg	by Richmond	54738-0469	Antihypertensive
SL469	Tab, SL/469	Propranolol HCl 40 mg	by Kaiser	62224-0339	Antihypertensive
SL469	Tab	Propranolol HCl 40 mg	by Quality Care	60346-0806	Antihypertensive
SL469	Tab	Propranolol HCl 40 mg	by Major	00904-0414	Antihypertensive
SL469	Tab	Propranolol HCl 40 mg	by Qualitest	00603-5491	Antihypertensive
SL469	Tab	Propranolol HCl 40 mg	by Geneva	00781-1364	Antihypertensive
SL469	Tab, Green, Round, Scored	Propranolol HCl 40 mg	Inderal by Sidmak	50111-0469	Antihypertensive
SL469	Tab, Light Green, Round, Scored, SL/469	Propranolol HCl 40 mg	by Allscripts	54569-0561	Antihypertensive
SL469	Tab, SL Over 469	Propranolol HCl 40 mg	by Baker Cummins	63171-1814	Antihypertensive
SL470	Tab	Propranolol HCl 60 mg	by Warner Chilcott	00047-0073	Antihypertensive
SL470	Tab	Propranolol HCl 60 mg	by Allscripts	54569-0442	Antihypertensive
SL470	Tab	Propranolol HCl 60 mg	by Richmond	54738-0470	Antihypertensive
SL470	Tab, Pink, Round, Scored, SL/470	Propranolol HCl 60 mg	by Roberts	54092-0189	Antihypertensive
SL470	Tab	Propranolol HCl 60 mg	by Quality Care	60346-0431	Antihypertensive
SL470	Tab	Propranolol HCl 60 mg	by Geneva	00781-1374	Antihypertensive
SL470	Tab	Propranolol HCl 60 mg	by HL Moore	00839-7117	Antihypertensive
SL470	Tab	Propranolol HCl 60 mg	by Qualitest	00603-5492	Antihypertensive
SL470	Tab, Pink, Round, Scored	Propranolol HCl 60 mg	Inderal by Sidmak	50111-0470	Antihypertensive
SL471	Tab, SL Over 471	Propranolol HCl 80 mg	by Baker Cummins	63171-1815	Antihypertensive
SL471	Tab, SL/471	Propranolol HCl 80 mg	by Warner Chilcott	00047-0074	Antihypertensive
SL471	Tab	Propranolol HCl 80 mg	by Zenith Goldline	00182-1762	Antihypertensive
SL471	Tab, SL/471 Debossed, Compressed	Propranolol HCl 80 mg	by Kaiser	00179-1091	Antihypertensive
SL471	Tab	Propranolol HCl 80 mg	by Richmond	54738-0471	Antihypertensive
SL471	Tab	Propranolol HCl 80 mg	by Quality Care	60346-0967	Antihypertensive
SL471	Tab, SL/471	Propranolol HCl 80 mg	by Kaiser	62224-0335	Antihypertensive
SL471	Tab	Propranolol HCl 80 mg	by Geneva	00781-1384	Antihypertensive
SL471	Tab, Yellow, Round, Scored	Propranolol HCl 80 mg	Inderal by Sidmak	50111-0471	Antihypertensive
SL471	Tab	Propranolol HCl 80 mg	by Qualitest	00603-5493	Antihypertensive
SL472	Tab	Propranolol HCl 90 mg	by Sidmak	50111-0472	Antihypertensive
SL473	Tab, White, Round, Scored	Hydrochlorothiazide 25 mg, Propranolol HCl 40 mg	Inderide by Sidmak	50111-0473	Diuretic; Antihypertensive
SL473	Tab	Hydrochlorothiazide 25 mg, Propranolol HCl 40 mg	by Qualitest	00603-5503	Diuretic; Antihypertensive
SL474	Tab	Hydrochlorothiazide 25 mg, Propranolol HCl 80 mg	by Zenith Goldline	00182-1834	Diuretic; Antihypertensive
SL474	Tab, White, Round, Scored	Hydrochlorothiazide 25 mg, Propranolol HCl 80 mg	Inderide by Sidmak	50111-0474	Diuretic; Antihypertensive
SL474	Tab	Hydrochlorothiazide 25 mg, Propranolol HCl 80 mg	by Qualitest	00603-5504	Diuretic; Antihypertensive

ID FRONT <> BACK	DESCRIPTION FRONT <> BACK	INGREDIENT & STRENGTH	BRAND (OR EQUIV.) & FIRM	NDC#	CLASS; SCH.
SL475	Tab, Film Coated	Methyldopa 125 mg	by Sidmak	50111-0475	Antihypertensive
SL476	Tab, Film Coated	Methyldopa 250 mg	by Sidmak	50111-0476	Antihypertensive
SL477	Tab, Film Coated	Methyldopa 500 mg	by Sidmak	50111-0477	Antihypertensive
SL477 <> Z2932	Tab, Film Coated, Sidmak Labs <> Zenith Goldline	Methyldopa 500 mg	by United Res	00677-0974	Antihypertensive
SL478	Tab, Brown, Round	Methyldopa 250 mg, Hydrochlorothiazide 15 mg	Aldoril by Sidmak		Antihypertensive
SL479	Tab, White, Round	Methyldopa 250 mg, Hydrochlorothiazide 25 mg	Aldoril by Sidmak		Antihypertensive
SL480	Tab, Brown, Oval	Methyldopa 500 mg, Hydrochlorothiazide 30 mg	Aldoril by Sidmak		Antihypertensive
SL481	Tab, White, Oval	Methyldopa 500 mg, Hydrochlorothiazide 50 mg	Aldoril by Sidmak		Antihypertensive
SL482	Tab, ER	Theophylline Anhydrous 200 mg	by Warner Chilcott	00047-0659	Antiasthmatic
SL482	Tab	Theophylline Anhydrous 200 mg	by Heartland	61392-0016	Antiasthmatic
SL482	Tab, White, Oval, Scored	Theophylline Anhydrous 200 mg	Theo-Dur by Sidmak	50111-0482	Antiasthmatic
SL482	Tab, ER	Theophylline Anhydrous 200 mg	by DEY LP	49502-0432	Antiasthmatic
SL482	Tab, ER	Theophylline Anhydrous 200 mg	by Geneva	00781-1004	Antiasthmatic
SL482	Tab, Ex Release	Theophylline 200 mg	by Physicians Total Care	54868-0028	Antiasthmatic
SL482	Tab, Ex Release, Sidmak Lab	Theophylline 200 mg	by Pharmedix	53002-0330	Antiasthmatic
SL482	Tab, Debossed	Theophylline 200 mg	by Quality Care	60346-0669	Antiasthmatic
SL482	Tab, ER	Theophylline 200 mg	by Qualitest	00603-5945	Antiasthmatic
SL482	Tab, Ex Release, Sidmak Lab	Theophylline 200 mg	by United Res	00677-0846	Antiasthmatic
SL482	Tab, White, Oval, Scored	Theophylline Anhydrous 200 mg	Theo-Dur by Martec	52555-0703	Antiasthmatic
SL483	Tab, ER	Theophylline Anhydrous 100 mg	by Warner Chilcott	00047-0657	Antiasthmatic
SL483	Tab	Theophylline Anhydrous 100 mg	by Quality Care	60346-0713	Antiasthmatic
SL483	Tab, White, Round, Scored	Theophylline Anhydrous 100 mg	Theo-Dur by Sidmak	50111-0483	Antiasthmatic
SL483	Tab, ER	Theophylline Anhydrous 100 mg	by Geneva	00781-1003	Antiasthmatic
SL483	Tab, ER	Theophylline Anhydrous 100 mg	by Dey LP	49502-0431	Antiasthmatic
SL483	Tab, ER	Theophylline 100 mg	by Qualitest	00603-5944	Antiasthmatic
SL484	Tab, Yellow, Round	Sulindac 150 mg	Clinoril by Sidmak		NSAID
SL485	Tab, Yellow, Round	Sulindac 200 mg	Clinoril by Sidmak		NSAID
SL485	Tab, Film Coated	Verapamil HCl 80 mg	by Quality Care	60346-0813	Antihypertensive
SL486	Tab, Film Coated	Verapamil HCl 80 mg	by Warner Chilcott	00047-0328	Antihypertensive
SL486	Tab, Film Coated	Verapamil HCl 80 mg	by Qualitest	00603-6357	Antihypertensive
SL486	Tab, White, Round, Film Coated, Scored	Verapamil HCl 80 mg	Isoptin by Sidmak	50111-0486	Antihypertensive
SL487	Tab, White, Round, Film Coated, Scored	Verapamil HCl 120 mg	Isoptin by Sidmak	50111-0487	Antihypertensive
SL487	Tab, Film Coated	Verapamil HCl 120 mg	by Qualitest	00603-6358	Antihypertensive
SL487	Tab, Film Coated	Verapamil HCl 120 mg	by Warner Chilcott	00047-0329	Antihypertensive
SL488	Tab, Green, Oblong	Verapamil SR 240 mg	Isoptin SR by Sidmak		Antihypertensive
SL491	Tab	Albuterol Sulfate	by Geneva	00781-1671	Antiasthmatic
SL491	Tab, White, Round, Scored	Albuterol Sulfate 2 mg	Ventolin by Sidmak	50111-0491	Antiasthmatic
SL491	Tab	Albuterol Sulfate 2.4 mg	by Martec	52555-0491	Antiasthmatic
SL492	Tab, White, Round, Scored	Albuterol Sulfate 4 mg	Ventolin by Sidmak	50111-0492	Antiasthmatic
SL492	Tab, Coated	Albuterol Sulfate 4.8 mg	by Quality Care	60346-0285	Antiasthmatic
SL492	Tab, Coated	Albuterol Sulfate 4.8 mg	by Martec	52555-0492	Antiasthmatic
SL493	Tab, White, Oval	Aspirin Controlled Release 800 mg	ZORprin by Sidmak		Analgesic
SL497	Tab, Yellow, Oblong	Fenoprofen Calcium 600 mg	Nalfon by Sidmak		NSAID
SL505	Tab	Hydrochlorothiazide 50 mg, Triamterene 75 mg	by Zenith Goldline	00182-1872	Diuretic
SL505	Tab	Hydrochlorothiazide 50 mg, Triamterene 75 mg	by Richmond	54738-0127	Diuretic
SL505	Tab, Yellow, Rectangular, Scored	Hydrochlorothiazide 50 mg, Triamterene 75 mg	Maxzide by Sidmak	50111-0505	Diuretic
SL505	Tab	Hydrochlorothiazide 50 mg, Triamterene 75 mg	by Qualitest	00603-6182	Diuretic
SL506	Tab	Atenolol 50 mg	by Sidmak	50111-0506	Antihypertensive
SL507	Tab	Atenolol 100 mg	by Sidmak	50111-0507	Antihypertensive
SL508	Tab	Atenolol 50 mg, Chlorthalidone 25 mg	by Sidmak	50111-0508	Antihypertensive; Diuretic

ID FRONT <> BACK	DESCRIPTION FRONT <> BACK	INGREDIENT & STRENGTH	BRAND (OR EQUIV.) & FIRM	NDC#	CLASS; SCH.
SL509	Tab	Atenolol 100 mg, Chlorthalidone 25 mg	by Sidmak	50111-0509	Antihypertensive; Diuretic
SL514	Tab, Blue & Yellow, Round	Meclizine HCl 50 mg	Antivert by Sidmak		Antiemetic
SL515	Tab, Sugar Coated, SL/515	Hydroxyzine HCl 100 mg	by Sidmak	50111-0515	Antihistamine
SL516	Tab, White, Round, Film Coated, Scored	Verapamil HCl 40 mg	Isoptin by Sidmak	50111-0516	Antihypertensive
SL516	Tab, Film Coated, Debossed	Verapamil HCl 40 mg	by Qualitest	00603-6356	Antihypertensive
SL517	Tab, Light Green	Metoclopramide HCl 5 mg	by Rugby	00536-5902	Gastrointestinal
SL517	Tab, Debossed	Metoclopramide HCl 5 mg	by Martec	52555-0657	Gastrointestinal
SL517	Tab, Light Green, Round	Metoclopramide HCl 5 mg	Reglan by Sidmark	51285-0585	Gastrointestinal
SL517	Tab	Metoclopramide HCl 5 mg	by Richmond	54738-0517	Gastrointestinal
SL517	Tab, Debossed	Metoclopramide HCl 5 mg	by Quality Care	60346-0880	Gastrointestinal
SL517	Tab	Metoclopramide HCl 5 mg	by HL Moore	00839-7530	Gastrointestinal
SL517	Tab, Light Green, Round	Metoclopramide HCl 5 mg	Reglan by Sidmak	50111-0517	Gastrointestinal
SL517	Tab	Metoclopramide 5 mg	by Zenith Goldline	00182-1898	Gastrointestinal
SL517	Tab	Metoclopramide 5 mg	by United Res	00677-1323	Gastrointestinal
SL517	Tab	Metoclopramide HCl	by Qualitest	00603-4616	Gastrointestinal
SL518	Tab, Ex Release	Theophylline Anhydrous 450 mg	by Warner Chilcott	00047-0593	Antiasthmatic
SL518	Tab, Ex Release	Theophylline Anhydrous 450 mg	by Zenith Goldline	00182-1941	Antiasthmatic
SL518	Tab, White, Oblong, Scored	Theophylline Anhydrous 450 mg	by Qualitest Pharms	00603-5747	Antiasthmatic
SL518	Tab, White, Cap Shaped, Debossed, Scored	Theophylline Anhydrous ER 450 mg	Theo-Dur by Sidmak	50111-0518	Antiasthmatic
SL520	Tab, Orange, Oblong	Phenylephrine 25 mg, Chlorpheniramine 8 mg, Pyrilamine 25 mg	Rynatan by Sidmak		Cold Remedy
SL521	Tab, Pink, Oblong	Carbetapentane 60 mg, Chlorpheniramine 5 mg, Ephedrine 10 mg, PhenEph. 10 mg	Rynatuss by Sidmak		Cold Remedy
SL522	Tab, Green, Oval, Film Coated, Scored	Guaifenesin 400 mg, Phenylpropanolamine HCl 75 mg	Entex La by Sidmak	50111-0522	Cold Remedy
SL523	Tab, Film Coated	Protriptyline HCl 5 mg	by Zenith Goldline	00182-2643	Antidepressant
SL523	Tab, Film Coated, Debossed	Protriptyline HCl 5 mg	by Martec	52555-0655	Antidepressant
SL523	Tab, Film Coated	Protriptyline HCl 5 mg	by Qualitest	00603-5531	Antidepressant
SL524	Tab, Golden Yellow, Film Coated	Protriptyline HCl 10 mg	by Zenith Goldline	00182-2644	Antidepressant
SL524	Tab, Film Coated, Debossed	Protriptyline HCl 10 mg	by Martec	52555-0656	Antidepressant
SL524	Tab, Film Coated	Protriptyline HCl 10 mg	by Qualitest	00603-5532	Antidepressant
SL524	Tab, Yellow, Oblong, Film Coated	Protriptyline HCl 10 mg	Vivactil by Sidmak	50111-0524	Antidepressant
SL528	Tab, Yellow, Film Coated	Choline Magnesium 500 mg	Trililsate by Geneva	00781-1637	NSAID
SL528	Tab, Yellow, Cap Shaped, Film Coated, Scored	Choline Magnesium Trisalicylate 500 mg	by Allscripts	54569-4733	NSAID
SL528	Tab, Yellow, Cap Shaped, Film Coated, Scored	Choline Magnesium Trisalicylate 500 mg	Trilisate by Sidmak	50111-0528	NSAID
SL528	Tab, Yellow, Oblong	Choline Magnesium Trisalicylate 500 mg	Trilisate by Sidmak		NSAID
SL528	Tab, Film Coated, SL/528	Choline Magnesium Trisalicylate 500 mg	Choline Magnesium Trisalicylate by Kaiser	00179-1218	NSAID
SL528	Tab, Film Coated	Choline Magnesium Trisalicylate 500 mg	Choline Magnesium Trisalicylate by Zenith Goldline	00182-1899	NSAID
SL528	Tab, Yellow, Oblong, Scored, Film Coated	Choline Magnesium Trisalicylate 500 mg	by Compumed	00403-0759	NSAID
SL528	Tab, Yellow, Oblong, Film Coated	Choline Magnesium Trisalicylate 500 mg	by Compumed	00403-0532	NSAID
SL528	Tab, Yellow, Oblong, Scored, Film Coated	Choline Magnesium Trisalicylate 500 mg	by Compumed	00403-0318	NSAID
SL528	Tab, Yellow, Oblong, Film Coated	Choline Magnesium Trisalicylate 500 mg	Choline Magnesium Trisalicylate by United Res	00677-1390	NSAID
SL529	Tab, Blue	Choline Magnesium 750 mg	Trilisate by Geneva	00781-1638	NSAID
SL529	Tab, Blue, Oblong	Choline Magnesium Trisalicylate 750 mg	Trilisate by Sidmak		NSAID
SL529	Tab, Film Coated, SL/529	Salicylate 750 mg	Choline Magnesium Trisalicylate by Kaiser	00179-1219	NSAID
SL529	Tab, Film Coated	Salicylate 750 mg	Choline Magnesium Trisalicylate by Zenith Goldline	00182-1895	NSAID
SL529	Tab, Film Coated	Salicylate 750 mg	Choline Magnesium Trisalicylate by PDRX	55289-0282	NSAID
SL529	Tab, Film Coated	Salicylate 750 mg	by Martec	52555-0529	NSAID

ID FRONT <> BACK	DESCRIPTION FRONT <> BACK	INGREDIENT & STRENGTH	BRAND (OR EQUIV.) & FIRM	NDC#	CLASS; SCH.
SL529	Tab, Film Coated	Salicylate 750 mg	Choline Magnesium Trisalicylate by Medirex	57480-0402	NSAID
SL529	Tab, Film Coated	Salicylate 750 mg	Choline Magnesium Trisalicylate by Heartland	61392-0181	NSAID
SL529	Tab, Film Coated	Salicylate 750 mg	Choline Magnesium Trisalicylate by United Res	00677-1391	NSAID
SL529	Tab, Blue, Cap Shaped, Film Coated, Scored	Salicylate 750 mg	Choline Magnesium Trisalicylate by Sidmak	50111-0529	NSAID
SL530	Tab, Pink, Oblong	Choline Magnesium Trisalicylate 1000 mg	Trilisate by Sidmak		NSAID
SL530	Tab, Film Coated, Debossed	Salicylate 1000 mg	Choline Magnesium Trisalicylate by Zenith Goldline	00182-2604	NSAID
SL530	Tab, Film Coated	Salicylate 1000 mg	by Martec	52555-0530	NSAID
SL530	Tab, Film Coated	Salicylate 1000 mg	CMT by HL Moore	00839-7619	NSAID
SL530	Tab, Pink, Cap Shaped, Film Coated, Scored	Salicylate 1000 mg	Choline Magnesium Trisalicylate by Sidmak	50111-0530	NSAID
SL534	Tab	Hydrochlorothiazide 25 mg, Triamterene 37.5 mg	by Zenith Goldline	00182-1903	Diuretic
SL534	Tab	Hydrochlorothiazide 25 mg, Triamterene 37.5 mg	by Richmond	54738-0117	Diuretic
SL534	Tab, Debossed	Hydrochlorothiazide 25 mg, Triamterene 37.5 mg	by Major	00904-5281	Diuretic
SL534	Tab, Orange, Rectangular, Scored	Hydrochlorothiazide 25 mg, Triamterene 37.5 mg	Maxzide 25 by Sidmak	50111-0534	Diuretic
SL534	Tab	Hydrochlorothiazide 25 mg, Triamterene 37.5 mg	by Qualitest	00603-6180	Diuretic
SL535	Tab, White, Oblong, Scored	Guaifenesin 600 mg	by Phy Total Care	54868-1778	Expectorant
SL535	Tab, White, Oblong, Scored	Guaifenesin 600 mg	by Lilly	00110-4415	Expectorant
SL535	Tab, White, Cap Shaped, Scored	Guaifenesin 600 mg	Humibid LA by Sidmak	50111-0535	Expectorant
SL549	Tab, Film Coated	Cimetidine 200 mg	by Sidmak	50111-0549	Gastrointestinal
SL550	Tab, White, Round, SL over 550	Cimetidine 300 mg	by ESI Lederle	59911-5550	Gastrointestinal
SL550	Tab, Film Coated, Round, Film Coated	Cimetidine 300 mg	Cimetidine USP by Compumed	00403-1068	Gastrointestinal
SL550	Tab, White, Round, Film Coated	Cimetidine 300 mg	Tagament by Sidmak	50111-0550	Gastrointestinal
SL551	Tab, White, Oblong, Scored	Cimetidine 400 mg	by Va Cmop	65243-0021	Gastrointestinal
SL551	Tab, White, Cap Shaped	Cimetidine 400 mg	by ESI Lederle	59911-5551	Gastrointestinal
SL551	Tab, White, Oblong, Scored, Film Coated	Cimetidine 400 mg	Cimetidine USP by Compumed	00403-1083	Gastrointestinal
SL551	Tab, White, Oblong, Film Coated, Scored	Cimetidine 400 mg	by Dixon Shane	17236-0447	Gastrointestinal
SL551	Tab, White, Cap Shaped, Film Coated, Scored	Cimetidine 400 mg	Tagamet by Sidmak	50111-0551	Gastrointestinal
SL552	Tab, White, Cap Shaped	Cimetidine 800 mg	by ESI Lederle	59911-5552	Gastrointestinal
SL552	Tab, White, Oblong, Scored, Film Coated	Cimetidine 800 mg	Cimetidine USP by Compumed	00403-1091	Gastrointestinal
SL552	Tab, Film Coated	Cimetidine 800 mg	by Richmond	54738-0114	Gastrointestinal
SL552	Tab, White, Cap Shaped, Film Coated, Scored	Cimetidine 800 mg	Tagamet by Sidmak	50111-0552	Gastrointestinal
SL553	Tab	Atenolol 25 mg	by Sidmak	50111-0553	Antihypertensive
SL555	Tab	Naproxen 250 mg	by Sidmak	50111-0555	NSAID
SL556	Tab	Naproxen 375 mg	by Sidmak	50111-0556	NSAID
SL558	Tab, Film Coated	Naproxen Sodium 275 mg	by Sidmak	50111-0558	NSAID
SL559	Tab, Film Coated	Naproxen Sodium 550 mg	by Sidmak	50111-0559	NSAID
SL563	Tab, Coated	Cyclobenzaprine HCl 10 mg	by Warner Chilcott	00047-0057	Muscle Relaxant
SL563	Tab, Coated	Cyclobenzaprine HCl 10 mg	by Qualitest	00603-3077	Muscle Relaxant
SL563	Tab, Coated	Cyclobenzaprine HCl 10 mg	by United Res	00677-1429	Muscle Relaxant
SL563	Tab, Yellow, Round, Film Coated	Cyclobenzaprine HCl 10 mg	by Allscripts	54569-3193	Muscle Relaxant
SL563	Tab, Yellow, Round, Film Coated	Cyclobenzaprine HCl 10 mg	by Allscripts	54569-2573	Muscle Relaxant
SL584	Tab	Glipizide 5 mg	by Sidmak	50111-0584	Antidiabetic
SL585	Tab	Glipizide 10 mg	by Sidmak	50111-0585	Antidiabetic
SL604	Tab, Green, Oval	Pseudoephedrine HCl 120 mg, Guaifenesin 600 mg	Entex PSE by Sidmak		Cold Remedy
SL605	Tab, Coated, SL over 605	Flurbiprofen 50 mg	by Sidmak	50111-0605	NSAID
SL606	Tab, Coated	Flurbiprofen 100 mg	by Sidmak	50111-0606	NSAID
SL609	Tab, Yellow, Oblong, Film Coated	Pentoxifylline 400 mg	by Pharmafab	62542-0743	Anticoagulent

ID FRONT <> BACK	DESCRIPTION FRONT <> BACK	INGREDIENT & STRENGTH	BRAND (OR EQUIV.) & FIRM	NDC#	CLASS; SCH.
SL609	Tab, Yellow, Cap Shaped, Film Coated	Pentoxifylline ER 400 mg	Trental by Sidmak	50111-0609	Anticoagulent
SL614	Tab, Green, Oblong, Film Coated	Naproxen 375 mg	by Novopharm	43806-0397	NSAID
SL614	Tab, Light Green, Cap Shaped, Film Coated	Naproxen DR 375 mg	Ec Naprosyn by Sidmak	50111-0614	NSAID
SL615	Tab, Green, Oblong, Film Coated	Naproxen 500 mg	by Novopharm	43806-0399	NSAID
SL615	Tab, Green, Cap Shaped, Film Coated	Naproxen DR 500 mg	Ec Naprosyn by Sidmak	50111-0615	NSAID
SL621	Tab, White, Round, Scored	Ketoconazole 200 mg	Nizoral by Sidmak	50111-0621	Antifungal
SL621	Tab, White, Round, Scored	Ketoconazole 200 mg	by Murfreesboro	51129-1595	Antifungal
SL66	Tab, Coated, SL Over 66	Amitriptyline HCl 10 mg	by Quality Care	60346-0354	Antidepressant
SL66	Tab, Round, Film Coated	Amitriptyline HCl 10 mg	by Apothecon	59772-2592	Antidepressant
SL66	Tab, Film Coated	Amitriptyline HCl 10 mg	by Zenith Goldline	00182-1018	Antidepressant
SL66	Tab, Film Coated, SL/66	Amitriptyline HCl 10 mg	by Qualitest	00603-2212	Antidepressant
SL66	Tab, Film Coated	Amitriptyline HCl 10 mg	by HJ Harkins Co	52959-0008	Antidepressant
SL66	Tab, Film Coated, SL/66	Amitriptyline HCl 10 mg	by Major	00904-0200	Antidepressant
SL66	Tab, Coated	Amitriptyline HCl 10 mg	by Heartland	61392-0143	Antidepressant
SL67	Tab, Coated, SL Over 67	Amitriptyline HCl 25 mg	by Quality Care	60346-0027	Antidepressant
SL67	Tab, Film Coated	Amitriptyline HCl 25 mg	by Prescription Dispensing	61807-0129	Antidepressant
SL67	Tab, Green, Round, Film Coated	Amitriptyline HCl 25 mg	Amitriptyline by Apothecon	59772-0377	Antidepressant
SL67	Tab, Green, Round, Film Coated	Amitriptyline HCl 25 mg	by Apothecon	59772-2593	Antidepressant
SL67	Tab, Film Coated	Amitriptyline HCl 25 mg	by St Marys Med	60760-0367	Antidepressant
SL67	Tab, Film Coated, SL/67	Amitriptyline HCl 25 mg	by Amerisource	62584-0614	Antidepressant
SL67	Tab, Film Coated	Amitriptyline HCl 25 mg	by Baker Cummins	63171-1019	Antidepressant
SL67	Tab, Film Coated, SL/67	Amitriptyline HCl 25 mg	by Qualitest	00603-2213	Antidepressant
SL67	Tab, Film Coated, SL/67	Amitriptyline HCl 25 mg	by Allscripts	54569-0175	Antidepressant
SL67	Tab, Film Coated, SL/67	Amitriptyline HCl 25 mg	by Med Pro	53978-0023	Antidepressant
SL67	Tab, Film Coated	Amitriptyline HCl 25 mg	by HJ Harkins Co	52959-0348	Antidepressant
SL67	Tab, Film Coated, SL/67	Amitriptyline HCl 25 mg	by Apotheca	12634-0401	Antidepressant
SL67	Tab, Film Coated, SL/67	Amitriptyline HCl 25 mg	by Major	00904-0201	Antidepressant
SLFKJ10	Tab, Film Coated	Lithium Carbonate 450 mg	Eskalith CR by Physicians Total Care	54868-2557	Antipsychotic
SLOBID100MG	Cap, Opaque & White, Slo-Bid 100 mg	Theophylline 100 mg	Slo-Bid by Rhone-Poulenc Rorer	Canadian	Antiasthmatic
SLOBID100MG <> RPR	Cap, Slo-Bid 100 mg, RPR Logo	Theophylline 100 mg	Slo Bid by RPR	00075-0100	Antiasthmatic
SLOBID125MG <> RPR	Cap, White	Theophylline 125 mg	Slo Bid by Murfreesboro Ph	51129-1668	Antiasthmatic
SLOBID125MG <> RPR	Cap, Slo-Bid 125 mg, RPR Logo	Theophylline 125 mg	Slo Bid by RPR	00075-1125	Antiasthmatic
SLOBID200MG	Cap, Opaque & White, Slo-Bid 200 mg	Theophylline 200 mg	Slo-Bid by Rhone-Poulenc Rorer	Canadian	Antiasthmatic
SLOBID200MG <> RPR	Cap, Slo-Bid 200 mg, RPR Logo	Theophylline 200 mg	Slo Bid by RPR	00075-0200	Antiasthmatic
SLOBID300MG	Cap, Opaque & White, Slo-Bid 300 mg	Theophylline 300 mg	Slo-Bid by Rhone-Poulenc Rorer	Canadian	Antiasthmatic
SLOBID300MG <> RPR	Cap, Slo-Bid 300 mg, RPR Logo	Theophylline 300 mg	Slo Bid by RPR	00075-0300	Antiasthmatic
SLOBID50MG	Cap, White, Slo-Bid 50 mg	Theophylline 50 mg	Slo-Bid by Rhone-Poulenc Rorer	Canadian	Antiasthmatic
SLOBID50MG <> RPR	Cap	Theophylline 50 mg	Slo Bid by RPR	00075-0057	Antiasthmatic
SLOBID75MG <> RPR	Cap, Slo-Bid 75 mg	Theophylline 75 mg	Slo Bid by RPR	00075-1075	Antiasthmatic
SLOWK	Tab, Light Orange, Round, Sugar Coated	Potassium Chloride 600 mg	Slow-K by Ciba	Canadian DIN# 00074225	Electrolytes
SLV <> ACEON4	Tab, Pink, Oblong	Perindopril Erbumine 4 mg	Aceon by Solvay Pharms	00032-1102	Antihypertensive
SLV <> ACEON8	Tab, Orange, Oblong, Scored	Perindopril Erbumine 8 mg	Aceon by Rhone Poulenc (PR)	00801-1103	Antihypertensive
SLVSLV <> ACEON4	Tab, Pink, Oblong, Scored	Perindopril Erbumine 4 mg	Aceon by Rhone Poulenc (PR)	00801-1102	Antihypertensive
SLVSLV <> ACEON8	Tab, Round, Oblong, Scored, SLV Score SLV<>Aceon 8	Perindopril Erbumine 8 mg	Aceon by Pharmafab	62542-0790	Antihypertensive
SMP <> I	Tab, Coated	Sumatriptan Succinate 25 mg	Imitrex by Glaxo	00173-0460	Antimigraine
SMS	Cap	Acetaminophen 250 mg, Dextromethorphan 10 mg, Guaifenesin 100 mg, Pseu 30 mg	Sudafed by Warner Wellcome	Canadian	Cold Remedy
SOLI3NT	Tab, Tan, Round, Soli/3NT	Thyroid 194.4 mg	Nature Thyroid by Jones		Thyroid
SOLINT3	Tab, Soli/NT3	Thyroid 3 gr	Parloid Thyroid Rn3 by JMI Canton	00252-3312	Thyroid
SOLVAY <> 1022	Tab, Sugar Coated	Estrogens, Esterified 0.625 mg	by Apotheca	12634-0509	Hormone
SOLVAY <> 1205	Cap, Gelatin	Amylase 16600 Units, Lipase 5000 Units, Protease 18750 Units	Creon 5 by Solvay	00032-1205	Gastrointestinal

ID FRONT <> BACK	DESCRIPTION FRONT <> BACK	INGREDIENT & STRENGTH	BRAND (OR EQUIV.) & FIRM	NDC#	CLASS; SCH.
SOLVAY <> 1210	Cap	Amylase 33200 Units, Lipase 10000 Units, Protease 37500 Units	Creon 10 by Solvay	00032-1210	Gastrointestinal
SOLVAY <> 1220	Cap	Amylase 66400 Units, Lipase 20000 Units, Protease 75000 Units	Creon 20 by Solvay	00032-1220	Gastrointestinal
SOLVAY <> 1472	Tab, Coated	Ascorbic Acid 70 mg, Calcium 200 mg, Cyanocobalamin 2.2 mcg, Folic Acid 1 mg, Iodine 175 mcg, Iron 65 mg, Magnesium 100 mg, Niacin 17 mg, Pyridoxine HCl 2.2 mg, Riboflavin 1.6 mg, Thiamine Mononitrate 1.5 mg, Vitamin A 3000 Units, Vitamin D 400 Units, Vitamin E 10 Units, Zinc 15 mg	Zenate by Leiner	59606-0497	Vitamin
SOLVAY <> 1472	Tab, Coated	Ascorbic Acid 70 mg, Calcium 200 mg, Cyanocobalamin 2.2 mcg, Folic Acid 1 mg, Iodine 175 mcg, Iron 65 mg, Magnesium 100 mg, Niacin 17 mg, Pyridoxine HCl 2.2 mg, Riboflavin 1.6 mg, Thiamine Mononitrate 1.5 mg, Vitamin A 3000 Units, Vitamin D 400 Units, Vitamin E 10 Units, Zinc 15 mg	Zenate by Solvay	00032-1472	Vitamin
SOLVAY <> 5046	Tab, White, Oblong	Eprosartan Mesylate 600 mg	Teveten by Halsey Drug	00904-5343	Antihypertensive
SOLVAY0840	Cap, Yellow	Acetaminophen 325 mg, Codeine 16 mg, Phenylephrine 10 mg, Chlorphen. 2 mg	Colrex by Solvay		Analgesic; C III
SOLVAY1007	Tab	Medroxyprogesterone Acetate 10 mg	Curretab by Solvay	00032-1007	Progestin
SOLVAY1014	Tab, Blue, Round	Estrogen Esterified 0.3 mg	Estratab by Heartland	61392-0318	Hormone
SOLVAY1014	Tab, Sugar Coated	Estrogens, Esterified 0.3 mg	by Solvay	00032-1014	Hormone
SOLVAY1022	Tab, Sugar Coated, Imprinted in Black	Estrogens, Esterified 0.625 mg	by Amerisource	62584-0022	Hormone
SOLVAY1022	Tab, Sugar Coated	Estrogens, Esterified 0.625 mg	by Solvay	00032-1022	Hormone
SOLVAY1023	Tab, Sugar Coated, Solvay 1023	Estrogens, Esterified 0.625 mg, Methyltestosterone 1.25 mg	by Quality Care	60346-0852	Hormone
SOLVAY1023	Tab, Sugar Coated	Estrogens, Esterified 0.625 mg, Methyltestosterone 1.25 mg	by Solvay	00032-1023	Hormone
SOLVAY1023	Tab, Sugar Coated	Estrogens, Esterified 0.625 mg, Methyltestosterone 1.25 mg	by Physicians Total Care	54868-3564	Hormone
SOLVAY1024	Tab, Red, Round	Esterified Estrogens 1.25 mg	Estratab by Solvay		Hormone
SOLVAY1025	Tab, Sugar Coated	Estrogens, Esterified 2.5 mg	by Solvay	00032-1025	Hormone
SOLVAY1026	Tab, Sugar Coated	Estrogens, Esterified 1.25 mg, Methyltestosterone 2.5 mg	Estratest by Nat Pharmpak Serv	55154-6501	Hormone
SOLVAY1026	Tab, Sugar Coated	Estrogens, Esterified 1.25 mg, Methyltestosterone 2.5 mg	Estratest by Solvay	00032-1026	Hormone
SOLVAY1026	Tab, Sugar Coated	Estrogens, Esterified 1.25 mg, Methyltestosterone 2.5 mg	Estratest by Physicians Total Care	54868-3565	Hormone
SOLVAY1039	Tab, White & Blue Specks, Oblong	Phenylpropanolamine 50 mg, Pyrilamine 25 mg, Chlorphen 4 mg, Phenylep 10 mg	Histalet Forte by Solvay		Cold Remedy
SOLVAY1050	Tab, White & Green Specks, Round	Pseudoephedrine HCl 120 mg, Guaifenesin 400 mg	Histalet X by Solvay		Cold Remedy
SOLVAY1082	Cap, Orange & Clear	Phendimetrazine tartrate 105 mg	Melfiat-105 by Solvay		Anorexiant; C III
SOLVAY1088	Tab, Peach, Oblong	Hydrocodone Bitartrate 5 mg, Phenindamine 25 mg, Guaifenesin 200 mg	P-V-Tussin by Solvay		Analgesic; C III
SOLVAY1091	Tab, Peach, Oblong	Hydrocodone bitartrate 5 mg, Pseudoephedrine HCl 60 mg	P-V-Tussin by Solvay		Analgesic; C III
SOLVAY1132	Tab, Yellow, Round	Hydralazine 25 mg, Reserpine 0.1 mg, Hydrochlorothiazide 15 mg	Unipres by Solvay		Antihypertensive
SOLVAY1146	Tab, Blue, Oblong	Prenatal Vitamin	Zenate by Solvay		Vitamin
SOLVAY1200	Cap, Brown & Clear	Pancreatin, Lipase, Protease, Amylase	Creon by Solvay		Gastrointestinal
SOLVAY1210	Cap, Brown & Clear	Lipase 10,000 Units, Protease 37,500 Units, Amylase 33,200 Units	Creon 10 by Murfreesboro	51129-1671	Gastrointestinal
SOLVAY1210	Cap, Brown & Clear	Lipase, Protease, Amylase	Creon-10 by Solvay		Gastrointestinal
SOLVAY1216	Cap, Brown	Vitamin Combination	Vio-Bec by Solvay		Vitamin
SOLVAY1220	Cap, Brown & Clear	Lipase 20000 Unt, Protease 75000 Unt, Amylase 66400 Unt	Creon by Phy Total Care	54868-3475	Gastrointestinal
SOLVAY1220	Cap, Brown & Clear	Lipase, Protease, Amylase	Creon-20 by Solvay		Gastrointestinal
SOLVAY1225	Cap, Orange & Yellow	Pancreatin, Lipase, Protease, Amylase	Creon-25 by Solvay		Gastrointestinal
SOLVAY1611	Tab, Peach, Oval	Vitamin, Mineral Comb.	Norlac RX by Solvay		Vitamin
SOLVAY2808	Tab	Prednisone 1 mg	Orasone by Solvay	00032-2808	Steroid
SOLVAY2810	Tab	Prednisone 5 mg	Orasone by Solvay	00032-2810	Steriod
SOLVAY2812	Tab	Prednisone 10 mg	Orasone by Solvay	00032-2812	Steriod
SOLVAY2814	Tab	Prednisone 20 mg	Orasone by Solvay	00032-2814	Steroid
SOLVAY2816	Tab, Coated	Prednisone 50 mg	Orasone by Solvay	00032-2816	Steroid
SOLVAY3205	Tab	Dexamethasone 0.5 mg	Dexone by Solvay	00032-3205	Steroid
SOLVAY3210	Tab	Dexamethasone 0.75 mg	Dexone by Solvay	00032-3210	Steroid
SOLVAY3215	Tab	Dexamethasone 1.5 mg	Dexone by Solvay	00032-3215	Steroid
SOLVAY3220	Tab	Dexamethasone 4 mg	Dexone by Solvay	00032-3220	Steroid
SOLVAY4020	Cap, Clear	Quinidine Sulfate 300 mg	Cin-Quin by Solvay		Antiarrhythmic
SOLVAY4028	Tab, White, Round	Quinidine Sulfate 200 mg	Cin-Quin by Solvay		Antiarrhythmic
SOLVAY4032	Tab, White, Round	Quinidine Sulfate 300 mg	Cin-Quin by Solvay		Antiarrhythmic

ID FRONT <> BACK	DESCRIPTION FRONT <> BACK	INGREDIENT & STRENGTH	BRAND (OR EQUIV.) & FIRM	NDC#	CLASS; SCH.
SOLVAY4120	Cap, Orange, Oval	Valproic Acid 250 mg	Depakene by Solvay		Anticonvulsant
SOLVAY4202	Tab, Film Coated	Fluvoxamine Maleate 25 mg	Luvox by Solvay	00032-4202	OCD
SOLVAY4205	Tab, Film Coated, Solvay 4205	Fluvoxamine Maleate 50 mg	Luvox by Pharm Utilization	60491-0810	OCD
SOLVAY4205	Tab, Yellow, Oval, Scored	Fluvoxamine Maleate 50 mg	Luvox by Heartland Healthcare	61392-0849	OCD
SOLVAY4205	Tab, Film Coated	Fluvoxamine Maleate 50 mg	Luvox by Solvay	00032-4205	OCD
SOLVAY4210	Tab, Film Coated, Solvay 4210	Fluvoxamine Maleate 100 mg	Luvox by Pharm Utilization	60491-0811	OCD
SOLVAY4210	Tab, Film Coated	Fluvoxamine Maleate 100 mg	Luvox by Solvay	00032-4210	OCD
SOLVAY4210	Tab, Yellow, Oval, Scored	Fluvoxamine Maleate 50 mg	Luvox by Heartland Healthcare	61392-0849	OCD
SOLVAY4492	Tab, Film Coated, In Red Ink	Lithium Carbonate 300 mg	Lithobid by Solvay	00032-4492	Antipsychotic
SOLVAY7512	Cap, Peach	Lithium Carbonate 300 mg	Lithonate by Solvay		Antipsychotic
SOLVAY7516	Tab, Embossed, Coated	Lithium Carbonate 300 mg	Lithotabs by Solvay	00032-7516	Antipsychotic
SOMA <> 37WALLACE	Tab	Carisoprodol 350 mg	Soma by Nat Pharmpak Serv	55154-4102	Muscle Relaxant
SOMA <> 37WALLACE2001	Tab, White, Round	Carisoprodol 350 mg	Soma by Rightpac	65240-0738	Muscle Relaxant
SOMA <> 37WALLACE2001	Tab, White, Round	Carisoprodol 350 mg	Soma by Thrift Services	59198-0361	Muscle Relaxant
SOMA <> 37WALLACE2001	Tab, White, Round, Soma <> 37-Wallace 2001	Carisoprodol 350 mg	Soma by Wallace	00037-2001	Muscle Relaxant
SOMA <> 37WALLACE2001	Tab, White, Round, Soma <> 37-Wallace 2001	Carisoprodol 350 mg	Soma by Caremark	00339-6143	Muscle Relaxant
SOMA37 <> WALLACE2001	Tab	Carisoprodol 350 mg	Soma by Quality Care	60346-0149	Muscle Relaxant
SOMAC <> WALLACE2103	Tab, Yellow & Light Orange, Round, Soma C <> Wallace 2103	Aspirin 325 mg, Carisoprodol 200 mg	Soma Compound by Wallace	00037-2103	Analgesic; Muscle Relaxant
SOMACC <> WALLACE24	Tab	Aspirin 325 mg, Carisoprodol 200 mg, Codeine Phosphate 16 mg	Soma Compound by Pharmedix	53002-0124	Analgesic; C III
SOMACC <> WALLACE2403	Tab, Soma CC <> Wallace over 2403	Aspirin 325 mg, Carisoprodol 200 mg, Codeine Phosphate 16 mg	Soma Compound by Quality Care	60346-0894	Analgesic; C III
SOMACC <> WALLACE2403	Tab, White & Yellow, Oval	Aspirin 325 mg, Carisoprodol 200 mg, Codeine Phosphate 16 mg	Soma Compound with Codeine by Wallace	00037-2403	Analgesic; C III
SONATA <> 10MG	Cap, Green	Zaleplon 10 mg	Sonata by Wyeth Pharms	52903-0926	Sedative/Hypnotic; C IV
SONATA <> 10MG	Cap, Green	Zaleplon 10 mg	Sonata by Wyeth Labs	00008-0926	Sedative/Hypnotic; C IV
SONATA <> 5MG	Cap, Green	Zaleplon 5 mg	Sonata by Wyeth Labs	00008-0925	Sedative/Hypnotic; C IV
SORIATANE10ROCH <> SORIATANE10ROCH	Tab, Brown, Soriatane 10 Roche	Acitretin 10 mg	Soriatane by Amerisource	62584-0075	Dermatologic
SORIATANE10ROCH <> SORIATANE10ROCH	Cap, Gelatin	Acitretin 10 mg	Soriatane by Hoffmann La Roche	00004-0213	Dermatologic
SORIATANE25ROCH <> SORIATANE25ROCH	Tab, Brown, Oval, Soriatane 25 Roche	Acitretin 25 mg	Soriatane by Amerisource	62584-0096	Dermatologic
SORIATANE25ROCH <> SORIATANE25ROCH	Cap, Gelatin	Acitretin 25 mg	Soriatane by Hoffmann La Roche	00004-0214	Dermatologic
SOTACORBL160	Tab, Light Blue, Oblong, Sotacor/BL/160	Sotalol 160 mg	Sotacor by Bristol	Canadian	Antiarrhythmic
SOTACORBL240	Tab, Light Blue, Oblong, Sotacor/BL/240	Sotalol 240 mg	Sotacor by Bristol	Canadian	Antiarrhythmic
SOTACORBL80	Tab, Light Blue, Oblong, Sotacor/BL/80	Sotalol 80 mg	Sotacor by Bristol	Canadian	Antiarrhythmic
SP <> 111	Tab, White, Round	Hyoscyamine Sulfate 0.125 mg	NuLev by Schwarz	00091-3111	Gastrointestinal
SP <> 712	Tab, Yellow, Film Coated, Scored	Hydrochlorothiazide 12.5 mg, Moexipril HCl 7.5 mg	Uniretic by Schwarz Pharma	00091-3712	Diuretic; Antihypertensive
SP <> 725	Tab, Yellow, Film Coated, S and P	Hydrochlorothiazide 25 mg, Moexipril HCl 15 mg	Uniretic by Schwarz	51217-3725	Diuretic; Antihypertensive
SP <> 725	Tab, Yellow, Film Coated, Scored	Hydrochlorothiazide 25 mg, Moexipril HCl 15 mg	Uniretic by Schwarz Pharma	00091-3725	Diuretic; Antihypertensive
SP006	Tab, Green, Hexagonal	Chlorzoxazone 250 mg, Acetaminophen 300 mg	Parafon Forte by Superpharm		Muscle Relaxant

ID FRONT <> BACK	DESCRIPTION FRONT <> BACK	INGREDIENT & STRENGTH	BRAND (OR EQUIV.) & FIRM	NDC#	CLASS; SCH.
SP01	Tab, White, Round	Furosemide 40 mg	Lasix by Superpharm		Diuretic
SP02	Tab, White, Oval	Furosemide 20 mg	Lasix by Superpharm		Diuretic
SP062	Tab, White, Round	Acetaminophen 300 mg, Codeine Phosphate 60 mg	Tylenol w/Codeine by Superpharm		Analgesic; C III
SP063	Tab, White, Round	Acetaminophen 300 mg, Codeine Phosphate 30 mg	Tylenol w/Codeine by Superpharm		Analgesic; C III
SP091	Tab, White, Round	Allopurinol 100 mg	Zyloprim by Superpharm		Antigout
SP092	Tab, Peach, Round	Allopurinol 300 mg	Zyloprim by Superpharm		Antigout
SP094	Tab, White, Round	Chlorpropamide 100 mg	Diabinese by Superpharm		Antidiabetic
SP095	Tab, White, Round	Chlorpropamide 250 mg	Diabinese by Superpharm		Antidiabetic
SP100	Tab, Yellow, Round	Doxycycline 100 mg	Vibramycin by Superpharm		Antibiotic
SP101	Cap, Blue & White	Doxycycline 50 mg	Vibramycin by Superpharm		Antibiotic
SP102	Cap, Blue	Doxycycline 100 mg	Vibramycin by Superpharm		Antibiotic
SP103	Tab, Peach, Round	Hydralazine 10 mg	Apresoline by Superpharm		Antihypertensive
SP104	Tab, Peach, Round	Hydralazine 25 mg	Apresoline by Superpharm		Antihypertensive
SP105	Tab, Peach, Round	Hydralazine 50 mg	Apresoline by Superpharm		Antihypertensive
SP106	Tab, Lavender, Round	Hydroxyzine HCl 10 mg	Atarax by Superpharm		Antihistamine
SP107	Tab, Violet, Round	Hydroxyzine HCl 25 mg	Atarax by Superpharm		Antihistamine
SP108	Tab, Purple, Round	Hydroxyzine HCl 50 mg	Atarax by Superpharm		Antihistamine
SP109	Cap, Orange & Yellow	Tetracycline HCl 250 mg	Achromycin V by Superpharm		Antibiotic
SP110	Cap, Black & Yellow	Tetracycline HCl 500 mg	Achromycin V by Superpharm		Antibiotic
SP111	Tab, White, Round	Tolbutamide 500 mg	Orinase by Superpharm		Antidiabetic
SP112	Tab, Pink, Round	Amitriptyline HCl 10 mg	Elavil by Superpharm		Antidepressant
SP113	Tab, Green, Round	Amitriptyline HCl 25 mg	Elavil by Superpharm		Antidepressant
SP114	Tab, Brown, Round	Amitriptyline HCl 50 mg	Elavil by Superpharm		Antidepressant
SP115	Tab, Purple, Round	Amitriptyline HCl 75 mg	Elavil by Superpharm		Antidepressant
SP116	Tab, Orange, Round	Amitriptyline HCl 100 mg	Elavil by Superpharm		Antidepressant
SP118	Cap, Dark Green & Light Green	Hydroxyzine Pamoate 25 mg	Vistaril by Sidmak		Antihistamine
SP119	Cap, Dk.Green & White	Hydroxyzine Pamoate 50 mg	Vistaril by Superpharm		Antihistamine
SP120	Cap, Dk.Green & Gray	Hydroxyzine Pamoate 100 mg	Vistaril by Superpharm		Antihistamine
SP121	Tab, Salmon, Round	Prednisolone 5 mg	by Superpharm		Steroid
SP122	Tab, White, Round	Prednisone 5 mg	Deltasone by Superpharm		Steroid
SP123	Tab, White, Round	Prednisone 10 mg	Deltasone by Superpharm		Steroid
SP124	Tab, Peach, Round	Prednisone 20 mg	Deltasone by Superpharm		Steroid
SP126	Cap, Green & Yellow	Chlordiazepoxide HCl 5 mg	Librium by Superpharm		Antianxiety; C IV
SP127	Cap, Black & Green	Chlordiazepoxide HCl 10 mg	Librium by Superpharm		Antianxiety; C IV
SP128	Cap, Green & White	Chlordiazepoxide HCl 25 mg	Librium by Superpharm		Antianxiety; C IV
SP129	Tab, Peach, Round	Hydrochlorothiazide 25 mg	Hydrodiuril by Superpharm		Diuretic
SP130	Tab, Peach, Round	Hydrochlorothiazide 50 mg	Hydrodiuril by Superpharm		Diuretic
SP131	Tab, Peach, Round	Hydrochlorothiazide 100 mg	Hydrodiuril by Superpharm		Diuretic
SP132	Tab, White, Round	Quinidine Sulfate 200 mg	by Superpharm		Antiarrhythmic
SP136	Tab, Orange, Round	Thioridazine 10 mg	Mellaril by Superpharm		Antipsychotic
SP137	Tab, Orange, Round	Thioridazine 25 mg	Mellaril by Superpharm		Antipsychotic
SP138	Tab, Orange, Round	Thioridazine 50 mg	Mellaril by Superpharm		Antipsychotic
SP14	Tab, White, Round	Diazepam 2 mg	Valium by Superpharm		Antianxiety; C IV
SP140	Tab, White, Round	Quinidine Gluconate SR 324 mg	Quinaglute by Superpharm		Antiarrhythmic
SP141	Tab, White, Round	Diphenoxylate HCl 2.5 mg, Atropine 0.025 mg	Lomotil by Superpharm		Antidiarrheal; C V
SP142	Cap, Clear & Pink	Diphenhydramine HCl 25 mg	Benadryl by Superpharm		Antihistamine
SP143	Cap, Pink	Diphenhydramine HCl 50 mg	Benadryl by Superpharm		Antihistamine
SP144	Tab, Blue & White, Oval	Meclizine HCl 12.5 mg	Antivert by Superpharm		Antiemetic
SP145	Tab, Yellow & White, Oval	Meclizine HCl 25 mg	Antivert by Superpharm		Antiemetic
SP146	Tab, White, Round	Sulfamethoxazole 400 mg, Trimethoprim 80 mg	Septra by Superpharm		Antibiotic
SP147	Tab, White	Sulfamethoxazole 800 mg, Trimethoprim DS 160 mg	Septra DS by Superpharm		Antibiotic
SP148	Tab, Yellow, Round	Sulfasalazine 500 mg	Azulfidine by Superpharm		Gastrointestinal

ID FRONT <> BACK	DESCRIPTION FRONT <> BACK	INGREDIENT & STRENGTH	BRAND (OR EQUIV.) & FIRM	NDC#	CLASS; SCH.
SP15	Tab, Yellow, Round	Diazepam 5 mg	Valium by Superpharm		Antianxiety; C IV
SP15 <> 715	Tab, Salmon, Film Coated, Scored	Moexipril HCl 15 mg	Univasc by Schwarz Pharma	00091-3715	Antihypertensive
SP15 <> 715	Tab, Salmon, Film Coated, SP Above & 15 Below the Score <> Both Sides	Moexipril HCl 15 mg	Univasc by Allscripts	54569-4276	Antihypertensive
SP152	Cap, Green	Indomethacin 25 mg	Indocin by Superpharm		NSAID
SP153	Cap, Green	Indomethacin 50 mg	Indocin by Superpharm		NSAID
SP154	Tab, White, Round	Spironolactone 25 mg, Hydrochlorothiazide 25 mg	Aldactazide by Superpharm		Diuretic
SP16	Tab, Blue, Round	Diazepam 10 mg	Valium by Superpharm		Antianxiety; C IV
SP161	Tab, White, Round	Metoclopramide 10 mg	Reglan by Superpharm		Gastrointestinal
SP164	Cap, Blue & Scarlet	Disopyramide Phosphate 100 mg	Norpace by Superpharm		Antiarrhythmic
SP165	Cap, Buff & Scarlet	Disopyramide Phosphate 150 mg	Norpace by Superpharm		Antiarrhythmic
SP166	Tab, White, Round	Spironolactone 25 mg	Aldactone by Superpharm		Diuretic
SP170	Tab, White, Round	Ibuprofen 400 mg	Motrin by Superpharm		NSAID
SP171	Tab, White, Oval	Ibuprofen 600 mg	Motrin by Superpharm		NSAID
SP175	Tab, Pink, Oblong	Propoxyphene Napsylate 100 mg, Acetaminophen 650 mg	Darvocet N 100 by Superpharm		Analgesic; C IV
SP181	Tab, White, Round	Lorazepam 0.5 mg	Ativan by Superpharm		Sedative/Hypnotic; C IV
SP182	Tab, White, Round	Lorazepam 1 mg	Ativan by Superpharm		Sedative/Hypnotic; C IV
SP183	Tab, White, Round	Lorazepam 2 mg	Ativan by Superpharm		Sedative/Hypnotic; C IV
SP184	Cap, Blue & White	Flurazepam HCl 15 mg	Dalmane by Superpharm		Hypnotic; C IV
SP185	Cap, Blue	Flurazepam HCl 30 mg	Dalmane by Superpharm		Hypnotic; C IV
SP189	Tab, Orange, Round	Propranolol HCl 10 mg	Inderal by Superpharm		Antihypertensive
SP190	Tab, Blue, Round	Propranolol HCl 20 mg	Inderal by Superpharm		Antihypertensive
SP191	Tab, Green, Round	Propranolol HCl 40 mg	Inderal by Superpharm		Antihypertensive
SP192	Tab, Yellow, Round	Propranolol HCl 80 mg	Inderal by Superpharm		Antihypertensive
SP20	Tab, White, Round	Pseudoephedrine HCl 60 mg	Sudafed by Superpharm		Decongestant
SP2055 <> GUAIMAXD	Tab, White to Off-White, Scored	Guaifenesin 600 mg, Pseudoephedrine HCl 120 mg	Guaimax-D by Schwarz Pharma	00131-2055	Cold Remedy
SP2104 <> 5005	Tab, White, Scored	Acetaminophen 500 mg, Hydrocodone Bitartrate 5 mg	Co Gesic by Schwarz Pharma	00131-2104	Analgesic; C III
SP2164 <> 750MG	Tab, Pink, Scored	Salsalate 750 mg	Mono-Gesic by Schwarz Pharma	00131-2164	NSAID
SP2164750MG	Tab, Pink, Round, SP 2164/750 mg	Salsalate 750 mg	Mono-Gesic by Schwarz		NSAID
SP22	Tab, Yellow, Coated, Scored	Penbutolol Sulfate 20 mg	Levatol by Schwarz Pharma	00091-4500	Antihypertensive
SP2200	Tab, Brown, Round	Polysaccharide Iron Complex 50 mg	Niferex Tablets by Schwarz Pharma	00131-2200	Vitamin
SP2209 <> 13105	Tab, Blue, Film Coated, SP 2209 <> 131/05	Calcium Carbonate, Cyanocobalamin 3 mcg, Vitamin D 400 Units, Polysaccharide Iron Complex, Folic Acid 1 mg, Niacinamide 10 mg, Pyridoxine HCl 2 mg, Riboflavin 3 mg, Sodium Ascorbate 50, Thiamine Mononitrate 3 mg, Vitamin A 4000 Units, Zinc Sulfate Monohydrate	Niferex PN by Schwarz Pharma	00131-2209	Vitamin/Mineral
SP23	Tab, Peach, Round	Chlorthalidone 25 mg	Hygroton by Superpharm		Diuretic
SP2309 <> 10	Tab, White, Cap Shaped, Film Coated, Scored	Ascorbic Acid, Calcium Carbonate, Cupric Oxide, Cyanocobalamin 12 mcg, Ergocalciferol, Ferric Polysaccharide Complex, Folic Acid 1 mg, Magnesium Oxide, Niacinamide 20 mg, Potassium Iodide, Pyridoxine HCl, Riboflavin 3.4 mg, Thiamine Mononitrate, Vitamin A Acetate, Vitamin E Acetate, Zinc Sulfate	Niferex PN Forte by Schwarz Pharma	00131-2309	Vitamin
SP24	Tab, Blue, Round	Chlorthalidone 50 mg	Hygroton by Superpharm		Diuretic
SP26	Tab, White, Round	Methocarbamol 500 mg	Robaxin by Superpharm		Muscle Relaxant
SP27	Tab, White, Oblong	Methocarbamol 750 mg	Robaxin by Superpharm		Muscle Relaxant
SP38	Cap, Green	Hydralazine 25 mg, Hydrochlorothiazide 25 mg	Apresazide by Superpharm		Antihypertensive
SP39	Cap, Dark Green & Light Green	Hydralazine 50 mg, Hydrochlorothiazide 50 mg	Apresazide by Superpharm		Antihypertensive
SP41	Tab, White, Round	Cyproheptadine HCl 4 mg	Periactin by Superpharm		Antihistamine
SP4220	Cap, Clear & Orange, Opaque w/ Brown Beads	Polysaccharide-Iron Complex 150 mg	Niferex-150 by Schwarz Pharma	00131-4220	Vitamin
SP43	Tab, White, Round	Dipyridamole 25 mg	Persantine by Superpharm		Antiplatelet
SP431	Tab, White, White, Film, Schering Plough Trademark and 431	Albuterol Sulfate 4 mg	Proventil Repetabs by Amerisource	62584-0895	Antiasthmatic
SP431	Tab, White, Film Coated, Schering Logo 431	Albuterol Sulfate ER 4 mg	Proventil by Schering	00085-0431	Antiasthmatic
SP4330	Cap, Clear & Red, Opaque, White Print, Brown Beads	Cyanocobalamin 25 mcg, Polysaccharide-Iron Complex 150 mg, Folic Acid 1 mg	Niferex-150 Forte by Schwarz Pharma	00131-4330	Vitamin
SP4330	Cap, Clear & Red	Cyanocobalamin 25 mcg; Ferric Polysaccharide Complex; Folic Acid 1 mg	Niferex Forte by Phy Total Care	54868-2600	Vitamin

ID FRONT <> BACK	DESCRIPTION FRONT <> BACK	INGREDIENT & STRENGTH	BRAND (OR EQUIV.) & FIRM	NDC#	CLASS; SCH.
SP44	Tab, White, Round	Dipyridamole 50 mg	Persantine by Superpharm		Antiplatelet
SP45	Tab, White, Round	Dipyridamole 75 mg	Persantine by Superpharm		Antiplatelet
SP49	Tab, White, Round	Triprolidine 2.5 mg, Pseudoephedrine 60 mg	Actifed by Superpharm		Cold Remedy
SP52	Tab, Pink, Round	Isosorbide Dinitrate 5 mg	Isordil by Superpharm		Antianginal
SP53	Tab, White, Round	Isosorbide Dinitrate 10 mg	Isordil by Superpharm		Antianginal
SP538	Tab, Orange, Oblong, Scored	Hyoscyamine Sulfate 0.375 mg	Levbid by Natl Pharmpak	55154-0951	Gastrointestinal
SP538	Tab, Light Orange, Scored	Hyoscyamine Sulfate 0.375 mg	Levbid by Schwarz Pharma	00091-3538	Gastrointestinal
SP538	Tab, ER	Hyoscyamine Sulfate 0.375 mg	Levbid by Caremark	00339-5930	Gastrointestinal
SP538	Tab, Orange, Oblong, Scored	Hyoscyamine Sulfate 0.375 mg	Levbid by Murfreesboro	51129-1490	Gastrointestinal
SP538	Tab, ER	Hyoscyamine Sulfate 0.375 mg	Levbid by Amerisource	62584-0019	Gastrointestinal
SP538	Tab, Orange, Oblong, Scored	Hyoscyamine Sulfate 0.375 mg	Levbid by Schwarz Pharma Mfg	00131-3538	Gastrointestinal
SP538	Tab, ER	Hyoscyamine Sulfate 0.375 mg	Levbid by Eckerd Drug	19458-0850	Gastrointestinal
SP538	Tab, Orange, Oblong, Scored	Hyoscyamine Sulfate 0.375 mg	Levbid by Thrift Services	59198-0321	Gastrointestinal
SP54	Tab, Green, Round	Isosorbide Dinitrate 20 mg	Isordil by Superpharm		Antianginal
SP57	Tab, White, Round	Tolazamide 250 mg	Tolinase by Superpharm		Antidiabetic
SP58	Tab, White, Round	Tolazamide 500 mg	Tolinase by Superpharm		Antidiabetic
SP62	Tab, White, Round	Acetaminophen 300 mg, Codeine Phosphate 60 mg	Tylenol # 4 by Superpharm		Analgesic; C III
SP63	Tab, White, Round	Acetaminophen 300 mg, Codeine Phosphate 30 mg	Tylenol # 3 by Superpharm		Analgesic; C III
SP64	Tab, White, Round	Acetaminophen 300 mg, Codeine 15 mg	Tylenol #2 by Superpharm		Analgesic; C III
SP74	Cap, Clear & Green	Chlordiazepoxide HCl 5 mg, Clidinium 2.5 mg	Librax by Superpharm		Gastrointestinal; C IV
SP75 <> 707	Tab, Pink, Film Coated, Scored, SP 7.5 <> 707	Moexipril HCl 7.5 mg	Univasc by Schwarz Pharma	00091-3707	Antihypertensive
SP78	Tab, White, Round	Ergoloid Mesylates Oral 1 mg	Hydergine by Superpharm		Ergot
SP84	Tab, White, Round	Quinine Sulfate 260 mg	Quinamm by Superpharm		Antimalarial
SP89	Tab, White, Oval	Ergoloid Mesylates SL 1 mg	Hydergine by Superpharm		Ergot
SP90	Tab, White, Round	Ergoloid Mesylates SL 0.5 mg	Hydergine by Superpharm		Ergot
SP96	Tab, White, Round	Metronidazole 250 mg	Flagyl by Superpharm		Antibiotic
SP97	Tab, White, Round	Metronidazole 500 mg	Flagyl by Superpharm		Antibiotic
SP98	Tab, White, Round	Chlorthalidone 100 mg	Hygroton by Superpharm		Diuretic
SPORANOX100 <> JANSSEN	Cap	Itraconazole 100 mg	Sporanox by Physicians Total Care	54868-3706	Antifungal
SPORANOX100 <> JANSSEN	Cap	Itraconazole 100 mg	Sporanox by Janssen	50458-0290	Antifungal
SPORANOX100 <> JANSSEN	Cap	Itraconazole 100 mg	Sporanox by Nat Pharmpak Serv	55154-1404	Antifungal
SPORANOX100 <> JANSSEN	Cap	Itraconazole 100 mg	Sporanox by Johnson & Johnson	59604-0290	Antifungal
SPORANOX100 <> JANSSEN	Cap, Sporanox 100	Itraconazole 100 mg	Sporanox by Janssen	12578-0290	Antifungal
SPRONAOX100 <> JANSSEN	Cap, Blue & Pink	Itraconazole 100 mg	Sporanox by Allscripts	54569-4869	Antifungal
SQUIBB <> 138	Tab, White, Round, Scored	Sulfamethoxazole 400 mg, Trimethoprim 80 mg	by Mutual	53489-0145	Antibiotic
SQUIBB <> 138	Tab	Sulfamethoxazole 400 mg, Trimethoprim 80 mg	SMZ TMP 400/80 by Apothecon	59772-0139	Antibiotic
SQUIBB <> 171	Tab, White, Oval Shaped, Scored	Sulfamethoxazole 800 mg, Trimethoprim 160 mg	by Mutual	53489-0146	Antibiotic
SQUIBB <> 171	Tab	Sulfamethoxazole 800 mg, Trimethoprim 160 mg	SMZ TMP 800/160 by Apothecon	59772-0174	Antibiotic
SQUIBB <> 239	Cap	Cephalexin Monohydrate	by Quality Care	60346-0055	Antibiotic
SQUIBB <> 655	Cap	Tetracycline HCl	by Prepackage Spec	58864-0493	Antibiotic
SQUIBB <> 655	Cap	Tetracycline HCl 250 mg	by Quality Care	60346-0609	Antibiotic
SQUIBB <> UNILOG181	Cap, Swedish Orange, Squibb and Unilog 181, Swedish	Cephalexin Monohydrate	by Quality Care	60346-0441	Antibiotic
SQUIBB <> W028	Cap	Cloxacillin Sodium	by Apothecon	59772-6028	Antibiotic
SQUIBB <> W048	Cap	Dicloxacillin Sodium	by Golden State	60429-0059	Antibiotic
SQUIBB <> W048	Cap, Blue	Dicloxacillin Sodium Monohydrate 250 mg	by DRX	55045-2727	Antibiotic
SQUIBB 622	Cap	Meclofenamate 50 mg	Meclomen by Squibb		NSAID

ID FRONT <> BACK	DESCRIPTION FRONT <> BACK	INGREDIENT & STRENGTH	BRAND (OR EQUIV.) & FIRM	NDC#	CLASS; SCH.
SQUIBB113	Cap, Light Blue	Cephradine 250 mg	Velosef by Bristol Myers Barcelaneta	55961-0113	Antibiotic
SQUIBB113	Cap, White Print	Cephradine 250 mg	Velosef by ER Squibb	00003-0113	Antibiotic
SQUIBB114	Cap	Cephradine 500 mg	Velosef by Bristol Myers Barcelaneta	55961-0114	Antibiotic
SQUIBB114	Cap, White Print	Cephradine 500 mg	Velosef by ER Squibb	00003-0114	Antibiotic
SQUIBB138	Tab, White, Round	Sulfamethoxazole, Trimethoprim	by ER Squibb	00003-0138	Antibiotic
SQUIBB154	Tab, White, Round	Pravastatin Sodium 10 mg	Pravachol by BMS		Antihyperlipidemic
SQUIBB15410	Tab, White, Round, Squibb 154/10	Pravastatin Sodium 10 mg	Pravachol by Squibb	Canadian	Antihyperlipidemic
SQUIBB15410	Tab, White, Round, Squibb 154/10	Pravastatin Sodium 10 mg	Pravachol by Bristol		Antihyperlipidemic
SQUIBB158M	Tab, White, Diamond	Fosinopril Sodium 10 mg	Monopril by Squibb		Antihypertensive
SQUIBB160	Tab	Erythromycin Stearate 250 mg	Ethril by Squibb		Antibiotic
SQUIBB161	Tab	Erythromycin Stearate 500 mg	Ethril by Squibb		Antibiotic
SQUIBB164	Tab	Penicillin G Potassium 125 mg	Pentids by Squibb		Antibiotic
SQUIBB165	Tab	Penicillin G Potassium 250 mg	Pentids 400 by Squibb		Antibiotic
SQUIBB168	Tab	Penicillin G Potassium 500 mg	Pentids 800 by Squibb		Antibiotic
SQUIBB171	Tab, White, Oval-Shaped	Sulfamethoxazole, Trimethoprim	by ER Squibb	00003-0171	Antibiotic
SQUIBB17820	Tab, White, Round, Squibb 178/20	Pravastatin Sodium 20 mg	Pravachol by Squibb	Canadian	Antihyperlipidemic
SQUIBB17820	Tab, White, Round, Squibb 178/20	Pravastatin Sodium 20 mg	Pravachol by BMS		Antihyperlipidemic
SQUIBB181	Cap	Cephalexin Monohydrate	by Med Pro	53978-5020	Antibiotic
SQUIBB181	Cap, Black Print	Cephalexin Monohydrate	by Bristol Myers Barcelaneta	55961-0749	Antibiotic
SQUIBB181	Cap, Black Print, Squibb 181	Cephalexin Monohydrate	by ER Squibb	00003-0749	Antibiotic
SQUIBB193	Tab	Perphenazine 2 mg, Amitriptyline HCl 10 mg	Triavil by Squibb		Antipsychotic; Antidepressant
SQUIBB19440	Tab, White, Round, Squibb 194/40	Pravastatin Sodium 40 mg	Pravachol by BMS		Antihyperlipidemic
SQUIBB195	Tab	Tolazamide 100 mg	Tolinase by Squibb		Antidiabetic
SQUIBB202	Cap	Dicloxacillin Sodium 250 mg	Dynapen by Squibb		Antibiotic
SQUIBB203	Cap	Dicloxacillin Sodium 500 mg	Dynapen by Squibb		Antibiotic
SQUIBB207	Tab, Blue, Round	Nadolol 40 mg	Corgard by Princeton		Antihypertensive
SQUIBB208	Tab, Blue, Oblong	Nadolol 120 mg	Corgard by Princeton		Antihypertensive
SQUIBB211	Cap	Cloxacillin Sodium 250 mg	Tegopen by Squibb		Antibiotic
SQUIBB212	Cap	Cloxacillin Sodium 500 mg	Tegopen by Squibb		Antibiotic
SQUIBB230	Cap, Green	Amoxicillin 250 mg	Trimox by Squibb		Antibiotic
SQUIBB231	Cap, Green & Light Green	Amoxicillin 500 mg	Trimox by Squibb		Antibiotic
SQUIBB232	Tab, Blue, Round	Nadolol 20 mg	Corgard by Princeton		Antihypertensive
SQUIBB239	Tab, Coated	Cephalexin Monohydrate	by Med Pro	53978-5021	Antibiotic
SQUIBB239	Cap, Black Print	Cephalexin Monohydrate	by Bristol Myers Barcelaneta	55961-0874	Antibiotic
SQUIBB239	Cap, Black Print, Squibb 239	Cephalexin Monohydrate	by ER Squibb	00003-0874	Antibiotic
SQUIBB241	Tab, Blue, Round	Nadolol 80 mg	Corgard by Princeton		Antihypertensive
SQUIBB246	Tab, Blue, Oblong	Nadolol 160 mg	Corgard by Princeton		Antihypertensive
SQUIBB259	Tab	Perphenazine 2 mg, Amitriptyline HCl 25 mg	Triavil by Squibb		Antipsychotic; Antidepressant
SQUIBB267	Tab	Perphenazine 4 mg, Amitriptyline HCl 10 mg	Triavil by Squibb		Antipsychotic; Antidepressant
SQUIBB271	Tab	Perphenazine 4 mg, Amitriptyline HCl 25 mg	Triavil by Squibb		Antipsychotic; Antidepressant
SQUIBB277	Tab	Tolazamide 250 mg	Tolinase by Squibb		Antidiabetic
SQUIBB279	Tab	Isosorbide Dinitrate SA 40 mg	Isordil SA by Squibb		Antianginal
SQUIBB283	Tab, White & Blue Specks, Round	Nadolol 40 mg, Bendroflumethiazide 5 mg	Corzide by Princeton		Antihypertensive
SQUIBB284	Tab, White & Blue Specks, Round	Nadolol 80 mg, Bendroflumethiazide 5 mg	Corzide by Princeton		Antihypertensive
SQUIBB286	Tab	Quinidine Gluconate 324 mg	Quinaglute by Squibb		Antiarrhythmic
SQUIBB288	Tab, Round	Allopurinol 300 mg	Zyloprim by Squibb		Antigout
SQUIBB429	Tab, Light Pink	Fludrocortisone Acetate 0.1 mg	Florinef Acetate by ER Squibb	00003-0429	Steroid
SQUIBB431	Tab, Yellow, Oblong	Procainamide HCl 250 mg	Pronestyl by Princeton		Antiarrhythmic

ID FRONT ⟺ BACK	DESCRIPTION FRONT ⟺ BACK	INGREDIENT & STRENGTH	BRAND (OR EQUIV.) & FIRM	NDC#	CLASS; SCH.
SQUIBB434	Tab, Gold, Oblong	Procainamide HCl 375 mg	Pronestyl by Princeton		Antiarrhythmic
SQUIBB438	Tab, Orange, Oblong	Procainamide HCl 500 mg	Pronestyl by Princeton		Antiarrhythmic
SQUIBB450	Tab, White, Oblong	Captopril 12.5 mg	Capoten by Squibb		Antihypertensive
SQUIBB452	Tab	Captopril 25 mg	by Pharmedix	53002-0431	Antihypertensive
SQUIBB455	Cap, Squibb over 455	Ipodate Sodium 500 mg	by Banner Pharmacaps	10888-1051	Diagnostic
SQUIBB457	Tab, Beige, Oval	Nystatin 100,000 Units	Mycostatin Vaginal by Squibb		Antifungal
SQUIBB482	Tab, White, Oval	Captopril 50 mg	Capoten by Squibb		Antihypertensive
SQUIBB485	Tab, White, Oval	Captopril 100 mg	Capoten by Squibb		Antihypertensive
SQUIBB512	Tab	Triamcinolone 4 mg	Kenacort by Squibb		Steroid
SQUIBB518	Tab	Triamcinolone 8 mg	Kenacort by Squibb		Steroid
SQUIBB535	Tab, Coated, Black Print, Squibb over 535	Calcium Pantothenate 11.7 mg, Cupric Sulfate, Anhydrous 1.675 mg, Cyanocobalamin 50 mcg, Ergocalciferol 3.3 mcg, Ferrous Fumarate 66.7 mg, Folic Acid 0.33 mg, Magnesium Carbonate 41.7 mg, Niacinamide 33.3 mg, Pyridoxine HCl 3.3 mg, Riboflavin 3.3 mg, Sodium Ascorbate 113 mg, Thiamine Mononitrate 3.3 mg, Tocopheryl Succinate 4.13 mg, Vitamin A Acetate 8333 Units, Vitamin E Acetate 5 mg	Theragran Hematinic by ER Squibb	00003-0535	Vitamin/Mineral
SQUIBB537	Tab, White, Round	Niacin 500 mg	Niacin by BMS		Vitamin
SQUIBB537	Tab, White, Round	Niacin 500 mg	Niacin by ER Squibb	00003-0537	Vitamin
SQUIBB573	Tab	Fluoxymesterone 5 mg	Ora-Testryl by Squibb		Steroid; C III
SQUIBB580	Tab, Light Yellow to Light Brown	Nystatin 500000 Units	Mycostatin by ER Squibb	00003-0580	Antifungal
SQUIBB603	Tab, Squibb over 603 in Black Ink	Tetracycline HCl 500 mg	Sumycin 500 by ER Squibb	00003-0603	Antibiotic
SQUIBB606	Tab, Green, Round	Bendroflumethiazide 5 mg	Naturetin by Princeton		Diuretic
SQUIBB611	Tab, White, Round	Niacin 50 mg	Niacin by BMS		Vitamin
SQUIBB611	Tab, White, Round	Niacin 50 mg	Niacin by ER Squibb	00003-0611	Vitamin
SQUIBB612	Tab, White, Round	Niacin 100 mg	Niacin by BMS		Vitamin
SQUIBB612	Tab, White, Round	Niacin 100 mg	Niacin by ER Squibb	00003-0612	Vitamin
SQUIBB618	Tab, Peach, Round	Bendroflumethiazide 10 mg	Naturetin by Princeton		Diuretic
SQUIBB623	Cap	Chloral Hydrate 250 mg	Noctec by Squibb		Sedative/Hypnotic; C IV
SQUIBB626	Cap	Chloral Hydrate 500 mg	Noctec by Squibb		Sedative/Hypnotic; C IV
SQUIBB629	Cap	Meclofenamate 100 mg	Meclomen by Squibb		NSAID
SQUIBB637	Tab	Isoniazid 100 mg	Nydrazid by Squibb		Antimycobacterial
SQUIBB647	Cap, White	Doxycycline Hyclate 50 mg	Vibramycin by BMS		Antibiotic
SQUIBB648	Tab, White, Oblong	Penicillin V Potassium 500 mg	Veetids by Squibb		Antibiotic
SQUIBB655	Cap	Tetracycline HCl	by Golden State	60429-0208	Antibiotic
SQUIBB655	Cap	Tetracycline HCl	Sumycin by Quality Care	60346-0484	Antibiotic
SQUIBB655	Cap	Tetracycline HCl 500 mg	by Med Pro	53978-5048	Antibiotic
SQUIBB655	Cap	Tetracycline HCl	Sumycin 250 by ER Squibb	00003-0655	Antibiotic
SQUIBB663	Tab, Light Pink, Coated	Tetracycline HCl	Sumycin 250 by ER Squibb	00003-0663	Antibiotic
SQUIBB674	Cap	Doxycycline Hyclate 50 mg	Vibramycin by Squibb		Antibiotic
SQUIBB684	Tab, Peach, Oblong	Penicillin V Potassium 250 mg	Veetids by Squibb		Antibiotic
SQUIBB690	Tab, Squibb over 690	Testolactone 50 mg	Teslac by ER Squibb	00003-0690	Hormone
SQUIBB713	Tab, Red, Round	Rauwolfia Serpentina 50 mg	Raudixin by Princeton		Antihypertensive
SQUIBB723	Cap	Phenytoin 100 mg	by Squibb		Anticonvulsant
SQUIBB726	Tab	Procainamide HCl SR 250 mg	Pronestyl by Squibb		Antiarrhythmic
SQUIBB738	Cap	Temazepam 15 mg	Restoril by Squibb		Sedative/Hypnotic; C IV
SQUIBB742	Tab	Procainamide HCl SR 500 mg	Pronestyl by Squibb		Antiarrhythmic
SQUIBB747	Cap	Temazepam 30 mg	Restoril by Squibb		Sedative/Hypnotic; C IV
SQUIBB749	Cap	Cephalexin 250 mg	Keflex by Squibb		Antibiotic
SQUIBB756	Cap, White & Orange	Procainamide HCl 375 mg	Pronestyl by Princeton		Antiarrhythmic
SQUIBB757	Cap, Yellow & Orange	Procainamide HCl 500 mg	Pronestyl by Princeton		Antiarrhythmic
SQUIBB758	Cap, Yellow & Orange	Procainamide HCl 250 mg	Pronestyl by Princeton		Antiarrhythmic
SQUIBB763	Cap	Tetracycline HCl	by Golden State	60429-0209	Antibiotic
SQUIBB763	Cap	Tetracycline HCl 500 mg	by Quality Care	60346-0435	Antibiotic

ID FRONT <> BACK	DESCRIPTION FRONT <> BACK	INGREDIENT & STRENGTH	BRAND (OR EQUIV.) & FIRM	NDC#	CLASS; SCH.
SQUIBB763	Cap	Tetracycline HCl	Sumycin 500 by ER Squibb	00003-0763	Antibiotic
SQUIBB769	Tab, Green, Round	Rauwolfia Serpentina 50 mg, Bendroflumethiazide 4 mg	Rauzide by Princeton		Antihypertensive
SQUIBB775	Tab, Yellow, Oval	Procainamide HCl SR 500 mg	Pronestyl-SR by Princeton		Antiarrhythmic
SQUIBB776	Tab, Red, Round	Rauwolfia Serpentina 100 mg	Raudixin by Princeton		Antihypertensive
SQUIBB777	Tab	Procainamide HCl SR 750 mg	Pronestyl by Squibb		Antiarrhythmic
SQUIBB779	Cap	Tetracycline 250 mg, Amphotericin B 50 mg	Mysteclin-F by Squibb		Antibiotic
SQUIBB788	Tab, Round	Allopurinol 300 mg	Zyloprim by Squibb		Antigout
SQUIBB812	Tab, Tan, Round	Doxycycline Hyclate 100 mg	Vibramycin by BMS		Antibiotic
SQUIBB830	Cap, Pink & Green	Hydroxyurea 500 mg	Hydrea by Squibb		Antineoplastic
SQUIBB834	Tab	Multivitamin, Iron, Biotin	Theragran Stress by Squibb		Vitamin
SQUIBB842	Tab	Multivitamin	Theragran by Squibb		Vitamin
SQUIBB845	Tab, Round	Allopurinol 100 mg	Zyloprim by Squibb		Antigout
SQUIBB849	Tab	Multivitamin, Minerals	Theragran M by Squibb		Vitamin
SQUIBB863	Tab, Pink, Round	Fluphenazine HCl 1 mg	Prolixin by BMS		Antipsychotic
SQUIBB864	Tab, Yellow, Round	Fluphenazine HCl 2.5 mg	Prolixin by Princeton		Antipsychotic
SQUIBB874	Cap	Cephalexin 500 mg	Keflex by Squibb		Antibiotic
SQUIBB877	Tab, Green, Round	Fluphenazine HCl 5 mg	Prolixin by Princeton		Antipsychotic
SQUIBB940	Cap, White	Doxycycline Hyclate 100 mg	Vibramycin by BMS		Antibiotic
SQUIBB956	Tab, Dark Pink, Round	Fluphenazine HCl 10 mg	Prolixin by Princeton		Antipsychotic
SQUIBB971	Cap, Gray	Ampicillin 250 mg	Principen by Squibb		Antibiotic
SQUIBB974	Cap, Dark Gray & Gray	Ampicillin 500 mg	Principen by Squibb		Antibiotic
SQUIBBW028	Cap, Squibb and W028	Cloxacillin Sodium	by Quality Care	60346-0345	Antibiotic
SQUIBBW038	Cap, Orange, Opaque, Squibb/W 038	Cloxacillin Sodium 500 mg	Tegopen by BMS		Antibiotic
SQUIBBW048	Cap, Blue	Dicloxacillin Sodium 250 mg	by Apothecon	57783-6048	Antibiotic
SQUIBBW048	Cap, Blue	Dicloxacillin Sodium 250 mg	by Apothecon	59772-6048	Antibiotic
SQUIBBW048	Cap	Dicloxacillin Sodium 250 mg	by Quality Care	60346-0480	Antibiotic
SQUIBBW058	Cap, Squibb W058	Dicloxacillin Sodium	by Quality Care	60346-0229	Antibiotic
SQUIBBW058	Cap, Blue	Dicloxacillin Sodium 500 mg	by Apothecon	57783-6058	Antibiotic
SQUIBBW058	Cap, Blue	Dicloxacillin Sodium 500 mg	by Apothecon	59772-6058	Antibiotic
SR	Cap, Orange, SR over Abbott Logo	Fenofibrate Micronized 200 mg	TriCor by Abbott	00074-6415	Antihyperlipidemic
SR <> NASABID	Tab, S/R <> Nasabid	Guaifenesin 600 mg, Pseudoephedrine HCl 90 mg	Nasabid Sr by Anabolic	00722-6356	Cold Remedy
SR <> NASABID	Tab, Yellow, Oval, Scored	Guaifenesin 600 mg, Pseudoephedrine HCl 90 mg	Nasabid Sr by Jones	52604-0600	Cold Remedy
SR100	Tab, Pink, Round, SR/100	Diclofenac Sodium 100 mg	Novo Difenac by Novopharm	Canadian	NSAID
SR100NOVO	Tab, White, Round, SR/100/Novo	Diclofenac Sodium 100 mg	by Novopharm	Canadian	NSAID
SR120 <> CALAN	Tab, Light Violet, Film Coated	Verapamil HCl 120 mg	Calan Sr by Quality Care	60346-0298	Antihypertensive
SR120 <> CALAN	Tab, Light Violet, Oval, Film Coated Tab	Verapamil HCl 120 mg	Calan Sr by GD Searle	00025-1901	Antihypertensive
SR180 <> 7711	Tab, Film Coated	Verapamil 180 mg	by Qualitest	00603-6359	Antihypertensive
SR180 <> 7711	Tab, Off White, Film Coated	Verapamil HCl 180 mg	by Quality Care	60346-0781	Antihypertensive
SR180 <> CALAN	Cap, Light Pink, Oval, Film Coated	Calan SR 180 mg	by Allscripts	54569-8555	Antihypertensive
SR180 <> CALAN	Tab, Light Pink	Verapamil HCl 180 mg	Calan Sr by GD Searle	00025-1911	Antihypertensive
SR180 <> CALAN	Tab, Tab Ex Release	Verapamil HCl 180 mg	Calan Sr by Nat Pharmpak Serv	55154-3616	Antihypertensive
SR180 <> CALAN	Tab, Tab Ex Release	Verapamil HCl 180 mg	Calan Sr by Allscripts	54569-3802	Antihypertensive
SR180 <> Z4286	Tab, Film Coated	Verapamil 180 mg	by Qualitest	00603-6359	Antihypertensive
SR180 <> Z4286	Tab, Film Coated	Verapamil HCl 180 mg	by Warner Chilcott	00047-0472	Antihypertensive
SR180 <> Z4286	Tab, Film Coated	Verapamil HCl 180 mg	by Major	00904-7956	Antihypertensive
SR200	Tab, White, Round	Theophylline 200 mg	Theolair by 3M Pharmaceuticals	Canadian	Antiasthmatic
SR200 <> 3M	Tab, Tab Ex Release	Theophylline 200 mg	by Urgent Care Ctr	50716-0505	Antiasthmatic
SR200 <> 3M	Tab, White, Round, Scored	Theophylline 200 mg	Theolair SR by 3M	00089-0341	Antiasthmatic
SR240 <> 7722	Tab, Off White, Film Coated	Verapamil HCl 240 mg	by DRX	55045-2321	Antihypertensive
SR240 <> 7722	Tab, Film Coated	Verapamil HCl 240 mg	by Qualitest	00603-6360	Antihypertensive
SR240 <> 7722	Tab, Film Coated	Verapamil HCl 240 mg	by United Res	00677-1453	Antihypertensive
SR240 <> 7722	Tab, Off-White, Film Coated	Verapamil 240 mg	by Quality Care	60346-0959	Antihypertensive

ID FRONT <> BACK	DESCRIPTION FRONT <> BACK	INGREDIENT & STRENGTH	BRAND (OR EQUIV.) & FIRM	NDC#	CLASS; SCH.
SR240 <> CALAN	Tab, Green, Oblong, Film Coated, Scored	Verapamil HCl 240 mg	Calan SR by Rx Pac	65084-0141	Antihypertensive
SR240 <> CALAN	Tab, Light Green, Cap-Shaped, Film Coated Tab, SR/240	Verapamil HCl 240 mg	Calan Sr by GD Searle	00014-1891	Antihypertensive
SR240 <> CALAN	Tab, Light Green, Film Coated	Verapamil HCl 240 mg	Calan Sr by Nat Pharmpak Serv	55154-3615	Antihypertensive
SR240 <> CALAN	Tab, SR/240, Film Coated	Verapamil HCl 240 mg	by Med Pro	53978-0588	Antihypertensive
SR240 <> CALAN	Tab, Light Green, Cap-Shaped, Film Coated Tab	Verapamil 240 mg	Calan Sr by GD Searle	00025-1891	Antihypertensive
SR240 <> Z4280	Tab, Film Coated	Verapamil HCl 240 mg	by Warner Chilcott	00047-0474	Antihypertensive
SR240 <> Z4280	Tab, Film Coated	Verapamil HCl 240 mg	by Med Pro	53978-2029	Antihypertensive
SR240 <> Z4280	Tab, Film Coated	Verapamil HCl 240 mg	by Major	00904-7957	Antihypertensive
SR240 <> Z4280	Tab, Film Coated	Verapamil HCl 240 mg	by Qualitest	00603-6360	Antihypertensive
SR240 <> Z4280	Tab, Off-White, Film Coated	Verapamil HCl 240 mg	by HL Moore	00839-7670	Antihypertensive
SR250	Tab, White, Round	Verapamil 240 mg	by Quality Care	60346-0959	Antihypertensive
SR250 <> 3M	Tab, White, Round, Scored	Theophylline 250 mg	Theolair by 3M Pharmaceuticals	Canadian	Antiasthmatic
SR300	Tab, White, Oval	Theophylline 250 mg	Theolair SR by 3M	00089-0345	Antiasthmatic
SR300 <> 3M	Tab, White, Oval, Scored	Theophylline 300 mg	Theolair by 3M Pharmaceuticals	Canadian	Antiasthmatic
SR500	Tab, White, Oblong	Theophylline 300 mg	Theolair SR by 3M	00089-0343	Antiasthmatic
SR500 <> 3M	Tab, White, Cap Shaped, Scored	Theophylline 500 mg	Theolair by 3M Pharmaceuticals	Canadian	Antiasthmatic
SR672	Tab, Tab Ex Release	Theophylline 500 mg	Theolair SR by 3M	00089-0347	Antiasthmatic
SR672	Tab, Tab Ex Release	Hyoscyamine Sulfate 0.375 mg	Symax Sr by Sovereign	58716-0672	Gastrointestinal
SR75	Tab, Pink, Triangular, SR/75	Hyoscyamine Sulfate 0.375 mg	Symax Sr by ION	11808-0112	Gastrointestinal
SR75 <> VOLTAREN	Tab, Light Pink, Triangular, Film Coated	Diclofenac Sodium 75 mg	Novo Difenac by Novopharm	Canadian	NSAID
		Diclofenac Sodium 75 mg	Voltaren SR by Novartis	Canadian DIN# 00782459	NSAID
SR75NOVO	Tab, White, Triangular, SR/75/Novo	Diclofenac Sodium 75 mg	by Novopharm	Canadian	NSAID
SRNASABID	Tab, Yellow, Oval, SR/Nasabid	Guaifenesin 600 mg, Pseudoephedrine 90 mg	Nasabid SR by Jones		Cold Remedy
SS	Tab, Orange, Round, S/S	Sennoside 8.6 mg, Docusate NA 50 mg	Senokot-S by Purdue Frederick	Canadian	Gastrointestinal
SS121	Tab, White, Round	Tiopronin 100 mg	Thiola by Mission		Urinary Tract
SSANDOZ7852	Tab, White, Round	Mephenytoin 100 mg	Mesantoin by Sandoz		Anticonvulsant
ST3 <> 2243850	Cap, Blue & Pink, ST-3 <> 224 3850	Ephedra, White Willow Bark, Grapefruit, Kola Nut, Chitosan	Stacker 3 by NVE Pharm		Supplement
STAGESIC	Cap, in Blue Ink	Acetaminophen 500 mg, Hydrocodone Bitartrate 5 mg	Stagesic by Huckaby	58407-0091	Analgesic; C III
STAHIST	Tab, STA/Hist	Atropine Sulfate 40 mcg, Chlorpheniramine Maleate 8 mg, Hyoscyamine Sulfate 190 mcg, Phenylephrine HCl 25 mg, Phenylpropanolamine HCl 50 mg, Scopolamine Hydrobromide 10 mcg	Stahist by Anabolic	00722-6243	Cold Remedy
STARLIX <> 120	Tab, Yellow, Oval	Nateglinide 120 mg	Starlix by Novartis	00078-0352	Antidiabetic
STARLIX <> 60	Tab, Pink, Round	Nateglinide 60 mg	Starlix by Novartis	00078-0351	Antidiabetic
STASON <> 1011	Tab, 10/11	Captopril 12.5 mg	by Stason	60763-1011	Antihypertensive
STASON <> 1012	Tab, Off-White, Diamond, Cross Scored	Captopril 25 mg	by Stason Pharms	60763-1012	Antihypertensive
STASON <> 1013	Tab, White, Diamond Shaped, Stason <> 10/13	Captopril 50 mg	by Duramed	51285-0957	Antihypertensive
STASON <> 1013	Tab, White, Diamond, Scored	Captopril 50 mg	by Stason Pharms	60763-1013	Antihypertensive
STASON <> 1014	Tab, Oblong, Scored	Captopril 100 mg	by Stason Pharms	60763-1014	Antihypertensive
STASON <> 10X12	Tab, White, Diamond Shaped	Captopril 25 mg	by Duramed	51285-0956	Antihypertensive
STASON1020	Tab, Off-White, Round, Stason-1020	Selegiline HCl 5 mg	Eldepryl by Stason	51285-0020	Antiparkinson
STDS911	Tab, White, Oval, S/T DS 911	Sulfamethoxazole 800 mg, Trimethoprim 160 mg	Septra DS by Lemmon		Antibiotic
STSS <> 910	Tab, White, ST/SS, Round	Sulfamethoxazole 400 mg, Trimethoprim 80 mg	by Teva	00093-0088	Antibiotic
STUART021	Tab, Yellow, Oblong	Multivitamin, Multimineral combination	Stuartnatal 1+1 by Zeneca		Vitamin
STUART071	Tab, Pink, Oblong	Multivitamin, Multimineral combination	Stuart Prenatal by Zeneca		Vitamin
STUART145 <> ZESTORETIC	Tab	Hydrochlorothiazide 25 mg, Lisinopril 20 mg	Zestoretic 20 25 by Caremark	00339-5848	Diuretic; Antihypertensive
STUART220	Tab, White, Oval	Belladonna Alkaloids, Phenobarbital	Kinesed by Zeneca		Gastrointestinal; C IV
STUART380	Cap, Brown	Docusate Potassium 240 mg	Kasof by Zeneca		Laxative
STUART41	Tab, Film Coated	Amitriptyline HCl 50 mg	Elavil by Leiner	59606-0638	Antidepressant
STUART41	Tab, Film Coated	Amitriptyline HCl 50 mg	Elavil by Prestige Packaging	58056-0292	Antidepressant

ID FRONT <> BACK	DESCRIPTION FRONT <> BACK	INGREDIENT & STRENGTH	BRAND (OR EQUIV.) & FIRM	NDC#	CLASS; SCH.
STUART45	Tab, Film Coated	Amitriptyline HCl 25 mg	Elavil by Prestige Packaging	58056-0291	Antidepressant
STUART450	Tab, White, Round	Simethicone 40 mg	Mylicon by Zeneca		Antiflatulent
STUART455	Tab, Pink, Round	Simethicone 125 mg	Mylicon-125 by Zeneca		Antiflatulent
STUART470	Cap, Pink	Docusate Potassium 100 mg	Dialose by Zeneca		Laxative
STUART475	Cap, Yellow	Docusate Potassium 100 mg, Casanthranol 30 mg	Dialose Plus by Zeneca		Laxative
STUART620	Tab, White & Yellow, Round	Aluminum 200 mg, Magnesium Hydroxide 200 mg, Simethicone 20 mg	Mylanta by Zeneca		Gastrointestinal
STUART650	Tab, Brown & Yellow, Round	Chewable Hematinic	Ferancee by Zeneca		Vitamin
STUART651	Tab, Green & White, Round	Aluminum 400 mg, Magnesium Hydroxide 400 mg, Simethicone 40 mg	Mylanta II by Zeneca		Gastrointestinal
STUART710	Tab, Orange, Round	Fluoride, Multivitamins	Mulvidren-F by Zeneca		Vitamin/Mineral
STUART858	Tab, Pink, Round	Simethicone 80 mg	Mylicon-80 by Zeneca		Antiflatulent
STUART864	Tab, Yellow, Round	Buclizine HCl 50 mg	Bucladin-S Softab by Zeneca		Antiemetic
SUDAFED12HOUR	Cap, White	Pseudoephedrine HCl 120 mg	Sudafed by Warner Wellcome	Canadian	Decongestant
SUDAFEDA7C	Cap, WhiteSudafed/A7C	Psuedoephedrine 60 mg, Acetaminophen 50 mg	Sudafed by Warner Wellcome	Canadian	Cold Remedy
SUDAFEDS7A	Tab, White, Biconvex	Pseudoephedrine HCl 60 mg	Sudafed by Warner Wellcome	Canadian	Decongestant
SUDAL120	Tab, Yellow, Oblong	Pseudoephedrine HCl 120 mg, Guaifenesin 600 mg	SUDAL 120/600 by Atley		Cold Remedy
SUDAL60	Tab, White	Pseudoephedrine HCl 60 mg, Guaifenesin 500 mg	SUDAL 60/500 by Atley		Cold Remedy
SUDAL60 <> AP	Tab, White, Tab Ex Release, Cap Shaped	Guaifenesin 500 mg, Pseudoephedrine HCl 60 mg	Sudal by Atley	59702-0060	Cold Remedy
SUDAL60 <> AP	Tab, Sudal 60 <> A over P	Guaifenesin 500 mg, Pseudoephedrine HCl 60 mg	Sudal by Anabolic	00722-6395	Cold Remedy
SUDAL60 <> AP	Tab, White, Oblong, Scored, Sudal 60 <> A over P	Guaifenesin 500 mg, Pseudoephedrine HCl 60 mg	GFN 500 PSEH 60 by Martec		Cold Remedy
SUDALDM	Tab, White, Oblong	Dextromethorphan Hydrobromide 30 mg, Guaifenesin 500 mg	SUDAL DM by Atley		Cold Remedy
SUDALDM <> AP	Tab, White, Oblong, Scored, Sudal DM <> A over P	Guaifenesin 500 mg, Dextromethorphan Hydriodide 30 mg	GFN 500 DTMH 30 by Martec		Cold Remedy
SUDALDMA <> P	Tab, White, Cap Shaped, P Scored	Dextromethorphan 30 mg, Guaifenesin 500 mg	Sudal DM by Atley	59702-0305	Cold Remedy
SULCRATEMMDC	Tab, White, Oblong, Sulcrate/MMDC	Sucralfate 1 g	by Hoechst Marion Roussel	Canadian	Gastrointestinal
SULFAMETHOXAZO <> TRIMETHOPRIM160	Tab	Sulfamethoxazole 800 mg, Trimethoprim 160 mg	by HL Moore	00839-6406	Antibiotic
SUPERMINI	Tab, Dark Brown, Round	Ephedra 250 mg 10%	Super Mini by BDI		Supplement
SUPRAX <> LL200	Tab, Film Coated	Cefixime 200 mg	Suprax by Quality Care	60346-0220	Antibiotic
SUPRAX <> LL400	Tab, Coated	Cefixime 400 mg	Suprax by PDRX	55289-0954	Antibiotic
SUPRAX <> LL400	Tab, Coated, Scored	Cefixime 400 mg	Suprax by Quality Care	60346-0846	Antibiotic
SUPRAX <> LL400	Tab, Coated	Cefixime 400 mg	Suprax by Lederle	00005-3897	Antibiotic
SUPRAX <> LL400	Tab, Coated, Scored	Cefixime 400 mg	Suprax by Physicians Total Care	54868-1383	Antibiotic
SUPRAX <> LL400	Tab, Coated	Cefixime 400 mg	Suprax by Allscripts	54569-2861	Antibiotic
SUPRAX <> LL400	Tab, Coated	Cefixime 400 mg	Suprax by Dept Health Central Pharm	53808-0062	Antibiotic
SUPROPD	Cap, Opaque, Supro/PD	Gabapentin 100 mg	Neurontin by Parke-Davis	Canadian	Anticonvulsant
SUPROPD	Cap, Yellow & Opaque, Supro/PD	Gabapentin 300 mg	Neurontin by Parke-Davis	Canadian	Anticonvulsant
SUPROPD	Cap, Orange & Opaque, Supro/PD	Gabapentin 400 mg	Neurontin by Parke-Davis	Canadian	Anticonvulsant
SURGAM200	Tab, White, Biconvex, Surgam/200	Tiaprofenic 200 mg	Surgam by Hoechst Roussel	Canadian	NSAID
SURGAM300	Tab, White, Biconvex, Surgam/300	Tiaprofenic 300 mg	Surgam by Hoechst Roussel	Canadian	NSAID
SURGAMSR	Cap, Pink & Maroon	Tiaprofenic 300 mg	Surgam by Hoechst Roussel	Canadian	NSAID
SUSTIVA <> 100MG	Cap, White	Efavirenz 100 mg	Sustiva by Dupont Pharma	00056-0473	Antiviral
SUSTIVA <> 200MG	Cap, Gold	Efavirenz 200 mg	Sustiva by Dupont Pharma	00056-0474	Antiviral
SUSTIVA <> 50MG	Cap, Gold & White	Efavirenz 50 mg	Sustiva by Dupont Pharma	00056-0470	Antiviral
SV	Cap, Peach	Progesterone 100 mg	Prometrium by West Pharm	52967-0290	Progestin
SV	Cap, Peach, Round	Progesterone 100 mg	Prometrium by Solvay	00032-1708	Progestin
SV	Cap, Cap Gelatin Coated	Progesterone 100 mg	Prometrium by RP Scherer	11014-0856	Progestin
SV	Cap, Peach	Progesterone 100 mg	Prometrium by Schering	00085-0869	Progestin
SV2	Cap, Yellow	Progesterone 200 mg	Prometrium by Scherer Rp North	11014-1147	Progestin
SV2	Cap, Yellow	Progesterone 200 mg	Prometrium by Solvay Pharms	00032-1711	Progestin
SW <> 200	Tab	Tiludronate Disodium 240 mg	Skelid by Sanofi	00024-1800	Bisphosphonate
SW <> 200	Tab	Tiludronate Disodium 240 mg	Skelid by Sanofi Winthrop	53360-1800	Bisphosphonate
SYC B	Tab, White, Oval	Bromocriptine Mesylate 2.5 mg	by SynCare	Canadian	Antiparkinson
SYC B 5MG	Cap, Caramel & White	Bromocriptine Mesylate 5 mg	by SynCare	Canadian	Antiparkinson

ID FRONT <> BACK	DESCRIPTION FRONT <> BACK	INGREDIENT & STRENGTH	BRAND (OR EQUIV.) & FIRM	NDC#	CLASS; SCH.
SYC160	Tab, Light Blue, Oblong	Sotalol HCl 160 mg	by AltiMed	Canadian DIN# 02084236	Antiarrhythmic
SYC80	Tab, Light Blue, Oblong	Sotalol HCl 80 mg	by AltiMed	Canadian DIN# 02084228	Antiarrhythmic
SYCAMSYCAM	Tab, Peach, Diamond, Syc/AM/Syc-AM	Hydrochlorothiazide 50 mg, Amiloride 5 mg	by MSD	Canadian DIN# 02174596	Diuretic; Antihypertensive
SYCBMZ15	Tab, White, Cylindrical, Syc-BMZ/1.5	Bromazepam 1.5 mg	by AltiMed	Canadian	Sedative
SYCBMZ3	Tab, Pink, Cylindrical, Syc-BMZ/3	Bromazepam 3 mg	by AltiMed	Canadian	Sedative
SYCBMZ6	Tab, Green, Cylindrical, Syc-BMZ/6	Bromazepam 6 mg	by AltiMed	Canadian	Sedative
SYCC125	Tab, White, Oblong, Syc/C12.5	Captopril 12.5 mg	by SynCare	Canadian	Antihypertensive
SYCC25	Tab, White, Square, Syc/C25	Captopril 25 mg	by SynCare	Canadian	Antihypertensive
SYCCL05	Tab, Pale Peach, Cylindrical, Syc-CL 0.5	Clonazepam 0.5 mg	by AltiMed	Canadian DIN# 02103656	Anticonvulsant
SYCCL05	Tab, Orange, Cylindrical, Syc-CL 0.5	Clonazepam 0.5 mg	by Altimed	Canadian	Anticonvulsant
SYCCL2	Tab, White, Cylindrical, Syc-CL 2	Clonazepam 2 mg	by AltiMed	Canadian DIN# 02103737	Anticonvulsant
SYCCY10	Tab, Yellow, D-Shaped, Syc/CY 10	Cyclobenzaprine 10 mg	by AltiMed	Canadian DIN# 02174618	Muscle Relaxant
SYCCYU10	Tab, White, Syc/CYü10	LL A minocaproic Acid, A10 A minocaproic Acid	by Bristol	Canadian	Hemostatic
SYCD30	Tab, Green, Syc-D30	Diltiazem 30 mg	by Altimed	Canadian DIN# 00888524	Antihypertensive
SYCD60	Tab, Yellow, Syc-D60	Diltiazem 60 mg	by Altimed	Canadian DIN# 00888532	Antihypertensive
SYCN160	Tab, Blue, Oblong, Syc/N160	Nadolol 160 mg	by AltiMed	Canadian	Antihypertensive
SYCN40	Tab, Off-White, Round, Syc/N40	Nadolol 40 mg	by Altimed	Canadian	Antihypertensive
SYCN40	Tab, White, Round, Scored	Nadolol 40 mg	by Altimed	Canadian DIN# 00851663	Antihypertensive
SYCN80	Tab, White, Round, Syc/N80	Nadolol 80 mg	by AltiMed	Canadian	Antihypertensive
SYCT100	Tab, White, Round, Syc/T100	Trazodone 100 mg	by AltiMed	Canadian DIN# 02053195	Antidepressant
SYCT50	Tab, Orange, Round, Syc/T50	Trazadone HCl 50 mg	by AltiMed	Canadian DIN# 02053187	Antidepressant
SYCT50	Tab, Orange, Round, Syc/T50	Trazodone 50 mg	by Altimed	Canadian	Antidepressant
SYCT75	Tab, Orange, Rectangular, Syc-T/75	Trazodone 150 mg	by Altimed	Canadian DIN# 02053209	Antidepressant
SYCTCP <> 250	Tab, White, Oval, Film Coated, Syc-TCP <> 250	Ticlopidine HCl 250 mg	by Altimed	Canadian DIN# 02194422	Anticoagulant
SYMMETREL	Tab, Orange, Triangular	Amantadine HCl 100 mg	Symmetrel by Endo		Antiviral
SYMMETREL	Tab	Amantadine HCl 100 mg	by Du Pont Pharma	00056-0108	Antiviral

ID FRONT <> BACK	DESCRIPTION FRONT <> BACK	INGREDIENT & STRENGTH	BRAND (OR EQUIV.) & FIRM	NDC#	CLASS; SCH.
SYMMETREL	Tab, Light Orange, Triangular	Amantadine HCl 100 mg	Symmetrel by Endo Labs	63481-0108	Antiviral
SYMMETREL <> DUPONTPHARMA	Cap	Amantadine HCl 100 mg	by Dupont Pharma	00056-0315	Antiviral
SYNCAREM2MIN50MG	Cap, Orange, SynCare M2/Min 50 mg	Minocycline HCl 50 mg	by AltiMed	Canadian	Antibiotic
SYNCAREM4MIN100MG	Cap, Orange & Purple, SynCare M4/Min 100 mg	Minocycline HCl 100 mg	by AltiMed	Canadian	Antibiotic
SYNCARESYC100	Tab, White, Oval, SynCare/Syc/100	Captopril 100 mg	by SynCare	Canadian	Antihypertensive
SYNCARESYC50	Tab, White, Oval, SynCare/Syc/50	Captopril 50 mg	by SynCare	Canadian	Antihypertensive
SYNCARESYCC100	Tab, White, Oval, Syncare/Syc/C100	Captopril 100 mg	by Altimed	Canadian DIN# 00851655	Antihypertensive
SYNCARESYCC50	Tab, White, Oval, SynCare/Syc/C50	Captopril 50 mg	by Altimed	Canadian DIN# 00851647	Antihypertensive
SYNCARESYCN160	Tab, Blue, Oblong, SynCare/Syc/N160	Nadolol 160 mg	by Altimed	Canadian DIN# 00851698	Antihypertensive
SYNCARESYCN80	Tab, Off-White, Round, SynCare/Syc/N80	Nadolol 80 mg	by Altimed	Canadian DIN# 00851671	Antihypertensive
SYNFLEX	Tab, Blue, Oval	Naproxen Sodium 275 mg	by AltiMed	Canadian DIN# 00675369	NSAID
SYNFLEX DS	Tab, Blue, Oval	Naproxen Sodium 550 mg	by AltiMed	Canadian DIN# 01900897	NSAID
SYNTEC	Tab, Blue, Round	Norethindrone 0.5 mg, Ethinyl Estradiol 35 mcg	Brevicon by Searle	Canadian	Oral Contraceptive
SYNTEX	Tab, Yellow, Oblong	Naproxen 500 mg	Naprosyn by Roche	Canadian	NSAID
SYNTEX	Tab, Peach, Oblong	Naproxen 375 mg	Naprosyn by Roche	Canadian	NSAID
SYNTEX	Tab, Film Coated	Naproxen Sodium 275 mg	Anaprox by Amerisource	62584-0274	NSAID
SYNTEX <> 274	Tab, Film Coated	Naproxen Sodium 275 mg	Anaprox by Allscripts	54569-0264	NSAID
SYNTEX <> 274	Tab, Light Blue, Film Coated	Naproxen Sodium 275 mg	Anaprox by Quality Care	60346-0727	NSAID
SYNTEX <> ANAPROXDS	Tab, Anaprox DS, Film Coated	Naproxen Sodium 550 mg	Anaprox DS by Quality Care	60346-0035	NSAID
SYNTEX <> NAPROSYN250	Tab	Naproxen 250 mg	Naprosyn by Quality Care	60346-0092	NSAID
SYNTEX <> NAPROXEN250	Tab	Naproxen 250 mg	by Pharmedix	53002-0324	NSAID
SYNTEX <> TORADOL	Tab, Red Print, Film Coated	Ketorolac Tromethamine 10 mg	Toradol by Quality Care	60346-0446	NSAID
SYNTEX1	Tab, White, Round	Norethindrone 1 mg, Mestranol 0.05 mg	Norinyl by Syntex		Oral Contraceptive
SYNTEX110	Tab, Blue, Round	Norethindrone 0.5 mg, Ethinyl Estradiol 0.035 mg	Brevicon by Syntex		Oral Contraceptive
SYNTEX111	Tab, Green, Round	Norethindrone 1 mg, Ethinyl Estradiol 0.035 mg	Norinyl by Syntex		Oral Contraceptive
SYNTEX2437 CARDENE20MG	Cap, White	Nicardipine HCl 20 mg	Cardene by Roche	Canadian	Antihypertensive
SYNTEX2438 CARDENE30MG	Cap, Blue	Nicardipine HCl 30 mg	Cardene by Roche	Canadian	Antihypertensive
SYNTEX2440 <> CARDENESR30MG	Cap	Nicardipine HCl 30 mg	Cardene Sr by Physicians Total Care	54868-3817	Antihypertensive
SYNTEX272	Tab, Yellow, Round	Naproxen 250 mg	Naprosyn by Syntex		NSAID
SYNTEX273	Tab, Peach, Oblong	Naproxen 375 mg	Naprosyn by Syntex		NSAID
SYNTEX277	Tab, Yellow, Oblong	Naproxen 500 mg	Naprosyn by Syntex		NSAID
SYNTEX2902	Tab, White, Round	Oxymetholone 50 mg	Anadrol-50 by Syntex		Steroid
SYNTEX3	Tab, Yellow, Round	Norethindrone 1 mg, Mestranol 0.08 mg	Norinyl by Syntex		Oral Contraceptive

ID FRONT ⟷ BACK	DESCRIPTION FRONT ⟷ BACK	INGREDIENT & STRENGTH	BRAND (OR EQUIV.) & FIRM	NDC#	CLASS; SCH.
SYNTEX50	Tab, White, Syntex/50	Oxymethelone 50 mg	Syntex by Roche	Canadian	Steroid
SYNTEX50	Tab, White, Round	Oxymetholone 50 mg	Anapolon by Syntex		Steroid
SYNTEXBX	Tab, Blue, Circular, Syntex/BX	Norethindrone 0.5 mg, Ethinyl Estradiol 0.035 mg	by Searle	Canadian	Oral Contraceptive
T	Tab, Lavender, Round	Acetaminophen 80 mg	Tempra by MJ	Canadian	Antipyretic
T	Tab, Orange, Round	Aspirin 325 mg	Ecotrin by Geneva		Analgesic
T	Cap, Round Ball Shaped, Cap Gelatin Coated	Benzonatate 100 mg	by Quality Care	60346-0101	Antitussive
T	Cap	Benzonatate 100 mg	Tessalon Perles by Quality Care	60346-0766	Antitussive
T	Cap, Clear & Yellow, Round Perle, Gelatin	Benzonatate 100 mg	Tessalon Perles by Forest	00456-0688	Antitussive
T	Cap	Benzonatate 100 mg	Tessalon by Allscripts	54569-0618	Antitussive
T	Cap, Gelatin Coated	Benzonatate 100 mg	by Allscripts	54569-4091	Antitussive
T	Cap	Benzonatate 100 mg	Tessalon Perles by RP Scherer	11014-0732	Antitussive
T	Tab, Orange, Round	Iodinated Glycerol 30 mg	Organidin by Trinity		Expectorant
T	Tab, Green, Round	Potassium Bicarbonate 2.5g	Effervescent by Tower Labs.		Electrolytes
T	Tab, Orange, Round	Potassium Bicarbonate 2.5g	Effervescent by Tower Labs.		Electrolytes
T	Tab, Tab Efferv	Potassium Bicarbonate 2500 mg	K Efferv Potassium by Qualitest	00603-4170	Electrolytes
T	Tab, Tab Efferv	Potassium Bicarbonate 2500 mg	Efferv Potassium by Bajamar Chem	44184-0024	Electrolytes
T	Tab, Tab Efferv	Potassium Bicarbonate 2500 mg	Efferv Potassium by Tower	50201-2400	Electrolytes
T	Tab, Tab Efferv	Potassium Bicarbonate 2500 mg	Efferv Potassium by Tower	50201-2401	Electrolytes
T ⟷ 100MG	Tab, Yellow, Round, Coated	Carbamazepine XR 100 mg	Tegretol XR by Novartis	00083-0061	Anticonvulsant
T ⟷ 100MG	Tab, Yellow, Round	Carbamazepine 100 mg	Tegretol XR by Caremark	00339-6131	Anticonvulsant
T ⟷ 107	Tab, White, Round	Atenolol 25 mg	Tenormin by AstraZeneca	00310-0107	Antihypertensive
T ⟷ 109	Tab	Carbamazepine 200 mg	by Baker Cummins	63171-1233	Anticonvulsant
T ⟷ 200MG	Tab, Pink, Round, Coated	Carbamazepine XR 200 mg	Tegretol XR by Novartis	00083-0062	Anticonvulsant
T ⟷ 400MG	Tab, Film Coated	Carbamazepine 400 mg	by Physicians Total Care	54868-3862	Anticonvulsant
T ⟷ 400MG	Tab, Brown, Round, Coated	Carbamazepine XR 400 mg	Tegretol XR by Novartis	00083-0060	Anticonvulsant
T 109	Tab, Coated	Carbamazepine 200 mg	by Physicians Total Care	54868-0147	Anticonvulsant
T013	Tab, White, Round, Scored, T over 013	Hyoscyamine Sulfate 0.125 mg	by Murfreesboro	51129-1498	Gastrointestinal
T024	Tab, White, Round	Colchicine 0.6 mg	by DRX Pharm Consults	55045-2420	Antigout
T024	Tab	Colchicine 0.6 mg	by Qualitest	00603-3052	Antigout
T024	Tab	Colchicine 0.6 mg	by Major	00904-2047	Antigout
T024	Tab, White, Round, Scored, T over 024	Colchicine 0.6 mg	by Dixon	17236-0635	Antigout
T03	Tab, Pale Blue, Round	Hyoscyamine SL 0.125 mg	Levsin by Trinity		Gastrointestinal
T03	Tab, Greenish White	Hyoscyamine Sulfate 0.125 mg	by Zenith Goldline	00182-2603	Gastrointestinal
T03	Tab, Green, Round, Scored, T over 03	Hyoscyamine Sulfate 0.125 mg	by Murfreesboro	51129-1499	Gastrointestinal
T04	Tab, Light Blue, T/04	Hyoscyamine 0.15 mg	by Shire Richwood	58521-0295	Gastrointestinal
T04	Tab, Blue, Round, Scored	Hyoscyamine Sulfate 0.15 mg	by Murfreesboro	51129-1497	Gastrointestinal
T04	Tab, Blue, Round	Meperidine HCl 50 mg	Cytospaz by Trinity		Analgesic; C II
T05	Tab, White, Round	Yohimbine HCl 5.4 mg	Yocon by Trinity		Impotence Agent
T1 ⟷ LL	Tab, Dark Red, Coated	Ascorbic Acid 600 mg, Cobalamin Concentrate 25 mcg, Docusate Sodium 50 mg, Ferrous Fumarate 350 mg, Folic Acid 1 mg, Intrinsic Factor 75 mg, Tocopheryl Succinate 30 Units	Trihemic 600 by Lederle	00005-4590	Vitamin
T1 ⟷ NU	Tab, White, Round	Terazosin HCl 1 mg	by Nu Pharm	Canadian DIN# 02233047	Antihypertensive
T10	Tab, Aqua, Round	Haloperidol 10 mg	Peridol by Technilab	Canadian	Antipsychotic
T10	Tab, Aquamarine, Round, Scored	Haloperidol 10 mg	by Altimed	Canadian DIN# 00728306	Antipsychotic
T10	Tab, White, Round, T/10	Tamoxifen Citrate 10 mg	Tamofen by Rhone-Poulenc Rorer	Canadian	Antiestrogen
T10 ⟷ NU	Tab, Blue, Round	Terazosin HCl 10 mg	by Nu Pharm	Canadian DIN# 02233050	Antihypertensive

ID FRONT <> BACK	DESCRIPTION FRONT <> BACK	INGREDIENT & STRENGTH	BRAND (OR EQUIV.) & FIRM	NDC#	CLASS; SCH.
T109	Tab, T/109	Carbamazepine 200 mg	by Zenith Goldline	00182-1233	Anticonvulsant
T109	Tab, White, Round, Scored, T over 109	Carbamazepine 200 mg	by Teva	00093-0109	Anticonvulsant
T109	Tab	Carbamazepine 200 mg	by Caremark	00339-5941	Anticonvulsant
T109	Tab, White, Round	Carbamazepine 200 mg	Epitol by Caremark	00339-6133	Anticonvulsant
T109	Tab	Carbamazepine 200 mg	by Allscripts	54569-2655	Anticonvulsant
T109	Tab	Carbamazepine 200 mg	by Med Pro	53978-1070	Anticonvulsant
T109	Tab, T Over 109	Carbamazepine 200 mg	by Quality Care	60346-0777	Anticonvulsant
T109	Tab, White to Off-White, Round, Scored, T over 109	Carbamazepine 200 mg	Tegretol by UDL	51079-0385	Anticonvulsant
T11	Tab, White, Round, T-11	Carbamazepine 200 mg	Tegretol by Taro	52549-4005	Anticonvulsant
T11	Tab, White, Round, T-11	Carbamazepine 200 mg	Tegretol by Taro	51672-4005	Anticonvulsant
T121	Tab, Blue, Round	Atro, Hyoscy, Methenamine, M.Blue, Phenyl Sal, Benz. Ac	Urised by Trinity		Urinary Tract
T142	Tab, Burgundy, Round	Phenazopyridine HCl 200 mg	Pyridium by Trinity		Urinary Analgesic
T147	Tab, Burgundy, Round	Phenazopyridine HCl 200 mg	Pyridium by Trinity		Urinary Analgesic
T17	Tab, White, Oval	Aspirin 800 mg	Zorprin by Interpharm		Analgesic
T2	Tab, Pink, Round	Haloperidol 2 mg	Peridol by Technilab	Canadian	Antipsychotic
T2	Tab, Pink, Round, Scored	Haloperidol 2 mg	by Altimed	Canadian DIN# 00728292	Antipsychotic
T2 <> NU	Tab, Orange, Round	Terazosin HCl 2 mg	by Nu Pharm	Canadian DIN# 02233048	Antihypertensive
T20	Tab, White, Round, T/20	Tamoxifen Citrate 20 mg	Tamofen by Rhone-Poulenc Rorer	Canadian	Antiestrogen
T27 <> WINTHROP	Tab	Aspirin 325 mg, Pentazocine HCl	Talwin Compound by Sanofi	00024-1927	Analgesic; C IV
T27 <> WINTHROP	Tab	Aspirin 325 mg, Pentazocine HCl	Talwin Compound by Searle	00966-1927	Analgesic; C IV
T3 <> M	Tab, White, Round, Film Coated	Trifluoperazine HCl 1 mg	Stelazine by UDL	51079-0572	Antipsychotic
T3 <> M	Tab, White, Film Coated, Beveled Edge	Trifluoperazine HCl	by Mylan	00378-2401	Antipsychotic
T31	Tab, Pink, Oblong, Flat, Scored	Warfarin Sodium 1 mg	Warfarin Sodium USP by Thrift Drug	59198-0351	Anticoagulant
T31	Tab, Pink, Oblong, Scored	Warfarin Sodium 1 mg	by Goldline Labs	00182-2671	Anticoagulant
T31	Tab, Light Pink, Cap-Shaped	Warfarin Sodium 1 mg	Coumadin by Taro	51672-4027	Anticoagulant
T31 <> W	Tab, T and 31, Tab Coated	Iopanoic Acid 500 mg	Telepaque by Nycomed	00407-1931	Diagnostic
T32	Tab, Pink, Round	Amobarbital 100 mg	Amytal by Lilly		Sedative/Hypnotic; C II
T32	Tab, Lavender, Cap-Shaped	Warfarin Sodium 2 mg	Coumadin by Taro	51672-4028	Anticoagulant
T32	Tab, Purple, Oblong, Flat, Scored	Warfarin Sodium 2 mg	Warfarin Sodium by Thrift Drug	59198-0352	Anticoagulant
T32	Tab, Purple, Oblong, Scored	Warfarin Sodium 2 mg	by Goldline Labs	00182-2672	Anticoagulant
T33	Tab, Green, Oblong, Flat, Scored	Warfarin Sodium 2.5 mg	Warfarin Sodium by Thrift Drug	59198-0353	Anticoagulant
T33	Tab, Green, Cap-Shaped	Warfarin Sodium 2.5 mg	Coumadin by Taro	51672-4029	Anticoagulant
T33	Tab, Green, Oblong, Scored	Warfarin Sodium 2.5 mg	by Goldline Labs	00182-2673	Anticoagulant
T34	Tab, Blue, Cap-Shaped	Warfarin Sodium 4 mg	Coumadin by Taro	51672-4031	Anticoagulant
T34	Tab, Blue, Oblong, Flat, Scored	Warfarin Sodium 4 mg	Warfarin Sodium by Thrift Drug	59198-0357	Anticoagulant
T34	Tab, Blue, Oblong, Scored	Warfarin Sodium 4 mg	by Goldline Labs	00182-2675	Anticoagulant
T35	Tab, White, Round	Calcium Carbonate 10 gr	by Lilly		Vitamin/Mineral
T35	Tab, Peach, Cap-Shaped	Warfarin Sodium 5 mg	Coumadin by Taro	51672-4032	Anticoagulant
T35	Tab, Peach, Oblong, Flat, Scored	Warfarin Sodium 5 mg	Warfarin Sodium by Torpharm	62318-0018	Anticoagulant
T35	Tab, Peach, Oblong, Scored	Warfarin Sodium 5 mg	by Goldline Labs	00182-2676	Anticoagulant
T36	Tab, Yellow, Cap-Shaped	Warfarin Sodium 7.5 mg	Coumadin by Taro	51672-4034	Anticoagulant
T36	Tab, Yellow, Oblong, Flat, Scored	Warfarin Sodium 7.5 mg	Warfarin Sodium by Torpharm	62318-0020	Anticoagulant
T36	Tab, Yellow, Oblong, Scored	Warfarin Sodium 7.5 mg	by Goldline Labs	00182-2678	Anticoagulant
T37	Tab	Acetaminophen 650 mg, Pentazocine HCl	Talacen by Pharmedix	53002-0514	Analgesic; C IV
T37	Tab, Orange, Round	Amobarbital 50 mg	Amytal by Lilly		Sedative/Hypnotic; C II
T37	Tab, White, Cap-Shaped	Warfarin Sodium 10 mg	Coumadin by Taro	51672-4035	Anticoagulant
T37	Tab, White, Oblong, Flat, Scored	Warfarin Sodium 10 mg	Warfarin Sodium by Torpharm	62318-0021	Anticoagulant
T37	Tab, White, Oblong, Scored	Warfarin Sodium 10 mg	by Goldline Labs	00182-2679	Anticoagulant

ID FRONT <> BACK	DESCRIPTION FRONT <> BACK	INGREDIENT & STRENGTH	BRAND (OR EQUIV.) & FIRM	NDC#	CLASS; SCH.
T37 <> WINTHROP	Tab, Light Blue	Acetaminophen 650 mg, Pentazocine HCl	Talacen by Quality Care	60346-0985	Analgesic; C IV
T38	Tab, Tan, Cap-Shaped	Warfarin Sodium 3 mg	Coumadin by Taro	51672-4030	Anticoagulant
T38	Tab, Tan, Oblong, Flat, Scored	Warfarin Sodium 3 mg	Warfarin Sodium by Thrift Drug	59198-0354	Anticoagulant
T38	Tab, Tan, Oblong, Scored	Warfarin Sodium 3 mg	by Goldline Labs	00182-2674	Anticoagulant
T39	Tab, Greenish-Yellow, Cap-Shaped	Warfarin Sodium 6 mg	Coumadin by Taro	51672-4033	Anticoagulant
T39	Tab, Yellow, Oblong, Flat, Scored	Warfarin Sodium 6 mg	Warfarin Sodium by Torpharm	62318-0019	Anticoagulant
T39	Tab, Green, Oblong, Scored	Warfarin Sodium 6 mg	by Goldline Labs	00182-2677	Anticoagulant
T4 <> M	Tab, White, Round, Film Coated	Trifluoperazine HCl 2 mg	Stelazine by UDL	51079-0573	Antipsychotic
T4 <> M	Tab, White, Round, Film Coated	Trifluoperazine HCl 2 mg	by Dixon Shane	17236-0293	Antipsychotic
T4 <> M	Tab, White, Film Coated, Beveled Edge	Trifluoperazine HCl	by Mylan	00378-2402	Antipsychotic
T41	Tab, Burgundy, Round	Phenazopyridine HCl 100 mg	Pyridium by Trinity		Urinary Analgesic
T45	Tab, Purple, Round, Scored	Clorazepate Dipotassium 3.75 mg	by Taro Pharms (US)	51672-4042	Antianxiety; C IV
T45	Tab, Purple, Round, Scored	Clorazepate Dipotassium 3.75 mg	by Taro Pharm (IS)	52549-4042	Antianxiety; C IV
T46	Tab, Purple, Round, Scored	Clorazepate Dipotassium 15 mg	by Taro Pharm (IS)	52549-4044	Antianxiety; C IV
T46	Tab, Orange, Round, Scored	Clorazepate Dipotassium 7.5 mg	by Taro Pharms (US)	51672-4043	Antianxiety; C IV
T46	Tab, Orange, Round, Scored	Clorazepate Dipotassium 7.5 mg	by Taro Pharm (IS)	52549-4043	Antianxiety; C IV
T46	Tab, White, Round	Sulfapyridine 500 mg	by Lilly		Dermatitis Herpetifornis Suppressant
T47	Tab, Pink, Round, Scored	Clorazepate Dipotassium 15 mg	by Taro Pharms (US)	51672-4044	Antianxiety; C IV
T5	Tab, Green, Round	Haloperidol 5 mg	Peridol by Technilab	Canadian	Antipsychotic
T5	Tab, Green, Round, Scored	Haloperidol 5 mg	by Altimed	Canadian DIN# 00647969	Antipsychotic
T5 <> M	Tab, Lavender, Round, Film Coated	Trifluoperazine HCl 5 mg	Stelazine by UDL	51079-0574	Antipsychotic
T5 <> M	Tab, Purple, Round, Film Coated	Trifluoperazine HCl 5 mg	by Dixon Shane	17236-0296	Antipsychotic
T5 <> M	Tab, Lavender, Film Coated, Beveled Edge	Trifluoperazine HCl	by Mylan	00378-2405	Antipsychotic
T5 <> NU	Tab, Tan, Round	Terazosin HCl 5 mg	by Nu Pharm	Canadian DIN# 02233049	Antihypertensive
T51 <> W	Tab, T.51	Naloxone HCl 0.5 mg, Pentazocine HCl	Talwin Nx by Allscripts	54569-0022	Analgesic; C IV
T51 <> W	Tab, T 51	Naloxone HCl 0.5 mg, Pentazocine HCl 50 mg	Talwin Nx by Sanofi	00024-1951	Analgesic; C IV
T51 <> W	Tab, T 51	Naloxone HCl 0.5 mg, Pentazocine HCl 50 mg	Talwin Nx by Searle	00966-1951	Analgesic; C IV
T51 <> W	Tab, Yellow, Oblong, Scored	Naloxone HCl 50 mg	by Novartis	17088-0005	Analgesic; C IV
T52	Tab, White, Round	Acetazolamide 125 mg	Diamox by Taro	51672-4022	Diuretic
T52	Tab, White, Round	Acetazolamide 125 mg	Diamox by Taro	52549-4022	Diuretic
T53	Tab, White, Round	Acetazolamide 250 mg	Diamox by Taro	51672-4023	Diuretic
T53	Tab, White, Round	Acetazolamide 250 mg	Diamox by Taro	52549-4023	Diuretic
T54	Tab, White, Round	Sulfadiazine 500 mg	by Lilly		Antibiotic
T55	Tab, White, Round	Papaverine HCl 100 mg	by Lilly		Vasodilator
T56	Tab, Yellow, Round	Amobarbital 30 mg	Amytal by Lilly		Sedative/Hypnotic; C II
T57	Tab, T Over 57, Tab Ex Release	Atropine Sulfate 0.04 mg, Chlorpheniramine Maleate 8 mg, Hyoscyamine Sulfate 0.19 mg, Phenylephrine HCl 25 mg, Phenylpropanolamine HCl 50 mg, Scopolamine Hydrobromide 0.01 mg	Pro Tuss by Quality Care	60346-0287	Cold Remedy
T57	Tab	Atropine Sulfate 0.04 mg, Chlorpheniramine Maleate 8 mg, Hyoscyamine Sulfate 0.19 mg, Phenylephrine HCl 25 mg, Phenylpropanolamine HCl 50 mg, Scopolamine Hydrobromide 0.01 mg	Phenchlor Sha by Rugby	00536-4410	Cold Remedy
T57	Tab	Atropine Sulfate 0.04 mg, Chlorpheniramine Maleate 8 mg, Hyoscyamine Sulfate 0.19 mg, Phenylphrine HCl 25 mg, Phenylpropanolamine HCl 50 mg, Scopolamine Hydrobromide 0.01 mg	Pro Tuss by United Res	00677-1418	Cold Remedy
T57	Tab, T/57	Atropine Sulfate 40 mcg, Chlorpheniramine Maleate 8 mg, Hyoscyamine Sulfate 190 mcg, Phenylphrine HCl 25 mg, Phenylpropanolamine HCl 50 mg, Scopolamine Hydrobromide 10 mcg	Pro Tuss by Anabolic	00722-6073	Cold Remedy

ID FRONT <> BACK	DESCRIPTION FRONT <> BACK	INGREDIENT & STRENGTH	BRAND (OR EQUIV.) & FIRM	NDC#	CLASS; SCH.
T57	Tab, White, Round, Flat, Scored	Ketoconazole 200 mg	Ketoconazole by Murfreesboro	51129-1593	Antifungal
T57	Tab, Off-White, Round	Ketoconazole 200 mg	Nizoral by Taro	51672-4026	Antifungal
T6 <> M	Tab, Purple, Round, Film Coated	Trifluoperazine HCl 10 mg	by Dixon Shane	17236-0334	Antipsychotic
T6 <> M	Tab, Lavender, Round, Film Coated	Trifluoperazine HCl 5 mg	Stelazine by UDL	51079-0575	Antipsychotic
T6 <> M	Tab, Lavender, Film Coated, Beveled Edge	Trifluoperazine HCl	by Mylan	00378-2410	Antipsychotic
T66	Tab	Carbinoxamine Maleate 8 mg, Pseudoephedrine HCl 120 mg	Carbodec by Rugby	00536-4453	Cold Remedy
T67	Tab, Film Coated, T-67	Carbinoxamine Maleate 8 mg, Pseudoephedrine HCl 120 mg	Andec TR by Anabolic	00722-6077	Cold Remedy
T73	Tab, White, Round	Papaverine HCl 200 mg	P 200 by Lilly		Vasodilator
T750 <> PF	Tab, Film Coated	Choline Magnesium Trisalicylate 750 mg	Trilisate by Purdue Frederick	00034-0505	NSAID
T750 <> PF	Tab, Film Coated	Choline Magnesium Trisalicylate 750 mg	Trilisate 750 by Allscripts	54569-2493	NSAID
T77	Tab, Coated	Carbinoxamine Maleate 4 mg, Pseudoephedrine HCl 60 mg	Cardec by Zenith Goldline	00182-1199	Cold Remedy
T77	Tab, Coated	Carbinoxamine Maleate 4 mg, Pseudoephedrine HCl 60 mg	Carbodec by Rugby	00536-4452	Cold Remedy
T77	Tab, Coated, T-77	Carbinoxamine Maleate 4 mg, Pseudoephedrine HCl 60 mg	Andec by Anabolic	00722-6082	Cold Remedy
T88	Tab, Peach, Oval, Film Coated	Etodolac 400 mg	by Taro Pharms (US)	51672-4018	NSAID
T88	Tab, Peach, Oval, Film Coated	Etodolac 400 mg	by Taro Pharm (IS)	52549-4018	NSAID
T93	Tab, White, Round	Isoniazid 100 mg	by Lilly		Antimycobacterial
T95	Tab, White, Round	Sulfamerazine 167 mg, Sulfamethazine 167 mg	Neotrizine by Lilly		Antibiotic
T96	Tab, White, Round	Neomycin Sulfate 500 mg	by Lilly		Antibiotic
T99	Tab, Yellow, Round	Paramethasone Acetate 1 mg	Haldrone by Lilly		Steroid
TA	Tab, Pink, Round, Chewable	Acetaminophen 80 mg, Pseudoephedrine HCl 7.5 mg, Diphenhydramine HCl 6.25 mg	Children's Tylenol Allergy- ChewableTablets by McNeil	Canadian DIN# 02240560	Cold Remedy
TA	Tab, Pink, Round	Metronidazole 250 mg	Childrens Tylenol Allergy D Chewable by McNeil	50580-0827	Antibiotic
TAGAMET <> 300SB	Tab, Light Green, Film Coated	Cimetidine 300 mg	Tagamet by Quality Care	60346-0001	Gastrointestinal
TAGAMET <> 300SKF	Tab, Film Coated	Cimetidine 300 mg	by Pharmedix	53002-0328	Gastrointestinal
TAGAMET <> 400SB	Tab, Light Green, Film Coated	Cimetidine 400 mg	Tagamet by Quality Care	60346-0706	Gastrointestinal
TAGAMET300B	Tab, Light Green, Round, Tagamet/300/SB	Cimetidine 300 mg	Tagamet by SKB	00108-5013	Gastrointestinal
TAGAMET400SB	Tab, Light Green, Round, Tagamet/400/SB	Cimetidine 400 mg	Tagamet by SKB	00108-5026	Gastrointestinal
TAGAMET400SB	Tab, Film Coated, Tagamet/400/SB	Cimetidine 400 mg	Tagamet by Kaiser	00179-1108	Gastrointestinal
TAGAMET800SB	Tab, Light Green, Round, Tagamet/800/SB	Cimetidine 800 mg	Tagamet by SKB	00108-5027	Gastrointestinal
TAGAMETSB <> 300	Tab, Film Coated	Cimetidine 300 mg	Tagamet by HJ Harkins Co	52959-0270	Gastrointestinal
TAGAMETSB300	Tab, Light Green, Film Coated, Tagamet-SB-300	Cimetidine 300 mg	Tagamet by Kaiser	00179-0156	Gastrointestinal
TAGAMETSB300	Tab, Film Coated	Cimetidine 300 mg	Tagamet by Allscripts	54569-0438	Gastrointestinal
TAGAMETSB400	Tab, Film Coated	Cimetidine 400 mg	Tagamet by Allscripts	54569-0439	Gastrointestinal
TAP <> PREVACID15	Cap, Green & Pink	Lansoprazole 15 mg	Prevacid by Abbott	00074-1541	Gastrointestinal
TAP <> PREVACID30	Cap, Black & Pink	Lansoprazole 30 mg	Prevacid by Va Cmop	65243-0044	Gastrointestinal
TAP <> PREVACID30	Cap, Pink & Black, Tap <> Prevacid over 30	Lansoprazole 30 mg	Prevacid by PDRX	55289-0451	Gastrointestinal
TAP <> PREVACID30	Cap, Black & Pink, Hard Gel	Lansoprazole 30 mg	Prevacid by Abbott	00074-3046	Gastrointestinal
TAP <> PREVACID30	Cap, Black & Pink	Lansoprazole 30 mg	Prevacid by Compumed	00403-2121	Gastrointestinal
TARGRETIN	Cap, White	Bexarotene 75 mg	Targretin by Scherer Rp North	11014-1263	Antineoplastic - Retinoid
TARGRETIN	Cap, White	Bexarotene 75 mg	Targretin by Ligand	64365-0502	Antineoplastic - Retinoid
TARKA <> 242	Tab, Light Orange, Oblong, Coated	Verapamil HCL 240 mg, Trandolapril 2 mg	by Knoll		Antihypertensive
TARO	Tab, White, Round	Carbamazepine 200 mg	by Taro	Canadian	Anticonvulsant
TARO <> 89	Tab, Blue, Oval, Film Coated	Etodolac 500 mg	by Taro Pharm (IS)	52549-4036	NSAID
TARO <> 89	Tab, Blue, Oval, Film Coated	Etodolac 500 mg	by Taro Pharms US	51672-4036	NSAID
TARO25	Cap, Blue	Clomipramine 25 mg	Anafranil by Taro	51672-4011	OCD
TARO50	Cap, Yellow	Clomipramine 50 mg	Anafranil by Taro	51672-4012	OCD
TARO75	Cap, White	Clomipramine 75 mg	Anafranil by Taro	51672-4013	OCD
TAS <> 500	Cap, Yellow, Film Coated	Acetaminophen 500 mg, Chlorpheniramine Maleate 2mg, Pseudoephedrine HCl 30 mg	Extra Strength Tylenol Allergy Sinus by McNeil	Canadian DIN# 01933728	Cold Remedy

ID FRONT <> BACK	DESCRIPTION FRONT <> BACK	INGREDIENT & STRENGTH	BRAND (OR EQUIV.) & FIRM	NDC#	CLASS; SCH.
TASMAR100	Tab, Beige, Hexagon, Convex, Film	Tolcapone 100 mg	Tasmar by Teva	00480-0100	Antiparkinson
TASMAR100 <> ROCHE	Tab, Film Coated	Tolcapone 100 mg	Tasmar by Hoffmann La Roche	00004-5920	Antiparkinson
TASMAR200 <> ROCHE	Tab, Reddish-Brown, Film Coated	Tolcapone 200 mg	Tasmar by Hoffmann La Roche	00004-5921	Antiparkinson
TAVISTD	Tab	Clemastine Fumarate 1.34 mg, Phenylpropanolamine HCl 75 mg	Tavist D by Pharmedix	53002-0371	Cold Remedy
TC	Tab, White, Round, Abbott Logo	Methamphetamine HCl 2.5 mg	Desoxyn by Abbott		Stimulant; C II
TCL <> 019	Cap	Papaverine HCl 150 mg	by UDL	51079-0010	Vasodilator
TCL <> 019	Cap, in Black Ink, Cap Ex Release	Papaverine HCl 150 mg	Para Time by Time Caps	49483-0019	Vasodilator
TCL <> 022	Tab, Engraved	Thyroid 65 mg	by Time Caps	49483-0022	Thyroid
TCL <> 036	Cap, Black Print	Chlorpheniramine Maleate 4 mg, Phenylephrine HCl 20 mg, Phenyltoloxamine Citrate 50 mg	Com Time by Time Caps	49483-0036	Cold Remedy; C III
TCL <> 038	Tab, Engraved	Thyroid 195 mg	by Time Caps	49483-0038	Thyroid
TCL <> 039	Tab, Sugar Coated, White Print	Brompheniramine Maleate 12 mg, Phenylephrine HCl 15 mg, Phenylpropanolamine HCl 15 mg	Dime Time by Time Caps	49483-0039	Cold Remedy
TCL <> 041	Cap, Blue-Green, White Print	Chlorpheniramine Maleate 8 mg	by Time Caps	49483-0041	Antihistamine
TCL <> 043	Cap, Blue-Green, Black Print	Chlorpheniramine Maleate 12 mg	by Time Caps	49483-0043	Antihistamine
TCL <> 1221	Cap	Nitroglycerin 2.5 mg	by Schein	00364-0174	Vasodilator
TCL <> 1221	Cap, Lavender, in Black Ink, Lavendered, Cap Ex Release	Nitroglycerin 2.5 mg	Nitro Time by Time Caps	49483-0221	Vasodilator
TCL <> 1222	Cap	Nitroglycerin 6.5 mg	by Schein	00364-0432	Vasodilator
TCL <> 1222	Cap, in Black Ink, Cap Ex Release	Nitroglycerin 6.5 mg	Nitro Time by Time Caps	49483-0222	Vasodilator
TCL <> 1223	Cap	Nitroglycerin 9 mg	by Schein	00364-0664	Vasodilator
TCL <> 1223	Cap, in Black Ink, Cap Ex Release	Nitroglycerin 9 mg	Nitro Time by Time Caps	49483-0223	Vasodilator
TCL001	Tab, Orange, Round	Aspirin Enteric Coated 325 mg	Ecotrin by Time-Caps		Analgesic
TCL002	Tab, Red, Round	Aspirin Enteric Coated 650 mg	Ecotrin by Time-Caps		Analgesic
TCL003	Tab, Yellow, Round	Bisacodyl 5 mg	Dulcolax by Time-Caps		Gastrointestinal
TCL005	Tab, Orange, Round	Aspirin 500 mg	by Perrigo	00113-0511	Analgesic
TCL019	Cap	Papaverine HCl 150 mg	by Schein	00364-0181	Vasodilator
TCL019	Cap	Papaverine HCl 150 mg	by Qualitest	00603-5043	Vasodilator
TCL021	Tab, Tan, Round	Thyroid 30 mg	by Time-Caps		Thyroid
TCL023	Tab, Tan, Round	Thyroid 130 mg	Thyroid by Time-Caps		Thyroid
TCL025	Tab, Yellow, Round	Aspirin 81 mg	by Perrigo	00113-0535	Analgesic
TCL027	Tab, Red, Round, TCL/027	Ferrous Sulfate 324 mg	Feosol by Time-Cap		Mineral
TCL028	Cap, Banded	Phenylpropanolamine HCl 4 mg, Chlorphen Mal (Time Rel) 75 mg	Aler-Releaf by Reese	10956-0703	Cold Remedy
TCL032	Tab, Red, Round	Aspirin Enteric Coated 325 mg	Ecotrin Max-Strength by Time-Caps		Analgesic
TCL036	Cap	Chlorpheniramine Maleate 4 mg, Phenylephrine HCl 20 mg, Phenyltoloxamine Citrate 50 mg	Q Hist LA by Qualitest	00603-5537	Cold Remedy; C III
TCL041	Cap	Chlorpheniramine Maleate 8.8 mg	by Qualitest	00603-2784	Antihistamine
TCL043	Cap, Blue-Green & Clear with Black Ink, ER	Chlorpheniramine Maleate 12 mg	by Quality Care	60346-0782	Antihistamine
TCL050	Cap, White	Brompheniramine 4 mg, Pseudoephedrine 60 mg	by Time-Caps		Cold Remedy
TCL050	Cap	Guaifenesin 250 mg, Pseudoephedrine HCl 120 mg	by Zenith Goldline	00182-2601	Cold Remedy
TCL050	Cap	Guaifenesin 250 mg, Pseudoephedrine HCl 120 mg	by Qualitest	00603-3776	Cold Remedy
TCL050	Cap	Guaifenesin 250 mg, Pseudoephedrine HCl 120 mg	Pseudo Guaifed by Time Caps	49483-0050	Cold Remedy
TCL051	Cap, Blue & Clear	Bromopheniramine 6 mg, Pseudoephedrine 60 mg	by Time-Caps		Cold Remedy
TCL051	Cap, Blue, Opaque	Guaifenesin 300 mg, Pseudoephedrine HCl 60 mg	by Zenith Goldline	00182-2602	Cold Remedy
TCL051	Cap	Guaifenesin 300 mg, Pseudoephedrine HCl 60 mg	by Qualitest	00603-3777	Cold Remedy
TCL051	Cap	Guaifenesin 300 mg, Pseudoephedrine HCl 60 mg	Pseudo Guiafed by Time Caps	49483-0051	Cold Remedy
TCL103	Tab, Film Coated	Salsalate 500 mg	by Zenith Goldline	00182-1802	NSAID
TCL1221	Cap	Nitroglycerin 2.5 mg	by United Res	00677-0485	Vasodilator
TCL1222	Cap	Nitroglycerin 6.5 mg	by United Res	00677-0486	Vasodilator
TCL1222	Cap, Dark Blue	Nitroglycerin 6.5 mg	by Qualitest	00603-4783	Vasodilator
TCL1223	Cap, TCL-1223	Nitroglycerin 9 mg	by Baker Cummins	63171-1670	Vasodilator
TCL1223	Cap	Nitroglycerin 9 mg	by United Res	00677-0967	Vasodilator
TCL1223	Cap	Nitroglycerin 9 mg	by Qualitest	00603-4784	Vasodilator

ID FRONT <> BACK	DESCRIPTION FRONT <> BACK	INGREDIENT & STRENGTH	BRAND (OR EQUIV.) & FIRM	NDC#	CLASS; SCH.
TCLO50	Cap	Guaifenesin 250 mg, Pseudoephedrine HCl 120 mg	by Zenith Goldline	00182-2601	Cold Remedy
TCLO51	Cap	Guaifenesin 300 mg, Pseudoephedrine HCl 60 mg	by Zenith Goldline	00182-2602	Cold Remedy
TCM <> 325	Cap, Yellow, Film Coated	Acetaminophen 325 mg, Chlorpheniramine Maleate 2mg, Pseudoephedrine HCl 30 mg, Dextromethorphan Hydrobromide 15 mg	Regular Tylenol Cold Nighttime	Canadian DIN# 00574007	Cold Remedy
TCM <> 500	Cap, Yellow, Film Coated	Acetaminophen 500 mg, Chlorpheniramine Maleate 2mg, Pseudoephedrine HCl 30 mg, Dextromethorphan Hydrobromide 15 mg	Extra Strength Tylenol Cold Nighttime	Canadian DIN# 00743275	Cold Remedy
TCM 325	Cap, Yellow	Acetaminophen 325 mg, Chlorphen 2 mg, Pseudoephed 30 mg, Dextrmeth 15 mg	Tylenol Cold by McNeil	Canadian	Cold Remedy
TCMDM <> 160	Tab, Purple, Round, Scored, Chewable	Acetaminophen 160 mg, Chlorpheniramine Maleate 1 mg, Pseudoephedrine HCl 15 mg, Dextromethorphan Hydrobromide 7.5 mg	Junior Strength Tylenol Cold DM	Canadian DIN# 00890677	Cold Remedy
TCMND <> 325	Cap, Yellow, Film Coated	Acetaminophen, Pseudoephedrine HCl 30 mg, Dextromethorphan Hydrobromide 15 mg	Regular Tylenol Daytime	Canadian DIN# 00743283	Cold Remedy
TCMND <> 500	Cap, Yellow, Film Coated	Acetaminophen 500 mg, Pseudoephedrine HCl 30 mg, Dextromethorphan Hydrobromide 15 mg	Extra Strength Tylenol Cold Daytime by McNeil	Canadian DIN# 00743267	Cold Remedy
TD <> A	Tab	Levothyroxine 19 mcg, Liothyronine 4.5 mcg	Armour Thyroid by Amerisource	62584-0457	Antithyroid
TD <> CG	Tab, Yellow, Oval, Film Coated, Scored	Oxcarbazepine 150 mg	Trileptal FCT by Novartis Pharm AG	17088-0010	Anticonvulsant
TD <> CG	Tab, Yellow, Oval, Film Coated, Scored, T/D <> C/G	Oxcarbazepine 150 mg	Tripeptal by Novartis Pharms	00078-0336	Anticonvulsant
TE	Tab, Tan, Round, Convex, Debossed with A Mortar and Pestle	Levothyroxine 38 mcg, Liothyronine 9 mcg	Armour Thyroid by Murfreesboro	51129-1637	Antithyroid
TE	Tab, White, Round, Abbott Logo	Methamphetamine HCl 5 mg	Desoxyn by Abbott	00074-3317	Stimulant; C II
TE	Tab, White, Round, TE <> Abbott Logo	Methamphetamine HCl 5 mg	Desoxyn by Abbott	00074-3377	Stimulant; C II
TEC	Cap, Orange & White, Scored	Acetaminophen 325 mg, Codeine Phosphate 16.2 mg, Methocarbamol 400 mg	by Altimed	Canadian DIN# 01966367	Analgesic
TEC	Cap, Peach & White, Scored	Acetaminophen 325 mg, Codeine Phosphate 32.4 mg, Methocarbamol 400 mg	by Altimed	Canadian DIN# 01966375	Analgesic
TEC	Cap, Light Blue & White, Scored	Acetaminophen 325 mg, Codeine Phosphate 8 mg, Methocarbamol 400 mg	by Altimed	Canadian DIN# 02236872	Analgesic
TEC	Cap, Yellow & White, Scored	Acetaminophen 325 mg, Codeine Phosphate 8 mg, Methocarbamol 400 mg	by Altimed	Canadian DIN# 01941895	Analgesic
TEC	Cap, Light Green & White, Scored	Acetaminophen 325 mg, Methocarbamol 400 mg	by Altimed	Canadian DIN# 02230521	Muscle Relaxant
TEC	Cap, Pink & White, Scored	Acetaminophen 325 mg, Methocarbamol 400 mg	by Altimed	Canadian DIN# 00868868	Muscle Relaxant
TEC	Tab, Yellow, Scored	Acetaminophen 325 mg, Oxycodone HCl 5 mg	by Altimed	Canadian DIN# 00608157	Analgesic
TEC	Tab, White, Round, Scored	Acetaminophen 325 mg, Oxycodone HCl 5 mg	by Altimed	Canadian DIN# 00608165	Analgesic
TEC	Tab, White, Round	Acetaminophen 330 mg, Butalbital 50 mg, Caffeine 40 mg	by Altimed	Canadian DIN # 00608211	Analgesic

ID FRONT <> BACK	DESCRIPTION FRONT <> BACK	INGREDIENT & STRENGTH	BRAND (OR EQUIV.) & FIRM	NDC#	CLASS; SCH.
TEC	Tab, Pink, Round	Chlorzoxazone 250 mg, Acetaminophen 300 mg, Codeine Phosph 8 mg	Acetazone Forte C8 by Technilab	Canadian DIN# 00834319	Muscle Relaxant
TEC	Tab, Green, Round	Chlorzoxazone 250 mg, Acetaminophen 300 mg	Acetazone Forte by Technilab	Canadian DIN# 00834300	Muscle Relaxant
TEC	Cap, Red, Gelatin	Docusate Calcium 100 mg	by Altimed	Canadian DIN# 00870196	Laxative
TEC	Cap, Red, Gelatin	Docusate Calcium 240 mg	by Altimed	Canadian DIN# 00809055	Laxative
TEC	Tab, White, Oval, Scored	Metformin HCl 850 mg	by Altimed	Canadian DIN# 02242931	Antidiabetic
TEC	Tab, Yellowish, Oval	Nystatin 100,000 Units	by Altimed	Canadian DIN# 02194171	Antifungal
TEC	Tab, Pink, Round, Film Coated	Nystatin 500,000 units	by Altimed	Canadian DIN# 02194198	Antifungal
TEC <> 10	Tab, Yellow, Pentagonal, Film Coated	Cyclobenzaprine HCl 10 mg	by Altimed	Canadian DIN# 02236506	Muscle Relaxant
TEC <> 203A	Tab, White to Off-White, Round, Scored	Doxazosin Mesylate 1 mg	by Altimed	Canadian DIN# 02243215	Antihypertensive
TEC <> 203B	Tab, White to Off-White, Rectangular, Scored	Doxazosin Mesylate 2 mg	by Altimed	Canadian DIN# 02243216	Antihypertensive
TEC <> 79B	Tab, Beige, D-Shaped, Film Coated, Scored	Famotidine 20 mg	by Altimed	Canadian DIN# 02242327	Gastrointestinal
TEC <> 79B	Tab, Brown, D-Shaped, Film Coated, Scored	Famotidine 40 mg	by Altimed	Canadian DIN# 02242328	Gastrointestinal
TEC 1	Tab, Yellow, Round	Haloperidol 1 mg	Peridol by Technilab	Canadian	Antipsychotic
TEC05	Tab, White, Round, TEC 0.5	Haloperidol 0.5 mg	Peridol by Technilab	Canadian	Antipsychotic
TEC050	Tab, White, Pentagonal, Scored, TEC 0.50	Dexamethasone 0.50 mg	by Altimed	Canadian DIN# 02240684	Steroid
TEC075	Tab, White, Pentagonal, Scored, TEC 0.75	Dexamethasone 0.75 mg	by Altimed	Canadian DIN# 02240685	Steroid
TEC1	Cap, White	Acetaminophen 300 mg, Caffeine 15 mg, Codeine Phosphate 8 mg	Lenoltec 1 by Technilab	Canadian	Analgesic
TEC1	Tab, White, Round	Acetaminophen 300 mg, Caffeine 15 mg, Codeine Phosphate 8 mg	Lenoltec 1 by Technilab	Canadian	Analgesic
TEC100	Cap, Blue, Opaque, Gelatin w/ Light Yellow Powder	Doxycycline Hyclate 100 mg	by Altimed	Canadian DIN# 02093103	Antibiotic
TEC102A	Tab, White, Cap Shaped, Scored	Baclofen 10 mg	by Altimed	Canadian DIN# 02236507	Muscle Relaxant

ID FRONT <> BACK	DESCRIPTION FRONT <> BACK	INGREDIENT & STRENGTH	BRAND (OR EQUIV.) & FIRM	NDC#	CLASS; SCH.
TEC102B	Tab, White, Cap Shaped, Scored	Baclofen 20 mg	by Altimed	Canadian DIN# 02236508	Muscle Relaxant
TEC137A	Cap, Green & Grey	Fluoxetine HCl 11.18 mg	by Altimed	Canadian DIN# 02241371	Antidepressant
TEC137B	Cap, Green & Ivory	Fluoxetine HCl 22.36 mg	by Altimed	Canadian DIN# 02241374	Antidepressant
TEC145	Tab, White, Round, Scored	Metformin HCl 500 mg	by Altimed	Canadian DIN# 02242974	Antidiabetic
TEC15	Tab, White, Round	Codeine Phosphate 15 mg	by Altimed	Canadian DIN# 00593435	Analgesic
TEC173A	Cap, White & Yellow, Opaque w/ White Powder	Nortriptyline HCl 10 mg	by Altimed	Canadian DIN# 02240789	Antidepressant
TEC173B	Cap, White & Yellow, Opaque w/ White Powder	Nortriptyline HCl 25 mg	by Altimed	Canadian DIN# 02240790	Antidepressant
TEC177X	Tab, Blue, Scored	Sotalol HCl 80 mg	by Altimed	Canadian DIN# 02238415	Antiarrhythmic
TEC177Y	Tab, Blue, Scored	Sotalol HCl 160 mg	by Altimed	Canadian DIN# 02238416	Antiarrhythmic
TEC185A	Cap, Maroon & Peach, Gelatin	Temazepam 15 mg	by Altimed	Canadian DIN# 02243023	Sedative/Hypnotic
TEC185B	Cap, Maroon & Peach, Gelatin	Temazepam 30 mg	by Altimed	Canadian DIN# 02243024	Sedative/Hypnotic
TEC186B	Tab, White, Square, Quadrisected	Captopril 25 mg	by Altimed	Canadian DIN# 02237862	Antihypertensive
TEC186C	Tab, White, Oval, Scored	Captopril 50 mg	by Altimed	Canadian DIN# 02237863	Antihypertensive
TEC186D	Tab, White, Oval, Scored	Captopril 100 mg	by Altimed	Canadian DIN# 02237864	Antihypertensive
TEC2	Tab, White, Round	Acetaminophen 300 mg, Caffeine 15 mg, Codeine Phosphate 15 mg	Lenoltec 2 by Technilab	Canadian	Analgesic
TEC203C	Tab, White to Off-White, Diamond Shaped, Scored	Doxazosin Mesylate 4 mg	by Altimed	Canadian DIN# 02243217	Antihypertensive
TEC250	Cap, Orange w/ Yellowish Liquid	Valproic Acid 250 mg	b Altimed	Canadian DIN# 02217414	Anticonvulsant
TEC3	Tab, White, Round	Acetaminophen 300 mg, Caffeine 15 mg, Codeine Phosphate 30 mg	Lenoltec 3 by Technilab	Canadian	Analgesic

ID FRONT <> BACK	DESCRIPTION FRONT <> BACK	INGREDIENT & STRENGTH	BRAND (OR EQUIV.) & FIRM	NDC#	CLASS; SCH.
TEC30	Tab, White, Round, Scored	Codeine Phosphate 30 mg	by Altimed	Canadian DIN# 00593451	Analgesic
TEC39	Tab, White, Round, Coated	Domperidone Maleate 12.72 mg	by Altimed	Canadian DIN# 02230473	Gastrointestinal
TEC4	Tab, White, Round	Acetaminophen 300 mg, Codeine Phosphate 60 mg	Lenoltec 4 by Technilab	Canadian	Analgesic
TEC4	Tab, White, Pentagonal, Scored	Dexamethasone 4 mg	by Altimed	Canadian DIN# 02240687	Steroid
TEC90	Tab, White to Brownish-White, Oval, Scored	Buspirone HCl 10 mg	by Altimed	Canadian DIN# 02237858	Antianxiety
TECNALC12TECHNILAB	Cap, Blue & Light Blue, Tecnal C 1/2: Technilab	Acetaminophen 330 mg, Butalbital 50 mg, Caffeine 40 mg, Codeine Phosphate 30 mg	by Altimed	Canadian DIN# 00608181	Analgesic
TECNALC14 TECHNILAB	Cap, Light Blue & White, Opaque, Tecnal C 1/4: Technilab	Acetaminophen 330 mg, Butalbital 50 mg, Caffeine 40 mg, Codeine Phosphate 15 mg	by Altimed	Canadian DIN# 00608203	Analgesic
TECNALTECHNILAB	Cap, Light Blue & Violet, Tecnal:Technilab	Acetaminophen 330 mg, Butalbital 50 mg, Caffeine 40 mg	Tecnal by Technilab	Canadian DIN # 00608238	Analgesic
TECZEM5180	Tab, Film Coated, Teczem 5/180	Diltiazem Malate 219 mg, Enalapril Maleate 5 mg	Teczem by Merck	00006-0764	Antihypertensive
TECZEM5180	Tab, Gold, Film Coated	Diltiazem Malate 219 mg, Enalapril Maleate 5 mg	Teczem by Hoechst Roussel	00088-1765	Antihypertensive
TEGRETOL <> 2727	Tab, Pink, Cap Shaped, Scored, Tegretol <> 27/27	Carbamazepine 200 mg	Tegretol by Novartis	00083-0027	Anticonvulsant
TEGRETOL <> 2727	Tab	Carbamazepine 200 mg	by Quality Care	60346-0777	Anticonvulsant
TEGRETOL <> 2727	Tab	Carbamazepine 200 mg	by Nat Pharmpak Serv	55154-1012	Anticonvulsant
TEGRETOL <> 52	Tab, Tab Chewable	Carbamazepine 100 mg	by Basel	58887-0052	Anticonvulsant
TEGRETOL <> 52	Tab, Pink, Round, Scored	Carbamazepine 100 mg	Tegretol Chewable by Allscripts	54569-0165	Anticonvulsant
TEGRETOL <> 5252	Tab, Red Specks, Scored, Chewable	Carbamazepine 100 mg	by Nat Pharmpak Serv	55154-1011	Anticonvulsant
TEGRETOL <> 5252	Tab, Pink, Round, Scored	Carbamazepine 100 mg	Tegretol by Neuman Distbtrs	64579-0325	Anticonvulsant
TEGRETOL <> 5252	Tab, Pink with Red Specks, Round, Scored	Carbamazepine 100 mg	by Novartis	00083-0052	Anticonvulsant
TEMAZEPAM15MG <> 272	Cap, in Red Ink, 272 Creighton Logo	Temazepam 15 mg	Tem by Kaiser	00179-1106	Sedative/Hypnotic; C IV
TEMAZEPAM15MG <> 272CP	Cap	Temazepam 15 mg	Tem by Creighton Prod	50752-0272	Sedative/Hypnotic; C IV
TEMAZEPAM15MG <> 272CP	Cap	Temazepam 15 mg	Tem by Quality Care	60346-0668	Sedative/Hypnotic; C IV
TEMAZEPAM30MG <> 273CP	Cap	Temazepam 30 mg	Tem by Creighton Prod	50752-0273	Sedative/Hypnotic; C IV
TEMAZEPAM30MG <> 273CP	Cap, in Red Ink	Temazepam 30 mg	Tem by Quality Care	60346-0005	Sedative/Hypnotic; C IV
TEMPRA	Tab, Light Purple, Round	Acetaminophen 80 mg	Tempra by MJ	Canadian	Antipyretic
TEMPRA160	Tab, Purple, Rectangular	Acetaminophen 160 mg	Tempra by MJ	Canadian	Antipyretic
TEMPRA160	Tab, Purple, Tempra/160	Acetaminophen 160 mg	Tempra by Sanofi	Canadian	Antipyretic
TEMPRA80	Tab, Purple, Tempra/80	Acetaminophen 80 mg	Tempra by Mead Johnson	Canadian	Antipyretic
TENAKE <> SEATRACE	Cap, Green Print	Acetaminophen 325 mg, Butalbital 50 mg, Caffeine 40 mg	Tenake by Seatrace	00551-0181	Analgesic
TENEX <> 1AHR	Tab	Guanfacine HCl 1.15 mg	Tenex by Leiner	59606-0748	Antihypertensive
TENEX <> 1AHR	Tab, 1 and AHR	Guanfacine HCl 1.15 mg	Tenex by Amerisource	62584-0901	Antihypertensive
TENEX <> 1AHR	Tab, Light Pink, Tenex <> #1 AHR	Guanfacine HCl 1.15 mg	Tenex by A H Robins	00031-8901	Antihypertensive
TENEX <> AHR	Tab, Pink, Diamond	Guanfacine HCl 1.15 mg	Tenex by Rightpac	65240-0748	Antihypertensive
TENEX <> AHR1	Tab	Guanfacine HCl 1.15 mg	Tenex by Nat Pharmpak Serv	55154-3008	Antihypertensive

ID FRONT <> BACK	DESCRIPTION FRONT <> BACK	INGREDIENT & STRENGTH	BRAND (OR EQUIV.) & FIRM	NDC#	CLASS; SCH.
TENOLIN 100	Tab, White, Biconvex	Atenolol 100 mg	by Technilab	Canadian	Antihypertensive
TENOLIN50	Tab, White, Biconvex	Atenolol 50 mg	by Technilab	Canadian	Antihypertensive
TENORETIC <> 115	Tab, White, Round	Atenolol 50 mg, Chlorthalidone 25 mg	Tenoretic 50 by AstraZeneca	00310-0115	Antihypertensive; Diuretic
TENORETIC <> 115	Tab	Atenolol 50 mg, Chlorthalidone 25 mg	Tenoretic 50 by Physicians Total Care	54868-0321	Antihypertensive; Diuretic
TENORETIC <> 117	Tab, White, Round	Atenolol 100 mg, Chlorthalidone 25 mg	Tenoretic 100 by AstraZeneca	00310-0117	Antihypertensive; Diuretic
TENORETIC115	Tab	Atenolol 50 mg, Chlorthalidone 25 mg	Tenoretic by Allscripts	54569-0596	Antihypertensive; Diuretic
TENORMIN	Tab, White, Biconvex	Atenolol 100 mg	Tenormin by Zeneca	Canadian	Antihypertensive
TENORMIN <> 101	Tab, Debossed	Atenolol 100 mg	Tenormin by Pharm Utilization	60491-0629	Antihypertensive
TENORMIN <> 101	Tab, White, Round	Atenolol 100 mg	Tenormin by AstraZeneca	00310-0101	Antihypertensive
TENORMIN <> 105	Tab, Debossed, Bisected	Atenolol 50 mg	Tenormin by Pharm Utilization	60491-0627	Antihypertensive
TENORMIN <> 105	Tab	Atenolol 50 mg	Tenormin by Wal Mart	49035-0166	Antihypertensive
TENORMIN <> 105	Tab, White, Round	Atenolol 50 mg	Tenormin by AstraZeneca	00310-0105	Antihypertensive
TENORMIN 50	Tab, White, Biconvex	Atenolol 50 mg	Tenormin by Zeneca	Canadian	Antihypertensive
TENUATE25	Tab, White, Round	Diethylpropion HCl 25 mg	Tenuate Dospan by Hoechst Marion Roussel	00068-0697	Antianorexiant; C IV
TENUATE75	Tab, Tenuate 75, Tab Ex Release	Diethylpropion HCl 75 mg	Tenuate Dospan by Quality Care	60346-0973	Antianorexiant; C IV
TENUATE75	Tab, White, Cap Shaped	Diethylpropion HCl 75 mg	Tenuate Dospan by Hoechst Marion Roussel	00068-0698	Antianorexiant; C IV
TEQUIN200 <> BMS	Tab, White, Almond Shaped, Film Coated	Gatifloxacin 200 mg	by Bristol Myers Squibb	00015-1117	Antibiotic
TEQUIN200 <> BMS	Tab, White, Film Coated	Gatifloxacin 200 mg	Tequin by Squibb Mfg	12783-0117	Antibiotic
TEQUIN400 <> BMS	Tab, White, Film Coated	Gatifloxacin 400 mg	by Bristol Myers Squibb	00015-1177	Antibiotic
TEQUIN400 <> BMS	Tab, White, Film Coated	Gatifloxacin 400 mg	Tequin by Squibb Mfg	12783-0177	Antibiotic
TERF60	Tab, White, Round, Terf/60	Terfenadine 60 mg	Novo Terfenadine by Novopharm	Canadian	Antihistamine
TETE <> CGCG	Tab, Yellow, Oval, Film Coated, Scored, TE/TE <> CG/CG	Oxcarbazepine 300 mg	Tripeptal by Novartis Pharms	00078-0337	Anticonvulsant
TETE <> CGCG	Tab, Yellow, Oval, Film Coated, Scored	Oxcarbazepine 300 mg	Trileptal FCT by Novartis Pharm AG	17088-0011	Anticonvulsant
TF	Tab, Abb. Logo	Metharbital 100 mg	Gemonil by Abbott		Sedative
TF <> A	Tab	Levothyroxine 76 mcg, Liothyronine 18 mcg	Armour Thyroid by Amerisource	62584-0461	Antithyroid
TFTF <> CGCG	Tab, Yellow, Oval, Film Coated, Scored	Oxcarbazepine 600 mg	Trileptal FCT by Novartis Pharm AG	17088-0012	Anticonvulsant
TFTF <> CGCG	Tab, Yellow, Oval, Film Coated, Scored, TF/TF <> CG/CG	Oxcarbazepine 600 mg	Tripeptal by Novartis Pharms	00078-0338	Anticonvulsant
TFTFCGCG	Tab, Yellow, Oval, Slightly Biconvex, Film Coated, Scored, TF/TF <> CG/CG	Oxcarbazepine 600 mg	Trileptal by Novartis	00078-0339	Anticonvulsant
TH	Tab, White, Round, TH <> Abbott Logo	Pemoline 18.75 mg	Cylert by Abbott	00074-6025	Stimulant; C IV
TH1 <> MYLAN	Tab, Green, TH/1, Beveled Edge	Hydrochlorothiazide 25 mg, Triamterene 37.5 mg	by Mylan	00378-1352	Diuretic
TH1 <> MYLAN	Tab, Green, TH Over 1	Hydrochlorothiazide 25 mg, Triamterene 37.5 mg	by Mylan	55160-0126	Diuretic
TH2	Tab, Yellow, Round	Triamterene 75 mg, Hydrochlorothiazide 50 mg	Maxide by Mylan		Diuretic
TH2 <> MYLAN	Tab, Yellow, Round, Scored, TH over 2 <> Mylan	Hydrochlorothiazide 50 mg, Triamterene 75 mg	Maxide by UDL	51079-0433	Diuretic
TH2 <> MYLAN	Tab, Yellow, TH/2, Beveled Edge	Hydrochlorothiazide 50 mg, Triamterene 75 mg	by Mylan	00378-1355	Diuretic
TH2 <> MYLAN	Tab, Yellow, TH Over 2	Hydrochlorothiazide 50 mg, Triamterene 75 mg	by Mylan	55160-0127	Diuretic
THCA09	Tab, White, Round, THC over A09	Ephedrine 12.5 mg, Guaifenesin 200 mg	by Hammer		Expectorant
THCP07	Tab, White, Round	Ephedrine 20 mg, Guaifenesin 100 mg	by The Hammer Corp.		Cold Remedy
THE 200	Tab, White, Oval	Anhydrous Theophylline 200 mg	Theo LA by Apotex	Canadian	Antiasthmatic
THE 300	Tab, White, Oblong	Anhydrous Theophylline 300 mg	Theo LA by Apotex	Canadian	Antiasthmatic
THE100	Tab, White, Round, The/100	Anhydrous Theophylline 100 mg	Theo LA by Apotex	Canadian	Antiasthmatic
THEO24100MGUCB <> 2832	Cap, Clear & Orangish Yellow, Theo-24 100 mg ucb <> 2832	Theophylline Anhydrous ER 100 mg	Theo-24 by UCB Pharma	50474-0100	Antiasthmatic
THEO24200MG <> 2842	Cap, Orange Red, Cap Ex Release	Theophylline Anhydrous 200 mg	Theo 24 ER by DRX	55045-2354	Antiasthmatic

ID FRONT <> BACK	DESCRIPTION FRONT <> BACK	INGREDIENT & STRENGTH	BRAND (OR EQUIV.) & FIRM	NDC#	CLASS; SCH.
THEO24200MG <> UCB2842	Cap, Orange & Clear, Theo 24 Over 200 MG <> UCB Over 2842	Theophylline Anhydrous 200 mg	THEO 24 by Taro	52549-4028	Antiasthmatic
THEO24200MGUCB <> 2842	Cap, Clear & Orangish Red, Theo-24 200 mg ucb <> 2842	Theophylline Anhydrous ER 300 mg	Theo-24 by UCB Pharma	50474-0200	Antiasthmatic
THEO24300MG <> UCB2852	Cap, Red & Clear, Theo 24 Over 300 MG <> UCB Over 2852	Theophylline Anhydrous 300 mg	THEO 24 by Taro	52549-4029	Antiasthmatic
THEO24300MG <> UCB2852	Cap, Red & Clear, Theo-24 300MG <> UCB Over 2852	Theophylline Anhydrous 300 mg	THEO 24 by Taro	52549-4026	Antiasthmatic
THEO24300MGUCB <> 2852	Cap, Clear & Red, Theo-24 300 mg ucb <> 2852	Theophylline Anyhdrous ER 300 mg	Thea-24 by UCB Pharma	50474-0300	Antiasthmatic
THEO24400MGUCB <> 2902	Cap, Clear & Pink, Theo-24 400 mg ucb <> 2902	Theophylline Anhydrous ER 400 mg	Theo 24 by UCB	50474-0400	Antiasthmatic
THEOBID260	Cap, ER, Black Ink, Filled with White Beads	Theophylline Anhydrous 260 mg	Theobid by	00131-4748	Antiasthmatic
THEODOR300	Tab, Tab Ex Release	Theophylline Anhydrous 300 mg	Theo-Dur by Rite Aid	11822-5278	Antiasthmatic
THEODUR100	Tab, Theo-Dur 100, Tab Ex Release	Theophylline Anhydrous 100 mg	Theo Dur by Allscripts	54569-0318	Antiasthmatic
THEODUR100	Tab, White to Off-White, Theo-Dur 100, Debossed, ER	Theophylline Anhydrous 100 mg	Theo Dur by Thrift Drug	59198-0235	Antiasthmatic
THEODUR100	Tab, Theo-Dur 100, Debossed, Tab Ex Release	Theophylline Anhydrous 100 mg	Theo Dur by Amerisource	62584-0487	Antiasthmatic
THEODUR100	Tab, Off White, Round	Theophylline Anhydrous 100 mg	Theo-Dur by Schering	00085-0487	Antiasthmatic
THEODUR100	Tab, White, Round, Scored, Theo-Dur 100	Theophylline Anhydrous 100 mg	THEO DUR by Takeda	64764-0301	Antiasthmatic
THEODUR200	Tab, White, Oval, Scored	Theophylline Anhydrous 200 mg	Theo Dur by Rightpac	65240-0750	Antiasthmatic
THEODUR200	Tab, Off White, Oval	Theophylline Anhydrous 200 mg	Theo-Dur ER by Schering	00085-0933	Antiasthmatic
THEODUR200	Tab, Theo-Dur/200, Compressed Ex Release	Theophylline Anhydrous 200 mg	Theo Dur by Kaiser	00179-1047	Antiasthmatic
THEODUR200	Tab, Theo-Dur Over 200, Tab Ex Release	Theophylline Anhydrous 200 mg	Theo Dur by Med Pro	53978-0243	Antiasthmatic
THEODUR200	Tab, Debossed, Tab Ex Release	Theophylline Anhydrous 200 mg	Theo Dur by CVS	51316-0018	Antiasthmatic
THEODUR200	Tab, Tab Ex Release	Theophylline Anhydrous 200 mg	Theo Dur by Nat Pharmpak Serv	55154-1502	Antiasthmatic
THEODUR200	Tab, Theo-Dur 200 Embossed, Slightly Speckled, Tab Ex Release	Theophylline Anhydrous 200 mg	Theo Dur by Thrift Drug	59198-0108	Antiasthmatic
THEODUR200	Tab, Theo-Dur 200, Debossed, Tab Ex Release	Theophylline Anhydrous 200 mg	Theo Dur by Amerisource	62584-0933	Antiasthmatic
THEODUR200	Tab, White, Oval, Theo-Dur 200	Theophylline 200 mg	Theo-Dur by Astra	Canadian	Antiasthmatic
THEODUR200	Tab, Theo-Dur 200, Tab Ex Release	Theophylline 200 mg	by Med Pro	53978-0319	Antiasthmatic
THEODUR300	Tab, Theo-Dur 300, Debossed, Tab Ex Release	Theophylline Anhydrous 300 mg	Theo Dur by Amerisource	62584-0584	Antiasthmatic
THEODUR300	Tab, White to Off-White, Slightly Speckled, Theo-Dur 300 Debossed, ER	Theophylline Anhydrous 300 mg	Theo Dur by Thrift Drug	59198-0109	Antiasthmatic
THEODUR300	Tab, Off-White, Cap Shaped	Theophylline Anhydrous 300 mg	Theo-Dur by Schering	00085-0584	Antiasthmatic
THEODUR300	Tab, White, Oblong, Scored	Theophylline Anhydrous 300 mg	Theo Dur by Rightpac	65240-0751	Antiasthmatic
THEODUR300	Tab, White with Specks, Theo-Dur/300, Tab Ex Release	Theophylline Anhydrous 300 mg	Theo Dur by Kaiser	00179-0365	Antiasthmatic
THEODUR300	Tab, White to Off-White, Tab Ex Release	Theophylline Anhydrous 300 mg	Theo Dur by Caremark	00339-5395	Antiasthmatic
THEODUR300	Tab, Theo-Dur 300, Tab Ex Release	Theophylline Anhydrous 300 mg	Theo Dur by Allscripts	54569-0062	Antiasthmatic
THEODUR300	Tab, Tab Ex Release	Theophylline Anhydrous 300 mg	Theodur by Pharmedix	53002-0575	Antiasthmatic
THEODUR300	Tab, Debossed, Tab Ex Release	Theophylline Anhydrous 300 mg	Theo Dur by Nat Pharmpak Serv	55154-1503	Antiasthmatic
THEODUR300	Tab, Theo-Dur 300, Tab Ex Release	Theophylline Anhydrous 300 mg	by Med Pro	53978-0320	Antiasthmatic
THEODUR300	Tab, Theo-Dur 300, Tab Ex Release	Theophylline Anhydrous 300 mg	Theo-Dur by Med Pro	53978-0343	Antiasthmatic
THEODUR300	Tab, White, Theo-Dur 300, Oblong, Scored	Theophylline Anhydrous 300 mg	Theo-Dur by Taro	52549-4027	Antiasthmatic
THEODUR300	Tab, White, Theo-Dur/300	Theophylline 300 mg	Theo-Dur by Astra	Canadian	Antiasthmatic
THEODUR300	Tab, White, Theo-Dur 300	Theophylline 300 mg	Theo-Dur by Astra	Canadian	Antiasthmatic
THEODUR450	Tab, Off White, Cap Shaped	Theophylline 450 mg	Theo-Dur by Schering	00085-0806	Antiasthmatic
THEODUR450	Tab, White, Theo-Dur 450	Theophylline 450 mg	Theo-Dur by Astra	Canadian	Antiasthmatic
THEODUR450MG	Tab, Tab Ex Release	Theophylline Anhydrous 450 mg	Theo Dur by Pharmedix	53002-1042	Antiasthmatic
THEODUR75	Cap, ER	Theophylline Anhydrous 75 mg	Theo Dur by Pharmedix	53002-1058	Antiasthmatic
THEOLAIR250	Tab, White, Oblong	Theophylline Anhydrous 250 mg	by Theolair	Canadian	Antiasthmatic
THEOLAIR250 <> 3M	Tab, White, Cap-Shaped, Scored	Theophylline 250 mg	Theolair by 3M	00089-0344	Antiasthmatic
THEOPHYLLINE200	Tab, Debossed, Tab Ex Release	Theophylline 200 mg	by Repack Co	55306-1660	Antiasthmatic
THEOPHYLLINE300	Tab, Theophylline/300 Debossed, Tab Ex Release	Theophylline 300 mg	by Quality Care	60346-0596	Antiasthmatic

ID FRONT <> BACK	DESCRIPTION FRONT <> BACK	INGREDIENT & STRENGTH	BRAND (OR EQUIV.) & FIRM	NDC#	CLASS; SCH.
THEOPHYLLINEXR <> ARCOLA	Cap, Theophylline-XR 100, Cap Ex Release	Theophylline Anhydrous 100 mg	by Arcola	00070-2340	Antiasthmatic
THEOPHYLLINEXR <> ARCOLA	Cap, Theophylline-XR 125, Cap Ex Release	Theophylline Anhydrous 125 mg	by Arcola	00070-2341	Antiasthmatic
THEOPHYLLINEXR <> ARCOLA	Cap, Cap Ex Release	Theophylline Anhydrous 200 mg	by DRX	55045-2279	Antiasthmatic
THEOPHYLLINEXR1 <> ARCOLA	Cap, White, Cap Ex Release	Theophylline Anhydrous 100 mg	Theophylline by RPR	00801-2340	Antiasthmatic
THEOPHYLLINEXR1 <> ARCOLA	Cap, White	Theophylline Anhydrous 125 mg	by Murfreesboro Ph	51129-1670	Antiasthmatic
THEOPHYLLINEXR1 <> ARCOLA	Cap, White, Cap Ex Release	Theophylline Anhydrous 125 mg	Theophylline by RPR	00801-2341	Antiasthmatic
THEOPHYLLINEXR2 <> ARCOLA	Cap, Theophylline-XR 200, Cap Ex Release	Theophylline Anhydrous 200 mg	by Arcola	00070-2342	Antiasthmatic
THEOPHYLLINEXR2 <> ARCOLA	Cap, White, Cap Ex Release	Theophylline Anhydrous 200 mg	Theophylline by RPR	00801-2342	Antiasthmatic
THEOPHYLLINEXR3 <> ARCOLA	Cap, White, Cap Ex Release	Theophylline Anhydrous 300 mg	Theophylline by RPR	00801-2343	Antiasthmatic
THEOPHYLLINEXR3 <> ARCOLA	Cap, Theophylline-XR 300, Cap Ex Release	Theophylline Anhydrous 300 mg	by Arcola	00070-2343	Antiasthmatic
THERRX <> 014	Tab, Yellow, Diamond Shaped, Film Coated	Ascorbic Acid 60 mg; Calcium Carbonate 200 mg; Iron 30 mg; Vitamin E 30 unt; Thiamine Mononitrate 3 mg; Riboflavin 3.4 mg; Niacinamide 20 mg; Pyridoxine HCl 50 mg; Folic Acid 1 mg; Magnesium Oxide 100 mg; Cyanocobalamin 12 mcg; Zinc Oxide 15 mg; Cupric Ox	Precare Conceive by Ther Rx	64011-0014	Vitamins/Minerals
THERRX <> 019	Tab, Blue, Oval, Film Coated	Calcium 200 mg, Folic Acid 1 mg, Vitamin B6 75 mg, Vitamin B12 12 mcg	by KV Pharmaceutical	64011-0019	Vitamin/Mineral
THERRX <> 025	Tab, Peach, Cap Shaped, Film Coated, Scored	Ascorbic Acid 50 mg; Calcium Carbonate 250 mg; Cyanocobalamin12 mcg; Cholecalciferol 6 mcg; Thiamine Mononitrate 3 mg; Riboflavin 3.4 mg; Niacinamide 20 mg; Pyridoxine HCl 20 mg; Folic Acid 1 mg; Magnesium Oxide 50 mg; Zinc Sulfate 15 mg; Cupric Sulfate 2	Precare Prenatal by Ther Rx	64011-0025	Vitamin
THERRX <> 14	Tab, Yellow, Diamond, Film Coated	Ascorbic Acid 60 mg; Calcium Carbonate 200 mg; Iron 30 mg; Vitamin E 30 Unt; Thiamine Mononitrate 3 mg; Riboflavin 3.4 mg; Niacinamide 20 mg; Pyridoxine HCl 50 mg; Folic Acid 1 mg; Magnesium Oxide 100 mg; Cyanocobalamin 12 mcg; Zinc Oxide 15 mg	Precare Conceive by KV Pharm	10609-1433	Vitamin
THERRX <> 19	Tab, Blue, Oval	P 75 mg, Cyanocobalamin 12 mcg, Folic Acid 1 mg, Calcium 200 mg	Premesisrx by KV Pharm	10609-1444	Vitamin
THERRX <> 25	Tab, Peach, Oblong, Film Coated, Scored	Ascorbic Acid 50 mg; Calcium Carbonate 250 mg; Cyanocobalamin 12 mcg; Cholecalciferol 6 mcg; Thiamine Mononitrate 3 mg; Riboflavin 3.4 mg; Niacinamide 20 mg; Pyridozine HCl 20 mg; Folic Acid 1 mg; Magnesium Oxide 50 mg; Zinc Sulfate 15 mg; Cupric sulfate	Precare Prenatal by KV Pharm	10609-1445	Vitamin
THERRX009 <> MICROK10	Cap, Light Orange & White, Ther-Rx 009 <> Micro-K 10	Potassium Chloride 750 mg	by Allscripts	54569-0660	Electrolyte
THERRX009 <> MICROK10	Cap, Orange & White, Opaque, Gelatin, Ther-Rx 009 <> Micro-K 10	Potassium Chloride 750 mg	Micro K by Ther Rx	64011-0009	Electrolyte
THERRX010 <> MICROK	Cap, Orange, Gelatin, Ther-Rx 010 <> Micro-K	Potassium Chloride 600 mg	by KV Pharmaceutical	64011-0010	Electrolyte
THISENDUP <> PFMSIR30	Cap	Morphine Sulfate 30 mg	Msir by PF	48692-0001	Analgesic; C II
THISENDUP <> PFMSIR30	Cap, Lavender	Morphine Sulfate 30 mg	Msir by Purdue Frederick	00034-1026	Analgesic; C II
THX <> 024	Tab, Mottled Orange, Oval, Film Coated, Dimple w/ 024	Calcium 250 mg, Copper 2 mg, Folic Acid 1 mg, Iron 40 mg, Magnesium 50 mg, Vitamin B6 2 mg, Vitamin C 50 mg, Vitamin D3 6 mcg, Vitamin E 3.5 mg, Zinc 15 mg	by KV Pharmaceutical	64011-0024	Vitamin/Mineral
TI	Tab, Orange, Round, Scored, TI <> Abbott Logo	Pemoline 37.5 mg	Cylert by Abbott	00074-6057	Stimulant; C IV

ID FRONT <> BACK	DESCRIPTION FRONT <> BACK	INGREDIENT & STRENGTH	BRAND (OR EQUIV.) & FIRM	NDC#	CLASS; SCH.
TIAFEN200	Tab, White	Tiaprofenic Acid 200 mg	Tiafen by Altimed	Canadian DIN# 01924613	NSAID
TIAFEN200	Tab, White	Tiaprofenic Acid 200 mg	Albert Tiafen by Albert Pharma	Canadian	NSAID
TIAFEN300	Tab, White	Tiaprofenic Acid 300 mg	Tiafen by Altimed	Canadian DIN# 01924621	NSAID
TIAFEN300	Tab, White	Tiaprofenic Acid 300 mg	Albert Tiafen by Albert Pharma	Canadian	NSAID
TIAMATE120	Tab	Diltiazem Malate 146 mg	Tiamate by Merck	00006-0760	Antihypertensive
TIAMATE120	Tab, Off-White, Cap Shaped	Diltiazem Malate 146 mg	Tiamate by Hoechst Roussel	00088-1760	Antihypertensive
TIAMATE180	Tab	Diltiazem Malate 219 mg	Tiamate by Merck	00006-0762	Antihypertensive
TIAMATE180	Tab, Off-White, Cap Shaped	Diltiazem Malate 219 mg	Tiamate by Hoechst Roussel	00088-1761	Antihypertensive
TIAMATE240	Tab	Diltiazem Malate 292 mg	Tiamate by Merck	00006-0763	Antihypertensive
TIAMATE240	Tab, Off-White, Cap Shaped	Diltiazem Malate 292 mg	Tiamate by Hoechst Roussel	00088-1762	Antihypertensive
TIAZAC <> 180	Cap	Diltiazem HCl 180 mg	Tiazac by CVS	51316-0244	Antihypertensive
TIAZAC <> 240	Cap	Diltiazem HCl 240 mg	Tiazac by CVS	51316-0243	Antihypertensive
TIAZAC <> 300	Cap, Purple & White	Diltiazem HCl 300 mg	Tiazac by Rx Pac	65084-0134	Antihypertensive
TIAZAC120	Cap	Diltiazem HCl 120 mg	Tiazac by Biovail	55542-0001	Antihypertensive
TIAZAC120	Cap, Purple	Diltiazem HCl 120 mg	Tiazac by Rx Pac	65084-0227	Antihypertensive
TIAZAC120	Cap, Cap Ex Release	Diltiazem HCl 120 mg	Tiazac by Biovail	62660-0001	Antihypertensive
TIAZAC120	Cap, Purple	Diltiazem HCl 120 mg	Tiazac by Rx Pac	65084-0227	Antihypertensive
TIAZAC120	Cap, Lavender	Diltiazem HCl 120 mg	Tiazac by Forest	00456-2612	Antihypertensive
TIAZAC120	Cap, Lavender	Diltiazem HCl 120 mg	Tiazac Er by Physicians Total Care	54868-3774	Antihypertensive
TIAZAC120	Cap, Lavender	Diltiazem HCl 120 mg	Tiazac by Wal Mart	49035-0160	Antihypertensive
TIAZAC120	Cap	Diltiazem HCl 120 mg	Tiazac by Eckerd Drug	19458-0860	Antihypertensive
TIAZAC120	Cap, Purple, Tiazac Over 120	Diltiazem HCl 120 mg	Tiazac	63941-0642	Antihypertensive
TIAZAC180	Cap, Blue-Green	Diltiazem HCl 180 mg	Tiazac by Eckerd Drug	19458-0861	Antihypertensive
TIAZAC180	Cap	Diltiazem HCl 180 mg	Tiazac by Biovail	55542-0002	Antihypertensive
TIAZAC180	Cap, Green & White	Diltiazem HCl 180 mg	Tiazac by Phy Total Care	54868-3956	Antihypertensive
TIAZAC180	Cap, White	Diltiazem HCl 180 mg	Tiazac by Rx Pac	65084-0226	Antihypertensive
TIAZAC180	Cap, Blue & White	Diltiazem HCl 180 mg	Tiazac by Thrift Services	59198-0350	Antihypertensive
TIAZAC180	Cap, White & Green	Diltiazem HCl 180 mg	Tiazac Extended Release	63941-0282	Antihypertensive
TIAZAC180	Cap, White & Green	Diltiazem HCl 180 mg	Tiazac Extended Release	63941-0183	Antihypertensive
TIAZAC180	Cap, Cap Ex Release	Diltiazem HCl 180 mg	Tiazac by Biovail	62660-0002	Antihypertensive
TIAZAC180	Cap, Blue-Green & White	Diltiazem HCl 180 mg	Tiazac by Forest	00456-2613	Antihypertensive
TIAZAC180	Cap, Blue-Green	Diltiazem HCl 180 mg	Tiazac by Wal Mart	49035-0161	Antihypertensive
TIAZAC240	Cap	Diltiazem HCl 240 mg	Tiazac by Biovail	55542-0003	Antihypertensive
TIAZAC240	Cap, Blue & Purple	Diltiazem HCl 240 mg	Tiazac Extended Release	63941-0416	Antihypertensive
TIAZAC240	Cap, Cap Ex Release	Diltiazem HCl 240 mg	Tiazac by Biovail	62660-0003	Antihypertensive
TIAZAC240	Cap, Blue	Diltiazem HCl 240 mg	Tiazac by Rx Pac	65084-0228	Antihypertensive
TIAZAC240	Cap, Blue-Green & Lavender	Diltiazem HCl 240 mg	Tiazac by Forest	00456-2614	Antihypertensive
TIAZAC240	Cap, Blue-Green & Lavender	Diltiazem HCl 240 mg	Tiazac by Wal Mart	49035-0162	Antihypertensive
TIAZAC240	Cap, Green & Purple	Diltiazem HCl 240 mg	Tiazac Extended Release by Egis	48581-6124	Antihypertensive
TIAZAC240	Cap, Blue-Green & Lavender	Diltiazem HCl 240 mg	Tiazac by Eckerd Drug	19458-0862	Antihypertensive
TIAZAC240 <> TIAZAC240	Cap, Blue & Purple, Tiazac over 240	Diltiazem HCl 240 mg	Tiazac Extended Release by Geneva	00781-1514	Antihypertensive
TIAZAC300	Cap	Diltiazem HCl 300 mg	Tiazac by Biovail	55542-0004	Antihypertensive
TIAZAC300	Cap, Cap Ex Release	Diltiazem HCl 300 mg	Tiazac by Biovail	62660-0004	Antihypertensive
TIAZAC300	Cap, Lavender & White	Diltiazem HCl 300 mg	Tiazac by Forest	00456-2615	Antihypertensive
TIAZAC300	Cap, Lavender	Diltiazem HCl 300 mg	Tiazac by Wal Mart	49035-0163	Antihypertensive
TIAZAC300	Cap, Lavender	Diltiazem HCl 300 mg	Tiazac by Nat Pharmpak Serv	55154-4607	Antihypertensive
TIAZAC300	Cap	Diltiazem HCl 300 mg	Tiazac by Eckerd Drug	19458-0863	Antihypertensive

ID FRONT <> BACK	DESCRIPTION FRONT <> BACK	INGREDIENT & STRENGTH	BRAND (OR EQUIV.) & FIRM	NDC#	CLASS; SCH.
TIAZAC300	Cap, White & Purple, Tiazac over 300	Diltiazem HCl 300 mg	Tiazac by Fujisawa	61276-0607	Antihypertensive
TIAZAC300	Cap, Purple & White	Diltiazem HCl 300 mg	Tiazac by Thrift Services	59198-0323	Antihypertensive
TIAZAC360	Cap	Diltiazem HCl 360 mg	Tiazac by Biovail	55542-0005	Antihypertensive
TIAZAC360	Cap, Cap Ex Release	Diltiazem HCl 360 mg	Tiazac by Biovail	62660-0005	Antihypertensive
TIAZAC360	Cap, Blue	Diltiazem HCl 360 mg	Tiazac Extended Release	63941-0479	Antihypertensive
TIAZAC360	Cap, Blue-Green	Diltiazem HCl 360 mg	Tiazac by Forest	00456-2616	Antihypertensive
TIAZAC360	Cap, Blue-Green	Diltiazem HCl 360 mg	Tiazac by Wal Mart	49035-0164	Antihypertensive
TIAZAC360	Cap, Blue-Green	Diltiazem HCl 360 mg	Tiazac by Eckerd Drug	19458-0864	Antihypertensive
TIAZAC360	Cap, Blue, Tiazac over 360	Diltiazem HCl 360 mg	Tiazac Extended Release by Geneva	00781-2051	Antihypertensive
TIAZAC420	Cap, White	Diltiazem HCl 420 mg	Tiazac	63941-0447	Antihypertensive
TIAZAC420	Cap, White	Diltiazem HCl 420 mg	Tiazac 420 by Forest	00456-2617	Antihypertensive
TICLID <> 250	Tab, Printed in Blue, Film Coated	Ticlopidine HCl 250 mg	Ticlid by Wal Mart	49035-0165	Anticoagulant
TICLID <> 250	Tab, Printed in Blue, Film Coated	Ticlopidine HCl 250 mg	Ticlid by Physicians Total Care	54868-3783	Anticoagulant
TICLID <> 250	Tab, Printed in Blue, Film Coated	Ticlopidine HCl 250 mg	by Med Pro	53978-3027	Anticoagulant
TICLID <> 250	Tab, Printed in Blue Ink, Film Coated	Ticlopidine HCl 250 mg	Ticlid by Quality Care	60346-0702	Anticoagulant
TICLID <> 250	Tab, Printed in Blue Ink, Tab Coated	Ticlopidine HCl 250 mg	Ticlid by Syntex	18393-0431	Anticoagulant
TICLID <> 250	Tab, Printed in Blue Ink, Film Coated	Ticlopidine HCl 250 mg	Ticlid by Hoffmann La Roche	00004-0018	Anticoagulant
TICLID250	Tab, White, Oval	Ticlopidine 250 mg	Ticlid by Roche	Canadian	Anticoagulant
TIGAN <> M187	Cap, Blue, Opaque	Trimethobbenzamide HCl 250 mg	Tigan by King	54092-0186	Antiemetic
TIGAN <> M187	Cap, Blue, Opaque	Trimethobbenzamide HCl 250 mg	Tigan by King	61570-0187	Antiemetic
TIGAN <> ROBERTS186	Cap	Trimethobenzamide HCl 100 mg	Tigan by Roberts	54092-0186	Antiemetic
TIGAN <> ROBERTS187	Cap	Trimethobenzamide HCl 250 mg	Tigan by King	60793-0885	Antiemetic
TIGAN <> TIGAN	Cap, Blue & White	Trimethobenzamide HCl 100 mg	Tigan by Murfreesboro Ph	51129-1432	Antiemetic
TIGAN <> TIGAN	Cap	Trimethobenzamide HCl 100 mg	Tigan by King	60793-0857	Antiemetic
TIGAN100MG	Cap, Blue & White	Trimethobenzamide HCl 100 mg	Tigan by Monarch	54092-0186	Antiemetic
TIGAN200MG	Cap, Blue	Trimethobenzamide HCl 100 mg	Tigan by Monarch	54092-0187	Antiemetic
TIGAN250MG	Cap	Trimethobenzamide HCl 250 mg	Tigan by Roberts	54092-0187	Antiemetic
TIGAN250MG	Cap	Trimethobenzamide HCl 250 mg	Tigan by Thrift Drug	59198-0273	Antiemetic
TIMEHIST <> MCR	Cap, TIME HIST Printed in Red, Cap Ex Release	Chlorpheniramine Maleate 8 mg, Pseudoephedrine HCl 120 mg	Time Hist by Sovereign	58716-0016	Cold Remedy
TIMEHISTMCR	Cap, Clear, Time-Hist MCR	Chlorpheniramine Maleate 8 mg, Pseudoephedrine HCl 120 mg	CPM PSEH 05 by Compumed	00403-0010	Cold Remedy
TISH3712	Tab, Green, Triangular, Tish/3712	Ferrous Sulfate 324 mg	Feosol by ADH Health Products		Mineral
TJ	Tab, Logo TJ	Levothyroxine 57 mcg, Liothyronine 13.5 mcg	Armour Thyroid by Allscripts	54569-4471	Antithyroid
TJ	Tab, Tan, Round, Scored, TJ <> Abbott Logo	Pemoline 75 mg	Cylert by Abbott	00074-6073	Stimulant; C IV
TK	Tab, Orange, Square, Scored, TK <> Abbott Logo	Pemoline 37.5 mg	Cylert Chewable by Abbott	00074-6088	Stimulant; C IV
TKN500PFIZER	Cap, Peach & White	Dofetilide 0.5 mg	Tikosyn by Pfizer Labs	00069-5820	Antiarrhythmic
TL	Tab, Blue, _/ Shaped, Scored, TL over Abbott Logo	Clorazepate Dipotassium 3.75 mg	Tranxene by Abbott	00074-4389	Antianxiety; C IV
TL	Tab, Blue, T-Tab, Scored, TL over Abbott Logo	Clorazepate Dipotassium 3.75 mg	Tranxene T-Tab by Abbott	00074-4389	Antianxiety; C IV
TL001	Tab, White, Oval, Scored, Film	Methylprednisolone 4 mg	Methylprednisolone by Neuman Distr	64579-0042	Steroid
TL001	Tab, White, Oval, Double Scored	Methylprednisolone 4 mg	by Trigen	59746-0001	Steroid
TL113	Tab, Yellow, Round, Scored, Film	Prochlorperazine Maleate 5 mg	Prochlorperazine by Ranbaxy	63304-0512	Antiemetic
TL113	Tab, Yellow, Round, Film	Prochlorperazine Maleate 5 mg	by Ranbaxy	54907-6540	Antiemetic
TL115	Tab, Yellow, Round, Scored, Film	Prochlorperazine Maleate 10 mg	Prochlorperazine USP by Ranbaxy	63304-0654	Antiemetic
TL115	Tab, Yellow, Round, Scored, Film	Prochlorperazine Maleate 10 mg	by Ranbaxy	54907-6550	Antiemetic
TLC <> 023	Tab, Engraved	Thyroid 130 mg	by Time Caps	49483-0023	Thyroid
TLC037	Cap, Blue & Clear Cap with Blue & White Beads, ER	Phenylpropanolamine 75 mg	Mini Thin Diet Aid by BDI		Decongestant; Appetite Suppressant
TLC1221	Cap, ER	Nitroglycerin 2.5 mg	by Zenith Goldline	00182-0702	Vasodilator
TLC1222	Cap, ER	Nitroglycerin 6.5 mg	by Zenith Goldline	00182-0703	Vasodilator
TLC1223	Cap, ER	Nitroglycerin 9 mg	by Zenith Goldline	00182-1670	Vasodilator
TM	Tab, Peach, Scored	Clorazepate Dipotassium 7.5 mg	Tranxene by Abbott Hlth	60692-4390	Antianxiety; C IV

ID FRONT <> BACK	DESCRIPTION FRONT <> BACK	INGREDIENT & STRENGTH	BRAND (OR EQUIV.) & FIRM	NDC#	CLASS; SCH.
TM	Tab, Peach, _/ Shaped, Scored, TM over Abbott Logo	Clorazepate Dipotassium 7.5 mg	Tranxene T-Tab by Abbott	00074-4390	Antianxiety; C IV
TM	Tab, Abbott Logo	Clorazepate Dipotassium 7.5 mg	Tranxene by Med Pro	53978-3079	Antianxiety; C IV
TN	Tab, Lavender, _/ Shaped, Scored, TN over Abbott Logo	Clorazepate Dipotassium 15 mg	Tranxene T-Tab by Abbott	00074-4391	Antianxiety; C IV
TN10G	Tab, White, Biconvex, TN 10/G	Tamoxifen Citrate 10 mg	Gen Tamoxifen by Genpharm	Canadian	Antiestrogen
TN20G	Tab, White, Octagonal, TN-20/G	Tamoxifen Citrate 20 mg	Gen Tamoxifen by Genpharm	Canadian	Antiestrogen
TO	Tab, White, Round, Biconvex, Film-Coated Tab, with arcs above and below the letters TO	Tolterodine 1 mg	Detrol by Pharmacia & Upjohn	00009-4541	Urinary Tract
TO	Tab, White, Round, Film Coated	Tolterodine 1 mg	by Pharmacia	Canadian DIN# 02239064	Urinary Tract
TO	Tab, White, Round	Tolterodine Tartrate 1 mg	Detrol by Pharmacia Upjohn (It)	10829-4541	Urinary Tract
TO60	Tab, White, Round	Toremifene 60 mg	Fareston by Schering	00085-1126	Antiestrogen
TO60	Tab, White, Round	Toremifene Citrate 60 mg	Fareston by Roberts Labs	54092-0170	Antiestrogen
TOA1	Tab, White, Cylindrical, T/O/A1	Glyburide 2.5 mg	by Boehringer Mannheim	Canadian	Antidiabetic
TOLECTIN200 <> MCNEIL	Tab, White	Tolmetin Sodium 200 mg	Tolectin by McNeil	00045-0412	NSAID
TOLECTIN200MCNEIL	Tab, Cream, Round, Tolectin/200 McNeil	Tolmetin Sodium 200 mg	Tolectin by McNeil	Canadian	NSAID
TOLECTIN600 <> MCNEIL	Tab, Orange, Film Coated	Tolmetin Sodium 600 mg	Tolectin by McNeil	00045-0416	NSAID
TOLECTIN600 <> MCNEIL	Tab, Film Coated	Tolmetin Sodium 738 mg	by Pharmedix	53002-0597	NSAID
TOLECTIN600MCNE	Tab, Tolectin 600 Over McNeil, Film Coated	Tolmetin Sodium 738 mg	Tolectin 600 by Amerisource	62584-0416	NSAID
TOLECTIN600MCNEIL	Cap, Orange & Opaque, Tolectin/600/McNeil	Tolmetin Sodium 400 mg	Tolectin by McNeil	Canadian	NSAID
TOLECTINDS <> MCNEIL	Cap	Sodium 36 mg, Tolmetin Sodium 490 mg	Tolectin Ds by Thrift Drug	59198-0127	NSAID
TOLECTINDS <> MCNEIL	Cap, Gray Band, Gray Band	Tolmetin Sodium 492 mg	Tolectin Ds by McNeil	00045-0414	NSAID
TOLECTINDS <> MCNEIL	Cap	Tolmetin Sodium 492 mg	by Pharmedix	53002-0318	NSAID
TOLECTINDS <> MCNEIL	Cap, Parallel Bands	Tolmetin Sodium 492 mg	Tolectin Ds by Amerisource	62584-0414	NSAID
TOLECTINDSMCNEIL	Cap, Parallel Bands	Tolmetin Sodium 492 mg	Tolectin Ds by Allscripts	54569-1467	NSAID
TOLMENTIN600	Tab, Film Coated	Tolmetin Sodium 738 mg	by Major	00904-5149	NSAID
TOLMETIN <> 400	Cap	Tolmetin Sodium 492 mg	by Quality Care	60346-0615	NSAID
TOLMETIN200	Tab	Sodium 18 mg, Tolmetin Sodium 245 mg	by McNeil	52021-0846	NSAID
TOLMETIN200	Tab, White, Round	Sodium 18 mg, Tolmetin Sodium 245 mg	by Duramed	51285-0846	NSAID
TOLMETIN400	Cap, Orange, Parallel Bands	Sodium 36 mg, Tolmetin Sodium 490 mg	by Duramed	51285-0847	NSAID
TOLMETIN400	Cap, Parallel Bands	Sodium 36 mg, Tolmetin Sodium 490 mg	by McNeil	52021-0847	NSAID
TOLMETIN600	Tab, Orange, Coated, Football Shaped	Sodium 54 mg, Tolmetin Sodium 735 mg	by Duramed	51285-0848	NSAID
TOLMETIN600	Tab, Tab Coated	Sodium 54 mg, Tolmetin Sodium 735 mg	by McNeil	52021-0848	NSAID
TOP <> 15MG	Cap	Topiramate 15 mg	Topamax Sprinkles by McNeil	00045-0647	Anticonvulsant
TOP <> 25	Tab, White, Tab Coated	Topiramate 25 mg	Topamax by McNeil	00045-0639	Anticonvulsant
TOP <> 25	Tab, Tab Coated	Topiramate 25 mg	Topamax by Ortho	00062-0639	Anticonvulsant
TOP <> 25	Tab, Tab Coated	Topiramate 25 mg	Topamax by McNeil	52021-0639	Anticonvulsant
TOP <> 25MG	Cap	Topiramate 25 mg	Topamax Sprinkles by McNeil	00045-0645	Anticonvulsant
TOP25	Tab, White, Round, Top/25	Topiramate 25 mg	by Janssen	Canadian	Anticonvulsant
TOP25MG	Cap, White & Clear, Opaque	Topiramate 25 mg	Topamax Sprinkle by Teva	00480-0109	Anticonvulsant
TOPAMAX <> 100	Tab, Tab Coated	Topiramate 100 mg	Topamax by Ortho	00062-0641	Anticonvulsant
TOPAMAX <> 100	Tab, Yellow, Tab Coated	Topiramate 100 mg	Topamax by McNeil	00045-0641	Anticonvulsant
TOPAMAX <> 100	Tab, Tab Coated	Topiramate 100 mg	Topamax by McNeil	52021-0641	Anticonvulsant
TOPAMAX <> 200	Tab, Tab Coated	Topiramate 200 mg	Topamax by Ortho	00062-0642	Anticonvulsant
TOPAMAX <> 200	Tab, Salmon, Tab Coated	Topiramate 200 mg	Topamax by McNeil	00045-0642	Anticonvulsant

ID FRONT <> BACK	DESCRIPTION FRONT <> BACK	INGREDIENT & STRENGTH	BRAND (OR EQUIV.) & FIRM	NDC#	CLASS; SCH.
TOPAMAX <> 200	Tab, Tab Coated	Topiramate 200 mg	Topamax by McNeil	52021-0642	Anticonvulsant
TOPAMAX100	Tab, Yellow, Round, Topamax/100	Topiramate 100 mg	by Janssen	Canadian	Anticonvulsant
TOPAMAX200	Tab, Yellow, Round, Topamax/200	Topiramate 200 mg	by Janssen	Canadian	Anticonvulsant
TORADOL	Tab, in Red Ink, Film Coated	Ketorolac Tromethamine 10 mg	Toradol by Hoffmann La Roche	00004-0273	NSAID
TORADOL <> ROCHE	Tab, Toradol in T Logo <> Roche in T Logo, Film Coated	Ketorolac Tromethamine 10 mg	Toradol by Murfreesboro	51129-1151	NSAID
TORADOL <> ROCHE	Tab, Film Coated	Ketorolac Tromethamine 10 mg	Toradol by Quality Care	60346-0446	NSAID
TORADOL <> SYNTEX	Tab, Red Print, Film Coated	Ketorolac Tromethamine 10 mg	Toradol by Quality Care	60346-0446	NSAID
TOURLA <> DP636	Tab, White, Oblong	Guaifenesin 525 mg; Pseudoephedrine HCl 120 mg	Touro LA by Dartmouth Pharms	58869-0636	Cold Remedy
TOURO <> AH	Cap, A&H, Cap Ex Release	Brompheniramine Maleate 6 mg, Pseudoephedrine HCl 60 mg	Touro A & H by Sovereign	58716-0030	Cold Remedy
TOURO <> ALLERGY	Cap, Cap Ex Release	Brompheniramine Maleate 5.75 mg, Pseudoephedrine HCl 60 mg	Touro Allergy by Pharmafab	62542-0106	Cold Remedy
TOUROAH	Cap, Orange & White, Touro A & H	Pseudophedrine HCl 60 mg, Brompheniramine Maleate 6 mg	TOURO A&H by Dartmouth	58869-0301	Cold Remedy
TOUROALLERGY	Cap, Orange & White	Pseudophedrine HCl 60 mg, Brompheniramine Maleate 5.75 mg	TOURO Allergy by Dartmouth	58869-0401	Cold Remedy
TOUROCC <> DP	Tab, White, Oblong	Guaifenesin 575 mg; Pseudoephedrine HCl 60 mg; Dextromethorphan Hydrobromide 30 mg	by Pfab	62542-0770	Cold Remedy
TOUROCC <> DP	Tab, White	Pseudoephedrine HCl 60 mg, Dextromethorphan 30 mg, Guaifenesin 575 mg	Touro CC by Dartmouth	58869-0441	Cold Remedy
TOURODM <> DP311	Tab, Touro DM, DP 311	Dextromethorphan Hydrobromide 30 mg, Guaifenesin 600 mg	Touro DM by Anabolic	00722-6297	Cold Remedy
TOURODM <> DP311	Tab, Blue, Oblong, Scored, DP over 311	Guaifenesin 575 mg, Dextromethorphan Hydriodide 30 mg	by Martec		Cold Remedy
TOUROEX <> DP321	Tab, White, Tab Ex Release, Touro EX <> DP/321	Guaifenesin 575 mg	Touro EX by Dartmouth	58869-0421	Expectorant
TOUROEX <> DP321	Tab, Touro EX <> DP/321	Guaifenesin 575 mg	Touro EX by Anabolic	00722-6394	Expectorant
TOUROEX <> DP321	Tab, Touro EX, DP/321	Guaifenesin 600 mg	Touro EX by Anabolic	00722-6282	Expectorant
TOUROEX <> DP421	Tab, White, Oblong, Scored	Guaifenesin 575 mg	by Pfab	62542-0705	Expectorant
TOUROLA <> DP436	Tab, Touro LA, DP/436	Guaifenesin 500 mg, Pseudoephedrine HCl 120 mg	Touro LA by Anabolic	00722-6284	Cold Remedy
TOUROLA <> DP436	Cap, White	Pseudoephedrine HCl 120 mg, Guaifenesin 500 mg	Touro LA by Dartmouth	58869-0536	Cold Remedy
TOUROLA <> DP636	Tab, White, Oblong, Scored	Guaifenesin 525 mg; Pseudoephedrine HCl 120 mg	by Pfab	62542-0755	Cold Remedy
TP305	Tab, White, Round	Colchicine 648 mcg	by Towne Paulsen		Antigout
TP352	Cap, Pink	Zinc Sulfate 220 mg	Orazinc by Towne Paulsen		Mineral Supplement
TP403	Tab, Peach, Round	Hydrochlorothiazide 100 mg	Hydrodiuril by Towne Paulsen		Diuretic
TP404	Tab, Peach, Round	Hydrochlorothiazide 25 mg	Hydrodiuril by Towne Paulsen		Diuretic
TP405	Tab, Peach, Round	Hydrochlorothiazide 50 mg	Hydrodiuril by Towne Paulsen		Diuretic
TP4214	Tab, White, Round, TP421/4	Aspirin 325 mg, Codeine 60 mg	Empirin #4 by Towne Paulsen		Analgesic; C III
TP4243	Tab, White, Round	Aspirin 325 mg, Codeine 30 mg	Empirin #3 by Towne Paulsen		Analgesic; C III
TP4653	Tab, White, Round, TP 465/3	Acetaminophen 300 mg, Codeine 30 mg	Tylenol #3 by Towne Paulsen		Analgesic; C III
TP4664	Tab, White, Round, TP 466-4	Acetaminophen 300 mg, Codeine 60 mg	Tylenol #4 by Towne Paulsen		Analgesic; C III
TP520	Tab, White, Round	Meprobamate 400 mg	Miltown by Towne Paulsen		Sedative/Hypnotic; C IV
TP522	Tab, White, Round	Meprobamate 200 mg	Miltown by Towne Paulsen		Sedative/Hypnotic; C IV
TP601	Tab, White, Round	Colchicine 540 mcg	by Towne Paulsen		Antigout
TP604	Tab, White, Round	Cortisone Acetate 25 mg	Cortone by Towne Paulsen		Steroid
TP606	Tab, White, Round	Hydrocortisone 20 mg	Cortef by Towne Paulsen		Steroid
TP608	Tab, White, Round	Hydrocortisone 10 mg	by Towne Paulsen		Steroid
TP758	Tab, White, Round, TP-758	Acetaminophen 325 mg	Tylenol by Rosemont		Antipyretic
TP783	Tab, Bluish Green, Round	Butabarbital 30 mg	Butisol by Towne Paulsen		Sedative; C III
TP816	Tab, Yellow, Round	Chlorpheniramine Maleate 4 mg	Chlor-trimeton by Towne Paulsen		Antihistamine
TP827	Cap, Pink	Diphenhydramine 50 mg	Benadryl by Towne Paulsen		Antihistamine
TP833	Cap, Pink & White	Diphenhydramine 25 mg	Benadryl by Towne Paulsen		Antihistamine
TP865	Tab, Yellow, Round	Isoniazid 100 mg	by Towne Paulsen		Antimycobacterial
TP873	Tab, Yellow, Round	Folic Acid 1 mg	Folvite by Rosemont		Vitamin
TP900	Tab, White, Octagonal	Quinidine Sulfate 200 mg	Quinidine Sulfate by Towne Paulsen		Antiarrhythmic
TP913	Tab, White, Round	Prednisone 10 mg	Deltasone by Towne Paulsen		Steroid
TP922	Tab, Orange, Round	Prednisone 5 mg	by Towne Paulsen		Steroid
TP924	Tab, White, Round	Prednisone 5 mg	Deltasone by Towne Paulsen		Steroid
TP925	Tab, Peach, Round	Prednisone 20 mg	Deltasone by Towne Paulsen		Steroid
TP926	Tab, Peach, Round	Prednisone 2.5 mg	Deltasone by Towne Paulsen		Steroid

ID FRONT <> BACK	DESCRIPTION FRONT <> BACK	INGREDIENT & STRENGTH	BRAND (OR EQUIV.) & FIRM	NDC#	CLASS; SCH.
TR100 <> 3M	Tab, White, Round, Scored	Flecainide 100 mg	Tambocor by 3M	00089-0307	Antiarrhythmic
TR125 <> G	Tab	Triazolam 0.125 mg	by Par	49884-0453	Sedative/Hypnotic; C IV
TR125 <> G	Tab, TR/125	Triazolam 0.125 mg	by Qualitest	00603-6186	Sedative/Hypnotic; C IV
TR150 <> 3M	Tab, White, Oval, Scored	Flecainide 150 mg	Tambocor by 3M	00089-0314	Antiarrhythmic
TR250 <> G	Tab	Triazolam 0.25 mg	by Par	49884-0454	Sedative/Hypnotic; C IV
TR250 <> G	Tab, TR/250	Triazolam 0.25 mg	by Quality Care	60346-0886	Sedative/Hypnotic; C IV
TR250 <> G	Tab, TR/250	Triazolam 0.25 mg	by Qualitest	00603-6187	Sedative/Hypnotic; C IV
TR4 <> ORGANON	Tab, Film Coated, TR over 4 <> Organon	Desogestrel 0.15 mg, Ethinyl Estradiol 0.02 mg, Ethinyl Estradiol 0.01 mg	Mircette by Organon	00052-0281	Oral Contraceptive
TR4 <> ORGANON	Tab, Film Coated, T R over 4 <> Organon	Desogestrel 0.15 mg, Ethinyl Estradiol 0.02 mg, Ethinyl Estradiol 0.01 mg	Mircette by NV Organon	12860-0281	Oral Contraceptive
TR5 <> ORGANON	Tab, TR Over 5	Desogestrel 0.15 mg, Ethinyl Estradiol 0.03 mg	Desogen by Organon	60889-0261	Oral Contraceptive
TR5 <> ORGANON	Tab, White, Round	Desogestrel 0.15 mg, Ethinyl Estradiol 0.03 mg	Marvelon 21 by Organon	Canadian DIN# 02042487	Oral Contraceptive
TR5 <> ORGANON	Tab, White, Round	Desogestrel 0.15 mg, Ethinyl Estradiol 0.03 mg	Marvelon 28 by Organon	Canadian DIN# 02042479	Oral Contraceptive
TR5 <> ORGANON	Tab	Desogestrel 0.15 mg, Ethinyl Estradiol 0.03 mg	Desogen by Organon	00052-0261	Oral Contraceptive
TR50 <> 3M	Tab, White, Round	Flecainide 50 mg	Tambocor by 3M	00089-0305	Antiarrhythmic
TR50 <> 3M	Tab, White, Round	Flecainide Acetate 50 mg	Tambocor by Murfreesboro Ph	51129-1378	Antiarrhythmic
TRANDATE100	Tab, Orange, Oblong	Labetalol 100 mg	by Roberts	Canadian	Antihypertensive
TRANDATE100	Tab, Orange, Round, Scored	Labetalol HCl 100 mg	Trandate by Med-Pro	53978-3374	Antihypertensive
TRANDATE100	Tab, Light Orange, Light Orange	Labetalol HCl 100 mg	Trandate by Glaxo Wellcome		Antihypertensive
TRANDATE100	Tab, Orange, Round, Scored	Labetalol HCl 100 mg	Trandate by Faro Pharms	60976-0346	Antihypertensive
TRANDATE100	Tab, Orange, Round, Scored	Labetalol HCl 100 mg	Trandate by Rightpac	65240-0754	Antihypertensive
TRANDATE100	Tab, Light Orange, Tab Coated	Labetalol HCl 100 mg	Trandate by Glaxo	00173-0346	Antihypertensive
TRANDATE100	Tab, Orange, Round, Scored, Film Coated	Labetalol HCl 100 mg	Trandate by Murfreesboro	51129-1615	Antihypertensive
TRANDATE100	Tab, Tab Coated	Labetalol HCl 100 mg	Trandate by Drug Distr	52985-0219	Antihypertensive
TRANDATE100	Tab, Tab Coated	Labetalol HCl 100 mg	Trandate by Nat Pharmpak Serv	55154-1100	Antihypertensive
TRANDATE100	Tab, Tab Coated	Labetalol HCl 100 mg	Trandate by Leiner	59606-0754	Antihypertensive
TRANDATE100	Tab, Light Orange, Coated	Labetalol HCl 100 mg	Trandate by Thrift Drug	59198-0284	Antihypertensive
TRANDATE100	Tab, Tab Coated	Labetalol HCl 100 mg	Trandate by Amerisource	62584-0346	Antihypertensive
TRANDATE200	Tab, White, Oblong	Labetalol HCl 200 mg	Trandate by Roberts	Canadian	Antihypertensive
TRANDATE200	Tab, White, Round	Labetalol HCl 200 mg	Trandate by Glaxo Wellcome		Antihypertensive
TRANDATE200	Tab, White, Round, Scored	Labetalol HCl 200 mg	Trandate by Rightpac	65240-0755	Antihypertensive
TRANDATE200	Tab, White, Round, Scored	Labetalol HCl 200 mg	Trandate by Med-Pro	53978-3388	Antihypertensive
TRANDATE200	Tab, Film Coated	Labetalol HCl 200 mg	Trandate by Glaxo	00173-0347	Antihypertensive
TRANDATE200	Tab, White, Round, Scored, Film Coated	Labetalol HCl 200 mg	Trandate by Murfreesboro	51129-1616	Antihypertensive
TRANDATE200	Tab, Film Coated	Labetalol HCl 200 mg	Trandate by Amerisource	62584-0347	Antihypertensive
TRANDATE200	Tab, Film Coated	Labetalol HCl 200 mg	Trandate by Nat Pharmpak Serv	55154-1101	Antihypertensive
TRANDATE200	Tab, Film Coated	Labetalol HCl 200 mg	Trandate by Thrift Drug	59198-0285	Antihypertensive
TRANDATE200	Tab, Film Coated	Labetalol HCl 200 mg	Trandate by Leiner	59606-0755	Antihypertensive
TRANDATE300	Tab, Peach, Round, Film Coated, Scored	Labetalol HCl 300 mg	Trandate by Neuman Distbtrs	64579-0386	Antihypertensive
TRANDATE300	Tab, Peach, Round	Labetalol HCl 300 mg	Trandate by Glaxo Wellcome		Antihypertensive
TRANDATE300	Tab, Peach, Round, Scored	Labetalol HCl 300 mg	Trandate by Rightpac	65240-0770	Antihypertensive
TRANDATE300	Tab, Film Coated	Labetalol HCl 300 mg	Trandate by Glaxo	00173-0348	Antihypertensive
TRANDATE300	Tab, Film Coated	Labetalol HCl 300 mg	Trandate by Leiner	51947-3332	Antihypertensive
TRANDATE300	Tab, Film Coated	Labetalol HCl 300 mg	Trandate by Leiner	59606-0770	Antihypertensive
TRANDATE300	Tab, Film Coated	Labetalol HCl 300 mg	Trandate by Thrift Drug	59198-0286	Antihypertensive
TRAZODONE	Tab, White, Biconvex, Scored	Trazodone HCl 100 mg	by Pharmascience	Canadian	Antidepressant
TRAZODONE	Tab, Orange, Round, Scored	Trazodone HCl 50 mg	by Pharmascience	Canadian	Antidepressant
TRENTAL	Tab, Film Coated	Pentoxifylline 400 mg	Trental by Merrell	00068-0780	Anticoagulent
TRENTAL	Tab, Film Coated, Encircled R Logo	Pentoxifylline 400 mg	Trental by DRX	55045-2327	Anticoagulent

ID FRONT <> BACK	DESCRIPTION FRONT <> BACK	INGREDIENT & STRENGTH	BRAND (OR EQUIV.) & FIRM	NDC#	CLASS; SCH.
TRENTAL	Tab, Film Coated	Pentoxifylline 400 mg	Trental by Nat Pharmpak Serv	55154-1205	Anticoagulent
TRENTAL	Tab, Film Coated	Pentoxifylline 400 mg	Trental by Amerisource	62584-0078	Anticoagulent
TRENTAL	Tab, Film Coated	Pentoxifylline 400 mg	Trental by Quality Care	60346-0750	Anticoagulent
TRENTAL <> HOECHST	Tab, Film Coated, Oblong	Pentoxifylline 400 mg	Trental by Hoechst Roussel	00039-0078	Anticoagulent
TRENTAL <> HOECHST	Tab, Film Coated	Pentoxifylline 400 mg	Trental by Allscripts	54569-0668	Anticoagulent
TRENTAL <> HOECHST	Tab, Film Coated	Pentoxifylline 400 mg	Trental by Pharmedix	53002-1040	Anticoagulent
TRENTALHOECHST	Tab, Film Coated	Pentoxifylline 400 mg	by Med Pro	53978-0374	Anticoagulent
TREXAN <> DUPONT	Tab, Debossed	Naltrexone HCl 50 mg	Trexan by Du Pont Pharma	00056-0080	Opiod Antagonist
TRIAD <> UAD305	Cap, White, Triad <> UAD Logo 305	Acetaminophen 325 mg, Butalbital 50 mg, Caffeine 40 mg	Triad by UAD	00785-2305	Analgesic
TRIADUAD305	Cap, Red, Triad/UAD 305	Butalbital 50 mg, Acetaminophen 325 mg, Caffeine 40 mg	Triad (old) by Forest		Analgesic
TRIADUAD305	Cap, Off-White, Opaque	Butalbital 50 mg, Acetaminophen 325 mg, Caffeine 40 mg	Triad (current) by Forest	00785-2305	Analgesic
TRIANAL	Cap, Blue	Butalbital 50 mg, Caffeine 40 mg, Aspirin 330 mg	by Trianon	Canadian	Analgesic
TRIANAL	Tab, White	Butalbital 50 mg, Caffeine 40 mg, Aspirin 330 mg	by Trianon	Canadian	Analgesic
TRIANALC12	Cap, Blue, Trianal C 1/2	Butalbital 50 mg, Caffeine 40 mg, Aspirin 330 mg	by Trianon	Canadian	Analgesic
TRIANALC14	Cap, Blue, Trianal C 1/4	Butalbital 50 mg, Caffeine 40 mg, Aspirin 330 mg	by Trianon	Canadian	Analgesic
TRIANGLE	Tab, Off-White, Round, Debossed Modied Square	Rizatriptan Benzoate 10 mg	Maxalt-MLT by Merck	00006-3801	Antimigraine
TRIANGLE	Tab, Off-White, Round, Debossed Modied Triangle	Rizatriptan Benzoate 5 mg	Maxalt-MLT by Merck	00006-3800	Antimigraine
TRIANGLE <> ZOVIRAX	Tab	Acyclovir 400 mg	Zovirax by Quality Care	62682-1013	Antiviral
TRIANGLE150	Tab, White, Round	Propafenone HCl 150 mg	Rythmol by Knoll		Antiarrhythmic
TRIANGLE168	Tab, White, Cylindrical	Nilutamide 50 mg	Nilandron by Hoechst Marion Roussel		Antiandrogen
TRIANGLE182 <> TARKA	Tab, Pink, Oval	Trandolapril 2 mg, Verapamil 180 mg	Tarka by Knoll Pharm	00048-5921	Antihypertensive
TRIANGLE225	Tab, White, Round	Propafenone HCl 225 mg	Rythmol by Knoll		Antiarrhythmic
TRIANGLE241 <> TARKA	Tab, White, Oval	Trandolapril 1 mg, Verapamil 240 mg	Tarka by Knoll Pharm	00048-5912	Antihypertensive
TRIANGLE242 <> TARKA	Tab, Yellow, Oval	Trandolapril 2 mg, Verapamil 240 mg	Tarka by Knoll Pharm	00048-5922	Antihypertensive
TRIANGLE244 <> TARKA	Tab, Brown, Oval	Trandolapril 4 mg, Verapamil 240 mg	Tarka by Knoll Pharm	00048-5942	Antihypertensive
TRIANGLE300	Tab, White, Round	Propafenone HCl 300 mg	Rythmol by Knoll		Antiarrhythmic
TRIMETHOPRIM160 <> SULFAMETHOXAZO	Tab	Sulfamethoxazole 800 mg, Trimethoprim 160 mg	by HL Moore	00839-6406	Antibiotic
TRINALIN703	Tab, Coral, Tab Sugar Coated	Azatadine Maleate 1 mg, Pseudoephedrine Sulfate 120 mg	Trinalin by Quality Care	60346-0274	Cold Remedy
TRINALIN703	Tab, Coral, Sugar Coated, Black Print	Azatadine Maleate 1 mg, Pseudoephedrine Sulfate 120 mg	Trinalin by Caremark	00339-5411	Cold Remedy
TRINITY <> 60030	Tab, Film Coated, Scored	Dextromethorphan Hydrobromide 30 mg, Guaifenesin 600 mg	by United Res	00677-1486	Cold Remedy
TRITEC	Tab, Blue, Octagonal, Stomach Logo	Ranitidine Bismuth Citrate 400 mg	Tritec by Glaxo Wellcome	00173-0488	Gastrointestinal
TRM5MG	Tab, White, Round, TRM/5 mg	Trihexyphenidyl HCl 2 mg	by Pharmascience	Canadian	Antiparkinson
TROCHE <> TTORADOL	Tab, Film Coated, Red Print	Ketorolac Tromethamine 10 mg	Toradol by Allscripts	54569-3539	NSAID
TROCHE <> TTORADOL	Tab, White, Round, Film Coated	Ketorolac Tromethamine 10 mg	Toradol by HJ Harkins	52959-0224	NSAID
TROCHE <> TTORADOL	Tab, Film Coated, Red Print	Ketorolac Tromethamine 10 mg	Toradol by Syntex	18393-0435	NSAID
TRYPTAN <> 500MG	Tab, White, Oval, Film Coated	L-Tryptophan 500 mg	by Altimed	Canadian DIN# 02240333	Supplement
TS	Tab, Red, Round, Chewable	Acetaminophen 80 mg, Pseudoehedrine HCl 7.5 mg	Children's Tylenol Sinus Chewable Tablets By McNeil	Canadian DIN# 02240419	Cold Remedy
TT	Tab, Pink, Oblong	Pseudoephedrine 60 mg, Chlorpheniramine 4 mg, Acetaminophen 650 mg	Singlet by Trinity		Cold Remedy
TT <> 207	Tab	Guaifenesin 600 mg, Pseudoephedrine HCl 60 mg	by United Res	00677-1487	Cold Remedy
TT10110	Tab, White, Round, TT/101 10	Isoxsuprine HCl 10 mg	Vasodilan by Trinity		Vasodilator
TT10220	Tab, White, Round, TT/102 20	Isoxsuprine HCl 20 mg	Vasodilan by Trinity		Vasodilator
TT177	Tab, Yellow, Oblong, T/T 177	Pseudoephedrine HCl 120 mg, Guaifenesin 600 mg	Entex PSE by Trinity		Cold Remedy

ID FRONT <> BACK	DESCRIPTION FRONT <> BACK	INGREDIENT & STRENGTH	BRAND (OR EQUIV.) & FIRM	NDC#	CLASS; SCH.
TT207	Tab	Guaifenesin 600 mg, Pseudoephedrine HCl 60 mg	by Major	00904-5150	Cold Remedy
TT60075	Tab, White, Oblong, TT 600/75	Phenylpropanolamine HCl 75 mg, Guaifenesin 600 mg	Duravent by Trinity		Cold Remedy
TTC <> G600	Tab, Light Green	Guaifenesin 600 mg	by Quality Care	60346-0863	Expectorant
TTC <> G600	Tab	Guaifenesin 600 mg	by United Res	00677-1475	Expectorant
TTC40075	Tab, Blue, Oblong, TTC 400/75	Phenylpropanolamine HCl 75 mg, Guaifenesin LA 400 mg	Entex LA by Trinity		Cold Remedy
TTG200	Tab, Pink, Round, TT/G200	Guaifenesin 200 mg	Organidin NR by Trinity		Expectorant
TTG200	Tab, Pink, Round, Scored, TT over G200	Guaifenesin 200 mg	by Mallinckrodt Hobart	00406-1121	Expectorant
TTORADOL <> TROCHE	Tab, White, Round, Film Coated	Ketorolac Tromethamine 10 mg	Toradol by HJ Harkins	52959-0224	NSAID
TTORADOL <> TROCHE	Tab, Film Coated, Red Print	Ketorolac Tromethamine 10 mg	Toradol by Allscripts	54569-3539	NSAID
TTORADOL <> TROCHE	Tab, Film Coated, Red Print	Ketorolac Tromethamine 10 mg	Toradol by Syntex	18393-0435	NSAID
TTS500	Tab, Blue, Round	Salsalate 500 mg	Disalcid by Trinity		NSAID
TTS750	Tab, Blue, Oblong	Salsalate 750 mg	Disalcid by Trinity		NSAID
TUMS	Tab, Purple, Round	Calcium Carbonate 1000 mg	Tums Ultra Maximum Strength Antacid by Caremark	00339-5423	Vitamin/Mineral
TUSSIGON <> DP082	Tab, DP/082	Homatropine Methylbromide 1.5 mg, Hydrocodone Bitartrate 5 mg	Tussigon by Quality Care	60346-0947	Cold Remedy; C III
TUSSIGON <> DP082	Tab, Blue, Round, Scored, Tussigon <> dp/082	Homatropine Methylbromide 1.5 mg, Hydrocodone Bitartrate 5 mg	Tussigon by JMI Daniels	00689-0082	Cold Remedy; C III
TVN100 <> PFIZER	Tab, Blue, Round	Trovafloxacin 100 mg	Trovan by Pfizer	Canadian DIN# 02239191	Antibiotic
TVN200 <> PFIZER	Tab, Blue, Oval	Trovafloxacin 200 mg	Trovan by Pfizer	Canadian DIN# 02239192	Antibiotic
TX	Tab, Blue, Round, TX over Abbott Logo	Clorazepate Dipotassium 11.25 mg	Tranxene-SD by Abbott	00074-2699	Antianxiety; C IV
TY	Tab, Tan, Round, TY over Abbott Logo	Clorazepate Dipotassium 22.5 mg	Tranxene-SD by Abbott	00074-2997	Antianxiety; C IV
TY <> 160	Tab, Pink or Purple, Round, Scored, Chewable	Acetaminophen 160 mg	Jr. Streng Tylenol by McNeil	Canadian DIN# 02241361	Antipyretic
TY80	Tab, Pink or Purple, Round, Chewable	Acetaminophen 80 mg	Junior Strength Tylenol by McNeil	Canadian DIN# 02238295	Antipyretic
TYCOF <> 500	Cap, Red, Film Coated	Acetaminophen 500 mg, Dextromethorphan Hydrobromide	Extra Strength Tylenol Cough	Canadian DIN# 02017377	Cold Remedy
TYLCODEINE3 <> MCNEIL	Tab, TYL Over Codeine 3	Acetaminophen 300 mg, Codeine Phosphate 30 mg	Tylenol Codeine No 3 by Quality Care	60346-0853	Analgesic; C III
TYLENOL <> 500	Tab, White, Round	Acetaminophen 500 mg	ES Tylenol by McNeil	Canadian DIN# 00559407	Antipyretic
TYLENOL <> 325	Tab, White, Round, Scored	Acetaminophen 325 mg	Tylenol by McNeil	Canadian DIN# 00559393	Antipyretic
TYLENOL <> 325	Cap, White, Film Coated, Scored	Acetaminophen 325 mg	Tylenol by McNeil	Canadian DIN# 00723894	Antipyretic
TYLENOL <> 500	Cap, White, Film Coated	Acetaminophen 500 mg	ES Tylenol by McNeil	Canadian DIN# 00723908	Antipyretic

ID FRONT <> BACK	DESCRIPTION FRONT <> BACK	INGREDIENT & STRENGTH	BRAND (OR EQUIV.) & FIRM	NDC#	CLASS; SCH.
TYLENOL <> 80	Tab, Pink or Purple, Round, Scored, Chewable	Acetaminophen	Children's Tylenol Chewable by McNeil	Canadian DIN# 02229539	Antipyretic
TYLENOL160	Tab, Pink or Purple, Round, Scored, Chewable	Acetaminophen	Junior Strength Tylenol Chewable By McNeil	Canadian DIN# 01967819	Antipyretic
TYLENOL3CODEINE <> MCNEIL	Tab	Acetaminophen 300 mg, Codeine Phosphate 30 mg	Tylenol Codeine No 3 by McNeil	00045-0513	Analgesic; C III
TYLENOL4CODEINE <> MCNEIL	Tab	Acetaminophen 300 mg, Codeine Phosphate 60 mg	Tylenol Codeine No 4 by McNeil	00045-0515	Analgesic; C III
TYLENOL500	Cap, Red & Yellow, Film Coated	Acetaminophen 500 mg	ES Tylenol by McNeil	Canadian DIN# 00863270	Antipyretic
TYLENOLAS	Cap, Light Blue, Film Coated, Tylenol A/S	Acetaminophen 500 mg, Pseudoephedrine 30 mg, Diphenhdramine HCl	Extra Strength Tylenol Alergy Sinus, Nighttime	Canadian DIN# 02237483	Cold Remedy
TYLENOLCODEINE2 <> MCNEIL	Tab	Acetaminophen 300 mg, Codeine Phosphate 15 mg	Tylenol Codeine No 2 by McNeil	00045-0511	Analgesic; C III
TYLENOLCODEINE2 <> MCNEIL	Tab	Acetaminophen 300 mg, Codeine Phosphate 15 mg	Tylenol Codeine No 2 by Murfreesboro	51129-1393	Analgesic; C III
TYLENOLCODEINE3 <> MCNEIL	Tab	Acetaminophen 300 mg, Codeine Phosphate 30 mg	Tylenol Codeine No 3 by Allscripts	54569-0024	Analgesic; C III
TYLENOLCODEINE3 <> MCNEIL	Tab	Acetaminophen 300 mg, Codeine Phosphate 30 mg	Tylenol Codeine No 3 by Med Pro	53978-3087	Analgesic; C III
TYLENOLCODEINE4 <> MCNEIL	Tab	Acetaminophen 300 mg, Codeine Phosphate 60 mg	Tylenol Codeine No 4 by Med Pro	53978-3094	Analgesic; C III
TYLENOLCODEINE4 <> MCNEIL	Tab, White, Round	Codeine Phosphate 60 mg; Acetaminophen 300 mg	by Natl Pharmpak	55154-1916	Analgesic; C III
TYLENOLCOLD <> 80	Tab, Pink or Orange, Round, Scored, Chewable	Acetaminophen 80 mg, Chlorpheniramine Maleate 0.5 mg, Pseudoephedrine HCl 7.5 mg	Children's Tylenol by McNeil	Canadian DIN# 00743224	Cold Remedy
TYLENOLCOLDDM <> 80	Tab, Pink or Purple, Round, Chewable	Acetaminophen 80 mg, Chlorpheniramine Maleate 0.5 mg, Pseudoephedrine HCl 7.5 mg, Dextrometh 3.75 mg	Children's Tylenol by McNeil	Canadian DIN# 00870455	Cold Remedy
TYLENOLCOLDSC	Cap, Yellow, Film Coated	Acetaminophen 325 mg, Pseudoephedrine HCl 30 mg, Dextromethorphan Hydrobromide 15 mg, Guaifenesin 200 mg	Regular Strength Tylenol Cold Chest Congestion	Canadian DIN# 02240277	Cold Remedy
TYLENOLER	Cap, White, Film Coated	Acetaminophen 650 mg	Tylenol Arthritis Pain Extended Relief	Canadian DIN# 02238885	Antipyretic
TYLENOLFLU	Cap, Dark Red & White, Film Coated	Acetaminophen 500 mg, Pseudoephedrine HCl 30 mg, Dextromethorphan Hydrobromide 15 mg	Extra Strength Tylenol Flu Daytime by McNeil	Canadian DIN# 02241526	Cold Remedy
TYLENOLFLUNT	Cap, Blue & White, Gelatin, Film-Coated	Acetaminophen 500 mg, Diphenhydramine HCl 25 mg, Pseudoephedrine HCl 30 mg	Extra Strength Tylenol Flu Nighttime	Canadian DIN# 02167670	Cold Remedy
TYLENOLSINUSNT	Cap, Teal, Film Coated	Acetaminophen 500 mg, Pseudoephedrine HCl 30 mg, Doxylamine Succinate 6.25 mg	Extra Strength Tylenol Sinus Nighttime by McNeil	Canadian DIN# 02240302	Cold Remedy
TYLOXMCNEIL	Cap, Black Print	Acetaminophen 500 mg, Oxycodone HCl 5 mg	Tylox by McNeil	00045-0526	Analgesic; C II

ID FRONT <> BACK	DESCRIPTION FRONT <> BACK	INGREDIENT & STRENGTH	BRAND (OR EQUIV.) & FIRM	NDC#	CLASS; SCH.
TYME <> 500	Cap, Peach, Film Coated	Acetaminophen 500 mg, Pamabrom 25 mg, Pyrilamine Maleate15 mg	Extra Strength Tylenol Menstrual	Canadian DIN# 02231239	Cold Remedy
TZ	Tab, Mauve, Oval	Triazolam 0.125 mg	Gen Triazolam by Genpharm	Canadian	Sedative/Hypnotic
TZ	Tab, Blue, Oval	Triazolam 0.25 mg	Gen Triazolam by Genpharm	Canadian	Sedative/Hypnotic
TZ3 <> ORGANON	Tab, Yellow, Oval	Mirtazapine 15 mg	Remeron by Neuman Distbtrs	64579-0390	Antidepressant
TZ3 <> ORGANON	Tab, Film Coated	Mirtazapine 15 mg	Remeron by Organon	00052-0105	Antidepressant
TZ3 <> ORGANON	Tab, Film Coated	Mirtazapine 15 mg	Remeron by NV Organon	12860-0105	Antidepressant
TZ5 <> ORGANON	Tab, Red-Brown, Film Coated	Mirtazapine 30 mg	Remeron by Organon	00052-0107	Antidepressant
TZ5 <> ORGANON	Tab, Red-Brown, Film Coated	Mirtazapine 30 mg	Remeron by NV Organon	12860-0107	Antidepressant
TZ7 <> ORGANON	Tab, Film Coated	Mirtazapine 45 mg	Remeron by Organon	00052-0109	Antidepressant
TZ7 <> ORGANON	Tab, White, Oval, Film Coated	Mirtazapine 45 mg	Remeron by Nv Organon	12860-0109	Antidepressant
TZD100832	Tab, White, Round	Trazodone HCl 100 mg	Desyrel by Rosemont		Antidepressant
TZD50832	Tab, White, Round	Trazodone HCl 50 mg	Desyrel by Rosemont		Antidepressant
U	Tab, Light Yellow, Elliptical, Film Coated	Colestid 1 gm	by Pharmacia & Upjohn	Canadian DIN# 02132680	Lipid Lower Agent
U	Tab, White	Prednisone 50 mg	Deltasone by Upjohn	Canadian	Steroid
U <> 2	Tab	Pramipexole DiHCl 0.125 mg	Mirapex by Pharmacia & Upjohn	00009-0002	Antiparkinson
U <> 2	Tab	Pramipexole DiHCl 0.125 mg	Mirapex by Promex Med	62301-0026	Antiparkinson
U <> 201	Tab	Acetaminophen 650 mg, Hydrocodone Bitartrate 7.5 mg	Lorcet Plus by Amerisource	62584-0028	Analgesic; C III
U <> 201	Tab	Acetaminophen 650 mg, Hydrocodone Bitartrate 7.5 mg	Lorcet Plus by Med Pro	53978-2071	Analgesic; C III
U <> 201	Tab	Acetaminophen 650 mg, Hydrocodone Bitartrate 7.5 mg	by Mikart	46672-0025	Analgesic; C III
U <> 3774	Tab, Blue, Oblong	Estropipate 2.5 mg	Ogen by Heartland	61392-0500	Hormone
U <> 76	Tab, White, Rectangular	Dinoprostone 0.5 mg	by Pharmacia	Canadian DIN# 00400688	Oxytocic
U01	Tab, Orange, Round	Paramethasone Acetate 2 mg	Haldrone by Lilly		Steroid
U03	Tab, White, Cap Shaped	Acetohexamide 250 mg	Dymelor by Lilly		Antidiabetic
U05	Tab, Pink, Square	Erythromycin Estolate Chewable 125 mg	Ilosone by Lilly		Antibiotic
U07	Tab, Yellow, Oblong	Acetohexamide 500 mg	Dymelor by Lilly		Antidiabetic
U09	Tab, Blue, Oblong	Cyclothiazide 2 mg	Anhydron by Lilly		Diuretic
U121	Tab, White, Round	Minoxidil 2.5 mg	Loniten by Upjohn	Canadian	Antihypertensive
U121 <> 25	Tab, White, Round, Scored, U 121 <> 2.5	Minoxidil 2.5 mg	by Pharmacia	Canadian DIN# 00514497	Antihypertensive
U12125	Tab, White, Round, U/121 2.5	Minoxidil 2.5 mg	Loniten by Upjohn		Antihypertensive
U137	Tab, White, Round	Minoxidil 10 mg	Loniten by Upjohn	Canadian	Antihypertensive
U137 <> 10	Tab, White, Round, Scored	Minoxidil 10 mg	by Pharmacia	Canadian DIN# 00514500	Antihypertensive
U2	Tab, White, Round	Pramipexole DiHCl 0.125 mg	Mirapex by Upjohn		Antiparkinson
U201	Tab, White, Scored	Acetaminophen 650 mg, Hydrocodone Bitartrate 7.5 mg	by Forest Pharma	00785-1122	Analgesic; C III
U201	Tab, White, U/201	Hydrocodone Bitartrate 7.5 mg, Acetaminophen 650 mg	by Forest Pharma	0785-1122	Analgesic; C III
U23	Tab, White, Round	Isoniazid 300 mg	by Lilly		Antimycobacterial
U25	Tab, Pink, Square	Erythromycin Estolate Chewable 250 mg	Ilosone by Lilly		Antibiotic
U26	Tab, Salmon, Oblong	Erythromycin Estolate 500 mg	Ilosone by Lilly		Antibiotic
U286	Tab, Blue, Round, Scored	Medroxyprogesterone Acetate 5 mg	Provera by Upjohn	Canadian DIN# 00030937	Progestin
U29	Tab, Green, Round	Reserpine 0.25 mg	Sandril by Lilly		Antihypertensive
U3617	Tab, Film Coated	Cefpodoxime Proxetil 100 mg	Vantin by Pharmacia & Upjohn	00009-3617	Antibiotic

ID FRONT <> BACK	DESCRIPTION FRONT <> BACK	INGREDIENT & STRENGTH	BRAND (OR EQUIV.) & FIRM	NDC#	CLASS; SCH.
U3617	Tab, Film Coated	Cefpodoxime Proxetil 100 mg	Vantin by Allscripts	54569-4058	Antibiotic
U3618	Tab, Coral Red, Elliptical Shaped, Film Coated	Cefpodoxime Proxetil	Vantin by Quality Care	60346-0981	Antibiotic
U3618	Tab, Film Coated	Cefpodoxime Proxetil	Vantin by Pharmacia & Upjohn	59267-3618	Antibiotic
U3618	Tab, Film Coated	Cefpodoxime Proxetil	Vantin by Pharmacia & Upjohn	00009-3618	Antibiotic
U3761	Tab	Delavirdine Mesylate 100 mg	Rescriptor by Pharmacia & Upjohn	00009-3761	Antiviral
U3772	Tab	Estropipate 0.75 mg	Ogen by Quality Care	60346-0319	Hormone
U3772	Tab	Estropipate 0.75 mg	Ogen by Wal Mart	49035-0175	Hormone
U3772	Tab, Yellow, Oblong, Scored	Estropipate 0.75 mg	Ogen by Apotheca	12634-0512	Hormone
U3772	Tab	Estropipate 0.75 mg	Ogen by Eckerd Drug	19458-0873	Hormone
U3772	Tab, Yellow, Oval, U/3772	Estropitate 0.75 mg	by Pharmacia	Canadian	Hormone
U3772	Tab, Yellow, Oval, Scored	Estropipate 0.625 mg	by Pharmacia	Canadian DIN# 02089793	Hormone
U3772	Tab	Estropipate 0.75 mg	Ogen by Abbott	60692-3943	Hormone
U3772 <> U3772	Tab	Estropipate 0.75 mg	Ogen by Pharmacia & Upjohn	00009-3772	Hormone
U3773	Tab, Peach, Oval, Scored	Estropipate 1.25 mg	by Pharmacia	Canadian DIN# 02089769	Hormone
U3773	Tab	Estropipate 1.5 mg	Ogen by Abbott	60692-3946	Hormone
U3773	Tab	Estropipate 1.5 mg	Ogen by Wal Mart	49035-0174	Hormone
U3773	Tab	Estropipate 1.5 mg	Ogen by Eckerd Drug	19458-0874	Hormone
U3773	Tab, Peach, Oval, U/3773	Estropitate 1.5 mg	by Pharmacia	Canadian	Hormone
U3773 <> U3773	Tab, Peach, Oval, Tab, Scored	Estropipate 1.25 mg	Ogen by Heartland	61392-0492	Hormone
U3774	Tab, Blue, Oval, Scored	Estropipate 2.5 mg	by Pharmacia	Canadian DIN# 02089777	Hormone
U3774	Tab	Estropipate 3 mg	Ogen by Abbott	60692-3951	Hormone
U3774	Tab	Estropipate 3 mg	Ogen by Wal Mart	49035-0173	Hormone
U3774	Tab	Estropipate 3 mg	Ogen by Eckerd Drug	19458-0875	Hormone
U3774	Tab, Blue, Oval, U/3774	Estropitate 3 mg	by Pharmacia	Canadian	Hormone
U3775 <> U3775	Tab	Estropipate 1.5 mg	Ogen by Pharmacia & Upjohn	00009-3773	Hormone
U3B <> WELLCOME	Tab	Thioguanine 40 mg	Thioguanine by Catalytica	63552-0880	Antineoplastic
U400 <> PF	Tab	Theophylline Anhydrous 400 mg	Uniphyl by Purdue Frederick	00034-7004	Antiasthmatic
U400PF	Tab, White, Round, U/400/PF	Theophylline 400 mg	Uniphyl by Purdue Frederick	Canadian	Antiasthmatic
U400PF	Tab	Theophylline 400 mg	Uniphyl by Pharmedix	53002-1076	Antiasthmatic
U467	Tab, White, Round, Scored	Medroxyprogesterone Acetate 100 mg	Provera by Upjohn	Canadian DIN# 00030945	Progestin
U4AZYLOPRIM	Tab, White, Round, U4A/Zyloprim	Allopurinol 100 mg	by Glaxo	Canadian	Antigout
U53	Tab, Peach, Square	Methadone HCl Chewable 40 mg	Methadone Disket by Lilly		Analgesic; C II
U56	Tab, Yellow, Round	Folic Acid 1 mg	Folvite by Lilly		Vitamin
U60	Tab, Green, Oblong	Cephalexin 1 g	Keflex by Lilly		Antibiotic
U600 <> PF	Tab	Theophylline Anhydrous 600 mg	Uniphyl by PF	48692-0004	Antiasthmatic
U600 <> PF	Tab, P, Vertical Score, F,	Theophylline Anhydrous 600 mg	Uniphyl by Purdue Frederick	00034-7006	Antiasthmatic
U600PF	Tab, White, Oblong, U 600/PF	Theophylline 600 mg	Uniphyl by Purdue Frederick	Canadian	Antiasthmatic
U64	Tab, Orange, Round, Scored	Medroxyprogesterone Acetate 2.5 mg	Provera by Upjohn	Canadian DIN# 00708917	Progestin
U76	Tab, White, Rectangular, U/76	Dinoprostone 0.5 mg	by Pharmacia	Canadian	Oxytocic
UAD <> 204	Tab, White, Oblong	Guaifenesin 300 mg, Phenylephrine HCl 20 mg	Endal Time Release by Martec	52555-0161	Cold Remedy
UAD <> 204	Tab	Guaifenesin 300 mg, Phenylephrine HCl 20 mg	by Mikart	46672-0145	Cold Remedy
UAD <> 204	Tab, White, Oblong	Phenylephrine HCl 20 mg, Guasifenesin 300 mg	Endal by Physicians Total Care	54868-4094	Cold Remedy

ID FRONT <> BACK	DESCRIPTION FRONT <> BACK	INGREDIENT & STRENGTH	BRAND (OR EQUIV.) & FIRM	NDC#	CLASS; SCH.
UAD <> 6350	Tab	Acetaminophen 650 mg, Hydrocodone Bitartrate 10 mg	Lorcet by Nat Pharmpak Serv	55154-7301	Analgesic; C III
UAD <> 6350	Tab	Acetaminophen 650 mg, Hydrocodone Bitartrate 10 mg	Lorcet by Amerisource	62584-0021	Analgesic; C III
UAD <> 6350	Tab	Acetaminophen 650 mg, Hydrocodone Bitartrate 10 mg	Lorcet by Quality Care	60346-0955	Analgesic; C III
UAD <> 6350	Tab	Acetaminophen 650 mg, Hydrocodone Bitartrate 10 mg	Lorcet 10-650 by Allscripts	54569-3782	Analgesic; C III
UAD <> 6350	Tab	Acetaminophen 650 mg, Hydrocodone Bitartrate 10 mg	Lorcet by Med Pro	53978-2068	Analgesic; C III
UAD <> 6350	Tab, 63 50	Acetaminophen 650 mg, Hydrocodone Bitartrate 10 mg	Lorcet 10-650 by DRX	55045-2122	Analgesic; C III
UAD <> 6350	Tab	Acetaminophen 650 mg, Hydrocodone Bitartrate 10 mg	by Mikart	46672-0103	Analgesic; C III
UAD <> 6350	Tab, Blue, Oblong, Scored	Hydrocodone Bitartrate 10 mg, Acetaminophen 650 mg	by Southwood Pharms	58016-0232	Analgesic; C III
UAD111	Tab, Orange, Oblong	Propoxyphene HCl 65 mg, Acetaminophen 650 mg	Wygesic by Forest		Analgesic; C IV
UAD111	Tab, Orange, UAD/111	Propoxyphene HCl 65 mg, Acetaminophen 650 mg	E-Lor by Forest	00785-1117	Analgesic; C IV
UAD111	Tab, Orange, UAD/111	Propoxyphene HCl 65 mg, Acetaminophen 650 mg	by Forest Pharma	00785-1117	Analgesic; C IV
UAD1120	Cap, UAD/1220	Acetaminophen 500 mg, Hydrocodone Bitartrate 5 mg	Lorcet HD by UAD	00785-1120	Analgesic; C III
UAD1120	Cap, Maroon, Opaque, UAD/1120	Acetaminophen 500 mg, Hydrocodone Bitartrate 5 mg	by Forest Pharma	00785-1120	Analgesic; C III
UAD1120	Cap, Maroon, UAD Forest Logo 1120	Hydrocodone Bitartrate 5 mg, Acetaminophen 500 mg	Lorcet HD by Forest	00785-1120	Analgesic; C III
UAD202	Tab, Yellow, UAD/202	Acetaminophen 325 mg, Hydrocodone 2.5 mg	by Forest		Analgesic; C III
UAD204	Tab, White, Cap Shaped, UAD/204	Guaifenesin 300 mg, Phenylephrine HCl 20 mg	Endal by UAD	00785-2204	Cold Remedy
UAD204	Tab, White, Cap Shaped, UAD/204	Phenylephrine HCl 20 mg, Guaifenesin 300 mg	by Forest Pharma	00785-2204	Cold Remedy
UAD207	Tab, Red, UAD/207	Acetaminophen 325 mg, Hydrocodone 7.5 mg	by Forest		Analgesic; C III
UAD210	Tab, Burgandy, UAD/210	Acetaminophen 325 mg, Hydrocodone 10 mg	by Forest		Analgesic; C III
UAD2404	Cap, Blue, Opaque, UAD/2404	Dimenhydrinate 50 mg	by Forest Pharma	00785-2404	Antiemetic
UAD2404	Cap, Blue	Dimenhydrinate 50 mg	Vertab by Forest	00785-2404	Antiemetic
UAD305 <> TRIAD	Cap, White, UAD Logo 305 <> Triad	Acetaminophen 325 mg, Butalbital 50 mg, Caffeine 40 mg	Triad by UAD	00785-2305	Analgesic
UAD308	Tab, Peach, UAD/308	Acetaminophen 150 mg, Aspirin 180 mg, Hydrocodone 5 mg	by Forest		Analgesic; C III
UAD309	Tab, Purple, UAD/309	Acetaminophen 150 mg, Aspirin 180 mg, Hydrocodone 7.5 mg	by Forest		Analgesic; C III
UAD310	Tab, Red, UAD/310	Acetaminophen 150 mg, Aspirin 180 mg, Hydrocodone 10 mg	by Forest		Analgesic; C III
UAD400	Tab, White, Scored, UAD/400	Guaifenesin 400 mg, Pseudoephedrine 120 mg	by Forest Pharma	00785-6301	Cold Remedy
UAD400	Tab, White, UAD/400	Guaifenesin 400 mg, Pseudoephedrine HCl 120 mg	Eudal Sr by UAD	00785-6301	Cold Remedy
UAD405	Tab, White, UAD/405	Acetaminophen 650 mg, Hydrocodone 5 mg	by Forest		Analgesic; C III
UAD505	Cap, Red, UAD/505	Acetaminophen 325 mg, Hydrocodone 5 mg	by Forest		Analgesic; C III
UAD63 <> 50	Tab, Light Blue, UAD/63	Acetaminophen 650 mg, Hydrocodone Bitartrate 10 mg	Lorcet by UAD	00785-6350	Analgesic; C III
UAD6350	Tab, Light Blue, Scored	Acetaminophen 650 mg, Hydrocodone Bitartrate 10 mg	by Forest Pharma	00785-6350	Analgesic; C III
UAD6350	Tab, Blue	Hydrocodone Bitartrate 10 mg, Acetaminophen 650 mg	Lorcet by Forest	00785-6350	Analgesic; C III
UADCEZINS811	Cap, Yellow, UAD Cezin-S/811	Vitamin A, DD, E, Ascorbic Acid	Cezin-S by Forest	00785-4811	Vitamin
UADCEZINS811	Cap, Yellow, UAD Cezin-S/811	Vitamin A, Vitamin DD, Vitamin E, Ascorbic acid, Nicotinamide (Niacinamide), Thiamine Mononitrate, d-Calcium Pantothenate, Riboflavin, Magnesium Chloride, Pyridoxine HCl, Folic Acid, Magnesium Sulfate, Zinc Sulfate	by Forest Pharma	00785-4811	Vitamin
UADENDAFED206	Cap, Blue & Clear, UAD/Endafed 206	Pseudoephedrine HCl 120 mg, Brompheniramine Maleate 12 mg	Endafed by Forest	00785-2206	Cold Remedy
UC	Tab, White, Rectangular, Abbott Logo	Estazolam 1 mg	Prosom by Abbott	Canadian	Sedative/Hypnotic
UC	Tab, White, Round, Abbott Logo	Estazolam 1 mg	ProSom by Abbott	00074-3735	Sedative/Hypnotic; C IV
UC	Tab, White, Rectangular, Scored, UC over Abbott Logo	Estazolam 1 mg	ProSom by Abbott	00074-3735	Sedative/Hypnotic; C IV
UC5337 <> A625	Tab, Green, Round, Scored	Pergolide Mesylate 0.25 mg	Epermax by Phcy Care	65070-0513	Antiparkinson
UC5364	Tab, Tab Delayed Release	Dirithromycin 250 mg	Dynabac by Promex Med	62301-0012	Antibiotic
UC5364	Tab, Coated	Dirithromycin 250 mg	Dynabac by Sanofi	00024-0490	Antibiotic
UC5364 <> DYNABAC	Tab, White, Oval, Coated	Dirithromycin 250 mg	Dynabac by Eli Lilly	00002-0490	Antibiotic
UC5391	Tab, Blue	Cefaclor 375 mg	Ceclor CD by Dura	51479-0036	Antibiotic
UC5391	Tab	Cefaclor Monohydrate 375 mg	Ceclor CD by DURA		Antibiotic
UC5392	Tab, Blue	Cefaclor 500 mg	Ceclor CD by Dura	51479-0035	Antibiotic
UC5392	Tab, Tab Ex Release	Cefaclor Monohydrate	Ceclor CD by Promex Med	62301-0028	Antibiotic
UC5392	Tab	Cefaclor Monohydrate 500 mg	Ceclor CD by DURA		Antibiotic
UC5395	Tab, Dark Green, Elliptical	Cephalexin HCl 500 mg	KEFTAB by DURA		Antibiotic
UCB <> 250	Tab, Blue, Oblong, Scored, Film Coated	Levetiracetam 250 mg	Keppra by UCB Pharma	50474-0591	Anticonvulsant

ID FRONT <> BACK	DESCRIPTION FRONT <> BACK	INGREDIENT & STRENGTH	BRAND (OR EQUIV.) & FIRM	NDC#	CLASS; SCH.
UCB <> 315	Cap, Black & Orange	Niacinamide 25 mg, Vitamin A 8000 unt, Magnesium Sulfate 70 mg, Zinc Sulfate 80 mg; Ascorbic Acid 150 mg; Vitamin E 50 unt; Thiamine Mononitrate 10 mg; Calcium Pantothenate 10 mg; Riboflavin 5 mg; Manganese Chloride 4 mg, Pyridoxine HCl 2 mg, Folic Acid	Vicon Forte by Rx Pac	65084-0211	Vitamin
UCB <> 316	Cap	Ascorbic Acid 150 mg, Calcium Pantothenate 10 mg, Cyanocobalamin 10 mcg, Folic Acid 1 mg, Magnesium Sulfate 70 mg, Manganese Chloride 4 mg, Niacinamide 25 mg, Pyridoxine HCl 2 mg, Riboflavin 5 mg, Thiamine Mononitrate 10 mg, Vitamin A 8000 Units, Vitamin E 50 Units, Zinc Sulfate 80 mg	Vicon Forte by Eckerd Drug	19458-0847	Vitamin
UCB <> 500	Tab	Aspirin 500 mg, Hydrocodone Bitartrate 5 mg	Lortab ASA by UCB	50474-0500	Analgesic; C III
UCB <> 500	Tab, Yellow, Oblong, Scored, Film Coated	Levetiracetam 500 mg	Keppra by UCB Pharma	50474-0592	Anticonvulsant
UCB <> 612	Tab, White, Oval, Tab, Scored, Film Coated	Guaifenesin 600 mg, Pseudoephedrine HCl 120 mg	Duratuss by Med Pro	53978-3355	Cold Remedy
UCB <> 612	Tab, Film Coated	Guaifenesin 600 mg, Pseudoephedrine HCl 120 mg	by Mikart	46672-0126	Cold Remedy
UCB <> 612	Tab, White, Oval, Scored, Film Coated	Guaifenesin 600 mg, Pseudoephedrine 120 mg	Duratuss by Med Pro	53978-3340	Cold Remedy
UCB <> 612	Tab, Film Coated	Guaifenesin 600 mg, Pseudoephedrine HCl 120 mg	Duratuss by Nat Pharmpak Serv	55154-7203	Cold Remedy
UCB <> 612	Tab, White, Oval, Film Coated, Scored	Guaifenesin 600 mg, Pseudoephedrine HCl 120 mg	Duratuss by UCB Pharma	50474-0612	Cold Remedy
UCB <> 612	Tab, Film Coated	Guaifenesin 600 mg, Pseudoephedrine HCl 120 mg	Duratuss by Paco	53668-0237	Cold Remedy
UCB <> 612	Tab, White, Oval, Scored	Pseudoephedrine HCl 120 mg; Guaifenesin 600 mg	Duratuss by Phy Total Care	54868-3943	Cold Remedy
UCB <> 750	Tab, Orange, Oblong, Scored, Film Coated	Levetiracetam 750 mg	Keppra by UCB Pharma	50474-0593	Anticonvulsant
UCB <> 901	Tab, White, Pink Specks, Cap Shaped, Scored	Acetaminophen 500 mg, Hydrocodone Bitartrate 10 mg	Lortab 10/500 by UCB	50474-0925	Analgesic; C III
UCB <> 901	Tab, White, Oblong, Bisected	Acetaminophen 500 mg, Hydrocodone Bitartrate 2.5 mg	Lortab by Alphagen	59743-0028	Analgesic; C III
UCB <> 901	Tab, White, Pink Specks, Cap Shaped, Scored	Acetaminophen 500 mg, Hydrocodone Bitartrate 2.5 mg	Lortab 2.5/500 by UCB	50474-0925	Analgesic; C III
UCB <> 901	Tab, White, Oblong, Scored	Hydrocodone Bitartrate 2.5 mg, Acetaminophen 500 mg	Lortab by Murfreesboro Ph	51129-1399	Analgesic; C III
UCB <> 902	Tab, White, Blue Specks, Cap Shaped, Scored	Acetaminophen 500 mg, Hydrocodone Bitartrate 5 mg	Lortab 5/500 by UCB	50474-0902	Analgesic; C III
UCB <> 902	Tab, White, Blue Specks, Oblong, Scored	Acetaminophen 500 mg, Hydrocodone Bitartrate 5 mg	by Allscripts	54569-0956	Analgesic; C III
UCB <> 903	Tab, White, Green Specks, Cap Shaped, Scored	Acetaminophen 500 mg, Hydrocodone Bitartrate 7.5 mg	by Allscripts	54569-0957	Analgesic; C III
UCB <> 903	Tab, White, Green Specks, Cap Shaped, Scored	Acetaminophen 500 mg, Hydrocodone Bitartrate 7.5 mg	Lortab 7.5 500 by UCB	50474-0907	Analgesic; C III
UCB <> 903	Tab, White, Oblong, Scored	Acetaminophen 500 mg, Hydrocodone Bitartrate 7.5 mg	Lortab by Allscripts	54569-4750	Analgesic; C III
UCB <> 910	Tab, Pink, Cap Shaped, Scored	Acetaminophen 500 mg, Hydrocodone Bitartrate 10 mg	Lortab 10/500 by UCB	50474-0910	Analgesic; C III
UCB <> 935	Tab, White, Oblong, Scored, with Orange Specks	Hydrocodone Bitartrate 5 mg, Acetaminophen 325 mg	by Murfreesboro	51129-1452	Analgesic; C III
UCB316	Cap	Ascorbic Acid 150 mg, Calcium Pantothenate 10 mg, Cyanocobalamin 10 mcg, Folic Acid 1 mg, Magnesium Sulfate 70 mg, Manganese Chloride 4 mg, Niacinamide 25 mg, Pyridoxine HCl 2 mg, Riboflavin 5 mg, Thiamine Mononitrate 10 mg, Vitamin A 8000 Units, Vitamin E 50 Units, Zinc Sulfate 80 mg	Vicon Forte by D M Graham	00756-0235	Vitamin
UCB316	Cap, Black & Orange, UCB/316	Ascorbic Acid 150 mg, Calcium Pantothenate 10 mg, Cyanocobalamin 10 mcg, Folic Acid 1 mg, Magnesium Sulfate 70 mg, Manganese Chloride 4 mg, Niacinamide 25 mg, Pyridoxine HCl 2 mg, Riboflavin 5 mg, Thiamine Mononitrate 10 mg, Vitamin A 8000 Units, Vitamin E 50 Units, Zinc Sulfate 80 mg	Vicon Forte by UCB	50474-0316	Vitamin
UCB316	Cap, Black & Orange	Niacinamide 25 mg, Vitamin A 8000 unt, Magnesium Sulfate 70 mg, Zinc Sulfate 80 mg; Ascorbic Acid 150 mg; Vitamin E 50 unt; Thiamine Mononitrate 10 mg; Calcium Pantothenate 10 mg; Riboflavin 5 mg; Manganese Chloride 4 mg, Pyridoxine HCl 2 mg, Folic Acid	Vicon Forte by Rightpac	65240-0780	Vitamin
UCB364	Cap, Dark Pink & Dark Red, UCB/364	Ascorbic Acid 75 mg, Cyanocobalamin 15 mcg, Ferrous Fumarate 110 mg, Folic Acid 0.5 mg, Liver With Stomach 240 mg	Trinsicon by UCB	50474-0364	Vitamin
UCB620	Tab, Film Coated, UCB/620	Guaifenesin 1200 mg	Duratuss G by Nat Pharmpak Serv	55154-7205	Expectorant
UCB620	Tab, White, Oblong, Film Coated, Scored	Guaifenesin 1200 mg	Duratuss G by Thrift Services	59198-0329	Expectorant
UCB620	Tab, White, Oblong, Scored	Guaifenesin 1200 mg	Duratuss G by Rx Pac	65084-0224	Expectorant
UCB620	Tab, White, Oblong, Scored, Film Coated, UCB/620	Guaifenesin 1200 mg	Duratuss G by Lilly	00110-0895	Expectorant
UCB620	Tab, White, Cap Shaped, Scored, Film Coated, UCB/620	Guaifenesin 1200 mg	Duratuss G by UCB	50474-0620	Expectorant
UCB620	Tab, Film Coated, UCB/620	Guaifenesin 1200 mg	by Mikart	46672-0163	Expectorant
UCB620	Tab, Film Coated, UCB/620	Guaifenesin 1200 mg	Duratuss G by Eckerd Drug	19458-0869	Expectorant
UCB640	Tab, White, Cap Shaped, Film Coated, Scored	Guaifenesin 1200 mg, Pseudoephedrine HCl 120 mg	Duratuss by UCB Pharma	50474-0640	Cold Remedy
UCB902	Tab, White, Blue Specks, UCB/902	Acetaminophen 500 mg, Hydrocodone Bitartrate 5 mg	Lortab 5/500 by Nat Pharmpak Serv	55154-7204	Analgesic; C III

ID FRONT <> BACK	DESCRIPTION FRONT <> BACK	INGREDIENT & STRENGTH	BRAND (OR EQUIV.) & FIRM	NDC#	CLASS; SCH.
UCB902	Tab, UBC/902	Acetaminophen 500 mg, Hydrocodone Bitartrate 5 mg	Lortab by Quality Care	60346-0991	Analgesic; C III
UCB902	Tab, White, Oblong, Scored	Acetaminophen 500 mg; Hydrocodone Bitartrate 5 mg	Lortab by HJ Harkins	52959-0185	Analgesic; C III
UCB902	Tab, White, Oblong, Scored, UCB Over 902	Hydrocodene Bitartrate 5 mg, Acetaminophen 500 mg	Lortab by Murfreesboro	51129-1434	Analgesic; C III
UCB903	Tab, White, Green Specks, ucb/903	Acetaminophen 500 mg, Hydrocodone Bitartrate 7.5 mg	Lortab by Amerisource	62584-0907	Analgesic; C III
UCB903	Tab, UCB/903	Acetaminophen 500 mg, Hydrocodone Bitartrate 7.5 mg	Lortab by Med Pro	53978-2069	Analgesic; C III
UCB903	Tab, White, Oblong, Scored	Acetaminophen 500 mg; Hydrocodone Bitartrate 7.5 mg	Lortab by HJ Harkins	52959-0186	Analgesic; C III
UCB903	Tab, White, Green Specks, UCB/903	Atropine Sulfate 0.025 mg, Diphenoxylate HCl 2.5 mg	Lortab by Nat Pharmpak Serv	55154-7201	Antidiarrheal; C V
UCB903	Tab, White with Green Specks, Oblong	Hydrocodone Bitartrate 7.5 mg, Acetaminophen 500 mg	Lortab by UCB Pharma		Analgesic; C III
UCB910	Tab, ucb/910	Acetaminophen 500 mg, Hydrocodone Bitartrate 10 mg	Lortab by Amerisource	62584-0016	Analgesic; C III
UCB910	Tab	Acetaminophen 500 mg, Hydrocodone Bitartrate 10 mg	Lortab 10 500 by D M Graham	00756-0249	Analgesic; C III.
UCB910	Tab, Pink, Oblong, Scored	Acetaminophen 500 mg; Hydrocodone Bitartrate 10 mg	Lortab by HJ Harkins	52959-0453	Analgesic; C III
UCBUCB	Cap, Orange & Yellow, Blue Band, ucb/ucb	High Potency Multivitamin; Mineral Supplement	by UCB	50474-0273	Vitamin
UCBUCB	Cap, Orange, Blue Band, ucb/ucb	High Potency Vitamin C, E, Zinc Supplement	by UCB	50474-0292	Vitamin
UCBUCB	Cap, Light Yellow & Red with Blue Band, ucb/ucb	Multivitamin; Mineral Supplement	by UCB	50474-0305	Vitamin
UCY500	Tab, Beige, Oval	Sodium Phenylbutyrate 500 mg	Buphenyl by Pharmaceutics	61916-0496	Pharmaceutical Aids
UCY500	Tab, Beige, Oval	Sodium Phenylbutyrate 500 mg	Buphenyl by Ucyclyd	62592-0496	Pharmaceutical Aids
UD	Tab, Coral, Round, Scored, UD over Abbott Logo	Estazolam 2 mg	ProSom by Abbott	00074-3736	Sedative/Hypnotic; C IV
UD	Tab, Mottled Pink, Rectangular, Scored, UD over Abbott Logo	Estazolam 2 mg	ProSom Reformulated by Abbott	00074-3736	Sedative/Hypnotic; C IV
UD	Tab, Pink, Rectangular, Abbott Logo	Estazolam 2 mg	Prosom by Abbott	Canadian	Sedative/Hypnotic
UDANL5347	Tab, White, Round, U:DAN L:5347	Minoxidil 10 mg	Loniten by Danbury		Antihypertensive
ULTRADOL200MG	Cap, Light Gray w/ Two Red Bands	Etodolac 200 mg	Ultradol by Procter & Gamble	Canadian DIN# 02142023	NSAID
ULTRADOL300MG	Cap, Light Gray w/ Red Bands	Etodolac 300 mg	Ultradol by Procter & Gamble	Canadian DIN# 02142031	NSAID
ULTRASE	Cap, White	Lipase 4,500 units, Amylase 20,000 units, Protease 25,000 units	Ultrase by Scandipharm	58914-0045	Gastrointestinal
ULTRASE <> MT20	Cap, Gray & Yellow	Pancrelipase (Amylase 65000 U, Lipase 20000 U, Protease 65000 U)	Ultrase MT 20 by Eurand	57298-0052	Gastrointestinal
ULTRASEMT12	Cap, White & Yellow	Lipase 12,000 units, Amylase 39,000 units, Protease 39,000 units	Ultrase MT by Scandipharm	58914-0002	Gastrointestinal
ULTRASEMT18	Cap, White & Gray	Lipase 18,000 units, Amylase 58,500 units, Protease 58,500 units	Ultrase MT by Scandipharm	58914-0018	Gastrointestinal
UNIGEN601	Tab, Purple, Oblong, Scored	Carbetapentane Tannate 60 mg; Chlorpheniramine Tannate 5 mg; Ephedrine Tannate 10 mg; Phenylephrine Tannate 10 mg	Quadratuss by Unigen	62305-0601	Cold Remedy
UNIGEN601	Tab, Pink, Oblong, Scored	Carbetapentane Tannate 60 mg; Chlorpheniramine Tannate 5 mg; Ephedrine Tannate 10 mg; Phenylephrine Tannate 10 mg	Ry Tuss by Cypress Pharm	60258-0271	Cold Remedy
UNILOG181 <> SQUIBB	Cap, Swedish Orange	Cephalexin Monohydrate	by Quality Care	60346-0441	Antibiotic
UNIMED	Tab, Mottled Pink, Round, Scored	Betahistine Dihydrochloride 4 mg	by Solvay	Canadian DIN# 02222035	Antivertigo
UPJOHN	Tab, Green, Round, Scored	Fluoxymesterone 5 mg	Halotestin by Upjohn	Canadian DIN# 00030902	Steroid
UPJOHN	Cap, Light Blue	Lincomycin HCl 500 mg	by Pharmacia	Canadian	Antibiotic
UPJOHN10	Tab, Violet	Triazolam 0.125 mg	by Pharmacia	Canadian	Sedative/Hypnotic
UPJOHN15	Tab, White, Round	Cortisone Acetate 5 mg	by Upjohn		Steroid
UPJOHN17	Tab, Powder Blue, Scored	Triazolam 0.25 mg	by Pharmacia	Canadian DIN# 00443158	Sedative/Hypnotic
UPJOHN18	Tab, Yellow, Round	Benzphetamine HCl 25 mg	Didrex by Upjohn		Sympathomimetic; C III
UPJOHN225	Cap, Lavender & Maroon, Gelatin	Clindamycin HCl 150 mg	by Pharmacia	Canadian DIN# 00030570	Antibiotic
UPJOHN23	Tab, White, Round	Cortisone Acetate 10 mg	by Upjohn		Steroid

ID FRONT <> BACK	DESCRIPTION FRONT <> BACK	INGREDIENT & STRENGTH	BRAND (OR EQUIV.) & FIRM	NDC#	CLASS; SCH.
UPJOHN29	Tab, White, Scored	Alprazolam 0.25 mg	Xanax by Upjohn	Canadian DIN# 00548359	Antianxiety
UPJOHN34	Tab, White, Round	Cortisone Acetate 25 mg	by Upjohn		Steroid
UPJOHN395	Cap, Light Blue, Gelatin	Clindamycin HCl 300 mg	by Pharmacia	Canadian DIN# 02182866	Antibiotic
UPJOHN45	Tab, White	Prednisone 5 mg	Deltasone by Upjohn	Canadian	Steroid
UPJOHN50	Tab, White, Round, Scored	Medroxyprogesterone Acetate 10 mg	Provera by Upjohn	Canadian DIN# 00729973	Progestin
UPJOHN55	Tab, Peach, Scored	Alprazolam 0.5 mg	by Upjohn	Canadian DIN# 00548367	Antianxiety
UPJOHN56	Tab, White, Elliptical, Scored	Methylprednisolone 4 mg	by Upjohn	Canadian DIN# 00030988	Steroid
UPJOHN90	Tab, Lavender, Scored	Alprazolam 1 mg	Xanax by Upjohn	Canadian DIN# 00723770	Antianxiety
UPJOHN949	Cap, Yellow & Blue	Uracil Mustard 1 mg	by Upjohn		Antineoplastic
URECHOLINE <> MSD403	Tab, White	Bethanechol Chloride 5 mg	Urecholine by Merck	00006-0403	Urinary Tract
URECHOLINE <> MSD412	Tab, Pink	Bethanechol Chloride 10 mg	Urecholine by Merck	00006-0412	Urinary Tract
URECHOLINE <> MSD457	Tab, Yellow	Bethanechol Chloride 25 mg	Urecholine by Merck	00006-0457	Urinary Tract
URECHOLINE <> MSD460	Tab, Yellow	Bethanechol Chloride 50 mg	Urecholine by Merck	00006-0460	Urinary Tract
URETRONDS	Tab, Sugar Coated, Uretron D/S	Hyoscyamine Sulfate 0.12 mg, Methenamine 81.6 mg, Methylene Blue 10.8 mg, Phenyl Salicylate 36.2 mg, Sodium Phosphate, Monobasic 40.8 mg	Uretron DS by A G Marin	12539-0144	Gastrointestinal
URETRONDS	Tab, Purple, Round, Uretron D/S	Phenyl Phosphate 36.2 mg, Methylene Blue 10.8 mg, Methenamine 81.6, Hyoscyamine Sulfate 0.12 mg	Uretron DS by Physicians Total Care		Urinary
UREX <> 3M	Tab, White, Cap-Shaped, Scored	Methenamine Hippurate 1 g	Urex by 3M	00089-0371	Antibiotic; Urinary Tract
UREX <> VP	Tab, White, Oblong, Scored	Methenamine Hippurate 1 gm	Urex by Virco Pharms	65199-1201	Antibiotic; Urinary Tract
UREX3M	Tab, White, Oblong, Urex/3M	Methenamine Hippurate 1g	Urex by 3M		Antibiotic; Urinary Tract
URIMAX	Tab, Purple, Round	Sodium Phosphate 0.8 mg, Methylene Blue 36.2 mg, Methenamine 81.6, Hyoscyamine Sulfate 0.12 mg	Urimax	00091-9108	Electrolyte
URISPAS <> SKF	Tab, White, Round, Film Coated	Flavoxate HCl 100 mg	Urispas by Integrity	64731-0860	Antispasmodic
URISPASSKF	Tab, White, Round, Urispas/SKF	Flavoxate HCl 100 mg	Urispas by SKB		Antispasmodic
UROKPNEUTRAL	Cap, Light Peach, Film Coated Cap, URO-KP-Neutral	Phosphorous 250 mg, Potassium 49.4 mg, Sodium 250.5 mg	Uro-KP-Neutral by Star	00076-0109	Supplement
UROLENEBLUE	Tab, Blue	Methylene Blue 65 mg	Urolene Blue by Star	00076-0501	Analgesic
URS785	Tab, White	Ursodeoxycholic Acid 250 mg	Urso by Schwarz Pharma		Gastrointestinal
URS785	Tab	Ursodiol 250 mg	Urso by Global	55983-0785	Gastrointestinal
URSODIOL300MG <> COPLEY380	Cap, Red & White	Ursodiol 300 mg	Ursodiol by Copley Pharm	38245-0380	Gastrointestinal
US	Tab, Yellow	B Complex, E.C., Folic Acid, Trace Minerals	Mediplex- Ultra	52747-0305	Vitamin
US	Tab, Red, Round	Ferrous Fumarate 324 mg	Hemocyte by US	52747-0307	Mineral
US	Tab, Maroon, Round	Ferrous Fumarate, Folic Acid	Hemocyte-F by US	52747-0306	Mineral
US	Tab, Maroon, Debossed, Round	Iron Vitamin Mineral Complex	Hemocyte Plus by US	52747-0308	Vitamin/Mineral
US <> 017	Tab, Green, Round	Folic Acid 800 mcg~10 mg, Vitamin B 115 mcg, Vitamin B-6 10 mg	Folgard by Upsher-Smith	00245-0017	Vitamin
US <> A	Tab, White, Round	Amiodarone HCl 200 mg	by Heartland Hlthcare	61392-0935	Antiarrhythmic

ID FRONT ⟷ BACK	DESCRIPTION FRONT ⟷ BACK	INGREDIENT & STRENGTH	BRAND (OR EQUIV.) & FIRM	NDC#	CLASS; SCH.
US ⟷ US	Cap, in Green	Acetaminophen 325 mg, Butalbital 50 mg, Caffeine 40 mg	Medigesic by US	52747-0600	Analgesic
US ⟷ US	Cap, Black Print	Acetaminophen 325 mg, Chlorpheniramine Maleate 4 mg, Phenylpropanolamine HCl 25 mg, Phenyltoloxamine Citrate 25 mg	Norel Plus by US	52747-0128	Cold Remedy
US0147 ⟷ P200	Tab, Pink, Round, Scored, U-S over 0147 ⟷ P200	Amidarone HCl 200 mg	Pacerone by Apotheca	12634-0549	Antiarrhythmic
US0147 ⟷ P200	Tab, Pink, Round, Scored	Amiodarone HCl 200 mg	Pacerone by Thrift Services	59198-0362	Antiarrhythmic
US0147 ⟷ P200	Tab, U-S over 0147	Amiodarone HCl 200 mg	Pacerone by Upsher Smith	00245-0147	Antiarrhythmic
US027	Tab, Pink, Oblong, Film Coated	Pentoxifylline 400 mg	Pentopak by Zoetica Pharm	64909-0001	Anticoagulent
US027	Tab, Light Pink, Cap Shaped, U-S 027	Pentoxifylline 400 mg	Pentoxil by Upsher-Smith		Anticoagulent
US027	Tab, Pink, Oblong, Film, U-S 027	Pentoxifylline 400 mg	Pentoxil by Pharmafab	62542-0751	Anticoagulent
US027	Tab, Pink, Oblong, Film Coated	Pentoxifylline 400 mg	Pentoxil by Upsher Smith	00245-0027	Anticoagulent
US047P200	Tab, Pink, Round, U-S 047/P200	Amidarone HCl 200 mg	Pacerone by Upsher-Smith	00245-0147	Antiarrhythmic
US200 ⟷ A	Tab, White, Round	Amiodarone 200 mg	Cordarone by Geneva	00781-1203	Antiarrhythmic
US200 ⟷ A	Tab, White, Round, Flat, Scored, Uncoated, U-S/200	Amiodarone HCl 200 mg	Pacerone by Apothecon	59772-0352	Antiarrhythmic
US200 ⟷ A	Tab, White, Round, Scored	Amiodarone HCl 200 mg	by Upsher Smith	00245-1480	Antiarrhythmic
US411	Tab, Green Mottled	Nitroglycerin ER 2.6 mg	Nitrong by RPR		Vasodilator
US412	Tab, Orange Mottled	Nitroglycerin ER 6.5 mg	Nitrong by RPR		Vasodilator
US500	Tab, Blue, Round	Salsalate 500 mg	Salsitab by Upsher		NSAID
US750	Tab, Blue, Oblong	Salsalate 750 mg	Salsitab by Upsher		NSAID
USB001 ⟷ HEXALEN50MG	Cap, Clear	Altretamine 50 mg	Hexalen by US Bioscience	58178-0001	Antineoplastic
USB001 ⟷ HEXALEN50MG	Cap	Altretamine 50 mg	Hexalen by AAI	27280-0001	Antineoplastic
USE ⟷ 411	Tab, Scored, US Over E ⟷ 411	Nitroglycerin 2.6 mg	Nitrong by RPR	00075-0221	Vasodilator
USE ⟷ 412	Tab, US Over E ⟷ 412, Film Coated, Scored	Nitroglycerin 6.5 mg	Nitrong by RPR	00075-0274	Vasodilator
USL ⟷ 8	Tab, Dark Blue, Film Coated	Potassium Chloride 600 mg	by Quality Care	60346-0453	Electrolyte
USL10	Tab, Film Coated	Potassium Chloride 750 mg	by Zenith Goldline	00182-1840	Electrolyte
USL10	Tab, Film Coated	Potassium Chloride 750 mg	by Rugby	00536-4311	Electrolyte
USL10	Tab, Tab, Film Coated	Potassium Chloride 750 mg	by Qualitest	00603-5241	Electrolyte
USL10	Tab	Potassium Chloride 750 mg	by Med Pro	53978-2060	Electrolyte
USL10	Tab, White, Round	Potassium Chloride Er 750 mg	by Upsher-Smith		Electrolyte
USL8	Tab, Film Coated	Potassium Chloride 600 mg	by Qualitest	00603-5237	Electrolyte
USL8	Tab, Film Coated	Potassium Chloride 600 mg	by Zenith Goldline	00182-1839	Electrolyte
USL8	Tab, Dark Blue, Round	Potassium Chloride ER 600 mg	by Upsher-Smith		Electrolyte
USL80	Cap, Pink	Zinc Sulfate 220 mg	by Upsher	00245-0080	Mineral Supplement
USV2835	Cap, Black & Clear	Nicotinic Acid Time Release 125 mg	Nicobid by RPR		Vitamin
USV2840	Cap, Green & Clear	Nicotinic Acid Time Release 250 mg	Nicobid by RPR		Vitamin
USV2841	Cap, Blue & White	Nicotinic Acid Time Release 500 mg	Nicobid by RPR		Vitamin
USVHK	Tab, Orange, Round, USV Logo HK	Levothyroxine Sodium 25 mcg	Levothroid by USV		Antithyroid
USVLP	Tab, Turquoise, Round, USV Logo LP	Levothyroxine Sodium 175 mcg	Levothroid by Forest	00456-0326	Antithyroid
UU ⟷ 201	Tab	Acetaminophen 650 mg, Hydrocodone Bitartrate 7.5 mg	Lorcet Plus by Quality Care	60346-0759	Analgesic; C III
UU ⟷ 201	Tab, U/U ⟷ 201	Acetaminophen 650 mg, Hydrocodone Bitartrate 7.5 mg	Lorcet Plus by Nat Pharmpak Serv	55154-7302	Analgesic; C III
UU ⟷ 201	Tab	Acetaminophen 650 mg, Hydrocodone Bitartrate 7.5 mg	Lorcet Plus by Murfreesboro	51129-0053	Analgesic; C III
UU ⟷ 201	Tab, U-U ⟷ 201	Acetaminophen 650 mg, Hydrocodone Bitartrate 7.5 mg	Lorcet Plus by Allscripts	54569-0916	Analgesic; C III
UU ⟷ 201	Tab, U/U	Acetaminophen 650 mg, Hydrocodone Bitartrate 7.5 mg	Lorcet Plus by UAD	00785-1122	Analgesic; C III
UU ⟷ 3737	Tab	Pramipexole DiHCl 1.5 mg	Mirapex by Pharmacia & Upjohn	00009-0037	Antiparkinson
UU ⟷ 44	Tab, White, Oval, Scored	Pramipexole DiHCl 0.25 mg	Mirapex by Purdue Pharma	59011-0105	Antiparkinson
UU ⟷ 44	Tab	Pramipexole DiHCl 0.25 mg	Mirapex by Pharmacia & Upjohn	00009-0004	Antiparkinson
UU ⟷ 66	Tab	Pramipexole DiHCl 1 mg	Mirapex by Pharmacia & Upjohn	00009-0006	Antiparkinson
UU ⟷ 88	Tab	Pramipexole DiHCl 0.5 mg	Mirapex by Pharmacia & Upjohn	00009-0008	Antiparkinson
UU33	Tab, White, Oval	Pramipexole DiHCl 1.25 mg	Mirapex by Pharmacia & Upjohn		Antiparkinson
UU37	Tab, White, Round	Pramipexole DiHCl 1.5 mg	Mirapex by Pharmacia & Upjohn		Antiparkinson
UU4	Tab, White, Oval	Pramipexole DiHCl 0.25 mg	Mirapex by Pharmacia & Upjohn		Antiparkinson

ID FRONT <> BACK	DESCRIPTION FRONT <> BACK	INGREDIENT & STRENGTH	BRAND (OR EQUIV.) & FIRM	NDC#	CLASS; SCH.
UU6	Tab, White, Round	Pramipexole DiHCl 1.5 mg	Mirapex by Pharmacia & Upjohn		Antiparkinson
UU8	Tab, White, Oval	Pramipexole DiHCl 0.5 mg	by Pharmacia & Upjohn		Antiparkinson
V <> 2732	Cap	Chlordiazepoxide HCl 5 mg, Clidinium Bromide 2.5 mg	by Quality Care	60346-0780	Gastrointestinal; C IV
V <> 3186	Tab, Coated	Codeine Phosphate 10 mg, Guaifenesin 300 mg	by Vintage	00254-3186	Cold Remedy; C III
V <> 3186	Tab, Red, Oblong	Guaifenesin 300 mg; Codeine Phosphate 10 mg	by Qualitest Pharms	00603-3781	Analgesic; C III
V <> 3592	Tab, 35 92	Acetaminophen 500 mg, Hydrocodone Bitartrate 5 mg	by Quality Care	60346-0442	Analgesic; C III
V <> 3592	Tab, 35/92	Acetaminophen 500 mg, Hydrocodone Bitartrate 5 mg	by Kaiser	00179-1026	Analgesic; C III
V <> 3592	Tab, White, Oblong, Scored	Hydrocodone Bitartrate 5 mg, Acetaminophen 500 mg	by Vangard Labs	00615-0400	Analgesic; C III
V <> 3913	Tab, Bluish Purple, Round, Scored	Levothyroxine Sodium 0.075 mg	by Allscripts	54569-4157	Antithyroid
V <> 4140	Tab, Double Layered	Meclizine HCl 12.5 mg	by Qualitest	00603-4319	Antiemetic
V <> 5012	Tab, White, Round	Phenobarbital 30 mg	by Vangard Labs	00615-0463	Sedative/Hypnotic; C IV
V <> 5051	Tab, Blue, Oblong	Guaifenesin 400 mg, Phenylpropanolamine HCl 75 mg	Guaitex LA by Vintage		Cold Remedy
V <> 5053	Tab	Guaifenesin 600 mg, Phenylpropanolamine HCl 75 mg	Guaivent by Qualitest	00603-3778	Cold Remedy
V <> 5053	Tab, V <> 50/53	Guaifenesin 600 mg, Phenylpropanolamine HCl 75 mg	Guaivent by Vintage	00254-5053	Cold Remedy
V <> 5112	Tab, Coated	Acetaminophen 650 mg, Propoxyphene Napsylate 100 mg	by Vintage	00254-5112	Analgesic; C IV
V <> 5112	Tab, Coated	Acetaminophen 650 mg, Propoxyphene Napsylate 100 mg	by Qualitest	00603-5466	Analgesic; C IV
V <> 5113	Tab, Coated	Acetaminophen 650 mg, Propoxyphene Napsylate 100 mg	by Vintage	00254-5113	Analgesic; C IV
V <> 5114	Tab, Coated	Acetaminophen 650 mg, Propoxyphene Napsylate 100 mg	by Vintage	00254-5114	Analgesic; C IV
V <> 5114	Tab, Coated	Acetaminophen 650 mg, Propoxyphene Napsylate 100 mg	by Qualitest	00603-5468	Analgesic; C IV
V <> 5812	Tab, Turquoise, 58 to Left, 12 to Right, Tab Coated	Salsalate 750 mg	by Quality Care	60346-0034	NSAID
V <> NT	Tab, N/T	Ascorbic Acid 40 mg, Biotin 300 mcg, Cyanocobalamin 6 mcg, Docusate Sodium 75 mg, Ferrous Fumarate 200 mg, Folic Acid 1 mg, Niacinamide 20 mg, Pantothenic Acid 10 mg, Pyridoxine HCl 10 mg, Riboflavin 1.7 mg, Thiamine Mononitrate 1.5 mg	Nephron Fa by Nephro Tech	59528-4456	Vitamin
V1 <> BL	Tab	Penicillin V Potassium	by Quality Care	60346-0414	Antibiotic
V2063	Tab	Acetaminophen 300 mg, Codeine Phosphate 15 mg	by Qualitest	00603-2337	Analgesic; C III
V2063	Tab, White, V-Scored, Round	Acetaminophen 300 mg, Codeine Phosphate 15 mg	Tylenol #2 by Vintage	00254-2063	Analgesic; C III
V2064	Tab, V-Scored	Acetaminophen 300 mg, Codeine Phosphate 30 mg	by Vintage	00254-2064	Analgesic; C III
V2064	Tab	Acetaminophen 300 mg, Codeine Phosphate 30 mg	by Qualitest	00603-2338	Analgesic; C III
V2065	Tab, V-Scored	Acetaminophen 300 mg, Codeine Phosphate 60 mg	by Vintage	00254-2065	Analgesic; C III
V2065	Tab	Acetaminophen 300 mg, Codeine Phosphate 60 mg	by Qualitest	00603-2339	Analgesic; C III
V2732	Cap, Light Green	Chlordiazepoxide HCl 5 mg, Clidinium Bromide 2.5 mg	by Qualitest	00603-2714	Gastrointestinal; C IV
V3592	Tab	Acetaminophen 500 mg, Hydrocodone Bitartrate 5 mg	by Vintage	00254-3592	Analgesic; C III
V3592	Tab	Acetaminophen 500 mg, Hydrocodone Bitartrate 5 mg	by Qualitest	00603-3881	Analgesic; C III
V3594	Tab, White, Green Specks	Acetaminophen 500 mg, Hydrocodone Bitartrate 7.5 mg	by Qualitest	00603-3882	Analgesic; C III
V3595	Tab	Acetaminophen 650 mg, Hydrocodone Bitartrate 7.5 mg	by Qualitest	00603-3884	Analgesic; C III
V3596	Tab	Acetaminophen 750 mg, Hydrocodone Bitartrate 7.5 mg	by Qualitest	00603-3883	Analgesic; C III
V3611	Tab	Hydromorphone HCl 2 mg	by Qualitest	00603-3925	Analgesic; C II
V3612	Tab	Hydromorphone HCl 4 mg	by Qualitest	00603-3926	Analgesic; C II
V3911	Tab	Levothyroxine Sodium 25 mcg	by Qualitest	00603-4192	Antithyroid
V3912	Tab, White, Round	Levothyronine 50 mcg	Levothyronine by Vintage		Antithyroid
V3912	Tab	Levothyroxine Sodium 50 mcg	by Qualitest	00603-4193	Antithyroid
V3913	Tab	Levothyroxine Sodium 75 mcg	by Qualitest	00603-4194	Antithyroid
V3914	Tab	Levothyroxine Sodium 100 mcg	by Qualitest	00603-4195	Antithyroid
V3915	Tab	Levothyroxine Sodium 150 mcg	by Vintage	00254-3915	Antithyroid
V3915	Tab	Levothyroxine Sodium 150 mcg	by Qualitest	00603-4196	Antithyroid
V3916	Tab	Levothyroxine Sodium 200 mcg	by Qualitest	00603-4197	Antithyroid
V3917	Tab	Levothyroxine Sodium 300 mcg	by Qualitest	00603-4198	Antithyroid

ID FRONT <> BACK	DESCRIPTION FRONT <> BACK	INGREDIENT & STRENGTH	BRAND (OR EQUIV.) & FIRM	NDC#	CLASS; SCH.
V4130	Tab, Coated	Ascorbic Acid 100 mg, Biotin 30 mcg, Calcium 250 mg, Cholecalciferol 400 Units, Chromium 25 mcg, Copper 2 mg, Cyanocobalamin 12 mcg, Folic Acid 1 mg, Iron 60 mg, Magnesium 25 mg, Manganese 5 mg, Molybdenum 25 mcg, Niacinamide 20 mg, Pantothenic Acid 10 mg, Potassium Iodide 150 mcg, Pyridoxine HCl 10 mg, Riboflavin 3.4 mg, Thiamine Mononitrate 3 mg, Vitamin A 5000 Units, Vitamin E Acetate 30 Units, Zinc 25 mg	Maternity by Qualitest	00603-4304	Vitamin
V4206	Cap, Red	Meperidine HCl 50 mg, Promethazine HCl 25 mg	Mepergan by Wyeth Ayerst		Analgesic; C II
V4206	Cap	Meperidine HCl 50 mg, Promethazine HCl 25 mg	Meprozine by Vintage	00254-4206	Analgesic; C II
V4206	Cap	Meperidine HCl 50 mg, Promethazine HCl 25 mg	by Qualitest	00603-4424	Analgesic; C II
V4839	Tab, White, Round	Oxycodone HCl 5 mg, Acetaminophen 325 mg	Percocet by Vintage		Analgesic; C II
V4971	Tab, Tab Coated	Phenazopyridine HCl 100 mg	by Vintage	00254-4971	Urinary Analgesic
V4971	Tab, Tab Coated	Phenazopyridine HCl 100 mg	by Qualitest	00603-5141	Urinary Analgesic
V4972	Tab, Tab Sugar Coated	Phenazopyridine HCl 200 mg	by Vintage	00254-4972	Urinary Analgesic
V4972	Tab, Tab Sugar Coated	Phenazopyridine HCl 200 mg	by Qualitest	00603-5142	Urinary Analgesic
V5011	Tab, Bisected V	Phenobarbital 17.01 mg	by Vintage	00254-5011	Sedative/Hypnotic; C IV
V5011	Tab	Phenobarbital 17.01 mg	by Qualitest	00603-5165	Sedative/Hypnotic; C IV
V5012	Tab	Phenobarbital 30 mg	by Zenith Goldline	00182-0292	Sedative/Hypnotic; C IV
V5012	Tab, Bisected V	Phenobarbital 30 mg	by Vintage	00254-5012	Sedative/Hypnotic; C IV
V5012	Tab	Phenobarbital 30 mg	by Qualitest	00603-5166	Sedative/Hypnotic; C IV
V5013	Tab, Bisected V	Phenobarbital 64.8 mg	by Vintage	00254-5013	Sedative/Hypnotic; C IV
V5013	Tab	Phenobarbital 64.8 mg	by Zenith Goldline	00182-0590	Sedative/Hypnotic; C IV
V5013	Tab	Phenobarbital 64.8 mg	by Qualitest	00603-5167	Sedative/Hypnotic; C IV
V5013	Tab, White, Round	Phenobarbital 65 mg	by Vintage		Sedative/Hypnotic; C IV
V5014	Tab, Bisected V	Phenobarbital 100 mg	by Vintage	00254-5014	Sedative/Hypnotic; C IV
V5014	Tab	Phenobarbital 100 mg	by Qualitest	00603-5168	Sedative/Hypnotic; C IV
V5051	Tab, Film Coated, V-Scored	Guaifenesin 400 mg, Phenylpropanolamine HCl 75 mg	Guaitex LA by Vintage	00254-5051	Cold Remedy
V5051	Tab	Guaifenesin 400 mg, Phenylpropanolamine HCl 75 mg	by Qualitest	00603-5214	Cold Remedy
V5052	Tab, Film Coated	Guaifenesin 400 mg, Phenylpropanolamine HCl 75 mg	by Qualitest	00603-5215	Cold Remedy
V5097	Tab, Coated	Ascorbic Acid 80 mg, Beta-Carotene, Biotin 0.03 mg, Calcium Carbonate, Cholecalciferol 400 Units, Cupric Oxide, Cyanocobalamin 2.5 mcg, Ferrous Fumarate, Folic Acid 1 mg, Magnesium Oxide, Niacinamide 17 mg, Pantothenic Acid 7 mg, Pyridoxine HCl 4 mg, Riboflavin 1.6 mg, Thiamine Mononitrate 1.5 mg, Vitamin A Acetate, Vitamin E Acetate 15 mg, Zinc Oxide	Prenatal Rx by Qualitest	00603-5359	Vitamin
V5098	Tab, Coated	Ascorbic Acid 120 mg, Calcium 250 mg, Cholecalciferol 400 Units, Copper 2 mg, Cyanocobalamin 12 mcg, Docusate Sodium 50 mg, Folic Acid 1 mg, Iodine 150 mcg, Iron 90 mg, Niacinamide 20 mg, Pyridoxine HCl 20 mg, Riboflavin 3.4 mg, Thiamine HCl 3 mg, Vitamin A 4000 Units, Vitamin E 30 Units, Zinc 25 mg	Maternity 90 Prenatal Vit & Min by Qualitest	00603-5355	Vitamin
V5099	Tab, Coated	Ascorbic Acid 80 mg, Calcium Carbonate, Precipitated, Cholecalciferol 400 Units, Cyanocobalamin 12 mcg, Ferrous Fumarate, Folic Acid 1 mg, Magnesium Oxide, Niacinamide 20 mg, Potassium Iodide, Pyridoxine HCl 10 mg, Riboflavin 3 mg, Thiamine Mononitrate 3 mg, Vitamin A Palmitate 5000 Units, Vitamin E Acetate 30 mg, Zinc Oxide	Z Plus Prenatal by Qualitest	00603-6475	Vitamin
V5100	Tab, Coated	Ascorbic Acid 120 mg, Calcium Sulfate, Cupric Oxide, Cyanocobalamin 12 mcg, Ferrous Fumarate, Folic Acid 1 mg, Niacin 20 mg, Pyridoxine HCl 10 mg, Riboflavin 3 mg, Thiamine HCl 1.5 mg, Vitamin A 4000 Units, Vitamin D 400 Units, Vitamin E 11 mg, Zinc Oxide	Prenatal 1 Plus Iron by Qualitest	00603-5357	Vitamin
V5101	Tab, Yellow	Prenatal Vitamin	Prenatal Improved by Vintage		Vitamin
V5311	Tab, Light Green, Film Coated	Dextromethorphan Hydrobromide 30 mg, Guaifenesin 600 mg	by Zenith Goldline	00182-1042	Cold Remedy
V5311	Tab, Film Coated	Dextromethorphan Hydrobromide 30 mg, Guaifenesin 600 mg	Q-Bid DM by Qualitest	00603-5542	Cold Remedy
V5312	Tab	Guaifenesin 600 mg	by Zenith Goldline	00182-1188	Expectorant
V5312	Tab	Guaifenesin 600 mg	Q-Bid LA by Qualitest	00603-5543	Expectorant
V5312	Tab, Green, Oblong, Scored	Guaifenesin 600 mg	Q Bid LA Sustained Release by Mason	11845-0975	Expectorant

ID FRONT <> BACK	DESCRIPTION FRONT <> BACK	INGREDIENT & STRENGTH	BRAND (OR EQUIV.) & FIRM	NDC#	CLASS; SCH.
V5811	Tab, Film Coated	Salsalate 500 mg	by Qualitest	00603-5754	NSAID
V5812	Tab, Film Coated	Salsalate 750 mg	by Qualitest	00603-5755	NSAID
V5935	Tab, Coated	Choline Magnesium Trisalicylate 500 mg	Tricosal by Qualitest	00603-6215	NSAID
V5936	Tab, Coated	Choline Magnesium Trisalicylate 986.835 mg	Tricosal by Qualitest	00603-6216	NSAID
V5937	Tab, Film Coated	Choline Magnesium Trisalicylate 1000 mg	Tricosal by Qualitest	00603-6217	NSAID
V6211	Tab, Film Coated	Guaifenesin 600 mg, Pseudoephedrine HCl 120 mg	by Zenith Goldline	00182-1740	Cold Remedy
V6211	Tab, Film Coated	Guaifenesin 600 mg, Pseudoephedrine HCl 120 mg	Guaifen PSE by Vintage	00254-6211	Cold Remedy
V6211	Tab, Film Coated	Guaifenesin 600 mg, Pseudoephedrine HCl 120 mg	Quaifen PSE by Qualitest	00603-5668	Cold Remedy
V6377	Tab	Yohimbine HCl 5.4 mg	by Vintage	00254-6377	Impotence Agent
V6377	Tab	Yohimbine HCl 5.4 mg	by Qualitest	00603-6430	Impotence Agent
VA250	Cap, Orange	Valproic Acid 250 mg	by Genpharm	Canadian	Anticonvulsant
VAD <> 6330	Tab, Blue, Oblong, Scored	Acetaminophen 650 mg; Hydrocodone Bitartrate 10 mg	Lorcet by HJ Harkins	52959-0403	Analgesic; C III
VALPRC250	Cap, Off White, Valprc./250	Valproic Acid 250 mg	by RP Scherer	11014-0879	Anticonvulsant
VALPROIC250 <> 0364	Cap, Off-White	Valproic Acid 250 mg	by Schein	00364-0822	Anticonvulsant
VALPROIC2500364	Cap, Valproic 250-0364	Valproic Acid 250 mg	by Vangard	00615-1325	Anticonvulsant
VALTREX1GRAM	Tab, Blue, Oblong, Film Coated	Valacyclovir HCl 1 gm	Valtrex by Catalytica Pharms	63552-0565	Antiviral
VALTREX1GRAM	Tab, Blue, Cap-Shaped	Valacyclovir HCl 1 gm	Valtrex by Glaxo Wellcome	00173-0565	Antiviral
VALTREX1GRAM	Tab, Film Coated	Valacyclovir HCl 1 gm	Valtrex by Glaxo Wellcome	00173-0565	Antiviral
VALTREX500MG	Tab, Blue	Valacyclovir HCl 500 mg	Valtrex by Glaxo Wellcome	Canadian	Antiviral
VALTREX500MG	Tab, Film Coated	Valacyclovir HCl 500 mg	Valtrex by Catalytica	63552-0933	Antiviral
VALTREX500MG	Tab, Blue, Oblong, Film Coated	Valacyclovir HCl 500 mg	Valtrex by Promex Medcl	62301-0040	Antiviral
VALTREX500MG	Tab, Film Coated	Valacyclovir HCl 500 mg	Valtrex by Glaxo Wellcome	00173-0933	Antiviral
VALTREX500MG	Cap, Blue, Cap-Shaped	Valacyclovir HCl 500 mg	Valtrex by Glaxo Wellcome	00173-0933	Antiviral
VALTREX500MG	Tab, Film Coated	Valacyclovir HCl 500 mg	Valtrex by Physicians Total Care	54868-3804	Antiviral
VALTREX500MG	Cap, Film Coated	Valacyclovir HCl 500 mg	Valtrex by Allscripts	54569-4280	Antiviral
VALTREX500MG	Tab, Film Coated	Valacyclovir HCl 500 mg	Valtrex by PDRX	55289-0926	Antiviral
VALTREX500MG	Tab, Film Coated	Valacyclovir HCl 500 mg	Valtrex by Quality Care	62682-1012	Antiviral
VANCOCINHCL125MG <> 3125	Cap	Vancomycin HCl	by Eli Lilly	00002-3125	Antibiotic
VANCOCINHCL125MG <> 3126	Cap	Vancomycin HCl	by Eli Lilly	00002-3126	Antibiotic
VANCOCINHCL125MG <> LILLY3125	Cap	Vancomycin HCl	by Nat Pharmpak Serv	55154-1805	Antibiotic
VANCOCINHCL250MG <> 3216	Cap, Blue & Purple, Opaque	Vancocin HCl 250 mg	by Teva	00480-0778	Antibiotic
VASCOR200	Tab, Blue, Film Coated, Scored	Bepridil HCl 200 mg	Vascor by Mcneil Pharm	52021-0682	Antianginal
VASCOR200	Tab, Light Blue, Film Coated, Scored	Bepridil HCl 200 mg	Vascor by McNeil	00045-0682	Antianginal
VASCOR300	Tab, Blue, Film Coated	Bepridil HCl 300 mg	Vascor by McNeil	00045-0683	Antianginal
VASCOR300	Tab, Coated	Bepridil HCl 300 mg	Vascor by McNeil	52021-0683	Antianginal
VASCOR400	Tab, Dark Blue, Film Coated	Bepridil HCl 400 mg	Vascor by McNeil	00045-0684	Antianginal
VASERETIC <> MSD720	Tab, Rust, Squared Cap Shape	Enalapril Maleate 10 mg, Hydrochlorothiazide 25 mg	Vaseretic by Merck	00006-0720	Antihypertensive; Diuretic
VASOTEC <> 712	Tab	Enalapril Maleate 5 mg	by Med Pro	53978-0176	Antihypertensive
VASOTEC <> MSD14	Tab, Yellow, Oblong, Scored	Enalapril Maleate 2.5 mg	Vasotec by Southwood Pharms	58016-0882	Antihypertensive
VASOTEC <> MSD14	Tab	Enalapril Maleate 2.5 mg	Vasotec by Amerisource	62584-0482	Antihypertensive
VASOTEC <> MSD14	Tab, Yellow, Barrel Shaped	Enalapril Maleate 2.5 mg	Vasotec by Merck	00006-0014	Antihypertensive
VASOTEC <> MSD14	Tab	Enalapril Maleate 2.5 mg	Vasotec by Allscripts	54569-3258	Antihypertensive
VASOTEC <> MSD14	Tab	Enalapril Maleate 2.5 mg	Vasotec by Nat Pharmpak Serv	55154-5008	Antihypertensive
VASOTEC <> MSD14	Tab	Enalapril Maleate 5 mg	Vasotec by Caremark	00339-5413	Antihypertensive
VASOTEC <> MSD712	Tab, Barrel Shape	Enalapril Maleate 5 mg	Vasotec by PDRX	55289-0622	Antihypertensive
VASOTEC <> MSD712	Tab, Barrel Shaped	Enalapril Maleate 5 mg	Vasotec by Quality Care	60346-0612	Antihypertensive
VASOTEC <> MSD712	Tab	Enalapril Maleate 5 mg	Vasotec by Amerisource	62584-0483	Antihypertensive

ID FRONT <> BACK	DESCRIPTION FRONT <> BACK	INGREDIENT & STRENGTH	BRAND (OR EQUIV.) & FIRM	NDC#	CLASS; SCH.
VASOTEC <> MSD712	White, Oblong, Scored	Enalapril Maleate 5 mg	Vasotec by Southwood Pharms	58016-0572	Antihypertensive
VASOTEC <> MSD712	Tab, White, Barrel Shaped	Enalapril Maleate 5 mg	Vasotec by Merck	00006-0712	Antihypertensive
VASOTEC <> MSD712	Tab, Barrel Shaped	Enalapril Maleate 5 mg	Vasotec by DRX	55045-2319	Antihypertensive
VASOTEC <> MSD712	Tab	Enalapril Maleate 5 mg	Vasotec by Nat Pharmpak Serv	55154-5001	Antihypertensive
VASOTEC <> MSD712	Tab, Barrel Shaped	Enalapril Maleate 5 mg	Vasotec by Allscripts	54569-0606	Antihypertensive
VASOTEC <> MSD713	Tab, Salmon, Barrel Shaped	Enalapril Maleate 10 mg	Vasotec by Quality Care	60346-0901	Antihypertensive
VASOTEC <> MSD713	Pink, Oblong	Enalapril Maleate 10 mg	Vasotec by Southwood Pharms	58016-0569	Antihypertensive
VASOTEC <> MSD713	Tab, Salmon	Enalapril Maleate 10 mg	Vasotec by Amerisource	62584-0484	Antihypertensive
VASOTEC <> MSD713	Tab, Salmon, Barrel Shaped	Enalapril Maleate 10 mg	Vasotec by Merck	00006-0713	Antihypertensive
VASOTEC <> MSD713	Tab, Salmon	Enalapril Maleate 10 mg	Vasotec by Nat Pharmpak Serv	55154-5003	Antihypertensive
VASOTEC <> MSD713	Tab, Salmon, Barrel Shaped	Enalapril Maleate 10 mg	Vasotec by Allscripts	54569-0607	Antihypertensive
VASOTEC <> MSD713	Tab	Enalapril Maleate 10 mg	by Med Pro	53978-3013	Antihypertensive
VASOTEC <> MSD714	Tab	Enalapril Maleate 10 mg	Vasotec by Caremark	00339-5415	Antihypertensive
VASOTEC <> MSD714	Tab	Enalapril Maleate 20 mg	Vasotec by Quality Care	60346-0534	Antihypertensive
VASOTEC <> MSD714	Tab, Peach, Oblong	Enalapril Maleate 20 mg	Vasotec by Southwood Pharms	58016-0571	Antihypertensive
VASOTEC <> MSD714	Tab, Yellow, Barrel Shaped	Enalapril Maleate 20 mg	Vasotec by Merck	00006-0714	Antihypertensive
VASOTEC <> MSD714	Tab, Barrel Shaped	Enalapril Maleate 20 mg	Vasotec by Allscripts	54569-0612	Antihypertensive
VASOTEC <> MSD714	Tab	Enalapril Maleate 20 mg	Vasotec by DRX	55045-2364	Antihypertensive
VASOTEC <> MSD714	Tab	Enalapril Maleate 20 mg	by Med Pro	53978-3016	Antihypertensive
VASOTEC <> MSD714	Tab	Enalapril Maleate 20 mg	Vasotec by Nat Pharmpak Serv	55154-5013	Antihypertensive
VASOTEC 712	Tab, White, Barrel Shaped	Enalapril Maleate 5 mg	Vasotec by Frosst	Canadian	Antihypertensive
VASOTEC 713	Tab, Red, Barrel Shaped	Enalapril Maleate 10 mg	Vasotec by Frosst	Canadian	Antihypertensive
VASOTEC 714	Tab, Peach, Barrel Shaped	Enalapril Maleate 20 mg	Vasotec by Frosst	Canadian	Antihypertensive
VASOTEC14	Tab, Yellow, Barrel Shaped, Vasotec/14	Enalapril Maleate 2.5 mg	Vasotec by Frosst	Canadian	Antihypertensive
VC5364 <> DYNABAC	Tab, Tab Delayed Release	Dirithromycin 250 mg	Dynabac by Quality Care	60346-0601	Antibiotic
VCILLINK250	White, V-Cillin K 250	Penicillin V Potassium 250 mg	V-Cillin by Lilly		Antibiotic
VCILLINK250LILL	Tab, V-Cillin K 250, Lilly	Penicillin V Potassium	V-Cillin K by Eli Lilly	00002-0329	Antibiotic
VCILLINK500LILL	Tab, V-Cillin K 500, Lilly	Penicillin V Potassium	V-Cillin K by Eli Lilly	00002-0346	Antibiotic
VECTRIN100MG	Cap	Minocycline HCl 100 mg	Vectrin by Warner Chilcott	00047-0688	Antibiotic
VECTRIN100MG	Cap	Minocycline HCl 100 mg	Vectrin by Parke Davis	00071-0688	Antibiotic
VECTRIN50MG	Cap	Minocycline HCl 50 mg	Vectrin by Warner Chilcott	00047-0687	Antibiotic
VECTRIN50MG	Cap	Minocycline HCl 50 mg	Vectrin by Parke Davis	00071-0687	Antibiotic
VENTOLIN2 <> GLAXOGLAXO	Tab, Ventolin over 2, Glaxo over Glaxo	Albuterol Sulfate	Ventolin by Glaxo	00173-0341	Antiasthmatic
VENTOLIN200GLAXO	Cap, Light Blue, Ventolin 200/Glaxo	Albuterol Sulfate 200 mcg	Ventolin Rotacaps by Glaxo Wellcome		Antiasthmatic
VENTOLIN4 <> GLAXOGLAXO	Tab, Ventolin over 4, Glaxo over Glaxo	Albuterol Sulfate	Ventolin by Glaxo	00173-0342	Antiasthmatic
VERELAN120 <> LEDERLEV8	Cap, Verelan over 120 on Right, Lederle over V8 on Left	Verapamil HCl 120 mg	Verelan by Elan Hold	60274-0120	Antihypertensive
VERELAN120MG <> SCHWARZ2490	Cap, Yellow, Schwarz over 2490 <> Verelan over 120 mg	Verapamil HCl 120 mg	Verelan by Schwarz Pharma	00091-2490	Antihypertensive
VERELAN180 <> LEDERLEV7	Cap, Verelan over 180 on Right, Lederle over V7 on Left	Verapamil HCl 180 mg	Verelan by Elan Hold	60274-0180	Antihypertensive
VERELAN180MG <> SCHWARZ2489	Cap, Gray & Yellow, Schwarz over 2489 <> Verelan over 180 mg	Verapamil HCl 180 mg	Verelan by Schwarz Pharma	00091-2489	Antihypertensive
VERELAN240 <> LEDERLEV9	Cap, Verelan over 240 on Right, Lederle over V9 on Left	Verapamil HCl 240 mg	Verelan by Elan Hold	60274-0240	Antihypertensive
VERELAN240MG <> SCHWARZ2491	Cap, Blue & Yellow, Schwarz over 2491 <> Verelan over 240 mg	Verapamil HCl 240 mg	Verelan by Schwarz Pharma	00091-2491	Antihypertensive
VERELAN360 <> LEDERLEV6	Cap, Verelan over 360 on Right, Lederle over V6 on Left	Verapamil HCl 360 mg	Verelan by Elan Hold	60274-0360	Antihypertensive

ID FRONT <> BACK	DESCRIPTION FRONT <> BACK	INGREDIENT & STRENGTH	BRAND (OR EQUIV.) & FIRM	NDC#	CLASS; SCH.
VERELAN360MG <> SCHWARZ2495	Cap, Lavender & Yellow, Schwarz over 2495 <> Verelan over 360 mg	Verapamil HCl 360 mg	Verelan by Schwarz Pharma	00091-2495	Antihypertensive
VERMOX <> JANSSEN	Tab, Pink, Round	Mebendazole 100 mg	Vermox by HJ Harkins	52959-0160	Anthelmintic
VERMOX <> JANSSEN	Tab, Chewable	Mebendazole 100 mg	Vermox by Janssen	50458-0110	Anthelmintic
VERMOX <> JANSSEN	Tab, Chewable	Mebendazole 100 mg	Vermox C by Johnson & Johnson	59604-0110	Anthelmintic
VERSACAP <> 2AMPM	Cap, White to Off White Beads, 2-AM over PM, Cap Ex Release	Guaifenesin 300 mg, Pseudoephedrine HCl 60 mg	Versacaps by Pharmafab	62542-0403	Cold Remedy
VERSACAPS2AMPM	Cap, Versacap/2-AM/PM	Guaifenesin 300 mg, Pseudoephedrine HCl 60 mg	Versacaps by Seatrace	00551-0173	Cold Remedy
VESANOID <> 10ROCHE	Cap	Tretinoin 10 mg	Vesanoid by Hoffmann La Roche	00004-0250	Retinoid
VESANOID10ROCHE	Cap, Orange & Red	Tretinoin 10 mg	Vesanoid by Teva	00480-0537	Retinoid
VGR100 <> PFIZER	Tab, Blue, Diamond Shaped	Sildenafil 100 mg	Viagra by Pfizer	Canadian DIN# 02239768	Impotence Agent
VGR100 <> PFIZER	Tab, Blue, Diamond	Sildenafil Citrate 100 mg	Viagra by Southwood Pharms	58016-0371	Impotence Agent
VGR100 <> PFIZER	Tab, Blue, Rounded Diamond Shape, Film Coated	Sildenafil Citrate 100 mg	Viagra by Pfizer	00069-4220	Impotence Agent
VGR100 <> PFIZER	Tab, Blue, Diamond	Sildenafil Citrate 100 mg	Viagra		Impotence Agent
VGR100 <> PFIZER	Tab, Rounded Diamond Shape, Film Coated	Sildenafil Citrate 100 mg	Viagra by Allscripts	54569-4570	Impotence Agent
VGR100 <> PFIZER	Tab, Blue, Diamond, Film Coated	Sildenafil Citrate 100 mg	Viagra by Compumed	00403-1989	Impotence Agent
VGR25	Tab, Blue, Diamond, Scored, Film, VGR 25	Sildenafil Citrate 25 mg	Viagra		Impotence Agent
VGR25 <> PFIZER	Tab, Blue, Diamond Shaped	Sildenafil 25 mg	Viagra by Pfizer	Canadian DIN# 02239766	Impotence Agent
VGR25 <> PFIZER	Tab, Blue, Rounded-Diamond-Shaped, Film Coated	Sildenafil Citrate 25 mg	by Allscripts	54569-4568	Impotence Agent
VGR25 <> PFIZER	Tab, Blue, Rounded Diamond Shape, Tab Delayed Release	Sildenafil Citrate 25 mg	Viagra by Pfizer	00069-4200	Impotence Agent
VGR50 <> PFIZER	Tab, Blue, Diamond Shaped	Sildenafil 50 mg	Viagra by Pfizer	Canadian DIN# 02239767	Impotence Agent
VGR50 <> PFIZER	Tab, Blue, Diamond	Sildenafil Citrate 50 mg	Viagra by Southwood Pharms	58016-0355	Impotence Agent
VGR50 <> PFIZER	Tab, Blue, Rounded Diamond Shape, Film Coated	Sildenafil Citrate 50 mg	Viagra by Pfizer	00069-4210	Impotence Agent
VGR50 <> PFIZER	Tab, Rounded Diamond Shape, Film Coated	Sildenafil Citrate 50 mg	Viagra by Allscripts	54569-4569	Impotence Agent
VGR50 <> PFIZER	Tab, Blue, Diamond, Film Coated	Sildenafil Citrate 50 mg	Viagra by Compumed	00403-1947	Impotence Agent
VIBRA <> PFIZER095	Cap, Light Blue	Doxycycline Hyclate	Vibramycin by Pfizer	00069-0950	Antibiotic
VIBRATA3 <> PFIZER099	Tab, Salmon, Round, Film Coated, Vibra TA3 <> Pfizer 099	Doxycycline Hyclate	Vibra by Pfizer	00069-0990	Antibiotic
VIBRATAB <> PFIZER099	Tab, Orange, Film Coated	Doxycycline Hyclate 100 mg	Vibra-Tabs by Pfizer	Canadian DIN# 00578452	Antibiotic
VICODIN	Tab	Acetaminophen 500 mg, Hydrocodone Bitartrate 5 mg	Vicodin by PDRX	55289-0116	Analgesic; C III
VICODIN	Tab	Acetaminophen 500 mg, Hydrocodone Bitartrate 5 mg	Vicodin by DRX	55045-2464	Analgesic; C III
VICODIN	Tab	Acetaminophen 500 mg, Hydrocodone Bitartrate 5 mg	Vicodin by Quality Care	60346-0657	Analgesic; C III
VICODIN	Tab	Acetaminophen 500 mg, Hydrocodone Bitartrate 5 mg	Vicodin by Amerisource	62584-0023	Analgesic; C III
VICODIN	Tab, White, Cap Shaped, Scored	Acetaminophen 500 mg, Hydrocodone Bitartrate 5 mg	Vicodin by Knoll	00044-0727	Analgesic; C III
VICODIN	Tab	Acetaminophen 500 mg, Hydrocodone Bitartrate 5 mg	by Caremark	00339-4072	Analgesic; C III
VICODIN	Tab	Acetaminophen 500 mg, Hydrocodone Bitartrate 5 mg	Vicodin by Allscripts	54569-0032	Analgesic; C III
VICODIN	Tab, Scored	Acetaminophen 500 mg, Hydrocodone Bitartrate 5 mg	Vicodin by Nat Pharmpak Serv	55154-1603	Analgesic; C III
VICODIN	Tab	Acetaminophen 500 mg, Hydrocodone Bitartrate 5 mg	Vicodin by Med Pro	53978-3093	Analgesic; C III
VICODINES	Tab	Acetaminophen 750 mg, Hydrocodone Bitartrate 7.5 mg	Vicodin ES by Quality Care	60346-0943	Analgesic; C III
VICODINES	Tab	Acetaminophen 750 mg, Hydrocodone Bitartrate 7.5 mg	Vicodin ES by Amerisource	62584-0025	Analgesic; C III
VICODINES	Tab, White, Oval, Scored	Acetaminophen 750 mg, Hydrocodone Bitartrate 7.5 mg	Vicodin ES by Amerisource	62584-0039	Analgesic; C III
VICODINES	Tab, White, Oval, Scored	Acetaminophen 750 mg, Hydrocodone Bitartrate 7.5 mg	Vicodin ES by Knoll	00044-0728	Analgesic; C III
VICODINES	Tab	Acetaminophen 750 mg, Hydrocodone Bitartrate 7.5 mg	Vicodin ES by Allscripts	54569-2736	Analgesic; C III
VICODINES	Tab, Scored	Acetaminophen 750 mg, Hydrocodone Bitartrate 7.5 mg	Vicodin ES by Nat Pharmpak Serv	55154-1604	Analgesic; C III

ID FRONT <> BACK	DESCRIPTION FRONT <> BACK	INGREDIENT & STRENGTH	BRAND (OR EQUIV.) & FIRM	NDC#	CLASS; SCH.
VICODINHP	Tab, White, Oval, Scored	Acetaminophen 660 mg, Hydrocodone Bitartrate 10 mg	Vicodin HP by Knoll	00044-0725	Analgesic; C III
VICODINHP	Tab	Acetaminophen 660 mg, Hydrocodone Bitartrate 10 mg	Vicodin HP by Nat Pharmpak Serv	55154-1607	Analgesic; C III
VICODINHP	Tab	Acetaminophen 660 mg, Hydrocodone Bitartrate 10 mg	Vicodin HP by Eckerd Drug	19458-0872	Analgesic; C III
VICODINHP	Tab, White, Oval, Scored	Hydrocodone Bitartrate	by Murfreesboro	51129-1441	Analgesic; C III
VIDEX <> 100	Tab, Mottled Off-White to Light Orange & Yellow, Orange Specks, Chewable	Didanosine 100 mg	Videx T by Bristol Myers Squibb	00087-6652	Antiviral
VIDEX <> 150	Tab, Mottled Off-White to Light Orange & Yellow, Orange Specks, Chewable	Didanosine 150 mg	Videx T by Bristol Myers Squibb	00087-6653	Antiviral
VIDEX <> 200	Tab, Mottled Off-White to Light Orange & Yellow, Orange Specks, Round, Chewable	Didanosine 200 mg	Videx T by Bristol Myers Squibb	00087-6665	Antiviral
VIDEX <> 25	Tab, Mottled Off-White to Light Orange & Yellow, Orange Specks, Chewable	Didanosine 25 mg	Videx T by Bristol Myers Squibb	00087-6650	Antiviral
VIDEX <> 50	Tab, Mottled Off-White to Light Orange & Yellow, Orange Specks, Round, Chewable	Didanosine 50 mg	Videx T by Bristol Myers Squibb	00087-6651	Antiviral
VIDEX100	Tab, White, Orange, Orange, Round, Videx/100	Didanosine 100 mg	by Bristol	Canadian	Antiviral
VIDEX150	Tab, White, Orange, Orange, Round, Videx/150	Didanosine 150 mg	by Bristol	Canadian	Antiviral
VIDEXBL	Tab, White, Round, Videx/BL	Didanosine 25 mg	by Bristol	Canadian	Antiviral
VIDEXBL	Tab, White, Round, Videx/BL	Didanosine 50 mg	by Bristol	Canadian	Antiviral
VIOKASE <> 9111	Tab	Amylase 30000 Units, Lipase 8000 Units, Protease 30000 Units	Viokase by Paddock	00574-9111	Gastrointestinal
VIOKASE <> 9111	Tab	Amylase 30000 Units, Lipase 8000 Units, Protease 30000 Units	Viokase by Eckerd Drug	19458-0871	Gastrointestinal
VIOXX <> MRK74	Tab, Cream, Round	Rofecoxib 12.5 mg	Vioxx by Allscripts	54569-4758	NSAID
VIOXX <> MRK74	Tab, Cream, Round	Rofecoxib 12.5 mg	Vioxx by Phy Total Care	54868-4148	NSAID
VIOXX <> MRK74	Tab, Beige, Round	Rofecoxib 12.5 mg	Vioxx by DRX Pharm Consults	55045-2720	NSAID
VIRACEPT <> 250MG	Tab	Nelfinavir Mesylate	Viracept by Physicians Total Care	54868-3947	Antiviral
VIRACEPT <> 250MG	Tab, Light Blue	Nelfinavir Mesylate	Viracept by MOVA	55370-0560	Antiviral
VIRACEPT <> 250MG	Tab, Blue, Oblong	Nelfinavir Mesylate 250 mg	Viracept by Allscripts	54569-4543	Antiviral
VIRACEPT <> 250MG	Tab, Blue, Oblong	Nelfinavir Mesylate 250 mg	Viracept by Par	49884-0578	Antiviral
VIRACEPT <> 250MG	Tab, Blue, Oblong	Nelfinavir Mesylate 250 mg	Viracept by Par	49884-0575	Antiviral
VIRACEPT <> 250MG	Tab	Nelfinavir Mesylate 292.25 mg	Viracept by Patheon	63285-0010	Antiviral
VIRACEPT <> 250MG	Tab	Nelfinavir Mesylate 292.25 mg	Viracept by Circa	71114-4206	Antiviral
VIRACEPT <> 250MG	Tab, Light Blue	Nelfinavir Mesylate 292.25 mg	Viracept by Agouron	63010-0010	Antiviral
VIRACEPT250MG	Tab, Light Blue, Oblong, Viracept/250 mg	Nelfinavir Mesylate 250 mg	Viracept by Agouron		Antiviral
VIRILON	Cap, Opaque Black, Gray & White Beads	Methyltestosterone 10 mg	Virilon by Star	00076-0301	Hormone; C III
VIRILON 10MG	Cap, Black & Clear	Methyltestosterone 10 mg	Virilon by Star Pharm		Hormone; C III
VIRILON10MG	Cap, Black & Clear	Methyltestosterone 10 mg	Virilon by Schwarz Pharma Mfg	00131-4950	Hormone; C III
VISKAZIDES <> 10251025	Tab, Peach, Round, Scored, Viskazide S in a triangle <> 10/25	Hydrochlorothiazide 25 mg, Pindolol 10 mg	Viskazide by Sandoz	Canadian DIN# 00568627	Diuretic; Antihypertensive
VISKAZIDES <> 10501050	Tab, Orange, Round, Scored, Viskazide S in a triangle <> 10/50	Pindolol 10 mg, Hydrochlorothiazide 50 mg	Viskazide by Sandoz	Canadian DIN# 00568635	Antihypertensive
VISKEN10	Tab, White	Pindolol 10 mg	Visken by Sandoz	Canadian	Antihypertensive
VISKEN10	Tab, White, Round, Scored	Pindolol 10 mg	Visken by Novartis	Canadian DIN# 00443174	Antihypertensive
VISKEN10 <> V	Tab, White, Round	Pindolol 10 mg	Visken by Prepackage Spec	58864-0489	Antihypertensive
VISKEN15 <> JU	Tab, White, Round, Scored	Pindolol 15 mg	Visken by Novartis	Canadian DIN# 00417289	Antihypertensive
VISKEN5 <> LB	Tab, White, Round, Scored	Pindolol 5 mg	Visken by Sandoz	Canadian DIN# 00417270	Antihypertensive

ID FRONT <> BACK	DESCRIPTION FRONT <> BACK	INGREDIENT & STRENGTH	BRAND (OR EQUIV.) & FIRM	NDC#	CLASS; SCH.
VISKEN5 <> V	Tab, White, Round	Pindolol 5 mg	Visken by Prepackage Spec	58864-0488	Antihypertensive
VISTA065 <> 20	Tab, White, Round, Scored	Isoxsuprine HCl 20 mg	by Vista Pharms	61970-0066	Vasodilator
VISTA065 <> 20	Tab, Tab Coated, Embossed	Isoxsuprine HCl 20 mg	Tri Soxsuprine by Vista	61970-0065	Vasodilator
VISTARIL <> PFIZER541	Cap, Light Green & Dark Green	Hydroxyzine Pamoate	Vistaril by Pfizer	00069-5410	Antihistamine
VISTARIL <> PFIZER542	Cap, Dark Green	Hydroxyzine Pamoate	Vistaril by Pfizer	00069-5420	Antihistamine
VJ <> SANDOZ	Tab, White, Round	Ergoloid Mesylates 1 mg	Hydergine by Novartis	Canadian DIN# 00176176	Ergot
VOCODINES	Tab	Acetaminophen 750 mg, Hydrocodone Bitartrate 7.5 mg	Vicodin ES by Med Pro	53978-1104	Analgesic; C III
VOLMAX <> 4	Tab, Blue, Hexagonal	Albuterol Sulfate 4 mg	Volmax by Med-Pro	53978-2026	Antiasthmatic
VOLMAX <> 4	Tab, Blue, Hexagon, Dark Blue Print	Albuterol Sulfate 4 mg	Volmax Extended Release by Anabolic	00722-6429	Antiasthmatic
VOLMAX <> 4	Tab, Dark Blue Print	Albuterol Sulfate 4.8 mg	Volmax by Muro	00451-0398	Antiasthmatic
VOLMAX <> 4	Tab, Dark Blue Print	Albuterol Sulfate 4.8 mg	Volmax by Nat Pharmpak Serv	55154-4304	Antiasthmatic
VOLMAX <> 4	Tab, Dark Blue Print	Albuterol Sulfate 4.8 mg	Volmax by CVS	51316-0240	Antiasthmatic
VOLMAX <> 4	Tab	Albuterol Sulfate 4.8 mg	Volmax by Wal Mart	49035-0159	Antiasthmatic
VOLMAX <> 4	Tab, Dark Blue Print	Albuterol Sulfate 4.8 mg	Volmax by Eckerd Drug	19458-0848	Antiasthmatic
VOLMAX <> 8	Tab, White, Hexagon	Albuterol Sulfate 8 mg	Volmax by Thrift Services	59198-0355	Antiasthmatic
VOLMAX <> 8	Tab, White, Hexagon, 8 in Dark Blue	Albuterol Sulfate 8 mg	Volmax ER by Amerisource	62584-0873	Antiasthmatic
VOLMAX <> 8	Tab, White, Hexagon, Dark Blue Ink	Albuterol Sulfate 8 mg	Volmax by Amerisource	62584-0874	Antiasthmatic
VOLMAX <> 8	Tab	Albuterol Sulfate 9.6 mg	Volmax by Muro	00451-0399	Antiasthmatic
VOLMAX <> 8	Tab, Dark Blue Print	Albuterol Sulfate 9.6 mg	Volmax by Eckerd Drug	19458-0849	Antiasthmatic
VOLTAREN <> 25	Tab, Yellow, Round, Enteric Coated	Diclofenac Sodium 25 mg	Voltaren by Novartis	Canadian DIN# 00514004	NSAID
VOLTAREN <> 50	Tab, Light Brown, Round, Enteric Coated	Diclofenac Sodium 50 mg	Voltaren by Novartis	Canadian DIN# 00514012	NSAID
VOLTAREN <> RAPIDE50	Tab, Reddish-Brown, Round, Sugar Coated	Diclofenac Potassium 50 mg	Voltaren Rapide by Novartis	Canadian DIN# 00881635	NSAID
VOLTAREN <> SR75	Tab, Light Pink, Triangular, Film Coated	Diclofenac Sodium 75 mg	Voltaren SR by Novartis	Canadian DIN# 00782459	NSAID
VOLTAREN25	Tab, Yellow, Triangular	Diclofenac Sodium 25 mg	Voltaren by Novartis	00028-0258	NSAID
VOLTAREN50	Tab, Tab Coated	Diclofenac Potassium 50 mg	Cataflam by Prescription Dispensing	61807-0084	NSAID
VOLTAREN50	Tab, Brown, Triangle	Diclofenac Potassium 50 mg	by Novartis Pharms (Ca)	61615-0109	NSAID
VOLTAREN50	Tab, Light Brown, Biconvex, is Light Brown, Tab DR	Diclofenac Sodium 50 mg	Voltaren by Pharm Utilization	60491-0705	NSAID
VOLTAREN50	Tab, Tab Delayed Release	Diclofenac Sodium 50 mg	Voltaren by Quality Care	60346-0477	NSAID
VOLTAREN50	Tab, Brown, Triangular	Diclofenac Sodium 50 mg	Voltaren DR by DRX	55045-2691	NSAID
VOLTAREN50	Tab	Diclofenac Sodium 50 mg	Voltaren by Nat Pharmpak Serv	55154-1008	NSAID
VOLTAREN50	Tab, Light Brown, Triangular	Diclofenac Sodium 50 mg	Voltaren by Novartis	00028-0262	NSAID
VOLTAREN50	Tab, Light Brown	Diclofenac Sodium 50 mg	Voltaren by Med Pro	53978-1059	NSAID
VOLTAREN50	Tab	Diclofenac Sodium 50 mg	by Pharmedix	53002-0537	NSAID
VOLTAREN50	Tab	Diclofenac Sodium 50 mg	Voltaren by Allscripts	54569-2155	NSAID
VOLTAREN75	Tab, Light Pink, Triangular	Diclofenac Sodium 75 mg	Voltaren by Novartis	00028-0264	NSAID
VOLTAREN75	Tab,	Diclofenac Sodium 75 mg	Voltaren by Allscripts	54569-2156	NSAID
VOLTAREN75	Tab	Diclofenac Sodium 75 mg	Voltaren by Med Pro	53978-1049	NSAID
VOLTAREN75	Tab	Diclofenac Sodium 75 mg	by Pharmedix	53002-0536	NSAID
VOLTAREN75	Tab	Diclofenac Sodium 75 mg	Voltaren by Nat Pharmpak Serv	55154-1007	NSAID
VOLTAREN75	Tab, Geigy, Tab Delayed Release	Diclofenac Sodium 75 mg	Voltaren by Prescription Dispensing	61807-0049	NSAID
VOLTAREN75	Tab, Light Pink, Biconvex, Tab Delayed Release	Diclofenac Sodium 75 mg	Voltaren by Quality Care	60346-0743	NSAID
VOLTAREN75	Tab, Pink, Triangle	Diclofenac Sodium 75 mg	Voltaren by Rx Pac	65084-0119	NSAID

ID FRONT <> BACK	DESCRIPTION FRONT <> BACK	INGREDIENT & STRENGTH	BRAND (OR EQUIV.) & FIRM	NDC#	CLASS; SCH.
VOLTARENSR <> 100	Tab, Pink, Round, Film Coated	Diclofenac Sodium 100 mg	Voltaren SR by Novartis	Canadian DIN# 00590827	NSAID
VOLTARENXR <> 100	Tab, Pink, Round, Film Coated	Diclofenac Sodium 100 mg	Voltaren by HJ Harkins	52959-0472	NSAID
VOLTARENXR <> 100	Tab, Light Pink, Round, Coated, Voltaren-XR <> 100	Diclofenac Sodium 100 mg	Voltaren-XL by Novartis	00028-0205	NSAID
VOLTARENXR <> 100	Tab, Voltaren-XR	Diclofenac Sodium 100 mg	Voltaren by Caremark	00339-6091	NSAID
VOLTARENXR <> 100	Tab, Voltaren-XR	Diclofenac Sodium 100 mg	Voltaren XR by Allscripts	54569-4513	NSAID
VOLTARENXR <> 100	Tab, Film Coated	Diclofenac Sodium 100 mg	Voltaren XR by Novartis	17088-0205	NSAID
VOO31	Tab	Acetaminophen 500 mg	by Diversified	55887-0945	Antipyretic
VP	Tab, White, Round, Film Coated, VP over Knoll Triangle	Hydrocodone Bitartrate 7.5 mg, Ibuprofen 200 mg	Vicoprofen by Knoll	00044-0723	Analgesic; C III
VP	Tab, White, Round, Convex, Film, VP Over the Knoll Triangle	Hydrocodone Bitartrate 7.5 mg, Ibuprofen 200 mg	Vicoprofen by Murfreesboro	51129-1457	Analgesic; C III
VP	Tab, White, Round, Convex, Film, Knoll Triangle	Hydrocodone Bitartrate 7.5 mg, Ibuprofen 200 mg	Vicoprofen by Murfreesboro	51129-1459	Analgesic; C III
VP	Tab, White, Round, Convex, Film, VP Over the Knoll Triangle	Hydrocodone Bitartrate 7.5 mg, Ibuprofen 200 mg	Vicoprofen by Murfreesboro	51129-1458	Analgesic; C III
VP	Tab, White, Round, Convex, Film, Knoll Triangle	Hydrocodone Bitartrate 7.5 mg, Ibuprofen 200 mg	Vicoprofen by Murfreesboro	51129-1456	Analgesic; C III
VP	Tab, VP Over Knoll Triangle	Hydrocodone Bitartrate 7.5 mg, Ibuprofen 200 mg	Vicoprofen by Quality Care	62682-2007	Analgesic; C III
VP	Tab, White, Round, Film Coated	Hydrocodone Bitartrate 7.5 mg, Ibuprofen 200 mg	Vicoprofen by Phy Total Care	54868-4035	Analgesic; C III
VP	Tab, White, Round	Hydrocodone Bitartrate 7.5 mg, Ibuprofen 200 mg	Vicoprofen by Southwood Pharms	58016-0442	Analgesic; C III
VP	Tab, White, Round, Convex, Film, VP Over Knoll Triangle	Hydrocondone Bitartrate 7.5 mg, Ibuprofen 200 mg	Vicoprofen by Murfreesboro	51129-1463	Analgesic; C III
VP <> 11	Tab, White, Round	Ethambutol HCl 100 mg	by Versapharm	61748-0011	Antituberculosis
VP <> 11	Tab, White, Round, Film Coated	Ethambutol HCl 100 mg	by WestWard Pharm	00143-9100	Antituberculosis
VP <> 14	Tab, White, Round, Film Coated	Ethambutol HCl 400 mg	by WestWard Pharm	00143-9101	Antituberculosis
VP <> UREX	Tab, White, Oblong, Scored	Methenamine Hippurate 1 gm	Urex by Virco Pharms	65199-1201	Antibiotic; Urinary Tract
VP11	Tab, White, Round	Ethambutol HCl 400 mg	by Versapharm	61748-0014	Antituberculosis
VT1052	Cap, Brown & Clear, VT-1052	Theophylline SR 260 mg	by Eon		Antiasthmatic
VT5720	Cap, Red & Clear, VT-5720	Phendimetrazine Tartrate 35 mg	by Eon		Anorexiant; C III
VT76	Tab, Yellow, Round	Phendimetrazine Tartrate 35 mg	Plegine by Eon		Anorexiant; C III
VT77	Tab, Pink, Oblong, VT-77	Phendimetrazine Tartrate 35 mg	by Eon		Anorexiant; C III
W	Tab, White, Round	Chloroquine Phosphate 250 mg	Aralen by Sanofi	Canadian	Antimalarial
W	Cap, Yellow	Danazol 100 mg	Cyclomen by Sanofi	Canadian	Steroid
W	Cap, Orange	Danazol 200 mg	Cyclomen by Sanofi	Canadian	Steroid
W	Cap, Orange & White	Danazol 50 mg	Cyclomen by Sanofi	Canadian	Steroid
W	Cap, Brown	Dihydrotachysterol 0.125 mg	Hytakerol by Sanofi	Canadian	Vitamin
W	Cap, Brown	Dihydrotachysterol 0.125 mg	Hytakerol by Sanofi		Vitamin
W	Cap, Brown & Gray, Opaque	Dihydrotachysterol 170 mg	Hytakerol by RP Scherer	11014-0300	Vitamin
W	Tab, White, Round	Floctafenine 200 mg	Idarac by Sanofi	Canadian	Anti-Inflammatory
W	Tab, White, Round	Floctafenine 400 mg	Idarac by Sanofi	Canadian	Anti-Inflammatory
W	Tab	Lead 12 X	Scleron by Weleda	00164-1193	Homeopathic
W	Tab	Lead 12 X	Scleron by Weleda	55946-0396	Homeopathic
W	Tab, Maroon, Round	Phenazopyridine HCl 95 mg	by Able		Urinary Analgesic
W <> 1605	Tab, Branded in Blue, Sugar Coated	Perphenazine 8 mg	by Schein	00364-2625	Antipsychotic
W <> 901	Tab, Film Coated	Naproxen Sodium 412.5 mg	Naprelan 375 by Wyeth Labs	00008-0901	NSAID
W <> 901	Tab, Film Coated	Naproxen Sodium 412.5 mg	Naprelan by Physicians Total Care	54868-3974	NSAID
W <> 901	Tab, Film Coated	Naproxen Sodium 412.5 mg	Naprelan by Quality Care	62682-2000	NSAID
W <> 902	Tab, Film Coated	Naproxen Sodium 550 mg	Naprelan by Physicians Total Care	54868-3973	NSAID
W <> 902	Tab, Film Coated	Naproxen Sodium 550 mg	Naprelan by Quality Care	62682-2001	NSAID
W <> 902	Tab, White, Oblong	Naproxen Sodium 500 mg	Naprelan 500 by Par	49884-0498	NSAID
W <> 902	Tab, White, Oblong	Naproxen Sodium 550 mg	Naprelan by PDRX Pharms	55289-0304	NSAID
W <> 902	Tab, Film Coated	Naproxen Sodium 550 mg	Naprelan by Wyeth Labs	00008-0902	NSAID
W <> 902	Tab, Film Coated	Naproxen Sodium 550 mg	Naprelan 500 by Caremark	00339-6102	NSAID
W <> A77	Tab, Film Coated, Black Print	Chloroquine Phosphate 500 mg	Aralen Phosphate by Sanofi	00024-0084	Antimalarial
W <> A77	Tab, Film Coated, Black Print	Chloroquine Phosphate 500 mg	Aralen Phosphate by Bayer	00280-0084	Antimalarial
W <> A77	Tab, Film Coated	Chloroquine Phosphate 500 mg	Aralen by Allscripts	54569-3777	Antimalarial

ID FRONT ⬦ BACK	DESCRIPTION FRONT ⬦ BACK	INGREDIENT & STRENGTH	BRAND (OR EQUIV.) & FIRM	NDC#	CLASS; SCH.
W ⬦ D35	Tab, D/35	Meperidine HCl 50 mg	Demerol Hydrochloride by Sanofi	00024-0335	Analgesic; C II
W ⬦ D35	Tab, D/35, Tab Coated	Meperidine HCl 50 mg	Demerol by Bayer	00280-0335	Analgesic; C II
W ⬦ D37	Tab, D/37	Meperidine HCl 100 mg	Demerol Hydrochloride by Sanofi	00024-0337	Analgesic; C II
W ⬦ D37	Tab, D/37, Tab Coated	Meperidine HCl 100 mg	Demerol by Bayer	00280-0337	Analgesic; C II
W ⬦ D92	Cap, White Print, W in Circle ⬦ D92	Ergocalciferol 1.25 mg	Drisdol by Sanofi	00024-0392	Vitamin
W ⬦ D92	Cap, White Print, W in a Circle	Ergocalciferol 1.25 mg	Drisdol by Bayer	00280-0392	Vitamin
W ⬦ EFFEXORXR	Cap, Orange	Venlafaxine HCl 150 mg	Effexor ER by Ayerst Lab (Div Wyeth)	00046-0836	Antidepressant
W ⬦ EFFEXORXR	Cap, Gray & Peach	Venlafaxine HCl 37.5 mg	Effexor ER by Ayerst Lab (Div Wyeth)	00046-0837	Antidepressant
W ⬦ M87	Tab, Coated, W⬦ M/87	Ambenonium Chloride 10 mg	Mytelase by Bayer	00280-1287	Myasthenia Gravis
W ⬦ M87	Tab, W ⬦ M/87	Ambenonium Chloride 10 mg	Mytelase Chloride by Sanofi	00024-1287	Myasthenia Gravis
W ⬦ N21	Tab, Light Buff, N/21	Nalidixic Acid 250 mg	Neggram by Sanofi	00024-1321	Antibiotic
W ⬦ N22	Tab, Light Buff, N/22	Nalidixic Acid 500 mg	Neggram by Sanofi	00024-1322	Antibiotic
W ⬦ N23	Tab, Light Buff, N/23	Nalidixic Acid 1 gm	Neggram by Sanofi	00024-1323	Antibiotic
W ⬦ P97	Tab, in Black Ink, Tab Coated	Primaquine Phosphate 26.3 mg	by Sanofi	00024-1596	Antimalarial
W ⬦ P97	Tab, in Black Ink, Tab Coated	Primaquine Phosphate 26.3 mg	by Bayer	00280-1596	Antimalarial
W ⬦ T31	Tab, T and 31, Tab Coated	Iopanoic Acid 500 mg	Telepaque by Nycomed	00407-1931	Diagnostic
W ⬦ T51	Tab, T.51	Naloxone HCl 0.5 mg, Pentazocine HCl	Talwin Nx by Allscripts	54569-0022	Analgesic; C IV
W ⬦ T51	Tab, T 51	Naloxone HCl 0.5 mg, Pentazocine HCl 50 mg	Talwin Nx by Sanofi	00024-1951	Analgesic; C IV
W ⬦ T51	Tab, T 51	Naloxone HCl 0.5 mg, Pentazocine HCl 50 mg	Talwin Nx by Searle	00966-1951	Analgesic; C IV
W028 ⬦ SQUIBB	Cap	Cloxacillin Sodium	by Apothecon	59772-6028	Antibiotic
W038	Cap, Orange, in White Ink	Cloxacillin Sodium 500 mg	by Apothecon	59772-6038	Antibiotic
W048 ⬦ SQUIBB	Cap	Dicloxacillin Sodium	by Golden State	60429-0059	Antibiotic
W05	Tab, White, Round, W/0.5	Lorazepam 0.5 mg	by Wyeth-Ayerst	Canadian	Sedative/Hypnotic; C IV
W1	Tab, Yellow, Round	Isosorbide Dinitrate 2.5 mg	Isordil by West Ward	00143-1765	Antianginal
W1	Tab	Isosorbide Dinitrate 2.5 mg	Wesorbide by West Ward	00143-9403	Antianginal
W1	Tab, W-1	Isosorbide Dinitrate 2.5 mg	by Qualitest	00603-4122	Antianginal
W1	Tab, Yellow, Round	Isosorbide Dinitrate Sublingual 2.5 mg	Isordil by West-ward		Antianginal
W10	Tab, White, Round, W/10	Isosorbide Dinitrate SL 10 mg	Isordil by Wyeth		Antianginal
W1600	Tab, Gray, Round	Perphenazine 2 mg	Trilafon by Warrick		Antipsychotic
W1600	Tab, Sugar Coated	Perphenazine 2 mg	by Warrick	59930-1600	Antipsychotic
W1600	Tab, Tab Sugar Coated	Perphenazine 2 mg	by Qualitest	00603-5090	Antipsychotic
W1600 ⬦ W1600	Tab, Sugar Coated, Black Print	Perphenazine 2 mg	by Martec	52555-0569	Antipsychotic
W1603	Tab, Gray, Round	Perphenazine 4 mg	Trilafon by Warrick		Antipsychotic
W1603	Tab, Sugar Coated, Green Print	Perphenazine 4 mg	by Warrick	59930-1603	Antipsychotic
W1603	Tab, Sugar Coated, Green Print	Perphenazine 4 mg	by Qualitest	00603-5091	Antipsychotic
W1603 ⬦ W1603	Tab, Sugar Coated	Perphenazine 4 mg	by Martec	52555-0570	Antipsychotic
W1605	Tab, Sugar Coated	Perphenazine 8 mg	by Qualitest	00603-5092	Antipsychotic
W1605	Tab, Gray	Perphenazine 8 mg	Trilafon by Warrick		Antipsychotic
W1606 ⬦ W1606	Tab, Sugar Coated	Perphenazine 8 mg	by Martec	52555-0571	Antipsychotic
W1610	Tab, Gray	Perphenazine 16 mg	Trilafon by Warrick		Antipsychotic
W1610 ⬦ W1610	Tab, Sugar Coated	Perphenazine 16 mg	by Martec	52555-0572	Antipsychotic
W16WYETH92	Tab, White, Pentagonal, W16/Wyeth 92	Guanabenz Acetate 16 mg	Wytensin by Wyeth		Antihypertensive
W200	Tab, Orange, Round	Cyclandelate 200 mg	by Wyeth-Ayerst	Canadian	Vasodilator
W200	Tab, Orange, Round, W/200	Peripheral Vasodilator 200 mg	Cyclospasmol by Wyeth-Ayerst	Canadian	Vasodilator
W2183	Tab, Purple, Round	Atro, Hyoscy, Methenamine, M.Blue, Phenyl Sali, Benz. A	Urised by Webcon		Urinary Tract
W2183	Tab, Dark Blue, Round	Phenyl Salicylate 18.1 mg; Methylene Blue 5.4 mg; Atropine Sulfate 0.03 mg; Benzoic Acid 4.5 mg; Hyoscyamine 0.03 mg; Methenamine 40.8 mg	Urised by Polymedica Pharms	61451-2183	Urinary
W2225	Tab, Light Blue, Round	Hyoscyamine 0.15 mg	Cystospaz by Polymedica	61451-2225	Gastrointestinal
W2225	Tab	Hyoscyamine 0.15 mg	Cystospaz by Pegasus	55246-0956	Gastrointestinal
W2260	Cap, Clear Blue	Hyoscyamine Sulfate 0.375 mg	by Eon	00185-5322	Gastrointestinal
W2260	Cap, Light Blue	Hyoscyamine Sulfate 0.375 mg	Cystospaz-M by Polymedica	61451-2260	Gastrointestinal
W23	Tab, White, W/23	D-Norgestrel 250 mcg, Ethinyl Estradiol 50 mcg	by Wyeth-Ayerst	Canadian	Oral Contraceptive

ID FRONT <> BACK	DESCRIPTION FRONT <> BACK	INGREDIENT & STRENGTH	BRAND (OR EQUIV.) & FIRM	NDC#	CLASS; SCH.
W23	Tab, White, W/23	Norgestrel 250 mcg	Orval 21 by Wyeth-Ayerst	Canadian	Oral Contraceptive
W25	Tab, Yellow, Round, W/2.5	Isosorbide Dinitrate SL 2.5 mg	Isordil by Wyeth		Antianginal
W3	Tab, White, Round	Isosorbide Dinitrate 5 mg	Isordil by West Ward	00143-1767	Antianginal
W3	Tab	Isosorbide Dinitrate 5 mg	Wesorbide by West Ward	00143-9404	Antianginal
W3	Tab	Isosorbide Dinitrate 5 mg	by United Res	00677-0409	Antianginal
W3	Tab, W-3	Isosorbide Dinitrate 5 mg	by Qualitest	00603-4123	Antianginal
W300	Tab	Furosemide 20 mg	by Qualitest	00603-3736	Diuretic
W302	Tab	Furosemide 80 mg	by Qualitest	00603-3738	Diuretic
W332	Tab	Ascorbic Acid 500 mg, Biotin 0.15 mg, Calcium Pantothenate, Chromic Nitrate, Cupric Oxide, Cyanocobalamin 50 mcg, Ferrous Fumarate, Folic Acid 0.8 mg, Magnesium Oxide, Manganese Dioxide, Niacinamide, Pyridoxine HCl 25 mg, Riboflavin 20 mg, Thiamine Mononitrate, Vitamin A Acetate, Vitamin E Acetate, Zinc Oxide	Vitalize Plus by West Ward	00143-2332	Vitamin
W363	Tab	Clorazepate Dipotassium 3.75 mg	by Qualitest	00603-3004	Antianxiety; C IV
W365	Tab	Clorazepate Dipotassium 15 mg	by Qualitest	00603-3006	Antianxiety; C IV
W365	Tab	Clorazepate Dipotassium 7.5 mg	by Qualitest	00603-3005	Antianxiety; C IV
W369	Cap	Loxapine Succinate	by Qualitest	00603-4268	Antipsychotic
W371	Cap	Loxapine Succinate	by Qualitest	00603-4270	Antipsychotic
W372	Cap	Loxapine Succinate	by Qualitest	00603-4271	Antipsychotic
W373	Tab, Film Coated	Maprotiline HCl 25 mg	by Qualitest	00603-4294	Antidepressant
W379	Tab	Amoxapine 25 mg	by Qualitest	00603-2240	Antidepressant
W380	Tab, Salmon	Amoxapine 50 mg	by Qualitest	00603-2241	Antidepressant
W381	Tab	Amoxapine 100 mg	by Qualitest	00603-2242	Antidepressant
W382	Tab	Amoxapine 150 mg	by Qualitest	00603-2243	Antidepressant
W4	Tab, White, Round	Trihexyphenidyl 2 mg	by West Ward Pharm	00143-1764	Antiparkinson
W4 <> WYETH73	Tab, Coated, W 4 <> Wyeth 73	Guanabenz Acetate 4 mg	Wytensin by Wyeth Labs	00008-0073	Antihypertensive
W400	Tab, Film Coated	Ibuprofen 400 mg	by Quality Care	60346-0430	NSAID
W404	Tab, Film Coated, Debossed	Verapamil HCl 40 mg	by Qualitest	00603-6356	Antihypertensive
W414	Tab	Estropipate 0.75 mg	by Qualitest	00603-3559	Hormone
W415	Tab	Estropipate 1.5 mg	by Qualitest	00603-3560	Hormone
W416	Tab	Estropipate 3 mg	by Qualitest	00603-3561	Hormone
W424	Tab	Hydrochlorothiazide 25 mg, Triamterene 37.5 mg	by Qualitest	00603-6180	Diuretic
W425	Cap	Aspirin 325 mg, Butalbital 50 mg, Caffeine 40 mg, Codeine Phosphate 30 mg	by Qualitest	00603-2549	Analgesic; C III
W431	Tab, White, Round	Lorazepam 0.5 mg	Ativan by Watson		Sedative/Hypnotic; C IV
W451	Tab	Guanabenz Acetate	by Qualitest	00603-3779	Antihypertensive
W452	Tab	Guanabenz Acetate	by Qualitest	00603-3780	Antihypertensive
W454	Tab, Film Coated	Gemfibrozil 600 mg	by Qualitest	00603-3750	Antihyperlipidemic
W460	Tab	Glipizide 5 mg	by Qualitest	00603-3755	Antidiabetic
W462	Tab	Metoprolol Tartrate 50 mg	by Qualitest	00603-4627	Antihypertensive
W463	Tab	Metoprolol Tartrate 100 mg	by Qualitest	00603-4628	Antihypertensive
W480	Tab, White, Round	Propylthiouracil 50 mg	by Rondex		Antithyroid
W49	Tab, Pink, Round	Aluminum 180 mg, Magnesium Hydroxide 160 mg	Wingel by Sanofi		Gastrointestinal
W5	Tab, Pink, Round, W/5	Isosorbide Dinitrate SL 5 mg	Isordil by Wyeth		Antianginal
W53	Tab, W Over 53	Stanozolol 2 mg	Winstrol by Sanofi	00024-2253	Anabolic Steroid; C III
W53	Tab, W Over 53	Stanozolol 2 mg	Winstrol by Searle	00966-2253	Anabolic Steroid; C III
W587 <> 120	Tab, White, Oval, Scored	Isosorbide Mononitrate 120 mg	by Warrick Pharms	59930-1587	Antianginal
W587 <> 120	Tab, White, Oval, W-587	Isosorbide Mononitrate ER 120 mg	by Murfreesboro	51129-1581	Antianginal
W587 <> 120	Tab, White, Oval, Scored	Isosorbide Mononitrate 120 mg	by Murfreesboro	51129-1569	Antianginal
W641	Tab, Coated	Ethinyl Estradiol 0.03 mg, Ethinyl Estradiol 0.04 mg, Ethinyl Estradiol 0.03 mg, Levonorgestrel 0.05 mg, Levonorgestrel 0.075 mg, Levonorgestrel 0.125 mg	Triphasil 28 by Dept Health Central Pharm	53808-0060	Oral Contraceptive
W641	Tab	Ethinyl Estradiol 0.03 mg, Ethinyl Estradiol 0.04 mg, Ethinyl Estradiol 0.03 mg, Levonorgestrel 0.05 mg, Levonorgestrel 0.125 mg, Levonorgestrel 0.075 mg	Triphasil 28 Day by Physicians Total Care	54868-0518	Oral Contraceptive

ID FRONT <> BACK	DESCRIPTION FRONT <> BACK	INGREDIENT & STRENGTH	BRAND (OR EQUIV.) & FIRM	NDC#	CLASS; SCH.
W642	Tab, Coated	Ethinyl Estradiol 0.03 mg, Ethinyl Estradiol 0.04 mg, Ethinyl Estradiol 0.03 mg, Levonorgestrel 0.05 mg, Levonorgestrel 0.075 mg, Levonorgestrel 0.125 mg	Triphasil 28 by Dept Health Central Pharm	53808-0060	Oral Contraceptive
W642	Tab	Ethinyl Estradiol 0.03 mg, Ethinyl Estradiol 0.04 mg, Ethinyl Estradiol 0.03 mg, Levonorgestrel 0.05 mg, Levonorgestrel 0.125 mg, Levonorgestrel 0.075 mg	Triphasil 28 Day by Physicians Total Care	54868-0518	Oral Contraceptive
W643	Tab	Ethinyl Estradiol 0.03 mg, Ethinyl Estradiol 0.04 mg, Ethinyl Estradiol 0.03 mg, Levonorgestrel 0.05 mg, Levonorgestrel 0.125 mg, Levonorgestrel 0.075 mg	Triphasil 28 Day by Physicians Total Care	54868-0518	Oral Contraceptive
W643	Tab, Coated	Ethinyl Estradiol 0.03 mg, Ethinyl Estradiol 0.04 mg, Ethinyl Estradiol 0.03 mg, Levonorgestrel 0.05 mg, Levonorgestrel 0.075 mg, Levonorgestrel 0.125 mg	Triphasil 28 by Dept Health Central Pharm	53808-0060	Oral Contraceptive
W650	Tab	Ethinyl Estradiol 0.03 mg, Ethinyl Estradiol 0.04 mg, Ethinyl Estradiol 0.03 mg, Levonorgestrel 0.05 mg, Levonorgestrel 0.125 mg, Levonorgestrel 0.075 mg	Triphasil 28 Day by Physicians Total Care	54868-0518	Oral Contraceptive
W650	Tab, Coated	Ethinyl Estradiol 0.03 mg, Ethinyl Estradiol 0.04 mg, Ethinyl Estradiol 0.03 mg, Levonorgestrel 0.05 mg, Levonorgestrel 0.075 mg, Levonorgestrel 0.125 mg	Triphasil 28 by Dept Health Central Pharm	53808-0060	Oral Contraceptive
W650	Tab, Green, Round	Inert	Alesse by Wyeth		Placebo
W650	Tab, Green, Round, Scored	Levonorgestrel 0.1 mg, Ethinyl Estradiol 0.02 mg	Alesse 28 by Wyeth Labs	00008-2576	Oral Contraceptive
W650	Tab, Green, Round, Scored	Levonorgestrel 0.1 mg, Ethinyl Estradiol 0.02 mg	Alesse 28 by Wyeth Pharms	52903-2576	Oral Contraceptive
W7	Tab, White, Round	Captopril 12.5 mg	by ESI Lederle	59911-5832	Antihypertensive
W7	Tab, White, Round	Captopril 12.5 mg	Capoten by West Ward	00143-1171	Antihypertensive
W7300	Tab, Pink, Round	Methdilazine 3.6 mg	Tacaryl Chewable by Westwood		Antihistamine
W7400	Tab, Peach, Round	Methdilazine HCl 8 mg	Tacaryl by Westwood		Antihistamine
W75 <> 704	Tab, W 75, Shield-Shaped	Venlafaxine HCl	Effexor by Allscripts	54569-4132	Antidepressant
W791	Tab	Allopurinol Sulphate 4 mg	by Squibb		Antigout
W8WYETH74	Tab, Gray, Pentagonal, W8/Wyeth 74	Guanabenz Acetate 8 mg	Wytensin by Wyeth		Antihypertensive
W901	Tab, White, Debossed with 901, Round,	Niacin 500 mg	Niacor by Upsher Smith	00245-0067	Vitamin
W906	Tab, Peach, Oval, Film Coated	Ranitidine HCl 150 mg	by Wockhardt Americas	64679-0906	Gastrointestinal
W906	Tab, White, Hexagonal, Film-Coated, W over 906	Ranitidine 150 mg	Zantac by Sidmak	50111-0899	Gastrointestinal
W906	Tab, Peach, Oval, Film Coated, W Over 906	Ranitidine 150 mg	Ranitidine by RX PAK	65084-0155	Gastrointestinal
W906	Tab, Peach, Oval, Film Coated, W Over 906	Ranitidine 150 mg	Ranitidine by RX PAK	65084-0158	Gastrointestinal
W906	Tab, Peach, Oblong, Film Coated, W Over 906	Ranitidine 150 mg	by RX PAK	65084-0161	Gastrointestinal
W906	Tab, Peach, Oblong, Film Coated	Ranitidine 150 mg	Ranitidine by RX PAK	65084-0152	Gastrointestinal
W907	Tab, Yellow, Oblong, Film Coated, W Over 907	Ranitidine 300 mg	Ranitidine by RX PAK	65084-0154	Gastrointestinal
W907	Tab, Yellow, Oblong, Film, W Over 907	Ranitidine 300 mg	Ranitidine by RX PAK	65084-0157	Gastrointestinal
W907	Tab, Yellow, Oblong, Film Coated, W Over 907	Ranitidine 300 mg	by RX PAK	65084-0162	Gastrointestinal
W907	Tab, White, Cap Shaped, Film Coated	Ranitidine 300 mg	Zantac by Sidmak	50111-0900	Gastrointestinal
W907	Tab, Yellow, Oblong, Film Coated	Ranitidine HCl 300 mg	by Wockhardt Americas	64679-0907	Gastrointestinal
W907	Tab, Yellow, Oblong, Film Coated	Ranitidine 300 mg	Ranitidine USP by RX PAK	65084-0164	Gastrointestinal
W912	Tab, Pink, Round	Levonorgestrel 0.1 mg, Ethinyl Estradiol 0.02 mg	Alesse by Wyeth		Oral Contraceptive
W912	Tab, Pink, Round, Scored	Levonorgestrel 0.1 mg, Ethinyl Estradiol 0.02 mg	Alesse 21 by Wyeth Labs	00008-0912	Oral Contraceptive
W912	Tab, Pink, Round, Scored	Levonorgestrel 0.1 mg, Ethinyl Estradiol 0.02 mg	Alesse 28 by Wyeth Pharms	52903-2576	Oral Contraceptive
W912	Tab, Pink, Round, Scored	Levonorgestrel 0.1 mg, Ethinyl Estradiol 0.02 mg	Alesse 28 by Wyeth Labs	00008-2576	Oral Contraceptive
W912	Tab, Pink, Round, Scored	Levonorgestrel 0.1 mg, Ethinyl Estradiol 0.02 mg	Alesse 21 by Wyeth Pharms	52903-0912	Oral Contraceptive
W921 <> BMS	Tab	Metoprolol Tartrate 50 mg	by Apothecon	59772-3692	Antihypertensive
W921 <> BMS	Tab, Film Coated	Metoprolol Tartrate 50 mg	by Quality Care	60346-0523	Antihypertensive
W923	Tab, White, Round, Scored, W over 923	Enalapril Maleate 2.5 mg	Vasotec by Sidmak	50111-0891	Antihypertensive
W923	Tab, White, Round, Scored, W over 923	Enalapril Maleate 2.5 mg	Vasotec by Sidmak	50111-0891	Antihypertensive
W924	Tab, White, Round, Scored, W over 924	Enalapril Maleate 5 mg	Vasotec by Sidmak	50111-0892	Antihypertensive
W924	Tab, White, Round, Scored, W over 924	Enalapril Maleate 5 mg	Vasotec by Sidmak	50111-0892	Antihypertensive
W925	Tab, Light Salmon, Round, W over 925	Enalapril Maleate 10 mg	Vasotec by Sidmak	50111-0893	Antihypertensive
W926	Tab, Light Beige, Round, W over 926	Enalapril Maleate 20 mg	Vasotec by Sidmak	50111-0894	Antihypertensive
W933 <> BMS	Tab	Metoprolol Tartrate 100 mg	by Apothecon	59772-3693	Antihypertensive
W933 <> BMS	Tab	Metoprolol Tartrate 100 mg	by Quality Care	60346-0514	Antihypertensive
WA77	Tab, Pink, Round	Chloroquine Phosphate 500 mg	Aralen by Sanofi		Antimalarial
WA79	Tab, Orange, Round	Chloroquine Phosphate 500 mg, Primaquine Phosphate 79 mg	Aralen / Primaquine by Sanofi		Antimalarial

ID FRONT <> BACK	DESCRIPTION FRONT <> BACK	INGREDIENT & STRENGTH	BRAND (OR EQUIV.) & FIRM	NDC#	CLASS; SCH.
WA82	Tab, Yellow, Round	Quinacrine HCl 100 mg	Atabrine by Sanofi		Antimalarial
WALLACE <> 0430	Tab, Yellow, Cap Shaped, Scored	Felbamate 400 mg	Felbatol by Wallace	00037-0430	Anticonvulsant
WALLACE <> 0431	Tab, Peach, Cap Shaped, Scored	Felbamate 600 mg	Felbatol by Wallace	00037-0431	Anticonvulsant
WALLACE <> 371001	Tab, White, Round, Scored, Wallace <> 37-1001	Meprobamate 400 mg	Miltown by Wallace	00037-1001	Sedative/Hypnotic; C IV
WALLACE <> 371101	Tab, White, Round, Sugar Coated, Wallace 37-1101	Meprobamate 200 mg	Miltown by Wallace	00037-1101	Sedative/Hypnotic; C IV
WALLACE <> 374401	Tab, White, Oval, Scored, Wallace <> 37 Over 4401	Penicillamine 250 mg	Depen Titratable by Wallace	00037-4401	Chelating Agent
WALLACE0430	Tab, Yellow, Oval	Felbamate 400 mg	Felbatol by Wallace		Anticonvulsant
WALLACE0640	Tab, Mauve, Cap Shaped, Scored	Carbetapentane Tannate 60 mg, Chlorpheniramine Tannate 5 mg, Phenylephrine Tannate 10 mg	Tussi-12 by Wallace	00037-0640	Cold Remedy
WALLACE0640	Tab, Purple, Oblong, Scored	Carbetapentane Tannate 60 mg; Chlorpheniramine Tannate 5 mg; Phenylephrine Tannate 10 mg	by Allscripts	54569-4902	Cold Remedy
WALLACE153	Tab, Peach, Rectangular	Methyclothiazide 5 mg	Aquatensen by Wallace	00037-0153	Diuretic
WALLACE2001 <> SOMA37	Tab	Carisoprodol 350 mg	Soma by Quality Care	60346-0149	Muscle Relaxant
WALLACE2103 <> SOMAC	Tab, Yellow & Light Orange, Round, Wallace 2103 <> Soma C	Aspirin 325 mg, Carisoprodol 200 mg	Soma Compound by Wallace	00037-2103	Analgesic; Muscle Relaxant
WALLACE24 <> SOMACC	Tab	Aspirin 325 mg, Carisoprodol 200 mg, Codeine Phosphate 16 mg	Soma Compound by Pharmedix	53002-0124	Analgesic; C III
WALLACE2403 <> SOMACC	Tab, Wallace over 2403 <> Soma CC	Aspirin 325 mg, Carisoprodol 200 mg, Codeine Phosphate 16 mg	Soma Compound by Quality Care	60346-0894	Analgesic; C III
WALLACE2403 <> SOMACC	Tab, White & Yellow, Oval	Aspirin 325 mg, Carisoprodol 200 mg, Codeine Phosphate 16 mg	Soma Compound with Codeine by Wallace	00037-2403	Analgesic; C III
WALLACE272	Tab, White, Round	Cryptenamine 2 mg, Methyclothiazide 2.5 mg	Diutensen by Wallace		Antihypertensive
WALLACE274	Tab, Pink & White, Round	Methyclothiazide 2.5 mg, Reserpine 0.1 mg	Diutensen-R by Wallace	00037-0274	Diuretic; Antihypertensive
WALLACE3001	Tab, Pink, Round	Meprobamate 400 mg, Benactyzine HCl 1 mg	Deprol by Wallace		Sedative/Hypnotic; C IV
WALLACE301	Tab, White, Round, Scored	Atropine Sulfate 0.025 mg, Hyoscyamine Sulfate 0.1286 mg, Phenobarbital 16 mg, Scopolamine Hydrobromide 0.0074 mg	Barbidonna by Wallace	00037-0301	Gastrointestinal; C IV
WALLACE311	Tab, Light Brown, Round, Scored	Atropine Sulfate 0.025 mg, Hyoscyamine Sulfate 0.1286 mg, Phenobarbital 32 mg, Scopolamine Hydrobromide 0.0074 mg	Barbidonna No. 2 by Wallace	00037-0311	Gastrointestinal; C IV
WALLACE370120	Tab, Orange & White, Cap Shaped, Wallace 37-0120	Aspirin 325 mg, Meprobamate 200 mg	Micrainin by Wallace	00037-0120	Analgesic; C IV
WALLACE370120	Tab, Orange & White, Oblong, Wallace 37-0120	Meprobamate 200 mg, Aspirin 325 mg	Micrainin by Wallace		Sedative/Hypnotic; C IV
WALLACE371001	Tab, White, Round	Meprobamate 400 mg	Miltown by Wallace		Sedative/Hypnotic; C IV
WALLACE371101	Tab, White, Round	Meprobamate 200 mg	Miltown by Wallace		Sedative/Hypnotic; C IV
WALLACE371601 <> 600	Tab, Wallace over 37-1601	Meprobamate 600 mg	Miltown by Wallace	00037-1601	Sedative/Hypnotic; C IV
WALLACE374224	Tab, Rose, Round	Guaifenesin 200 mg	Organidin NR by Wallace		Expectorant
WALLACE374224	Tab, Rose, Round	Iodinated Glycerol 30 mg	Organidin by Wallace		Expectorant
WALLACE472	Tab, White, Round	Potassium Iodide 130 mg	Thyro-Block by Wallace	00037-0472	Antithyroid
WALLACE521	Tab, White, Rectangular, Scored	Dyphylline 200 mg	Lufyllin by Wallace	00037-0521	Antiasthmatic
WALLACE541	Tab, Light Yellow, Round, Scored	Dyphylline 200 mg, Guaifenesin 200 mg	Lufyllin-GG by Wallace	00037-0541	Antiasthmatic
WALLACE561	Tab, Pink, Round, Scored	Dyphylline 100 mg, Ephedrine HCl 16 mg, Guaifenesin 200 mg, Phenobarbital 16 mg	Lufyllin-EPG by Wallace	00037-0561	Antiasthmatic; C IV
WALLACE713	Tab	Chlorpheniramine Tannate 8 mg, Phenylephrine Tannate 25 mg, Pyrilamine Tannate 25 mg	Rynatan by Caremark	00339-5495	Cold Remedy
WALLACE713	Tab	Chlorpheniramine Tannate 8 mg, Phenylephrine Tannate 25 mg, Pyrilamine Tannate 25 mg	Rynatan by Nat Pharmpak Serv	55154-4105	Cold Remedy
WALLACE713	Tab	Chlorpheniramine Tannate 8 mg, Phenylephrine Tannate 25 mg, Pyrilamine Tannate 25 mg	Rynatan by Leiner	59606-0732	Cold Remedy
WALLACE713	Tab, Buff	Chlorpheniramine Tannate 8 mg, Phenylephrine Tannate 25 mg, Pyrilamine Tannate 25 mg	Rynatan by Amerisource	62584-0713	Cold Remedy
WALLACE713	Tab	Chlorpheniramine Tannate 8 mg, Phenylephrine Tannate 25 mg, Pyrilamine Tannate 25 mg	Rynatan by Wallace	00037-0713	Cold Remedy

ID FRONT <> BACK	DESCRIPTION FRONT <> BACK	INGREDIENT & STRENGTH	BRAND (OR EQUIV.) & FIRM	NDC#	CLASS; SCH.
WALLACE717	Tab, Mauve, Cap Shaped, Scored	Carbetapentane Tannate 60 mg, Chlorpheniramine Tannate 5 mg, Ephedrine Tannate 10 mg, Phenylephrine Tannate 10 mg	Rynatuss by Wallace	00037-0717	Cold Remedy
WALLACE731	Tab, White, Cap Shaped, Scored	Dyphylline 400 mg	Lufyllin-400 by Wallace	00037-0731	Antiasthmatic
WARRICK <> 1520	Tab, White, Round, Scored	Albuterol Sulfate 2 mg	by Allscripts	54569-3409	Antiasthmatic
WARRICK <> 1520	Tab, White, Round, Scored	Albuterol Sulfate 2 mg	by Southwood Pharms	58016-0473	Antiasthmatic
WARRICK <> 1620	Tab, White, Scored	Griseofulvin ULT 250 mg	by Lederle	59911-5811	Antifungal
WARRICK1520	Tab, White, Round	Albuterol Sulfate 2 mg	Proventil by Warrick		Antiasthmatic
WARRICK1530	Tab, White, Round	Albuterol Sulfate 4 mg	Proventil by Warrick		Antiasthmatic
WARRICK1620	Tab, White, Round	Griseofulvin Ultramicrosize 125 mg	Fulvicin P/G by Warrick		Antifungal
WARRICK1620	Tab, White, Round, Scored	Griseofulvin, Ultramicrosize 125 mg	Fulvicin P/G by Martec	52555-0583	Antifungal
WARRICK1621	Tab, White, Round, Scored	Griseofulvin, Ultramicrosize 250 mg	Fulvicin P/G by Martec	52555-0584	Antifungal
WARRICK1624	Tab, Off-White, Oval	Griseofulvin Ultramicrosize 330 mg	Fulvicin P/G by Warrick		Antifungal
WARRICK1624	Tab, Off-White, Oval, Scored	Griseofulvin, Ultramicrosize 330 mg	Fulvicin P/G by Martec	52555-0585	Antifungal
WARRICK16421	Tab, White, Round	Griseofulvin Ultramicrosize 250 mg	Fulvicin P/G by Warrick		Antifungal
WARRICK1648	Tab, White, Round	Griseofulvin 250 mg	Fulvicin by Warrick	59930-1648	Antifungal
WARRICK1649	Tab, White, Round	Griseofulvin 500 mg	Fulvicin by Warrick	59930-1649	Antifungal
WARRICK1653 <> 300	Tab, Blue, Round	Labetolol 300 mg	by Warrick		Antihypertensive
WARRICK1670	Tab, Tab Ex Release	Theophylline 300 mg	by Repack Co	55306-1670	Antiasthmatic
WATSON	Tab, Peach, Round	Desipramine HCl 50 mg	by Blue Ridge	59273-0010	Antidepressant
WATSON	Tab, Peach, Round	Desipramine HCl 25 mg	by Blue Ridge	59273-0009	Antidepressant
WATSON	Tab, Peach, Round	Desipramine HCl 100 mg	by Blue Ridge	59273-0012	Antidepressant
WATSON	Tab	Furosemide 40 mg	by United Res	00677-0659	Diuretic
WATSON <> 12530	Tab, Pink, Round, Watson <> 125/30	Ethinyl Estradiol 30 mcg; Levonorgestrel 0.25 mg	Trivora-28 by Watson	52544-0291	Oral Contraceptive
WATSON <> 12530	Tab, Pink, Round, Flat, 125/30	Levonorgestrel 0.03 mg, Ethinyl Estradiol 0.125 mg	Trivora 125 30 by Murfreesboro	51129-1632	Oral Contraceptive
WATSON <> 1530	Tab, White, Round, Watson <> 15/30	Levora 0,15 mg, 30 mcg	Nordette by Watson	52544-0279	Oral Contraceptive
WATSON <> 235	Tab, Yellow	Nor-QD 0.35 mg	by Watson	52544-0235	Hormone
WATSON <> 24005	Tab, Watson <> 240 Over 0.5	Lorazepam 0.51 mg	by Watson	52544-0240	Sedative/Hypnotic; C IV
WATSON <> 2411	Tab, Watson <> 241 Over 1	Lorazepam 1 mg	by Watson	52544-0241	Sedative/Hypnotic; C IV
WATSON <> 2422	Tab, Watson <> 242 Over 2	Lorazepam 2 mg	by Watson	52544-0242	Sedative/Hypnotic; C IV
WATSON <> 25650	Tab, Light Aqua, Cap-Shaped, Watson <> 25/650	Pentazocine 25 mg, Acetaminohen 650 mg	Talacen by Watson	52544-0396	Analgesic; C IV
WATSON <> 300	Tab, White, Round	Furosemide 20 mg	by Allscripts	54569-0572	Diuretic
WATSON <> 301	Tab, White, Round	Furosemide 40 mg	by Allscripts	54569-0574	Diuretic
WATSON <> 311	Tab	Furosemide 20 mg	by Golden State	60429-0078	Diuretic
WATSON <> 311	Tab	Furosemide 20 mg	Delone by Macnary	55982-0010	Diuretic
WATSON <> 311	Tab	Furosemide 20 mg	by DRX	55045-1553	Diuretic
WATSON <> 311	Tab	Furosemide 20 mg	by Watson	52544-0311	Diuretic
WATSON <> 311	Tab	Furosemide 20 mg	by Major	00904-1580	Diuretic
WATSON <> 33205	Tab, Watson <> 332 Over 0.5	Lorazepam 0.5 mg	by UDL	51079-0417	Sedative/Hypnotic; C IV
WATSON <> 33205	Tab, White, Round, Scored	Lorazepam 0.5 mg	by Murfreesboro Ph	51129-1410	Sedative/Hypnotic; C IV
WATSON <> 33310	Tab, Watson <> 333 1.0	Lorazepam 1 mg	by Quality Care	60346-0047	Sedative/Hypnotic; C IV
WATSON <> 33310	Tab, Watson <> 333 Over 1.0	Lorazepam 1 mg	by UDL	51079-0386	Sedative/Hypnotic; C IV
WATSON <> 33420	Tab, Watson <> 334 Over 2.0	Lorazepam 2 mg	by UDL	51079-0387	Sedative/Hypnotic; C IV
WATSON <> 349	Tab	Acetaminophen 500 mg, Hydrocodone Bitartrate 5 mg	by Quality Care	60346-0442	Analgesic; C III
WATSON <> 387	Tab	Acetaminophen 750.6 mg, Hydrocodone Bitartrate 7.5 mg	by Quality Care	60346-0106	Analgesic; C III
WATSON <> 3955005	Tab, Green, Oblong, Watson <> 395/50-0.5	Pentazocine 50 mg, Naloxone HCl 0.5 mg	by Watson	52544-0394	Analgesic; C IV
WATSON <> 3955005	Tab, Green, Oblong, Scored	Pentazocine HCl 50 mg, Naloxone HCl 0.5 mg	by Watson Labs	52544-0395	Analgesic; C IV
WATSON <> 418	Tab, Film Coated	Cyclobenzaprine HCl 10 mg	by DHHS Prog	11819-0069	Muscle Relaxant
WATSON <> 418	Tab, Film Coated	Cyclobenzaprine HCl 10 mg	by Major	00904-7809	Muscle Relaxant
WATSON <> 418	Tab, Film Coated	Cyclobenzaprine HCl 10 mg	by Prepackage Spec	58864-0128	Muscle Relaxant
WATSON <> 418	Tab, Film Coated	Cyclobenzaprine HCl 10 mg	by Quality Care	60346-0581	Muscle Relaxant
WATSON <> 418	Tab, Film Coated	Cyclobenzaprine HCl 10 mg	by Watson	52544-0418	Muscle Relaxant
WATSON <> 418	Tab, White, Round	Cyclobenzaprine HCl 10 mg	by Apotheca	12634-0528	Muscle Relaxant

ID FRONT <> BACK	DESCRIPTION FRONT <> BACK	INGREDIENT & STRENGTH	BRAND (OR EQUIV.) & FIRM	NDC#	CLASS; SCH.
WATSON <> 425	Cap	Aspirin 325 mg, Butalbital 50 mg, Caffeine 40 mg, Codeine Phosphate 30 mg	by Watson	52544-0425	Analgesic; C III
WATSON <> 425	Cap	Aspirin 325 mg, Butalbital 50 mg, Caffeine 40 mg, Codeine Phosphate 30 mg	by Rugby	00536-5754	Analgesic; C III
WATSON <> 425	Cap	Aspirin 325 mg, Butalbital 50 mg, Caffeine 40 mg, Codeine Phosphate 30 mg	by HL Moore	00839-6689	Analgesic; C III
WATSON <> 425	Cap	Aspirin 325 mg, Butalbital 50 mg, Caffeine 40 mg, Codeine Phosphate 30 mg	by Major	00904-5140	Analgesic; C III
WATSON <> 425	Cap, Blue & Yellow	Butalbital 50 mg, Aspirin 325 mg, Caffeine 50 mg, Codeine Phosphate 30 mg	by Caremark	00339-5120	Analgesic; C III
WATSON <> 425	Cap, Blue & Yellow	Butalbital 50 mg; Aspirin 325 mg; Caffeine 40 mg; Codeine Phosphate 30 mg	by Phy Total Care	54868-1037	Analgesic; C III
WATSON <> 5030	Tab, Blue, Round, Watson <> 50/30	Ethinyl Estradiol 30 mcg; Levonorgestrel 0.05 mg	Trivora-28 by Watson	52544-0291	Oral Contraceptive
WATSON <> 5030	Tab, Blue, Round, Flat	Levonorgestrel 0.03 mg, Ethinyl Estradiol 0.05 mg	Trivora 50 30 by Murfreesboro	51129-1631	Oral Contraceptive
WATSON <> 507	Tab	Ethinyl Estradiol 0.035 mg, Norethindrone 0.5 mg	Necon 0.5 35 21 by Watson	52544-0507	Oral Contraceptive
WATSON <> 507	Tab	Ethinyl Estradiol 0.035 mg, Norethindrone 0.5 mg	Necon 0.5 35 28 by Watson	52544-0550	Oral Contraceptive
WATSON <> 507	Tab	Ethinyl Estradiol 0.035 mg, Norethindrone 0.5 mg, Norethindrone 1 mg	Necon 10 11 21 by Watson	52544-0553	Oral Contraceptive
WATSON <> 507	Tab	Ethinyl Estradiol 0.035 mg, Norethindrone 0.5 mg, Norethindrone 1 mg	Necon 10 11 28 by Watson	52544-0554	Oral Contraceptive
WATSON <> 508	Tab	Ethinyl Estradiol 0.035 mg, Norethindrone 0.5 mg, Norethindrone 1 mg	Necon 10 11 21 by Watson	52544-0553	Oral Contraceptive
WATSON <> 508	Tab	Ethinyl Estradiol 0.035 mg, Norethindrone 0.5 mg, Norethindrone 1 mg	Necon 10 11 28 by Watson	52544-0554	Oral Contraceptive
WATSON <> 508	Tab	Ethinyl Estradiol 0.035 mg, Norethindrone 1 mg	Necon 1 35 21 by Watson	52544-0508	Oral Contraceptive
WATSON <> 508	Tab	Ethinyl Estradiol 0.035 mg, Norethindrone 1 mg	Necon 1 35 28 by Watson	52544-0552	Oral Contraceptive
WATSON <> 510	Tab	Mestranol 0.05 mg, Norethindrone 1 mg	Necon 1 50 21 by Watson	52544-0510	Oral Contraceptive
WATSON <> 510	Tab	Mestranol 0.05 mg, Norethindrone 1 mg	Necon 1 50 28 by Watson	52544-0556	Oral Contraceptive
WATSON <> 510	Tab, Blue, Round	Norethindrone 1 mg, Mestranol 0.05 mg	Necon by DRX Pharm Consults	55045-2722	Oral Contraceptive
WATSON <> 639500	Tab	Chlorzoxazone 500 mg	by Martec	52555-0263	Muscle Relaxant
WATSON <> 667400	Tab, Watson <> 667 over 400	Etodolac 400 mg	by Rugby	00536-3623	NSAID
WATSON <> 667400	Tab, Watson <> 667 over 400	Etodolac 400 mg	by Qualitest	00603-3570	NSAID
WATSON <> 667400	Tab, Watson <> 667 over 400	Etodolac 400 mg	by Watson	52544-0667	NSAID
WATSON <> 667400	Tab, Watson <> 667 over 400	Etodolac 400 mg	by Major	00904-5246	NSAID
WATSON <> 682025	Tab, White, Oval, Scored, Watson <> 682 0.25	Alprazolam 0.25 mg	by Allscripts	54569-3755	Antianxiety; C IV
WATSON <> 682025	Tab, Watson <> 682 over 0.25	Alprazolam 0.25 mg	by Watson	52544-0682	Antianxiety; C IV
WATSON <> 68305	Tab, Peach, Oval, Scored	Alprazolam 0.5 mg	by Allscripts	54569-3756	Antianxiety; C IV
WATSON <> 68305	Tab, Scored, Watson <> 683 over 0.5	Alprazolam 0.5 mg	by Watson	52544-0683	Antianxiety; C IV
WATSON <> 68410	Tab, Scored, Watson <> 684 over 1.0	Alprazolam 1 mg	by Watson	52544-0684	Antianxiety; C IV
WATSON <> 68410	Tab, Blue, Oval, Scored, Watson <> 684-1.0	Alprazolam 1 mg	by Allscripts	54569-4619	Antianxiety; C IV
WATSON <> 685550	Tab	Amiloride HCl 5 mg, Hydrochlorothiazide 50 mg	by Qualitest	00603-2188	Diuretic
WATSON <> 685550	Tab, Scored, Watson <> 685 over 5-50	Amiloride HCl 5 mg, Hydrochlorothiazide 50 mg	by Watson	52544-0685	Diuretic
WATSON <> 685550	Tab, Watson <> 685 over 5-50	Amiloride HCl 5 mg, Hydrochlorothiazide 50 mg	by Martec	52555-0338	Diuretic
WATSON <> 685550	Tab	Amiloride HCl 5 mg, Hydrochlorothiazide 50 mg	by Major	00904-2114	Diuretic
WATSON <> 68610	Tab, White, Oval, Scored	Baclofen 10 mg	by Murfreesboro Ph	51129-1409	Muscle Relaxant
WATSON <> 68610	Tab, White, Oval, Scored	Baclofen 10 mg	by DRX Pharm Consults	55045-2724	Muscle Relaxant
WATSON <> 68610	Tab, 686 Over 10	Baclofen 10 mg	by Supremus Med	62114-0120	Muscle Relaxant
WATSON <> 68610	Tab, Watson <> 686/10	Baclofen 10 mg	by Watson	52544-0686	Muscle Relaxant
WATSON <> 68610	Tab, Watson <> 686/10	Baclofen 10 mg	by Major	00904-5216	Muscle Relaxant
WATSON <> 68610	Tab, Watson <> 686/10	Baclofen 10 mg	by HL Moore	00839-7472	Muscle Relaxant
WATSON <> 68720	Tab, 687/20	Baclofen 20 mg	by Supremus Med	62114-0122	Muscle Relaxant
WATSON <> 68720	Tab, Watson <> 687/20	Baclofen 20 mg	by Watson	52544-0687	Muscle Relaxant
WATSON <> 68720	Tab, Watson <> 687/20	Baclofen 20 mg	by Major	00904-5222	Muscle Relaxant
WATSON <> 688125	Tab, White, Oblong, Scored	Captopril 12.5 mg	by Allscripts	54569-4593	Antihypertensive
WATSON <> 688125	Tab, Watson <> 688 12.5	Captopril 12.5 mg	by Qualitest	00603-2555	Antihypertensive
WATSON <> 688125	Tab, Watson <> 688 12.5	Captopril 12.5 mg	by Watson	52544-0688	Antihypertensive
WATSON <> 688125	Tab, Watson <> 688 12.5	Captopril 12.5 mg	by Major	00904-5045	Antihypertensive
WATSON <> 68925	Tab	Captopril 25 mg	by Qualitest	00603-2556	Antihypertensive
WATSON <> 68925	Tab	Captopril 25 mg	by Watson	52544-0689	Antihypertensive
WATSON <> 68925	Tab	Captopril 25 mg	by Major	00904-5046	Antihypertensive
WATSON <> 69050	Tab	Captopril 50 mg	by Qualitest	00603-2557	Antihypertensive
WATSON <> 69050	Tab, Football Shaped	Captopril 50 mg	by Watson	52544-0690	Antihypertensive

ID FRONT <> BACK	DESCRIPTION FRONT <> BACK	INGREDIENT & STRENGTH	BRAND (OR EQUIV.) & FIRM	NDC#	CLASS; SCH.
WATSON <> 69050	Tab	Captopril 50 mg	by Major	00904-5047	Antihypertensive
WATSON <> 691	Tab	Captopril 100 mg	by Major	00904-5048	Antihypertensive
WATSON <> 691100	Tab	Captopril 100 mg	by Watson	52544-0691	Antihypertensive
WATSON <> 693500	Tab, Green, Cap Shaped, Scored, Watson <> 693,500	Chlorzoxazone 500 mg	by Allscripts	54569-1970	Muscle Relaxant
WATSON <> 693500	Tab, Scored	Chlorzoxazone 500 mg	by Watson	52544-0693	Muscle Relaxant
WATSON <> 693500	Tab	Chlorzoxazone 500 mg	by Major	00904-0302	Muscle Relaxant
WATSON <> 698200	Tab, White, Oval, Scored	Hydroxychloroquine Sulfate 201 mg	by Allscripts	54569-4981	Antimalarial
WATSON <> 698200	Tab, Coated	Hydroxychloroquine Sulfate 201 mg	by Martec	52555-0642	Antimalarial
WATSON <> 698200	Tab, Coated	Hydroxychloroquine Sulfate 201 mg	by Watson	52544-0698	Antimalarial
WATSON <> 698200	Tab, Coated	Hydroxychloroquine Sulfate 201 mg	by Major	00904-5107	Antimalarial
WATSON <> 698200	Tab, Coated	Hydroxychloroquine Sulfate 201 mg	by HL Moore	00839-7963	Antimalarial
WATSON <> 698200	Tab, Coated	Hydroxychloroquine Sulfate 201 mg	by Qualitest	00603-3944	Antimalarial
WATSON <> 69910	Tab	Hydroxyzine HCl 10 mg	by Watson	52544-0699	Antihistamine
WATSON <> 69910	Tab	Hydroxyzine HCl 10 mg	Rezine by Martec	52555-0557	Antihistamine
WATSON <> 70025	Tab	Hydroxyzine HCl 25 mg	by Martec	52555-0558	Antihistamine
WATSON <> 70025	Tab	Hydroxyzine HCl 25 mg	by Watson	52544-0700	Antihistamine
WATSON <> 70450	Tab	Hydroxyzine HCl 50 mg	by Martec	52555-0559	Antihistamine
WATSON <> 70450	Tab	Hydroxyzine HCl 50 mg	by Watson	52544-0704	Antihistamine
WATSON <> 706210	Tab, Blue, Round, Watson <> 706 2-10	Perphenazine 2 mg, Amitriptyline HCl 10 mg	Etrafon by Watson	52544-0706	Antipsychotic; Antidepressant
WATSON <> 707225	Tab, Light Orange, Watson <> 707 2-25	Amitriptyline HCl 25 mg, Perphenazine 2 mg	by Watson	52544-0707	Antipsychotic
WATSON <> 707225	Tab	Amitriptyline HCl 25 mg, Perphenazine 2 mg	by Major	00904-1825	Antipsychotic
WATSON <> 708410	Tab, Beige, Round, Watson <> 708 4-10	Perphenazine 4 mg, Amitriptyline HCl 10 mg	Etrafon by Watson	52544-0708	Antipsychotic; Antidepressant
WATSON <> 709425	Tab, Yellow, Round, Watson <> 709 4-25	Perphenazine 4 mg, Amitriptyline HCl 25 mg	Etrafon by Watson	52544-0709	Antipsychotic; Antidepressant
WATSON <> 7105	Tab, Watson <> 710 Over 5	Pindolol 5 mg	by Qualitest	00603-5220	Antihypertensive
WATSON <> 7105	Tab, Watson <> 710 Over 5	Pindolol 5 mg	by Major	00904-7893	Antihypertensive
WATSON <> 7105	Tab, Watson <> 710 Over 5	Pindolol 5 mg	by HL Moore	00839-7761	Antihypertensive
WATSON <> 7105	Tab, Watson <> 710 over 5	Pindolol 5 mg	by Watson	52544-0710	Antihypertensive
WATSON <> 71110	Tab, Watson <> 711 Over 10	Pindolol 10 mg	by Watson	52544-0711	Antihypertensive
WATSON <> 71465650	Tab, Orange, Cap Shaped, Film Coated	Acetaminophen 650 mg, Propoxyphene HCl 6.5 mg	by Allscripts	54569-2588	Analgesic; C IV
WATSON <> 71465650	Tab, 714/65 650	Acetaminophen 650 mg, Propoxyphene HCl 65 mg	by Qualitest	00603-5463	Analgesic; C IV
WATSON <> 71465650	Tab, Watson <> 714 65 over 650	Acetaminophen 650 mg, Propoxyphene HCl 65 mg	by Watson	52544-0714	Analgesic; C IV
WATSON <> 715250	Tab	Quinine Sulfate 260 mg	by Watson	52544-0715	Antimalarial
WATSON <> 71754	Tab, Watson <> 717 5.4	Yohimbine HCl 5.4 mg	by Martec	52555-0538	Impotence Agent
WATSON <> 71754	Tab, Watson <> 717 Over 5.4	Yohimbine HCl 5.4 mg	by Watson	52544-0717	Impotence Agent
WATSON <> 72650	Tab, Watson <> 726 Over 50	Meperidine HCl 50 mg	by Watson	52544-0726	Analgesic; C II
WATSON <> 727100	Tab, Watson <> 727 Over 100	Meperidine HCl 100 mg	by Watson	52544-0727	Analgesic; C II
WATSON <> 728500	Tab, Blue, Oblong, Film Coated	Etodolac 500 mg	by Watson Labs	52544-0728	NSAID
WATSON <> 7441	Tab, White, Diamond Shaped, Scored, Watson <> 744/1	Estazolam 1 mg	Prosom by Watson	52544-0744	Sedative/Hypnotic; C IV
WATSON <> 7452	Tab, Pink, Diamond Shaped, Scored, Watson <> 745/2	Estazolam 2 mg	Prosom by Watson	52544-0745	Sedative/Hypnotic; C IV
WATSON <> 749	Tab, White, Round	Oxycodone 5 mg, Acetaminophen 325 mg	Percocet by Watson	52544-0749	Analgesic; C II
WATSON <> 7540	Tab, White, Round, Watson <> 75/40	Ethinyl Estradiol 40 mcg; Levonorgestrel 0.075 mg	Trivora-28 by Watson	52544-0291	Oral Contraceptive
WATSON <> 7540	Tab, White, Round, Flat	Levonorgestrel 0.04 mg, Ethinyl Estradiol 0.075 mg	Trivora 75 40 by Murfreesboro	51129-1633	Oral Contraceptive
WATSON <> 760	Tab, Beige, Round	Ranitidine 150 mg	Zantac By Watson	52544-0760	Gastrointestinal
WATSON <> 761	Tab, Beige, Cap-Shaped	Ranitidine 300 mg	Zantac By Watson	52544-0761	Gastrointestinal
WATSON <> 7711875	Tab, White, Round, Scored, Watson <> 771 over 18.75	Pemoline 18.75 mg	by Watson	52544-0771	Stimulant; C IV
WATSON <> 772375	Tab, Peach, Round, Scored, Watson <> 772 over 37.5	Pemoline 37.5 mg	by Watson	52544-0772	Stimulant; C IV
WATSON <> 7731875	Tab, Yellow, Round, Scored, Watson <> 773 over 18.75	Pemoline 75 mg	by Watson	52544-0773	Stimulant; C IV
WATSON <> 774	Tab, White, Round, Scored	Oxycodone HCl 5 mg	Percolone by Watson	52544-0774	Analgesic; C II
WATSON <> 775	Tab, Blue, Round	Diltiazem HCl 30 mg	Cardizem by Watson	52544-0775	Antihypertensive

ID FRONT ⬥ BACK	DESCRIPTION FRONT ⬥ BACK	INGREDIENT & STRENGTH	BRAND (OR EQUIV.) & FIRM	NDC#	CLASS; SCH.
WATSON ⬥ 776	Tab, White, Round	Diltiazem HCl 60 mg	Cardizem by Watson	52544-0776	Antihypertensive
WATSON ⬥ 777	Tab, Blue, Oblong	Diltiazem HCl 90 mg	Cardizem by Watson	52544-0777	Antihypertensive
WATSON ⬥ 778	Tab, White, Oblong	Diltiazem HCl 120 mg	Cardizem by Watson	52544-0778	Antihypertensive
WATSON ⬥ 779	Tab, Blue, Round	Oxybutynin Chloride 5 mg	Ditropan by Watson	52544-0779	Urinary
WATSON ⬥ 780	Tab, Light Blue, Oblong	Sucralfate 1 gm	Carafate by Watson	52544-0780	Gastrointestinal
WATSON ⬥ 782	Tab, White, Oblong	Diethylpropion HCl 75 mg	Tenuate Dosepan by Watson	52544-0782	Antianorexiant; C IV
WATSON ⬥ 783	Tab, White, Round	Diethylpropion HCl 25 mg	by Blue Ridge	59273-0007	Antianorexiant; C IV
WATSON ⬥ 783	Tab, White, Round	Diethylpropion HCl 25 mg	by Dupont Pharma	00056-0698	Antianorexiant; C IV
WATSON ⬥ 783	Tab, White, Round	Diethylpropion HCl 25 mg	Tenuate by Watson	52544-0783	Antianorexiant; C IV
WATSON ⬥ 784	Tab, White, Round	Carisoprodol 350 mg	Soma by Watson	52544-0784	Muscle Relaxant
WATSON ⬥ 785	Cap, Green & Yellow, Opaque	Chlordiazepoxide HCl 5 mg	by CCA	61543-0017	Antianxiety; C IV
WATSON ⬥ 785	Cap, Green & Yellow	Chlordiazepoxide HCl 5 mg	by Blue Ridge	59273-0045	Antianxiety; C IV
WATSON ⬥ 785	Cap, Green & Yellow	Chlordiazepoxide HCl 5 mg	Librium by Watson	52544-0785	Antianxiety; C IV
WATSON ⬥ 786	Cap, Black & Green	Chlordiazepoxide HCl 10 mg	Librium by Watson	52544-0786	Antianxiety; C IV
WATSON ⬥ 787	Cap, Green & White	Chlordiazepoxine HCl 25 mg	Librium by Watson	52544-0787	Antianxiety; C IV
WATSON ⬥ 793	Tab, White	Naproxen Sodium 550 mg	by Blue Ridge	59273-0041	NSAID
WATSON ⬥ 793	Tab, White	Naproxen Sodium 550 mg	by Par	49884-0544	NSAID
WATSON ⬥ 79410	Cap, Dark Blue	Dicyclomine HCl 10 mg	Bentyl by Watson	52544-0794	Gastrointestinal
WATSON ⬥ 79520	Tab, Blue, Round	Dicyclomine HCl 20 mg	Bentyl by Watson	52544-0795	Gastrointestinal
WATSON ⬥ 801	Cap, Green & White	Hydroxyzine Pamoate 50mg	by Blue Ridge	59273-0044	Antihistamine
WATSON ⬥ 80150	Cap, Green & White, Watson ⬥ 801/50	Hydroxyzine Pamoate 50 mg	Vistaril by Watson	52544-0801	Antihistamine
WATSON ⬥ 802125	Tab, Blue & White, Oval, Watson ⬥ 802/12.5	Meclizine HCl MLT 12.5 mg	Antivert/Bonnie by Watson	52544-0802	Antiemetic
WATSON ⬥ 80325	Tab, Yellow & White, Oval, Watson ⬥ 803/25	Meclizine HCl MLT 25 mg	Antivert/Bonnie by Watson	52544-0803	Antiemetic
WATSON ⬥ 804	Tab, White, Round	Meprobamate 200 mg	Equanil by Watson	52544-0804	Sedative/Hypnotic; C IV
WATSON ⬥ 805	Tab, White, Round	Meprobamate 400 mg	Equanil by Watson	52544-0805	Sedative/Hypnotic; C IV
WATSON ⬥ 808	Tab, Yellow, Round	Desipramine HCl 25 mg	Norpramin by Watson	52544-0808	Antidepressant
WATSON ⬥ 809	Tab, Green, Round	Desipramine HCl 50 mg	Norpramin by Watson	52544-0809	Antidepressant
WATSON ⬥ 820	Tab, Yellow, Round	Oxycodone 4.5 mg, Aspirin 325 mg	Percodan by Watson	52544-0820	Analgesic; C II
WATSON ⬥ 831	Tab, White, Round	Prednisone 10 mg	Merticorten by Watson		Steroid
WATSON ⬥ 835375	Tab, Blue, Triangular, Scored	Clorazepate Dipotassium 3.75 mg	by Watson Labs	52544-0835	Antianxiety; C IV
WATSON ⬥ 835375	Tab, Blue, T-Shaped, Scored, Watson ⬥ 835 3.75	Clorazepate Dipotassium 3.75 mg	Tranxene by DHHS Prog	11819-0135	Antianxiety; C IV
WATSON ⬥ 835375	Tab, Blue, Triangle, Scored, Watson ⬥ 8353.75	Clorazepate Dipotassium 3.75 mg	Clorazepate Dipotassium by DHHS Prog	11819-0156	Antianxiety; C IV
WATSON ⬥ 83675	Tab, Peach, Triangle, Scored, Watson ⬥ 8367.5	Clorazepate Dipotassium 7.5 mg	Clorazepate Dipotassium by DHHS Prog	11819-0160	Antianxiety; C IV
WATSON ⬥ 83675	Tab, Peach, Triangle, Scored, Watson ⬥ 836 7.5	Clorazepate Dipotassium 7.5 mg	Tranxene by DHHS Prog	11819-0137	Antianxiety; C IV
WATSON ⬥ 836750	Tab, Peach, Triangular, Scored	Clorazepate Dipotassium 7.5 mg	by Watson Labs	52544-0836	Antianxiety; C IV
WATSON ⬥ 83715	Tab, Purple, Triangular, Scored	Clorazepate Dipotassium 15 mg	by Watson Labs	52544-0837	Antianxiety; C IV
WATSON ⬥ 83715	Tab, Purple, Triangle, Scored	Clorazepate Dipotassium 15 mg	Tranxene by DHHS Prog	11819-0139	Antianxiety; C IV
WATSON ⬥ 83715	Tab, Purple, Triangle, Scored	Clorazepate Dipotassium 15 mg	Clorazepate Dipotassium by DHHS Prog	11819-0162	Antianxiety; C IV
WATSON ⬥ 913	Tab, White, Orange Specks, Cap Shaped, Scored	Acetaminophen 325 mg, Hydrocodone Bitartrate 5 mg	Norco 5/325 by Watson	52544-0913	Analgesic; C III
WATSON ⬥ LOXATANE25MG	Cap, Dark Green & Light Green, Opaque, Logo over Watson ⬥ Loxitane over 25 mg	Loxapine Succinate 25 mg	Loxitane by Watson	52544-0496	Antipsychotic
WATSON ⬥ LOXITANE10MG	Cap, Yellow & Dark Green, Opaque, Logo over Watson ⬥ Loxitane over 10 mg	Loxapine Succinate 10 mg	Loxitane by Watson	52544-0495	Antipsychotic
WATSON ⬥ LOXITANE50MG	Cap, Blue & Dark Green, Opaque, Logo over Watson ⬥ Loxitane over 50 mg	Loxapine Succinate 50 mg	Loxitane by Watson	52544-0497	Antipsychotic
WATSON ⬥ LOXITANE5MG	Cap, Dark Green, Opaque, Logo over Watson ⬥ Loxitane over 5 mg	Loxapine Succinate 5 mg	Loxitane by Watson	52544-0494	Antipsychotic
WATSON ⬥ P	Tab	Ethinyl Estradiol 0.035 mg, Norethindrone 0.5 mg	Necon 0.5 35 28 by Watson	52544-0550	Oral Contraceptive
WATSON ⬥ P	Tab	Ethinyl Estradiol 0.035 mg, Ethynodiol Diacetate 1 mg	Zovia 1 35E 28 by Watson	52544-0383	Oral Contraceptive
WATSON ⬥ P	Tab	Ethinyl Estradiol 0.035 mg, Norethindrone 0.5 mg, Norethindrone 1 mg	Necon 10 11 28 by Watson	52544-0554	Oral Contraceptive
WATSON ⬥ P	Tab	Ethinyl Estradiol 0.035 mg, Norethindrone 1 mg	Necon 1 35 28 by Watson	52544-0552	Oral Contraceptive
WATSON ⬥ P	Tab	Ethinyl Estradiol 0.05 mg, Ethynodiol Diacetate 1 mg	by Watson	52544-0384	Oral Contraceptive

ID FRONT <> BACK	DESCRIPTION FRONT <> BACK	INGREDIENT & STRENGTH	BRAND (OR EQUIV.) & FIRM	NDC#	CLASS; SCH.
WATSON <> P	Tab	Mestranol 0.05 mg, Norethindrone 1 mg	Necon 1 50 28 by Watson	52544-0556	Oral Contraceptive
WATSON <> P	Tab, White	Norethindrone 1 mg, Mestranol 0.05 mg	Necon by DRX Pharm Consults	55045-2722	Oral Contraceptive
WATSON 300	Tab	Furosemide 20 mg	by Quality Care	60346-0761	Diuretic
WATSON 301	Tab, White, Round, Scored	Furosemide 40 mg	by JB	51111-0479	Diuretic
WATSON 301	Tab	Furosemide 40 mg	by Kaiser	62224-1222	Diuretic
WATSON 302	Tab	Furosemide 80 mg	by Quality Care	60346-0061	Diuretic
WATSON 302	Tab	Furosemide 80 mg	by Amerisource	62584-0711	Diuretic
WATSON 302	Tab	Furosemide 80 mg	by Physicians Total Care	54868-2180	Diuretic
WATSON 349	Tab	Acetaminophen 500 mg, Hydrocodone Bitartrate 5 mg	by Amerisource	62584-0738	Analgesic; C III
WATSON 363 <> 375	Tab, Watson 363 <> 3.75	Clorazepate Dipotassium 3.75 mg	by Quality Care	60346-0409	Antianxiety; C IV
WATSON 385	Tab, Watson over 385	Acetaminophen 500 mg, Hydrocodone Bitartrate 7.5 mg	by Quality Care	60346-0012	Analgesic; C III
WATSON 385	Tab	Acetaminophen 500 mg, Hydrocodone Bitartrate 7.5 mg	by Heartland	61392-0729	Analgesic; C III
WATSON 385	Tab	Acetaminophen 500 mg, Hydrocodone Bitartrate 7.5 mg	by Direct Dispensing	57866-3915	Analgesic; C III
WATSON 385	Tab	Acetaminophen 500 mg, Hydrocodone Bitartrate 7.5 mg	by HL Moore	00839-7781	Analgesic; C III
WATSON 387	Tab	Acetaminophen 750 mg, Hydrocodone Bitartrate 7.5 mg	by Zenith Goldline	00182-0681	Analgesic; C III
WATSON 387	Tab	Acetaminophen 750 mg, Hydrocodone Bitartrate 7.5 mg	by Schein	00364-2505	Analgesic; C III
WATSON 387	Tab	Acetaminophen 750 mg, Hydrocodone Bitartrate 7.5 mg	by HL Moore	00839-7728	Analgesic; C III
WATSON 460	Tab, White, Round, Scored	Glipizide 5 mg	by Kaiser	00179-1300	Antidiabetic
WATSON 487	Tab, Gray, Round, Scored	Estradiol 1 mg	by Heartland	61392-0024	Hormone
WATSON 487	Tab	Estradiol 1 mg	by Haines	59564-0121	Hormone
WATSON 502	Tab	Acetaminophen 650 mg, Hydrocodone Bitartrate 7.5 mg	by Zenith Goldline	00182-0692	Analgesic; C III
WATSON 503	Tab, Light Green	Acetaminophen 650 mg, Hydrocodone Bitartrate 10 mg	by Allscripts	54569-4272	Analgesic; C III
WATSON 503	Tab, Green, Oblong	Acetaminophen 650 mg, Hydrocodone Bitartrate 10 mg	by Amerisource	62584-0068	Analgesic; C III
WATSON 503	Tab, Green, Oblong, Scored	Acetaminophen 650 mg, Hydrocodone Bitartrate 11 mg	by Amerisource	62584-0072	Analgesic; C III
WATSON 540	Tab	Acetaminophen 500 mg, Hydrocodone Bitartrate 10 mg	by St Marys Med	60760-0540	Analgesic; C III
WATSON137	Cap, Aqua Blue/Light Blue	Selegiline HCl 5 mg	Eldepryl by Watson	52544-0137	Antiparkinson
WATSON213	Tab, Blue, Round	Estropipate 3 mg	Ogen by Watson		Hormone
WATSON24005	Tab, White, Round, Watson 240/0.5	Lorazepam 0.5 mg	Ativan by Watson		Sedative/Hypnotic; C IV
WATSON2411	Tab, White, Round, Watson 241/1	Lorazepam 1 mg	Ativan by Watson		Sedative/Hypnotic; C IV
WATSON2422	Tab, White, Round, Watson 242/2	Lorazepam 2 mg	Ativan by Watson		Sedative/Hypnotic; C IV
WATSON300	Tab	Furosemide 20 mg	by Golden State	60429-0078	Diuretic
WATSON300	Tab	Furosemide 20 mg	by Kaiser	62224-1220	Diuretic
WATSON300	Tab	Furosemide 20 mg	by Amerisource	62584-0709	Diuretic
WATSON300	Tab	Furosemide 20 mg	by Kaiser	00179-0380	Diuretic
WATSON300	Tab, Watson/300	Furosemide 20 mg	by Watson	52544-0300	Diuretic
WATSON300	Tab	Furosemide 20 mg	by Major	00904-1480	Diuretic
WATSON301	Tab	Furosemide 40 mg	by Watson	52544-0301	Diuretic
WATSON301	Tab	Furosemide 40 mg	by Major	00904-1481	Diuretic
WATSON301	Tab	Furosemide 40 mg	by Golden State	60429-0079	Diuretic
WATSON301	Tab	Furosemide 40 mg	by Macnary	55982-0011	Diuretic
WATSON301	Tab	Furosemide 40 mg	by Quality Care	60346-0487	Diuretic
WATSON301	Tab	Furosemide 40 mg	by Amerisource	62584-0710	Diuretic
WATSON301	Tab, Watson/301	Furosemide 40 mg	by Kaiser	00179-0381	Diuretic
WATSON302	Tab	Furosemide 80 mg	by Murfreesboro	51129-1161	Diuretic
WATSON302	Tab	Furosemide 80 mg	by Kaiser	00179-0382	Diuretic
WATSON302	Tab	Furosemide 80 mg	by Zenith Goldline	00182-1736	Diuretic
WATSON302	Tab	Furosemide 80 mg	by United Res	00677-0976	Diuretic
WATSON302	Tab	Furosemide 80 mg	by Rugby	00536-3835	Diuretic
WATSON302	Tab	Furosemide 80 mg	by Watson	52544-0302	Diuretic
WATSON302	Tab	Furosemide 80 mg	by HL Moore	00839-6777	Diuretic
WATSON302	Tab	Furosemide 80 mg	by Major	00904-1482	Diuretic
WATSON303	Cap	Indomethacin 25 mg	by Warner Chilcott	00047-0887	NSAID

ID FRONT <> BACK	DESCRIPTION FRONT <> BACK	INGREDIENT & STRENGTH	BRAND (OR EQUIV.) & FIRM	NDC#	CLASS; SCH.
WATSON304	Cap	Indomethacin 50 mg	by Warner Chilcott	00047-0888	NSAID
WATSON305	Tab, Watson Over 305	Propranolol HCl 10 mg	by UDL	51079-0277	Antihypertensive
WATSON305	Tab	Propranolol HCl 10 mg	by Watson	52544-0305	Antihypertensive
WATSON305	Tab, Watson 305	Propranolol HCl 10 mg	by Amerisource	62584-0842	Antihypertensive
WATSON305	Tab, Watson 305	Propranolol HCl 10 mg	by Quality Care	60346-0570	Antihypertensive
WATSON306	Tab, Watson Over 306	Propranolol HCl 20 mg	by UDL	51079-0278	Antihypertensive
WATSON306	Tab	Propranolol HCl 20 mg	by Watson	52544-0306	Antihypertensive
WATSON306	Tab	Propranolol HCl 20 mg	by Quality Care	60346-0598	Antihypertensive
WATSON306	Tab	Propranolol HCl 20 mg	by Amerisource	62584-0843	Antihypertensive
WATSON307	Tab	Propranolol HCl 40 mg	by Amerisource	62584-0844	Antihypertensive
WATSON307	Tab	Propranolol HCl 40 mg	by Apotheca	12634-0472	Antihypertensive
WATSON307	Tab, Watson Over 307	Propranolol HCl 40 mg	by UDL	51079-0279	Antihypertensive
WATSON308	Tab, Watson Over 308	Propranolol HCl 80 mg	by UDL	51079-0280	Antihypertensive
WATSON308	Tab	Propranolol HCl 80 mg	by Watson	52544-0308	Antihypertensive
WATSON308	Tab	Propranolol HCl 80 mg	by Amerisource	62584-0845	Antihypertensive
WATSON308	Tab	Propranolol HCl 80 mg	by Nat Pharmpak Serv	55154-5538	Antihypertensive
WATSON308	Tab	Propranolol HCl 80 mg	by Major	00904-0418	Antihypertensive
WATSON309	Cap, Green	Doxycycline Monohydrate 50 mg	Monodox by Watson	52544-0309	Antibiotic
WATSON310	Cap, Green	Doxycycline Monohydrate 100 mg	Monodox by Watson	52544-0310	Antibiotic
WATSON312	Tab	Metoclopramide 10 mg	by Watson	52544-0312	Gastrointestinal
WATSON312	Tab, Watson/312	Metoclopramide 10 mg	by Nat Pharmpak Serv	55154-5804	Gastrointestinal
WATSON312	Tab, Watson/312	Metoclopramide HCl	by Zenith Goldline	00182-1789	Gastrointestinal
WATSON332	Tab	Lorazepam 0.5 mg	by Zenith Goldline	00182-1806	Sedative/Hypnotic; C IV
WATSON332	Tab	Lorazepam 0.5 mg	by Watson	52544-0332	Sedative/Hypnotic; C IV
WATSON332	Tab	Lorazepam 0.5 mg	by Major	00904-1500	Sedative/Hypnotic; C IV
WATSON332	Tab	Lorazepam 0.51 mg	by Qualitest	00603-4243	Sedative/Hypnotic; C IV
WATSON33205	Tab, White, Round, Watson 332/0.5	Lorazepam 0.5 mg	Ativan by Watson		Sedative/Hypnotic; C IV
WATSON333	Tab	Lorazepam 1 mg	by Watson	52544-0333	Sedative/Hypnotic; C IV
WATSON333	Tab	Lorazepam 1 mg	by Med Pro	53978-5008	Sedative/Hypnotic; C IV
WATSON333	Tab	Lorazepam 1 mg	by PDRX	55289-0487	Sedative/Hypnotic; C IV
WATSON333	Tab	Lorazepam 1 mg	by Amerisource	62584-0770	Sedative/Hypnotic; C IV
WATSON333	Tab	Lorazepam 1 mg	by Major	00904-1501	Sedative/Hypnotic; C IV
WATSON333	Tab	Lorazepam 1 mg	by United Res	00677-1057	Sedative/Hypnotic; C IV
WATSON333	Tab	Lorazepam 1 mg	by Qualitest	00603-4244	Sedative/Hypnotic; C IV
WATSON33310	Tab, White, Watson 333 1.0	Lorazepam 1 mg	by Nat Pharmpak Serv	55154-0550	Sedative/Hypnotic; C IV
WATSON33310	Tab, White, Round, Watson 333/1.0	Lorazepam 1 mg	Ativan by Watson		Sedative/Hypnotic; C IV
WATSON334	Tab	Lorazepam 2 mg	by Zenith Goldline	00182-1808	Sedative/Hypnotic; C IV
WATSON334	Tab	Lorazepam 2 mg	by Watson	52544-0334	Sedative/Hypnotic; C IV
WATSON334	Tab	Lorazepam 2 mg	by Amerisource	62584-0771	Sedative/Hypnotic; C IV
WATSON334	Tab, White, Round, Uncoated	Lorazepam 2 mg	by Nat Pharmpak Serv	55154-0914	Sedative/Hypnotic; C IV
WATSON334	Tab	Lorazepam 2 mg	by PDRX	55289-0594	Sedative/Hypnotic; C IV
WATSON334	Tab, White, Round, Scored	Lorazepam 2 mg	by Compumed	00403-0012	Sedative/Hypnotic; C IV
WATSON334	Tab	Lorazepam 2 mg	by Major	00904-1502	Sedative/Hypnotic; C IV
WATSON334	Tab, Watson Over 334, Tab Coated	Verapamil HCl 80 mg	by UDL	51079-0682	Antihypertensive
WATSON334 <> 20	Tab, Watson 334 <> 2.0	Lorazepam 2 mg	by Quality Care	60346-0800	Sedative/Hypnotic; C IV
WATSON33420	Tab, White, Round, Watson 334/2.0	Lorazepam 2 mg	Ativan by Watson		Sedative/Hypnotic; C IV
WATSON335	Tab, White, Oval	Acyclovir 400 mg	Zovirax by Watson	52544-0335	Antiviral
WATSON336	Tab, White, Oval	Acyclovir 800 mg	Zovirax by Watson	52544-0336	Antiviral
WATSON338	Tab, White, Round	Diclofenac Sodium DR 50 mg	Voltaren by Watson	52544-0338	NSAID
WATSON339	Tab, White, Round	Diclofenac Sodium DR 75 mg	Voltaren by Watson	52544-0339	NSAID
WATSON343	Tab, White, Round, Scored	Verapamil HCl 80 mg	by Allscripts	54569-0639	Antihypertensive
WATSON343	Tab, White, Scored	Verapamil HCl 80 mg	by Kaiser Fdn Hlth	62224-8558	Antihypertensive

ID FRONT <> BACK	DESCRIPTION FRONT <> BACK	INGREDIENT & STRENGTH	BRAND (OR EQUIV.) & FIRM	NDC#	CLASS; SCH.
WATSON343	Tab, Tab Coated	Verapamil HCl 80 mg	by Zenith Goldline	00182-1300	Antihypertensive
WATSON343	Tab, Tab Coated	Verapamil HCl 80 mg	by Watson	52544-0343	Antihypertensive
WATSON343	Tab, Film Coated	Verapamil HCl 80 mg	by Quality Care	60346-0813	Antihypertensive
WATSON343	Tab, White, Oval, Scored	Verapamil HCl 80 mg	by Thrift Drug	59198-0251	Antihypertensive
WATSON343	Tab, Tab Coated, Debossed	Verapamil HCl 80 mg	by United Res	00677-1130	Antihypertensive
WATSON343	Tab, Tab Coated	Verapamil HCl 80 mg	by Major	00904-2920	Antihypertensive
WATSON344	Tab, Film Coated	Verapamil HCl 80 mg	by Med Pro	53978-7001	Antihypertensive
WATSON344	Tab, Light Peach, Film Coated	Verapamil HCl 80 mg	by Quality Care	60346-0813	Antihypertensive
WATSON344	Tab, Peach, Scored	Verapamil HCl 80 mg	by Caremark	00339-6174	Antihypertensive
WATSON345	Tab, Tab Coated	Verapamil HCl 120 mg	by Watson	52544-0345	Antihypertensive
WATSON345	Tab, Tab Coated, Debossed	Verapamil HCl 120 mg	by Major	00904-2924	Antihypertensive
WATSON345	Tab, White, Round, Scored, Coated	Verapamil HCl 120 mg	by Allscripts	54569-0646	Antihypertensive
WATSON345	Tab, Tab Coated	Verapamil HCl 120 mg	by Zenith Goldline	00182-1301	Antihypertensive
WATSON346	Tab, Watson Over 346, Film Coated	Verapamil HCl 120 mg	by UDL	51079-0683	Antihypertensive
WATSON347	Cap, Teal & White, Opaque	Hydrochlorothiazide 12.5 mg	Microzide by Watson	52544-0347	Diuretic
WATSON348	Tab	Hydrochlorothiazide 50 mg, Triamterene 75 mg	by Baker Cummins	63171-1872	Diuretic
WATSON348	Tab, Watson Over 348	Hydrochlorothiazide 50 mg, Triamterene 75 mg	by UDL	51079-0433	Diuretic
WATSON348	Tab	Hydrochlorothiazide 50 mg, Triamterene 75 mg	by Warner Chilcott	00047-0833	Diuretic
WATSON348	Tab, Yellow, Round, Scored	Hydrochlorothiazide 50 mg, Triamterene 75 mg	Maxzide by Martec	52555-0974	Diuretic
WATSON348	Tab	Hydrochlorothiazide 50 mg, Triamterene 75 mg	by Watson	52544-0348	Diuretic
WATSON348	Tab	Hydrochlorothiazide 50 mg, Triamterene 75 mg	by Par	49884-0017	Diuretic
WATSON348	Tab, Yellow, Round, Scored	Hydrochlorothiazide 50 mg, Triamterene 75 mg	Digoxin HCTZ by Murfreesboro	51129-1420	Diuretic
WATSON348	Tab	Hydrochlorothiazide 50 mg, Triamterene 75 mg	by Quality Care	60346-0704	Diuretic
WATSON348	Tab	Hydrochlorothiazide 50 mg, Triamterene 75 mg	by HL Moore	00839-7422	Diuretic
WATSON348	Tab	Hydrochlorothiazide 50 mg, Triamterene 75 mg	by Apotheca	12634-0270	Diuretic
WATSON348	Tab, Yellow, Round, Scored	Triamterene 75 mg; Hydrochlorothiazide 50 mg	by Allscripts	54569-2545	Diuretic
WATSON349	Tab	Acetaminophen 500 mg, Hydrocodone Bitartrate 5 mg	by Nat Pharmpak Serv	55154-5549	Analgesic; C III
WATSON349	Tab, White, Cap Shaped, Scored, Watson over 349	Acetaminophen 500 mg, Hydrocodone Bitartrate 5 mg	Vicodin by UDL	51079-0420	Analgesic; C III
WATSON349	Tab	Acetaminophen 500 mg, Hydrocodone Bitartrate 5 mg	by Zenith Goldline	00172-5643	Analgesic; C III
WATSON349	Tab	Acetaminophen 500 mg, Hydrocodone Bitartrate 5 mg	by Warner Chilcott	00047-0448	Analgesic; C III
WATSON349	Tab	Acetaminophen 500 mg, Hydrocodone Bitartrate 5 mg	by Geneva	00781-1606	Analgesic; C III
WATSON349	Tab	Acetaminophen 500 mg, Hydrocodone Bitartrate 5 mg	by United Res	00677-1184	Analgesic; C III
WATSON349	Tab	Acetaminophen 500 mg, Hydrocodone Bitartrate 5 mg	by PDRX	55289-0137	Analgesic; C III
WATSON349	Tab	Acetaminophen 500 mg, Hydrocodone Bitartrate 5 mg	by Allscripts	54569-0303	Analgesic; C III
WATSON349	Tab	Acetaminophen 500 mg, Hydrocodone Bitartrate 5 mg	by Watson	52544-0349	Analgesic; C III
WATSON349	Tab	Acetaminophen 500 mg, Hydrocodone Bitartrate 5 mg	by Pharmedix	53002-0119	Analgesic; C III
WATSON349	Tab, Debossed	Acetaminophen 500 mg, Hydrocodone Bitartrate 5 mg	by Major	00904-3440	Analgesic; C III
WATSON349	Tab	Acetaminophen 500 mg, Hydrocodone Bitartrate 5 mg	by HL Moore	00839-7176	Analgesic; C III
WATSON349	Tab	Acetaminophen 500 mg, Hydrocodone Bitartrate 5 mg	by Talbert Med	44514-0413	Analgesic; C III
WATSON349	Tab	Acetaminophen 500 mg, Hydrocodone Bitartrate 5 mg	by Apotheca	12634-0514	Analgesic; C III
WATSON349	Tab, White, Oblong, Scored	Hydrocodone 5 mg, Acetaminophen 500 mg	by Murfreesboro	51129-1439	Analgesic; C III
WATSON349	Tab, White, Oblong, Scored	Hydrocodone Bitartrate 5 mg, Acetaminophen 500 mg	by Murfreesboro	51129-1448	Analgesic; C III
WATSON352	Tab, Pink, Round	Propranolol 60 mg	Inderal by Watson		Antihypertensive
WATSON353	Tab, Lavender, Round	Propranolol 90 mg	Inderal by Watson		Antihypertensive
WATSON357	Tab, White, Round	Methyldopa 250 mg, Hydrochlorothiazide 15 mg	Aldoril 15 by Watson		Antihypertensive
WATSON358	Tab, White, Round	Methyldopa 250 mg, Hydrochlorothiazide 25 mg	Aldoril 25 by Watson		Antihypertensive
WATSON359	Tab, White, Round	Methyldopa 500 mg, Hydrochlorothiazide 30 mg	Aldoril by Watson		Antihypertensive
WATSON360	Tab, White, Round	Methyldopa 500 mg, Hydrochlorothiazide 50 mg	Aldoril by Watson		Antihypertensive
WATSON363	Tab	Clorazepate Dipotassium 3.75 mg	by Zenith Goldline	00182-0009	Antianxiety; C IV
WATSON363	Tab	Clorazepate Dipotassium 3.75 mg	by Watson	52544-0363	Antianxiety; C IV
WATSON363	Tab	Clorazepate Dipotassium 3.75 mg	by Major	00904-3970	Antianxiety; C IV
WATSON364	Tab	Clorazepate Dipotassium 7.5 mg	by Quality Care	60346-0866	Antianxiety; C IV

ID FRONT <> BACK	DESCRIPTION FRONT <> BACK	INGREDIENT & STRENGTH	BRAND (OR EQUIV.) & FIRM	NDC#	CLASS; SCH.
WATSON364	Tab	Clorazepate Dipotassium 7.5 mg	by Zenith Goldline	00182-0010	Antianxiety; C IV
WATSON364	Tab	Clorazepate Dipotassium 7.5 mg	by Watson	52544-0364	Antianxiety; C IV
WATSON364	Tab	Clorazepate Dipotassium 7.5 mg	by Major	00904-5160	Antianxiety; C IV
WATSON365	Tab	Clorazepate Dipotassium 15 mg	by Zenith Goldline	00182-0014	Antianxiety; C IV
WATSON365	Tab	Clorazepate Dipotassium 15 mg	by Major	00904-5159	Antianxiety; C IV
WATSON365 <> 15	Tab, Watson over 365	Clorazepate Dipotassium 15 mg	by Watson	52544-0365	Antianxiety; C IV
WATSON366	Tab	Fenoprofen Calcium 691.8 mg	by Pharmedix	53002-0367	NSAID
WATSON366	Tab, Coated	Fenoprofen Calcium 692 mg	by Physicians Total Care	54868-0775	NSAID
WATSON366	Tab	Fenoprofen Calcium 692 mg	by Watson	52544-0366	NSAID
WATSON367	Cap, White & Yellow	Fenoprofen Calcium 200 mg	Nalfon by Watson		NSAID
WATSON368	Cap, Yellow	Fenoprofen Calcium 300 mg	Nalfon by Watson		NSAID
WATSON369	Cap	Loxapine Succinate	by Geneva	00781-2710	Antipsychotic
WATSON369 <> 5MG	Cap, White	Losapine Succinate 5 mg	by Dixon Shane	17236-0698	Antipsychotic/Antimanic
WATSON369 <> 5MG	Cap, White, Opaque, Watson over 369 <> 5 mg	Loxapine 5 mg	Loxitane by UDL	51079-0900	Antipsychotic
WATSON369 <> 5MG	Cap, White, Opaque, Hard Gel	Loxapine 5 mg	by Nat Pharmpak Serv	55154-4605	Antipsychotic
WATSON369 <> 5MG	Cap, White, Opaque	Loxapine Succinate 5 mg	by Nat Pharmpak Serv	55154-4611	Antipsychotic
WATSON369 <> 5MG	Cap	Loxapine Succinate	by Watson	52544-0369	Antipsychotic
WATSON369 <> 5MG	Cap, Watson Over 369 <> 5 mg	Loxapine Succinate	by Zenith Goldline	00182-1305	Antipsychotic
WATSON369 <> 5MG	Cap	Loxapine Succinate	by UDL	51079-0677	Antipsychotic
WATSON369 <> 5MG	Cap	Loxapine Succinate	by HL Moore	00839-7495	Antipsychotic
WATSON370 <> 10MG	Cap, White & Yellow	Loxapine Succinate 10 mg	by Major	00904-2310	Antipsychotic
WATSON370 <> 10MG	Cap, White & Yellow, Opaque, Watson over 370 <> 10 mg	Loxapine 10 mg	by Dixon Shane	17236-0694	Antipsychotic
WATSON370 <> 10MG	Cap, White & Yellow, Opaque, Hard Gel	Loxapine 10 mg	Loxitane by UDL	51079-0901	Antipsychotic
WATSON370 <> 10MG	Cap	Loxapine Succinate	by Nat Pharmpak Serv	55154-4606	Antipsychotic
WATSON370 <> 10MG	Cap	Loxapine Succinate	by Watson	52544-0370	Antipsychotic
WATSON370 <> 10MG	Cap, Watson Over 370 <> 10 mg	Loxapine Succinate	by Zenith Goldline	00182-1306	Antipsychotic
WATSON370 <> 10MG	Cap	Loxapine Succinate	by UDL	51079-0678	Antipsychotic
WATSON370 <> 10MG	Cap	Loxapine Succinate	by Physicians Total Care	54868-2327	Antipsychotic
WATSON370 <> 10MG	Cap	Loxapine Succinate	by Qualitest	00603-4269	Antipsychotic
WATSON370 <> 10MG	Cap	Loxapine Succinate	by HL Moore	00839-7496	Antipsychotic
WATSON370 <> 10MG	Cap	Loxapine Succinate	by Geneva	00781-2711	Antipsychotic
WATSON371	Cap	Loxapine Succinate	by Major	00904-2311	Antipsychotic
WATSON371 <> 25	Cap	Loxapine Succinate	by Zenith Goldline	00182-1307	Antipsychotic
WATSON371 <> 25MG	Cap, Green & White	Loxapine Succinate 25 mg	by Major	00904-2312	Antipsychotic
WATSON371 <> 25MG	Cap, Green & White, Opaque, Watson over 371 <> 25 mg	Loxapine 25 mg	by Dixon Shane	17236-0695	Antipsychotic
WATSON371 <> 25MG	Cap, White & Green, Opaque, Hard Gel	Loxapine 25 mg	Loxitane by UDL	51079-0902	Antipsychotic
WATSON371 <> 25MG	Cap, Watson Over 371 <> 25 mg	Loxapine Succinate	by Nat Pharmpak Serv	55154-4609	Antipsychotic
WATSON371 <> 25MG	Cap	Loxapine Succinate	by UDL	51079-0679	Antipsychotic
WATSON371 <> 25MG	Cap	Loxapine Succinate	by Physicians Total Care	54868-2478	Antipsychotic
WATSON371 <> 25MG	Cap	Loxapine Succinate	by Geneva	00781-2712	Antipsychotic
WATSON371 <> 25MG	Cap	Loxapine Succinate	by HL Moore	00839-7497	Antipsychotic
WATSON372	Cap	Loxapine Succinate	by United Res	00677-1320	Antipsychotic
WATSON372 <> 50	Cap	Loxapine Succinate	by United Res	00677-1321	Antipsychotic
WATSON372 <> 50MG	Cap, Blue & White	Loxapine Succinate 50 mg	by Major	00904-2313	Antipsychotic
WATSON372 <> 50MG	Cap, Blue & White	Loxapine Succinate 50 mg	by Murfreesboro Ph	51129-1351	Antipsychotic
WATSON372 <> 50MG	Cap, Blue & White, Opaque, Watson over 372 <> 50 mg	Loxapine 50 mg	by Dixon Shane	17236-0696	Antipsychotic
WATSON372 <> 50MG	Cap, White & Blue, Opaque, Hard Gel	Loxapine 50 mg	Loxitane by UDL	51079-0903	Antipsychotic
WATSON372 <> 50MG	Cap	Loxapine Succinate	by Nat Pharmpak Serv	55154-4610	Antipsychotic
WATSON372 <> 50MG	Cap	Loxapine Succinate	by Watson	52544-0372	Antipsychotic
WATSON372 <> 50MG	Cap	Loxapine Succinate	by Zenith Goldline	00182-1308	Antipsychotic
WATSON372 <> 50MG	Cap, Watson Over 372 <> 50 mg	Loxapine Succinate	by UDL	51079-0680	Antipsychotic
WATSON372 <> 50MG	Cap	Loxapine Succinate	by Physicians Total Care	54868-2479	Antipsychotic

ID FRONT <> BACK	DESCRIPTION FRONT <> BACK	INGREDIENT & STRENGTH	BRAND (OR EQUIV.) & FIRM	NDC#	CLASS; SCH.
WATSON372 <> 50MG	Cap	Loxapine Succinate	by Geneva	00781-2713	Antipsychotic
WATSON372 <> 50MG	Cap	Loxapine Succinate	by HL Moore	00839-7498	Antipsychotic
WATSON373	Tab, Film Coated	Maprotiline HCl 25 mg	by Watson	52544-0373	Antidepressant
WATSON373	Tab, Film Coated	Maprotiline HCl 25 mg	by Zenith Goldline	00182-1882	Antidepressant
WATSON373	Tab, Film Coated	Maprotiline HCl 25 mg	by Medirex	57480-0493	Antidepressant
WATSON373	Tab, Film Coated	Maprotiline HCl 25 mg	by Geneva	00781-1631	Antidepressant
WATSON374	Tab, Tab Coated	Maprotiline HCl 50 mg	by Watson	52544-0374	Antidepressant
WATSON374	Tab, Tab Coated	Maprotiline HCl 50 mg	by Zenith Goldline	00182-1883	Antidepressant
WATSON374	Tab, Tab Coated	Maprotiline HCl 50 mg	by Medirex	57480-0494	Antidepressant
WATSON374	Tab, Tab Coated	Maprotiline HCl 50 mg	by Geneva	00781-1632	Antidepressant
WATSON375	Tab, White, Oval	Maprotiline 75 mg	Ludiomil by Watson	52544-0375	Antidepressant
WATSON375	Tab, White, Oval	Maprotiline HCl 75 mg	Ludiomil by Watson		Antidepressant
WATSON379	Tab	Amoxapine 25 mg	by Medirex	57480-0480	Antidepressant
WATSON379	Tab, White, Round	Amoxapine 25 mg	Asendin by Watson		Antidepressant
WATSON379	Tab, White, Round, Scored	Amoxapine 25 mg	by Dixon Shane	17236-0888	Antidepressant
WATSON380	Tab, Salmon	Amoxapine 50 mg	by Major	00904-3995	Antidepressant
WATSON380	Tab, Orange, Round, Scored	Amoxapine 50 mg	by Dixon Shane	17236-0889	Antidepressant
WATSON380	Tab	Amoxapine 50 mg	by Medirex	57480-0481	Antidepressant
WATSON380	Tab, Pink, Salmon	Amoxapine 50 mg	by Watson	52544-0380	Antidepressant
WATSON380	Tab, Salmon	Amoxapine 50 mg	by United Res	00677-1378	Antidepressant
WATSON381	Tab	Amoxapine 100 mg	by Zenith Goldline	00182-1045	Antidepressant
WATSON381	Tab	Amoxapine 100 mg	by United Res	00677-1379	Antidepressant
WATSON381	Tab, Blue, Round, Scored	Amoxapine 100 mg	by Dixon Shane	17236-0890	Antidepressant
WATSON382	Tab, Peach, Round	Amoxapine 150 mg	Asendin by Watson		Antidepressant
WATSON382	Tab, Peach, Round, Scored	Amoxapine 150 mg	by Dixon Shane	17236-0891	Antidepressant
WATSON383	Tab	Ethinyl Estradiol 0.035 mg, Ethynodiol Diacetate 1 mg	Zovia 1 35E 28 by Watson	52544-0383	Oral Contraceptive
WATSON383	Tab	Ethinyl Estradiol 35 mcg, Ethynodiol Diacetate 1 mg	Zovia 1 35E 21 by Watson	52544-0532	Oral Contraceptive
WATSON384	Tab	Ethinyl Estradiol 0.05 mg, Ethynodiol Diacetate 1 mg	by Watson	52544-0384	Oral Contraceptive
WATSON384	Tab	Ethinyl Estradiol 50 mcg, Ethynodiol Diacetate 1 mg	Zovia 1 50E 21 by Watson	52544-0533	Oral Contraceptive
WATSON385	Tab	Acetaminophen 500 mg, Hydrocodone Bitartrate 7.5 mg	by Watson	52544-0385	Analgesic; C III
WATSON385	Tab	Acetaminophen 500 mg, Hydrocodone Bitartrate 7.5 mg	by Zenith Goldline	00182-0691	Analgesic; C III
WATSON385	Tab	Acetaminophen 500 mg, Hydrocodone Bitartrate 7.5 mg	by Warner Chilcott	00047-0319	Analgesic; C III
WATSON385	Tab	Acetaminophen 500 mg, Hydrocodone Bitartrate 7.5 mg	by Qualitest	00603-3882	Analgesic; C III
WATSON385	Tab	Acetaminophen 500 mg, Hydrocodone Bitartrate 7.5 mg	by Martec	52555-0699	Analgesic; C III
WATSON385	Tab	Acetaminophen 500 mg, Hydrocodone Bitartrate 7.5 mg	by Allscripts	54569-3911	Analgesic; C III
WATSON385	Tab	Acetaminophen 500 mg, Hydrocodone Bitartrate 7.5 mg	by PDRX	55289-0268	Analgesic; C III
WATSON385	Tab	Acetaminophen 500 mg, Hydrocodone Bitartrate 7.5 mg	by Major	00904-7631	Analgesic; C III
WATSON385	Tab	Acetaminophen 750 mg, Hydrocodone Bitartrate 7.5 mg	by PDRX	55289-0360	Analgesic; C III
WATSON385	Tab, White, Capsule-Shaped, Bisected, Watson over 385	Hydrocodone Bitartrate 7.5 mg, Acetaminophen 500 mg	Lortab by Watson	51079-0867	Analgesic; C III
WATSON385	Tab, White, Oblong, Scored	Hydrocodone Bitartrate 7.5 mg, Acetaminophen 500 mg	by Southwood Pharms	58016-0195	Analgesic; C III
WATSON385	Tab, White, Oblong, Bisected	Hydrocodone Bitartrate 7.5 mg, Acetaminophen 500 mg	by Geneva Pharms	00781-1513	Analgesic; C III
WATSON387	Tab	Acetaminophen 750 mg, Hydrocodone Bitartrate 7.5 mg	by Watson	52544-0387	Analgesic; C III
WATSON387	Tab	Acetaminophen 750 mg, Hydrocodone Bitartrate 7.5 mg	by Warner Chilcott	00047-0486	Analgesic; C III
WATSON387	Tab	Acetaminophen 750 mg, Hydrocodone Bitartrate 7.5 mg	by United Res	00677-1504	Analgesic; C III
WATSON387	Tab	Acetaminophen 750 mg, Hydrocodone Bitartrate 7.5 mg	by Qualitest	00603-3883	Analgesic; C III
WATSON387	Tab	Acetaminophen 750 mg, Hydrocodone Bitartrate 7.5 mg	by Geneva	00781-1532	Analgesic; C III
WATSON387	Tab, White, Oblong, Scored, Watson over 387	Acetaminophen 750 mg, Hydrocodone Bitartrate 7.5 mg	Vicodin by UDL	51079-0748	Analgesic; C III
WATSON387	Tab	Acetaminophen 750 mg, Hydrocodone Bitartrate 7.5 mg	by Martec	52555-0701	Analgesic; C III
WATSON387	Tab	Acetaminophen 750 mg, Hydrocodone Bitartrate 7.5 mg	by Allscripts	54569-3909	Analgesic; C III
WATSON387	Tab	Acetaminophen 750 mg, Hydrocodone Bitartrate 7.5 mg	by Major	00904-7632	Analgesic; C III
WATSON387	Tab	Acetaminophen 750.6 mg, Hydrocodone Bitartrate 7.5 mg	by Rugby	00536-5508	Analgesic; C III
WATSON387	Tab, White, Oblong, Scored	Hydrocodone 7.5 mg, Acetaminophen 750 mg	Murfreesboro	51129-1440	Analgesic; C III

ID FRONT ⇔ BACK	DESCRIPTION FRONT ⇔ BACK	INGREDIENT & STRENGTH	BRAND (OR EQUIV.) & FIRM	NDC#	CLASS; SCH.
WATSON387	Tab, White, Oblong, Scored	Hydrocodone Bitartrate 7.5 mg, Acetaminophen 750 mg	by Southwood Pharms	58016-0758	Analgesic; C III
WATSON388	Tab	Acetaminophen 500 mg, Hydrocodone Bitartrate 2.5 mg	by Watson	52544-0388	Analgesic; C III
WATSON388	Tab	Acetaminophen 500 mg, Hydrocodone Bitartrate 2.5 mg	by Warner Chilcott	00047-0318	Analgesic; C III
WATSON403	Tab, Peach, Round	Verapamil 40 mg	Isoptin by Watson		Antihypertensive
WATSON404	Tab, Film Coated, Debossed	Verapamil HCl 40 mg	by Watson	52544-0404	Antihypertensive
WATSON404	Tab, Film Coated, Debossed	Verapamil HCl 40 mg	by Rugby	00536-5624	Antihypertensive
WATSON404	Tab, Film Coated	Verapamil HCl 40 mg	by Zenith Goldline	00182-1601	Antihypertensive
WATSON404	Tab, Film Coated, Debossed	Verapamil HCl 40 mg	by HL Moore	00839-7921	Antihypertensive
WATSON404	Tab, Film Coated, Debossed	Verapamil HCl 40 mg	by Major	00904-7799	Antihypertensive
WATSON414	Tab, Yellow, Round	Estropipate 0.75 mg	Ogen by Watson	52544-0414	Hormone
WATSON414	Tab	Estropipate 0.75 mg	by Zenith Goldline	00182-1976	Hormone
WATSON415	Tab, Peach, Round	Estropipate 1.5 mg	Ogen by Watson	52544-0415	Hormone
WATSON415	Tab, Peach, Round	Estropipate 1.5 mg	Ogen by Watson		Hormone
WATSON416	Tab, Blue, Round	Estropipate 3 mg	Ogen by Watson	52544-0416	Hormone
WATSON416	Tab, Blue, Round	Estropipate 3 mg	Ogen by Watson		Hormone
WATSON417	Tab, Green, Round	Estropipate 6 mg	Ogen by Watson		Hormone
WATSON418	Tab, Coated	Cyclobenzaprine HCl 10 mg	by Med Pro	53978-1035	Muscle Relaxant
WATSON424	Tab	Hydrochlorothiazide 25 mg, Triamterene 37.5 mg	by Watson	52544-0424	Diuretic
WATSON424	Tab	Hydrochlorothiazide 25 mg, Triamterene 37.5 mg	by Rugby	00536-5665	Diuretic
WATSON424	Tab	Hydrochlorothiazide 25 mg, Triamterene 37.5 mg	by Zenith Goldline	00182-1903	Diuretic
WATSON424	Tab	Hydrochlorothiazide 25 mg, Triamterene 37.5 mg	by Major	00904-7873	Diuretic
WATSON424	Tab, Green, Round, Scored	Triamterene 37.5 mg, Hydrochlorothiazide 25 mg	Digoxin HCTZ by Teva	00480-0670	Diuretic
WATSON425 ⇔ 425	Cap	Aspirin 325 mg, Butalbital 50 mg, Caffeine 40 mg, Codeine Phosphate 30 mg	by Zenith Goldline	00182-0036	Analgesic; C III
WATSON430	Tab, Blue, Round	Carbidopa 10 mg, Levodopa 100 mg	Sinemet by Watson		Antiparkinson
WATSON431	Tab, Tan, Round	Carbidopa 25 mg, Levodopa 100 mg	Sinemet by Watson		Antiparkinson
WATSON432	Tab, Blue, Round	Carbidopa 25 mg, Levodopa 250 mg	Sinemet by Watson		Antiparkinson
WATSON437	Cap	Acebutolol HCl	by Qualitest	00603-2046	Antihypertensive
WATSON437	Cap	Acebutolol HCl	by Zenith Goldline	00182-2629	Antihypertensive
WATSON437	Cap	Acebutolol HCl	by Major	00904-5138	Antihypertensive
WATSON437	Cap, Gray & Red	Acebutolol HCl 200 mg	Sectral by Watson	52544-0437	Antihypertensive
WATSON438	Cap	Acebutolol HCl	by Qualitest	00603-2047	Antihypertensive
WATSON438	Cap	Acebutolol HCl	by Zenith Goldline	00182-2630	Antihypertensive
WATSON438	Cap	Acebutolol HCl	by Major	00904-5139	Antihypertensive
WATSON438	Cap, Green & Maroon	Acebutolol HCl 400 mg	Sectral by Watson	52544-0438	Antihypertensive
WATSON444	Tab, Pink, Round	Guanfacine HCl 1 mg	Tenex by Watson	52544-0444	Antihypertensive
WATSON444	Tab	Guanfacine HCl 1 mg	by Warner Chilcott	00047-0312	Antihypertensive
WATSON444	Tab	Guanfacine HCl 1 mg	by Zenith Goldline	00182-2641	Antihypertensive
WATSON444	Tab	Guanfacine HCl 1 mg	by HL Moore	00839-8046	Antihypertensive
WATSON444	Tab	Guanfacine HCl 1 mg	by Geneva	00781-1366	Antihypertensive
WATSON444	Tab	Guanfacine HCl 1 mg	by Rugby	00536-5756	Antihypertensive
WATSON444	Tab	Guanfacine HCl 1 mg	by Caremark	00339-6089	Antihypertensive
WATSON444	Tab, Pink, Round	Guanfacine HCl 1 mg	by Qualitest	00603-3774	Antihypertensive
WATSON444	Tab	Guanfacine HCl 1 mg	by Med Pro	53978-3365	Antihypertensive
WATSON444	Tab	Guanfacine HCl 1 mg	by Major	00904-5133	Antihypertensive
WATSON451	Tab	Guanabenz Acetate	by Warner Chilcott	00047-0560	Antihypertensive
WATSON451	Tab, Orange, Round	Guanabenz Acetate 4 mg	Wytensin by Watson	52544-0451	Antihypertensive
WATSON452	Tab	Guanabenz Acetate	by Warner Chilcott	00047-0561	Antihypertensive
WATSON452	Tab, Grey, Round	Guanabenz Acetate 8 mg	Wytensin by Watson	52544-0452	Antihypertensive
WATSON453	Tab	Guanfacine HCl	by HL Moore	00839-8047	Antihypertensive
WATSON453	Tab	Guanfacine HCl	by Zenith Goldline	00182-2642	Antihypertensive
WATSON453	Tab	Guanfacine HCl	by Geneva	00781-1373	Antihypertensive
WATSON453	Tab	Guanfacine HCl	by Qualitest	00603-3775	Antihypertensive

ID FRONT <> BACK	DESCRIPTION FRONT <> BACK	INGREDIENT & STRENGTH	BRAND (OR EQUIV.) & FIRM	NDC#	CLASS; SCH.
WATSON453	Tab	Guanfacine HCl	by Rugby	00536-5757	Antihypertensive
WATSON453	Tab	Guanfacine HCl	by Major	00904-5134	Antihypertensive
WATSON453	Tab, Peach, Round	Guanfacine HCl 2 mg	Tenex by Watson	52544-0453	Antihypertensive
WATSON453	Tab	Guanfacine HCl	by Warner Chilcott	00047-0313	Antihypertensive
WATSON453	Tab	Guanfacine HCl	by Caremark	00339-6090	Antihypertensive
WATSON454	Tab, White, Oval	Gemfibrozil 600 mg	Lopid by Watson		Antihyperlipidemic
WATSON460	Tab	Glipizide 5 mg	by Watson	52544-0460	Antidiabetic
WATSON460	Tab	Glipizide 5 mg	by Warner Chilcott	00047-0463	Antidiabetic
WATSON460	Tab	Glipizide 5 mg	by HL Moore	00839-7939	Antidiabetic
WATSON460	Tab	Glipizide 5 mg	by United Res	00677-1544	Antidiabetic
WATSON460	Tab, White, Round, Scored	Glipizide 5 mg	by Compumed	00403-0920	Antidiabetic
WATSON460	Tab	Glipizide 5 mg	by Major	00904-7924	Antidiabetic
WATSON460	Tab	Glipizide 5 mg	by PDRX	55289-0806	Antidiabetic
WATSON461	Tab	Glipizide 10 mg	by PDRX	55289-0976	Antidiabetic
WATSON461	Tab	Glipizide 10 mg	by Watson	52544-0461	Antidiabetic
WATSON461	Tab, White, Round, Scored	Glipizide 10 mg	by Kaiser	00179-1315	Antidiabetic
WATSON461	Tab	Glipizide 10 mg	by Warner Chilcott	00047-0464	Antidiabetic
WATSON461	Tab	Glipizide 10 mg	by United Res	00677-1545	Antidiabetic
WATSON461	Tab	Glipizide 10 mg	by Schein	00364-2605	Antidiabetic
WATSON461	Tab	Glipizide 10 mg	by HL Moore	00839-7940	Antidiabetic
WATSON461	Tab	Glipizide 10 mg	by Qualitest	00603-3756	Antidiabetic
WATSON461	Tab	Glipizide 10 mg	by Major	00904-7925	Antidiabetic
WATSON462	Tab, Pink, Round, Scored	Metoprolol Tartrate 50 mg	by Allscripts	54569-3787	Antihypertensive
WATSON462	Tab	Metoprolol Tartrate 50 mg	by Major	00904-5110	Antihypertensive
WATSON462	Tab	Metoprolol Tartrate 50 mg	by Watson	52544-0462	Antihypertensive
WATSON463	Tab	Metoprolol Tartrate 100 mg	by Watson	52544-0463	Antihypertensive
WATSON463	Tap, Light Blue, Round, Scored	Metoprolol Tartrate 100 mg	by Allscripts	54569-3788	Antihypertensive
WATSON463	Tab	Metoprolol Tartrate 100 mg	by Major	00904-5111	Antihypertensive
WATSON485	Tab, White, Round	Butalbital 50 mg, Acetaminophen 325 mg, Caffeine 40 mg	Fioricet by Watson	52544-0485	Analgesic
WATSON487	Tab, Gray, Round, Scored	Estradiol 1 mg	by Allscripts	54569-4907	Hormone
WATSON487	Tab	Estradiol 1 mg	by Watson	52544-0487	Hormone
WATSON487	Tab	Estradiol 1 mg	by HL Moore	00839-8077	Hormone
WATSON487	Tab	Estradiol 1 mg	by Geneva	00781-1898	Hormone
WATSON487	Tab	Estradiol 1 mg	by Rugby	00536-3848	Hormone
WATSON487	Tab	Estradiol 1 mg	by Zenith Goldline	00182-2649	Hormone
WATSON487	Tab	Estradiol 1 mg	by Qualitest	00603-3557	Hormone
WATSON487	Tab	Estradiol 1 mg	by Martec	52555-0650	Hormone
WATSON487	Tab	Estradiol 1 mg	by Major	00904-5178	Hormone
WATSON488	Tab	Estradiol 2 mg	by Watson	52544-0488	Hormone
WATSON488	Tab	Estradiol 2 mg	by Qualitest	00603-3558	Hormone
WATSON488	Tab	Estradiol 2 mg	by Rugby	00536-3849	Hormone
WATSON488	Tab	Estradiol 2 mg	by HL Moore	00839-8078	Hormone
WATSON488	Tab	Estradiol 2 mg	by Geneva	00781-1899	Hormone
WATSON488	Tab	Estradiol 2 mg	by Zenith Goldline	00182-2650	Hormone
WATSON488	Tab	Estradiol 2 mg	by Martec	52555-0651	Hormone
WATSON488	Tab	Estradiol 2 mg	by Major	00904-5179	Hormone
WATSON491 <> 150MG	Cap, Light Brown, Cap Ex Release	Mexiletine HCl 150 mg	by Watson	52544-0491	Antiarrhythmic
WATSON492 <> 200MG	Cap	Mexiletine HCl 200 mg	by Watson	52544-0492	Antiarrhythmic
WATSON493 <> 250MG	Cap	Mexiletine HCl 250 mg	by Watson	52544-0493	Antiarrhythmic
WATSON498	Cap, Blue, Opaque	Doxycycline Hyclate 100 mg	Vibramycin by Watson	52544-0498	Antibiotic
WATSON499	Tab, Beige, Round, Film Coated	Doxycycline Hyclate 100 mg	Vibra Tabs by Watson	52544-0499	Antibiotic
WATSON500	Cap, Blue & White, Opaque	Doxycycline Hyclate 50 mg	Vibramycin by Watson	52544-0500	Antibiotic

ID FRONT <> BACK	DESCRIPTION FRONT <> BACK	INGREDIENT & STRENGTH	BRAND (OR EQUIV.) & FIRM	NDC#	CLASS; SCH.
WATSON502	Tab	Acetaminophen 650 mg, Hydrocodone Bitartrate 7.5 mg	by Watson	52544-0502	Analgesic; C III
WATSON502	Tab	Acetaminophen 650 mg, Hydrocodone Bitartrate 7.5 mg	by Warner Chilcott	00047-0355	Analgesic; C III
WATSON502	Tab	Acetaminophen 650 mg, Hydrocodone Bitartrate 7.5 mg	by Rugby	00536-5731	Analgesic; C III
WATSON502	Tab	Acetaminophen 650 mg, Hydrocodone Bitartrate 7.5 mg	by Geneva	00781-1523	Analgesic; C III
WATSON502	Tab	Acetaminophen 650 mg, Hydrocodone Bitartrate 7.5 mg	by Major	00904-5158	Analgesic; C III
WATSON502	Tab, Pink, Oblong, Scored	Hydrocodone Bitartrate 7.5 mg, Acetaminophen 650 mg	by Murfreesboro Ph	51129-1690	Analgesic; C III
WATSON502	Tab, Pink, Oblong, Scored	Hydrocodone Bitartrate 7.5 mg, Acetaminophen 650 mg	by Direct Dispensing	57866-5507	Analgesic; C III
WATSON502	Tab, Pink, Oblong, Scored	Hydrocodone Bitartrate 7.5 mg, Acetaminophen 650 mg	Hydrocodone by Compumed	00403-5196	Analgesic; C III
WATSON503	Tab	Acetaminophen 650 mg, Hydrocodone Bitartrate 10 mg	by Watson	52544-0503	Analgesic; C III
WATSON503	Tab	Acetaminophen 650 mg, Hydrocodone Bitartrate 10 mg	by Warner Chilcott	00047-0164	Analgesic; C III
WATSON503	Tab	Acetaminophen 650 mg, Hydrocodone Bitartrate 10 mg	by Zenith Goldline	00182-0034	Analgesic; C III
WATSON503	Tab	Acetaminophen 650 mg, Hydrocodone Bitartrate 10 mg	by Geneva	00781-1524	Analgesic; C III
WATSON503	Tab	Acetaminophen 650 mg, Hydrocodone Bitartrate 10 mg	by Physicians Total Care	54868-3729	Analgesic; C III
WATSON503	Tab	Acetaminophen 650 mg, Hydrocodone Bitartrate 10 mg	by Major	00904-5288	Analgesic; C III
WATSON503	Tab, Green, Oblong, Scored	Hydrocodone Bitartrate 10 mg, Acetaminophen 650 mg	Hydrocodone by Compumed	00403-5306	Analgesic; C III
WATSON503	Tab, Green, Oblong, Scored	Hydrocodone Bitartrate 7.5 mg, Acetaminophen 650 mg	by Southwood Pharms	58016-0239	Analgesic; C III
WATSON504	Tab	Indapamide 2.5 mg	by Watson	52544-0504	Diuretic
WATSON527	Tab	Estradiol 0.5 mg	by HL Moore	00839-8076	Hormone
WATSON527	Tab, Film Coated, Debossed	Indapamide 1.25 mg	by Physicians Total Care	54868-3885	Diuretic
WATSON527	Tab, Film Coated	Indapamide 1.25 mg	by Watson	52544-0527	Diuretic
WATSON528	Tab	Estradiol 0.5 mg	by Qualitest	00603-3556	Hormone
WATSON528	Tab	Estradiol 0.5 mg	by Zenith Goldline	00182-2648	Hormone
WATSON528	Tab	Estradiol 0.5 mg	by Geneva	00781-1897	Hormone
WATSON528	Tab	Estradiol 0.5 mg	by Martec	52555-0649	Hormone
WATSON528	Tab	Estradiol 0.5 mg	by Watson	52544-0528	Hormone
WATSON528	Tab	Estradiol 0.5 mg	by Major	00904-5177	Hormone
WATSON540	Tab	Acetaminophen 500 mg, Hydrocodone Bitartrate 10 mg	by Murfreesboro	51129-1104	Analgesic; C III
WATSON540	Tab	Acetaminophen 500 mg, Hydrocodone Bitartrate 10 mg	by Watson	52544-0540	Analgesic; C III
WATSON540	Tab, Blue, Scored	Hydrocodone Bitartrate 10 mg, Acetaminophen 500 mg	by Southwood Pharms	58016-0229	Analgesic; C III
WATSON544	Tab, Orange, Round	Desipramine HCl 75 mg	Norpramin by Watson		Antidepressant
WATSON545	Tab, Peach, Round, Watson/545	Desipramine HCl 25 mg	by DRX	55045-2308	Antidepressant
WATSON545	Tab, Peach, Watson over 545	Desipramine HCl 100 mg	by DRX	55045-2576	Antidepressant
WATSON545	Tab, Peach	Desipramine HCl 100 mg	by Blue Ridge	59273-0012	Antidepressant
WATSON545	Tab, Peach, Round	Desipramine HCl 100 mg	Norpramin by Watson	52544-0545	Antidepressant
WATSON575	Tab, White, Round, Scored	Trihexyphenidyl HCl 2 mg	by Watson Labs	52544-0575	Antiparkinson
WATSON576	Tab, White, Round, Scored	Trihexyphenidyl HCl 5 mg	by Watson Labs	52544-0576	Antiparkinson
WATSON576	Tab, White, Round, Scored	Trihexyphenidyl HCl 5 mg	by Teva	00480-0755	Antiparkinson
WATSON582	Tab, White, Round, Film Coated, Scored	Propafenone HCl 150 mg	by Watson	52544-0582	Antiarrhythmic
WATSON583	Tab, White, Round, Film Coated, Scored	Propafenone HCl 225 mg	by Watson	52544-0583	Antiarrhythmic
WATSON585	Tab, Brown, Round, Film Coated	Diclofenac Potassium 50 mg	by Watson Labs	52544-0585	NSAID
WATSON594	Cap, Blue	Clomipramine 25 mg	Anafranil by Watson		OCD
WATSON594 <> 25MG	Cap	Clomipramine HCl 25 mg	by Watson	52544-0594	OCD
WATSON595 <> 50MG	Cap, Yellow, Opaque	Clomipramine HCl 50 mg	by CTEX	62022-0088	OCD
WATSON595 <> 50MG	Cap, Gelatin	Clomipramine HCl 50 mg	by Watson	52544-0595	OCD
WATSON596 <> 75MG	Cap, Gelatin	Clomipramine HCl 75 mg	by Watson	52544-0596	OCD
WATSON605	Tab, Tab Coated, Debossed	Labetalol HCl 100 mg	by Watson	52544-0605	Antihypertensive
WATSON605100	Tab, Beige, Round, Watson 605/100	Labetolol HCl 100 mg	Normodyne by Watson		Antihypertensive
WATSON606	Tab, Tab Coated	Labetalol HCl 200 mg	by Watson	52544-0606	Antihypertensive
WATSON606200	Tab, White, Round, Watson 606/200	Labetolol HCl 200 mg	Normodyne by Watson		Antihypertensive
WATSON607	Tab, Tab Coated, Debossed	Labetalol HCl 300 mg	by Watson	52544-0607	Antihypertensive
WATSON607300	Tab, Blue, Round, Watson 607/300	Labetolol HCl 300 mg	Normodyne by Watson		Antihypertensive
WATSON613	Tab, Blue, Oval	Butabital 50 mg, Acetaminophen 500 mg, Caffeine 40 mg	Esgic-Plus by Watson		Analgesic

ID FRONT <> BACK	DESCRIPTION FRONT <> BACK	INGREDIENT & STRENGTH	BRAND (OR EQUIV.) & FIRM	NDC#	CLASS; SCH.
WATSON613	Tab, Blue, Oblong, Scored	Butalbital 50 mg; Acetaminophen 500 mg; Caffeine 40 mg	by Watson	52544-0613	Analgesic
WATSON613	Tab, Blue, Oblong, Scored	Butalbital 50 mg; Acetaminophen 500 mg; Caffeine 40 mg	by Allscripts	54569-4935	Analgesic
WATSON637	Tab, Red, Oblong, Film Coated, Scored	Pentoxifylline 400 mg	by Watson	52544-0637	Anticoagulent
WATSON637	Tab, Red, Oblong, Film Coated	Pentoxifylline 400 mg	Pentoxifyline ER by Andrx	62037-0951	Anticoagulent
WATSON637	Tab, Red, Oblong	Pentoxifylline ER 400 mg	Trental by Watson		Anticoagulent
WATSON667400	Tab, Yellow, Oblong, Watson 667/400	Etodolac 400 mg	Lodine by Watson		NSAID
WATSON667400	Tab, Yellow, Oblong, Watson/667/400	Etodolac 400 mg	by Watson		NSAID
WATSON682	Tab, White, Oval	Alprazolam 0.25 mg	Xanax by Watson		Antianxiety; C IV
WATSON683	Tab, Peach, Oval	Alprazolam 0.5 mg	Xanax by Watson		Antianxiety; C IV
WATSON684	Tab, Blue, Oval	Alprazolam 1 mg	Xanax by Watson		Antianxiety; C IV
WATSON685	Tab, Peach, Round	Amiloride HCl 5 mg, Hydrochlorothiazide 50 mg	Moduretic 5/50 by Watson		Diuretic
WATSON686	Tab, White, Oval	Baclofen 10 mg	Lioresal by Watson		Muscle Relaxant
WATSON687	Tab, White, Oval	Baclofen 20 mg	Lioresal by Watson		Muscle Relaxant
WATSON688	Tab, White, Oblong	Captopril 12.5 mg	Capoten by Watson		Antihypertensive
WATSON689	Tab, White, Round	Captopril 25 mg	Capoten by Watson		Antihypertensive
WATSON690	Tab, White, Oval	Captopril 50 mg	Capoten by Watson		Antihypertensive
WATSON692	Tab, White, Round	Carisoprodol 350 mg	Soma by Watson	52544-0692	Muscle Relaxant
WATSON693	Tab, Green, Oblong	Chlorzoxazone 500 mg	Parafon by Watson		Muscle Relaxant
WATSON69410	Tab, Dark Yellow, Round, Watson/694/10	Cyclobenzaprine 10 mg	by Watson		Muscle Relaxant
WATSON695 <> 10MG	Cap	Doxepin HCl 11.25 mg	by Watson	52544-0695	Antidepressant
WATSON696 <> 25MG	Cap, Blue, Opaque	Doxepin HCl 25 mg	by H J Harkins Co	52959-0351	Antidepressant
WATSON696 <> 25MG	Cap	Doxepin HCl 28.35 mg	by Watson	52544-0696	Antidepressant
WATSON696 <> 25MG	Cap	Doxepin HCl 28.35 mg	by Martec	52555-0295	Antidepressant
WATSON697 <> 50MG	Cap, Pink, Opaque	Doxepin HCl 50 mg	by H J Harkins Co	52959-0361	Antidepressant
WATSON697 <> 50MG	Cap	Doxepin HCl 56.7 mg	by Martec	52555-0296	Antidepressant
WATSON697 <> 50MG	Cap	Doxepin HCl 56.7 mg	by Watson	52544-0697	Antidepressant
WATSON698	Tab, White, Oval	Hydroxychloroquine Sulfate 200 mg	Plaquenil by Watson		Antimalarial
WATSON699	Tab, Orange, Round	Hydroxyzine HCl 10 mg	Atarax by Watson		Antihistamine
WATSON700	Tab, Green, Round	Hydroxyzine HCl 25 mg	Atarax by Watson		Antihistamine
WATSON704	Tab, Yellow, Round	Hydroxyzine HCl 50 mg	Atarax by Watson		Antihistamine
WATSON707	Tab, Orange, Round	Perphenazine 2 mg, Amitriptyline HCl 25 mg	Etrafon by Watson		Antipsychotic; Antidepressant
WATSON710	Tab, White, Round	Pindolol 5 mg	Visken by Watson		Antihypertensive
WATSON711	Tab, White, Round	Pindolol 10 mg	Visken by Watson		Antihypertensive
WATSON712 <> 10MG	Cap, Light Blue & White	Piroxicam 10 mg	by Allscripts	54569-3974	NSAID
WATSON712 <> 10MG	Cap, Filled with Off White to Yellow Powder	Piroxicam 10 mg	by Watson	52544-0712	NSAID
WATSON713 <> 20MG	Cap, Filled with Off White to Yellow Powder, Cap	Piroxicam 20 mg	by Watson	52544-0713	NSAID
WATSON714	Tab, Orange, Oblong	Propoxyphene HCl 65 mg, Acetaminophen 650 mg	Wygesic by Watson		Analgesic; C IV
WATSON715260	Tab, Off White, Round, Watson/715/260	Quinine Sulfate 260 mg	by Watson		Antimalarial
WATSON715260	Tab, White, Round, Watson 715/260	Quinine Sulfate 260 mg	by Watson		Antimalarial
WATSON716 <> 325MG	Cap, Filled with White Powder	Quinine Sulfate 325 mg	by Watson	52544-0716	Antimalarial
WATSON716 <> 325MG	Cap	Quinine Sulfate 325 mg	by Golden State	60429-0242	Antimalarial
WATSON716 <> 325MG	Cap, White, Opaque	Quinine Sulfate 325 mg	by RX PAK	65084-0137	Antimalarial
WATSON716325	Cap, White, Watson/716/325	Quinine Sulfate 325 mg	by Watson		Antimalarial
WATSON716325	Cap, White, Watson 716/325	Quinine Sulfate 325 mg	by Watson		Antimalarial
WATSON717	Tab, White, Round	Yohimbine HCl 5.4 mg	Yocon by Watson		Impotence Agent
WATSON72650	Tab, White, Round, Watson/726/50	Meperidine HCl 50 mg	by Watson		Analgesic; C II
WATSON72650	Tab, White, Round, Watson 726/50	Meperidine HCl 50 mg	Demerol by Watson		Analgesic; C II
WATSON727100	Tab, White, Round, Watson/727/100	Meperidine HCl 100 mg	by Watson		Analgesic; C II
WATSON72750	Tab, White, Round, Watson 727/50	Meperidine HCl 100 mg	Demerol by Watson		Analgesic; C II
WATSON735 <> 200MG	Cap, Light Gray & Brown	Etodolac 200 mg	Lodine by Watson	52544-0735	NSAID
WATSON736 <> 300MG	Cap, Light Gray & Orange	Etodolac 300 mg	Lodine by Watson	52544-0736	NSAID

ID FRONT <> BACK	DESCRIPTION FRONT <> BACK	INGREDIENT & STRENGTH	BRAND (OR EQUIV.) & FIRM	NDC#	CLASS; SCH.
WATSON736300MG	Cap, Gray & Red, Watson 736/300 mg	Etodolac 300 mg	by Watson		NSAID
WATSON737 <> 5500MG	Cap, Watson over 737 <> 5-500 mg	Acetaminophen 500 mg, Oxycodone HCl 5 mg	by Watson	52544-0737	Analgesic; C II
WATSON7375500MG	Cap, White & Red, Watson 737/5-500 mg	Oxycodone 5 mg, Acetaminophen 500 mg	Tylox by Watson		Analgesic; C II
WATSON746	Tab, Yellow, Round	Clonazepam 0.5 mg	by Watson		Anticonvulsant; C IV
WATSON746	Tab, Yellow, Round, Watson/746	Clonazepam 0.5 mg	by Watson		Anticonvulsant; C IV
WATSON746	Tab, Watson over 746	Clonazepam 0.5 mg	by Watson	52544-0746	Anticonvulsant; C IV
WATSON747	Tab, Aqua, Round	Clonazepam 1 mg	Anafranil by Watson		Anticonvulsant; C IV
WATSON747	Tab, Aqua, Round, Watson/747	Clonazepam 1 mg	by Watson		Anticonvulsant; C IV
WATSON747	Tab, Watson over 747	Clonazepam 1 mg	by Watson	52544-0747	Anticonvulsant; C IV
WATSON748	Tab, White, Round	Clonazepam 2 mg	Anafranil by Watson		Anticonvulsant; C IV
WATSON748	Tab, White, Round, Watson/748	Clonazepam 2 mg	by Watson		Anticonvulsant; C IV
WATSON748	Tab, Watson over 748	Clonazepam 2 mg	by Watson	52544-0748	Anticonvulsant; C IV
WATSON749	Tab, White, Round, Watson/749	Oxycodone 5 mg, Acetaminophen 325 mg	by Watson		Analgesic; C II
WATSON760	Tab, Beige, Round	Ranitidine 150 mg	Zantac by Watson		Gastrointestinal
WATSON761	Tab, Beige, Oblong	Ranitidine 300 mg	Zantac by Watson		Gastrointestinal
WATSON775	Tab, Blue, Round	Diltiazem HCl 30 mg	by Endo	60951-0653	Antihypertensive
WATSON775	Tab, Light Blue, Round, Coated	Diltiazem HCl 30 mg	by Allscripts	54569-3665	Antihypertensive
WATSON775	Tab, Blue, Round, Scored	Diltiazem HCl 30 mg	by Blue Ridge	59273-0002	Antihypertensive
WATSON776	Tab, White, Scored	Diltiazem HCl 60 mg	by Endo	63481-0652	Antihypertensive
WATSON776	Tab, White, Scored	Diltiazem HCl 60 mg	by Blue Ridge	59273-0003	Antihypertensive
WATSON776	Tab, White, Round, Scored	Diltiazem HCl 60 mg	by Allscripts	54569-3667	Antihypertensive
WATSON777	Tab, Blue, Oblong, Scored	Diltiazem HCl 120 mg	by Blue Ridge	59273-0005	Antihypertensive
WATSON777	Tab, Blue, Oblong, Scored	Diltiazem HCl 90 mg	by Endo		Antihypertensive
WATSON777	Tab, Blue, Oblong, Scored	Diltiazem HCl 90 mg	by Blue Ridge	59273-0004	Antihypertensive
WATSON777 <> 3103	Tab, Blue, Oblong	Diltiazem HCl 30 mg	by Elan Hold	60274-0886	Antihypertensive
WATSON777 <> 3103	Tab, Blue, Oblong, Scored	Diltiazem HCl 30 mg	by Blue Ridge	59273-0002	Antihypertensive
WATSON777 <> 3103	Tab, Blue, Oblong, Scored	Diltiazem HCl 120 mg	by Endo		Antihypertensive
WATSON777 <> 3103	Tab, Blue, Oblong, Scored	Diltiazem HCl 60 mg	by Endo		Antihypertensive
WATSON777 <> 3103	Tab, Blue, Oblong, Scored	Diltiazem HCl 60 mg	by Blue Ridge	59273-0003	Antihypertensive
WATSON778	Tab, White, Oblong, Scored	Diltiazem HCl 120 mg	by Blue Ridge	59273-0005	Antihypertensive
WATSON778	Tab, White, Oblong, Scored	Diltiazem HCl 120 mg	by Excellium	64125-0104	Antihypertensive
WATSON778 <> 3104	Tab, White, Oblong, Scored	Diltiazem HCl 30 mg	by Endo	60951-0652	Antihypertensive
WATSON778 <> 3104	Tab, White, Oblong, Scored	Diltiazem HCl 30 mg	by Blue Ridge	59273-0002	Antihypertensive
WATSON778 <> 3104	Tab, White, Oblong, Scored	Diltiazem HCl 120 mg	by Excellium	64125-0103	Antihypertensive
WATSON778 <> 3104	Tab, White, Oblong, Scored	Diltiazem HCl 60 mg	by Endo		Antihypertensive
WATSON778 <> 3104	Tab, White, Oblong, Scored	Diltiazem HCl 60 mg	by Blue Ridge	59273-0003	Antihypertensive
WATSON780	Tab, Blue, Oblong, Scored	Sucralfate 1 gm	by Blue Ridge	59273-0001	Gastrointestinal
WATSON780	Tab, Blue, Oblong, Scored	Sucralfate 1 gm	Carafate by SKB	00135-0181	Gastrointestinal
WATSON781	Tab, Off White, Round	Clomiphene Citrate 50 mg	Serophene by Watson	52544-0781	Infertility
WATSON781	Tab, White, Round	Clomiphene Citrate 50 mg	Serophene by Watson		Infertility
WATSON782	Tab, White, Oblong	Diethylpropion HCl 75 mg	by Blue Ridge	59273-0008	Antianorexiant; C IV
WATSON782	Tab, White, Cap Shaped	Diethylpropion HCl 75 mg	by Allscripts	54569-0396	Antianorexiant; C IV
WATSON782	Tab, White, Oblong	Diethylpropion HCl 75 mg	by Dupont Pharma	00590-0627	Antianorexiant; C IV
WATSON783	Tab, White, Round, Watson over 783	Diethylpropion 25 mg	by Allscripts	54569-2059	Antianorexiant; C IV
WATSON790	Tab, White, Oval, Quadrisect	Methylprednisolone 4 mg	Medrol by Watson	52544-0790	Steroid
WATSON790	Tab, White, Oval	Methylprednisolone 4 mg	Medrol by Watson		Steroid
WATSON791	Tab, White, Capsule Shaped	Naproxen 500 mg	Naprosyn by Watson	52544-0791	NSAID
WATSON791	Tab, White, Oblong	Naproxen 500 mg	Naprosyn by Watson		NSAID
WATSON792	Tab, White, Oval	Naproxen Sodium 275 mg	Anaprox by Watson	52544-0792	NSAID
WATSON792	Tab, White, Oval	Naproxen Sodium 275 mg	Anaprox by Watson		NSAID
WATSON793	Tab, Green, Oval	Naproxen Sodium 550 mg	Anaprox DS by Watson	52544-0793	NSAID
WATSON793	Tab, Green, Oval, Film Coated	Naproxen Sodium 550 mg	by Allscripts	54569-3762	NSAID

ID FRONT <> BACK	DESCRIPTION FRONT <> BACK	INGREDIENT & STRENGTH	BRAND (OR EQUIV.) & FIRM	NDC#	CLASS; SCH.
WATSON795	Tab, Blue, Round	Dicyclomine 20 mg	by Allscripts	54569-0419	Gastrointestinal
WATSON795	Tab, Blue, Round, Flat	Ketorolac Tromethamine 10 mg	by Watson	54569-4494	NSAID
WATSON796	Tab, Butterscotch, Round	Sulfaslsazine 500 mg	Azulfidine by Watson		Gastrointestinal
WATSON796	Tab, Mustard, Round, Scored	Sulfasalazine 500 mg	by Allscripts	54569-0313	Gastrointestinal
WATSON796	Tab, Mustard, Round Bisect	Sulfasalazine 500 mg	Azulfidine by Watson	52544-0796	Gastrointestinal
WATSON797	Tab, White, Round, Scored	Prednisone 50 mg	by Allscripts	54569-0333	Steroid
WATSON797	Tab, White, Round	Prednisone 50 mg	Merticorten by Watson		Steroid
WATSON80025	Cap, Green, Watson 800/25	Hydroxyzine Pamoate 25 mg	Vistaril by Watson	52544-0800	Antihistamine
WATSON806	Tab, White, Round, Scored	Methocarbamol 500 mg	Robaxin by Watson	52544-0806	Muscle Relaxant
WATSON806	Tab, White, Oblong	Methocarbamol 500 mg	Robaxin by Watson		Muscle Relaxant
WATSON807	Tab, White, Capsule Shaped, Scored	Methocarbamol 750 mg	Robaxin by Watson	52544-0807	Muscle Relaxant
WATSON807	Tab, White, Oblong	Methocarbamol 750 mg	Robaxin by Watson		Muscle Relaxant
WATSON808	Tab, Yellow, Watson over 808	Desipramine HCl 25 mg	by DRX	55045-2339	Antidepressant
WATSON808	Tab, Yellow	Desipramine HCl 25 mg	by Blue Ridge	59273-0009	Antidepressant
WATSON809	Tab, Green, Watson over 809	Desipramine HCl 50 mg	by DRX	55045-2565	Antidepressant
WATSON809	Tab, Green	Desipramine HCl 50 mg	by Blue Ridge	59273-0010	Antidepressant
WATSON819	Cap, Green, Oblong	Indomethacin 50 mg	Indocin by Watson		NSAID
WATSON821	Tab, White, Round	Naproxen 250 mg	Naprosyn by Watson	52544-0821	NSAID
WATSON821	Tab, White, Round	Naproxen 250 mg	Naprosyn by Watson		NSAID
WATSON822	Tab, Grey, Capsule Shaped	Naproxen 375 mg	Naprosyn by Watson	52544-0822	NSAID
WATSON822	Tab, Gray, Cap-Shaped	Naproxen 375 mg	by Allscripts	54569-3759	NSAID
WATSON822	Tab, Gray, Oblong	Naproxen 375 mg	Naprosyn by Watson		NSAID
WATSON830	Tab, White, Round	Prednisone 5 mg	by Allscripts	54569-2785	Steroid
WATSON830	Tab, White, Round	Prednisone 5 mg	Merticorten by Watson		Steroid
WATSON832	Tab, White, Round	Prednisone 20 mg	Merticorten by Watson		Steroid
WATSON835375	Tab, Blue, Triangular, Scored	Clorazepate Dipotassium 3.75 mg	by Allscripts	54569-0952	Antianxiety; C IV
WATSON841	Tab, Yellow, Round	Bisoprolol Fumarate 2.5 mg, Hydrochlorthiazide 6.25 mg	Ziac by Watson	52544-0841	Antihypertensive; Diuretic
WATSON842	Tab, Pink, Round	Bisoprolol Fumarate 5 mg, Hydrochlorthiazide 6.25 mg	Ziac by Watson	52544-0842	Antihypertensive; Diuretic
WATSON843	Tab, White, Round	Bisoprolol Fumarate 10 mg, Hydrochlorthiazide 6.25 mg	Ziac by Watson	52544-0843	Antihypertensive; Diuretic
WATSON847	Tab, White, Round	Low-Ogestrel (Norgestrel 0.3 mg and Ethinyl Estradiol 0.03 mg)	Lo-Ovral by Watson	52544-0847	Oral Contraceptive
WATSON850	Tab, White, Round, Watson/850	Acetaminophen 15 mg, Codeine Phosphate 300 mg	by Watson		Analgesic; C III
WATSON850	Tab, White, Round, Scored	Acetaminophen 300 mg, Codeine Phosphate 15 mg	Tylenol with Codeine by Watson	52544-0850	Analgesic; C III
WATSON851	Tab, White, Round, Watson/851	Acetaminophen 30 mg, Codeine Phosphate 300 mg	by Watson		Analgesic; C III
WATSON851	Tab, White, Round, Scored	Acetaminophen 300 mg, Codeine Phosphate 30 mg	Tylenol with Codeine by Watson	52544-0851	Analgesic; C III
WATSON852	Tab, White, Round, Scored	Acetaminophen 300 mg, Codeine Phosphate 60 mg	Tylenol with Codeine by Watson	52544-0852	Analgesic; C III
WATSON853	Tab, Yellow, Capsule-Shaped	Hydrocodone Bitartrate 10 mg, Acetaminophen 325 mg	Norco by Watson	52544-0853	Analgesic; C III
WATSONDILACOR120	Cap, Gold & White, Watson/Dilacor/120	Diltazem 120 mg	Dilacor XR by Watson		Antihypertensive
WATSONDILACOR180	Cap, Gold & White, Watson/Dilacor/180	Diltazem 180 mg	Dilacor XR by Watson		Antihypertensive
WATSONDILACOR240	Cap, Gold & White, Watson/Dilacor/240	Diltazem 240 mg	Dilacor XR by Watson		Antihypertensive
WATSONP	White, Round, Watson>P	Placebo	by Watson		Placebo
WATSONP	Tab, White, Round	Placebo	Zovia by Watson		Placebo
WATSONP1	Tab, Peach, Round, Watson>P1	Placebo	by Watson		Placebo
WB34	Cap, Tan & Cream	Tyropanoate 750 mg	Bilopaque by Sanofi		Diagnostic
WBS	Tab, Blue & White, Round, Schering Logo WBS	Dexbrompheniramine Maleate 2 mg, Pseudoephedrine Sulf 60 mg	Disophrol by Schering		Cold Remedy
WC <> 084	Tab, White, Oval, Film Coated	Gemfibrozil 600 mg	by Allscripts	54569-3695	Antihyperlipidemic
WC <> 084	Tab, Elliptical, Film Coated	Gemfibrozil 600 mg	by Warner Chilcott	00047-0084	Antihyperlipidemic
WC <> 084	Tab, Film Coated, Blue Print	Gemfibrozil 600 mg	by Kaiser	00179-1171	Antihyperlipidemic

ID FRONT <> BACK	DESCRIPTION FRONT <> BACK	INGREDIENT & STRENGTH	BRAND (OR EQUIV.) & FIRM	NDC#	CLASS; SCH.
WC <> 227	Tab, Light Buff, Round	Vitamin A 1000 Unt, Cholecalciferol 400 Unt, Vitamin E 11 Unt, Ascorbic Acid 120 mg; Folic Acid 1 mg; Thiamine Mononitrate 2 mg; Riboflavin 3 mg; Niacinamide 20 mg; Cyanocobalamin 12 mcg, Pyridoxine HCl 10 mg, Iron 29 mg	Natachew by Warner Chilcott W C	00430-0227	Vitamin
WC <> 227	Tab, Round	Vitamin A 1000 Unt, Cholecalciferol 400 Unt, Vitamin E 11 Unt, Ascorbic Acid 120 mg; Folic Acid 1 mg; Thiamine Mononitrate 2 mg; Riboflavin 3 mg; Niacinamide 20 mg; Cyanocobalamin 12 mcg; Pyridoxine HCl 10 mg, Iron 29 mg	Natachew by Amide Pharm	52152-0210	Vitamin
WC 084	Tab, Film Coated	Gemfibrozil 600 mg	by Kaiser	62224-1226	Antihyperlipidemic
WC014	Tab, White, Round	Propranolol 40 mg, Hydrochlorothiazide 25 mg	Inderide by WC		Antihypertensive
WC015	Tab, White, Round	Propranolol 80 mg, Hydrochlorothiazide 25 mg	Inderide by WC		Antihypertensive
WC030	Tab, Green, Round	Methyldopa 250 mg, Hydrochlorothiazide 15 mg	Aldoril by WC		Antihypertensive
WC031	Tab, White, Oblong	Methyldopa 250 mg, Hydrochlorothiazide 25 mg	Aldoril by WC		Antihypertensive
WC032	Tab, Maroon	Methyldopa 500 mg, Hydrochlorothiazide 30 mg	Aldoril by WC		Antihypertensive
WC033	Tab, Gray	Methyldopa 500 mg, Hydrochlorothiazide 50 mg	Aldoril by WC		Antihypertensive
WC038	Tab, Off-White	Amoxicillin Chewable 250 mg	Amoxil by WC		Antibiotic
WC048	Cap, Yellow	Benzonatate 100 mg	Tessalon by WC		Antitussive
WC049	Tab, White, Round	Butalbital 50 mg, Aspirin 325 mg, Caffeine 40 mg	Fiorinal by WC		Analgesic
WC057	Tab, White, Round	Cyclobenzaprine HCl 10 mg	Flexeril by WC		Muscle Relaxant
WC070	Tab, Orange, Round	Propranolol 10 mg	Inderal by WC		Antihypertensive
WC071	Tab, Blue, Round	Propranolol 20 mg	Inderal by WC		Antihypertensive
WC072	Tab, Green, Round	Propranolol 40 mg	Inderal by WC		Antihypertensive
WC073	Tab, Pink, Round	Propranolol 60 mg	Inderal by WC		Antihypertensive
WC074	Tab, Yellow, Round	Propranolol 80 mg	Inderal by WC		Antihypertensive
WC077	Tab, Peach, Oval	Fenoprofen 600 mg	Nalfon by WC		NSAID
WC078	Cap, Yellow	Nifedipine 10 mg	Procardia by WC		Antihypertensive
WC079	Cap, Orange & Red & Brown	Nifedipine 20 mg	Procardia by WC		Antihypertensive
WC081	Cap, Yellow	Fenoprofen 300 mg	Nalfon by WC		NSAID
WC084	Tab, Film Coated	Gemfibrozil 600 mg	by HL Moore	00839-7787	Antihyperlipidemic
WC084	Tab, Film Coated	Gemfibrozil 600 mg	by Sidmak	50111-0857	Antihyperlipidemic
WC091	Cap, Blue & Yellow	Doxycycline Hyclate Coated Pellets 100 mg	by WC		Antibiotic
WC121	Tab, Blue, Round	Chlorthalidone 50 mg	Hygroton by WC		Diuretic
WC123	Tab, Orange, Round	Chlorthalidone 25 mg	Hygroton by WC		Diuretic
WC124	Tab, Yellow, Round	Estropipate 00.75 mg	Ogen by WC		Hormone
WC126	Tab, Peach, Round	Estropipate 1.5 mg	Ogen by WC		Hormone
WC128	Tab, Blue, Round	Estropipate 3 mg	Ogen by WC		Hormone
WC141	Tab, White, Oval	Diazepam 2 mg	Valium by WC		Antianxiety; C IV
WC142	Tab, White, Triangular	Diazepam 5 mg	Valium by WC		Antianxiety; C IV
WC143	Tab, White, Round	Diazepam 10 mg	Valium by WC		Antianxiety; C IV
WC180	Tab, Sugar Coated	Phenazopyridine HCl 100 mg	Pyridium by Warner Chilcott	00430-0180	Urinary Analgesic
WC180	Tab, Sugar Coated	Phenazopyridine HCl 100 mg	Pyridium by Murfreesboro	51129-1346	Urinary Analgesic
WC181	Tab, Maroon, Round	Phenazopyridine HCl 200 mg	by Allscripts	54569-0089	Urinary Analgesic
WC181	Tab, Brown, Round	Phenazopyridine HCl 200 mg	Pyridium by Warner Chilcott	00430-0181	Urinary Analgesic
WC181	Tab, Sugar Coated	Phenazopyridine HCl 200 mg	by Amide	52152-0004	Urinary Analgesic
WC181	Tab, Maroon, Round	Phenazopyridine HCl 200 mg	by Physicians Total Care	54868-0878	Urinary Analgesic
WC181	Tab, Maroon, Round, Film Coated	Phenazopyridine HCl 200 mg	Pyridium by Pharmafab	62542-0919	Urinary Analgesic
WC182	Tab, Maroon, Oval, Coated	Phenazopyridine HCl 150 mg, Hyoscyamine HBr 0.3 mg, Butabarbital 15 mg	Pyridium Plus by Warner Chilcott	00430-0182	Urinary
WC196	Cap, Clear & White	Theophylline CR 100 mg	SloBid by WC		Antiasthmatic
WC197	Cap, Clear	Theophylline CR 125 mg	SloBid by WC		Antiasthmatic
WC198	Cap, Clear & White	Theophylline CR 200 mg	SloBid by WC		Antiasthmatic
WC199	Cap, Clear & White	Theophylline CR 300 mg	SloBid by WC		Antiasthmatic
WC214	Tab, Film Coated	Oxtriphylline 400 mg	Choledyl SA by Warner Chilcott	00430-0214	Antiasthmatic
WC214	Tab, Pink, Oblong	Oxtriphylline ER 400 mg	Choledyl SA by Warner Chilcott	00430-0214	Antiasthmatic
WC221	Tab, Film Coated	Oxtriphylline 600 mg	Choledyl SA by Warner Chilcott	00430-0221	Antiasthmatic

ID FRONT <> BACK	DESCRIPTION FRONT <> BACK	INGREDIENT & STRENGTH	BRAND (OR EQUIV.) & FIRM	NDC#	CLASS; SCH.
WC221	Tab, Tan, Oblong	Oxtriphylline ER 600 mg	Choledyl SA by Warner Chilcott	00430-0221	Antiasthmatic
WC242	Tab, Pink, Round	Carbamazepine Chewable 100 mg	Tegretol by WC		Anticonvulsant
WC243	Tab, White	Carbamazepine 200 mg	Tegretol by WC		Anticonvulsant
WC271	Tab, Mustard, Round	Amitriptyline 100 mg	Elavil by WC		Antidepressant
WC272	Tab, Tan, Round, W-C 272	Amitriptyline 10 mg	Elavil by WC		Antidepressant
WC273	Tab, Coral, Round, W-C 273	Amitriptyline 25 mg	Elavil by WC		Antidepressant
WC274	Tab, Blue, Round, W-C274	Amitriptyline 50 mg	Elavil by WC		Antidepressant
WC275	Tab, Green, Round, W-C 275	Amitriptyline 75 mg	Elavil by WC		Antidepressant
WC278	Tab, Orange, Round	Amitriptyline 150 mg	Elavil by WC		Antidepressant
WC314	Tab, White, Round	Amoxapine 25 mg	Asendin by WC		Antidepressant
WC315	Tab, Salmon, Round	Amoxapine 50 mg	Asendin by WC		Antidepressant
WC316	Tab, Salmon, Round	Amoxapine 100 mg	Asendin by WC		Antidepressant
WC317	Tab, Peach, Round	Amoxapine 150 mg	Asendin by WC		Antidepressant
WC318	Tab, White, Oblong	Acetaminophen 500 mg, Hydrocodone 2.5 mg	by WC		Analgesic; C III
WC319	Tab, White, Oblong	Hydrocodone Bitartrate 7.5 mg, Acetaminophen 500 mg	Vicodin by WC		Analgesic; C III
WC323	Tab, White, Round	Methyldopa 250 mg	Aldomet by WC		Antihypertensive
WC324	Tab, White, Round	Methyldopa 500 mg	Aldomet by WC		Antihypertensive
WC328	Tab, White, Round	Verapamil HCl 80 mg	Isoptin, Calan by WC		Antihypertensive
WC329	Tab, White, Round	Verapamil HCl 120 mg	Isoptin, Calan by WC		Antihypertensive
WC334	Tab, Orange, Round	Levothyroxine Sodium 0.25 mg	Synthroid by WC		Antithyroid
WC336	Tab, White, Round	Levothyroxine Sodium 0.5 mg	Synthroid by WC		Antithyroid
WC338	Tab, Violet, Round	Levothyroxine Sodium 0.075 mg	Synthroid by WC		Antithyroid
WC341	Tab, Yellow, Round	Levothyroxine Sodium 0.1 mg	Synthroid by WC		Antithyroid
WC343	Tab, Brown, Round	Levothyroxine Sodium 0.125 mg	Synthroid by WC		Antithyroid
WC344	Tab, Blue, Round	Levothyroxine Sodium 0.15 mg	Synthroid by WC		Antithyroid
WC347	Tab, Pink, Round	Levothyroxine Sodium 0.2 mg	Synthroid by WC		Antithyroid
WC348	Tab, Green, Round	Levothyroxine Sodium 0.3 mg	Synthroid by WC		Antithyroid
WC402	Cap	Ampicillin Trihydrate	by Pharmedix	53002-0230	Antibiotic
WC402	Cap, Blue & Gray	Ampicillin 250 mg	Polycillin by Mova	55370-0880	Antibiotic
WC402	Cap, Light Blue, WC Over 402	Ampicillin Trihydrate	by Quality Care	60346-0082	Antibiotic
WC402	Cap	Ampicillin Trihydrate	by Clonmell	55190-0402	Antibiotic
WC404	Cap	Ampicillin Trihydrate	by Clonmell	55190-0404	Antibiotic
WC404	Cap	Ampicillin Trihydrate	by Pharmedix	53002-0231	Antibiotic
WC404	Cap, Blue & Gray	Ampicillin Trihydrate 500 mg	Polycillin by Mova	55370-0881	Antibiotic
WC404	Cap	Ampicillin Trihydrate	by Quality Care	60346-0593	Antibiotic
WC407	Cap, Yellow & Orange	Tetracycline HCl 250 mg	Achromycin V by WC		Antibiotic
WC420	Tab, White, Round	Quinine Sulfate 325 mg	by WC		Antimalarial
WC431	Tab, White, Round	Lorazepam 0.5 mg	Ativan by WC		Sedative/Hypnotic; C IV
WC432	Tab, White, Round	Lorazepam 1 mg	Ativan by WC		Sedative/Hypnotic; C IV
WC433	Tab, White, Round	Lorazepam 2 mg	Ativan by WC		Sedative/Hypnotic; C IV
WC440	Tab, White, Oval	Furosemide 20 mg	Lasix by WC		Diuretic
WC441	Tab, White, Round	Furosemide 40 mg	Lasix by WC		Diuretic
WC442	Tab, White, Round	Furosemide 80 mg	Lasix by WC		Diuretic
WC443	Tab, Pink, Round	Clonidine HCl 0.1 mg	Catapres by WC		Antihypertensive
WC444	Tab, White, Round	Clonidine HCl 0.2 mg	Catapres by WC		Antihypertensive
WC445	Tab, White, Round	Clonidine HCl 0.3 mg	Catapres by WC		Antihypertensive
WC448	Tab, White, Oblong	Hydrocodone Bitartrate 5 mg, Acetaminophen 500 mg	Vicodin by WC		Analgesic; C III
WC451	Tab, Blue, Round	Clorazepate 30.75 mg	Tranxene by WC		Antianxiety; C IV
WC452	Tab, Beige, Round	Clorazepate 7.5 mg	Tranxene by WC		Antianxiety; C IV
WC453	Tab, Pink, Round	Clorazepate 15 mg	Tranxene by WC		Antianxiety; C IV
WC463	Tab, White, Round	Glipizide 5 mg	Glucotrol by WC		Antidiabetic
WC464	Tab, White, Round	Glipizide 10 mg	Glucotrol by WC		Antidiabetic

ID FRONT ⟷ BACK	DESCRIPTION FRONT ⟷ BACK	INGREDIENT & STRENGTH	BRAND (OR EQUIV.) & FIRM	NDC#	CLASS; SCH.
WC472	Tab, White, Oval	Verapamil HCl SR 180 mg	Calan by WC		Antihypertensive
WC474	Tab, White, Oval	Verapamil HCl SR 240 mg	Calan by WC		Antihypertensive
WC486	Tab, White, Oblong	Hydrocodone Bitartrate 7.5 mg, Acetaminophen 750 mg	by WC		Analgesic; C III
WC508	Tab, Green, Oval	Cimetidine 800 mg	Tagamet by WC		Gastrointestinal
WC515	Tab, White, Round	Allopurinol 100 mg	Zyloprim by WC		Antigout
WC516	Tab, White, Elongated	Ibuprofen 400 mg	Motrin by WC		NSAID
WC517	Tab, Peach, Round	Allopurinol 300 mg	Zyloprim by WC		Antigout
WC528	Cap, Blue	Ketoprofen 50 mg	Orudis by WC		NSAID
WC538	Cap, Blue & Yellow	Cefadroxil 500 mg	Duricef by WC		Antibiotic
WC548	Tab, White, Round	Cephalexin 250 mg	Keflex by WC		Antibiotic
WC549	Tab, White, Round	Cephalexin 500 mg	Keflex by WC		Antibiotic
WC551	Tab, Yellow, Round	Oxazepam 15 mg	Serax by WC		Sedative/Hypnotic; C IV
WC557	Tab, White, Round	Verapamil 80 mg	Isoptin by WC		Antihypertensive
WC558	Cap, Purple & Yellow	Disopyramide Phosphate CR 100 mg	Norpace CR by WC		Antiarrhythmic
WC560	Tab, Orange, Round	Guanabenz Acetate 4 mg	Wytensin by WC		Antihypertensive
WC561	Tab, Gray, Round	Guanabenz Acetate 8 mg	Wytensin by WC		Antihypertensive
WC566	Cap, Blue & White	Ketoprofen 75 mg	Orudis by WC		NSAID
WC573	Tab, White, Round	Verapamil 120 mg	Isoptin by WC		Antihypertensive
WC575	Cap, Orange & Clear	Danazol 200 mg	Danocrine by WC		Steroid
WC577	Tab, White, Round	Trazodone 50 mg	Desyrel by WC		Antidepressant
WC578	Tab, White, Round	Trazodone 100 mg	Desyrel by WC		Antidepressant
WC592	Tab, White, Round	Theophylline CR 300 mg	Theo-Dur by WC		Antiasthmatic
WC593	Tab, White, Oval	Theophylline CR 450 mg	Theo-Dur by WC		Antiasthmatic
WC594	Tab, Green, Round	Desipramine 25 mg	Norpramin by WC		Antidepressant
WC594	Tab, Yellow, Round	Desipramine 25 mg	Norpramin by WC		Antidepressant
WC595	Tab, Green, Round	Desipramine 50 mg	Norpramin by WC		Antidepressant
WC596	Tab, Orange, Round	Desipramine 75 mg	Norpramin by WC		Antidepressant
WC606	Tab, White, Round	Aspirin 325 mg	Aspirin by WC		Analgesic
WC607	Tab, White, Round	Phenobarbital 60 mg	by WC		Sedative/Hypnotic; C IV
WC611	Tab, White, Round	Baclofen 10 mg	Lioresal by WC		Muscle Relaxant
WC612	Tab, White, Round	Baclofen 20 mg	Lioresal by WC		Muscle Relaxant
WC615	Cap	Minocycline HCl	by Pharmedix	53002-0288	Antibiotic
WC615	Cap, Olive Green	Minocycline HCl 50 mg	by Parke Davis	00071-0615	Antibiotic
WC615	Cap, Olive and Brown	Minocycline HCl 50 mg	by Quality Care	60346-0830	Antibiotic
WC616	Cap, Olive Green	Minocycline HCl 100 mg	by Parke Davis	00071-0616	Antibiotic
WC617	Tab, White, Round	Quinidine Gluconate 324 mg	Quinaglute by WC		Antiarrhythmic
WC621	Cap, White	Loxapine 5 mg	Loxitane by WC		Antipsychotic
WC630	Tab, White, Round	Pindolol 5 mg	Visken by WC		Antihypertensive
WC631	Tab, White, Round	Pindolol 10 mg	Visken by WC		Antihypertensive
WC632	Cap, Yellow & White	Loxapine 10 mg	Loxitane by WC		Antipsychotic
WC634	Tab, White, Round, W-C 634	Acetaminophen 300 mg, Codeine 15 mg	Tylenol #2 by WC		Analgesic; C III
WC635	Tab, White, Round, W-C 635	Acetaminophen 300 mg, Codeine 30 mg	Tylenol #3 by WC		Analgesic; C III
WC637	Tab, White, Round, W-C 637	Acetaminophen 300 mg, Codeine 60 mg	Tylenol #4 by WC		Analgesic; C III
WC640	Tab, White, Round	Acetaminophen 325 mg	Tylenol by WC		Antipyretic
WC648	Tab	Penicillin V Potassium	by Urgent Care Ctr	50716-0648	Antibiotic
WC648	Tab	Penicillin V Potassium	by Pharmedix	53002-0201	Antibiotic
WC648	Tab	Penicillin V Potassium	by Clonmell	55190-0648	Antibiotic
WC650	Cap, Green & White	Loxapine 25 mg	Loxitane by WC		Antipsychotic
WC651	Cap, Blue & White	Loxapine 50 mg	Loxitane by WC		Antipsychotic
WC657	Tab, White, Round	Theophylline CR 100 mg	Theo-Dur by WC		Antiasthmatic
WC659	Tab, White, Oval	Theophylline CR 200 mg	Theo-Dur by WC		Antiasthmatic
WC665	Cap, Natural, Natural	Oxazepam 15 mg	Serax by WC		Sedative/Hypnotic; C IV

ID FRONT <> BACK	DESCRIPTION FRONT <> BACK	INGREDIENT & STRENGTH	BRAND (OR EQUIV.) & FIRM	NDC#	CLASS; SCH.
WC667	Cap, Orange & White	Oxazepam 30 mg	Serax by WC		Sedative/Hypnotic; C IV
WC672	Tab, Yellow, Round	Erythromycin Stearate 250 mg	Erythrocin by WC		Antibiotic
WC673	Tab, White, Oval	Penicillin V Potassium 500 mg	V-Cillin K by WC		Antibiotic
WC690	Cap, Blue & White	Oxazepam 10 mg	Serax by WC		Sedative/Hypnotic; C IV
WC696 <> ERYC	Cap, Clear & Orange	ErythroMycin 250 mg	ERYC DR by Halsey Drug	00904-5394	Antibiotic
WC697	Cap	Tetracycline HCl 500 mg	by Pharmedix	53002-0217	Antibiotic
WC698	Tab, White, Round	Phenobarbital 100 mg	by WC		Sedative/Hypnotic; C IV
WC699	Tab, White, Round	Phenobarbital 15 mg	by WC		Sedative/Hypnotic; C IV
WC700	Tab, White, Round	Phenobarbital 30 mg	by WC		Sedative/Hypnotic; C IV
WC702	Tab, White, Round	Hydrochlorothiazide 25 mg	Hydrodiuril by WC		Diuretic
WC710	Tab, White, Round	Hydrochlorothiazide 50 mg	Hydrodiuril by WC		Diuretic
WC712	Tab, White, Round	Spironolactone 25 mg, Hydrochlorothiazide 25 mg	Aldactazide by WC		Diuretic
WC713	Tab, White, Round	Spironolactone 25 mg	Aldactone by WC		Diuretic
WC716	Tab, White	Trazodone 150 mg	Desyrel by WC		Antidepressant
WC720	Cap, Orange & Purple	Disopyramide Phosphate CR 150 mg	Norpace CR by WC		Antiarrhythmic
WC724	Tab, White, Oblong	Timolol Maleate 20 mg	Blocadren by WC		Antihypertensive
WC725	Tab, White, Round	Aspirin 325 mg, Codeine Phosphate 15 mg	Empirin #2 by WC		Analgesic; C III
WC726	Tab, White, Round	Aspirin 325 mg, Codeine Phosphate 30 mg	Empirin #3 by WC		Analgesic; C III
WC727	Tab, White, Round	Aspirin 325 mg, Codeine Phosphate 60 mg	Empirin #4 by WC		Analgesic; C III
WC728	Tab, White, Round	Timolol Maleate 10 mg	Blocadren by WC		Antihypertensive
WC729	Tab, White, Round	Timolol Maleate 5 mg	Blocadren by WC		Antihypertensive
WC730	Cap, Orange & Peach	Amoxicillin Trihydrate	by Clonmell	55190-0730	Antibiotic
WC730	Cap	Amoxicillin Trihydrate	by Compumed	00403-0254	Antibiotic
WC730	Cap	Amoxicillin Trihydrate	by Pharmedix	53002-0208	Antibiotic
WC730	Cap, Orange & Peach	Amoxicillin Trihydrate 250 mg	by HJ Harkins	52959-0011	Antibiotic
WC730	Cap, Pink & Red	Amoxicillin Trihydrate 250 mg	Amoxil by Mova	55370-0884	Antibiotic
WC731	Cap, Orange & Peach	Amoxicillin 500 mg	by Barr	00555-0887	Antibiotic
WC731	Cap, Orange & Peach	Amoxicillin Trihydrate	by Clonmell	55190-0731	Antibiotic
WC731	Cap	Amoxicillin Trihydrate	by Compumed	00403-0260	Antibiotic
WC731	Cap	Amoxicillin Trihydrate	by Pharmedix	53002-0216	Antibiotic
WC731	Cap	Amoxicillin Trihydrate	by Apotheca	12634-0182	Antibiotic
WC731	Cap, Orange & Peach	Amoxicillin Trihydrate 500 mg	by HJ Harkins	52959-0020	Antibiotic
WC731	Cap, Pink & Red	Amoxicillin Trihydrate 500 mg	Amoxil by Mova	55370-0885	Antibiotic
WC759	Tab, White, Round	Acetaminophen 500 mg	Tylenol by WC		Antipyretic
WC765	Tab, Green, Oval	Cimetidine 400 mg	Tagamet by WC		Gastrointestinal
WC768	Tab, Green, Oval	Cimetidine 300 mg	Tagamet by WC		Gastrointestinal
WC773	Tab	Sulindac 150 mg	by Warner Chilcott	00047-0773	NSAID
WC773	Tab, Gold, WC/773	Sulindac 150 mg	by Kaiser	00179-1144	NSAID
WC773	Tab	Sulindac 150 mg	by Parke Davis	00071-0773	NSAID
WC773	Tab	Sulindac 150 mg	by Zenith Goldline	00182-1705	NSAID
WC773	Tab	Sulindac 150 mg	by Kaiser	62224-8119	NSAID
WC774	Tab, Elliptical Shaped	Sulindac 200 mg	by Warner Chilcott	00047-0774	NSAID
WC774	Tab, Gold	Sulindac 200 mg	by Kaiser	00179-1145	NSAID
WC774	Tab	Sulindac 200 mg	by Parke Davis	00071-0774	NSAID
WC774	Tab	Sulindac 200 mg	by Kaiser	62224-8117	NSAID
WC774	Tab, Elliptical Shaped	Sulindac 200 mg	by Quality Care	60346-0686	NSAID
WC784	Tab, Yellow, Round	Potassium Chloride ER 10 mEq	K-Tab by WC		Electrolyte
WC785	Tab, Blue, Round	Alprazolam 1 mg	Xanax by WC		Antianxiety; C IV
WC786	Tab, White, Round	Alprazolam 0.5 mg	Xanax by WC		Antianxiety; C IV
WC787	Tab, Orange, Round	Alprazolam 0.25 mg	Xanax by WC		Antianxiety; C IV
WC788	Cap, Pink & Yellow	Nitrofurantoin 50 mg	Macrodantin by WC		Antibiotic
WC789	Cap, Pink	Nitrofurantoin 100 mg	Macrodantin by WC		Antibiotic

ID FRONT <> BACK	DESCRIPTION FRONT <> BACK	INGREDIENT & STRENGTH	BRAND (OR EQUIV.) & FIRM	NDC#	CLASS; SCH.
WC790	Tab, Peach, Round	Maprotiline 25 mg	Ludiomil by WC		Antidepressant
WC791	Tab, Peach, Round	Maprotiline 50 mg	Ludiomil by WC		Antidepressant
WC795	Tab, White, Round	Maprotiline 75 mg	Ludiomil by WC		Antidepressant
WC796	Tab, White, Round	Fluphenazine 1 mg	Prolixin by WC		Antipsychotic
WC797	Tab, Beige, Round	Fluphenazine 2.5 mg	Prolixin by WC		Antipsychotic
WC798	Tab, Blue, Round	Fluphenazine 5 mg	Prolixin by WC		Antipsychotic
WC799	Tab, Red, Round	Fluphenazine 10 mg	Prolixin by WC		Antipsychotic
WC808	Cap, Green & Pink	Cephradine 250 mg	Velosef by WC		Antibiotic
WC809	Cap, Green, & Green	Cephradine 500 mg	Velosef by WC		Antibiotic
WC813	Tab, Beige, Round	Doxycycline Hyclate 100 mg	Vibra-Tab by WC		Antibiotic
WC829	Cap, Blue & White	Doxycycline Hyclate 50 mg	Vibramycin by WC		Antibiotic
WC830	Cap, Blue	Doxycycline Hyclate 100 mg	Vibramycin by WC		Antibiotic
WC832	Tab, Yellow, W-C 832	Amiloride 5 mg, Hydrochlorothiazide 50 mg	Moduretic by WC		Diuretic
WC833	Tab, Yellow, Round	Triamterene 75 mg, Hydrochlorothiazide 50 mg	Maxzide by Watson		Diuretic
WC834	Cap, Red	Triamterene 50 mg, Hydrochlorothiazide 25 mg	Dyazide by WC		Diuretic
WC843	Cap, Ivory & Opaque	Prazosin 1 mg	Minipress by WC		Antihypertensive
WC844	Cap, Pink & Opaque	Prazosin 2 mg	Minipress by WC		Antihypertensive
WC845	Cap, Blue & Opaque	Prazosin 5 mg	Minipress by WC		Antihypertensive
WC849	Tab, White, Round	Quinidine Sulfate 200 mg	Quinidine by WC		Antiarrhythmic
WC850	Tab, White, Round	Quinidine Gluconate 330 mg	Duraquin by WC		Antiarrhythmic
WC853	Cap, Red, W-C 853	Amantadine 100 mg	Symmetrel by WC		Antiviral
WC865	Tab, Blue, Round	Methyldopa 250 mg	Aldomet by WC		Antihypertensive
WC866	Tab, Blue, Round	Methyldopa 500 mg	Aldomet by WC		Antihypertensive
WC868	Cap, Green	Hydralazine 25 mg, Hydrochlorothiazide 25 mg	Apresazide by WC		Antihypertensive
WC871	Cap, Green	Hydralazine 50 mg, Hydrochlorothiazide 50 mg	Apresazide by WC		Antihypertensive
WC872	Tab, Green, Round	Fluoxymesterone 10 mg	Halotestin by WC		Steroid; C III
WC874	Tab, White, Round	Medroxyprogesterone 10 mg	Provera by WC		Progestin
WC875	Cap, Clear & Lavender w/ White Beads	Indomethacin 75 mg	by Inwood	00258-3607	NSAID
WC875	Cap, Lavender/Clear	Indomethacin SR 75 mg	Indocin by WC		NSAID
WC878	Tab, White, Round	Metoclopramide 10 mg	Reglan by Watson		Gastrointestinal
WC887	Cap, Blue & Aqua	Indomethacin 25 mg	Indocin by WC		NSAID
WC888	Cap, Blue & Aqua	Indomethacin 50 mg	Indocin by WC		NSAID
WC914	Tab, White, Elongated	Ibuprofen 800 mg	Motrin by WC		NSAID
WC919	Tab, Yellow, Oval	Erythromycin Stearate 500 mg	Erythrocin by WC		Antibiotic
WC922	Tab, White, Elongated	Ibuprofen 600 mg	Motrin by WC		NSAID
WC926	Tab, Yellow, Round	Norethindrone 0.5 mg, Ethinyl Estradiol 35 mcg	Nelova by WC		Oral Contraceptive
WC927	Tab, Yellow, Round	Norethindrone 1 mg, Ethinyl Estradiol 35 mcg	Nelova by WC		Oral Contraceptive
WC929	Tab, Yellow, Round	Norethindrone 0.5 mg, Ethinyl Estradiol 35 mcg	Nelova 0.5/35 E by WC		Oral Contraceptive
WC930	Tab, Yellow, Round	Norethindrone 1 mg, Ethinyl Estradiol 35 mcg	Nelova 1/35 by WC		Oral Contraceptive
WC938	Cap, Gray & Orange	Cephalexin 250 mg	Keflex by WC		Antibiotic
WC939	Cap, Orange	Cephalexin 500 mg	Keflex by WC		Antibiotic
WC940	Tab, Beige, Oblong	Phenylephrine 25 mg, Chlorpheniramine 8 mg, Pyrilamine 25 mg	Rynatan by WC		Cold Remedy
WC941	Tab, White, Round	Norethindrone 0.5 mg, Ethinyl Estradiol 35 mcg	Nelova 10/11 by WC		Oral Contraceptive
WC942	Tab, Blue, Round	Norethindrone 1 mg, Mestranol 50 mcg	Nelova 1/50 by WC		Oral Contraceptive
WC944	Tab, Yellow, Round	Norethindrone 10 mg, Mestranol 11 mg	Nelova by WC		Oral Contraceptive
WC945	Cap, Green	Dicloxacillin 250 mg	Dynapen by WC		Antibiotic
WC946	Cap, Green	Dicloxacillin 500 mg	Dynapen by WC		Antibiotic
WC947	Tab, Yellow, Round	Norethindrone 10 mg, Mestranol 11 mg	Nelova by WC		Oral Contraceptive
WC949	Cap, Green & Red	Cloxacillin 250 mg	Tegopen by WC		Antibiotic
WC950	Cap, Green & Red	Cloxacillin 500 mg	Tegopen by WC		Antibiotic
WC951	Tab, Peach, Round	Potassium Chloride ER 8 mEq	Slow K by WC		Electrolytes
WC951	Tab, Blue, Round	Potassium Chloride ER 8 mEq	Slow K by WC		Electrolytes

ID FRONT <> BACK	DESCRIPTION FRONT <> BACK	INGREDIENT & STRENGTH	BRAND (OR EQUIV.) & FIRM	NDC#	CLASS; SCH.
WC954	Tab, White, Oblong	Metoprolol Tartrate 50 mg	Lopressor by WC		Antihypertensive
WC954	Tab, Pink, Round	Metoprolol Tartrate 50 mg	Lopressor by WC		Antihypertensive
WC955	Tab, Blue, Round	Metoprolol Tartrate 100 mg	Lopressor by WC		Antihypertensive
WC955	Tab, White, Oblong	Metoprolol Tartrate 100 mg	Lopressor by WC		Antihypertensive
WC956	Tab, White, Round	Albuterol Sulfate 2 mg	Proventil by WC		Antiasthmatic
WC957	Tab, White, Round	Albuterol Sulfate 4 mg	Proventil by WC		Antiasthmatic
WC966	Tab, Orange, Round	Thioridazine HCl 10 mg	Mellaril by WC		Antipsychotic
WC967	Tab, Orange, Round	Thioridazine HCl 25 mg	Mellaril by WC		Antipsychotic
WC968	Tab, Orange, Round	Thioridazine HCl 50 mg	Mellaril by WC		Antipsychotic
WC969	Tab, Orange, Round	Thioridazine HCl 100 mg	Mellaril by WC		Antipsychotic
WC970	Cap	Thiothixene 1 mg	Navane by WC		Antipsychotic
WC971	Cap, Caramel & Yellow	Thiothixene 2 mg	Navane by WC		Antipsychotic
WC972	Cap, Caramel & White	Thiothixene 5 mg	Navane by WC		Antipsychotic
WC973	Tab, White, Round	Placebo	by WC		Placebo
WC975	Cap, Caramel & Peach	Thiothixene 10 mg	Navane by WC		Antipsychotic
WC977	Cap, Green & White	Temazepam 15 mg	Restoril by WC		Sedative/Hypnotic; C IV
WC978	Cap, White	Temazepam 30 mg	Restoril by WC		Sedative/Hypnotic; C IV
WC979	Tab, Orange, Oblong	Propoxyphene 65 mg, Acetaminophen 650 mg	Wygesic by WC		Analgesic; C IV
WC980	Tab, Pink	Propoxyphene Napsylate 100 mg, Acetaminophen 650 mg	Darvocet N by WC		Analgesic; C IV
WC981	Tab, Orange, Round	Haloperidol 0.5 mg	Haldol by WC		Antipsychotic
WC982	Tab, Orange, Round	Haloperidol 1 mg	Haldol by WC		Antipsychotic
WC983	Tab, Orange, Round	Haloperidol 2 mg	Haldol by WC		Antipsychotic
WC984	Tab, Orange, Round	Haloperidol 5 mg	Haldol by WC		Antipsychotic
WC985	Tab, Yellow, Round	Clonidine HCl 0.1 mg, Chlorthalidone 15 mg	Combipres by WC		Antihypertensive; Diuretic
WC986	Tab, Yellow, Round	Clonidine HCl 0.2 mg, Chlorthalidone 15 mg	Combipres by WC		Antihypertensive; Diuretic
WC987	Tab, Yellow, Round	Clonidine HCl 0.3 mg, Chlorthalidone 15 mg	Combipres by WC		Antihypertensive; Diuretic
WC988	Cap, Blue & White	Flurazepam 15 mg	Dalmane by WC		Hypnotic; C IV
WC988	Cap, Peach & Orange	Flurazepam 15 mg	Dalmane by WC		Hypnotic; C IV
WC989	Cap, Blue	Flurazepam 30 mg	Dalmane by WC		Hypnotic; C IV
WC989	Cap, Peach & Red	Flurazepam 30 mg	Dalmane by WC		Hypnotic; C IV
WD03	Cap, Orange & White	Danazol 50 mg	Danocrine by Sanofi		Steroid
WD04	Cap, Yellow	Danazol 100 mg	Danocrine by Sanofi		Steroid
WD05	Cap, Orange	Danazol 200 mg	Danocrine by Sanofi		Steroid
WD35	Tab, White, W/D/35	Meperdine HCl 50 mg	Demerol by Sanofi	Canadian	Analgesic
WD35	Tab, White, Round	Meperidine HCl 50 mg	Demerol by Sanofi		Analgesic; C II
WD37	Tab, White, Round, W/D37	Meperidine HCl 100 mg	Demerol by Sanofi		Analgesic; C II
WD92 <> WD92	Cap, Clear & Forest Green	Ergocalciferol 50000 Units	Drisdol by RP Scherer	11014-0890	Vitamin
WDILACORXR120MG	Cap, Peach & Pink	Diltiazem HCl 120 mg	Dilacor XR by Rx Pac	65084-0241	Antihypertensive
WDILACORXR120MG	Cap, Yellow & White, Watson Logo	Diltiazem HCl 120 mg	Dilacor XR by Excellium	64125-0128	Antihypertensive
WDR	Tab, Orange, Oval, Schering Logo WDR	Fluphenazine HCl 2.5 mg	Permitil by Schering	00085-0442	Antipsychotic
WE <> 04	Cap, Cap Ex Release	Brompheniramine Maleate 6 mg, Pseudoephedrine HCl 60 mg	Ultrabrom PD by Sovereign	58716-0026	Cold Remedy
WE <> 06	Cap, Cap Ex Release	Brompheniramine Maleate 12 mg, Pseudoephedrine HCl 120 mg	Ultrabrom by Sovereign	58716-0025	Cold Remedy
WE01	Tab, WE/01, Tab Ex Release	Guaifenesin 600 mg, Phenylpropanolamine HCl 75 mg	Sinuvent by Sovereign	58716-0631	Cold Remedy
WE02	Tab, WE/02, Tab Ex Release	Chlorpheniramine Maleate 8 mg, Methscopolamine Nitrate 2.5 mg, Phenylephrine HCl 20 mg	Omnihist LA by Sovereign	58716-0620	Cold Remedy
WE03	Tab, WE/03, Tab Chew	Chlorpheniramine Maleate 2 mg, Methscopolamine Nitrate 1.25 mg, Phenylephrine HCl 10 mg	AH Chew by Sovereign	58716-0619	Cold Remedy
WE05	Tab, WE/05, Tab Ex Release	Guaifenesin 600 mg, Pseudoephedrine HCl 60 mg	by Kiel	59063-0110	Cold Remedy
WE05	Tab, WE/05, Tab Ex Release	Guaifenesin 600 mg, Pseudoephedrine HCl 60 mg	D Feda II by Sovereign	58716-0625	Cold Remedy

ID FRONT <> BACK	DESCRIPTION FRONT <> BACK	INGREDIENT & STRENGTH	BRAND (OR EQUIV.) & FIRM	NDC#	CLASS; SCH.
WE05	Tab, WE/05, Tab Ex Release	Guaifenesin 600 mg, Pseudoephedrine HCl 60 mg	D Feda II by WE	59196-0005	Cold Remedy
WE07	Tab, Scored, Chewable	Phenylephrine HCl 10 mg	AH Chew D by WE	59196-0007	Decongestant
WE07	Tab, Tab Chew	Phenylephrine HCl 10 mg	AH Chew D by Nadin	14836-0007	Decongestant
WEFFEXORXR <> 150	Cap, Orange	Venlafaxine HCl 150 mg	Effexor XR by Wyeth Pharms	52903-0836	Antidepressant
WEFFEXORXR <> 150	Cap, Orange	Venlafaxine HCl 150 mg	Effexor XR by Murfreesboro Ph	51129-1677	Antidepressant
WEFFEXORXR <> 150	Cap, Orange	Venlafaxine HCl 150 mg	Effexor XR by Wyeth Labs	00008-0836	Antidepressant
WEFFEXORXR <> 375	Cap, Gray & Peach	Venlafaxine HCl 37.5 mg	Effexor XR by Wyeth Pharms	52903-0837	Antidepressant
WEFFEXORXR <> 375	Cap, Gray & Peach	Venlafaxine HCl 37.5 mg	Effexor XR by Murfreesboro Ph	51129-1678	Antidepressant
WEFFEXORXR <> 375	Cap, Gray & Peach	Venlafaxine HCl 37.5 mg	Effexor XR by Wyeth Labs	00008-0837	Antidepressant
WEFFEXORXR <> 75	Cap, Peach	Venlafaxine HCl 75 mg	Effexor XR by Wyeth Pharms	52903-0833	Antidepressant
WEFFEXORXR <> 75	Cap, Peach	Venlafaxine HCl 75 mg	Effexor XR by Wyeth Labs	00008-0833	Antidepressant
WEFFEXORXR <> 75	Cap, Peach	Venlafaxine HCl 75 mg	Effexor ER by Ayerst Lab (Div Wyeth)	00046-0833	Antidepressant
WELLBUTRIN <> 75	Tab	Bupropion HCl 75 mg	Wellbutrin by Catalytica	63552-0177	Antidepressant
WELLBUTRIN <> 75	Tab	Bupropion HCl 75 mg	Wellbutrin by Glaxo Wellcome	00173-0177	Antidepressant
WELLBUTRIN SR 100	Tab, Blue, Round	Bupropion HCl 100 mg	by Glaxo Wellcome	Canadian	Antidepressant
WELLBUTRIN SR 100	Tab, Blue, Round	Bupropion HCl 100 mg	Wellbutrin SR by Glaxo Wellcome	00173-0947	Antidepressant
WELLBUTRIN SR 150	Tab, Purple, Round	Bupropion HCl 150 mg	by Glaxo Wellcome	Canadian	Antidepressant
WELLBUTRIN100	Tab, Film Coated	Bupropion HCl 100 mg	Wellbutrin by Quality Care	60346-0242	Antidepressant
WELLBUTRIN100	Tab	Bupropion HCl 100 mg	Wellbutrin by Catalytica	63552-0178	Antidepressant
WELLBUTRIN100	Tab, Film Coated	Bupropion HCl 100 mg	Wellbutrin by Allscripts	54569-3190	Antidepressant
WELLBUTRIN75	Tab, Gold, Wellbutrin 75, Tab Coated	Bupropion HCl 75 mg	Wellbutrin by Quality Care	60346-0070	Antidepressant
WELLBUTRIN75	Tab, Coated	Bupropion HCl 75 mg	Wellbutrin by Allscripts	54569-3573	Antidepressant
WELLBUTRINSR100	Tab, Wellbutrin SR 100, Film Coated	Bupropion HCl 100 mg	Wellbutrin SR by Catalytica	63552-0947	Antidepressant
WELLBUTRINSR150	Tab, Wellbutrin SR 150, Film Coated	Bupropion HCl 150 mg	Wellbutrin SR by Catalytica	63552-0135	Antidepressant
WELLBUTRINSR150	Tab, Purple, Round	Bupropion HCl 150 mg	Wellbutrin SR by Direct Dispensing	57866-0901	Antidepressant
WELLBUTRINSR150	Tab, Purple, Round, Film Coated	Bupropion HCl 150 mg	Wellbutrin Sr by Glaxo Wellcome	00173-0135	Antidepressant
WELLBUTRINSR150	Tab, Purple, Round, Film Coated	Bupropion HCl 150 mg	Wellbutrin SR by Caremark	00339-4032	Antidepressant
WELLBUTRINSR150	Tab, Film Coated	Bupropion HCl 150 mg	Wellbutrin SR by Physicians Total Care	54868-3984	Antidepressant
WELLCOME <> U3B	Tab	Thioguanine 40 mg	Thioguanine by Catalytica	63552-0880	Antineoplastic
WELLCOME <> Y9C100	Cap, Dark Blue Band, Unicorn Logo	Zidovudine 100 mg	Retrovir by Catalytica	63552-0108	Antiviral
WELLCOME <> Y9C100	Cap, White with Dark Blue Band	Zidovudine 100 mg	Retrovir by Allscripts	54569-1772	Antiviral
WELLCOME <> Y9C100	Cap, Dark Blue Band, Unicorn Logo	Zidovudine 100 mg	Zidovudine by Med Pro	53978-2098	Antiviral
WELLCOME <> Y9C100	Cap, Blue Band, Y9C Over 100	Zidovudine 100 mg	Retrovir by Quality Care	62682-1015	Antiviral
WELLCOME <> Y9C100	Cap, Wellcome and Unicorn Logo, Y9C 100, White with Dark Blue Band	Zidovudine 100 mg	Retrovir by Amerisource	62584-0464	Antiviral
WELLCOME <> Y9C100	Cap, Unicorn Logo	Zidovudine 100 mg	Retrovir by Prepackage Spec	58864-0462	Antiviral
WELLCOME <> Y9C100	Cap, and Unicorn Logo, with Dark Blue Band, Y9C 100 with Dark Blue Band	Zidovudine 100 mg	Retrovir by Pharm Utilization	60491-0561	Antiviral
WELLCOME <> Y9C100	Cap, White, Wellcome Unicorn Logo <> Y9C 100 Dark Blue Band	Zidovudine 100 mg	Retrovir by United Res	00677-1701	Antiviral
WELLCOME <> Y9C100	Cap, White, Opaque, Blue Band Unicorn Logo	Zidovudine 100 mg	Retrovir by United Res	00677-1698	Antiviral
WELLCOME <> Y9C100	Cap, White, Opaque, Dark Blue Band	Zidovudine 100 mg	Retrovir by United Res	00677-1699	Antiviral
WELLCOME <> Y9C100	Cap, White, Opaque, Wellcome and Unicorn Logo	Zidovudine 100 mg	Retrovir by United Res	00677-1700	Antiviral
WELLCOME <> ZOVIRAX200	Cap	Acyclovir 200 mg	Zovirax by Quality Care	60346-0006	Antiviral
WELLCOME <> ZOVIRAX200	Cap	Acyclovir 200 mg	Zovirax by Prepackage Spec	58864-0563	Antiviral
WELLCOME <> ZOVIRAX200	Cap	Acyclovir 200 mg	Zovirax by Allscripts	54569-0091	Antiviral
WELLCOMEP4B	Tab, White	Triprolidine 4 mg, Pseudoephedrine 60 mg, Codeine Phosphate 20 mg	by Glaxo	Canadian	Cold Remedy
WELLCOMEU3B	Tab	Thioguanine 40 mg	Thioguanine by Glaxo	00173-0880	Antineoplastic
WELLCOMEU3B	Tab, Greenish-Yellow, Round	Thioguanine 40 mg	Tabloid by Glaxo Wellcome		Antineoplastic

ID FRONT <> BACK	DESCRIPTION FRONT <> BACK	INGREDIENT & STRENGTH	BRAND (OR EQUIV.) & FIRM	NDC#	CLASS; SCH.
WELLCOMEUNICORN <> Y9C100	Cap, Unicorn Logo, Dark Blue Band	Zidovudine 100 mg	Retrovir by Glaxo	00173-0108	Antiviral
WELLCOMEX2F	Cap, White	Pseudoephedrine 60 mg, Dextromethorphan 30 mg, Acetaminophen 500 mg	Sudafed by Warner Wellcome	Canadian	Cold Remedy
WELLCOMEZOVIRA2	Cap	Acyclovir 200 mg	Zovirax by Glaxo	00173-0991	Antiviral
WELLCOMEZOVIRAX	Cap, Blue	Acyclovir 200 mg	Zovirax by Amerisource Health	62584-0494	Antiviral
WELLCOMEZOVIRAX <> 200	Cap	Acyclovir 200 mg	Zovirax by Catalytica	63552-0991	Antiviral
WESTWARD	Tab, White, Round	Metoclopramide 10 mg	Reglan by West-ward		Gastrointestinal
WESTWARD <> 020	Tab	Aminophylline 100 mg	by Schein	00364-0004	Antiasthmatic
WESTWARD <> 025	Tab	Aminophylline 200 mg	by Schein	00364-0005	Antiasthmatic
WESTWARD <> 260	Tab, White, Round, West-ward <> 260	Isoniazid 100 mg	by Allscripts	54569-2942	Antimycobacterial
WESTWARD <> 260	Tab	Isoniazid 100 mg	Isoniazid by West Ward	00143-1260	Antimycobacterial
WESTWARD <> 260	Tab	Isoniazid 100 mg	Isoniazid by Versapharm	61748-0016	Antimycobacterial
WESTWARD <> 260	Tab	Isoniazid 100 mg	Isoniazid by Amerisource	62584-0759	Antimycobacterial
WESTWARD <> 261	Tab	Isoniazid 300 mg	Isoniazid by Versapharm	61748-0013	Antimycobacterial
WESTWARD <> 30	Cap	Flurazepam HCl 30 mg	by Quality Care	60346-0762	Hypnotic; C IV
WESTWARD <> 3142	Cap	Doxycycline Hyclate	by Quality Care	60346-0109	Antibiotic
WESTWARD <> 473	Tab	Prednisone 10 mg	by Quality Care	60346-0058	Steroid
WESTWARD <> 785	Tab	Aspirin 325 mg, Butalbital 50 mg, Caffeine 40 mg	by Quality Care	60346-0619	Analgesic; C III
WESTWARD <> 785	Tab	Aspirin 325 mg, Butalbital 50 mg, Caffeine 40 mg	by Schein	00364-0677	Analgesic; C III
WESTWARD <> FLURAZEPAM15	Cap, Black Print	Flurazepam HCl 15 mg	by Kaiser	00179-1098	Hypnotic; C IV
WESTWARD <> FLURAZEPAM15	Cap, Blue & White	Flurazepam HCl 15 mg	Dalmane by Invamed	52189-0375	Hypnotic; C IV
WESTWARD <> FLURAZEPAM15	Tab, Blue & White, Oblong	Flurazepam HCl 15 mg	by Southwood Pharms	58016-0811	Hypnotic; C IV
WESTWARD <> FLURAZEPAM30	Tab, Blue, Oblong	Flurazepam HCl 30 mg	by Southwood Pharms	58016-0812	Hypnotic; C IV
WESTWARD <> FLURAZEPAM30	Cap, Black Print	Flurazepam HCl 30 mg	by Kaiser	00179-1099	Hypnotic; C IV
WESTWARD <> FLURAZEPAM30	Cap, Blue	Flurazepam HCl 30 mg	Dalmane by Invamed	52189-0383	Hypnotic; C IV
WESTWARD004	Tab, White, Round	Acetaminophen 300 mg, Codeine Phosphate 30 mg	Tylenol #3 by West-ward		Analgesic; C III
WESTWARD005	Tab, White, Round	Acetaminophen 300 mg, Codeine Phosphate 60 mg	Tylenol #4 by West-ward		Analgesic; C III
WESTWARD010	Tab, White, Round	Allopurinol 100 mg	Zyloprim by West-ward		Antigout
WESTWARD013	Tab, Orange, Round	Allopurinol 300 mg	Zyloprim by West-ward		Antigout
WESTWARD020	Tab	Aminophylline 100 mg	by Quality Care	60346-0328	Antiasthmatic
WESTWARD020	Tab, White, Round	Aminophylline 100 mg	by West Ward	00143-1020	Antiasthmatic
WESTWARD020	Tab	Aminophylline 100 mg	by United Res	00677-0003	Antiasthmatic
WESTWARD025	Tab, White, Round	Aminophylline 200 mg	by West Ward	00143-1025	Antiasthmatic
WESTWARD025	Tab	Aminophylline 200 mg	by United Res	00677-0007	Antiasthmatic
WESTWARD045	Tab, Pink, Round, West-ward 045	Amitriptyline HCl 10 mg	Elavil by West-ward		Antidepressant
WESTWARD046	Tab, Green, Round, West-ward 046	Amitriptyline HCl 25 mg	Elavil by West-ward		Antidepressant
WESTWARD047	Tab, Brown, Round, West-ward 047	Amitriptyline HCl 50 mg	Elavil by West-ward		Antidepressant
WESTWARD048	Tab, Purple, Round, West-ward 048	Amitriptyline HCl 75 mg	Elavil by West-ward		Antidepressant
WESTWARD049	Tab, Orange, Round, West-ward 049	Amitriptyline HCl 100 mg	Elavil by West-ward		Antidepressant
WESTWARD050	Tab, Peach, Round, West-ward 050	Amitriptyline HCl 150 mg	Elavil by West-ward		Antidepressant
WESTWARD060	Tab, White, Round, West-ward 060	Ascorbic Acid 500 mg	by West-ward		Vitamin
WESTWARD074	Tab, Blue, Round, West-ward 074	Bro-Phen Time Release	by West-ward		Antihistamine
WESTWARD087	Tab, Butterscotch Yellow, Round, West-ward 087	Chlorpromazine HCl 100 mg	Thorazine by West-ward		Antipsychotic
WESTWARD090	Cap, Green & Yellow, West-ward 090	Chlordiazepoxide HCl 5 mg	Librium by West-ward		Antianxiety; C IV
WESTWARD090	Tab, Butterscotch Yellow, Round, West-ward 090	Chlorpromazine HCl 200 mg	Thorazine by West-ward		Antipsychotic

ID FRONT <> BACK	DESCRIPTION FRONT <> BACK	INGREDIENT & STRENGTH	BRAND (OR EQUIV.) & FIRM	NDC#	CLASS; SCH.
WESTWARD093	Cap, Black & Green, West-ward 093	Chlordiazepoxide HCl 10 mg	Librium by West-ward		Antianxiety; C IV
WESTWARD095	Cap, Green & White, West-ward 095	Chlordiazepoxide HCl 25 mg	Librium by West-ward		Antianxiety; C IV
WESTWARD107	Tab, White, Round, West-ward 107	Dipyridamole 25 mg	Persantine by West-ward		Antiplatelet
WESTWARD109	Tab, White, Round, West-ward 109	Dipyridamole 50 mg	Persantine by West-ward		Antiplatelet
WESTWARD110	Cap, Green, Oval, West-ward 110	Chloral Hydrate 500 mg	Noctec by West-ward		Sedative/Hypnotic; C IV
WESTWARD111	Tab, White, Round, West-ward 111	Dipyridamole 75 mg	Persantine by West-ward		Antiplatelet
WESTWARD136	Cap, Clear & Pink, West-ward 136	Diphenhydramine HCl 25 mg	Benadryl by West-ward		Antihistamine
WESTWARD137	Cap, Pink, West-ward 137	Diphenhydramine HCl 50 mg	Benadryl by West-ward		Antihistamine
WESTWARD140	Tab	Atropine Sulfate 0.0194 mg, Hyoscyamine Sulfate 0.1037 mg, Phenobarbital 16.2 mg, Scopolamine Hydrobromide 0.0065 mg	Haponal by United Res	00677-0074	Gastrointestinal; C IV
WESTWARD140	Tab	Atropine Sulfate 0.0194 mg, Hyoscyamine Sulfate 0.1037 mg, Phenobarbital 16.2 mg, Scopolamine Hydrobromide 0.0065 mg	Belladonna PB by Quality Care	60346-0042	Gastrointestinal; C IV
WESTWARD140	Tab	Atropine Sulfate 0.0194 mg, Hyoscyamine Sulfate 0.1037 mg, Phenobarbital 16.2 mg, Scopolamine Hydrobromide 0.0065 mg	Belladonna Phenobarb by Kaiser	00179-0027	Gastrointestinal; C IV
WESTWARD140	Tab, White, Round	Atropine Sulfate 0.0194 mg, Hyoscyamine Sulfate 0.1037 mg, Phenobarbital 16.2 mg, Scopolamine Hydrobromide 0.0065 mg	Belladonna Phenobarb by West Ward	00143-1140	Gastrointestinal; C IV
WESTWARD140	Tab	Atropine Sulfate 0.0194 mg, Hyoscyamine Sulfate 0.1037 mg, Phenobarbital 16.2 mg, Scopolamine Hydrobromide 0.0065 mg	Belladonna Phenobarb by Kaiser	00179-1276	Gastrointestinal; C IV
WESTWARD140	Tab, White, Round, Scored	Hyoscyamine Sulfate 0.1037 mg, Phenobarbital 16.2 mg, Atropine Sulfate 0.0194 mg, Scopolamine Hydrobromide 0.0065 mg	by HJ Harkins	52959-0023	Gastrointestinal
WESTWARD143	Tab, White, Round, West-ward 143	Benztropine Mesylate 1 mg	Cogentin by West-ward		Antiparkinson
WESTWARD144	Tab, White, Round	Benztropine Mesylate 2 mg	Cogentin by West-ward		Antiparkinson
WESTWARD147	Tab, Rust, Round	Imipramine HCl 25 mg	Tofranil by West-ward		Antidepressant
WESTWARD15	Cap	Flurazepam HCl 15 mg	by Geneva	00781-2806	Hypnotic; C IV
WESTWARD150	Tab, Green, Round	Imipramine HCl 50 mg	Tofranil by West-ward		Antidepressant
WESTWARD153	Tab, White, Round	Methyldopa 250 mg	Aldomet by West-ward		Antihypertensive
WESTWARD155	Tab, Lavender, Round	Butabarbital Sodium 15 mg	Butisol Sodium by West-ward		Sedative; C III
WESTWARD155	Tab, White, Oblong	Methyldopa 500 mg	Aldomet by West-ward		Antihypertensive
WESTWARD157	Tab, Lavender, Round	Butabarbital Sodium 30 mg	Butisol Sodium by West-ward		Sedative; C III
WESTWARD178	Tab, White, Round	Propoxyphene Napsylate 50 mg, Acetaminophen 325 mg	Darvocet N by West-ward		Analgesic; C IV
WESTWARD179	Tab, White, Oblong	Propoxyphene Napsylate 100 mg, Acetaminophen 650 mg	Darvocet N by West-ward		Analgesic; C IV
WESTWARD181	Tab, White, Round, West-ward 181	Carbamazepine 200 mg	Tegretol by West-ward		Anticonvulsant
WESTWARD183	Tab, Blue, Round, West-ward 183	Chlorpropamide 100 mg	Diabinese by West-ward		Antidiabetic
WESTWARD185	Tab, Blue, Round, West-ward 185	Chlorpropamide 250 mg	Diabinese by West-ward		Antidiabetic
WESTWARD186	Tab, Yellow, Round, West-ward 186	Clonidine HCl 0.1 mg	Catapres by West-ward		Antihypertensive
WESTWARD187	Tab, White, Round, West-ward 187	Clonidine HCl 0.2 mg	Catapres by West-ward		Antihypertensive
WESTWARD195	Tab	Chloroquine Phosphate 250 mg	by West Ward	00143-1195	Antimalarial
WESTWARD200	Tab, Yellow, Round, West-ward 200	Chlorpheniramine Maleate 4 mg	Chlor-Trimeton by West-ward		Antihistamine
WESTWARD201	Tab	Colchicine 0.6 mg	by Quality Care	60346-0683	Antigout
WESTWARD201	Tab, White, Round	Colchicine 0.6 mg	by Allscripts	54569-0236	Antigout
WESTWARD201	Tab	Colchicine 0.6 mg	by Zenith Goldline	00182-0174	Antigout
WESTWARD201	Tab, White, Round	Colchicine 0.6 mg	by West Ward	00143-1201	Antigout
WESTWARD201	Tab	Colchicine 0.6 mg	by Rugby	00536-3494	Antigout
WESTWARD201	Tab	Colchicine 0.6 mg	by United Res	00677-0040	Antigout
WESTWARD201	Tab, West-ward 201	Colchicine 0.6 mg	by Caremark	00339-5450	Antigout
WESTWARD201	Tab, White, Round	Colchicine 0.6 mg	by Dixon	17236-0668	Antigout
WESTWARD201	Tab	Cortisone Acetate 25 mg	by Zenith Goldline	00182-1648	Steroid
WESTWARD202	Tab, White, Round, Scored	Cortisone Acetate 25 mg	by DJ Pharma	64455-0008	Steroid
WESTWARD202	Tab, White, Round	Cortisone Acetate 25 mg	Cortone by West Ward	00143-1202	Steroid
WESTWARD202	Tab	Cortisone Acetate 25 mg	by Qualitest	00603-3062	Steroid
WESTWARD202	Tab	Cortisone Acetate 25 mg	by United Res	00677-0046	Steroid
WESTWARD205	Tab, Butterscotch Yellow, Round, West-ward 205	Chlorpromazine HCl 25 mg	Thorazine by West-ward		Antipsychotic

ID FRONT ⟷ BACK	DESCRIPTION FRONT ⟷ BACK	INGREDIENT & STRENGTH	BRAND (OR EQUIV.) & FIRM	NDC#	CLASS; SCH.
WESTWARD207	Tab, Butterscotch Yellow, Round, West-ward 207	Chlorpromazine HCl 50 mg	Thorazine by West-ward		Antipsychotic
WESTWARD209	Tab	Chlorothiazide 250 mg	by West Ward	00143-1209	Diuretic; Antihypertensive
WESTWARD209	Tab	Chlorothiazide 500 mg	by Zenith Goldline	00182-0790	Diuretic
WESTWARD210	Tab, White, Round	Chlorothiazide 500 mg	Diuril by West Ward	00143-1210	Diuretic
WESTWARD210	Tab	Chlorothiazide 500 mg	by Physicians Total Care	54868-0672	Diuretic
WESTWARD210	Cap	Oxytetracycline HCl 250 mg	by West Ward	00143-3210	Antibiotic
WESTWARD217	Tab, Pink, Round	Reserpine 0.125 mg, Chlorothiazide 250 mg	Diupres by West-ward		Antihypertensive
WESTWARD218	Tab, Pink, Round	Reserpine 0.125 mg, Chlorothiazide 500 mg	Diupres by West-ward		Antihypertensive
WESTWARD220	Tab, White, Round, West-ward 220	Diazepam 2 mg	Valium by West-ward		Antianxiety; C IV
WESTWARD222	Tab, Yellow, Round, West-ward 222	Diazepam 5 mg	Valium by West-ward		Antianxiety; C IV
WESTWARD225	Tab, Blue, Round, West-ward 225	Diazepam 10 mg	Valium by West-ward		Antianxiety; C IV
WESTWARD227	Cap, White	Prazosin HCl 1 mg	Minipress by West-ward		Antihypertensive
WESTWARD228	Cap, Pink	Prazosin HCl 2 mg	Minipress by West-ward		Antihypertensive
WESTWARD229	Cap, Blue	Prazosin HCl 5 mg	Minipress by West-ward		Antihypertensive
WESTWARD235	Cap, Opaque Pink	Propoxyphene HCl 65 mg	Davon by West Ward	00143-3235	Analgesic; C IV
WESTWARD235	Cap, Coated	Propoxyphene HCl 65 mg	by Qualitest	00603-5459	Analgesic; C IV
WESTWARD239	Tab, White, Round, West-ward 239	Dimenhydrinate 50 mg	Dramamine by West-ward		Antiemetic
WESTWARD245	Tab, White, Round, West-ward 245	Diphenoxylate HCl 2.5 mg, Atropine Sulfate 0.025 mg	Lomotil by West-ward		Antidiarrheal; C V
WESTWARD247	Tab, White, Round, West-ward 247	Ergoloid Mesylates 1 mg	Hydergine by West-ward		Ergot
WESTWARD248	Tab	Folic Acid 1 mg	by Quality Care	60346-0697	Vitamin
WESTWARD248	Tab	Folic Acid 1 mg	by Golden State	60429-0212	Vitamin
WESTWARD248	Tab	Folic Acid 1 mg	by Heartland	61392-0244	Vitamin
WESTWARD248	Tab, Yellow, Round	Folic Acid 1 mg	Folvite by West Ward	00143-1248	Vitamin
WESTWARD248	Tab	Folic Acid 1 mg	by Caremark	00339-5564	Vitamin
WESTWARD248	Tab	Folic Acid 1 mg	by United Res	00677-0449	Vitamin
WESTWARD248	Tab	Folic Acid 1 mg	by Nat Pharmpak Serv	55154-5502	Vitamin
WESTWARD248	Tab, Yellow, Round, Scored	Folic Acid 1 mg	by Janssen	50458-0301	Vitamin
WESTWARD248	Tab, Yellow, Round, Scored	Folic Acid 1 mg	by Janssen	50458-0302	Vitamin
WESTWARD248	Tab, Yellow, Round, Scored	Folic Acid 1 mg	Folvite by UDL	51079-0041	Vitamin
WESTWARD248	Tab	Folic Acid 1 mg	by Med Pro	53978-0913	Vitamin
WESTWARD249	Tab, White, Round, West-ward 249	Furosemide 20 mg	Lasix by West-ward		Diuretic
WESTWARD250	Tab, White, Round, West-ward 250	Furosemide 40 mg	Lasix by West-ward		Diuretic
WESTWARD253	Tab, White, Round, West-ward 253	Furosemide 80 mg	Lasix by West-ward		Diuretic
WESTWARD254	Tab, White, Round	Hydrocortisone 20 mg	Hydrocortisone by West Ward	00143-1254	Steroid
WESTWARD254	Tab	Hydrocortisone 20 mg	Hydrocortisone by Rugby	00536-3913	Steroid
WESTWARD254	Tab, White, Round, Scored	Hydrocortisone 20 mg	by Murfreesboro	51129-1464	Steroid
WESTWARD254	Tab	Hydrocortisone 20 mg	Hydrocortisone by Physicians Total Care	54868-1743	Steroid
WESTWARD254	Tab	Hydrocortisone 20 mg	Hydrocortisone by United Res	00677-0076	Steroid
WESTWARD256	Tab, Peach, Round	Hydrochlorothiazide 25 mg	Hydrodiuril by West-ward		Diuretic
WESTWARD257	Tab, Peach, Round	Hydrochlorothiazide 50 mg	Hydrodiuril by West-ward		Diuretic
WESTWARD258	Tab, White, Round	Isoxsuprine HCl 10 mg	Vasodilan by West-ward		Vasodilator
WESTWARD259	Tab, White, Round	Isoxsuprine HCl 20 mg	Vasodilan by West-ward		Vasodilator
WESTWARD261	Tab, White, Round, Scored	Isoniazid 300 mg	by Allscripts	54569-2509	Antimycobacterial
WESTWARD261	Tab, White, Round	Isoniazid 300 mg	Isoniazid by West Ward	00143-1261	Antimycobacterial
WESTWARD261	Tab	Isoniazid 300 mg	Isoniazid by Golden State	60429-0115	Antimycobacterial
WESTWARD261	Tab	Isoniazid 300 mg	Isoniazid by Heartland	61392-0803	Antimycobacterial
WESTWARD261	Tab	Isoniazid 300 mg	Isoniazid by Amerisource	62584-0760	Antimycobacterial
WESTWARD265	Tab, Green, Round	Reserpine 0.125 mg, Hydrochlorothiazide 50 mg	Hydropres 50 by West-ward		Antihypertensive
WESTWARD269	Tab, Orange, Round, West-ward 269	Hydralazine HCl 25 mg	Apresoline by West-ward		Antihypertensive
WESTWARD271	Tab, Orange, Round, West-ward 271	Hydralazine HCl 50 mg	Apresoline by West-ward		Antihypertensive
WESTWARD272	Tab, White, Round	Lorazepam 0.5 mg	Ativan by West-ward		Sedative/Hypnotic; C IV

ID FRONT <> BACK	DESCRIPTION FRONT <> BACK	INGREDIENT & STRENGTH	BRAND (OR EQUIV.) & FIRM	NDC#	CLASS; SCH.
WESTWARD273	Tab, White, Round	Lorazepam 1 mg	Ativan by West-ward		Sedative/Hypnotic; C IV
WESTWARD274	Tab, White, Round	Lorazepam 2 mg	Ativan by West-ward		Sedative/Hypnotic; C IV
WESTWARD279	Tab, White, Pink Specks	Chlorpheniramine Maleate 5 mg, Phenylephrine HCl 10 mg, Phenylpropanolamine HCl 40 mg, Phenyltoloxamine Citrate 15 mg	Decongestant by Qualitest	00603-3120	Cold Remedy
WESTWARD285	Tab, White, Oblong	Hydrocodone Bitartrate 5 mg, Acetaminophen 500 mg	Vicodin by West-ward		Analgesic; C III
WESTWARD285	Cap, Orange	Sulfinpyrazone 200 mg	Anturane by West-ward		Uricosuric
WESTWARD290	Tab	Methocarbamol 500 mg	by Kaiser	00179-1268	Muscle Relaxant
WESTWARD290	Tab	Methocarbamol 500 mg	by Zenith Goldline	00182-0572	Muscle Relaxant
WESTWARD290	Tab, White, Round	Methocarbamol 500 mg	Robaxin by West Ward	00143-1290	Muscle Relaxant
WESTWARD290	Tab	Methocarbamol 500 mg	by HJ Harkins Co	52959-0167	Muscle Relaxant
WESTWARD290	Tab	Methocarbamol 500 mg	by DRX	55045-1531	Muscle Relaxant
WESTWARD290	Tab	Methocarbamol 500 mg	by Amerisource	62584-0780	Muscle Relaxant
WESTWARD290	Tab	Methocarbamol 500 mg	by Quality Care	60346-0080	Muscle Relaxant
WESTWARD290	Tab, White, Round, Scored	Methocarbamol 500 mg	by Compumed	00403-1836	Muscle Relaxant
WESTWARD290	Tab, White, Round, Scored	Methocarbamol 500 mg	by Neuman Distr	64579-0004	Muscle Relaxant
WESTWARD290	Tab, White, Round, Scored	Methocarbamol 500 mg	by Neuman Distr	64579-0006	Muscle Relaxant
WESTWARD290	Tab, White, Round, Scored	Methocarbamol 500 mg	by Neuman Distr	64579-0007	Muscle Relaxant
WESTWARD290	Tab, White, Round, Scored	Methocarbamol 500 mg	by Neuman Distr	64579-0013	Muscle Relaxant
WESTWARD290	Tab, White, Round, Scored, West-ward 290	Methocarbamol 500 mg	by Allscripts	54569-0852	Muscle Relaxant
WESTWARD292	Tab, White, Oblong, Scored	Methocarbamol 750 mg	by Neuman Distr	64579-0005	Muscle Relaxant
WESTWARD292	Tab, White, Cap-Shaped, Scored, West-ward 292	Methocarbamol 750 mg	by Allscripts	54569-0843	Muscle Relaxant
WESTWARD292	Tab, White, Oblong, Scored	Methocarbamol 750 mg	by Southwood Pharms	58016-0258	Muscle Relaxant
WESTWARD292	Tab, White, Oblong, Scored	Methocarbamol 750 mg	by Bryant Ranch Phcy	63629-1292	Muscle Relaxant
WESTWARD292	Tab, White, Oblong, Scored	Methocarbamol 750 mg	by Kaiser	00179-1279	Muscle Relaxant
WESTWARD292	Tab, White, Oblong, Scored	Methocarbamol 750 mg	by Zenith Goldline	00182-0573	Muscle Relaxant
WESTWARD292	Tab, White, Oblong, Scored	Methocarbamol 750 mg	Robaxin by West Ward	00143-1292	Muscle Relaxant
WESTWARD292	Tab, White, Oblong, Scored	Methocarbamol 750 mg	by Pharmedix	53002-0359	Muscle Relaxant
WESTWARD292	Tab, White, Oblong, Scored	Methocarbamol 750 mg	by HJ Harkins Co	52959-0099	Muscle Relaxant
WESTWARD292	Tab, White, Oblong, Scored	Methocarbamol 750 mg	by Quality Care	60346-0063	Muscle Relaxant
WESTWARD292	Tab, White, Oblong, Scored	Methocarbamol 750 mg	by Amerisource	62584-0781	Muscle Relaxant
WESTWARD292	Tab, White, Oblong, Scored	Methocarbamol 750 mg	by Qualitest	00603-4488	Muscle Relaxant
WESTWARD292	Tab, White, Oblong, Scored	Methocarbamol 750 mg	by United Res	00677-0431	Muscle Relaxant
WESTWARD295	Tab, White, Round	Metronidazole 250 mg	Flagyl by West-ward		Antibiotic
WESTWARD295	Cap, Orange & Yellow	Tetracycline HCl 250 mg	Tetracyn by West-ward		Antibiotic
WESTWARD296	Tab, Beige, Round	Thioridazine HCl 10 mg	Mellaril by West-ward		Antipsychotic
WESTWARD297	Tab, White, Oblong	Metronidazole 500 mg	Flagyl by West-ward		Antibiotic
WESTWARD297	Tab, Blue, Round	Thioridazine HCl 15 mg	Mellaril by West-ward		Antipsychotic
WESTWARD298	Tab, Yellow, Round	Thioridazine HCl 25 mg	Mellaril by West-ward		Antipsychotic
WESTWARD299	Tab, Pink, Round	Thioridazine HCl 50 mg	Mellaril by West-ward		Antipsychotic
WESTWARD30	Cap	Flurazepam HCl 30 mg	by Geneva	00781-2807	Hypnotic; C IV
WESTWARD300	Tab, White, Round	Ibuprofen 400 mg	Motrin by West-ward		NSAID
WESTWARD3001	Cap, Pink & Red, White, Print	Butalbital 50 mg, Acetaminophen 500 mg, Caffeine 40 mg	by Caremark	00339-4112	Analgesic
WESTWARD3001	Cap, Pink & Red	Butalbital 50 mg; Acetaminophen 500 mg; Caffeine 40 mg	by WestWard Pharm	00143-3001	Analgesic
WESTWARD302	Tab, White, Oblong	Ibuprofen 600 mg	Motrin by West-ward		NSAID
WESTWARD302	Tab, White, Round	Thioridazine HCl 100 mg	Mellaril by West-ward		Antipsychotic
WESTWARD303	Tab, Green, Round	Thioridazine HCl 150 mg	Mellaril by West-ward		Antipsychotic
WESTWARD304	Tab, White, Oblong	Ibuprofen 800 mg	Motrin by West-ward		NSAID
WESTWARD304	Tab, Orange, Round	Thioridazine HCl 200 mg	Mellaril by West-ward		Antipsychotic
WESTWARD307	Tab, Lavender, Round	Trifluoperazine HCl 1 mg	Stelazine by West-ward		Antipsychotic
WESTWARD309	Tab, Lavender, Round	Trifluoperazine HCl 2 mg	Stelazine by West-ward		Antipsychotic
WESTWARD311	Tab, Lavender, Round	Trifluoperazine HCl 5 mg	Stelazine by West-ward		Antipsychotic
WESTWARD3126	Cap, Dark Blue	Decyclomine HCl 10 mg	by Heartland	61392-0182	Gastrointestinal

ID FRONT <> BACK	DESCRIPTION FRONT <> BACK	INGREDIENT & STRENGTH	BRAND (OR EQUIV.) & FIRM	NDC#	CLASS; SCH.
WESTWARD3126	Cap, Blue, West-ward 3126	Decyclomine HCl 10 mg	Bentyl by West Ward	00143-3126	Gastrointestinal
WESTWARD3126	Cap, West-ward 3126,	Decyclomine HCl 10 mg	by Warner Chilcott	00047-0403	Gastrointestinal
WESTWARD3126	Cap	Decyclomine HCl 10 mg	by Qualitest	00603-3265	Gastrointestinal
WESTWARD3126	Cap	Decyclomine HCl 10 mg	by United Res	00677-0341	Gastrointestinal
WESTWARD313	Tab, Lavender, Round	Trifluoperazine HCl 10 mg	Stelazine by West-ward		Antipsychotic
WESTWARD3136	Cap, Clear & Pink, West-ward 3136	Diphenhydramine HCl 25 mg	Benadryl by West-ward		Antihistamine
WESTWARD3141	Cap, West-ward 3141	Doxycycline Hyclate 50 mg	by Warner Chilcott	00047-0829	Antibiotic
WESTWARD3141	Cap, Blue & White	Doxycycline Hyclate 50 mg	Vibramycinby West Ward	00143-3141	Antibiotic
WESTWARD3142	Cap	Doxycycline Hyclate 100 mg	Doxal by West Ward	00143-9410	Antibiotic
WESTWARD3142	Cap	Doxycycline Hyclate 100 mg	by Rugby	00536-0230	Antibiotic
WESTWARD3142	Cap, Blue	Doxycycline Hyclate 100 mg	Vibramycin by West Ward	00143-3142	Antibiotic
WESTWARD3142	Cap	Doxycycline Hyclate 100 mg	by Comm Action	59214-0839	Antibiotic
WESTWARD3142	Cap, Opaque	Doxycycline Hyclate 100 mg	by Prepackage Spec	58864-0190	Antibiotic
WESTWARD3145	Cap, Pink, West-ward 3145	Ephedrine Sulfate 25 mg	by West-ward		Antiasthmatic
WESTWARD320	Cap, Ivory & Fuchsia	Hydroxyzine Pamoate 25 mg	Vistaril by West-ward		Antihistamine
WESTWARD325	Cap, Ivory & Red	Hydroxyzine Pamoate 50 mg	Vistaril by West-ward		Antihistamine
WESTWARD325	Cap, Green & White	Temazepam 15 mg	Restoril by West-ward		Sedative/Hypnotic; C IV
WESTWARD327	Cap, White	Temazepam 30 mg	Restoril by West-ward		Sedative/Hypnotic; C IV
WESTWARD329	Cap, Maroon	Triamterene 50 mg, Hydrochlorothiazide 25 mg	Dyazide by West-ward		Diuretic
WESTWARD330	Cap, Ivory & Fuchsia	Hydroxyzine Pamoate 100 mg	Vistaril by West-ward		Antihistamine
WESTWARD330	Tab, Yellow, Round	Methyltestosterone 25 mg	by West-ward		Hormone; C III
WESTWARD332	Tab, Yellow, Oblong	Vitamin B Complex	Berocca Plus by West-ward		Vitamin
WESTWARD336	Tab, White, Round, West-ward 336	Acetaminophen 325 mg	Tylenol by West-ward		Antipyretic
WESTWARD339	Tab, White, Round, West-ward 339	Acetaminophen 500 mg	Tylenol by West-ward		Antipyretic
WESTWARD367	Cap, Blue & White, West-ward 367	Flurazepam HCl 15 mg	Dalmane by West-ward		Hypnotic; C IV
WESTWARD370	Cap, Blue, West-ward 370	Flurazepam HCl 30 mg	Dalmane by West-ward		Hypnotic; C IV
WESTWARD445	Tab, White, Round	Phenobarbital 15 mg	by West Ward	00143-1445	Sedative/Hypnotic; C IV
WESTWARD445	Tab, West-ward 445	Phenobarbital 15 mg	by Allscripts	54569-0937	Sedative/Hypnotic; C IV
WESTWARD445	Tab, White, Round	Phenobarbital 15 mg	by United Res	00677-1667	Sedative/Hypnotic; C IV
WESTWARD445	Tab	Phenobarbital 15 mg	by Geneva	00781-1091	Sedative/Hypnotic; C IV
WESTWARD445	Tab, White, Round	Phenobarbital 100 mg	by WestWard Pharm	00143-1458	Sedative/Hypnotic; C IV
WESTWARD450	Tab, White, Round	Phenobarbital 30 mg	by West Ward	00143-1450	Sedative/Hypnotic; C IV
WESTWARD450	Tab	Phenobarbital 30 mg	by Geneva	00781-1110	Sedative/Hypnotic; C IV
WESTWARD450	Tab, White, Round, Scored	Phenobarbital 30 mg	by United Res	00677-1666	Sedative/Hypnotic; C IV
WESTWARD455	Tab, White, Round	Phenobarbital 60 mg	by West-ward		Sedative/Hypnotic; C IV
WESTWARD473	Tab	Prednisone 10 mg	by Baker Cummins	63171-1334	Steroid
WESTWARD473	Tab	Prednisone 10 mg	Predone by West Ward	00143-9412	Steroid
WESTWARD473	Tab, White, Round	Prednisone 10 mg	Deltasone by West Ward	00143-1473	Steroid
WESTWARD473	Tab, Coated	Prednisone 10 mg	by Qualitest	00603-5333	Steroid
WESTWARD473	Tab	Prednisone 10 mg	by Zenith Goldline	00182-1334	Steroid
WESTWARD473	Tab, Westward/473	Prednisone 10 mg	by UDL	51079-0033	Steroid
WESTWARD473	Tab	Prednisone 10 mg	by Geneva	00781-1500	Steroid
WESTWARD475	Tab, White, Round	Prednisone 5 mg	Deltasone by West Ward	00143-1475	Steroid
WESTWARD475	Tab	Prednisone 5 mg	by Qualitest	00603-5332	Steroid
WESTWARD475	Tab	Prednisone 5 mg	by Zenith Goldline	00182-0201	Steroid
WESTWARD475	Tab	Prednisone 5 mg	by Med Pro	53978-0060	Steroid
WESTWARD475	Tab	Prednisone 5 mg	by Allscripts	54569-0330	Steroid
WESTWARD475	Tab, Westward/475	Prednisone 5 mg	by UDL	51079-0032	Steroid
WESTWARD475	Tab	Prednisone 5 mg	by Quality Care	60346-0515	Steroid
WESTWARD475	Tab	Prednisone 5 mg	by Geneva	00781-1495	Steroid
WESTWARD477	Tab	Prednisone 20 mg	by Geneva	00781-1485	Steroid
WESTWARD477	Tab	Prednisone 20 mg	by United Res	00677-0427	Steroid

ID FRONT <> BACK	DESCRIPTION FRONT <> BACK	INGREDIENT & STRENGTH	BRAND (OR EQUIV.) & FIRM	NDC#	CLASS; SCH.
WESTWARD477	Tab, Peach, Round	Prednisone 20 mg	Deltasone by West Ward	00143-1477	Steroid
WESTWARD477	Tab	Prednisone 20 mg	Predone by West Ward	00143-9413	Steroid
WESTWARD477	Tab	Prednisone 20 mg	by Zenith Goldline	00182-1086	Steroid
WESTWARD477	Tab, Westward/477	Prednisone 20 mg	by UDL	51079-0022	Steroid
WESTWARD477	Tab	Prednisone 20 mg	by Quality Care	60346-0094	Steroid
WESTWARD477	Tab	Prednisone 20 mg	by Baker Cummins	63171-1086	Steroid
WESTWARD480	Tab, White, Round, Scored	Propylthiouracil 50 mg	by DRX Pharm Consults	55045-2747	Antithyroid
WESTWARD480	Tab, White, Round	Propylthiouracil 50 mg	by West Ward	00143-1480	Antithyroid
WESTWARD481	Tab, White, Round	Prednisone 50 mg	Deltasone by West-ward		Steroid
WESTWARD485	Tab, White, Round	Pseudophedrine HCl 60 mg	by Pharmascience	Canadian	Decongestant
WESTWARD485	Tab, White, Round	Pseudoephedrine HCl 60 mg	Sudafed by West-ward		Decongestant
WESTWARD485	Tab, White, Round	Pseudoephedrine HCl 60 mg	by West-ward	00143-1485	Decongestant
WESTWARD502	Tab, Peach, Round	Propranolol 10 mg	Inderal by West-ward		Antihypertensive
WESTWARD503	Tab, Blue, Round	Propranolol 20 mg	Inderal by West-ward		Antihypertensive
WESTWARD504	Tab, Green, Round	Propranolol 40 mg	Inderal by West-ward		Antihypertensive
WESTWARD505	Tab, Pink, Round	Propranolol 60 mg	Inderal by West-ward		Antihypertensive
WESTWARD506	Tab, Yellow, Round	Propranolol 80 mg	Inderal by West-ward		Antihypertensive
WESTWARD508	Tab, White, Round	Quinidine Gluconate 324 mg	Quinaglute by West-ward		Antiarrhythmic
WESTWARD510	Cap, Clear	Quinidine Sulfate 200 mg	by West-ward		Antiarrhythmic
WESTWARD530	Tab, White, Round	Reserpine 0.1 mg	Serpasil by West-ward		Antihypertensive
WESTWARD535	Tab, White, Round	Reserpine 0.25 mg	Serpasil by West-ward		Antihypertensive
WESTWARD625	Tab, White, Oval	Sulfamethoxazole 800 mg, Trimethoprim 160 mg	Bactrim DS by West-ward		Antibiotic
WESTWARD680	Tab, White, Round	Sulfinpyrazone 100 mg	Anturane by West-ward		Uricosuric
WESTWARD683	Tab, White, Round	Sulfisoxazole 500 mg	Gantrisin by West-ward		Antibiotic
WESTWARD689	Tab, White, Oval	Theophylline Anhydrous CR 200 mg	Theo-Dur by West-ward		Antiasthmatic
WESTWARD690	Tab, White, Oblong	Theophylline Anhydrous CR 300 mg	Theo-Dur by West-ward		Antiasthmatic
WESTWARD695	Tab, White, Round	Theophylline 118 mg, Ephedrine HCl 24 mg, Phenobarbital 8 mg	Tedral by West-ward		Antiasthmatic
WESTWARD737	Tab, West-ward 737	Acetaminophen 325 mg, Butalbital 50 mg, Caffeine 40 mg	by West Ward	00143-1737	Analgesic
WESTWARD737	Tab	Acetaminophen 325 mg, Butalbital 50 mg, Caffeine 40 mg	by Qualitest	00603-2547	Analgesic
WESTWARD737	Tab, White, Round, West-ward 737	Caffeine 40 mg, Butalbital 50 mg, Acetaminophen 325 mg	Fioricet by Westward		Analgesic
WESTWARD737	Tab, White, Round	Butalbital 50 mg; Acetaminophen 325 mg; Caffeine 40 mg	by United Res Tabs	00677-1748	Analgesic
WESTWARD750	Tab, Round	Triamterene 75 mg, Hydrochlorothiazide 50 mg	Maxzide by West-ward		Diuretic
WESTWARD769	Tab	Isosorbide Dinitrate 5 mg	Wesorbide by West Ward	00143-9400	Antianginal
WESTWARD769	Tab, White, Round	Isosorbide Dinitrate 5 mg	Isordil by West Ward	00143-1769	Antianginal
WESTWARD769	Tab	Isosorbide Dinitrate 5 mg	by Heartland	61392-0311	Antianginal
WESTWARD769	Tab	Isosorbide Dinitrate 5 mg	by Qualitest	00603-4116	Antianginal
WESTWARD769	Tab	Isosorbide Dinitrate 5 mg	by Vangard	00615-1564	Antianginal
WESTWARD771	Tab	Isosorbide Dinitrate 10 mg	Wesorbide by West Ward	00143-9401	Antianginal
WESTWARD771	Tab	Isosorbide Dinitrate 10 mg	by Quality Care	60346-0577	Antianginal
WESTWARD771	Tab	Isosorbide Dinitrate 10 mg	by PDRX	55289-0667	Antianginal
WESTWARD771	Tab	Isosorbide Dinitrate 10 mg	by Vangard	00615-1560	Antianginal
WESTWARD771	Tab	Isosorbide Dinitrate 10 mg	by Talbert Med	44514-0465	Antianginal
WESTWARD771	Tab	Isosorbide Dinitrate 10 mg	by Qualitest	00603-4117	Antianginal
WESTWARD772	Tab	Isosorbide Dinitrate 20 mg	Wesorbide by West Ward	00143-9402	Antianginal
WESTWARD772	Tab	Isosorbide Dinitrate 20 mg	by Quality Care	60346-0798	Antianginal
WESTWARD772	Tab	Isosorbide Dinitrate 20 mg	by Vangard	00615-1575	Antianginal
WESTWARD772	Tab	Isosorbide Dinitrate 20 mg	by Qualitest	00603-4118	Antianginal
WESTWARD772	Tab	Isosorbide Dinitrate 20 mg	by Talbert Med	44514-0477	Antianginal
WESTWARD785	Tab, White, Round	Aspirin 325 mg, Butalbital 50 mg, Caffeine 40 mg	by Allscripts	54569-0339	Analgesic; C III
WESTWARD785	Tab	Aspirin 325 mg, Butalbital 50 mg, Caffeine 40 mg	by Kaiser	00179-1042	Analgesic; C III
WESTWARD785	Tab	Aspirin 325 mg, Butalbital 50 mg, Caffeine 40 mg	by Zenith Goldline	00182-1631	Analgesic; C III
WESTWARD785	Tab, White, Round	Aspirin 325 mg, Butalbital 50 mg, Caffeine 40 mg	Fiorinal by West Ward	00143-1785	Analgesic; C III

ID FRONT <> BACK	DESCRIPTION FRONT <> BACK	INGREDIENT & STRENGTH	BRAND (OR EQUIV.) & FIRM	NDC#	CLASS; SCH.
WESTWARD785	Tab	Aspirin 325 mg, Butalbital 50 mg, Caffeine 40 mg	by Geneva	00781-1435	Analgesic; C III
WESTWARD785	Tab	Aspirin 325 mg, Butalbital 50 mg, Caffeine 40 mg	Fiormor by Med Pro	53978-3164	Analgesic; C III
WESTWARD785	Tab	Aspirin 325 mg, Butalbital 50 mg, Caffeine 40 mg	by Talbert Med	44514-0088	Analgesic; C III
WESTWARD785	Tab	Aspirin 325 mg, Butalbital 50 mg, Caffeine 40 mg	Fiormor by HL Moore	00839-6733	Analgesic; C III
WESTWARD787	Tab, Blue, Round, West-ward over 787	Acetaminophen 325 mg, Butalbital 50 mg, Caffeine 40 mg	by Teva	00093-0854	Analgesic
WESTWARD787	Tab, Blue, Round	Acetaminophen 325 mg, Butalbital 50 mg, Caffeine 40 mg	Fioricet by West Ward	00143-1787	Analgesic
WESTWARD787	Tab	Acetaminophen 325 mg, Butalbital 50 mg, Caffeine 40 mg	by Zenith Goldline	00182-2659	Analgesic
WESTWARD787	Tab	Acetaminophen 325 mg, Butalbital 50 mg, Caffeine 40 mg	by HL Moore	00839-7831	Analgesic
WESTWARD900	Tab, Round	Triprolidine HCl 2.5 mg, Pseudoephedrine HCl 60 mg	Actifed by West-ward		Cold Remedy
WESTWARD FLURAZEPAM	Cap, Blue & White	Flurazepam HCl 15 mg	Dalmane by West Ward	00143-3367	Hypnotic; C IV
WESTWARD FLURAZEPAM <> 15	Cap	Flurazepam HCl 15 mg	by Quality Care	60346-0239	Hypnotic; C IV
WESTWARD FLURAZEPAM15	Cap, Blue & White, Gelatin	Flurazepam 15 mg	by Invamed	52189-0315	Hypnotic; C IV
WESTWARD FLURAZEPAM30	Cap, Blue	Flurazepam HCl 30 mg	Dalmane by West Ward	00143-3370	Hypnotic; C IV
WFF	Tab, Pinkish Purple, Oval, Schering Logo WFF	Fluphenazine HCl 5 mg	Permitil by Schering	00085-0550	Antipsychotic
WFG	Tab, Red, Oval, Schering Logo WFG	Fluphenazine HCl 10 mg	Permitil by Schering	00085-0316	Antipsychotic
WFHC101	Tab, White, Diamond, Scored	Estropipate 0.75 mg	Ortho EST by Women First Hlthcare	64248-0101	Hormone
WFHC101	Tab, White, Diamond, Scored	Estropipate 0.625 mg	Ortho EST by Heartland	61392-0557	Hormone
WFHC102	Tab, Purple, Diamond, Scored	Estropipate 1.5 mg	Ortho EST by Women First Hlthcare	64248-0102	Hormone
WG1503328	Cap, Blue & Green	Clindamycin HCl 150 mg	by Copley	38245-0217	Antibiotic
WHITBY <> 612	Tab, Film Coated	Guaifenesin 600 mg, Pseudoephedrine HCl 120 mg	Duratuss by UCB	50474-0612	Cold Remedy
WHITBY <> 612	Tab, Film Coated	Guaifenesin 600 mg, Pseudoephedrine HCl 120 mg	Duratuss by CVS	51316-0238	Cold Remedy
WHITBY <> 901	Tab, White, Oblong, Pink Specks	Acetaminophen 500 mg, Hydrocodone Bitartrate 2.5 mg	Lortab by Alphapharm	57315-0009	Analgesic; C III
WHITBY <> 902	Tab, White, Blue Specks	Acetaminophen 500 mg, Hydrocodone Bitartrate 5 mg	Lortab 5/500 by UCB	50474-0902	Analgesic; C III
WHITBY <> 903	Tab, White, Oblong, Green Specks	Acetaminophen 500 mg, Hydrocodone Bitartrate 7.5 mg	Lortab by Allscripts	54569-4761	Analgesic; C III
WHITBY500	Tab, Pink, Oblong	Hydrocodone Bitartrate 5 mg, Aspirin 500 mg	Lortab ASA by UCB Pharma		Analgesic; C III
WHITBY901	Tab, White, Tab/Pink Specks, Oblong	Hydrocodone Bitartrate 2.5 mg, Acetaminophen 500 mg	Lortab by UCB Pharma		Analgesic; C III
WHITBY902	Tab, White, Blue Specks, Whitby/902	Acetaminophen 500 mg, Hydrocodone Bitartrate 5 mg	Lortab 5 by Allscripts	54569-0956	Analgesic; C III
WHITBY903	Tab, White with Green Specks, Whitby/903	Acetaminophen 500 mg, Hydrocodone Bitartrate 7.5 mg	Lortab by Quality Care	60346-0679	Analgesic; C III
WHITBY903	Tab, White, Green Specks, Whitby/903	Acetaminophen 500 mg, Hydrocodone Bitartrate 7.5 mg	Lortab 7 by Allscripts	54569-0957	Analgesic; C III
WHITBY903	Tab, White, Green Specks, Whitby/903	Atropine Sulfate 0.025 mg, Diphenoxylate HCl 2.5 mg	Lortab by Nat Pharmpak Serv	55154-7201	Antidiarrheal; C V
WHITE <> RELAFEN500	Tab, Film Coated	Nabumetone 500 mg	Relafen by Prescription Dispensing	61807-0051	NSAID
WHITEHALLLOGO	Tab, Pink	Aspirin 325 mg, Caffeine 32 mg, Codeine Phosphate 8 mg	Anacin by Whitehall-Robbins	Canadian	Analgesic
WHR100	Cap, Clear & White	Theophylline 100 mg	Slo-Bid Gyrocaps by RPR		Antiasthmatic
WHR125	Cap, White	Theophylline 125 mg	Slo-Bid Gyrocaps by RPR		Antiasthmatic
WHR1354	Cap, White	Theophylline 60 mg	Slophyllin Gyrocaps by Rorer		Antiasthmatic
WHR1355	Cap, Brown	Theophylline 125 mg	Slophyllin Gyrocaps by Rorer		Antiasthmatic
WHR1356	Cap, Purple	Theophylline 250 mg	Slophyllin Gyrocaps by Rorer		Antiasthmatic
WHR200	Cap, Clear & White	Theophylline 200 mg	Slo-Bid Gyrocaps by RPR		Antiasthmatic
WHR300	Cap, Clear & White	Theophylline 300 mg	Slo-Bid Gyrocaps by RPR		Antiasthmatic
WHR50MG	Cap, Clear & White	Theophylline 50 mg	Slo-Bid Gyrocaps by RPR		Antiasthmatic
WHR75MG	Cap, Clear & White	Theophylline 75 mg	Slo-Bid Gyrocaps by RPR		Antiasthmatic
WI200	Tab, White, Round, W/I/200	Floctafenine 200 mg	Idarac by Sanofi	Canadian	Anti-Inflammatory
WI400	Tab, White, Round, W/I/400	Floctafenine 400 mg	Idarac by Sanofi	Canadian	Anti-Inflammatory
WINTHROP <> T27	Tab	Aspirin 325 mg, Pentazocine HCl	Talwin Compound by Sanofi	00024-1927	Analgesic; C IV
WINTHROP <> T27	Tab	Aspirin 325 mg, Pentazocine HCl	Talwin Compound by Searle	00966-1927	Analgesic; C IV
WINTHROP <> T37	Tab, Light Blue	Acetaminophen 650 mg, Pentazocine HCl	Talacen by Quality Care	60346-0985	Analgesic; C IV
WINTHROPT37	Tab, Blue, Oblong	Pentazocine HCl 25 mg, Acetaminophen 500 mg	Talacen by Sanofi		Analgesic; C IV

ID FRONT <> BACK	DESCRIPTION FRONT <> BACK	INGREDIENT & STRENGTH	BRAND (OR EQUIV.) & FIRM	NDC#	CLASS; SCH.
WL	Tab, Yellow, Round, Scored, W.L. Logo	Colchicine 0.6 mg	by Altimed	Canadian DIN# 00287873	Antigout
WL	Tab, Pink, Round, Scored, W.L. Logo	Colchicine 1 mg	by Altimed	Canadian DIN# 00206032	Antigout
WL	Tab, Pink, Round	Digitoxin 0.1 mg	by Welcker-Lyster	Canadian	Cardiac Agent
WL	Tab, Pink, Round, Scored	Quinidine Phenylethylbarbiturate 100 mg	by Altimed	Canadian DIN# 00249424	Antiarrhythmic
WL53	Tab, White, Round	Talbutal 120 mg	Lotusate by Sanofi		Hypnotic
WM31	Tab, White, Round	Mephobarbital 32 mg	Mebaral by Sanofi		Sedative/Hypnotic; C IV
WM32	Tab, White, Round	Mephobarbital 50 mg	Mebaral by Sanofi		Sedative/Hypnotic; C IV
WM33	Tab, White, Round	Mephobarbital 100 mg	Mebaral by Sanofi		Sedative/Hypnotic; C IV
WM87	Tab, White, Round	Ambenonium 10 mg	Mytelase by Sanofi		Myasthenia Gravis
WM9060MG	Cap, Black & Pink, W M-90 60 mg	Trilostane 60 mg	Modrastane by Sanofi		Steroid Inhibitor
WM9130MG	Cap, Pink, W M-91 30 mg	Trilostane 30 mg	Modrastane by Sanofi		Steroid Inhibitor
WMERRELL547	Tab, White, White	Quinine Sulfate 260 mg	Quinamm by Merrell		Antimalarial
WMO	Tab, White, W/M-O	Levonogestrel 150 mcg, Ethinyl Estradiol 30 mcg	by Wyeth-Ayerst	Canadian	Oral Contraceptive
WMP	Cap, Green	Atropine Sulfate 0.195 mg, Phenobarbital 16 mg	Anthrocol by Poythress		Gastrointestinal; C IV
WMP9525	Cap, Brown & Yellow	Phenobarbital 16 mg	Solfoton by Poythress		Sedative/Hypnotic; C IV
WN21	Tab, Tan, Oblong	Nalidixic Acid 250 mg	NegGram by Sanofi		Antibiotic
WN22	Tab, Tan, Oblong	Nalidixic Acid 500 mg	NegGram by Sanofi		Antibiotic
WN23	Tab, Tan, Oval	Nalidixic Acid 1000 mg	NegGram by Sanofi		Antibiotic
WP101	Tab	Carbinoxamine Maleate 8 mg, Pseudoephedrine HCl 120 mg	Biohist LA by Anabolic	00722-6250	Cold Remedy
WP102	Tab, Tab Ex Release	Dextromethorphan Hydrobromide 30 mg, Guaifenesin 600 mg, Phenylpropanolamine HCl 37.5 mg	Profen II DM by Wakefield	59310-0110	Cold Remedy
WP102	Tab	Dextromethorphan Hydrobromide 30 mg, Guaifenesin 600 mg, Phenylpropanolamine HCl 37.5 mg	Profen II DM by Anabolic	00722-6385	Cold Remedy
WP12	Tab, White, WP/12, Film Coated, White, Elliptical	Guaifenesin 1200 mg	Muco Fen 1200 by Wakefield	59310-0120	Expectorant
WP12	Tab, Film Coated, WP/12	Guaifenesin 1200 mg	Muco Fen by Anabolic	00722-6412	Expectorant
WP61	Tab, White, Round	Hydroxychloroquine Sulfate 200 mg	Plaquenil by Sanofi		Antimalarial
WP97	Tab, Pink & Orange, W/P97	Primaquine Phosphate 26.3 mg	Primaquine by Sanofi	Canadian	Antimalarial
WP97	Tab, White, Round	Primaquine Phosphate 26.3 mg	Primaquine by Sanofi		Antimalarial
WPHH <> 170	Tab	Sulindac 150 mg	by Merck Sharp & Dohme	62904-0170	NSAID
WPI3111	Tab, Mottled White to Off-White, Oval	Methylphenidate 20 mg	ER by Danbury	00591-3111	Stimulant; C II
WPN325	Tab, White, Round	Phenylpropanolamine HCl 37.5 mg	Revive by NVE Pharm		Decongestant; Appetite Suppressant
WPN375	Tab, White, Round, WPN/37.5	Phenylpropanolamine 37.5 mg	Revive Diet Aid by NVE		Decongestant; Appetite Suppressant
WPPH <> 152	Tab, Film Coated	Methyldopa 250 mg	by Quality Care	60346-0459	Antihypertensive
WPPH <> 152	Tab, Yellow, Round, Film Coated	Methyldopa 250 mg	by Endo	60951-0776	Antihypertensive
WPPH <> 153	Tab, Film Coated	Hydrochlorothiazide 25 mg, Methyldopa 250 mg	by Merck	00006-0153	Diuretic; Antihypertensive
WPPH <> 153	Tab, White, Round, Film Coated	Hydrochlorothiazide 25 mg, Methyldopa 250 mg	by Endo	60951-0779	Diuretic; Antihypertensive
WPPH <> 153	Tab, Film Coated	Hydrochlorothiazide 25 mg, Methyldopa 250 mg	by West Point	59591-0153	Diuretic; Antihypertensive
WPPH <> 154	Tab	Sulindac 200 mg	by Merck Sharp & Dohme	62904-0154	NSAID
WPPH <> 154	Tab, Bright Yellow, Hexagonal, Scored	Sulindac 200 mg	by Endo	60951-0781	NSAID
WPPH <> 154	Tab	Sulindac 200 mg	by Quality Care	60346-0686	NSAID
WPPH <> 154	Tab	Sulindac 200 mg	by West Point	59591-0154	NSAID

ID FRONT <> BACK	DESCRIPTION FRONT <> BACK	INGREDIENT & STRENGTH	BRAND (OR EQUIV.) & FIRM	NDC#	CLASS; SCH.
WPPH <> 156	Tab, Butterscotch Yellow-Colored, D-Shaped, Film Coated	Cyclobenzaprine HCl 10 mg	by Quality Care	60346-0581	Muscle Relaxant
WPPH <> 156	Tab, D Shape, Film Coated	Cyclobenzaprine HCl 10 mg	by West Point	59591-0156	Muscle Relaxant
WPPH <> 156	Tab, Yellow, D-Shaped, Film Coated	Cyclobenzaprine HCl 10 mg	by Endo	60951-0767	Muscle Relaxant
WPPH <> 156	Tab, D-Shaped, Film Coated	Cyclobenzaprine HCl 10 mg	by PDRX	55289-0567	Muscle Relaxant
WPPH <> 157	Cap, Blue and White Pellets, Blue and White Pellets, ER	Indomethacin 75 mg	by West Point	59591-0157	NSAID
WPPH <> 157	Cap	Indomethacin 75 mg	by Quality Care	60346-0687	NSAID
WPPH <> 159	Cap, Blue	Indomethacin 50 mg	by Southwood Pharms	58016-0236	NSAID
WPPH <> 159	Cap	Indomethacin 50 mg	by West Point	59591-0159	NSAID
WPPH <> 162	Tab	Amiloride HCl 5 mg, Hydrochlorothiazide 50 mg	by West Point	59591-0162	Diuretic
WPPH <> 162	Tab, Peach, Diamond Shaped, Scored	Amiloride HCl 5 mg, Hydrochlorothiazide 50 mg	by Endo	60951-0764	Diuretic
WPPH <> 170	Tab	Sulindac 150 mg	by Quality Care	60346-0044	NSAID
WPPH <> 170	Tab	Sulindac 150 mg	by West Point	59591-0170	NSAID
WPPH <> 170	Tab, Bright Yellow, Round	Sulindac 150 mg	by Endo	60951-0780	NSAID
WPPH <> 172	Cap	Indomethacin 25 mg	by West Point	59591-0172	NSAID
WPPH <> 174	Tab, Yellow, Round, Film Coated	Methyldopa 125 mg	Aldomet by Endo	60951-0775	Antihypertensive
WPPH <> 176	Tab, Film Coated	Methyldopa 500 mg	by Merck	00006-0176	Antihypertensive
WPPH <> 176	Tab, Yellow, Round, Film Coated	Methyldopa 500 mg	by Endo	60951-0777	Antihypertensive
WPPH <> 179	Tab, Film Coated	Hydrochlorothiazide 15 mg, Methyldopa 250 mg	by Merck	00006-0179	Diuretic; Antihypertensive
WPPH <> 179	Tab, Salmon, Round, Film Coated	Hydrochlorothiazide 15 mg, Methyldopa 250 mg	by Endo	60951-0778	Diuretic; Antihypertensive
WPPH <> 192	Tab	Timolol Maleate 5 mg	by West Point	59591-0192	Antihypertensive
WPPH <> 192	Tab, Light Blue, Round	Timolol Maleate 5 mg	by Endo	60951-0782	Antihypertensive
WPPH <> 194	Tab	Timolol Maleate 10 mg	by West Point	59591-0194	Antihypertensive
WPPH <> 194	Tab, Light Blue, Round	Timolol Maleate 10 mg	by Endo	60951-0783	Antihypertensive
WPPH <> 195	Tab, Peach, Cap Shaped, Film Coated	Diflunisal 250 mg	by Endo	60951-0768	NSAID
WPPH <> 196	Tab, Film Coated	Diflunisal 500 mg	by Quality Care	60346-0053	NSAID
WPPH <> 196	Tab, Orange, Cap Shaped, Film Coated	Diflunisal 500 mg	by Endo	60951-0769	NSAID
WPPH <> 196	Tab, Orange, Oblong, Film Coated	Diflunisal 500 mg	by HJ Harkins	52959-0379	NSAID
WPPH <> 196	Tab, Orange, Oblong, Film Coated, WPPH <> 196 underlined	Diflunisal 500 mg	by Duramed	51285-0503	NSAID
WPPH <> 240	Tab, White, Round, Scored	Chlorothiazide 250 mg	by Endo	60951-0765	Diuretic
WPPH <> 240	Tab	Chlorothiazide 250 mg	by Merck	00006-0240	Diuretic
WPPH <> 241	Tab	Hydrochlorothiazide 25 mg	by Merck	00006-0241	Diuretic
WPPH <> 241	Tab	Hydrochlorothiazide 25 mg	by Endo	60951-0770	Diuretic
WPPH <> 243	Tab	Hydrochlorothiazide 50 mg	by Merck	00006-0243	Diuretic
WPPH <> 243	Tab	Hydrochlorothiazide 50 mg	by Endo	60951-0771	Diuretic
WPPH <> 243	Tab	Hydrochlorothiazide 50 mg	Hctz by Quality Care	60346-0675	Diuretic
WPPH <> 245	Tab, White, Round, Scored	Chlorothiazide 500 mg	by Endo	60951-0766	Diuretic
WPPH196	Tab, Film Coated	Diflunisal 500 mg	by Pharmedix	53002-0303	NSAID
WPPH245	Tab, White, Round	Chlorothiazide 500 mg	Diuril by Endo		Diuretic
WR	Tab, Blue, Round, W-R	Brom Mal 12 mg, Phenyl Hydro 15 mg, Phenylpro Hydr 15 mg	Dimetapp by Whitehall-Robbins		Cold Remedy
WR	Tab, Peach, Round, Scored, W-R	Brom Mal 4 mg, Phenyl Hydro 5 mg	Dimetapp by Whitehall-Robbins		Cold Remedy
WR	Tab, Peach, W-R	Brompheniramine Maleate 4 mg	by Whitehall-Robins	Canadian	Antihistamine
WR	Tab, White, Oblong	Methocarbamol 750 mg	Robaxin-750 by Whitehall-Robbins	Canadian	Muscle Relaxant
WR	Tab, White, Oblong, Scored	Methocarbamol 750 mg	Robaxin by Whitehall-Robbins		Muscle Relaxant
WR	Cap, Green & White	Methocarbamol 400 mg, Acetaminophen 325 mg	Robaxacet by Whitehall-Robbins	Canadian	Muscle Relaxant
WR	Tab, Green/White	Methocarbamol 400 mg, Acetaminophen 325 mg	Robaxacet by Whitehall-Robbins	Canadian	Muscle Relaxant
WR	Cap, Green & White, Cap Layers, Scored	Methocarbamol 400 mg, Acetaminophen 325 mg	Robaxacet by Whitehall-Robbins		Muscle Relaxant
WR	Tab, Green/White, Round, Scored	Methocarbamol 400 mg, Acetaminophen 325 mg	Robaxacet by Whitehall-Robbins		Muscle Relaxant
WR	Tab, Blue/White, Round	Methocarbamol 400 mg, Acetaminophen 325 mg, Codeine Phosphate 8 mg	Robaxacet 8 by Whitehall-Robbins	Canadian	Muscle Relaxant
WR	Tab, Blue/White, Round, Scored	Methocarbamol 400 mg, Acetaminophen 325 mg, Codeine Phosphate 8 mg	Robaxacet by Whitehall-Robbins		Muscle Relaxant
WR	Cap, White/Pink, Scored, W-R	Methocarbamol 400 mg, Acetylsalicylic 325 mg	Robaxisal by Whitehall-Robbins		Muscle Relaxant

ID FRONT <> BACK	DESCRIPTION FRONT <> BACK	INGREDIENT & STRENGTH	BRAND (OR EQUIV.) & FIRM	NDC#	CLASS; SCH.
WR	Tab, White, Tab/Pink Layers, Round, Scored, W-R	Methocarbamol 400 mg, Acetylsalicylic 325 mg	Robaxisal by Whitehall-Robbins		Muscle Relaxant
WR	Tab, White, Tab/Yellow Layers, Round, Scored, W-R	Methocarbamol 400 mg, Acetylsalicylic Acid 325 mg, Codeine Phosph 8 mg	Robaxisal by Whitehall-Robbins		Muscle Relaxant
WR	Tab, Coral & White, Round, Scored, W-R	Methocarbamol 400 mg, Acetylsalicylic Acid 325 mg, Codeine Phosph 32.4 mg	Robaxisal by Whitehall-Robbins		Muscle Relaxant
WR	Tab, Orange & White, Round, Scored, W-R	Methocarbamol 400 mg, Acetylsalicylic Acid 325 mg, Codeine Phosph 16.2 mg	Robaxisal by Whitehall-Robbins		Muscle Relaxant
WR	Tab, Orange & White	Methocarbamol 400 mg, Aspirin 325 mg, Codeine Phosphate 16.2 mg	Robaxisal-C by Whitehall-Robbins	Canadian	Muscle Relaxant
WR	Tab, Coral & White	Methocarbamol 400 mg, Aspirin 325 mg, Codeine Phosphate 32.4 mg	by Whitehall-Robbins	Canadian	Muscle Relaxant
WR	Tab, Yellow with White	Methocarbamol 400 mg, Aspirin 325 mg, Codeine Phosphate 8 mg	Robaxisal-C by Whitehall-Robbins	Canadian	Muscle Relaxant
WR	Tab, White	Methocarbamol 500 mg	Robaxin by Whitehall-Robbins	Canadian	Muscle Relaxant
WR	Tab, White, Round, Scored	Methocarbamol 500 mg	Robaxin by Whitehall-Robbins		Muscle Relaxant
WRP1	Cap, Mauve, WR/P-1	Multivitamins	Paramettes by Whitehall-Robbins		Vitamin
WRP2	Cap, Lime, WR/P-2	Multivitamins	Paramettes by Whitehall-Robbins		Vitamin
WRS1	Tab, Orange, Oval, W-R/S1	Multi Vitamins	by Whitehall-Robins	Canadian	Vitamin
WRS1	Tab, Orange & Red, Oval, W-R/S/1	Vitamin B Complex Vitamins C & E & Iron	Stresstabs by Whitehall-Robbins		Vitamin
WRS2	Tab, Red, Oval, W-R/S2	Multi Vitamins	by Whitehall-Robins	Canadian	Vitamin
WRS3	Tab, Peach, Oval, W-R/S3	Multi Vitamins	by Whitehall-Robins	Canadian	Vitamin
WRS3	Tab, Light Apricot, Oval, W-R/S/3	Vitamin B Complex Vitamins C & E Zinc	Stresstabs by Whitehall-Robbins		Vitamin
WRS4	Tab, Orange, Oval, W-R/S4	Multi Vitamins	by Whitehall-Robins	Canadian	Vitamin
WRS4	Tab, Light Orange, Oval, WR/S/4	Vitamin B Complex Vitamins C & E	Stresstabs by Whitehall-Robbins		Vitamin
WRU10	Tab, Orange, Oval, WR/U/10	Multimineral Multivitamin	Centrum by Whitehall-Robbins		Vitamin
WRU12	Tab, Peach, Oval, W-R/U/12	Multimineral Multivitamin	Centrum by Whitehall-Robbins		Vitamin
WRU23	Tab, Orange, Oval, W-R/U/23	Multimineral Multivitamin	Centrum by Whitehall-Robbins		Vitamin
WRU7	Tab, Light Peach, Oval, W-R/U/7	18 Multimineral Multivitamin	Centrum by Whitehall-Robbins		Vitamin
WRWR	Cap, Green & Yellow, WR/WR	Therapeutic B-Complex with Vitamin C	Allbee by Whitehall-Robbins		Vitamin
WRWR	Cap, Yellow, WR/WR	Therapeutic B-Complex with Vitamin C 550 mg	Allbee by Whitehall-Robbins		Vitamin
WT21	Tab, Peach, W/T/21	Pentazocine HCl 50 mg	Talwin Tablets by Sanofi	Canadian	Analgesic
WT31	Tab, White, Doscoid, W/T/31	Iopanoic Acid 500 mg	Telepaque by Sanofi	Canadian	Diagnostic
WT31	Tab, Yellow, Round	Iopanoic Acid 500 mg	Telepaque by Sanofi		Diagnostic
WT4111	Tab, White, Oblong, W-T 4111	Magnesium Salicylate 500 mg	Efficin by Adria		Analgesic
WT51	Tab	Naloxone HCl 0.5 mg, Pentazocine HCl	Talwin Nx by Pharmedix	53002-0381	Analgesic; C IV
WV22	Tab, Speckled Buff, Oblong	Stanozolol 2 mg	Winstrol-V Chewable by Sanofi		Anabolic Steroid; C III
WW	Tab, Red with Specks	Chlorpheniramine Maleate 5 mg, Phenylephrine HCl 10 mg, Phenylpropanolamine HCl 40 mg, Phenyltoloxamine Citrate 15 mg	De Con by Patient	57575-0034	Cold Remedy
WW115	Tab, White, Oblong, WW-115	Butalbital 50 mg, Acetaminophen 500 mg, Caffeine 40 mg	by West-Ward	00143-1115	Analgesic
WW115	Tab, White, Oblong, Scored	Butalbital 50 mg; Acetaminophen 500 mg; Caffeine 40 mg	by United Res Tabs	00677-1738	Analgesic
WW125	Tab, Pink, Round, Film Coated	Chloroquine Phosphate 500 mg	by West Ward Pharm	00143-2125	Antimalarial
WW172	Tab, WW-172	Captopril 25 mg	by ESI Lederle	59911-5833	Antihypertensive
WW172	Tab, White, Round	Captopril 25 mg	by West Ward	00143-1172	Antihypertensive
WW173	Tab, WW-173	Captopril 50 mg	by ESI Lederle	59911-5834	Antihypertensive
WW173	Tab, White, Oblong	Captopril 50 mg	by West Ward	00143-1173	Antihypertensive
WW174	Tab, White, Oval, WW/174	Captopril 100 mg	by ESI Lederle	59911-5835	Antihypertensive
WW174	Tab, White, Oblong	Captopril 100 mg	by West Ward	00143-1174	Antihypertensive
WW176	Tab	Carisoprodol 350 mg	by Amerisource	62584-0644	Muscle Relaxant
WW176	Tab	Carisoprodol 350 mg	by Zenith Goldline	00182-1079	Muscle Relaxant
WW176	Tab, White, Round	Carisoprodol 350 mg	by West Ward	00143-1176	Muscle Relaxant
WW27	Tab	Decyclomine HCl 20 mg	by Novopharm	55953-0667	Gastrointestinal
WW27	Tab	Decyclomine HCl 20 mg	by Heartland	61392-0041	Gastrointestinal
WW27	Tab, Embossed	Decyclomine HCl 20 mg	by Kaiser	62224-9222	Gastrointestinal
WW27	Tab	Decyclomine HCl 20 mg	by Amerisource	62584-0671	Gastrointestinal
WW27	Tab	Decyclomine HCl 20 mg	by Warner Chilcott	00047-0405	Gastrointestinal
WW27	Tab, Blue, Round	Decyclomine HCl 20 mg	Bentyl by West Ward	00143-1227	Gastrointestinal
WW27	Tab	Decyclomine HCl 20 mg	by HL Moore	00839-8099	Gastrointestinal
WW27	Tab	Decyclomine HCl 20 mg	by Qualitest	00603-3266	Gastrointestinal

ID FRONT <> BACK	DESCRIPTION FRONT <> BACK	INGREDIENT & STRENGTH	BRAND (OR EQUIV.) & FIRM	NDC#	CLASS; SCH.
WW27	Tab	Decyclomine HCl 20 mg	by United Res	00677-0498	Gastrointestinal
WW27	Tab, Blue, Round, WW-27	Decyclomine HCl 20 mg	by Novopharm	43806-0667	Gastrointestinal
WW27	Tab, Blue, Round	Dicyclomine HCl 20 mg	by UDL	51079-0119	Gastrointestinal
WW27	Tab, Blue, Round	Dicyclomine HCl 20 mg	by Direct Dispensing	57866-3377	Gastrointestinal
WW27	Tab, Blue, Round	Dicyclomine HCl 20 mg	Bentyl by Mova	55370-0879	Gastrointestinal
WW279	Tab, Red Specks	Chlorpheniramine Maleate 5 mg, Phenylephrine HCl 10 mg, Phenylpropanolamine HCl 40 mg, Phenyltoloxamine Citrate 15 mg	Decongestant by Kaiser	62224-9116	Cold Remedy
WW279	Tab, Red Specks	Chlorpheniramine Maleate 5 mg, Phenylephrine HCl 10 mg, Phenylpropanolamine HCl 40 mg, Phenyltoloxamine Citrate 15 mg	Tri Phen Mine Sr by Zenith Goldline	00182-1094	Cold Remedy
WW279	Tab	Chlorpheniramine Maleate 5 mg, Phenylephrine HCl 10 mg, Phenylpropanolamine HCl 40 mg, Phenyltoloxamine Citrate 15 mg	West Decon by Kaiser	00179-1217	Cold Remedy
WW279	Tab	Chlorpheniramine Maleate 5 mg, Phenylephrine HCl 10 mg, Phenylpropanolamine HCl 40 mg, Phenyltoloxamine Citrate 15 mg	West-Decon by West Ward	00143-1279	Cold Remedy
WW279	Tab	Chlorpheniramine Maleate 5 mg, Phenylephrine HCl 10 mg, Phenylpropanolamine HCl 40 mg, Phenyltoloxamine Citrate 15 mg	Tri-Phen-Chlor by Rugby	00536-5655	Cold Remedy
WW279	Tab	Chlorpheniramine Maleate 5 mg, Phenylephrine HCl 10 mg, Phenylpropanolamine HCl 40 mg, Phenyltoloxamine Citrate 15 mg	Uni Decon by United Res	00677-0472	Cold Remedy
WW279	Tab, Pink Specks	Chlorpheniramine Maleate 5 mg, Phenylephrine HCl 10 mg, Phenylpropanolamine HCl 40 mg, Phenyltoloxamine Citrate 15 mg	Decongest by Pharmedix	53002-0306	Cold Remedy
WW455	Tab, White, Round	Phenobarbital 60 mg	by WestWard Pharm	00143-1455	Sedative/Hypnotic; C IV
WW455	Tab, White, Round	Phenobarbital 60 mg	by Physicians Total Care	54868-3997	Sedative/Hypnotic; C IV
WW456	Tab, White, Round	Phenobarbital 90 mg	by WestWard Pharm	00143-1456	Sedative/Hypnotic; C IV
WW456	Tab, White, Round	Phenobarbital 90 mg	by Physicians Total Care	54868-3998	Sedative/Hypnotic; C IV
WW53	Tab, Pink, Round	Stanozolol 2 mg	Winstrol by Sanofi		Anabolic Steroid; C III
WW771	Tab	Isosorbide Dinitrate 10 mg	by Heartland	61392-0305	Antianginal
WW772	Tab	Isosorbide Dinitrate 20 mg	by Heartland	61392-0321	Antianginal
WWW <> 771	Tab, White, Round	Isosorbide Dinitrate 10 mg	Isordil by West Ward	00143-1771	Antianginal
WWW <> 772	Tab, Green, Round	Isosorbide Dinitrate 20 mg	Isordil by West Ward	00143-1772	Antianginal
WYETH <> 227	Tab, Pink, Scored	Promethazine HCl 50 mg	Phenargan by Wyeth Pharms	52903-0227	Antiemetic; Antihistamine
WYETH <> 261	Cap, Red	Meperidine HCl 50 mg, Promethazine HCl 25 mg	Mepergan Fortis by Ayerst	00046-0261	Analgesic; C II
WYETH <> 390	Tab	Penicillin V Potassium	Pen Vee K by Casa De Amigos	62138-0390	Antibiotic
WYETH <> 4125	Tab, Light Green, Tab Ex Release	Isosorbide Dinitrate 40 mg	Isordil by Wyeth Labs	00008-4125	Antianginal
WYETH <> 4130	Tab, Orange, Round	Ethionamide 250 mg	Trecator SC by Ayerst	00046-4130	Antituberculosis
WYETH <> 4191	Cap	Aspirin 356.4 mg, Caffeine 30 mg, Dihydrocodeine Bitartrate 16 mg	Synalgos DC by Quality Care	60346-0303	Analgesic; C III
WYETH <> 4191	Cap	Aspirin 356.4 mg, Caffeine 30 mg, Dihydrocodeine Bitartrate 16 mg	Synalgos DC by Wyeth Labs	00008-4191	Analgesic; C III
WYETH <> 56	Tab	Ethinyl Estradiol 0.05 mg, Norgestrel 0.5 mg	Ovral by Quality Care	60346-0715	Oral Contraceptive
WYETH <> 56	Tab	Ethinyl Estradiol 0.05 mg, Norgestrel 0.5 mg	Ovral by PDRX	55289-0245	Oral Contraceptive
WYETH <> 56	Tab	Ethinyl Estradiol 0.05 mg, Norgestrel 0.5 mg	Ovral by MS Dept Hlth	50596-0026	Oral Contraceptive
WYETH <> 560	Cap	Amoxicillin Trihydrate	Wymox by Allscripts	54569-1509	Antibiotic
WYETH <> 59	Tab, Flat-faced, Beveled Edges	Penicillin V Potassium	by Kaiser	00179-0081	Antibiotic
WYETH <> 78	Tab	Ethinyl Estradiol 0.03 mg, Norgestrel 0.3 mg	Lo Ovral by PDRX	55289-0246	Oral Contraceptive
WYETH <> 78	Tab	Ethinyl Estradiol 0.03 mg, Norgestrel 0.3 mg	Lo Ovral 28 by Dept Health Central Pharm	53808-0028	Oral Contraceptive
WYETH <> 85	Tab, Coated	Acetaminophen 650 mg, Propoxyphene HCl 65 mg	Wygesic by Wyeth Labs	00008-0085	Analgesic; C IV
WYETH1	Tab, White, Round	Meprobamate 400 mg	Equanil by Wyeth		Sedative/Hypnotic; C IV
WYETH19	Tab, Orange, Round	Promethazine 12.5 mg	Phenergan by Wyeth		Antiemetic; Antihistamine
WYETH2	Tab, White, Pentagonal	Meprobamate 200 mg	Equanil by Wyeth		Sedative/Hypnotic; C IV
WYETH200	Tab, Pink, Round	Promazine 100 mg	Sparine by Wyeth		Antipsychotic
WYETH227	Tab, Pink, Round	Promethazine 50 mg	Phenergan by Wyeth		Antiemetic; Antihistamine

ID FRONT <> BACK	DESCRIPTION FRONT <> BACK	INGREDIENT & STRENGTH	BRAND (OR EQUIV.) & FIRM	NDC#	CLASS; SCH.
WYETH27	Tab, Tab Coated	Promethazine HCl 25 mg	Phenergan by Allscripts	54569-0358	Antiemetic; Antihistamine
WYETH27	Tab, Tab Coated	Promethazine HCl 25 mg	Phenergan by Wyeth	52903-0027	Antiemetic; Antihistamine
WYETH28	Tab, Red, Round	Promazine 50 mg	Sparine by Wyeth		Antipsychotic
WYETH29	Tab, Yellow, Round	Promazine 25 mg	Sparine by Wyeth		Antipsychotic
WYETH309	Cap, Pink & Purple	Ampicillin 500 mg	Omnipen by Wyeth		Antibiotic
WYETH33	Tab, Yellow, Round	Meprobamate 400 mg	Equanil by Wyeth		Sedative/Hypnotic; C IV
WYETH360	Cap, Purple & White	Dicloxacillin Sodium Monohydrate 250 mg	Pathocil by Wyeth		Antibiotic
WYETH389	Cap, Yellow & Blue	Tetracycline HCl 250 mg	Achromycin V by Wyeth		Antibiotic
WYETH390	Tab, White, Round	Penicillin V Potassium 500 mg	Pen Vee K by Wyeth		Antibiotic
WYETH4132	Cap, Blue & Yellow	Trimipramine Maleate 25 mg	Surmontil by Wyeth		Antidepressant
WYETH4133	Cap, Blue & Yellow	Trimipramine Maleate 50 mg	Surmontil by Wyeth		Antidepressant
WYETH4140	Cap, Blue & Clear	Isosorbide Dinitrate SA 40 mg	Isordil by Wyeth		Antianginal
WYETH4152	Tab, Pink, Round	Isosorbide Dinitrate 5 mg	Isordil by Wyeth Pharms	52903-4152	Antianginal
WYETH4152	Tab, Pink, Round	Isosorbide Dinitrate Oral 5 mg	Isordil by Wyeth		Antianginal
WYETH4153	Tab, White, Round, Scored	Isosorbide Dinitrate 10 mg	Isordil by Amerisource Health	62584-0061	Antianginal
WYETH4153	Tab, White, Round, Scored	Isosorbide Dinitrate 10 mg	Isordil by Rx Pac	65084-0214	Antianginal
WYETH4153	Tab, Wyeth over 4153	Isosorbide Dinitrate 10 mg	Isordil by Wyeth Labs	00008-4153	Antianginal
WYETH4153	Tab	Isosorbide Dinitrate 10 mg	Isordil Titradose by Thrift Drug	59198-0283	Antianginal
WYETH4154	Tab	Isosorbide Dinitrate 20 mg	Isordil by Wyeth Labs	00008-4154	Antianginal
WYETH4154	Tab	Isosorbide Dinitrate 20 mg	Isordil Titradose by Thrift Drug	59198-0146	Antianginal
WYETH4158	Cap, Blue & Yellow	Trimipramine Maleate 100 mg	Surmontil by Wyeth		Antidepressant
WYETH4159	Tab	Isosorbide Dinitrate 30 mg	Isordil Titradose by Wyeth Labs	00008-4159	Antianginal
WYETH4177 <> SECTRAL200	Cap, Orange & Purple	Acebutolol HCl 200 mg	Sectral by Wyeth Pharms	52903-4177	Antihypertensive
WYETH4179 <> SECTRAL400	Cap, Brown & Orange, Opaque	Acebutolol HCl 400 mg	Sectral by Abbott	60692-3871	Antihypertensive
WYETH4179 <> SECTRAL400	Cap, Brown & Orange	Acebutolol HCl 400 mg	Sectral by Wyeth Pharms	52903-4179	Antihypertensive
WYETH4181 <> ORUDIS50	Cap, Dark Green & Light Green	Ketoprofen 50 mg	Orudis by Allscripts	54569-2178	NSAID
WYETH4181 <> ORUDIS50	Cap, Dark Green & Light Green	Ketoprofen 50 mg	Orudis by Quality Care	60346-0253	NSAID
WYETH4187 <> ORUDIS75	Cap, Coated	Ketoprofen 75 mg	Orudis by Wyeth Labs	00008-4187	NSAID
WYETH4187 <> ORUDIS75	Cap	Ketoprofen 75 mg	Ketoprofen by Pharmedix	53002-0531	NSAID
WYETH4187 <> ORUDIS75	Cap	Ketoprofen 75 mg	Orudis by Nat Pharmpak Serv	55154-4201	NSAID
WYETH4187 <> ORUDIS75	Cap, Dark Green	Ketoprofen 75 mg	Orudis by Thrift Drug	59198-0087	NSAID
WYETH4187 <> ORUDIS75	Cap, Dark Green	Ketoprofen 75 mg	Orudis by Amerisource	62584-0187	NSAID
WYETH4187 <> ORUDIS75	Cap, Dark-Green and White, Coated	Ketoprofen 75 mg	Orudis by Quality Care	60346-0443	NSAID
WYETH4188 <> C200	Tab	Amiodarone HCl 200 mg	Cordarone by Amerisource	62584-0345	Antiarrhythmic
WYETH4188 <> C200	Tab, Wyeth/4188 <> C/200	Amiodarone HCl 200 mg	Cordarone by Wyeth Labs	00008-4188	Antiarrhythmic
WYETH4188 <> C200	Tab, Wyeth/4188 <> C 200	Amiodarone HCl 200 mg	Cordarone by Caremark	00339-6082	Antiarrhythmic
WYETH4188 <> C200	Tab	Amiodarone HCl 200 mg	Cordarone by Nat Pharmpak Serv	55154-4202	Antiarrhythmic
WYETH4188 <> C200	Tab	Amiodarone HCl 200 mg	by Med Pro	53978-2092	Antiarrhythmic
WYETH4191	Cap	Aspirin 356.4 mg, Caffeine 30 mg, Dihydrocodeine Bitartrate 16 mg	Synalgos DC by Pharmedix	53002-0118	Analgesic; C III

ID FRONT <> BACK	DESCRIPTION FRONT <> BACK	INGREDIENT & STRENGTH	BRAND (OR EQUIV.) & FIRM	NDC#	CLASS; SCH.
WYETH4192	Tab, Green, Round	Isosorbide Dinitrate Oral 40 mg	Isordil by Wyeth		Antianginal
WYETH434	Tab, Orange & White, Round	Promethazine 6.25 mg, Pseudoephedrine 60 mg	Phenergan D by Wyeth		Cold Remedy
WYETH445	Tab, Pink, Round	Inert	Ovral 28 by Wyeth		Placebo
WYETH464	Tab, White, Oblong	Nafcillin Sodium 500 mg	Unipen by Wyeth		Antibiotic
WYETH471	Cap, Yellow & Blue	Tetracycline HCl 500 mg	Achromycin V by Wyeth		Antibiotic
WYETH486	Tab, Pink, Round	Inert	Lo Ovral 28 by Wyeth		Placebo
WYETH486 <> WYETH78	Tab	Ethinyl Estradiol 0.03 mg, Norgestrel 0.3 mg	Lo Ovral 28 by Pharm Utilization	60491-0367	Oral Contraceptive
WYETH51 <> SERAX10	Cap, Wyeth-51 x 3 with 10 triangles <> Serax 10 x 5, Coated	Oxazepam 10 mg	Serax by Wyeth Labs	00008-0051	Sedative/Hypnotic; C IV
WYETH53	Cap, Pink & Purple	Ampicillin 250 mg	Omnipen by Wyeth		Antibiotic
WYETH559	Cap	Amoxicillin Trihydrate	Wymox by Allscripts	54569-1508	Antibiotic
WYETH56	Tab	Ethinyl Estradiol 0.05 mg, Norgestrel 0.5 mg	Ovral by Apotheca	12634-0480	Oral Contraceptive
WYETH560	Cap, Gray & Green	Amoxicillin 500 mg	Wymox by Wyeth		Antibiotic
WYETH57	Cap, Green & Yellow	Nafcillin Sodium 250 mg	Unipen by Wyeth		Antibiotic
WYETH576	Tab, Pink, Round	Erythromycin Ethylsuccinate 250 mg	Wyamycin S by Wyeth		Antibiotic
WYETH578	Tab, Pink, Oval	Erythromycin Ethylsuccinate 500 mg	Wyamycin S by Wyeth		Antibiotic
WYETH59	Tab	Penicillin V Potassium	by Med Pro	53978-5042	Antibiotic
WYETH593	Cap, Purple & White	Dicloxacillin Sodium Monohydrate 500 mg	Pathocil by Wyeth		Antibiotic
WYETH6 <> SERAX15	Cap, Wyeth-6 x 3 with 10 Triangles <> Serax 10 x 5, Coated	Oxazepam 15 mg	Serax by Wyeth Labs	00008-0006	Sedative/Hypnotic; C IV
WYETH614	Tab, Yellow, Oblong	Cyclacillin 250 mg	Cyclapen-W by Wyeth		Antibiotic
WYETH615	Tab, Yellow, Oblong	Cyclacillin 500 mg	Cyclapen-W by Wyeth		Antibiotic
WYETH62	Tab, Yellow, Round	Norgestrel 0.075 mg	Ovrette by Wyeth		Oral Contraceptive
WYETH64 <> A	Tab	Lorazepam 1 mg	Ativan by Physicians Total Care	54868-1339	Sedative/Hypnotic; C IV
WYETH64 <> A	Tab	Lorazepam 1 mg	Ativan by Med Pro	53978-3086	Sedative/Hypnotic; C IV
WYETH64 <> A	Tab, White, Scored	Lorazepam 1 mg	Ativan by Natl Pharmapk	55154-4204	Sedative/Hypnotic; C IV
WYETH64 <> A	Tab	Lorazepam 1 mg	Ativan by Wyeth Labs	00008-0064	Sedative/Hypnotic; C IV
WYETH641	Tab, Brown, Round	Levonorgestrel 0.05 mg, Ethinyl Estradiol 0.03 mg	Triphasil by Wyeth		Oral Contraceptive
WYETH642	Tab, White, Round	Levonorgestrel 0.075 mg, Ethinyl Estradiol 0.04 mg	Triphasil by Wyeth		Oral Contraceptive
WYETH643	Tab, Yellow, Round	Levonorgestrel 0.125 mg, Ethinyl Estradiol 0.03 mg	Triphasil by Wyeth		Oral Contraceptive
WYETH65 <> A	Tab	Lorazepam 2 mg	Ativan by Wyeth Labs	00008-0065	Sedative/Hypnotic; C IV
WYETH650	Tab, Blue, Round	Inert	Triphasil 28 by Wyeth		Placebo
WYETH71	Tab, White, Round	Mazindol 1 mg	Mazanor by Wyeth		Anorexiant
WYETH73 <> W4	Tab, Coated	Guanabenz Acetate 4 mg	Wytensin by Wyeth Labs	00008-0073	Antihypertensive
WYETH75	Tab, Orange, Round	Levonorgestrel 0.15 mg, Ethinyl Estradiol 0.03 mg	Nordette by Wyeth		Oral Contraceptive
WYETH78	Tab,	Ethinyl Estradiol 0.03 mg, Norgestrel 0.3 mg	Lo Ovral 28 by Physicians Total Care	54868-0428	Oral Contraceptive
WYETH78	Tab, White, Round	Ethinyl Estradiol 0.03 mg; Ferrous Fumarate 75 mg; Norgestrel 0.3 mg	by Wyeth Pharms	52903-2542	Oral Contraceptive
WYETH78 <> WYETH486	Tab	Ethinyl Estradiol 0.03 mg, Norgestrel 0.3 mg	Lo Ovral 28 by Pharm Utilization	60491-0367	Oral Contraceptive
WYETH81 <> A	Tab	Lorazepam 0.5 mg	Ativan by Wyeth Labs	00008-0081	Sedative/Hypnotic; C IV
WYETH81 <> A	Tab	Lorazepam 0.5 mg	Ativan by Med Pro	53978-3085	Sedative/Hypnotic; C IV
WYETH91	Tab, Pink, Tab/Yellow, Round	Meprobamate 200 mg, Aspirin 325 mg	Equagesic by Wyeth		Sedative/Hypnotic; C IV
X <> 35	Tab, White, Round	Phendimetrazine Tartrate 35 mg	by Allscripts	54569-2668	Anorexiant; C III
X <> 7301	Tab, Hourglass Logo, Film Coated	Verapamil HCl 180 mg	by Heartland	61392-0345	Antihypertensive
X3A <> LANOXIN	Tab	Digoxin 0.25 mg	Lanoxin by Catalytica	63552-0249	Cardiac Agent
X3A <> LANOXIN	Tab	Digoxin 0.25 mg	Lanoxin by Amerisource	62584-0249	Cardiac Agent
X3A <> LANOXIN	Tab, White, Scored	Digoxin 0.25 mg	Lanoxin by Va Cmop	65243-0024	Cardiac Agent
X3A <> LANOXIN	Tab	Digoxin 0.25 mg	by Med Pro	53978-3060	Cardiac Agent
X7300	Tab, Ivory, Oblong	Verapamil HCl ER 240 mg	Isoptin,Calan SR by Baker		Antihypertensive
XANAX <> 2	Tab, White, Oblong, Coated	Alprazolam 2 mg	Xanax by Pharmacia & Upjohn	00009-0094	Antianxiety; C IV
XANAX 10	Tab, Xanax 1.0	Alprazolam 1 mg	Xanax by Nat Pharmpak Serv	55154-3920	Antianxiety; C IV
XANAX025	Tab, Xanax 0.25	Alprazolam 0.25 mg	Xanax by Amerisource	62584-0035	Antianxiety; C IV
XANAX025	Tab, Xanax 0.25	Alprazolam 0.25 mg	Xanax by Quality Care	60346-0051	Antianxiety; C IV

ID FRONT <> BACK	DESCRIPTION FRONT <> BACK	INGREDIENT & STRENGTH	BRAND (OR EQUIV.) & FIRM	NDC#	CLASS; SCH.
XANAX025	Tab, White, Oval, Xanax 0.25	Alprazolam 0.25 mg	Xanax by Pharmacia & Upjohn	00009-0029	Antianxiety; C IV
XANAX025	Tab, Coated, Xanax 0.25	Alprazolam 0.25 mg	by Med Pro	53978-1300	Antianxiety; C IV
XANAX025	Tab, Xanax over 0.25	Alprazolam 0.25 mg	Xanax by Allscripts	54569-0953	Antianxiety; C IV
XANAX025	Tab, Xanax 0.25	Alprazolam 0.25 mg	Xanax by Nat Pharmpak Serv	55154-3921	Antianxiety; C IV
XANAX025	Tab	Alprazolam 0.25 mg	Xanax by Nat Pharmpak Serv	55154-3921	Antianxiety; C IV
XANAX025	Tab, Xanax 0.25	Alprazolam 0.25 mg	Xanax by Med Pro	53978-3091	Antianxiety; C IV
XANAX05	Tab, Xanax 0.5	Alprazolam 0.5 mg	Xanax by Amerisource	62584-0036	Antianxiety; C IV
XANAX05	Tab, Xanax 0.5	Alprazolam 0.5 mg	Xanax by Quality Care	60346-0567	Antianxiety; C IV
XANAX05	Tab, Peach, Oval, Xanax 0.5	Alprazolam 0.5 mg	Xanax by Pharmacia & Upjohn	00009-0055	Antianxiety; C IV
XANAX05	Tab, Xanax 0.5	Alprazolam 0.5 mg	Xanax by Caremark	00339-4041	Antianxiety; C IV
XANAX05	Tab, Xanax 0.5	Alprazolam 0.5 mg	Xanax by Allscripts	54569-0954	Antianxiety; C IV
XANAX05	Tab	Alprazolam 0.5 mg	Xanax by Nat Pharmpak Serv	55154-3919	Antianxiety; C IV
XANAX05	Tab, Xanax 0.5	Alprazolam 0.5 mg	by Pharmedix	53002-0395	Antianxiety; C IV
XANAX10	Tab, Xanax 1.0	Alprazolam 1 mg	Xanax by Med Pro	53978-3090	Antianxiety; C IV
XANAX10	Tab	Alprazolam 1 mg	Xanax by Med Pro	53978-3089	Antianxiety; C IV
XANAX10	Tab, Xanax 1.0	Alprazolam 1 mg	Xanax by Allscripts	54569-1769	Antianxiety; C IV
XANAX10	Tab, Light Blue, Oval, Xanaz 1.0	Alprazolam 1 mg	Xanax by Amerisource	62584-0037	Antianxiety; C IV
XELODA <> 150	Tab, Film Coated	Capecitabine 150 mg	Xanax by Pharmacia & Upjohn	00009-0090	Antianxiety; C IV
XELODA <> 500	Tab, Film Coated	Capecitabine 500 mg	Xeloda by Hoffmann La Roche	00004-1100	Antineoplastic
XELODA150	Tab, Light Peach, Oblong, Xeloda/150	Capecitabine 150 mg	Xeloda by Hoffmann La Roche	00004-1101	Antineoplastic
XENICAL120 <> ROCHE	Cap, Blue, Hard Gel	Orlistat 120 mg	Xeloda by Roche	Canadian	Antineoplastic
XENICAL120 <> ROCHE	Cap, Blue, Opaque, Hard Gel	Orlistat 120 mg	Xenical by PDRX	55289-0544	Lipase Inhibitor
XPMS1	Tab, Salmon, Round, x/PMS-1	Benztropine Mesylate 1 mg	Xenical by PDRX	55289-0521	Lipase Inhibitor
Y	Tab, Pink, Round	Yohimbine HCl 2 mg	by Pharmascience	Canadian	Antiparkinson
Y3B <> LANOXIN	Tab, Yellow, Scored	Digoxin 0.125 mg	by Pharmascience	Canadian	Impotence Agent
Y3B <> LANOXIN	Tab	Digoxin 0.125 mg	Lanoxin by Va Cmop	65243-0023	Cardiac Agent
Y3B <> LANOXIN	Tab	Digoxin 0.125 mg	Lanoxin by Amerisource	62584-0242	Cardiac Agent
Y3B <> LANOXIN	Tab	Digoxin 0.125 mg	Lanoxin by Catalytica	63552-0242	Cardiac Agent
Y3B <> LANOXIN	Tab	Digoxin 0.125 mg	by Med Pro	53978-3061	Cardiac Agent
Y3B <> LANOXIN	Tab	Digoxin 0.125 mg	Lanoxin by Quality Care	60346-0396	Cardiac Agent
Y3B <> LANOXIN	Tab	Digoxin 125 mcg	Lanoxin by Thrift Drug	59198-0232	Cardiac Agent
Y9C100 <> WELLCOME	Cap, Dark Blue Band, Unicorn Logo	Zidovudine 100 mg	Retrovir by Catalytica	63552-0108	Antiviral
Y9C100 <> WELLCOME	Cap, Dark Blue Band, Unicorn Logo	Zidovudine 100 mg	Zidovudine by Med Pro	53978-2098	Antiviral
Y9C100 <> WELLCOME	Cap, White with Dark Blue Band	Zidovudine 100 mg	Retrovir by Allscripts	54569-1772	Antiviral
Y9C100 <> WELLCOME	Cap, Dark Blue Band, Y9C 100 with Dark Blue Band, and Unicorn Logo, with Dark Blue Band	Zidovudine 100 mg	Retrovir by Pharm Utilization	60491-0561	Antiviral
Y9C100 <> WELLCOME	Cap, Blue Band, Y9C Over 100 <> Wellcome	Zidovudine 100 mg	Retrovir by Quality Care	62682-1015	Antiviral
Y9C100 <> WELLCOME	Cap, PLUS Logo	Zidovudine 100 mg	Retrovir by Prepackage Spec	58864-0462	Antiviral
Y9C100 <> WELLCOME	Cap, White, Dark Blue Band, Y9C 100 <> Wellcome Unicorn Logo	Zidovudine 100 mg	Retrovir by Amerisource	62584-0464	Antiviral
Y9C100 <> WELLCOMEUNICORN	Cap, Dark Blue Band, Dark Blue Band, Unicorn Logo	Zidovudine 100 mg	Retrovir by Glaxo	00173-0108	Antiviral
YELLOW780	Tab	Isosorbide Dinitrate 10 mg	Sorbitrate by Pharmedix	53002-1047	Antianginal
YF	Tab, Forest Logo YF	Levothyroxine Sodium 100 mcg, Liothyronine Sodium 25 mcg	Thyrolar 2 by Allscripts	54569-3640	Antithyroid
YJ2243850	Cap, Lime Green with Black Stripes	Ephedra Extract 300 mg, Colanut, Ginseng	Yellow Jacket #87 by NVE Pharm		Supplement
YJ244385	Black & Yellow, with 3 Black Stripes	Ephedra Extract 300 mg, Colanut, Ginseng	by NVE Pharm		Supplement
YOCON53	Tab	Yohimbine HCl 5.4 mg	Yocon by Thrift Drug	59198-0116	Impotence Agent
YOCON53	Tab, Yocon/53	Yohimbine HCl 5.4 mg	Yocon by Nat Pharmpak Serv	55154-6001	Impotence Agent
YUTOPAR	Tab, Yellow, Round	Ritodrine HCl 10 mg	by Bristol	Canadian	Urinary Relaxant
Z <> 2416	Cap	Tetracycline HCl 250 mg	by Quality Care	60346-0609	Antibiotic
Z <> 2908	Tab	Furosemide 20 mg	by Quality Care	60346-0761	Diuretic
Z <> 2909	Cap	Hydroxyzine Pamoate	by Schein	00364-0484	Antihistamine
Z <> 2985	Cap, Light Blue	Doxycycline Hyclate	by Quality Care	60346-0109	Antibiotic

ID FRONT ⟨⟩ BACK	DESCRIPTION FRONT ⟨⟩ BACK	INGREDIENT & STRENGTH	BRAND (OR EQUIV.) & FIRM	NDC#	CLASS; SCH.
			by Quality Care	60346-0507	Antibiotic
Z ⟨⟩ 3007	Tab, Zenith Logo, Tab Coated	Metronidazole 500 mg	by Quality Care	60346-0449	Antibiotic
Z ⟨⟩ 3626	Cap	Doxycycline Hyclate	by Quality Care	60346-0684	NSAID
Z ⟨⟩ 4029	Cap	Indomethacin 25 mg	by Quality Care	60346-0733	NSAID
Z ⟨⟩ 4030	Cap	Indomethacin 50 mg	Keflex by Zenith Goldline	00172-4073	Antibiotic
Z ⟨⟩ 4073	Cap, Gray & Red	Cephalexin Monohydrate 250 mg	by Quality Care	60346-0055	Antibiotic
Z ⟨⟩ 4074	Cap, Logo	Cephalexin Monohydrate	Keflex by Zenith Goldline	00172-4074	Antibiotic
Z ⟨⟩ 4074	Cap, Red	Cephalexin Monohydrate 500 mg	by Quality Care	60346-0816	NSAID
Z ⟨⟩ 4107	Tab	Naproxen 250 mg	by Novartis	61615-0017	NSAID
Z ⟨⟩ 4107	Tab, White, Round, Uncoated	Naproxen 250 mg	Wytensin by Zenith Goldline	00172-4226	Antihypertensive
Z ⟨⟩ 4226	Tab, Peach, Round	Guanabenz Acetate 4 mg	Wytensin by Zenith Goldline	00172-4227	Antihypertensive
Z ⟨⟩ 4227	Tab, Gray, Round	Guanabenz Acetate 8 mg	Bumex by Zenith Goldline	00172-4232	Diuretic
Z ⟨⟩ 423205	Tab, Green, Round, Z ⟨⟩ 4232 0.5	Bumetanide 0.5 mg	Bumex by Zenith Goldline	00172-4233	Diuretic
Z ⟨⟩ 42331	Tab, Yellow, Round, Z ⟨⟩ 4233 1	Bumetanide 1 mg	Bumex by Zenith Goldline	00172-4234	Diuretic
Z ⟨⟩ 42342	Tab, Peach, Round, Z ⟨⟩ 4234 2	Bumetanide 2 mg	Lozol by Zenith Goldline	00172-4259	Diuretic
Z ⟨⟩ 4259	Tab, White, Round, Coated	Indapamide 2.5 mg	by Physicians Total Care	54868-3106	Diuretic
Z ⟨⟩ 4259	Tab, Tab Coated, Debossed	Indapamide 2.5 mg	by Qualitest	00603-4061	Diuretic
Z ⟨⟩ 4259	Tab, Tab Coated	Indapamide 2.5 mg	by Major	00904-5074	Diuretic
Z ⟨⟩ 4259	Tab, Tab Coated, Debossed	Indapamide 2.5 mg	by Qualitest	00603-4161	Diuretic
Z ⟨⟩ 4259	Tab, Tab Coated, Debossed	Indapamide 2.5 mg	by Geneva	00781-1051	Diuretic
Z ⟨⟩ 4259	Tab, Tab Coated, Debossed	Indapamide 2.5 mg	Glycron by Mova Pharms	55370-0592	Antidiabetic
Z ⟨⟩ M0315	Tab, White, Oval, Scored	Glyburide 1.5 mg	Glycron by Mova Pharms	55370-0594	Antidiabetic
Z ⟨⟩ M0430	Tab, Blue, Oval, Scored	Glyburide 3 mg	Glycron by Mova Pharms	55370-0595	Antidiabetic
Z ⟨⟩ M0645	Tab, Green, Oval, Scored	Glyburide 4.5 mg	Glycron by Mova Pharms	55370-0596	Antidiabetic
Z ⟨⟩ M0760	Tab, Yellow, Oval, Scored	Glyburide 6 mg	Robaxisal by Zenith Goldline	00182-1911	Analgesic; Muscle Relaxant
Z 2813	Tab, Pink & White, Round	Aspirin 325 mg, Methocarbamol 400 mg	Stelazine by Zenith Goldline		Antipsychotic
Z12916	Tab, Lavender, Round, Z-1 2916	Trifluoperazine HCl 1 mg	by Zenith Goldline	00172-7111	Gastrointestinal
Z200 ⟨⟩ 7111	Tab, Tab Coated	Cimetidine 200 mg	Colchicine by Zenith Goldline		Antigout
Z2047	Tab, White, Round	Colchicine 0.6 mg	Benadryl byZenith Goldline		Antihistamine
Z2055	Cap, Clear & Pink	Diphenhydramine HCl 25 mg	Benadryl by Zenith Goldline		Antihistamine
Z2056	Cap, Pink	Diphenhydramine HCl 50 mg	by Zenith Goldline	00172-2057	Anticonvulsant
Z2057	Cap, Natural	Phenytoin Sodium 100 mg	Lanoxin by Zenith Goldline		Cardiac Agent
Z2058	Tab, White, Round	Digoxin 0.25 mg	by Allscripts	54569-0547	Diuretic
Z2083	Tab, Light Orange, Round, Scored	Hydrochlorothiazide 25 mg	Hydrodiuril by Zenith Goldline	00182-0556	Diuretic
Z2083	Tab, Peach, Round	Hydrochlorothiazide 25 mg	Hydrodiuril by Zenith Goldline	00172-2083	Diuretic
Z2083	Tab, Peach, Round	Hydrochlorothiazide 25 mg	Hctz by Quality Care	60346-0184	Diuretic
Z2083	Tab	Hydrochlorothiazide 25 mg	by Kaiser	62224-1441	Diuretic
Z2083	Tab, Debossed	Hydrochlorothiazide 25 mg	by Baker Cummins	63171-0556	Diuretic
Z2083	Tab, Debossed	Hydrochlorothiazide 25 mg	by Allscripts	54569-0549	Diuretic
Z2089	Tab, Light Orange, Round, Scored	Hydrochlorothiazide 50 mg	Hydrodiuril by Zenith Goldline	00172-2089	Diuretic
Z2089	Tab, Peach, Round	Hydrochlorothiazide 50 mg	Hydrodiuril by Zenith Goldline	00182-0557	Diuretic
Z2089	Tab, Peach, Round	Hydrochlorothiazide 50 mg	by DRX	55045-1431	Diuretic
Z2089	Tab	Hydrochlorothiazide 50 mg	by Murfreesboro	51129-1312	Diuretic
Z2089	Tab, Orange, Round, Scored	Hydrochlorothiazide 50 mg	by Pharmedix	53002-0362	Diuretic
Z2089	Tab	Hydrochlorothiazide 50 mg	by Kaiser	62224-1445	Diuretic
Z2089	Tab, Debossed	Hydrochlorothiazide 50 mg	by Baker Cummins	63171-0557	Diuretic
Z2089	Tab	Hydrochlorothiazide 50 mg	Hctz by Quality Care	60346-0675	Diuretic
Z2089	Tab, Light Orange	Hydrochlorothiazide 50 mg	by Golden State	60429-0213	Diuretic
Z2089	Tab	Hydrochlorothiazide 50 mg	by Compumed	00403-1026	Diuretic
Z2089	Tab, Peach, Round, Scored	Hydrochlorothiazide 50 mg	Macrodantin by Zenith Goldline	00172-2130	Antibiotic
Z2130	Cap, Pink & White	Nitrofurantoin 50 mg	by Qualitest	00603-4776	Antibiotic
Z2130	Cap	Nitrofurantoin 50 mg			

ID FRONT <> BACK	DESCRIPTION FRONT <> BACK	INGREDIENT & STRENGTH	BRAND (OR EQUIV.) & FIRM	NDC#	CLASS; SCH.
Z2130	Cap, Pink & White	Nitrofurantoin Macrocrystallines 50 mg	Macrodantin by Zenith	00172-1944	Antibiotic
Z2130	Cap, White	Nitrofurantoin Macrocrystalline 50 mg	by Goldline Labs	00182-1944	Antibiotic
Z2131	Cap, Pink, Macro Caps	Nitrofurantoin 100 mg	Macrodantin by Zenith Goldline	00182-1945	Antibiotic
Z2131	Cap, Pink	Nitrofurantoin 100 mg	Macrodantin by Zenith Goldline	00172-2131	Antibiotic
Z2131	Cap	Nitrofurantoin 100 mg	by United Res	00677-1225	Antibiotic
Z2131	Cap	Nitrofurantoin 100 mg	by Qualitest	00603-4777	Antibiotic
Z2168	Tab, Green, Round	Hydrochlorothiazide 50 mg, Reserpine (Hydroserpine #2) 0.125 mg	Hydropres by Zenith Goldline		Diuretic; Antihypertensive
Z2169	Tab, Green, Round	Hydrochlorothiazide 25 mg, Reserpine (Hydroserpine #1) 0.125 mg	Hydropres by Zenith Goldline		Diuretic; Antihypertensive
Z2184	Cap, Clear	Quinine Sulfate 325 mg	Quinine Sulfate by Zenith Goldline	00172-4172	Antimalarial
Z2186	Cap, Pink, Z-2186	Propoxyphene HCl 65 mg	Daryon-65 by Zenith Goldline	00172-2186	Analgesic; C IV
Z2186	Cap, Pink	Propoxyphene HCl 65 mg	Daryon-65 by Zenith Goldline	00182-0698	Analgesic; C IV
Z2186	Cap, Pale Pink, Cap Coated	Propoxyphene HCl 65 mg	by Quality Care	60346-0693	Analgesic; C IV
Z2190	Tab, Yellow, Oblong, Tab Coated	Probenecid 500 mg	Benemid by Zenith Goldline	00172-2190	Antigout
Z2190	Tab, Film Coated	Probenecid 500 mg	by Quality Care	60346-0768	Antigout
Z2190	Tab, Tab Coated	Probenecid 500 mg	by Qualitest	00603-5381	Antigout
Z2190	Tab, Tab Coated	Probenecid 500 mg	by Geneva	00781-1021	Antigout
Z2193	Tab, White, Oblong	Colchicine 0.5 mg, Probenecid 500 mg	Colbenemid by Zenith Goldline	00172-2193	Antigout
Z2193	Tab	Colchicine 0.5 mg, Probenecid 500 mg	by Geneva	00781-1023	Antigout
Z2201	Tab, White, Round	Quinidine Sulfate 200 mg	Quinamm by Zenith Goldline	00172-4171	Antiarrhythmic
Z2218	Tab, White, Round	Sulfisoxazole 500 mg	Gantrisin by Zenith Goldline	00172-2218	Antibiotic
Z2218	Tab	Sulfisoxazole 500 mg	by Physicians Total Care	54868-1535	Antibiotic
Z2218	Tab	Sulfisoxazole 500 mg	by DRX	55045-1450	Antibiotic
Z2218	Tab, Z-2218	Sulfisoxazole 500 mg	by Quality Care	60346-0671	Antibiotic
Z2245 <> G1084	Tab, White, Round	Tolbutamide 500 mg	Orinase by Zenith Goldline	00172-2245	Antidiabetic
Z22940	Tab, Lavender, Round, Z-2 2940	Trifluoperazine HCl 2 mg	Stelazine by Zenith Goldline		Antipsychotic
Z2335	Tab, White, Round	Hydrochlorothiazide 15 mg, Hydralazine 25 mg, Reserpine (Hydroserpine Plus) 0.1 mg	Ser-Ap-Es by Zenith Goldline		Antihypertensive
Z2338	Tab, Orange, Round	Hydralazine HCl 10 mg	Apresoline by Zenith Goldline		Antihypertensive
Z2339	Tab, Orange, Round	Hydralazine HCl 25 mg	Apresoline by Zenith Goldline		Antihypertensive
Z2345	Cap, Yellow	Procainamide HCl 250 mg	Pronestyl by Zenith Goldline	00172-2345	Antiarrhythmic
Z2345	Cap	Procainamide HCl 250 mg	by Qualitest	00603-5404	Antiarrhythmic
Z2345 <> Z2345	Cap, Yellow	Procainamide HCl 250 mg	by Quality Care	62682-5020	Antiarrhythmic
Z2346	Cap, Orange & White	Procainamide HCl 375 mg	Pronestyl by Zenith Goldline	00172-2346	Antiarrhythmic
Z2346	Cap	Procainamide HCl 375 mg	Pronestyl by Zenith Goldline	00182-0925	Antiarrhythmic
Z2346	Cap	Procainamide HCl 375 mg	by Qualitest	00603-5405	Antiarrhythmic
Z2347	Cap	Procainamide HCl 500 mg	Pronestyl by Zenith Goldline	00182-0521	Antiarrhythmic
Z2347	Cap, Orange & Yellow	Procainamide HCl 500 mg	Pronestyl by Zenith Goldline	00172-2347	Antiarrhythmic
Z2347	Cap	Procainamide HCl 500 mg	by Qualitest	00603-5406	Antiarrhythmic
Z2348	Tab, White, Round	Nylidrin HCl 6 mg	Arlidin by Zenith Goldline		Vasodilator
Z2349	Tab, White, Round	Nylidrin HCl 12 mg	Arlidin by Zenith Goldline		Vasodilator
Z2350	Tab, Yellow with White, Oval	Meclizine HCl 25 mg	Antivert by Zenith Goldline		Antiemetic
Z2359	Cap, Natural	Quinine Sulfate 200 mg	Quinamm by Zenith Goldline	00172-4171	Antimalarial
Z2384	Tab, Blue/White, Oval	Meclizine HCl 12.5 mg	Antivert by Zenith Goldline		Antiemetic
Z2387	Tab, White, Round	Isoxsuprine HCl 10 mg	Vasodilan by Zenith Goldline		Vasodilator
Z2388	Tab, White, Round	Isoxsuprine HCl 20 mg	Vasodilan byZenith Goldline		Vasodilator
Z2407	Cap	Tetracycline HCl	by Allscripts	54569-2501	Antibiotic
Z2407	Cap, Black & Yellow	Tetracycline HCl 500 mg	Tetrex by Zenith Goldline	00172-2407	Antibiotic
Z2407	Cap, Zenith Logo	Tetracycline HCl 500 mg	by Quality Care	60346-0435	Antibiotic
Z2407	Cap	Tetracycline HCl 500 mg	by Baker Cummins	63171-0679	Antibiotic
Z2407	Cap, Black & Yellow	Tetracycline HCl 500 mg	Tetrex BID by Zenith Goldline	00182-0679	Antibiotic
Z2407 <> G0112	Cap, Orange & Yellow	Tetracycline HCl 250 mg	Tetrex by Zenith Goldline	00182-0112	Antibiotic

ID FRONT <> BACK	DESCRIPTION FRONT <> BACK	INGREDIENT & STRENGTH	BRAND (OR EQUIV.) & FIRM	NDC#	CLASS; SCH.
Z2407 <> G0679	Cap, Black & Yellow	Tetracycline HCl 500 mg	Tetrex by Zenith Goldline	00182-0679	Antibiotic
Z2407 <> G0679	Cap, Black & Yellow	Tetracycline HCl 500 mg	Tetrex by Zenith Goldline	00172-2407	Antibiotic
Z2416	Cap	Tetracycline HCl	by Allscripts	54569-2279	Antibiotic
Z2416	Cap, Orange & Yellow	Tetracycline HCl 250 mg	Tetrex by Zenith Goldline	00182-0112	Antibiotic
Z2416	Cap	Tetracycline HCl 250 mg	by Quality Care	60346-0609	Antibiotic
Z2416	Cap	Tetracycline HCl 250 mg	by Baker Cummins	63171-0112	Antibiotic
Z2416	Cap	Tetracycline HCl 250 mg	by Apotheca	12634-0186	Antibiotic
Z2416 <> G0112	Cap, Orange & Yellow	Tetracycline HCl 250 mg	Tetrex by Zenith Goldline	00172-2416	Antibiotic
Z2416 <> Z2416	Cap, in Black Ink	Tetracycline HCl 250 mg	by Kaiser	00179-1020	Antibiotic
Z2430	Cap, Purple/Yellow	Tetracycline HCl 250 mg	Achromycin V by Zenith Goldline		Antibiotic
Z2458	Tab, Pink, Round	Erythromycin Stearate 250 mg	Erythrocin by Zenith Goldline		Antibiotic
Z2485	Tab, Light Orange, Round, Coated, Z-2485	Hydrochlorothiazide 100 mg	Hydrodiuril by Zenith Goldline	00172-2485	Diuretic
Z2493	Tab, Orange, Round	Hydralazine HCl 50 mg	Apresoline by Zenith Goldline		Antihypertensive
Z2507	Tab, Green, Round	Reserpine 0.125 mg, Hydroflumethiazide 50 mg	Salutensin by Zenith Goldline		Antihypertensive
Z2813	Tab, Tab Layered	Aspirin 325 mg, Methocarbamol 400 mg	by Quality Care	60346-0956	Analgesic; Muscle Relaxant
Z2813	Tab, Pink & White, Round	Aspirin 325 mg, Methocarbamol 400 mg	Robaxisal by Zenith Goldline	00172-2813	Analgesic; Muscle Relaxant
Z2814	Cap, Orange	Cyclandelate 200 mg	Cyclospasmol by Zenith Goldline		Vasodilator
Z2815	Cap, Green & White	Cyclandelate 400 mg	Cyclospasmol by Zenith Goldline		Vasodilator
Z2823	Tab, Pink, Oval	Erythromycin Stearate 500 mg	Erythrocin by Zenith Goldline		Antibiotic
Z2902	Tab, Blue, Round	Chlorpropamide 250 mg	Diabinese by Zenith Goldline		Antidiabetic
Z2903	Tab, White, Round	Spironolactone 25 mg	Aldactone by Zenith Goldline		Diuretic
Z2904	Tab, White, Round	Chlorthalidone 100 mg	Hygroton by Zenith Goldline		Diuretic
Z2907	Tab	Furosemide 40 mg	by Pharmedix	53002-0430	Diuretic
Z2907	Tab	Furosemide 40 mg	by Quality Care	60346-0487	Diuretic
Z2907	Tab	Furosemide 40 mg	by Nat Pharmpak Serv	55154-5803	Diuretic
Z2907	Tab	Furosemide 40 mg	by Baker Cummins	63171-1161	Diuretic
Z2907	Tab, White, Round, Z-2907	Furosemide 40 mg	Lasix by Zenith Goldline	00172-2907	Diuretic
Z2907	Tab, White, Round	Furosemide 40 mg	Lasix by Zenith Goldline	00182-1161	Diuretic
Z2907	Tab	Furosemide 40 mg	by Qualitest	00603-3737	Diuretic
Z2907	Tab	Furosemide 40 mg	by DRX	55045-1217	Diuretic
Z2907	Tab	Furosemide 40 mg	by Med Pro	53978-5032	Diuretic
Z2908	Tab, Debossed	Furosemide 20 mg	by Baker Cummins	63171-1170	Diuretic
Z2908	Tab, White, Oval, Z-2908	Furosemide 20 mg	Lasix by Zenith Goldline	00172-2908	Diuretic
Z2908	Tab, White, Oval	Furosemide 20 mg	Lasix by Zenith Goldline	00182-1170	Diuretic
Z2909	Cap, Zenith Logo 2909	Hydroxyzine Pamoate	by Quality Care	60346-0797	Antihistamine
Z2909	Cap	Hydroxyzine Pamoate	by Medirex	57480-0396	Antihistamine
Z2909	Cap	Hydroxyzine Pamoate	by Baker Cummins	63171-1099	Antihistamine
Z2909	Cap, Green & White	Hydroxyzine Pamoate 50 mg	Vistaril by Zenith Goldline	00182-1099	Antihistamine
Z2909	Cap, Green & White	Hydroxyzine Pamoate 50 mg	Vistaril by UDL	51079-0078	Antihistamine
Z2909	Cap	Hydroxyzine Pamoate 85 mg	by HL Moore	00839-6271	Antihistamine
Z2909	Cap	Hydroxyzine Pamoate 85 mg	by United Res	00677-0597	Antihistamine
Z2909	Cap	Hydroxyzine Pamoate 85 mg	by Geneva	00781-2254	Antihistamine
Z2909 <> G1099	Cap, Green & White	Hydroxyzine Pamoate 50 mg	Vistaril by Zenith Goldline	00172-2909	Antihistamine
Z2909 <> Z2909	Cap	Hydroxyzine Pamoate	by Heartland	61392-0010	Antihistamine
Z2911	Cap, Dark Green & Light Green	Hydroxyzine Pamoate	by PDRX	55289-0226	Antihistamine
Z2911	Cap	Hydroxyzine Pamoate	by Medirex	57480-0395	Antihistamine
Z2911	Cap, Dark Green & Light Green	Hydroxyzine Pamoate	by Nat Pharmpak Serv	55154-5564	Antihistamine
Z2911	Cap	Hydroxyzine Pamoate	by Baker Cummins	63171-1098	Antihistamine
Z2911	Cap	Hydroxyzine Pamoate	by Geneva	00781-2252	Antihistamine
Z2911	Cap, Light Green & Dark Green	Hydroxyzine Pamoate 25 mg	Vistaril by UDL	51079-0077	Antihistamine

ID FRONT <> BACK	DESCRIPTION FRONT <> BACK	INGREDIENT & STRENGTH	BRAND (OR EQUIV.) & FIRM	NDC#	CLASS; SCH.
Z2911	Cap, Light Green & Dark Green, Zenith Logo 2911	Hydroxyzine Pamoate 43 mg	by Quality Care	60346-0208	Antihistamine
Z2911	Cap	Hydroxyzine Pamoate 43 mg	by United Res	00677-0596	Antihistamine
Z2911 <> G1098	Cap, Dark Green & Light Green	Hydroxyzine Pamoate 25 mg	Vistaril by Zenith Goldline	00172-2911	Antihistamine
Z2929	Tab, Debossed	Cyproheptadine 4 mg	by Baker Cummins	63171-1132	Antihistamine
Z2929	Tab	Cyproheptadine 4 mg	by Major	00904-1145	Antihistamine
Z2929	Tab, White, Round, Z-2929	Cyproheptadine HCl 4 mg	Periactin by Zenith Goldline	00172-2929	Antihistamine
Z2929	Tab, White, Round, Z-2929	Cyproheptadine HCl 4 mg	Periactin by Zenith Goldline	00182-1132	Antihistamine
Z2931	Tab, Film Coated	Methyldopa 250 mg	by Baker Cummins	63171-1732	Antihypertensive
Z2931	Tab, Zenith Logo, Film Coated	Methyldopa 250 mg	by Kaiser	00179-1061	Antihypertensive
Z2931	Tab, White, Round	Methyldopa 250 mg	Aldomet by Zenith Goldline	00182-1732	Antihypertensive
Z2931	Tab, White, Round	Methyldopa 250 mg	Aldomet by Zenith Goldline	00172-2931	Antihypertensive
Z2931	Tab, Film Coated	Methyldopa 250 mg	by Allscripts	54569-0508	Antihypertensive
Z2931	Tab, Film Coated	Methyldopa 250 mg	by Quality Care	60346-0459	Antihypertensive
Z2932	Tab, Film Coated	Methyldopa 250 mg	by Qualitest	00603-4536	Antihypertensive
Z2932	Tab, Zenith Logo, Film Coated	Methyldopa 500 mg	by Baker Cummins	63171-1733	Antihypertensive
Z2932	Tab, White, Round	Methyldopa 500 mg	by Kaiser	00179-1062	Antihypertensive
Z2932	Tab, White, Round	Methyldopa 500 mg	Aldomet by Zenith Goldline	00172-2932	Antihypertensive
Z2932	Tab, Film Coated	Methyldopa 500 mg	Aldomet by Zenith Goldline	00182-1733	Antihypertensive
Z2932	Tab, Film Coated	Methyldopa 500 mg	by Med Pro	53978-0003	Antihypertensive
Z2932 <> SL477	Tab, Zenith Logo, Film Coated	Methyldopa 500 mg	by Qualitest	00603-4537	Antihypertensive
Z2936	Tab, Blue, Round	Methyldopa 500 mg	by United Res	00677-0974	Antihypertensive
Z2937	Tab, Orange, Round	Perphenazine 2 mg, Amitriptyline HCl 10 mg	Triavil by Zenith Goldline		Antipsychotic; Antidepressant
Z2938	Tab, Salmon, Round	Perphenazine 2 mg, Amitriptyline HCl 25 mg	Triavil by Zenith Goldline		Antipsychotic; Antidepressant
Z2939	Tab, Yellow, Round	Perphenazine 4 mg, Amitriptyline HCl 10 mg	Triavil by Zenith Goldline		Antipsychotic; Antidepressant
Z2942	Tab, Lavender, Round	Perphenazine 4 mg, Amitriptyline HCl 25 mg	Triavil by Zenith Goldline		Antipsychotic; Antidepressant
Z2950	Cap, Maroon, Opaque	Trifluoperazine HCl 10 mg	Stelazine by Zenith Goldline		Antipsychotic
Z2950	Cap	Hydrochlorothiazide 25 mg, Triamterene 50 mg	Triamterene/ HCTZ by Zenith Goldline	00172-2950	Diuretic
Z2950	Cap	Hydrochlorothiazide 25 mg, Triamterene 50 mg	by Martec	52555-0648	Diuretic
Z2950	Cap	Hydrochlorothiazide 25 mg, Triamterene 50 mg	by Major	00904-5016	Diuretic
Z2950	Tab, Maroon, Scored	Hydrochlorothiazide 25 mg, Triamterene 50 mg	by HL Moore	00839-8043	Diuretic
Z2950	Cap, Maroon, Z-2950	Hydrochlorothiazide 50 mg	by Murfreesboro	51129-1308	Diuretic
Z2958	Tab, White, Round	Triamterene 50 mg, Hydrochlorothiazide 25 mg	Triamterene / HCTZ by Zenith Goldline	00182-1750	Diuretic
Z2959	Tab, White, Oval	Ergoloid Mesylates sublingual 0.5 mg	Hydergine SL by Zenith Goldline		Ergot
Z2960	Cap, White	Dihydroergocristine Mesylate 0.333 mg, Dihydroergocryptine Mesylate 0.333 mg, Ergoloid Mesylates Sublingual 1 mg	Hydergine SL by Zenith Goldline	00172-2959	Ergot;Cardiovascular
Z2962	Tab, White, Round	Chloramphenicol 250 mg	Chloromycetin by Zenith Goldline		Antibiotic
Z2963	Cap, Amethyst/Natural	Ephedrine 25 mg, Theophylline 130 mg, Hydroxyzine HCl 10 mg	Marax by Zenith Goldline		Antiasthmatic
Z2964	Cap, Blue & Yellow	Nitroglycerin TD 2.5 mg	Nitrobid by Zenith Goldline		Antianginal
Z2969	Cap	Nitroglycerin TD 6.5 mg	Nitrobid by Zenith Goldline		Antianginal
Z2970	Tab, White, Round	Sulfinpyrazone 200 mg	by Zenith Goldline	00172-2969	Uricosuric
Z2971	Tab, White, Round	Sulfinpyrazone 100 mg	Anturane by Zenith Goldline		Uricosuric
Z2971	Tab	Metronidazole 250 mg	Flagyl by Zenith Goldline	00172-2971	Antibiotic
Z2971	Tab	Metronidazole 250 mg	by Kaiser	00179-0690	Antibiotic
Z2971	Tab, Zenith Logo	Metronidazole 250 mg	by Med Pro	53978-0215	Antibiotic
Z2971	Tab	Metronidazole 250 mg	by Pharmedix	53002-0221	Antibiotic
Z2971	Tab, Zenith Logo	Metronidazole 250 mg	by UDL	51079-0122	Antibiotic
Z2971	Tab	Metronidazole 250 mg	by Quality Care	60346-0592	Antibiotic
Z2971	Tab	Metronidazole 250 mg	by Nat Pharmpak Serv	55154-5509	Antibiotic

ID FRONT <> BACK	DESCRIPTION FRONT <> BACK	INGREDIENT & STRENGTH	BRAND (OR EQUIV.) & FIRM	NDC#	CLASS; SCH.
Z2971	Tab, White, Round	Metronidazole 250 mg	Flagyl by Zenith Goldline	00182-1330	Antibiotic
Z2971 <> G1330	Tab, White, Round	Metronidazole 250 mg	Flagyl by Zenith Goldline	00172-2971	Antibiotic
Z2974	Tab	Chlorthalidone 25 mg	by Zenith Goldline	00172-2974	Diuretic
Z2976	Tab, White, Round	Dipyridamole 50 mg	Persantine by Zenith Goldline		Antiplatelet
Z2977	Tab, White, Round	Dipyridamole 75 mg	Persantine by Zenith Goldline		Antiplatelet
Z2978	Tab, White, Round, Z-2978	Tolazamide 100 mg	Tolinase by Zenith Goldline		Antidiabetic
Z2978	Tab, White, Round	Tolazamide 100 mg	Tolinase by Zenith Goldline	00172-2978	Antidiabetic
Z2978	Tab	Tolazamide 100 mg	by Qualitest	00603-6096	Antidiabetic
Z2979	Tab, Off-White to White, Round	Tolazamide 250 mg	Tolinase by Zenith Goldline	00172-2979	Antidiabetic
Z2979	Tab	Tolazamide 250 mg	by Apotheca	12634-0490	Antidiabetic
Z2980	Tab	Tolazamide 500 mg	by Zenith Goldline	00182-1679	Antidiabetic
Z2980	Tab, Off-White to White, Round	Tolbutamide 500 mg	Tolinase by Zenith Goldline	00172-2980	Antidiabetic
Z2982	Cap, White	Chlordiazepoxide 5 mg, Clindinium 2.5 mg	Librax by Zenith Goldline		Gastrointestinal; C IV
Z2984	Cap, Light Blue & White	Doxycycline Hyclate 50 mg	Vibramycin by Zenith Goldline	00172-2984	Antibiotic
Z2984	Cap	Doxycycline Hyclate	by PDRX	55289-0502	Antibiotic
Z2985	Cap, Light Blue	Doxycycline Hyclate 100 mg	Vibramycin by Zenith Goldline	00172-2985	Antibiotic
Z2985	Cap, Light Blue	Doxycycline Hyclate 100 mg	Vibramycin by Zenith Goldline	00182-1035	Antibiotic
Z2985	Cap	Doxycycline Hyclate	by Darby Group	66467-0230	Antibiotic
Z2985	Cap, Yellow Powder	Doxycycline Hyclate	by Baker Cummins	63171-1035	Antibiotic
Z2985	Cap	Doxycycline Hyclate	by Apotheca	12634-0169	Antibiotic
Z2986	Tab, Light Orange	Methyclothiazide 2.5 mg	by Zenith Goldline	00172-2986	Diuretic
Z2987	Tab, Salmon, Round	Methyclothiazide 5 mg	Enduron by Zenith Goldline		Diuretic
Z2994	Tab, White, Round	Dipyridamole 25 mg	Persantine by Zenith Goldline		Antiplatelet
Z2999	Tab	Chlorthalidone 50 mg	by Zenith Goldline	00172-2999	Diuretic
Z300 <> 7117	Tab, Film Coated	Cimetidine 300 mg	by Quality Care	60346-0944	Gastrointestinal
Z300 <> 7117	Tab, White, Round, Coated	Cimetidine 300 mg	Tagamet by Zenith Goldline	00172-7117	Gastrointestinal
Z300 <> 7117	Tab, White, Round	Cimetidine 300 mg	Tagamet by Zenith Goldline	00182-1984	Gastrointestinal
Z3001	Tab, White, Round	Quinine Sulfate 260 mg	Quinamm by Zenith Goldline		Antimalarial
Z3001	Tab, White, Round	Quinine Sulfate 260 mg	by Vangard Labs	00615-1579	Antimalarial
Z3007	Tab	Metronidazole 500 mg	by UDL	51079-0126	Antibiotic
Z3007	Tab	Metronidazole 500 mg	by Kaiser	00179-1227	Antibiotic
Z3007	Tab, White, Oval	Metronidazole 500 mg	Flagyl by Zenith Goldline	00172-3007	Antibiotic
Z3007	Tab	Metronidazole 500 mg	by Allscripts	54569-0967	Antibiotic
Z3007	Tab, Zenith Logo	Metronidazole 500 mg	by Pharmedix	53002-0247	Antibiotic
Z3007	Tab	Metronidazole 500 mg	by Med Pro	53978-3056	Antibiotic
Z3007	Tab, Zenith Logo, Coated	Metronidazole 500 mg	by Quality Care	60346-0507	Antibiotic
Z3007	Tab, White, Oval	Metronidazole 500 mg	Flagyl by Zenith Goldline	00182-1517	Antibiotic
Z3007117	Tab, White, Round, Z300/7117	Cimetidine 300 mg	Tagamet by Zenith Goldline	00172-7117	Gastrointestinal
Z3606	Tab, Orange, Round	Thioridazine HCl 10 mg	Mellaril by Zenith Goldline		Antipsychotic
Z3607	Tab, Orange, Round	Thioridazine HCl 15 mg	Mellaril by Zenith Goldline		Antipsychotic
Z3608	Tab, Orange, Round	Thioridazine HCl 25 mg	Mellaril by Zenith Goldline		Antipsychotic
Z3609	Tab, Orange, Round	Thioridazine HCl 50 mg	Mellaril by Zenith Goldline		Antipsychotic
Z3610	Tab, White, Round	Thioridazine HCl 100 mg	Mellaril by Zenith Goldline		Antipsychotic
Z3614	Tab, Orange, Round	Propranolol HCl 10 mg	Inderal by Zenith Goldline		Antihypertensive
Z3615	Tab, Blue, Round	Propranolol HCl 20 mg	Inderal by Zenith Goldline		Antihypertensive
Z3616	Tab, Green, Round	Propranolol HCl 40 mg	Inderal by Zenith Goldline		Antihypertensive
Z3617	Tab, Yellow, Round	Propranolol HCl 80 mg	Inderal by Zenith Goldline		Antihypertensive
Z3626	Tab, Peach, Round, Film Coated	Doxycycline Hyclate 100 mg	Vibramycin by Zenith Goldline	00182-1535	Antibiotic
Z3626	Tab, Peach, Round, Film Coated	Doxycycline Hyclate 100 mg	Vibramycin by Zenith Goldline	00172-3626	Antibiotic
Z3626	Tab, Film Coated	Doxycycline Hyclate	by Prepackage Spec	58864-0189	Antibiotic
Z3626	Tab, Film Coated	Doxycycline Hyclate	by Golden State	60429-0069	Antibiotic
Z3626	Tab, Film Coated, Debossed	Doxycycline Hyclate	by Baker Cummins	63171-1535	Antibiotic

ID FRONT ⟷ BACK	DESCRIPTION FRONT ⟷ BACK	INGREDIENT & STRENGTH	BRAND (OR EQUIV.) & FIRM	NDC#	CLASS; SCH.
Z3626	Tab, Film Coated, Z over 3626	Doxycycline Hyclate	by UDL	51079-0554	Antibiotic
Z3626	Tab, Film Coated	Doxycycline Hyclate	by Pharmedix	53002-0271	Antibiotic
Z3626	Cap	Doxycycline Hyclate	by Apotheca	12634-0167	Antibiotic
Z3638	Tab, Red, Round	Propranolol HCl 60 mg	Inderal by Zenith Goldline		Antihypertensive
Z3643	Cap, Green & Yellow	Nitroglycerin TD 9 mg	Nitrobid by Zenith Goldline		Antianginal
Z3657	Tab, Blue, Round	Chlorpropamide 100 mg	Diabinese by Zenith Goldline		Antidiabetic
Z3667	Tab, Gray, Round, Sugar Coated	Perphenazine 2 mg	Trilafon by Zenith Goldline	00172-3667	Antipsychotic
Z36672	Tab, Gray, Round, Sugar Coated	Perphenazine 2 mg	Trilafon by UDL	51079-0738	Antipsychotic
Z36672	Tab, Zenith Logo over 3667 over 2, Sugar Coated	Perphenazine 2 mg	by Quality Care	60346-0834	Antipsychotic
Z36672	Tab, Gray, Round, Z Over 3667 Over 2	Perphenazine 2 mg	by Pharmafab	62542-0905	Antipsychotic
Z3668	Tab, Gray, Round, Sugar Coated	Perphenazine 4 mg	Trilafon by Zenith Goldline	00172-3668	Antipsychotic
Z36684	Tab, Gray, Round, Sugar Coated	Perphenazine 4 mg	Trilafon by UDL	51079-0739	Antipsychotic
Z36684	Tab, Z Over 3668 Over 4, Tab Sugar Coated	Perphenazine 4 mg	by Med Pro	53978-3168	Antipsychotic
Z36684	Tab, Gray, Round, Z Over 3668 Over 4	Perphenazine 4 mg	by Pharmafab	62542-0910	Antipsychotic
Z36684 ⟷ 4	Tab, Zenith Logo over 3668 over 4, Film Coated	Perphenazine 4 mg	by Quality Care	60346-0835	Antipsychotic
Z3669	Tab, Gray, Round, Sugar Coated	Perphenazine 8 mg	Trilafon by Zenith Goldline	00172-3669	Antipsychotic
Z3669	Tab, Gray, Round, Tab Sugar Coated	Perphenazine 8 mg	Trilafon by Zenith Goldline	00182-1867	Antipsychotic
Z36698	Tab, Gay, Round, Sugar Coated	Perphenazine 8 mg	Trilafon by UDL	51079-0740	Antipsychotic
Z36698 ⟷ 8	Tab, Zenith Logo over 3669 over 8, Tab Sugar Coated	Perphenazine 8 mg	by Quality Care	60346-0990	Antipsychotic
Z3670	Tab, Gray, Round, Sugar Coated	Perphenazine 16 mg	Trilafon by Zenith Goldline	00172-3670	Antipsychotic
Z3670	Tab, Gray, Round, Tab Sugar Coated	Perphenazine 16 mg	Trilafon by Zenith Goldline	00182-1868	Antipsychotic
Z3670	Tab, Gray, Round, Tab Sugar Coated	Perphenazine 2 mg	Trilafon by Zenith Goldline	00182-1865	Antipsychotic
Z367016	Tab, Gray, Round	Perphenazine 16 mg	by Direct Dispensing	57866-1058	Antipsychotic
Z367016	Tab, Z Over 3670 Over 16, Tab Sugar Coated	Perphenazine 16 mg	by Physicians Total Care	54868-2857	Antipsychotic
Z367016	Tab, Gray, Round, Tab Sugar Coated	Perphenazine 16 mg	Trilafon by UDL	51079-0823	Antipsychotic
Z367016	Tab, Gray, Round, Tab, Z Over 3670 Over 16	Perphenazine 16 mg	by Pharmafab	62542-0912	Antipsychotic
Z3671	Tab, Orange, Round	Perphenazine 4 mg, Amitriptyline HCl 50 mg	Triavil by Zenith Goldline		Antipsychotic; Antidepressant
Z3690 ⟷ 5	Tab, Gold, Round	Prochlorperazine Mal 5 mg	Compazine by Zenith Goldline	00182-8210	Antiemetic
Z3691 ⟷ 10	Tab, Gold, Round	Prochlorperazine Mal 10 mg	Compazine by Zenith Goldline	00182-8211	Antiemetic
Z3747	Tab, White, Round	Phenobarbital 8 mg, Theophylline 130 mg, Ephedrine (Azpan) 24 mg	Tedral by Zenith Goldline		Antiasthmatic; C IV
Z3904	Tab, White, Round	Meprobamate 400 mg	Miltown by Zenith Goldline		Sedative/Hypnotic; C IV
Z3905	Tab, White, Round	Meprobamate 200 mg	Miltown by Zenith Goldline		Sedative/Hypnotic; C IV
Z3915	Tab, White, Round	Acetaminophen 300 mg, Codeine 30 mg	Tylenol #3 by Zenith Goldline		Analgesic; C III
Z3916	Tab, White, Round	Acetaminophen 300 mg, Codeine 60 mg	Tylenol #4 by Zenith Goldline		Analgesic; C III
Z3925 ⟷ 2	Tab	Diazepam 2 mg	by Quality Care	60346-0579	Antianxiety; C IV
Z3925 ⟷ 2	Tab, White, Round	Diazepam 2 mg	Valium by Zenith Goldline	00172-3925	Antianxiety; C IV
Z3925 ⟷ 2	Tab, Z over 3925 ⟷ 2	Diazepam 2 mg	by Kaiser	00179-1085	Antianxiety; C IV
Z39252	Tab, White, Round	Diazepam 2 mg	Valium by Zenith Goldline	00182-1755	Antianxiety; C IV
Z3926 ⟷ 5	Tab	Diazepam 5 mg	by Quality Care	60346-0478	Antianxiety; C IV
Z3926 ⟷ 5	Tab, Yellow, Round	Diazepam 5 mg	Valium by Zenith Goldline	00172-3926	Antianxiety; C IV
Z3926 ⟷ 5	Tab	Diazepam 5 mg	by Qualitest	00603-3217	Antianxiety; C IV
Z3926 ⟷ 5	Tab	Diazepam 5 mg	by Pharmedix	53002-0334	Antianxiety; C IV
Z3927	Tab	Diazepam 5 mg	by PDRX	55289-0091	Antianxiety; C IV
Z3927 ⟷ 10	Tab, Light Blue	Diazepam 10 mg	by Quality Care	60346-0033	Antianxiety; C IV
Z3927 ⟷ 10	Tab, Light Blue, Round	Diazepam 10 mg	Valium by Zenith Goldline	00172-3927	Antianxiety; C IV
Z392710	Tab, Light Blue, Round	Diazepam 10 mg	Valium by Zenith Goldline	00182-1757	Antianxiety; C IV
Z3964	Tab	Aspirin 325 mg, Codeine Phosphate 30 mg	by Qualitest	00603-2361	Analgesic; C III
Z3981	Tab, Tab Coated	Acetaminophen 650 mg, Propoxyphene Napsylate 100 mg	Propoxy N APAP by Quality Care	60346-0610	Analgesic; C IV
Z3981	Tab, Coated	Acetaminophen 650 mg, Propoxyphene Napsylate 100 mg	by Zenith Goldline	00172-3981	Analgesic; C IV
Z3981	Tab, Film Coated	Acetaminophen 650 mg, Propoxyphene Napsylate 100 mg	by Talbert Med	44514-0750	Analgesic; C IV
Z3984	Tab, White, Round	Aspirin 325 mg, Codeine Phosphate 30 mg	Empirin w/ Codeine by Zenith Goldline	00172-3984	Analgesic; C III

ID FRONT <> BACK	DESCRIPTION FRONT <> BACK	INGREDIENT & STRENGTH	BRAND (OR EQUIV.) & FIRM	NDC#	CLASS; SCH.
Z3984	Tab	Aspirin 325 mg, Codeine Phosphate 30 mg	by United Res	00677-0647	Analgesic; C III
Z3984	Tab	Aspirin 325 mg, Codeine Phosphate 30 mg	by Qualitest	00603-2361	Analgesic; C III
Z3984 <> 3	Tab	Aspirin 325 mg, Codeine Phosphate 30 mg	by Quality Care	60346-0560	Analgesic; C III
Z3984 <> 3	Tab	Aspirin 325 mg, Codeine Phosphate 30 mg	by Allscripts	54569-0300	Analgesic; C III
Z3984 <> 3	Tab	Aspirin 325 mg, Codeine Phosphate 30 mg	by Pharmedix	53002-0109	Analgesic; C III
Z3985	Tab, White, Round	Aspirin 325 mg, Codeine Phosphate 60 mg	Empirin w/ Codeine by Zenith Goldline	00172-3985	Analgesic; C III
Z3985	Tab	Aspirin 325 mg, Codeine Phosphate 60 mg	by United Res	00677-0676	Analgesic; C III
Z3985	Tab	Aspirin 325 mg, Codeine Phosphate 60 mg	by Qualitest	00603-2362	Analgesic; C III
Z3996	Tab, White, Round	Butalbital 50 mg, Aspirin 325 mg, Caffeine (Butalbital Compound) 40 mg	Fiorinal by Zenith Goldline		Analgesic; C III
Z400 <> 7171	Tab, Film Coated	Cimetidine 400 mg	by Golden State	60429-0047	Gastrointestinal
Z400 <> 7171	Tab, Film Coated, Zenith Logo	Cimetidine 400 mg	by Quality Care	60346-0945	Gastrointestinal
Z400 <> 7171	Tab, White, Cap Shaped, Film Coated	Cimetidine 400 mg	Tagamet by Zenith Goldline	00172-7171	Gastrointestinal
Z400 <> 7171	Tab, White, Cap Shaped	Cimetidine 400 mg	Tagamet by Zenith Goldline	00182-1985	Gastrointestinal
Z400 <> 7171	Tab, Film Coated	Cimetidine 400 mg	by Med Pro	53978-2009	Gastrointestinal
Z400 <> 7171	Tab, Film Coated	Cimetidine 400 mg	by Murfreesboro	51129-1336	Gastrointestinal
Z4007171	Tab, White, Cap Shaped, Film Coated, Z400/7171	Cimetidine 400 mg	Tagamet by Zenith Goldline	00172-7171	Gastrointestinal
Z4029	Cap	Indomethacin 25 mg	by Baker Cummins	63171-1681	NSAID
Z4029	Cap, Green	Indomethacin 25 mg	by Allscripts	54569-4123	NSAID
Z4029	Cap, Green	Indomethacin 25 mg	Indocin by Zenith Goldline	00182-1681	NSAID
Z4029	Cap, Green	Indomethacin 25 mg	Indocin by Zenith Goldline	00172-4029	NSAID
Z4029	Cap	Indomethacin 25 mg	by Mova	55370-0858	NSAID
Z4029	Cap, Zenith Logo	Indomethacin 25 mg	by Pharmedix	53002-0305	NSAID
Z4029	Cap	Indomethacin 25 mg	by Allscripts	54569-0277	NSAID
Z4029	Cap	Indomethacin 25 mg	by Med Pro	53978-0039	NSAID
Z4029	Cap	Indomethacin 25 mg	by Kaiser	62224-3446	NSAID
Z4029	Cap	Indomethacin 25 mg	by Qualitest	00603-4067	NSAID
Z4029	Cap	Indomethacin 25 mg	by HL Moore	00839-6762	NSAID
Z4030	Cap	Indomethacin 50 mg	by Baker Cummins	63171-1682	NSAID
Z4030	Cap, Green	Indomethacin 50 mg	Indocin by Zenith Goldline	00182-1682	NSAID
Z4030	Cap, Green	Indomethacin 50 mg	Indocin by Zenith Goldline	00172-4030	NSAID
Z4030	Cap	Indomethacin 50 mg	by Allscripts	54569-0275	NSAID
Z4030	Cap	Indomethacin 50 mg	by Mova	55370-0859	NSAID
Z4030	Cap	Indomethacin 50 mg	by Med Pro	53978-5037	NSAID
Z4030	Cap, Zenith Logo	Indomethacin 50 mg	by Pharmedix	53002-0350	NSAID
Z4030	Cap, Zenith Logo	Indomethacin 50 mg	by Prescription Dispensing	61807-0041	NSAID
Z4030	Cap	Indomethacin 50 mg	by PDRX	55289-0663	NSAID
Z4030	Cap	Indomethacin 50 mg	by Kaiser	62224-3557	NSAID
Z4030	Cap	Indomethacin 50 mg	by Quality Care	60346-0733	NSAID
Z4030	Cap	Indomethacin 50 mg	by Qualitest	00603-4068	NSAID
Z4030	Cap	Indomethacin 50 mg	by HL Moore	00839-6763	NSAID
Z4051	Cap, Blue & Clear	Disopyramide Phosphate 100 mg	Norpace by Zenith Goldline		Antiarrhythmic
Z4052	Cap, Blue & Clear	Disopyramide Phosphate 150 mg	Norpace by Zenith Goldline		Antiarrhythmic
Z4058	Cap, Clear & White	Cefadroxil 500 mg	Duricef by Zenith Goldline		Antibiotic
Z4058	Cap, Red & White	Cefadroxil 500 mg	Duricef by Zenith Goldline		Antibiotic
Z4058500MG	Cap, Clear & White	Cefadroxil Hemihydrate 500 mg	Duricef by Zenith Goldline	00172-4058	Antibiotic
Z4059	Tab, White, Oval	Cefadroxil 1000 mg	Duricef by Zenith Goldline		Antibiotic
Z4059	Tab, White, Cap Shaped	Cefadroxil Hemihydrate 1000 mg	Duricef by Zenith Goldline	00172-4059	Antibiotic
Z4063	Cap, Maroon	Cephradine 250 mg	Anspor by Zenith Goldline		Antibiotic
Z4064	Cap, Pink	Cephradine 500 mg	Anspor by Zenith Goldline		Antibiotic
Z4067	Cap, Ivory	Prazosin HCl 1 mg	Minipress by Zenith Goldline	00172-4067	Antihypertensive
Z4067	Cap	Prazosin HCl 1 mg	by Quality Care	60346-0572	Antihypertensive
Z4068	Cap, Pink	Prazosin HCl 2 mg	Minipress by Zenith Goldline	00172-4068	Antihypertensive

ID FRONT <> BACK	DESCRIPTION FRONT <> BACK	INGREDIENT & STRENGTH	BRAND (OR EQUIV.) & FIRM	NDC#	CLASS; SCH.
Z4069	Cap, Blue	Prazosin HCl 5 mg	Minipress by Zenith Goldline	00182-1257	Antihypertensive
Z4069	Cap, Blue	Prazosin HCl 5 mg	Minipress by Zenith Goldline	00172-4069	Antihypertensive
Z4069	Cap, Zenith Logo 4069	Prazosin HCl	by Quality Care	60346-0206	Antihypertensive
Z4073	Cap, Gray & Red, Zenith Labs	Cephalexin Monohydrate	by Quality Care	60346-0441	Antibiotic
Z4073	Cap	Cephalexin Monohydrate 250 mg	Keflex by Zenith Goldline	00182-1278	Antibiotic
Z4073	Cap, Gray & Red, Z-4073	Cephalexin Monohydrate 250 mg	Keflex by Zenith Goldline	00172-4073	Antibiotic
Z4074	Cap, Red	Cephalexin 500 mg	Keflex by Zenith Goldline		Antibiotic
Z4074	Cap	Cephalexin Monohydrate 500 mg	Keflex by Zenith Goldline	00182-1279	Antibiotic
Z4074	Cap, Red, Z-4074	Cephalexin Monohydrate 500 mg	Keflex by Zenith Goldline	00172-4074	Antibiotic
Z4077	Cap, Blue & Red	Piroxicam 10 mg	Feldene by Zenith Goldline	00172-4077	NSAID
Z4079	Cap, Red	Piroxicam 20 mg	Feldene by Zenith Goldline	00172-4079	NSAID
Z4079	Cap, Red & Opaque	Piroxicam 20 mg	Feldene by Zenith Goldline	00182-1934	NSAID
Z4079	Cap, Goldline	Piroxicam 20 mg	by HJ Harkins Co	52959-0232	NSAID
Z4079	Cap	Piroxicam 20 mg	by Quality Care	60346-0676	NSAID
Z4079	Cap, Red, Opaque	Piroxicam 20 mg	by Promeco SA	64674-0007	NSAID
Z4096 <> 10	Tab, Z over 4096	Baclofen 10 mg	by Baker Cummins	63171-1295	Muscle Relaxant
Z4096 <> 10	Tab, White, Round	Baclofen 10 mg	Lioresal by Zenith Goldline	00172-4096	Muscle Relaxant
Z4096 <> 10	Tab, Z over 4096	Baclofen 10 mg	by Caremark	00339-5834	Muscle Relaxant
Z4096 <> G129510	Tab, White, Round	Baclofen 10 mg	Lioresal by Zenith Goldline	00172-4096	Muscle Relaxant
Z409610	Tab, White, Round	Baclofen 10 mg	Lioresal by Zenith Goldline	00182-1295	Muscle Relaxant
Z4097 <> 20	Tab, Film Coated	Baclofen 20 mg	by Prescription Dispensing	61807-0131	Muscle Relaxant
Z4097 <> 20	Tab, Z over 4097, Film Coated	Baclofen 20 mg	by Baker Cummins	63171-1296	Muscle Relaxant
Z4097 <> 20	Tab, White, Round, Film Coated	Baclofen 20 mg	Lioresal by Zenith Goldline	00172-4097	Muscle Relaxant
Z4097 <> 20	Tab, Film Coated, Z over 4097 <> 20	Baclofen 20 mg	by Med Pro	53978-3167	Muscle Relaxant
Z4097 <> 20	Tab, Film Coated, Z over 4097 <> 20	Baclofen 20 mg	by UDL	51079-0669	Muscle Relaxant
Z4097 <> G129620	Tab, White, Round, Film Coated	Baclofen 20 mg	Lioresal by Zenith Goldline	00172-4097	Muscle Relaxant
Z409720	Tab, White, Round	Baclofen 20 mg	Lioresal by Zenith Goldline	00182-1296	Muscle Relaxant
Z4107	Tab	Naproxen 250 mg	by Zenith Goldline	00182-1971	NSAID
Z4108	Tab	Naproxen 375 mg	by Zenith Goldline	00182-1972	NSAID
Z4109	Tab	Naproxen 500 mg	by Zenith Goldline	00182-1973	NSAID
Z4116275	Tab, White, Oval, Z 4116/275	Naproxen Sodium 275 mg	Anaprox by Zenith Goldline		NSAID
Z4141	Tab, Peach, Oblong, Coated	Fenoprofen Calcium 600 mg	Nalfon by Zenith Goldline	00172-4141	NSAID
Z4141	Tab, Coated	Fenoprofen Calcium 691.8 mg	by Zenith Goldline	00182-1902	NSAID
Z4141 <> 600	Tab, Film Coated, Zenith Logo Z 4141 <> 600	Fenoprofen Calcium 691.8 mg	by Quality Care	60346-0233	NSAID
Z4141600	Tab, Coated	Fenoprofen Calcium 691.8 mg	by Zenith Goldline	00182-1902	NSAID
Z4171	Cap, Clear	Quinidine Sulfate 200 mg	Quinamm by Zenith Goldline	00172-4171	Antiarrhythmic
Z4171	Cap, Natural	Quinine Sulfate 200 mg	Quinamm by Zenith Goldline	00172-4171	Antimalarial
Z4217	Tab, White, Round, Z/4217	Pindolol 5 mg	Visken by Zenith Goldline	00172-4217	Antihypertensive
Z4218	Tab, White, Round, Z/4218	Pindolol 10 mg	Visken by Zenith Goldline	00172-4218	Antihypertensive
Z4219	Tab, White, Round	Diltiazem 30 mg	Cardizem by Zenith Goldline		Antihypertensive
Z4220	Tab, White, Round	Diltiazem 60 mg	Cardizem by Zenith Goldline		Antihypertensive
Z4221	Tab, White, Oblong	Diltiazem 90 mg	Cardizem by Zenith Goldline		Antihypertensive
Z4222	Tab, White, Oblong	Diltiazem 120 mg	Cardizem by Zenith Goldline		Antihypertensive
Z4226	Tab, Peach, Round	Guanabenz Acetate 4 mg	Wytensin by Zenith Goldline		Antihypertensive
Z4226	Tab, Peach, Round	Guanabenz Acetate 4 mg	Wytensin by Zenith Goldline	00172-4226	Antihypertensive
Z4227	Tab, Gray, Round	Guanabenz Acetate 8 mg	Wytensin by Zenith Goldline		Antihypertensive
Z4227	Tab, Gray, Round	Guanabenz Acetate 8 mg	Wytensin by Zenith Goldline	00172-4227	Antihypertensive
Z4229	Cap, Red	Triamterene 50 mg, Hydrochlorothiazide 25 mg	Dyazide by Zenith Goldline		Diuretic
Z4232 <> 05	Tab, Scored, Z over 4232 <> 0.5	Bumetanide 0.5 mg	by HL Moore	00839-8011	Diuretic
Z4232 <> 05	Tab, Scored, Z 4232 <> 0.5	Bumetanide 0.5 mg	by Geneva	00781-1821	Diuretic
Z4232 <> 05	Tab, Green, Round, Z4232 <> 0.5	Bumetanide 0.5 mg	Bumex by Zenith Goldline	00182-2615	Diuretic
Z4232 <> 05	Tab, Scored, Z over 4232 <> 0.5	Bumetanide 0.5 mg	by Major	00904-5102	Diuretic

ID FRONT <> BACK	DESCRIPTION FRONT <> BACK	INGREDIENT & STRENGTH	BRAND (OR EQUIV.) & FIRM	NDC#	CLASS; SCH.
Z4232 <> 5	Tab, Green, Round, Scored	Bumetanide 0.5 mg	by Vangard Labs	00615-4541	Diuretic
Z423205	Tab, Green, Round, Z 4232 0.5	Bumetanide 0.5 mg	Bumex by Zenith Goldline		Diuretic
Z4233 <> 1	Tab, Scored, Z over 4233 <> 1	Bumetanide 1 mg	by Nat Pharmpak Serv	55154-5819	Diuretic
Z4233 <> 1	Tab, Z over 4233 <> 1	Bumetanide 1 mg	by Geneva	00781-1822	Diuretic
Z4233 <> 1	Tab, Z over 4233 <> 1	Bumetanide 1 mg	by HL Moore	00839-8012	Diuretic
Z4233 <> 1	Tab, Yellow, Round	Bumetanide 1 mg	Bumex by Zenith Goldline	00182-2616	Diuretic
Z4233 <> 1	Tab, Z over 4233 <> 1	Bumetanide 1 mg	by Murfreesboro	51129-1337	Diuretic
Z4233 <> 1	Tab, Z over 4233 <> 1	Bumetanide 1 mg	by Major	00904-5103	Diuretic
Z4234 <> 2	Tab, Peach, Round, Scored	Bumetanide 2 mg	by Murfreesboro Ph	51129-1383	Diuretic
Z4234 <> 2	Tab, Scored	Bumetanide 2 mg	by Geneva	00781-1823	Diuretic
Z4234 <> 2	Tab, Peach, Round	Bumetanide 2 mg	Bumex by Zenith Goldline	00182-2617	Diuretic
Z4234 <> 2	Tab, Scored, Z over 4234 <> 2	Bumetanide 2 mg	by Major	00904-5104	Diuretic
Z4235 <> 20	Tab, White, Round, Z/4235 <> 20	Nadolol 20 mg	Corgard by Zenith Goldline	00182-2632	Antihypertensive
Z423520	Tab, White, Round, Z 4235/20	Nadolol 20 mg	Corgard by Zenith Goldline		Antihypertensive
Z4236 <> 40	Tab, White, Round, Z/4236 <> 40	Nadolol 40 mg	Corgard by Zenith Goldline	00182-2633	Antihypertensive
Z423640	Tab, White, Round, Z 4236/40	Nadolol 40 mg	Corgard by Zenith Goldline		Antihypertensive
Z4237 <> 80	Tab, White, Round, Z/4237 <> 80	Nadolol 80 mg	Corgard by Zenith Goldline	00182-2634	Antihypertensive
Z423780	Tab, White, Round, Z 4237/80	Nadolol 80 mg	Corgard by Zenith Goldline		Antihypertensive
Z4238 <> 120	Tab, White, Cap-Shaped	Nadolol 120 mg	Corgard by Zenith Goldline	00172-4238	Antihypertensive
Z4239 <> 160	Tab, White, Cap-Shaped	Nadolol 160 mg	Corgard by Zenith Goldline	00172-4239	Antihypertensive
Z4259	Tab, White, Round, Z-4259	Indapamide 2.5 mg	Lozol by Zenith Goldline	00182-2610	Diuretic
Z4259	Tab, White, Round, Coated, Z-4259	Indapamide 2.5 mg	Lozol by Zenith Goldline	00172-4259	Diuretic
Z4262 <> 125	Tab, Orange, Round, Z4262 <> 1.25	Indapamide 1.25 mg	Lozol by Zenith Goldline	00182-8201	Diuretic
Z4262125	Tab, Orange, Round, Z4262/1.25	Indapamide 1.25 mg	Lozol by Zenith Goldline	00172-4262	Diuretic
Z4275550	Tab, White, Oval, Z 4275/550	Naproxen Sodium 550 mg	Anaprox by Zenith Goldline		NSAID
Z4280 <> SR240	Tab, Film Coated	Verapamil HCl 240 mg	by Warner Chilcott	00047-0474	Antihypertensive
Z4280 <> SR240	Tab, Film Coated	Verapamil HCl 240 mg	by Med Pro	53978-2029	Antihypertensive
Z4280 <> SR240	Tab, Film Coated	Verapamil HCl 240 mg	by Qualitest	00603-6360	Antihypertensive
Z4280 <> SR240	Tab, Film Coated	Verapamil HCl 240 mg	by HL Moore	00839-7670	Antihypertensive
Z4280 <> SR240	Tab, Film Coated	Verapamil HCl 240 mg	by Major	00904-7957	Antihypertensive
Z4280 <> SR240	Tab, Off-White, Film Coated	Verapamil 240 mg	by Quality Care	60346-0959	Antihypertensive
Z4286 <> SR180	Tab, Film Coated	Verapamil HCl 180 mg	by Warner Chilcott	00047-0472	Antihypertensive
Z4286 <> SR180	Tab, Film Coated	Verapamil HCl 180 mg	by Major	00904-7956	Antihypertensive
Z4286 <> SR180	Tab, Film Coated	Verapamil 180 mg	by Qualitest	00603-6359	Antihypertensive
Z4361	Tab, White, Oval, Coated, Z-4361	Flurbiprofen 50 mg	Ansaid by Zenith Goldline	00172-4361	NSAID
Z4362	Tab, Green, Oval, Coated, Z-4362	Flurbiprofen 100 mg	Ansaid by Zenith Goldline	00172-4362	NSAID
Z4362 <> 100	Tab, Green, Oval	Flurbiprofen 100 mg	Ansaid by Zenith Goldline	00182-2621	NSAID
Z4760CEFACLOR <> 250MG	Cap, Zenith Logo 4760 Cefaclor <> 250 mg	Cefaclor Monohydrate 250 mg	by Allscripts	54569-3901	Antibiotic
Z4761CEFACLOR <> 500MG	Cap	Cefaclor Monohydrate 500 mg	by Zenith Goldline	00172-4761	Antibiotic
Z4761CEFACLOR <> 500MG	Cap, Zenith Logo 4761 Cefaclor <> 500 mg	Cefaclor Monohydrate 500 mg	by Allscripts	54569-3902	Antibiotic
Z4804	Cap, Blue & White	Oxazepam 10 mg	Serax by Zenith Goldline	00172-4804	Sedative/Hypnotic; C IV
Z4804	Cap	Oxazepam 10 mg	by Qualitest	00603-4950	Sedative/Hypnotic; C IV
Z4805	Cap, Clear w/ White Powder	Oxazepam 15 mg	Serax by UDL	51079-0478	Sedative/Hypnotic; C IV
Z4805	Cap, Clear	Oxazepam 15 mg	Serax by Zenith Goldline	00182-1231	Sedative/Hypnotic; C IV
Z4805	Cap, Clear	Oxazepam 15 mg	Serax by Zenith Goldline	00172-4805	Sedative/Hypnotic; C IV
Z4805	Cap	Oxazepam 15 mg	by Qualitest	00603-4951	Sedative/Hypnotic; C IV
Z4806	Cap, Orange & White, Z4806	Oxazepam 30 mg	Serax by UDL	51079-0479	Sedative/Hypnotic; C IV
Z4806	Cap, Orange & White	Oxazepam 30 mg	Serax by Zenith Goldline	00172-4806	Sedative/Hypnotic; C IV
Z4806	Cap	Oxazepam 30 mg	by Qualitest	00603-4952	Sedative/Hypnotic; C IV

ID FRONT <> BACK	DESCRIPTION FRONT <> BACK	INGREDIENT & STRENGTH	BRAND (OR EQUIV.) & FIRM	NDC#	CLASS; SCH.
Z4811	Cap, Red/Gray	Propoxyphene 65 mg, Aspirin 389 mg, Caffeine 32.4 mg	Darvon Compound 65 by Zenith Goldline		Analgesic; C IV
Z4835	Tab	Alprazolam 0.25 mg	by Zenith Goldline	00182-0027	Antianxiety; C IV
Z4835025	Tab, White, Round, Z 4835/0.25	Alprazolam 0.25 mg	Xanax by Zenith Goldline		Antianxiety; C IV
Z483605	Tab, Peach, Round, Z 4836/0.5	Alprazolam 0.5 mg	Xanax by Zenith Goldline		Antianxiety; C IV
Z48371	Tab, Blue, Round, Z 4837/1	Alprazolam 1 mg	Xanax by Zenith Goldline		Antianxiety; C IV
Z4845ZENITH	Tab, White, Rectangular, Z 4845/Zenith	Alprazolam 2 mg	Xanax by Zenith Goldline		Antianxiety; C IV
Z500MG <> 4058	Cap	Cefadroxil Hemihydrate	by Pharmedix	53002-0229	Antibiotic
Z50MG2130	Cap, Zenith Logo	Nitrofurantoin 50 mg	by Apotheca	12634-0181	Antibiotic
Z52941	Tab, Lavender, Round, Z-5 2941	Trifluoperazine HCl 5 mg	Stelazine by Zenith Goldline		Antipsychotic
Z5600	Tab, White, Round	Lorazepam 0.5 mg	Ativan by Zenith Goldline		Sedative/Hypnotic; C IV
Z5800	Tab, White, Round	Lorazepam 1 mg	Ativan by Zenith Goldline		Sedative/Hypnotic; C IV
Z6000	Tab, White, Round	Lorazepam 2 mg	Ativan by Zenith Goldline		Sedative/Hypnotic; C IV
Z6100	Tab, Lavender, Round	Hydroxyzine HCl 10 mg	Atarax by Zenith Goldline		Antihistamine
Z6200	Tab, Magenta, Round	Hydroxyzine HCl 25 mg	Atarax by Zenith Goldline		Antihistamine
Z6300	Tab, Purple, Round	Hydroxyzine HCl 50 mg	Atarax by Zenith Goldline		Antihistamine
Z7301	Tab, Orange, Oblong	Verapamil HCl SR 180 mg	Calan SR/Isoptin SR by Zenith Goldline		Antihypertensive
Z800 <> 7711	Tab, Tab Coated	Cimetidine 800 mg	by Golden State	60429-0048	Gastrointestinal
Z800 <> 7711	Tab, White, Oval, Coated	Cimetidine 800 mg	Tagamet by Zenith Goldline	00172-7711	Gastrointestinal
Z8007711	Tab, White, Oval, Coated	Cimetidine 800 mg	Tagamet by Zenith Goldline	00182-1986	Gastrointestinal
Z8007711	Tab, White, Oval, Z800/7711	Cimetidine 800 mg	Tagamet by Zenith Goldline	00172-7711	Gastrointestinal
ZA <> 74	Tab, White	Terazosin 1 mg	by Altimed	Canadian DIN# 02218941	Antihypertensive
ZADITEN	Tab, White, Round, Scored	Ketotifen Fumarate 1 mg	Zaditen by Novartis	Canadian DIN# 00577308	Antiasthmatic
ZANTAC150 <> 427	Tab, Tab Efferv	Ranitidine HCl 168 mg	Zantac Efferdose by Glaxo	00173-0427	Gastrointestinal
ZANTAC150 <> 427	Tab, Tab Efferv	Ranitidine HCl 168 mg	Zantac Efferdose by Glaxo	60937-0427	Gastrointestinal
ZANTAC150 <> GLAXO	Tab, Film Coated	Ranitidine HCl	by Med Pro	53978-2075	Gastrointestinal
ZANTAC150 <> GLAXO	Tab, Film Coated	Ranitidine HCl 150 mg	Zantac by Nat Pharmpak Serv	55154-1107	Gastrointestinal
ZANTAC150 <> GLAXO	Tab, Film Coated	Ranitidine HCl 150 mg	Zantac by Pharmedix	53002-0552	Gastrointestinal
ZANTAC150 <> GLAXO	Tab, Film Coated	Ranitidine HCl 150 mg	Zantac by Allscripts	54569-0445	Gastrointestinal
ZANTAC150 <> GLAXO	Tab, Peach, Pentagon, Film Coated	Ranitidine HCl 150 mg	Zantac by RX PAK	65084-0183	Gastrointestinal
ZANTAC150 <> GLAXO	Tab, Film Coated	Ranitidine HCl 150 mg	Zantac by Kaiser	00179-1079	Gastrointestinal
ZANTAC150 <> GLAXO	Tab, Film Coated	Ranitidine HCl 150 mg	Zantac by Glaxo	00173-0344	Gastrointestinal
ZANTAC150 <> GLAXO	Tab, Film Coated	Ranitidine HCl 150 mg	Zantac by Amerisource	62584-0488	Gastrointestinal
ZANTAC150 <> GLAXO	Cap, Imprinted in Blue	Ranitidine HCl 150 mg	by Nat Pharmpak Serv	55154-1110	Gastrointestinal
ZANTAC150 <> GLAXO	Tab, Film Coated	Ranitidine HCl 150 mg	Zantac by Quality Care	60346-0729	Gastrointestinal
ZANTAC150 <> GLAXO	Tab, Film Coated	Ranitidine HCl 150 mg	Zantac by Prescription Dispensing	61807-0054	Gastrointestinal
ZANTAC150 <> GLAXOWELLCOME	Cap, Blue Ink, Blue Ink	Ranitidine HCl 150 mg	Zantac Geldose by Glaxo	00173-0428	Gastrointestinal
ZANTAC150 <> GLAXOWELLCOME	Cap, Blue Ink, Blue Ink	Ranitidine HCl 150 mg	Zantac Geldose by Glaxo	00173-0481	Gastrointestinal
ZANTAC150427	Tab, White, Tab-Yellow, Round, Zantac 150/427	Ranitidine HCl 150 mg	Zantac 150 EFFER by Glaxo Wellcome		Gastrointestinal
ZANTAC150GLAXO	Cap, Beige, Zantac 150/Glaxo	Ranitidine HCl 150 mg	Zantac 150 Gel by Glaxo Wellcome		Gastrointestinal
ZANTAC150GLAXO	Tab, Peach, Pentagonal, Zantac 150/Glaxo	Ranitidine HCl 150 mg	Zantac 150 by Glaxo Wellcome		Gastrointestinal
ZANTAC300 <> GLAXO	Tab, Film Coated	Ranitidine HCl 300 mg	Zantac by Kaiser	00179-1211	Gastrointestinal
ZANTAC300 <> GLAXO	Tab	Ranitidine HCl 336 mg	Zantac by Pharmedix	53002-1028	Gastrointestinal
ZANTAC300 <> GLAXO	Tab	Ranitidine HCl 336 mg	Zantac by Allscripts	54569-0444	Gastrointestinal
ZANTAC300 <> GLAXO	Tab, Embossed	Ranitidine HCl 336 mg	Zantac by Amerisource	62584-0393	Gastrointestinal

ID FRONT <> BACK	DESCRIPTION FRONT <> BACK	INGREDIENT & STRENGTH	BRAND (OR EQUIV.) & FIRM	NDC#	CLASS; SCH.
ZANTAC300 <> GLAXOWELLCOME	Cap, Blue Ink	Ranitidine HCl 300 mg	Zantac Geldose by Glaxo	00173-0429	Gastrointestinal
ZANTAC300 <> GLAXOWELLCOME	Tab	Ranitidine HCl 336 mg	Zantac by Glaxo	00173-0393	Gastrointestinal
ZANTAC300GLAXO	Tab, Yellow, Oblong, Zantac 300/Glaxo	Ranitidine HCl 300 mg	Zantac 300 by Glaxo Wellcome		Gastrointestinal
ZANTAC300GLAXO	Cap, Beige, Zantac 300/Glaxo	Ranitidine HCl 300 mg	Zantac 300 GEL by Glaxo Wellcome		Gastrointestinal
ZANTACC150	Cap, Beige, Zantac-C/150	Ranitidine HCl 168 mg	Zantac by Glaxo	Canadian	Gastrointestinal
ZANTACC300	Cap, Beige, Zantac-C/300	Ranitidine HCl 300 mg	Zantac by Glaxo	Canadian	Gastrointestinal
ZAROXOLYN	Tab, Blue	Metolazone 5 mg	by Rhone-Poulenc Rorer	Canadian	Diuretic
ZAROXOLYN <> 10	Tab, Yellow	Metolazone 10 mg	Zaroxolyn by Medeva	53014-0835	Diuretic
ZAROXOLYN <> 212	Tab, Pink, Round, Convex	Metolazone 2.5 mg	Zaroxolyn by Neuman Distr	64579-0053	Diuretic
ZAROXOLYN <> 212	Tab, Zaroxolyn <> 2 1/2	Metolazone 2.5 mg	Zaroxolyn by Caremark	00339-5426	Diuretic
ZAROXOLYN <> 212	Tab, Zaroxolyn <> 2 1/2	Metolazone 2.5 mg	Zaroxolyn by Medeva	53014-0975	Diuretic
ZAROXOLYN <> 212	Tab, Zaroxolyn <> 2 1/2	Metolazone 2.5 mg	Zaroxolyn by Nat Pharmpak Serv	55154-2504	Diuretic
ZAROXOLYN <> 212	Tab, Zaroxolyn <> 2 1/2	Metolazone 2.5 mg	Zaroxolyn by Prestige Packaging	58056-0355	Diuretic
ZAROXOLYN <> 212	Tab, Zaroxolyn <>2 1/2	Metolazone 2.5 mg	Zaroxolyn by Amerisource	62584-0975	Diuretic
ZAROXOLYN <> 212	Tab, Pink, Round	Metolazone 2.5 mg	Zaroxolyn by Compumed	00403-1597	Diuretic
ZAROXOLYN <> 25	Tab, Pink, Zaroxolyn <> 2.5	Metolazone 2.5 mg	Zaroxolyn by Medeva	53014-0975	Diuretic
ZAROXOLYN <> 25	Tab, Zaroxolyn <> 2.5	Metolazone 2.5 mg	Zaroxolyn by Drug Distr	52985-0218	Diuretic
ZAROXOLYN <> 5	Tab, Blue, Round, Convex	Metolazone 5 mg	Zaroxolyn by Neuman Distr	64579-0057	Diuretic
ZAROXOLYN <> 5	Tab	Metolazone 5 mg	Zaroxolyn by Nat Pharmpak Serv	55154-2505	Diuretic
ZAROXOLYN <> 5	Tab, Blue	Metolazone 5 mg	Zaroxolyn by Medeva	53014-0850	Diuretic
ZAROXOLYN <> 5	Tab	Metolazone 5 mg	Zaroxolyn by Quality Care	62682-6023	Diuretic
ZAROXOLYN <> 5	Tab	Metolazone 5 mg	Zaroxolyn by Prestige Packaging	58056-0356	Diuretic
ZAROXOLYN <> 5	Tab, Debossed	Metolazone 5 mg	Zaroxolyn by Amerisource	62584-0850	Diuretic
ZAROXOLYN <> 5	Tab, Blue, Round	Metolazone 5 mg	by Compumed	00403-1603	Diuretic
ZAROXOLYN <> 5	Tab, Blue, Round, Scored	Metolazone 5 mg	Zaroxolyn by Caremark	00339-5428	Diuretic
ZB <> 74	Tab, Orange	Terazosin 2 mg	by Altimed	Canadian DIN# 02218968	Antihypertensive
ZBECAHR	Tab, Green, Elliptical, Zbec/AHR	Therapeutic B-Complex Zinc & Vitamin E	Zbec by Whitehall-Robbins		Vitamin
ZBN	Tab, White, Round	Leflunomide 10 mg	Arava by Hoechst Marion Roussel	00088-2160	Antiarthritic
ZBN	Tab, White, Round, Film Coated	Leflunomide 10 mg	Arava by Hoechst Marion (FR)	12579-0509	Antiarthritic
ZBO	Tab, Light Yellow, Round	Leflunomide 20 mg	Arava by Hoechst Marion Roussel	00088-2161	Antiarthritic
ZBO	Tab, Yellow, Triangle, Film Coated	Leflunomide 20 mg	Arava by Hoechst Marion (FR)	12579-0510	Antiarthritic
ZBP	Tab, White, Round	Leflunomide 100 mg	Arava by Hoechst Marion Roussel	00088-2162	Antiarthritic
ZBP	Tab, White, Round, Film Coated	Leflunomide 100 mg	Arava by Hoechst Marion (FR)	12579-0511	Antiarthritic
ZC <> 74	Tab, Tan	Terazosin 5 mg	by Altimed	Canadian DIN# 02218976	Antihypertensive
ZD <> 74	Tab, Blue	Terazosin 10 mg	by Altimed	Canadian DIN# 02218984	Antihypertensive
ZE <> 74	Tab, Film Coated	Erythromycin 500 mg	by Quality Care	60346-0646	Antibiotic
ZE4760	Cap, Zenith Logo	Cefaclor Monohydrate 250 mg	by Quality Care	60346-0202	Antibiotic
ZELODA500	Tab, Peach, Oblong, Zeloda/500	Capecitabine 500 mg	by Roche	Canadian	Antineoplastic
ZEN50MG2130	Cap, Zenith Logo	Nitrofurantoin 50 mg	by Quality Care	60346-0616	Antibiotic
ZENECA <> ACCOLATE10	Tab, White, Round, Coated Tab	Zafirlukast 10 mg	Accolate by AstraZeneca	00310-0401	Antiasthmatic
ZENECA <> ACCOLATE20	Tab, White, Round, Film Coated	Zafirlukast 20 mg	Accolate by AstraZeneca	00310-0402	Antiasthmatic

ID FRONT <> BACK	DESCRIPTION FRONT <> BACK	INGREDIENT & STRENGTH	BRAND (OR EQUIV.) & FIRM	NDC#	CLASS; SCH.
ZENECA <> ACCOLATE20	Tab, Film Coated	Zafirlukast 20 mg	Accolate by IPR	54921-0402	Antiasthmatic
ZENECA <> ACCOLATE20	Tab, White, Round, Convex, Scored, Film	Zafirlukast 20 mg	Accolate by United Res	00677-1651	Antiasthmatic
ZENECA10 <> 891	Tab, Oyster, Tab Ex Release, Round	Nisoldipine 10 mg	Sular by AstraZeneca	00310-0891	Antihypertensive
ZENECA10 <> 891	Tab, Tab Ex Release	Nisoldipine 10 mg	Sular by Bayer AG	12527-0891	Antihypertensive
ZENECA20 <> 892	Tab, Yellow Cream, Tab Ex Release, Round	Nisoldipine 20 mg	Sular by AstraZeneca	00310-0892	Antihypertensive
ZENECA20 <> 892	Tab,	Nisoldipine 20 mg	Sular ER by Murfreesboro	51129-1278	Antihypertensive
ZENECA20 <> 892	Tab, Tab Ex Release	Nisoldipine 20 mg	Sular by Bayer AG	12527-0892	Antihypertensive
ZENECA30 <> 893	Tab, Mustard, Tab Ex Release, Round	Nisoldipine 30 mg	Sular by AstraZeneca	00310-0893	Antihypertensive
ZENECA30 <> 893	Tab, Mustard Yellow, Zeneca 30 <> 893 Underlined	Nisoldipine 30 mg	Sular Er by Murfreesboro	51129-1334	Antihypertensive
ZENECA30 <> 893	Tab	Nisoldipine 30 mg	Sular by Bayer AG	12527-0893	Antihypertensive
ZENECA40 <> 894	Tab	Nisoldipine 40 mg	Sular by Bayer AG	12527-0894	Antihypertensive
ZENECA40 <> 894	Tab, Burnt Orange, Tab Ex Release, Round	Nisoldipine 40 mg	Sular by AstraZeneca	00310-0894	Antihypertensive
ZENITH <> 500MG	Cap, Yellowish White Powder	Cefadroxil Hemihydrate	by Physicians Total Care	54868-3742	Antibiotic
ZENITH100 <> 2131	Cap	Nitrofurantoin 103 mg	by Prepackage Spec	58864-0371	Antibiotic
ZENITH100MG <> 2131	Cap	Nitrofurantoin 100 mg	by Quality Care	60346-0008	Antibiotic
ZENITH100MG <> 2131	Cap, Zenith Logo	Nitrofurantoin 100 mg	by Medirex	57480-0817	Antibiotic
ZENITH100MG <> 2131	Cap, Zenith Logo Zenith over 100 mg	Nitrofurantoin 100 mg	Nitrofurant Macrcrys by HJ Harkins Co	52959-0405	Antibiotic
ZENITH100MG <> 2131	Cap, 3 Bands	Nitrofurantoin 100 mg	by Thrift Drug	59198-0243	Antibiotic
ZENITH2131	Cap, Pink	Nitrofurantoin Macrocrystallines 100 mg	Macrodantin by Zenith		Antibiotic
ZENITH4058 <> 500	Cap, Zenith Logo	Cefadroxil Monohydrate	by Prescription Dispensing	61807-0123	Antibiotic
ZENITH4171 <> 200MG	Cap	Quinine Sulfate 200 mg	by Quality Care	60346-0808	Antimalarial
ZENITH4266 <> 200	Cap, Zenith Logo Zenith 4266 <> 200	Acyclovir 200 mg	by Murfreesboro	51129-1252	Antiviral
ZENITH4280	Tab, Off-White, Oblong	Verapamil SR 240 mg	Isoptin,Calan by Zenith		Antihypertensive
ZENITH4286	Tab, Off-White, Oval	Verapamil SR 180 mg	Isoptin,Calan by Zenith		Antihypertensive
ZENITH4760 <> CEFACLOR250	Cap	Cefaclor Monohydrate 250 mg	by PDRX	55289-0749	Antibiotic
ZENITH4761	Cap, Gray & White	Cefaclor 500 mg	Ceclor by Zenith		Antibiotic
ZENITH50MG <> 2130	Cap, Zenith Logo	Nitrofurantoin 50 mg	by Caremark	00339-6037	Antibiotic
ZENITH50MG <> 2130	Cap	Nitrofurantoin 50 mg	by Allscripts	54569-0181	Antibiotic
ZENITH50MG <> 2130	Cap, Zenith Logo	Nitrofurantoin 50 mg	by Medirex	57480-0816	Antibiotic
ZENITH50MG <> 2130	Cap, 2 Bands	Nitrofurantoin 50 mg	by Thrift Drug	59198-0242	Antibiotic
ZESTORETIC	Tab, White, Round	Lisinopril 20 mg, Hydrochlorothiazide 12.5 mg	by Zeneca	Canadian	Antihypertensive
ZESTORETIC	Tab, Peach, Round	Lisinopril 20 mg, Hydrochlorothiazide 25 mg	by Zeneca	Canadian	Antihypertensive
ZESTORETIC <> 141	Tab, Peach, Round, Debossed	Hydrochlorothiazide 12.5 mg, Lisinopril 10 mg	Zestoretic by AstraZeneca	00310-0141	Diuretic; Antihypertensive
ZESTORETIC <> 141	Tab, Debossed	Hydrochlorothiazide 12.5 mg, Lisinopril 10 mg	Zestoretic by IPR	54921-0141	Diuretic; Antihypertensive
ZESTORETIC <> 142	Tab, White, Round, Debossed	Hydrochlorothiazide 12.5 mg, Lisinopril 20 mg	Zestoretic 20 1 2.5 by AstraZeneca	00310-0142	Diuretic; Antihypertensive
ZESTORETIC <> 142	Tab, Debossed	Hydrochlorothiazide 12.5 mg, Lisinopril 20 mg	Zestoretic by IPR	54921-0142	Diuretic; Antihypertensive
ZESTORETIC <> 145	Tab, Peach, Round, Debossed	Hydrochlorothiazide 25 mg, Lisinopril 20 mg	Zestoretic 20 25 Mg by Zeneca	00310-0145	Diuretic; Antihypertensive
ZESTORETIC <> 145	Tab, Debossed	Hydrochlorothiazide 25 mg, Lisinopril 20 mg	Zestoretic by IPR	54921-0145	Diuretic; Antihypertensive
ZESTORETIC <> STUART145	Tab	Hydrochlorothiazide 25 mg, Lisinopril 20 mg	Zestoretic 20 25 by Caremark	00339-5848	Diuretic; Antihypertensive
ZESTRIL <> 130	Tab, Pink, Oblong	Lisinopril 5 mg	Zestril by Heartland Healthcare	61392-0929	Antihypertensive
ZESTRIL <> 130	Tab	Lisinopril 5 mg	Zestril by Caremark	00339-5618	Antihypertensive
ZESTRIL <> 130	Tab, Pink, Cap-Shaped	Lisinopril 5 mg	Zestril by Zeneca	00310-0130	Antihypertensive

ID FRONT <> BACK	DESCRIPTION FRONT <> BACK	INGREDIENT & STRENGTH	BRAND (OR EQUIV.) & FIRM	NDC#	CLASS; SCH.
ZESTRIL <> 130	Tab, Debossed	Lisinopril 5 mg	Lisinopril by Kaiser	00179-1168	Antihypertensive
ZESTRIL <> 130	Tab	Lisinopril 5 mg	Lisinopril by Med Pro	53978-3063	Antihypertensive
ZESTRIL <> 130	Tab	Lisinopril 5 mg	Zestril by Allscripts	54569-3771	Antihypertensive
ZESTRIL <> 130	Tab, Biconvex	Lisinopril 5 mg	Zestril by Pharm Utilization	60491-0711	Antihypertensive
ZESTRIL <> 130	Tab, Scored	Lisinopril 5 mg	Lisinopril by Talbert Med	44514-0480	Antihypertensive
ZESTRIL10	Tab, Pink, Round, Zestril/10	Lisinopril 10 mg	Zestril by Zeneca	Canadian	Antihypertensive
ZESTRIL10 <> 131	Tab, Pink, Round, Film Coated	Ketorolac Tromethamine 10 mg	by Compumed	00403-4136	NSAID
ZESTRIL10 <> 131	Tab, Pink, Round	Lisinopril 10 mg	Zestril by PDRX Pharms	55289-0509	Antihypertensive
ZESTRIL10 <> 131	Tab, Pink, Round	Lisinopril 10 mg	Zestril by Heartland Healthcare	61392-0930	Antihypertensive
ZESTRIL10 <> 131	Tab	Lisinopril 10 mg	Zestril by Murfreesboro	51129-1105	Antihypertensive
ZESTRIL10 <> 131	Tab	Lisinopril 10 mg	Zestril by Caremark	00339-5638	Antihypertensive
ZESTRIL10 <> 131	Tab	Lisinopril 10 mg	Lisinopril by Kaiser	00179-1157	Antihypertensive
ZESTRIL10 <> 131	Tab, Pink, Round	Lisinopril 10 mg	Zestril by Zeneca	00310-0131	Antihypertensive
ZESTRIL10 <> 131	Tab	Lisinopril 10 mg	Zestril by IPR	54921-0131	Antihypertensive
ZESTRIL10 <> 131	Tab	Lisinopril 10 mg	Zestril by Med Pro	53978-1000	Antihypertensive
ZESTRIL10 <> 131	Tab, Debossed	Lisinopril 10 mg	Zestril by Drug Distr	52985-0216	Antihypertensive
ZESTRIL10 <> 131	Tab, Debossed	Lisinopril 10 mg	Zestril by Repack Co of Amer	55306-0131	Antihypertensive
ZESTRIL10 <> 131	Tab	Lisinopril 10 mg	Zestril by Quality Care	60346-0871	Antihypertensive
ZESTRIL10 <> 131	Tab, Debossed	Lisinopril 10 mg	Zestril by DRX	55045-2389	Antihypertensive
ZESTRIL10 <> 131	Tab	Lisinopril 10 mg	Zestril by Nat Pharmpak Serv	55154-6901	Antihypertensive
ZESTRIL10 <> 131	Tab	Lisinopril 10 mg	Zestril by Eckerd Drug	19458-0835	Antihypertensive
ZESTRIL10MG <> 131	Tab, Pink, Round	Lisinopril 10 mg	Zestril by Promex Medcl	62301-0044	Antihypertensive
ZESTRIL20	Tab, Pink, Round, Zestril/20	Lisinopril 20 mg	Zestril by Zeneca	Canadian	Antihypertensive
ZESTRIL20 <> 132	Tab, Red, Round	Lisinopril 20 mg	Zestril by Heartland Healthcare	61392-0931	Antihypertensive
ZESTRIL20 <> 132	Tab, Red, Round	Lisinopril 20 mg	Zestril by Zeneca	00310-0132	Antihypertensive
ZESTRIL20 <> 132	Tab	Lisinopril 20 mg	Lisinopril by Kaiser	00179-1169	Antihypertensive
ZESTRIL20 <> 132	Tab	Lisinopril 20 mg	Zestril by Caremark	00339-5632	Antihypertensive
ZESTRIL20 <> 132	Tab, Red-Pink	Lisinopril 20 mg	Zestril by Murfreesboro	51129-1330	Antihypertensive
ZESTRIL20 <> 132	Tab	Lisinopril 20 mg	Zestril by Med Pro	53978-1017	Antihypertensive
ZESTRIL20 <> 132	Tab, Debossed	Lisinopril 20 mg	Zestril by Drug Distr	52985-0217	Antihypertensive
ZESTRIL20 <> 132	Tab	Lisinopril 20 mg	Zestril by Repack Co of Amer	55306-0132	Antihypertensive
ZESTRIL20 <> 132	Tab, Debossed	Lisinopril 20 mg	Zestril by PDRX	55289-0106	Antihypertensive
ZESTRIL20 <> 132	Tab	Lisinopril 20 mg	Zestril by Quality Care	60346-0537	Antihypertensive
ZESTRIL20 <> 132	Tab	Lisinopril 20 mg	Zestril by Nat Pharmpak Serv	55154-6902	Antihypertensive
ZESTRIL20 <> 132	Tab	Lisinopril 20 mg	Zestril by Eckerd Drug	19458-0830	Antihypertensive
ZESTRIL20132	Tab, Zestril 20-132	Lisinopril 20 mg	Zestril by Allscripts	54569-2665	Antihypertensive
ZESTRIL212 <> 135	Tab, Zestril 2 1/2 <> 135	Lisinopril 2.5 mg	Zestril by Zeneca	00310-0135	Antihypertensive
ZESTRIL30 <> 133	Tab, Red, Round, Biconvex, Uncoated Tab	Lisinopril 30 mg	Zestril by AstraZeneca	00310-0133	Antihypertensive
ZESTRIL40 <> 134	Tab, Yellow, Round	Lisinopril 40 mg	Zestril by Heartland Healthcare	61392-0932	Antihypertensive
ZESTRIL40 <> 134	Tab	Lisinopril 40 mg	Lisinopril by Kaiser	00179-1203	Antihypertensive
ZESTRIL40 <> 134	Tab, Yellow, Round	Lisinopril 40 mg	Zestril by Zeneca	00310-0134	Antihypertensive
ZESTRIL40 <> 134	Tab, Yellow, Round	Lisinopril 40 mg	Zestril by Mylan	00378-0341	Antihypertensive
ZESTRIL40 <> 134	Tab	Lisinopril 40 mg	Zestril by Caremark	00339-5636	Antihypertensive
ZESTRIL40 <> 134	Tab, Debossed	Lisinopril 40 mg	Zestril by Quality Care	60346-0595	Antihypertensive
ZG20MG <> 4288	Cap, White, Opaque	Nicardipine HCl 20 mg	Cardene by Zenith Goldline	00172-4288	Antihypertensive
ZG30MG <> 4289	Cap, Light Blue, Opaque	Nicardipine HCl 30 mg	Cardene by Zenith Goldline	00172-4289	Antihypertensive
ZITHROMAXPFIZER	Cap, Red, Zithromax/Pfizer	Azithromycin Dihydrate 250 mg	by Pfizer	Canadian	Antibiotic
ZL <> 600	Tab, White, Oval, Film Coated, Scored	Zileuton 600 mg	Zyflo by Murfreesboro Ph	51129-1380	Antiasthmatic
ZL <> 600	Tab, White, Ovaloid, Scored, ZL over Abbott Logo <> 600	Zileuton 600 mg	Zyflo by Abbott	00074-8036	Antiasthmatic
ZLA <> BOCK	Tab, Z/LA	Guaifenesin 600 mg, Pseudoephedrine HCl 120 mg	Zephrex LA by		Cold Remedy
ZLA <> BOCK	Tab, Film Coated	Guaifenesin 600 mg, Pseudoephedrine HCl 120 mg	Zephrex LA by Sanofi	00024-2627	Cold Remedy
ZOCOR <> MSD726	Tab, Buff, Shield-Shaped, Film Coated	Simvastatin 5 mg	Zocor by Merck	00006-0726	Antihyperlipidemic

ID FRONT <> BACK	DESCRIPTION FRONT <> BACK	INGREDIENT & STRENGTH	BRAND (OR EQUIV.) & FIRM	NDC#	CLASS; SCH.
ZOCOR <> MSD735	Tab, Peach	Simvastatin 10 mg	Zocor by Va Cmop	65243-0064	Antihyperlipidemic
ZOCOR <> MSD735	Tab, Peach	Simvastatin 10 mg	Zocor by Southwood Pharms	58016-0364	Antihyperlipidemic
ZOCOR <> MSD735	Tab, Peach, Shield-Shaped, Film Coated	Simvastatin 10 mg	Zocor by Merck	00006-0735	Antihyperlipidemic
ZOCOR <> MSD735	Tab, Film Coated	Simvastatin 10 mg	Zocor by Caremark	00339-5795	Antihyperlipidemic
ZOCOR <> MSD735	Tab, Film Coated	Simvastatin 10 mg	Simvastatin by Med Pro	53978-3069	Antihyperlipidemic
ZOCOR <> MSD735	Tab, Shield-Shaped, Film Coated	Simvastatin 10 mg	Zocor by DRX	55045-2316	Antihyperlipidemic
ZOCOR <> MSD735	Tab, Shield-Shaped, Film Coated	Simvastatin 10 mg	Zocor by Allscripts	54569-4180	Antihyperlipidemic
ZOCOR <> MSD735	Tab, Film Coated	Simvastatin 10 mg	Zocor by Nat Pharmpak Serv	55154-5012	Antihyperlipidemic
ZOCOR <> MSD740	Tab, Tan	Simvastatin 20 mg	Zocor by Southwood Pharms	58016-0385	Antihyperlipidemic
ZOCOR <> MSD740	Tab, Tan	Simvastatin 20 mg	Zocor by Va Cmop	65243-0065	Antihyperlipidemic
ZOCOR <> MSD740	Tab, Tan	Simvastatin 20 mg	Simvastatin by Med-Pro	53978-3370	Antihyperlipidemic
ZOCOR <> MSD740	Tab, Tan, Shield-Shaped, Film Coated	Simvastatin 20 mg	Zocor by Merck	00006-0740	Antihyperlipidemic
ZOCOR <> MSD740	Tab, Shield Shaped, Film Coated	Simvastatin 20 mg	Zocor by Physicians Total Care	54868-3104	Antihyperlipidemic
ZOCOR <> MSD749	Tab, Red	Simvastatin 40 mg	Zocor by Va Cmop	65243-0082	Antihyperlipidemic
ZOCOR <> MSD749	Tab, Film Coated	Simvastatin 40 mg	Zocor by Caremark	00339-5798	Antihyperlipidemic
ZOCOR <> MSD749	Tab, Red, Film Coated	Simvastatin 40 mg	Zocor by Kaiser Fdn	00179-1331	Antihyperlipidemic
ZOFRAN <> 4	Tab, White, Oval, Film	Ondasetron 4 mg	Zofran by PDRX	55289-0480	Antiemetic
ZOFRAN <> 4	Tab, White, Oval, Film Coated	Ondansetron HCl	Zofran by Glaxo Wellcome	00173-0446	Antiemetic
ZOFRAN <> 8	Tab, Yellow, Oval	Ondansetron HCl 8 mg	Zofran by Glaxo Wellcome	00173-0447	Antiemetic
ZOFRAN <> 8	Tab, Yellow, Oval, Film	Ondasetron 8 mg	Zofran by PDRX	55289-0478	Antiemetic
ZOFRAN <> SAMPLE	Tab	Ondansetron HCl 8 mg	Zofran by Glaxo Wellcome	00173-0447	Antiemetic
ZOFRAN <> SAMPLE	Tab, Film Coated	Ondansetron HCl	Zofran by Glaxo Wellcome	00173-0446	Antiemetic
ZOFRAN4	Tab, White, Oval, Zofran/4	Ondansetron HCl 4 mg	Zofran by Glaxo Wellcome	00173-0446	Antiemetic
ZOFRAN8	Tab, Yellow, Oval, Zofran/8	Ondansetron HCl 8 mg	Zofran by Glaxo Wellcome	00173-0447	Antiemetic
ZOLOFT	Tab, Yellow, Oblong, Scored	Sertraline HCl 100 mg	Zoloft by Heartland Healthcare	61392-0939	Antidepressant
ZOLOFT	Tab, Yellow, Oblong, Scored	Sertraline HCl 100 mg	Zoloft by Va Cmop	65243-0063	Antidepressant
ZOLOFT <> 100	Tab, Yellow, Oblong	Sertraline HCl 100 mg	Zoloft by PDRX Pharms	55289-0550	Antidepressant
ZOLOFT <> 100MG	Tab, Yellow, Oblong, Film Coated, Scored	Sertraline HCl 100 mg	Zoloft by Natl Pharmpak	55154-2712	Antidepressant
ZOLOFT <> 100MG	Tab, Film Coated, Engraved	Sertraline HCl 100 mg	Zoloft by Physicians Total Care	54868-2637	Antidepressant
ZOLOFT <> 100MG	Tab, Film Coated	Sertraline HCl 100 mg		54569-3575	Antidepressant
ZOLOFT <> 100MG	Tab, Film Coated	Sertraline HCl 100 mg	Zoloft by Direct Dispensing	57866-6305	Antidepressant
ZOLOFT <> 100MG	Tab, Film Coated	Sertraline HCl 100 mg	Zoloft by Amerisource	62584-0910	Antidepressant
ZOLOFT <> 25MG	Tab, Light Green, Film Coated, Cap Shaped	Sertraline HCl	Zoloft by Roerig	00049-4960	Antidepressant
ZOLOFT <> 25MG	Tab, Light Green, Film Coated	Sertraline HCl	Zoloft by Murfreesboro	51129-1333	Antidepressant
ZOLOFT <> 25MG	Tab, Film Coated	Sertraline HCl	Zoloft by Allscripts	54569-4529	Antidepressant
ZOLOFT <> 25MG	Tab, Light Green, Oblong, Scored	Sertraline HCl 25 mg	Zoloft by Phcy Care	65070-0210	Antidepressant
ZOLOFT <> 25MG	Tab, Light Green, Oblong, Scored	Sertraline HCl 25 mg	Zoloft by Direct Dispensing	57866-1057	Antidepressant
ZOLOFT <> 50MG	Tab, Light Blue, Film Coated, Cap Shaped	Sertraline HCl	Zoloft by Roerig	00049-4900	Antidepressant
ZOLOFT <> 50MG	Tab, Film Coated	Sertraline HCl	Zoloft by Nat Pharmpak Serv	55154-2709	Antidepressant
ZOLOFT <> 50MG	Tab, Film Coated	Sertraline HCl	by Med Pro	53978-3019	Antidepressant
ZOLOFT <> 50MG	Tab, Film Coated	Sertraline HCl	Zoloft by Allscripts	54569-3724	Antidepressant
ZOLOFT <> 50MG	Tab, Light Blue, Film Coated	Sertraline HCl	Zoloft by Amerisource	62584-0900	Antidepressant
ZOLOFT <> 50MG	Tab, Film Coated	Sertraline HCl	Zoloft by Direct Dispensing	57866-6304	Antidepressant
ZOLOFT <> 50MG	Tab, Blue, Oblong, Film Coated, Scored	Sertraline HCl 50 mg	Zoloft by Heartland Healthcare	61392-0629	Antidepressant
ZOLOFT <> 50MG	Tab, Blue, Oblong, Film Coated, Scored	Sertraline HCl 50 mg	Zoloft by Compumed	00403-4721	Antidepressant
ZOLOFT <> 50MG	Tab, Blue, Oblong, Scored	Sertraline HCl 50 mg	Zoloft by Phcy Care	65070-0035	Antidepressant
ZOLOFT <> 50MG	Tab, Blue, Scored	Sertraline HCl 50 mg	Zoloft by Southwood Pharms	58016-0366	Antidepressant
ZOLOFT <> 50MG	Tab, Blue, Scored, Film	Sertraline HCl 50 mg	Zoloft by Scherer	11014-1215	Antidepressant
ZOLOFT <> 50MG	Tab, Blue, Scored, Film	Sertraline HCl 50 mg	Zoloft by Scherer	11014-1216	Antidepressant
ZOLOFT100MG	Tab, Light Yellow, Film Coated	Sertraline HCl 100 mg	Zoloft by Quality Care	60346-0707	Antidepressant
ZOLOFT100MG	Tab, Film Coated	Sertraline HCl 100 mg	Zoloft by DRX	55045-2208	Antidepressant
ZOLOFT50MG	Tab, Light Blue, Film Coated	Sertraline HCl 50 mg	Zoloft by Quality Care	60346-0516	Antidepressant

ID FRONT <> BACK	DESCRIPTION FRONT <> BACK	INGREDIENT & STRENGTH	BRAND (OR EQUIV.) & FIRM	NDC#	CLASS; SCH.
ZOMIG25	Tab, Yellow, Film Coated, Scored	Zolmitriptan 2.5 mg	Zomig by Promex Medcl	62301-0041	Antimigraine
ZOMIG25	Tab, Yellow, Round, Zomig 2.5, Film Coated	Zolmitriptan 2.5 mg	Zomig by AstraZeneca	00310-0210	Antimigraine
ZOMIG25	Tab, Zomig 2.5, Film Coated	Zolmitriptan 2.5 mg	Zomig by IPR	54921-0210	Antimigraine
ZOMIG5	Tab, Pink, Round, Film Coated	Zolmitriptan 5 mg	Zomig by AstraZeneca	00310-0211	Antimigraine
ZOMIG5	Tab, Film Coated	Zolmitriptan 5 mg	Zomig by IPR	54921-0211	Antimigraine
ZOVIRAX	Tab, Blue, Shield	Acyclovir 200 mg	by Glaxo	Canadian	Antiviral
ZOVIRAX	Tab, Triangle Logo	Acyclovir 400 mg	Zovirax by Catalytica	63552-0949	Antiviral
ZOVIRAX	Tab, Triangle Logo	Acyclovir 400 mg	Zovirax by Glaxo	00173-0949	Antiviral
ZOVIRAX	Tab, Shield Shaped, Triangle Logo	Acyclovir 400 mg	Zovirax by Murfreesboro	51129-1289	Antiviral
ZOVIRAX	Tab, Shield-Shaped, Triangle Logo	Acyclovir 400 mg	Zovirax by Allscripts	54569-4192	Antiviral
ZOVIRAX <> 800	Tab, Light Blue	Acyclovir 800 mg	Zovirax by Quality Care	60346-0735	Antiviral
ZOVIRAX	Tab, Shield Shaped, Zovirax <> Triangle	Acyclovir 400 mg	Zovirax by DRX	55045-2293	Antiviral
ZOVIRAX	Tab, Zovirax <> Triangle	Acyclovir 400 mg	Zovirax by Quality Care	62682-1013	Antiviral
ZOVIRAX 400	Tab, Pink, Shield	Acyclovir 400 mg	by Glaxo	Canadian	Antiviral
ZOVIRAX 800	Tab, Blue, Elongated	Acyclovir 800 mg	by Glaxo	Canadian	Antiviral
ZOVIRAX200	Cap	Acyclovir 200 mg	Zovirax by Nat Pharmpak Serv	55154-0706	Antiviral
ZOVIRAX200	Cap	Acyclovir 200 mg	by Pharmedix	53002-0245	Antiviral
ZOVIRAX200	Cap	Acyclovir 200 mg	Zovirax by Apotheca	12634-0180	Antiviral
ZOVIRAX200 <> WELLCOME	Cap	Acyclovir 200 mg	Zovirax by Prepackage Spec	58864-0563	Antiviral
ZOVIRAX200 <> WELLCOME	Cap	Acyclovir 200 mg	Zovirax by Quality Care	60346-0006	Antiviral
ZOVIRAX200 <> WELLCOME	Cap	Acyclovir 200 mg	Zovirax by Allscripts	54569-0091	Antiviral
ZOVIRAX800	Tab	Acyclovir 800 mg	Zovirax by Glaxo	00173-0945	Antiviral
ZOVIRAX800	Tab	Acyclovir 800 mg	Zovirax by PDRX	55289-0564	Antiviral
ZOVIRAX800	Tab	Acyclovir 800 mg	Zovirax by Nat Pharmpak Serv	55154-0708	Antiviral
ZOVIRAX800	Tab	Acyclovir 800 mg	Zovirax by Catalytica	63552-0945	Antiviral
ZT10	Tab, Peach, Round, Zt/10	Lisinopril 10 mg, Hydrochlorothiazide 12.5 mg	Zestoretic by Zeneca	Canadian	Antihypertensive
ZYBAN150	Tab, Zyban 150, Film Coated	Bupropion HCl 150 mg	Zyban by Catalytica	63552-0556	Antidepressant
ZYBAN150	Tab, Purple, Round, Film Coated	Bupropion HCl 150 mg	Zyban by Glaxo Wellcome	00173-0556	Antidepressant
ZYBAN150	Tab	Bupropion HCl 150 mg	Zyban by Murfreesboro	51129-1340	Antidepressant
ZYDONE	Cap, White	Hydrocodone Bitartrate 5 mg, Acetaminophen 500 mg	Zydone by Endo		Analgesic; C III
ZYLOPRIM100	Tab, Zyloprim 100 on Raised Hexagon	Allopurinol 100 mg	Zyloprim by Catalytica	63552-0996	Antigout
ZYLOPRIM100	Tab	Allopurinol 100 mg	Zyloprim by Glaxo	00173-0996	Antigout
ZYLOPRIM300	Tab, Zyloprim 300 on Raised Hexagon	Allopurinol 300 mg	Zyloprim by Catalytica	63552-0998	Antigout
ZYLOPRIM300	Tab	Allopurinol 300 mg	Zyloprim by Glaxo	00173-0998	Antigout
ZYLOPRIM300	Tab, Peach & White, Oval, Flat, Scored	Allopurinol 300 mg	Zyloprim by Apotheca	12634-0520	Antigout
ZYRTEC <> 10	Tab, White, Oblong, Film Coated	Cetirizine HCl 10 mg	Zyrtec by Catalytica	63552-0032	Antihistamine
ZYRTEC <> 10	Tab, White, Rectangle, Film Coated	Cetirizine HCl 10 mg	Zyrtec by Murfreesboro Ph	51129-1379	Antihistamine
ZYRTEC <> 10	Tab, White, Rectangle, Film Coated	Cetirizine HCl 10 mg	Zyrtec by Catalytica	63552-0033	Antihistamine
ZYRTEC <> 5	Tab, White, Rectangular, Film Coated	Cetirizine HCl 5 mg	Zyrtec by Murfreesboro Ph	51129-1192	Antihistamine
ZYVOX600MG	Tab, White, Oblong	Linezolid 600 mg	Zyvox by Pharmacia And Upjohn	00009-5135	Antibiotic
ZZENITH4058	Cap, Zenith Logo Zentih 4058	Cefadroxil Hemihydrate	by Major	00904-7878	Antibiotic
ZZENITH4058	Cap, Clear & White	Cefadroxil Hemihydrate 500 mg	Duricef by Zenith Goldline	00172-4058	Antibiotic

Get additional copies of

IDENT-A-DRUG

R E F E R E N C E

3816 P99

❑ I want to START a new subscription to *Ident-A-Drug Reference.*

  ❑ Printed version $39.50

  ❑ Web version $39.50 per year for one computer or one person.

  ❑ BOTH versions $59.50 (This is the best deal.)

❑ I want to EXTEND my subscription to *Ident-A-Drug Reference.*

  ❑ Send me the newest printed version $39.50

  ❑ Extend my web subscription $39.50 per year

  ❑ Give me BOTH a new printed version and one more year of the web version for $59.50

In California add 7.50% sales tax. For printed versions shipped outside the U.S. add $18.

Contact the publisher for information on licensing opportunities for portions of **identadrug.com** as an addition to consumer health-related websites. **Identadrug.com** allows consumers to assure that their medication, or the medication they are administering to a loved one, is correct.

If you prefer, you can subscribe online at www.identadrug.com.

❑ Payment enclosed (make check payable to Ident-A-Drug)

❑ Please charge my VISA, Mastercard, American Express, or Discover

Card number _____ Exp date _____

Signature _____

❑ Bill my business or institution on this purchase order number _____

Ship to:

Name _____

Address _____

City _____ State _____ Zip Code _____

Phone _____ E-mail _____

Send this order form to:

Ident-A-Drug Reference
Pharmacist's Letter / Prescriber's Letter
3120 W. March Lane
P.O. Box 8190
Stockton, CA 95208

Telephone: 209-472-2240 • Fax: 209-472-2249
E-mail: mail@identadrug.com • Website: www.identadrug.com

Get additional copies of

IDENT-A-DRUG
R E F E R E N C E

☐ I want to START a new subscription to *Ident-A-Drug Reference.*
- ☐ Printed version $39.50
- ☐ Web version $39.50 per year for one computer or one person.
- ☐ BOTH versions $59.50 (This is the best deal.)

☐ I want to EXTEND my subscription to *Ident-A-Drug Reference.*
- ☐ Send me the newest printed version $39.50
- ☐ Extend my web subscription $39.50 per year
- ☐ Give me BOTH a new printed version and one more year of the web version for $59.50

In California add 7.50% sales tax. For printed versions shipped outside the U.S. add $18.

Contact the publisher for information on licensing opportunities for portions of **identadrug.com** as an addition to consumer health-related websites. **Identadrug.com** allows consumers to assure that their medication, or the medication they are administering to a loved one, is correct.

If you prefer, you can subscribe online at www.identadrug.com.

☐ Payment enclosed (make check payable to Ident-A-Drug)
☐ Please charge my VISA, Mastercard, American Express, or Discover

Card number _____ Exp date _____

Signature _____

☐ Bill my business or institution on this purchase order number _____

Ship to:

Name _____

Address _____

City _____ State _____ Zip Code _____

Phone _____ E-mail _____

Send this order form to:

Ident-A-Drug Reference
Pharmacist's Letter / Prescriber's Letter
3120 W. March Lane
P.O. Box 8190
Stockton, CA 95208

Telephone: 209-472-2240 • Fax: 209-472-2249
E-mail: mail@identadrug.com • Website: www.identadrug.com

Since you already have purchased the Ident-A-Drug Reference book you can

ADD-ON access to

www.identadrug.com

This printed version of *Ident-A-Drug Reference* was current the day the data were extracted from **identadrug.com**, but the site is constantly updated with new data.

If you have not yet purchased your access to **identadrug.com**, now is a good time to do so. You can sign up by phone, mail, fax, or by going to the site.

If you have already purchased a printed version you can add-on the Web access for only $20.00. Access lasts one year and is for either one user or one computer.

ONE-THIRD OFF!

Only $20 for one year of access to identadrug.com

Price valid on orders placed prior to March 31, 2002.

☐ **YES,** please send me an access code so I can use www.identadrug.com

☐ Payment enclosed (make check payable to Ident-A-Drug)

☐ Please charge my VISA, Mastercard, American Express, or Discover

Card number _____ Exp date _____

Signature _____

☐ Bill my business or institution on this purchase order number _____

Ship to:

Name _____ Member # _____

Address _____

City _____ State _____ Zip Code _____

Phone _____ E-mail _____

If you have not yet purchased Ident-A-Drug Reference book, you can get the web access, or the book for $39.50, or the combination of both the book AND access to identadrug.com for $59.50. Sign up using the order form on the previous page, or send your order to the address below.

Send this order form to:

Ident-A-Drug Reference
Pharmacist's Letter / Prescriber's Letter
3120 W. March Lane
P.O. Box 8190
Stockton, CA 95208

Telephone: 209-472-2240 • Fax: 209-472-2249

E-mail: mail@identadrug.com • Website: www.identadrug.com